DEVELOPMENTAL-BEHAVIORAL PEDIATRICS

DEVELOPMENTAL-BEHAVIORAL PEDIATRICS

FOURTH EDITION

William B. Carey, MD
Clinical Professor of Pediatrics
University of Pennsylvania
School of Medicine
Director of Behavioral Pediatrics
Division of General Pediatrics
Children's Hospital of Philadelphia
Philadelphia, Pennsylvania

Allen C. Crocker, MD
Associate Professor of Pediatrics
Harvard Medical School
Associate Professor of Maternal and Child Health
Harvard School of Public Health
Program Director, Institute for Community Inclusion
Children's Hospital
Boston, Massachusetts

William L. Coleman, MD
Professor of Pediatrics
The Clinical Center for the Study of Development and Learning
University of North Carolina
Chapel Hill, North Carolina

Ellen Roy Elias, MD
Professor of Pediatrics
University of Colorado School of Medicine
Director, Special Care Clinic
The Children's Hospital
Denver, Colorado

Heidi M. Feldman, MD, PhD
Ballinger-Swindells Professor of Developmental and Behavioral Pediatrics
Stanford University School of Medicine
Stanford, California
Medical Director
Mary L. Johnson Developmental and Behavioral Pediatric Programs
Lucile Packard Children's Hospital
Palo Alto, California

SAUNDERS

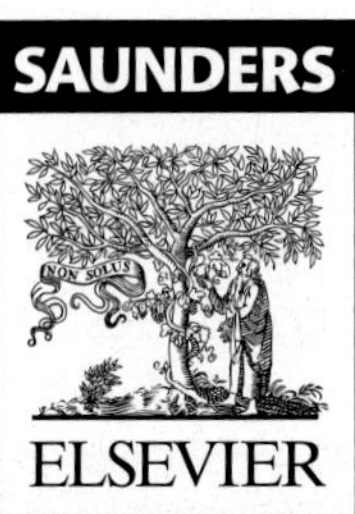

ELSEVIER

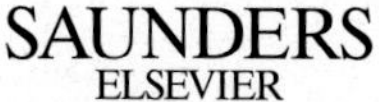

SAUNDERS
ELSEVIER

1600 John F. Kennedy Blvd.
Ste 1800
Philadelphia, PA 19103-2899

DEVELOPMENTAL-BEHAVIORAL PEDIATRICS, FOURTH EDITION ISBN: 978-1-4160-3370-7

Cover image: Detail of Family Group 1944 (LH 2237a). Photo: The Henry Moore Foundation archive. Reproduced by permission of The Henry Moore Foundation. Original work is held at the Scottish National Gallery of Modern Art.

Notice

Knowledge and best practice in this field are constantly changing. As new research and experience broaden our knowledge, changes in practice, treatment and drug therapy may become necessary or appropriate. Readers are advised to check the most current information provided (i) on procedures featured or (ii) by the manufacturer of each product to be administered, to verify the recommended dose or formula, the method and duration of administration, and contraindications. It is the responsibility of the practitioner, relying on their own experience and knowledge of the patient, to make diagnoses, to determine dosages and the best treatment for each individual patient, and to take all appropriate safety precautions. To the fullest extent of the law, neither the Publisher nor the Editors assumes any liability for any injury and/or damage to persons or property arising out of or related to any use of the material contained in this book.

The Publisher

Library of Congress Cataloging-in-Publication Data
Developmental-behavioral pediatrics / [edited by] William B. Carey ... [et al.]. — 4th ed.
p. ; cm.
ISBN 978-1-4160-3370-7
1. Pediatrics. 2. Pediatrics—Psychological aspects. 3. Child development. 4. Child psychology. 5. Child development deviations. 6. Pediatric neuropsychiatry. I. Carey, William B.
[DNLM: 1. Child Development. 2. Child Behavior Disorders. 3. Child Behavior. 4. Developmental Disabilities. WS 105 D48912 2009]

RJ47.D48 2009
618.92—dc22 2008032777

Acquisitions Editor: Judith Fletcher
Developmental Editor: Melissa Dudlick
Publishing Services Manager: Frank Polizzano
Project Manager: Rachel Miller
Design Direction: Ellen Zanolle
Illustration Direction: Lesley Frazier
Marketing Manager: Courtney Ingram

Printed in China

Last digit is the print number: 9 8 7 6 5 4 3 2 1

CONTRIBUTORS

Marilee C. Allen, MD Professor of Pediatrics, The Johns Hopkins School of Medicine; Neonatologist, The Johns Hopkins Hospital; Neurodevelopmental Pediatrician, The Johns Hopkins Bayview Medical Center; Codirector of the NICU Development Clinic, Kennedy Krieger Institute, Baltimore, Maryland
Neurodevelopmental Consequences of Preterm Birth: Causes, Assessment, and Management

Tanni L. Anthony, PhD, Ed.S. Supervisor of Low-Incidence Programs/State Consultant on Blindness and Low Vision, Denver, Colorado
Blindness and Visual Impairment

Marilyn Augustyn, MD Associate Professor of Pediatrics, Division of Developmental and Behavioral Pediatrics, Boston University School of Medicine, Boston, Massachusetts
Infancy and Toddler Years

William J. Barbaresi, MD Associate Professor of Pediatrics, College of Medicine, Mayo Clinic; Chair, Division of Developmental and Behavioral Pediatrics, Codirector, Mayo Clinic–Dana Child Development and Learning Disorders Program, Mayo Clinic, Rochester, Minnesota
Oppositional Behavior/Noncompliance

Jane Holmes Bernstein, PhD Associate Professor in Psychology (Psychiatry), Harvard Medical School; Senior Associate in Psychology/Neuropsychology, Children's Hospital Boston, Boston, Massachusetts
Neuropsychologic Assessment of the Developing Child

Nathan J. Blum, MD Associate Professor of Pediatrics, University of Pennsylvania School of Medicine; Director, Section of Behavioral Pediatrics, Division of Child Development, Rehabilitation, and Metabolic Disease, The Children's Hospital of Philadelphia, Philadelphia, Pennsylvania
Repetitive Behaviors and Tics

Terrill Bravender, MD, MPH Associate Professor of Clinical Pediatrics, The Ohio State University; Chief, Adolescent Medicine, Nationwide Children's Hospital, Columbus, Ohio
Adaptation and Maladaptation to School

Carolyn Bridgemohan, MD Assistant Professor of Pediatrics, Harvard Medical School; Associate in Medicine, Children's Hospital Boston, Boston, Massachusetts
Bowel Function, Toileting, and Encopresis

Gray M. Buchanan, PhD Assistant Professor of Clinical Pediatrics, University of South Carolina School of Medicine, Columbia, South Carolina; Staff Psychologist, Greenville Hospital System–Children's Hospital, Greenville, South Carolina
Behavior Management

Jane E. Caplan, MD Psychiatrist, Private Practice, Scottsdale, Arizona
Psychotherapy with Children and Adolescents

William B. Carey, MD Clinical Professor of Pediatrics, University of Pennsylvania, School of Medicine; Director of Behavioral Pediatrics, Division of General Pediatrics, Children's Hospital of Philadelphia, Philadelphia, Pennsylvania
Normal Individual Differences in Temperament and Behavioral Adjustment; Acute Minor Illness; "Colic": Prolonged or Excessive Crying in Young Infants; Assessment of Behavioral Adjustment and Behavioral Style; Comprehensive Formulation of Assessment; The Right to Be Different

John E. Carr, PhD Professor Emeritus, Psychiatry and Behavioral Sciences, Psychology, University of Washington, Seattle, Washington
Coping Strategies

Jane Case-Smith, EdD, MOT Professor, The Ohio State University School of Allied Medical Professions; Director, Occupational Therapy, The Ohio State University, Columbus, Ohio
Other Sensory Problems

Patrick H. Casey, MD Professor of Pediatrics, University of Arkansas for Medical Sciences; Harvey and Bernice Jones Professor of Developmental Pediatrics, Arkansas Children's Hospital, Little Rock, Arkansas
Failure-to-Thrive

Donna Madden Chadwick, MT-BC, MS, LMHC Associate Professor of Music Therapy (Adjunct), Berklee College of Music, Boston, Massachusetts; Music Therapist, Crotched Mountain Rehabilitation Center, Greenfield, New Hampshire; Director, Music Therapy Clinical Services, Westford, Massachusetts
The Arts Therapies

Thomas D. Challman, MD Assistant Professor of Pediatrics, Jefferson Medical College, Philadelphia, Pennsylvania; Director, Pediatric Subspecialties, Geisinger Medical Center, Danville, Pennsylvania
Alternative Therapies

Diego Chaves-Gnecco, MD, MPH Assistant Professor, University of Pittsburgh, School of Medicine; Developmental-Behavioral Pediatrician, Program Director and Founder, Salud Para Niños Children's Hospital of Pittsburgh of UPMC, Pittsburgh, Pennsylvania
Special Education Services

Amy Cheung, MD, MSc Assistant Professor of Psychiatry, University of Toronto; Staff Physician, Department of Psychiatry, Sunnybrook Health Sciences Centre, Toronto, Canada
Major Disturbances of Emotion and Mood

Jeffrey M. Chinsky, MD, PhD Assistant Professor of Pediatrics, Johns Hopkins University School of Medicine; Attending Physician, Johns Hopkins Hospital; Associate, McKusick-Nathans Institute of Genetic Medicine, Johns Hopkins University School of Medicine; Director, Inpatient Pediatrics and Attending, St. Agnes Hospital, Baltimore, Maryland
Inborn Errors of Metabolism

Mary Ann Chirba-Martin, JD, MPH Assistant Professor, Boston College Law School, Newton, Massachusetts
Legal Issues

Thomas Chun, MD Assistant Professor of Emergency Medicine and Pediatrics, The Warren Alpert Medical School, Brown University; Attending Physician, Emergency Department, Hasbro Children's Hospital, Providence, Rhode Island
Crisis Management

William I. Cohen, MD Professor of Pediatrics and Psychiatry, University of Pittsburgh School of Medicine; Developmental-Behavioral Pediatrician and Director, Down Syndrome Center, Children's Hospital of Pittsburgh of UPMC, Pittsburgh, Pennsylvania
Critical Family Events; Down Syndrome: Care of the Child and Family

William Lord Coleman, MD Professor of Pediatrics, The Clinical Center for the Study of Development and Learning, University of North Carolina, Chapel Hill, North Carolina
After the Death of a Child: Helping Bereaved Parents and Brothers and Sisters; The Right to Be Different

Allen C. Crocker, MD Associate Professor of Pediatrics, Harvard Medical School; Associate Professor of Maternal and Child Health, Harvard School of Public Health; Program Director, Institute for Community Inclusion, Children's Hospital Boston, Boston, Massachusetts
Intellectual Disability; The Right to Be Different

Timothy Culbert, MD Assistant Professor of Clinical Pediatrics, University of Minnesota Medical School; Medical Director, Integrative Medicine Program, Children's Hospitals and Clinics of Minnesota, Minneapolis, Minnesota
Pediatric Self-Regulation

Richard E. D'Alli, ScM, MD Associate Professor of Psychiatry and Pediatrics, Duke University Medical Center; Medical Director, Child and Adolescent Psychiatry Services, Duke University Medical Center; Division Chief, Division of Child Development and Behavioral Health, Department of Pediatrics, Duke University Medical Center, Durham, North Carolina
Child and Adolescent Psychopharmacology

Howard Dubowitz, MD, MPH Professor of Pediatrics, University of Maryland School of Medicine; Director, Center for Families, University of Maryland Hospital, Baltimore, Maryland
Social Withdrawal and Isolation

Carol S. Dweck, PhD Lewis and Virginia Eaton Professor of Psychology, Stanford University, Stanford, California
Self-Concept

Paul H. Dworkin, MD Professor and Chair, Department of Pediatrics, University of Connecticut School of Medicine, Farmington, Connecticut; Physician-in-Chief, Connecticut Children's Medical Center, Hartford, Connecticut
Schools as Milieu

Ellen Roy Elias, MD Professor of Pediatrics, University of Colorado School of Medicine; Director, Special Care Clinic, The Children's Hospital, Denver, Colorado
Biomedical Basis of Development and Behavior; Genetic Syndromes and Dysmorphology; Intellectual Disability; Children with Multiple Disabilities and Special Health Care Needs; The Right to Be Different

Kathleen Selvaggi Fadden, MD Clinical Assistant Professor of Pediatrics, University of Medicine and Dentistry–New Jersey Medical School, Newark, New Jersey; Medical Director, Child Development Center, Goryeb Children's Hospital, Morristown, New Jersey
Developmental Assessment of the School-Age Child

Mirna Farah, MD Associate Professor of Clinical Pediatrics, University of Pennsylvania School of Medicine; Attending Physician, Department of Pediatrics, Division of Emergency Medicine, The Children's Hospital of Philadelphia, Philadelphia, Pennsylvania
Crisis Management

John Farley, MD, MPH Associate Professor, Pediatrics, Epidemiology, and Preventive Medicine, University of Maryland School of Medicine; Deputy Director, Division of Epidemiology and Prevention, Institute of Human Virology at the University of Maryland School of Medicine, Baltimore, Maryland
Human Immunodeficiency Virus Infection in Children

Heidi M. Feldman, MD, PhD Ballinger-Swindells Professor of Developmental and Behavioral Pediatrics, Stanford University School of Medicine, Stanford, California; Medical Director, Mary L. Johnson Developmental and Behavioral Pediatric Programs, Lucile Packard Children's Hospital, Palo Alto, California
The History of Developmental-Behavioral Pediatrics; Influences of Experience in the Environment on Human Development and Behavior; Language and Speech Disorders; The Laying on of Hands: The Physical Examination in Developmental and Behavioral Assessment; The Right to Be Different

Marianne E. Felice, MD Professor and Chair, Department of Pediatrics, University of Massachusetts Medical School; Physician-in-Chief, UMass Memorial Children's Medical Center, Worcester, Massachusetts
Adolescence

Brian W. C. Forsyth, MB, ChB Professor of Pediatrics, Child Study Center, Yale University School of Medicine, New Haven, Connecticut
Early Health Crises and Vulnerable Children

Deborah A. Frank, MD Professor of Pediatrics and Assistant Professor of Public Health, Boston University School of Medicine; Developmental and Behavioral Pediatrician, Boston Medical Center, Boston, Massachusetts
Infancy and Toddler Years

Craig Garfield, MD, MAPP Assistant Professor of Pediatrics, Northwestern University's Feinberg School of Medicine, Chicago, Illinois; Pediatrician, Evanston Northwestern Healthcare, Evanston, Illinois
Variations in Family Composition

William Garrison, PhD Professor of Pediatrics, University of Massachusetts Medical School; Director of Developmental and Behavioral Pediatrics, UMass Memorial Children's Medical Center, Worcester, Massachusetts
Adolescence

Dale Sussman Gertz, MD Adjunct Assistant Professor of Pediatrics, University of North Carolina School of Medicine, Chapel Hill, North Carolina; Courtesy Staff, Pediatrics, Moses Cone Health System, Greensboro, North Carolina
Pediatric Self-Regulation

Andrew R. Gilbert, MD Assistant Professor of Psychiatry, University of Pittsburgh School of Medicine, Western Psychiatric Institute and Clinic, Pittsburgh, Pennsylvania
Schizophrenia, Phobias, and Obsessive-Compulsive Disorder

Laurie Glader, MD Instructor in Pediatrics, Harvard Medical School; Medical Director, Cerebral Palsy Program, Assistant in Medicine, Children's Hospital Boston, Boston, Massachusetts
Cerebral Palsy

Peter A. Gorski, MD, MPA Professor of Public Health, Pediatrics, and Psychiatry, University of South Florida; Director of Research and Innovation, The Children's Board of Hillsborough County, Tampa, Florida
Pregnancy, Birth, and the First Days of Life

Judith Greeley, MA Program Coordinator and Teacher, Anchor Center for Blind Children, Denver, Colorado
Blindness and Visual Impairment

Linda S. Gudas, PhD Assistant Clinical Professor of Psychology, Harvard Medical School, Boston, Massachusetts; Associate Scientific Staff, Children's Hospital Boston, Boston, Massachusetts; Therapist, Needham Psychotherapy Associates, Needham, Massachusetts
Palliative and End of Life Care for Children and Families

Joseph F. Hagan, Jr., MD Clinical Professor in Pediatrics, The University of Vermont College of Medicine; Attending Physician in Pediatrics, The Vermont Children's Hospital at Fletcher Allen Health Care, Burlington, Vermont
Disasters, War, and Terrorism

Randi Hagerman, MD Professor of Pediatrics, University of California, Davis; Medical Director, M.I.N.D. Institute, University of California, Davis, Sacramento, California
Chromosomal Disorders and Fragile X Syndrome

Sara C. Hamel, MD Associate Professor of Pediatrics, University of Pittsburgh Medical School; Developmental-Behavioral Pediatrician, Child Development Unit, Children's Hospital of Pittsburgh, Pittsburgh, Pennsylvania
Preschool Years

Lawrence D. Hammer, MD Professor of Pediatrics, Stanford University School of Medicine; Medical Director, Ambulatory Services, Lucile Packard Children's Hospital, Palo Alto, California
Child and Adolescent Obesity

Robin L. Hansen, MD Professor of Pediatrics, Director of Clinical Programs, M.I.N.D. Institute; Director, Center for Excellence in Developmental Disabilities, University of California, Davis, Sacramento, California
The Spectrum of Social Cognition

Antonio Y. Hardan, MD Assistant Professor of Psychiatry, Department of Psychiatry and Behavioral Sciences, Stanford University School of Medicine, Palo Alto, California
Schizophrenia, Phobias, and Obsessive-Compulsive Disorder

John J. Hardt, PhD Assistant Professor, Loyola University Chicago, Stritch School of Medicine, Maywood, Illinois
Ethics

Sara Harkness, PhD, MPH Professor of Human Development, Pediatrics, Public Health, and Anthropology, University of Connecticut, Storrs, Connecticut
Culture and Ethnicity

Penny Hauser-Cram, EdD Professor, Boston College, Lynch School of Education, Chestnut Hill, Massachusetts
Early Intervention Services

Fred M. Henretig, MD Professor of Pediatrics and Emergency Medicine, University of Pennsylvania School of Medicine; Director, Clinical Toxicology, Children's Hospital of Philadelphia, Philadelphia, Pennsylvania
Toxins

Pamela C. High, MS, MD Professor of Pediatrics, The Warren Alpert Medical School of Brown University; Director, Developmental-Behavioral Pediatrics, Hasbro Children's Hospital/Rhode Island Hospital, Providence, Rhode Island
Behavior Management

Jennifer B. Hillman, MD Assistant Professor of Pediatrics, University of Cincinnati College of Medicine; Division of Adolescent Medicine, Cincinnati Children's Hospital Medical Center, Cincinnati, Ohio
Sexuality: Its Development and Direction

Lynne C. Huffman, MD Associate Professor of Pediatrics, Stanford University, Stanford, California; Director, Division of Outcomes Measurement and Research, Children's Health Council, Palo Alto, California
Neighborhood and Community

Michael S. Jellinek, MD Professor of Pediatrics and Psychiatry, Massachusetts General Hospital, Harvard Medical School, Boston, Massachusetts; Chief, Child Psychiatry Service, Massachusetts General Hospital, Boston, Massachusetts; President, CEO, Newton Wellesley Hospital, Newton, Massachusetts
Psychotherapy with Children and Adolescents

Peter Jensen, MD President and CEO, The REACH Institute, Resource for Advancing Children's Health, New York, New York
Major Disturbances of Emotion and Mood

Louise Kaczmarek, PhD Associate Professor, Department of Instruction and Learning, School of Education, University of Pittsburgh, Pittsburgh, Pennsylvania
Special Education Services

James R. Kallman, PhD Clinical Associate Professor, Department of Pediatrics and Human Development, College of Human Medicine, Michigan State University; School Psychologist, Ingham Intermediate School District, East Lansing, Michigan
Middle Childhood

Constance H. Keefer, MD Assistant Professor of Pediatrics, Harvard Medical School; Faculty, Brazelton Institute and Brazelton Touchpoints Center, Boston, Massachusetts
Culture and Ethnicity

Desmond P. Kelly, MD Professor of Clinical Pediatrics, University of South Carolina School of Medicine, Columbia, South Carolina; Medical Director, Division of Developmental-Behavioral Pediatrics, Gardner Family Center for Developing Minds, Children's Hospital, Greenville Hospital System, Greenville, South Carolina
Hearing Impairment

Perri Klass, MD Professor of Journalism and Pediatrics, New York University, New York, New York
Brothers and Sisters

John R. Knight, MD Associate Professor of Pediatrics, Harvard Medical School; Director, Center for Adolescent Substance Abuse Research, Children's Hospital Boston, Boston, Massachusetts
Substance Use, Abuse, and Dependence and Other Risk-Taking Behaviors

Kelly Knupp, MD Senior Instructor of Pediatrics, University of Colorado Denver School of Medicine, Denver, Colorado; Codirector, Clinical Program, Neurology, The Children's Hospital, Aurora, Colorado
Nervous System Disorders

Gerald P. Koocher, PhD, ABPP Professor and Dean, School of Health Sciences, Simmons College; Lecturer in Psychology, Harvard Medical School; Senior Associate in Psychology, Children's Hospital Boston, Boston, Massachusetts
Palliative and End of Life Care for Children and Families

Mary C. Kral, PhD Assistant Professor of Pediatrics, Medical University of South Carolina, Charleston, South Carolina
The Gifted Child

Nancy F. Krebs, MD, MS Professor of Pediatrics, University of Colorado Denver School of Medicine, Denver, Colorado; Medical Director, Clinical Nutrition, The Children's Hospital, Aurora, Colorado
Nutrition Assessment and Support

Stephen S. Leff, PhD Associate Professor of Clinical Psychology in Pediatrics, University of Pennsylvania School of Medicine; Associate Professor of Clinical Psychology in Pediatrics/Licensed Psychologist, Pennsylvania, The Children's Hospital of Philadelphia, Philadelphia, Pennsylvania
Aggression, Violence, and Delinquency

Mary Leppert, MB, BCh, BAO Assistant Professor of Pediatrics, Johns Hopkins University School of Medicine; Attending Physician, Neurodevelopmental Pediatrics, Kennedy Krieger Institute, Baltimore, Maryland
Neurodevelopmental Consequences of Preterm Birth: Causes, Assessment, and Management

Melvin D. Levine, MD Professor of Pediatrics, University of North Carolina, Chapel Hill, North Carolina
Differences in Learning and Neurodevelopmental Function in School-Age Children

Paul H. Lipkin, MD Associate Professor of Pediatrics, Johns Hopkins University School of Medicine; Director, Center for Development and Learning, Kennedy Krieger Institute, Baltimore, Maryland
Motor Development and Dysfunction

Irene M. Loe, MD Instructor, Stanford University School of Medicine, Stanford, California; Developmental-Behavioral Pediatrician, Lucile Packard Children's Hospital, Palo Alto, California
Influences of Experience in the Environment on Human Development and Behavior

Stephen Ludwig, MD Professor of Pediatrics and Emergency Medicine, University of Pennsylvania School of Medicine; Associate Physician-in-Chief for Education, Children's Hospital of Philadelphia, Philadelphia, Pennsylvania
Family Function and Dysfunction

Meghan Korey Lukasik, PhD Clinical Psychologist, Developmental Evaluation Clinic, Rady Children's Hospital, San Diego, California
Developmental Screening and Assessment: Infants, Toddlers, and Preschoolers

Allison Master, MA PhD Candidate, Teaching Assistant, and Instructor, Stanford University, Stanford, California
Self-Concept

Cheryl Messick, PhD Assistant Professor, Director of Clinical Education, Communication Sciences, and Disorders, School of Health and Rehabilitation Sciences, University of Pittsburgh, Pittsburgh, Pennsylvania
Language and Speech Disorders

Laurie C. Miller, MD Associate Professor of Pediatrics, Tufts University School of Medicine; Director, International Adoption Clinic, Floating Hospital for Children, Tufts Medical Center, Boston, Massachusetts
Adoption and Foster Family Care

John B. Moeschler, MD Professor of Pediatrics, Dartmouth Medical School, Hanover, New Hampshire; Director, Clinical Genetics, Dartmouth Hitchcock Medical Center, Lebanon, New Hampshire
Health Care Systems

Daniel Moran, MD Clinical Assistant Professor, Clinical Center for the Study of Development and Learning, University of North Carolina at Chapel Hill, Chapel Hill, North Carolina
Childcare

John A. Nackashi, MD, PhD Professor and Chief, Division of General Pediatrics, Department of Pediatrics, College of Medicine, University of Florida; Attending Physician, Shands at the University of Florida, Shands Children's Hospital, Gainesville, Florida
Peers

Ramzi Nasir, MD Instructor, Harvard Medical School; Assistant in Medicine, Children's Hospital Boston, Boston, Massachusetts
Urinary Function and Enuresis

Jack H. Nassau, PhD Clinical Assistant Professor of Psychiatry and Human Behavior, The Warren Alpert Medical School of Brown University; Staff Psychologist, Bradley Hasbro Children's Research Center, Child and Adolescent Psychiatry, Hasbro Children's Hospital/Rhode Island Hospital, Providence, Rhode Island
Behavior Management

Robert Needlman, MD Associate Professor of Pediatrics, Case Western Reserve University School of Medicine; Attending Physician, Department of Pediatrics, Metro Health Medical Center, Cleveland, Ohio
Adjustment and Adjustment Disorders

Sharon Nichols, PhD Assistant Professor of Neurosciences, University of California, San Diego, School of Medicine, La Jolla, California; Pediatric Neuropsychologist, University of California, San Diego, Medical Center, San Diego, California
Human Immunodeficiency Virus Infection in Children

Karen Olness, MD Professor of Pediatrics, Family Medicine, and Global Health, Case Western Reserve University, Cleveland, Ohio
Self-Control and Self-Regulation: Normal Development to Clinical Conditions

Judith A. Owens, MD, MPH Associate Professor of Pediatrics, Warren Alpert Medical School of Brown University; Director, Pediatric Sleep Disorders Clinic, Rhode Island Hospital, Providence, Rhode Island
Sleep and Sleep Disorders in Children

Tonya M. Palermo, PhD Associate Professor of Anesthesiology and Perioperative Medicine and Psychiatry; Chief, Division of Clinical Pain and Regional Anesthesia Research; Director, Anesthesiology Clinical Research and Training, Oregon Health and Science University, Portland, Oregon
Recurrent and Chronic Pain

Judith S. Palfrey, MD T. Berry Brazelton Professor, Harvard Medical School; Director, Children's International Pediatric Center, Children's Hospital Boston, Boston, Massachusetts
Legislation for the Education of Children With Disabilities

Julie Parsons, MD Assistant Professor, University of Colorado Medical School, Denver, Colorado; Child Neurology Residency Director, The Children's Hospital, Aurora, Colorado
Nervous System Disorders

Amanda Pelphrey, PsyD Adjunct Instructor, Chatham University; Psychologist, Child Development Unit, Children's Hospital of Pittsburgh, Pittsburgh, Pennsylvania
Preschool Years

Ellen C. Perrin, MA, MD Professor of Pediatrics, Tufts University School of Medicine; Director, Division of Developmental-Behavioral Pediatrics, The Floating Hospital for Children, Tufts Medical Center, Boston, Massachusetts
Hospitalization, Surgery, and Medical and Dental Procedures

James M. Perrin, MD Professor of Pediatrics, Harvard Medical School; Director, Massachusetts General Hospital for Children, Center for Child and Adolescent Health Policy; Associate Chair for Research, Massachusetts General Hospital for Children, Boston, Massachusetts
Chronic Health Conditions

Randall Phelps, MD, PhD Assistant Professor of Pediatrics, Oregon Health and Science University; Developmental and Behavioral Pediatrician, Child Development and Rehabilitation Center, Eugene, Oregon
The Laying on of Hands: The Physical Examination in Developmental and Behavioral Assessment

Laura Pickler, MD, MPH Assistant Professor, University of Colorado Health Science Center; Director, Oral Feeding Clinic, University of Colorado Health Sciences Center, Aurora, Colorado
Chromosomal Disorders and Fragile X Syndrome

Daniela Plesa-Skwerer, PhD Instructor, Department of Anatomy and Neurobiology, Boston University School of Medicine, Boston, Massachusetts
Assessment of Intelligence

Jill C. Posner, MD Assistant Professor of Pediatrics, University of Pennsylvania School of Medicine; Attending Physician, Pediatric Emergency Medicine, The Children's Hospital of Philadelphia, Philadelphia, Pennsylvania
Aggression, Violence, and Delinquency

Lisa Albers Prock, MD, MPH Assistant Professor, Harvard Medical School; Director, Developmental-Behavioral Pediatric Services, Developmental Medicine Center, Children's Hospital Boston, Boston, Massachusetts
Attention and Deficits of Attention

Virginia Kent Proud, BA, MS, MD Professor of Pediatrics and Clinical Genetics, Eastern Virginia Medical School; Director, Division of Medical Genetics and Metabolism, Children's Hospital of the King's Daughters, Department of Pediatrics, Eastern Virginia Medical School, Norfolk, Virginia
Genetic Syndromes and Dysmorphology

Leonard Rappaport, MS, MD Mary Deming Scott Professor of Pediatrics, Harvard Medical School; Director, Developmental Medicine Center, Children's Hospital Boston, Boston, Massachusetts
Attention and Deficits of Attention

Marsha D. Rappley, MD Professor of Pediatrics and Human Development; Dean, College of Human Medicine, Michigan State University, East Lansing, Michigan
Middle Childhood

Karen Ratliff-Schaub, MD Assistant Professor, Medical Director, Nisonger Center, The Ohio State University; Developmental Pediatrician, Nationwide Children's Hospital, Columbus, Ohio
Other Sensory Problems

Martha S. Reed, BA, MEd Educational Specialist, Chapel Hill, North Carolina
Educational Assessment

Julius Benjamin Richmond, MD John D. MacArthur Professor of Health Policy, Emeritus, Department of Social Medicine, Harvard University, Boston, Massachusetts
After the Death of a Child: Helping Bereaved Parents and Brothers and Sisters

Thomas N. Robinson, MD, MPH Irving Schulman, MD, Endowed Professor in Child Health, Stanford University School of Medicine, Stanford, California; Director, Center for Healthy Weight, Lucile Packard Children's Hospital, Palo Alto, California
Child and Adolescent Obesity

Anthony Rostain, MS, MD Professor of Psychiatry and Pediatrics, University of Pennsylvania School of Medicine; Director of Education, Department of Psychiatry, University of Pennsylvania Health System, Philadelphia, Pennsylvania
Family Function and Dysfunction

Olle Jane Z. Sahler, MD Professor of Pediatrics, Psychiatry, and Medical Humanities, University of Rochester School of Medicine and Dentistry; Director, Psychosocial Oncology Services and Research, Director, Long-term Cancer Survivors Program, Golisano Children's Hospital at Strong, Rochester, New York
Coping Strategies

Barton D. Schmitt, MD Professor of Pediatrics, University of Colorado School of Medicine; Medical Director, Sleep Disorder Clinic and Enuresis-Encopresis Clinic, The Children's Hospital, Aurora, Colorado
Pediatric Counseling

Alison Schonwald, MD Assistant Professor, Harvard Medical School; Assistant in Medicine, Children's Hospital Boston, Boston, Massachusetts
Urinary Function and Enuresis

Deborah Shipman, MD Developmental-Behavioral Pediatrician, Floating Hospital for Children, Tufts Medical Center, Boston, Massachusetts
Hospitalization, Surgery, and Medical and Dental Procedures

Eric Sigel, MD Associate Professor of Pediatrics, University of Colorado Denver School of Medicine, Denver, Colorado; Fellowship Director, Adolescent Medicine, The Children's Hospital, Aurora, Colorado
Disordered Eating Behaviors: Anorexia Nervosa and Bulimia Nervosa

Peter J. Smith, MD, MA Assistant Professor of Pediatrics, University of Chicago; Program Director, Fellowship in Developmental and Behavioral Pediatrics, Chief of the Medical Staff, La Rabida Children's Hospital, Chicago, Illinois
Ethics

Michael G. Spigarelli, MD, PhD Assistant Professor of Pediatrics and Internal Medicine, Division of Adolescent Medicine; Fellowship Director, Adolescent Medicine, Cincinnati Children's Hospital Medical Center, University of Cincinnati, Cincinnati, Ohio
Sexuality: Its Development and Direction

Raymond H. Starr, Jr., PhD Professor Emeritus, University of Maryland Baltimore County, Baltimore, Maryland
Social Withdrawal and Isolation

Martin T. Stein, MD Professor of Pediatrics, University of California, San Diego, School of Medicine, La Jolla, California; Pediatrician, Rady Children's Hospital San Diego, San Diego, California
Common Issues in Feeding; Developmental Screening and Assessment: Infants, Toddlers, and Preschoolers

Robert D. Steiner, MD Professor of Pediatrics and Molecular and Medical Genetics, Oregon Health and Science University; Attending Physician, Doernbecher Children's Hospital, Portland, Oregon
Inborn Errors of Metabolism

Marilyn Stevenson, RD, CSP Registered Dietitian, The Children's Hospital, Aurora, Colorado
Nutrition Assessment and Support

Eric A. Storch, PhD Associate Professor of Pediatrics and Psychiatry, University of South Florida, St. Petersburg, Florida
Peers

Victor C. Strasburger, MD Professor of Pediatrics, Professor of Family and Community Medicine, University of New Mexico School of Medicine; Chief, Division of Adolescent Medicine, University of New Mexico School of Medicine, Albuquerque, New Mexico
Media

Raymond Sturner, MD Associate Professor of Pediatrics, Johns Hopkins University School of Medicine; Codirector, Center for Promotion of Child Development Through Primary Care, Baltimore, Maryland
General Principles of Psychological Testing

Stephen Sulkes, MD Professor of Pediatrics, University of Rochester School of Medicine and Dentistry; Director, Strong Center for Developmental Disabilities, Golisano Children's Hospital at Strong, Rochester, New York
Transition to Adulthood for Youth with Developmental Disabilities

Charles M. Super, PhD Professor of Human Development and Pediatrics, University of Connecticut, Storrs, Connecticut
Culture and Ethnicity

Trenna L. Sutcliffe, MD Instructor, Stanford University School of Medicine, Stanford, California; Developmental-Behavioral Pediatrician, Lucile Packard Children's Hospital, Palo Alto, California
The History of Developmental-Behavioral Pediatrics

Ludwik S. Szymanski, MD Associate Professor of Psychiatry, Harvard Medical School; Senior Associate in Psychiatry, Director Emeritus of Psychiatry, Institute for Community Inclusion, Children's Hospital Boston, Boston, Massachusetts
Behavioral Challenges and Mental Disorders in Children and Adolescents with Intellectual Disability

Helen Tager-Flusberg, PhD Professor of Anatomy and Neurobiology, Professor of Pediatrics, Boston University School of Medicine; Professor of Psychology, Boston University, Boston, Massachusetts
Assessment of Intelligence

J. Lane Tanner, MD Clinical Professor of Pediatrics, University of California, San Francisco, California; Associate Director, Division of Developmental and Behavioral Pediatrics, Children's Hospital and Research Center at Oakland, Oakland, California
Separation, Divorce, and Remarriage

Nicole Tartaglia, MD Assistant Professor of Pediatrics, University of Colorado Denver School of Medicine, Denver, Colorado; Developmental-Behavioral Pediatrician, Child Development Unit, The Children's Hospital, Aurora, Colorado
Chromosomal Disorders and Fragile X Syndrome

Stuart W. Teplin, MD Associate Professor Emeritus, University of North Carolina School of Medicine, Chapel Hill, North Carolina; Developmental-Behavioral Pediatrician, Developmental and Behavioral Pediatrics of the Carolinas, CMC-NorthEast Medical Center, Concord, North Carolina
Blindness and Visual Impairment

Melissa Thingvoll, MD Developmental-Behavioral Pediatrician, Mission Children's Hospital–Olson Huff Center, Asheville, North Carolina
Transition to Adulthood for Youth with Developmental Disabilities

Ute Thyen, MD Professor of Pediatrics, University of Lübeck; Director, Social Pediatric Center, Department of Pediatrics and Adolescent Medicine, University Hospital Schleswig-Holstein, Campus Lübeck, Lübeck, Germany
Chronic Health Conditions

Ann Tilton, MD Professor of Neurology and Pediatrics, Louisiana State University Health Sciences Center–New Orleans; Codirector, Rehabilitation Center, Children's Hospital of New Orleans, New Orleans, Louisiana
Cerebral Palsy

Anne Chun-Hui Tsai, MD Associate Professor, University of Colorado at Denver Health Science Center, Denver, Colorado; Attending Physician, Section of Clinical Genetics and Metabolism, The Children's Hospital, Aurora, Colorado
Chromosomal Disorders and Fragile X Syndrome

Callista Tulleners, BA Graduate Student in Nursing, Brandywine School of Nursing, Coatesville, Pennsylvania; Former Research Assistant, The Children's Hospital of Philadelphia, Philadelphia, Pennsylvania
Aggression, Violence, and Delinquency

Gordon L. Ulrey, PhD Associate Clinical Professor of Psychiatry, University of California, Davis, California
The Spectrum of Social Cognition

David K. Urion, MD Associate Professor of Neurology, Harvard Medical School; Director, Learning Disabilities/Behavioral Neurology Program, Director of Education, Department of Neurology, Children's Hospital Boston, Boston, Massachusetts
Diagnostic Methods for Disorders of the Central Nervous System

Craigan T. Usher, MD Assistant Professor of Child and Adolescent Psychiatry, Oregon Health and Science University; Child and Adolescent Psychiatrist, Oregon Health and Science University, Doembecher Children's Hospital, Portland, Oregon
Psychotherapy with Children and Adolescents

Fred Volkmar, MD Director, Yale Child Study Center; Irving B. Harris Professor of Child Psychiatry, Pediatrics, and Psychology, Yale University School of Medicine; Chief, Child Psychiatry, Children's Hospital at Yale–New Haven, New Haven, Connecticut
Autism and Related Disorders

Marji Erickson Warfield, PhD Senior Scientist, Brandeis University, Waltham, Massachusetts
Early Intervention Services

Lynn Mowbray Wegner, MD Clinical Associate Professor of Pediatrics, University of North Carolina School of Medicine, Chapel Hill, North Carolina
School Achievement and Underachievement

Laura Weissman, MD Instructor in Pediatrics, Harvard Medical School; Assistant in Medicine, Children's Hospital Boston, Boston, Massachusetts
Bowel Function, Toileting, and Encopresis

Esther H. Wender, MD Clinical Professor of Pediatrics, University of Washington School of Medicine, Seattle, Washington
Interviewing: A Critical Skill

Lisa Wiesner, MD Assistant Clinical Professor of Pediatrics, Yale University School of Medicine; Attending Physician, Yale–New Haven Hospital, New Haven, Connecticut
Autism and Related Disorders

Paul H. Wise, MD, MPH Richard E. Behrman Professor of Child Health and Society, Stanford University School of Medicine, Stanford, California; Director, Center for Policy Outcomes and Prevention, Department of Pediatrics, Lucile Packard Children's Hospital, Palo Alto, California
Neighborhood and Community

Lise M. Youngblade, PhD Professor and Department Head, Department of Human Development and Family Studies, Colorado State University, Fort Collins, Colorado
Peers

Lonnie K. Zeltzer, MD Professor of Pediatrics, Anesthesiology, Psychiatry, and Biobehavioral Sciences, David Geffen School of Medicine, University of California, Los Angeles; Director, Pediatric Pain Program, Associate Director, Patients and Survivors Program, Mattel Children's Hospital, University of California, Los Angeles, Division of Cancer Prevention and Control Research, UCLA Jonsson Comprehensive Cancer Center, Los Angeles, California
Recurrent and Chronic Pain

Barry S. Zuckerman, MD Professor and Chair, Department of Pediatrics, Boston University School of Medicine, Boston, Massachusetts
Infancy and Toddler Years

PREFACE

Welcome to the fourth edition of *Developmental-Behavioral Pediatrics*. We editors have attempted to insure that this new version maintains the high standards of the previous three. In addition to the necessary updates of the changing science and practice, it adds even further to the breadth, depth, and clarity of the coverage of this vital aspect of comprehensive pediatric care.

The first edition appeared twenty-six years ago, in 1983. It came at a time when developmental and behavioral pediatrics had grown independently over preceding decades and were still regarded as largely disconnected enterprises. Our 1983 edition was the first text to integrate the two strands in the same book. The hyphenated title, *Developmental-Behavioral Pediatrics,* was the simplest term we could contrive to describe the full contents of the unified field. This name was eventually taken by the American Board of Pediatrics as the official designation for the newly recognized subspecialty. The hyphen has not been just a punctuation mark but also a declaration of the acceptance of the professional common ground.

From the outset we were determined to produce a volume with sufficient theory and science for the academic specialist and enough description of diagnosis and management for the clinician. We have attempted to emphasize the broad range of "normal" and to acknowledge children's strengths as well as deficits.

The second edition in 1992 and the third in 1999 aimed both to revise evolving subject areas and to add significant topics not previously described.

Between 1999 and 2009 the field has matured in several ways besides the acceptance by the American Board of Pediatrics of this vital independent subspecialty with its own certifying examination of competence. Other significant developments are the wide range of new techniques for understanding the origins of developmental and behavioral differences, an enhanced appreciation of the nature of dysfunctions and disorders, and advances in management.

This fourth edition of this text strives to integrate theory, science, and practice and to maintain interdisciplinary collaboration. The Table of Contents informs the reader that we have maintained our original unique and logical arrangement of the chapters. We have substantially updated the section on Biological Influences to incorporate new information from genetics and neuroscience and about inborn errors of metabolism. The previous Part V with its mixture of Outcomes during Childhood has now been organized better and subdivided into separate sections on behavioral and emotional status, school performance, physical functions, and developmental outcomes. Within each of these areas there is an increased emphasis on children's assets as well as weaknesses, on dimensional as opposed to categorical diagnoses, on cultural variations, and on scientifically based approaches to diagnosis and management.

The publisher is again our original colleagues at Saunders, although that firm has now been incorporated with others under the management of Elsevier in Philadelphia. Instead of looking out on historic, late Georgian Independence Hall, their offices now are a few steps from the center of the city and the monumental Victorian City Hall with plain Quaker leader, William Penn, on top.

The editors of the first edition were Drs. Melvin D. Levine of Boston, William B. Carey of Philadelphia, Allen C. Crocker of Boston, and Ruth T. Gross of Stanford. Dr. Gross retired after the first edition. Dr. Levine, now in Chapel Hill, who was our lead editor for the first three editions, has withdrawn this time in order to devote himself fully to his important work on children's learning. The two remaining original editors, Drs. Carey and Crocker, have now been joined by three younger ones: Drs. William L. Coleman of Chapel Hill, Ellen R. Elias of Denver, and Heidi M. Feldman of Palo Alto, all of whom are distinguished pediatricians in both the academic and practical worlds.

Many of the outstanding authors of chapters in previous editions are back again. Many new authors are helping us to achieve our more ambitious goals for this one. A variety of new chapters will be evident, for example: self-esteem, self-control, coping, and the death of the child.

Our hope is that this volume will meet the needs of a varied and interdisciplinary readership. For the specialist in developmental-behavioral pediatrics, who is involved in teaching pediatric and general medical trainees and performing special consultations, it should provide a reliable resource for the best information available in this broad and complex field. For the generalist clinician, struggling to understand the spectrum from normal development and behavior to difficult childhood problems, it should offer guidance that is clear and practical. For the researcher in pursuit of significant issues for investigation there should be clear indications about the areas where our knowledge needs most urgently to be improved or augmented. We hope that the text may prove useful not only to pediatricians and general physicians but also to psychiatrists, psychologists, other therapists, educators, and others in the United States and from other countries who are actively engaged in health care and welfare of infants, children, and adolescents.

In all three previous editions of this volume the Preface began with a poem by Robert Frost, a selection made by our lead editor, Mel Levine. This time our new chief editor continues the tradition by selecting as a conclusion to this Preface a few pertinent one-liners from his favorite American author, Mark Twain:

"A baby is an inestimable blessing and bother."

—Letter to Annie Webster, September 1, 1876

"Training is everything. The peach was once a bitter almond; the cauliflower is nothing but cabbage with a college education."

—*Pudd'nhead Wilson's Calendar*, Chapter 5

"Loyalty to petrified opinion never yet broke a chain or freed a human soul."

—Inscription beneath his bust in the Hall of Fame

May our efforts bring you enlightenment, high performance, and satisfaction.

The Editors

CONTENTS

PART VII
OUTCOMES—PHYSICAL FUNCTIONING

PART VIII
OUTCOMES—DEVELOPMENTAL

PART IX
ASSESSMENT

PART X
MANAGEMENT AND TREATMENT

PART XI

LEGAL, ADMINISTRATIVE, AND ETHICAL ISSUES

1 THE HISTORY OF DEVELOPMENTAL-BEHAVIORAL PEDIATRICS

Heidi M. Feldman and Trenna L. Sutcliffe

Developmental-behavioral pediatrics is a recent addition to the growing list of subspecialties of Western medicine. This textbook explores the breadth and depth of the field. We begin with a brief history, highlighting many strands of medicine, social thought, political action, and scientific discovery that have shaped the creation and direction of this young discipline.

The field of developmental-behavioral pediatrics is distinctive among health care disciplines because it serves individuals who, for centuries, had been excluded from traditional medical care—children, individuals with disabilities and mental health disorders, and children at risk for these disorders on the basis of poverty and other adverse environmental conditions. Given that medical practices derive from prevailing social and cultural philosophies, it is not surprising that in the late 18th century, when philosophers of the Enlightenment asserted the fundamental value of all individuals, Western allopathic medicine began to address the needs of these underserved populations. Even then, medical approaches vacillated between promoting habilitation and education and supporting institutionalization or neglect.

This chapter recounts the history of developmental-behavioral pediatrics from the ancient era through the Enlightenment to the 21st century. We review key events in the origins of care for individuals with disabilities and mental health disorders. We describe the differentiation of pediatrics from medicine and the origins of psychology, because both disciplines interact to shape this interdisciplinary field. We examine events in the United States over the last 2 decades of the 20th century when developmental-behavioral pediatrics differentiated from general pediatrics. Finally, we come to the current era in which developmental-behavioral pediatrics has a vibrant interdisciplinary professional society, a respected journal, subspecialty status within pediatrics, and enormous promise for a future serving children developing typically, children with developmental and behavioral disorders, children at risk for such problems, and the families of all these groups.

A LONG HISTORY OF NEGLECT: ANTIQUITY THROUGH THE SEVENTEENTH CENTURY

Health Care of Children

Throughout ancient history, health care for children had been the province of families and midwives. Children were conceptualized as the property of families. Infanticide, abandonment, and child maltreatment were widespread in many cultures (Kanner, 1964). Literature and art portrayed children as miniature adults, paying no attention to their distinctive physical or psychological characteristics.

Treatises on the health care of children were limited through the 17th century. Table 1-1 lists notable contributors to the literature on children's health. Physicians avoided the care of children because of prevailing social beliefs, limited medical training about children's health, and the poor prognosis of many childhood diseases.

Medical Care of Individuals with Disabilities

From antiquity through the Middle Ages in the West, disabilities were usually interpreted from a metaphysical as opposed to a biomedical perspective (Kanner, 1964). Because they were understood to represent a punishment for sin or the work of evil forces, care for individuals with disabilities, such as it was, was relegated to the realm of religion. Infants with obvious physical defects were often abandoned by their families with the implicit understanding that if they did not die, they might end up in slavery or prostitution. Individuals with intellectual disability who were not socially isolated might be sold for the amusement of the rich (Biasini et al, 1999).

Medical Care of Individuals with Mental Illness

Mental illness at various times was attributed to environmental causes, such as loss of status or money; physiologic causes; astrologic alterations, particularly regarding the moon; possession by the devil; moral weakness; or divine punishment. Approaches to treatment were predicated on the underlying theory.

Table 1-1. **Important Contributions to Child Health from Antiquity to the Seventeenth Century**

Individual	Dates	Contributions
Hippocrates	460-377 B.C.	Considered the father of medicine; wrote about epilepsy, cerebral palsy, and other disorders differentially affecting children
Aristotle	384-322 B.C.	Wrote about physiology of the newborn
Soranus of Ephesus (Fig. 1-1)	Practiced 98-138 A.D.	Wrote extensively about gynecology, fetal development, perinatal medicine, and care of newborns
Claudius Galenus of Pergamum	129-200 A.D.	Studied fetal growth and development
Ibn-Zakariya, al-Razi or Rhazes (Fig. 1-2)	860-925	Persian physician; described measles and smallpox; devoted a textbook to childhood diseases
Ibu-e-Sina, or Avicenna	980-1037	Persian physician and philosopher; described many disorders, including several diseases of childhood; preserved Greco-Roman tradition
Paulo Bagellardo	1472	Wrote one of first medical treatises to be printed; focused on the teachings of Rhazes
Bartholomaeus Metlinger	1473	Published a pediatric book for the general public
Thomas Phaer	1544	Wrote the first book in English rather than Latin, called *The Boke of Chyldren*
Gabriel Miron (Le Jeune)	1544	Physician to Louis XII; introduced term "pedenimice," possible origin of term pediatrics

Data from Mahnke CB: The growth and development of a specialty: The history of pediatrics. Clin Pediatr 39:705-714, 2000.

Regardless of the explanation, however, blame for the condition rested on the individual and justified isolation. Approaches to individuals with mental illness were frequently cruel. Incarceration was mandatory in many societies. In colonial America, medical procedures for mental health disorders involved catharsis to expel the evil forces, including submerging patients in ice baths, inducing vomiting, or bleeding.

Concepts of Poverty and Social Disadvantage

Throughout history, poverty has resulted from not only limitations in available resources, but also the uneven distribution of power, limitations of property ownership, excessive taxation, political injustice, and corruption. The poor have remained highly vulnerable to famine, natural disasters, and illness. Nonetheless, in many societies, poverty was ascribed to laziness, idleness, and incompetence.

Interactions among Adverse Conditions

Throughout history, poverty, disabilities, mental health disorders, and youth have been inextricably linked. Poverty is a risk factor for disabilities and mental health disorders through poor nutrition, unfavorable environmental conditions, accidents, illness, and limited access to health care. Individuals from the middle or upper classes who develop disabilities or mental health disorders might descend to the lower classes. The birth rate is typically higher among the poor than the middle and upper classes, increasing demand on limited resources.

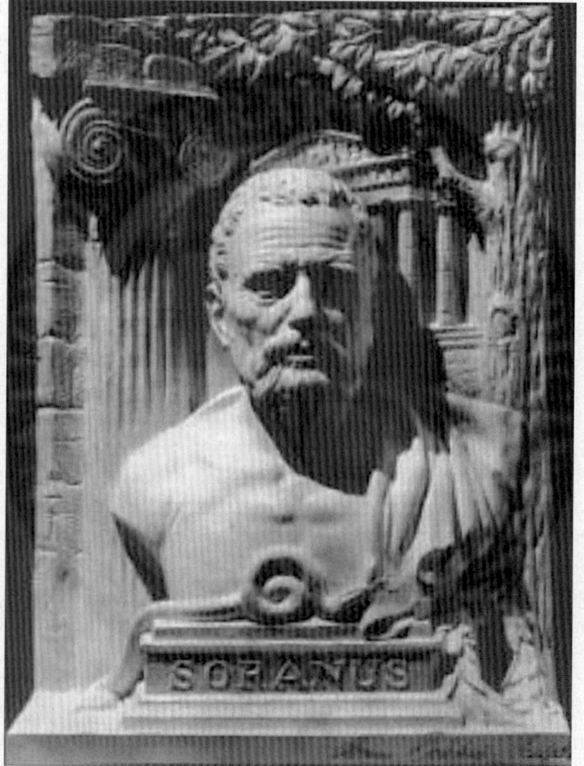

Figure 1-1. Soranus, considered the first pediatrician. (From greciantiga.org/img/esc/nlm-soranus.jpg.)

CHANGING SOCIAL CONDITIONS, PHILOSOPHY, AND MEDICINE: THE EIGHTEENTH AND NINETEENTH CENTURIES

Urbanization

Beginning in the late Middle Ages and continuing through the Renaissance and Industrial Revolution, peasants migrated to towns in search of freedom and prosperity. With increasing urbanization, poverty, disability, and mental illness evolved from isolated individual or family issues to visible social problems.

Life in the cities was extremely difficult for the poor. The cost of living was high. Women, who needed to work to support their families, required child care and artificial formulas. Desperately poor women sometimes resorted to prostitution to earn a living. The infant mortality rate was extremely high, at about 20% to 25%

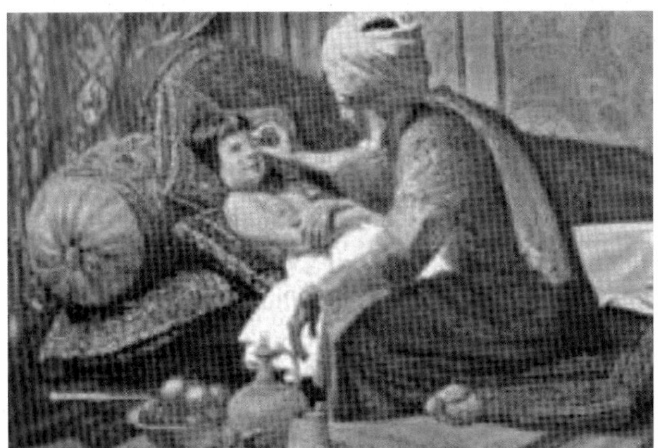

Figure 1-2. Ibn-Zakariya, al-Razi, Persian physician who described measles. (From http://222.ishim.net/alrazi2.jpg.)

in Western Europe into the 19th century. Infectious epidemics ravaged large populations of children and adults (Mahnke, 2000).

The Enlightenment

In the late 17th century and early 18th century, a new social philosophy rejected the absolute authority of the church and monarchy and, in so doing, reframed basic concepts of human experience and human worth. The Enlightenment rested on the supposition that the universe could be understood through the use of reason. One of the early contributors was the British philosopher John Locke (1632-1704), who argued that ideas and moral thought were not innate, but rather acquired through experience. The mind, in his philosophy, could be conceptualized as a blank slate on which sensations stamp simple ideas, which are processed through reflection to form complex ideas. Another highly influential thinker of the era was Jean-Jacques Rousseau (1712-1778). He articulated another influence of environment: humans were good by nature and corrupted by their experiences in society. He argued that the role of government was freedom, equality, and justice for all. The Enlightenment inspired the origins of democracy on the political sphere.

Treatment of Children with Disabilities

A pivotal social change in Western medicine occurred when a physician, Jean-Marc-Gaspard Itard (1775-1835), undertook the education of Victor, the Wild Boy of Aveyron (Kanner, 1964). Victor was a young adolescent who had apparently lived in the mountains outside of human society until his capture by townspeople. Itard made a commitment to educate him, based on Enlightenment concepts that an enriched environment could compensate for the severe deprivation. An intensive 5-year individualized program of rehabilitation had better results than many of the time predicted, although Victor was never able to participate fully in society (Kanner, 1964). Itard's student, Eduard Séguin (1812-1880), a French physician, further popularized this concept of a comprehensive individualized educational program for children with intellectual disability, deafness, and other disabilities. Séguin has been called the father of special education. Maria Montessori, the first woman physician in Italy (1870-1952), based her educational philosophy on Séguin's contributions.

The usual goal of the Enlightenment physicians was normality, the cure of intellectual deficits. To this end, beautiful residential educational centers were built in mountain settings where intensive instruction could be enhanced through fresh air and healthy diets. These pioneers oversold their capabilities, however. When the centers failed to deliver the promise of cured citizens, they quickly evolved from educational programs to custodial institutions (Kanner, 1964). In the second half of the 19th century, residential institutions flourished throughout Western Europe and America. Many physicians abandoned their role in habilitation and participated in euthanasia and sterilization.

Treatment of Mental Health Disorders

The Enlightenment also dramatically altered the care of individuals with mental health disorders. Philippe Pinel (1745-1826) is often regarded as the father of modern psychiatry. Rather than harsh, punitive care, he promoted "moral management," or what might be better referred to as psychological management. The method included intense observation and conversation with individuals with mental disorders. In this model, supportive care was offered in homelike settings (Weiner, 1992). Hypnosis and relaxation were introduced. Work programs also were developed on the assumption that such programs could facilitate a transition from asylum to community. Attractive asylums were built that promised humane and effective treatments (Weiner, 1992).

Despite noble intentions, the institutions gradually became overcrowded. Soldiers returning from war often required psychological care. Families brought elderly individuals to the institutions when their care exceeded the family's capacities. Crowding and inadequate staffing led to a return to restraints and shock therapies. The asylum population remained very high and the conditions deplorable until the 1950s.

EMERGENCE OF PEDIATRICS: EIGHTEENTH TO TWENTIETH CENTURIES

In the early 18th century, the diseases of children garnered increasing attention. William Cadogan (1711-1797), an English physician, wrote an influential text, "Essay upon Nursing and the Management of Children" in 1748, and George Armstrong (1719-1789), another English physician, established the first dispensary for children in London, in 1769. In 1802, the first children's hospital, L'hôpital des Enfants-Malades, was founded in Paris, the center of Western medicine at the time (Mahnke, 2000). After unrelenting advocacy on the part of Charles West (1816-1898), The Hospital for Sick Children at No. 49 Great Ormond Street opened in London in 1852.

The same period witnessed major changes in the United States. A leading physician, Benjamin Rush (1745-1813), lectured on the diseases of children in the late 18th and early 19th centuries. Eli Ives (1779-1861) was appointed the Professor of the Diseases of Children in 1820 at the Medical Institution of Yale College and offered formal courses in pediatrics for 40 years (Strain, 2004). The first children's hospital in the United States was established in Philadelphia in 1855, about the same time as the New York Nursing and Child Hospital opened in New York City (American Academy of Pediatrics Historical Archives Advisory Committee, 2001). Pioneering work by Pasteur, Koch, and Lister began to increase the range of possible treatments for childhood disorders. In addition, public health advances, such as sewage and clean water, substantially improved the health of children.

Abraham Jacobi (1830-1919) (Fig. 1-3) is often considered the father of American pediatrics (Strain, 2004). He organized the first children's clinic at the New York Medical College in 1860. He also organized the pediatric subsections for the American Medical Association in 1880. He collaborated on public health efforts, such as the creation of pasteurization plants and milk stations to provide safe milk for poor infants in New York (Mahnke, 2000).

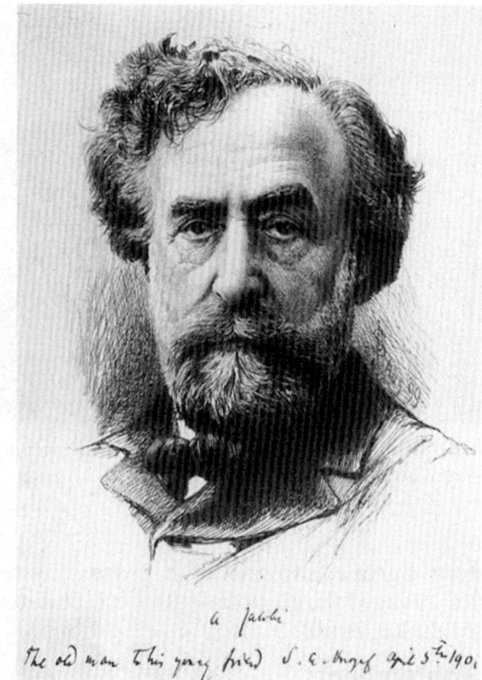

Figure 1-3. Abraham Jacobi, often considered the Father of Pediatrics.

The *Archives of Pediatrics,* the first journal in the United States to be devoted exclusively to children, was first published in 1884, and the American Pediatric Society was founded in 1888. By 1900, about half of the medical schools in the United States had chairs of pediatrics (American Academy of Pediatrics Historical Archives Advisory Committee, 2001).

A highly relevant feature of the emerging field of pediatrics in the United States was its commitment not only in understanding and treating the diseases of childhood, but also in advocating for preventive public health efforts and legal protections for children. This public health perspective led to the differentiation of pediatrics from adult medicine. In 1922, the Section on the Diseases of Children of the American Medical Association voted in support of the Sheppard-Towner Act, a modest federal maternal and child health program. On the same day, the American Medical Association House of Delegates passed a resolution condemning the act. The conflict that followed ultimately led to creation of the American Academy of Pediatrics (AAP) in 1930. Shortly thereafter, the American Board of Pediatrics (ABP) formed, effectively severing administrative ties between pediatrics and medicine within the United States (Strain, 2004).

Sociopolitical movements occurring simultaneously validated the importance of distinctive health care for children. The child welfare movement began in the 19th century in France. Societies began that encouraged breastfeeding, free medical care, and well-baby visits. The movement spread to the United States and linked up with the public health movement. In 1908, the New York City Health Department founded a Bureau of Child Hygiene to address public health concerns of children, including prenatal care, infant mortality, school inspections, and child labor laws. As a result of these efforts, infant mortality rates decreased by half (Mahnke, 2000). In addition, the public school movement in the United States began in the mid-19th century. Until then, education was available only to the wealthy. Public education was seen as a way to integrate poor immigrant children and former slaves into the mainstream American culture (Kanner, 1964). Early textbooks emphasized moral education and industry. Influential leaders, such as Horace Mann (1796-1859), promoted public education. Near the end of the 19th century, mandatory school attendance laws were passed in many states. The public school movement generally favored the education of all children, including children with disabilities, in the local community.

DEVELOPMENT OF PSYCHOLOGY: THE NINETEENTH AND TWENTIETH CENTURIES

The core concepts and approaches of developmental-behavioral pediatrics are as solidly rooted in psychology as they are in pediatrics. The following brief summary highlights major developments in psychology that were particularly relevant to current practice and research.

Charles Darwin (1809-1882) has been credited with introducing the study of human behavioral development, which evolved into the psychology of children (Kessen, 1999). His essay, entitled, "A Biographical Sketch of an Infant" was a meticulous account of the capacities of his infant son. He carefully described developments in a variety of domains—movement, vision, emotions (anger, fear, and pleasure), reasoning, moral sense, and communication. This inventory presaged the domains of functioning further described and studied by subsequent contributors and formed the basis of how we view child development in the current era.

Francis Galton (1822-1911), Darwin's cousin, launched the study of human intelligence. He was particularly interested in the variation among individuals. Galton's legacy is developmental and intelligence testing, a foundation of current developmental-behavioral pediatric practice (Kessen, 1999). Alfred Binet (1857-1911) collaborated with Theodore Simon in designing a carefully constructed scale that could be used to differentiate children who were developing typically from children who required special education because of slow development. The Binet-Simon test was first published in 1905. Lewis Terman (1877-1956) standardized the Simon-Binet test on a large sample of U.S. children, creating the Stanford-Binet test of intelligence. Arnold Gesell (1880-1961) used a similar empirical approach to create an evaluation of the development of young children. His book, entitled *An Atlas of Infant Behavior* and published in 1934, described the typical developmental milestones. Although the developers of these assessments were clear about the limitations of the quantitative approach to measuring intelligence, the Eugenics Movement used the work of Galton and results of intelligence testing to support their claims about the superiority of white race and inferiority of African Americans, immigrants, and individuals with disabilities and mental health disorders. Eugenics advocated for improvements in the human race through selective breeding, prenatal testing, birth control, sterilization, and euthanasia (Kanner, 1964). This history emphasizes the ethical obligations of professionals in assessing the capacities of young children.

In a concurrent but independent tradition of psychology, Sigmond Freud (1856-1939) described the development of emotions and emotional disorders (Kessen, 1999). Freud proposed a three-part structure of the mind: the id, the ego, and the superego. He described five stages of psychosexual development: the oral, anal, phallic, latency, and genital stages. Freud also articulated the concept of the unconscious. Psychoanalysis became the method for helping patients acquire insights into the unconscious conflicts in their upbringing that caused emotional disorders. Most of these concepts have been severely criticized or reworked throughout the 20th and 21st centuries. Erik Erikson (1902-1994) later reconceptualized Freudian stages in psychosocial rather than psychosexual terms. The major tasks that children face at various points in development are still described in Erikson's terms.

James Mark Baldwin (1861-1934) was a leading figure in the area of sensation and perception. His experimental work on infant development strongly influenced Jean Piaget (1896-1980), whose intense observation of his three children formed the foundation of an integrated theory of cognitive development. In Piaget's theory, the sensorimotor stage of development preceded the preoperational, operational, and formal operational stages. Children progressed through these stages through processes of assimilation of environmental experiences and accommodations to those experiences. These concepts remain a foundation in experimental cognitive development.

Another influential tradition within psychology that emerged in the 19th century was the study of learning. Ivan Pavlov (1849-1936), a Russian physiologist, psychologist, and physician, described what he called the "conditioned reflex." The conditioned reflex is the ability of a once neutral stimulus, such as a bell, to cause a physiologic reaction, such as salivation, in an animal or human based on pairings of the neutral stimulus with a motivating stimulus, such as food. These concepts are current in areas such as the causes and treatments of phobias. In the United States, James B. Watson (1878-1958) was an early behaviorist, who argued for cutting out consciousness and other intangibles from the dialogue of psychology. His hope was to control children's emotions through conditioning. B. F. Skinner (1904-1990) elaborated on operant conditioning, the ability of a reinforcing stimulus to change the probability of the appearance of behaviors. Operant conditioning still plays a central role in behavior management of children developing typically and children with disabilities. Following Skinner, behavioral approaches scrutinize antecedent conditions, behaviors, and consequences in the search for reinforcers. In addition, the frequency and pattern of reinforcement are still considered important to the maintenance of behavior change.

ACCELERATED SOCIAL CHANGE: THE TWENTIETH CENTURY

Social and Legal Conditions

By the 20th century, pediatrics had a foothold in medical schools around the Western world, and children's hospitals were proliferating. The plight of children had finally commanded the attention of public leaders. There remained, however, huge gaps in understanding the needs of children and meeting those needs through public programs. President Theodore Roosevelt convened a White House conference on children and youth in 1909. The ultimate consequences of the meeting was the establishment of the U.S. Children's Bureau in 1912, which evolved into the Maternal and Child Health Bureau (MCHB) in 1935. The establishment of the MCHB was included in the Social Security Act. One of its first programs was Crippled Children Services. Eventually, the MCHB migrated to Health Resources and Services Administration, reflecting the shift from conceptualizing child health strictly as a set of social service issues to a set of public health and medical issues.

In 1930, President Herbert Hoover hosted the White House Conference on Child Health and Protection. The purpose of the conference was to develop appropriate services to address the problems of dependent children, including regular medical examination, school or public clinics for children, hospitalization, adequate milk supplies, community nurses, maternity instruction and nurses, teaching of health in the schools, facilities for playgrounds and recreation, child labor laws, and scores of related issues. Among its recommendations, the conference concluded that all children, including children with disabilities, regardless of condition, should be educated in their home communities (Hoover, 1930).

Progress on health care and social services for children, including children with disabilities and other conditions, came to a sudden halt during the Great Depression. Limited fiscal resources were diverted into other programs, such as employment. World War II followed, again redirecting human and fiscal resources to the military. Rather than the recommended moves toward inclusion and habilitation, care of children and adults with disabilities and mental disorders moved increasingly to institutionalization. The association of the Eugenics Movement with the human rights catastrophes of Nazi Germany ended the potency of the movement.

Advocacy after World War II

In the aftermath of World War II, families and friends, not physicians or educators, championed the cause of disabilities (Kanner, 1964). In the 1950s, these individuals established advocacy organizations to educate the public, impact local schools and communities, and have a presence at the national stage. One particularly successful parent group, formed in 1950, was the National Association of Parents and Friends of Mentally Retarded Children, which went through subsequent name changes and is now known simply as The Arc (Segal, 1974). The Arc advocated for equal rights, improved education, and improved health care for individuals with disabilities; taught skills that are important for independence and employment to individuals with disabilities; and encouraged research in the area of disability. In addition, a self-advocacy movement originated in the 1960s in Sweden, England, and Canada. Individuals with intellectual disability were supported in creating their own organizations, many of which initially focused on developing leisure activities. The concept of self-advocacy became known in the United States in the early 1970s.

Advocacy groups for individuals with physical impairments also became active during this time. In 1958, the President's Commission on Employment of the Handicapped, the National Easter Seal Society, and the American National Standards Institute (ANSI) met to discuss accessibility to public buildings. Voluntary building standards were developed over the next few years, including reserved parking spaces close to buildings; accessible elevators, ramps, and toilet stalls to accommodate wheelchairs; and extra hand rails for support. The limited progress through voluntary standards led to the Architectural Barriers Act, passed by the U.S. Congress in 1968. Enforcement of building standards in the 1970s and beyond facilitated the integration of individuals with disabilities into the workforce, education systems, and public domain.

The civil rights movement of the 1960s provided the organizing framework for these fledgling advocacy efforts. The "disability rights movement," a grass roots effort, formulated a political agenda that closely resembled that of the civil rights movement: overcoming the oppression experienced by individuals with disabilities, promoting independence and self-sufficiency, and advocating for social change. A distinctive concept of the disability rights movement group was that individuals with disabilities faced more barriers because of social and political norms than because of actual physical or mental impairment. The social model of disability contrasts with the medical model, which assumes that the main issue is the limitation of the individual. The social model favors social and political change to allow individuals with disabilities to participate fully in community life.

Building an Infrastructure for Care and Services for Individuals with Disabilities

The field of developmental-behavioral pediatrics owes much of the current infrastructure for research and training in disabilities and mental health disorders to President John F. Kennedy (Wolraich and Bennett, 2003). Rosemary Kennedy, his oldest sister, had a cognitive impairment and behavioral disorder, which was worsened by a therapeutic lobotomy. Eunice Shriver, sister of Rosemary and John, published the story of the family's experience in *The Saturday Evening Post* in 1962 (Shriver, 1962). Figure 1-4 shows the Kennedy children.

In 1963, President Kennedy convened the President's Panel on Mental Retardation. Recognizing the lack of programs training professionals to work with children and adults with intellectual disability, the panel proposed federal funding for the development of University-Affiliated Facilities. These new centers were designed to support training programs, university-based research, and clinical services to benefit individuals with disabilities. Federal funding supported the development of 18 University-Affiliated Facilities and 12 Mental Retardation Centers (Association of University Centers on Disabilities, 2004). After the initial phase of construction, the University-Affiliated Facilities were continued as University-Affiliated Programs (UAPs). The UAP mission included moving research and technology forward, improving government policies, measuring outcomes,

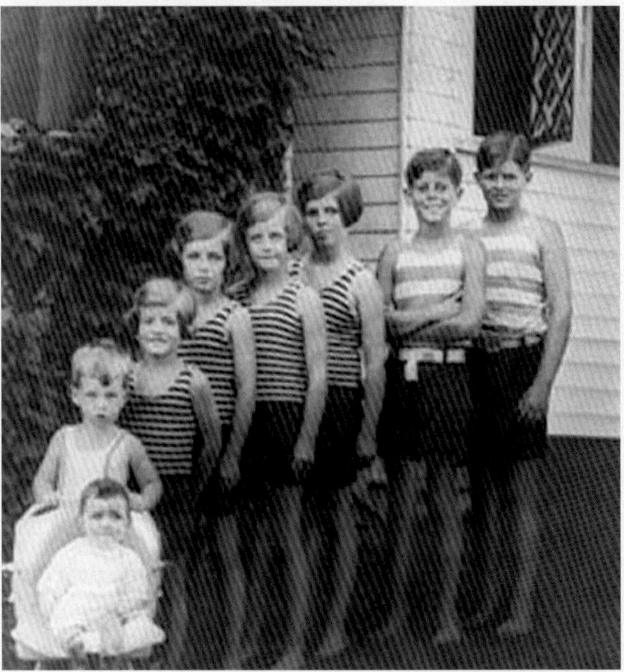

Figure 1-4. John F. Kennedy and his siblings as children. (From www.john-f-kennedy.net/jfksiblings.jpg.)

developing and evaluating social and community programs for individuals with disabilities, training clinicians and researchers involved in disability care and science, and communicating with the community to determine needs. The programs were interdisciplinary, requiring representatives from a wide range of disciplines, including psychology, nursing, social work, occupational and physical therapy, and public health.

The UAPs were funded by one of two sources. UAPs funded by the Administration for Developmental Disabilities are now known as University Centers for Excellence for Developmental Disabilities; there are 61 centers nationally. These centers are associated with major universities and work closely with community-based organizations, services, and self-advocacy groups. This community collaboration has many advantages, including ensuring that individuals with disabilities contribute to the policies and programs that affect them, stimulating leadership in the community, and ensuring that academic and research programs are relevant and respectful. UAPs funded by the MCHB are now known as Leadership Education in Neurodevelopmental and Related Disabilities (LEND); there are 36 programs nationally. These programs, also associated with major universities, emphasize interdisciplinary clinical and leadership training. They also promote community participation to improve communication, coordination, and shared leadership at all levels. Developmental Disabilities Research Centers, funded by the National Institute of Child Health and Human Development, were established initially in 1963, charged with using basic, clinical, and translational research to understand the causes and provide treatments for disabilities. All of these university programs are members of the Association of University Centers on Disability, an advocacy network for disabilities and the programs themselves (Association of University Centers on Disabilities, 2004).

Legal Protections for Individuals with Disabilities

The laws of the 1970s to the present have ensured equality for individuals with disabilities and mental health disorders. We emphasize here just a few examples that are particularly relevant to developmental-behavioral pediatrics. The Rehabilitation Act of 1973, borrowing concepts and language from the Civil Rights Act, was primarily designed to provide job opportunities and training to adults with disabilities. Section 504 of the Rehabilitation Act prohibited discrimination on the basis of disability in service availability, accessibility, or delivery in organizations that receive federal funding. As applied to schools, the language served to prohibit schools and districts from denying public education on the basis of a student's disability. The Education for All Handicapped Children Act (P.L. 94-142), a landmark education bill, was passed in 1975. This law mandated a free and public education for all children as befitting their needs. The law also required that the education occur in the least restrictive environment, a provision specifically designed to combat the social and educational isolation that many children with disabilities faced. The law has been reauthorized on several occasions and is now known as the Individuals with Disabilities Education Act (IDEA). An important revision passed in 1986 lowered the mandated age for educational services to 3 years and provided states with incentives to establish programs for children from birth to age 3 years.

In the United States, the capstone of legislative protections is the Americans with Disabilities Act (ADA). Conservative and progressive politicians collaborated to move forward policies ensuring equality for all individuals with disabilities. The bill was drafted by Ronald Reagan appointees to the National Council on Disability and passed by the U.S. Congress in 1990 under the administration of George H. W. Bush. It significantly expanded protection laws against discrimination on the basis of disability.

New Paradigms for Care of Individuals with Mental Illness

In parallel to the changes in care of individuals with disabilities, new approaches to the care of children and adults with mental health disorders emerged in the second half of the 20th century. During World War II, conscientious objectors assigned to the Civilian Public Service ushered in an era of reform by publishing the abuses they witnessed in Byberry Hospital in Philadelphia. They stimulated an exposé in *Life* magazine in 1946 and the formation of the Mental Hygiene Project, which later became the National Mental Health Foundation. Eleanor Roosevelt sat on the board of the foundation (Sareyan, 1994).

A major shift in the care of individuals with mental illness was the discovery of psychoactive medications in the mid-1950s. In the 1940s and 1950s, the prevailing treatments for individuals included electroconvulsive shock therapy, insulin shock therapy, and frontal lobotomy. In 1952, Henri Laborit (1914-1995), a French surgeon, inadvertently discovered that chlorpromazine could calm without completely sedating individuals. He encouraged its use in patients with mental and emotional disorders. When the drug was approved by the U.S. Food and Drug Administration in 1954, it rapidly revolutionized the care of individuals with mental health disorders, particularly in state institutions. It also gradually shifted concepts of the origins of mental disorders and ushered in an emphasis on biologic treatments for mental disorders.

President John F. Kennedy proposed a national mental health program with a strong emphasis on reducing the number of individuals in custodial care, eliminating hazardous conditions in institutions, and discarding outmoded and cruel methods of care. He endorsed the concept of comprehensive community mental health centers with the full spectrum of services from diagnosis through emergency care. Deinstitutionalization gradually gained momentum. The ability of communities to support individuals with mental health disorders adequately was not sufficiently supported, however. Problems such as homelessness and crime continue to be visible indications of the limitations of community-based programs.

Another major advance in psychiatry was the publication of the *Diagnostic and Statistical Manual of Mental Disorders* (DSM) in 1952. This manual clarified diagnostic criteria for mental and emotional disorders. In the first edition, only one pediatric diagnosis was included—adjustment reaction of childhood/adolescence. The second and third editions of DSM were published in 1968 and 1987 and included significantly more pediatric diagnoses. Changes in the fourth and revised fourth editions from 1994 and 2000 have resulted in increased prevalence of childhood diagnoses such as attention-deficit/hyperactivity disorder and autism. The DSM has improved the quality of research in that diagnosis is standardized according to strict criteria. The strictly symptom-based, nontheoretical approach of the DSM also has severe limitations, however, for understanding complex interactions of biologic predispositions and environmental forces and the changing nature of disorders with development (Jensen and Mrazek, 2006).

New Paradigms for Children at Risk on the Basis of Poverty

Pediatrics began to play a pivotal role in changing approaches to children living in poverty. In the mid-1960s, Julius Richmond (1916-2008), head of the Office of Employment Opportunities, launched Project Head Start, a program of free, community-based preschool programs for children from low-income families. The objectives of Head Start were to meet the emotional, developmental, health, social, and nutritional needs of the children and to stimulate employment and empowerment of the communities in which these children lived. Positive and long-lasting impacts of high-quality early education have been documented in school-age children (Lee et al, 1990) to young adults (Campbell et al, 2002). In the 21st century, Head Start has remained an important resource for children who live in poverty. Richmond later became Assistant Secretary for Health, U.S. Department of Health and Human Services, and Surgeon General in 1977 (Fig. 1-5). One of his many important contributions in that role was the publication of *Healthy People: The Surgeon General's Report on Health Promotion and Disease Prevention*. This publication stressed the importance of quantitative research in public health and promoted healthy lifestyle as an important public health measure.

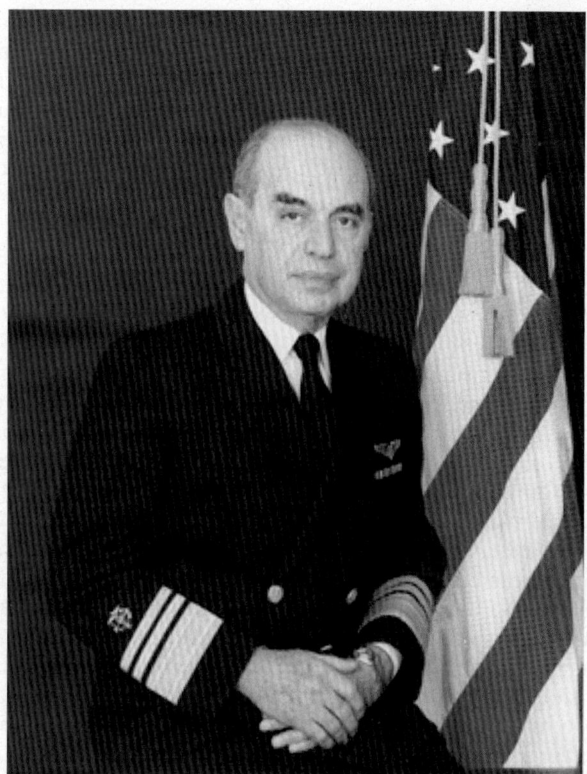

Figure 1-5. Julius Richmond as Surgeon General. (From profiles.nlm.nih.gov/NN/B/K/B/K/_/nnbdbk_.jpg.)

BIRTH OF DEVELOPMENTAL-BEHAVIORAL PEDIATRICS

Changing Demographics

The prevalence of children with developmental and behavioral disorders or at risk for such disorders increased dramatically in the second half of the 20th century, creating a need for specialists in the care of these children. A major factor in the shifting demographics was advances in medical science and technology. In 1960, the survival rate for an infant weighing 1 kg was 5%, and an infant born at less than 28 weeks' gestation was considered nonviable. The development of neonatal intensive care units, specialized respirators, and the use of surfactant dramatically altered survival rates. In 2000, the survival rate of the infant weighing 1 kg was 95%, and 50% of infants born at 24 weeks' gestation are viable (Philip, 2005). These infants often experience medical complications, however, and remain at high risk for developmental and behavioral disorders, including cerebral palsy, hearing impairment, vision impairment, cognitive deficits, learning disorders, and school problems. The population of children born prematurely has steadily increased over the last several decades, while the proportion of that population with disabilities has remained essentially unchanged, leading to an increasing number of children with disabilities.

A second example is that infants born with previously fatal complex congenital heart disease now undergo lifesaving surgeries. Repair of atrioventricular canal defects has contributed to improved survival rates for children with Down syndrome from less than 50% (Record and Smith, 1955) to greater than 90% (Yang et al, 2002). Improvements in medical and social services have contributed to the median age of survival for individuals with Down syndrome increasing from 25 years in 1983 to 49 years in 1997 (Yang et al, 2002).

Increased Awareness of Developmental and Behavioral Problems

The second half of the 20th century witnessed a substantial increase in the prevalence of families reporting behavioral issues to pediatricians and other health care providers (Haggerty and Friedman, 2003). The exact reasons for the increase are unclear, but have been related to a decrease in serious infectious diseases, increased parental awareness in the baby boom era,

Table 1-2. Early Centers for Developmental-Behavioral Pediatrics in 1960-1970

University Center	Contributions and Features
University of California San Francisco	Program required pediatric residents to train in mental health issues; early fellowship training program
Harvard University	Julius Richmond encouraged pediatricians to establish expertise in development and behavior; Allen Crocker studied children with neurologic disorders and established Developmental Evaluation Center; T. Berry Brazelton developed a neonatal assessment tool; Melvin D. Levine focused on problems of attention and learning, and established training program and clinical service; Eli Newberger launched program in child abuse
Rochester University	Robert Haggerty and Stanford Friedman began training fellows in behavioral pediatrics and adolescent medicine
Yale University	Arnold Gesell founded Yale Child Study Center; initial focus was child development; Milton Senn and Albert Solnit brought psychoanalytic focus
Children's Hospital of Philadelphia	Henry Cecil began program in psychological pediatrics, funded by William T. Grant Foundation; William B. Carey was first fellow
Johns Hopkins University	Leo Kanner and Leon Eisenberg began fellowship training through department of psychiatry; Kennedy Center focused on children with disabilities; Arnold Capute was first fellow

changes in family structure, and increasing expectations for children (Haggerty and Friedman, 2003).

During that same period, expectations regarding education also were changing. In the 1960s, many young adolescents, including those with academic and behavioral problems, never graduated from high school. As the importance of literacy and higher education has increased, rates of high school graduation also have increased. Public education is being held accountable to show that children can read and write at grade-appropriate levels, or that they should receive special accommodations. Many children come to medical and psychological attention for evaluations that allow them to access special education services and other potentially useful therapies.

Evolving Pediatric Practice

In 1972, the AAP articulated standards of care that stated that supporting families so that their children could achieve optimal growth and development was central to the pediatrician's role (American Academy of Pediatrics, 1972). Pediatricians were encouraged to offer anticipatory guidance to the family and assess the developmental and behavioral status of the child (American Academy of Pediatrics, 1972). Practicing pediatricians recognized that they did not have the necessary skills to fulfill this recommendation (Dworkin et al, 1979; Shonkoff et al, 1979). In 1978, the AAP Task Force on Pediatric Education again raised concerns that medical education in the United States was providing insufficient teaching and training around biopsychosocial aspects of child health and child development to support future roles for pediatricians in managing emotional disorders, learning problems, and chronic conditions (Haggerty and Friedman, 2003). Their report included recommendations for curriculum. Recommendations for developmental surveillance continue to be published (Committee on Children with Disabilities American Academy of Pediatrics, 2001).

Establishment of Training Programs

Given the changing demographics and the changing paradigm in pediatrics, medical professionals trained in child development, child behavior, and developmental and behavioral disorders were clearly needed. The AAP established the Section on Mental Health in 1949, which became the Section for Developmental and Behavioral Pediatrics in 1960 (Haggerty and Friedman, 2003). In an oral history, William B. Carey, an original and current editor of this textbook, states that in 1959, the only places offering fellowship training were the Yale Child Study Center, the Syracuse University, Johns Hopkins University, and Children's Hospital of Philadelphia. Table 1-2 lists several of the major university centers that subsequently began residency and fellowship training in the next decade. The MCHB provided financial support for training through the UAPs and through developmental-behavioral pediatrics fellowships.

A contentious issue at that time was whether training in behavioral pediatrics should most appropriately fall under the domain of child psychiatrists or pediatricians (Haggerty and Friedman, 2003). Some of the initial pioneers in the field, such as Benjamin Spock (1903-1998), and T. Berry Brazelton, were trained in programs led by child psychiatry. Others, including William Carey, who studied at Children's Hospital of Philadelphia, trained in a program led by pediatrics. The emerging consensus was that pediatrics, rather than child psychiatry, was more suitable for this training for many reasons, such as its ability to put emphasis on the full range of issues from normal function to severe disorder, the ability to understand and intervene in the complex interplay of psychosocial factors and physical health, and the potential for pediatrics to coordinate the care of psychosocial issues and behavioral health with routine health supervision and treatment of physical disorders (Haggerty and Friedman, 2003).

The concept of behavioral pediatrics was slowly recognized through an emergence of literature related to the topic and funding grants to support the training. In 1970, Friedman wrote about the challenges of behavioral pediatrics (Haggerty and Friedman, 2003). In 1975, the August issue of *Pediatric Clinics of North America* was dedicated to behavioral pediatrics. The William T. Grant Foundation provided grant support for behavioral pediatrics training programs, beginning in 1959 with support of programs in Baltimore and Philadelphia and expanding in the 1970s to sites across the United States (Carey, 2003).

Establishment of a Journal and Society

Marvin Gottlieb (1928-2008) had a vision for a journal of developmental and behavioral issues from the early 1950s (Haggerty and Friedman, 2003). The *Journal of Developmental and Behavioral Pediatrics* was initially published in 1980. The journal has provided a prominent forum to present research and commentary on topics related to the field. Its impact factor is relatively high among pediatric subspecialty journals.

The Society of Behavioral Pediatrics was established in 1982, after discussion and collaboration of behavioral pediatric program directors who met at the Society of Pediatric Research annual meeting. Initially, the name of the group was Society of Behavioral and Developmental Pediatrics; however, because of potential legal challenges from an already existing society referred to as the Society for Developmental Pediatrics (see later), the name was initially changed to the Society of Behavioral Pediatrics. In 1994, it changed its name to the Society for Developmental and Behavioral Pediatrics in recognition of the substantial overlap of developmental and behavioral issues in childhood and the scope of practice of its members. The society prides itself on its interdisciplinary membership. Shortly after its formation, the new organization applied for and was granted editorial sponsorship of *Journal of Developmental and Behavioral Pediatrics*. Stanford Friedman became the editor in 1985. *Developmental-Behavioral Pediatrics* was chosen as the title for the first comprehensive textbook in the field, published in 1983 with editors Melvin D. Levine, William B. Carey, Allen C. Crocker, and Ruth T. Gross.

Path to Board Certification

Within pediatrics, board certification for subspecialties provides recognition of a distinctive scope of practice and public assurance regarding the quality of practitioners. The detailed history of board certification for developmental-behavioral pediatrics has been described in detail in other sources (Haggerty and Friedman, 2003; Perrin et al, 2000).

Important in this history is that two professional groups with overlapping interests chose to follow separate paths for certification through the American Board of Medical Specialties. One group was headed by Arnold Capute (1923-2003) and included many of his trainees, some of whom were project directors of UAPs (Wolraich and Bennett, 2003). Capute left a busy private pediatric practice on Staten Island, NY, in 1965 to become the first fellow in Developmental Pediatrics at the Johns Hopkins University School of Medicine at the newly opened John F. Kennedy Institute, now called the Kennedy-Krieger Institute. He served as the director of the training program in developmental pediatrics, educating numerous subspecialists for roles in education and research. He formed the Society for Developmental Pediatrics in 1978. Focusing on the issues of children with developmental disorders rather than on the broader issues of development and behavior in normal children, children at risk, and children with disorders, this society successfully created a second section within the AAP in 1990 called the Section on Children with Disabilities. The Society for Developmental Pediatrics made the first application for subspecialty board certification. Their application focused on children with developmental disabilities and, in particular, on the neurobiology of these disorders.

The Society of Behavioral Pediatrics Executive Council voted to pursue board certification in 1991. Attempts to combine efforts with a single application, given the overlapping scope of practice of the two groups, failed.

The ABP was initially hesitant to support a subspecialty in development and behavior because of concerns that the new specialty would have too much overlap with the practice of general pediatrics and would reduce the responsibilities of general pediatricians. The ABP heard strong support, however, from the developmental and behavioral section of the AAP and numerous academic and community pediatricians. In particular, general pediatricians wanted subspecialists who would teach, train, study, and practice child development and behavior. In 1994, the ABP declared that they would support the creation of a developmental-behavioral pediatrics subspecialty.

The Society for Developmental Pediatrics subspecialty ultimately called itself Neurodevelopmental Disabilities (NDD) and sought primary certification from the American Board of Psychiatry and Neurology. The ABP agreed to support the application and cosponsor subspecialty certification during the initial years, while pediatricians in practice could become board certified on the basis of their previous experience. NDD also was recognized as a subspecialty by American Board of Medical Subspecialties in 1999. As of 2007, training in child neurology is a prerequisite for board certification in NDD.

The developmental-behavioral pediatrics subspecialty was supported by the ABP. It encountered resistance from the American Board of Psychiatry and Neurology, however, which was concerned that the role of the developmental-behavioral pediatrician was not sufficiently distinct from that of the child psychiatrist. The ABP stipulates that a subspecialty must improve on the care of children, supplement the role of the general pediatrician, and teach the subspecialty field to trainees and other professionals before it can be considered for subspecialty status (Stockman, 2000). The Society for Developmental and Behavioral Pediatrics addressed the American Board of Psychiatry and Neurology concerns in a subsequent application. Training in child neurology and child psychiatry was integrated into the training requirements for developmental-behavioral pediatrics at the same time that developmental-behavioral pediatrics was recognized as a distinct subspecialty. Participation of psychologists in training also was required to show the commitment to an interdisciplinary field. In 1999, developmental-behavioral pediatrics was approved as a subspecialty by the American Board of Medical Specialties.

Board certification for NDD was first granted in 2001. Board certification in developmental-behavioral pediatrics was first granted in 2002. In 2006, after three certification examinations, there were 520 board-certified developmental-behavioral pediatricians in the United States. In 2007, there were 31 accredited fellowship training programs and 76 fellows in training. As of 2005, there were 241 board-certified NDD specialists. In 2007, there were seven training programs and six fellows in training.

CURRENT ERA

Developmental-behavioral pediatrics is securely embedded as a subspecialty within pediatrics. At the same time, it remains an interdisciplinary field integrating psychology, pediatrics, and related disciplines. The field of developmental-behavioral pediatrics plays many key roles in academic medicine, clinical practice, and community advocacy.

Developmental-behavioral pediatrics is an important element in the education of general pediatricians. At the time of this writing, general pediatric residencies are required by the Residency Review Committee of the Accreditation Council of Graduate Medical Education to provide residents with a 1-month dedicated rotation and a longitudinal component, the equivalent of a second month spread throughout residency. Through developmental-behavioral pediatrics, many residents learn an approach to the so-called new morbidities, which continue to evolve with shifting demographic trends (Haggerty, 2006). Through these experiences, residents also learn an approach to the care of children with disabilities and other special health care needs. It is often in this rotation that pediatric residents experience interdisciplinary clinical practice and learn about leadership and teamwork.

The number of fellowship programs is growing. As in other pediatric subspecialties, fellowship requirements include a scholarly project. Developmental-behavioral pediatrics is beginning to expand the types of research it encompasses, branching out to genomics and neuroscience, in addition to traditional clinical medicine and psychology. Evidence-based practice guidelines are now available for many of the disorders treated within the discipline.

Clinical practice in developmental-behavioral pediatrics generally uses a family-centered approach. Families are invited to participate in the clinical encounter, not only providing history, but also sharing in the decision making about clinical care. Clinical practice also seeks to be culturally and linguistically competent. The field recognizes the important role that culture plays in the manifestations and understanding of illness and disability and in decisions about the acceptability of approaches to treatment. Care is generally compassionate, recognizing the unique strengths of these young patients and their needs. Finally, developmental-behavioral pediatrics recognizes that care of children developing typically, at risk for developmental disorders, or with clinical conditions requires the close collaboration of the health care system with community resources and services. Developmental-behavioral pediatricians are frequently the ones within the pediatric health care systems who link children and families to appropriate community-based agencies and services.

Based on these characteristics of the clinical practice, it is not surprising that many developmental-behavioral pediatricians also are active in advocacy for children. Many developmental-behavioral pediatricians serve on local, regional, state, and national committees and organizations that address the fundamental and often unmet needs of children and families.

SUMMARY

Developmental-behavioral pediatrics is a relatively young interdisciplinary field that contributes to the care of children who are developing normally, children at risk for developmental and behavioral disorders on the basis of medical conditions and adverse environments, and children with developmental disabilities and mental health disorders. The field traces its roots to the Enlightenment, the developments within psychology, and the differentiation of pediatrics from medicine. In the United States, it became a distinct subspecialty in the late 20th century, the time of great advances in social and political thinking about civil rights, disabilities, and mental health. The history includes development of a society, journal, training programs, and subspecialty board certification. In the 21st century, developmental-behavioral pediatrics plays key roles in academic medicine, clinical service, and community advocacy.

REFERENCES

American Academy of Pediatrics, Committee on Standards of Child Health: Standards of Child Health Care, 2nd edition. Evanston, IL: American Academy of Pediatrics, 1972.

American Academy of Pediatrics Historical Archives Advisory Committee: Committee report: American pediatrics: Milestones at the millennium. Pediatrics 107:1482-1491, 2001.

Association of University Centers on Disabilities: AUCD history. June 7, 2004. Available at: http://www.aucd.org/about/history.htm. Accessed January 29, 2007.

Biasini FJ, Grupe L, Huffman L, Bray NW: Mental retardation: A symptom and a syndrome. *In* Netherton S, Holmes D, Walker CE (eds): Child and Adolescent Psychological Disorders: A Comprehensive Textbook. New York, Oxford University Press, 1999, pp 2-23.

Campbell FA, Ramey CT, Pungello E, et al: Early childhood education: Young adult outcomes from the abecedarian project. Appl Dev Sci 6:42-57, 2002.

Carey WB: History of developmental-behavioral pediatrics. J Dev Behav Pediatr 24:215, 2003.

Committee on Children with Disabilities American Academy of Pediatrics: Developmental surveillance and screening of infants and young children. Pediatrics 108:192-196, 2001.

Dworkin PH, Shonkoff JP, Leviton A, Levine MD: Training in developmental pediatrics: How practitioners perceive the gap. Am J Dis Child 133:709-712, 1979.

Haggerty RJ: Some steps needed to ensure the health of America's children: Lessons learned from 50 years in pediatrics. Ambulat Pediatr 6:123, 2006.

Haggerty RJ, Friedman SB: History of developmental-behavioral pediatrics. J Dev Behav Pediatr 24(1 Suppl):S1-S18, 2003.

Hoover HR: Address to the White House Conference on Child Health and Protection, 1930. *In* Woolley J, Peters G (eds): The American Presidency Project [online]. Santa Barbara, CA, University of California (hosted) Gerhard Peters database. Available at www.presidency.ucsb.edu/ws/?pid-22442. Accessed September 3, 2008.

Jensen PS, Mrazek DA: Introduction. *In* Pensen PS, Knapp P, Mrazek DA (eds): Toward a New Diagnostic System for Child Psychopathology: Moving Beyond the DSM. New York, NY: Guilford Publications, 2006, pp 1-10.

Kanner L: A History of the Care and Study of the Mentally Retarded. Springfield, IL: Charles C Thomas, 1964.

Kessen W: The development of behavior. *In* Levine MD, Carey WB, Crocker AC (eds): Developmental-Behavioral Pediatrics, 3rd ed. Philadelphia, WB Saunders, 1999, pp 1-13.

Lee VE, Brooks-Gunn J, Schnur E, Liaw F-R: Are Head Start effects sustained? A longitudinal follow-up comparison of disadvantaged children attending Head Start, no preschool, and other preschool programs. Child Dev 81(2, Spec Iss):495-507, 1990.

Mahnke CB: The growth and development of a specialty: The history of pediatrics. Clin Pediatr 39:705-714, 2000.

Perrin EC, Bennett FC, Wolraich ML: Subspecialty certification in developmental-behavioral pediatrics: Past and present challenges. J Dev Behav Pediatr 21:130-132, 2000.

Philip, AGS: The evolution of neonatology. Pediatr Res 58:799-815, 2005.

Record RG, Smith A: Incidence, mortality, and sex distribution of mongoloid defectives. Br J Prev Soc Med 9:10-15, 1955.

Sareyan A: The Turning Point: How Persons of Conscience Brought Major Change in the Care of America's Mentally Ill. Scottdale, PA, Herald Press, 1994.

Segal R: The national association for retarded citizens. 1974. Available at: http://www.thearc.org/history/segal.htm. Accessed January 29, 2007.

Shonkoff JP, Dworkin PH, Leviton A, Levine MD: Primary care approaches to developmental disabilities. Pediatrics 64:506-514, 1979.

Shriver EK: Hope for retarded children. The Saturday Evening Post 234:71, 1962.

Stockman JA III: Developmental-behavioral pediatrics: The American Board of Pediatrics' perspective. J Dev Behav Pediatr 21:133-135, 2000.

Strain JE: Celebrating 75 years: Founding members laid strong foundation for Academy. AAP News 2004, p 180.

Weiner DB: Philippe Pinel's "memoir on madness" of December 11, 1794: A fundamental text of modern psychiatry. Am J Psychiatry 149:725-732, 1992.

Wolraich ML, Bennett FC: History of developmental-behavioral pediatrics. J Dev Behav Pediatr 24:215-216; author reply 216, 2003.

Yang Q, Rasmussen SA, Friedman JM: Mortality associated with Down's syndrome in the USA from 1983 to 1997: A population-based study. Lancet 359:1019-1025, 2002.

Part I LIFE STAGES

2 PREGNANCY, BIRTH, AND THE FIRST DAYS OF LIFE

Peter A. Gorski

"After the initial surprise and the long, bumpy ride of pregnancy, I finally had my baby home with me. I couldn't believe how tiny she was. She needed me for everything—she had to learn about me, about our family, and our home. Even after all our planning and expectation, I felt totally unprepared to become her parent. That first week at home I went in to check her sleep every couple of hours to make sure she was breathing. I tried to prevent her from crying—yet she seemed to cry all the time she was awake. She fed every couple of hours at first, and we both had to learn how to use my breasts for feeding. I had so many questions about what to do with and for my baby. I felt constantly exhausted, worried, and nervous. But she was mine, I had worked hard to have her home with me, and I felt so happy and proud."

—Words of a postpartum primiparous mother of a 1-week-old, full-term, appropriate weight for gestational age healthy newborn.

PREGNANCY

Fetal life marks the emergence and initial growth of the infant organism and the infant-parent relationship. As the fetus grows in size, draws increasingly from the mother's supply systems, initiates autonomous activity and discrete reactivity, and ultimately demands to begin extrauterine life, so too the developing pregnancy gives shape to a growing sense of emotional connection, relationship, upheaval, and commitment in the expectant parents. Although stressful biologic or psychological conditions can overwhelm and disturb this natural process of somatopsychic development of the child and of the child's primary caregiving relationships, childbearing offers every parent the chance to start over, to make a profound contribution to others, and, ultimately, to feel human.

The work of pregnancy involves at least five psychological domains and social circumstances. All contribute to perinatal outcome and to parents' will and capacity to support long-term health and development. Pediatricians who meet with expectant parents can use these five subject areas to engage quickly with them in discovering their stage of preparedness and use of support.

1. Attachments and commitments, past and future. Pregnancy causes expectant parents to reconsider and renegotiate relationships with each other, with older children, with family of origin (parents and siblings), with career, with friends, with community, and with culture. In the dawning light of anticipating energy increasingly directed to the new infant, existing ties and commitments necessarily open, although they do not necessarily loosen. New insights and attachments may strengthen relationships with individual and institutional sources of support. The history and current nature of relationships with parents' own parents become central for expectant parents and for helping professionals to understand the sources of support and conflict that will likely influence the interactive relationship with the fetus and newborn. As is the case in many other nations, American couples are bearing and raising children outside of marriage in increasing numbers. To date, there are no convincing

data about if and how this trend affects emotional attachments between children and their parents.

2. Forming a mental representation of the unborn infant. Expectant mothers and fathers begin early in pregnancy to identify increasingly specific behavioral characteristics, temperamental attributes, and intentionality in their child. Prenatal ultrasound augments the process biologically triggered by the perception of fetal movement, activity states, and motor reactivity to intrauterine and environmental sensory stimuli. The direction and shape of such mental representations, or personifications, are influenced equally by fetal behavior patterns and by parents' self-concept, self-esteem, temperamental world view, physical condition, mood, sense of hope, doubts, dreams, and fears. Especially during the last trimester, the health professional has a uniquely accessible opportunity to elicit powerful personal insights from parents and to interpret and anticipate jointly caregiving possibilities or consequences.
3. Social and professional support—past history. Expectant parents' use of and need for social and professional support reflect their past history of dependence, interdependence, connectedness, isolation, or alienation. The health professional has a chance to gather insight into the way to structure professional interventions after the infant's birth. Questions concerning this issue also can stimulate the expectant parents to consider and plan actively their future childcare support needs.
4. History of loss. The parents' history of personal loss can take many forms. Each can affect a person's sense of vulnerability about life in general and about human attachments in particular. The physical and emotional stretching and unknown consequences of pregnancy open expectant parents to a heightened sensitivity to potential (and universally inevitable) loss. Add to physical losses the symbolic loss of one's imagined, hoped for, idealized infant, and you have a rich menu to sample with parents that can help identify, distinguish, and organize important influences on and interferences with parents' developing perceptions and interactions with their infant. Examples of past losses might include death of a family member (especially if it occurred just before or during pregnancy, or if pregnancy or delivery coincides with an anniversary associated with the birth or death of a departed loved one); marital separation or divorce; previous pregnancy losses; onset of disease or disability (loss of one's good health); and departure from a relative, friend, community, or job.
5. Parents' sense of security. This is a sadly crucial contemporary subject for concern. Beyond the timeless developmental challenge of acquiring a basic sense of trust in one's own and others' will and ability to provide care, many parents, and half of all women, have suffered some form of violent threat or action against them. Family or domestic violence and impersonal violations by strangers endanger the safety of adults and children alike. Beyond any real ongoing threat, perceived danger can paralyze a new parent's trust and modeling of intimate relationships. Health professionals who inquire about the expectant parent's sense of safety can organize protection that might enable the parent to communicate the hope of unconditional love to her newborn infant.

Pediatric Prenatal Interview—Format and Questions

Pediatric clinicians who start their relationship with families during the poignant developmental transition of pregnancy gain a distinct advantage toward supporting later stages of healthy development and facing physical, behavioral, or emotional crises as they arise. The prenatal interview should be scheduled for 20 to 30 minutes sometime after the 30th week of gestation. Regardless of the parents' marital status, the father is always invited to attend the visit. If conducted by a pediatric primary care provider, the visit with expectant parents can introduce them to the staff, philosophy, and policies of the practice. The following guidelines are intended to offer a structured approach to obtaining medical and personal histories so as to identify the psychological stage and issues in preparing for parenting. Equally importantly, such questions are intended to stimulate further parents' own mental process of creating and individuating their infant. The suggested sets of questions direct the health professional's attention to the five clinically applied conceptual domains previously discussed.

The health professional opens the interview with welcomes, congratulations, and general questions such as "How are you feeling?"; "When are you due?"; "How has the pregnancy gone so far?" Answers to these questions may lead naturally into further explorations along any of the five psychological domains that follow. Asking openly, "How difficult was it to get pregnant?" may lead comfortably to a question as to whether the parents had planned to have a child at this time and from there into a conversation about how pregnancy will affect their current activities and plans.

1. Attachments and Commitments, Past and Future

Ask the expectant parents where they live and how they each currently occupy their time. Are they planning any changes around the birth of the new baby? How much time off will mother and father take from commitments outside of parenting? Where do their families live? How close are they to family members, physically and emotionally? How did their own parents rear them? What roles did parents and children play in their family of origin? These questions should spark insights by, as well as issues for, the expectant parents regarding possible changes in the direction, intensity, and commitment of their relationships to specific individuals and pursuits.

2. Forming a Mental Representation of the Unborn Child

Questions might include: Do you know whether you're having a girl or a boy? How do you feel about that? What gender would you want more? Tell me about your baby. How active is the baby? Can you recognize any patterns of fetal activity and rest? How do these correlate with your own activity and rest cycles? When you dream about your baby, what thoughts, hopes, or anxieties come to mind? What were you like as a child? How would you describe yourself and your partner now? What's your worst fear about your baby's health or personality? How are you planning to feed your infant? How did you make that choice?

These sample questions are designed to open conversation about parents' identification with their child. Emotional valence might be alternately directed positively, negatively, or ambivalently. Your professional interest, sympathy, and effort to understand and support the full range of possible affect help begin to secure a therapeutic alliance and a safe base for engaging future conflicts.

3. Social and Professional Support—Past History

Questions should include: Who will help you care for your baby at home? What kind of support do you imagine you will want? What are your thoughts about sharing childcare responsibilities with other family members or hired substitutes in your home or at a childcare center? Will your family's help be welcome with or without some reservations?

Explain your own professional availability, schedule of planned office visits, and access to your staff during day and night hours. Explore how that feels to the expectant parents—too frequent? not often enough? Inquire about the parents' access to transportation and communication (telephone, Internet). Have they met and formed an enduring connection with other expectant parents? This discussion should help you consider individual needs and benefits of specific community-based resources during the initial adjustment to parenting (e.g., nurse home visitation, community parent drop-in center, professional counseling, childcare resource network, lactation consultant, more frequent pediatric office and telephone contact).

4. History of Loss

At this time, or earlier in the interview when opportune, express sympathy for expressed losses and sensitively inquire further into the timing, emotional significance, and resolution or active influence of particular experiences with personal loss. Examples, if relevant, might include asking: How old were you when your mother died? How do you feel now that you are pregnant and expecting to become a mother yourself? How much do you miss your mother at this time? What month did that happen? How much do you still miss living in that community? What about those times do you miss most? Who helps you? Whom do you turn to when these strong feelings rise up in you? Tell me about your previous attempts to have a baby? How does that experience affect your sense of your baby's fragility or vulnerability? When do you think you will be able to trust that the baby will survive? How will you know when to stop worrying whether that might happen to this baby?

Do not be afraid to accept parents' invitations to learn more deeply how to care about them; how the past influences the present and the future; how, when, and why they may feel most comfortable with specific offers of professional support.

5. Parents' Sense of Security

After you begin to establish rapport with the expectant parents, ask directly how safe they feel. If you suspect vulnerability here, find a time and way to arrange for a confidential conversation about personal safety. At that time, inquire specifically whether the individual has ever been hit or threatened. Do they feel that they and their baby will be protected from harm where they live? How careful does the parent have to be about what he or she says to the other parent, partner, family member, or boss? If appropriate, would he or she like to speak to someone outside the family about this concern? You can offer names and telephone numbers at any time that a parent feels ready and able to use such help.

GESTATIONAL INFLUENCES ON NEWBORN BEHAVIOR

Newborn behavior develops over the course of gestation under the influence of genetics and exposure to maternal metabolic and psychological states and placental circulation. The developing brain and nervous system are constantly exposed and responsive to various conditions, substances, and stimuli within the fetal-placental circulation and from the external environment. Among the known fetal environmental influences on newborn behavior and development, the most studied include maternal metabolic imbalance, in utero drug exposure, hypoxic-ischemic encephalopathy, and maternal stress and depression.

Metabolic Influences

Studies of the effects on newborn behavior of antepartum maternal metabolism have focused on gestational and pregestational diabetes as an exemplary model. Although influence on long-term neurodevelopmental outcome is inconclusive, direct effects on the behavioral organization of newborns are measurable (Pressler et al, 1999; Rizzo et al, 1990; Silverman et al, 1991). Compared with infants matched for gestational age, birth weight, perinatal complications, socioeconomic status, and ethnicity, but whose mothers were in better glucose regulation, study infants showed poorer physiologic control, more immature motor processes, and weaker interactive capacities. Important questions remain to be answered concerning whether these neurobehavioral deficits mark teratogenic influences that will challenge behavioral processes throughout development, or whether these differences are transient effects dependent on active exposure to maternal fuels. Nonetheless, clinicians must recognize and respond to the potential for initial parental difficulty understanding the behavioral cues of these newborns.

The potential concerns for the neurobehavioral effects of maternal glucose dysregulation loom large as the public health consequences of the metabolic syndrome affect an increasingly pervasive cross section of the U.S. population at ever younger ages. Increasing rates of obesity in children and adults in the United States have caused a concomitant increase in rates of gestational diabetes.

Substance Exposure

The developing brain and nervous system are constantly exposed and responsive to various conditions, substances, and stimuli from the external environment. Perinatal medical risks and intrauterine exposure to chemicals used by, prescribed to, or passively experienced by women during pregnancy and birthing contribute to newborn behavioral characteristics and risks. Among the more pervasive (yet underrecognized) toxicants to fetal and infant growth and development is tobacco smoke. Studies converge on dose-related neurobehavioral effects on visual orienting and motor excitability (Garcia-Algar et al, 2001; Law et al, 2003; MacArthur and Knox, 1988) and newborn length and weight (Andres and Day, 2000). Smoking during pregnancy is responsible for 20% to 30% of all low-birth-weight infants. Exposed infants weigh an average of 150 to 250 g less than infants born to nonsmoking mothers. Two mechanisms are postulated for the negative effect of intrauterine tobacco exposure. Metabolites of cigarette smoke pass through the placenta and act as vasoconstrictors, reducing uterine blood flow as much as 38% and causing fetal hypoxia-ischemia and malnutrition (Suzuki et al, 1980). In addition, nicotine is a neurotoxicant that directly alters synaptic cell proliferation, differentiation, and activity (Levin and Slotkin, 1998). Chemical and behavioral tobacco addiction treatment modalities have proven efficacy and safety when used during pregnancy (Rayburn and Bogenschutz, 2004).

Fetal alcohol syndrome represents the tip of an iceberg of physical, developmental, and neuropsychologic sequelae that can result from maternal alcohol use during pregnancy (Hoyme et al, 2005; Johnson et al, 1996; Mattson et al, 1996). Coles and colleagues (2002) reported on longitudinal correlations between neonatal findings associated with fetal alcohol syndrome and global intelligence and academic functioning into early adolescence. Infants with more dysmorphic features tend to have lower birth weights and a range of behavioral deficits of arousal, motor organization, state regulation, and orientation as newborns, and lower IQ, academic deficits, and less visual attention as adolescents (Coles et al, 2002).

The behavioral effects of narcotic drugs on the developing fetus have been a long-standing concern. Heroin-addicted newborns are at high risk for sleep disturbances (with abnormal electroencephalograms), growth retardation, central nervous system (CNS) irritability associated with narcotic withdrawal, sudden infant death syndrome, and behavioral disorganization of state and alerting and motor processes (Desmond and Wilson, 1975; Strauss et al, 1975). Similar findings have been reported for infants prenatally exposed to methadone and numerous other narcotic and non-narcotic drugs. Quality of prenatal care, maternal nutrition, and home environment compound, or even exceed, the developmental risks associated with maternal drug addiction.

The potential neurodevelopmental and behavioral effects of cocaine on infants are of serious concern, ranging from perinatal cerebral infarction to intrauterine growth retardation, abnormal sleep and feeding patterns, irritability, and tremulousness (Chasnoff, 1988; Chiriboga et al, 1993; Mayes et al, 1993; Oro and Dixon, 1987; Scafidi et al, 1996). More recently, studies find that cocaine may have less direct neurobehavioral teratogenicity than associated or synergistic influence along with an impoverished, depressed, polydrug caregiving environment (Brooks-Gunn et al, 1994; Coles and Platzman, 1993; Volpe, 1992; Zuckerman and Frank, 1994). Still, the subtle influence of intrauterine cocaine exposure on newborn infant interactive behavior and infant-mother engagement could have a deleterious cumulative effect on the infant's later development and quality of relationships (Tronick et al, 2005).

Other substances that cross the placental circulation may contribute to neonatal behavioral disturbances and later developmental dysfunction. These include caffeine (Emory et al, 1985), and lead (Patel et al, 2006). We often cannot discriminate the extent to which drugs directly cause long-term CNS damage, whether they act primarily to contribute to hypoxic-ischemic conditions, or whether they serve as a proxy for a suboptimal social environment.

A subset of the new science of environmental health focuses concern on exposure to neurotoxicants during pregnancy and the possible causal association with CNS malformations and behavioral teratology. Even as research begins to identify links between pathologic neurogenesis and exposure to heavy metals and other chemicals in the ambient environment of pregnant women and infants, governmental regulatory oversight remains minimal (Rodier, 2004). As toxic waste dumps and other sources of hazardous effluents into the water, air, and soil tend to concentrate in poor neighborhoods where residents have marginal political influence, social inequities contribute to disparities in the risks and untoward consequences of perinatal and lifespan exposure to environmental pollution.

Compounds that create regional depression of sensory pathways during labor may cross the placental circulation and cause CNS depression in the delivered newborn. Studies that carefully control for the effects of parity and length of labor indicate, however, that when applied in tightly controlled dosage, using the minimum quantities needed to achieve anesthesia, behavioral signs of neurologic depression are minimal and short-lived (Kraemer et al, 1972; Tronick et al, 1976). This finding has been replicated across studies that tested the effects of a variety of drugs and routes of administration (Lester et al, 1982; Murray et al, 1981; Sepokoski et al, 1992). Current clinical concern centers, however, on the possibly disorganizing effect of obstetric medication on newborn sucking and feeding (Kuhnert et al, 1985; Sanders-Phillps et al, 1988). Neonatal medical procedures may affect newborn behavior during the first days or weeks of life. Research on the disorganizing effects of phototherapy cautions about the prudent use of this therapeutic intervention in cases of mild-to-moderate nonhemolytic hyperbilirubinemia (Ju and Lin, 1991).

A burgeoning field of research is examining the impact of emotional stress and support during pregnancy and childbirth on newborn behavior, parental mood, infant-parent relationship, and infant health and development. In studies using primates, sustained stress during pregnancy has been associated with impaired newborn neurobehavior, specifically immature motor abilities, impaired equilibrium reactions and vestibular functioning, and shorter episodes of looking and visual attention (Schneider and Coe, 1993). In addition, increased incidence of low birth weight has been found to be associated with mothers who report stress or clinical depression or both during pregnancy (Edwards et al, 1994). Several causal mechanisms could explain the newborn neurobehavioral effects of emotional stress during pregnancy. Recurrent maternal sympathetic activation can alter placental blood flow and create transient fetal hypoxia. The flood of stress-induced corticoids chronically engages the pituitary-adrenal axis. In fetal monkeys treated with dexamethasone for 3 days at midgestation, the size of the newborn's hippocampus is diminished. An alternative explanatory model suggests that infant behavior may become modified by stress-induced increases in tryptophan production with consequent increases in serotonin in the fetal cortex (Gennaro and Fehder, 1996; Herrenkohl, 1986; Moyer et al, 1977). Although definitive understanding of causality awaits further research, intervention programs offering social-emotional support to expectant women have successfully reduced the numbers of low-birth-weight and small-for-gestational-age infants born to these women (Edwards et al, 1994).

More recent concern about an association between the use of selective serotonin reuptake inhibitors during the third trimester of pregnancy and the subsequent appearance of symptoms suggestive of poor neonatal adaptation has caused the U.S. Food and Drug Administration to issue warnings about perinatal complications associated with the use of antidepressants. At this time, no consensus has been reached about the relative benefits and risks from treatment on newborn behavioral and physiologic adaptation. Questions remain as to whether the constellation of symptoms not specific to use of selective serotonin reuptake inhibitors is the consequence of drug withdrawal or serotonin toxicity (Koren et al, 2005).

Emotional support for expectant women during labor and delivery itself can have a positive influence on pregnancy outcome. Whether provided by trained professional obstetric staff or lay companions, also known as doulas, social support during labor has been found to be associated with improved physical outcomes for women and newborns, more positive childbirth experiences for laboring women, more physiologically stable and behaviorally organized infants, and more satisfying breastfeeding interactions (Kennell et al, 1991; Zhang et al, 1996).

NEUROLOGIC BASIS AND CLINICAL IMPORTANCE OF NEWBORN BEHAVIOR

Ontogeny of Behavioral Systems

Intrinsic Activity Cycles

Much research has concentrated on the search for a basic cycle of human movement, rest, and alerting that might describe a fundamental characteristic of behavioral organization and underlying brain activity that exists from early fetal life. Robertson (1987) documented the existence of spontaneous motility cycles in human newborns across all behavioral states of sleep and wakefulness. This cyclic variation in spontaneous movement every 1 to 10 minutes is observed in utero in human fetuses during the second half of gestation and perhaps earlier (deVries et al, 1982, 1985; Robertson, 1985). These patterns of human cyclic motility are weaker and less regular during less organized behavioral states of active sleep and may be influenced by alterations in the metabolic environment of the fetus and newborn (Robertson and Drierker, 1986). Most importantly, the finding of remarkable stability of these cycles of spontaneous movement from midgestation through the first 10 weeks of post-term life adds evidence for a dramatic shift in brain organization and behavioral self-regulation, not around 40 weeks at the time of birth, but after 50 postconceptual weeks. Previous studies of electrophysiologic organization of the CNS, structural maturation of the cerebral cortex, and behavioral development of infant crying and sleep patterns indicate relative CNS immaturity during the first 2 to 4 months post-term with respect to fundamental organization of cortical activity and higher perceptual and cognitive processes (Brazelton, 1962; Conel, 1947; Parmelee, 1977; Parmelee et al, 1964). Despite substantial environmental and physiologic changes that accompany birth, the human fetus and newborn share basic continuities of behavior and responsiveness.

Healthy full-term infants display a regular series of distinct states over time, first described and systematized byWolff (1959, 1966). Numerous other classification schemes have been published (Brazelton, 1995; Prechtl, 1974; Thoman, 1985). Brazelton proposed a system with the following six states: (1) quiet sleep, (2) active sleep, (3) drowsiness, (4) alert inactivity, (5) active awake, and (6) crying. Each state is distinguished on the basis of many distinct clusters of behavior (Table 2-1).

The study of behavioral states in infants has attracted wide interest as an indicator of the functional integrity of the CNS during the fetal, neonatal, and infant periods of development. Maturational changes in sleep-wake cycles have been studied, and neonatal state periodicities have been correlated with later neurodevelopmental, especially mental, outcome. These investigations have found that earlier maturation of electrophysiologic and behavioral patterns of quiet sleep in the newborn period predict higher performance on cognitive tests at preschool and school age (Anders and Keener, 1985; Nijhuis et al, 1982; Scher, 2005; Thoman et al, 1981; Whitney and Thoman, 1993).

Sleeping and waking states in infancy reflect the competency of the CNS, and they modulate the infant's interactions with the external environment (Thoman et al, 1979). Many studies have documented the influence that an infant's state has on his or her response to stimulation; the response may differ depending on whether the infant is in a sleep, drowsy, or alert state (Berg and Berg, 1979; Korner, 1972; Pomerleau-Malcuit and Clifton, 1973). A visual stimulus that captures the attention of a quietly awake infant does not elicit a response from a more aroused, crying infant. This arousal distinction applies not only between states, but also within

Table 2-1. Neonatal State Classification Scale

State	Characteristics
Quiet sleep	Regular breathing, eyes closed; spontaneous activity confined to startles and jerky movements at regular intervals. Responses to external stimuli are partially inhibited, and any response is likely to be delayed. No eye movements, and state changes are less likely after stimuli or startles than in other states.
Active sleep	Irregular breathing patterns, sucking movements, eyes closed, but rapid eye movements can be detected underneath the closed lids. Infants also have some low-level and irregular motor activity. Startles occur in response to external stimuli and can produce a change of state.
Drowsiness	While the newborn is semidozing, eyes may be open or closed; eyelids often flutter; activity level variable and interspersed with mild startles. Drowsy newborns are responsive to sensory stimuli, but with some delay, and state change frequently follows stimulation.
Alert inactivity	A bright alert look, with attention focused on sources of auditory or visual stimuli; motor activity is inhibited while attending to stimuli.
Active awake	Eyes open, considerable motor activity, thrusting movements of extremities, and occasional startles set off by activity; reactive to external stimulation with an increase in startles or motor activity. Discrete responses are difficult to distinguish because of general high activity level.
Crying	Intense irritability in the form of sustained crying, and jerky limb movement. This state is difficult to break through with stimulation.

Data from Brazelton TB: Neonatal Behavioral Assessment Scale, 2nd ed. London, Heinemann, 1984.

a particular state. A newborn displays a different pattern of responsiveness at the beginning of an alert period compared with the end of the period. This difference is analogous to the daytime pattern of adults who commonly go through periods of higher and lower arousal while awake. This pattern, called the basic rest-activity cycle by Aserinsky and Kleitman (1955), is distinct from the sleep-wake cycle and is theoretically related to the cyclic activity of the autonomic nervous system. The autonomic nervous system mediates the infant's responsivity to the external environment and is responsible for regulating numerous homeostatic functions.

Neonatal behavioral and psychophysiologic measures of state organization are now among the most frequently applied methods in neonatal behavioral research. These techniques highlight maturational differences between preterm and term infants that could affect their responses to caregiving and treatment practices. Research findings suggest that the underlying difference in CNS organization between premature and full-term infants lies in an unevenness in the development of premature infants. Aspects of greater CNS maturity (more alertness and less sleep) coexist with characteristics of less CNS maturity (more nonalert waking activity and more frequent sleep-wake transitions). As Davis and Thoman (1987) conclude, premature infants exhibit irregular state development compared with full-term infants, rather than either increased maturity or immaturity.

These early neurobehavioral differences between infants of different gestational ages could reflect significant changes in brain organization that may continue throughout childhood development. Long-term follow-up studies of preterm infants tend to find that the mental development and neurologic status of medically uncompromised preterm infants at school age does not differ from that of full-terms (Bakeman and Brown, 1980; Saint-Anne Dargassies, 1979), yet these same children are more likely to show visuomotor and spatial difficulties, with associated school underachievement (Hack et al, 1994; Hunt et al, 1982; Klein et al, 1985). More recent reports of 25- to 30-year follow-up of developmental and behavioral functioning among very-low-birth-weight infants in adulthood reveal decided disadvantage with respect to educational achievement and neurosensory impairments (Hack et al, 2002). Infants who experience severe perinatal medical complications, such as bronchopulmonary dysplasia or severe intracranial hemorrhage, are more vulnerable to continued long-term neurodevelopmental disabilities (Brazy et al, 1991; Vohr et al, 1991).

The infant cry state is attracting interest in the effort to develop predictive measures of CNS functioning based on newborn behavior. Successful prediction of developmental outcome from neonatal cry analyses corroborates a relationship between the characteristics of the infant's cry and the functional integrity of the infant's nervous system (Lester, 1987).

Sensory-Perceptual Functions

Infant behavior is premised on sensory processes that serve as avenues of communication between the infant and the world. Sensory systems undergo rapid changes during the last trimester of pregnancy and the first several months after birth.

There seems to be an orderly sequence in the functional development of the sensory systems of infants. This sequence unfolds starting with the cutaneous (somesthetic or tactile) in the third month of gestation and proceeding through vestibular, auditory (becoming functional between the 25th and 27th weeks of gestation), and visual (maturing 3 to 6 months post-term) (Anand and Hickey, 1987; Banks, 1980; Gottlieb, 1971; Rubel, 1985). How remarkable that the visual system, which is usually dominant in our everyday interactions with our environment, is the last system to start functioning during gestation and the least well developed at birth. Still, the healthy full-term newborn can fixate visually with a variety of stimuli, exhibiting differential attention to inanimate versus animate stimuli.

Temperament

The preceding discussion highlighted aspects of behavioral and neurobiologic development that are common to all infants. Differences in development were noted to

Table 2-2. **Temperament Categories**

Category	Description
Activity level	Motor level of a child's functioning. The ratio of active to inactive periods each day (e.g., infant may move often even during sleep)
Intensity of reaction	General magnitude of response, regardless of affective direction (e.g., cries loudly for all needs, also vocalizes with audible vigor)
Quality of mood	Predominance of contented, positive behavior versus irritable, negative disposition, regardless of intensity (e.g., generally calm, smiling, easily engaged versus fussy)
Rhythmicity or regularity	Predictability or unpredictability of biologic or behavioral patterns (e.g., sleep-wake cycle, hunger, feeding pattern, elimination schedule, crying, and alerting)
Threshold of responsiveness	Amount of stimulation required to elicit a response (e.g., rapidity of buildup to full cry when handled)
Approach or withdrawal	Initial response to a new stimulus (e.g., new food, toy, person, or room). Responses are observed through mood (e.g., smiling, grimacing, or crying) or activity (e.g., in infancy, by calming, squirming, or spitting)
Adaptability	Eventual response to a new or changed environment or condition (e.g., acceptance of bottle or babysitter)
Attention span and persistence	Two related categories describing the duration of effort at a task or activity and the continuation at task, despite attention to distractions (e.g., prolonged visual fixation and orienting)
Distractibility	Infant's susceptibility to changing attention or activity when presented with interfering stimuli (e.g., diverted from visual attention by extraneous sound stimulus)

Adapted from Chess S, Thomas A: Temperament in Clinical Practice. New York, Guilford Press, 1986, pp 273-278.

be caused by idiosyncrasies of gestational age at birth or other medical risk factors. How, then, can we account for the range and stability of differences in the behavior of infants born at the same gestation, and with similar medical courses? The pattern of behavioral and psychophysiologic responses to animate and inanimate stimuli that characterize each newborn is often referred to as temperament. Temperament describes the style without supplying the explanation of individual patterns of behavior (see Chapter 7).

Researchers tend to agree that temperamental dimensions reflect behavioral styles rather than discrete behavioral acts, have biologic underpinnings, and enjoy continuity of expression relative to other aspects of behavior (Goldsmith et al, 1987; Tirosh et al, 1992). Infancy is commonly regarded as the time of clearest expression of temperamental characteristics, before the link between temperament and behavior becomes more complex as the child matures.

Disagreements exist about the extent to which an infant's behavior can be attributed to temperament, whether temperament is stable within individuals regardless of social contexts, and the nature of its inheritance. Formal neonatal behavioral examination, standardized psychological assessment, and parents' reports all identify behavioral traits that together compose an image of the nature each infant brings into interaction with the caregiving world (Brazelton, 1995; Carey and McDevitt, 1978; Rothbart, 1981; Thomas et al, 1963). According to Chess and Thomas (1986), caregivers learn to relate to infants through nine behavioral categories of individual differences that compose temperament (Table 2-2).

Caregivers and children bring their individual temperaments into the relationship they create with each other. Similarities or differences can produce understanding and comfort or confusion and conflict. Whether stable or changed over time, temperament influences the ease, harmony, and pleasure between the child and his or her environment at each stage of development. In return, the child continuously learns to find those environments and relationships that best support his or her needs and style. These lessons begin immediately through the new relationship between newborn and parent. The neonatal period serves to launch parents' perceptions and infants' expectations in the direction of contented anticipation of the future or toward frustration and learned helplessness (Goldberg, 1979; Seligman, 1975; Sroufe, 1986).

Culture

Culture may influence newborn behavior, growth, and development, representing the biobehavioral nexus of the developing nervous system within an evolving society. Generational exposure to child rearing, dietary, environmental, and health care practices and conditions may genetically shape infant behavior. Culturally mandated parental expectations and guidance can influence patterns of caregiver-infant interactions, molding each individual's developmental trajectory within acceptable or imaginable bounds. Culturally specific and cross-cultural investigations help to inform an appreciation of the impact of the caregiving environment on the biologic expression of our genetic code and the evolving expression of human behavior (Cole, 1999; Nugent et al, 1989, 1991).

NEWBORN BEHAVIORAL ASSESSMENT

Brazelton (1995) elaborated on earlier assessments of newborn behavior to complement and potentially enrich basic neurologic assessment of motor tone and reflexes. Framed within the matrix of observing and manipulating changes in states of arousal of newborns, the Neonatal Behavioral Assessment Scale (NBAS) follows the newborn through sleep, drowsiness, bright and active alertness, and crying while the examiner interacts with the infant. The examination elicits 20 neurologic reflex behaviors. It also scores 26 behavioral responses to unique stimuli and common caregiving routines, such as cuddling, consoling, and visual and auditory stimulation.

An important concept of the NBAS lies in assessing the infant's capacities to initiate support from the environment, modulate or terminate his or her response to excess outside stimulation, and rely on self for coping with a rewarding or distressing situation. Reflecting the range of behavioral capacities of the normal newborn, the behavioral items assess the infant's ability to (1) organize states of consciousness, (2) habituate reactions to disturbing events, (3) attend to and process simple and complex environmental stimuli, (4) control motor tone and activity while attending to these stimuli, and (5) perform integrated motor acts for self-defense and social interaction.

The NBAS is designed and validated to elicit the behavioral capacities of full-term infants from birth to 2 months of age. Although attempts have been made to apply this tool to premature infants (Field et al, 1978), results are not wholly satisfying because the neurologic organization of these infants is qualitatively different. Responses to stimuli are often uninterpretable using the scoring system of the full-term scale.

Als and associates (1982) have developed a complex set of assessment techniques packaged to evaluate quality of behavioral organization at various ages in preterm and high-risk full-term newborns. The Assessment of Preterm Infant Behavior (APIB), and its related clinical observation method called the Newborn Individualized Developmental Care and Assessment Program (NIDCAP) (Als et al, 1994), is an extension of the NBAS that provides a comprehensive description of the range of behavioral functions in the less mature infant. APIB scores indicate functional maturity and the infant's degree of fragility and ability to tolerate sensory activity during caregiving and handling. From this information, an individualized developmental care plan can be generated. Preliminary research results of clinical trials using the NIDCAP show positive hope toward stabilizing infants' initial physiologic fragility, improving developmental outcome after premature birth, and reducing costs of neonatal hospitalization (Als et al, 1986, 1994; Buehler et al, 1995).

CLINICAL OPPORTUNITIES IN THE NEWBORN PERIOD

Powerful circumstances combine during the perinatal period to heighten the child health professional's opportunities to support healthy infant development effectively. The birth family is exceptionally exposed with respect to their emotional anticipation and uncertainty. The newborn comes remarkably equipped to communicate interests and needs through physiologic and behavioral signal systems. Capitalizing on the parents' open availability and the infant's compelling responsivity, the clinician's visits during the newborn hospitalization can cement a lasting relationship built on trust, honesty, and optimism. By examining newborns together with the parents at the mother's bedside, the practitioner can show the range of a newborn's physical and behavioral competencies and individual behavioral reactions. As the infant moves from sleep to increasingly wakeful, active, and even irritable states, the clinician can observe the parents' personal responses to each behavior. Newborn infants not only are hard to resist, but also parents can hardly resist projecting intentionality about the infant's movements, sounds, and sleep-wake states. An observant practitioner can make use of such affect, whether positive or not, for diagnostic and therapeutic advantage. The infant is a most effective psychotherapeutic agent in the hands of an attentive pediatric professional who uses the newborn assessment to engage the family's love and attention for their child.

Atypical Infant Behavior

Although birth is almost always a magnificent celebration of life, occasionally perinatal circumstances for the infant or mother or both are distressing or life-threatening. This chapter has already discussed the disorganizing or disabling effects on behavior often associated with prematurity and gestational insult or stress. Another group of infants born at risk for atypical patterns of behavioral development are infants born small for gestational age, whether preterm or full-term. These infants, who are born at less than the 10th percentile by ponderal index (weight in grams divided by the cube of length in centimeters), are unusually likely to exhibit the effects of sleep state disorganization and extremely low sensory thresholds (Als et al, 1976; Feldman and Eidelman, 2006). Their nervous systems have difficulty organizing adaptive responses to more than one or two concurrent sources of stimulation from the ambient sensory environment. They present with clinical concerns such as frequent gaze aversion from face-to-face interaction; disjointed movement patterns and frequent startles and tremors; mottling or wild fluctuations of skin color, including acrocyanosis; and, rarely, dyspnea or apnea.

Follow-up studies find this population of infants to be at higher risk for failure-to-thrive; behavioral disturbances, particularly of self-regulation (e.g., colic and inattention) and activity; educational underachievement; and child abuse and neglect (Pryor et al, 1995; Walther, 1988). Early diagnosis through newborn behavioral assessment and attention to parental frustration can direct effective therapeutic strategies for diminishing sensory overload and providing external organization until the infant can develop higher sensory limits and consistent behavioral self-regulation.

Even when no medical risks occur, the fragile faith of newborn parents can be wounded by seemingly minor or even tangential disappointments, tensions, or misfortunes. All too easily, parents may transfer the real vulnerability of the moment or of another person into the mental representation of the newborn infant. These infants' normal behavioral signals may get misinterpreted by anxious or depressed parents who imagine that their child is physically vulnerable. Overprotecting or overindulging the child from infancy onward, distressed parents often fail to guide these infants toward healthy social autonomy. A classic syndrome, known as the vulnerable child syndrome, can develop (Gorski, 1988; Green and Solnit, 1964). These children often present with prolonged separation anxiety well beyond early childhood; prolonged infantile, often aggressive, behaviors; sleep and feeding problems; psychosomatic disorders; or school underachievement months or years after the signal event that triggered the parents' malaise. Over time, the young child internalizes the caregivers' insecurities into his or her own self-concept, avoiding the risks all children must take to stretch beyond what is comfortable to develop new abilities and relationships. Pediatricians, through their early and frequent encounters with newborn families, can identify and sympathetically help shift the family's perception of their child from vulnerable to adaptive and strong.

Breastfeeding

Increasingly, American women are choosing to breastfeed their newborns. By 2004, 70% of newborns were breastfed, a 25% increase over the previous 10 years (National Immunization Survey, 2004). Less than half of the original number continue to be breastfed 6 months after birth (Neifert, 1996), despite empirical evidence that human milk is nutritionally superior to synthetically prepared formula and significantly reduces the risk of many common illnesses, including diarrheal diseases, lower respiratory infections, otitis media, bacteremia, meningitis, and allergies (Lawrence, 1994). New studies support the health benefits of human milk for hospitalized preterm infants (Schanler and Hurst, 1994). The composition of milk expressed from postpartum women changes over time and over the course of each feeding. Protein and lipid content of human milk adapts to the needs and capacities of the infant's intestinal and immunologic systems at each stage of development.

Efforts to guide and support successful initiation of breastfeeding are extremely challenged by the current practice of discharging healthy newborns and mothers from the hospital 1 to 2 days after birth. Few women have begun lactating confidently by then. Many return home without help for childcare or social support. While lobbying hospitals for postpartum stays determined by the needs of individual families, health providers should augment the traditional pediatric care of newborns with early office and home visits as necessary.

SOCIAL SIGNIFICANCE OF NEWBORN BEHAVIOR

A newborn can perceive, respond to, and communicate with his or her environment. Newborns help adults succeed as caregivers by being readable, predictable, and responsive. No longer can professionals allow parents to feel totally responsible for all of their infant's behavior. The newborn, previously thought to be a "blank slate to be written upon by his environment, his world a blooming, buzzing confusion" (James, 1890), now is respected as a social partner who can effectively engage and, to some extent, guide caregivers to support his or her growth and development.

Not all infants are born after a full intrauterine gestation, without CNS pathology or behavioral dysfunction. Premature and other high-risk newborns, born with disorganized signaling systems, challenge their caregivers to understand their behavior and support their physiologic and psychological development (DiVitto and Goldberg, 1979). Similarly, families stressed by untoward pregnancy outcome, social isolation, insecure spousal relationship, a history of child abuse or neglect, or emotional depression may be unable to cope with a behaviorally disorganized, or even an alert, self-regulated, infant.

Early intervention, through the physician-patient relationship and other community-based family resources, which provides emotional support and developmental counseling for parents of high-risk newborns at home and in the hospital, can help prevent negative outcomes and foster positive infant growth and family relationships (Gilkerson et al, 1990; Olds et al, 1994; Rauh et al, 1990). Health professionals have a distinct opportunity to note the psychological condition of the parents in addition to the medical status and behavior of the newborn. By offering attention and support to the family and the newborn, health professionals can contribute most effectively to the quality of infant health and development.

REFERENCES

Als H, Lawhon G, Brown E, et al: Individualized behavioral and environmental care for the very low birth weight preterm infant at high risk for bronchopulmonary dysplasia: Neonatal intensive care unit and developmental outcome. Pediatrics 78:1123-1132, 1986.

Als H, Lawhon G, Duffy FH, et al: Individualized developmental care for the very low birth weight preterm infant: Medical and neurofunctional effects. JAMA 272:853-858, 1994.

Als H, Lester BM, Tronick EZ, et al: Manual for the assessment of preterm infants' behavior (APIB). *In* Fitzgerald HE, Yogman MW (eds): Theory and Research in Behavioral Pediatrics. New York, Plenum Press, 1982, pp 35-63.

Als H, Tronick EZ, Adamson L, Brazelton TB: The behavior of the full-term but underweight newborn infant. Dev Med Child Neurol 18:590-602, 1976.

Anand KJS, Hickey PR: Pain and its effects in the human neonate and fetus. N Engl J Med 317:1321-1329, 1987.

Anders TF, Keener MA: Developmental course of nighttime sleep-wake patterns in full-term and premature infants during the first year of life, I. Sleep 8:173-192, 1985.

Andres RI, Day MC: Perinatal complications associated with maternal tobacco use. Semin Neonatol 5:231-241, 2000.

Aserinsky E, Kleitman N: A motility cycle in infants as manifested by ocular and gross bodily activity. J Appl Physiol 8:11-18, 1955.

Bakeman R, Brown JV: Early interaction: Consequences for social and mental development at three years. Child Dev 51:437-447, 1980.

Banks MS: The development of visual accommodation during early infancy. Child Dev 51:646-666, 1980.

Berg WK, Berg KM: Psychophysiologic development in infancy: State, sensory function, and attention. *In* Osofsky JD (ed): Handbook of Infant Development. New York, John Wiley, 1979, pp 283-343.

Brazelton TB: Crying in infancy. Pediatrics 4:579-588, 1962.

Brazelton TB: Neonatal Behavioral Assessment Scale, 3rd ed. London, Mac Keith Press, 1995.

Brazy JE, Eckerman CO, Oehler JM, et al: Nursery neurobiologic risk score: Important factors in predicting outcome in very low birth weight infants. J Pediatr 118:783-792, 1991.

Brooks-Gunn J, McCarton C, Hawley T: Effects of in utero drug exposure on children's development. Arch Pediatr Adolesc Med 148:33-39, 1994.

Buehler DM, Als H, Duffy FH, et al: Effectiveness of individualized developmental care for low-risk preterm infants: Behavioral and electrophysiologic evidence. Pediatrics 96:923-932, 1995.

Carey WB, McDevitt SC: Revision of the infant temperament questionnaire. Pediatrics 61:735-739, 1978.

Chasnoff IJ: Newborn infants with drug withdrawal symptoms. Pediatr Rev 9:273-277, 1988.

Chess S, Thomas A: Temperament in Clinical Practice. New York, Guilford Press, 1986, pp 273-281.

Chiriboga CA, Bateman DA, Brust JC, Hauser WA: Neurologic findings in neonates with intrauterine cocaine exposure. Pediatr Neurol 9:115-119, 1993.

Cole M: Culture and development. *In* Bornstein MH, Lamb ME (eds): Developmental Psychology, 4th ed. Hillsdale, NJ, Lawrence Erlbaum, 1999.

Coles CD, Platzman KA: Behavioral development in children prenatally exposed to drugs and alcohol. Int J Addict 28:1393-1433, 1993.

Coles CD, Platzman KA, Lynch ML, Freides D: Auditory and visual sustained attention in adolescents prenatally exposed to alcohol. Alcohol Clin Exp Res 26:263-271, 2002.

Conel JL: The Postnatal Development of the Human Cerebral Cortex. Cambridge, MA, Harvard University Press, 1947.

Davis DH, Thoman EB: Behavioral states of premature infants: Implications for neural and behavioral development. Dev Psychobiol 20:25-38, 1987.

Desmond MM, Wilson GS: Neonatal abstinence syndrome: Recognition and diagnosis. Addict Dis 2:113-121, 1975.

deVries JIP, Vissar GHA, Prechtl HFR: The emergence of fetal behaviour, I: Qualitative aspects. Early Hum Dev 7:301-322, 1982.

deVries JIP, Vissar GHA, Prechtl HFR: The emergence of fetal behaviour, II: Quantitative aspects. Early Hum Dev 12:99-120, 1985.

DiVitto B, Goldberg S: The effects of newborn medical status on early parent-infant interaction. *In* Field TM, Sostek AS, Goldberg S, Shuman HH (eds): Infants Born at Risk. New York, Spectrum, 1979.

Edwards CH, Cole OJ, Oyemade UJ, et al: Maternal stress and pregnancy outcome in a prenatal clinic population. J Nutr 124:1006s-1021s, 1994.

Emory EK, Konopka S, Hronsky S, et al: Salivary caffeine and neonatal behavior: Assay modification and functional significance. Psychopharmacology 76:145-153, 1985.

Feldman R, Eidelman A: Neonatal state organization, neuromaturation, mother-infant interaction, and cognitive development in small-for-gestational-age premature infants. Pediatrics 118:e869-e878, 2006.

Field TM, Hallock N, Ting G, et al: A first follow-up of high-risk infants: Formulating a cumulative risk index. Child Dev 49:173-192, 1978.

Garcia-Algar O, Puig C, Vall O, et al:Neonatal nicotine withdrawal syndrome. J Epidemiol Community Health 55:687-688, 2001.

Gennaro S, Fehder WP: Stress, immune function and relationship to pregnancy outcome. Nurs Clin North Am 31:293-303, 1996.

Gilkerson L, Gorski PA, Panitz P: Hospital-based intervention for preterm infants and their families. *In* Meisels SJ, Shonkoff JP (eds): Handbook of Early Intervention: Theory, Practice, and Analysis. Cambridge, Cambridge University Press, 1990.

Goldberg S: Premature birth: Consequences for the parent-infant relationship. Am Sci 67:214-220, 1979.

Goldsmith HH, Buss AH, Plomin R, et al: Roundtable: What is temperament? Four approaches. Child Dev 58:505-529, 1987.

Gorski PA: Fostering family development following preterm hospitalization. *In* Ballard RA (ed): Pediatric Care of the ICN Graduate. Philadelphia, WB Saunders, 1988, pp 27-32.

Gottlieb G: Ontogenesis of sensory function in birds and mammals. *In* Tobach E, Aronson LR, Shaw E (eds): The Biopsychology of Development. New York, Academic Press, 1971, pp 67-126.

Green M, Solnit A: Reactions to the threatened loss of a child: A vulnerable child syndrome. Pediatrics 34:58-66, 1964.

Hack M, Flannery DJ, Schluchter M, et al: Outcomes in young adulthood for very-low-birthweight infants. N Engl J Med 346:149-157, 2002.

Hack M, Taylor G, Klein N, et al: School-age outcomes in children with birth weights under 750 g. N Engl J Med 331:753-759, 1994.

Herrenkohl LR: Prenatal stress disrupts reproductive behavior and physiology in offspring. Ann N Y Acad Sci 474:120-128, 1986.

Hoyme HE, May PA, Kalberg WO, et al: A practical clinical approach to diagnosis and of fetal alcohol spectrum disorders: Clarification of the 1996 Institute of Medicine criteria. Pediatrics 115:39-47, 2005.

Hunt JV, Tooley WH, Harvin D: Learning disabilities in children with birth weights <1500 grams. Semin Perinatol 6:280-287, 1982.

James W: Principles of Psychology, Vol 1. Burkhardt F (ed). Cambridge, Harvard University Press, 1981 (1890).

Johnson VP, Swayze VW, Sato Y Andreasen NC: Fetal alcohol syndrome: Craniofacial and central nervous system manifestations. Am J Med Genet 61:329-339, 1996.

Ju SH, Lin CH: The effect of moderate non-hemolytic jaundice and phototherapy on newborn behavior. Acta Paediatr Sin 32:31-41, 1991.

Kennell J, Klaus M, McGrath S, et al: Continuous emotional support during labor in a US hospital. JAMA 265:2197-2201, 1991.

Klein N, Hack M, Gallagher J, et al: Preschool performance of children with normal intelligence who were very low birth weight infants. Pediatrics 75:531-537, 1985.

Koren G, Matsui D, Einarson A, et al: Is maternal use of selective serotonin reuptake inhibitors in the third trimester of pregnancy harmful to neonates? Can Med Assoc J 172:1457-1459, 2005.

Korner AF: State as variable, as obstacle, and as mediator of stimulation in infant research. Merrill-Palmer Q 18:77-94, 1972.

Kraemer H, Korner A, Thoman E: Methodological considerations in evaluating the influence of drugs used during labor and delivery on the behavior of the newborn. Developmental Psychosoc 6:128-134, 1972.

Kuhnert BR, Linn PL, Kuhnert PM: Obstetric medication and neonatal behavior: Current controversies. Clin Perinatol 12:423-440, 1985.

Law KL, Stroud KR, LeGasse L, et al: Smoking during pregnancy and newborn neurobehavior. Pediatrics 111:1318-1323, 2003.

Lawrence PB: Breast milk: Best source of nutrition for term and preterm infants. Pediatr Clin North Am 41:925-941, 1994.

Lester BM: Developmental outcome prediction from acoustic cry analysis in term and preterm infants. Pediatrics 80:529-534, 1987.

Lester BM, Als H, Brazelton TB: Regional obstetric anesthesia and newborn behavior: A reanalysis toward synergistic effects. Child Dev 53:687-692, 1982.

Levin ED, Slotkin TA: Developmental neurotoxicity of nicotine. *In* Slikker W, Chang LW (eds): Handbook of Developmental Neurotoxicity. New York, Academic Press, 1998, pp 587-615.

MacArthur C, Knox EG: Smoking in pregnancy: Effects of stopping at different stages. Br J Obstet Gynaecol 95:551-555, 1988.

Mattson SN, Rilet EP, Delis DC, et al: Verbal learning and memory in children with fetal alcohol syndrome. Alcoholism Clin Exp Res 20:810-816, 1996.

Mayes LC, Granger RH, Frank MA, et al: Neurobehavioral profiles of neonates exposed to cocaine prenatally. Pediatrics 91:778-783, 1993.

Moyer JA, Herrenkohl LR, Jacobowitz DM: Effects of stress during pregnancy on catecholamines in discrete brain regions. Brain Res 121:385-393, 1977.

Murray AD, Dolby RM, Nation RL, et al: Effects of epidural anesthesia on newborns and their mothers. Child Dev 52:71-82, 1981.

National Immunization Survey. 2004 Available at: http://www.cdc.gov/breastfeeding/data/NIS_data/data_2004.htm.

Neifert M: Early assessment of the breastfeeding infant. Contemp Pediatr 13:142-166, 1996.

Nijhuis J, Prechtl H, Martin C, et al: Are there behavioral states in the human fetus? Early Hum Dev 6:177-195, 1982.

Nugent KJ, Lester BM, Brazelton TB: The Cultural Context of Infancy, Vol I: Biology, Culture and Infant Development. Norwood, NJ, Ablex,1989.

Nugent KJ, Lester BM, Brazelton TB: The Cultural Context of Infancy, Vol II: Multicultural and Interdisciplinary Approaches to Parent-Infant Relations. Norwood, NJ, Ablex, 1991.

Olds DI, Henderson CR, Kitzman H: Does prenatal and infancy nurse home visitation have enduring effects on qualities of parental caregiving and child health at 25 to 50 months of life? Pediatrics 93:89-98, 1994.

Oro AS, Dixon SD: Perinatal cocaine and methamphetamine exposure: Maternal and neonatal correlates. J Pediatr 111:571-578, 1987.

Parmelee AH: Remarks on receiving the C. Anderson Aldrich Award. Pediatrics 59:389-395, 1977.

Parmelee AH, Wenner WH, Akiyama Y, et al: Infant sleep patterns from birth to 16 weeks of age. J Pediatr 65:576-582, 1964.

Patel AB, Mamtani MR, Thakre TP, Kulkarni H: Association of umbilical cord blood lead with neonatal behavior at varying levels of exposure. Behav Brain Functions 2:22, 2006.

Pomerleau-Malcuit A, Clifton RK: Neonatal heart rate response to tactile, auditory, and vestibular stimulation in different states. Child Dev 44:485, 1973.

Prechtl HRF: The behavioral states of the newborn infant: A review. Brain Res 76:1304-1311, 1974.

Pressler JL, Hepworth JT, La Montagne L, et al: Behavioral responses of newborns of insulin-dependent and nondiabetic, healthy mothers. Clin Nurs Res 8:103-118, 1999.

Pryor J, Silva PA, Brooke M: Growth, development and behaviour in adolescents born small-for-gestational-age. J Paediatr Child Health 31:403-407, 1995.

Rayburn WF, Bogenschutz MP: Pharmacotherapy for pregnant women with addictions. Am J Obstet Gynecol 191:1885-1897, 2004.

Rauh VA, Nurcombe B, Achenbach T, Howell C: The mother-infant transaction program: The content and implications of an intervention for the mothers of low-birthweight infants. Clin Perinatol 17:31-45, 1990.

Rizzo T, Freinkel N, Metzger BE, et al: Correlations between antepartum maternal metabolism and newborn behavior. Am J Obstet Gynecol 163:1458-1464, 1990.

Robertson SS: Cyclic motor activity in the human fetus after midgestation. Dev Psychobiol 18:411-419, 1985.

Robertson SS: Human cyclic motility: Fetal-newborn continuities and newborn state differences. Dev Psychobiol 20:425-442, 1987.

Robertson SS, Drierker LJ: The development of cyclic motility in fetuses of diabetic mothers. Dev Psychobiol 19:223-234, 1986.

Rodier P: Environmental causes of central nervous system maldevelopment. Pediatrics 113:1076-1083, 2004.

Rothbart MK: Measurement of temperament in infancy. Child Dev 52:569-578, 1981.

Rubel EW: Auditory system development. *In* Gottlieb G, Krasnegor NA (eds): Measurement of Audition and Vision in the First Year of Postnatal Life: A Methodological Overview. Norwood, NJ, Ablex, 1985, pp 53-89.

Saint-Anne Dargassies S: Normality and normalization as seen in a long-term neurological follow-up of 286 truly premature infants. Neuropediatrics 10:226-244, 1979.

Sanders-Phillips K, Strauss ME, Gutberlet RL: The effect of obstetric medication on newborn infant feeding behavior. Infant Behav Dev 11:251-263, 1988.

Scafidi FA, Field TM, Wheeden MS, et al: Cocaine-exposed preterm neonates show behavioral and hormonal differences. Pediatrics 97:851-855, 1996.

Schanler RJ, Hurst NM: Human milk for the hospitalized preterm infant. Semin Perinatol 18:476-484, 1994.

Scher A: Infant sleep at 10 months of age as a window to cognitive development. Early Hum Dev 81:289-292, 2005.

Schneider ML, Coe CL: Repeated social stress during pregnancy impairs neuromotor development of the primate infant. J Dev Behav Pediatr 14:81-87, 1993.

Seligman MR: Helplessness: On Development, Depression, and Death. San Francisco, WH Freeman, 1975.

Sepokoski CM, Lester BM, Ostheimer GW, Brazelton TB: The effects of maternal epidural anesthesia on neonatal behavior during the first month. Dev Med Child Neurol 34:1072-1080, 1992.

Silverman BL, Rizzo T, Green OC, et al: Long-term prospective evaluation of offspring of diabetic mothers. Diabetes 40:121-125, 1991.

Sroufe A: Attachment and the construction of relationships. *In* Hartup WW, Rubin Z (eds): Relationships and Development. Hillsdale, NJ, Lawrence Erlbaum, 1986, pp 51-71.

Strauss ME, Lessen-Firestine JK, Starr RH, et al: Behavior of narcotic-addicted newborns. Child Dev 46:887-893, 1975.

Suzuki K, Minei LJ, Johnson EE: Effect of nicotine upon uterine blood flow in the pregnant rhesus monkey. Am J Obstet Gynecol 136:1009-1013, 1980.

Thoman EB: Sleep and Waking States of the Neonate, rev ed. 1985. (Available from EB Thoman, Box U-154, Dept of Psychology/Behavioral Neuroscience, 3107 Horsebarn Hill Rd, University of Connecticut, Storrs, CT 06268.)

Thoman EB, Acebo C, Dreyer CA, et al: Individuality in the interactive process. *In* Thoman EB (ed): Origins of the Infant's Social Responsiveness. Hillsdale, NJ, Lawrence Erlbaum, 1979, pp 305-338.

Thoman EB, Denenberg VH, Sieval J, et al: State organization in neonates: Developmental inconsistency indicates risk for developmental dysfunction. Neuropediatrics 12:45-54, 1981.

Thomas A, Chess S, Birch HG, et al: Behavioral individuality in early childhood. New York, New York University Press, 1963.

Tirosh E, Harel J, Abad J, et al: Relationship between neonatal behavior and subsequent temperament. Acta Paediatr 81:829-831, 1992.

Tronick E, Wise S, Als H, et al: Regional obstetric anesthesia and newborn behavior: Effect over the first ten days of life. Pediatrics 58:94-100, 1976.

Tronick EZ, Messinger DS, Weinberg MK, et al: Cocaine exposure is associated with subtle compromises of infants' and mothers' social-emotional behavior and dyadic features of their interaction in the face-to-face still-face paradigm. Dev Psychol 41:711-722, 2005.

Vohr BR, Coll CG, Lobato D, et al: Neurodevelopmental and medical status of low-birthweight survivors of bronchopulmonary dysplasia at 10 to 12 years of age. Dev Med Child Neurol 33:690-697, 1991.

Volpe JJ: Effect of cocaine use on the fetus. N Engl J Med 327:399-407, 1992.

Walther FJ: Growth and development of term disproportionate small-for-gestational age infants at the age of 7 years. Early Hum Dev 18:1-11, 1988.

Whitney MP, Thoman EB: Early sleep patterns of premature infants are differentially related to later developmental disabilities. J Dev Behav Pediatr 14:71-80, 1993.

Wolff PH: Observations on newborn infants. Psychosom Med 221:110-118, 1959.

Wolff PH: The causes, controls, and organization of behavior in the neonate. Psychol Issues 5:1-105, 1966.

Zhang J, Bernasko JW, Leybovich E, et al: Continuous labor support from labor attendant for primiparous women: A meta-analysis. Obstet Gynecol 88:739-744, 1996.

Zuckerman B, Frank DA: Prenatal cocaine exposure: Nine years later. J Pediatr 124:731-733, 1994.

3 INFANCY AND TODDLER YEARS

Marilyn Augustyn, Deborah A. Frank, and Barry S. Zuckerman

At birth, a child's biologic endowment includes sensory, motor, and neurologic capacities, intact or impaired for organizing experience and interacting with the environment. Initially, infants are totally dependent on the adults in their world. In the first 2 years of life, highly integrated multiple streams of development flow with extraordinary swiftness. These rapid changes integrate infants into their social world and simultaneously allow them to function autonomously, if only in limited domains.

The transactional model (Sameroff and Chandler, 1974) is a useful framework with which to view the child and family in this highly dynamic period of development. The model explains various phenomena and facilitates informed clinical supervision of children's behavior and development from birth to age 2 years. The transactional model of development assumes that infants, caregivers, and their environment determine the child's developmental and behavioral outcome. This model differs from other models in which the child or the caregivers or the environment unilaterally determines outcome. The transactional model of development holds that the child and the caregiving environment tend to alter each other mutually. Seen in these terms, child development is more than a two-way street; it is an intimate and complex interaction.

This approach is supported by emerging research on brain development showing that caregiving and social factors (as mediated by vision, hearing, smell, touch, and taste) as well as genetic influences shape the developing brain's architecture associated with changes in development and behavior (see Chapter 8). An enriched environment ensures growth and maintenance of synaptic connections during the period of early development, when central nervous system connections are being formed at a rapid rate, and simultaneous pruning of unused connections is occurring. Certain stimuli, such as significant stressful experiences, result in neurochemical changes that can lead to structural changes in the brain.

This chapter discusses the multiple developmental processes that occur during the first 2 years of life across all the classic "streams of development": social and emotional development, sensory and motor maturation, cognitive development, communication, and physical growth. For each developmental process, possible normal variations and indications for clinical concern are described.

SOCIAL-EMOTIONAL DEVELOPMENT

Clinical expectations for adaptive sequential social-emotional and interactive patterns have been formulated based on progressive understanding of how infants form relationships and interact with their caregiver as described in the transactional model. The process by which parents support a child's attempts at self-regulation can be understood further as mutual regulation—a process by which infants thrive through the support and responsive interactions provided by their caregivers. Similarly, the infant's response to the caregiver (e.g., whether enthusiastic or flat) shapes the parent's behavior. Three theoretical constructs—attachment/separation, joint attention/social referencing, and autonomy/mastery—provide a framework for additional understanding of social-emotional development on a clinical level.

Attachment

Attachment describes the discriminating, enduring, and specific affective bond that children develop with caregivers. Some authors use the term *bonding* to describe the comparable bonds that caregivers develop with infants, but we use the term *attachment* for both aspects of the relationship. Attachment is bidirectional; there is attachment of the primary caregiver to the infant and attachment of the infant to the primary caregiver, although they can be asymmetric. Although infant behaviors that create and maintain this bond vary from one developmental stage to the next, they serve to maintain the child's internal security.

The process of attachment begins in utero. With quickening, parents begin to perceive the fetus as a separate individual and enter into an intense relationship with the imagined child-to-be. Newborns and even fetuses know their own mother's voice. Non-nutritive sucking (Mehler et al, 1978) and fetal heart rate increase (Kisilevsky et al, 2003) in response to their mother's voice compared with the voice of a stranger. After birth, parents modify the expectations, hopes, and fears that evolved during the pregnancy as they become acquainted with the real infant. Parents who are emotionally available, sensitive, perceptive, and effective at meeting the needs of their infant throughout the early months of life are likely to have securely attached infants.

The infant also contributes to the relationship. An alert infant who reacts readily to parents' faces and responds promptly to consoling maneuvers enhances parents' positive feelings and a sense of competence. Conversely, a drowsy, relatively hypotonic infant who provides less satisfying feedback may disappoint parents anticipating emotional satisfaction from their infant.

Empirical studies and meta-analyses have shown security of attachment to be predicted by (1) caregivers' current representations of their own childhood experiences as expressed by their attachment experiences and (2) caregivers' sensitive responsivity to their infants' cues during the first year of life (Meins, 1999). Self-understanding for parents comes through a long process, in which they review their upbringing on their own and with their spouse or partner, relatives, friends, other parents, and professionals (Siegel and Hartzell, 2003). Parents' self-understanding greatly enhances their ability to be good parents and to foster the best possible development in their child (van Ijzendoorn, 1995).

Most families require several months before they feel they know their infant. During this initial attachment period, parents strive through trial and error to understand their infant's needs for food, rest, or social interaction. Parents begin to show an intuitive understanding of how to enhance their child's social responsiveness. In face-to-face interactions, parents exaggerate their facial expressions (eyebrows go up, mouths open wide) and slow their vocalizations ("parent-ese"—conversation consists of "aahs" and "oohs.") in response to the infant's limited ability to process social information. In response to such maneuvers, the infant's eyelids widen, the pupils dilate, and mouths become rounded. These signs of social interest occur long before the development of responsive smiling at 6 to 8 weeks of age. A newborn has all the necessary neurologic coordination to perform the seven universal facial expressions (happiness, sadness, surprise, interest, disgust, fear, and anger) and is able to produce them; these expressions are much more readily identifiable at 2 to 3 months of age and are responsive to environmental cues by 6 months of age (Walker-Andrews, 1998).

By 3 months of age, the child and parents achieve social synchrony manifested by reciprocal vocal and affective exchanges. Parental displays of pleasure are followed by smiling, cooing, and movement in the infant. When the excitement peaks, the infant transiently disengages to reorganize for another cycle of excitement. Infants also initiate these pleasurable exchanges.

The next important step in the attachment process is the development of a clear preference for primary caregivers. By 3 to 5 months of age, an infant stops crying more readily for familiar caregivers than for strangers. Infants smile sooner and more brightly for their parents, and this clear behavioral preference enhances the parents' formation of positive emotional ties to their infants. As recall memory for absent objects emerges between 7 and 9 months of age, the infant's preference for primary caregivers produces the well-recognized phenomena of separation protest and stranger awareness or anxiety. If these normal developmental milestones are misattributed by caregivers or others to "spoiling," inappropriately punitive responses may be made, increasing the infant's distress further.

Attachment involves close proximity and provides a secure base, which allows infants to explore their world. Initially, attachment figures provide a sense of security by their physical presence. Later in the first year, infants internalize their relationship with attachment figures, leading to an internal model of security. By 18 months of age, infants have the ability to conjure an image of the attachment figure in their mind (memory), which helps comfort them in times of stress. An example, commonly observed when children are dropped off at childcare, is a child who walks around aimlessly repeating "Mommy, mommy, mommy." The child is working to maintain the image of the mother and a sense of security by repeating her name in the face of her leaving.

The two behavioral hallmarks of a secure attachment relationship in the first 2 years of life are security and exploration (Sroufe, 1979). Infants must have a secure attachment to explore their environment. Without a secure "home base," infants cannot move outward effectively. This sense of self and other as different and important beings embodies core expectations about the trustworthiness and dependability of others in one's world; these concepts are often referred to as an internalized working model and can be seen in infants' behavior as they use their parents as a secure base to explore the world progressively.

The creation of a secure relationship of attachment requires consistent availability of adults who are affectionate and responsive to the child's physical and emotional needs—although sensitivity is not the only factor contributing to attachment security. Other factors to consider include mutuality and synchrony, stimulation, positive attitude, and emotional support (de Wolff and van Ijzendoorn, 1997). Children given the opportunity to develop a secure relationship possess a foundation on which to build positive relationships with peers and unrelated adults. Children's secure attachment to caregivers also is associated at a later age with more effective coping with stress and better performance at school (Sroufe, 1988; Waters et al, 1979). The possibility of forming these relationships with more than one caring adult has been tested in studies of adoptive families and communal living situations. Most adoptive mothers and their infants adopted before 6 months of age develop warm and secure attachment relationships (Singer et al, 1985). In the community relationship of the kibbutz or in African villages, children form attachment relationships of similar quality with nonfamilial caregivers (Sagi et al, 1995).

Studying Attachment

The research method commonly used to describe infant attachment is called the "strange situation" (Ainsworth, 1979). The purpose of the paradigm is to assess the quality of infants' attachment to parents and to evaluate infants' capacities for coping with stress. The separation of the child from his or her attachment figure activates the child's behavioral attachment system, which can be studied during the reunion by assessing the proximity to the primary caregiver and the ease of being soothed and return to play. Attachment theory describes four categories of response at the time of reunion with the caregiver.

Infants with *secure attachment* are able to use their caregiver to become calmed and return to play quickly. This behavioral pattern suggests that the child has experienced responsive caregiving with communication contingent to the child's emotional signals. Infants with *avoidant attachment* show no overt response to the return of their caregiver and continue to play as though their caregiver did not leave and return. This pattern suggests the child's signals are rarely perceived or responded to in an effective manner (e.g., when a parent is consistently emotionally distant). Avoidant attachment predicts later difficulty relating to peers and the emergence of a poorly developed sense of self. Infants with *ambivalent attachment* turn to their mother, but are not easily soothed and do not return to play. Such attachment predicts a later level of uncertainty and anxiety in social situations. Finally, infants with *disorganized attachment* show chaotic or self-destructive behavior or both. For example, the child first approaches and then backs away from the parent. Disorganized attachment is ascribed to recurring situations when a parent repeatedly causes a state of fear in a child—by expressing excessive anger, withdrawing, or creating a setting in which the child is offered no hope of comfort or safety, or no relief from distress.

Separation

On the flip side of maintaining attachment, negotiation of separation, both psychological and physical, poses a continuous challenge to parents and children. In psychiatric theory, best outlined by Mahler and associates (1975), separation refers to the internal processes by which the child evolves a satisfying identity as an individual distinct from the parents. Depending on the psychological context, actual physical separations can enhance or impede the child's ability to develop a comfortable individuality. As the reliable physical availability to responsive caregivers encourages the infant's efforts toward independence, a complementary process of acceptance of the child's internal separation must occur within the parents. Some parents accept an infant's total dependence, but have difficulty tolerating a toddler's striving for an independent identity.

Cultural Variations in Separation and Attachment

The above-discussed theory primarily reflects a Western framework. Does this reflect the situation across the world? Evidence from Japan suggests that extremely close ties between mother and child are perceived as adaptive and are more common, and that children experience less adverse effects from such relationships than do children in the West (Rothbaum et al, 2002). In a study comparing Anglo and Puerto Rican mothers, researchers found that Anglo mothers place greater emphasis on socialization goals and child-rearing strategies consonant with an individualistic orientation, whereas Puerto Rican mothers place greater focus on goals and strategies consistent with a sociocentric orientation. Puerto Rican mothers were more likely than Anglo mothers to structure their infants' behaviors directly (Harwood et al, 1999).

One of the most intriguing studies on cultural variations in infancy involved comparing American and Chinese mothers telling stories to their young children (Wang et al, 2000). American mothers and children showed a highly elaborative, independently oriented conversational style in which they co-constructed their memories and stories by elaborating on each other's responses, focusing on the child's direction. Chinese mother-child dyads employed a less elaborative, interdependently oriented conversational style in which mothers frequently posed and repeated factual questions and showed great concern with moral rules and behavioral standards. The impact of these differences in mother-child interaction on later memory, storytelling, and cultural identification is the focus of active research.

Clinical Implications

Parental sensitivity is a necessary but insufficient condition of attachment security (de Wolff and van Ijzendoorn, 1997). Parents burdened by illness, psychiatric impairment, drug abuse, or other crises may find it particularly difficult to respond warmly and consistently to an infant's frequent demands. Infants and toddlers who have experienced chronically inconsistent nurturing may seem uninterested in exploring the surrounding world, even in the caregiver's presence. Some of these children appear clingy without the presence of obvious stress. Others appear actively angry and distrustful of their primary caregivers, ignoring or resisting caregivers' efforts to comfort them after brief separations or other stress (Sroufe, 1979). The possible role of behavioral genetics in attachment and temperament is a topic of current research (Hobcraft, 2006).

A serious disturbance of the attachment process may be suspected when otherwise typically developing infants between the ages of 9 months and 2 years fail to show a behavioral preference for familiar caregivers in response to stress. Lack of discriminate attachment behaviors toward familiar caregivers can be an ominous sign requiring the clinician to search for developmental delay in the child, serious family dysfunction, neglect, or abuse (Gaensbauer and Sands, 1979). Long separation from parents and disorganized patterns of multiple caregiving—conditions that occur in many prolonged hospitalizations and separations—also can produce indiscriminate attachment behaviors. These are not immutable. When a child exhibits indiscriminate, avoidant, or resistant attachment behaviors, caregivers' continuous availability, warmth, and responsiveness, whether the child is at home, in childcare, or in the hospital, may restore a more secure attachment pattern (Zuckerman et al, 2005). Hospital and childcare personnel should provide the child with one or two nurses or teachers who are assigned consistently to augment parents' efforts to restore the child's sense of internal security.

If the child's avoidant, resistant, or indiscriminate attachment behaviors persist, mental health referral for the family is indicated.

The child's and parents' responses to everyday experiences of physical separation, such as bedtime, childcare, parental travel, or hospitalization of the parent or child, can vary widely. In assessing the developmental progress of the child's internal process of separation, the parents and the child show mixed feelings about separations. Brief, predictable physical separations from the parents facilitate successful psychological separation for young children. The first such separation occurs when the infant is put to bed alone at night. The next occurs the first time parents leave their infant with a relative or babysitter. Most parents are uncomfortable with these first separations. When parents express apparently disproportionate anxiety about their child's well-being during routine separations, they are often expressing ambivalence about the child's evolution of independence. Explicit discussion of the parents' feelings about internal and external separations can be more effective than reassurance about the ostensible concern. For example, the clinician might suggest, "it's not easy for parents to be away from their babies."

Initial difficulties with separation subside only to become acute again when, at 7 to 9 months of age, children begin to show separation distress by crying whenever the caregiver leaves their presence. Clinicians can help parents recognize that the separation distress that results from normal cognitive phenomena diminishes as the child learns from multiple brief separations and reunions that parents reliably return.

As the psychological process of separation proceeds, the child develops the ability to form relationships with caregivers other than the parents. Parents can facilitate the formation of these new relationships by their physical availability to the child as the relationship is first formed. A new babysitter should be introduced with a parent present for at least 1 day, as is the best practice when the child is starting at a new childcare center. Slowly increasing the duration of separation may aid the child in a smooth transition, but regressive behavior on reunion with the parent should be expected and should trigger verbalization and comfort ("We missed each other, didn't we"), rather than scolding ("Big girls don't cry")

Overwhelming stress, such as physical illness and the painful experiences entailed in hospitalization, exceeds any infant's capacity to tolerate physical separation from parents. When the child is tired or ill or has recently sustained a prolonged separation from caregivers, the physical presence of the parent paradoxically supports the process of internal separation by preventing the child from becoming overwhelmed by internal or external stress. The clinician should recommend that a parent or other familiar caregiver remain with a young child during hospitalization (see Chapter 33).

Because the separation process is mutual, clinicians should be alert to parental issues that can unintentionally sabotage the child's establishment of a separate identity. This process is particularly in jeopardy when the parents perceive the child as unusually "vulnerable" because of past illness or other factors that make a child special (e.g., only boy, only girl, last child). A recent loss in the parents' lives, such as a death or divorce, also can threaten the normal separation process.

When parents regard their child as uniquely susceptible to harm or illness, they can become overprotective, leading to the "vulnerable child syndrome" with separation difficulties, insufficient setting of limits, somatic concerns, and overuse of the health care system (Pearson and Boyce, 2004). Overprotection is a disturbance in the parent-child relationship associated with the parents' difficulty in supporting age-appropriate, socioculturally concordant separation and individuation in the child. A clinician who encourages parents to discuss their real or imagined losses and their ambivalence about separation can help to liberate the parent and the child. The process of internal separation does not end in infancy for either parent or child, but must be negotiated repeatedly throughout the life cycle (see Chapter 34).

Social Referencing and Joint Attention

Infants look to their primary caregiver for signals (smile, comfort, fear) showing how to deal with new experiences, a reliable phenomenon referred to as social referencing. When approached by a stranger, whether a relative who visits infrequently or the physician at an office visit, a 7-month-old infant looks to the mother to see if it is okay to allow this stranger to approach. If the mother smiles comfortably, the infant is more likely to remain calm. If the mother herself is upset, either about the person or about the possible pain the child will experience with immunizations, the child is more likely to cry.

The classic experiment showing social referencing is the finding that the mother's facial expression of comfort or fear was related to the 6-month-old infant's propensity to crawl over or avoid a "visual cliff" (Gibson and Walk, 1960). The initial studies with young children showed that most human infants can discriminate depth as soon as they can crawl. When a caregiver was introduced into the paradigm, the child was willing to crawl over the cliff if the caregiver's facial expression was encouraging and refused to crawl if the caregiver looked worried. Vocal cues, even without a visual reference, have been found to be more potent than facial cues in guiding infants' behavior (Vaish and Striano, 2004). This social referencing is a critical milestone in the formation of "theory of the mind" (i.e., recognition of self versus other). Children often develop social referencing between 6 and 18 months of age.

In parallel, joint attention emerges. The development of joint attention is considered to be critical to early social, cognitive, and language development. Joint attention refers to the capacity to coordinate attention with others regarding objects and events. Although infants and toddlers display systematic, age-related gains in joint attention between birth and 18 months of age, they also may display considerable individual differences in the development of this skill. In children 2 to 14 months of age, joint attention becomes "triadic"—the child is able to engage one parent, while maintaining the attention of the other. By 18 months of age, the child is able to direct the attention of one person actively to share in the child's experience of another person or object, often a toy. In this "directing of attention," children show that they recognize that *their* experience is not automatically the experience of another, and, by this intentional redirection of the "other" to what they are interested in, children show an understanding that others may have their *own* interests and behaviors. Joint attention is a fundamental skill to individuation that continues to develop throughout childhood and is critical to all the developmental streams.

Clinical Implications

Encouraging parents to engage their child in conversation, song, and natural eye contact is important from the first days of life. Monitoring for the appearance of social referencing and joint attention in the first 2 years of life has become a focus of great attention in efforts for earlier identification of social and emotional disorders, such as autism spectrum disorders. At approximately 1 year of age, a typically developing child attempts to obtain an object out of reach by getting the caregiver's attention through pointing, verbalizing, and making eye contact. This behavior is often labeled "protoimperative pointing." The child looks alternatively at the object and the caregiver in an effort to communicate his or her desire. A few months later, the typically developing child shows "protodeclarative pointing." The child points to an interesting object, verbalizes, and looks alternatively between the object and the caregiver simply to direct the adult's attention to the object or event of interest. At about the same time, typically developing children also begin bringing objects to adults just to show them, an example of social referencing. Children with autism spectrum disorder show impairments in some or all of these joint attention and social referencing activities (see Chapter 69).

Autonomy and Mastery

Autonomy refers to the achievement of behavioral independence. Mastery describes the child's quest for ever-increasing competence. These complementary processes require that caregivers and infants continually renegotiate control of the infant's bodily functions and social interactions.

Self-consoling behavior marks the beginning of autonomy. From the earliest days after birth, a crying infant tries to bring the hand to the mouth. When the hand is inserted, the infant begins to suck and stops crying. Sucking facilitates the infant's ability to regulate his or her level of arousal. Brazelton (1962) found that during the first 3 months of life, infants who engage in frequent hand sucking cry less than other infants. Sucking on sucrose may reduce further a reaction to a painful stimulus possibly through a neurally mediated pathway (Bucher et al, 1995).

As infants mature, the repertoire for self-consolation expands to include rhythmic behaviors such as body rocking (20% of all children) and head banging or rolling (6% of all children); these behaviors usually begin between 6 and 10 months of age. In the second year of life, toddlers employ favored possessions such as blankets (transitional objects) and repetitive rituals (e.g., saying goodnight to stuffed animals in a fixed order) to cope autonomously with bedtime and other stressful situations (see also Chapter 65). In addition, this is a time when "first fears" may emerge, often revolving around themes of separation, such as fear of the dark, fear of strangers, and fear of being alone.

The infant's drive to master the environment serves as an important motivating force in itself, independent of the need for food, warmth, sleep, and social approval. This intense striving for competence and independence can lead to struggles with caregivers over feeding, sleep, toileting, and exploration. Many 9-month-old infants are so intent on practicing new fine motor skills that they insist on feeding themselves with their fingers, refusing to allow parents to feed them. Like the legendary explorer, an 18-month-old child will repetitively scale a forbidden sofa simply "because it's there." Similarly, a toddler insists on repetition of stories and games multiple times, tiring out even the most tolerant grandparent, all on a mission of mastery.

Clinical Implications

The child's struggles for autonomy and mastery produce varying degrees of discord depending on the temperamental style of the child and the characteristics of the caregivers. Clinicians' use of the construct of temperament or "the how of behavior" can facilitate successful negotiation of this developmental stage. Temperamentally persistent youngsters delight parents by working at a new task until they have mastered it. Such persistent children also may infuriate parents, however, by refusing to abandon unsafe explorations of the kitchen stove.

Parental concerns about thumb sucking, temper tantrums, and toilet training provide three common clinical examples of autonomy issues. Sucking, the first organized behavior under the infant's control, is used to obtain nutrition and to achieve self-regulation by sucking on a pacifier, a hand, or on nothing. Parents, unaware of the self-regulatory function of non-nutritive sucking, may interpret it as a sign of hunger and inadvertently overfeed the infant (Friman, 1990). To add to the complexity, the American Academy of Pediatrics has revised its policy statement on reducing the incidence of sudden infant death syndrome, making the controversial recommendation that use of pacifiers be encouraged to reduce this risk (American Academy of Pediatrics Task Force on SIDS, 2005). Non-nutritive sucking of any object (body part or pacifier) may serve not only a soothing, but also a survival protecting role in the first year of life. If parents ignore the harmless (and potentially helpful) self-regulating behavior of thumb or finger sucking, most children spontaneously relinquish it between the ages of 4 and 5 years, as other strategies for coping develop. If parents try to discourage finger sucking through criticism or restraint, a positive coping mechanism becomes an occasion for a negative struggle over who controls the child's body. To assert their autonomy, children may stubbornly persist in thumb sucking longer than they would otherwise. Clinicians can help parents perceive the positive functions of non-nutritive sucking and alleviate unnecessary anxiety about orthodontic problems or digital deformity, which arises only if thumb sucking persists past the age at which permanent teeth erupt (American Association of Pediatric Dentistry, 2006).

Tantrums, common in the second year of life, arise from the child's efforts to exercise mastery and autonomy. Clinicians and caregivers can better devise appropriate management if they understand the developmental issues that give rise to tantrums. Some tantrums result from the child's frustration at failing to master a task. Distracting the child and permitting success in a more manageable activity can be a helpful maneuver to alleviate this type of tantrum. Most toddlers respond with tantrums as parents impose limits that restrict their autonomy. Parental response to such tantrums should encourage self-control. Young children may need to be held so that they can regain control. Older children should be left alone in a safe place until they have calmed themselves. In using a "time out" procedure, parents should not attempt to inflict a rigid number of minutes of isolation, but rather use this time of lost positive attention to help the child develop self-regulation (see Chapter 87). As soon as the tantrum subsides, isolation should end, and the child should receive praise for the quieter state.

An appropriate balance between necessary limits and support for independence requires frequent renegotiation as the child develops. Generally, successful limits are firm, consistent, explicit, and selective. Children thrive on routine and structure. Setting limits should include more praise for desired behavior ("time in") than the also necessary disapproval for or removal from an undesired behavior. Parents of toddlers often need help in choosing which issues are worth a battle. Breaking the child's will should never become an end in itself. Constant tantrum behavior indicates that the family and child have lost control. Such families may benefit from counseling or mental health referral (see Chapter 86).

Toilet training proceeds optimally when parents appreciate the child's need for autonomy and mastery. Anticipatory guidance around toilet training should begin toward the end of the first year because many parents plan to initiate toilet training the first birthday. If toilet training is begun on an arbitrary schedule, before the child has shown an interest in mastery of this skill, unnecessary tension can be created between the parent and child (see Chapter 63). By respecting the child's autonomy and pride in mastery, parents can make toilet training an occasion for growth rather than conflict.

SENSORY AND MOTOR MATURATION

Maturing sensory and motor abilities progressively refine the quality of information available to the growing infant. To learn about the social and inanimate world, the infant must actively coordinate the three systems that result in (1) regulation of state (i.e., level of arousal), (2) reception and processing of sensory stimuli, and (3) voluntary control of fine and gross motor movements. Neuromaturation of these regulatory systems in conjunction with mutual regulation with the caregiver forms the basis of social and emotional development.

State Control

The newborn's level of arousal creates six organized clusters of behaviors called states (see Chapter 2). During the first 3 months of life, neurophysiologic changes (doubling of quiet sleep and diminishing latency of the visual evoked potential) and neuroanatomic changes (rapid myelinization and increased dendritic branching) progressively permit the infant to regulate the state of arousal. This improved regulation of arousal produces increased sustained alertness, decreased crying, and longer periods of sleep. Research spearheaded by the "Back to Sleep" campaign found that prone REM (active) sleep was associated with lower frequencies of short arousals, body movements, and sighs, and a shorter duration of apneas than supine REM sleep at 2½ and 5 months (Skadberg and Markestad, 1997). At 2½ months, there were less frequent episodes of periodic breathing during prone sleep in non-REM (quiet) and REM sleep. Heart rate and peripheral skin temperature were higher in the prone position during both sleep states at both ages. This observation of decreased variation in behavior and respiratory pattern may indicate that young infants are less able to maintain adequate respiratory and metabolic homeostasis during prone sleep than supine sleep.

Sensory abilities in infants mature rapidly during the first year of life. Although immature, the infant's innate visual capacities are preset to select socially relevant stimuli. The newborn's visual field is relatively narrow, and only objects at the fixed focal distance of 19 cm are perceived clearly. Infants ignore visual stimuli that are too close or too distant; the mother's face is seen more clearly by the newborn than are his or her own hands. By 2 to 3 months of age, visual accommodation matures. The infant discovers hands and other near objects. In the first month of life, the infant has a visual acuity of about 20/120 (Norcia et al, 1990). By 8 months of age, the nervous system has matured enough to improve acuity to 20/30, now nearly as good as normal adult acuity (20/20). Over the next several years, acuity improves gradually to adult levels; but the most dramatic change is over that first 8 months.

Very young infants modify their behavior in response to information gathered by smell and taste. By 7 days of age, infants reliably discriminate between their own mother's breast pads and those of other nursing mothers (MacFarlane, 1975). Infants vary their sucking patterns in response to the taste of breast milk, formula, and salty or sweet liquid. The flavor aspects of food eaten by mothers are transmitted through their milk to their infants; the odor of garlic is an example. Infants suck less on an unsweetened liquid, such as breast milk, after they have tasted a sweet solution. Newborns respond to dilute sweet solutions and can differentiate varying degrees of sweetness and different kinds of sugars. Eye contact and sweet taste induce face preference in 9- and 12-week-old infants, introducing the potential role of taste in inducing facial recognition (Blass and Camp, 2001).

Clinical Implications

As underlined by the old quip "people who say they sleep like a baby usually don't have one," sleep is a major issue for the caregivers of young children. Promoting sleep hygiene from the first days of life can help ward off problems by improving sleep-onset associations (Garcia and Wills, 2000). The wide variations in infant sleep-wake cycles make this a challenge. The infant's first social responses consist of attaining or maintaining an alert slate in response to caregiving maneuvers. A crying infant who quiets down when picked up or a drowsy one who becomes wide-eyed at the sound of mother's voice delights caregivers.

There are wide individual variations in the infant's control of state, responsiveness to environmental input, and sleep-wake patterns. Some infants spontaneously rouse from active sleep into quiet alertness. Others move directly from sleep to crying, becoming alert only after being consoled. When roused, many infants independently inhibit their movements to attend to an interesting sound or sight. Some infants cannot sustain an alert, receptive state, however, unless assisted by an adult who swaddles them or gently restrains their hands. These inattentive infants can be frustrating to caregivers. Methods to help such infants maintain alertness include not only swaddling, but also minimizing extraneous sounds and images when the infant is trying to focus. Successful application of such methods can alleviate parents' distress by pointing out that the infant's inattentiveness reflects immaturity and will improve with time.

Similar to inattentive infants, colicky infants have a disorder of state control that improves with maturation. Colic, or "paroxysmal fussiness," tends to occur in infants with low sensory thresholds (Barr et al, 2000). Parents who try to soothe an inexplicably crying infant may inadvertently overstimulate the infant further and prolong the crying bout. Chapter 57 discusses potential techniques for managing colic. Communication about what therapies a parent is trying is critical, and the safety of individual approaches must be discussed. Colic is a diagnosis of exclusion, and the condition resolves in a predictable time course with or without out medical therapy in most cases. The most important role of the health care professional in colic is to educate, reassure, and support families (Fireman, 2006).

Clinical supervision of sleep disorders requires an understanding of the normal developmental and individual variability in children's sleep patterns. Newborns typically sleep 16½ hours per day, including naps; by age 6 months, the amount of sleep declines to approximately 14¼ hours. Children 1 to 2 years old sleep approximately 13 hours a day including naps, and 3-year-olds sleep 12 hours per day on average (Ferber, 2006). Duration of sleep depends on the maturation of the infant's central nervous system and on parental handling. The clinician can help parents devise strategies that can gradually mold the infant's innate biologic rhythms into more socially convenient patterns. By 9 months of age (and particularly during the second year), children are motivated to control their bodies and the environment. Letting go of daytime exploration and excitement is difficult, leading to resistance to sleep as an autonomy and self-regulatory issue.

Some new parents require help with distinguishing active sleep from wakefulness. Active sleep occurs every 50 to 60 minutes during a sleep cycle. If parents rush to check or feed the infant at every rustle or moan made during active sleep, the development of sustained sleep may be delayed. The clinician who suspects this to be the case can advise parents to wait until the infant seems fully awake before picking him or her up.

Parents subliminally monitor their infant's responses to sensory input and modulate that input to enhance the infant's responsiveness. A mother may move her head slowly back and forth until the infant's expression signals that her face is now in focus. When the infant is startled by the father's deep voice, the father switches to falsetto, also known as "parent-ese." Clinicians may need to provide explicit guidance for families whose infants are unusually hypersensitive or unresponsive. Some premature or small-for-gestational-age infants have low sensory thresholds. Sounds and sights that are attractive to most infants are aversive to hypersensitive infants. Although most infants prefer to track a moving face that is making sounds, a hypersensitive infant may avert his or her gaze, vomit, or startle when confronted with this simultaneous visual and auditory stimulation. With these infants, stimulation can be adaptively offered to only one of the infant's senses at a time. Extraneous stimuli, such as bright lights and loud radios, should be decreased.

Healthy infants should turn to voices and track faces with their eyes. Parents are exquisitely sensitive to their infant's responses. When parents express concern that their infant does not seem to hear or see, the infant should be formally assessed. No child is too young for audiologic testing, and the Joint Committee on Infant Hearing and Testing recommended in 1994 universal newborn screening (see Chapter 70).

Fine Motor Development

It is in large part through motor acts that infants develop and express perception, emotion, and cognition. Between 2 and 3 months of age, the weakening of the obligatory asymmetric tonic neck reflex and expansion of accommodative abilities permit infants to look at their hands and touch one hand with the other. By furnishing simultaneous information to the senses of vision and touch, this mutual hand grasp provides a foundation for later visual motor skills. During the third month of life, as the world of close proximity comes into focus, infants begin swiping at objects with loosely fisted hands. At this stage, infants swipe with one hand only at objects in front of one shoulder or the other. By 6 months of age, they reach persistently toward objects in the midline, at first with both hands and then with one.

Between 3 and 6 months of age, the coordination of grasping and reaching gradually comes under visual guidance and voluntary control. During early reaching efforts, grasping may occur, but only after the hand has contacted the object. After 6 months of age, infants begin to shape their hands for grasping in the horizontal or vertical plane of the desired object immediately before touching it. By 9 months of age, shaping of the hand occurs before the object is reached. At 1 year old, children orient the hand in the appropriate plane when starting to reach for an object (Twitchell, 1965).

When the infant can reliably obtain an object, clumsy whole-hand grasping becomes progressively refined. At 4 months of age, the infant holds an object between fingers and palm; at 5 months of age, the thumb becomes involved. By 7 months of age, thumb and fingers can grasp and retain an object without resting on the palm at all. At this time, the infant uses a raking motion between the thumb and several fingers to scoop up small objects. By 9 months of age, the infant manipulates small objects with a neat pincer grasp, using thumb and forefinger perpendicular to the surface. Every nook and cranny is now accessible to the infant's exploration. During the second year of life, toddlers develop a palmar grasp and wrist supination that permits them to use tools such as spoons and pencils.

Gross Motor Development

Three processes enable the infant to attain upright posture and the ability to move the limbs across the body's midline: (1) balance of flexor and extensor tone, (2) decline of obligatory primary reflexes, and (3) evolution of protective and equilibrium responses. First, the infant's muscle tone progresses from the neonatal state of predominant flexion to a balance in the tone of flexor and extensor muscles. The flexed newborn posture gradually unfolds until by 6 months of age; infants can extend their legs so far that they can put their toes in their mouths. Second, the decline and integration into voluntary patterns of initially obligatory primary reflexes (e.g., the Moro or asymmetric tonic neck reflex) permit the infant more flexible movement. A 1-month-old infant cannot look to one side or the other without assuming the fencing posture of the asymmetric tonic neck reflex. As this reflex disappears, the infant develops the ability to bring the hands toward the midline. Third, to sit and walk, the infant must establish equilibrium and protective responses. These responses are the automatic changes in trunk and extremity positions that the infant uses to balance and keep from falling. The familiar parachute response of 9-month-old infants who extend arms or legs to catch themselves when dropped toward the ground is an example of such protective reactions. Table 3-1 summarizes the age ranges for acquisition of selected milestones in motor development.

Clinical Implications

As Table 3-1 illustrates, the age range for normal development of gross motor skills is wide. An important tenet a clinician can follow in promoting development is not to focus on a rigid timetable of motor milestones, but to appreciate the ongoing process. Generally, infants learn to maintain new positions weeks to months before they can attain them voluntarily. Many infants at 6 months of age sit briefly unsupported if placed in that position, but cannot get themselves into a sitting position until 8 months of age. Coordinated motion from a new posture takes even longer to develop. Most children cannot walk independently until 4 to 5 months after they have learned to pull themselves up to a standing position.

Table 3-1. Median Age and Range* in Acquisition of Skills

Skill	Range (mo)
Fixates on disappearance of ball	4-5
Uses whole hand to grasp	3-6
Sits alone while playing with toy	3-6
Uses partial thumb opposition to grasp pellet	7-9
Supports weight momentarily	6-8
Grasps pencil at farthest end	8-12
Walks alone with good coordination	10-16
Runs with coordination	14-25
Uses eye-hand coordination in tossing ring	29-42

*5th to 95th percentile.

Adapted from Bayley N: Manual for the Bayley Scales of Infant Development, 2nd ed.

The developmental route to walking varies with the child's tone and temperament. Temperamentally inactive children or children who adapt slowly may not attempt independent walking until long after they are neurologically able to do so. Conversely, very active infants start taking steps as soon as they can stand. During the second year of life, these active infants rarely walk if they can run.

Parents are often relieved to know that within the wide range of normal variation, there is no correlation between intelligence and the age at which gross motor skills are acquired. No single motor skill can be used as an indicator of neurologic integrity or dysfunction. Generally, the clinician should investigate when delayed milestones are associated with global delays, opisthotonic posturing, persistent fisting of the hands, consistent disuse of a limb or side of the body, obligatory and prolonged infantile reflexes, or failure to develop a neat pincer grasp by the first birthday. The early diagnosis of cerebral palsy and other motor disabilities is described in Chapter 67.

COGNITIVE DEVELOPMENT

The developmental theories of Jean Piaget, as outlined by Ginsberg and Opper (1979), provide a useful clinical framework for understanding infant cognitive growth. Piaget believed that infants are active initiators, not passive recipients, in learning; infants are aware of the environment and begin to modify behavior in response to environmental demands. Infants can take in (assimilate) information and use it to revise (accommodate) existing mental structures, which Piaget called schemas—structures that have evolved from primitive reflex responses and were created in response to interactions with the environment. When confronted with a novel situation, the infant can create new schemas or change existing ones to revise or "accommodate" the new information that does not conform to existing schemas.

Piaget organized cognitive development during the sensorimotor period (birth to 2 years of age) into six stages (Table 3-2). Each stage represents a temporary equilibrium between the infant's skills and the environment's challenges. A toy that is too familiar no longer

Table 3-2. **Cognition, Play, and Language**

Piagetian Stage	Age	Object Permanence	Causality	Play	Receptive Language	Expressive Language
I	Birth-1 mo	Shifting images	Generalization of reflexes		Turns to voice	Range of cries (hunger, pain)
II	1-4 mo	Stares at spot from which object disappeared (looks at hand after yarn drops)	Primary circular reactions (thumb sucking)		Searches for speaker with eyes	Cooing; vocal contagion
III	4-8 mo	Visually follows dropped object through vertical trajectory (tracks dropped yarn to floor)	Secondary circular reactions (recreates accidentally discovered environmental effects, e.g., kicks mattress to shake mobile)	Same behavioral repertoire for all objects (bangs, shakes, puts in mouth, drops)	Responds to own name and to tones of voice	Babbling; four distinct syllables
IV	9-12 mo	Finds an object after watching it hidden	Coordination of secondary circular reactions	Visual motor inspection of objects; peek-a-boo	Listens selectively to familiar words; responds to "no" and other verbal requests	First real word; "jargoning"; symbolic gestures (shakes head "no")
V	12-18 mo	Recovers hidden object after multiple visible changes of position	Tertiary circular reactions (deliberately varies behavior to create novel effects)	Awareness of social function of objects; symbolic play centered on own body (drinks from toy cup)	Can bring familiar object from another room; points to parts of body	Many single words—uses words to express needs; acquires 10 words by 18 mo
VI	18 mo-2 yr	Recovers hidden object after invisible changes in position	Spontaneously uses nondirect causal mechanisms (uses key to move wind-up toy)	Symbolic play directed toward doll (gives doll a drink)	Follows series of two or three commands; points to picture when named	Telegraphic 2-word sentence

engages the toddler, who prefers the greater challenges posed by the contents of the kitchen cupboard. Conversely, a completely insoluble problem (e.g., a crayon presented for a 9-month-old infant to use) does not hold the infant's interest. Cognitive development requires opportunities for exploration and manipulation that are neither too easy nor too hard. Piaget believed that infants and young toddlers are active in this learning process; infants use all sensory modalities and emerging motor skills to explore the world and the people in it. In the following sections, we describe core concepts of infant cognition—object permanence, causality, recognition memory, and habituation of attention.

Object Permanence

Newborns behave as though the world consists of shifting images that cease to exist when they are no longer perceived. "Out of sight, out of mind" is a description of the infant's world during the first stage of sensorimotor development (stage I). Gradually, stable mental images of absent objects and people develop. By 2 months of age, infants continue to look expectantly at a person's empty hand after an object has been dropped from sight (stage II). Between 4 and 8 months of age, infants locate a partly hidden object and visually track objects through a vertical trajectory. If infants see an object being hidden, however, they do not search for it (stage III). Between 9 and 12 months of age, infants can find an object that they see hidden (stage IV). At this age, however, infants cannot retrieve an object that is moved in plain view from one hiding place to another. By 18 months of age, infants reliably find objects after multiple changes of position as long as those changes are observed, but they cannot deduce the whereabouts of an object if they do not see it being moved (stage V). Finally, by age 2 years, toddlers have sufficient symbolic abilities to infer a hidden object's position from other cues without actually observing it being moved to that position (stage VI). People and things now reliably exist for toddlers as stable entities whether or not they are perceptually present—an important achievement that has implications for separation and attachment behaviors. Behaviors characteristic of each stage of the child's understanding of object permanence are outlined in Table 3-2.

Causality

Piaget observed an orderly sequence of changes in the child's understanding of causal relationships over the first 2 years of life. First, infants learn to recreate satisfying bodily sensations by maneuvers such as thumb sucking (primary circular reaction). At about 3 months of age, infants begin to use causal behaviors to recreate accidentally discovered, interesting effects (secondary circular reaction). Infants at this age repeatedly kick the mattress once they have discovered by chance that this behavior sets in motion a mobile above the bed. Infants' understanding of cause and effect gradually leads to increasingly specific behavior patterns aimed at particular environmental effects. During the second year of life, toddlers become experimenters, intent on causing novel events rather than reinstituting familiar ones (tertiary circular reactions). At the same time, children begin to comprehend that apparently unrelated behaviors can be combined to created a desired effect. By age 2 years, a child spontaneously winds up a toy to make it move.

Recognition Memory and Habituation of Attention

An infant's capacity for memory begins very early, perhaps as early as 6 months, by means of deferred imitation (Collie and Hayne, 1999). The research paradigm used to assess infant memory consists of the presentation of a stimulus and subsequent observation of whether the infant spends more time attending to a novel rather than a familiar stimulus (recognition memory and habituation of attention) (Bornstein and Sigman, 1986). Preference for novelty is believed to represent a "hard-wired" predisposition for exploring stimuli that leads to developmental progression. Learning by habituation refers to a decrease in response to a stimulus after repeated presentations when the stimulus is no longer perceived as novel.

Many more recent studies have shown that periodic reminders can maintain early memories over significant periods of development and challenge popular claims that preverbal human infants cannot maintain memories over the long-term because of neural immaturity or an inability to rehearse experiences by talking about them (Rovee-Collier et al, 1999; Saffran et al, 2000). Maturation in recall begins late in the first year of life, and by the end of the second year long-term memory is reliable and robust, but can be elicited only nonverbally (Bauer, 2006).

Play

"Play is a window through which we come to understand the child from both inside and outside" (Sheridan, 1995). Peek-a-boo signals the emergence of object permanence. An elaborate detour to retrieve a ball rolled under the couch shows that the child understands invisible displacements, and repetitive dropping of food from the high chair at different heights and angles completes many tertiary circular reactions in a child's learning process, as long as someone is there to pick up the food and close the circle. See Table 3-2 for further examples.

An infant's handling of objects also reflects his or her progressive understanding of the world. At 5 to 6 months of age, an infant can reliably reach and grasp attractive objects. At this stage, the infant subjects all toys to the same behavioral repertoire, regardless of their particular properties. A toy car, a bell, and a spoon all are mouthed, shaken, banged, and dropped. By 9 months of age, the infant systematically manipulates the object to inspect it with eyes and hands in all orientations, showing the cognitive ability to process information simultaneously instead of sequentially.

By the first birthday, the infant shows understanding of the socially assigned function of objects. A toy car is pushed on its wheels; a bell is rung. Next, early representational play, which reflects stable concept of objects, appears. At first, such play centers on the child's own body as the child "drinks" from a toy cup or puts a toy telephone to his or her ear. Between 17 and 24 months of age, the child's thought and play become less egocentric. Now a doll is offered a drink. When the child becomes facile in the use of symbols (24 to 30 months of age), truly imaginative play begins with the onset of symbolic play. In such play, the child uses one object to represent another (e.g., putting bits of paper on a plate to symbolize food).Table 3-2 outlines the concurrent development of object permanence, causality, and play.

Clinical Implications

Each cognitive transformation alters the infant's social behavior. Although 2- to 3-month-old infants can recognize their parents, they have no recall memory—that is, no internal symbolic representation of their parents—until they attain stage IV object permanence (the stage at which they search for a completely hidden object). The child's recall memory for parents evolves before memory for inanimate objects (Bell, 1970). The child's experience of "missing" the parent after separation results from the discrepancy between the recalled image of the parent and the parent's absence from the child's perceptual field. For a 4-month-old infant, the parent does not exist when not seen. A 10-month-old infant knows that parents still exist when they are not there, but infants of this age cannot imagine where they might be. No wonder these infants vigorously protest separation and anxiously track parents even into the bathroom. Not until they attain stage V object permanence (at 15 to 18 months of age) can children predict the position of an object from a series of unseen displacements. When this cognitive capacity emerges, children have the ability to infer parents' whereabouts in their absence, and separation protest diminishes.

The ability to deal simultaneously with several pieces of information develops at the same time children achieve stage IV object permanence. Stranger awareness results because children now can actively compare unfamiliar with familiar people. A 4-month-old infant smiles at any smiling adult. A 7- to 9-month-old child glances warily from parent to stranger to parent and howls. The child health professional can reduce parents' bewilderment at separation protest and stranger anxiety by explaining these behaviors as positive signs of normal cognitive development rather than as results of inexplicable emotional disturbance or indications that the child is "spoiled."

COMMUNICATION

Communication consists of speech and language and all the complex nonverbal and pragmatic pieces that complicate and enrich our lives and are present from the moment of birth. Speech is produced by precise coordinated muscle actions in the head, neck, chest, and abdomen. Language is the expression of human communication through which knowledge, belief, and behavior can be experienced, explained, and shared. Nonverbal communication includes smiles, body positions, tones, and points and gestures. This section focuses more on the development of language. Similar to other developmental phenomena, the infant's acquisition of language follows a predictable sequence. Infants communicate actively from birth. Lacking words, infants communicate through numerous sensory channels with three major purposes to their communication efforts: (1) to regulate another person's behavior, (2) to attract or maintain another person's attention for social interaction, (3) to draw joint attention to objects and events. In addition, communicating is inherently pleasurable.

Infants can acquire reciprocal language only through interaction with responsive sources. Television and radio have negligible effects on language learning in infants. Children's experiences with language cannot be separated from their experiences with interaction because parent-child talk is saturated with affect. Long before they begin using words, children begin learning about how families interact in their culture, what people are like, and who and how valued the children themselves are. This knowledge permeates the language system itself and influences children's motivation to learn and use words. Children who are sung to throughout the day often learn these "musical words" earlier because of the strong affect with which they are presented as well as the addition of melody. Parents and infants begin to construct the basis for later language acquisition long before infants can understand or produce a single word.

During the first year, through games and caregiving rituals, children learn to take turns communicating. With vocalization and nonverbal cues, caregivers and infants learn to direct each other's attention to interesting environmental events, to signal needs and feelings, and to interpret each other's intentions. During the second year of life, children begin to extend the rules of communication learned in action to the use of spoken words.

The actual production of meaningful communication is the result of cognitive, oral-motor, and social processes. Infant crying and parental response is the first communication of the new dyadic relationship (LaGasse et al, 2005). By 1 month of age, the infant has a range of cries that parents may associate with hunger, pain, and fatigue. Between 1 and 3 months of age, the infant develops a range of nondistress vocalizations, onomatopoietically described as "cooing." When the caregiver imitates the infant, the infant's production of sound is prolonged. The caregiver's contingent responses to these early vocalizations shape the infant's vocalization into conversation-like patterns. Adult speech elicits and reinforces infant communication (Bloom, 1977).

By 3 to 4 months of age, infants can produce repetition of all vowel sounds and some consonants, although some of these sounds are opportunistic. At least two distinct syllables are produced. As babbling matures, infants produce repetitive two-syllable combinations, such as mama and dada, although at this time these combinations have no symbolic reference.

The emergence of actual words, or sounds used as symbols, depends on the infant's attainment of rudimentary object permanence. Before a person or object can be named, it must have a stable existence in the infant's mind. Not surprisingly, the first true words usually refer to parents and other family members because the infant's concept of object permanence occurs for people before inanimate objects. Between 10 and 15 months of age, infants speak their first real words. During this time, infants also begin to use symbolic gestures, such as shaking the head to indicate no. "Jargoning"—long utterances that sound like statements or questions, but contain no real words—also occurs initially around the first birthday.

Receptive language ability precedes expressive ability during the toddler years. When asked to do so, children can point to pictures or objects before they can name them. Most 1-year-old infants respond to simple commands, such as "bye-bye" or "no-no," and most 15-month-old children can point to one or two body parts.

During the second and third years of life, expressive vocabulary expands exponentially. Infants have acquired a mean of 10 words by age 18 months and about 1000 words by age 3 years. At the same time, the child begins to construct two-word telegraphic sentences, first to comment on his or her own needs ("more cookie") and then to comment on events in the immediate environment ("mommy go"). By conversing with children and expanding statements ("mommy's going out"), caregivers help children to become generally competent speakers of their native language by the age of 5 years.

Clinical Implications

The rate and quality of the infant's progression through linguistic development can be more sensitive to caregiving practices than are other sensorimotor skills. Children who hear more language develop it more quickly (Bornstein et al, 1998). During physical examinations, clinicians can provide a model for talking to even the youngest infant. Clinicians should be able to differentiate between immaturity and pathologic conditions in children's language abilities. Pronunciation should not be a focus of concern for children younger than 3 years of age. At this age, children frequently make sound substitutions and omit final consonants. Parents should provide a model and not demand correct speech.

Clinicians must distinguish difficulties with speech (sound production) from difficulties with language (use of symbols). Ability to use symbols can be easily observed in children's representational and symbolic play. Receptive language skills are another indication of symbolic skill development. Isolated speech difficulties from either anatomic or neurologic abnormalities may be seen in children with normal symbolic skills (see Chapter 72). Such children often have difficulty with other oral-motor behaviors, such as eating or blowing kisses, or with other fine motor skills. If half a child's speech output is unintelligible by age 3 years, referral to a speech pathologist and audiologist for evaluation is appropriate.

True delay in acquisition of language constitutes a serious developmental dysfunction. An 18-month-old child who uses no single words other than mama or dada, a 24-month-old child without multiple real words, or a 30-month-old child without two-word phrases should undergo evaluation. Language delays of this magnitude do not result from spoiling or laziness, as parents sometimes suggest (e.g., "He never has to ask for anything"). Chapter 72 describes full evaluation and treatment of language impairments.

Literacy also may begin during infancy (McLane and McNamee, 1991). Through exposure to books, signs, and a world of readers, infants gradually become increasingly aware of the importance of written language. Infants use their keen powers of observation and their desire to imitate activity to learn about books and written language long before they can read and write. Sharing books with children can start interest at 6 months of age when infants may merely pat the faces in a picture book. Book sharing enhances parent-child relationships by establishing an enjoyable joint activity that persists through early childhood (Needlman et al, 2005).

PHYSICAL GROWTH

Caregivers must provide infants with nutrients to sustain the rapid growth of body and brain, which is greater during the first 2 years of life than at any other time after birth. An infant's own feeding behavior also affects the intake of adequate nutrition. At birth, an infant has a rooting reflex that helps in locating the nipple. An extrusion reflex pushes out solids to prevent ingestion of inappropriate foods. The infant's small, elongated mouth, combined with forward and backward movements of the tongue, squeeze the nipple so that milk is suckled.

Extrusion and rooting reflexes disappear after 4 months of age. By 3 months, as the mouth enlarges, neuromaturation of the cheek and tongue allows the infant to become progressively efficient at true sucking, which employs negative pressure to obtain milk from the nipple. By 6 to 8 months of age, infants begin chewing motions and are able to close their lips over the rim of a cup and drink. By 9 to 12 months of age, the development of the pincer grasp permits the child to eat finger foods. During the second year of life, infants acquire the ability to use a spoon and hold a cup or bottle. Parental concerns about messiness, decreased appetite, and selective tastes emerge at this time.

Infant nutrition affects concurrent and future growth patterns. Overfeeding and underfeeding can jeopardize the infant's later well-being. During this period of rapid growth, the brain is uniquely vulnerable to nutritional insult. Seventy percent of adult brain weight is attained by 2 years of age.

Although growth of the brain is the most critical organic achievement of infancy, most adult attention focuses on the rapid growth of the infant's body. For infants born at term between 2500 and 4000 g, birth weight should approximately double by 5 months of age, triple by 1 year of age, and quadruple by 2 years of age. Length at birth increases 50% in the first year of life and doubles by age 4 years. The rate of growth and consequent caloric requirement per unit of body weight decline gradually over the first 2 years of life. As caloric needs change during maturation, so does the infant's capacity to ingest and digest an increasing variety of foods.

Clinical Implications

Newborn boys are larger than newborn girls at birth, and they continue to grow at a faster rate during the first 3 to 6 months of life. After the first 6 months of life, there are no sex differences in infant growth rate. A severely decreased rate of weight gain in young children during the first 2 years of life should be investigated because it usually reflects inadequate nutrition or complicating illness, not immutable genetic potential.

The rate of increase in the length of a child during the first 2 years of life varies. Two thirds of normal infants cross percentile measurements (Smith, 1977). An infant's genotype for height is expressed by 2 years of age. A child's height can be evaluated, by means of standard charts, as a function of midparental height (Gohlke and Stanhope, 2002).

Premature infants should be evaluated according to their corrected age (current postnatal age minus the number of weeks the child was premature). A statistically significant difference in growth percentiles is found without such correction in head circumference until 18 months postnatal age, in weight until 24 months postnatal age, and in length until 40 months postnatal age (Brandt, 1979). Even after such correction, infants with very low birth weights (<1501 g) may remain smaller than infants born at term for at least the first 3 years of life (Casey et al, 1991). Although the field lacks clear guidelines, preterm infants born before 34 weeks generally should receive a premature formula until they are at least 2000 g, and then an enriched "post discharge formula," higher in calories and micronutrients per ounce than that designed for term infants. Enriched formulas are more expensive than term formula and may be difficult for economically stressed families to afford, unless the family receives a physician's prescription to Special Supplemental Nutrition for Women, Infants, and Children (WIC). Generally, these post-discharge formulas should be continued until 9 to 12 months corrected age or at least until the infant's weight for length is maintained above the 25th percentile (Nieman, 2006). Formerly premature children who show depressed weight-for-height progressively deviating from a channel parallel to the National Center for Health Statistics (NCHS) norms should be assessed for potentially correctable (and sometimes iatrogenic) causes of growth failure.

Small-for-gestational-age infants show unpredictable growth patterns, depending on the timing, severity, and cause of their intrauterine failure to grow. Infants who show growth acceleration in the first 6 months of life have the best prognosis for later outcome, whereas infants whose growth deviates downward from a previously established trajectory parallel to, if not on, the NCHS reference standards should be evaluated.

Neuromaturation, cognitive and social development, and temperament all influence feeding during infancy. Lethargic infants are difficult to feed. Management should focus on maintaining alertness. A hyperresponsive extrusion reflex (tongue thrusting) or dyskinetic tongue movements or both result in difficult and prolonged feeding, These responses warrant further evaluation and often referral to a feeding therapist (whether an occupational or speech therapist) because they are often associated with dysfunction of the central nervous system.

Anticipatory guidance at the 6- and 9-month visits should address potential feeding conflicts. Children's need for autonomy may result in their refusing food from parents. In this case, parents can present finger foods to facilitate independent feeding. Parents also should be warned that most children at this age explore by banging and dropping. Most parents do not mind when infants repetitively drop toys, but may become annoyed when food is dropped. Parents can be told that this behavior is not intentionally provocative, but reflects the child's need to practice new cognitive and motor abilities.

Some feeding problems need to be seen in the context of development and temperament because newly acquired skills can present difficulties. Parents should anticipate that new gross motor abilities will make eating less interesting to most toddlers. The clinician can help parents by pointing out the contribution of the child's temperament to feeding behavior. A child with a high activity level may have difficulty sitting long enough to complete a meal. Children who are distractible and nonpersistent also are unlikely to finish a meal. Children with a habitual withdrawal response are often unwilling to try unfamiliar foods. Children who respond intensely scream if forced to accept new foods. Toddlers who adapt slowly have a selective diet because they do not readily learn to like new foods. The clinician can work with parents to devise specific strategies for dealing with such feeding problems.

SUMMARY

An understanding of infant and toddler development and behavior provides a framework for child care during the first 2 years of life. To promote or assess a child's development, aspects of "nature" and "nurture" need to be identified and understood. Surveillance and referral about infant behavior has two goals: (1) to nurture the child's primary attachment and promote its development (internal security, self-control, and adaptive autonomy), while decreasing parent-child conflicts and increasing the parents' understanding and empathy for the child, and (2) to identify remediable disabilities and problems. This knowledge can be organized by a transactional model for child development, which stresses the contributions of the child and caregiver to developmental outcome. Usually, the child health professional is the only professional involved with families of young children, and he or she may be able to prevent unnecessary parental concerns or parent-child conflicts that can contribute to later behavior disturbances. When developmental delays, sensory deficits, or serious behavioral problems already exist, the clinician can minimize their long-term impact by early identification and appropriate management and referral and providing ongoing support to the family. Changing the delivery method of primary care to families may be necessary to make this change a reality (Bethell et al, 2004; Kuo et al, 2006; Zuckerman et al, 2004).

REFERENCES

Ainsworth MDS: Infant-mother attachment. Am Psychol 33:932, 1979.

American Association of Pediatric Dentistry: Available at:http://www.aapd.org/publications/brochures/content/tfphabits.html. Accessed October 6, 2006.

American Academy of Pediatrics Task Force on SIDS: The changing concept of SIDS: Diagnostic coding shifts, controversies regarding the sleeping environment, and new variables to consider in reducing risk. Pediatrics 116:1245-1255, 2005.

Barr RG, Hopkins B, Green JA (eds): Crying as a Sign, a Symptom, and a Signal: Clinical, Emotional, and Developmental Aspects of Infant and Toddler Crying. Clinics in Developmental Medicine No. 152. London: Mac Keith Press, 2000.

Bauer PJ: Constructing a past in infancy: A neuro-developmental account. Trends Cogn Sci 10:175-181, 2006.

Bell SM: The development of the concept of object as related to infant-mother attachment. Child Dev 41:291, 1970.

Bethell C, Reuland CH, Halfon N, Schor EL: Measuring the quality of preventive and developmental services for young children: National estimates and patterns of clinicians' performance. Pediatrics 113(6 Suppl):1973-1983, 2004.

Blass EM, Camp CA: The ontogeny of face recognition: Eye contact and sweet taste induce face preference in 9- and 12-week-old human infants. Dev Psychol 37:762-774, 2001.

Bloom K: Patterning of infant vocal behavior. J Child Psychol 23:367, 1977.

Bornstein MH, Sigman MD: Continuity in mental development from infancy. Child Dev 57:251, 1986.

Bornstein MH, Haynes MO, Painter KM: Sources of child vocabulary competence: A multivariate model. J Child Lang 25:367-393, 1998.

Brandt I: Growth dynamics of low birthweight infants with emphasis on the prenatal period. *In* Falkner F, Tanner J (eds): Human Growth, Neurobiology and Nutrition, New York. Plenum Press, 1979.

Brazelton TB: Crying in infancy. Pediatrics 29:579, 1962.

Bucher H, Moser T, von Siebenthal K, et al: Sucrose reduces pain reaction to heel lancing in preterm infants: A placebo controlled, randomized and masked study. Pediatr Res 38:332, 1995.

Casey PH, Kraemer HC, Bernbaum J, et al: Growth status and growth rates of a varied sample of low birth weight preterm infants: A longitudinal cohort from birth to three years of age. J Pediatr 119:559-605, 1991.

Collie R, Hayne H: Deferred imitation by 6- and 9-month-old infants: More evidence for declarative memory. Dev Psychobiol 35:83-90, 1999.

de Wolff M, van Ijzendoorn M: Sensitivity and attachment: A meta-analysis on parental antecedents of infant attachment. Child Dev 68:571-591, 1997.

Ferber R: Solve Your Child's Sleep Problems: New, Revised, and Expanded Edition. New York: Simon & Schuster, 2006.

Fireman L: Colic. Pediatr Rev 27:357-358, 2006.

Friman P: Concurrent habits. Am J Dis Child 144:1316, 1990.

Gaensbauer TJ, Sands K: Distorted affective communications in abused/neglected infants and their potential impact on caretakers. J Am Acad Child Psychiatry 18:236-250, 1979.

Garcia J, Wills L: Sleep disorders in children and teens: Helping patients and their families get some rest. Postgrad Med 107:161-178, 2000.

Gibson EJ, Walk RD: The "visual cliff." Sci Am 202:67-71, 1960.

Ginsberg H, Opper S: Piaget's Theory of Intellectual Development. Englewood Cliffs, NJ, Prentice-Hall, 1979.

Gohlke BC, Stanhope R: Final height in psychosocial short stature: Is there complete catch-up? Acta Paediatr 91:961-965, 2002.

Harwood RL, Schoelmerich A, Schulze PA, et al: Cultural differences in maternal beliefs and behaviors: A study of middle-class Anglo and Puerto Rican mother-infant pairs in four everyday situations. Child Dev 70:1005-1016, 1999.

Hobcraft J: The ABC of demographic behavior: How the interplays of alleles, brains, and contexts over the life course should shape research aimed at understanding population processes. Population Studies 60:153-187, 2006.

Kisilevsky BS, Hains SM, Lee K, et al: Effects of experience on fetal voice recognition. Psychol Sci 14:220-224, 2003.

Kuo AA, Inkelas M, Lotstein DS, et al: Rethinking well-child care in the United States: An international comparison. Pediatrics 118:1692-1702, 2006.

LaGasse LL, Neal AR, Lester BM: Assessment of infant cry: Acoustic cry analysis and parental perception. Ment Retard Dev Disabil Res Rev 11:83-93, 2005.

MacFarlane JA: Olfaction in the development of social preferences in the human neonate. *In* Parent-Infant Interactions. CIBA Foundation Symposium 33. New York, Elsevier, 1975, p 103.

Mahler M, Pine F, Bergman A: The Psychological Birth of the Human Infant. New York: Basic Books, 1975.

McLane JB, McNamee GD: Early Literacy. Cambridge, MA: Harvard University Press, 1991.

Mehler J, Bertoncini J, Barriere M: Infant recognition of mother's voice. Perception 7:491-497, 1978.

Meins E: Sensitivity, security and internal working models: Bridging the transmission gap. Attach Hum Dev 1:325-342, 1999.

Needlman R, Toker KH, Dreyer BP, et al: Effectiveness of a primary care intervention to support reading aloud: A multicenter evaluation. Ambul Pediatr 5:209-215, 2005.

Nieman L: Follow up nutrition after discharge from the neonatal intensive care unit. Building Block for Life 29:8, 2006.

Norcia AM, Tyler CW, Hamer RD: Development of contrast sensitivity in the human infant. Vision Res 30:1475-1486, 1990.

Pearson SR, Boyce TW: The vulnerable child. Pediatr Rev 25:345-349, 2004.

Rothbaum F, Rosen K, Ujiie T, Uchida N: Family systems theory, attachment theory, and culture. Family Process 41:328-350, 2002.

Rovee-Collier C, Hartshorn K, DiRubbo M: Long-term maintenance of infant memory. Dev Psychobiol 35:91-102, 1999.

Saffran JR, Loman MM, Robertson RR: Infant memory for musical experiences. Cognition 77:B15-B23, 2000.

Sagi A, van Ijzendoorn MH, Aviezer O, et al: Attachments in a Multiple-Caregiver and Multiple Infant Environment: The Case of the Israeli Kibbutzim. Monograph of the SRCD. Chicago: University of Chicago Press, 1995.

Sameroff AJ, Chandler MJ: Reproductive risk and the continuum of caretaking causality. Rev Child Dev Res 4:187-244, 1974.

Sheridan MK, Foley GM, Radlinski SH: Using the Supportive Play Model: Individualized Intervention in Early Childhood Practice. New York: Teachers College Press, 1995.

Siegel DJ, Hartzell M: Parenting from the Inside Out: How a Deeper Self-understanding Can Help You Raise Children Who Thrive. New York, Penguin Putnam, 2003.

Singer LM, Brodzinsky DM, Ramsay D, et al: Mother-infant attachment in adoptive families. Child Dev 56:1543-1551, 1985.

Skadberg BT, Markestad T: Behaviour and physiological responses during prone and supine sleep in early infancy. Arch Dis Child 76:320-324, 1997.

Smith DW: Growth and its Disorders. Philadelphia, WB Saunders, 1977.

Sroufe LA: The coherence of individual development: Early care, attachment, and subsequent developmental issues. Am Psychol 34:834, 1979.

Sroufe LA: The role of infant-caregiver attachment in development. *In* Belsky J, Nezworski T (eds): Clinical Implications of Attachment. New York: Erlbaum, 1988, p 18.

Twitchell T: The automatic grasping responses of infants. Neuropsychologia 3:247, 1965.

Vaish A, Striano T: Is visual reference necessary? Contributions of facial versus vocal cues in 12-month-olds' social referencing behavior. Dev Sci 7:261-269, 2004.

van Ijzendoorn MH: Adult attachment representations, parental responsiveness, and infant attachment: A meta-analysis on the predictive validity of the adult attachment interview. Psychol Bull 117:387, 1995.

Walker-Andrews AS: Emotions and social development: Infants' recognition of emotions in others. Pediatrics 102(5 Suppl E):1268-1271, 1998.

Wang Q, Leichtman MD, Davies KI: Sharing memories and telling stories: American and Chinese mothers and their 3-year-olds. Memory 8:159-177, 2000.

Waters E, Wippman J, Sroufe LA: Attachment, positive affect and competence in the peer group: Two studies in construct validation. Child Dev 50:821, 1979.

Zuckerman B, Parker S, Kaplan-Sanoff M, et al: Healthy Steps: A case study of innovation in pediatric practice. Pediatrics 114:820-826, 2004.

Zuckerman B, Zuckerman P, Siegel D: Promoting self-understanding in parents—for the great good of your patients. Contemp Pediatrics, April 1, 2005.

4 PRESCHOOL YEARS

Sara C. Hamel and Amanda Pelphrey

Vignette

Annie has recently turned 3 years old, and her parents have brought her for a well-child visit. They are concerned about her speech because they cannot understand some of the things that she says. Annie's parents further question whether she is ready for preschool, which will be starting in 2 months, because she seems "immature" for her age. Annie was adopted from China at age 21 months. She appeared healthy and well grown at that time, but had very little expressive language. She was evaluated by an international adoptions specialist after arriving in the United States and was deemed healthy. Her parents were reassured that she would "catch up" with her development, and she was speaking in English at age-appropriate levels within 6 months. Currently, Annie has age-appropriate gross motor coordination; feeds herself; likes to scribble; and loves playing with dolls, kitchen sets, stuffed animals, and doctor kits. She has just achieved consistent toilet use with only an occasional wetting episode, although she still wears Pull-ups at night. Annie speaks in full sentences, but has trouble with the pronunciation of *r* and *l* sounds. Sleep is marked by preferring to have someone stay with her when she falls asleep, and she wakes two or three times each night calling for her parents or visiting them in their bed. Annie can be clingy when she goes to her dance class and usually needs extra encouragement to participate. She also can be demanding, crying and whining when her wishes are not immediately honored.

Is Annie "immature" for her age? Should she go to preschool? What other advice or discussion might Annie's parents benefit from at the well-child visit?

MAJOR TASKS

This chapter covers the period between 2 years and 5 years, which is divided into two parts: (1) 2- to 3-year-old children (pre-preschoolers) and (2) 3- to 5-year-old children (more truly preschool).

The period between ages 2 and 3 also could be termed *late toddlerhood* and is a time when children are still consolidating the basic skills needed to participate optimally in a preschool setting. The hallmark of this age is the miraculously rapid development of functional language; improved gross motor coordination; refinement of basic fine motor skills for eating and manipulating objects; increased knowledge about concepts of shapes, colors, and daily routines; and social skills, such as sharing or saying "please" and "thank you." These skills are necessary for children to achieve a measure of functional autonomy or independence with respect to eating, drinking, playing, toileting, dressing, and getting along with others. This is an age of tremendous developmental growth and is usually accompanied by some degree of emotional reactivity as children strive to gain increasing self-control. Autonomy and self-control are the two most important psychological tasks of 2- to 3-year-old children, and they are occurring in conjunction with unprecedented development of language and cognition.

Preschoolers 3 to 5 years old should possess the basic skills of a functioning individual, including conversational language; gross and fine motor skills; and adaptive functioning, such as independent eating, sleeping, and toileting skills. With this solid foundation, the major tasks of the era involve understanding the larger world beyond one's family and home and interacting with people outside of the family in community venues, such as preschools, dance class, church, or the playground. Preschool-age children continue to refine issues of self-regulation and sense of self with an emerging understanding of others' perspectives and emotional reactions. Children of this age are delightfully enthusiastic about all they do and endlessly curious, imaginative, and creative. This is the time of life when children say the darnedest things and think that anything is possible. This is a time for total fun, playing doctor with the pets, dressing in fabulous clothes pretending to be a king or queen, and rejoicing in every new skill acquired. Exclamations such as, "I did it, mom! Clap your hands!" are examples of mastery that should be heard frequently during this age.

Under most circumstances, this is a joyful time for children and families, but specific risk factors have been identified for children and families that can affect development and behavior during the preschool years. This chapter discusses the basic developmental and behavioral achievements of the era, issues for families of preschool children, cultural and societal issues that affect children of this age, and key tasks for the primary health care clinician in supporting children of this age and their families.

DEVELOPMENTAL DOMAINS

Biophysical Maturation: Basis of Developmental Change

In recent years, great advances in neuroscience have contributed substantial new information to the understanding of brain development throughout childhood. We now know that the brain continues to establish neural networks well into adolescence. Most neurodevelopment occurs in the fetus, infancy, and early childhood periods, however. Brain development follows a biologically or genetically prescribed sequence for all humans and includes growth; differentiation and migration of cells; sprouting of new axons and formation of connections; refining synapses; and formation of supporting tissues, such as the glial cells and myelin (Aylward, 1997).

Although much of the influence of this process is under genetic control, there is increasing evidence primarily from animal studies of the significant impact of the environment on early brain development; the notion of nature versus nurture has been replaced by transactional and ecologic theories that seek to define the roles of nature and nurture working in tandem (see Chapter 8) (Shonkoff and Phillips, 2000). These researchers indicate evidence for the presence of sensitive periods for the development of specific systems in the brain, such as vision and language, which rely on specific kinds and amounts of environmental input to proceed normally. Additionally, there are increasing data on how environmental stressors can alter brain function. Most children live in environments that provide sufficient nurture and stimulation for optimal brain growth. Certain types of experiences, however, or lack of experiences, have been determined to represent significant risk for the developing brain (Table 4-1). Genetic risks include specific disorders or conditions that can be identified in the laboratory as discrete gene abnormalities or a strong family history of a developmental or behavioral disorder, with an as yet unidentified gene site or sites. Outcomes for all of these children can be significantly affected by providing early intervention in the form of enhanced stimulation and specific therapies.

In the toddler and preschool years, the development of various domains of skills occurs simultaneously and reciprocally, with the domains influencing each other. Language function may significantly contribute to cognitive development and vice versa. Similarly, the attainment of motor control allows a child to gain an increasing sense of mastery of the environment, which is a key influence on self-esteem and self-regulation. Wide individual differences also are observed in the sequence of developmental achievement, and this is likely the result of the interface of the individuals' unique biologic or genetic predispositions interacting with environmental events and conditions unique to an individual child.

In the case example of Annie (see vignette), having lived the first 21 months of life in an orphanage would represent a considerable risk factor for the emergence of developmental or behavioral differences. Since her adoption, however, she has been living in an environment that has provided optimal stimulation from her parents and caregivers. Data from long-term studies of various at-risk infants, such as children from orphanages, have shown that the more optimal the environment of the child, the greater the developmental gains (Rutter and the English and Romanian Adoptees Study Team, 1998). The fact of Annie's adoption makes it more likely, however, that her parents view her as vulnerable, and they may be more likely to interpret any behavior as something that warrants concern or that indicates immaturity. In displaying increased protectiveness of her, they also may be more likely to give in to Annie's desire to sleep with them or offer her increased reassurance. Ideally, such parental attributes or responses could be explored during well care visits, and a useful discussion might ensue regarding how to help Annie and her parents overcome the sense of vulnerability for her because she is actually doing quite well.

Table 4-1. Environmental Risk Factors and the Developing Brain

Neonatal exposure to psychoactive drugs (tobacco, alcohol, cocaine)
Lead
Malnourishment
Chemical exposure

Motor Development

Gross motor skills at age 2 years should allow a child to walk with good balance and fluidity, turn, pivot, and run. Table 4-2 summarizes development in this domain. A 2-year-old would be tentative on stairs, able to go up better than down, initially using two feet together on each stair. Children at this age also are beginning to climb with better balance. By age 3 years, children can negotiate stairs, going up and down with alternating feet, and can ride a tricycle, run, jump, climb, and slide with little likelihood of falling (Fig. 4-1). They are capable of relatively independent motor functioning in a playground situation. Between 3 and 5 years, most children learn how to hop and skip and can learn more complex gross motor skills, such as roller skating, dancing, riding a two-wheeler, and pumping their feet to swing.

There is wide variation in how children display balance, coordination, and overall quality of movement, some of which is due to familial genetic factors. Some variation may be influenced by environmental factors, such as how much children have the opportunity to practice and perform. Generally, all children advance in these areas during the preschool years, so any loss of balance, coordination, or gross motor skills during this age would constitute a significant abnormality in need of assessment by a physician.

With regard to fine motor skills, 2- to 3-year-olds can use their hands for holding utensils and feeding themselves, and they gain dexterity throughout the year. Additionally, most children master downward zipping and taking shoes and socks off first, stacking blocks,

Table 4-2. **Motor Milestones for Preschoolers**

2 Years Old	3 Years Old	4 Years Old
Drinks from a straw	Feeds self with spilling	Feeds self, uses fork
Feeds self with a spoon	Opens doors	Holds pencil; tries to write
Helps in washing hands	Holds glass with one hand	Draws circle, face
Puts arms in sleeves with help	Holds crayon well	Cuts with small scissors
Builds a tower of 3-4 blocks	Throws a ball overhead	Brushes teeth with help
Tosses or rolls a large ball	Dresses self with help	Unbuttons
Opens cabinets, drawers, boxes	Uses toilet with help	Uses toilet alone
Walks up steps with help	Alternates feet on steps	Tries to skip
Takes steps backwards	Jumps with both feet	Catches a bouncing ball
	Kicks ball forward	Swings
	Pedals tricycle	

Reprinted with permission from the National Network for Child Care—NNCC: Powell J, Smith CA: The first year. *In* Developmental Milestones: A Guide for Parents. Manhattan, KS: Kansas State University Cooperative Extension Service, 1994.

fitting simple shapes into puzzles, and dressing dolls. A 2-year-old may be able to imitate a line or scribble a crude circle. Between 3 and 5 years, rapid advancement is made in drawing and copying skills, with a 3-year-old capable of copying a simple circle, a 4-year-old capable of copying a square, and a 5-year-old capable of printing the letters of her or his name. During this time, a child progresses in ability to draw a picture by adding details to the figure drawing. Use of scissors to cut simple shapes also begins at 3 years and is much refined by 5 years.

These advancing skills are necessary for mastery of many preschool craft activities and are the precursors for handwriting skills. Children having difficulty in these areas may refuse to participate in a craft, or may display avoidance behavior or defiance during the activity. It is important to recognize fine motor problems and provide appropriate referrals for evaluation and treatment by occupational therapists or educators to advance a child's skill set during the preschool years. Primary care clinicians should routinely screen fine and gross motor milestones in preschoolers at well-child visits (see Table 4-2).

Social and Emotional Development

Young preschoolers (2 to 3 years old) experience an array of intense emotions, but are not consistently able to regulate these experiences, often resulting in impulsive reactions. As a result, parents often express concern about their children's increasing behavioral "acting out" (e.g., tantrum behaviors) or emotional sensitivity (e.g., frequent tearfulness). Emotions in toddlers and older preschoolers are short-lived, but can be intense. This is a time that may include typical fears (e.g., the dark, separation, dogs), but also a time of increased self-confidence, establishment of love attachments possibly to comfort objects (e.g., blanket, teddy bear), and development of empathic awareness. During the preschool years, much advancement is made in emotional regulation, and most children are successfully able to implement basic, but effective, strategies for coping by the end of the preschool years.

Psychosocial development is characterized by a unique combination of increased individuation and independence with increased social reciprocity and

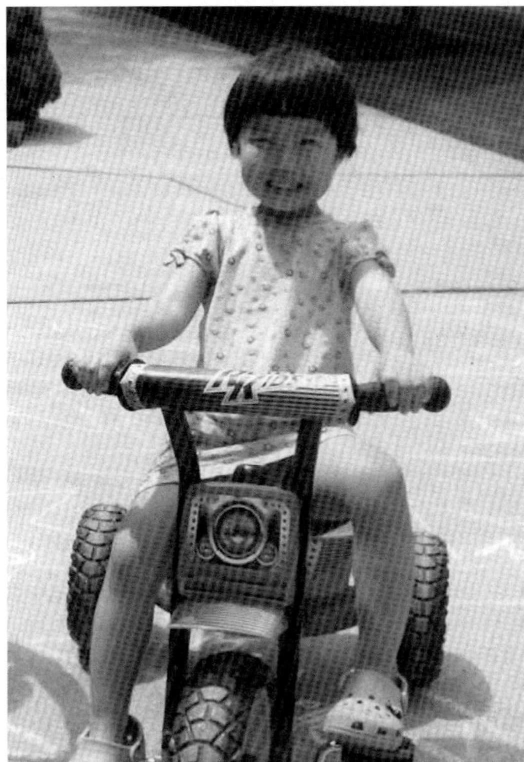

Figure 4-1. Three-year-old girl demonstrating mastery of riding the tricycle.

awareness of self in relation to others. This developmental period involves increased initiative in approaching new tasks and experiences, and preschoolers are proud of their accomplishments and actively seek approval from caregivers (Fig. 4-2). At the same time, there may be increasing awareness and heightened sensitivity to self-perceptions of failing. The degree of resolution of this internal conflict influences development of self-concept and aspects of personality.

The emerging self is deeply rooted within the sociocultural context, including interactions with family and community environments. During the preschool years, children become well identified with their specific gender roles as a result of interacting biologic and sociocultural experiences. As with learning of aggression

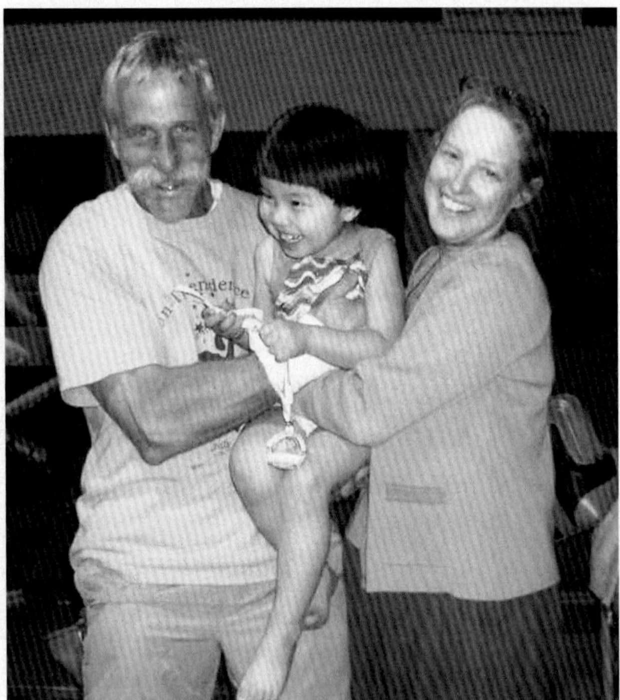

Figure 4-2. A preschooler seeks active approval and affection from her proud parents.

or fear, observational learning influences acquisition of expectations for gender-specific behaviors. Gender differences are seen in preschool play patterns, including choice of toys, group play behavior, and gender-specific language, which all are integrated in emerging self-identity (Weintraub et al, 1984). At this time, children become increasingly aware of physical attributes of others and of self as young as age 3 years, and by age 5 would have a clear understanding of why some people look alike or not. For adoptive families, as with Annie, particularly where children are from other countries and may have a dramatically different physical appearance, explanations to the child about this phenomenon are very important, as is an explanation about the adoption concept in general.

Cognitive Development

During the first 2 years of life, children rely heavily on sensorimotor functioning for learning acquisition, by manipulating objects, studying them, putting them in their mouths, and beginning to experiment with objects and developing simple concepts. Cognitive development during the preschool period is characterized by less reliance on direct sensory experience of the world, however, and movement toward cognition governed by principles based on symbolic thought. Although children at this time have not yet acquired skills for concrete reasoning, cognition in preschoolers begins to include emergence of categorization in efforts toward building causal reasoning skills characteristic of school-age thinking.

Often referred to as the preoperational stage of development, children at this age rely heavily on their own growing personal perspective of reality to make sense of events and relationships. They have a markedly difficult time taking the perspective of others or even anticipating consequences of their behaviors, displaying difficulty holding multiple rules, remembering sequences, and delaying gratification (Diamond et al, 2002). This tendency toward egocentrism is readily seen in play with peers and in language patterns of preschoolers, who take turns reciprocally, but do not seem to grasp or necessarily build on the thoughts of others in play or conversations.

Children at this stage do not yet display ability for rational thought operations. One way they make sense of and assimilate new information is by reliance on appearance of physical characteristics and associated assumptions. For these reasons, bigger toys are better toys.

Socialized gender awareness begins to solidify at this time in development, a function of their experiences in the world and their improved cognitive functioning. Children rely on assumptions they have about what boys and girls should and should not do in processing information based on visible appearance. Similarly, reality often is confused with fantasy or pretend. When asked, "What do you want to be when you grow up," 3- or 4-year-olds may say, "a princess" or "a superhero." Their vivid imagination encourages creativity, identity development, and fears. Shadows on the bedroom wall readily are interpreted as monsters despite parents' insistence that monsters do not exist.

Sociocultural norms are integrated into learning experiences, and children at this age readily participate in joint learning activities, relying on imitation, social support, and guidance for advancements in skills sets. When presented with a new or complex task, preschool children learn best if provided structure; assistance in breaking tasks into smaller, more attainable pieces; and ample encouragement and praise. These strategies parallel theories on guided participation in cognitive development, suggesting that children develop scripts or schemas for how given experiences should proceed, which they apply to similar situations in the future (Wood and Wood, 1996).

Play Development

One of the most important advancements during the preschool years is the development of meaningful, creative, and interactive play. Play is the activity in which children practice new skills in cognition and motor development, and in the process negotiate social relationships and explore emerging characteristics of self-identity. Infant play is characterized primarily by object exploration and manipulation and serves to allow the child to discover basic cause-and-effect relationships and relationships between themselves and objects in the world. Preschool play represents emergence of pretend play skills, such as using a block as a telephone, or having a tea party with parents, or playing the piano (Fig. 4-3). Through observational learning, preschoolers rehearse gender role behaviors, such as sweeping, washing pretend dishes, and feeding baby dolls for girls, and using tools, driving construction vehicles, or mowing the grass for boys. Older preschoolers enjoy dressing up as imaginary characters, such as princesses or cartoon characters, as well as in their parents' clothes. In the world of

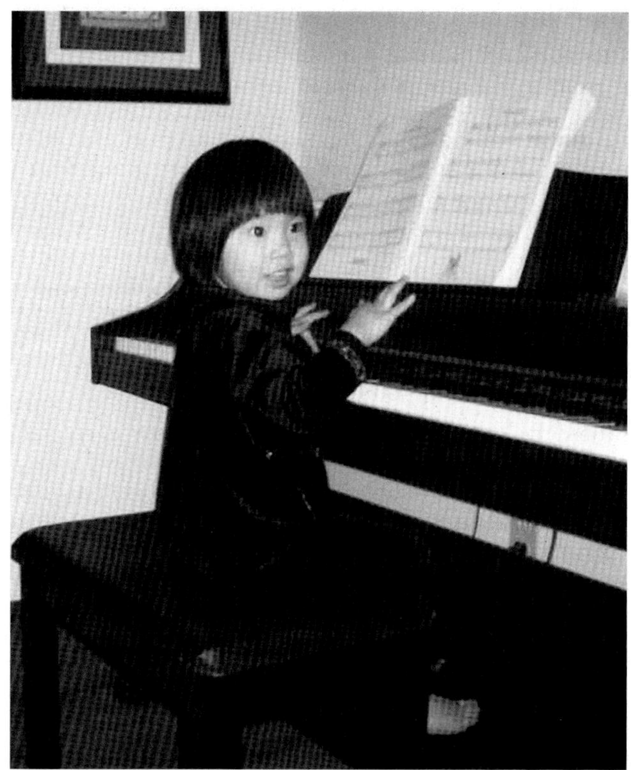

Figure 4-3. A three-year-old pretends to be a concert pianist.

pretend play, preschoolers practice gender-specific behaviors encouraged by their sociocultural environment.

Two-year-olds are known for resistance or indifference toward interactive or cooperative play, generally maintaining parallel play with others. They tolerate or even welcome the presence of other children next to them, but generally do not play cooperatively. Increased social reciprocity emerges by age 3 and becomes increasingly refined during the preschool years. Skills in sharing, turn taking, and cooperation improve markedly by the start of the school years, and meaningful and reciprocal peer relationships are established. Encouraging parents to engage in daily interactive and creative play with their children and encouraging them to schedule frequent play dates with same-age peers help ensure development of play skills progresses smoothly for their preschooler.

Language Development

At 24 months old, children have a basic expressive vocabulary of at least 50 words, mostly nouns and verbs, and they begin to make combinations with these words, such as "ride car," "mama up," and "see baby." Two-year-olds also should be masters of nonverbal communication, regularly pointing and often mimicking other commonly seen instrumental and descriptive gestures in their environment. Shortly after age 2, children start to form short sentences, stringing more and more words together and playing with phrases, particularly noun phrases, such as "the dirty car" or "mama's green hat." They also frequently mimic common household phrases, such as "Oh, my goodness!" or "I knew it!" which they exclaim with the same degree of enthusiasm as the original speaker. Gestures and facial expressions accompany much of this new language, usually to the delight of their audience. As children advance from age 2 to 3, the length of sentences increases, and expressive vocabulary increases very rapidly (Table 4-3). It is easiest to remember that 2-year-olds have two-word combinations, and 3-year-olds have three-word combinations; however, this general rule may underestimate the actual fluency and mastery of speech of preschoolers.

Preschool children should be fully conversational (i.e., able to answer and ask questions) by age 3. The hallmark of this stage is the repetitive use of "Wh" questions (what, who, when, and why) to learn about the world and how it works. Accompanying this insatiability for questioning is a rapidly progressing ability to tell a story or to relate what has happened. A 2-year-old may answer the question, "How was your day?" by saying "Go park. See Leila," whereas a 5-year-old should be able to describe in detail several activities that he or she participated in during kindergarten. Children seem to acquire grammatical correctness naturally as they learn to talk—they seem to know the correct sequences or syntax of sentences (Gropen et al, 1991).

Articulation is typically incomplete for 2-year-olds, in whom speech is commonly characterized by various sound deletions or substitutions, but improves rapidly along with length of sentences during the preschool years. Typical developmental articulation errors at 2 years of age include substituting one consonant for another. A common sound substitution is *t* for *c*, where "kitty cat" becomes "titty tat." The most difficult consonants to pronounce are *l* and *r*, with many children still having difficulty at age 5. Dysfluency also is fairly common for 3- to 5-year-old children, usually lasting only a few months before resolving spontaneously. It is differentiated from stuttering by a preponderance of repetitions of whole words and phrases, rather than sounds and syllables (see Chapter 72).

Receptive language skills involve ability to process spoken language and concept formation. At 2 years of age, most children understand two-step commands, such as "Go in the kitchen and get your shoes." They also can follow sequences, such as "First, we'll have lunch; then you can take a nap," and they can comprehend consequences, such as "You must sit on that chair because you hit that boy." As children enter the years between 3 and 5, they are able to understand longer explanations of how things function as well as answers to those dreaded "Wh" questions.

Moral Development

Through social learning and imitation as well as from rewards and consequences during the preschool period, a foundation emerges for establishing norms and values regarding concepts of right versus wrong, empathic awareness of others, and altruism or helping of others. The balance for any individual child is the result of a complex interaction of the child's capacities and the family's teaching approach. There is a unique interaction between elements of cognitive development and psychosocial development with establishment of

Table 4-3. Speech and Language Milestones for Preschoolers

2 Years Old	3 Years Old	4 Years Old
Uses 2-3 word sentences	Uses 3-5 word sentences	Has large vocabulary
Inquires about objects	Asks short questions	Uses good grammar often
Imitates parents	Uses plurals	Uses articles (a, the, an)
Refers to self by name	Repeats simple rhymes	Uses past tenses of verbs
Verbalizes desires and feelings	Knows first and last name	Asks why and how
Points to eyes, ears, nose	Understands pronouns	Relates personal experience
	Knows gender for self	Understands spatial concept

Reprinted with permission from the National Network for Child Care—NNCC: Powell J, Smith CA: The first year. *In* Developmental Milestones: A Guide for Parents. Manhattan, KS: Kansas State University Cooperative Extension Service, 1994.

moral reasoning skills, often depicted in how children approach and resolve daily dilemmas. By 2 years of age, children show an understanding of basic behavior rules (i.e., good versus bad), and by 4 years of age, children display a basic understanding of motives behind other people's behaviors or reasons for behavior rules (i.e., you do not hit others because it will hurt them). Also by 4 years, children begin to use judgments of fairness or justness; although often egocentric in perspective, they display emerging awareness of emotional reactions of others, such as questioning why a baby might be crying and making some efforts to help.

PSYCHOSOCIAL CONTEXT OF PRESCHOOL DEVELOPMENT

Child development occurs within the context of the micro and macro social systems. Early childhood is a time when children often experience an initial shift from being fully embedded within the family system to participation in external community systems. Influences from family and community contexts provide opportunity for developmentally enriching experiences and possibly anxiety-provoking stressors, such as separation anxiety, parental divorce, or the birth of a new sibling.

Family Systems

The developmental trajectory during the preschool years is determined by a combination of internal biologic influences with environmental influences. The family context and parenting in particular have a major influence on preschoolers' emotional and behavioral functioning. Preschoolers learn the norms of their family's way of communicating thoughts and feelings and the individual roles each member plays in the family. Parenting styles may differ with respect to degree of nurturance and discipline. Classic theories classify parenting styles as "authoritarian," which is characterized by high demands and low nurturance; "permissive," which is characterized by low demands and high nurturance; or "authoritative," which is characterized by firm but democratic style combined with high nurturance (Baumrind, 1966). Optimal child outcomes are generally associated with an authoritative approach, where parents provide warmth and support to their children and allow children to have input in the decision making process, although parents optimally have the final say. Expectations and consequences for children's behaviors should be clear, fair, and consistent across caregivers and across situations.

Although family support is a protective factor against psychosocial problems, changes in the family system also may be a source of psychological distress for the preschooler. During the preschool years, children may experience the arrival of a sibling, which may arouse feelings of jealousy, displacement, or rejection. Additionally, parental separation or divorce may be associated with deleterious psychological or behavioral consequences. The research on postdivorce outcomes on emotional and behavioral functioning is unclear. Nearly 1 million children each day are affected by parental divorce. The 2005 U.S. Census Bureau reports that only 33.9% of preschool children age 5 years and younger live in a married couple family household. Amato (2000) summarized the negative consequences of divorce on children to include decreased academic achievement, increased conduct problems, psychological maladjustment, and compromised self-concept and social competence, although numerous protective factors also were identified, including coping skills, family support, and therapy. The degree to which children experience the emotional content of the conflict between their parents, whether they are married or divorced, seems to be primary contributor to psychosocial distress.

Preschool and Daycare

There is an increasing trend for children to participate in preschool programs, which may be associated with positive developmental outcomes and successful adjustment to major life transitions. This is particularly true for at-risk children. With the increase of children's participation in formal preschool and daycare programs, children at this age are often faced with the anxiety-provoking task of separating from their parents. Separation anxiety issues may be exacerbated if enrollment in a school or daycare co-occurs with the primary caregiver beginning a new job. Research has long documented benefits of increased social competence for children participating in structured preschool, however (Peisner-Feinberg et al, 2001). The NICHD Child Care Study followed more than 1300 children from 10 different sites nationally and looked at developmental and behavioral outcomes of children in relation to types and duration of childcare. The study's main conclusions were that the quality of home and childcare environments is important for optimal child outcomes. High-quality childcare environments had low adult-to-child ratios, had caregivers with higher levels of education, and provided stimulating and structured environments (NICHD Study of Early Child Care and Youth Development).

Of particular interest at this time is the increasing participation in Project Head Start, which provides comprehensive preschool programming for disadvantaged children. Project Head Start provides a structured setting for enrichment in early learning skills acquisition similar to other traditional preschool programs. Head Start is unique, however, in the support also provided for physical health, social-emotional development, and family education outreach, providing such services as nutrition education and developmental and health screens. Research has found that improvement of general and mental health in preschoolers is associated with high academic achievement (Spernak et al, 2006) as studied in children previously enrolled in Head Start. Other research has suggested a decline in initially measured gains in the Head Start population, however, with few differences found in long-term comparison between Head Start and non–Head Start preschoolers (Lee et al, 1990).

Psychosocial Stressors

The preschool years are a time of vast developmental growth, but they also may be a time marked by challenges and risk factors affecting physical, cognitive, and psychosocial developmental trajectories. One such factor is poverty. In 2000, 16% of children in the United States lived in poverty, and this number increased to 39% for children living in mother-only households (Lugaila and Overturf, 2004). The effects of poverty on the developing child span across global domains of functioning, including physical health, cognitive development, language development, and academic achievement.

There is a positive correlation for rates of poverty and rates of child abuse or maltreatment. Additionally, children living in poverty are more likely than children living above the poverty line to experience lead poisoning, low birth weight, hospitalization, growth retardation owing to nutritional deficiency, developmental delay and learning disability, grade retention, and eventual school drop out (Duncan et al, 1998). These effects may be particularly evident for preschoolers. These researchers found that preschool-age and early school–age children living in poverty have lower rates of school completion than children who experience onset of poverty in later years.

CLINICAL IMPLICATIONS: THE ROLE OF PRIMARY CARE

From a developmental-behavioral pediatrics perspective, the most important tasks for the primary health care provider include screening for significant developmental and behavioral problems, supporting parents with information on typical child development and behavior, and providing anticipatory guidance on issues with regulation. Actively monitoring developmental progress is essential in providing accurate parenting advice and is essential in early detection of developmental or behavioral pathology.

Developmental and Behavioral Screening

Clinicians in primary care often use informal techniques to decide if children are experiencing developmental delays or behavioral problems significant enough to warrant referral, relying on clinical judgment of whether a child has reached certain milestones, or whether a behavior may be abnormal. These informal assessments are generally weak in reliability and validity and often lead to under-referral of children who are experiencing significant difficulty. The task of identifying delays becomes more challenging as the children enter the preschool years because cognitive and language milestones are more difficult to assess in casual interactions with preschoolers than were motor milestones with infants. The use of standardized screening instruments for detection of developmental delays or behavioral abnormalities is highly recommended.

Screening for Developmental Delay

The American Academy of Pediatrics recommends that screening for developmental delay should occur at least three times at well-care visits for children between infancy and age 3 years. The current literature documents limited sensitivity and specificity of the various tools often used in the primary care setting for identifying developmental delays (Glascoe, 2005), and a survey reported that nearly half of all preschoolers had ever received a single developmental assessment (Halfon et al, 2004). Barriers to screening include time, knowledge of the use of a particular screen, reimbursement, and a clear understanding of the importance of early identification and intervention. The most likely areas of developmental concern to be identified in the preschool age group are delays in expressive or receptive language skills, fine motor or gross motor coordination skills, and rate of acquisition of early learning concepts.

The clinician should give special consideration to children in at-risk groups who may have subtle undetected problems, such as premature infants or children whose parents have learning disabilities (Aylward, 1997). Although the primary care physician can use information from common red flags often associated with developmental delay, accuracy of evaluation of developmental progression improves with use of standardized assessment tools with proven validity and reliability. Assessment tools should cover global domains of communication, gross and fine motor skills, problem solving, and personal-social skills development. Information obtained from such tools can be used to document and monitor developmental progress and to guide clinical decision making for further evaluation and intervention if needed. Glascoe (2005) provides a thorough summary of suggested tools for screening developmental and behavioral problems in the primary care setting, including the Ages and Stages Questionnaires and the Parents Evaluation of Developmental Status.

The clinician may wish to consult websites that provide up-to-date information about screening instruments or recommendations for parent consultation (Table 4-4). Additionally, in most communities, Early Intervention programs are in place and available to assess

Table 4-4. Primary Care Physician Resources for Screening and Consultation*

American Academy of Pediatrics	www.aap.org
Developmental Behavioral Pediatrics Online	www.dbpeds.org
Bright Futures (Georgetown University)	www.brightfuture.org
First Signs	www.firstsigns.org
Centers for Disease Control and Prevention	www.cdc.gov
National Network for Child Care	www.nncc.org

*The websites provide useful resources for developmental milestones, screening tools, and parent handouts.

children from birth to 5 years of age for free. Primary care clinicians who have no ability to offer their own screening or who want a secondary screening method are advised to become familiar with the contact information for Early Intervention and mention to families that their services are home or community based, making them very accessible, and they are of no or low cost to all families.

Behavioral Screening

Standardized instruments also are available for assessing the degree of abnormality of a child's behavior and are recommended over the use of informal clinical judgment. Instruments that can be used as routine screens include the Ages and Stages SE, the Pediatric Symptom Checklist, and the Child Behavior Checklist. It is especially important to perform an assessment or provide a referral for any child for whom the parent voices a concern about a behavior problem.

Parent Support and Guidance

Parent support and anticipatory guidance around developmental and behavioral issues, even for children who have no indicators of delays or significant dysfunction, are a major focus of the primary care visit. In several studies, parents have indicated that they want advice about how to promote their child's development, and they want behavioral advice. Additionally, parents often have questions about what they should expect of their child at a particular age. With regard to promotion of optimal behavioral health for typically developing preschoolers, the task is to achieve good behavioral regulation, which parents can promote by establishing guidelines or rules of behavior and enforcing them consistently. A step-by-step approach to promote optimal parenting would include a discussion of (1) setting up a good environment with clear expectations and good modeling, (2) education of what is desirable behavior, (3) identification and rewards for desirable behavior, (4) negative reinforcement for undesirable behavior, and (5) punishment.

1. Setting up a good environment for preschoolers: Structuring a home environment in a way that promotes exploration of toys, books, and music, and encourages talk with others and discussion of actions and feelings is ideal. Having a relatively set mealtime and bedtime also provides an environment that minimizes stress for a young child.
2. Education of what is desirable behavior: Preschoolers do best if they know what is going to happen next for them, and parents talk them through confusing or difficult situations. Parents need to use simple, clear language to explain what they want preschoolers to do, and they may have to go over the information several times before the child has absorbed the information. Having the child repeat back to the parent what he or she heard also is a good strategy. Examples include saying, "After we eat, you can go sit on your potty and I'll read you a book. If you make a poop, you can get a big sticker on your chart. What can happen if you make a poop on your potty?" Parents and siblings who model desired behavior for preschoolers are a very powerful influence because preschoolers generally watch everything that goes on in a household to determine how they should behave.
3. Rewards for desirable behavior: For preschool children, the rewards should be given immediately because their concept of time is poor. A preschooler prefers something tangible—a hug, kiss, sticker, or small prize of some other nature—and it is reinforcing to discuss several times why a reward was given and what a good job was done. Provision of frequent rewards keeps the child motivated to perform the desired behavior until it becomes routine. Usually at that point, the rewards can be phased out without any complaint from the child because performing the behavior has become rewarding in and of itself. This is important to explain to parents, who often worry that they will need to continue rewarding their child for every good behavior he or she performs well into the future.
4. Negative reinforcements: These strategies include the use of time out, where a child is removed from a situation with the goal of decreasing unwanted behavior, or taking away a privilege. These can be quite powerful and should be reserved for that kind of use.
5. Punishment: Although punishment strategies may be effective in changing undesirable behaviors under particular circumstances, reinforcement strategies are often preferred because of harmful consequences associated with physical punishment. Research has shown that spanking often leads to increased fear, anxiety, and aggression, and is not any more powerful than the above-mentioned strategies. Spanking is not recommended.

The challenge is for parents to maintain consistency with regard to monitoring the child's behavior and providing immediate and appropriate consequences, whether positive or negative, and the difficulty is that the need to respond to children of this age is frequent and intense. Children of this age can wear parents out to the point where they give up trying to maintain consistency and give up dealing with difficult behaviors. Primary caregivers can empathize with parents regarding the work they are doing and provide support for their continued efforts.

Regulatory Issues

Parents of preschoolers often seek advice about regulatory issues such as toilet training, sleeping, or eating. Parenting children of this age requires patience, understanding, constant communication, and reinforcement. Power struggles must be avoided. Because the clinician has only 10 to 15 minutes in a typical well-child visit, written advice for parents is highly recommended. Parenting books also are plentiful, and the clinician is advised to stay up-to-date on what parents are reading.

Toileting

Most children indicate readiness for toileting between the ages of 18 and 24 months, and complete toilet training is generally accomplished by 3 years for typically developing children, although boys may be a bit slower than girls in being completely toilet trained by 3 years. Readiness first includes an interest in sitting on the toilet. Secondary readiness signs are dislike of being soiled or wet, ability to get to the toilet and pull down pants and underwear, and having a word for urination and stooling. The use of a child-sized model is a recommended approach to minimize fearfulness and to allow the child to plant his or her feet on the ground to facilitate the Valsalva maneuver, although some children may be willing to sit on an adult-sized toilet with a stool for their feet. Children of this age cannot be expected to understand their internal signaling system and consistently indicate their need to go to the bathroom, although this skill does come in time. Parents must first help to set a typical toileting schedule, such as once every hour or within the first hour after eating or drinking, when elimination typically occurs. The first step is to become familiar with the toilet itself and with the expectations of toilet use. Parents should cue children to sit and try to eliminate in the toilet and should reward children for their cooperation, including just sitting.

Toileting problems at this age are most commonly characterized by behavioral struggles between parent and child. If minimal progress in toilet training has occurred by age 3 years, however, further evaluation and intervention may be warranted. Diagnostically, enuresis is not technically an appropriate diagnosis until children reach 5 years of age or older, given wetting accidents are developmentally common occurrences for preschoolers. Preschool children who experience complications with bowel movements may warrant clinical attention. Children often withhold bowel movements at this age, even when they are fairly well toilet trained, and the development of constipation is of concern. Often adding a laxative and using it regularly for some period of time resolves the situation. Encopresis may be a diagnostic consideration in children at least 4 years or older who display repeated overflow incontinence either with or without constipation.

Sleeping

Most preschool-age children have developed regulated sleep patterns, displaying the ability to fall asleep on their own and sleep uninterrupted throughout the night. Although it is common for preschoolers to display problems with nightmares, night terrors, sleepwalking, or sleep talking, generally these occurrences are infrequent, not functionally impairing, and not representative of a sleep disorder. Most sleep concerns in children in this age group are behavioral in nature, specifically bedtime avoidance, which may be a symptom of a more global issue with compliance or power struggles between parents and preschoolers. The clinician's role is often guidance on establishing a consistent sleep schedule and implementation of a structured behavior plan regarding bedtime routine. Many parenting books and websites provide strategies to combat bedtime behavior problems. Ferber's (1985) book for the lay public is extremely popular and offers support and guidance for many sleep difficulties. In the event of increased nighttime fears or anxiety in preschoolers (e.g., the dark or monsters), usually gentle reassurance from parents is all that is needed to prevent an escalation in sleep problems. Creating circumstances for children when they fall off to sleep initially that can be replicated if they awaken in the night increases the likelihood that toddlers and preschoolers can fall back to sleep after nighttime awakening without requiring parental assistance.

Eating and Diet

Preschoolers often become pickier in their diet habits than they were when they were younger. One reason for this change in eating behavior is that their rate of growth slows dramatically, and they require less food. Another reason is a result of socialization and their emerging sense of self, exaggerating their need to assert their right to choose. Parents should offer a variety of foods, not make a special meal for the picky child, and establish rules about healthy foods versus junk or desserts. Providing structure in the form of regular mealtimes also is helpful because it avoids the child's desire to eat only snacks. As is seen across all other age groups, preschoolers too are becoming accustomed to a more sedentary lifestyle, which has increasing public health concerns. With the current increase in the prevalence of childhood obesity, parents should proactively incorporate physical activity into each day, such as walking, dancing to music, visiting a playground, or riding a tricycle. It is generally recommended that preschoolers get at least an hour daily of active play provided at home and in preschool programs.

Advising on Kindergarten Readiness

With the large percentage of preschool children attending a formal preschool program, most parents now receive guidance about kindergarten readiness directly from the preschool personnel. So-called kindergarten readiness assessments include preacademic or academic skills, motor abilities, and language development. Other important predictors of success in school include the child's attentional and social abilities and self-regulation (see Chapter 46). These domains are more difficult to assess in a quick screening than preacademic and motor abilities. There also is increased attention to safety concerns, such as stranger and danger awareness, and encouragement that the child knows his or her telephone number and address as a part of kindergarten preparedness.

Table 4-5. **Red Flags for Autism Spectrum Disorders**

Language/Communication	Social Development	Atypical Behaviors
Delayed speech milestones	Limited eye contact	Preoccupation with interests
Limited expression of needs	Lack of initiating play	Sensory-oriented play
Lack of sustaining conversation	Lack of interest in peers	Stereotyped movements
Stereotyped speech or echolalia	Limited empathy	Fixed routines or rituals
Limited nonverbal communication	Not seeking others for shared enjoyment	Insistence on sameness
	Primarily independent or parallel play	

Children are entering kindergartens at later ages with more preschools handling early academic skills, such as letter and number identification.

Children previously identified with developmental delays who have been attending early intervention preschools or programs (see Chapter 92) must now transition into elementary school programs, and their services may or may not need to be continued (see Chapter 93). In most states, a transition assessment of the child is completed by the school district, and parents meet with school providers to discuss the best placement for their children (see Chapter 93).

DEVELOPMENTAL AND BEHAVIORAL PATHOLOGY

There is a wide range of normal development and behavior in this age range. It is often difficult to differentiate extremes of normal from clinical conditions. At the same time, specific pathologic conditions exist that are important to identify and discuss with parents of preschoolers. Currently, autism spectrum disorders represent a neurodevelopmental disability that is increasing in frequency, and identification of these disorders is crucial to facilitate early intervention and optimal outcome. Additionally, certain specific behavioral problems are most likely to emerge in the preschool period, such as anxiety and attention-deficit/hyperactivity disorder (ADHD) behaviors.

Autism Spectrum Disorders

Although autism spectrum disorders were previously considered rare, more recent accounts indicate dramatically increased prevalence rates, from 4 to 5 children per 10,000 to an estimated range from 3.4 to 6.7 per 1000 children (Kolevzon et al, 2007). As prevalence rates have increased, there has been increased attention directed toward the role of the primary care practitioner in early identification efforts. Parents' concerns about language and social development in their toddler and preschool-age children need to be seriously considered, and referral for developmental evaluation by a specialist should be done if warranted (see Chapter 69).

Red flags associated with autism spectrum disorders include qualitative impairments in social and communicative functioning, including delayed speech milestones (e.g., not talking by or displaying limited speech at 2 years of age); presence of echolalic or scripted speech; pronoun confusion; lack of response to name when called; limited eye contact with others; lack of seeking out others for play or to communicate needs; and delayed play development, often characterized by lack of pretend play and propensity toward repetitive or nonfunctional play behaviors (e.g., spinning wheels, lining up play objects, fixated play interests). If one or more red flags are present at 2 to 2½ years of age, a referral should be made to the early intervention services of the county and to a developmental behavioral pediatrician (Table 4-5).

Attention-Deficit/Hyperactivity Disorder

Attentional skills build gradually during the preschool years, with increasing ability to maintain concentration to tasks. Although parents of preschoolers may broach concerns during well-child visits about possible emerging attention-deficit disorders or emerging learning difficulties, with few exceptions, learning achievement and executive functions are not well solidified during the preschool years and are more reliably assessed during the school-age years (see Chapter 54). Even so, symptoms of ADHD are often present in preschool children and must be present at least before age 7 years. Because of caution regarding labeling behavioral pathology in very young children, clinicians may be unresponsive to parents' concerns about how to deal with their child's high activity levels or aggressive behaviors. Primary care clinicians do not need to diagnose children in this age group, but they should address parents' concerns and refer families for behavioral therapy when hyperactivity, impulsivity, or tantrum behaviors present consistent and frequent challenges to parenting. Table 4-6 presents common symptoms of ADHD that often emerge during the preschool years.

Anxiety

Anxiety symptoms are common in preschool children, often manifesting into specific fears, such as separating from the primary caregiver during the transition into preschool. Generally, it is recommended that parents be patient and understanding to childhood fears, providing acceptance and understanding of their preschoolers' feelings, while offering support with coping. Anxiety responses are often conditioned responses that can be reduced with careful and gentle exposure to the feared situation or object. Separation anxiety can be helped by increasing transition times and allowing use of a transition object in the new setting.

Selective mutism is an anxiety disorder that may be seen in children at this age especially when entering the preschool setting or becoming increasingly a part of other community systems. Selective mutism is characterized by failure to speak in social settings, while speaking

Table 4-6. Red Flags for Emerging Attention-Deficit/Hyperactivity Disorder

Inattention	Hyperactivity	Impulsivity
Not following directions	Runs or climbs excessively	Darting away from family
Not listening when spoken to	Loud play and loud talk	Not waiting turn
Easily distractible	Talking excessively	Intrudes on others
Shifting quickly from one activity to the next	Acts as if "driven by a motor"	Lack of consideration for danger situations

normally in comfortable settings, such as at home with the family. Selective mutism is considered a precursor to social phobia, which may emerge in older children, adolescents, or adults. It is essential that children suspected to have this disorder be evaluated and treated for underlying components of anxiety. Increased expectation that the child speak can make the symptoms worse because there is also a strong component of performance anxiety involved with selective mutism. With proper diagnosis and treatment, prognosis rates are quite good for full recovery.

SUMMARY

We have attempted to capture the essence of the preschool years by describing the developmental skills of children of this age, the issues facing families, the larger sociocultural issues, and the nature of support and guidance that should be available to families in the context of the well-child visit. Preschoolers are much more complex than we can describe in one chapter. They are at an exciting age full of wondrous exploration of the world and fantastic imaginary experiences, but also an age where if something goes wrong it can be the end of the world. Parents need support and guidance from well care providers to help them understand these complex individuals and to interpret any possible developmental and behavioral concerns.

REFERENCES

Amato PR: The consequences of divorce for adults and children. J Marriage Fam 62:1269-1287, 2000.

Aylward G: Infant and Early Childhood Neuropsychology. New York: Plenum Press, 1997.

Baumrind D: Effects of authoritative control on child behavior. Child Dev 37:887-907, 1966.

Diamond A, Kirkham N, Amso D: Conditions under which young children can hold two rules in mind and inhibit a proponent response. Dev Psychol 38:352-362, 2002.

Duncan G, Yeung W, Brooks-Gunn J, Smith J: How much does childhood poverty affect the life changes of children? Am Sociol Rev 63:406-423, 1998.

Ferber R: Solving Your Child's Sleep Problems. New York: Simon & Schuster, 1985.

Glascoe F: Screening for developmental and behavioral problems. Ment Retard Dev Disabil Res Rev 11:173-179, 2005.

Gropen J, Pinker S, Hollander M: Affectedness and direct objects: The role of lexical semantics in the acquisition of verb argument structure. Cognition 41:153-195, 1991.

Halfon N, Regalado M, Sareen H, et al: Assessing development in the pediatric office. Pediatrics 113:1926-1933, 2004.

Kolevzon A, Gross R, Reichenberg A: Prenatal and perinatal risk factors for autism. Arch Pediatr Adolesc Med 161:326-333, 2007.

Lee V, Brooks-Gunn J, Schnur E, Liaw F: Are Head Start effects sustained? A longitudinal follow up comparison of disadvantaged children attending Head Start no preschool, and other preschool programs. Child Dev 61:495-507, 1990.

Lugaila T, Overturf J: Children and the Households They Live in: 2000. Census 2000 Special Reports. Washington, DC: U.S. Census Bureau, 2004.

NICHD Study of Early Child Care and Youth Development. Available at: http://public.rti.org/secc/home.cfm. Accessed October 5, 2008.

Peisner-Feinberg E, Burchinal M, Clifford R, et al: The relation of preschool child-care quality to children's cognitive and social developmental trajectories through second grade. Child Dev 72:1534-1553, 2001.

Rutter M; and the English Romanian Adoptees Study Team: Developmental catch-up and deficit, following adoption after severe global early privation. J Child Psychol Psychiatry 39:465-476, 1998.

Shonkoff J, Phillips D (eds): From Neurons to Neighborhoods: The Science of Early Child Development. Washington, DC: National Academy Press, 2000.

Spernak S, Schottenbauer M, Ramey S, Ramey C: Child health and academic achievement among former Head Start children. Children and Youth Services Review 28:1251-1261, 2006.

Weintraub M, Clemens C, Sockloff A, et al: The development of sex stereotypes in the third year: Relationships to gender labeling, gender identity, sex-typed toy preference, and family characteristics. Child Dev 55:1493-1503, 1984.

Wood D, Wood H: Vygotsky, tutoring, and learning. Oxford Review of Education 22:5-16, 1996.

5 MIDDLE CHILDHOOD

Marsha D. Rappley and James R. Kallman

Vignette

Sean is a 10-year-old boy about to enter fifth grade who presents to his pediatrician for a physical examination required for his soccer team. He is excited about playing soccer on a travel team, but tells you that his mother will not let him play if he doesn't do better in school. Teachers have expressed concern that he doesn't finish his work in school, preferring to be the "class clown." His mother complains that he avoids homework, causing many battles with his parents. The pediatrician determines that he is healthy, excels as a soccer goalie, has several good friends, enjoys participating in a faith-based youth group, and considers himself "not one of the smarter ones" in his class. Sean's mother confirms that he is "on probation"—either he completes all of his school work and homework without reminders, or he will be pulled from the soccer team. How can the pediatrician be useful to this school-age child?

Middle childhood traditionally has been described as a period of quiescence, marking time between the rapid development of early childhood and the dramatic changes of puberty and adolescence. Freud described middle childhood as "the latency period," in which the psychodynamics of relationships with important others, especially parents, are characterized by the sublimation of sexual feelings into age-appropriate activities. Erikson characterized the activities of middle childhood as a dynamic tension between industry and inferiority, in which over time the child develops a sense of mastery and competency. Piaget described discrete achievements in learning and understanding, which develop in a predictable sequence. Through advances in neuroimaging, we are now able to witness tremendous growth and change in the central nervous system (CNS) occurring between the ages of 5 and 12 years. What emerges from the diverse concepts of middle childhood, new information about cognition and relationships, and advances in neuroimaging is a rich understanding of the profound transformation that brings the kindergarten-age child into adolescence.

This chapter first explores physical growth and motor development during middle childhood. Next, the rapid development of cognition, language, and executive functions is described, followed by academic milestones and social and emotional development. Insight gained from imaging techniques illustrates the phenomenal developmental changes of the brain throughout middle childhood. The context of cultural and psychosocial variation provides a frame. Finally, clinical implications are explored, and the case of Sean and his family is reviewed (see vignette), tying together the multiple layers of development that must be considered in evaluation and treatment of problems of middle childhood.

PHYSICAL AND MOTOR GROWTH

Growth and development during middle childhood occurs in discontinuous spurts—three to six per year—lasting approximately 8 weeks each. Average yearly growth is approximately 7 lb and 2.5 inches per year. By age 7 years, the ratio for the upper and lower body reaches 1 and remains stable thereafter. Dental development includes exfoliation of deciduous teeth from ages 6 through 12 years. Eruption of permanent teeth may be immediate or follow exfoliation by 4 to 5 months. The paranasal sinuses continue to develop through middle childhood; the frontal sinuses are apparent on imaging studies by approximately 6 years of age, and the ethmoid sinuses reach maximum size during this time. Lymphoid tissue also develops to adult size and hypertrophies, reaching maximum size between 6 and 8 years of age, and subsequently receding to adult proportions.

The lean body habitus of many children between 6 and 10 years of age is reflected in the nadir of body mass index at age 5 to 7 years for boys and age 5 years for girls (Kuczmarski et al, 2000). Skin folds also are least thick between ages 6 and 9 years. Height velocity peaks for girls between 11 and 12 years, and later for boys, between 13 and 14 years. The physiologic increase in alkaline phosphatase during middle childhood reflects this period of rapid bone growth. Sexual maturation begins for girls with breast budding, on average, at a mean age of 10.9 years, with 8.9 to 14.8 years representing

2 standard deviations below and above the mean. Sexual maturation begins for boys with growth of the penis, on average at a mean age of 10.5 years, with 9.2 to 13.7 years representing 2 standard deviations above and below the mean (Tanner and Davies, 1985). Respiratory rate and pulse decline through childhood. Diastolic blood pressure begins to increase toward adult levels at age 6 years. Gastric emptying time is increased during early and middle childhood compared with adults and may affect the absorption of some medications.

Middle childhood is marked by significant improvement in neuromotor control. This development is illustrated by an elegant study of 662 Swiss children from age 5 to 18 years describing speed of performing tasks such as repetitive hand movements, sequential finger movements, and pegboard placement (Largo et al, 2003). A steady increase in speed was noted, with a plateau by age 13 to 15 years. The more complicated the task, the older the age at which the plateau occurred. A wide variation was noted among children in the ability to perform these tasks, indicative of the wide range of normal development (Fig. 5-1). Associated movements, sometimes referred to as overflow movements, were assessed as well. More complex tasks were characterized by more associated movements at all ages than simple tasks and showed more variability among individuals. The largest difference among individual children in intensity of associated movements occurred during kindergarten and early school years; the difference narrowed thereafter. Girls carried out complex tasks more rapidly than boys did, but the difference did not achieve significance; girls also had fewer associated movements. The authors speculate that these gender differences lead to a more harmonious appearance in the performance of neuromotor tasks for girls.

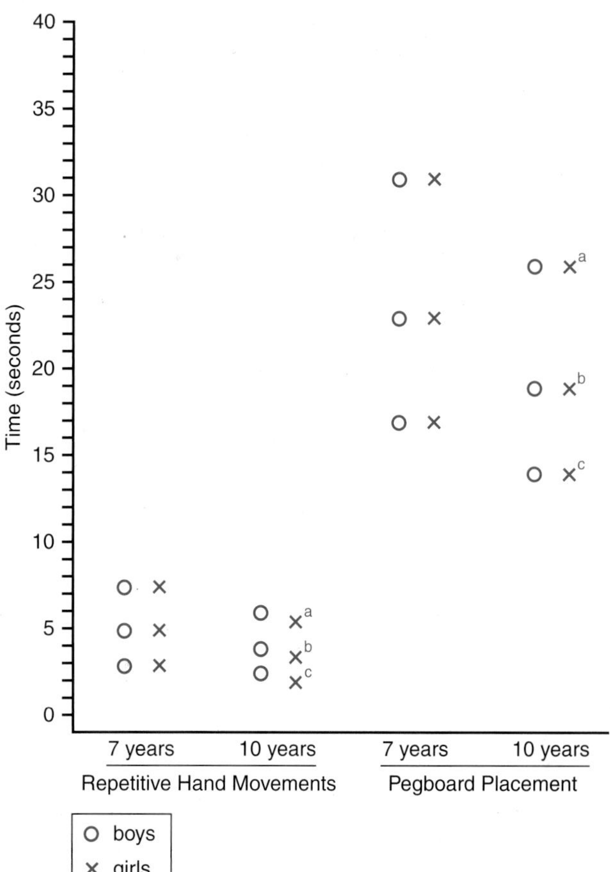

Figure 5-1. Variability of performance of neuromotor tasks as a function of age. *a*, 97th percentile; *b*, 50th percentile; *c*, 3rd percentile. (From Largo RH, Fischer JE, Rousson V: Neuromotor development from kindergarten age to adolescence: Developmental course and variability. Swiss Med Wkly 133(13-14):193-199, 2003.)

Sports are an important part of life for most children. Approximately 30 million children participate in sports each year, including more than half of children 5 to 18 years old in the United States. The ability to compare oneself with others emerges sometime after 6 years, an understanding of the competitive nature of sports occurs around 9 years, and the comprehension and mastery of skill needed for complex sports occurs about 12 years of age (Patel et al, 2002). The rate of visits to emergency departments for sports-related injuries is highest for the age group 5 to 12 years; 34% of middle school children may sustain an injury related to physical activity that is treated by a physician or nurse (Adirim and Cheng, 2003). Children 5 to 11 years old are more likely to sustain a fracture and to experience heat-related injuries than older children (Taylor and Attia, 2000). The sports most often associated with injury in this age group are football, baseball, and soccer. The average age of injury for rollerblading and in-line skating occurs at 10 years. This is the only sport among the top six associated with injury that has an average injury at an age younger than 12 years (Taylor and Attia, 2000). When injuries in general were examined for 5- to 19-year-olds, children 5 to 9 years old accounted for approximately one quarter of injuries, and 10- to 14-year-olds represented one third to almost one half of injuries sustained in and out of school (Linakis et al, 2006).

The rapid growth and development of middle childhood likely contributes to this high prevalence of sports-related injury. Compared with older children, these children have a larger ratio of surface area to mass, a proportionally larger head, and a larger variation in size within a given group and so experience poor fit in activity and protective equipment. They have open growth plates at epiphyses and growing cartilage. Finally, mastery of complex motor skills, judgment, planning abilities, and self-awareness all mature at a later age than that at which these children enter sports (Adirim and Cheng, 2003).

DEVELOPMENT OF COGNITION, THINKING, AND LANGUAGE

During middle childhood, children develop increasingly complex ways to handle and process information, moving from thinking that depends on concrete experiences to thinking that uses abstract and conceptual understanding. The influence of genetics on intelligence follows a developmental trajectory. Heritability describes the extent to which differences in IQ within a population are explained best by genetics or environment (but does not address how to understand an individual's IQ).

A review of twin studies calculated the heritability of intelligence as 0.22 at age 5 years, increasing to 0.85 at 12 years, and remaining stable thereafter (Bouchard, 2006). This finding suggests that the effect of shared environment is strongest among younger children, and the heritability of intelligence increases with age.

Profound changes in understanding and use of language occur in middle childhood. Metalinguistic skills develop as the child becomes increasingly aware of language. A major shift in the ability to recognize components of language and the speed of response to these components occurs at about 7 to 8 years (Edwards and Kirkpatrick, 1999). This is the time at which grammatical rules are explicitly recognized and consciously applied. Increasing phonologic awareness is evident in how children understand the esthetics of language. The love of puns, plays on words, jokes, and fill-in-the-blank silly word games illustrates this increasing awareness. The ability to define words has a developmental trajectory between the ages of 5 and 11 years, and is thought to be related to metalinguistic awareness (Benelli et al, 2006). An increase in creative and figurative expressions and the use of novel metaphors increases during middle childhood and peaks in adolescence (Levorato and Cacciari, 2002). The growth in syntax, which peaks in early adulthood, is shown in the child's increasing ability to employ complex sentences, conversation, and discourse, particularly in creating narrative or expository discourse. It is common for a child to be articulate and fluent in explaining a project, but stumbling and hesitant with casual conversation. It is speculated that the developing complexity of thought is driving the developing complexity in language (Nippold et al, 2005).

Piaget was among the first to study cognitive development of children. He described the intuitive substage of preoperational thinking as occurring between 4 and 7 years. During this time, children are capable of organizing and categorizing according to certain attributes without awareness of underlying principles. According to Piaget, children this age have difficulty discriminating between parts and the whole. More recent studies indicate, however, that children this age can understand, for example, that dogs are animals, and that dogs are different from other animals, indicating a greater capability to understand an overarching concept than might otherwise be predicted (Hetherington et al, 2006).

Piaget also described an increasing capacity to understand conservation that progresses from number and mass at 7 years, to weight at 8 to 10 years, and to volume at 11 to 12 years. Studies in various cultures show that the age at which a child acquires a grasp of conservation varies to a moderate degree with the cultural milieu. For example, children raised in a community in Mexico in which pottery making is essential to the economic wellbeing of the community develop a sense of conservation of volume earlier than the European children studied by Piaget.

Semilogical and inconsistent thinking is characteristic of children 4 to 7 years of age, whereas children 7 to 11 years move into the phase Piaget described as concrete operations. They become more flexible in their thinking. The concept of reversibility seems to inform thinking after 6 years of age. A child can reverse steps mentally, attend to more than one dimension of a subject, and think deductively. Piaget described children at this age as best able to problem solve when the elements of the problem are physically evident, as opposed to when the elements are presented in the auditory mode, and problem solving must occur mentally. After memory training, however, children are able to remember elements of a problem and solve it mentally at this age, even when the objects are not physically present (Bryant and Trabasso, 1971).

Memory is critical to cognitive development. Adults and 5-year-olds have similar capacity to store sensory input in memory. The ability to encode that information into a mental representation and working memory increases with age, however; this is partly a result of increasing speed of pronunciation and rehearsal in memorization between the ages of 5 and 11 years (Siegler and Alibali, 2005). Working memory is present by age 6 years and increases in functional capacity as the child grows (Gathercole et al, 2004).

The development of executive control, or the ability to direct information through perception and attention, steadily increases between the ages of 3 and 12 years. Before sophisticated images of brain development were available, a "connectionist theory" of information processing described neural networks as the premise for simultaneous and parallel distributed processing of sensory input. The premise that children learn to suppress selectively irrelevant information, and with age increasingly focus on detail important to the task at hand, whether physically present or not, is in keeping with the imaging studies of the CNS (described later). As children show an increased ability to perform neuropsychologic tasks that represent these abilities, and as this is studied with images of the brain while children perform these tasks, it is noted that the developmental trajectories of the brain, behavior, and cognition are parallel and supportive of one another.

DEVELOPMENT OF ACADEMIC SKILLS

Language, memory, and attention are critical to the academic skills, which facilitate achievement in school. Decoding is recognition and use of symbols in reading, writing, and mathematics. Encoding requires a different set of skills to apply to the symbols and derive meaning and comprehension. Detailed studies of how children learn to read yield conflicting results about the relative predictive value of general language competency, metalinguistic awareness, working memory, phonologic awareness, and semantic skills. Most studies reinforce the importance of the development of these discrete skills during middle childhood as essential to meeting the academic challenges of each successive grade in school.

The environment plays an important role in the development of reading skills; improvements in environment is an important strategy of intervention (Molfese et al, 2003). Learning to read is a language process, a psychological and affective process, and a social and cultural process. Children in late preschool and kindergarten show evidence of emerging literacy in their interest in picture books and in scribbling. With maturation, they

Table 5-1. General "Checkpoints" of Development of Reading Skills

Grade	Typical Reading Activity
Kindergarten	
	Knows that print carries meaning
	Turns pages to find out what happens next
	Writes (scribbles) a message
	Uses language and voice of a story
	Knows written language
	Recognizes that letters together make words
	Identifies letters in unfamiliar words
	Knows letters of alphabet
	Knows letters are associated with sounds
	Knows that words serve a purpose
	Knows how books work
	Can link what is read to previous experience
	Shows understanding by talking about the story
	Enjoys being read to and reading
Grade 3	
	Comprehension is improving
	Asks questions while reading
	Creates and changes mental pictures
	Rereads when confused
	Applies word analysis skills
	Understands elements of literature
	Explains characters
	Aware of different genres: humor, poetry, fiction
	Uses appropriate conventions of language
	Spells high-frequency words correctly
	Completes sentences
Grade 6	
	Uses strategies to figure out unfamiliar words
	Reads a variety of texts: science, math, social studies
	Summarizes what is read
	Reads critically, draws conclusions
	Improves comprehension
	Rereads, questions, discusses
	Understands elements of literature
	Names author, characters, themes
	Uses appropriate conventions of language
	No significant spelling errors
	Writes legibly
	Provides detail in discussion and writing

Adapted from Council for Educational Development and Research; and Hopkins G: Checkpoints in Reading. 2004. Available at: www.education-world.com/a_curr/curr009.shtml. Accessed February 2, 2007.

become interested in books and writing. Children approach reading as a functional activity that allows them to do things. Oral and written skills influence one another. Table 5-1 presents activities and behaviors that are typical of the progressive development of reading skills (Hopkins, 2004).

The specific language skills of listening comprehension, oral expression, reading comprehension, and written expression are developmentally stable over time and moderately correlated with one another (Berninger et al, 2006). A comparison of fluency in drawing and writing from age 4 to 12 years indicates that a shift occurs at approximately age 6 years, in which writing becomes more fluent for most children (Adi-Japha and Freeman, 2001). A fascinating illustration of the juxtaposition of culture and language is found in the study of reading development among Chinese children. Although the relationship between phonologic awareness and reading is strong in Western countries, it is weak for Chinese children. The ability to read in Chinese languages is strongly related to the child's ability to write. It is speculated that this is because Chinese logographic characters are based on meaning, rather than phonology (Tan et al, 2005).

Skill in arithmetic and mathematics begins to develop at approximately age 3 years. By 5 to 6 years, many children cannot yet link counting with quantity. A child might count correctly from 1 to 5, but not recognize that 5 is greater than 2. The awareness of conservation, as described by Piaget, and the ability to shift from concrete to mental representation are important in the development of math skills (Gersten et al, 2005). Early research illustrated that for young children, simple arithmetic problems are complex problems to solve and require effort and coordination of nascent executive function. Fluency and mastery of arithmetic combinations (e.g., 5 + 3) require effective counting strategies. Verbal counting and computation, as opposed to finger counting, is a key developmental step. Lack of these skills in first through third grade may indicate opportunity for intervention and prevention of mathematic difficulties or disabilities (Gersten et al, 2005).

Boys are more competent in spatial skills and geometry than girls, whereas girls are more competent in computation than boys. Computation is a more verbal skill than is geometry. Boys and girls do equally well on basic math knowledge and algebra (Hyde et al, 1990). Math skills are influenced by the development of reading skills, and computational skills are linked to phonologic processing (Hecht et al, 2001).

The overall prevalence of mathematic disability is estimated at 5%. In Wake County Public Schools, North Carolina, from 1999 to 2000, 13% of students in the first grade and 22% of children in third through fifth grade were found to have deficiencies in math skills (Speas, 2001). Because this study reports deficiencies rather than disabilities, the prevalence rates are likely to be relevant for other populations using different definitions of disability. The heritability of mathematic difficulty, as reported by teachers, was found to be 0.6 to 0.7 among twins, and consistent from ages 7 to 9 years (Haworth et al, 2007). Genetic syndromes, such as Prader-Willi syndrome, fragile X syndrome, and Turner syndrome, illustrate how specific genetic defects can result in specific mathematic difficulties (Butler et al, 2004; Mazzocco, 2001).

The influence of culture on development of math skills is illustrated in a study of urban children in Brazil. Children 9 to 15 years old successfully applied mental computation strategies to solve rapid commercial transactions while engaged in the street economy of Brazilian cities, but these children could not then successfully complete the same problem in the traditional academic, written context (Hetherington et al, 2006; Nunes and Bryant, 1996). In the United States, children of lower socioeconomic status (SES) have more difficulty with math than children of middle and upper SES (Jordan and Hanich, 2003). It is unclear if this difference reflects lack of exposure to effective strategies. Considering the development of executive function and cognitive control between ages 3 and 12 years, it is not surprising that self-regulation of affect, behavior, and inhibitory control in kindergarten-age children has been shown to be related to the development of math and reading skills (Blair and Razza, 2007). Figure 5-2 relates SES and neurocognitive functions.

SOCIAL AND EMOTIONAL DEVELOPMENT

Children become aware of their own feelings and experiences as private and distinct from those of others at about 7 to 8 years of age. A significant increase in the ability to describe others in psychological terms occurs around 8 years of age. Half of children 8 to 10 years old are able to see themselves through the eyes of another person, and anticipate and consider the thoughts and feelings of another. Approximately 10% to 20% of children this age are able to consider a third view, perhaps that of a teacher, a classmate, and oneself. The ability to understand the role of another is moderately related to intelligence, prosocial behavior, and altruism. In addition, the ability to understand and refer to stereotypes increases between ages 6 and 10 years and is stronger among children of stigmatized ethnic groups than among majority groups (Hetherington et al, 2006; McKown and Weinstein, 2003).

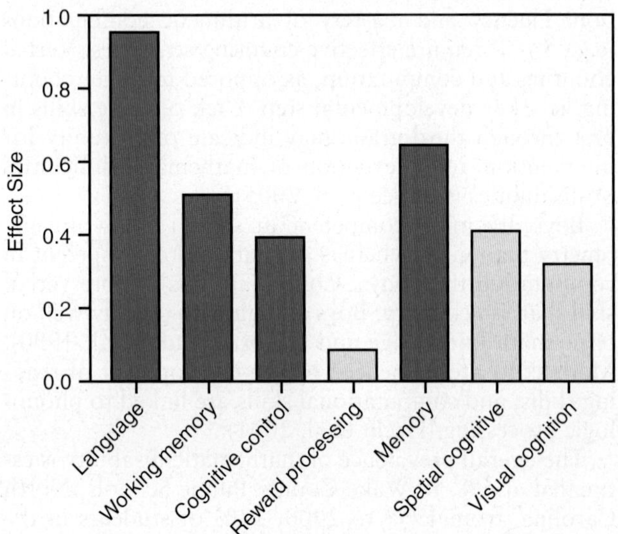

Figure 5-2. Effect sizes, measured in standard deviations of separation between low and middle socioeconomic status group performance, on the composite measures of the seven different neurocognitive systems. *Dark blue bars* represent effect sizes for statistically significant effects; *light blue bars* represent effect sizes for nonsignificant effects. (From Farah MJ, Shera DM, Savage JH, et al: Childhood poverty: Specific associations with neurocognitive development. Brain Res 1110:166-174, 2006.)

This marked shift away from egocentric thinking accompanies the development of mature communication skills and of moral standards and empathy (Eisenberg et al, 2006; Hetherington et al, 2006). Piaget described the ages of 5 to 11 years as characterized by moral realism, which is an absolute sense of rules, and the notion of immanent justice, which is the belief that deviation from the rules inevitably results in punishment. Piaget described that at approximately age 11 years, children understand moral reciprocity. They understand that rules can be arbitrary and are subject to question, and that intent is important in judging right and wrong. More recent research indicates that if presented with information in a variety of ways, with clear depictions of intent, and videotaped as opposed to oral or written description, 6-year-olds can evaluate and consider intent in a moral judgment (Hetherington et al, 2006). Kohlberg's classic depiction of six stages of moral development, acquired at various ages, but in the same developmental progression, is affirmed by more recent studies. A sense of justice is likely to be culturally bound, however, especially as it is predicated on the premise of obligations to help others and one's community or is based on individual rights and obligations (Miller and Bersoff, 1992).

Prosocial behavior is associated with the ability to take another's point of view, with moderation of expressions of emotions and insight, all mediated through the development of empathy (Fig. 5-3) (Roberts and Strayer, 1996). Studies of twins indicate that prosocial behavior and empathy may be rooted in genetics and

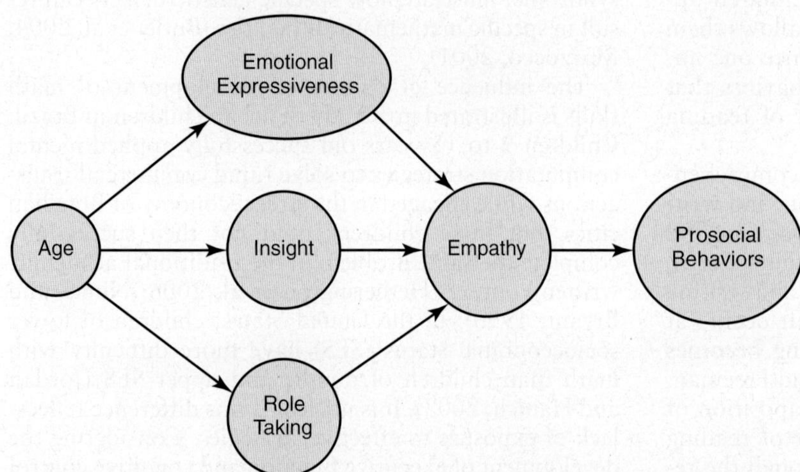

Figure 5-3. Empathy and variables related to prosocial behavior. (From Strayhorn JM, Jr., Bickel DD: A randomized trial of individual tutoring for elementary school children with reading and behavior difficulties. Psychological Rep 92:427-444, 2003.)

environment (Deater-Deckard et al, 2001; Hetherington et al, 2006). A striking example is found in children with Williams syndrome, which is caused by a deletion of an allele of chromosome subunit 7q11.23, who are observed to be more empathetic and prosocial than other children of the same age. Parents influence the development of prosocial behavior through parenting and modeling. Some television programming, such as *Mister Rogers* and *Sesame Street,* also may influence prosocial behavior, especially for children whose parents watch with them (Hetherington et al, 2006; Mares and Woodward, 2001).

Children form intimate and fast friendships over the years of elementary school. In the early school years, friendships are characterized by a desire to maximize enjoyment through coordinating play, managing conflict, and managing emotions. Young school-age children often define friendship in terms of what they themselves might gain. Later elementary years are characterized by a desire to be included and admired, a sharing of gossip through which acceptable and unacceptable behaviors are shaped, and developing a further sense of appropriate expression of feelings (Hetherington et al, 2006) (Table 5-2). Older school-age children, especially girls, often cite emotional support and benefit to the friend as a reason to be friends. Children with friendships in middle childhood have more success as adults in relationships with family and peers than children without such friendships (Hetherington et al, 2006).

Within the context of family and school, the child develops a sense of competency and mastery of concrete skills and relationships. The rapid progression and joy of mastery create a time of excitement and gratification for many children and parents, although this is often described in hindsight. Erikson's description of the dynamic tension between the industrious nature of middle childhood and the need to overcome the sense of inferiority is evident in academic skills, friendships, sibships, relationships with parents, and relationships with other adults. The explosion of neuroscience also makes more evident the interplay and dependency of what was previously considered a dichotomy between "nature" and "nurture" (Oliver and Plomin, 2007). The dependent and evolving relationship of genetics and experience for an individual is increasingly shown.

Table 5-2. Characteristics of Friendship

Grades 2-3	Reward-cost stage	Friends expected to offer help, share common activities, join organized play, offer judgments, be physically near, demographically similar
Grades 4-5	Normative stage	Friends expected to accept and admire one another, express loyalty and commitment, share values and attitudes
Grades 6-7	Empathetic stage	Friends expect genuineness and intimacy, self-disclosure

Data from Hetherington EM, Parke RD, Gauvain M, Locke VO: Child Psychology: A Contemporary View, 6th ed. Boston: McGraw-Hill, 2006.

DEVELOPMENT OF THE BRAIN

Observations and studies of behavior are increasingly supplemented by imaging technology, which allows a window on the maturation of the CNS. Anatomic studies of growth, morphology, and mass are accomplished through computed tomography and magnetic resonance imaging (MRI). Functional studies provide images of blood flow (functional MRI) or of positron emission from glucose uptake or other metabolic activity (positron emission tomography). Diffusion tensor imaging creates images by contrasting water diffusion in the CNS, allowing a fine discrimination of gray and white matter, elucidation of fiber tracts, and estimation of myelination and conductivity. These sophisticated imaging techniques do not establish causality, but rather allow observations of development that are linked with what we learn about genetics, behavior, and experience (see Chapter 8).

The concept of differential growth is critical to understanding developmental changes in the CNS as children grow. Some areas of the brain undergo selective thinning, whereas other areas undergo selective thickening. This modeling of the brain continues well into young adult years.

After birth, the brain develops most rapidly during the early years of life; significant maturation continues through middle childhood. Myelination of white matter continues into young adult years, particularly in areas associated with higher cognitive function. The increase in white matter from age 5 to 12 continues into the third decade of life. Developmental changes also are noted in subcortical areas of the brain. The corpus callosum is shown to grow in a front-to-back wave between 5 and 13 years as myelination increases, allowing increased conduction speed and transmission between the right and left hemispheres.

The developmental peak in cortical gray matter occurs at about 12 years of age (Geidd et al, 1999). The brain of a 5-year-old child has grown rapidly in gray matter, with different regions growing at different rates. Over the next several years before puberty, the brain undergoes selective loss and thinning of gray matter. This is a mark of the maturing brain (Fig. 5-4) (Evans, 2006). The pattern of gray matter loss between 4 and 8 years appears first in the areas associated with the most basic functions of sensory perception and movement. Areas of spatial orientation mature with decline of the thinning process at about 11 to 13 years. Prefrontal areas associated with executive functions mature later in adolescence. The cortical gray matter thinning and the growth of white matter observed with imaging correlate with postmortem histology and support the concept of synaptic pruning as a maturational process (Barnea-Goraly et al, 2005; Toga et al, 2006).

While loss and thinning are occurring in these areas, thickening of gray matter is occurring in the cortex of the temporal and frontal areas associated with language (Fig. 5-5) (Toga et al, 2006). This pattern found in imaging studies corroborates histologic studies of the cytoarchitecture of Broca's region (Amunts et al, 2003). The thickening also seems to be correlated with performance

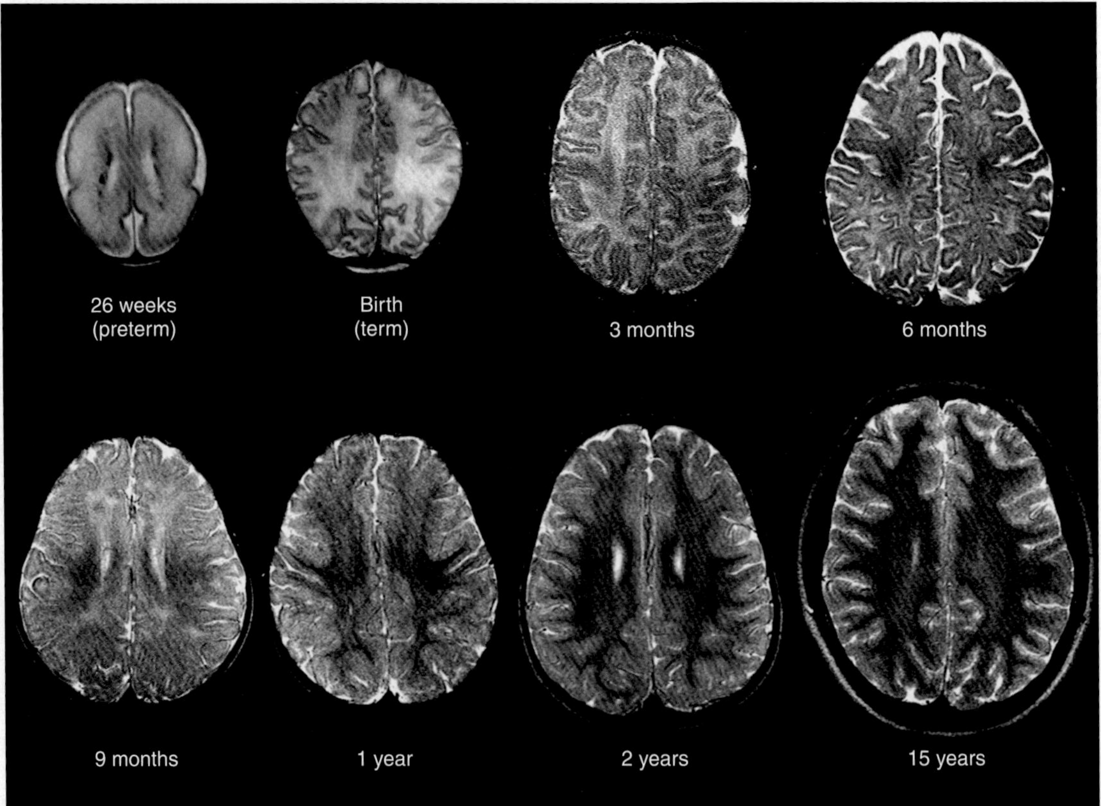

Figure 5-4. Contrast changes in the brain from birth through adolescence. (From Evans AC: The NIH MRI study of normal brain development. Neuroimage 30:184-202, 2006.)

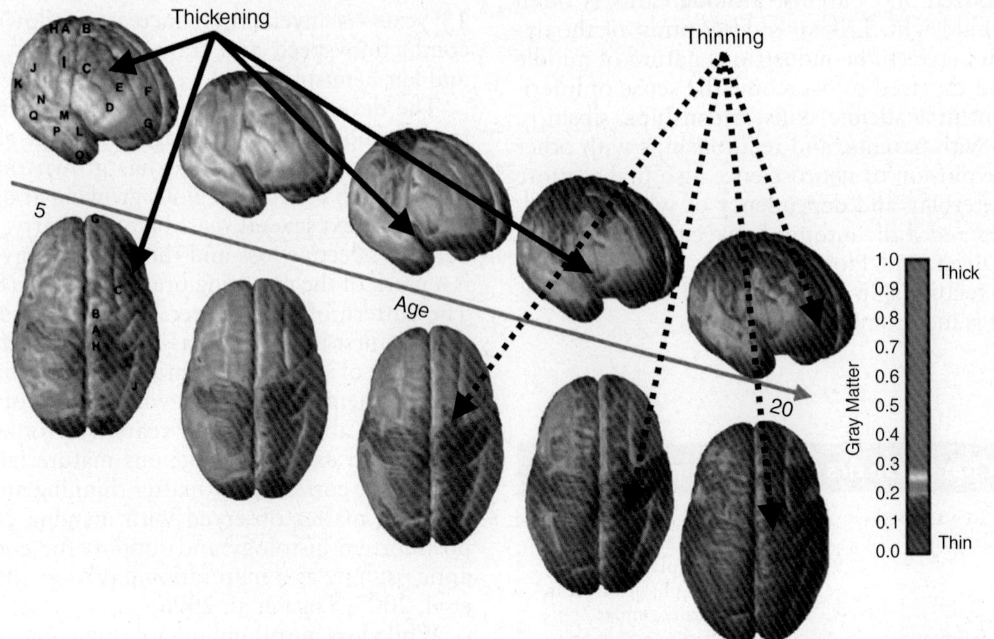

Figure 5-5. Maturation and thickening of temporal and frontal areas associated with language. (From Toga AW, Thompson PM, Sowell ER: Mapping brain maturation. Trends Neurosci 29:148-159, 2006.)

on verbal tests of intelligence. It is speculated that thickening represents the differential growth process (Toga et al, 2006); slower maturation and continued molding of the language areas of the frontal and temporal cortex into adolescence underlies the developmental progression during middle childhood of language and metalinguistic awareness. It may be that this physiologic process allows the positive influence of stimulation and practice on language development during childhood (Szaflarski et al, 2006).

Activation and engagement of the brain also occurs in a pattern that follows a developmental and differential sequence. Relevant studies combine imaging techniques with neuropsychologic testing of children at different ages. Children perform specific tasks while they are in a scanner, and the images that are created show areas of the brain that are activated during performance of that specific task. Generally, across tasks, young children show a pattern of diffuse and widespread activation as they execute the task. As children get older, they show more focused and discrete activations of specific areas of the brain. An important part of this maturational process is a selective process that attenuates activity in certain areas of the brain, while engaging activity in other areas. With age, fewer and more select regions of the brain are activated for specific tasks.

A parallel in behavior is seen in the developmental progression of attention, with an increasing ability to suppress information and actions between ages 4 and 12 years (see Chapter 54). Younger children are susceptible to interference of irrelevant stimuli; the capacity to respond selectively matures at approximately 12 years or older (Durston and Casey, 2006). A corollary also is observed in neuromotor development. Younger children have more extraneous, or overflow, movements, which recede as they grow older (Largo et al, 2003). Lack of the maturational effect was noted in imaging studies of children diagnosed with attention-deficit/hyperactivity disorder (ADHD). Subjects were challenged with a task in which they had to suppress a response. The children with ADHD had a more diffuse activation pattern and did not attenuate activation in certain areas of the brain compared with control children without ADHD (Durston et al, 2003).

Feedback loops and changes in connectivity between the forebrain and the midbrain also have a developmental trajectory. The theory of cognitive control examines how flexible regulation of thoughts and actions occurs in the presence of competing stimuli. Functional MRI studies show increased blood flow to the prefrontal cortex and substantia nigra in the midbrain during tasks requiring cognitive control. These studies support theories that link the executive functions of the frontal lobe with the dopamine-rich areas of the substantia nigra. Diffusion tensor imaging further shows activation of white matter fibers projecting from the ventral prefrontal cortex to the caudate nucleus while subjects perform neuropsychologic measures of cognitive control, lending credence to this feedback loop between the prefrontal areas of the brain and the nigrostriatum (Fig. 5-6) (Durston and Casey, 2006). Diffusion, which provides the basis for the image, becomes more restricted to these white matter tracts between ages 7 and 30 years, in association with increased efficiency in performing the task.

These findings support a theory of the development of cognitive control based on the increasing ability to respond selectively to stimuli and the increase in processing speed observed in physiology and behavior. This maturational process of the brain underlies the ability, as well as the variability among individuals, in the capacity to act selectively on stimuli.

The developmental process captured in neuroimaging and studies of behavior is influenced by genetics and experience. Studies of twins suggest that the greatest genetic influence is in the growth processes of the frontal cortex (Toga et al, 2006). Studies of twins in large registries also indicate a strong contribution of genetics to the phenotype associated with the diagnosis of ADHD (Larsson et al, 2006). The impact of experience and especially environmental insults, such as lead poisoning, is shown in many studies to result in similar impairments (Neuman et al, 2006; Schettler, 2001; Stein et al, 2002).

CULTURE AND PSYCHOSOCIAL VARIATION

Children begin to interact with a larger world and develop new relationships between the ages of 5 and 12 years. The influence of the child's interaction with the community and society is described by the theories of Vygotsky. Children acquire language and the ability to work with symbols as they grow, developing in close alignment with their culture. Basic functions, such as memory and attention, are transformed by interaction with the community and the world into higher order functions of voluntary attention and logical and abstract thinking. As the role of society is considered in child development, the possibility of guidance, or discrete intervention, becomes evident. Concepts of educational interventions that evolved from this model include scaffolding, reciprocal learning, guided participation, and community of learners (Hetherington et al, 2006).

Vygotsky emphasized the role of the institutions of a society in shaping cognitive development. Schools provide formal instruction in literacy, which becomes a tool to further the growth of intelligence. Vygotsky also maintained that understanding the cultural context of a child is imperative to fully estimating the child's capability at any given age. This idea is supported by studies from around the world that show advanced skill in areas of importance within a particular cultural milieu (Price-Williams et al, 1969).

SES is a composite of psychosocial, environmental, experiential, and genetic influences. Despite the fact that this complex interplay of elements is expressed in a simple measure of income and type of employment, SES is found to be associated with discrete aspects of development of language and cognitive control. Among kindergarten children, lower SES was found to be associated with lower performance in testing of language and executive control (Noble et al, 2005). Among children 10 to 13 years old, lower SES was significantly correlated with neuropsychologic measures of language,

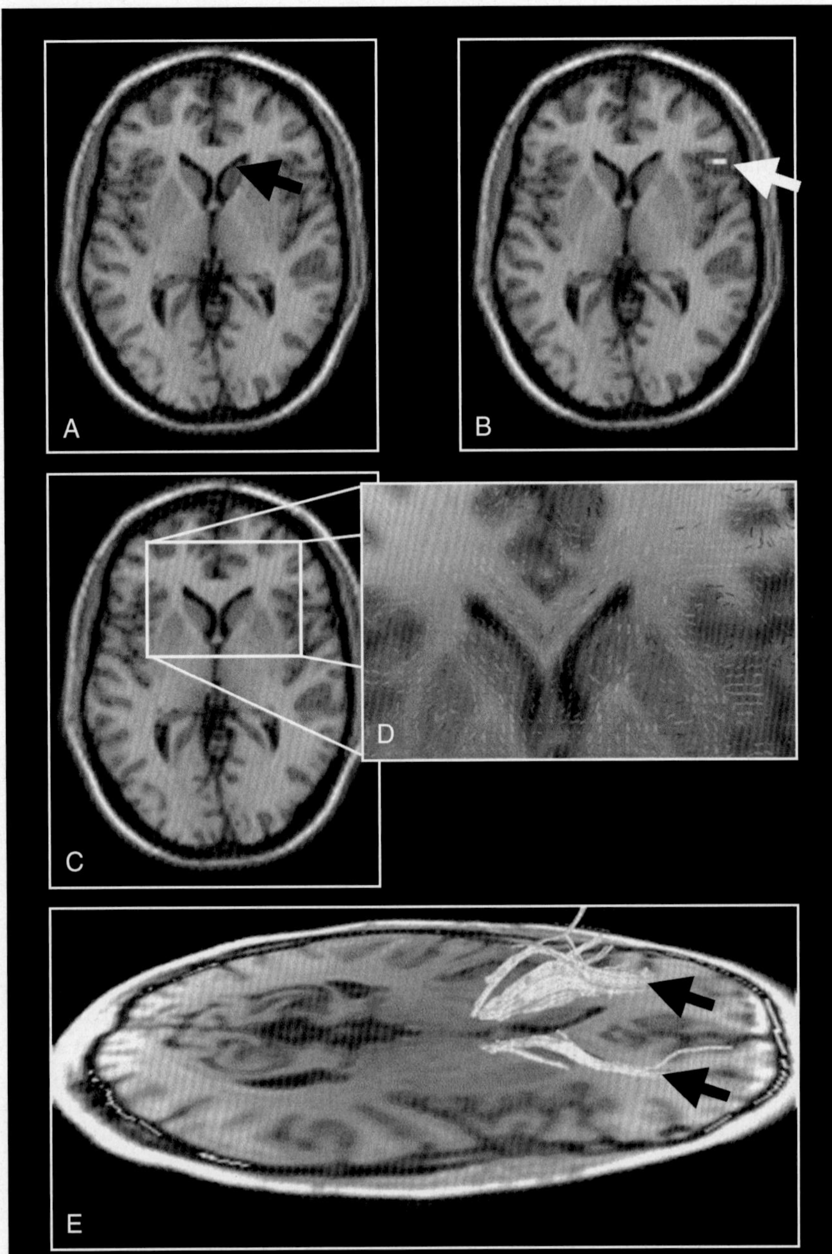

Figure 5-6. Diffusion tensor imaging and anatomic and functional MRI to investigate functional networks. **A,** *Arrow* indicates the caudate nucleus, which is defined on anatomic MRI as a seedpoint for fiber tracking. **B,** Functional activation maps from a single subject during a cognitive control task, overlaid on the anatomic MRI. *Arrow* indicates an area of activation. **C** and **D,** Vectors calculated from the diffusion tensor imaging scan, where the faint lines represent the direction of the vector, overlaid on a section of the anatomic scan. **E,** Fibers, indicated by *arrows,* tracked on the basis of the vectors in **D,** connecting both caudate nuclei with regions in the frontal cortex, including the frontal region activated in **B.** (From Durston S, Casey BJ: What have we learned about cognitive development for neuroimaging? Neuropsychologia 44:2149-2157, 2006.)

memory, and cognitive control, but not with measures of reward processing and visual and spatial cognition (see Fig. 5-2) (Farah et al, 2006). This differential, as opposed to more uniform, adverse effects of poverty on discrete areas of cognitive development, suggests different pathways and opportunities for intervention.

CLINICAL IMPLICATIONS

Evidence from imaging studies, observations of behavior within the context of a social milieu, and the differential growth of cognition and language all strongly suggest that, during middle childhood, interventions that change the environment or provide new experiences for the child can support development (Noble et al, 2005). It seems that language develops continually throughout this period, and that the adverse impact of lower SES on language development persists from early childhood to early puberty (Farah et al, 2006). Interventions for behavioral and reading problems are successful for children identified in early elementary school (Chard et al, 2002; Smolkowski et al, 2005). The understanding of how children rapidly grow and develop cognitive, social, and neuromotor skills during middle childhood suggests important interventions for safety, especially associated with sports (Washington et al, 2001).

In addition, the middle childhood achievement of recognition of feelings and perceptions of others and understanding of social stigma and stereotypes suggest important times for supporting the development of prosocial behavior and empathy. This is the underlying premise of programs that show the effectiveness of teachers as coaches and training of parents and teachers together to promote prosocial behavior (Barrera et al, 2002; Grossman et al, 1997; Hetherington et al, 2006; Olweus, 1993). Studies of family functioning and resiliency indicate that children who perceive their parents and teachers as supportive are more resilient and empathetic (Rigby, 1993; Stewart and Sun, 2004). These findings strongly suggest that community, education, and health system supports for families directly benefit school-age children.

During middle childhood, visits to the physician often concern a specific illness or need, such as the sports physical in the vignette at the beginning of the chapter featuring Sean. Because health maintenance visits are fewer than in early childhood, and because the focus shifts to more pragmatic issues, it is possible inadvertently to neglect opportunities for prevention and intervention. Height and weight continue to be salient markers of overall health and should be monitored regularly. Neuromuscular development and participation in sports provides an opportunity to explore self-esteem, impulse control, and expectations of self and family. Lack of participation in sports may provide an opportunity for validation from a respected authority figure for an alternative avenue for industry and mastery. The elementary grades are critical times for intervention with academic skill development. Although children are typically supported in their development by social and cultural institutions, many families are in transition among cultures, either ethnic or socioeconomic. A visit to the physician for episodic illness may be one of few opportunities a parent or child has to explore the difficulties that occur with these transitions.

In the case of Sean, the physician has several opportunities to make an impact. One opportunity is to discuss safety issues related to sports, such as properly fitting equipment, especially for a goalie, and adequate hydration. Equally important, the physician must make a decision about whether or not to respond to the child's statement that things are not going very well in school and the mother's strategy of putting him on probation. The issues raised in this family are common: a child must do well in school to participate in sports; a teacher focuses on a child's role as class clown, rather than on the child's academic skills; and parents battle with a child over homework. Although these issues could be easily dismissed as ordinary family problems, 20% of visits of children for primary care involve problems related to development, learning, and behavior. The problems are common, that they are raised with the physician is common, and the conditions they suggest are common. In this case, it is important to explore learning (see Chapter 51), attention (see Chapter 54), adjustment (see Chapter 42), anxiety and depression (see Chapter 47), and family relationships (see Chapter 10).

The pediatrician took up the challenge. Further history revealed that Sean is a very poor reader and has trouble getting his ideas on paper. He is demoralized about school and his inability to be successful with school work. He believes it is better to not try (see Chapter 44), and to be funny so that others will like him. His parents have focused on the fact that he is not trying his best, but they are beginning to wonder if the solution is simply to get him to try harder. His mother wonders if he might have ADHD.

The pediatrician realized it would require a series of visits to sort the issues out. The physician gave the parents standardized checklists for the parents, Sean, and his teacher to complete. He arranged a mutual agreement between the parents and child that Sean would remain in soccer, and that he would do 30 minutes of homework 5 days per week without arguing, although he might need reminders. He would read material of his own choosing to complete the 30 minutes if he should not have homework. A return appointment was scheduled for 1 month.

At the return visit, the physician reviewed the checklists with Sean and his mother. The behavior checklists did not note problems with attention, hyperactivity, aggression, defiance, anxiety, or other emotional problems. His teacher noted that he was reading well below fifth grade level, and his written work was more like that of a second grader. The physician suggested that Sean and his mother request a psychoeducational evaluation for a learning disability and described what his mother must do to initiate this request at the school. The physician provided a written report of her recommendation that this evaluation be done, along with copies of the checklists, history, and physical examination. Sean remained in soccer and complied with his terms of the agreement during the evaluation process. This "demystification" (i.e., bringing the history to open problem solving among the family, child, teacher, and physician, rather than keeping matters in the realm of hidden feelings of inadequacy and failure on the part of parents and child) was an important key to the success of the intervention.

The evaluation revealed that Sean had a high average IQ and learning disability in reading and written expression. The school suggested resource room assistance for Sean. The physician helped to shift the family, including Sean, from a position of blaming to a proactive plan for addressing these problems. Sports participation became viewed as a legitimate and important source of positive feedback and success for Sean. All acknowledged that extra effort would be required to make progress in academics, and that everyone has an important role in making this success happen. The family connected with resources for families and young people with learning disabilities so that Sean and his parents could understand that they are not alone and that the future is very bright for children like Sean. The physician assumed a supportive role in monitoring progress by offering visits every 3 to 4 months or as needed, at which the family could discuss challenges, struggles, and success. The physician also alerted Sean and his parents to other conditions and problems, such as difficulty with attention that might persist after appropriate measures are in place for the learning disability, social isolation as a result of peer teasing for "special education," anxiety or depression as a result of falling farther behind in academics, and family discord or stress. The office visits themselves became therapeutic because they provided an experience in which the child felt respected, accepted, and understood; the parents felt respected and supported in their parenting; and all family members trusted that they could raise issues of concern and seek guidance regarding Sean's growth, development, learning, behavior, and adaptation to his learning disability (see Chapter 89).

SUMMARY

Middle childhood is a dynamic and exciting time of change. The spirit of industry and the mastery of one significant challenge after another are truly awesome to witness. Improvements in neuromotor control lead to increased participation in sports. Changes in cognition and language support abstract reasoning and the development of academic skills. Children become aware of their own feelings and develop a moral sense. Differential thinning and thickening of the areas of the brain are thought to be the neural substrate of many of these changes. Clinical evaluations of children in middle childhood require surveying these diverse domains of functioning. Management of difficulties requires close collaboration of parents, children, teachers, and physicians. Optimally, a sense of competency in the world and with the self emerges for the child, laying the foundation for the developmental work of the years ahead.

REFERENCES

Adi-Japha E, Freeman NH: Development of differentiation between writing and drawing systems. Dev Psychol 37:101-114, 2001.

Adirim TA, Cheng TL: Overview of injuries in the young athlete. Sports Med 33:75-81, 2003.

Amunts K, Schleicher A, Ditterich A, Zilles K: Broca's region: Cytoarchitectonic asymmetry and developmental changes. J Comp Neurol 465:72-89, 2003.

Barnea-Goraly N, Menon V, Eckert M, et al: White matter development during childhood and adolescence: a cross-sectional diffusion tensor imaging study. Cereb Cortex 15:1848-1854, 2005.

Barrera M Jr, Biglan A, Taylor TK, et al: Early elementary school intervention to reduce conduct problems: A randomized trial with Hispanic and non-Hispanic children. Prev Sci 3:83-94, 2002.

Benelli B, Belacchi C, Gini G, Lucangeli D: "To define means to say what you know about things": The development of definitional skills as metalinguistic acquisition. J Child Lang 33:71-97, 2006.

Berninger VW, Abbott RD, Jones J, et al: Early development of language by hand: composing, reading, listening, and speaking connections; three letter-writing modes; and fast mapping in spelling. Dev Neuropsychol 29:61-92, 2006.

Blair C, Razza RP: Relating effortful control, executive function, and false belief understanding to emerging math and literacy ability in kindergarten. Child Dev 78:647-663, 2007.

Bouchard TJ: Genetic influence on human psychological traits. *In* Duffy KG (ed): Psychology 2006/2007, 36th ed. Dubuque, IA: McGraw-Hill, 2006, pp 27-31.

Bryant PE, Trabasso J: Transitive inferences and memory in young children. Nature 232:456-458, 1971.

Butler MG, Bittel DC, Kibiryeva N, et al: Behavioral differences among subjects with Prader-Willi syndrome and type I or type II deletion and maternal disomy. Pediatrics 113(3 Pt 1):565-573, 2004.

Chard DJ, Vaughn S, Tyler BJ: A synthesis of research on effective interventions for building reading fluency with elementary students with learning disabilities. J Learn Disabil 35:386-406, 2002.

Deater-Deckard K, Pike A, Petrill SA, et al: Nonshared environmental processes in social-emotional development. Dev Sci 4:F1-F6, 2001.

Durston S, Casey BJ: What have we learned about cognitive development for neuroimaging? Neuropsychologia 44:2149-2157, 2006.

Durston S, Tottenham NT, Thomas KM, et al: Differential patterns of striatal activation in young children with and without ADHD. Biol Psychiatry 53:871-878, 2003.

Edwards HT, Kirkpatrick AG: Metalinguistic awareness in children: A developmental progression. J Psycholinguist Res 28:313-329, 1999.

Eisenberg N, Fabes RA, Spinrad T: Prosocial development. *In* Damon W, Lerner RM, Eisenberg N (eds): Handbook of Child Psychology, 6th ed. Vol 3. New York: Wiley, 2006.

Evans AC: The NIH MRI study of normal brain development. Neuroimage 30:184-202, 2006.

Farah MJ, Shera DM, Savage JH, et al: Childhood poverty: Specific associations with neurocognitive development. Brain Res 1110: 166-174, 2006.

Gathercole SE, Pickering SJ, Ambridge B, Wearing H: The structure of working memory from 4 to 15 years of age. Dev Psychol 40:177-190, 2004.

Gersten R, Jordan NC, Flojo JR: Early identification and interventions for students with mathematics difficulties. J Learn Disabil 38:293-304, 2005.

Giedd JN, Blumenthal J, Jeffries NO, et al: Brain development during childhood and adolescence: A longitudinal MRI study. Nat Neurosci 2:861-863, 1999.

Grossman DC, Neckerman HJ, Koepsell TD, et al: Effectiveness of a violence prevention curriculum among children in elementary school: A randomized controlled trial. JAMA 277:1605-1611, 1997.

Haworth CM, Kovas Y, Petrill SA, Plomin R: Developmental origins of low mathematics performance and normal variation in twins from 7 to 9 years. Twin Res Hum Genet 10:106-117, 2007.

Hecht SA, Torgesen JK, Wagner RK, Rashotte CA: The relations between phonological processing abilities and emerging individual differences in mathematical computation skills: A longitudinal study from second to fifth grades. J Exp Child Psychol 79:192-227, 2001.

Hetherington EM, Parke RD, Gauvain M, Locke VO: Child Psychology: A Contemporary View, 6th ed. Boston: McGraw-Hill, 2006.

Hopkins G: Checkpoints in Reading. 2004. Available at: www.educationworld.com/a_curr/curr009.shtml. Accessed February 2, 2007.

Hyde JS, Fennema E, Lamon SJ: Gender differences in mathematics performance: A meta-analysis. Psychol Bull 107:139-155, 1990.

Jordan N, Hanich L: Characteristics of children with moderate mathematics deficiencies. Learn Disabil Res and Pract 18:213-221, 2003.

Kuczmarski RJ, Ogden CL, Grummer-Strawn LM, et al: CDC growth charts: United States. Adv Data 314:1-27, 2000.

Largo RH, Fischer JE, Rousson V: Neuromotor development from kindergarten age to adolescence: Developmental course and variability. Swiss Med Wkly 133(13-14):193-199, 2003.

Larsson H, Lichtenstein P, Larsson JO: Genetic contributions to the development of ADHD subtypes from childhood to adolescence. J Am Acad Child Adolesc Psychiatry 45:973-981, 2006.

Levorato MC, Cacciari C: The creation of new figurative expressions: Psycholinguistic evidence in Italian children, adolescents and adults. J Child Lang 29:127-150, 2002.

Linakis JG, Amanullah S, Mello MJ: Emergency department visits for injury in school-aged children in the United States: A comparison of non-fatal injuries occurring within and outside of the school environment. Acad Emerg Med 13:567-570, 2006.

Mares M, Woodward EH: Prosocial effects on children's interactions. *In* Singer DG, Singer J (eds): Handbook of Children and the Media. Thousand Oaks, CA: Sage, 2001.

Mazzocco MM: Math learning disability and math LD subtypes: Evidence from studies of Turner syndrome, fragile X syndrome, and neurofibromatosis type 1. J Learn Disabil 34:520-533, 2001.

McKown C, Weinstein RS: The development and consequences of stereotype consciousness in middle childhood. Child Dev 74: 498-515, 2003.

Miller JG, Bersoff DM: Culture and moral judgment: How are conflicts between justice and interpersonal responsibilities resolved? J Person Soc Psychol 62:541-554, 1992.

Molfese V, Modglin A, Molfese D: The role of environment in the development of reading skills: A longitudinal study of preschool and school-age measures. J Learn Disabil 36:59-67, 2003.

Neuman RJ, Lobos E, Reich W, et al: Prenatal smoking exposure and dopaminergic genotypes interact to cause a severe ADHD subtype. Biol Psychiatry 61:1320-1328, 2006.

Nippold MA, Hesketh LJ, Duthie JK, Mansfield TC: Conversational versus expository discourse: A study of syntactic development in children, adolescents, and adults. J Speech Lang Hear Res 48:1048-1064, 2005.

Noble KG, Norman MF, Farah MJ: Neurocognitive correlates of socioeconomic status in kindergarten children. Dev Sci 8:74-87, 2005.

Noble KG, Tottenham NT, Casey BJ: Neuroscience perspectives on disparities in school readiness and cognitive achievement. Future Child 15:71-89, 2005.

Nunes T, Bryant P: Children Doing Mathematics. Oxford: Blackwell, 1996.

Oliver BR, Plomin R: Twins' Early Development Study (TEDS): A multivariate, longitudinal genetic investigation of language, cognition and behavior problems from childhood through adolescence. Twin Res Hum Genet 10:96-105, 2007.

Olweus D: Bullying and School: What We Know and What We Can Do. Oxford: Blackwell, 1993.

Patel DR, Pratt HD, Greydanus DE: Pediatric neurodevelopment and sports participation: When are children ready to play sports? Pediatr Clin North Am 49:505-531, v-vi, 2002.

Price-Williams DR, Gordon W, Ramirez M III: Skill and conversation: A study of pottery-making children. Dev Psychol 1:769, 1969.

Rigby K: School children's perceptions of their families and parents as a function of peer relations. J Genet Psychol 154:501-513, 1993.

Roberts W, Strayer J: Empathy, emotional responsiveness, and prosocial behavior. Child Dev 67:449-470, 1996.

Schettler T: Toxic threats to neurologic development of children. Environ Health Perspect 109(Suppl 6):813-816, 2001.

Siegler RS, Alibali MW: Children's Thinking, 4th ed. Upper Saddle River, NJ: Prentice Hall, 2005.

Smolkowski K, Biglan A, Barrera M, et al: Schools and Homes in Partnership (SHIP): Long-term effects of a preventive intervention focused on social behavior and reading skill in early elementary school. Prev Sci 6:113-125, 2005.

Speas C: Wake County Public School System Grades K-12 Literacy and Mathematics Assessment Results 1999-2000 (No. E&R-R-01.05). Raleigh, NC: Wake County Public School System, 2001.

Stein J, Schettler T, Wallinga D, Valenti M: In harm's way: Toxic threats to child development. J Dev Behav Pediatr 23(1 Suppl):S13-S22, 2002.

Stewart D, Sun J: How can we build resilience in primary school aged children? The importance of social support from adults and peers in family, school and community settings. Asia Pacif J Public Health 16(Suppl):S37-S41, 2004.

Szaflarski JP, Schmithorst VJ, Altaye M, et al: A longitudinal functional magnetic resonance imaging study of language development in children 5 to 11 years old. Ann Neurol 59:796-807, 2006.

Tan LH, Spinks JA, Eden GF, et al: Reading depends on writing, in Chinese. Proc Natl Acad Sci U S A 102:8781-8785, 2005.

Tanner JM, Davies PS: Clinical longitudinal standards for height and height velocity for North American children. J Pediatr 107:317-329, 1985.

Taylor BL, Attia MW: Sports-related injuries in children. Acad Emerg Med 7:1376-1382, 2000.

Toga AW, Thompson PM, Sowell ER: Mapping brain maturation. Trends Neurosci 29:148-159, 2006.

Washington RL, Bernhardt DT, Gomez J, et al: Organized sports for children and preadolescents. Pediatrics 107:1459-1462, 2001.

6 ADOLESCENCE

William Garrison and
Marianne E. Felice

Vignette

Johnny P., a 15-year-old boy, is a long-standing patient of Dr. K., a primary care physician. His mother brings him to the office now with a variety of parental concerns. After earning average grades throughout his previous school years, his achievement in his sophomore year of high school has been deteriorating rapidly. In the same time period, conflict with his parents, now divorced but living in the same large city, has escalated dramatically. His mother brings him to see Dr. K. so that she can "talk some sense into him." Mother describes Johnny as more oppositional than in previous years, secretive and withdrawn from the family, and more involved with his peer group, who are also mysterious to Johnny's parents. In addition to the expected pubertal physical changes in her son, the mother reports an increase in angry outbursts, lower frustration tolerance, a "whatever" attitude to the tasks of everyday life, a growing obsession with video games, and near-constant computer or cell phone contact with peers.

When alone with Dr. K., Johnny gradually admits to engaging in several risky behaviors, including initiating sexual activity with one or more female friends ("hooking up"), weekly marijuana and alcohol use ("it relaxes me"), occasional school truancy, and at least one incident of shoplifting with friends. At this point, Johnny becomes silent and looks to his pediatric provider as if to say, "OK, so what are you going to do about it?"

Dr. K. realizes quickly that she must sort out what is normal versus abnormal adolescent behavior and hatch a plan to address the teen's high-risk behaviors.

Adolescence is a transitional period between childhood and adulthood marked by dramatic growth in physical, psychological, social, cognitive, and moral development. G. S. Hall, a psychologist, coined the term *adolescence* in the early 1900s from the Latin derivative *adolescere,* which means, "to grow up." Some historians believe that the concept of adolescence is a relatively recent phenomenon since the Industrial Revolution. Margaret Mead's description of girls growing up in Samoa a century ago indicates, however, that even then common themes of a burgeoning awareness of sexuality and notable peer interactions were clearly present in this different culture. The observations of philosophers such as Socrates about the divide between youth and their parents could describe the arguments that occur in many homes today. In some of Shakespeare's plays (i.e., *Romeo and Juliet*; *A Winter's Tale*), the playwright laments many of the behaviors that we observe today, including sexuality, independence, and adolescent pregnancy. These examples support the argument that all young people undergo some universal developmental changes as they journey from childhood to adulthood, from immaturity to maturity. What is clearly different in modern times, however, is the relatively longer length of time adolescence consumes today compared with many generations ago.

Adolescence covers approximately one decade of life—roughly ages 10 to 20 years. Most experts do not view adolescence as one age group, but rather two or three distinct but overlapping phases: early adolescence (10 to 13 years old), mid adolescence (14 to 16 years old), and late adolescence (≥17 years old). Some authors prefer to use other terminology to describe these phases, such as preadolescent, adolescent, and youth. Regardless of the vocabulary, the concept is similar: A 13-year-old is different from a 19-year-old, and the social and psychological needs of younger adolescents differ from those of older adolescents. The age ranges noted are arbitrary and approximate and often overlap. Some 15-year-old teenagers may be grappling with early adolescent developmental tasks, others may be in mid adolescence, and a few may be ready for late adolescence. All three 15-year-old teenagers would be considered developmentally normal. Developmental phase also may depend on cultural variables and life events. A chronic illness may delay puberty and adolescence; a death of a parent may accelerate development and maturity. Psychosocial developmental age can be at variance with chronologic age, just as physical development may be at variance with chronologic age. An adolescent still can be completely within normal variants.

The term *adolescence* is sometimes used interchangeably with the term *pubescence*, but they are not the same. Pubescence refers to physiologic changes, particularly sexual maturity and reproductive capability. Adolescence refers to psychosocial growth and development. These two processes are interrelated and intertwined, however. Generally, pubescence heralds adolescence. Psychosocial attributes of the adolescent years usually are first noticed by parents, teachers, and siblings shortly after a child experiences the onset of puberty (described subsequently). The *beginning* of adolescence is easier to pinpoint than the *completion* of adolescence. Some individuals continue to grapple with adolescent issues well past the legal age of 21 years. Regardless of when adolescence ends, the transition to adulthood is complete when a physically and intellectually mature individual is able to formulate a distinct identity and develop the ability to respond to internal and external conflicts and challenges with a consistent and realistic value system.

PSYCHOSOCIAL GROWTH TASKS

The psychosocial growth tasks of adolescence have been described in various ways by many authorities and from different perspectives. Erikson (1968) characterized adolescence largely in terms of *identity formation*; Anna Freud (1966) marked adolescence as a time of struggles between a relatively strong *id* and a relatively weak *ego*; Blos (1967) wrote of adolescence as a second individuation process. Table 6-1 summarizes the developmental tasks commonly attributed to the adolescent age group (Felice and Friedman, 1982). These growth tasks occur concomitantly, but some tasks may be more prominent in different phases of adolescence than in others. Table 6-2 outlines the differences in the growth tasks in the three phases of adolescence.

Table 6-1. Psychosocial Growth Tasks of Adolescence

Gradual development as an independent individual
Mental evolvement of a satisfying, realistic body image
Harnessing appropriate control and expression of sexual drives
Expansion of relationships outside the home
Implementation of a realistic plan to achieve social and economic stability
Transition from concrete to abstract conceptualization
Integration of a value system applicable to life events

From Felice ME: Adolescence. In Levine MD, Carey WB, Crocker AC (eds): Developmental-Behavioral Pediatrics, 2nd ed. Philadelphia, WB Saunders, 1992, p 66.

Gradual Development as an Independent Individual

Before adolescence, most school-age children identify strongly with their families and look to one or both parents as role models. During early adolescence, young teenagers may begin to separate psychologically from their parents in an effort to establish their own identity. For many teens, this process may result in the adolescent taking issue with parental opinions, shunning parental viewpoints, and testing parental values. This verbal jousting with parents is an attempt to establish independence. In mid adolescence, teens may be ambivalent about the separation process as they experience unfamiliar situations. They may find themselves retreating to the comfort of the family and the familiar, and yet they can become angry with themselves for needing the comfort of the family. In some families, this ambivalence is expressed as hostility or bravado. By late adolescence, older teens are comfortable being away from home and in unfamiliar situations. In this later stage of development, many older adolescents are able to return to their parents and seek advice and counsel without feeling threatened or ashamed.

For many parents, the adolescent's efforts at separation are confusing and bewildering. They may be hurt that they no longer have the same closeness with their son or daughter that they perceived previously. They may be angry that the teen seems to contradict everything they say. Parents need reassurance about the normality of this process. They may be able to relate to a quotation attributed to Mark Twain: "At the age of 17, I could not believe how little my father knew. When I was 21, I could not believe how much he had learned in just 4 years."

Table 6-2. Growth Task Characteristics of the Three Phases of Adolescence

Tasks	Early: 10-13 Years	Mid: 14-16 Years	Late: ≥17 Years
1. Independence	Emotionally breaks from parents and prefers friends to family	Ambivalence about separation	Integration of independence issues
2. Body image	Adjustment to pubescent changes	"Trying on" different images to find real self	Integration of satisfying body image into personality
3. Sexual drives	Sexual curiosity; occasional masturbation	Sexual experimentation; individuals may be viewed as sex objects	Beginning of intimacy and caring
4. Relationships	Unisexual peer group; adult crushes	Begin heterosexual peer group; multiple adult role models	Individual relationships more important than peer group
5. Career plans	Vague and even unrealistic plans	Emerging plans may still be vague	Specific goals and specific steps to implement them
6. Conceptualization	Concrete thinking	Fascinated by new capacity for thinking	Ability to abstract
7. Value system	Decline in superego; testing of moral system of parents	Self-centered	Idealism; rigid concepts of right and wrong; other-oriented; asceticism

From Felice ME: Adolescence. *In* Levine MD, Carey WB, Crocker AC (eds): Developmental-Behavioral Pediatrics, 2nd ed. Philadelphia, WB Saunders, 1992, p 69.

Mental Evolvement of a Satisfying Realistic Body Image

In early adolescence, most teenagers are experiencing puberty and learning to adjust to the dramatic changes of pubescence. They are growing in height and weight; they are sprouting hair where it did not grow before. They have body odor and blemishes; breasts and genitalia have enlarged. Young adolescents are exquisitely self-conscious of their body's changes. They also are aware of changes in their classmates and friends and naturally compare their own changes with the changes of their friends. They worry that they may be developing too quickly or too slowly, and every adolescent needs reassurance about his or her physical development whether or not those concerns are expressed. By mid adolescence, most teenagers have already experienced puberty, but they may not yet be comfortable with the results. Young women and young men spend much time (and often money) trying to improve their faces and figures. These improvements can take the form of experimenting with different clothing styles to find a self-image that is comfortable to them. In late adolescence, most young people have begun to be comfortable with their bodies, although some young men (particularly so-called late bloomers) may continue to grow in height well into their early 20s. Although body image problems are not of major concern to most adolescents in their late teens, adolescents who have severe acne, a chronic illness, obesity, or anorexia nervosa may continue to have body image issues that are unresolved.

Harnessing Appropriate Control and Expression of Sexual Drives

Sexual and aggressive drives may be stronger during adolescence than at any other time of life. Learning to express and control these drives is a major and formidable task of the teenage years at a time when the young person may seem to be ill-equipped to master them. Becoming comfortable with one's sexuality is a major component of adolescent development. Early adolescence is mainly marked by sexual curiosity, and masturbation is common. In mid adolescence, teens begin further sexual experimentation, although not always full sexual intercourse. The percentage of high school students who have had sexual intercourse by age 16 years has decreased since the early 1990s; recent data indicate that about 50% of high school students report having had at least one voluntary sexual experience (Child Trends, 2005). These data may be obsolete in the next few years because more teenagers are engaging in a phenomenon known as "hooking up" or "friends with benefits," in which they have friendships solely for sex and not for romantic involvement, as in previous generations. Not all adolescents are heterosexual, and clinicians should be sensitive to and aware of the needs of homosexual and heterosexual teens. Some gay adolescents may delay the onset of sexual activity as they emotionally grapple with their sexual orientation.

During mid adolescence in both genders, there may be a tendency to view one's sexual partner as an opportunity for social gain. Late adolescence is distinguished by the ability to be intimate, that is, to care deeply for another person without the need for exploitation.

Expansion of Relationships Outside the Home

As adolescents move away emotionally from parents, they turn to relationships outside the home, which include a peer group and other adults. For most young adolescents, the peer group generally consists of members of the same gender. This unisexual peer group provides a psychological shelter in which youngsters can test out ideas and forge dyadic friendships without the often intense sexual tension created by proximity to the opposite sex (for heterosexual youth). Members of the peer group conform to certain group standards, such as dress, hairstyle, or even group rituals such as meeting at the same time at the same place every week. It also is common for young adolescents to develop friendships with adults outside the home (e.g., teacher, parent of a friend, another relative). Teens may prefer the company of extrafamilial adults (i.e., teachers, coaches) to the company of their own devoted parents. For many parents, this situation can cause hurt feelings and bewilderment. Such parents need reassurance that this can be normal behavior.

By mid adolescence, teenagers often expand their peer group to include heterosexual friendships, and for many teenagers, this period marks the beginning of dating patterns. Teens in mid adolescence also have a tendency to turn to adults outside the home as role models. Teens are exposed to family structures, religious beliefs, and lifestyles different from their own family, and this is an impetus for teens to "try on" different styles and philosophies. Parents may find this situation confusing and hurtful. In reality, most teenagers return to the family fold as young adults. For youth in late adolescence, individual relationships gradually assume more importance than the larger peer group relationships. Friendships are often more intense, and issues are discussed with more depth. The superficiality of previous years should be on the wane. The bonds of friendship are particularly strong among youth who are working toward a common goal for a common task, such as college roommates, sports team members, or military recruits.

Implementation of a Realistic Plan for Social and Economic Stability

Adolescents must decide what they want to do as adults to support themselves financially and socially. For young teens, this is a vague concept and may even be unrealistic. Teens in mid adolescence give more thought to this problem, but they may still be unrealistic. A typical 16-year-old may view a future job prospect as a way to escape from home or the opportunity to do something glamorous. For youths in late adolescence, the future is a serious issue, and they are often faced with hard decisions. This is a common problem among seniors in high school. Some teenagers find the final career choice so difficult that they avoid all decision making and simply go along with decisions made for them by parents or teachers. Eventually, these teens may pay an emotional price and end up resenting the adults who made the decisions for them. Clinical experience suggests that an adolescent who struggles with this decision making and does what he or she wants to do, rather than what someone else wants him or her to do, is more likely to achieve career satisfaction.

Transition from Concrete to Abstract Conceptualization

Cognitive development is a key component of adolescence and is described in more detail later in this chapter. Briefly, in terms of the described growth tasks, cognitive development is differentiated across the three phases of adolescence. A young adolescent thinks more concretely with limited abilities for abstraction; this has implications for health professionals who are taking a history from a 12-year-old in early adolescence. If a clinician wishes to discover if a young teenage girl has been sexually active, it may not be wise to ask, "Have you ever slept with a boy?" The answer, yes or no, may have nothing to do with sexual intercourse, just sleeping. Teens in mid adolescence have a greater capacity for abstraction and are usually more capable of introspection; mid adolescents can think about thinking. This is a giant step in mental development, and some teens become fascinated with this newfound intellectual tool. This aspect of adolescence may be another factor contributing to the self-centered behavior of teenagers in mid adolescence.

Teenagers in late adolescence are often capable of stretching their mental faculties immensely. Solutions to many problems are often thought through in great detail, but older teens often have a rigid value system that may limit their problem solving skills. Creative achievement may be quite remarkable at this age, particularly in the arts. The social implications of the cognitive development of late adolescents are many. Older adolescents can be very interesting and avid conversationalists with opinions on every issue. In addition, adolescents at this stage of development can now see a host of alternatives to parents' directions and may promptly point these out to a beleaguered mother or father.

Integration of a Value System Applicable to Life Events

Moral growth is a key concept to gaining maturity and is discussed in more detail later in this chapter. With respect to the developmental growth tasks, there are clear differences between early, mid, and late adolescence. In early adolescence, it is not unusual for young teens to experience a temporary decline in the superego as they make the transition from childhood under the watchful eye of parents to the more independent nature of adolescence when parents are not always present to tell teens what is right and wrong. The "collective conscience" of the peer group may be at odds with a teenager's parental standards. In some instances, a teen may feel the need to test the parent's moral code. An example of the decline in the superego in early adolescence could be the stealing of hubcaps in response to a group dare or as a group activity. Under ordinary circumstances, individual teens might never consider stealing hubcaps, but under group pressure, they may feel forced to do so. If such teens are caught in this activity, they are usually embarrassed and ashamed about their involvement.

Mid adolescence is marked by a narcissistic value system (i.e., "What is right is what makes me feel good"; "What is right is what I want"); this partially explains the sexual exploitation described previously. A clinical consequence of this type of thinking is that many teens in mid adolescence engage in activities impulsively with little thought about the consequences, such as unprotected intercourse. This self-serving behavior may be frightening and provoke anxiety in the adolescent. If there are no checks on impulses, the teenager may feel out of control. To guard against this outcome, he or she may develop severe moral standards with rigid concepts of right and wrong, particularly in late adolescence. Asceticism and idealism are common. Older adolescents are often very altruistic, and they may embrace moral causes with much zeal. Issues are often viewed in terms of black and white with self-righteous indignation and sometimes with self-imposed restrictions and prohibitions. Although a youth in late adolescence may champion "justice" and "rightness," there is little tolerance for opposing points of view. One could speculate that the transition to adulthood occurs when an individual finds that there are suddenly more "gray" issues in life than black-and-white ones.

CHARACTERISTICS OF THE THREE PHASES OF ADOLESCENT DEVELOPMENT

As noted previously, adolescents grapple with all seven growth tasks concomitantly, but some tasks are emphasized more clearly in one developmental phase than in others (see Table 6-2). Growth in some tasks may influence growth in other areas. Progression through all the tasks is necessary for healthy adulthood and emotional maturity.

Early Adolescence (10 to 13 Years Old)

The major developmental task of young adolescents is establishing independence from their parents. This process cannot occur in a vacuum, so adolescents turn to their peer group, who are usually members of the same gender. This is a normal phenomenon for heterosexual and homosexual adolescents. In addition, it is not unusual for young teenagers to have "crushes" on adults outside the home, or to idealize them compared with their all-too-familiar and imperfect parents. Early adolescents are usually in the throes of puberty and must adjust to a rapidly changing body and a changing body image. Although young teens are curious and fascinated with sexuality, most young teens have not yet begun to have sexual intercourse, even though they may reside within a larger society seemingly obsessed and titillated by sexual themes and innuendo. Young adolescents are concrete thinkers and may have vague and even unrealistic plans for a future career. There may be some testing of the parents' value system as the teenager struggles to develop a moral code. Early adolescence is marked by a unisexual peer group, concerns about puberty, and active establishment of independence from parents.

Mid Adolescence (14 to 16 Years Old)

The major developmental task in mid adolescence is sexual identity, that is, becoming comfortable with one's sexuality. This task includes the need to become comfortable with one's body and with one's body image. Many teens in mid adolescence "try on" different images in hopes of finding a "true" self; this may be expressed in their dress code or mannerisms and may change from week to week. Teens in mid adolescence generally begin heterosexual dating patterns. Gay or lesbian adolescents have the same developmental growth tasks as heterosexual adolescents, but the timing of their dating experiences may be delayed or influenced by other factors, such as self-acceptance of their homosexuality or perceived attitudes toward homosexuality in their environments. Teens in mid adolescence also begin to grapple with issues related to morality as their cognitive functions expand with the capacity and capability for abstraction. They begin to think about thinking. Career plans usually begin to take some shape, but may not be definite.

Late Adolescence (17 Years Old and Older)

The primary focus of late adolescence is planning a career or how one will contribute to society as a responsible adult. This planning is accompanied by high idealism, rigid concepts of right and wrong, and the newfound ability to think through problems with various alternatives. In addition, youth in late adolescence can shed the strong need to belong to a peer group in favor of a close, intimate, and caring relationship with another person. For many youngsters, finding a partner or significant other becomes a major search, and this is the usual time of falling in love for the first time.

BIOLOGIC BASIS FOR MAJOR DEVELOPMENTAL CHANGES

Hormonal Changes of Puberty

The onset of puberty marks the metamorphosis of a child into an adult capable of reproduction. The exact trigger that begins pubescence is unknown. It is known, however, that puberty is associated with specific changes in the hypothalamic-pituitary-adrenal axis. Sometime in late childhood, there is increased production of adrenal androgens before there are any physical signs of puberty. This increased production of adrenal androgens is followed by an increasing pulsatile secretion of gonadotropin-releasing hormone during sleep. Gonadotropin-releasing hormone secretion results in increasing levels of luteinizing hormone (LH) and to a lesser extent follicle-stimulating hormone (FSH). In males, LH stimulates the Leydig cells in the testes to produce testosterone, and later FSH stimulates testicular Sertoli cells to support the development of sperm. In females, FSH stimulates follicle growth in the ovary and the production of aromatase. LH stimulates ovarian thecal cells to produce androgens; aromatase converts androgens to estrogens in the FSH-stimulated granulosa cells. Later in puberty, under separate control mechanisms, a mid–menstrual cycle surge of estradiol results in an elevation of LH to trigger ovulation (Joffe and Blythe, 2003).

In addition to the above-mentioned gonadotropins, other hormones are released during puberty. The pituitary begins to secrete human growth hormone; this is regulated by growth hormone–releasing factor and somatostatin. Growth hormone–releasing factor is released in a pulsatile fashion during sleep. Insulin-like growth factor I (IGF-I or somatomedin C) and IGF-II are produced by the liver and influence growth, particularly growth rate, as does thyroxine and the corticosteroids. Parathyroid hormone, 1,25-dihydroxyvitamin D, and calcitonin affect skeletal mineralization. The release, surge, and interaction of all of these hormones result in the physical changes observed during adolescence.

Three areas show the dramatic changes of puberty: an increase in weight, an increase in height, and sexual development. Girls typically experience puberty about 2 years earlier than boys. The first sign of puberty in girls is usually the development of breast buds between the ages of 8 and 10 years. The start of pubic hair, further development of breasts, a height spurt, a weight spurt, and menarche then follow in a well-described pattern (Tanner, 1962). Menarche signifies the end of pubertal development in girls. In boys, puberty is signaled clinically by darkening of the scrotal skin, enlargement of the testes, and lengthening of the penis between the ages of 10 and 12 years. The proliferation of pubic hair, additional enlargement of the genitalia, and a height spurt follow over the next 2 to 6 years (Tanner, 1962). Other pubertal changes, such as acne, axillary hair, deepening of the voice, and the growth of chest hair in boys, also are characteristic, but vary from one individual to another, depending on genetic and cultural factors. The most dramatic changes of puberty usually occur in early adolescence, but it is common for young men, particularly "late bloomers," to continue to grow taller into their early 20s.

Neurologic Maturational Changes

In recent years, there has been a shift in how biologists view the process of puberty. Previously, the process of puberty was described solely by the hormonal aspects of puberty as related to reproduction. A large body of literature has developed, however, that has focused on the neural control of hormone secretion and a gradual awareness of extensive brain remodeling during adolescence. This literature has led to an emphasis on a neuronal basis for reproductive maturation (Sisk and Foster, 2004). In this model, the onset of puberty is viewed not as a gonadal event, but rather as a brain event.

Human adolescent development involves widespread changes in the gross morphology of the brain. The volume of white matter increases linearly as a result of increased myelination of cortical and subcortical fiber tracts. Gray matter volume takes an inverted U-shaped course, first increasing and then decreasing. The age of peak gray matter thickness varies by gender, occurring 1 year earlier in girls than in boys and correlating with the earlier average age of puberty onset in girls (Sisk and Zehr, 2005). The structural bases of adolescent changes in gross morphology of gray matter have not yet been determined, but many investigators interpret the adolescent reduction in gray matter volume as evidence for synaptic pruning (Sisk and Zehr, 2005). It is now generally accepted that steroids play an important role in brain development during the adolescent years. Steroid-dependent organization of neural circuits is a fundamental feature of adolescent brain development, broadening the influence of pubertal hormones beyond a purely activational role to agents of neural rearrangement (Sisk and Zehr, 2005). This area of neuromaturation of the adolescent brain is an exciting new topic that is being studied and debated in the field. More information is unfolding on a regular basis and is expected to add further to the body of literature on how and why puberty occurs.

DEVELOPMENTAL DOMAINS

Mastering the seven key psychosocial growth tasks listed in Table 6-1 typically determines the relative success or failure of teens as they transition into adulthood. Most teenagers do well in this transition. The adolescent years can be a time of elevated emotional vulnerability. Adolescence as a stage in human development is not as catastrophic or dire, however, as early developmental theorists, and many contemporary parents, might surmise. The reality is that most teens manage to steer successfully through the maze of adolescence, perhaps awkwardly at first, then more skillfully as they mature, and typically emerge as adults functioning well within the range of normal.

Pertinent to clinical work with teens, it seems that when adolescence becomes a persistently painful or problematic phase for a young individual, it is a clear sign that something has "gone wrong" in personal development or the environment itself, and it should not be categorized simplistically as just a symptom of *being a teenager*. To understand how things go awry in adolescence requires a familiarity with several major developmental domains, what should occur in those domains, and various factors that can derail normal development. These domains each represent essential ingredients necessary for the key tasks of adolescence cited earlier. Put in simpler terms, each domain represents a basic building block for successful human development during the second decade of life. These domains can be captured by three key questions:

1. "How well can I think, reason and decide?" (cognitive-developmental functioning)
2. "How well do I interact with others?" (moral and social development)
3. "Who am I, and do I like who I am?" (emergence of a sense of self)

In the following sections, we attempt to examine and discuss each of these topics in greater depth.

Cognitive-Developmental Functioning

Before the 1980s, much of the empiric work on cognitive development in adolescents was strongly influenced by the work of the major theorist Piaget. His "stage" theory of human cognitive development was a useful rubric for the study and understanding of how a child's burgeoning mental skills evolve over time from thought based solely on the outward appearances of things to concrete operations or mental skills that allow a child to solve problems mentally through steps from beginning to end. Piaget also theorized that a young adolescent's thought processes gradually evolved further, to a more abstract and multifactorial form of thinking Piaget called *formal operations*. Developmental research in the last 20 years has cast doubt, however, on the assumption that all adolescents (or adults, for that matter) actually achieve the stage Piaget labeled formal operations. Some research has suggested that less than half of adults found in industrialized societies achieve the formal operational stage Piaget described (Kuhn et al, 1977).

More recently, the field of developmental psychology has adopted an "information-processing approach" to the study of cognition in teenagers (Steinberg and Morris, 2001). In contrast to a Piagetian view, these studies would argue that there is wide variation in individual capacity to "think" and "process" information during adolescence. This variation is apparently due to a complex interaction between overall cognitive abilities and the accrual of environmental experience.

Two concepts regarding cognitive development in adolescents hold particular value for clinicians seeking to understand and help teenagers. First is *metacognition*, or the ability to "think about thoughts," a process that largely explains an adolescent's continuous growth in cognitive skills and the ability to draw on a useful store of knowledge accrued over time. Metacognition is the process whereby one is able to use knowledge from past experience and merge such knowledge with the challenges of a new task or problem, review and reflect on possible strategies, and eventually *solve or resolve* the tasks of everyday life, while navigating through the major social and emotional challenges of adolescence and adulthood. Metacognitive processes are thought to be largely responsible for helping adolescents successfully counterbalance an array of conflicting thoughts and emotions "new" to their experience, by virtue of rapid biologic growth and dramatically expanding life experiences.

Second, a *computational model* of cognitive developmental functioning in adolescents seems to be more useful than a "stage" model in explaining huge differences in the mental capacities of adolescents, which go beyond numerical differences in measurable intelligence (i.e., I.Q.). Generally, the effects of home milieu, schooling, and general life experience should combine to strengthen an adolescent's increasing mental capacities. The lack of appropriate stimulation in any of these life contexts, or the presence of considerable stress or trauma, also can act to limit or stultify individual cognitive development during adolescence.

According to the information-processing perspective, general intelligence remains stable during adolescence, but dramatic improvements evolve in the specific mental abilities that underlie intelligence. Verbal, mathematical, and spatial abilities increase, memory capacity grows, and adolescents are more adept at dividing their attention. In addition, their abstract and hypothetical thought grows; they know more about the world, and their store of knowledge increases (Feldman, 2006).

This contemporary view of adolescent cognitive development helps us to understand wide differences detectable in the overall cognitive and judgmental functioning of teenagers. If all adolescents were equally able to manipulate easily abstract concepts related to everyday life, we would expect far fewer problems arising from poor decision making in teens and young adults. Similarly, the broad variability in adolescent abilities to employ acquired knowledge and scientific reasoning helps to explain the real-life differences in achievement observed in teenagers.

Moral and Social Development in Adolescence

From the 1960s through the late 1970s, Kohlberg's theory of moral development dominated thinking about adolescent social decision making. To this day, the theory holds heuristic value for clinicians seeking to understand a young person's moral transition from childhood through the adolescent years (Kohlberg and Gilligan, 1972). This theory suggests that a child (4 to 10 years old) moves from evaluating morality largely from judgments about "good and bad" (essentially derived from the cues of adult authority figures) to moral decision making that relies on conventional definitions of "right and wrong," conventions that derive from an amalgam of parental, peer, and macrocultural influences. Much debate continues regarding the relative weight parental versus peer influence wields on adolescent moral and social decision making, with the bulk of empirical research supporting the view that most adolescents are affected by parents and peers in comparable measure, but in competing *and* concerted ways (Harris, 1998; Steinberg, 2001). A central problem in using Kohlberg's theory of moral development in clinical settings, however, is the fact that advanced-stage moral thinking is not always accompanied by advanced-stage moral behavior. In other words, it is clear that many people, including teenagers, often act or behave at odds with their capacity to recognize "right from wrong."

As we learn more about social, emotional, and moral growth during adolescence, we find that most adolescents do well in their journey from childhood to adulthood. Their social experiences appear rich and varied, and evolve rapidly from a view that is strongly influenced by peer influences to one that incorporates personal, familial, and societal/community values. Adolescents who do not fare well are the ones health care providers and others seek to help. Teens who need help in these areas are often those who have poor academic or work achievement, dysfunctional social relations, drug and alcohol abuse, chronic risk-taking, and antisocial behavior in general.

Emergence of Self

One reason psychological issues seem so dramatic during the adolescent years is simply due to the fact the issues are new to the experience of the teens and those around them, especially parents, teachers, and siblings. Biologic and cognitive changes give rise to a re-definition of the internal ("Who am I?") and the external ("What is the meaning of life?"). Too much has been written about this journey of self-discovery to be reviewed here. A synthesis of research and theory on the phenomenology of adolescence might provide the following key points:

1. Children generally evolve from a largely egocentric view of themselves, in terms of worldview and event causation, to a more realistic view during adolescence and adulthood that takes into account others' perspectives and allows for multiple-factor causation of events. A growing awareness of other people's perceptions can be a double-edged sword, however, heightening the adolescent's fears of being scrutinized and judged by peers or adults.
2. Self-esteem processes evolve from evaluation that stems largely from "What can I do/what am I good at" and "Who likes me/rejects me," to a more coalesced sense of identity that derives from an emerging self-appraisal based on past and current life experience. In Eriksonian terms, the child moves from the task of "Industry versus Inferiority" during the preadolescent years to one of "Identity versus Role Confusion" (Erikson, 1963). Less understood during this important developmental transition is the role of individual personality variables (at least partly due to biogenetic influences) on the expression of adolescent emotionality and self-appraisal. Although it is a given that we would see heightened emotionality in most teens, only personality differences seem to explain the wide range in variation adolescents show in negative emotions and poor coping with strong emotions.
3. Becoming comfortable with one's sexuality and accepting of one's body is a major component of adolescent development, but often extends into adulthood. Cultural and societal norms have a major influence in these areas of development. The emphasis on "thinness" in modern society as the ideal model for beauty is a different cultural norm today than it was in previous centuries and may be influencing the wave of eating disorders that is pervasive among many teenage girls in recent years. It is not unusual for women as well as adolescent girls to struggle with body image issues. Although modern society is more open about sexual activity and sexual orientation than it was in previous generations, there are many communities in which sex before marriage is unacceptable for adults and teenagers, and there are many areas of the United States in which gay and lesbian couples are not welcomed. These external factors have a strong influence on body image and sexual identity acceptance.

Much research is being done to understand adolescent development in all of its facets. Developmental theory and research seeks to help understand how it is that adolescents come to think about their internal and external world, and how they make meaning of their emotions, social relationships, and their emerging sense of selves as individuals in a crowded world of others. Developmental theory and research helps clinicians to see how adolescents come to hold values, beliefs, and attitudes that serve to guide their adult behavior, and how all these factors help to set the stage for the discovery of lifelong goals and loving relationships that seem necessary to achieve satisfying and well-adjusted adult development.

CULTURAL VARIATIONS IN ADOLESCENCE

Changes in the ethnic makeup of American youth during the past 20 years merit special attention in any contemporary chapter on adolescence. Understanding the diversity of American youth to develop healthcare and social intervention systems of care should be a high priority for all. As with other areas of psychosocial and medical research, most studies of normal adolescent development have involved only samples of European-American, heterosexual youth. In contrast, studies of teens judged at elevated risk for psychiatric and health problems often contain samples almost exclusively composed of ethnic minorities (Hagen et al, 2004). This schism in sampling techniques may underestimate levels of dysfunction in the general population of teens and overstate the case that most problems occur in "high-risk" youth in largely urban and poor communities.

Although it is clear that the risk-likelihood for mental health disorders and stressful life events increases dramatically with the presence of factors such as poverty and its concomitant lack of resources, adolescents from all social classes seem to be at elevated risk for adjustment issues. The sheer numbers of teens found within nonwhite groups is expected to continue to grow over the next 10 years, and these youth would be overrepresented among the poor (at rates of double to triple that of white youth). It has been estimated that the number of white juveniles will increase by 3% through 2015, whereas the number of Asian/Pacific-Islander, Hispanic, and African-American adolescents will increase by 75%, 59%, and 19% (Office of Juvenile Justice and Delinquency Prevention, 1999). At the same time, approximately one in four teens from Hispanic and African-American families live below the poverty level (National Association of Social Workers, 2001).

Studies of academic achievement in the United States are illustrative of how the risks of ethnic origins are largely mediated by socioeconomic status (SES).

> *On average, middle- and high-SES students earn higher grades, score higher on achievement tests, and complete more years of schooling than students from lower-SES homes. Several environmental factors explain this discrepancy including less adequate nutrition and health, crowded conditions, attending inadequate schools, fewer places to do homework, a lack of books and computers. In addition, parents living in poverty are less likely to be involved in their children's schooling. On average, African American and Hispanic students tend to perform at lower levels, receive lower grades, and score lower on achievement tests, than Caucasian students. When socioeconomic status is controlled for, achievement differences diminish (Feldman, 2000).*

Some research has suggested that "culture-bound disorders" also may exist, and that attitudes toward mental health problems vary by ethnic group, affecting how and what treatments adolescents from minority populations seek (Bains, 2001). Community-based prevention and intervention programs that begin well before adolescence have been identified as most likely to be effective in behavioral and mental health problem areas (Baruch, 2001).

CLINICAL IMPLICATIONS

Adolescents receive clinical care in various settings: private physician offices, adolescent clinics, public health clinics, and school-based health clinics. Regardless of the settings, there are commonly accepted guidelines for successful interactions and interventions with teens. First, the setting must be welcoming to the teen. For example, there are chairs big enough for teens in the waiting room; there are magazines appropriate for teens; there are brochures available and posters on the wall all reflecting the fact that adolescents are expected and welcomed.

Second, adolescents and parents must be interviewed separately so that the clinician can take a history concerning sexuality or drugs or both without the teenager being afraid to answer truthfully. When asking about drugs or sexuality, it may be helpful first to ask about friends' activities in these areas and then to ask about the teen's activities. This is one way that the questions may be less threatening. When asking about sexuality, it is important that the interviewer not presume that all adolescents are heterosexual and to ask questions in such a way that the homosexual adolescent would feel free to answer honestly. For example, the clinician may ask: "Do you have a boyfriend or girlfriend?" or "Everyone has sexual thoughts and feelings sometimes. With you, do you find yourself having sexual thoughts about sex with boys or girls or both?"

Third, adolescents should be told about confidentiality, and that the clinician will hold information in confidence except in those instances when the adolescent is a danger to self or others. Clinical sites should ensure that all staff, including the frontline staff, are educated about adolescents' rights to confidentiality and the site's expectations as to how adolescents should be treated. It is not unusual to find out that adolescents are reluctant to use a certain facility not because of the clinician, but because of an unpleasant experience they had with the person who answered the phone.

Fourth, all clinical sites should be familiar with the laws of the individual state concerning the rights of minors to receive health care without parental consent. In most states, these laws allow adolescents to be seen for the treatment of sexually transmitted infections or the prescribing of contraceptives without parental knowledge or consent. Although some parents may question these efforts, most parents understand the explanation that the clinician is helping the young person become more responsible for his or her own health care, and most parents are relieved that their son or daughter is receiving special attention from a trusted health care provider.

Returning briefly to the vignette described at the beginning of this chapter, we note that Dr. K. did interview Johnny P. alone. In doing so, she encountered a common clinical scenario—a patient who has minor problems that are not unusual during adolescence, but who also has some serious issues that need to be addressed soon. Johnny P. was not simply showing some of the normal psychological changes adolescents often display, he was also beginning to engage in a range of risky behaviors that had the clear potential to derail his development from typical to abnormal. The clinician's evaluation phase must attend to underlying changes attributable to adolescence per se and specific risky behaviors or attitudes that need intervention. Experimentation with drugs and alcohol, increasing sexual activity (often with multiple partners), and a strong, perhaps exclusive sphere of peer influence all foretell potential serious problems and may lead to significant psychosocial setbacks in a teenager.

As the child proceeds from the early adolescent to the mid and late adolescent phases, understanding how his or her individual development can be facilitated or derailed is crucial to early detection and intervention in teenagers' lives. As we have seen earlier, the complex interplay among the different but equally important domains of development—cognitive, emotional, social, moral, and emergence of "self"—can be daunting for the clinician to sort out. Imagine what it must be like for the adolescent! Significant disruption in any one or more of these areas can lead to psychological disorders or serious issues of maladjustment during adolescence and beyond.

Our fundamental view of the adolescent period is as an important developmental transition characterized by predictable change and overall stability in most youngsters, rather than a time of unmanageable or overwhelming "storm and stress." When adolescent development goes much awry in a young individual's life, it typically is due to the presence of one or more well-known factors known to put all humans at increased risk for psychological disorders, including (1) the powerful and insidious *effects of poverty,* which clearly affect minority and urban families at higher rates (especially as related to parenting practices, academic achievement, and overall quality of the community milieu); (2) the overall level of *family cohesion during and preceding the adolescent period*; and (3) the influence of *genetic history and biologic vulnerabilities* during adolescence.

Adolescence can be a time of heightened psychosocial vulnerability, but the onset of behavioral, emotional, and psychiatric problems in adolescents is more typically heralded by preexisting issues or problems that can be seen brewing during the early and preadolescent years. Adolescence does not occur de novo; it flows from infancy and childhood. These early problems, often magnified during adolescence and so more easily discerned, can be traced directly to family histories of similar dysfunction within the immediate and extended family pedigree. It has become too common and convenient to blame all clinical problems teens encounter on adolescence itself, rather than recognizing the larger biogenetic etiology of human psychological disorders and maladjustment to life.

Adolescents who encounter significant adjustment issues or come to the point where psychiatric diagnoses are appropriate often fall into broad categories of behavior description: *internalizing* and *externalizing* subtypes. Many of the teens encountered in health care settings may fall short of meeting all criteria for a formal psychiatric diagnosis, but present with significant problems of adjustment that merit attention and intervention. Some studies have estimated that 40% of adolescents show significant depressive symptoms, including dysphoric mood, low self-esteem, and suicidal ideation, at some point during the teen years (Steinberg, 1983), and about 15% of teens meet criteria for a depression diagnosis (Evans et al, 2005). Most of these teens improve with time and maturation, but all deserve evaluation and intervention.

The most intensive research efforts in this area have been focused on juvenile delinquency and its related behavioral manifestations of criminal behavior and substance abuse. This focus is understandable in light of the fact that conduct disorder is the most prevalent psychiatric diagnosis seen in clinical settings that treat teenagers (although anxiety and depressive disorders are more prevalent in the general population). Perhaps a reassuring finding from this body of work is that approximately 80% of adolescents cannot be formally labeled as "offenders" (i.e., defined as being apprehended and found guilty of a crime), although many of this group have and do engage in illegal behavior, strictly defined. One large, influential study of offending youth concluded that adolescent risk-taking was overly characterized as dangerous by adults, but that the more germane issues for teens involved increasing drug and alcohol use, problems associated with the dyad of heightened emotionality and impulsivity (i.e., anger/violence, suicidality), and antisocial behavior that fell considerably short of *criminality* (Offer and Boxer, 1991).

A high percentage of juvenile offenders, 80% (Kazdin, 2000), also meet criteria for one or more psychiatric diagnoses. Various studies suggest that 50% to 60% of juvenile offenders can be diagnosed with conduct disorder, followed by substance abuse (25% to 50%) and affective disorders (30% to 75%) (Grisso, 1998). Most juvenile offenders do not continue such behavior as adults (Grisso, 1998). There is evidence, however, that psychiatric issues continue in such youths as they enter the young adult years.

RISKY BEHAVIORS

The most common "risky behaviors" in youth are likely to be related to premature sexual activity, alcohol use, and poor impulse control in the operation of motor vehicles. Similar to Johnny P. in the opening vignette, most teens who engage in risky behaviors remain unknown to police or judicial authorities (similar to their risk-taking elders), but are more likely to come to the attention of parents, teachers, and often medical providers. Much less likely to be identified, although equally at risk, are the more prevalent number of youth with depressive and anxiety-based problems who are not or cannot be seen as conduct-disordered by the society at large. The fact remains that adolescents with psychiatric disorders are much more likely than normal adolescents to engage in risky behaviors with some frequency over longer duration (Flaherty, 1997), so screening for psychiatric issues often addresses both problem areas at once.

Teens engage in risky behaviors at alarming rates. It has been estimated that 12% of adolescents engage in heavy smoking, 15% engage in heavy drinking, 5% engage in frequent marijuana use, and 3% engage in frequent use of cocaine (Dryfoos, 1990). More recent studies in the United States and abroad suggest that some of these risky teen behaviors are dramatically increasing (Aggleton et al, 2000). Mean alcohol consumption by teens, ages 11 through 15 years, was estimated to increase 50% in Great Britain during a 10-year period in the 1990s. Similarly, behavioral epidemiology has identified illicit drug and alcohol use and teen sexual activity and its consequences as the key morbidities in the U.S. adolescent population (Friedman et al, 1998). Although teen birth rates have consistently decreased since the early 1990s, the United States still has the highest teen birth rates of all developed countries, and sexually transmitted infection rates have not decreased at all in that time period and may have increased (Child Trends, 2005).

ADOLESCENT CLINICAL SIGNS AND SYMPTOMS

How we approach the clinical evaluation of youth at risk can vary widely from setting to setting. Some providers now use screening techniques shown to be more accurate in identifying the full range of behavioral and emotional symptoms, and which place the individual child's symptoms in direct comparison with large samples of comparable youth (i.e., standardized norm-referenced checklists, questionnaires, and structured interviews where possible). These techniques have the advantage of saving time for busy practitioners, are usually more thorough during the initial evaluation phase, and provide a baseline for monitoring change over time, but are useful only in settings that are conducive to such questionnaires, such as middle-class practices that have English-speaking patients and parents. A good example of a screening questionnaire approach for teens is the BASC (*Behavior Assessment System for Children, Second Edition*), a general approach to measuring symptoms and strengths in children and adolescents (Reynolds and Kamphaus, 2004). Similarly, the *Beck Depression Inventory for Adolescents* (Beck, 1996) is an example of a disorder-specific instrument that can be administered and scored in the primary care setting. There are now many screening instruments to choose from, and questionnaires for a wide range of specific adolescent disorders or behaviors can be used.

The reality is that most health care and mental health providers use unstructured interview techniques to evaluate and diagnose most adolescents. A commonly used psychosocial interview tool that many clinicians find helpful is HEADSS (Table 6-3), which has been used successfully in many clinical settings (Cohen et al, 1991). Essentially all of these methods have the same goal: to identify and list the range of behavioral, emotional, and social "symptoms" for any given adolescent seen in a clinical setting and to gauge the severity of the presenting problems.

Table 6-3. HEADSS Interview Instrument

H	Home	Who lives with the teen? Own room? What are relationships like at home? How often has the family moved? Who does the teen turn to if problems? What happens if parents are angry?
E	Education/ Employment	What grade is the teen in? School grades? Favorite subjects? Best subjects? Worst? Any failures? Repeated classes? Truancy? Does the teen feel safe at school? Who does the teen turn to if problems? Future goals or ambitions?
A	Activities	What does the teen do for fun? Who are the teen's peers? Any organized sports? Clubs? Any hobbies? Church attendance? What does the teen do with peers? With family? Does teen have a car? Does teen use seatbelts?
D	Drugs	Used by peers? Used by teen? Alcohol? Cigarettes? Marijuana? How much? When? Where? With whom? Use by family members? Source? How paid for?
S	Sexuality	Orientation? Sexual experience? Number of partners? Masturbation? History of pregnancy or abortion? History of STIs? Contraception? Type? History of physical or sexual abuse?
S	Suicide/ Depression	Sleep disorders? Fatigue? Appetite changes? Feeling of hopelessness? Isolation? Boredom? Withdrawn? History of past suicide attempts? History of family suicides? History of recurrent accidents? Decreased affect? Preoccupation with death? Suicidal ideation?

Adapted from HEADSS for Adolescents.
Available at http://chipts.ucla.edu/assessment/Assessment_Instruments/Assessment_pdf_New/Assess_headss_pdf.pdf. Accessed August 26, 2008.

TREATMENT OVERVIEW: HELPING TODAY'S TEENS AND TOMORROW'S ADULTS

Ideally, there should be effective, comprehensive, prevention programs in place to help at-risk teens avoid harmful behavior. The cost and limitations in ability to penetrate the most at-risk teen populations before problems occur have hampered these efforts, however. Proactive, community-based interventions are more powerful than individually focused interventions, such as traditional psychotherapy, for adolescents. Because of logistical constraints on, and political resistance to, major overhaul of health care delivery to teens, public health attempts to make significant strides in prevention of social and psychiatric disorders in adolescence have been far less than successful. Only about half of all high schools in the United States offer on-site mental health services. Despite this, it has been estimated that 70% to 80% of teens who receive any mental health services are seen in such school-based clinical settings (Burns et al, 1995). This leaves a very large proportion of troubled youth who receive no professional mental health attention at all. Many critics of our current programs for youth have called for a major overhaul in the way mental health services are provided to American youth, starting with a merging of educational and health-related services, and the funding that drives both.

Psychopharmacologic interventions for troubled adolescents, although clearly often effective and important treatments, have increased exponentially during the past 20 years (see Chapter 90). This sudden surge in use of medications—particularly the burgeoning use of stimulant medications for attention-deficit and disruptive behavior disorders, and the expanding range and volume of antidepressant medications prescribed to American teenagers—has given rise to intense social critique and revised federal guidelines regarding psychotropic medication and youth. Although psychopharmacologic agents have a valuable place in the armamentarium of health care providers who help adolescents, they must not replace broader social, educational, and mental health interventions for teens. Medical and public health models that overly rely on the use of psychopharmacologic interventions typically miss the point of much of the social research concerning troubled youth over the past 50 to 60 years.

Identification and treatment of adolescents with substance abuse problems has overlap with internalizing and externalizing psychological symptoms and merits special attention in health care or school settings that see teenagers (see Chapter 45). Substance use/abuse rates in U.S. teens have been relatively stable since 1996, with minor decreases in some drug types and increases in others (Johnston et al, 2006). Alcohol abuse, in particular, has been described as increasing alarmingly in college-age youth in the last decade. One popular psychological view has proposed that substance use/abuse is a form of "self-medication" for troubled teens (and adults) who, for whatever reason, perceive no other treatment options readily available to them. Many adolescents and young adults begin to engage in substance abuse behaviors largely because of peer and perhaps larger societal pressures or influences to do so (e.g., the "smoking is cool" advertising campaigns of the 1950s and 1960s; the current symbiotic relationship between televised sporting events in the United States and the consumption of beer). The growing number of young individuals with various addictions is not simply a product of individual psychological processes or problems. Rather, substance abuse seems to be a problem that has a substantial basis within the common adolescent experience in many Western cultures today.

This discussion of substance use/abuse, one of the most common and vexing "risky behaviors" that clearly emerges during the teen years, provides a segue into some final comments. First, this chapter has been focused on the period of development identified as adolescence, but we must not forget that each developmental epoch is a function, to a degree, of what has come before. Many aspects of mature adult outcomes can be traced directly back to the adolescent years. Good adult outcomes and bad outcomes have a basis in periods of individual formation in childhood and adolescence. School or work failure, substance abuse, relationship disasters, and ultimately the individual's sense of self and satisfaction derive partly and importantly from the history that precedes the "here and now." As adolescence comes to a close—chronologically in the early 20s, although developmentally the actual end point is much more open-ended—the distinctions between immature and mature, between teenager and adult, become merged and difficult to discern. As in all clinical and educational work with youth, our attempts to promote the well-being of children and teens also represent a contribution to helping the adults that teens soon become.

ADOLESCENTS AS PARENTS

Although adolescent pregnancy and birth rates have decreased immensely over the last 15 years (Child Trends, 2005), most teenagers who give birth choose to keep their infants and do not give them up for adoption (Donnelly and Voydanoff, 1991). The clinician may care for two patients, the young mother and the infant, and both are at risk for certain problems. Teen parents often come from home situations that have a high incidence of poverty, violence, drug use, and pregnancy at a young age. In addition, these adolescent girls have a higher than average history of learning problems and school dropout (East and Felice, 1996), and some experience postpartum depression (Barnet et al, 1995). These issues alone may make their own adolescent development stunted, and the added responsibility of raising a child may lead to additional problems for themselves and their infants. Children born to teen mothers are at increased risk for behavioral, social, and learning problems (East and Felice, 1990, 1994) and for continuing the cycle of teen parenting. One cannot presume, however, that all adolescent mothers do poorly because some teen mothers do very well (Horwitz et al, 1991). Health care providers who are in the unique role of caring for a teen mother and her child should be certain to address the psychosocial problems of both youngsters and take the time to help the teenaged parent develop the parenting skills necessary to care for her child.

SUMMARY

Adolescence is a developmental period between childhood and adulthood marked by quantum leaps in physical, psychological, social, cognitive, and moral growth.

Although this developmental period transcends about one decade of life, it is often viewed as three distinct phases—early, mid, and late adolescence—that are characterized by specific growth tasks that must be attained for a healthy adulthood. *Pubescence* (the physiologic changes that unfold in the process of reproductive maturity) generally heralds *adolescence* (the psychosocial changes of the teen years). In past years, pubescence and adolescence were described in terms of hormonal activities. In recent years, studies in brain maturation have uncovered a new understanding of the phenomenon of puberty and adolescent development.

Contrary to popular views of adolescents, most teenagers do well in the transition from childhood to adulthood. This period of life is a vulnerable time for many adolescents, however, particularly individuals at risk for poor adjustment by virtue of internal or external factors. Clinicians who work with adolescents must be aware of the characteristics of normal development to recognize better when an adolescent's behavior is symptomatic of major dysfunction or problems.

REFERENCES

Aggleton P, Hurry J, Warwick I: Young People and Mental Health. London, John Wiley & Sons Ltd, 2000.

Bains R: Psychotherapy with young people from ethnic minority backgrounds in different community-based settings. *In* Baruch G (ed): Community Based Psychotherapy with Young People, Philadelphia. Taylor & Francis, 2001.

Barnet B, Duggan A, Wilson MD, Joffe A: Association between postpartum substance use and depressive symptoms, stress, and social support in adolescent mothers. Pediatrics 96:659-666, 1995.

Baruch G, (ed): Community Based Psychotherapy with Young People. Philadelphia. Taylor & Francis, 2001.

Beck A: The Beck Depression Inventory. San Antonio, TX, Psychological Corporation, 1996.

Blos P: The second individuation process of adolescence. Psychoanal Study Child 22:162-186, 1967.

Burns BJ, Costell EJ, Angold A, et al: Children's mental health service use across service sectors. Health Affairs 14:147-159, 1995.

Child Trends: Facts at a Glance. 2005. Available at:http://www.childtrends.org/_catdisp_page.cfm?LID=140.

Cohen E, Mackenzie RG, Yates GL: HEADSS, a psychosocial risk assessment instrument: Implications for designing effective intervention programs for runaway youth. J Adolesc Health 12:539-544, 1991.

Donnelly BW, Voydanoff P: Factors associated with releasing for adoption among adolescent mothers. Family Relations 40:404-410, 1991.

Dryfoos JG: Adolescents at Risk: Prevalence and Prevention. New York, Oxford University Press, 1990.

East PL, Felice ME: Outcomes and parent-child relationships of former adolescent mothers and their 12-year-old children. J Dev Behav Pediatr 11:175-183, 1990.

East PL, Felice ME: The psychosocial consequences of teenage pregnancy and childbearing. *In* Schenker R (ed): Adolescent Medicine. London, Harwood Academic Press, 1994, pp 73-92.

East PL, Felice ME: Adolescent Pregnancy and Parenting: Findings from a Racially Diverse Sample. Mahwah, NJ, Lawrence Erlbaum Associates, 1996.

Erikson E: Childhood and Society. New York, Norton & Co, 1963.

Erikson EH: Identity, Youth and Crisis. New York, WW Norton, 1968.

Evans DL, Foa EB, Gur RE, et al: Treating and preventing adolescent mental health disorders. Oxford, Oxford University Press, 2005.

Feldman R: Child Development, 3rd ed. Upper Saddle River, NJ, Prentice-Hall, 2006.

Felice ME, Friedman SB: Behavioral considerations in health care of adolescents. Pediatr Clin North Am 29:399-413, 1982.

Flaherty L: Risk-taking behaviors in adolescence. *In* Noshpitz JD (ed): Handbook of Child and Adolescent Psychiatry. Vol III, Adolescence: Development and Syndromes, New York, John Wiley & Sons, 1997.

Freud A: The Ego and the Mechanism of Defense. New York: International University Press, 1966.

Friedman SB, Fisher MM, Schonberg SK, et al: Comprehensive Adolescent Health Care. St Louis, Mosby-Year Book, 1998.

Grisso T: Forensic Evaluation of Juveniles. Sarasota, FL, Professional Resources Press, 1998.

Hagen JW, Nelson MJ, Velissaris N: Comparison of research in two major journals on adolescence. Presented at Biennial Meeting of the Society of Research in Adolescence, Baltimore, 2004.

Harris JR: The Nurture Assumption. New York, Free Press, 1998.

Horwitz SM, Klerman LV, Kuo HS, Jekel JF: School-age mothers: Predictors of long-term educational and economic outcomes. Pediatrics 87:862-868, 1991.

Joffe A, Blythe MJ: Biologic and psychosocial growth and development. Adolesc Med 14:231-262, 2003.

Johnston LD, O'Malley PM, Bachman JG, Schulenberg JE: Teen drug use continues down in 2006, particularly among older teens; but use of prescription-type drugs remains high. Ann Arbor, MI, University of Michigan News and Information Services, 2006. Available at: http://www.monitoringthefuture.org/data/06data.html#2006data-drugs.

Kazdin A: Adolescent development, mental disorders and decision-making in delinquent youths. *In* Grisso TG, Schwartz RG: Youths on Trial: A Developmental Perspective on Juvenile Justice. Chicago, University of Chicago Press, 2000.

Kohlberg L, Gilligan C: The adolescent as a philosopher: The discovery of the self in a post-conventional world. *In* Kagan J, Coles R (eds): 12 to 16: Early Adolescence. New York: Norton, 1972.

Kuhn D, Langer J, Kohlberg L, Haan NS: The development of formal operations. Genet Psychol Monogr 95:97-188, 1977.

National Association of Social Workers: Adolescent health and youths of color. Practice Update Vol 2, No. 3, 2001.

Offer D, Boxer AM: Normal adolescent development: Comprehensive research findings. *In* Lewis M (ed): Child and Adolescent Psychiatry: A Comprehensive Textbook. Baltimore, Williams & Wilkins, 1991.

Office of Juvenile Justice and Delinquency Prevention: Statistical Briefing Book. 1999. Available at www.ojjdp.ncjrs/ojstatbb/qa092.html.

Reynolds CR, Kamphaus RW: Behavior Assessment System for Children, 2nd ed. Circle Pines, MN: AGS Publishing, 2004.

Sisk CL, Foster DL: The neural basis of puberty and adolescence. Nat Neurosci 7:1040-1047, 2004.

Sisk CL, Zehr JL: Pubertal Hormones Organize the Adolescent Brain and Behavior. Front Neuroendocrinol 26:163-174, 2005.

Steinberg D: The Clinical Psychiatry of Adolescence. New York, J. Wiley & Sons, 1983.

Steinberg L: We know some things: Adolescent-parent relationships in retrospect and prospect. J Res Adolesc 11:1-19, 2001.

Steinberg L, Morris AS: Adolescent development. Annu Rev Psychol 52:83-110, 2001.

Tanner JM: Growth at Adolescence. Oxford, Blackwell Scientific Press, 1962.

7

NORMAL INDIVIDUAL DIFFERENCES IN TEMPERAMENT AND BEHAVIORAL ADJUSTMENT

William B. Carey

Vignette

At a kindergarten class, a group of 5- to 6-year-old children have finished their rest period and have been asked by the teacher to put their shoes back on. Tying shoes is a normal 5-year-old developmental milestone, and all these children can do it. All are sufficiently mature in the self-care component of behavioral adjustment that they want to do it. The children have different temperaments, however, and perform this task in various ways. Active, persistent, and negative Charlie carries it out rapidly with a frown on his face. Inactive, positive Barbara does it slowly, singing merrily all the while. Active, unadaptable, nonpersistent Kevin delays doing it until he has run around the room for a while. Distractible Carol ties her shoes partway, becomes diverted by the fascination of passing cars, but eventually returns to the job. The children's levels of development and motivation to cooperate are equal, but their performance is expressed by a multitude of normal behavioral styles.

Chapters 2 through 6 of this text presented a review of the stages of development through which a child normally passes in the course of growing from infancy through adolescence. Because the nervous system is maturing extensively over these years, it is necessary to describe the changes in what the human child is capable of doing during each of the several levels of the newborn period, infancy and toddlerhood, the preschool years, middle childhood, and adolescence. This chapter shifts the focus from development to behavior and presents the wide range of normal behavior that prevails during these 2 decades, including behavioral style or temperament and behavioral content or adjustment. The relatively greater continuity in the realm of behavior allows this briefer discussion in a single chapter.

INTERACTIONAL MODEL

At this point, we should attempt to tie these six chapters and the many more to come with the unifying concept of the interactional model of developmental-behavioral status. The basic assumption of this book is that the individual personality is the product of an ongoing interaction between biologic elements in the child and the influences of the environment (Chess and Thomas, 1996). The term *transactional* is sometimes used to emphasize that the interaction is bidirectional and continuing. The contribution of the child consists of his or her physical and neurologic condition, developmental and cognitive status, and temperament. The involvement of the environment includes the child's own family situation, the sociocultural circumstances, and the physical setting. The complex relationships among these diverse elements lead to the many different developmental, behavioral, emotional, functional, and physical outcomes, which are the concerns of Parts V through VIII of this book.

In the past century, theories of child development first favored the dominance of constitutional traits, then shifted to the supremacy of the environment, and more recently renewed the tendency to find explanations for variations and deviations in the nervous system of the child. The editors of this book agree regarding the value of the interactional or transactional model, and wish to avoid taking sides in the continuing battle between the proponents of the dominance of nature or nurture. "The findings call out for a better integration between genetic and psychosocial research … and investigations to identify the pathophysiological processes involved in genetic effects" (Rutter, 2003).

All of these etiologic factors and outcomes are discussed elsewhere in this book except for two: normal individual temperament differences and normal variations in behavioral adjustment—that is, the style and content of behavior that describe most children. These two subjects are discussed in this chapter. Comparable texts are likely to provide minimal coverage of what is normal and go straight to a catalog of abnormal outcomes. The editors of this text believe that an adequate presentation of the wide range of normal is indispensable for pediatricians and other professionals dealing with the whole population of children.

TEMPERAMENT

Definition

The term *temperament* means the behavioral style of the individual, the characteristic pattern of experiencing and reacting to the external and internal environment. Temperament can be thought of as the "how" of behavior, rather than the "what," which refers to developmental level and abilities, or the "why," which describes the individual's behavioral and emotional adjustment and motivations. Temperament is not the same as the individual's personality, but is a significant part of it (Chess and Thomas, 1984, 1996). Because at least with young children we cannot know for sure what children are feeling in these situations, we use the behavior observed by the caregivers for doing the ratings.

Historical Background

The word *temperament* is derived from the Latin verb *temperare,* which means "to mix." The most prominent Greco-Roman view of the origins of physical health and personality by Hippocrates and Galen was that they were derived from the variable mixture in the individual of the four humors: blood, black bile, yellow bile, and phlegm. Despite a complete lack of scientific evidence, this view and versions of it, such as the additional influence of the planets at the individual's birth and the alterations by purges and bloodletting, lasted until the 19th century and the dawn of modern scientific psychology and medicine. In the early 20th century, the pendulum swung to the opposite extreme in rejecting any ideas of inborn behavioral predispositions and in attributing virtually all normal and abnormal personality differences to the imprint of the environment. During that period, early modern insights about inborn temperament differences by the physicians Pavlov in Russia and Gesell in the United States and the psychologist Diamond went largely unnoticed or unaccepted by behavioral scientists and the general public.

In 1956, Chess and Thomas, wife and husband psychiatrists in New York City, and their associates began their New York Longitudinal Study (NYLS) of temperament and behavior problems in children (Thomas et al, 1963). Being parents as well as astute clinicians, Chess and Thomas knew that all children are not alike in their inborn behavioral tendencies. At first, many professionals in the mental health and academic behavioral science fields, contending that there is no such thing as congenital behavioral tendencies, greeted their findings with scorn. An exploration of the political and social reasons for this neglect and hostility is beyond the scope of this chapter. Recognition of the value of their contribution gradually increased, however, during the 1970s and 1980s. When these perceptive and courageous researchers called attention to this seriously neglected area of investigation and led the way, others in medicine, psychology, and education became involved.

With the advent of the "Decade of the Brain" in the late 20th century and its emphasis on the importance of brain physiology and pathology, the appreciation of the contribution of normal temperamental traits to behavioral adjustment spread less rapidly and for some was neglected. Even now in the 21st century, only about half of undergraduate and graduate students in medicine, psychology, and education have ever received any formal instruction about temperament differences. This chapter presents a concise summary of what the responsible child health professional should know. Various other publications are available for a more detailed review of the state of the art (see list at end of chapter).

Temperament Traits

Although the ancient Greco-Roman temperament traits were the result of mere speculation and no science, the traits introduced by the NYLS were empirically derived from discussions with parents and by direct observations of children. The aim was to select a set of "primary reactive patterns" that were present very early in life, with evidence of genetic determination, fairly stable over time and settings, and likely to affect the quality of parent-child interaction. The primary interest of the NYLS was in finding how these traits would influence the development of behavior problems through stressful interactions in the study population of 133 New York City children.

The traits the investigators selected (Table 7-1) were activity, biologic rhythmicity, approach/withdrawal (initial reaction), adaptability, intensity, mood, persistence/attention span, distractibility, and sensory threshold (sensitivity). These characteristics all were seen by the investigators as normal, even at their extremes. Since the presentation of these traits, some researchers and clinicians have questioned whether at least some of the traits, such as high activity or low attention span, may not become pathologic at their far extremes. No such quantitative cut-points have been established, however.

A variety of other conceptualizations have emerged subsequently primarily from the work of academic developmental psychologists. Some of these are by Rothbart, Strelau, Buss and Plomin, Eysenck, Kagan, and Zuckerman. Especially popular at present is Digman's "Big Five" for adults: extraversion, agreeableness, conscientiousness, emotional stability, and openness to experience. Most recently, we have been offered "The Really Big Two" of inhibition and impulsiveness (Kohnstamm et al, 1989; Strelau and Angleitner, 1991).

Although clinicians have preferred to maintain profiles of all traits with demonstrated practical implications, these later researchers have favored reducing the traits to as small a number as possible, even as few as two. These newer traits have been constructed by factor analysis of reported behaviors, rather than using the NYLS approach of identifying clinically observed and readily identified traits and then writing items to measure

Table 7-1. **Nine New York Longitudinal Study Dimensions of Temperament**

1. Activity	Amount of physical motion during sleep, eating, playing, dressing, and bathing
2. Rhythmicity	Regularity of physiologic functions, such as hunger, sleep, and elimination
3. Approach/withdrawal	Nature of initial responses to new stimuli—people, situations, places, foods, toys, procedures
4. Adaptability	Ease or difficulty with which reactions to stimuli can be modified in a desired way
5. Intensity	Energy level of responses, regardless of quality or direction
6. Mood	Amount of pleasant and friendly or unpleasant and unfriendly behavior in various situations (overt behavior, not assumed internal feelings)
7. Persistence/attention span	Length of time particular activities are pursued by the child, with or without obstacles
8. Distractibility	Effectiveness of extraneous stimuli in interfering with ongoing behaviors
9. Sensory threshold	Amount of stimulation, such as sounds or light, necessary to evoke discernible responses in the child

Adapted from Thomas A, Chess S: Temperament and Development. New York, Brunner/Mazel, 1977.

them with high internal consistency. These computer constructs have been used almost exclusively in theory-building research (Gartstein and Rothbart, 2003). Some of these derived traits, such as effortful control, impulsivity, and executive functions, may be helpful, but also may be more aspects of the resulting behavioral adjustment, rather than constituting largely inborn temperament traits. Some essential traits, such as adaptability, have been lost. The discussion in this chapter adheres to the original clinically derived and empirically supported NYLS conceptualization.

The proponents of sensory integration theory and practice (see Chapter 73) have described a set of variables that more recent research is showing to have a strong overlap with some of the temperament traits as described in this chapter. These variables include sensory threshold, intensity, mood, activity, and attention (Dunn, 2001). This matter warrants further scrutiny and clarification to bring closer the two lines of research.

Temperament Clusters

The NYLS group found it convenient for their research and clinically meaningful to define several clusters of their nine traits. The "difficult child," composing about 10% of their study population, was identified by the traits of low adaptability, low initial approach, largely negative mood, high intensity, and irregularity of biologic functions. The "easy child," with the opposite traits, accounted for a larger group of about 40%. The "slow-to-warm-up child," amounting to 15%, was similar to the "difficult child," but mild in intensity and less active.

At first, it seemed that the objective for clinical research and management should be to put one of these labels on every child under consideration. That system leaves almost half of the population without one of these designations, however. It soon became apparent that this practice could be derogatory and sometimes misleading. A resourceful, experienced parent might describe a child as exhibiting traits that would be regarded by most as difficult, but the parent might not think of the child as particularly aversive. It would be a conflict of terms to label a child as difficult if the parent were not regarding the child as such. This situation has resulted in the use of less pejorative terms, such as "spirited" and "challenging." The best policy seems to be to avoid use of labels entirely and to discuss the child's temperament with parents in terms of the individual traits, for example: "She takes a while to get used to changes and is not always very pleasant about it."

Gender differences have been investigated and shown to exist, but to be very small, at least before puberty. Boys are slightly more active than girls, and girls are slightly more withdrawing, but differences within the two sexes are far greater than between them. As for birth order differences, no differences have been noted in the actual ratings of firstborn compared with later born children, but firstborn children may be generally perceived as more challenging because of parental inexperience. Ethnic and cultural differences are noted frequently, but have proven elusive to verify because of the complexities of evaluating data in different languages. What is certain is that these traits may be differently valued in other social and cultural settings (see Chapter 19).

Temperament Risk Factors

Because the use of categorical cluster labels has proven to be unsatisfactory and incomplete, a different approach has been suggested. No one trait or combination or group of traits is always a source of harmonious or incompatible relationships. There are certain individual traits or groups of them, however, which tend to place children at risk for an abrasive association with their caregivers under certain circumstances. Particularly common is the combination of low adaptability and negative mood, which are probably responsible for more uncongenial interactions than any others at all ages and in most cultures. Some parents and other caregivers are not bothered by these children, however, and may even enjoy them. Similarly, some parents may enjoy a highly active child, whereas others may be unable to tolerate the amount of motion. The clinically significant issue here is the goodness or poorness of fit.

Goodness or Poorness of Fit

Goodness or poorness of fit is a concept introduced by the NYLS study group (Chess and Thomas, 1984, 1986). It describes whether there is compatibility or disharmony between the traits of the individual child and the values and expectations of the caregivers. Although the temperament pattern of the caregivers themselves may play a role in that interaction, what really matters to them is (1) their understanding of where the behavior is coming from (it is neither learned nor intentional); (2) their ability to tolerate the temperament even if they do not like it, which may be hard for them; and (3) their ability to manage the traits with a minimum of stress to prevent secondary or reactive behavior or functional problems arising in the child. Family and cultural factors are highly important in parental management.

Origins of Temperament

Evidence from family, twin, and adoption studies reveals that temperament is about 50% genetically determined. Multiple genes with small effects seem to be responsible, rather than one or two major ones. Associations with various chromosomal and genetic abnormalities have been explored, but only to a limited and inconclusive extent so far (Carey and McDevitt, 1995).

The rest of the input comes from nongenetic physical factors in the child, prenatal and postnatal, and from the psychosocial environment. The host of physical factors suspected or established includes pregnancy influences, such as maternal nutrition, toxins, alcohol and drug use, smoking, emotional stress, infections, prematurity (mostly if the infant is very small with neurologic insults) (Hughes et al, 2002), intrauterine growth retardation, and the season of birth. Postnatal conditions in the child could be anemia and other nutritional problems, toxins such as lead exposure and food additives, and traumatic brain injury. There is general agreement that psychosocial factors can and do modify the expression of the inborn traits, but little is documented as to how, when, and with whom it is likely to happen (Carey and McDevitt, 1995).

Some preliminary investigations have demonstrated support for a neuroanatomic basis for normal individual differences in temperament (Whittle et al, 2008).

Stability of Temperament

Behavioral differences are observable in newborns (see Chapter 2), but extensive research has shown that they are largely transient. The activity, reactivity, irritability, alertness, and soothability newborns may display are evidently the result of factors such as duration of pregnancy and labor and analgesic medication, the effects of which typically wear off in the coming days and weeks. Correlations with later behavioral findings have been negligible. If genetic influences have already begun their expression in the immediate newborn period, we have not yet developed ways to detect them.

Lack of appropriate research makes it hard to say exactly when the first appearance of stable temperament traits may occur, but by 3 to 4 months there begins to be measurable stability. From there on into adolescence, temperament traits become increasingly stable (Guerin et al, 2003). Temperament traits interact continually with the environment, but are not overwhelmed by it.

This evidence that temperament tends to be fairly stable should not mislead the reader into thinking that it never changes. Temperament is neither completely fixed nor completely changeable at any age. We know that it can and does change, but not how and when it happens. The question of whether some current psychopharmacologic agents are temporarily altering normal temperament rather than improving abnormal brain function is considered elsewhere (Carey and McDevitt, 1995).

The most important clinical consideration is whether in a poor fit and conflict situation between the child's temperament and the preferences of the caregivers it is possible to induce a change in the child's reactions. In brief, clinical experience has shown that by about 5 or 6 years of age some children can learn at least to modify the expression of some traits that are causing friction, such as shyness or high intensity. At this time, we cannot say with certainty how much change occurs within the child, or whether a lasting alteration has been achieved.

Before describing the clinical applications of this phenomenon, it is important to acknowledge that temperament-environment interactions are not just an interplay between two fixed elements. Not only may the environment alter the temperament, but also the reverse may be true. The temperamental genotype can alter the environment with which the child interacts in three main ways: (1) passively, through environments provided by biologically related parents, with whom the child shares multiple genes; (2) evocatively, as when the child's genetically determined style modifies the responses of others; and (3) actively, as when differently endowed children select different surroundings with which to interact (Shiner and Caspi, 2003).

Assessment of Temperament

In assessment of temperament, primary clinical reliance is on parent reports by interviewing or questionnaires, and less on observations by professionals. Laboratory tests, such as frontal electroencephalogram asymmetries, are of interest in research, but have no recognized diagnostic role at present (see Chapter 78).

Clinical Importance of Temperament

Temperament matters to caregivers and to children in a broad variety of ways (Carey and McDevitt, 1995).

Caregivers

For parents and other caregivers, there are two main areas of impact: (1) on themselves as individuals and (2) on their functioning as caregivers (Fig. 7-1). Although not broadly studied so far, an abundance of evidence supports the view that the child's temperament has a significant impact on the caregivers, especially the parents, as individuals. Whether the child is positive and flexible or negative and inflexible produces a very different experience for the adult caregiver. The experience may influence self-esteem, marital satisfaction, outside job performance, and general contentment with life. An irritable, hard-to-soothe infant may leave a mother believing that she is inept and unfulfilled, whereas a mild, pleasant one would be likely to make her feel content and competent.

The child's temperament may support or interfere with the caregiver's provision of the parenting benefits of physical care, emotional needs, developmental-behavioral needs, and socialization. All children are not equally able to evoke expressions of affection from parents. Inflexibility makes discipline harder to impose and may bring on more forceful measures from the parent. Shy children are harder to socialize and may leave

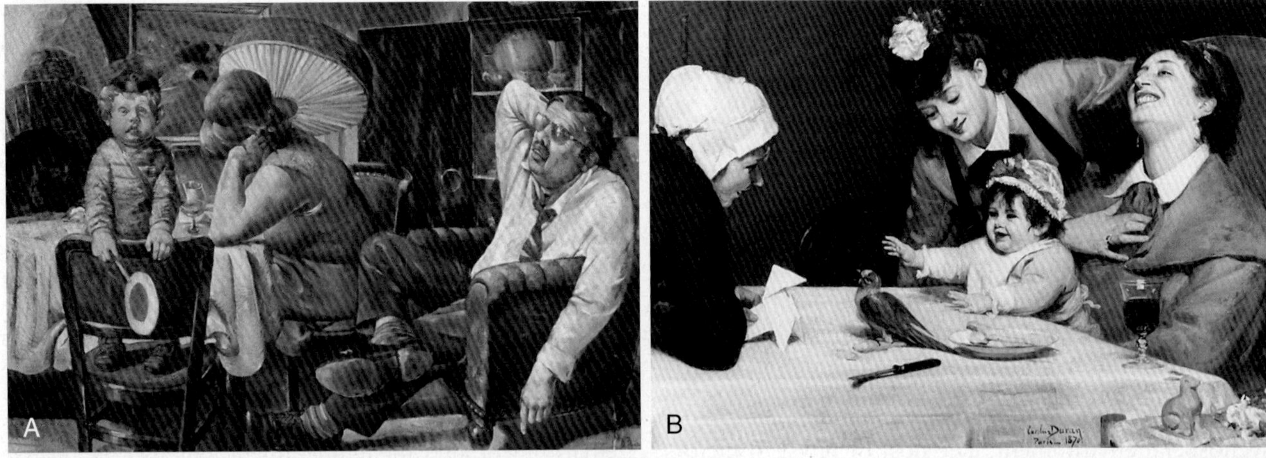

Figure 7-1. A and B, The varying impact of children's temperaments on their families. (A from Harald Duwe: Sonntagnachmittag. With permission of Hamburger Kunsthalle; B from Carolus-Duran: The Merrymakers. Founders Society Purchase, Robert H. Tannahill Foundation Fund. Photograph © The Detroit Institute of Arts, 1989.)

parents perplexed as to how much to coax them into unfamiliar situations. Children with low attention span and high distractibility tax the patience of parents and teachers trying to educate them.

Children

The impact on children is enormous, affecting most areas of their functioning, including general care, physical health, development, social behavior, school performance, and reactions to stressors. Every day of the child's existence, his or her general care is colored by the pattern of responses produced by the behavioral style: eating, sleeping, elimination, toilet training, dressing, playing, sibling relationships, and choice of peers and activities with them. It is hard to imagine an area of daily life unaffected by the child's reaction style.

Physical Problems

Several physical and functional conditions have an established or suspected connection with temperamental predispositions, including injuries, colic, weight gain in infants and older children, failure to thrive, child abuse, neglect, sleep disturbances, recurrent abdominal pains and headaches, bottle mouth caries, and constipation.

Regardless of what the physical condition may be and where it came from, the child's and the parents' reaction to it is affected by the child's general pattern of stress responses. The child could be mild, accepting, and uncomplaining, or loud, irritable, and intolerant. A quiet reaction is likely to produce a slower appeal to or response from the parents for help and may entail an underuse of medical care. A vigorous, reactive style would probably get parental attention more rapidly and hasten the seeking of medical care. These children may end up with too much medical intervention.

Development

Although temperament and development are conceptually quite separate, they have been shown to be interrelated to a significant degree. Because temperament consists of the style of interaction with the environment, it can be expected to affect the way in which the individual uses the positive and negative stimuli it offers. To some extent, temperament is independent of the quality of the environment, as with the way that more active infants have been shown to walk earlier than less active ones in various settings. Usually, however, the traits of approach and adaptability affect the rate with which the infant or child absorbs what the environment presents. Such a child would do well in an average or enriched setting, incorporating more rapidly the benefits available, as with new words and skills such as toilet training. The less approaching and adaptable child probably would pick up the benefits more slowly, but might be more resistant to the assumption of less socially desirable stimuli, such as bad language or antisocial behavior of neighbors. Later on, when it comes to learning in the preschool and school years, certain temperament traits play a major part in progress, as discussed later.

There is a question of a relationship between temperament and intelligence. When correlated with concurrently administered standardized tests of intelligence, the traits of mood, persistence/attention span, approach/withdrawal, and adaptability have shown correlations, but none greater than 0.40. Test-taking behavior was found to be a significant mediator (Guerin et al, 2003). Cognitive ability seems to have a bidirectional relationship with temperament. "That is, cognitive ability may serve to mediate the expression of temperament, and temperament may influence how intellectual energy is directed and expended" (Keogh, 2003).

Social Behavior Problems

The aim of the NYLS study was to investigate the role that temperament has in the onset and duration of reactive behavior problems in children, especially in the first decade of life. The investigators' work showed that most of the "difficult" and "slow-to-warm-up" children developed behavior problems during this period. Some children did not, however, apparently owing to skillful management of their challenging traits by their parents. Similarly, most of the "easy" children did well, but a few developed disorders because of unfavorable environmental factors, rather than their temperaments.

Since the NYLS study, numerous other studies have confirmed the predisposing effects of challenging behavioral style traits despite the use of other populations, different methods, and varied outcome measures (Carey and McDevitt, 1995; Rothbart, 2004; Shiner and Caspi, 2003). McDevitt, a clinical psychologist in community practice, has estimated that temperament is a significant part of the clinical picture in about half of the problem cases referred to him (McDevitt SC, personal communication, October 2000).

Although such behavioral problems may entail some preexisting condition in the child or parent, that is not necessary. Because the principal pathology described here is in the interaction, the parent and child may be functioning well apart from their abrasive relationship. The effectiveness of clinicians is greatly enhanced by the recognition that in such instances the appropriate management may lie in helping to modify just the caregiver interaction without any sort of individual therapy of the contending parties. For example, when a temperamentally challenging but previously normally functioning child becomes noncompliant and academically underachieving when advancing into first grade with a rigid, demanding, but generally respected teacher, the situation calls mainly for more individual, sensitive handling by the teacher. By this age, however, children may be able to learn to modify the expression of abrasive traits such as inflexibility to enhance the fit and reduce the conflict.

Because treatment of these problems entails altering the parent-child interactions as with most other behavior problems, one might wonder what is the benefit of being aware of the role of temperament in the situation. There are two advantages to note: One is that it helps to explain why this child, rather than an equally stressed sibling or fellow student, developed the signs of dysfunction more rapidly or extensively; the other is that it clarifies the objectives of the intervention. Although an appropriate improvement in the fit should cause the reactive symptoms to diminish and disappear, it would not change the underlying temperament. No amount of incentive or punishment would make an inflexible child resilient. The parents need to recognize the challenging behavioral style and learn to tolerate it better and deal with it more effectively to be ready when another stressor comes along and challenges the child.

Some clinicians have reported difficulty distinguishing between annoying temperament and a reactive behavior problem. If the concern is just about temperament, there would be an identifiable trait that the parent does not like, but no accompanying dysfunction. A behavioral problem involves some degree of dysfunction, as described in the second part of this chapter. Both a temperament issue and a dysfunction can be present. Low adaptability can be an annoying temperament trait. If it is not well managed, and the child becomes domineering, there is both a challenging trait and a behavior problem. In contrast, an unfavorable environment can make even an easy child dysfunctional.

Long-term predictions of adult outcome from childhood temperament have shown that such prognostications are hazardous. The NYLS found negligible correlations between preschool temperament and adult adjustment (Chess and Thomas, 1984). The Berkeley Guidance Study re-evaluated 30 years later children who had had temper tantrums or were shy at age 8 to 10 years and discovered more evidence of difficulties with job or marital status (Caspi et al, 1987). Another more recent study showed that "temperament in early and middle childhood accounted for an average of 32% of the variance in personality in late adolescence/early young adulthood" (Deal et al, 2005). Such studies are interesting, but what really matters is not that temperament determinations predict for the near or far future, but how they help in dealing with the current goodness or poorness of fit.

School Performance

The role of temperament in academic function in school remains controversial. There is no doubt that certain traits enhance or interfere with the performance of the tasks of learning, but much uncertainty remains as to how to differentiate between the normal traits of high activity and inattention and the seemingly identical ones now frequently diagnosed as the "neurodevelopmental disorder" of attention-deficit/hyperactivity disorder (ADHD).

Children's temperaments, by parent and by teacher ratings, have been confirmed to have an extensive influence on scholastic performance in normal elementary school children, as measured by grades and standard achievement tests. The characteristics most involved are in Keogh's "task orientation" cluster: persistence/attention span, distractibility, and activity. Keogh's analysis of the nine NYLS traits in the educational world found two other significant clusters: personal-social flexibility (adaptability, approach, and positive mood) and reactivity (intensity, threshold, and negative mood) (Keogh, 2003). All the other traits may play a part in the learning process, however. These conclusions apply to children at all levels of cognitive ability and in a broad range of socioeconomic situations. Much of the outcome depends on other elements of the fit between the child and the school situation, such as age, subject matter, curriculum and classroom arrangements, cognitive skills, motivation, and the flexibility of the teacher (Carey and McDevitt, 1995).

Temperament in the Classroom by Keogh (2003) contains the most comprehensive review of the research in this area. Keogh's conclusions from her own work and from that of Martin and others are as follows:

> *Children's temperament may affect their success in school in several ways such as how they approach, become involved in, and persist in learning tasks; their behavior in the classroom; and how teachers respond to them. The temperament dimensions of activity, persistence and distractibility that make up a broader factor of task orientation are especially important contributors to children's achievement and behavior. These dimensions appear to have real functional significance in school classrooms and to exert both direct and indirect influence on children's academic behaviors (Keogh, 2003).*

Are behavioral style and cognitive style the same? The components of behavioral style have been amply discussed earlier. Although there is no firm consensus, the cognitive style dimensions have been described as persistence, flexibility, and reflectivity (Gaskins and Barron, 1985). Although one deals with thinking and the other with behavior, the similarities are striking. One may be a part of the other, or they both may be components of an overall reactive style.

The indirect influence of temperament comes via teachers' response to the individual child:

Teachers' expectations about students are captured in the notion of teachability, and temperament is one of the contributors to teachers' views. Positive interactions are likely when there is a good fit between teachers' expectations and children's attributes, but negative interactions are often the product of a poor fit (Keogh, 2003).

Teachers find less active, less distractible, and more persistent children more enjoyable to work with and would like to remove children who are more active and more distractible from their classrooms. It might be hypothesized that teachers respond to more active, more distractible, less persistent children in a less warm and helpful manner (perhaps being more critical), which would further add to the burden these children face in the classroom (Martin, 1989; also in Carey and McDevitt, 1989, and in Harrison, 1998).

Finally, the child's temperament affects his or her social behavior in school.

We have no clear evidence that various learning differences or disabilities bring with them specific temperament traits. It is clear, however, that when such obstacles exist, children with certain temperament traits such as adaptability and persistence generally are more accepting of and make more diligent use of remedial measures.

Whether temperament affects test-taking skill as opposed to true academic achievement is an issue requiring further clarification, as suggested earlier. It has been argued and to some extent shown that the traits of approach, adaptability, and persistence may allow a child to process a test of ability or achievement with greater proficiency than another with lesser amounts of these traits and yield a false impression of status or accomplishment. Although undoubtedly true to some extent, the question requires further elucidation.

Temperament and Attention-Deficit/Hyperactivity Disorder

Probably the most common behavioral diagnosis given to children currently and the most confusing and in need of revision is ADHD. The overlap with normal temperament traits is particularly perplexing. The diagnosis is officially based on the *Diagnostic and Statistical Manual of Mental Disorders, Fourth Edition, Text Revision* (DSM-IV-TR) criteria of "6/9 inattention or 6/9 hyperactivity/impulsivity symptoms for 6 or more months, some of which have been present from before the age of 7 years, with impairment in two or more settings, and not due to other conditions" (American Psychiatric Association, 1994, 2000). Other assumptions include the beliefs that these behaviors are clearly distinguishable from normal, involve a neurodevelopmental disability, are not influenced by the environment, and can be adequately diagnosed by brief questionnaires.

Problems with this formulation include the following: (1) The current ADHD symptoms are not clearly distinguishable from normal behavior. The DSM system fails to acknowledge the existence of temperament and how it differs. The present diagnosis is based not on a determination of extremely high activity or extremely low attention span, but on an accumulation of normal or mildly to moderately annoying behaviors in these areas. (2) There is an absence of clear evidence that ADHD symptoms are related to brain malfunction. (3) The environment and interactions with it are neglected in the etiology. (4) The questionnaires presently used for the diagnosis are highly subjective and impressionistic. These issues are discussed elsewhere in greater detail (Carey, 2002). Children with a variety of non-neurologic disorders apparently are included erroneously presently under this diagnosis. Some of the misdiagnoses are likely to be as-yet-undetected learning differences or disabilities and temperament traits that are not understood, tolerated, or successfully managed by caregivers. Sleep deprivation, hunger, anxiety, and depression are some other conditions presently sometimes being misdiagnosed as ADHD.

Jensen and colleagues (2006) have suggested a major overhaul of the DSM system that would be less categorical and more developmental, adaptational, and cognizant of the context of the behavior (see Chapter 78). Attentive clinicians should be aware that the basis of the child's scholastic or behavioral problem might be a poor fit between the child's temperament and the preferences of the teacher, rather than a dysfunction of the child's nervous system.

Environmental Stressors and Crises

Children and adults are confronted by a wide variety of stressors in their environments, including fairly routine ones such as sibling births, school entry, and geographical moves, and increasing in magnitude up to parental separation and divorce, death of family members, and natural and civic disasters. Traditionally, reactions to these events and conditions have been attributed to the nature of the crisis, the prior adjustment of the child, the age and developmental level of the child, and the character and availability of the family supports. Because the child's temperament is the characteristic way the individual experiences and responds to the challenges of the environment, we should expect that it too would influence the type and extent of the reaction exhibited. Such differences have been well documented in several settings, such as sibling birth (see Chapters 11 and 14), parental divorce (see Chapter 12), and disasters (see Chapter 21). Allowing for the role of temperament in these situations helps the parent and clinician to recognize that the magnitude and type of the reaction displayed may be as much a reflection of the preexisting observed temperament as it is of the severity of the child's internal feelings. One child may scream whenever faced with a challenge, whereas another child may be more likely to withdraw and sulk (Carey, 2003).

In the case of chronic stress and deprivation, the qualities of activity, sociability, and emotionality have been shown to be among the various factors supporting positive adjustment (Werner and Smith, 2003). Kim-Cohen and associates (2004) stated, "Maternal warmth, stimulating activities, and children's outgoing temperament appeared to promote positive adjustment in children exposed to socioeconomic status deprivation."

Other Areas of Adjustment

Temperament likely plays a role in other areas of adjustment beside those discussed earlier: physical function, development, social behavior, school function and ADHD, and environmental stressors. Temperament even plays a role in the choice of friends. The quality of child-to-parent attachment, although thought by some experts to be solely a reflection of parental input, may be partly determined by the child's temperament. The self-relations components of self-care and self-esteem can be expected to reflect these individual differences in behavioral style. Some evidence suggests increased drug use by adolescents with "difficult" behavioral styles. Self-regulation or self-control, although assumed by some experts to be a primary innate trait, seems more likely to have contributions from the rearing experience and developmental stage in addition to temperament (Strayhorn, 2002). One would expect the formation of coping strategies, or "executive functions," to be similarly influenced. The child's internal status of feelings and thinking is another area awaiting exploration from this point of view.

Management of Temperament Concerns

The main point to remember about management of temperament is that it is different from what one attempts to accomplish with a reactive or learned behavior problem. Although one hopes with successful treatment, such as parent counseling, to lessen and get rid of the reactive behavior problem, that is not likely with annoying temperament traits. Traits are not learned and instead must be skillfully accommodated in younger children. Older children possibly can learn to modify their expression. The four stages of handling aversive temperament traits are discussed next.

Recognition of the Temperament by the Clinician or Teacher

No solution is possible unless the helping person first determines the true nature of the complaint, especially the temperament profile. Various techniques, detailed in Chapter 78, can be used usually fairly easily by knowledge of what the traits are and a few minutes of interviewing the parent.

Revising or Reframing the Caregiver's Understanding and Handling, Whether an Associated Behavior Problem Exists or Not

If it is an annoying temperament trait, the parent must understand that the behavior is something the child was apparently born with and is not a sign of some parenting failure or physical or social mishap. Use of descriptive terms such as "intense" or "slow to accept change" is much preferable to possibly unhelpful or disturbing labels such as "difficult." Freeing the parent of feelings of guilt, anger, or fear can be an enormous step toward establishing a cordial parent-child relationship.

The other part of this step is to help the parent to acquire more appropriate management techniques. The essence of the improved approach is to accommodate the child's aversive traits, but neither to surrender to them nor to try to overwhelm them. In other words, the strategy is to figure out ways to work with the temperament and not against it. Table 7-2 lists specific measures that have proven useful to many parents in this situation. Also, it is appropriate by the time the child is 5 or 6 years old to help the child at least modify the expression of the more aversive traits to reduce the friction at the time and later. (See the list of books for parents at the end of the chapter.)

Two different approaches have been suggested for how to proceed when an aversive temperament and a reactive behavior problem may be present. One approach recommends that the parent or clinician first should determine whether there is a temperament issue and manage it if present, and if not present then move on to investigate for a reactive behavior problem (Turecki and Tonner, 2000). The other approach proposes to find out first whether there is evidence of dysfunction in the child, then to see if temperament is playing a causal role in any dysfunction, and to find out whether the temperament itself may be the primary source of concern (see Chapter 78).

Relief for the Parents by Environmental Intervention

Most parents, but especially conscientious ones, try very hard to be good caregivers to all their children. Some children are clearly more pleasant and more immediately rewarding than others. In many cases, parents and challenging children would do better if the parents could take some recesses from the arduous task of parenting. Great relief, some rest, and a more balanced perspective can be achieved by an evening or a weekend away from home, and some help with the daily care from a friend, relative, or employee. Suggestion and encouragement from a trusted advisor such as the pediatrician or other health advisor can make a parent realize that he or she is not eternally indispensable, and that all of us do better with recreational time.

Referral

When, if at all, should challenging temperament traits be grounds for a referral to a psychologist or psychiatrist? The simple answer is that the clinician is dealing with normal behavior here, and that the child should be cared for by the general pediatrician, family physician, nurse practitioner, teacher, or other qualified caregiver. We are more acquainted with normal function and with the child and the family, and probably are in a better position to be helpful. Indications for referral would be only when there is an associated reactive problem that is greater than the generalist feels able to deal with, or when the parent has additional problems that make management more complex. The routine problems of a shy child can be dealt with at the primary care level. If withdrawal has been allowed to take over the shy child's

Table 7-2. Management of Temperament Differences

High Activity	***Low Activity***
Help the child find ample opportunity for physical activity Avoid unnecessary restrictions of activity Demand restraint of motion appropriate for age when necessary	Allow extra time to complete tasks Set realistic limits, such as meeting the school bus on time Do not criticize slow speed
High Regularity	***Low Regularity***
In an infant, plan feedings and other activities on a schedule In an older child, advise of expected disruptions of the schedule	In an infant, first try to accommodate the preference for irregularity, then gradually steer the infant toward a more regular schedule An older child can be expected increasingly to regularize eating and sleeping times, even if the child does not feel hungry or sleepy on schedule
Approaching or Bold Initial Reaction	***Withdrawing or Inhibited Initial Reaction***
Reinforce with praise if positive Remember that the initial positive reaction may not last Be aware of the child's boldness in dangerous situations	Avoid overload of new experiences Prepare the child for new situations and introduce the child to them slowly Do not push too hard Praise the child for overcoming fears of novelty Encourage self-management as the child grows older
High Adaptability	***Low Adaptability***
Look out for possible susceptibility to unfavorable influences in school and elsewhere	Avoid unnecessary requirements to adapt Reduce or spread out necessary adaptations, arranging for gradual changes in stages; do not push too hard or too quickly Give advance warnings about what to expect Teach social skills to expedite adaptation Maintain reasonable expectations for change Support and praise effort
High Intensity	***Low Intensity***
Intensity may exaggerate the apparent importance of response Avoid reacting to the child with the same intensity; try to read the child's real need, and respond calmly to that need Do not give in just to make peace Enjoy intense positive responses	Try to read the child's real need, and do not mistake it as trivial just because it is mildly expressed Take complaints seriously
Positive Mood	***Negative Mood***
Encourage positive and friendly responses Look out only for those situations in which the child's outward positive behavior may mask true distress, such as with pain, and situations in which being too friendly may be troublesome, such as with strangers	Remember that it is just the child's style, unless there is an underlying behavioral or emotional problem Do not let the child's mood make you feel guilty or angry; the child's mood is not your fault Ignore as many of the glum, unfriendly responses as possible; however, try to spot and deal with the real distress Advise an older child to try harder to be pleasant with people
High Persistence and Attention Span	***Low Persistence and Attention Span***
Redirect a persistent toddler whose persistence is annoying In an older child, warn about the need to end or interrupt activity when continued for too long Reassure the child that leaving some tasks unfinished is acceptable	The child may need help organizing tasks into shorter segments with periodic breaks; however, the responsibility for completion of the task belongs with the child Reward the adequate completion of the task and not the speed with which it is done
High Distractibility	***Low Distractibility***
If the problem involves an older child, try to eliminate or reduce competing stimuli Gently redirect the child to the task at hand when necessary; however, encourage the child to assume responsibility for doing this Praise adequately for completing the task	If the child ignores necessary interruptions, do not assume it is deliberate disobedience
High Sensitivity	***Low Sensitivity***
Avoid excessive stimulation Eliminate stimuli if disruptive Avoid overestimating extreme responses to stimuli Help the older child understand this trait in himself or herself Support and encourage the child's sensitivity to the feelings of others	Look out for underreporting of pain and other distress Help the child develop an awareness of important internal and external stimuli Help child to develop greater sensitivity to the feelings of others

From Carey WB: Understanding Your Child's Temperament, rev ed. Philadelphia, Xlibris, 2005.

life, however, and the child has become excessively withdrawn socially, a mental health specialist intervention may be necessary (see Chapter 41).

BEHAVIORAL ADJUSTMENT

The term *behavioral adjustment* is used here in the sense of the content of the child's behavior—that is, what he or she actually does and why, with some consideration of its "fit" with the environmental circumstances. Behavioral adjustment may interact with, and be to some extent derived from, the child's physical and developmental or cognitive status and temperament, but it is distinct from these other aspects of the child.

Lack of a Generally Accepted Profile of Normal Behavioral Adjustment

A curious condition of behavioral science today is that there is no comprehensive map of the full extent of normal behavior to guide physicians, psychologists, and educators. An odd feature of contemporary medical education is that we study normal anatomy and physiology before moving on to pathology in those areas. In the field of behavior, however, we typically go directly to abnormality even in the first year of medical school without having familiarized ourselves with what should be expected and acceptable as average or typical.

A thorough review of the literature of these three disciplines failed to discover any widely recognized comprehensive, dimensional profile of normal child adjustment. Establishing broad diagnostic profiles of function, which include positive and negative states in all significant areas, does not seem to have been a prominent interest of theorists in those disciplines. In clinical texts, one finds only lists of problems and background factors possibly leading to them. "Normal" is almost always assumed to be an absence of abnormality, rather than being described in terms of satisfactory or positive function. Even previous editions of this book had only a little to say on this matter.

Some Existing Partial Classifications

Probably the most truly comprehensive current classification is the International Classification of Functioning, Disability, and Health for Children and Youth (ICF-CY), which was published by the World Health Organization in 2001. Although broadly covering physical, developmental, cognitive, and personality status, the ratings are concerned only with impairments of function (Lollar and Simeonson, 2005). Another scheme is the Child Health and Illness Profile (Starfield et al, 1993) with 6 domains of activity, comfort, satisfaction, disorders, achievement of developmental expectations, and resilience, plus 25 subdomains. This instrument for 11- to 17-year-olds was intended for research use.

The most popular behavioral profile for adolescents is the HEADSS Assessment, in which the clinician asks the teenager about the situation with *H*ome, *E*ducation, *A*ctivities, *D*rugs (e.g., tobacco, alcohol, marijuana), *S*exuality, and *S*uicide (see Chapter 6) (see also Cohen et al, 1991). Some clinicians change the letters slightly to put *S*chool first, which makes it the SHADSS. This approach also is primarily a quest for problems, however, and is not suitable for prepubescent children.

A uniquely fruitful portrayal of normal behavior was produced in the course of a research project constructing an *Inventory of Child Individual Differences* (Halverson et al, 2003). Based on a collection of more than 50,000 parental descriptors of normal children in eight different countries, the researchers refined the analysis to 141 most commonly mentioned items. This number was reduced further by factor analysis to the 15 most robust items in three of the countries (China, Greece, and the United States) with numbers about 1000 in each of the countries. The resulting list of widely recognized traits was reported as achievement orientation, activity level, antagonism, compliance, considerate, distractible, fearful/insecure, intelligent/quick to learn, negative affect, openness, organized, positive emotions, shy, sociable/outgoing, and strong-willed. This is a unique survey of what parents in different parts of the world regard as normal constituents of children's behavior. Practical clinical applications were not attempted by the authors, who were more interested in matching these traits with the adult "Big Five" classification.

Eysenck (1994) offers his compromise structure of adult personality as consisting of: extraversion, agreeableness, conscientiousness, emotional stability, and culture. The five factor schemes have been popular in adult psychology, but have not found wide acceptance in the study of children.

Constructing a Practical Profile of Normal

A textbook such as this one cannot be without a survey of normal behavior. Because of the lack of a generally accepted comprehensive model, this chapter uses the BASICS approach as a working definition of normal until something better is developed. Two preliminary steps were followed to establish a new comprehensive and dimensional construct or profile of behavioral adjustment: (1) summarizing clinically recognized areas of abnormal function and (2) establishing the features of the corresponding normal and superior functions in those same areas.

First, from the standard lists of behavioral problems, one can assemble and organize an outline of areas with problems that are of concern to caregivers and clinicians. The *Diagnostic and Statistical Manual of Mental Disorders, Fourth Edition (DSM-IV)* (American Psychiatric Association, 1994) identifies such areas as (1) social adjustment problems—disruptive behavior disorders (e.g., conduct disorders and oppositional defiant disorders), adjustment disorders, attachment disorders, and selective mutism; (2) school performance difficulties—various learning disorders and ADHD; (3) self-relations troubles—substance abuse, impulse control issues; (4) internal concerns—mood and thinking disorders (e.g., anxiety, depression, obsessive-compulsive disorder); and (5) various body function issues—feeding, eating, elimination, tics, sleep, recurrent pains, and gender/sex.

The Diagnostic and Statistical Manual for Primary Care (DSM-PC) Child and Adolescent Version (American Academy of Pediatrics, 1996) generally followed the lead of the DSM-IV in identifying the domains of children's problem behavior with which we should concern ourselves. These descriptions of abnormality provide guidance as to what areas should be included on the negative end of the spectrum in a truly dimensional clinical appraisal of behavioral adjustment, but do not supply a view of what we should expect on the average or positive end.

The second step in establishing the conceptual basis for a comprehensive, dimensional behavioral adjustment profile was to match each of these broad areas of clinical concerns with descriptions of average and superior function to be used for ratings when they are appropriate. A subscale describing social relations having antisocial behavior at the negative end requires a consideration of such qualities as social competence, caring, and cooperation at the positive end. Such positive definitions of what a normal or outstanding child might look like are, as mentioned earlier, strikingly absent from the professional literature. A unique exception came from child psychiatrist Chess (personal communication, 1989):

> *As a working concept, keeping in mind its subjective nature, one may identify the following broad characteristics of normal children: They get along reasonably well with parents, sibs, and friends; have few overt manifestations of behavior disturbance; use their apparent intellectual potential to appropriate capacity; are interested in accomplishing developmentally appropriate tasks; and are contented a reasonable proportion of the time. This description covers a wide range of temperamental and personality patterns. One should not arbitrarily consider certain children to be abnormal because their conduct is identified with types of behavior that do not conform to an abstraction.*

Chess recommended thinking of positive adjustment in terms of the individual's relationships with other people, with tasks, and with oneself.

An earlier textbook chapter, which is repeated and revised in this volume (see Chapter 78), began to conceptualize a complete behavioral and emotional profile, putting together the areas regarded as significant clinical disorders with the positive counterparts derived from the Chess description. It conceives adjustment as involving six *BASICS* areas (Table 7-3):

1. *B*ehavior or relationships with people (parents, siblings, teachers, other adults, peers)—social competence versus undersocialization (aggressiveness or withdrawal)
2. *A*chievements or task performance in school, other tasks, and play—satisfactory achievement versus underachievement or excessive preoccupation with work or play
3. *S*elf-relations (self-regard, self-care, and self-regulation)—self-assurance versus poor self-esteem, poor self-care, or poor self-regulation or overconcern for oneself
4. *I*nternal status (feeling, thinking)—reasonable contentment versus distressing feelings or thoughts
5. *C*oping or problem solving patterns (strategies typically used to deal with crises and the other stressors confronted in daily life)—direct and appropriate engagement versus ineffective, maladaptive problem solving with overuse of "defense mechanisms" such as denial, avoidance, or repression
6. *S*ymptoms of body functions—eating, sleeping, elimination, gender/sex, unexplained physical complaints, and repetitive behaviors

All of these comprehensive aspects of adjustment can be rated on descriptive, dimensional scales ranging from (1) excellent—outstanding, (2) good—better than average, (3) satisfactory—minimal problems, (4) unsatisfactory—mild-to-moderate problems, (5) poor—major problems. The internal consistencies of these areas of function and their retest reliabilities have been established in a large standardization sample (see Chapter 78) (Carey and McDevitt, 2003).

The addition of an evaluation of coping strategies seemed appropriate in view of clinical evidence of its importance. Interpersonal problem solving is frequently

Table 7-3. BASICS Profile of Behavioral Adjustment

Area of Behavioral Adjustment	Concerns: Behavior, Emotions, Functions
Behavior competence in social relationships. Skills, success, caring, cooperation, involvement, reliance. Parents, sibs, peers, teachers, other adults.	Undersocialization—aggression, opposition, withdrawal.
Achievements—task performance and mastery in school, home, community. High or sufficient achievement, effort, motivation, satisfaction.	Poor achievement or failure. Excessive preoccupation with work or play.
Self-relations—self-assurance. Self esteem about academics, social worth, appearance, physical abilities. Self-care, good health and safety attitudes, practices, handling personal stress. Self-control or regulation, actions, feelings.	Poor self-esteem. Poor body image. Self-neglect, risk-taking. Overconcern for oneself. Overcontrol—inhibition—or under control—impulsivity.
Internal status—feeling and thinking. Reasonable contentment. Thought clarity.	Anxiety. Depression. Thought disturbance (e.g., obsessions).
Coping or problem solving patterns. Direct and appropriate engagement. Identifies problems; plans solutions; works on solutions; persists at solutions; revises solutions; gets help for solutions.	Ineffective, maladaptive problem solving with excessive use of denial, avoidance, or repression.
Symptoms of physical function. Comfortable function.	Moderate-to-severe symptoms in eating, sleep, elimination, gender/sex, unexplained physical complaints, repetitive behaviors.

the focus of behavioral intervention with children. Although some scales assess it separately, it stands out as an important outcome measure deserving inclusion in a comprehensive evaluation of behavioral adjustment. The DSM-IV mentions, "defense mechanisms or coping styles" only under "Proposed axes for further study." The newly popular concept of executive functions, although variously defined, probably fits best under this topic.

The phenomenon of self-control has been variously classified as a temperament trait of "effortful control" or as a component of the neurologically determined ADHD syndrome. Current evidence supports regarding it primarily as an outcome measure in behavioral adjustment (Strayhorn, 2002), and it is classified this way here.

At this point, it is useful to return to *The Inventory of Child Individual Differences* (Halverson et al, 2003) to see how closely this proposed profile of children's personality resembles what a large number of parents in many countries described as the most conspicuous components of their children's behavior. The nine temperament traits of Chess and Thomas and the six areas of behavioral adjustment proposed earlier are remarkably similar to the 15 items of *The Inventory of Child Individual Differences*. The temperament traits match as follows: activity (activity level); regularity (organized); approach (openness; shy); adaptability (strong willed; compliant); intensity (negative affect—quick tempered); mood (positive mood; negative affect—irritable); persistent and distractibility (distractibility; achievement oriented); and sensitivity (considerate—sensitive to others' feelings). The BASICS behavior profile outlined previously corresponds to the multinational parents' descriptions as follows: social behavior (antagonism; compliance; considerate; sociable); achievements (achievement oriented); self-relations (organized; strong-willed); internal status (fearful/insecure); coping (achievement oriented; intelligent—quick to learn); and symptoms of body function (no match).These two systems are not identical, and there is no parental reference to physical symptoms, which the parents may have been told not to include as a behavioral symptom. Lacking any comparable complete inventory of children's personality, however, we can conclude for now that the nine temperament and six adjustment variables are an adequate comprehensive summary of the real world of children's behavior.

The reader may observe that the outcomes sections and chapters of this book are organized approximately along these lines: Part V, behavioral and emotional; A, social relationships; B, self-relations; C, internal status; D, coping; Part VI, school function and other task performance; and Part VII, physical functioning. Chapter 85 offers a comprehensive formulation of assessment, a scheme for recording in one place these measures of outcome along with physical health, developmental function, temperament, and environmental transactions.

SUMMARY

Temperament or behavioral style differences are real, they matter extensively to caregivers and to children themselves in many ways, and their successful management requires the different approach of accommodation, rather than attempts to eradicate them. The present widespread lack of knowledge of these traits stands in the way of optimal care of children. These normal differences are too important to be ignored, trivialized, or pathologized. Consideration of them in diagnosis and management is essential for optimal care.

Current presentations of behavioral adjustment in children are limited to lists of problems and of factors leading to them. This chapter offers a unique profile of behavioral adjustment, which is comprehensive, dimensional, and descriptive. The suggested dimensions are (1) behavior or relationships with people; (2) achievements or task performance in school, other tasks, and play; (3) self-relations—self-regard, self-care, and self-regulation; (4) internal status—thinking and feeling; (5) coping or problem solving patterns; and (6) symptoms of physical functions, such as eating, sleeping, and elimination.

REFERENCES

American Academy of Pediatrics: The Classification of Child and Adolescent Mental Diagnoses in Primary Care (DSM-PC). Elk Grove Village, IL, American Academy of Pediatrics, 1996.

American Psychiatric Association: Diagnostic and Statistical Manual of Mental Disorders, 4th ed (DSM-IV). Washington, DC, American Psychiatric Association, 1994.

American Psychiatric Association: Diagnostic and Statistical Manual of Mental Disorders, 4th ed, Text Revision (DSM-IV-TR). Washington, DC, American Psychiatric Association, 2000.

Carey WB: Is ADHD a valid disorder? *In* Jensen P, Cooper J (eds): ADHD: State of the Science: Best Practices. Kingston, NJ, Civic Research Institute, 2002.

Carey WB: Children's temperaments influence the impact of environmental risks. J Child Health 1:181, 2003.

Carey WB, McDevitt SC (eds): Clinical and Educational Applications of Temperament Research. Amsterdam, Swets & Zeitlinger, 1989.

Carey WB, McDevitt SC: Coping with Children's Temperament: A Guide for Professionals. New York, Basic Books, 1995.

Carey WB, McDevitt SC: The BASICS Behavioral Adjustment Scale. Scottsdale, AZ, Behavioral-Developmental Initiatives, 2003.

Caspi A, Elder GH Jr, Bem DJ: Moving against the world: Life-course patterns of explosive children. Dev Psychol 23:308, 1987.

Chess S, Thomas A: Origins and Evolution of Behavior Disorders: From Infancy to Early Adult Life. New York, Brunner/Mazel, 1984.

Chess S, Thomas A: Temperament Theory and Practice. New York, Brunner/Mazel, 1996.

Cohen E, Mackenzie RG, Yates GL: HEADSS, a psycho-social risk assessment instrument. J Adol Health 12:539, 1991.

Deal JE, Halverson CF Jr, Havill V, Martin RP: Temperament factors as longitudinal predictors of young adult personality. Merrill-Palmer Q 51:315, 2005.

Dunn W: The sensations of everyday life: Empirical, theoretical, and pragmatic considerations. Am J Occup Ther 55:608, 2001.

Eysenck MW: Individual Differences: Normal and Abnormal. East Sussex, UK, Erlbaum, 1994.

Gartstein MA, Rothbart MK: Studying infant temperament via the Revised Infant Behavior Questionnaire. Infant Behav Dev 26:64, 2003.

Gaskins IW, Barron J: Teaching poor readers to cope the maladaptive cognitive styles: A training program. J Learn Disabil 18:390, 1985.

Guerin DW, Gottfried AW, Oliver PH, et al: Temperament: Infancy through Adolescence. The Fullerton Longitudinal Study. New York, Kluwer Academic, 2003.

Halverson CF, Havill V, Deal J, et al: Personality structure as derived from parental ratings of free descriptions of children: The Inventory of Child Individual Differences. J Pers 71:995, 2003.

Harrison PL (ed): Implications of Temperament for the Practice of School Psychology. School Psychol Rev 27: 475-486, 1998.

Hughes MB, Shults J, McGrath J, et al: Temperament characteristics of premature infants in the first year of life. J Dev Behav Pediatr 23:430, 2002.

Jensen PS, Knapp P, Mrazek DA: Toward a New Diagnostic System for Child Psychopathology: Moving Beyond the DSM. New York, Guilford, 2006.

Keogh BK: Temperament in the Classroom. Baltimore, Brookes, 2003.

Kim-Cohen J, Moffitt TE, Caspi A, Taylor A: Genetic and environmental processes in young children's resilience and vulnerability to socioeconomic deprivation. Child Dev 75:651, 2004.

Kohnstamm GA, Bates JE, Rothbart MK (eds): Temperament in Childhood. New York, Wiley, 1989.

Lollar DJ, Simeonson RJ: Diagnosis to function: Classification for children and youths. J Dev Behav Pediatr 26:323, 2005.

Martin RP: Activity level, distractibility, and persistence: Critical characteristics in early schooling. *In* Kohnstamm GA, Bates JE, Rothbart MK (eds): Temperament in Children. New York, Wiley, 1989, pp 451-461.

Rothbart MK: Commentary: Differentiated measures of temperament and multiple pathways to childhood disorders. J Clin Child Adolesc Psychol 33:82, 2004.

Rutter ML: Commentary: Nature-nurture interplay in emotional disorders. J Child Psychol Psychiatry 44:934, 2003.

Shiner R, Caspi A: Personality differences in childhood and adolescence: Measurement, development, and consequences. J Child Psychol Psychiatry 44:2, 2003.

Starfield B, Bergner M, Ensminger M, et al: Adolescent health status measurement: Development of the Child Health and Illness Profile. Pediatrics 91:430, 1993.

Strayhorn J: Self-control: Theory and research. J Am Acad Child Adolesc Psychiatry 41:7, 2002.

Strelau J, Angleitner A (eds): Explorations in Temperament: International Perspectives on Theory and Measurement. New York, Plenum, 1991.

Super CM, Harkness S, Axia G, et al: Culture, Temperament, and the "Difficult Child": A Study of Seven Western Cultures. In press.

Thomas A, Chess S, Birch HG, et al: Behavioral Individuality in Early Childhood. New York, New York University Press, 1963.

Turecki S, Tonner L: The Difficult Child, rev ed. New York, Bantam, 2000.

Werner EE, Smith RS: Journeys from Childhood to Midlife. Ithaca, NY, Cornell, 2003.

Whittle S, Yücel M, Fornito A, et al: Neuroanatomical correlates of temperament in earely adolescents. J Am Acad Child Adolesc Psychiatry 47:682-693, 2008.

BOOKS ON TEMPERAMENT FOR PROFESSIONALS

Carey WB, McDevitt SC: Coping with Children's Temperament: A Guide for Professionals. New York, Basic Books, 1995.

Chess S, Thomas A: Temperament in Clinical Practice. New York, Guilford, 1986.

Keogh BK: Temperament in the Classroom. Baltimore, Brookes, 2003.

Kohnstamm GA, Bates JE, Rothbart MK (eds): Temperament in Childhood. New York, Wiley, 1989.

Kristal J: The Temperament Perspective. Baltimore, Brookes, 2005.

Molfese VJ, Molfese DL (eds): Temperament and Personality Development across the Life Span. Mahway, NJ, Earlbaum, 2000.

BOOKS ON TEMPERAMENT FOR PARENTS

Carey WB, Jablow MM: Understanding Your Child's Temperament, rev ed. Philadelphia, Xlibris, 2005.

Chess S, Thomas A: Know Your Child (1987). Republished Northdale, NJ, Aronson, 1996.

Kurcinka MS: Raising Your Spirited Child. New York, HarperCollins, 1991.

Turecki S, Tonner L: The Difficult Child, rev ed. New York, Bantam, 2000.

Part II

ENVIRONMENTAL INFLUENCES—FAMILY AND SOCIAL

8 INFLUENCES OF EXPERIENCE IN THE ENVIRONMENT ON HUMAN DEVELOPMENT AND BEHAVIOR

IRENE M. LOE AND HEIDI M. FELDMAN

The chapters in this section address the influence of the social environment on human development and behavior. In the mid-20th century, the focus on behaviorism within psychological theory and practice emphasized aspects of the environment as the explanation for development and behavior. In the late 20th century to the present, the focus on genetic and neurobiologic mechanisms of development and behavior has sometimes overshadowed investigation into the role of the environment in shaping human behavior. The purpose of this chapter is to draw close attention to the chapters that follow in this section. We seek to show that the environment influences not only human behavior, but also the underlying neurobiologic and genetic mechanisms that create it. The nature versus nurture debate is no longer tenable as a contest between two extreme positions. Numerous molecular, animal, and human studies support the fundamental interaction of physiologic mechanisms and environmental inputs.

Environmental input is particularly important for species that are immature at birth. A cliff-dwelling bird must have strong innate abilities to fly because the environment is unlikely to provide any safe practice sites. Humans, by contrast, are extremely immature at birth. As such, the environment has more opportunity to influence the development of skills and behaviors. We now recognize that human infants rely on social structure not only for nurturance and protection, but also for the experiences that allow them to grow, develop, learn, and express their unique identity.

Environmental influences are bidirectional, with the child exerting influence on the environment as well. Many child characteristics, including genetics, temperament, and health status, shape the child's response to the environment. These interactions transform environmental features, for example, by creating stress or affecting parental emotions, family function, and social support. Topics related to child characteristics are highlighted in later chapters. The focus here is to highlight the role of the environment. This chapter documents through examples how experience influences (1) human behavior and development, (2) the human brain, and (3) gene expression.

DEFINITION

Environment can be defined as the circumstances, objects, or conditions by which one is surrounded; the complex of physical, chemical, and biotic factors that act on an organism or an ecologic community and ultimately determine its form and survival; or the aggregate of social and cultural conditions that influence the life of an individual or community. The environment is all-encompassing.

Environmental input must be stored in the brain to shape development and behavior. Greenough and colleagues (1987) have proposed two forms of storage dedicated to two distinct categories of environmental input. The first is input that is ubiquitous and common to all species members, or *experience-expectant*. The second is unique or idiosyncratic to the individual, or *experience-dependent*. Experience-expectant developmental processes imply that (1) there are required experiences covering a broad range of expected environments and (2) the lack of such experiences interferes with normal structural and functional development despite later exposure to appropriate environmental inputs. Experience-dependent processes also involve active changes among neural systems in response to an individual's unique and specific experiences. Learning could be considered an example of an experience-dependent process. These processes are crucial to individual survival because the timing and character of information needed vary widely among individuals within the species. The nervous system needs mechanisms to incorporate such experience whenever it becomes available.

Language development offers the opportunity to contrast the two types of processes. The organization of the language centers of the brain is an example of experience-expectant processes because almost every human reliably has early exposure to language in the environment. Learning the specific words and phrases of a language is an example of experience-dependent processes, based on the specific family and school experiences of an individual child.

ENVIRONMENTAL INFLUENCES OF DEVELOPMENT AND BEHAVIOR

Aspects of the physical environment, such as nutrition and toxins, have long been recognized to influence healthy growth and development. Folic acid deficiency during pregnancy has been associated with neural tube defects. Iodine deficiency remains the leading world cause of preventable intellectual disability, and neurologic damage from early fetal iodine deprivation is only minimally reversible with treatment. Iron deficiency in infancy, the most common nutritional deficiency, is associated with persistent lower scores on measures of mental and motor development. Exposure to environmental neurotoxins, such as lead, methyl mercury, and polychlorinated biphenyls, has been associated with significant developmental morbidity and mortality. The many adverse consequences of lead exposure, including inattention, learning problems, hyperactivity, decrease in IQ, aggression, impulsivity, encephalopathy, and anemia, have resulted in routine screening of blood lead levels and substantial public health efforts to eliminate lead exposure.

The impact of the psychosocial environment on development also is striking. In the 1940s, Spitz documented the devastating effects of extreme deprivation and institutionalization on motor, cognitive, and emotional development. The lack of a primary relationship with a human caregiver and the extreme social deprivation are considered mechanisms for poor developmental outcomes. Children from institutionalized settings not only are at high risk of poor developmental outcomes, but also exhibit continued behavioral difficulties in the form of aggression, indiscriminant sociability, hyperactivity, and peer relationship problems.

At far less severe levels of deprivation, the risk of unfavorable outcomes remains high. Children of lower socioeconomic status, who have increased exposure to medical illness, family stress, inadequate social support, and parental depression, have less favorable developmental and behavioral outcomes than children of the middle and upper classes. They also experience more serious consequences from these risks than children of higher socioeconomic status. A classic study by Werner (1989) found that poverty places children at greater risk from perinatal insults. Sameroff and colleagues (1993) found that the cumulative effects from multiple risk factors, such as maternal mental health problems, anxiety, low education, impaired mother-child interactions, unemployment, minority status, large family size, and stressful life events, increase the probability that development will be compromised.

Numerous studies document that parenting style and child rearing practices affect child development. Studies of developmental disorders, including attention-deficit/hyperactivity disorder, the most common neurobehavioral disorder, often focus on socioeconomic status, parenting style, and other factors in the environment as potential mediators or moderators of outcome. Similarly, research on attachment and personality focuses on the quality of the early caregiving environment and relationships to understand attachment quality and later behavioral adjustment. Current research shows that the connections between early experience and later behavior and personality are not direct (Schaffer, 2000).

Studies of children adopted from orphanages of the Ceaucescu regime in Romania have documented that the duration of deprivation, reflected in the age at the time of adoption, was more predictive of developmental outcome than weight and developmental status at the time of adoption. Children adopted after 2 years of age had the least favorable outcomes and were the most likely to have intellectual or behavioral impairments at follow-up compared with nonadopted peers. As a group, children adopted before 6 months of age had the most favorable outcomes and were similar to their nonadopted peers at age 4 or 6 years, whereas children adopted between 6 and 24 months were intermediate between the two groups.

ENVIRONMENTAL INFLUENCES ON NEURAL FUNCTION AND STRUCTURE

Current neurophysiologic and functional measures, in conjunction with more traditional assessments of behavior and development, allow for in-depth investigation of the impact of early experience and adversity on underlying neurobiologic mechanisms. The Bucharest Early Intervention Project is a randomized controlled trial of foster placement as an alternative to institutionalization of abandoned infants and toddlers in Bucharest, Romania (Zeanah et al, 2003). The study included assessment of the caregiving environment, physical growth, cognitive and language function, social communication and relatedness, and attachment, and measures of neural activity in the form of event-related potentials (ERPs) and brain electrophysiology (electroencephalography). ERPs are measured during repeated presentation of a stimulus, generating reliable patterns of brain activity that are believed to reflect the neurocognitive processes involved in processing a stimulus, such as a face. Responses to faces are believed to play an important role in social cognition. When presented with familiar (caregivers) and novel (strangers) faces, the ERPs measured in the institutionalized children differed from the noninstitutionalized children in overall amplitude and showed a group difference in face discrimination for one of the ERP components (Parker et al, 2005a). In another ERP study, the children were presented with four facial expressions—afraid, angry, happy, and sad (Parker et al, 2005b). The institutionalized children again showed group differences in amplitude of responses and different patterns of responding in early latency components of the ERPs compared with noninstitutionalized children. These findings suggest that early institutional rearing disrupts the neural structures and circuitry involved in facial and emotional processing.

Brain as a Self-Organizing System

Traditional views of the brain assumed that specific functions were located in restricted brain regions, and that each region contributed narrowly to isolated functions. The traditional view held that the localization of functions within specific regions of the brain was the result of genetic imprint, fixed and unchanging.

We now know that the brain holds enormous potential to self-organize in the face of experience and injury. Experience in the environment induces neural organization in sensory, motor, and higher cognitive systems. Basic functions are the result of multiple areas of brain collaborating. The connections between areas continue to evolve as a function of how often they are used and other experiential factors.

The classic example of how environmental deprivation affects neural structure and visual function was provided by Hubel and Wiesel (1965), who investigated visual development and critical periods in cats. They showed that not only visual behavior, but also the cytoarchitecture and physiology of the visual system of cats were based on specific visual inputs. Cats deprived of visual input did not develop the usual columnar organization of visual cortex. Similarly, patients with congenital cataracts who later recover vision have significant difficulty integrating newfound visual input (Fine et al, 2003). Such patients have described using touch with newly acquired visual input to perform a type of cross-modal transfer to "understand" what they see. Presumably, the cytoarchitecture of their visual system is unusual, as it was in the deprived cats.

At a less extreme level, the failure to correct strabismus in the first few years of life leads to abnormalities in binocular vision that are difficult, often believed to be impossible, to remediate. There is growing support, however, for more plasticity in the adult brain than previously believed, as evidenced by more recent case reports of the recovery of stereoscopic vision in adults with strabismus who received vision therapy in adulthood (Sacks, 2006). Extensive practice on a challenging visual task can improve perceptual performance in adults with amblyopia, and this improvement may transfer to improved visual acuity (Levi, 2005).

Animal studies offer strong evidence of alternative patterns of connectivity and profiles of neural organization as a function of experience. In the ferret, Sur and colleagues (1999) showed that lesioned neonatal sensory systems have the capacity to develop fundamentally different patterns of connectivity than the sensory systems found in unlesioned animals. Visual information was rerouted from visual to auditory cortex in the infant ferret. Although representations in the auditory cortex were not completely normal, the auditory tissue developed retinotopic maps. Schlaggar and O'Leary (1991) removed cortical tissue from one brain region in the rat (e.g., somatosensory cortex) and transplanted this tissue in another region (e.g., visual cortex). The transplanted tissue successfully integrated its functional connections within the host region and developed representations (cortical maps) appropriate for the new region in which they were located and not for the regions from which they originated.

In humans, numerous examples show cortical reorganization in the context of experience. After years of practice, violinists have reorganization of somatosensory cortex, with overrepresentation of the left fingers compared with the right fingers and with fingers of the left hands of nonviolinists (Elbert et al, 1995). Individuals who are blind and read Braille have an exceptionally large representation of the reading finger in tactile parts of the cortex. Adults with congenital blindness show activation of visual cortex when reading Braille (Pascual-Leone and Torres, 1993) or processing auditory stimuli, whereas deaf individuals show activation of auditory cortex when presented with visual input in the form of sign language (Fine et al, 2005). In amputees, mapping studies indicate that massive cortical reorganization occurs within days to weeks in response to amputation with expansion of functional representations of the remaining digits or limb into the amputated finger or limb space (Weiss et al, 2000).

Plasticity

Plasticity is the capacity of the brain to adapt or change in response to activity or experience, usually after injury or disease. Many of the examples in the previous section on cortical reorganization also are examples of plasticity. Other examples of plasticity in the human brain include the recovery of motor or language function after stroke or the sparing of language function after brain surgery for epilepsy. Modern imaging studies document that the brain is capable of novel organizations or reorganization after injury in response to learning. Reorganization may occur within brain regions or may involve recruitment of new regions to support function. Plasticity also can be observed at a cellular level, in which synapses show changes in communication or signaling with experience. Plasticity can occur in response to positive and negative events, conferring adaptability and vulnerability in young children.

The developmental timing of injury or experience can be crucial for outcome. In the animal literature, seminal work by Kennard (1938) showed that neonatal lesions of motor cortex in monkeys had minimal effect on the development of motor functions, whereas such lesions in adult monkeys resulted in severe and permanent motor impairment. Kennard also showed that such resilience did not apply to all neural systems, as illustrated by permanent blindness after bilateral ablation of occipital regions. More recent work by Webster and colleagues (1995) showed that more extensive lesions were required to disrupt performance of adult monkeys lesioned early in life, implying that alternative patterns of functional organization can develop after early lesions. In addition to timing, the site makes a difference. Lesions in subcortical systems that project to dorsolateral prefrontal cortex cause dramatic and lasting effects on performance, in contrast to early lesions made directly in the dorsolateral prefrontal cortex (Goldman, 1971).

Children who have had early focal lesions to what are considered left hemisphere language centers before learning language nonetheless learn language with only modest delays compared with normal learners. Functional imaging studies show that children with left hemisphere lesions or epilepsy with a left hemisphere focus frequently reorganize language into homologous regions of the right hemisphere (Booth et al, 2000). There are limits on plasticity, however, as shown by the fact that some injuries and exposures have greater impact the earlier they are sustained. Bilateral neural injury, traumatic brain injury, endocrine disorders such as hypothyroidism, and metabolic diseases such as phenylketonuria typically result in far worse outcomes when occurring or left untreated in early infancy than if acquired or untreated at an older age.

Mechanisms

It was previously believed that neurogenesis was complete at birth. More recent studies have documented that postnatal neurogenesis occurs in vertebrates ranging from birds to primates and persists through at least middle age in the hippocampus (Gould et al, 1999). Neurogenesis in the hippocampal dentate gyrus occurs in response to experience, including environmental complexity or enrichment, learning, and stress (Kempermann et al, 1997). Although these new neurons function similar to neurons formed prenatally, in that they form connections, are incorporated into existing circuitry, and show normal electrophysiologic profiles, they differ from prenatally derived neurons by having a shorter survival time. It is unclear if the postnatal neurons replace lost prenatal neurons or carry out some other function, such as functions involved with memory and learning (Leuner et al, 2006).

Synaptic sculpting is another neural mechanism that responds to experience. Initial overproduction of axons and dendrites is followed by retraction. Behaviorally, it has long been known that rats housed in complex learning environments outperform rats reared in isolation on motor, learning, and memory tasks (Hebb, 1947). In addition, rats in the complex environment had heavier and thicker regions of the dorsal neocortex, with more synapses per neuron, increased dendritic spines and branching patterns, and greater capillary branching, than rats raised in simple environments. Animal studies also show that exposure to a complex environment results in significant changes in dendritic field dimensions, synaptogenesis, and synaptic morphology compared with neural structures in animals housed in standard laboratory cages (Dong and Greenough, 2004). Even when the environmental exposure or training is discontinued, these neuronal changes persist for varying but substantial lengths of time.

Studies suggest that exposure to a complex environment does not induce a ubiquitous plastic response throughout the brain, but, rather, specific effects in the brain systems involved in processing specific components of the animal's experience. It is the learning experience that apparently is the cause of morphologic change in neurons, rather than other nonspecific global hormonal or metabolic effects.

Other mechanisms of learning and plasticity in the brain may involve non-neuronal elements, such as glial cells (astrocytes and oligodendrocytes), myelin, and vasculature. Myelination speeds nerve conduction velocity and has implications for serial and parallel processing in the brain. Exposure to an enriched environment increases myelination of subcortical pathways, increases the amounts of astrocytic material and the degree of contact between astrocytes and the surface of synapses, and dramatically increases the degree of capillary perfusion of the brain. Such non-neuronal plasticity often occurs in tandem spatially and temporally with neuronal plasticity. The effects of environmental manipulation on up-regulating processes, such as gliogenesis, neurogenesis, and structural interactions between neurons and glia, could have clinical implications for developmental brain disorders, such as autism and fragile X syndrome (Grossman et al, 2003; Irwin et al, 2005).

Implications for Therapy

New therapies are capitalizing on the role of experience in neural reorganization. In adults, constraint-induced movement therapy has been shown to improve motor function in hemiparesis owing to stroke. Traditional views of motor disability after stroke in adults included an assumption that functional improvement is unlikely beyond the first several months after stroke onset. Taub (1980) showed that in monkeys who developed chronic upper extremity nonuse after sectioning of the dorsal cervical and upper thoracic spinal nerve roots (somatosensory deafferentation), nonuse could be reversed several months to years later with 3 days of physical restraint applied to the contralateral, unaffected arm. Although the precision of movements was impaired, the limb function enabled self-care and routine daily living activities. When training was used, purposeful limb use also could be induced. A type of training called shaping, which involves incremental increases in the difficulty of task performance to achieve a reward, was especially effective.

Taub (1980) proposed the concept of "learned nonuse" to account for part of the persistent limb motor deficit after certain types of neurologic injury. An affected limb may have a potential but unrealized ability to move because of reliance on the unaffected limb. The individual either is unable to move the more affected limb or makes clumsy, inefficient movements, which discourages future attempts to use the more affected limb. At the same time, the individual learns to compensate by using only the uninvolved limb for most purposes. The individual eventually learns not to use the more affected limb, which is held in powerful inhibition. An important premise of constraint-induced movement therapy is that learned nonuse can be unlearned.

Applying these principles to rehabilitation after stroke, Taub (1980) showed that adults attain considerable recovery of function. Current constraint-induced movement therapy includes massed practice with the more affected arm on functional activities, shaping tasks in training exercises, and restraint of the less affected arm for a target of 90% of waking hours. Functional neuroimaging techniques enable study of training-induced plasticity in stroke patients. Some studies have shown bilateral activation of motor cortex before training and a subsequent shift in neural activation from the contralesional (unaffected hemisphere) to ipsilesional (affected hemisphere) motor areas after training. Some studies also have found activation in somatosensory cortex, similar to the findings in motor cortex, although laterality (contralesional versus ipsilesional) has varied in studies, suggesting interindividual variability or different reorganization mechanisms in different subjects (Hamzei et al, 2006).

Constraint therapy is now being used in children with cerebral palsy (Boyd et al, 2001), a nonprogressive syndrome of posture and motor impairment caused by a problem or injury in the developing central nervous system. Standard physical and occupational therapy in the treatment of cerebral palsy has shown only modest efficacy, and new skills often do not generalize to real-life situations. Adults with stroke lose previously mastered motor activities, whereas children with cerebral palsy fail to develop motor skills. Their motor impairments might more appropriately be labeled "developmental disregard," rather than learned nonuse (Taub et al, 2004). The same mechanisms that operate in adults likely create the same pattern in children, however—a behavioral tendency to inhibit use of the more affected arm and use the less affected arm because it is met with more success in daily activities. In a randomized, controlled trial of constraint-induced movement therapy in children with hemiparesis associated with cerebral palsy, Taub and colleagues (2004) found significant gains in motor function with benefits maintained over 6 months.

As we integrate neuroscience and developmental-behavioral pediatrics, we can anticipate that additional theory-driven therapies may emerge. Similar to constraint-induced movement therapy, they may vastly increase a set of experiences, allowing the individual to complete successive approximations to the goal successfully. Through the experiences of either the sensory or the motor systems, it is possible that experience would induce neural changes that subsequently improve the level of function. Imaging studies would allow investigation of whether neural reorganization occurred as a result of the intense experience. In this light, an early study of neural structure after developmentally enhanced experience in the neonatal intensive care unit suggests that some existing therapies also may change neural structure (Als et al, 2004). It is possible that some functions may recover better than others despite intensive therapeutic efforts, indicating limits on plasticity.

ENVIRONMENTAL INFLUENCES ON GENE EXPRESSION

In the same way that neural structure and function were traditionally conceptualized as fixed, gene expression was traditionally defined in simplistic terms. In the old model, genes coded a single trait, such as blonde hair or blue eyes, and those traits were stable features of an individual. What we have learned in the last decade is that gene action is far more complex. *Genomics* refers to the more ambitious study of all the genes in the genome, including their function, interaction, and role in various common disorders that are not due to single genes. Humans have fewer genes than previously estimated, essentially the same number as mice and only slightly more than twice that of *Drosophila*. The sequence of base pairs in human DNA seems insufficient, alone, to determine how gene products interact to produce an organism. Genes interact with each other, sometimes synergistically, sometimes antagonistically. Some gene expression is in a constant state of flux, responding to specific environmental inputs or experiences and allowing for the influence of phenomena, such as learning.

One strategy for identifying what a gene does is to see what happens to the organism when that gene is missing. Studying knockout mutant organisms that have acquired deletions in a given gene is a useful technique. The resulting distinctive appearance or behavior of the animal suggests the function of the gene. Analogous to the limitations of lesion studies to understand brain function, knockout experiments interrupt gene-gene interactions and related processes and may not accurately isolate the specific functions of that gene (Perrimon, 1998). Nevertheless, animal studies provide a mechanism for studying the role of environmental experience or enrichment on gene expression in the brain.

Gene expression has been studied in the rodent brain using oligonucleotide microarray hybridization to investigate molecular mechanisms underlying cognitive improvements after enrichment (Rampon et al, 2000). Mice were exposed to enriched environments for 3 hours to 14 days; changes in gene expression in the cortex were then examined. Enrichment training resulted in a significant change in the expression of multiple genes compared with control mice housed in standard laboratory conditions. Differential expression of genes occurred after short (3 and 6 hours of exploration) and long (2 and 14 days) periods of enrichment training, supporting early and longer term effects of enrichment. Although many of the expressed gene products are involved in neuronal structure, plasticity, and neurotransmission, the up-regulation of such proteins and their exact physiologic roles remain unclear and warrant further study. In another study of rats, exposure to an enriched environment resulted in increased levels of fragile X mental retardation protein levels in visual cortex and the hippocampal dentate gyrus compared with animals raised in standard laboratory cages (Irwin et al, 2005).

In humans, monozygotic twins show differences in disease susceptibility and phenotypic discordance despite having identical genotypes. Studies of monozygotic twins include investigation of the role of environmental influences on epigenetic information—genetic information that is heritable during cell division, but not contained within the DNA sequence itself. Such information causes changes in gene expression through mechanisms such as DNA methylation and chromatin modifications. A study of monozygotic twin pairs shows increasingly divergent patterns of epigenetic modifications as the pairs get older; the epigenetic markers studied were more distinct not only in monozygotic twins who were older, but also in twins who had different lifestyles and had spent less of their lives together, emphasizing the role of environmental factors (Fraga et al, 2005).

GENE-ENVIRONMENT INTERACTIONS

The study of genetic polymorphisms also provides another means of examining gene-environment interactions. The serotonin transporter gene (*5HTT*) is one of the most widely studied genes in relation to psychopathology. *5HTT* is involved in the regulation of the neurotransmitter serotonin via reuptake and the availability of serotonin in the synaptic cleft. The *5HTT* gene has two alleles, short (s) and long (l), resulting in three genotypes: homozygous short (s/s), homozygous long (l/l), and heterozygous (s/l). The short allele results in decreased *5HTT* transcription, lower transporter levels, and reduced serotonin reuptake (Verona et al, 2006). In adults, the short allele also has been associated with a predisposition to anxiety and negative emotionality (Munafo et al, 2003).

Numerous studies have investigated the interactions between *5HTT* alleles and the environment. In a prospective longitudinal study of a representative birth cohort of humans, the influence of stressful life events on depression was moderated by *5HTT* polymorphism (Caspi et al, 2003). Compared with individuals homozygous for the long allele, individuals with one or two copies of the short *5HTT* allele exhibited more depressive symptoms, diagnosable depression, and suicidality in relation to stressful life events. The *5HTT* short allele also has been associated with a predisposition for increased physiologic reactivity in response to stressors. In a functional magnetic resonance imaging experiment, Hariri and colleagues (2002) found that individuals with one or two copies of the short *5HTT* allele exhibited greater amygdala neuronal activity in response to fearful stimuli compared with individuals homozygous for the long allele.

Studies of associations of the short allele with temperamental traits in children have been less consistent than studies of psychopathology in adults. It may be that the timing and measure of behavioral characteristics determine the results of such association studies. It also is possible that the studies to date have failed to consider important environmental influences. Fox and colleagues (2005) found evidence for a gene-environment interaction with the presence of the short allele and low social support resulting in increased risk for behavioral inhibition in middle childhood.

Low levels of serotonin in the brain also have been implicated in the expression of aggressive behavior; however, it is unclear whether such correlations indicate causal relationships (Ferrari et al, 2005). The monoamine oxidase A (MAO-A) enzyme, which catalyzes the deamination of serotonin and norepinephrine, has been studied to investigate possible links between serotonin and aggression. MAO-A knockout mice show increased aggression despite high levels of brain serotonin (Cases et al, 1995), which contrasts with pharmacologic inhibitors of MAO enzymes, which reduce aggression in the mouse. The discrepancy highlights the importance of examining other secondary effects of the gene deletion, including potential environmental influences.

A study of maltreated boys followed from birth to adulthood found that a functional polymorphism of MAO-A moderated the effect of maltreatment (Caspi et al, 2002). Maltreated children with a genotype conferring high levels of MAO-A expression were less likely to develop antisocial problems. The neural mechanisms for these gene-environment interactions are still unknown and warrant further investigation. These studies of genetic polymorphisms and gene-environment interactions are new, and many require replication.

SUMMARY

In the current era, with rapid advances in neuroscience and genetics, the role of the environment in understanding human development and behavior remains central. In addition to a long and venerable history of studies documenting the effects of deprivation and enrichment on human development, we now have evidence that experiences in the environment can fundamentally affect neural organization through neurogenesis, synaptic sculpting, and changes in non-neural components of the brain. Studies of genetic polymorphisms show that environmental effects may operate differentially depending on the particular alleles an individual has in various systems. Future research must develop new methods for studying these interactions and identify other examples of environmental influences. With the advent of personalized medicine, therapies can be developed that capitalize on the ability of selected experiences to modify neural organization or genetic expression.

REFERENCES

Als H, Duffy FH, McAnulty GB, et al: Early experience alters brain function and structure. Pediatrics 113:846-857, 2004.

Booth JR, MacWhinney B, Thulborn KR, et al: Developmental and lesion effects in brain activation during sentence comprehension and mental rotation. Dev Neuropsychol 18:139-169, 2000.

Boyd RN, Morris ME, Graham HK: Management of upper limb dysfunction in children with cerebral palsy: A systematic review. Eur J Neurol 8(Suppl 5):150-166, 2001.

Cases O, Seif I, Grimsby J, et al: Aggressive behavior and altered amounts of brain serotonin and norepinephrine in mice lacking MAOA. Science 268:1763-1766, 1995.

Caspi A, McClay J, Moffitt TE, et al: Role of genotype in the cycle of violence in maltreated children. Science 297:851-854, 2002.

Caspi A, Sugden K, Moffitt TE, et al: Influence of life stress on depression: Moderation by a polymorphism in the 5-HTT gene. Science 301:386-389, 2003.

Dong WK, Greenough WT: Plasticity of nonneuronal brain tissue: Roles in developmental disorders. Ment Retard Dev Disabil Res Rev 10:85-90, 2004.

Elbert T, Pantev C, Wienbruch C, et al: Increased cortical representation of the fingers of the left hand in string players. Science 270:305-307, 1995.

Ferrari PF, Palanza P, Parmigiani S, et al: Serotonin and aggressive behavior in rodents and nonhuman primates: Predispositions and plasticity. Eur J Pharmacol 526(1-3):259-273, 2005.

Fine I, Finney EM, Boynton GM, Dobkins KR: Comparing the effects of auditory deprivation and sign language within the auditory and visual cortex. J Cogn Neurosci 17:1621-1637, 2005.

Fine I, Wade AR, Brewer AA, et al: Long-term deprivation affects visual perception and cortex. Nat Neurosci 6:915-916, 2003.

Fox NA, Nichols KE, Henderson HA, et al: Evidence for a gene-environment interaction in predicting behavioral inhibition in middle childhood. Psychol Sci 16:921-926, 2005.

Fraga MF, Ballestar E, Paz MF, et al: Epigenetic differences arise during the lifetime of monozygotic twins. Proc Natl Acad Sci U S A 102:10604-10609, 2005.

Goldman PS: Functional development of the prefrontal cortex in early life and the problem of neuronal plasticity. Exp Neurol 32:366-387, 1971.

Gould E, Reeves AJ, Fallah M, et al: Hippocampal neurogenesis in adult old world primates. Proc Natl Acad Sci U S A 96:5263-5267, 1999.

Greenough WT, Black JE, Wallace CS: Experience and brain development. Child Dev 58:539-559, 1987.

Grossman AW, Churchill JD, McKinney BC, et al: Experience effects on brain development: Possible contributions to psychopathology. J Child Psychol Psychiatry 44:33-63, 2003.

Hamzei F, Liepert J, Dettmers C, et al: Two different reorganization patterns after rehabilitative therapy: An exploratory study with fMRI and TMS. Neuroimage 31:710-720, 2006.

Hariri AR, Mattay VS, Tessitore A, et al: Serotonin transporter genetic variation and the response of the human amygdala. Science 297:400-403, 2002.

Hebb DO: The effect of early experience on problem solving at maturity. Am Psychol 2:737-745, 1947.

Hubel DH, Wiesel TN: Binocular interaction in striate cortex of kittens reared with artificial squint. J Neurophysiol 28:1041-1059, 1965.

Irwin SA, Christmon CA, Grossman AW, et al: Fragile X mental retardation protein levels increase following complex environment exposure in rat brain regions undergoing active synaptogenesis. Neurobiol Learn Memory 83:180-187, 2005.

Kempermann G, Kuhn HG, Gage FH: More hippocampal neurons in adult mice living in an enriched environment. Nature 386:493-495, 1997.

Kennard M: Reorganization of motor function in the cerebral cortex of monkeys deprived of motor and premotor areas in infancy. J Neurophysiol 1:477-496, 1938.

Leuner B, Gould E, Shors TJ: Is there a link between adult neurogenesis and learning? Hippocampus 16:216-224, 2006.

Levi DM: Perceptual learning in adults with amblyopia: A reevaluation of critical periods in human vision. Dev Psychobiol 46:222-232, 2005.

Munafo MR, Clark TG, Moore LR, et al: Genetic polymorphisms and personality in healthy adults: A systematic review and meta-analysis. Mol Psychiatry 8:471-484, 2003.

Parker SW, Nelson CA; Bucharest Early Intervention Project Core Group: An event-related potential study of the impact of institutional rearing on face recognition. Dev Psychopathol 17:621-639, 2005a.

Parker SW, Nelson CA; Bucharest Early Intervention Project Core Group: The impact of early institutional rearing on the ability to discriminate facial expressions of emotion: An event-related potential study. Child Dev 76:54–72, 2005b.

Pascual-Leone A, Torres F: Plasticity of the sensorimotor cortex representation of the reading finger in braille readers. Brain 116(Pt 1):39-52, 1993.

Perrimon N: New advances in *Drosophila* provide opportunities to study gene functions. Proc Natl Acad Sci U S A 95:9716-9717, 1998.

Rampon C, Jiang CH, Dong H, et al: Effects of environmental enrichment on gene expression in the brain. Proc Natl Acad Sci U S A 97:12880-12884, 2000.

Sacks O: Stereo Sue. The New Yorker 82(18), 2006.

Sameroff AJ, Seifer R, Baldwin A, Baldwin C: Stability of intelligence from preschool to adolescence: The influence of social and family risk factors. Child Dev 64:80-97, 1993.

Schaffer H: The early experience assumption: Past, present, and future. Int J Behav Dev 24:5-14, 2000.

Schlaggar BL, O'Leary DD: Potential of visual cortex to develop an array of functional units unique to somatosensory cortex. Science 252:1556-1560, 1991.

Sur M, Angelucci A, Sharma J: Rewiring cortex: The role of patterned activity in development and plasticity of neocortical circuits. J Neurobiol 41:33-43, 1999.

Taub E, (ed): Somatosensory Deafferentation Research with Monkeys: Implications for Rehabilitation Medicine. Baltimore, Williams & Wilkins, 1980.

Taub E, Ramey SL, DeLuca S, Echols K: Efficacy of constraint-induced movement therapy for children with cerebral palsy with asymmetric motor impairment. Pediatrics 113:305-312, 2004.

Verona E, Joiner TE, Johnson F, Bender TW: Gender specific gene-environment interactions on laboratory-assessed aggression. Biol Psychol 71:33-41, 2006.

Webster MJ, Bachevalier J, Ungerleider LG: Transient subcortical connections of inferior temporal areas TE and TEO in infant macaque monkeys. J Comp Neurol 352:213-226, 1995.

Weiss T, Miltner WH, Huonker R, et al: Rapid functional plasticity of the somatosensory cortex after finger amputation. Exp Brain Res 134:199-203, 2000.

Werner EE: Vulnerability and resiliency: A longitudinal perspective. *In* Brambring M, Losel F, Skowronek H, (eds): Children at Risk: Assessment, Longitudinal Research, and Intervention. Hawthorne, NY, Walter de Gruyter, 1989.

Zeanah CH, Nelson CA, Fox NA, et al: Designing research to study the effects of institutionalization on brain and behavioral development: The Bucharest Early Intervention Project. Dev Psychopathol 15:885-907, 2003.

9 VARIATIONS IN FAMILY COMPOSITION

CRAIG GARFIELD

In 2005, 73.5 million children younger than 18 years old resided in the United States, an increase from 64 million in 1990 (U.S. Bureau of the Census, 2006b). These 73.5 million children are being raised in a wide variety of different family structures. Children are living in married or unmarried families, being raised by one parent or two, by grandparents, or by adoptive or foster parents. Their parents may be gay or straight; they may live together or apart. Their parents may share the same religious, cultural, or race/ethnicity, or they may not. In some families, both parents may work, whereas in others, just one parent may work. In still others, neither parent may be able to find work, or parents may take turns in the breadwinner role. Each family structure provides a unique experience for children and may have an impact on their growth and development. For pediatricians, greater awareness of the diversity of family compositions and the strengths and concerns in each structure allows them to help optimize each child's development, and increases the ability of pediatricians to anticipate potential problems for their patients.

Family structure can play a role in child development partly by affecting family dynamics, such as how family members behave and interact. Family structures can facilitate families in providing basic economic and resource support and love, feelings of value and competence, companionship, and shared values. Families can connect their children to the community and teach children how to get along in the world and to cope with adversity. Additionally, successful families communicate with each other, spend time together, embrace a common spiritual/religious belief system, and deal with crises adeptly.

Regardless of family composition, a caring parent is the most important element to maximize optimal child health and development. Caring parents exhibit warmth, nurturance, affiliation, and responsiveness to a child's needs, which facilitates the development of a strong attachment bond between the child and parent. Not only do caring parents provide the basic needs for their child, such as food, clothing, safety, and shelter, and health care and education, but also quality parenting entails accessibility, responsibility, and setting structure and behavior limits, all with a close eye toward the child's best interests (see also Chapter 10).

Generally, descriptions of attachment bonds and parenting practices have focused on the primary caregiver, which has historically been the mother. A growing societal shift has seen greater involvement of the father throughout childhood and adolescence in many realms of family life (U.S. Department of Education National Center for Education Statistics, 2001). Positive and sustained paternal involvement has been associated with myriad positive outcomes for children, such as increased weight gain for premature infants, improved breastfeeding rates, higher receptive language skills, higher academic achievement, higher self-esteem, lower depression and anxiety, and lower delinquent behavior (Garfield and Isacco, 2006; U.S. Department of Education National Center for Education Statistics, 2001). Fathers and mothers who are committed to the well-being of their child, regardless of marital status, provide the most positive environment for their child to grow.

EVALUATING CHILDREN IN DIFFERENT FAMILY SITUATIONS

Pediatricians have a unique role in evaluating children who live in different family situations. To start with, pediatricians need to identify accurately who lives in the home, who is involved in childcare and at what locations, who provides emotional support for the parents, the extent of noncustodial or noncohabiting biologic parent involvement, adequacy of economic resources, and the underlying rewards or stresses of child rearing in the family (Table 9-1). These questions can be asked in a direct fashion of all families. Legal guardianship must always be clarified, and the role of any noncustodial or noncohabiting parent should be ascertained. The pediatrician can gain insight into family functioning and parenting competence by discussing how decisions are made in the family, evaluating the emotional support and discipline of the child, and evaluating the family response to stressful situations.

It is important that the pediatrician begin contact with a family with an expectation that the members of the family can effectively raise their children and recognize that it is the pediatrician's responsibility to support that commitment. Approached in this positive manner, families often develop a trusting relationship with the pediatrician and turn to the pediatrician for support when overwhelmed with child rearing. This chapter identifies the strengths and challenges for each of the various family compositions and the specific role pediatricians can play in working with children in these families.

MARRIED TWO PARENT FAMILY—THE "TRADITIONAL" FAMILY

The American Academy of Pediatrics' "Report of the Task Force on the Family" (Schor, 2003) reports that children do best when they live with two mutually committed parents. Ideally, the two mutually committed parents should respect and support one another with adequate social and financial resources and actively engage in the child's upbringing. In the United States, 46% of married couple households have at least one child living in the household (Simmons and O'Connell, 2003). This family composition is generally considered the "traditional" family, but its prevalence has been declining. There is an idealization of the traditional "nuclear" family as the happiest, healthiest, and best for children and parents.

Table 9-1. Pediatric Evaluation of Family Adequacy

Inquire about living situation
Inquire about who is involved in childcare
Inquire about where childcare is obtained and the quality of the care
Inquire about adequacy of economic support
Inquire about sources of emotional support for parents
Inquire about location and involvement of biologic parents
Review development, daily life, and peer activities of child
Review family responses to stressful situations or problems
Identify quality and appropriateness of emotional support and discipline for child
Review how important decisions are made in the family, and how differences in opinion are resolved
Inquire about particular needs the family has and how the family is addressing them

Adapted from Sargent J: Variations in family composition. *In* Levine MD, Carey WB, Crocker AC (eds): Developmental-Behavioral Pediatrics, 3rd ed. Philadelphia, WB Saunders, 1999.

These families tend to have stronger economic footing and parents with higher self-esteem and greater life satisfaction. In addition, there is more positive role modeling for male and female children (Table 9-2). For fathers, marriage seems to have potent meaning because married men have expressed greater commitment and involvement with their children (Garfield and Chung, 2006). The traditional family composition may not result in the highest levels of individual satisfaction for each parent, however. If a parent feels forced into predefined roles, the resulting stress can affect his or her parenting. In addition, low compatibility between parents can lead to fighting, aggression, and negative conflict resolution, which can adversely affect children. These stressors may represent some reasons for the continuing high levels of divorce (40% to 50%) in the United States (see Chapter 12).

Traditional nuclear families are changing. Economic shifts over the past few decades have resulted in 75% of married families living on two or more sources of income. Parents in these dual-earner families may experience feelings of guilt as they try to balance employment and family demands (see Table 9-2). This balancing may be particularly difficult for parents with young children or parents experiencing role conflicts at home. In addition, dual-earner families may have greater need for quality, flexible, and affordable childcare. Breastfeeding becomes more difficult for employed mothers, especially poorer, lower educated, young, or African American mothers who may have less on-the-job flexibility and support from employers. Fathers can play a critical role, however, in influencing and supporting a mother in breastfeeding (Wolfberg et al, 2004).

Work and family are interconnected domains, and the demands from each domain often result in stress and role conflicts for one or both parents. Role quality and performance in each domain depend on the amount of stress and the resources available to buffer against the experienced stress. Work-family conflict results when the demands of work and family roles are incompatible, which causes the participation in one role to be difficult because of participation in the other role. This conflict works both ways: work to family and family to work (Voydanoff, 2005).

Table 9-2. Strengths, Common Concerns, and the Role of the Pediatrician in Dual-Earner Families

Strengths	Common Concerns	Role of Pediatrician
Economic benefits	Stress on parents from role conflict and work-family balance tensions	Encourage time together as a couple, bidirectional spousal support, and positive methods of conflict resolution
Greater life satisfaction for both parents	Feelings of guilt for parents	Emphasize importance of a collaborative parenting style
Higher self-esteem for parents	Need for quality childcare	Educate both parents about benefits of breastfeeding, and how to work and breastfeed successfully (e.g., pumping, increasing feeds when at home)
Positive role modeling for children	Lower breastfeeding rates among employed mothers	Suggest creative employment strategies, such as workplace flexibility, telecommuting, flextime, and job sharing when possible to decrease work-family stress
	Irregular schedules	
	Impacts on children of less time with parents, more time in outside care	

Role conflict within families may arise from gender role reversal, in which fathers assume traditional maternal roles, and mothers assume traditional paternal roles. One example of gender role reversal that leads to role conflict is when the mother earns more income than the father. This situation may result in a father's self-esteem declining and a loss of purpose. Overall, the relationship between salary and marital stability may depend on the meanings that dual-career families attach to who makes the largest financial contributions. Today, fathers may be more willing to accept nontraditional familial roles beyond breadwinner than in the past. Research shows that fathers are spending more time with their children and assuming more childcare tasks in the home, some even taking on the role of primary caregiver for their children. Fathers and families that are more accepting of nontraditional gender roles may benefit through decreased role conflicts.

For children, the benefits of having two employed parents are substantial from a financial standpoint and in terms of future access to workforce networks. In addition to more money to spend on family and child needs, parents who are satisfied with their work and career are more satisfied with their lives and have higher self-esteem, both of which are related to positive child outcomes.

UNMARRIED PARENTS AND CHILDREN LIVING TOGETHER—COHABITATION

The U.S. Census Bureau acknowledges that in many cases, the "single parent" household is really a cohabitation family structure, creating some overlap in their statistics (Fields, 2003). Cohabitation is defined as two unmarried partners who live together; a single parent household is defined by a lack of the second partner residing in the house. Cohabitation has become an increasingly common living arrangement in the United States. The 2000 Census counted 5.5 million unmarried heterosexual couples sharing a household; in 1990, there were only 2.9 million (U.S. Bureau of the Census, 2006a). For most couples, cohabitation is a relatively short-term arrangement, with about 55% of cohabiting couples marrying and 40% dissolving within 5 years (Ciabattari, 2004).

In 2002, 1.8 million children lived in a household with their mother and her unmarried partner (Fields, 2003). Another 1.1 million children resided in a household with their father and his unmarried partner (Fields, 2003). Both of these living arrangements can be referred to as cohabiting family compositions. Children were more than four times as likely to live with a single mother (17 million) than a single father (3.5 million), but children living with a single parent were three times as likely to have their father cohabiting than their mother (Fields, 2003). Higher proportions of African American and Hispanic children live with single parents and cohabitating family structures than white children (Fields, 2003).

Cohabiting families benefit children compared with some alternative compositions, such as single parent households (Table 9-3). As in married parent families, the relationship quality between the cohabiting adults plays an important role in ensuring healthy child development. For all families, the ability to remain flexible and adaptable to stressors and to maintain open communication is beneficial to children as they grow. It is possible that cohabiting families with high-functioning parents and with positive relationships can provide children with many of the same benefits as similar married parent families. These families do present additional risks to some children, however, because they may be more likely to dissolve and often include parents with lower economic resources.

Children living with biologic cohabiting parents on average experience worse behavior, emotional, and educational outcomes compared with children living in two parent married families. This difference seems to be related to the level of economic resources a family can provide. For children 6 to 11 years old, economic resources and parental support attenuate differences between children in married and cohabiting families. As children enter the transitional time of adolescence, 12 to 17 years old, parental cohabitation is negatively associated with well-being and economic resources (Brown, 2004).

Cohabiting relationships are generally unstable and may involve repeated parental separations and family reconstitutions. The higher levels of conflict and the separations can be sources of stress for parents and children. Parents may receive less consistent social support from a cohabiting partner and may experience higher levels of stress because of the uncertainty of the cohabiting relationship. Cohabiting families often have higher

Table 9-3. Strengths, Common Concerns, and the Role of the Pediatrician in Cohabiting Families

Strengths	Common Concerns	Role of Pediatrician
Two unmarried parents living together can provide more resources and supports for each other and children than single parents	Cohabitation is an unstable family structure with potential for repeated separations and higher levels of conflict, which can lead to increased stress for parents and children	Promote ongoing and open discussion of family roles
Child rearing and household tasks may be shared by cohabiting parents	Lower levels of social support from cohabiting partners	Facilitate exploration of obtaining workplace benefits
	Ambiguity surrounding division of resources and assignment of responsibilities	Encourage the use of formal supports to facilitate focuses
	Lack of formal and informal societal and employer supports	
	Negative academic outcomes for child	

levels of ambiguity (and stress) surrounding issues such as sharing sources of income, division of household and childcare responsibilities, and the nature of each partner's commitment to the family. Higher levels of conflict and stress have a negative impact on children in these families. Finally, cohabiting parents are not typically provided with the same societal and employment benefits that married families receive, such as economic and tax benefits, health care benefits, and decision making capabilities regarding the child.

For cohabiting families, as for all families, the most important way to maximize children's health and development is to ensure that the child has loving, committed parents who put the child's interests first (see Table 9-3). This situation can be facilitated through ongoing, open discussions about family roles, transitions, and potential upcoming stressors. The use of formal supports, such as couples' counselors or child therapists, can facilitate these discussions and provide the structure and language for effective communication at home.

SINGLE PARENT FAMILIES

The number of single parent families, headed by single mothers and single fathers, has been increasing. In 1970, there were 3 million single parenting mothers and 393,000 single parenting fathers; in 2006, there are 10 million single parenting mothers and 2.3 million single parenting fathers (U.S. Bureau of the Census, 2005). More than 60% of U.S. children live some of their life in a single parent household (Simmons and O'Connell, 2003).

Although these households share many of the same concerns as families in different compositions, such as the need for quality daycare, some issues are unique to single parent families. Two parents usually share responsibility and monitoring of the child, and provide encouragement and discipline as needed. When only one parent is consistently present, that parent must be the sole economic and parenting resource and must stretch to cover both domains. Often, a single parent has less regular interaction and involvement in day-to-day activities of the child (Carlson and Corcoran, 2001). This situation may give children the opportunity to develop resiliency, to assist in household chores out of necessity, and to become motivated to succeed (Table 9-4). These families may experience greater economic concerns regarding the ability to provide materially for children. Single parent families are disproportionately poor; overall, 28% of families with children and a female head-of-household and no husband and 13% of families with children and a male head-of-household and no wife lived below the poverty level in 2005 (U.S. Bureau of the Census, 2002). Research shows that children reared in single parent families do not fare as well as children reared in two parent families, on average, regardless of race, education, or parental remarriage (McLanahan and Sandefur, 1994); they are more likely to experience increased academic difficulties and higher levels of emotional, psychological, and behavior problems (Hanson et al, 1997; Previti and Amato, 2003).

Single parents may be "stretched thin" financially and emotionally, and this can have a direct and indirect impact on their children (see Table 9-4). Children in single parent families are more likely to experience accidents—suggesting lower levels of child supervision—and to see a physician, to receive medical treatment for physical illnesses, and to be hospitalized than children from two parent families (O'Connor et al, 2000). Single parents have higher levels of mental health problems, which could result partly from the stress of trying to balance the needs of employment, home responsibilities, child rearing, and interactions with the child's school with limited time, personal, and social support (Cairney, 2003). Children in single parent families also are more likely to live with adults unrelated to them. This situation can be concerning because these children are eight times more likely to die of maltreatment than children in households with two biologic parents (O'Connor et al, 2000).

As in all families, single parents can maximize the likelihood of success for their children by establishing a quality home environment (see Table 9-4). Although this situation may be especially challenging for single parents, children benefit from an organized household with clear rules and expectations, appropriate consequences

Table 9-4. **Strengths, Common Concerns, and the Role of the Pediatrician in Single Parent Families**

Strengths	Common Concerns	Role of Pediatrician
Potential to develop resiliency and protective factors	Lower levels of economic resources	Encourage culturally relevant, accessible school-based and community-based prevention programs that focus on parent training and assist children in learning positive life and social skills
Potential for child to learn household skills through performing household work	Higher levels of mental health problems	Identify quality daycare settings
Potential for motivation to succeed	Increased risk of child maltreatment	Help children get involved with structured activities in the community, such as youth sport leagues, after-school programs, and mentoring programs
	Increased vulnerability to stress and little social support	Assist parent in establishing quality home environment (e.g., minimize disorganization, community violence)
	Little opportunity for social life	Emphasize the importance of providing emotional nurturance and consistent limits for children
	Children exhibit high rates of behavioral problems	

for misbehavior, and emotional nurturance from the parent. It is important to support single parents attempting to establish successful households.

The external community can play a major role in the health and development of children in single parent families. On the one hand, violence in the community can adversely affect the child's opportunities for growth and development, and dampen interactions outside the home for fear of injury. On the other hand, many community organizations and school-based prevention programs that are culturally relevant and focus on assisting adults in their parenting and children in their development are often available. For school-age children, involvement in structured activities available in the community, such as mentoring programs, after-school programs, and youth sport leagues, can help optimize healthy child development. This involvement may be especially important for children in single parent families.

Compared with most other family structures (i.e., two parent families and grandparent-headed households), children living in a single parent family are most at risk for school difficulties, behavior problems, poverty, maltreatment, and a host of other negative influences to their health and well-being. Pediatricians, as advocates for children in most need of quality health care, can use this knowledge to provide children from single parent families with an increased quality of care and referrals to other supports and local services. A referral to a social worker may help connect a child with youth programs in the community such as Big Brother/Big Sister, athletic teams, after-school programs, and Boy/Girl Scouts, which can provide opportunities for positive social development.

SAME-SEX PARENTS

Although exact figures for children being raised in gay or lesbian families are difficult to obtain because of possible reporting biases, estimates are that 2 to 10 million gay and lesbian parents are raising 6 to 14 million children in the United States (Dingfelder, 2005). There is wide variation in same-sex family compositions; there are domestic partnerships not dissimilar from married partnerships, single lesbian mother families, single gay father families, divorced lesbian mother families, divorced gay father families, civil unions, planned lesbian mother–led families, and planned gay father–led families. Planned families can come into existence through assisted reproduction (i.e., egg donation, sperm donation, artificial insemination), surrogacy, or adoption (Pawelski et al, 2006). Most children who have gay parents were born in the context of a heterosexual relationship; these children have experienced divorce or separation and may still have contact with another parent (Pawelski et al, 2006). Other children may be adopted by a gay or lesbian couple together or by one parent who then enters such a relationship. The adoptive rights of same-sex parents are not recognized in 11 states, however (Dingfelder, 2005).

As measured through self-esteem, personality measures, peer-group relationships, behavior difficulties, academic success, and warmth, no major differences have been found regarding children raised in homosexual and heterosexual families (Fig. 9-1 and Table 9-5) (Pawelski et al, 2006; Perrin and Committee on Psychosocial Aspects of Child and Family Health, 2006). Good parenting, regardless of sexual identity, leads to strong attachment bonds, minimal emotional and behavior problems, and minimal confusion over sexual identity (Lassiter et al, 2006; Sargent, 2001). Similar to all families, open communication between parents and children is important; in these families, open discussions about the parents' sexual orientation can strengthen the parent-child bond (Adams et al, 2004; Dingfelder, 2005). Children raised in same-sex families have been found to be more tolerant of diversity and more nurturing toward other children (Pawelski et al, 2006; Tasker, 2005).

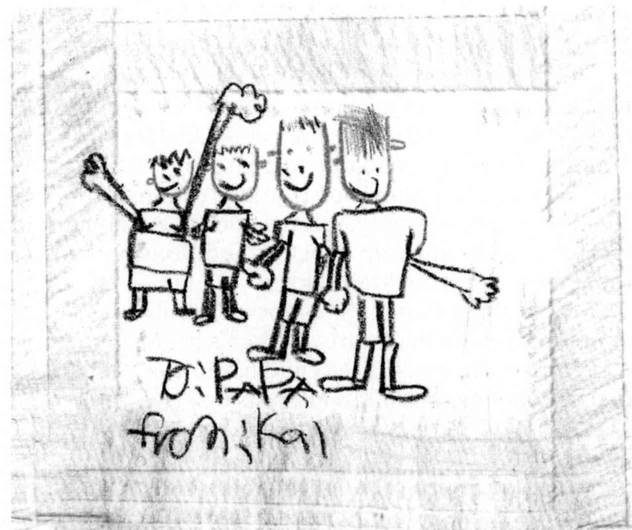

Figure 9-1. Child's drawing of his same-sex parent family.

Health care professionals need to be aware that children raised in same-sex families do have some concerns specific to this family structure (see Table 9-5). The social stigma of homosexuality and society's assumption that children of gay parents do not have healthy development can be hard on children and their parents. Children can become socially isolated from extended family if familial relationships were strained in their parents' "coming out" process. For children born into a heterosexual relationship that dissolved, negative interactions between their still-heterosexual biologic parent and their now-homosexual, bisexual or transgender parent can be especially stressful, and conflict between parents may be ongoing. For homosexual families working toward adoption, the legal process and associated societal stigma can be anxiety-provoking for parents and children (see Chapter 13) (Dingfelder, 2005). Finally, the cultural script for same-sex couples is more open to interpretation than for heterosexual couples and may result in greater role confusion among partners regarding financial, home, and childcare responsibilities (Adams et al, 2004). This greater ambiguity, as for cohabiting families, can increase conflict and be a source of stress for the entire family.

Table 9-5. Strengths, Common Concerns, and the Role of the Pediatrician in Same-Sex Families

Strengths	Common Concerns	Role of Pediatrician
No difference in child development exists between heterosexual and homosexual families as measured through peer-group relationships, personality measures, self-esteem, behavioral difficulties, academic success, warmth and quality of family relationships Good parenting, regardless of sexual identity, leads to strong attachment bonds, minimal emotional and behavioral problems, minimal confusion over sexual identity Open communication between parents and children about homosexuality strengthens parent-child bond Children are more tolerant of diversity and more nurturing toward other children	Social stigma of homosexuality and negative assumptions that children of gay parents do not have healthy development may create stress for child Children can become socially isolated from extended family if relationships were strained in their parents "coming out" process Parents may have their own issues in discussing their sexuality identity and development Prior heterosexual divorce and involvement of divorced parents may create higher levels of stress Child may have anxiety over legal adoption process Role confusion among partners with no set cultural script to follow regarding finances, chores, childcare responsibilities	Facilitate the use of formal and informal social supports (e.g., gay parenting and social groups) Advocate for greater parenting rights (e.g., adoptive, health care decision making) among same-sex parents Encourage open communication among parents and between parents and children about sexual identity, discrimination

INTERRACIAL AND INTERFAITH FAMILIES

Relationships outside one's own religion or race/ethnicity are becoming more common. From 1990 to 2000, biracial unions increased by 65%; interracial couples now constitute 1 in every 15 U.S. marriages. There are 3.7 million interracial marriages in the United States (Frey, 2003). The U.S. Census does not ask about religion, so religious intermarriages are more difficult to count; nevertheless, it is estimated that half of Catholics and Jews marry people outside their religion, and there is a reported 75% divorce rate for interfaith couples compared with divorce rates for Jewish and Catholic couples with shared faith of 30% and 21% (Lawlor, 1999). According to Myers (2006), religious homogamy—the extent to which husbands and wives hold similar religious beliefs and participate jointly in religious practices—seems to be one of the stronger religious predictors of marital quality.

Although these interracial and interfaith families may face many different issues, there are some commonalities. Children raised in these families are likely to have an increased awareness of the plurality of races and religions and an increased sensitivity toward different races, ethnicities, and religions (Fig. 9-2 and Table 9-6). These families are at risk, however, for stigmatization from their own extended families and from society in general. This lack of social support may be one element that makes these relationships more vulnerable to decreased marital satisfaction, family instability, and eventually divorce (Leslie and Letiecq, 2004). Children in these family structures may exhibit a decreased sense of belonging and identity confusion (Byrd and Garwick, 2006). Steps to avoid these issues include open discussion of historical racial or religious injustices and opportunities for each parent to express their worldview and thoughts about race and religion. Such families can find support through alliances with other like-minded families and individuals and through institutions with inclusive missions.

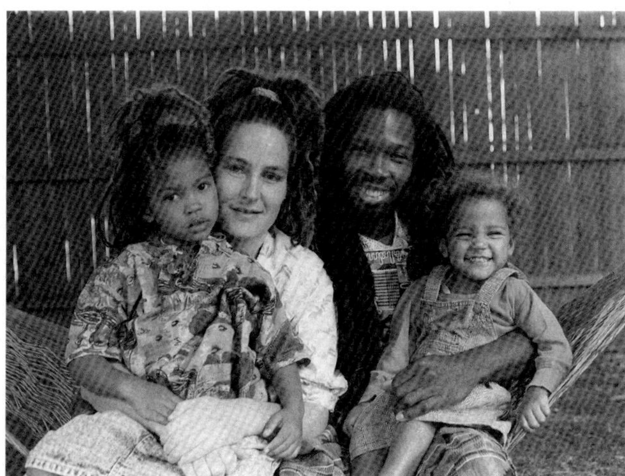

Figure 9-2. Multiracial family. (© Gigi Kaeser from the exhibits and books, "Of Many Colors: Portraits of Multiracial Families," produced and distributed by Family Diversity Projects, www.familydiv.org.)

GRANDPARENT-HEADED HOUSEHOLDS

Since 1990, there has been a 30% increase in the number of children living with grandparents (Hayslip and Kaminski, 2005). Although 5.5 million grandparents have grandchildren living with them and serve as the primary caregiver for the child, an additional 2.3 million grandparents provide basic needs (i.e., money, food, clothes) for their grandchildren, although the grandchildren do not live with them. Of these grandparents supporting grandchildren, 72% were younger than age 65.

Table 9-6. **Strengths, Common Concerns, and the Role of the Pediatrician in Interracial and Interfaith Families**

Strengths	Common Concerns	Role of Pediatrician
Children may have an increased awareness of plurality of races and religions Children may have higher sensitivity toward diversity of race, ethnicities, and religions	Racism, discrimination, and social stigma in larger society and in extended family Potential lack of social support and approval from family and society Child's own identity may be ambiguous or confused Children may have a decreased sense of belonging Families vulnerable to divorce, decreased marital satisfaction, and instability because of conflicting beliefs	Encourage discussion about historical injustices between racial/religious groups Facilitate better understanding of extended family of origin concerns regarding relationships outside own race/religion Support the parent in explaining each race/religion to child Encourage each parent to articulate own worldview Seek out like-minded individuals and institutions for support

Table 9-7. **Strengths, Common Concerns, and the Role of the Pediatrician in Grandparent-Headed Households**

Strengths	Common Concerns	Role of Pediatrician
Grandparents may enjoy a closer relationship with grandchild and having a second chance at parenting Grandparents may have enhanced sense of purpose Grandparents can maintain family identity and well-being Grandparents may have a low perception of stress Children have a positive role model Children have improved school performance, more autonomous decision making, and fewer deviant behaviors Children are less reliant on welfare Children benefit from love, security, and structure grandparents provide	Grandparents may have role overload and role confusion Grandparents may feel isolation from peer group Grandparent caregivers have poorer physical and mental health than noncaregiver grandparents Grandparent caregivers may lose income and have a higher chance of living at or below poverty line Grandparents may feel taken advantage of, disappointed, shameful, guilty, or resentful regarding their adult child Children may experience stress when biologic parent returns to family	Facilitate the use of formal supports such as community and professional services designed for grandparent caretakers to minimize impact of child-related caregiving stress Promote maintenance of informal supports, such as peer groups and friends, to continue with social connections Help family deal with the circumstances that resulted in grandparent being primary caretaker (i.e., death or incarceration of adult child) and experience of grief Anticipate when the parent may rejoin the family, and discuss the implications for the child

Most grandparent caregivers are female, and more than half of grandparents are married. More than 50% of grandparents caring for their children are white, 38% are African American, and 13% are Hispanic. Typically, grandparents become primary caregivers of grandchildren if the parents are young, incarcerated, financially restricted, ill, or dead.

Grandparents and grandchildren can benefit from living together, regardless of where the biologic parents reside (Table 9-7). Many grandparents enjoy this "second chance" at parenting and the chance to have a close relationship with their grandchild, and describe feeling an enhanced sense of purpose (Sands et al, 2005). Grandparents also may be motivated to care for their grandchildren because they want the opportunity to maintain family identity and well-being. Grandparents raising grandchildren typically have lower levels of perceived stress than grandparents not raising children. Children can benefit from this arrangement by having their grandparents as positive role models and love, security, encouragement, and structure in the form of supervision, rules, and expectations of behavior. These children have been found to have less reliance on federal aid programs, fewer deviant behaviors, more autonomous decision making, and improved school performance than children with physically or emotionally absent parents. Children from grandparent-headed households were as likely as children from single parent families to excel in school, but exhibited fewer behavior problems at school than children from single parents families (Hayslip and Kaminski, 2005).

This variation of family composition is not without its own difficulties (see Table 9-7). Grandparents may stop working to care for their grandchild, and consequently are more likely than grandparents not raising children to live at or below the poverty line; the mean income for grandparent caregivers is $20,000. In addition, grandparents who act as caregivers are at risk for becoming isolated from their peer group and are more likely to experience depression, diabetes, hypertension, heart disease, and insomnia than grandparents who are not caregivers (Hayslip and Kaminski, 2005).

Some grandparents may resent the imposition of having to care for their grandchild and may feel taken advantage of and disappointed by their lost freedom. Other grandparents may be upset with the failure of their own child to act as an appropriate parent figure. The circumstances that resulted in the grandparent becoming the primary caretaker (i.e., illness, protective services, jail, or death) also may weigh heavily on the family in general. Finally, the transition as a mother or father reenters the child's life can be stressful because the child will be used to one set of expectations and rules with the grandparents, and possibly another with the parent.

SUMMARY

Family composition continues to change, and even the diverse family formations discussed here are predicted to continue to change. Children will continue to develop and be raised in a variety of family structures, and may experience multiple family structures throughout their childhood. With continual change in family composition comes the need for clinicians working with families to know and understand the current strengths and concerns of each family structure to provide the highest quality of care to each patient. Likewise, knowing what steps can help to ensure the optimal healthy outcome for a child in a given family context is important for health care providers who work with children and families. Regardless of family composition, the necessary ingredients for a child to develop and flourish are a safe, nurturing environment created by nurturing and caring parents.

REFERENCES

Adams JL, Jaques JD, May KM: Counseling gay and lesbian families: Theoretical considerations. Family Journal: Counseling and Therapy for Couples and Families 12:40-42, 2004.

Brown SL: Family structure and child well being: The significance of parental cohabitation. J Marriage Fam 66:351-367, 2004.

Byrd MM, Garwick AW: Family identity: Black-white interracial family health experience. J Fam Nurs 12:22-37, 2006.

Cairney J, Boyle M, Offord DR, Racine Y: Stress, social support, and depression in single and married mothers. Soc Psychiatry Psychiatr Epidemiol 38:442-449, 2003.

Carlson MJ, Corcoran ME: Family structure and children's behavioral and cognitive outcomes. Journal of Marriage and Family 63: 779-792, 2001.

Ciabattari T: Cohabitation and housework: The effects of marital intentions. J Marriage Fam 66:118-125, 2004.

Dingfelder SF: The kids are all right. Monit Psychol 36:66-68, 2005.

Fields J: Children's Living Arrangements and Characteristics: March 2002. Current Population Reports (P20-547). Washington, DC: U.S. Census Bureau, 2003.

Frey WH: Charticle. Retrieved Third Quarter. 2003. Available at: http://www.frey-demographer.org/reports/Rainbownation.pdf#search=%22Frey%20interracial%20marriage%22. Accessed October 3, 2006.

Garfield C, Isacco AJ: Fathers and the well-child visit. Pediatrics 117:e637-e645, 2006.

Garfield CF, Chung P: A qualitative study of early differences in fathers' expectations of their child care responsibilities. Ambul Pediatr 6:215-220, 2006.

Hanson TL, McLanahan S, Thomson E, et al: Economic resources, parental practices, and children's well-being. *In*: Consequences of Growing Up Poor. New York, Russell Sage Foundation, 1997, pp 190-221.

Hayslip B, Kaminski PL: Grandparents raising their grandchildren: A review of the literature and suggestions for practice. Gerontologist 45:262-270, 2005.

Lassiter PS, Dew BJ, Newton K, et al: Self-defined empowerment for gay and lesbian parents: A qualitative examination. Family Journal: Counseling and Therapy for Couples and Families 14: 245-252, 2006.

Lawlor V: Is it OK for those of different faiths to wed? The Bergen Record, Hackensack, NJ, Marcull, 1999.

Leslie LA, Letiecq BL: Marital quality of African American and white partners in interracial couples. Personal Relationships 11:559-574, 2004.

McLanahan S, Sandefur GD: Which outcomes are most affected. *In*: Growing Up with a Single Parent: What Hurts, What Helps. Cambridge, MA, Harvard University Press, 1994, pp 39-63.

Myers SM: Religious homogamy and marital quality: Historical and generational patterns, 1980-1997. J Marriage Fam 68:292-304, 2006.

O'Connor TG, Davies L, Dunn J, et al: Distribution of accidents, injuries, and illnesses by family type. Pediatrics 106:68-72, 2000.

Pawelski JG, Perrin EC, Foy JM, et al: The effects of marriage, civil union, and domestic partnership laws on the health and well-being of children. Pediatrics 118:349-364, 2006.

Perrin EC: Committee on Psychosocial Aspects of Child and Family Health: Technical report: Coparent or second-parent adoption by same-sex parents. Pediatrics 109:341-344, 2006.

Previti D, Amato PR: Why stay married? Rewards, barriers, and marital stability. J Marriage Fam 65:561-573, 2003.

Sands RG, Goldberg-Glen R, Thornton PL: Factors associated with the positive well-being of grandparents caring for their grandchildren. J Gerontol Soc Work 45:65-82, 2005.

Sargent J: Variations in family composition. *In* Levine MD, Carey WB, Crocker AC (eds): Developmental-Behavioral Pediatrics, 3rd ed. Philadelphia, WB Saunders, 1999.

Sargent J: Variations in family composition: Implications for family therapy. Child Adolesc Psychiatr Clin N Am 10:577-599, 2001.

Schor EL: Family pediatrics: Report of the Task Force on the Family. Pediatrics 111(6 Pt 2):1541-1571, 2003.

Simmons T, O'Connell M: Married-couple and unmarried-partner households: 2000. 2003. Available at: http:www.census.gov/prod/2003pubs/censr-5.pdf. Accessed September 26, 2006.

Tasker F: Lesbian mothers, gay fathers, and their children: A review. J Dev Behav Pediatr 26:224-240, 2005.

U.S. Bureau of the Census: Detailed Poverty Tables, Table 16a: Poverty status of families by type of family, age of householder, and number of children: 2001. 2002. Available at: http://pubdb3census.gov/macro/032002/pov/new16a_000.htm. Accessed August 18, 2008.

U.S. Bureau of the Census: Facts for features: Mother's Day, May 8, 2005. 2005. Available at: http://www.census.gov/Press-Release/www/releases/archives/facts_for_features_special_editions/004109.html.

U.S. Bureau of the Census: America's Families and Living Arrangements: 2005. 2006a. Available at: http://www.census.gov/population/www/socdemo/hh-fam/cps2005.html. Accessed June 7, 2006.

U.S. Bureau of the Census: Annual Estimates of the Population by Selected Age Groups and Sex for the United States: April 1, 2000, to July 1, 2005. 2006b. Available at: www.census.gov/popest/national/asrh/NC-EST2006/NCEST 2006-02.xls. Accessed July 25, 2006.

U.S. Department of Education National Center for Education Statistics: Measuring father involvement in young children's lives: Recommendations for a fatherhood module for the ECLS-B (Working Paper No. 2001-02). Washington, DC, 2001.

Voydanoff P: Social integration, work-family conflict and facilitation, and job and marital quality. J Marriage Fam 67:666-679, 2005.

Wolfberg AJ, Michels KB, Shields W, et al: Dads as breastfeeding advocates: Results from a randomized controlled trial of an educational intervention. Am J Obstet Gynecol 191:708-712, 2004.

10 FAMILY FUNCTION AND DYSFUNCTION

STEPHEN LUDWIG AND ANTHONY ROSTAIN

Vignette

A 12-year-old girl is referred from her primary care pediatrician for a consultation. She has had intermittent abdominal pain for several months. The pain is moderate in quality, not localized, and does not relate to eating or stool patterns. She has neither lost nor gained weight. The primary care pediatrician has done a basic evaluation and has ruled out constipation, inflammatory bowel disease, celiac disease, or gynecologic cause. The child has yet to have menarche. The parents are very concerned and are looking for answers. The patient seems less concerned and has a flat affect.

After reviewing the history and performing a negative physical examination, the consultant takes a more in-depth social history. When asked about school, the child responds, "Which school?" With further questioning, it is revealed that this family is extremely wealthy. They own several homes in two cities in the United States and one in Switzerland. The family has domestic staff, clothes, and modes of transportation at each site. The family moves from place to place throughout the year, and the child travels with the family. She is enrolled in school in two locations. The child discussed the difficulty in finding and keeping a peer group in either location. Although she has all the material things a girl her age might want, she has not had a stable home. She has an excess of homes. The pain she has been experiencing is a psychophysiologic pain. It resulted from family dysfunction at a time in the child's life when she needed her family to provide stability for her to accomplish her adolescent developmental milestones. The child's parents were initially surprised by the diagnosis, but with discussion accepted it and determined to make appropriate lifestyle and family function changes.

A child's family is the primary influence of the psychosocial environment on her or his development and behavior. This chapter encourages the reader to think of the family's effects in terms of the specific tasks of supplying physical requirements; providing developmental, behavioral, and emotional needs; and socializing the child by furnishing and teaching about normal social relationships. This chapter also describes the consequences when there is a dysfunctional inadequacy or excess in the fulfillment of these roles, and their clinical management. The results of variations in family structure, rather than function, are discussed in Chapter 9.

The family's influence on a child is perhaps the most significant determinant of a child's development. There are important genetic and constitutional factors that are present at birth and that continue to influence the child throughout life. In the process of helping children grow and develop, the family and its functioning stand out as the strongest environmental factor. Although family structures, styles, and behavior patterns are varied in our culture (Bronfenbrenner, 1986) and around the world, the family is still the central social institution in all human societies.

A precise definition of family is difficult to construct because concepts are in a state of change. In 1965, a standard definition of family was "a social group characterized by common residence, economic cooperation, and reproduction" (Murdoch, 1965). The family includes adults of both sexes, at least two of whom maintain a socially accepted sexual relationship, and there are one or more children born to or adopted by the sexually cohabitant adults. This definition would not include many of the families rearing children today, however. This chapter does not explore the anatomy or structure of the family, but rather its physiology, or function. We explore the specific tasks of a family, and then review the nature and impact of various family dysfunctions on the child.

FAMILY FUNCTIONING

There are many variations not only in family form, but also in family functioning. All families have strengths and weaknesses. All families place different emphasis on different tasks at different points in the family's life cycle (Walsh, 1982).

Table 10-1. **Family Tasks in the Care of Children**

Supply Physical Needs
Protection
Food
Housing
Health care
Provide Developmental, Behavioral, and Emotional Needs
Stimulation—developmental and cognitive
Guidance—approval and discipline
Affection
Provide and Teach Social Relationships—Socialization
Training for family life
Training for citizenship

Table 10-2. **Family Dysfunction**

Task	Dysfunctional Inadequacy	Dysfunctional Excess
Supply Physical Needs		
Protection	Failure to protect Child abuse	Overprotection and overanxiety
Food	Underfeeding Failure to thrive	Overfeeding, obesity
Housing	Homelessness	Multiple residences "Yo-yo"/vagabond children
Health care	Medical neglect	Excessive medical care Munchausen syndrome by proxy
Providing Developmental, Behavioral, and Emotional Needs		
Stimulation—developmental and cognitive	Understimulation Neglect	Overstimulation "Hothousing" Parental perfectionism
Guidance—approval and discipline	Inadequate approval Overcriticism Psychological abuse	Overindulgence, "spoiled child"
Affection—acceptance, intimacy	Inadequate affection Emotional neglect Rejection Hostility	Sexual abuse Incest
Provide and Teach Social Relationships—Socialization		
Intrafamilial relationships	Attenuated family relationships Distanced parents	Parenting enmeshment Overinvolved relationships
Extrafamilial, community relationships	Boundary-less families Deficiency in training in extrafamilial relationships	Insular families Excessive restriction from extrafamilial relationships

Although there are many specific and specialized family functions, we can condense the functions pertaining to child rearing into three general categories: (1) to supply physical needs; (2) to provide developmental, behavioral, and emotional needs; and (3) to socialize or teach about relationships (Table 10-1). In the realm of supplying physical needs, the family must provide protection, food, shelter, health care, and other material goods. In the second area, the family should stimulate development and intellectual growth, provide guidance through approval and discipline, and meet needs for affection. The third category of function is socialization or teaching. This function involves helping the child relate initially with family members and later with external social networks (extended family, peers, school, and neighborhood) and with society in general. This last function may be termed the promotion of citizenship.

Some families are affected by pervasive parental dysfunction. The nature of this kind of dysfunction threatens all areas of family function and the integrity of the family unit.

Given the multitude of complex tasks that families strive to accomplish, it is reasonable to ask what constitutes normal family functioning. The answer depends on one's definition of the term *normal*. From the child's point of view, normal means that a family is meeting the child's needs.

SPECIFIC FORMS OF FAMILY DYSFUNCTION

The concept of dysfunction usually suggests lack of something important. With regard to the family function of providing food, inadequate function is considered to be lack of food, malnutrition, or failure to thrive. It is equally injurious to the child when there is excess—oversupplying food. Table 10-2 lists various forms of dysfunctional inadequacy and excess, such as too little or too much health care. There also can be a qualitative dimension; lack of protection may range from placing the child at risk for injury to active physical abuse by the parent. Although these forms are listed as distinct entities, they often overlap. A child who is physically abused also is likely to be psychologically abused. With each blow, there is an unspoken (and at times spoken) message to the child: You are bad, worthless, and unloved. An unknown factor in the effects of family dysfunction is the resilience of a given child. Ginsburg (2007) has detailed the elements and effects of individual resilience.

The factors responsible for and related to dysfunctional parenting are numerous, including personal problems of the parents, a variety of acute and chronic social stresses, and challenges presented by the child. Rather than present a list of these factors at once, we introduce them in the following sections, where they are most pertinent.

PHYSICAL NEEDS

Protection

Perhaps the most easily recognized and best documented form of family dysfunction is lack of protection. Lack of protection may range from parents who simply do not think of or provide a safe environment for their children (e.g., free of toxins, pests) (Hymel, 2006) to parents who are actively abusive. In this type of dysfunction, parents, rather than being protective, become destructive of their children.

Physical Abuse

Because there are state laws and sophisticated reporting systems for protecting children from physical abuse, we now have some idea of its incidence. The term *child abuse* is used as if it were a diagnosis, when it really describes a category or class of disorders that represent many different forms of family dysfunction. The 2006 report of the U.S. Department of Health and Human Services indicates that there were more than 3 million reports of abuse and more than 1 million substantiated reports. The rate of reports was 43 per 1000 population. Physical abuse was documented in 24.5% of the cases. It is believed, however, that there is gross underreporting of physical abuse, and that official reports may represent only half of the actual number of cases. The breakdown of the forms of abuse is shown in Figure 10-1. The American Academy of Pediatrics (Kellogg, 2007) has issued a statement on abuse evaluation.

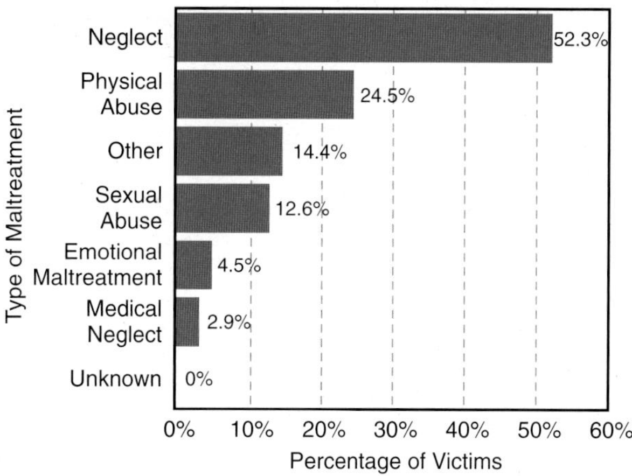

Figure 10-1. Types of maltreatment. N = 1,000,502 victims in 49 states. *Note*: Percentages total more than 100% because some states report more than one type of maltreatment per victim. *(From U.S. Department Health and Human Services, National Center on Child Abuse and Neglect: Child Maltreatment 1995: Report from the States to the National Child Abuse and Neglect Data System. Washington, DC, U.S. Government Printing Office, 1997.)*

Definition

Part of the problem of accurate reporting is the difficulty of uniformly defining physical abuse. Each state designates physical abuse in its own child protective laws. Each person may interpret abuse in his or her own way, based on numerous individual factors, such as age, sex, religion, cultural group, experiences as a child, experiences as an adult, and professional training. Giovannoni and Becerra (1979) showed that physicians and attorneys differ in their perceptions of abuse. Notions that child abuse exists and that each child has a right to societal protection from injury are evolving concepts. The first child abuse laws did not appear until the late 1960s. With all the nuances involved, clearly and precisely defining abuse as a risk factor is difficult. Child abuse is injury of a child by a parent or other caregiver either deliberately or by omission. Within a group of children captured by such a broad definition are children who have been murdered or repeatedly tortured by a deviant criminal parent and children who have been overzealously punished for a misbehavior on a single occasion (Fig. 10-2). At our current level of sophistication, it is difficult to define meaningfully the risk in terms of developmental or behavioral effects. We use the term *child abuse* as if it were a solitary diagnosis when in reality it reflects a spectrum of disorders.

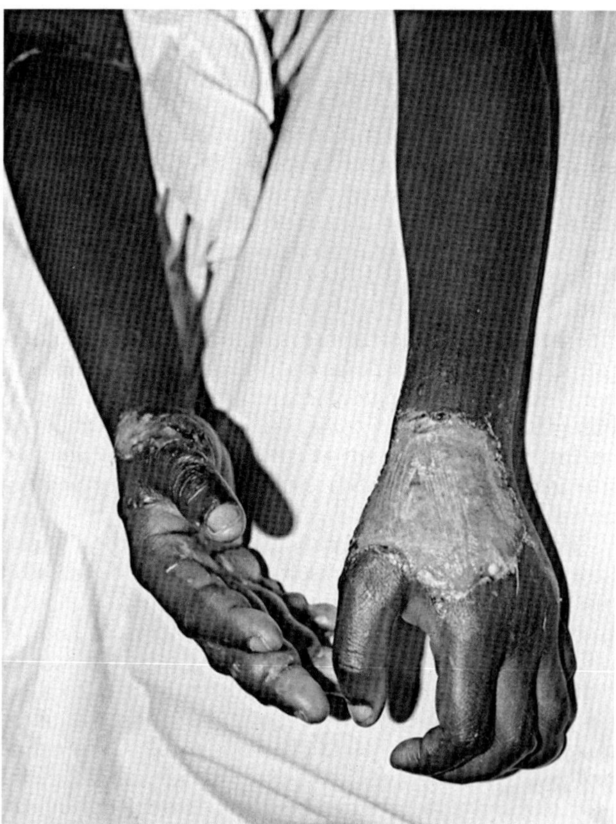

Figure 10-2. A 6-year-old boy with a history of fire setting who was overdisciplined by his mother's touching his hands to fire, producing second-degree burns of both hands.

Contributing Factors

Just as definitions and forms of abuse vary, so do reasons for child-harming behavior (Ludwig, 1993). Many factors are relevant. Why would a parent hurt a child? Table 10-3 lists these contributing factors and divides them into personal, familial, community-based, and society-based factors. Overall, parental stress stands out as the most important factor. The factors shown in Table 10-3 mediate through increasing parental stress levels. When stress becomes too great, the abuse-prone parent loses control. Children are always provocative and

Table 10-3. Factors Contributing to Physical Abuse

Parental Factors

Lack of knowledge about child development
Lack of preparation for parenting
Unrealistic expectations of child
Proclivity to violence in other forms—poor impulse control
Stress—marital, housing, economic
Use of drugs or alcohol
Emotional disorders—depression

Child Factors

Temperamental difficulty in the child
Child fails to meet parental expectations
Child is symbolic of something negative

Family Factors

Family pattern of physical violence
Isolation—absent or unhelpful extended family

Community Factors

Lack of support and community resources for parents
Factors that contribute to social isolation

Societal Factors

High rate of family mobility
Tolerance of corporal punishment
High level of violence in society
Devaluation of children

ready victims for parental explosive behavior. Physical injury results. Wu and colleagues (2004) have analyzed risk factors for infant maltreatment. The influence of societal violence also is an important contributing factor to the dynamics of violence against children.

Effects on the Child

The impact of physical abuse is physical and psychological. Each time a parent physically abuses the child, the potential exists for physical injury (e.g., broken bones, blindness, brain injury) (Fig. 10-3) and for psychological injury (e.g., "You are worthless; I can destroy you") that may seriously impede normal development and behavior (Table 10-4).

Most abuse victims do not die. In its worst form, however, physical abuse results in homicide. Studies by the Centers for Disease Control and Prevention (1982) show that the child homicide rate has increased sixfold since the 1930s. The 2008 NCANDS report indicates that 45 states reported 1530 child fatalities caused by abuse in 2006 (NCANDS, 2008). The report estimates the rate of 110 per 100,000 population. Of the homicides, 78% involved children younger than 3 years old. The consequences are experienced not only by the victim, but also by siblings and other family members. Schnitzer and Ewigman (2005) documented household risk factors. Studies of families that have lost a child show the profound effect of this type of loss even when the manner of death was other than homicide.

The number of physical manifestations that result from abuse are many and need not be detailed because they are described in references that focus on the diagnosis and physical management of abuse (Figs. 10-4 and 10-5) (Giardino et al, 1997; Kellogg, 2007; Ludwig, 1993; Ludwig and Kornberg, 1992; Reece, 1994; Wissow, 1990). Although any organ system or body part may be affected, numerous head and sensory organ injuries are reported. Some authors have suggested that the head is a prime target for abuse because it is the body part that cries, that talks back, and that holds the personality the parent wishes to injure. Head trauma carries with it the greatest potential for neurodevelopmental impairment. Martin's (1976) 5-year follow-up study of abused children found 53% of the 58 children studied to have some type of neurologic abnormality. Of children followed, 31% had moderate-to-severe injury that handicapped the everyday functioning of the child. Buchanan and Oliver (1979) estimated that 3% to 11% of children residing in hospitals for the retarded and handicapped were there as the result of violent abuse. Other studies

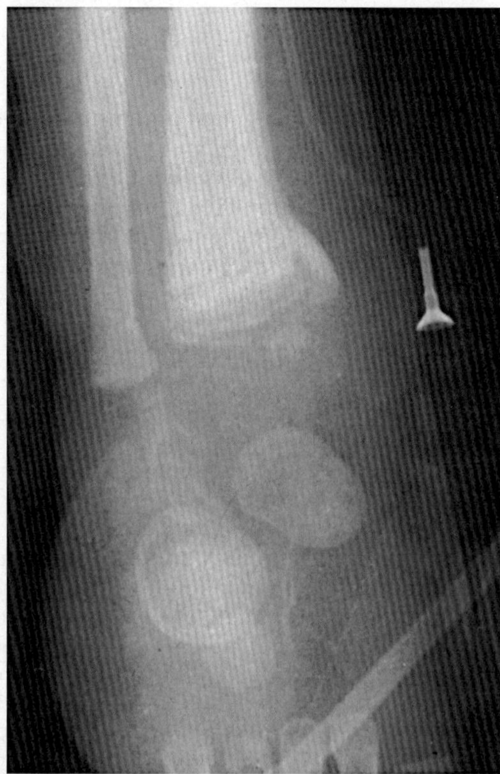

Figure 10-3. Bucket-handle fracture of distal tibia consistent with child abuse.

Table 10-4. Behavioral, Developmental, and Emotional Consequences of Physical Abuse

Situational, Short-term Consequences

Depression, anxiety
Avoidance behavior
Aggressive behavior
Scapegoating and self-pity behavior
Developmental delay
Academic difficulty
Social maladaptation

Profound, Long-term Consequences

Borderline personality
Distorted self-concept and self-esteem
Antisocial, delinquent behavior
Self-destructive behavior
Mental retardation

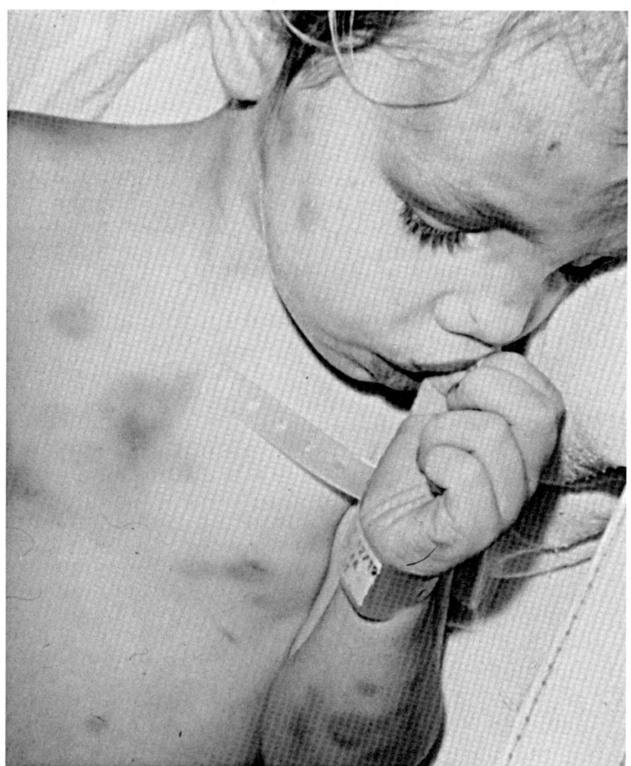

Figure 10-4. A child with multiple bruises secondary to inflicted trauma.

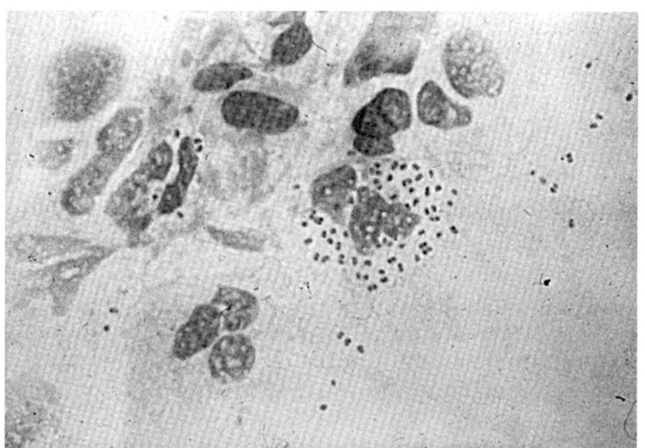

Figure 10-5. Gram stain of vaginal secretion showing gram-negative intracellular diplococci suggestive of sexual abuse.

(Appelbaum, 1977; Frank et al, 1985; Sandgrund et al, 1975) have documented similar findings. In addition to brain injury, there are many instances of damage inflicted on sensory organs, particularly the eyes (Fig. 10-6). The resulting sensory deficits have the potential for chronic, severe physical disability.

The developmental and behavioral consequences are extensive (Egeland et al, 1983). A long-standing belief in the concept of the "cycle of abuse" is well articulated by Helfer (1974) in his notion of "the abnormal rearing cycle." Widom (1989) showed that a cohort of abused children manifested more antisocial behaviors in adolescence and young adulthood than did a control group. Anecdotal studies have shown a high rate of histories of child abuse among the prison population and among individuals seeking psychiatric care in adulthood. It also seems that today's abused children have a greater chance of becoming tomorrow's abusing parents, although this is not an inevitable consequence. Children who are chronically abused seem either to accept the role of the victim or to become the aggressor themselves.

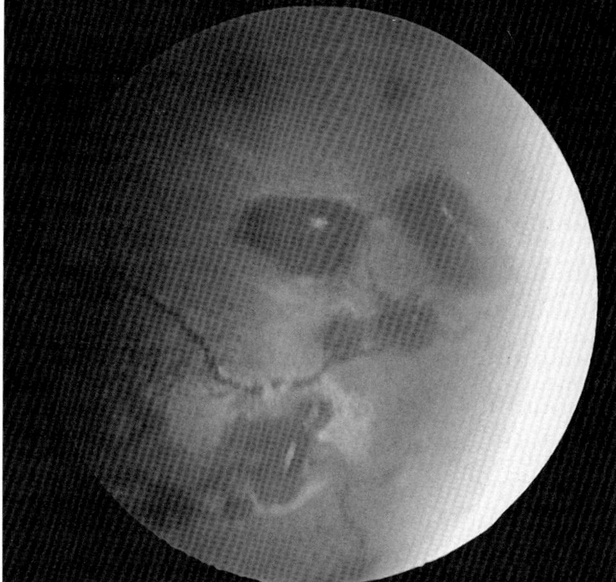

Figure 10-6. Retinal hemorrhages secondary to shaking.

The more immediate developmental and behavioral effects of physical abuse probably depend on several factors, including (1) the age of the child, (2) the severity and duration of abuse, (3) the extent of positive parenting behaviors that are present in nonabusive periods, and (4) individual strengths or vulnerabilities in the child. Some children tolerate extreme amounts of abuse yet seem intact. Other children may find one assault at the hands of a temporary family member quite devastating. The specific developmental and behavioral manifestations of physical abuse (Martin, 1976) are shown in Table 10-4. Some manifestations can be classified as specific psychiatric diagnoses, others are effects on speech and language development and intelligence, and still others represent abnormal or undesirable patterns of child behavior that may be attempts at adaptation (Kline, 1977).

Management

The first step in any management scheme is the identification of abuse. Health care providers need to be alert to the high incidence of abuse and to the fact that any traumatic injury must be suspected to be abuse if only for a moment's consideration (Ludwig, 1993). Some pediatricians may have difficulty in drawing the line between discipline and abuse. Most traumatic injuries are found to be nonintentional, but some injuries are more indicative of abuse. Evaluating a suspected injury encompasses (1) looking at it, (2) trying to match the injury to a plausible history, (3) using diagnostic tests and radiographs to understand it further, and (4) observing the interactions and interrelationships of family members. By using all four of these categories of information,

Table 10-5. Signs and Symptoms That Should Arouse Concern about Child Abuse or Neglect

Subnormal Growth
Weight, height, or both <5th percentile for age
Weight <5th percentile for height
Decreased velocity of growth
Head Injuries
Torn frenulum of upper or lower lip
Unexplained dental injury
Bilateral black eyes with history of single blow or fall
Traumatic hair loss
Retinal hemorrhage
Diffuse or severe central nervous system injury with history of minor-to-moderate fall (<3 m)
Skin Injuries
Bruise or burn in shape of an object
Bite marks
Burn resembling a glove or stocking or with some other distribution suggestive of an immersion injury
Bruises of various colors (in various stages of healing)
Injury to soft tissue areas that are normally protected (thighs, stomach, or upper arms)
Injuries of the Gastrointestinal or Genitourinary Tract
Bilious vomiting
Recurrent vomiting or diarrhea witnessed only by parent
Chronic abdominal or perineal pain with no identifiable cause
History of genital or rectal pain
Injury to genitals or rectum
Sexually transmitted disease
Bone Injuries
Rib fracture in the absence of major trauma (e.g., motor vehicle accident)
Complex skull fracture after a short fall (<1.2 m)
Metaphyseal long bone fracture in an infant
Femur fracture (any configuration) in a child <1 year old
Multiple fractures in various stages of healing
Laboratory Studies
Implausible or physiologically inconsistent laboratory results (polymicrobial contamination of body fluids, sepsis with unusual organisms, electrolyte disturbances inconsistent with the child's clinical state or underlying illness, wide and erratic variations in test results)
Positive toxicologic tests in the absence of a known ingestion or medication
Bloody cerebrospinal fluid (with xanthochromic supernatant) in an infant with altered mental status and no history of trauma

From Wissow LS: Child abuse and neglect. N Engl J Med 332:1423-1431, 1995.

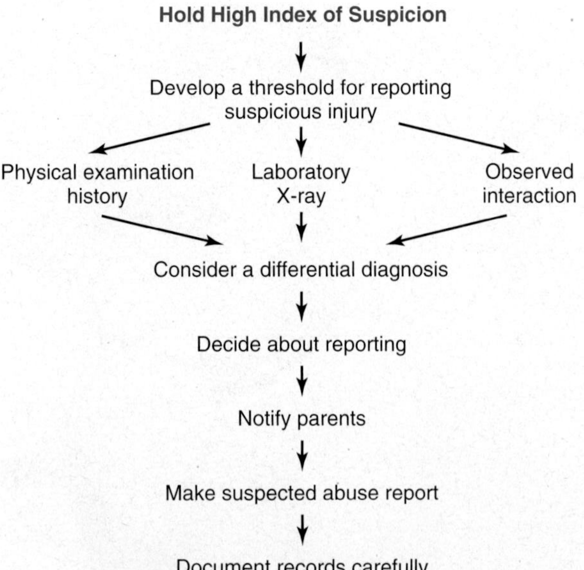

Figure 10-7. Steps in the management of child abuse.

the physician may arrive at a level of suspicion requiring a report of abuse. Wissow (1995) has published a compact list of the common signs and symptoms that should alert the clinician to consider the diagnosis of abuse (Table 10-5).

Each state has a reporting law mandating physicians to report suspected abuse and legally protecting them for doing so. The steps in case management are shown in Figure 10-7. The report of suspected abuse should be followed by an investigation by the local Child Protective Services (CPS) agency. It is the responsibility of CPS to evaluate the strengths and weaknesses of the family and to determine a plan for remediation. When the extent and nature of abuse has reached a criminal level, the physician needs to report this directly to the police to obtain immediate attention and protection for the child.

In addition to the identification and reporting of abuse, the physician must make an assessment of the child's safety. If the home is not safe, hospitalization is indicated, even without serious physical injury. Whether or not hospitalization is needed, the fact that the case is being reported to CPS should be explained directly to the parents. This step would be easy for the physician to omit, but such an omission sets up a difficult and nontherapeutic situation for the workers who must follow up.

Police, courts, and some CPS workers judge the severity of the child's abuse by the severity of the physical injury sustained. Such a relationship between extent of physical abuse and seriousness of family dysfunction does not exist, however. The physician also should assess the assets and deficits in other areas of family functioning. An assessment of the child's mental health and developmental level also is important. A child who has regressed, is developmentally delayed, and is bruised may be more at risk than a child with intact functioning who has sustained multiple fractures. The court may make the opposite determination because the number of broken bones is easy to count and constitutes concrete evidence.

The physician seeing a child for the developmental or behavioral manifestations of abuse may not know of the preexistent abuse. In the evaluation of any child with a developmental or behavioral problem, the physician should inquire about abuse. Abuse is so common a phenomenon that it warrants constant consideration in these settings, just as it does in situations in which acute trauma is the presenting sign.

Parental Overprotection and Overanxiety

Overprotective parents are pervasively afraid that some terrible disaster will befall their child. They call the physician for the most minor complaints, conveying tremendous anxiety about every physical symptom or ailment.

They express a great deal of concern about normal developmental transitions and behavioral variations in the child. There is often a history of an adverse event (or series of events) having affected the child (or another family member). Unresolved feelings about these stressful events leads to a general pattern of behavior first described by Green and Solnit (1964) as the vulnerable child syndrome (see Chapter 34). Perhaps a better term for this pattern of parental behavior would be the *overprotective parent syndrome*.

Overprotective parents often display an excessive preoccupation with bodily functioning and with potential threats to health, occasionally to the point of being hypochondriacal. Minor illness episodes become family crises, with the parents becoming incapable of carrying out their usual daily activities. Avoidance of all possible risks (and by extension, avoidance of conflict) is the general rule guiding family life. Such parents are themselves likely to be overanxious individuals who are insecure about their own parenting skills, who consult many experts for advice about parenting, and who are likely to have grown up in overprotective families with overanxious parents. Occasionally, these parents are overwhelmed, depressed, lonely, or unfulfilled. Their overprotectiveness brings them into close proximity with their children, who function as emotional supports. When there is marital distress, focusing on the child's vulnerability serves to defuse tensions between the spouses. Finally, in extreme cases, overprotective parents fail to formulate rules, set limits, or discipline their children for fear of hurting or upsetting them.

The primary care physician can play an important role in helping overprotective families become less fearful. When the overprotective pattern is recognized, the physician should invite the parents to discuss their concerns about their child and their own previous experiences with illness and other adverse events. The next step is to challenge gently but firmly the parents' perceptions that their child is sickly or at increased risk of harm. Such parents need a great deal of reassurance that they are doing a good job of caring for their child, but that their anxiety is unwarranted and potentially harmful. They also need education regarding the appropriate use of health care resources. This teaching may require repeated conversations over several months because some parents may have trouble believing medical opinion and need time to develop a trusting relationship with the physician.

The goal of these discussions is to get the parents to realize they are excessively fearful and to help them take steps to reduce their anxiety level. If they persist in their overprotectiveness, it may be necessary to confront them directly and to insist they change their inappropriate behaviors. Enlisting the help of another family member who views the behavior as overprotective and dysfunctional may stimulate the parents to reconsider their attitudes. In cases in which the parents are intransigent, referral for mental health intervention is indicated. If the parents resist this recommendation, it may be necessary for the physician to make this a major condition for continuing his or her relationship with the child and family.

Food

Underfeeding: Failure to Thrive and Starvation

Failure to thrive is a term that is used to describe children who are not growing according to normal standards. This problem, which is described in detail in Chapter 60, is often an outcome of family dysfunction. Block and Krebs (2005) authored an American Academy of Pediatrics statement about failure to thrive as a manifestation of child neglect.

Parents may underfeed children for various other reasons ranging from poverty to inappropriate selection, as in food fads (see Chapter 58). Some parents may be influenced by media stereotypes of beauty and strive to keep their child fashion-model thin. Underfeeding to the point of death is termed *starvation*. There are many clinical examples of this degree of family dysfunction.

Parental Overfeeding: Obesity

An undersupply of food is not the only form of family feeding dysfunction. The opposite is overprovision of food, leading to obesity in the child. As a society, we tend not to consider obesity in the same way we view failure to thrive or starvation, but to the child the consequences may be just as debilitating (see Chapter 61).

Housing

Homelessness

In recent years, the number of children being raised in families without housing has increased dramatically. It is estimated that single mothers and young children constitute more than one third of the 2.5 million homeless individuals in the United States (Bassuk and Rosenberg, 1990). The plight of these families has only more recently begun to be documented. Although the root causes of homelessness lie in society's failure to provide adequate economic assistance to families living in poverty, its dire effects on psychological well-being and social relationships are many. Family integrity is undermined, family life is disrupted, and family relationships are strained and torn apart. Life in homeless shelters is chaotic and stressful. Families are often crowded into a single room and are obliged to share toilet and eating facilities with dozens of other families in similar circumstances. Parents often feel inadequate, ineffective, and overwhelmed by a sense of powerlessness. Hopelessness, helplessness, apathy, confusion, and uncertainty also are common (see Chapter 18).

Multiple Homes

Children with an oversupply of homes have been described as "yo-yo" and "vagabond" children. These are children who have too many homes, as may occur in privileged wealthy families who may not appreciate the adverse effects of not having a single home. It also occurs while parents fight over who has custody and authority. Moore (1975) has described a series of 23 such cases, but the number of families experiencing this type of dysfunction is increasing as divorce rates increase.

The effects of such custody relationships are many. Children are unsettled, knowing neither where they live nor who is making the rules. Sometimes, a child is abducted from one parent by the other. Children feel themselves to be pawns in a parental chess game. The result is anxiety, frustration, and depression. No large or long-term studies of this phenomenon have been done.

The physician must be aware of marital status and custody arrangements and must serve as an active child advocate. Sometimes parental rights are placed at a higher level than what is good for the child; this is when the pediatrician must step forward to speak for the needs of the child. Parents who continue to be destructive to their child in the process of being destructive to one another may need to be reported to CPS or referred for counseling.

Health Care

Medical Neglect

The distinction between medical neglect and nonadherence is a fine one. Nonadherence is the act of not following medical advice. There may be a good reason (e.g., the wisdom of the patient), or it may simply be a lack of motivation, resources, or understanding. Studies of rates of compliance for simple antibiotic regimens show them to be quite low even for intelligent and educated parents consulting pediatricians in private practice. When lack of compliance results in actual injury to the child, it falls into the category of medical neglect. Because providing for a child's health is an important family function, failing to do so represents a form of dysfunction.

There are no official reports on the incidence of medical neglect. Increasing numbers of children do not receive regular well-child care. Immunizations also have been documented as being inadequate in substantial segments of the population. Some children die because their parents have not sought appropriate care for them. This pattern may begin in the prenatal period. Investigators have shown that women who do not get adequate prenatal care also are less likely to obtain care for their newborns postnatally.

In managing medical neglect, physicians need to explain their recommendations carefully to parents. Where nonadherence is occurring, the physician should document the treatment recommendation and clarify again the rationale for the therapy. Some physicians may wish to develop a formal contract with the parents. When a child is injured by medical neglect, the issue needs to be brought to CPS. In this circumstance, outside intervention is required to remediate the family dysfunction.

Parental Overuse of Medical Care: Munchausen Syndrome by Proxy

Munchausen syndrome by proxy (Rosenberg, 1987) refers to a parental fabrication or induction of illness in young children so that the parent gains recognition and support from a medical institution and its health care providers. The term is an outgrowth of a psychiatric disorder described in adults who subject themselves to multiple diagnostic evaluations and surgical treatments to derive the care and comfort extended to a patient. Munchausen syndrome by proxy may be seen as opposite of medical neglect. Instead of the family's underproviding medical services, it overprovides them, sometimes by exaggerating symptoms or sometimes by falsifying symptoms and laboratory findings. It is unclear whether Munchausen syndrome by proxy represents a distinct psychiatric problem, or whether it is the extreme end of a spectrum that begins with parents' prolonging an acute minor illness (Libow and Schreier, 1986), doctor shopping, making an excess number of physician visits, or using a child's illness to postpone their own return to work. Many forms of Munchausen syndrome by proxy have been reported, including administration of insulin, false hematuria, false fevers, suffocation, and intravenous administration of feces to cause polymicrobial infections (Levin and Sheridan, 1995). Meadow (1977) has named the syndrome the "hinterland of child abuse."

In its full-blown form, Munchausen syndrome by proxy is an extremely serious disorder that produces significant morbidity and mortality. Rosenberg (1987) reported 2 deaths in a series of 10 reported cases, along with 10 unexplained sibling deaths. Other authors described a 5% to 15% mortality. In less serious cases, morbidity takes the form of children learning the benefits of the "sick child role"; this may lead to future Munchausen behaviors or simply to hypochondriacal and dependent behaviors exhibited by many adults. Children may undergo unnecessary procedures, laboratory tests, and operations. They also may become involved in the falsification of signs, symptoms, and laboratory data. There have been few long-term studies of these children to document either the long-term manifestations or the possible cyclic nature of the problem.

As with the management of frankly abusive behavior, the clinician's first step is to suspect a medical problem that stumps all the experts. The parents involved usually are described as cooperative to excess. Usually there is a family pattern in which only one parent is an active caretaker, while the other is often absent, either physically or emotionally. Another clue may be that the parent may have a complex medical history or may have a professional background in nursing or in allied medical professions. If Munchausen syndrome by proxy is suspected, hospitalization may be required to finalize the diagnosis. It would not be difficult to convince the parent of the need for the hospitalization, because this ties in with the parent's existing needs. When the child is in the hospital, through close monitoring of the parent, through covert videotaping, or through restricting the parent's visiting pattern, a diagnosis can be confirmed. When the diagnosis is established, it must be presented to the parents and to CPS for the creation of a management plan. In some cases, separation of the child from the family may be necessary. The long-term outcome with therapy is unknown.

DEVELOPMENTAL, BEHAVIORAL, AND EMOTIONAL NEEDS

Stimulation—Developmental and Cognitive

Understimulation: Neglect

Pediatricians occasionally encounter parents who do not exhibit sufficient developmental or intellectual stimulation for their children. Such parents are likely to have been raised in families with similar difficulties. They may strike the physician as uncaring, uninvolved, indifferent, or intellectually impaired. They may appear to be unresponsive to their child's social cues, unaware of their emotional needs, or lacking in skills to play with or talk to their infants in ways that might promote intellectual development. They may seem preoccupied, apathetic, self-absorbed, depressed, or uninterested in caring for their children. At one extreme, such parents may be completely neglectful of their children's need for protection, nurturance, and guidance. This situation is generally easy to detect and requires the immediate attention of CPS.

In less severe cases, understimulating or neglectful parents may provide adequately for the child's physical needs, but are unable to engage in intellectually stimulating forms of interaction with their children. Hugging, kissing, holding, rocking, cuddling, and other forms of affectional exchange also may be rare or absent. Playing with age-appropriate toys and games, conversing about why and how things work, engaging in creative activities such as art and music, reading stories aloud, taking trips to explore the outdoor environment, and discussing issues that are interesting to the child may be missing from the parents' repertoire of behaviors. Strong dependence on television or radio also is typical of these families.

Children raised in understimulating or neglectful families may experience a host of adverse consequences immediately and over the long-term. Intellectually, such children are prone to become functionally mentally retarded or to exhibit learning difficulties. Emotionally, they may be prone to depression, anxiety, behavior disturbances, and personality disorders. Socially, these children may develop peer interaction difficulties, poor impulse control, or frank conduct disorders.

Children in understimulating or neglectful families may present to the pediatrician as dull, apathetic, emotionally bland, or indifferent. In severe cases, they can present with failure to thrive or developmental delay (see Chapter 60). In the office, the physician may observe limited or stilted parent-child interactions. There may be very little eye contact, spontaneous conversation, or signs of mutual emotional connection. The parents may perform their caregiving functions in a mechanical fashion or may interact with their children primarily around control of behavior and discipline. Indicators of this kind should prompt the physician to open a line of discussion with the parents regarding the child's needs for developmental and intellectual stimulation. If the parents show an interest in discussing these issues, it can be helpful to describe a few simple activities to promote parent-child interaction, to recommend a practical parenting guide, and to schedule a return visit in the near future to focus on the child's developmental and intellectual needs. If the situation is more severe, or if the parents are unwilling to discuss the concerns the physician is raising, referring the family to early intervention and childcare and parenting programs, and reporting the case to CPS may be indicated.

Parental Overstimulation or Perfectionism

In recent years, numerous social factors have contributed to "hothousing" (Katz and Becher, 1987), or overstructuring of the lives of children. Elkind (2001) wrote *The Hurried Child: Growing Up Too Fast Too Soon.* A suggested definition of this problem is inducing knowledge that is usually acquired at a later developmental level. In terms of family function, overstimulation of this kind may be just as deleterious as the understimulation discussed in the previous section. Several societal factors may play a part in the growth of this phenomenon, including the increase of parental age, number of two-career families, maternal career development, divorce rates, and competition in the educational system and society in general.

There have been no thorough studies of the effects of hothousing. Some authors (Katz and Becher, 1987; Rosenfeld and Wise, 2001) have pointed to the possible consequences. They suggest that overstructuring may be done by parents who feel inadequate and guilty about the amount of time they can spend with their children. Hothousing may result in even less time being spent together, however. A second consequence may be that the child gets the subtle message that achievement is important to receiving parental love. Hills (1987) has stated, "In affluent, upwardly striving middle-class families, children may be alternatively indulged and pressured for early, high, and sustained levels of achievement. Such children may come to believe that parental love and social acceptance are invariably conditional upon their achievement" (see Chapter 18). Structured learning also takes away from unstructured play, an activity that is vital for normal development.

It is important for the physician to assess how much of the child's life is being structured for him or her. When reviewing the child's growth and development, it is essential for the pediatrician to inquire about activities. Children should be asked about their own desires and inclinations and about nonschool undertakings. Parents who discuss their children in terms of their accomplishments rather than their qualities indicate possible overstructuring. School-age children who present with vague complaints such as fatigue or prolonged sleeping or toddlers with temper tantrums may be the victims of hothousing. If such symptoms are related to excessive parental pressure to achieve, the physician can help the family to attain a healthier equilibrium.

Guidance—Approval and Discipline

Inadequate Approval, Overcriticism, and Psychological Abuse

Psychological or emotional abuse involves a repeated pattern of disapproval, excessive discipline, hostility, criticism, scorn, and ridicule in the interactions among family members. In emotionally abusive families, relationships are charged with negative emotions, which are readily expressed or acted out in ways that undermine trust, self-esteem, and a sense of security. Psychological abuse can occur among spouses, siblings, parents, and children, or other family members. Relationships become marred by frequent and constant conflicts, arguments, "put-downs," scapegoating, blaming, and derision. There is often a history of substance abuse; inadequate parenting in the parents' families of origin; and physical abuse, abandonment, or both during periods of stress or emotional crisis.

It is common for individuals to state openly their hatred of and their wish to be rid of the individual with whom they have the greatest amount of conflict. Spouses may remark they wish they had never married, and parents may disclose to their children the wish that the children had never been born. Emotional abuse also may occur in school (Krugman and Krugman, 1984).

Children in psychologically abusive families may react in various ways. Children prone to internalize their feelings may present with generalized anxiety, clinginess, inhibitions, phobias, perfectionism, depression, and profound feelings of shame. They may be overly compliant and excessively self-controlled for fear of rejection or scorn. Children with a tendency to externalize may show aggressiveness, hyperactivity, defiance of rules and authority, irresponsibility, provocative behavior, and oversensitivity to criticism. These children may present as undersocialized, uncontrollable, and rebellious in social situations.

Children from abusive families may appear "starved for affection," may display an inappropriate need for acceptance and reassurance, and may be excessively eager to please adults, often going to great lengths to receive any positive attention they can solicit from others. If they can verbalize their emotions, these children may reveal deep-seated anger and resentment toward the emotionally abusive family members, along with profound feelings of shame, rejection, inadequacy, and self-doubt. Many express a sense of being unloved and unwanted. Some feel guilty for burdening their families with having to care for them. Children who are raised in emotionally abusive families tend to have chronic feelings of diminished self-worth and persistent problems with intimate personal relationships. They are at increased risk for developing marital and occupational difficulties, parenting problems, and psychiatric disorders.

When faced with evidence of emotional abuse within the family, the physician needs to respond in a straightforward and honest fashion. After expressing a deep concern for the emotional well-being of the child, the physician should emphasize that emotional abuse harms everyone in the family, and that it needs to be brought under control as quickly as possible. Parents may be unaware they are being critical of the child to a point that is harmful, or they may acknowledge the presence of tensions in the family that are causing them to be unsupportive. The prognosis for change is always better when there is eventual recognition of the problem. A referral for family therapy is strongly indicated in more serious cases. If there is evidence of moderate-to-severe psychological distress in the child, and if the physician's attempts to be helpful are met with strong resistance by the parents, consideration should be given to contacting CPS to pressure the family to seek help.

Parental Overindulgence

Parents in overindulgent families smother their children with an overabundance of love and nurturance, but are unable to set suitable limits or enforce restrictions. There is excessive approval and insufficient discipline. Whether out of fear of harming the child, anxiety about being disliked or rejected by the child, discomfort with being in authority, or discomfort with feelings of anger and aggression, or in reaction to a sense of being insufficiently loved by their own parents, overindulgent parents avoid conflicts with their children at all costs. They constantly give in to their children's demands and seem incapable of effectively setting limits on their children's behavior. This pattern is often seen in families in which parents are older, are working, are divorced or unmarried, or are not functioning effectively as a team. In families with marital distress, overindulgence of the children may function either to divert attention away from or to intensify the spousal conflict.

Commonly viewed as "spoiled" (McIntosh, 1989), overindulged children are able to exert tremendous control over their parents by whining, complaining, demanding, threatening, screaming, and throwing temper tantrums. They may not exhibit these behaviors with adults who can set limits effectively (e.g., grandparents or teachers), but they embarrass their parents in a variety of social settings (e.g., restaurants, stores, friends' homes) whenever their wishes or desires are not met instantly. When others express criticism of these manipulative behaviors, parents either agree with them (and feel terribly guilty and ineffective), or they defend their children and yield to their demands. Overindulged children tend to be immature, selfish, insecure, and easily bored and frustrated. They have trouble delaying gratification and give up easily when faced with difficult tasks. They may have grandiose opinions or unrealistic expectations of themselves and often become extremely disappointed when they fail to achieve their own goals. They have difficulty with self-control and are prone to misbehavior, particularly when conformity requires them to subordinate their wishes to those of others. They have problems with peers who may view them as "stuck-up," snobbish, and vain.

Physicians can help overindulgent parents by teaching them to become more assertive with their children. Techniques such as Parent Effectiveness Training have been successful in helping parents to feel less guilty, to overcome their sense of powerlessness, and to set limits effectively and enforce discipline with their children. After validating the parents' right to say "no" to their children's demands, and after emphasizing how important it is for children to learn to respect their parents' rules, skillful physicians can help overindulgent parents develop specific household rules with clear rewards and consequences. By starting with something simple and straightforward (e.g., picking up toys after playing with them), parents can be instructed to monitor the behavior they are trying to modify and to practice giving rewards and enforcing consequences around one particular rule before moving on to developing other ones. If the parents seem particularly ineffective or are unwilling to stick to their decisions in the face of their children's opposition, a referral for more intensive counseling is indicated.

Affection, Acceptance, and Intimacy

Emotional Neglect or Rejection

Emotional neglect can be defined as a relationship pattern in which an individual's affectional needs are consistently disregarded, ignored, invalidated, or unappreciated by a significant other. People in neglectful families are emotionally disconnected from one another, behaving as if they were living on different planets. Parents may have trouble understanding their children's needs for love, affection, closeness, and support, or they may feel too overwhelmed or powerless to meet these needs on a consistent basis. Neglectful parents usually come from families in which, as children, they were ignored or neglected by their parents. They also may lack emotionally satisfying adult relationships. Forced to rely on themselves for support, afraid of their own dependency needs, and reluctant to admit their pain, these parents are highly ambivalent about their children's needs, particularly when their children are hurting, crying, or looking for emotional support. They may feel jealous or resentful of their children and may perceive them as excessively demanding and impossible to satisfy. They may be so preoccupied with their own needs that they never consider the children's point of view. Alternatively, they may feel so angry and resentful about having children that they simply ignore them.

For children, affectional neglect may have devastating consequences, including failure to thrive, developmental delay, hyperactivity, aggression, depression, low self-esteem, running away from home, substance abuse, and a host of other emotional disorders. These children feel unloved and unwanted. They may strive to please others, or they may misbehave to receive the attention they crave. They may withdraw from people and appear uncaring and indifferent. They may be afraid of emotional closeness and may shun intimacy in relationships. They are at risk for emotional problems throughout the rest of their lives. The degree of neglect and the individual vulnerability apparently affect the magnitude of the consequences.

Severe cases of neglect are generally easy to spot (e.g., when the child's development is grossly delayed or shows evidence of failure to thrive), but more subtle examples are harder to detect. Emotional neglect should be suspected if the primary care practitioner observes a relative lack of spontaneous, positive, parent-child interactions in her or his office; if the parent seems uninformed and apathetic about the child's development and behavior; or if the child is exhibiting signs of emotional distress without an obvious cause. Questions about daily routines and sources of support to the parent should precede any direct queries into the parent-child relationship. Encouraging the parent to describe the child's positive attributes and focusing the discussion on these strengths can serve as an opening to raising matters of concern. It is important for the parent to hear these concerns directly from the practitioner. Vague, general, or indirect comments should be avoided, and specific recommendations should be made regarding the child's need for more sustained and positive interactions with the parent. How important the parent is to the child, and how vital it is for the parent to receive more support from his or her social network so as to be more emotionally available to the child also are important issues to emphasize. Most neglectful parents feel isolated and unsupported in their own families and feel that their own emotional needs are not being met. Encouraging the parent to talk directly with the physician about her or his view of parenting is another way of opening up the discussion.

Often it is helpful to obtain additional information from other family members, particularly other caregivers. This information enables the practitioner to assess the availability of emotional support to the parent and child from within the family system. Finally, whenever possible, a home visit and a family interview should be conducted. This interview may require the services of an experienced clinical social worker, who can help make the decision to contact CPS should emotional neglect be substantiated.

Sexual Abuse and Incest

The dysfunctional opposite of inadequate affection is what occurs when the family fails to maintain sexual boundaries between the generations. When this happens, there is an inappropriate excess, and sexual abuse or incest results. Sgroi (1984) has suggested that the term *sexual misuse* replace sexual abuse. This term more accurately reflects the misuse of the power of the perpetrator. The perpetrator is usually known to the child and has legitimate access to him or her. The child is coerced by positive rewards, destructive threats, or blackmail. The abuser begins by using casual touching, caressing, or kissing; this steadily increases to more advanced and overt sexual activities, often to the point of sexual intercourse. The type of sexual contact has been correlated with the age of the child victim. The victim may have a positive relationship with the abuser in many nonsexual realms of interaction. The victim may be told to "listen to your elders" and may repeatedly be placed in contact with the perpetrator.

Previously, many children tried to tell adults about their sexual contacts only to be unheard or ignored. Since the early 1980s, professionals have urged parents to listen to their children, and reports of child sexual abuse have increased strikingly. Several prevalence studies (Finkelhor, 1979; Russell, 1983) indicate that this form of family dysfunction is extremely common, involving up to 1 in 5 girls and 1 in 10 boys.

This form of family dysfunction is so societally unacceptable that its definition is established by the tenets of criminal law. All states have laws that define incest and other forms of sexual abuse.

The impact of child sexual abuse has never been fully or carefully documented. Paradise (personal communication, 1984) reviewed many of the existing studies and found that studies that have been published often lack the necessary scientific rigor. In the short-term, sexual abuse causes many varied physical and behavioral symptoms. Some of these symptoms are alleviated when the children disclose their histories of abuse. In addition, some studies document the long-term effects of this type of abuse through work with adult patients seeking psychiatric care. The effects of sexual abuse also may depend on several cofactors, such as the age of the child victim, the duration of the abuse, the disturbance of existing family life resulting from disclosure, the vulnerability of the child, and heterosexual versus homosexual abuse. Whether or not sexual abuse leaves a distinctive set of behavioral or developmental problems has yet to be proved. The consequences of sexual abuse may be confounded by other factors, such as parental divorce. When sexual abuse is intrafamilial, its disclosure may lead to parental divorce. Faller (1991) reported several distinct interaction patterns of these variables.

Finkelhor and Browne (1985) have characterized the aftermath of sexual abuse into four possible *traumagenic dynamics*. The first is *traumatic sexualization,* in which the child's introduction to sexuality becomes distorted, leaving the child with excessive fears or feelings about sexuality and sexual behavior. Second, the child may *feel powerless*. Third, some children indicate that they feel different from other children *(stigmatization)*. They may even feel that they can be picked out of a group of other children because of their experience. Fourth is a *sense of betrayal* and the feeling that adults cannot be trusted. These dynamics are clearly present in many victims of sexual abuse with whom we have worked. They are not constants, however. Issues of sexuality, power, stigmatization, and trust all are a part of the normal developmental process. One can easily imagine the tremendous impact an abusive experience might have on a child who is already struggling.

Some authors have suggested that there may be a sex difference in the way the risk factors affect boys compared with girls (Farber et al, 1984). The Minnesota Longitudinal Study (Erikson and Egeland, 1987) indicates that girls may react by becoming more quiet and dependent. Male victims may act out their abuse on younger children and identify with the aggressor. In our experience, numerous adolescent boys have been perpetrators of sexual abuse involving young girls. We hypothesize that this may result from the adolescents' being stimulated and "instructed" by readily available pornographic magazines, books, and films, and by having been victims of abuse themselves.

Beyond the developmental and behavioral effects of child sexual abuse, there are serious physical consequences. About 5% to 10% of child sexual abuse cases are diagnosed by the documentation of a sexually transmitted disease. Pregnancy also may be the result of sexual abuse. There are documented cases of human immunodeficiency virus infection as a consequence of sexual abuse.

In managing sexual abuse, the physician must open his or her mind to the possibility that the sexual abuse exists, and that it apparently is a common phenomenon in society. When one is willing to believe that sexual abuse of children occurs, the recognition of cases becomes easier. Children may draw attention to their diagnosis by telling about their abuse or more likely by showing their distress in trying to keep it secret. The signs and symptoms may be specific or may be nonspecific and vague. Many of the behavioral problems presented throughout this book may be manifestations of abuse. The list of nonspecific symptoms (Ludwig, 1993) includes enuresis, encopresis, school avoidance, runaway behavior, development of phobias, and others. When children manifest any change in behavior or personality, child sexual abuse should be considered.

When the suspicion of sexual abuse has been raised, the next step in management is its reporting. The reporting criteria for each state are determined by law. Reports may need to be made to the police, CPS, or both.

The child should undergo a complete physical examination, and cultures for sexually transmitted diseases should be obtained. Other aspects of evidence collection have been reviewed elsewhere. After the child reveals the "secret" of abuse, there may be a temporary relief of symptoms. When parents learn of the abuse, they are burdened with the terrible weight of the problem. The physician has a role in working with the parents and child to monitor their respective adjustments to the problem. In many cases, referral to mental health workers is necessary. The need for such services may be based on the continuation of existing symptoms or the development of new problems.

SOCIALIZATION

Intrafamilial Socialization

Dysfunctional Inadequacy in Socialization within the Family: Distant, Disengaged, or Absent Parents

Functional families provide and teach about family social relationships. Parental distancing or attenuated family relationships result from a variety of conditions. Parents may have psychiatric disorders, such as schizophrenia, manic-depressive illness, recurrent depressions, alcoholism, substance abuse, and a host of personality disorders. They may be emotionally unavailable to their children as a result of separation, divorce, abandonment, military service, incarceration, or physical illness. They may lack the ability to empathize with their children or to understand and respond to their basic emotional needs. They may be so consumed by excessively demanding jobs, by their own emotional difficulties, or by conflicts with their partners that they cannot provide their children with love and a sense of safety and security. Leaving aside situations of frank abuse or neglect (discussed in earlier sections), disengaged parents are frequently inconsistent, erratic, and ineffective in their approaches to child rearing. It is likely that this inconsistency itself is most detrimental to the child's development.

Children in families with distant or disengaged parents do not learn by experience about normal family social roles and are at heightened risk of developing emotional and behavioral problems. Gottman and DeClaire (1997) have written about the importance of raising an "emotionally intelligent" child. This risk is increased further if the child possesses a particularly difficult temperament, is physically disabled or intellectually limited, or has limited coping skills. Children may exhibit signs of depression, anxiety, somatization, hyperactivity, conduct problems, or emotional maladjustment in response to parental dysfunction. These signs tend to ameliorate when parental functioning improves and to worsen when parental dysfunction increases. When parents with psychiatric disorders experience an exacerbation of their symptoms, it is not unusual for their children to become more anxious or depressed. When children experience repeated separation from or abandonment by a particular parent, they usually exhibit signs of intense distress during the transition period immediately after the separation. Repeated loss of contact with a parent is generally extremely traumatic.

Physicians who encounter families with distanced or disengaged parents have three tasks: (1) to develop a helping relationship with the parents on behalf of providing care to the children, (2) to gain the trust of parents and learn about their difficulties, and (3) to support parents in their efforts to obtain treatment or help for their problems. Without gaining familiarity with the parents' issues, it is difficult to avoid becoming judgmental and critical of them. Parents who are dysfunctional usually appreciate the physician's efforts to help them become more effective in their parental roles. In situations when there is a serious split between the parents (e.g., where one parent is reporting on the dysfunctional behavior of the other), it is imperative that the clinician meet both parents and get to know their strengths and weaknesses. If their trust can be gained, it is easier to win their cooperation in efforts to improve their parenting. It also is important for the physician to have access to mental health and social service resources to refer dysfunctional parents for treatment. When making such referrals, it is important that the physician maintain an ongoing relationship with the family and continue to support them in their attempts to cope with the dysfunctional aspects of their lives.

Dysfunctional Excess of Relationships within the Family: Overinvolved or Enmeshed Families

Overinvolvement of parents with their children can create serious difficulties for all family members. The most extreme example of such overinvolvement is termed *enmeshment*; this is a situation in which the ego boundaries among individuals are so poorly defined that they cannot separate or individuate from one another without experiencing tremendous anxiety, anger, or other forms of emotional distress. The preconditions for overinvolvement include intergenerational patterns of overinvolvement, insufficient separation and individuation of parents from their own parents, parental disharmony, situational or developmental crises, perhaps temperamental predisposition, and other related factors. The primary characteristic of these families is the extreme emotional closeness that exists between parents and children. Although this may be a normative aspect of parenting during infancy, as the child begins to separate from the parents, they usually respond by "pulling back" emotionally and allowing the child to become a separate individual. If parents feel threatened by the child's move toward autonomy, they may undermine this process by focusing all their attention on the child, conveying to him or her the message that it is not all right to be a separate individual.

In some cases, the parents may continue to perform functions long past the age when the child is capable of self-care, such as feeding or dressing. In other situations, the child may withdraw from facing normal developmental tasks (e.g., going to school, sleeping over at friends' homes) and may exhibit overt signs of separation anxiety. As with other forms of dysfunction, this ranges from minimal to severe.

Children whose parents are overinvolved also do not experience and learn normal family roles. Anxiety about normal developmental tasks and preoccupation with their parents' emotional well-being leads some children to avoid developing friendships or to resist going to school. In the most severe cases, children can present with anxiety disorders, depression, and somatization disorders.

The physician's approach to overinvolved or enmeshed families is outlined in the section on overprotective families. The most important function the physician can perform is to challenge firmly the parents to invest their emotional energy in areas other than their children. Emphasizing that the children need to separate from them to become healthy, independent, and self-reliant adults can help parents to relax their grip and to allow their children some emotional freedom. If discussion of these issues fails to result in change, the family should be referred for psychotherapy.

Extrafamilial Socialization

Deficient Training in Extrafamilial Relationships: Undercontrolling, Boundary-less Families

Functional families provide experience and instruction in extrafamilial relationships: what they are and how they differ from intrafamilial ones. Undercontrolling families seem to have no boundaries with the outside world. There is a tendency for family members to be overly sociable, friendly, and emotionally accessible to nonfamily members. At times, relationships outside the family take precedence over those within the family. Romantic involvements, intense friendships, business relationships, neighbors, and acquaintances seem to occupy the bulk of family members' time. Parental roles and executive functions are de-emphasized, and children are given unusual freedom and latitude to come and go and do as they please. The term *hurried children* has been used to describe children with excessive freedom and insufficient supervision who become responsible for themselves before they are emotionally prepared.

Children in undercontrolling families do not experience and learn appropriate extrafamilial relationships. They are extremely conscious of their social standing and are constantly in search of social acceptance. At the same time, these relationships may be so numerous that they fail to form any deep attachments and ultimately end up without a foundation for true citizenship or friendship. Such children often experiment with sex, drugs, and alcohol at a young age and may first be exposed to these activities by observing their parents. Beneath their pseudomature appearance, children from unrestricted families are likely to be anxious, insecure, and unhappy. In severe cases, these children may become depressed, withdrawn, or apathetic about life. Family conflicts, school failure, indiscriminate sexual relations, and other forms of acting-out behavior also may be seen.

Excessive Restriction from Development of Extrafamilial Relationships: Isolated or Insular Families

Insular families have few external social supports and a very limited social network. Adults in these families have few friends and spend little time with nonfamily members. There is a tendency to see the outside world as unfriendly or threatening and to view outsiders in a way best described as "us against them." It is often difficult to learn what happens in these families because access to them is limited. Where there are excessively strong bonds of family loyalty, it is expected that children will stay in the household (or in the nearby vicinity) even as adults. At times, dysfunctional relationships and behavior patterns (e.g., incest or alcoholism) and health and psychosocial problems in these families are hidden and maintained through secrecy and denial. Although it would be incorrect to conclude that insular families have a higher incidence of disturbance than noninsular families, when dysfunctional relationships or psychosocial problems are present, these families are more difficult to treat.

Children in insular families do not learn appropriate extrafamilial relationships. They are usually discouraged from having friendships or from engaging in activities that take them out of the home. They may be shy or socially immature and may appear to others to be loners or marginal individuals. Problems may surface when the child attempts to separate from the family and starts to form friendships outside the home. If the family attempts to stifle these relationships, the child may begin to defy parental authority by going out without parental permission or even by running away from home.

Physicians who encounter insular families need to be aware of the difficulty involved in forming trusting relationships with them. If the child seems to be developing normally, is reasonably well adjusted, and is not exhibiting emotional or behavior problems, consistent encouragement of the child's developing peer relationships and outside activities is indicated. If there is evidence of family dysfunction or of a disturbance in the child, it is most helpful to begin by understanding the parents' views and concerns before offering any advice. If it seems that the parents are resisting the physician's recommendations, it is best to enlist help from other family members and to gain insight into the family's perceptions of the problem before proceeding to involve mental health professionals. By spending extra time winning the trust of key family members, the physician is more likely to succeed in getting the family to accept a recommendation for counseling or family therapy.

PERVASIVE PARENTAL DYSFUNCTION—THREATS TO FAMILY INTEGRITY

Clinicians commonly are faced with situations in which there is evidence of severe and pervasive parental dysfunction, often to the point where the integrity of the family is threatened. These situations include families in which parents have severe psychiatric disturbances, personality disorders, mental deficiency, or alcohol or substance abuse, and situations in which there is evidence of chronic and severe family discord leading to domestic violence. Although the incidence of serious psychopathology in parents is difficult to measure, epidemiologic studies report that 20% of the general population have alcoholism, 5% have other substance-related disorders, 6% have depression, 1% have bipolar affective disorder, 1% have schizophrenia, and 5% have mental deficiency. Given these statistics, it is reasonable to conclude that a substantial number of children are being raised by parents who are mentally ill or mentally impaired.

There is considerable evidence from research and clinical literature that mental disorders in parents have deleterious effects on child development. In an early study from the 1920s, children of parents with affective disorders or psychosis had a 21% incidence of behavior disorders, and children whose parents had antisocial personality disorders had a 45% incidence of problems (Minde, 1991). A more recent study of children of schizophrenics found the incidence of conduct disorder to be 9.5% compared with 1.6% of control subjects (Rutter and Quinton, 1984). Among children with parents with affective disorders, the rate of behavior problems when there was one affected parent was 24%; with two affected parents, the rate increased to 74% (Beardslee et al., 1983; Weissman et al, 1987). The combined effects of genetic loading, disordered parenting, and family discord seem to account for these childhood disturbances.

The precise mechanisms by which children in families with severe dysfunction themselves become afflicted with mental disorders is still the subject of intense research. Current theories emphasize several important aspects, including decreased parental responsiveness to the child's needs (owing to excessive preoccupation with themselves), inadequate protection of the child from extremes of affect (e.g., excitement, anger, distress), inconsistent supervision, ineffective disciplinary practices, excessive conflict and hostility in the family (much of which may be directed at the child), frequent separations and disruptions to family life (e.g., hospitalizations, departures from the family, migration), and unpredictable or erratic behavior. Regardless of the nature of the psychiatric disturbance itself, parenting is an extremely difficult responsibility for individuals who are mentally ill. The effects on the child are mediated by factors such as the duration and intensity of the parent's mental disorder, comorbid conditions (e.g., depression and alcoholism), the effectiveness of treatment, parent adherence to treatment, and the availability of social support. If the child does not have other parenting resources readily available, the negative is greater. It also seems that younger children and boys are at greater risk of developing psychiatric disorders.

Two patterns of parenting are particularly deleterious to child development: the detached and unresponsive pattern, and the hostile and overcontrolling pattern. In the former case, children are left neglected for long periods, often leading to an insecure pattern of attachment to the parent and to understimulation of cognitive functioning. In the latter case, children are frequently subjected to intense parental anger and to coercive forms of discipline, often leading to aggressive, defiant, and antisocial behavior. A third important pattern of pervasive parental dysfunction is the violence-prone family. Domestic violence between parents has been shown to have a pervasive deleterious effect on all the family members (Fantuzzo et al, 1991; Straus and Gelles, 1990). Even when not directly engaged in the physical conflict, children raised in a violent family experience severe long-term consequences.

It is important that clinicians recognize the signs of severe parental dysfunction as early as possible to assist the parents in getting treatment for themselves and to monitor the child closely for signs of developmental, emotional, or behavioral disturbances. If the pediatrician approaches these situations with a nonjudgmental but direct approach, there is a greater likelihood that positive steps will be taken by the family to ensure that the child's safety and well-being are not being compromised. In the most severe cases, collaboration with mental health and social service providers is required, especially when the family's survival is threatened.

SUMMARY

Physicians tend to speak in terms of "good families" and "bad families." In doing so, they are really applying a broad qualitative judgment about family function. In working with families, a more helpful approach is to look more precisely at family structure (anatomy) and function (physiology), and to evaluate for areas of strengths and areas of weakness. In doing so, we can build on the functional parts (i.e., the strengths) and aid in the correction of dysfunction. This chapter has addressed family function in a more detailed way, looking at three main functions of the family (1) as a supply agent for food, clothing, housing, and health care; (2) as a developer of behavioral and emotional needs; and (3) as a model for socialization inside the family and in relationships to the broader society. Families may have areas of dysfunction in one or more of these domains. Dysfunction can occur on one of two dimensions, inadequacy or excess; neither is good for promoting healthy and happy children. Dysfunction can be stark in the case of abuse or indolent as in the case of the child who feels rejection. As providers of health care for children, we also are providers of care for the family.

REFERENCES

Appelbaum AS: Developmental retardation in infants as a concomitant of physical child abuse. J Abnorm Child Psychol 5:417-422, 1977.

Bassuk EL, Rosenberg L: Psychosocial characteristics of homeless children and children with homes. Pediatrics 85:257-261, 1990.

Beardslee WR, Bemporad J, Keller MB, et al: Children of parents with major affective disorder: A review. Am J Psychiatry 140:825-832, 1983.

Block RW, Krebs NF: Failure to thrive as a manifestation of child neglect. American Academy of Pediatrics, Committee on Child Abuse and Neglect, Committee on Nutrition. Pediatrics 116:1234-1237, 2005.

Bronfenbrenner U: Ecology of the family as a context for human development: Research perspectives. Dev Psychol 12:723-742, 1986.

Buchanan A, Oliver JE: Abuse and neglect as a cause of mental retardation. Child Abuse Negl 3:467, 1979.

Centers for Disease Control and Prevention: Child homicide in US. MMWR Morb Mortal Wkly Rep 31:292-293, 1982.

Egeland B, Stroufe A, Erikson M: The developmental consequences of different patterns of maltreatment. Child Abuse Negl 7:459-469, 1983.

Elkind D: The Hurried Child: Growing Up Too Fast Too Soon, 3rd ed. Cambridge, MA, Perseus, 2001.

Erickson MR, Egeland B: A developmental view of the psychological consequences of maltreatment. School Psychol Rev 16:156-168, 1987.

Faller KC: Possible explanations for child sexual abuse: Allegations in divorce. Am J Orthopsychiatry 6:86-91, 1991.

Fantuzzo JW, DePaola LM, Lambert L, et al: Effects of interpersonal violence on the psychological adjustment and competencies of young children. J Consult Clin Psychol 59:1-8, 1991.

Farber ED, Showers J, Johnson CF: The sexual abuse of children: A comparison of male and female victims. J Clin Child Psychol 13:294-297, 1984.

Finkelhor D: Sexually Victimized Children. New York, Free Press, 1979.

Finkelhor D, Browne A: The traumatic impact of child sexual abuse. Am J Orthopsychiatry 55:530-541, 1985.

Frank Y, Zimmerman R, Leeds N: Neurologic manifestations in abused children who have been shaken. Day Med Child Neurol 27:312-316, 1985.

Giardino AP, Christian C, Giardino ER: A Practical Guide to the Evaluation of Child Abuse and Neglect. Thousand Oaks, Sage Publications, 1997.

Ginsburg KR. A Parent's Guide to Building Resilience in Children and Teens. Elk Grove Village, IL, American Academy of Pediatrics, 2007.

Giovannoni JM, Becerra RM: Defining Child Abuse. New York, Free Press, 1979.

Gottman JM, DeClaire J: The Heart of Parenting: Raising an Emotionally Intelligent Child. New York, Simon & Schuster, 1997.

Green M, Solnit AJ: Reactions to the threatened loss of a child: A vulnerable child syndrome. Pediatrics 34:58-64, 1964.

Helfer RE: World of Abnormal Rearing. Unit 1. Self-Instructional Program on Child Abuse. Elk Grove Village, IL, American Academy of Pediatrics, 1974.

Hills TW: Children in the fast lane. Early Child Res Q 2:265-273, 1987.

Hymel KP: When is lack of supervision neglect? American Academy of Pediatrics, Committee on Child Abuse and Neglect. Pediatrics 118:1296-1298, 2006.

Katz LG, Becher RM: Hothousing of young children. Early Child Res Q 2:1-299, 1987.

Kellogg ND: Evaluation of suspected child physical abuse. Committee on Child Abuse and Neglect. Pediatrics 119:1232-1241, 2007.

Kline DF: Educational and psychological problems, of abused children. Child Abuse Negl 1:301-308, 1977.

Krugman RD, Krugman MK: Emotional abuse in the classroom. Am J Dis Child 138:284-286, 1984.

Levin AV, Sheridan M: Munchausen Syndrome by Proxy. New York, Lexington, 1995.

Libow JA, Schreier HA: Three forms of factitious illness in children: When is it Munchausen syndrome by proxy? Am J Orthopsychiatry 56:602-611, 1986.

Ludwig S: Child abuse. *In* Fleisher G, Ludwig S (eds): Textbook of Pediatric Emergency Medicine, 3rd ed. Baltimore, Williams & Wilkins, 1993.

Ludwig S, Kornberg AE (eds): Child Abuse: A Medical Reference, 2nd ed. New York, Churchill Livingstone, 1992.

Martin HP: The Abused: A Multidisciplinary Approach to Developmental Issues and Treatment. Cambridge, Ballinger Publishers, 1976.

McIntosh BJ: Spoiled child syndrome. Pediatrics 83:108-115, 1989.

Meadow R: Munchausen syndrome by proxy: The hinterland of child abuse. Lancet 2:343-345, 1977.

Minde K: The effect of disordered parenting on the development of children. *In* Lewis M (ed): Child and Adolescent Psychiatry: A Comprehensive Textbook. Baltimore, Williams & Wilkins, 1991, pp 394-407.

Moore JG: "Yo Yo children," victims of matrimonial violence. Child Welfare 54:557-566, 1975.

Murdoch G: Social Structure. New York, Free Press, 1965.

National Child Abuse and Neglect Data System (NCANDS): Child Abuse and Neglect Fatalities: Statistics and Intervention. U.S. Department of Health and Human Services, 2008. Available at www.childwelfare.gov.

Reece RM (ed): Child Abuse: Medical Diagnosis and Management. Philadelphia, Lea & Febiger, 1994.

Rosenberg DA: Web of deceit: A literature review of Munchausen syndrome by proxy. Child Abuse Negl 11:547-563, 1987.

Rosenfeld AA, Wise N: The Over-Scheduled Child: Avoiding the Hyper-Parenting Trap. New York, St Martin's Griffin, 2001.

Russell D: The incidence and prevalence of intrafamiliar and extrafamiliar sexual abuse of female children. Child Abuse Negl 7:133-146, 1983.

Rutter M, Quinton D: Parental psychiatric disorder: Effects on children. Psychol Med 14:853-880, 1984.

Sandgrund A, Gaines RW, Green AH: Child abuse and mental retardation: A problem of cause and effect. J Ment Defic Res 19:327-336, 1975.

Schnitzer PG, Ewigman BG: Child deaths resulting from inflicted injuries: Household risk factors and perpetrator characteristics. Pediatrics 116:e687-e693, 2005.

Sgroi S (ed): Handbook of Clinical Intervention in Child Sexual Abuse. Lexington, KY, Lexington Books, 1984.

Straus MA, Gelles RJ: Physical Violence in American Families: Risk Factors and Adaptations to Violence in 8,145 Families. New Brunswick, NJ, Transaction Publications, 1990.

U.S. Department Health and Human Services: National Center on Child Abuse and Neglect: Child Maltreatment 1995: Report from the States to the National Child Abuse and Neglect Data System. Washington, DC, U.S. Government Printing Office, 1997.

U.S. Department of Health and Human Services: Administration on Children, Youth, and Families: Child Maltreatment 2004. Washington, DC, U.S. Government Printing Office, 2006.

Walsh F: Conceptualizations of normal family functioning. *In* Walsh (ed): Normal Family Processes. New York, Guilford Press, 1982.

Weissman MM, Gammon D, John K, et al: Children of depressed parents: Increased pathology and early onset of major depression. Arch Gen Psychiatry 44:847, 1987.

Widom LS: The cycle of violence. Science 244:160-166, 1989.

Wissow LS: Child Advocacy for the Clinician: An Approach to Child Abuse and Neglect. Baltimore, Williams & Wilkins, 1990.

Wissow LS: Child abuse and neglect. N Engl J Med 332:1423-1431, 1995.

Wu SS, Ma CX, Carter RL, et al: Risk factors for infant maltreatment: A population-based study. Child Abuse Negl 28:1253-1264, 2004.

11 BROTHERS AND SISTERS

PERRI KLASS

Vignette

At a 5-year-old boy's kindergarten checkup, his mother confides that she is very concerned about his relationship with his 8-year-old sister. He follows her constantly, especially when she is with friends, and she has begun to make fun of him for it; in return, he sometimes lashes out physically. Also, the boy has been assigned to the same kindergarten teacher that his sister had several years ago, who remembers her as a perfectly behaved, highly verbal student, and his parents, who feel that their son is "the noisier, rowdier, more athletic child," are worried that he will not measure up to the teacher's expectations.

It has been said that each child grows up in a different family; the same mother and father, shaped by time and experience, become slightly different parents with a slightly different marriage, and each successive child grows up in a unique domestic world. Sibling relationships have a great deal to do with shaping those different and specific families in which children grow and develop.

The sibling relationship is fraught with family tension, with historical, literary, and even biblical resonance. On the one hand, sibling status is a byword for love and loyalty, whether the closeness of a military "band of brothers," or the everlasting friendship vows of a sisterhood or sorority. Literature is full of brothers and sisters who protect one another, whether in a fairy tale, such as Hansel and Gretel, or a classic tragedy: In Sophocles' "Antigone," the heroine, who will incur her own death to give her brother's body a proper burial, declaims, "... A husband dead, there would be another for me, and a child from another man, if I lost this one, but with mother and father both hidden in the house of Hades, there is no brother who would be produced, ever" (translation, Tyrrell and Bennett, 1996).

On the other hand, siblinghood is so associated with hostility and competition that the word *sibling* seems almost automatically to evoke the word *rivalry*. Long before anyone used the term *sibling rivalry,* the first murder in the book of Genesis was committed out of anger when Abel's offering was preferred to Cain's. From the Mark of Cain to the evil sisters (and the feuding half-brothers) in "King Lear," the sibling relationship has long been associated with tension, competition, and lifelong antagonism.

In other words, siblings spend their childhood in close proximity, siblings often feel themselves closer and more similar than they are to anyone else, and siblings practice their earliest social strategies on one another—and against one another. Siblings often spend their entire lives in complex consciousness of one another, in competition, in reaction, in cooperation, and in context.

Although sibling relationships can shape daily life for young children, and although sibling events such as illness, disability, and death, can have huge impacts on the emotional and psychological states of pediatric patients, it is unusual for health care providers (with the exception of developmental-behavioral pediatricians and psychiatrists or other mental health practitioners) to inquire specifically about sibling dynamics as a routine part of a health care visit. Occasionally, sibling issues may be a chief complaint or part of a presenting concern, but even when they are not, sibling relationships are important in understanding a child's world and a child's sense of self. There are key clinical moments when sibling issues should routinely be addressed.

BIRTH ORDER

A tremendous amount has been written about birth order: birth order and personality, birth order and temperament, birth order and cognition, birth order and sexual orientation. Birth order effects, when delineated, have been attributed to environmental differences and to biologic effects on the developing fetus. Sometimes the literature on birth order can leave one with the sense that many traits can be handily explained by birth order—and that their inverses can be explained as well. An independent and resilient first-born child is identifying with the authority and autonomy of the parents, and exercising leadership and dominion over younger siblings; an independent and resilient younger child is defining a distinct niche as a way of differentiating from the older siblings. Nevertheless, there are some generally agreed-on personality traits—or perhaps tendencies—which assort with birth order, although all such effects are tempered and confounded by gender; social conditions; and the individual complexities of family life, happenstance, and history.

In 2007, the *New York Times* ran a front-page story with the following headline: "Research Finds Firstborns Gain the Higher I.Q." In this large study of 250,000 male Norwegian military conscripts, higher rank in the family was found to be associated with small but significant increases in IQ score (Kristensen and Bjerkedal, 2007). Second-born sons who had been reared as the oldest because a first-born child had died also had the higher IQ scores found in first-born sons. The tremendous attention paid to this study by the national press and the vigorous debate and discussion that followed served as a reminder of how immediate and personal these issues remain to many adults.

The study confirmed numerous earlier studies that showed a positive relationship between low birth order and IQ, and supported an environmental/family interaction mechanism in which the family environment in which the oldest surviving child develops accounts for the IQ difference (rather than, for example, a previously proposed mechanism in which maternal antibodies, which increase in successive pregnancies, affect the developing fetal brain with increasing severity). Other multilevel analyses of large samples in the past have attributed important intelligence differences to factors that vary between families, however, rather than within families. It also has been pointed out that many younger siblings develop special skills and talents that are not measured on traditional IQ tests, but that are important for success in school and in life.

Many researchers have argued that the most significant differences in cognitive development concern language. First-born children are exposed exclusively to adult parental language and generally receive more direct language stimulation from their parents; their vocabulary skills are consequently improved. The increased and often intense socializing that goes on among brothers and sisters can enhance communication skills, however, so that younger siblings may be able to use their language very effectively. In any case, individual developmental factors and home and family influences contribute to vast variation in language acquisition within any birth order group, and the milestones of normal language acquisition are the same for all children, regardless of birth order; parents may claim that a young child whose language is apparently delayed is able to communicate effectively with an older sibling, but that young child still warrants aggressive workup and intervention for the speech delay.

Another area of great controversy has been the effect of birth order on personality, achievement, and creativity. There are many popular beliefs about birth order and achievement, often focusing on the supposed drive and accomplishments of first-born children, explained sometimes as a result of their disproportionate share of parental attention, other times as part of their overidentification with parental roles, and sometimes as a relic of old systems of primogeniture and increased expectation of the oldest (especially because, according to some studies, the increased achievements of first children are a phenomenon in particular of families with higher socioeconomic status). A controversial book by Sulloway (1996) argued, based on the analysis of many historical figures in science, religion, and politics, that first-born children identify with their parents and accept existing authority, whereas younger brothers and sisters are more inclined to rebel and to manifest various kinds of revolutionary creativity.

There is some much-discussed research to suggest that sexual orientation may have a link to birth order, especially in males, and that more older brothers may increase the likelihood that a younger son will be homosexual (Bogaert and Liu, 2006). A biologic mechanism has been proposed involving a maternal immune effect engendered by male fetuses, with increasing intensity after sensitization by previous male fetuses. This mechanism would not account, however, for the link that some studies have found between birth order and female homosexuality. Other researchers have argued that any link is probably social and environmental.

With regard to birth order, there is no character trait and no important life thread for which birth order has been established as the most important determinant. Health care providers should discourage parents from generalizing on the basis of birth order (e.g., "first children are the superachievers," "younger siblings may be slower to start talking"). There is tremendous variability among first-born children—and among younger brothers and sisters—in every trait that has been studied, and there are multiple confounding factors, such as child's gender, sibling gender, birth spacing, culture, and family circumstances, all of which can figure in the ontogeny of personality, behavior, and life story. The many controversies over birth order serve to remind us, however, that in this very important respect, each child does grow up in a different family environment. There may not be simple predictive general rules of how birth order and sibling relationships will affect a child's life and character, but on an individual basis, those effects are powerful, unforgettable, and lifelong.

OTHER FAMILY FACTORS

Generally, the most intense rivalries seem to occur between children spaced about 2 years apart, which may be attributable partly to the developmental stage of the older child when the younger is born. When children are spaced more widely—at least 4 years apart—the older child is verbal and possibly able to articulate feelings when the younger is born. As the children grow up, rivalry issues may become more prominent (that 4-year difference will look less definitive in their teens, and still less so in their 20s).

Twins seem to be less prone to hostile and aggressive interactions. The literature describing the remarkable bonds and close relationships that form between twins, often while they are very young, and persist as they grow is considerable. Parents may find that their task with twins (or children of other multiple births) centers more on helping these children to develop individual identities, and to separate from one another. The older or younger brothers or sisters of twins or triplets (not part of the multiple birth) may experience a very particular form of jealousy, specifically because twins receive so much attention from family members and strangers. Parents can help minimize this jealousy on the part of the "non-multiples" and foster increased individual development by the "multiples" if they avoid the temptation to give similar or rhyming names, to dress the twins alike, or to draw attention from the crowd.

It also is important to remember, especially because twins and other multiple births are increasingly common as a result of the prevalence and success of assisted reproduction techniques, that the additional pressures that multiple births place on a family may exacerbate sibling conflicts. Families may be highly stressed in terms of time, money, and energy, meaning that children may be growing up under conditions that are physically and emotionally more difficult. Children may find themselves sharing rooms and possessions when they do not want to; caregivers may be sleep-deprived and anxious. Anything that alleviates some of this stress on the family may smooth out some of the sibling conflicts—or at least help parents to deal with the conflicts in a calmer and more measured manner. Finally, as twins grow up, they may evoke particularly invidious comparisons, within the family and from outside, and they may find themselves particularly vulnerable to being shaped by rivalries and being defined in relation to their brother or sister (the good twin, the big twin, the weak twin, the smart twin).

Family size is another important determinant of the individual child's environment and has been studied extensively as a determinant of outcomes. Many studies have suggested that a larger number of brothers and sisters is linked to poorer academic achievement, but there is still much debate about the mechanism of this effect (Steelman et al, 2002). It has been hypothesized that each child dilutes the family intellectual environment, and that with more children in a family, access to the various resources provided by parents (whether material or intellectual) becomes more problematic for all the children. Large family size, particularly in low socioeconomic status families, also can be a determinant of poverty or stressed and overstretched material and human resources. It may be for this reason that in some studies, large family size has been linked to poorer outcomes—especially among poorer people. Other economic analyses show no effect of family size on economic success.

All family relationships and parameters must be viewed in cultural, economic, and historical context. A family of five children could look large in certain contexts (modern, urban, nonreligious) and unremarkable in others (rural, farming, devoutly religious).

SIBLING RIVALRY

Antagonistic and competitive interactions between brothers and sisters have been perceived and understood and chronicled since ancient times and have been described in vastly different cultures, countries, and conditions. Although sibling rivalry probably would be recognized almost everywhere as part of "basic human nature," it was not until the 20th century that a specific biologic (and darwinian) mechanism was proposed to explain affection and hostility. Hamilton (1964) extended the darwinian notion of reproductive fitness, integrating into it what was increasingly understood about genetic inheritance. Fitness was not strictly the property of the individual: your inclusive reproductive fitness also comprised the fitness of those related to you—but only in proportion to the degree of that relatedness. In other words, you have a 100% interest in your own fitness because you are 100% related to yourself, but also a 50% interest in the fitness (and reproductive success) of a brother or sister, with whom you share, on average, 50% of your genetic material. It goes on from there: you have a 25% interest in your sibling's children (who carry one half of that one half of your shared genes), and a 12.5% interest in your first cousins; this is what gave rise to J.B.S. Haldane's famous line that he would lay down his life to save two brothers or eight cousins.

Hamilton's argument presumably would be that natural selection has built in a motivation for helping and supporting brothers and sisters to succeed in life, and ultimately in reproduction; their fitness is, in proportion, your fitness as well and perpetuates your genes. But you are most closely related to yourself, and it is with your brothers and sisters that you compete for the first and most basic resources that affect a young child: attention, love, and nurturing by your common parents, who are equally related to you and your brothers and sisters.

Sibling interaction as a force in child development is much more than a darwinian competition for scarce resources. It also is an ongoing exercise in socialization, negotiation, and conflict resolution. Differences in imaginative play of young children have been linked to sibling relationships and to parent-child relationships. Positive sibling relationships can contribute to successful adjustment to preschool programs and to school. A study of conflict delineated different strategies among older and younger brothers and sisters, but noted that for younger and older brothers and sisters, successful resolution depended on the ability to disregard old injuries and plan together (Ross et al, 2006).

BLENDED FAMILIES

When parents divorce and remarry, and families combine and recombine, children may need to adjust to step-parents, step-sisters, and step-brothers. The same problems can apply when older children come into a family as adoptive siblings or as foster children. Chapters 12 and 13 provide a full discussion of these situations.

CHILDREN WITH SPECIAL NEEDS

When families include children with special needs, the sibling issues can be particularly important. These issues are closely related to all the same sibling questions and tensions discussed previously, but they can be made more complex and more intense, and may require special thought and understanding on the part of parents and providers. Parents' coping abilities and family resilience are important for helping children cope with the stress of sibling disability and illness.

A child with special needs alters the family constellation; a brother or sister may experience the sense that all the parents' attentions and emotions are concentrated on the more "vulnerable" child and may deeply resent the time that the parents spend taking that child to medical or therapy appointments. Brothers and sisters of children with autistic spectrum disorders reported feeling anger at the aggressive behaviors associated with those disorders (Ross and Cuskelly, 2006). At the same time, as a child comes to understand that a brother or sister is struggling with illness or disability, there may be a great deal of guilt at having escaped the problem and concomitant guilt about feeling resentment. When there is a child in a family who faces extra struggles and extra limitations, other children may come to feel that they are being saddled with an extra weight of parental expectations and may react to this with a mixture of resentment, anxiety, and pride.

On the one hand, some children feel acute shame about a brother or sister who is visibly "different"—with obvious physical anomalies or with severe autism. This shame is often accompanied by guilt and a sense that the parents would be angry or disappointed if they knew. On the other hand, many children take on the roles of protector, guide, and major supporter for brothers and sisters with special needs. As with all sibling relationships, these different emotions and behavior patterns are not rigidly separated: a 9-year-old girl who has endless patience at home for her autistic brother and understands his limited communications better than anyone else may find herself hideously embarrassed when he has a meltdown at the mall just as a few of her classmates come along; she then may feel guilty and confused about her own embarrassment.

BROTHERS AND SISTERS THROUGH CHILDHOOD

As brothers and sisters grow and change, the pattern of their relationship and the degree of closeness vary, especially when the children are of different genders (Kim et al, 2006). The children's temperaments affect these evolving relationships profoundly (Brody, 1998).

Toddlers and preschoolers often show regressive behaviors (bed-wetting, demanding a bottle, throwing tantrums) with the advent of a new baby. School-age children have the advantage of segregation by age, so that a 12-year-old may live in a school-bound world quite distinct from that of a 9-year-old brother or sister. Everyone knows how complex the lot of the younger brother or sister can be, however, following through grade school a older brother or sister who leaves behind a stellar academic track record or a legend as a trouble-maker.

With the increased primacy of the peer group in adolescence, sibling issues often recede in importance, and conflicts decline after early adolescence. Health care providers should be sensitive to the situation of adolescents who find themselves compelled to function as family babysitters because the family is in difficult economic straits or, especially in immigrant families, because of cultural expectations that an older child should automatically take on this responsibility. High school students whose peers are not constrained by these expectations often believe that their sibling obligations are preventing participation in extracurricular activities, or in a "normal" social life, and this resentment can create substantial family stress.

SERIOUS ILLNESS OR DEATH OF A CHILD

The serious illness or death of a child is a tragedy and a terrible loss for the child's family. For the brother or sister of a child who dies, the loss is complicated by the grief of the parents, the individuals who in other circumstances would help the surviving child cope with grief. Chapter 37 provides a full discussion of this topic.

ADULT SIBLING RELATIONSHIPS

The sibling relationship shapes the individualized family in which a child grows and develops, but the relationship remains powerful in many individuals' lives long after childhood. A study of adult psychosocial development found that poor sibling relationships in childhood predicted major depression in adulthood, even after controlling for the quality of parent-child relationships (Waldinger et al, 2007). Many sisters and brothers carry the complex sibling balance of love and rivalry, affection and hostility, and pride and competition into their adult lives.

HEALTH CARE PROVIDER'S ROLE IN HELPING PARENTS COPE WITH SIBLING ISSUES

The most common sibling-related issues that are likely to be brought to the attention of the health care provider center around sibling rivalry and hostile interactions. Table 11-1 presents some strategies for providers in teasing out (no pun intended) the details and offering helpful strategies to parents. It can be particularly helpful to work with parents on the issue of labeling and typing siblings with relation to one another; probably nothing does as much to foment sibling hostility as the dread parental tendency to sort out and label their various childhood specimens. Labels such as "the smart one," "the pretty one," "the scientist," "the dreamer," "the athlete," "the artist," "the good eater" and "the picky one" all risk forcing children into patterns and into stereotypes that they may deeply resent. "The smart sister" always feels she is being told she is ugly, whereas "the pretty sister" is positive that her parents think she is dumb. Although it is impossible to avoid the fascinating activity of observing, analyzing, and categorizing one's own children (and marveling at the striking differences that appear among children with a common family heritage and a common genetic stock), it is important to fight against the temptation to sort children into easy and polarized types. Parents need to respect and appreciate sibling differences, without imprisoning children in rigid roles.

Table 11-1. Strategies for Providers When Parents Express Concerns about Sibling Behaviors

- Get a full description of the problematic behavior; elicit details about family practices and domestic arrangements
  - Where children sleep, where they do homework, where they play, where they store personal possessions
  - Specific precipitants and flashpoints for sibling conflict, including times of day, family context, and setting
  - How parents handle sibling conflicts
  - What strategies have worked in the past
  - The history of the sibling relationship; the birth of the younger child
- Talk to the child one-on-one; try to sort out what the child identifies as the particular problems, flashpoints, and "unfairnesses"
- Help parents see what is age-appropriate behavior; address the issue of older children, and whether they take on parental roles and responsibilities
- Offer developmentally appropriate strategies
  - Spend separate time with each child, structured around that individual child's needs and interests
  - Consider family meetings to deal with controversies and conflicts in an organized fashion and guarantee that everyone is heard
  - Avoid comparisons and contrasts between siblings; avoid labels such as "the smart one" or "the pretty one"
  - Encourage children to seek out different spheres of interest, activity, and achievement
  - Do not consistently sacrifice one child's interests, activities, or free time to the achievements of a sibling
  - Establish and follow codes of behavior and "fairness" so that arguments and conflicts can be settled with rules that apply to all children
    - Rotating some tasks by turns
    - Respecting the privacy of siblings' rooms (or their desks, or their backpacks)
  - Be wary of making a fetish of absolute equal treatment; do not promise exactly the same attention, gifts, special treats, or prerogatives
  - Set appropriate limits for sibling behavior
  - Younger siblings may need to be protected from physical harm
  - Older siblings need to know that they—and their belongings—also will be properly protected
  - Allow siblings some reasonable latitude to work out conflicts
- Reassure parents that sibling rivalry is not unusual and in particular is not a reflection of poor parenting

It also is important to remind parents that although children need to be protected, and serious issues need to be resolved, children can be allowed to arbitrate some of their own conflicts. For many children, sibling relationships are an early and valuable source of social conundrums and solutions. A child who is teased by an older brother or sister may learn how to handle it, whether by ignoring it or by answering back—and there are many older brothers and sisters who have experienced the unpleasant (although salutary) surprise of realizing that they have taught the basic lessons of teasing (how to find a weak point, how to exploit it) all too successfully. Unless a relationship is unusually difficult, or unless brothers and sisters are passing through a particularly rancorous phase, most children find in brothers and sisters early and important playmates; they need a little freedom and privacy to explore the possibilities.

Although most sibling hostilities fall within the range of normal family function, it is important for health care providers to keep in mind that there may be a larger problem within the family, such as marital difficulties or family violence, which is creating an atmosphere of stress and conflict. Also, extreme sibling conflict may be only part of a child's larger picture of aggression, violence, or dysfunction. It is always important to ask how the children are functioning in other spheres of their lives, and whether conflict or aggression is problematic in school or with friends. A child who is failing in school or manifesting explosive behaviors on the playground also may be fighting with a brother or sister, and the whole complex picture needs to be addressed.

Finally, providers should be aware that although sibling conflicts are common and even "normal," there are occasionally situations in which one brother or sister is repeatedly subject to physical injury by another. These must be considered situations of physical abuse in which a child is at risk and treated as such by physicians and social service agencies.

SUMMARY

Sibling relationships have powerful effects that shape the family environment in which a child grows up; the complexities of these relationships remain intense often into adulthood. Many different variables of birth order, family shape, and structure affect sibling dynamics and moderate the influence of those dynamics on behavior, development, and personality; birth order also has been linked to intelligence and sexual orientation. Sibling rivalry may be the most common issue that parents bring up at health care visits, but there are many other contexts in which clinicians may want to consider the power of sibling relationships and interactions, the strength and nature of the bonds, and the lasting influence of brothers and sisters.

REFERENCES

Bogaert AF, Liu J: Birth order and sexual orientation in men: Evidence for two independent interactions. J Biosoc Sci 38:811-819, 2006.

Brody GH: Sibling relationship quality: Its causes and consequences. Annu Rev Psychol 49:1-24, 1998.

Hamilton WD: The genetical evolution of social behavior. I and II. J Theor Biol 7:1-16. and 7-54, 1964.

Kim J-Y, McHale SM, Osgood W, Crouter D: Longitudinal course and family correlates of sibling relationships from childhood through adolescence. Child Dev 77:1746-1761, 2006.

Kristensen P, Bjerkedal T: Explaining the relation between birth order and intelligence. Science 316:1717, 2007.

Ross H, Ross M, Stein N, Trabasso T: How siblings resolve their conflicts: The importance of first offers, planning, and limited opposition. Child Dev 77:1730-1745, 2006.

Ross P, Cuskelly M: Adjustment, sibling problems and coping strategies of brothers and sisters of children with autistic spectrum disorder. J Intell Dev Disabil 31:77-86, 2006.

Steelman LC, Powell B, Werum R, Carter S: Reconsidering the effects of sibling configuration: Recent advances and challenges. Annu Rev Soc 28:243-266, 2002.

Sulloway FJ: Born to Rebel: Birth Order, Family Dynamics, and Creative Lives. New York, Pantheon Books, 1996.

Tyrell WB, Bennett LJ (trans.): Sophocles' Antigone. Translated with Introduction and Notes. 1996. Available at www.stoa.org/diotima/anthology/ant/. Accessed September 30, 2008.

Waldinger RJ, Vaillant GE, Orav EJ: Childhood sibling relationships as a predictor of major depression in adulthood: A 30-year prospective study. Am J Psychiatry 164:949-955, 2007.

BOOKS FOR PARENTS

Brazelton TB, Sparrow JD: Understanding Sibling Rivalry: The Brazelton Way. New York, Da Capo, 2005.

Faber A, Mazlich E: Siblings Without Rivalry: How to Help Your Children Live Together So You Can Live Too. New York, Collins (expanded edition), 2004.

Goldenthal P: Beyond Sibling Rivalry: How to Help Your Children Become Cooperative, Caring and Compassionate. New York, Owl Books, 2000.

Wolf A: "Mom, Jason's Breathing on Me!": The Solution to Sibling Bickering. New York, Ballantine Books, 2003.

BOOKS FOR CHILDREN

Alexander MG: Nobody Asked ME if I Wanted a Baby Sister and When the New Baby Comes, I'm Moving Out! Boston, Charlesbridge, 2005 and 2006 (reprints). These are humorous picture books suitable for young children.

Blume J: The Pain and the Great One. New York, Dragonfly, 1985. This is another picture book done with humor. By the same author, for older children, Tales of a Fourth-Grade Nothing, Fudge, and Superfudge are chapter books that school-age children find funny and recognizable as stories about family life with a younger sibling.

Henkes K: Julius, the Baby of the World. New York, Mulberry Books, 1990. This is a very funny picture book about an older sister and a new baby.

12 SEPARATION, DIVORCE, AND REMARRIAGE

J. LANE TANNER

Vignette

Eric, age 7, was referred to a developmental-behavioral pediatrician for evaluation of symptoms of attention-deficit/hyperactivity disorder. In completing the report-from-school form, Eric's second grade teacher had described Eric as the most hyperactive boy she had known in her 30 years of teaching. The pediatrician was surprised on his first meeting with Eric at how quiet and somber he seemed throughout their initial interview, never moving from his chair over the course of an hour-long meeting.

In discussing the family background with Eric's mother, including directly asking her about possible stressful experiences for Eric, the pediatrician learned that the parents' relationship had been growing increasingly conflictual over the past 2 years. Eric had witnessed many episodes of intense arguing, screaming, and name-calling between them. Periodically, such a fight would lead to the father storming out of the house, not to be seen again by Eric for a period that varied unpredictably between several days and a few months. Then the father would reappear, without explanation to his son, and a new period of tension and building conflict between the parents would ensue.

The pediatrician found no evidence for neurodevelopmental or learning disabilities in Eric. He requested meetings with each parent to discuss the emotional impact of their ongoing conflict on Eric. This led to a series of discussions between Eric and each parent, some of which were facilitated by the physician. Eventually, the parents separated and started divorce proceedings. Eric's behavior and attention in school was markedly improved in the subsequent year.

Nurture for the developing child begins with the family, and the health of the marital relationship has a direct impact on the care that parents provide. The stable presence of parents and other family members provides the foundation of understanding for growing children of who they are and how their world is configured. Disruptions in these relationships, including the loss of a parent through separation and divorce, or the creation of a step-family through remarriage, challenges the child's notions of this stable family universe and carries increased risk for short-term and long-term developmental and behavioral difficulties.

This chapter provides a description of the status of marital rearrangements in the United States today, current evidence regarding the short-term and long-term consequences for children whose parents separate or remarry, and a discussion of potential related roles and opportunities for pediatric clinicians. American children now grow up in a wide array of types of parental and family arrangements, including two parents, married to each other; two parents, not married; one parent and a step-parent, with or without step-brothers and step-sisters; single parents, never married; single parents, formerly married; grandparent-led and multigenerational families; gay or lesbian parents; adoptive parents; and foster parents. Today's extended families may include the new spouses of divorced parents, the new spouses' own parents, and the new spouses' children by former marriages.

The quality of parental relationships varies widely as well—from close and supportive to cold and distant. Children are the clear beneficiaries of a close, loving, and mutually appreciative parental relationship, and are unavoidably troubled when their parents grow apart. The ways in which parents define their roles as parents represents another spectrum of difference, with some couples intentionally sharing most parenting tasks, and others assuming more clearly defined and distinct roles with their children. Parents have their own unique histories of being parented and of experiencing relationships with their own parents, experiences that they may consciously or unconsciously want to replicate or change for their own children.

Cataloging the myriad possibilities of family structure and parent experience in this way provides ample reason why clinicians need to inquire routinely regarding (1) who are the parental figures for the child; (2) what is the quality of the parental relationship; and (3) how is each parent, and the parental relationship, adjusting to the child and his or her needs.

DEMOGRAPHICS OF SEPARATION, DIVORCE, AND REMARRIAGE

Permanent changes in the parental relationship—specifically, separation, divorce, and remarriage—are among the most common, significant family changes that children in the United States experience. The frequency with which American children experience these major redefinitions of their families is highlighted by the following demographic profile for families in the United States:

- The U.S. divorce rate has been fairly stable for the past 20 years. If this rate remains constant, it will result in an estimated 48% of all new marriages ending in divorce within 20 years (Bramlett and Mosher, 2002).
- In 2005, two thirds of all children 18 years old or younger were living with their two biologic parents. Slightly less than 25% were living with their mother and without their father, 4.8% were with their father without their mother, and 4.5% were living with neither parent (U.S. Bureau of the Census, 2005).
- By the age of 18 years, more than 55% of children are expected to spend some time in a single parent family—the result of parental separation and divorce in about half of cases and of growing up with a never-married parent in the other half (Hetherington, 2005).
- Of divorced adults, 50% remarry within 4 years, and approximately one third of American children eventually become members of a step-family (Hetherington, 2005).
- Of step-families, 86% are composed of the biologic mother and a step-father (Hetherington, 2005).
- The proportion of births that have occurred outside of marriage has steadily increased over the past 50 years (4% of births in 1950 versus 35% of births in 2003). It is estimated that approximately 40% of these births are to cohabiting couples.

Prevalence rates for permanent changes in parental relationships are underrepresented by marriage statistics (Bramlett and Mosher, 2002).

CONSEQUENCES OF SEPARATION, DIVORCE, AND REMARRIAGE

Separation, Divorce, and Remarriage as Family Processes

A key to understanding the impact of divorce and remarriage on children and families is to conceptualize such changes as ongoing processes as opposed to discrete events. For each family, marital separation or rearrangement carries with it a unique history and a new set of possibilities with respect to family life. By the time parents have separated from each other, it can be assumed that there has been a significant history of considered and attempted solutions for repairing the relationship, without success.

Marital conflict takes many forms, and the child's understanding of the conflict and his or her behavioral responses to it likewise vary. Clinicians benefit from understanding, as best they can, the course of the marital relationship before the separation and the experienced consequences of the change, as viewed by each parent and the child. The parents may see separation as the answer to their problems with each other, whereas children routinely experience it as the end of their family as they know it. The child's experience of grief for this loss, even when the marital relationship was highly dysfunctional, is an expectable consequence. How parents are able to respond to the child's experience of loss and mourning, while coping with the impact of the change for themselves, is predictive of how likely the child is to weather this major life change successfully (Wallerstein and Resnikoff, 1997).

Consequences for Parents

Central to an understanding of the impact of family change on the child is an inquiry into the substantive and emotional consequences for each parent, and for the resulting family units. Divorce carries direct economic consequences for families, including diminished household incomes and the expense of a second home for the parent who leaves. Economic necessity often leads to the custodial parent moving to a more affordable residence, with the associated displacement for the children from their familiar surroundings. Such moves often involve some compromise in the quality of the school and the "livability" of the community. Parents must rethink their work lives to satisfy new requirements for income. The balance between home and work responsibilities often must be renegotiated, with attendant requirements for changes in childcare and new dependencies on relatives and friends. New economic strains brought about by the divorce heighten tensions around financial settlements, which help to fuel ongoing, postdivorce conflict between the parents.

Separation and divorce routinely affect the emotional and mental health of parents, especially in the first year following the divorce. Parental depression, anxiety, low self-esteem, and grief reactions are frequent. A sense of profound loneliness, periods of intense anger, and general disorganization in psychological functioning are emotional states often reported by parents in the year or so following the separation (Wallerstein and Kelly, 1980). Physical illness, accidents, substance abuse, and antisocial behaviors also are commonly seen. The preoccupation that parents experience with their own emotional and circumstantial adjustments may lead to a diminished capacity to perceive and understand their child's experience. The quality of parenting may deteriorate subsequently until the parent has regained emotional balance and a new level of equilibrium regarding work, financial stability, and social support (Cohen, 2002). Effects on the parents vary widely, with some parents reporting emotional and psychological benefits after the separation, others showing serious but temporary declines in well-being, and others seeming never to recover fully (Amato, 2000).

For parents, the redefinition of themselves as single parents also has short-term and long-term effects. Newly separated parents must grapple with the immediate reality of being alone with the day-to-day responsibilities of home and family, and the emotional consequences of having no one to ask, "what do you think?" Long-term, single parents must forge a new set of priorities that permits them to "have a life" that includes adult friends, interests, exercise, respite from responsibility, and, especially, whether and when to form a new intimate, adult relationship.

Parents also must weather the legal consequences of divorce, including the division of property, determination of ongoing child support, and child custody or visiting schedules. This is a process that has variable consequences in terms of time, cost, and emotional turmoil for the parents—all of which depend on the level of ongoing conflict between the parents versus their ability to cooperate with each other. Conflicts regarding custody and financial support may be formally resolved by the parents working together with a divorce mediator, or in more adversarial fashion in court with each parent represented by an attorney. Mediation, when possible, holds the potential for each parent to feel more considered in the terms of their eventual agreement and to avoid some of the acrimony inevitable with adversarial confrontations in court. Divorce mediators are not yet licensed or board certified, however, so their qualifications may be less apparent. Parents may want to retain their own lawyer as well to review the terms developed in mediation before agreeing to them (Wallerstein, 2003). For a high-risk minority of parents, nonacceptance of the divorce may take the form of chronic conflict and persistent child custody battles with the ex-spouse (Sbarra and Emery, 2005).

Consequences for Children

General Considerations

Although the unique qualities of individual children, families, and divorce processes make general predictions regarding the effects of divorce tenuous for any given child, studies of the short-term and long-term consequences have shown an impact on cohorts of children and teens across a range of psychosocial and functional dimensions. Amato and Keith performed meta-analyses on 93 such studies published in the 1960s through 1980s, and another 67 studies conducted during the 1990s (Amato, 2001). This combined research has shown children of divorce to be worse off, overall, than children with continuously married parents on the following outcomes:

- Academic success, as measured by grades and standardized achievement tests
- Behavioral problems and aggression
- Psychological well-being, especially depressive symptoms
- Self-esteem, including positive feelings about themselves and perceptions of self-efficacy
- Peer relations, as measured by numbers of close friends and social support from peers
- Weaker emotional bonds with mothers and fathers (Amato, 1991, 2001, 2005).

In keeping with the wide variation of experience of children in these studies, overall differences, across each of the above-listed dimensions, between children of divorce and children of two parent families were *significant but modest*. Evidence supports the resiliency of most children to adjust successfully and be able to function competently after the divorce of their parents. Children of divorce face significant distress, however, and must cope with potent stressors. A significant minority are more seriously affected emotionally and psychologically (Emery and Forehand, 1994). For clinicians, the above-listed findings of measurable consequences in children provide a set of indicators of risk for more serious long-term dysfunction, rather than predictable areas of deficit.

Adding to the complexity in understanding this research, some longitudinal studies have highlighted childhood problems that existed before the parents' separation, finding that the long-term effects of divorce were less apparent when the educational and behavioral status of the child before the divorce was accounted for (Cherlin et al, 1991).

Nevertheless, a growing body of literature now exists to show significant long-term effects of divorce, at least for some children. Adults who experienced the divorce of their parents during childhood have been shown to have lower socioeconomic attainment, an increased risk of having a nonmarital birth, weaker bonds with their parents, lower psychological well-being, more difficulties in achieving intimate relationships, poorer marital quality, and a higher risk of having their own marriage end in divorce compared with peers with never-divorced parents (Amato, 2005; Wallerstein and Lewis, 2004). Young adults especially report distress regarding the distant relationship that developed after the divorce between them and their fathers, including the sense of loss and disappointment that their fathers were not more involved in their lives, and the loss of support, material and relational, for pursuing higher educational and career goals (Laumann-Billings and Emery, 2000; Wallerstein and Lewis, 2004).

What accounts for the variability of impact? The degree and chronicity of parental conflict before and after the separation is one such variable. Inevitably, children are aware of the predivorce parental problems and may see and hear far more of the conflict than the parents appreciate. In keeping with an understanding of divorce as a process, children are less likely to bounce back psychologically and developmentally when their parents are unable to leave behind the emotional intensity—including open arguments between parents, with screaming, yelling, belittling, or threats punctuating their ongoing conflict. Violence between parents, witnessed by the child, can be especially traumatizing (Buehler et al, 1997; Lieberman and Van Horn, 1998; Sbarra and Emery, 2005). Other qualities in the interaction between parent and child, before, during, and after the divorce, figure in the child's ability to weather the separation. These include the foundation of stable parenting provided to the child in early life, the qualities of parental warmth and praise toward the child throughout the divorce process, and the capacity of the parent to protect the child from the conflict and emotional intensity between the adults (Katz and Gottman, 1997).

Child factors also have been associated with effects of divorce. Individual characteristics that tend to elicit more positive responses from parents and others, such as an "easy" temperament, physical attractiveness, normal or above-average intelligence, higher self-esteem, and a sense of humor, seem to be protective for children experiencing parental divorce. Children with more difficult temperaments and children with behavior problems before the divorce tend to be more adversely affected (Hetherington, 2005; Tschann et al, 1989).

Consequences of divorce need not be seen as solely negative. Children and adults are likely to benefit when the separation and divorce marks a true decrease or cessation of tensions between the parents, and especially when the parents are able gradually to develop a more civil relationship with each other—one that can accommodate mutual discussion and decision making regarding the child. Research support exists, especially, for benefits to the child when a high-conflict marriage is ended. In addition, children of divorce often experience shifts in family roles that may support the development of self-reliance, a greater awareness of the needs of others, experience in responsibility taking and care for others, and, for some, an increase in emotional closeness with the custodial parent (Arditti, 1999).

Common Age-Related Behavior Changes

Children 0 to 3 Years Old

Behavior changes in children 0 to 3 years old tend to reflect the distress of the parents—the intensity of the parents' emotional preoccupation, continuing conflict, grief, and depression. A history of spousal conflict or separation during the pregnancy should alert the clinician to consider the degree to which the new mother feels abandoned and is depressed or otherwise preoccupied from a primary focus on the child. As with other circumstances in which parents must cope with significant personal distress and preoccupation, children younger than 3 years tend to react with increased irritability, crying, fearfulness, separation anxiety, sleep and gastrointestinal problems, aggression, and developmental regression (Cohen, 2002). When children of this age remain in stable attachment relationships that are caring and continuous, and do not experience significantly disruptive life changes, evidence exists to show minimal significant behavioral or developmental differences compared with children 0 to 3 years old of nondivorcing parents (Clarke-Stewart et al, 2000).

Children 3 to 5 Years Old

Preschool children may show an increase in clinginess and unhappiness, nightmares and fantasies, and fear of abandonment in response to the separation of their parents. The magical thinking typical of the age may result in a wide range of explanatory fantasies for the loss of a parent, including the belief that the child caused the breakup (Cohen, 2002). Longer term effects of parental separation at this age have been seen, including increases in anxious, hyperactive, and oppositional behaviors later in childhood (Japel et al, 1999; Pagani et al, 1997).

Children 6 to 12 Years Old

School-age children often have declining school performance associated with parental separation, most typically during the year following the separation. Irritability, moodiness, preoccupation, aggressive behaviors, and attention problems are frequently seen. Children of this age may feel personally rejected or deceived by the absent parent and may struggle with simultaneous feelings of anger, guilt, and loss. When the parents' conflict is persistent and evident after the separation, the child must negotiate, emotionally and interpersonally, how to divide and express his or her loyalties to each parent (Cohen, 2002). Moral development and behavior may be affected in children of this age as well, when the parents' own conduct is perceived by the child as at odds with the standards that had been the understood code for behavior and social relations to that point (Roseby and Johnston, 1998).

Adolescents

Teenagers who have experienced the separation, divorce, or remarriage of their parents must develop their own identity and goals for relationships with their parents' failed marriage as backdrop. Wallerstein and Lewis (2004) described a significant decrease in parental protection (i.e., fewer rules, more poorly enforced expectations, and greater personal responsibilities) for teenagers of divorced parents compared with nondivorced parents. Wallerstein and Lewis (2004) and others have found more acting out, earlier and more frequent sexual experiences in teen girls, depression, delinquency, and earlier and heavier use of drugs and alcohol among the teens of divorced families. Relationships between teens and their noncustodial fathers are often experienced by adolescents as more distant and strained, with many teens reporting feeling less accepted by their fathers and reporting less self-esteem (McCormick and Kennedy, 2000). Some teens, particularly boys, may idealize distant fathers and by mid adolescence become focused on reconnecting with or tying their identity to the idealized father.

Children in middle childhood and adolescence may find that parental separation brings with it new pressures to operate more independently and to fulfill new roles in support of the custodial parent and family. Some older children report a new emphasis, after divorce, on taking on more household chores, caring for brothers and sisters, and serving to a greater degree as the mother's companion and confidante. For some teens, this new role may propel them forward toward an earlier attainment of mature responsibility. Clinicians should be alert, however, for signs of stalled or derailed development because such "adultified" teens may suppress their own feelings and expressions of need, and may prematurely foreclose on experiences of exploration, personal challenge, and achievement of identity.

Consequences Associated with Gender

Early studies of effects of divorce found greater problems in adjustment, overall, in boys than in girls, with "sleeper effects" in some girls later on during adolescence. More recent studies have found more similarities than differences. Amato and Keith's meta-analysis of studies conducted before and during the 1990s showed some increase in conduct problems in boys compared with girls after a divorce, but no significant differences in academic achievement, overall conduct, or psychological adjustment (Amato, 2005).

Influence of Cultural Factors

The impact of parental separation on the child also must be seen within the context of community and cultural norms. How likely is the child to feel unique and stigmatized within his or her peer group? What are accepted norms for expression of feelings and needs? What extended family and community resources are available to assist the child to cope with the changes to his or her own family? Although research evidence for cross-cultural distinctions is still in early stages, clinicians would be well advised to ask questions regarding the cultural and religious beliefs surrounding marriage, separation, and divorce for any given child and family.

Consequences of Remarriage

Given that most divorcing adults remarry, and many never-married mothers marry men who are not the fathers of their children, life in a step-family has become commonplace, affecting an estimated one third of U.S. children (Hetherington, 2005). Adding a second parent to the household, in most cases, a step-father, provides the family with new resources, potentially an improved standard of living, and the availability of another supervising adult who, over time, may achieve parental qualities in his or her ability to nurture the child's development.

Studies consistently show greater numbers of problem behaviors in children in step-families compared with children raised by continuously married parents—20% to 25% of children in step-families versus 10% in two parent families. Whether such behavioral problems in step-families are connected more with an earlier parental separation than with the new family formation is unclear. Children in step-families and children being raised by single parents tend to have similar rates of behavior problems, however, indicating that the addition of a step-parent in most cases does not confer protection from emotional and behavioral problems for children in single parent families. Problem behaviors documented for children in step-families include, especially, externalizing disorders and lack of social responsibility, and to a lesser extent lower academic achievement (Amato, 2005; Hetherington et al, 1999). Stressors that typically attend a parent's remarriage, and that may help to explain these differences, include the following:

- The child's adjustment to changing family circumstances, often including a change of home and neighborhood and changing household rules and family routines
- Formation of a relationship with the step-parent, which especially for teenagers may feel imposed rather than desired
- The child's experience of having to share attention and affection for the parent with a new step-parent and potentially with step-brothers and step-sisters
- Loyalty conflicts, that is, the dilemma for the child of worrying that becoming close to the step-parent would be an act of disloyalty to the noncustodial biologic parent.

Relations between step-parents and children have a developmental course. If step-families survive the early stages of relationship building, step-parents may be of great importance in the child's long-term emotional and developmental well-being. The custodial biologic parent's role in this relationship building is vital and often difficult. The mother (in most cases) simultaneously must reassure the child of her continuing love and attention and mediate the inclusion of the step-father into progressively greater involvement with her children. The difficulties in this process are highlighted by the high frequency of divorce after remarriage, the tendency of step-parents to remain more detached over the long-term from their step-children, and the overrepresentation of step-children in official reports of child abuse (Amato, 2005; Hetherington et al, 1999).

Children adjusting to such a new family arrangement, including in some cases the addition of step-brothers and step-sisters, have been shown to do best when the style of parenting is authoritative (Hetherington et al, 1999). At the same time, a common error is for step-parents, most often step-fathers, to attempt to exert full parental authority at the start of the relationship with the step-child. If, instead, the mother is able to show that she retains the ultimate authority for the children and delegates authority to the step-father as needed (e.g., "I want you to listen to him while I'm away or you'll have to answer to me"), acceptance of the stepfather's parental role is enhanced.

ROLES AND OPPORTUNITIES FOR PEDIATRIC CLINICIANS

Primary Pediatric Care

Primary pediatric care that includes continuity of care in a medical home provides the opportunity for practicing "family pediatrics." This comprehensive care model includes the clinician's regular attention to the well-being of the family, as necessary to the health and well-being of the child (American Academy of Pediatrics, 2003). Marital difficulties are typically not brought, front and center, to the clinician's attention in the context of a pediatric urgent care or well-child visit. Parents who have, or expect to have, a longitudinal and trusting relationship with their child's pediatrician are responsive, however, to questions about their own well-being as parents

(Olson et al, 2004). The identification by the primary care clinician of marital difficulties or separation provides an opportunity for discussion regarding the child's experience and needs that may not be available to the parent from any other reliable and trusted source.

Primary care clinicians also have the unique opportunity to support the marital relationship from the time that parents first become parents. Even with the most wanted pregnancy, the arrival of the infant redefines life for new parents in practically every detail. The clinician's inquiries of parents regarding their adjustment to the infant is a routine, recommended component of well-child care. To ask further how the parents' relationship with each other is weathering the new demands connected with the care of their infant is easily included in this general inquiry regarding the family. In so doing, the pediatrician validates parental experiences, invites further discussion, and signals that attention to the health of the marriage is a priority during a time of major change and adjustment (Tanner, 2002).

This inquiry should not be restricted to infancy because challenges for parents accrue with each new developmental stage. Bantering with parents, especially when both are present at the visit, about when they last went out on a "date," if they ever get time alone, or if they remember romantic moments before children, may be a welcome springboard for talking about the importance of their lives as adults, partners, and lovers as well as parents. Writing them a "prescription for a date" may serve, lightheartedly, to emphasize the importance of caring for the relationship (Coleman, 2001).

For parents going through a separation and for patients who have experienced divorce or remarriage, primary care clinicians may provide important supportive counsel during the period immediately surrounding the family change and in connection with longer term adjustments. During the acute phase of a parental separation or divorce, the clinician may be able to assist the parent in refocusing on the child's possible interpretation of events and unattended needs at a time when parents are typically preoccupied by the meaning of the event to themselves.

Primary care clinicians may be consulted by parents wondering how they should tell their child about an incipient separation; Table 12-1 lists guidelines to suggest to parents. A difficult task for a parent going through the emotional upheavals of divorce is the avoidance of angry criticism of the ex-spouse in front of the child. Parents may be helped in gaining perspective on the impact of such name-calling, blame, or criticism on the child when they are reminded that the child "comes" 50% from one parent and 50% from the other, and needs to learn from the strengths, rather than the weaknesses, of each parent in growing to full potential.

Over time, the pediatrician's monitoring role also holds special importance for children of divorce and remarriage. Table 12-2 provides an approach to help in determining developmental risk and targeting needed counsel or therapy. Primary care clinicians and pediatric subspecialists have a vital role to play in determining when a child or the entire family should be referred for more specialized mental health care (Sammons and Lewis, 2001).

Table 12-1. Telling a Child about Divorce

Tell the child before the parent's departure
Reassure the child that relations with each parent will endure
Give reasons for the divorce, and convey that great thought was given before deciding
Allow time for several discussions before the separation, and encourage questions
Provide emphatic reassurance that the child will not be abandoned
Reassure that the departing spouse has a place to live and will be okay
Reassure that the child were not the cause of the divorce and cannot mend it
Reassure that neither parent expects the child to take sides against the other
Give the child permission to love both parents
Give the child permission to express fully feelings of sadness, anger, and disappointment
Express the expectation that order and routine will be restored in the future
Reassure, over time, that the parents' failed marriage has nothing to do with the child's own future intimate relationships

Adapted from Wallerstein JS: Separation, divorce, and remarriage. *In* Levine MD, Carey WB, Crocker AC (eds): Developmental-Behavioral Pediatrics, 2nd ed. Philadelphia, WB Saunders, 1992, pp 149-161.

Custodial arrangements strongly affect the experience and adaptation of the child, and pediatric clinicians may be asked to voice their opinion regarding what arrangement would be in the best interest of the child. Joint custody arrangements—especially those involving joint physical and legal custody—have proven to be particularly complex. Although appearing to represent an equitable and assured relationship for the child with each parent, a decision in favor of joint physical custody needs to be carefully thought through. Evidence for deterioration in the children has been found when joint custody is attempted in the context of parents who are locked in ongoing conflict, and when older children are given no say in the arrangements (Johnston et al, 1989; Pruett and Hoganbruen, 1998). Wallerstein (1992) has provided guidelines for advocacy for the child when joint custody is being considered (Table 12-3).

The tendency for fathers to become physically and emotionally disengaged from their children in the wake of divorce is a risk that primary care pediatricians and other involved clinicians may have a hand in preventing. For noncustodial fathers, physical distance with their child is an experience for which they have little preparation. Separation removes them from the day-to-day knowledge of their child's activities, challenges, moods, achievements, and needs. If the father's relationship with his child before the divorce was mediated to some degree by the mother, he may struggle after the divorce with knowing how to build a new father-to-child, only, relationship. By requesting the presence of the father for a visit soon after the separation, emphasizing his importance to his child, short-term and long-term, and offering a longitudinal relationship to support his parenting efforts, primary care clinicians may become valued counselors for fathers in their transition to single parenthood (Coleman and Garfield, 2004).

Table 12-2. Assessing Risk for Children of Divorce

Parent Factors

Parental mental health, current and past
Parent's capacity to distinguish own needs from those of child's
Degree of continuing conflict between parents
Impact of economic changes
Existence of supportive network—grandparents, other extended family, and friends especially
Parental coping responses that are active, not avoidant (Tein et al, 2000)
Religious/cultural beliefs strongly opposed to divorce (Booth and Amato, 1991)

Parent-Child Interaction Factors

Successful child adaptation more likely when the parent's relationship with the child is marked by
- A stable foundation of parent-child attachment before the divorce
- Warmth, encouragement, praise, and active guidance for the child
- Avoidance of behaviors or comments perceived by the child as rejecting
- Protection of the child from ongoing parental conflict
- Authoritative style of parenting, with consistency of discipline (Wolchick et al, 2000)
- Maintenance of parental expectations (Barber and Eccles, 1992)

Concerns to be explored
- Weakening of emotional bonds with either parent
- Significant loss of relationship with noncustodial parent

Child Factors

Signs of maladaptation to marital change
- Significant increase in behavior problems or aggression
- Changes of overall mood, including especially symptoms of depression or anxiety
- Decline in academic achievement
- Evidence for lowered self-esteem, self-efficacy
- Increased problems in making and maintaining friendships

Individual child factors that may confer increased vulnerability or resilience
- Temperament and personality
- Intelligence
- Appearance
- Behavioral difficulties
- Physical or mental disability
- Chronic health needs

Subspecialty Pediatric Care—Children with Special Health Care Needs

The parents of children with chronic disabilities or serious health conditions face stressors that often complicate or undermine the marital relationship. Examples of potential wedge issues between parents include feelings of self-blame and guilt regarding the child's condition; differing processes of emotional adjustment and coping, including significant grief reactions or depressive reactions or both; the assumption by one parent of most of the worry and responsibility for the child; sacrifices of work and earning capacity and career and personal goals; and conflict regarding interface roles with medical, educational, and other involved professionals. Biobehavioral conditions, including attention-deficit/hyperactivity disorder, depression, anxiety disorders, and highly impulsive or explosive behaviors, present an added level of complexity. When such behaviors exist, parents and professionals routinely attempt to understand whether the child's behavioral symptoms are mainly reactive to the stress of family change (the vignette at the beginning of the chapter is an example of this), are part of an underlying pathologic condition, or both simultaneously.

Table 12-3. Recommended Prerequisites for Joint Physical Custody

Both parents give high priority to their parenting roles
Both parents are sensitive observers of their child and respectful of the child's wishes
Both parents respect each other as parents and are able to communicate effectively with each other about the child
Both parents can live with the ambiguities and differences that arise, and can work cooperatively on such day-to-day issues as bedtime, homework, and television watching
Both parents can assist the child in making the transitions between households
The child is able to go back and forth between the two homes without disruption of psychological adjustment or social and educational activities

Adapted from Wallerstein JS: Separation, divorce, and remarriage. *In* Levine MD, Carey WB, Crocker AC (eds): Developmental-Behavioral Pediatrics, 2nd ed. Philadelphia, WB Saunders, 1992, pp 149-161.

The comprehensive care of children with special health care needs should include some regular monitoring of the health of the marital relationship. Clinicians may want to find an opportunity early on in the care of the child to have a frank discussion with both parents to raise awareness of the potential for the child's special needs to stress their relationship, and to discuss in advance ideas for proactively caring for their marriage and their child. This kind of counsel is especially warranted when risk factors, such as those listed in Table 12-2, are present.

Developmental-Behavioral Pediatricians and Developmental-Behavioral Problems

Developmental-behavioral pediatricians and related clinicians are often referred patients for whom separation, divorce, or remarriage plays a significant role in the referral problem. In some cases, parents are seeking help for difficulties in child adjustment that they understand and accept as primarily connected to the marital change. In other situations, the parents' separation becomes a major factor when the pediatrician is asked to adjudicate parent disagreements on some aspect of care. Psychopharmacologic treatments for attention-deficit/hyperactivity disorder and other behavioral disorders are an especially common source of conflict between separated parents, often fiercely contested between parents who have a history of a high-conflict postdivorce relationship. Most common of all are developmental-behavioral problems referred to specialty physicians in which the marital discord, separation, or family rearrangement is not recognized by the parents as strongly connected with the child's symptoms. Problems of anxiety, depressive symptoms, presumptive attention or learning disorders, and oppositional-defiant or conduct problems all may be consequences of parental distress and marital change, requiring careful focus on the family and the child.

General Clinical Guideposts

Table 12-2 provides a set of parent, parent-child interaction, and child factors that clinicians may use in assessing relative risk for children whose parents are undergoing separation and divorce. Review of these factors with the parent or child or both serves the dual purpose of (1) providing the clinician with insights regarding risk to the child of significant maladaptation, and (2) helping the parent focus on the emotional health and developmental needs of the child. To support parents who are struggling with marital change, it is often the case that clinicians first need to understand the parent's circumstances, stressors, and perspective. Empathic listening to the parent's story should include the elicitation of the parent's intentions and hopes for their child's adjustment and future. From a relationship of understanding and trust between the pediatrician and the parent, consideration of the child's experience and needs becomes more possible. Parental motivation is more easily established, and direction for effective support is clarified. Successful referrals for psychological therapy usually depend on this stepwise approach as well.

Referral for psychological therapy should be considered for any child whose distress over a change in their parents' relationship is particularly severe or longstanding, with deterioration in behavioral, academic, or social and emotional functioning. Individual therapy for children of divorce has been shown to have limited benefits on its own. Programs for the parents have been more successful, targeted at their own adjustment, including their management of ongoing interparental conflict, and their parenting practices. Programs for training newly single parents in an authoritative style of parenting, including noncoercive discipline, problem solving, monitoring, and positive involvement with the child, have been associated with declines in internalizing and externalizing behavior problems and drug and alcohol use and improvements in the academic performance of their children (Hetherington, 2005). In some communities, therapeutic groups for children of divorce have been developed to provide support especially during the difficult early phase after their parents' separation (see Kids' Turn website listed in Resources for Parents).

In the interest of gaining the views and concerns of each parent, custodial and noncustodial parents need to be invited for appointments. The parents and clinician need to consider whether the parents would be able, profitably, to attend appointments together. The goal of the clinician should be to develop a therapeutic relationship with each parent in an even-handed approach that avoids the perception of favoritism. Often these shifts in care relationships require limit-setting on the part of the clinician at the outset regarding who brings the child, at what intervals, and by whom payment or insurance coverage to the practice is to be provided.

Clinicians involved in monitoring the well-being of the child also should track the parental agreement regarding custody and visitation arrangements, the willingness of the noncustodial parent to contribute material support, and the involvement of court hearings and custody conflicts. To this end, the clinician might ask the parent if he or she has developed a "parenting plan" with the other parent. In some states, there are specific guidelines for such plans, typically centering on the decision making processes to be followed with respect to medical decisions and health care costs, insurance, current and long-term plans for education, and religious affiliation and practice (Wallerstein, 2003). In joint physical custody situations, the parents must live within reasonable proximity of each other, a requirement with implications for future changes in job and living circumstances for each spouse. Nonbiologic gay and lesbian parents, in states that do not permit co-parent adoption, face the added dilemma of not being able to rely on legal support for their claims of parenthood, even when the child has known them as their parent throughout their life (Pawelski et al, 2006).

When parents strongly disagree regarding an aspect of the clinician's treatment plan, in nonemergency cases, the dissenting parent's view must be respected. If discussion by the clinician with the dissenting parent regarding the importance of the treatment does not change his or her mind, the parent should be asked to write a letter formally withdrawing consent for the treatment. The letter may be shared with the assenting parent, and the clinician should withhold the treatment until the issue is resolved either in counseling sessions between the parents or through court mediation. When possible, the clinician should avoid testifying on behalf of one parent over the other, to maintain positive and therapeutic relationships with each in the service of the long-term care for the child (Wells and Stein, 2006).

SUMMARY

The separation of never-married and married parents and the divorce and remarriage of parents have become mainstream American phenomena. The high prevalence of these family change processes has not diminished their power, however, to disrupt the sense of security and the developmental trajectory of the affected child. Clinicians and families need to appreciate such family reorganizations as long-term processes, rather than as distinct events. With this understanding comes a realization of the potential to preserve and support the most important aspects of parent-child relationships and to mitigate the now well-documented potential risks, short-term and long-term, for the child. Pediatric clinicians, practicing family pediatrics, actively support parents and the marital relationship as a matter of course in the care of the child. From this foundation of comprehensive care, the impact of marital change, real and potential, is more easily assessed, and guidance is provided for parents to help in supporting the child's development and emotional health.

REFERENCES

Amato PR: Consequences of parental divorce for children's well-being: A meta-analysis. Psychol Bull 10:26-46, 1991.

Amato PR: The consequences of divorce for adults and children. J Marriage Fam 62:1269-1287, 2000.

Amato PR: Children of divorce in the 1990s: An update of the Amato and Keith (1991) meta-analysis. J Fam Psychol 15:355-370, 2001.

Amato PR: The impact of family formation change on the cognitive, social, and emotional well-being of the next generation. Future Children 15:75-96, 2005.

American Academy of Pediatrics: Report of the Task Force on the Family. Pediatrics 111:1541-1571, 2003.

Arditti JA: Rethinking relationships between divorced mothers and their children: Capitalizing on family strengths. Fam Relations Interdisciplinary J Appl Fam Stud 48:109-119, 1999.

Barber BL, Eccles JS: Long-term influence of divorce and single parenting on adolescent family- and work-related values, behaviors, and aspirations. Psychol Bull 111:118-126, 1992.

Booth A, Amato PR: Divorce and psychological stress. J Health Hum Behav 32:396-407, 1991.

Bramlett M, Mosher W: Cohabitation, Marriage, Divorce and Remarriage in the United States, series 22, no. 2. U.S. National Center for Health Statistics, Vital and Health Statistics, 2002. Available at: www.cdc.gov/nchs/data/series/sr_23/sr23_022.pdf.

Buehler C, Anthony C, Krishnakumar A, et al: Interparental conflict and youth problem behaviors: A meta-analysis. J Child Fam Stud 6:223-247, 1997.

Cherlin AJ, Furstenberg FF, Chase-Lansdale PL, et al: Longitudinal studies of effects of divorce on children in Great Britain and the United States. Science 252:1386-1389, 1991.

Clarke-Stewart KA, Vandell DL, McCartney K, et al: Effects of parental separation and divorce on very young children. J Fam Psychol 14:304-326, 2000.

Cohen GJ: Helping children and families deal with divorce and separation. AAP Committee on Psychosocial Aspects of Child and Family Health. Pediatrics 110:1019-1023, 2002.

Coleman WL: Family-Focused Behavioral Pediatrics. Philadelphia, Lippincott Williams & Wilkins, 2001, pp 224-233.

Coleman WL, Garfield C: Fathers and pediatricians: Enhancing men's roles in the care and development of their children. AAP Committee on Psychosocial Aspects of Child and Family Health. Pediatrics 113:1406-1411, 2004.

Emery RE, Forehand R: Parental divorce and children's well-being: A focus on resilience. *In* Haggerty RJ, Sherrod LR, Garmezy N, et al (eds): Stress, Risk, and Resilience in Children and Adolescents: Processes, Mechanisms and Interventions. New York, Cambridge University Press, 1994, pp 64-99.

Hetherington EM: Divorce and the adjustment of children. Pediatr Rev 26:163-169, 2005.

Hetherington EM, Henderson SH, Reiss D: Adolescent Siblings in Stepfamilies: Family Functioning and Adolescent Adjustment. Monographs of the Society for Research in Child Development Serial no. 259, Vol. 64, 1999.

Japel C, Tremblay RE, Vitaro F, et al: Early parental separation and the psychosocial development of daughters 6-9 years old. Am J Orthopsychiatry 69:49-60, 1999.

Johnston JR, Kline M, Tschann JM: Ongoing postdivorce conflict: Effects on children of joint custody and frequent access. Am J Orthopsychiatry 59:1-17, 1989.

Katz LF, Gottman JM: Buffering children from marital conflict and dissolution. J Clin Child Psychol 26:157-171, 1997.

Laumann-Billings L, Emery RE: Distress among young adults from divorced families. J Fam Psychol 14:671-687, 2000.

Lieberman AF: Van Horn P: Attachment, trauma, and domestic violence: Implications for child custody. Child Adolesc Psychiatr Clin North Am 7:423-444, 1998.

McCormick CB, Kennedy JH: Father-child separation, retrospective and current views of attachment relationship with father, and self-esteem in late adolescence. Psychol Rep 86:827-834, 2000.

Olson LM, Inkelas M, Halfon N, et al: The National Survey of Early Childhood Health: Overview of health supervision for young children: Reports from parents and pediatricians. Pediatrics 113(Suppl): 1907-1916, 2004.

Pagani L, Boulerice B, Tremblay RE, et al: Behavioral development in children of divorce and remarriage. J Child Psychol Psychiatry Allied Discipl 38:769-781, 1997.

Pawelski JG, Perrin EC, Foy JM, et al: The effects of marriage, civil union, and domestic partnership laws on the health and well-being of children. Pediatrics 118:349-364, 2006.

Pruett MK, Hoganbruen K: Joint custody and shared parenting. Child Adolesc Psychiatr Clin North Am 7:273-294, 1998.

Roseby V, Johnston J: Children of Armageddon: common developmental threats in high-conflict divorcing families. Child Adolesc Psychiatr Clin North Am 7:295-309, 1998.

Sammons WAH, Lewis J: Helping children survive divorce. Contemp Pediatr 18:103-114, 2001.

Sbarra DA, Emery RE: Coparenting conflict, nonacceptance, and depression among divorced adults: Results from a 12 year follow-up study of child custody mediation using multiple imputation. Am J Orthopsychiatry 75:63-75, 2005.

Tanner JL: Parental separation and divorce: Can we provide an ounce of prevention? AAP Committee on Psychosocial Aspects of Child and Family Health. Pediatrics 110:1007-1009, 2002.

Tein J-Y, Sandler IN, Zautra AJ: Stressful life events, psychological distress, coping and parenting of divorced mothers: a longitudinal study. J Fam Psychol 14:27-41, 2000.

Tschann JM, Johnston JR, Kline M, et al: Family process and children's functioning during divorce. J Marriage Fam 51:431-444, 1989.

U.S. Bureau of the Census: America's Families and Living Arrangements: 2005,Table C3. Living Arrangements of Children Under 18 Years and Marital Status of Parents. Available at: http://www.census.gov/population/socdemo/hh-fam/cps2005/tabC3-all.csv.

Wallerstein JS: Separation, divorce, and remarriage. *In* Levine MD, Carey WB, Crocker AC (eds): Developmental-Behavioral Pediatrics, 2nd ed. Philadelphia, WB Saunders, 1992, pp 149-161.

Wallerstein JS, Blakeslee S: What About the Kids?: Raising Your Children Before, During, and After Divorce. New York, Hyperion Books, 2003.

Wallerstein JS, Kelly JB: Surviving the Breakup: How Children and Parents Cope with Divorce. New York, Basic Books, 1980, pp 149-160.

Wallerstein JS, Lewis JM: The unexpected legacy of divorce: report of a 25 year study. Psychoanal Psychol 3:353-370, 2004.

Wallerstein JS, Resnikoff D: Parental divorce and developmental progression: an inquiry into their relationship. Int J Psychoanal 78(Pt 1):135-154, 1997.

Wells RD, Stein MS: Special families. *In*: Encounters with Children: Pediatric Behavior and Development, 4th ed. Philadelphia, Mosby/Elsevier, 2006, pp 628-635.

Wolchick SA, Wilcox KL, Tein J-Y, et al: Maternal acceptance and consistency of discipline as buffers of divorce stressors on children's psychological adjustment problems. J Abnormal Child Psychol 28:87-102, 2000.

RESOURCES FOR PARENTS

Kids' Turn. Available at: http://www.kidsturn.org/.

Stepfamily Association of America. Available at: www.saafamilies.org.

Wallerstein JS, Blakeslee S: What About the Kids?: Raising Your Children Before, During, and After Divorce. New York, Hyperion Books, 2003.

13 ADOPTION AND FOSTER FAMILY CARE

LAURIE C. MILLER

> "Our adopted daughter remains the sweet, kind-hearted, inquisitive person we met 9 years ago as a 5-year-old in Kazakhstan. She has struggled academically, but charms almost everyone she meets. Adults and children are drawn to her sweet, caring, and compassionate nature. She is a treasure and a wonderful example of how a person can survive and thrive despite hardships! Her dad and I have learned as much from her as she has from us! Over the last 2 months, she has become somewhat disrespectful to both of us parents, but I think it is the normal independence-seeking of teenagers."
>
> —The mother of a teenager adopted from Kazakhstan

Untold thousands of children throughout the world cannot be cared for by their birth parents, either permanently or temporarily. Parents may be neglectful or abusive, prompting authorities to remove children from parental custody. Parents may relinquish or abandon their children for reasons ranging from young age, poverty, substance abuse, mental or physical illness, or political constraints (e.g., the abandonment of infant girls in China). Parents may die, leaving their children as orphans (e.g., the 15 million children whose parents have died of AIDS).

In the United States, children who cannot be cared for by their families are placed with adoptive parents or in foster care. Some children are relinquished as newborns after careful adoption plans are made by their birth parents. Others are removed from neglectful or abusive homes and placed in foster care, where they may experience multiple placements. Some foster children eventually return to their birth families (reunification), others are adopted, and some enter long-term foster or residential care. Some children whose parents cannot care for them live with other relatives (kinship care), either under formal court sanctions or informally.

In other countries, children in need of out-of-family care usually reside in orphanages. Some of these children eventually are placed with adoptive families in their own countries or abroad (inter-country adoption). A few countries have well-developed foster care programs; sometimes this is available only to children for whom inter-country adoption is planned. Foster care and adoption greatly affect the child's health, emotional well-being, and social development. Physicians may assist families with many aspects of foster care and adoption (Table 13-1). This chapter reviews aspects of the health and development of foster and adopted children.

BIOLOGIC CONSEQUENCES OF EARLY NEGLECT

Many children who enter foster or adoptive families have had adverse experiences in early life. Prenatal exposures to drugs, alcohol, or other toxins may have long-term effects on child development and later brain function. Maternal stress or depression during pregnancy may impair the child's later emotional regulation. Inadequate care in early life may alter the child's stress responses, behavioral control, communication skills, emotional maturity, cognitive development, and physical growth. Abuse, neglect, and deprivation can hinder brain function and structural development (Chugani et al, 2001; Eluvathingal et al, 2006; Teicher et al, 2006), impair hypothalamic-pituitary-adrenal axis regulation of stress responses, and inhibit hormonal of emotional reactions control (oxytocin production and release) (Fries et al, 2005). Motor hyperactivity, anxiety, mood swings, impulsiveness, and sleep problems are common consequences of early child maltreatment. Children require a stable, loving, committed, protective family for optimal development. The child can "best overcome the stress of neglect and abuse if there is at least one adult who loves the child unconditionally and who is prepared to accept and value that child for a long time" (American Academy of Pediatrics Committee on Early Childhood and Adoption and Dependent Care, 2000).

ADOPTION

Adoption, the process by which a child legally joins a family, has always existed in human history. In the past 50 years in the United States, adoption has been transformed from a "shameful secret" to a widely recognized and accepted way to form a family. About one out of

Table 13-1. Role of the Physician Caring for Adopted and Foster Children

Learn about medical, emotional, and behavioral issues for adopted and foster children
Set up a preplacement visit with prospective parents to get acquainted and anticipate possible problem areas
Aid prospective adoptive or foster parents in review of child's medical dossier
Screen for and oversee care of specific health, emotional, and behavioral issues
Anticipatory guidance for "normative crises" throughout childhood and adolescence
Serve as knowledgeable source of information to parents and schools about the effects of adoption and foster care on child health and development
Aid adolescents with identity problems
Develop an appropriate network of community resources to assist in management of educational, emotional, and behavioral problems

Adapted from Nickman SL, Rosenfield AA, Fine P, et al: Children in adoptive families: Overview and update. J Am Acad Child Adolesc Psychiatry 44: 987-995, 2005.

six Americans has personal connections with adoption. Adoptive families are matter-of-factly featured in advertisements, television shows, and other media. Celebrities proudly introduce their newly adopted children. Pertman (2000), an adoption expert, wrote: "It's getting increasingly difficult to find a playground without at least one little girl from China, being watched lovingly by a white mother or father." Such changes coincide with large increases in the prevalence of adoption (especially international adoption); dramatic changes in adoption practices; and proliferation of information available on the Internet about waiting children, adoption issues, and related topics.

Because of these changes, virtually all U.S. pediatricians and family practitioners encounter adopted children in their practices. Adoption must be recognized as an important facet of health, emotional well-being, and psychological development for these children and their families. Health care professionals should be aware of the implications of adoption for these patients, understand the backgrounds of the children, and appreciate the experiences of adoptive parents.

Statistics, Types, and Terminology

Few quantitative data about domestic adoptions in the United States are tracked by official government agencies. The National Adoption Information Clearinghouse reported that 127,407 American children were adopted in the United States in 2001 (at least half by step-parents or relatives), and that about 2.5% (1,586,004) of all children younger than 18 years in the United States were adopted. The U.S. Census Bureau estimated that there are more than 2 million adopted individuals in the United States. These statistics do not reflect the many "quasi-adoption" situations that occur without specific legal sanction, such as grandparents caring for grandchildren and step-parents assuming responsibility for their partner's children, and they do not include adopted adults who have established their own households. In contrast, international adoptions are easily monitored through visas issued by the U.S. Citizenship and Immigration Services. These statistics show a 2.5-fold increase in the number of international adoptions in the past 10 years, with about 20,000 children from other countries joining U.S. families in 2007. Several other more recent trends in adoption also are notable (Table 13-2).

Table 13-2. Adoption Trends

Increased Numbers of
International adoptions
Transracial adoptions
Single parent adoptions
Gay or lesbian parent adoptions
Open adoptions
"Reunions" with birth relatives
Selection of adoptive parents by birth parents

Adapted from Nickman SL, Rosenfield AA, Fine P, et al: Children in adoptive families: Overview and update. J Am Acad Child Adolesc Psychiatry 44: 987-995, 2005.

There are many types of adoptions (Table 13-3), each with differing characteristics. Adoptions can be arranged by private or public agencies, private attorneys, or facilitators. Legal requirements vary among states. Domestic adoptions may be described as "closed," "open," or "semi-open," based on the amount of identifying information and contact shared between the birth family and adoptive family. International adoptions rarely (with the exception of Ethiopia) include any contact between the birth and adoptive families.

Adoption terminology has evolved to remove judgmental, hurtful, or archaic terms. The term "birth parents" is strongly preferred to "real," "natural," or "biologic" parents (with the connotations that the adoptive parents are "unreal" or "unnatural"). "International" or "intercountry" adoption is preferred to "foreign" adoption, with the connotation of distant or strange. The decision process is better described as "making an adoption plan" or "transferring parental rights," rather than "giving up" or "putting up" (recalling the orphan trains from 1850 through the 1920s where children were "put up" on platforms to be chosen or not chosen for adoption) (Adamec and Miller, 2006).

Process of Adoption for Families

Family preparation for adoption varies depending on the type of adoption pursued and legal requirements of the state of residence. Generally, prospective parents identify an adoption agency or facilitator who is responsible for placing the child. Parents undergo a "home study" to assess their suitability and readiness to adopt. Home studies conducted by licensed social workers address the prospective parent's motivation to adopt, personal histories, marital relationships, financial status, drug and alcohol use, child rearing philosophies, sexual orientation, physical and mental health, background criminal investigation, and other personal questions. The physical environment where the child would reside also is inspected. Parents also may be required to attend a series of preparatory educational classes. References from clergy, physicians, and other authorities may be required. The social worker prepares a detailed document, which recommends or disapproves the parents for adoption. Personal characteristics of the

Table 13-3. **Types of Adoptions**

Type of Adoption	Usual Scenario	Usual Time Frame	Typical Costs (Range)
Infant domestic adoption	*Agency:* Child assigned to prospective adoptive parents. Meeting and future contacts between adoptive and birth parents usually limited or none *Private:* Birth parents choose adoptive parents, sometimes with assistance of adoption facilitator (lawyer or other). Meetings and future contacts subject to personal preferences of all parties	≥1-2 yr	\$30,000-\$45,000
Adoption from foster care	Series of get-acquainted meetings between child and prospective parents, followed by placement. Ongoing relationship with birth relatives (or foster parents) may occur, sometimes legally mandated	Variable	Minimal
International adoption	Parents select agency with programs in desired country. Home study is forwarded to adoption officials in child's country, and eligible child matched. Parents travel to child's country, complete legal adoption there, assume custody of child. Child becomes American citizen on arrival in U.S.	8-15 mo	\$20,000-\$40,000

parents (e.g., age, marital status, religion, infertility) may determine which types of adoption can be pursued. State laws determine whether gay or lesbian individuals are permitted to adopt. Individuals who have undergone lengthy treatment for infertility may perceive the home study process as distressing and disheartening.

The process (and costs) vary considerably depending on the type of adoption. Most parents agree that the process is circuitous, laborious, and complex. Delays, frustrations, and uncertainty are commonplace. The process may take years longer than anticipated. For some parents, this process follows a lengthy and discouraging period of infertility treatment. International adoptions add the complexities of bureaucratic requirements of the U.S. Citizenship and Immigration Services, the child's country of origin, and international travel. Generally, children are adopted through the court system in their birth country, and then readopted in the United States.

Preadoptive Medical Evaluations

The offer of an individual child to prospective adoptive parents is known as the "referral." Increasingly, parents are seeking medical advice about the health and future well-being of the child from a pediatrician at the time they receive the referral. This preadoptive counseling often addresses issues such as risks of prenatal exposures to drugs or alcohol; lack of prenatal care; prematurity and low birth weight; and, for children placed after the newborn period, the potentially adverse effects of difficult early life experiences (e.g., abuse, neglect, multiple placements, institutionalizations). Lack of documentation of a problem should not be construed to mean the problem did not occur (e.g., prenatal exposure to alcohol). Evaluations are often conducted over the phone or via email. These conversations offer the pediatrician the opportunity to educate adopting parents about possible emotional, educational, and behavioral problems faced by some children after placement.

Incomplete medical histories are common for adopted children from abroad and children born in the United States. International adoption referrals usually include photographs; results of laboratory testing (likely outdated) for human immunodeficiency virus (HIV), hepatitis B, and syphilis; growth measurements; and (usually) cursory developmental and health reports. Chinese referrals lack any prenatal, birth, or family history; medical records routinely list all organ systems as "normal," and brief developmental reports bear little relationship to the child's actual skills. Limited maternal and only rare paternal information is available for children adopted from Russia, Kazakhstan, and other former Soviet Union countries. Alarming diagnoses, such as "perinatal encephalopathy," "hypertensive-hydrocephalic syndrome," or "spastic tetraparesis" appear regularly on these medical reports, although children have normal neurologic examinations when evaluated in the United States. Referrals from Ethiopia and Vietnam tend to provide brief reports of a single physical examination and laboratory test results; referrals from India and Philippines are more detailed and often include standardized developmental testing and social histories. Guatemalan referrals include a brief initial physical examination (usually the child is a newborn when the referral is made), followed by serial updates during the long waiting period for the adoption to be finalized. Detailed, carefully updated information is provided to parents adopting from South Korea, including social and medical histories of the birth parents.

More complete medical information is usually available for domestically adopted children. Birth parents are often young, however, and many health conditions may not yet be manifest. Mothers may not disclose information about substance abuse during pregnancy. Records of children adopted from foster care also may be incomplete (see later). Parents should make every effort to collect and record as much information as possible at the time of adoption; information becomes much more difficult to retrieve later.

Health of Children at Placement

Medical issues of the child at the time of adoption are specific to the prior life experiences of the individual. Children adopted as newborns do not share the medical and developmental risks of children who reside for prolonged periods in foster or institutional care

Table 13-4. Health Risks of Institutional and Inconsistent Foster Care

Exposure to infections
Emotional neglect
Poor nutrition/growth delays
Lack of medical care (including deficient immunizations)
Possible physical or sexual abuse
Delayed cognitive development
Toxic exposures (lead, radiation [e.g., Chernobyl])
Behavior problems
Attachment disorder

Data from Miller LC: Handbook of International Adoption Medicine. New York, Oxford University Press, 2005.

Table 13-5. Arrival Medical Evaluation for International Adoptees

Examination
Review of medical records (including vaccine records) from country of origin
Comprehensive physical examination
Hearing screen
Vision testing
Developmental assessment, with attention to gross and fine motor, personal-social, language, and cognitive milestones
Laboratory Testing
GENERAL HEALTH
Complete blood count
Lead level*
Urinalysis
Liver function tests
Thyroid function tests
Calcium, phosphorus
Ferritin
INFECTIOUS DISEASES
Hepatitis A IgM, IgG
Hepatitis B surface antigen, surface antibody, core antibody*
Hepatitis C antibody*
HIV ELISA (consider also PCR testing for infants <6 months old)*
Stool for ova and parasites, *Giardia* antigen
RPR (syphilis)
Tuberculin skin test (PPD)*
Vaccine titers to verify immunity for administered immunizations
ADDITIONAL TESTS TO CONSIDER BASED ON THE CLINICAL FINDINGS, COUNTRY OF ORIGIN, AND AGE OF THE CHILD
G6PD screen
H. pylori stool antigen
Stool cultures for bacterial pathogens
Newborn screen to State Board of Health (usually includes hemoglobin electrophoresis)
Malaria smear

*Repeat ≥6 months after arrival.
ELISA, enzyme-linked immunosorbent assay; HIV, human immunodeficiency virus; PCR, polymerase chain reaction; PPD, purified protein derivative; RPR, rapid plasma reagin.

(Table 13-4). Congenital or vertically transmitted infections may occur in any adopted child. Children adopted from other countries also may have infections that are unusual in U.S.-born children, including intestinal parasites (approximately 30% to 40% infected) and tuberculosis (5% to 10%). Other infections, such as congenital syphilis (1% to 2%), hepatitis B (3% to 5%), hepatitis C (1% to 2%), and HIV (<1%), are less common (Miller, 2005).

Table 13-6. Factors Contributing to Growth and Developmental Delays for Children with Difficult Early Life Experiences

Growth Delays
Insufficient food
Lack of nurturing physical contact
Illness
Improper feeding techniques
Developmental Delays
Swaddling
Lack of attention
Lack of stimulation and novelty
Long naps

Other medical risks related to international adoption include anemia (usually iron deficiency, but hemoglobinopathies also occur), lead poisoning (found most frequently in children arriving from China), and rickets (especially in children adopted from northern latitudes). Phenotypic changes suggesting prenatal exposure to alcohol were found among 58% of children residing in Russian orphanages (Miller et al, 2006); many children adopted from this region of the world also have these findings. Physical evidence suggesting prenatal exposure to alcohol may be found in children adopted from other countries as well. Many children arrive with deficient immunization records; the guidelines of the American Council on Immunization Practices address the management of these children. Newly arrived international adoptees benefit from detailed evaluation shortly after placement to identify potential health and development problems and to direct needed interventions (Table 13-5).

Growth delays are common in children who have lived in institutional care or other difficult circumstances in early life (Table 13-6). Growth measurements below the 5th percentile are found for height (approximately 45%), weight (35%), and head circumference (33%) of newly arrived international adoptees (Miller, 2005). Children with early deprivation also frequently have developmental delays. Motor delays are obvious because opportunities for physical exploration and play are limited. Delayed cognitive and language skills also reflect lack of nurturing care in early life. Social-emotional and self-care skills sometimes are preserved in some international adoptees because many orphanages encourage these abilities.

Immediate Behavioral Concerns after Adoption

Although parents spend considerable time and energy preparing for an adoption, children may have little or no opportunity to prepare for this major life transition. Although young infants superficially seem to adjust well to changes in caregivers, behavioral disturbances related to eating, sleeping, or bowel elimination are common. Older infants and toddlers may express fear and anxiety related to the transition by crying, tantrums, or withdrawal—often in combination. Self-comfort behaviors, such as rocking, thumb sucking, "hand staring," and ear or hair pulling, are frequent, but usually abate in the early weeks after placement. Many children grieve when leaving familiar caregivers and environments, even

Table 13-7. Challenges Faced by Some Adoptive Families

Unresolved feelings about infertility and adoption; diminished self-confidence as a parent
Attitudes toward adoption (celebration? secret?)
Uncertainties about the physical and psychosocial background of the child
Expectations of the child
Possible mismatches in temperament, interests, abilities
Reactions and acceptance of extended family
Delays in attachment
Misdirected support by professionals during family crises
Postadoption depression (Foli and Thompson, 2004)

if these were suboptimal situations. Age-appropriate preparation and explanations about adoption should be provided for any child old enough to understand. When possible, serial visits are helpful to prepare the child gradually for transition to a new family. Adjustments of internationally adopted children are complicated by the requirement of many countries for parents to make two or more visits often separated by several months.

Adoptive parents also must make the adjustment to their new family member. Parents should actively seek all possible facts about their child and his or her background at the time of placement and should write down information provided verbally. Despite all the planning and efforts, sometimes parents and children have difficulty adjusting to one another (Table 13-7). Attachment is rarely "instantaneous," but must build over time as parents care for children, and children come to trust in the security of their new homes. Although reactive attachment disorder occurs in some adopted children, most attach well to their new families. In some children, however, the attachment is "insecure" or "anxious." Inquiries about attachment are usually welcomed by adoptive parents, who otherwise may be reluctant to mention this as an area of concern. Likewise, postadoption depression is being recognized with increasing frequency; inquiries from physicians about whether "the adoption is everything you hoped for" may offer new adoptive parents the opportunity to express concerns about their own adjustment.

Health Outcomes of Adopted Children

Recovery of growth and developmental delays is frequently striking and rapid after adoptive placement in children who have been institutionalized (Fig. 13-1). Within 3 to 4 months, young malnourished children have often achieved normal growth. Many children with microcephaly at adoptive placement attain normal head circumference measurements. Developmental delays also improve dramatically within a short time; most investigators agree that younger children tend to improve more quickly than children who are older at placement. Less is known about the long-term health effects of early physical and emotional deprivation, although evidence suggests that children with this history may be more susceptible to medical (coronary artery disease, type 2 diabetes, hypertension) and behavioral (schizophrenia, cognitive dysfunction) difficulties as they age.

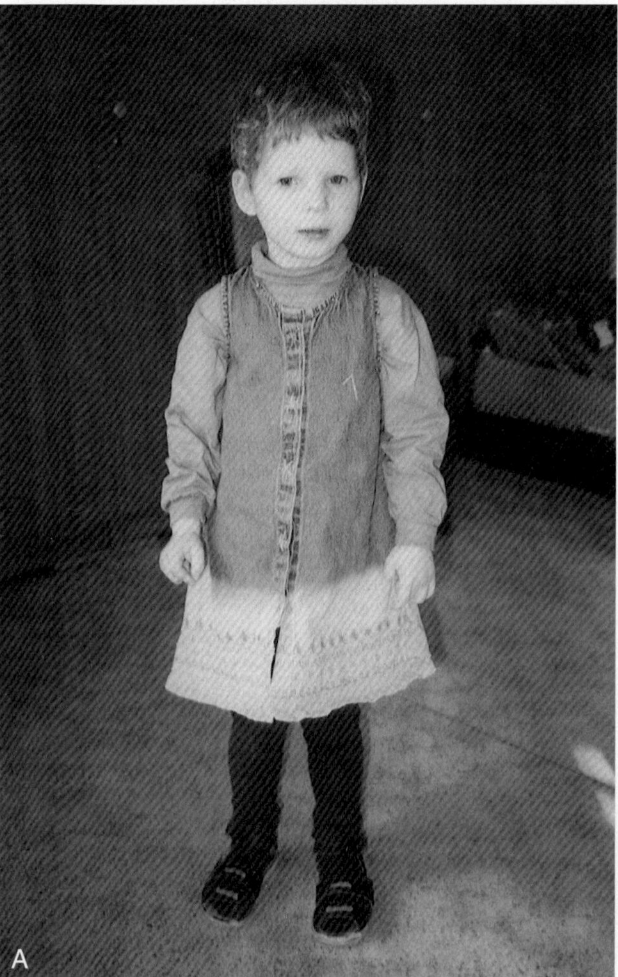

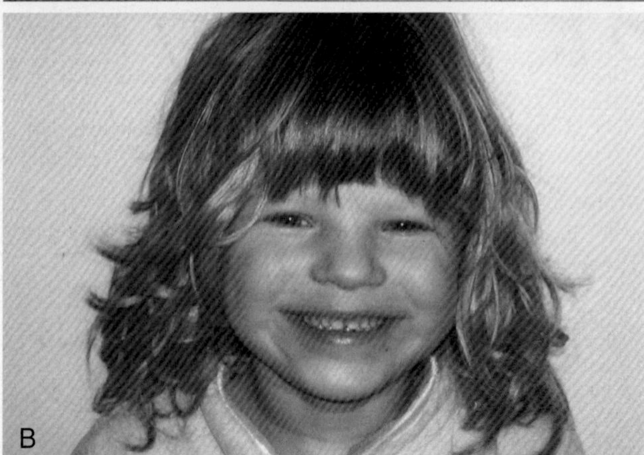

Figure 13-1. **A,** A child in a Russian orphanage, shortly before adoption, age 4.5 years. **B,** The same child after adoption, age 5.5 years.

School Problems

Numerous studies show that school problems, such as attention-deficit/hyperactivity disorder and learning disabilities, are more common in adopted children, likely reflecting genetic susceptibility, adverse prenatal exposures, and early environmental deprivation. A meta-analysis of the cognitive development of 17,767 adopted children found, however, that they scored higher on IQ tests and did better on school performance than children who remained in institutional care or with birth families. The adopted children's IQs did not differ from their nonadopted siblings and peers, although they had more learning problems, and delayed school performance and language ability (van Ijzendoorn et al, 2005). School problems may be overrepresented among internationally adopted children. A survey of children adopted from Eastern Europe found attention problems in 38%, learning disabilities in 36%, and multiple neurodevelopmental diagnoses in 35% (Tirella et al, 2006); parent demand for educational testing and remediation is likely higher in these families, possibly inflating the rates of these problems. Children adopted internationally by Dutch and Scandinavian families of higher socioeconomic backgrounds had more school-related problems than children adopted by parents of lower socioeconomic status, possibly because of unrealistic expectations and pressure from the higher socioeconomic families.

Behavior Problems and Mental Health Disorders

Research indicates that adopted children have more mental health problems than their nonadopted peers, although most adoptees are normal. For domestically adopted children, some researchers suggest that such mental health problems are about twice as common as the general population. Possible explanations include genetic susceptibility, the stress of separation from birth parents (and, in many cases, from other caregivers as well), the adoption itself, and various factors within the adoptive home. Some researchers speculate that adoptees may have an increased prevalence of genes for impulsive behaviors or mental health disorders, possibly inherited from both parents owing to assortative mating. Mental health statistics may be "boosted" in other ways as well: Adoptive parents may be more likely to seek professional guidance for their children, and it is plausible that professionals are more likely to "flag" an adopted child as having a mental health or behavior problem. Adoption experts note that health care professionals may not recognize "normative crises" in adoptive families, and that their lack of understanding can significantly disrupt the family bonds (Nickman and Lewis, 1994; Pavao, 1998).

A meta-analysis verified that internationally adopted children were referred for mental health services more often than nonadopted controls (Juffer and van Ijzendoorn, 2005), but international adoptees had fewer behavior problems and mental health referrals than domestically adopted children. A comprehensive follow-up study on mental health disorders (11,320 internationally adopted teens and young adults in Sweden) found that 85% of the boys and 92% of the girls had good social adjustment and no behavioral or mental health disorders (Hjern et al, 2002). Some problems may appear in later life, however (Stams et al, 2000).

Mental health problems in adopted children include internalizing disorders (anxiety and depression), externalizing disorders (attention disorders, conduct disorders, delinquency, aggressive and self-injurious behavior), and post-traumatic stress disorder. Unrecognized and untreated, these problems may cause lifelong disabilities. A subgroup of adopted children have severe neuropsychiatric problems; many of these children experienced extreme deprivation before adoption. Sadly, many of these adoptions have disrupted (i.e., ended). Some of these children have been placed in residential psychiatric treatment. Some adoptees, now older teens or young adults, enter the criminal justice system. These situations are among the most painful of all adoption stories; the precise extent of these problems is unknown.

Numerous studies address the outcome of adults who were adopted as children (Adamec and Miller, 2006). Most seem to be psychologically well adjusted; in one study, adults adopted as infants were more confident and viewed others more positively than nonadopted peers. In another study of adopted adults in Britain, 80% of interviewees reported "very" or "reasonably" satisfactory adoption experiences, and 70% had excellent or good adjustment. Outcomes are particularly favorable compared with children who are institutionalized or returned to dysfunctional birth families (Nickman et al, 2005). Likewise, most adoptive families report high levels of satisfaction with their adopted child.

Transracial Adoption and Cultural Identity

Transracial adoptions are increasing in frequency. More than 60% of international adoptions are transracial; the number is increasing as more children from China are adopted by white U.S. families (approximately 8000 in 2005). The adjustment and development of identity of these children likely encompasses different tasks and timelines than for children who racially match their parents. Nearly all international adoptions are transcultural. Adoption experts recommend that families embrace their new multiculturalism, celebrating the food, holidays, dress, and customs of their child's birth country. Homeland trips and language and dance lessons are now common activities for many families who have adopted internationally. Transracial adoption of American children also is gaining wider acceptance and increasing in numbers. Families are advised to acknowledge and celebrate their child's heritage to promote healthy identity formation.

Telling Children about Adoption

Adoption experts now concur that adoptive status and information should be disclosed early to children so that they never recollect time when they did not know this information. Although young children are unable to fathom the meaning of adoption, it is nonetheless important to introduce adoption vocabulary at an early age, and to reinforce concepts in an age-appropriate manner as children grow.

Some children are born as a result of artificial insemination or surrogacy; these children are raised by one biologically related and one unrelated parent. These families share some challenges with adoptive families, including facing public discussion of resemblances. Similar to adoptive families, parents who use gamete donors must emotionally reconcile their differences in biologic relatedness to the child, develop strategies for public and private disclosure of the child's heritage, and resolve lingering doubts about their psychological entitlement to the child. Despite the increasing ubiquity of families who use gamete donors, there is little research into these psychological issues for children and their parents.

Searching for Birth Parents

Some children who grow up in "closed adoptions" choose to search for their birth parents. Usually, states do not provide identifying information until the adopted individual is older than age 18. Numerous websites and organizations offer to assist in searches; some specialize in overseas searches (e.g., Russia, Romania). A more recent study found "... no evidence that the desire to search or searching behavior is the result of poor adoptive family relationships or adolescent maladjustments" (Miller Wrobel et al, 2004). Many adopted individuals cite curiosity or desire for family medical information (or, less commonly, occupations or interests) as the main impetus for their search; however, for others, the desire to search derives from dissatisfaction with their adoptive situations. Children provided with more information are generally less likely to wish to search for their birth parents.

FOSTER CARE

Demographics

In the United States on any given day, more than 500,000 children are residing in foster care. Over the course of a year, more than 800,000 children experience foster care. The average age of children in foster care is 10.2 years, with almost 50% between ages 6 and 15 years. About one third of children are in foster care for 30 months or longer; more than 10% reside in foster care for more than 5 years. Nearly half of these children live in nonrelative foster families, about one fourth live in kinship care (under control of the judicial system), and the remainder live in residential care or other settings.

Foster children in the United States undoubtedly have the "greatest combined needs of any group of children in our society" (Jee and Simms, 2006). These children "fare poorly despite large numbers of adults involved in their care, including biologic and foster parents, social workers, child advocates, lawyers and guardians ad litem, judges, teachers, and physicians" (Jee and Simms, 2006). It is no exaggeration to characterize the health care of foster children as "fragmented and crisis-oriented" (Jee and Simms, 2006).

The goal of foster care placement is usually to reunite biologic families, unless horrific abuse or neglect has occurred. After removal of children from the home, parents are given specific goals to meet, such as rehabilitation for substance abuse, obtaining employment, or attending parenting classes. Children usually are returned to their parents if these goals are met, although state supervision may continue. The Adoption and Safe Families Act of 1997 mandates that parental rights may be terminated if children have been in foster care for 15 out of the past 22 months, allowing the possibility of adoptive placement of the child. More recent research suggests that family reunification is not always in the best interest of the child, and that more rapid progression to adoption may serve the child's needs better.

Immediate Behavioral Concerns Related to Transition

Foster care placement usually occurs in a crisis situation. The sudden removal of children from their homes and placement in an unfamiliar environment with little preparation is often highly traumatic. At the time of removal, children may have experienced repeated abuse, emotional traumas, or prolonged neglect, and be in pain or distress from recent abuse or untreated medical conditions (Kerker and Dore, 2006; Simms et al, 2000). Such problems impede the child's ability to adjust emotionally to the new situation. Children often experience fear, guilt, and a sense of being punished. Although children may superficially seem to adapt well at first, within weeks or a few months they may display intense anger or depression. Atypical patterns of cortisol (stress hormone) production have been found in children living in foster care (Dozier et al, 2006).

Health Issues of Children in Foster Care

Children in foster care have increased prevalence of medical, mental health, and developmental problems. Most enter foster care in poor health because of poverty, poor prenatal care, prenatal infection, maternal substance abuse prenatally, family and neighborhood violence, or parental mental illness. Several surveys suggest that physical health problems are found in 87% to 95% of foster care children (Chernoff et al, 1994; Leslie et al, 2005; Simms et al, 2000), whereas developmental delays are found in 13% to 62% (compared with 4% to 10% of community controls). Mental health problems are even more prevalent, found in 48% to 80% of foster children (compared with 10% of community controls).

In a survey of 2419 children entering foster care in Baltimore, 92% had at least one abnormality on physical examination, 23% failed developmental screening, and 22% of school-age children were receiving special education services. In a large survey of young children (3 months to 6 years) entering foster care in San Diego, nearly 88% had physical, developmental, or mental health needs; more than 50% had two or more problems; and more than one third failed developmental testing. The medical and developmental problems of foster children exceed those of age-matched and gender-matched, Medicaid-eligible children living with their parents. The prevalence of fetal alcohol syndrome among children in foster care is approximately 10 to 15 per 1000, 10 to 15 times greater than in the general population (Astley et al, 2002). In addition, elevated blood lead levels are twice as likely in children entering foster care as their siblings (Chung et al, 2001).

Health assessment of children at the time of entry into care is often cursory and incomplete. A national survey of health units performing evaluations of children entering out of home care found that 94% addressed physical health, but only 58% assessed development, and 48% assessed mental health (Leslie et al, 2003). A survey of health care needs of foster children conducted by the U.S. General Accounting Office indicated that nearly one third of children had received no immunizations; one third had unmet identified health care needs; 12% had not received routine health care services; and only 9% had been tested

Table 13-8. Recommended Screening for Children Entering Foster Care

Review of all prior medical records
Physical examination with attention to signs of neglect or abuse and assessment of risk of prenatal alcohol exposure
Developmental assessment
Mental heath screen (e.g., Ages and Stages Questionnaire if <4 yr, Pediatric Symptom Checklist if >4 yr) (completed by foster parents)
Laboratory testing
Complete blood count
Lead
Sickle screen (as appropriate)
Hepatitis B
Hepatitis C
HIV
Tuberculosis (PPD)
Laboratory testing for adolescents or if suspected sexual abuse
RPR (syphilis)
Chlamydia
Gonorrhea
Vision and hearing screening
Referrals to Early Intervention (0-3 yr), dentists (>3 yr), other specialists (as needed)

HIV, human immunodeficiency virus; PPD, purified protein derivative.
Adapted from Sagor LD, Forkey H, Brooks S: FaCES (Foster Children Evaluation Services): A collaborative program to improve medical screening for children in foster care. Paper presented at the American Academy of Pediatrics, Atlanta, GA, October 9, 2006.

for HIV, although 78% were considered to be at risk (Simms et al, 2000). Several states have developed models that provide foster children with a "medical home." Current recommendations suggests that broad screening of children at entry into foster care can identify problems and needed treatments (Table 13-8); some experts recommend an initial screening visit within 7 days of placement, followed by a more comprehensive assessment within 30 days of placement (Sagor et al, 2006).

Emotional Problems

Children entering foster care have a high level of serious mental health problems—80% compared with 16% to 22% among children living with their parents (Kerker and Dore, 2006). Externalizing disorders (attention disorders, conduct disorders, delinquency, aggressive and self-injurious behavior) are most common, but depression and anxiety also occur. In one survey, 15% of children were suicidal, and 7% had homicidal ideation (Chernoff et al, 1994). The trauma of separation from the family undoubtedly contributes to the prevalence of mental health problems: It is difficult to differentiate mental health problems that precede foster placement from problems that result from placement.

Many children in foster care receive psychotropic medications. Most experts agree, however, that foster care children are probably undertreated and undermedicated for their mental health problems (Kerker and Dore, 2006; Simms et al, 2000). There are numerous barriers to care of children with these issues, including cost, unstable placements, and missing mental health histories.

Overall, the complex medical needs of children in foster care are frequently neglected, usually because of difficulties accessing health services. Care is often fragmented, as children move between placements, and medical records are unavailable to new providers. This situation may have serious health consequences for the child. Many foster children receive the bulk of their ambulatory care in emergency departments.

Foster Care Disruption

A serious difficulty for children in foster care is disruption of the placement. This is a common event in the lives of children consigned to foster care (Table 13-9). Behavior problems of the child account for few disruptions—only about 20% in a survey of 580 children, with 70% of disruptions resulting from system or policy changes (James, 2004). In an effort to predict disruption caused by child behavior problems, Chamberlain and colleagues (2006) supplied 246 foster parents with a "Parent Daily Report Checklist." Parents reported an average of 5.77 child problems a day. If child problems per day exceeded 6, the likelihood of disruption during the upcoming year increased significantly (Chamberlain et al, 2006). Other researchers found, however, that caseworkers' reports of child behavior problems better predicted placement disruption than parent reports. Overall, disrupted foster care is associated with many difficulties for the child, including diminished self-esteem, school problems, emotional disturbances, attachment problems, social adjustment difficulties, and delayed cognitive development.

Outcomes of Children in Foster Care

Foster care greatly benefits some children and is more beneficial for children than institutional care (Zeanah et al, 2003). In one study, foster care children did not differ from matched family children in their sense of well-being, self-esteem, or incidence of depression or behavior problems (Farruggia et al, 2006). Foster children had higher levels of work orientation, although lower levels of academic achievement. Factors cited that promote favorable outcomes of foster children include education, future orientation, family support, peer influence, and religion (Edmond et al, 2006). Despite the multiple health problems identified in many children entering foster care, medical and developmental status frequently improve after removal from a neglectful environment. Recovery of height is often notable.

Many foster children eventually are reunified with their parents. The outcomes of 149 reunified children were compared with the outcomes of children who remained in foster care (Taussig et al, 2001). The reunified children showed more self-destructive behaviors, substance use, internalizing behaviors, and total behavior problems, and lower total competence than the children who remained in foster care. The reunified youth also were more likely to have received a ticket or been arrested, to have dropped out of school, and to have lower grades. Reunification status significantly predicted many negative outcomes. Other studies suggest that foster care placement, rather than remaining with family members, after child maltreatment increases the likelihood of child behavior problems. Variables including the severity of family problems and availability of external resources may have differed among these and similar studies.

Some children are adopted from foster care. Factors reducing the likelihood of adoptive placement of foster

Table 13-9. **Child and Family Services Review National Data Indicators**

	Range	Median
Protection from Abuse and Neglect		
Abused children who were *not* victims of other substantiated or indicated maltreatment within 6 mo (%)	86-98	93.3
Timeliness of Reunification with Family (of Children Discharged from Foster Care to Reunification)		
Children in <12 mo (%)	44.3-92.5	69.9
Median length of stay in foster care (mo)	1.1-13.7	6.5
Children in foster care for the first time *who were discharged to reunification* in <12 mo (%)	17.7-68.9	39.4
Children who re-entered care within <12 mo (%)	1.6-29.8	15
Timeliness of Adoptions		
CHILDREN DISCHARGED FROM FOSTER CARE TO FINALIZED ADOPTION		
Discharged in <24 mo (%)	6.4-74.9	26.8
Median length of stay in foster care (mo)	16.2-55.7	32.4
CHILDREN LEGALLY FREE FOR ADOPTION		
Discharged to finalized adoption in <12 mo (%)	20-100	45.8
Stability of Placements		
CHILDREN WITH ≤2 PLACEMENTS		
In foster care <12 mo (%)	55-99.6	83.3
In foster care 12-24 mo (%)	27-99.8	59.9
In foster care >24 mo (%)	13.7-98.9	33.9

(Adapted from U.S. Department of Health and Human Services, Administration for Family and Children. Children's Bureau, Child and Family Services Reviews, Summary of Key Findings, Fiscal Years 2003 and 2004. September 23, 2004. Available at: www.acf.hhs.gov/programs/cb/cwmonitoring/results/keyfindings2003.pdf. Accessed September 19, 2008.

children include prior physical or sexual abuse, neglect, multiple foster care placements, severe behavioral problems, and older age at entry into foster care.

When studied as adults, former foster children have complicated outcomes. A Swedish study comparing more than 22,000 former foster children with their age-matched peers found that the former group had fourfold to fivefold higher risk of hospitalizations for suicide attempts, five to eight times more likely risk of psychiatric disorders, and excess risks for psychosis and depression (Vinnerljung et al, 2006). Children in long-term foster care fared worst. Prior foster care residence is associated with high-risk sexual behavior (Carpenter et al, 2001), incarceration (27% of males, 10% of females) (Jee and Simms, 2006), and disproportionately high rates of mental illness at age 17 years (McMillen et al, 2005). An outcome study of 659 former foster children found that 20% were doing well as adults, but 54% had one or more mental health problems (depression, post-traumatic stress disorder, anxiety, drug addition), 22% had experienced homelessness, and only 2% had graduated from college. Employment rate also was lower in the former foster children (80% versus 95%), and about 30% were living at or below the poverty level (Pecora, 2005).

SUMMARY

Children in the United States who cannot be cared for by their parents are placed in adoptive or foster families (or both). In other countries, children needing care often are consigned to orphanages. Many of these children have difficult experiences in early life, including neglect and abuse, health problems, and developmental delays. These traumatic experiences may increase the risk of behavioral and mental health disorders. Many children display remarkable resilience, however. Notable trends include increases in the number of international adoptions, adoptions by gay or lesbian or single parents, and transracial adoptions. Efforts to improve health monitoring and rapid resolution of legal quandaries of children in foster care need to expand; facilitation of adoption processes would benefit children in need of care. Medical practitioners can assist foster and adoptive families and the children in these placements by offering comprehensive, focused health care, anticipatory guidance related to potential problems, and emotional support.

REFERENCES

Adamec C, Miller LC: Encyclopedia of Adoption. New York, Facts on File, Inc, 2006.

American Academy of Pediatrics Committee on Early Childhood and Adoption and Dependent Care: Developmental issues for young children in foster care. Pediatrics 106:1145-1150, 2000.

Astley SJ, Stachowiak J, Clarren SK, Clausen C: Application of the fetal alcohol syndrome facial photographic screening tool in a foster care populations. J Pediatr 141:712-717, 2002.

Carpenter SC, Clyman RB, Davidson AJ, Steiner JF: The association of foster care or kinship care with adolescent sexual behavior and first pregnancy. Pediatrics 108:e46, 2001.

Chamberlain P, Price JM, Reid JB, et al: Who disrupts from placement in foster and kinship care? Child Abuse Negl 30:409-424, 2006.

Chernoff R, Combs-Orme T, Risley-Curtiss C: Assessing the health status of children entering foster care. Pediatrics 93:594-601, 1994.

Chugani HT, Behen ME, Muzik O, et al: Local brain functional activity following early deprivation: A study of postinstitutionalized Romanian orphans. Neuroimage 14:1290-1301, 2001.

Chung EK, Webb D, Clampet-Lundquist S, Campbell C: A comparison of elevated blood lead levels among children living in foster care, their siblings, and the general population. Pediatrics 107:e81, 2001.

Dozier M, Manni M, Gordon MK, et al: Foster children's diurnal production of cortisol: An exploratory study. Child Maltreat 11:189-197, 2006.

Edmond T, Auslander W, Elze D, Bowland S: Signs of resilience in sexually abused adolescent girls in the foster care system. J Child Sex Abus 15:1-28, 2006.

Eluvathingal TJ, Chugani HT, Behen ME, et al: Abnormal brain connectivity in children after early severe socioemotional deprivation: A diffusion tensor imaging study. Pediatrics 117:2093-2100, 2006.

Farruggia SP, Greenberger E, Chen C, Heckhausen J: Perceived social environment and adolescents' well-being and adjustment: Comparing a foster care sample with a matched sample. J Youth Adolesc 35:330-339, 2006.

Foli KJ, Thompson JR: The Post-Adoption Blues. Emmaus, PA, Rodale, 2004.

Fries AB, Ziegler TE, Kurian JR, et al: Early experience in humans is associated with changes in neuropeptides critical for regulating social behavior. Proc Natl Acad Sci U S A 102:17237-17240, 2005.

Hjern A, Lindblad F, Vinnerljung B: Suicide, psychiatric illness, and social maladjustment in intercountry adoptees in Sweden: A cohort study. Lancet 360:443-448, 2002.

James S: Why do foster care placements disrupt? Soc Serv Rev 78:601-627, 2004.

Jee SH, Simms MD: Health and well-being of children in foster care placement. Pediatr Rev 27:34-36, 2006.

Juffer F, van IJzendoorn MH: Behavior problems and mental health referrals of international adoptees: A meta-analytic approach. JAMA 293:2501-2515, 2005.

Kerker BD, Dore MM: Mental health needs and treatment of foster youth: Barriers and opportunities. Am J Orthopsychiatry 76:138-147, 2006.

Leslie LK, Gordon JN, Meneken L, et al: The physical, developmental, and mental health needs of young children in child welfare by initial placement type. J Dev Behav Pediatr 26:177-185, 2005.

Leslie LK, Hurlburt MS, Landsverk J, et al: Comprehensive assessments for children entering foster care: A national perspective. Pediatrics 112(1 Pt 1):134-142, 2003.

McMillen JC, Zima BT, Scott LD, et al: Prevalence of psychiatric disorders among older youths in the foster care system. J Am Acad Child Adolesc Psychiatry 44:88-95, 2005.

Miller LC: Handbook of International Adoption Medicine. New York, Oxford University Press, 2005.

Miller LC, Chan W, Litvinova A, et al: Boston-Murmansk Orphanage Research Team: Fetal alcohol spectrum disorders in children residing in Russian orphanages: A phenotypic survey. Alcohol Clin Exp Res 30:531-538, 2006.

Miller Wrobel G, Grotevant HD, McCoy RG: Adolescent search for birthparents: Who moves forward?. J Adolesc Res 19:132-151, 2004.

Nickman SL, Lewis RG: Adoptive families and professionals: When the experts make things worse. J Am Acad Child Adolesc Psychiatry 33:753-755, 1994.

Nickman SL, Rosenfield AA, Fine P, et al: Children in adoptive families: Overview and update. J Am Acad Child Adolesc Psychiatry 44:987-995, 2005.

Pavao JM: The Family of Adoption. Boston, Beacon Press, 1998.

Pecora PJ: Improving Family Foster Care: Findings from the Northwest Foster Care Alumni Study. Seattle, Casey Family Services, 2005.

Pertman A: Adoption Nation: How the Adoption Revolution Is Transforming America. New York, Basic Books, 2000.

Sagor LD, Forkey H, Brooks S: FaCES (Foster Children Evaluation Services): A collaborative program to improve medical screening for children in foster care. Paper presented at the American Academy of Pediatrics, Atlanta, GA, October 9, 2006.

Simms MD, Dubowitz H, Szilagyi MA: Health care needs of children in the foster care system. Pediatrics 106(4 Suppl):909-918, 2000.

Stams G-JJM, Juffer F, Rispens J, Hoksbergen RAC: The development and adjustment of 7-year-old children adopted in infancy. J Child Psychol Psychiatry 41:1025-1037, 2000.

Taussig HN, Clyman RB, Landsverk J: Children who return home from foster care: A 6-year prospective study of behavioral health outcomes in adolescence. Pediatrics 108:e10, 2001.

Teicher MH, Tomoda A, Andersen SL: Neurobiological consequences of early stress and childhood maltreatment: Are results from human and animal studies comparable? Ann N Y Acad Sci 1071:313-323, 2006.

Tirella LG, Chan W, Miller LC: Educational outcomes of post-institutionalized children adopted from Eastern Europe. J Res Child Educ 20:245-254, 2006.

van IJzendoorn MH, Juffer F, Poelhuis CW: Adoption and cognitive development: A meta-analytic comparison of adopted and nonadopted children's IQ and school performance. Psychol Bull 131:301-316, 2005.

Vinnerljung B, Hjern A, Lindblad F: Suicide attempts and severe psychiatric morbidity among former child welfare clients—a national cohort study. J Child Psychol Psychiatry 47:723-733, 2006.

Zeanah CH, Nelson CA, Fox NA, et al: Designing research to study the effects of institutionalization on brain and behavioral development: The Bucharest Early Intervention Project. Dev Psychopathol 15:885-907, 2003.

RECOMMENDED BOOKS FOR PARENTS

Brodzinsky DM, Schechter MD, Henig RM: Being Adopted: The Lifelong Search for Self. New York, Anchor Books, 1993.

Eldridge S: Twenty Things Adopted Kids Wish Their Adoptive Parents Knew. New York, Dell, 1999.

Pavao JM: The Family of Adoption. Boston, Beacon Press, 1998.

Pertman A: Adoption Nation: How the Adoption Revolution Is Transforming America. New York, Basic Books, 2000.

RECOMMENDED BOOKS FOR CHILDREN

Curtis JL: Tell Me Again About the Night I Was Born. New York, Harper Collins, 1996.

Koehler P: The Day We Met You. New York, Simon & Schuster, 1990.

Krementz J: How It Feels to Be Adopted. New York, Alfred A. Knopf, 2001.

Lewis R: I Love You Like Crazy Cakes. New York, Little, Brown, 2000.

14 CRITICAL FAMILY EVENTS

William I. Cohen (1947-2009)

Vignette

"The only constant is change"
—Heraclitus

Four-year-old Rebecca could not wait for her baby brother to arrive. She had helped her parents decorate the nursery, and she chose three of her favorite books and one stuffed animal to welcome him home. She became confused and frightened after he was born and had to stay in the hospital. Her parents would spend all day there, and although she loved being with her grandma and grandpa, they would sometimes whisper to each other after her parents called from the hospital. She began having trouble falling asleep, and she lost her appetite. Her brother was born with pulmonary hypertension and needed intensive treatment, including extracorporeal membrane oxygenation. It took quite a few days before her parents were able to explain what was happening, and it took quite a bit longer for Rebecca to get back on track after this episode.

Families are dynamic units that seek, absorb, and manage changes, such as additions and losses, to continue to nurture the individual members. Families function via the development of equilibrium or homeostasis. Any change destabilizes that balance. A delay in the establishment of a new balance point signals the need for thoughtful and careful intervention, starting with an assessment of the family's strengths and weaknesses. Some changes are normative (sometimes referred to as "on-time"), such as the birth of a child or the death of elderly, infirm grandparents. These changes can be anticipated, and appropriate preparations can be undertaken. Other changes, such as acute illness, disabling injury, or the death of a sibling or the early death of a parent or grandparent, can cause major disruption. Nevertheless, we should never take for granted that a normative change will go smoothly, or that a non-normative one will have devastating, long-lasting consequences. The particular structure and function of a given family, including its supportive social network and the personal resources of the individual members, is the best predictor of ultimate outcome.

The scope of these issues has been described in depth by Shonkoff and colleagues (1987). This discussion focuses on the addition of and the loss of a family member (Table 14-1). The addition of new family members most often occurs with the birth of a sibling, but includes the arrival emotionally or physically of parental partners or spouses (step-parents), grandparents, or other family members who join the household for economic or health reasons. The most significant loss a child experiences, that of a parent through separation and divorce, is discussed in Chapter 12. The other losses a child may experience include death of a brother or sister, parent, or grandparent. Additionally, the change in a family member's role because of illness or disability can have a significant impact on a child. The loss of community that occurs when a family moves as a result of the change in economic status related to divorce or loss of income from a parent who becomes disabled can be an additional source of difficulty for a child, as he or she leaves home, friends, and school.

A variety of modifying factors may magnify or diminish the impact of an event on a given child. As in all areas of development and behavior, the child's temperament plays an important role in the effect of the change. Often described as behavioral style, this qualitative description, along nine dimensions, helps explain the "how" of the child's behavior, rather than the "what." Appreciating these intrinsic factors provides a frame of reference that allows physicians to interpret behavioral difficulties as a reflection of individual differences and the "goodness of fit" between the parents and other caregivers and the child (Carey and McDevitt, 1995). In addition to the emotional resources of the parents, the cognitive abilities of the child affect how he or she experiences the changes. The lack of sufficient economic resources to address adequate housing and food provides another significant mitigating factor.

The other part of the "goodness of fit" equation is provided by the functional status of the family before the event. Optimally functioning families are structured with a clear hierarchy between the generations: The parental generation (partners or spouses) works well as

Table 14-1. Critical Family Events

Additions
CHILD
Birth of a brother or sister
Healthy
Medical problems
Developmental disabilities
Foster care
Adoption
Step-brothers and step-sisters
ADULT
Grandparent or other family member
Parental partner/spouse
Same-sex partner
Return from separation of parent/partner
Return of parent/partner from employment, military service, or incarceration
Losses
Death of brother or sister
Death of parent
Death of grandparent
Loss of parent/partner
Separation or divorce
Temporary loss of parent/partner
Move for employment
Military service
Incarceration
Loss of function (and attendant role) of family member
Acute or chronic illness
Injury

Table 14-2. Childhood Manifestations Related to Critical Life Events

Internalizing Symptoms
Withdrawal
Sadness
Sleep difficulties
Sleep initiation
Nighttime awakening
Nightmares
Appetite disturbances
Anxiety symptoms
Excessive worries
Externalizing Symptoms
Aggression
Anger
Defiance/noncompliance
Developmental Arrest/Regression
Self-care
Feeding
Toileting
Poor School Performance
Inattentiveness
Lack of motivation
Self-Medication
Alcohol
Prescription drugs
Illicit drugs

a team, with effective communication and robust problem solving. There are no cross-generational coalitions, such as a father-daughter alliance, which would short-circuit a more appropriate relationship between the spouses. Rules are clearly understood, and boundaries are clearly defined. Violations of the boundaries are quickly commented on and rectified. Another factor that supports optimal family functioning is support from the extended family and kinship networks.

An important ingredient that supports optimal family functioning is a rule that allows and encourages open communication about the wants and needs of each partner. In such an environment, each partner can report on his or her physical and emotional needs and expect to be listened to openly and generously. Statements of one's needs are offered in a manner that maximizes the likelihood that they will be accepted. In any given situation, it would be expected that such a couple would have the ability to respond to any untoward effect of a change in the structure of the family or the function of family members as soon as the negative effects of the change were recognized. Couples who do not have these skills, who are struggling with unfinished issues from their own childhood (e.g., blame, guilt, shame, sense of overresponsibility or underresponsibility) would be less likely to be able to activate the family's own resources and external resources from the community (Walsh, 2003).

Before discussing specific examples of critical events, their impact on children, and suggestions for management, a description of the family life cycle completes the framework of the underlying principles needed to help these children and their families. The *family life cycle* describes the progression of a couple through dating, marriage/committed relationship, birth of children, raising children, children leaving home, and re-establishment of the couple in the empty nest. Each of these changes in the structure of the family entails a change in roles for the family member. In becoming a couple, the individuals must cede some of their autonomy for the good of the partnership. Difficulties in family functioning frequently coincide with shifts from one stage to the next in the family life cycle (Carter and McGoldrick, 1988).

The adverse effects of these critical family events are associated with various behavioral manifestations (Table 14-2). The intrinsic coping mechanisms of the child and the coping mechanisms of the family serve to mitigate the impact. A single event may be absorbed without difficulty, whereas multiple changes can overwhelm the family. The challenge an 8-year-old experiences when her family moves as a unit to another city for a parent's change in employment may resolve quickly. When such a move occurs after a divorce, it is more likely to cause a major disruption. Not only must the child deal with the loss of friends, community, neighborhood, and school, but the child also is likely to face changes in economic status that typically occur after divorce and, most importantly, the loss of the relationship with the parent left behind (Boyce, 2005).

As with most behavior problems in pediatrics, the symptoms that a child manifests in response to intrinsic and extrinsic untoward events are not specific to the proximal event. The principle of *behavioral commonality* informs us that any given symptom can be related to numerous different conditions. Inattention is most often thought to represent attention-deficit/hyperactivity disorder, whereas it may be a manifestation of anxiety disorders, acute or post-traumatic stress disorder, bipolar disorder, or agitated depression. The incidence of significant behavior problems in primary care has been found to be 25%, suggesting that in addition to screening for developmental attainment, a screening protocol in primary care, such as using the Pediatric Symptom Checklist, can identify children at risk. In the high-risk situations discussed here, a prudent physician would administer a broader assessment of symptoms, such as the Child Behavior Checklist or the Behavior Assessment for Children (Stancin and Perrin, 2005).

ROLE OF THE PHYSICIAN

Frequent child health visits provide physicians a window into the life of the family, as long as the opportunity is used. Often, without formal assessments, primary care physicians develop an understanding of family structure and roles, beliefs, values, and aspirations. In addition, changes in a family's fortune, whether by illness, financial mishaps, or marital discord, become apparent to the office staff (by change of address or change in insurance coverage). Inasmuch as perhaps only 5% of families show optimal function, physicians should be alert for dysfunctional coping mechanisms in the face of critical life events. Using the relationship already established in the context of health care, the physician can monitor the passage of the family through each step of the family life cycle, intervening when the family seems to be stuck, which is often manifested as a symptomatic child.

ADDITIONS TO THE FAMILY

Birth of a Child

When families bring behavioral concerns to the physician, the physician characteristically seeks to identify events that may have precipitated the change. The birth of another child is seen as the archetype of such a change, and as such, it represents an important event in the family life cycle. The birth of the first child means that the partners/spouses must now add the additional role of parent. In a traditional family, the husband and wife now assume the additional roles of father and mother. These roles have certain culturally attached expectations related to providing an appropriate, secure environment for the child. These expectations inevitably change the relationship of the partners because energy solely directed to the partner must now be directed to the infant.

The addition of another child into the family is the prototype for a normative childhood experience, although according to the 2005 U.S. census, 15 million families had only one child. The predictable consequence for the child with the addition of a brother or sister is likely the loss of the parents' full engagement. This loss occurs in every situation—whether the caregiver is engaged in full-time childcare or provides the childcare after coming home from work. The new infant requires much more time and energy to meet his or her needs.

A young child (≤3 years old) may experience this change as a significant loss, whereas an older child, with greater autonomy, who is involved in preschool or school activities, may thrive in the role of the older, wiser, or helpful brother or sister. Grandparents, other members of the extended family, or daycare providers may be able to provide sufficient support for the older child, and if the child had been adequately parented in the first place, with attention to not only physical, but also emotional needs, one would expect only minor reactions, which would likely pass easily.

The parents' inabilities to provide for the new infant and meet the financial and emotional needs of the family may place undue expectations of childcare on an older child. Although the loss of the emotional connection with the parent would be expected to have a minimal effect on a school-age child, the shift of responsibility for caring for younger brothers or sisters or the assumption of other responsibilities or both may have significant consequences. This process, which frequently occurs in single parent families, has been called parentification and has the effect of depriving the child of the fun of childhood.

Role of the Physician

Regarding the birth of a brother or sister, physicians can provide significant anticipatory guidance as soon as they become aware of the pregnancy. The most acceptable interventions can occur by way of a gentle exploration of the family's expectation of the impact of the new infant on the household.

- Schedule a prenatal visit with both parents to discuss their experience as siblings. What do they remember about being an older (or younger) brother or sister? What was positive about their experiences? What would they like to do differently?
- Explore what the parents anticipate the impact the birth of a new child will be on their other child or children.
- Provide the parents information about available literature and online information (see references under Siblings at the end of the chapter).

Birth of a Child with an Acute Medical Problem or Developmental Disability

Prematurity or a complicated delivery with a prolonged nursery stay can prove as traumatic to the young child as to the parents, especially when it occurs unexpectedly. Likewise, the diagnosis of an acute medical problem requiring intensive treatment (e.g., congenital heart disease) should alert the primary care team to the potential for adjustment difficulties on the part of the older children. Parents may need to spend time with the new infant in the neonatal intensive care unit or in the acute care hospital. Caregiving roles may be spread among other family members. To the extent that these individuals (e.g., grandparents or close family friends) are well known to the child, one would expect a smooth transition. When less familiar relatives are involved in childcare, however, the child is likely to experience more difficulty. The exact nature of the new infant's medical problem and how the family relates to this affect the child's response.

The diagnosis of conditions associated with lifelong chronic illness or developmental disabilities (e.g., spina bifida, Down syndrome) presents another challenge to the family. The adults first face the task of quickly attempting to understand a complicated and confusing situation that has lifelong consequences, while dealing with the loss of the expected, healthy child. In the case of a child with a developmental disability identified at birth, fear, sadness, and sense of loss often make it difficult for the family to know how to announce the birth of this child to friends and family. Although adults seek to gather as much information as they can, what seems to help the siblings the most is a timely discussion that acknowledges that something is different. A discussion of the presence of the extra 21st chromosome in Down syndrome would likely confuse most children and not add anything to their understanding. A family that communicates early and openly creates the environment in which the children can question the parents when they are ready. Ultimately, in these situations, the success of the family rests on the ability first to make a place for the chronic condition in the family and then to put that condition in its place.

Role of the Physician

- Suggest that the family actively include the child in discussions about the infant using age-appropriate descriptions and avoiding too much detail: "Your sister was born early, and she is staying at the hospital so she can grow big enough to go home. This is not what we expected, and we were worried. We know the doctors are doing everything to get her healthy enough to come home as soon as she can."
- If possible, allow the child to visit the hospital, taking care to prepare for the experience. Children read the nonverbal behaviors and overhear adults talking and telephone calls, and quickly discern when the words of comfort directed to them are out of sync with the worried, whispered interactions on the phone, or the parent's tearful demeanor in the face of medical setbacks.
- In the case of a child with Down syndrome, the parents could be advised to say: "When your brother was born, the doctors noticed some things which make them think he may grow a little differently and develop a little slower than you. We will know more about this when they do some tests." After the diagnosis is confirmed, the discussion might continue, as follows: "The tests showed that your brother has Down syndrome, and we are going see some more doctors to make sure that he stays healthy. We are going to have people help to be sure that he develops as best as he can."
- Help the family connect with the specialized services for children (e.g., pediatric cardiology, spina bifida, cystic fibrosis, sickle cell, Down syndrome), which most often have team members available to provide support to parents. Local, family-run support groups are often most effective, offering practical suggestions and emotional support. The Parent-to-Parent organization has a national network that provides support for parents of children with physical and developmental disabilities, and special health care needs, behavioral or mental health issues, educational issues, and adoption/foster care questions (see Internet Resources).

Addition of Children via Adoption and Foster Care

It would be correct to anticipate that many of the previously discussed issues may occur as well in the case of foster children or adoptive children joining the family. In the case of foster children, the temporary nature of the placement may mitigate some of the issues, and many foster families are well organized in this type of short-term placement. Such an addition has the potential to stress the parents' financial, emotional, marital, and physical health. This stress affects the other children in the household (see Chapter 13). The addition of one or more step-brothers or step-sisters has the potential to evoke all of the above-described issues (see Chapter 11). The addition of a step-parent adds another confounding element, which is discussed subsequently.

Addition of Adults to the Family

When an adult joins the household, the key destabilizing issue is the change in role that occurs to the parents. As the population ages, many adults find themselves moving their parents into their home to provide shelter or health care. Young children would be expected to react to the change in role of their parents, who need to take on a caregiving role to their own parents and would be expected to be challenged in maintaining that role in the same way for their children. This loss of connection with their parents might be balanced, however, through the positive connection of children with their grandparents. Illness or infirmity of the grandparents can represent a loss to the children, especially in situations where the grandparents have lost memory (dementia) or functional abilities (after a stroke). There can be great richness in the participation of children in this part of the natural cycle of life and death, something that most children in urban cultures have not had an opportunity to experience.

The addition of a partner or spouse (which, for convenience sake, we refer to as step-parent) has many possible outcomes. In the best case, this individual can help support the parent to create an environment that optimizes the emotional life of the family. The addition of a step-parent can occur in several situations: after separation or divorce, after the death of a parent, or when a single parent marries. Even in the best situation, it would be prudent to anticipate that a period of adjustment will be needed. The longer this individual has been involved with the family before moving into the household, giving children the opportunity to develop a relationship with the individual, the more likely this may be a smoother transition. Nevertheless, the reality of a marriage or commitment ceremony may lead to the end of the "behavioral honeymoon," as the child realizes that this individual is here to stay.

After separation or divorce, when the parent moves a partner into the household, either emotionally or physically, powerful loyalty issues can be stimulated in the children. The wise partner assiduously avoids seeking to take the place of the absent biologic parent. Often parents are looking for someone to make up for the real or perceived faults or lapses of the absent parent, however. This scenario has two versions. In one, the step-father is brought in to be the stern disciplinarian to unruly children, a role that the mother was unable to perform. This is an unrealistic expectation: The mother is unable to invest the step-father with the authority to make him acceptable to a recalcitrant child, who may feel forced to obey this man, who may be seen as displacing a beloved father (see Chapter 12). In the second version, the step-mother is sought to attempt to make up for the real or perceived faults or lapses of the absent biologic parent, by nurturing and providing what she believes (or was told) was missing. In both cases, the tension set up between the step-parent and the absent biologic parent is a recipe for disaster for all involved.

The remarriage of a parent after the death of a spouse can represent a healing step for the family, depending on the timing. The perception of the children and other family members contributes greatly to the sense of the appropriateness of the interval. One would anticipate more problems should the marriage occur early, in the period of intense grief. Such an early marriage likely would lead to an increase in stressors for all involved, especially the younger child.

When a same-sex partner joins the household, several factors need to be assessed to be able to anticipate adequately the child's reaction. When the biologic parent is "out" to the extended family, community, and child, the major issues are those generic to the addition of any step-parent. If the addition of the same-sex partner represents the declaration of the biologic parent's sexual orientation, however, the child must deal with both issues at the same time. Younger children (infants through preschool) might experience little distress about the issue of having a gay parent. School-age children are influenced by negative reactions of other family members, especially their other biologic parent, and grandparents, aunts, and uncles. Older school-age children and especially adolescents often have absorbed society's homophobia and may develop understandable fears about their own sexuality and how they will be affected by their peers' knowledge of their parent's sexuality. The extended family's reaction mitigates or exacerbates the child's reaction, in parallel fashion. Accepting grandparents, aunts, and uncles can help normalize same-sex partnerships. Often, gay parents develop supportive "families by choice," which model healthy gay and lesbian parenting (American Academy of Pediatrics Committee on Psychosocial Aspects of Child and Family Health, 2002).

Although on the surface other "additions" to the family might be seen as positive events, the lens of family functioning can aid the physician in carefully assessing the process of these events. The return of a separated parent would likely be experienced by the child as a wish come true. All children pine for the reunification of the family, many years after a divorce is legally finalized. If the parents have had an opportunity to address the issues that led to the separation, the marital unit may be functionally improved. It would make sense to anticipate that the family might have improved function, although it there have been unhealthy, cross-generational coalitions, the children may find a new environment where their importance is diminished. Likewise, some single parents devote substantial energy to the children's needs, to the exclusion of their own. Similar to the step-family situation, the children may feel excluded as the returning spouse becomes the primary focus.

The return of parents from military service poses other potential problems. Many servicemen and servicewomen return home impaired. The loss of a parent's ability to be fully functional and employable (depending on the nature of the physical disability) tempers the joy and can place further burdens related to the need for extensive medical care, rehabilitation, and psychiatric care. A recent study documented that two thirds of married or cohabiting veterans returning from Afghanistan and Iraq "reported some type of family readjustment problem or conflict occurring several times a week: 42[%] felt like a guest in their household, 21.8[%] reported their children were not acting warmly or were afraid of them, and 35.7[%] were unsure about their role in regular household responsibilities. Veterans with depression or [post-traumatic stress disorder] were more likely to experience these readjustment problems" (Sayers et al, 2007). In addition to the immediate difficulties posed by individuals with clearly apparent disorders, the experience from the Persian Gulf War reveals excess injury mortality that the authors postulated "might be a consequence of depression, post-traumatic stress disorder and symptoms of other psychiatric conditions developed after the war." Another possibility is that the injuries were related to maladaptive coping mechanisms, such as drug or alcohol use (Bell et al, 2001). These later consequences can become an additional emotional wound to the child and family.

Role of the Physician

- Primary care providers have the opportunity to monitor the blending process. Assess the family's strengths and vulnerabilities, and monitor for the presence of symptomatic behavior in the children, which may be the first sign that the process may not be proceeding smoothly. It should become apparent when a referral to family counseling is indicated.
- When a same-sex partner joins a household, physicians who provide an environment that communicates an openness to diversity in all areas, and specifically in areas of sexual orientation, are able to listen carefully and sensitively, and to explore nonjudgmentally changes in the family structure. One need only inquire about how the child is faring during this transition, and offer assistance in the event that new difficulties arise. The physician and medical staff are most effective if they are able to create a welcoming environment in the office that signals

acceptance of diverse families (Perrin, 2002) (see Internet Resources).

- Be mindful of the acute and chronic stresses that affect children and families of deployed and returning members of the military. Use the available resources to guide yourself and the families to understand the typical reactions of all members of the family to the homecoming, which, although expected to be joyful, may be fraught with challenges (see Internet Resources).

LOSSES

Deaths in the Family

Death is inevitable. The loss we experience because of a death is modulated by the concept of "timeliness." The death of elderly grandparents occurs "on-time." The death of a young mother of breast cancer at age 34, 2 years after the birth of her child, clearly occurs "off-time" and has enormous repercussions for the family. In the same manner, the death of a brother or sister represents significant challenges to the child and family (see Chapter 37). The primary modulator for any child's experience is his or her conception of death, which relates, in typically developing children, to their age.

Children younger than 2 years of age do not have the ability to understand death cognitively. They experience the same feelings they do when an individual leaves for any reason. In the case of a parent, specifically, one who is involved in caregiving activities (as is typical in our society for mothers), the child experiences the loss as abandonment or desertion. It is almost impossible for the child to distinguish between temporary and permanent absences.

Between 2 and 6 years of age, death is equated with absence and is perceived as reversible. Sometimes death is understood as a faded continuation of life. The child does not understand that the dead family member cannot come back. Some children seem to understand that death is final as they watch their pet goldfish get flushed away. The same child, however, despite attending the funeral, may expect grandma to come home from the cemetery when she is tired or hungry. This is a time that children are engaged in magical thinking: Children may believe that their anger at their parent caused the parent's death, and thus they are being punished for bad thoughts or deeds. Death may be pictured as a person, such as a scary clown, or shadowy, threatening figure.

Between 6 and 11 years of age, children develop a sense of the fact that death is final and irreversible: Their parent, grandparent, or brother or sister will not be returning. Children's concrete reasoning (cause-and-effect thinking) serve them in making sense of what happened, especially in the face of a fatal illness.

Children 10 to 11 years old come to understand the inevitability of death for every living thing, including themselves. Children's abstract reasoning (described by Piaget as "formal operations") allows them to see and imagine circumstances they have not yet experienced. Although the latter can be a source of great satisfaction in anticipating how they will take control of the future, it also includes the possibility of their own death (American Academy of Pediatrics Committee on Psychosocial Aspects of Child and Family Health, 2000).

This framework also helps us understand some of the confusion that can occur in younger children in the face of separation and divorce. A very young child is likely to experience enormous distress if the primary caregiver must relocate temporarily for any reason (military service, employment, caring for an ill relative). The possibility of communication with the absent individual via telephone or Internet (webcam) can modulate the distress, at least for a child older than 2 years. Table 14-3 lists other factors that can influence a child's reaction to the death of a parent or caregiver.

Table 14-3. **Modulating Factors Regarding Death of a Parent or Family Member**
Traumatic death (e.g., motor vehicle accident)
Act of nature (e.g., lightning strike, flood, hurricane)
Self-inflicted—suicide
Accidental death related to specific behaviors (e.g., drug or alcohol use)
Overdose, driving while intoxicated
Member of police department, fire department, or armed forces killed in the line of duty

The death of a brother or sister causes great distress to the child, and given the child's developmental stage, can have significant consequences. This loss is most difficult for a family to manage. Ordinarily, we would expect the surviving children to turn to their parents for solace. The parents' grief may render them unable to provide this for their children, however. The loss of a brother or sister would lead to an imbalance in the family system, one that must be re-established as the mourning process proceeds. These issues are discussed in detail in Chapter 37. Likewise, the death of a friend or classmate can prove challenging to a child, although in both these instances, the child is not deprived of the nurturance of the parent.

All children take their cues from the adults in their life. The caregivers' availability to support the child provides a tempering effect on the child's experience. When the primary caregivers themselves are overwhelmed by the loss, younger children are especially vulnerable and are likely to become symptomatic.

In years past, children were discouraged from attending funerals, with the concern that this experience would be traumatic. With proper preparation and the presence of a family member to interpret the child's experience, there is great value in helping the child understand the reality and finality of death. It is wise to limit the amount of time that younger children spend at the funeral home. Older children and adolescents often can participate in the services in a way that assists in the grieving process with a remembrance or a reading of personal significance (American Academy of Pediatrics Committee on Psychosocial Aspects of Child and Family Health, 2000).

Role of the Physician

As daunting as it might seem, a more recent study showed that bereaving children are not as depressed as is commonly believed compared with community controls and with children diagnosed with a depressive disorder. The factors associated with more difficulty include parental depression, other life stressors for the family, and lower socioeconomic status (Cerel et al, 2006). The physician's interventions are best guided by understanding that the reaction to the acute loss and the aftermath evolves over time.

- Identify families with obvious risk, such as single parent families, families without extended support in the community, and families with marital separation or divorce, who may not have the resilience to meet the needs of the child.
- When parents bring in a symptomatic child, start by eliciting the story of the loss and the reactions of the child and family to understand where they are in the grieving process, and to assess that this painful process is progressing appropriately, or whether it is stalled and needs specific intervention.
- Empathically give permission for all members of the family to experience their emotions. Expect that the young child may be frightened by the abandonment and for the older child to lose interest in activities.
- Individuals of all ages must be allowed to use whatever coping mechanisms help them to survive the ordeal. Help support the child who does not seem in distress or refuses to answer repeated questions about their feelings, while monitoring the grieving process over time.
- In this case, as in all others, when you take the opportunity to see the family back to follow-up on their grieving process, you can discern when your interventions have not achieved the desired objective. At this point, in the face of a family that is stuck and unable to move through the healing stages, suggest consultation with a counselor or with an agency that assists grieving children and families. This last point is most important. Children follow their parents' lead: Parents who send their children to counseling without addressing their own issues see less benefit than parents who seek guidance for their own distress (American Academy of Pediatrics Committee on Psychosocial Aspects of Child and Family Health, 2000). (See Resources for Grieving Children and Families for information about support groups with grieving children in the United States and selected other countries.)

Other Losses Not Related to Deaths

In addition to the losses sustained by separation, divorce, and death, children experience similar, although perhaps temporary, loss when parents separate, move away for employment reasons, leave home for military service, or are incarcerated. Beyond the physical loss of the parent, illness and injury can rob an individual of his or her ability to work (inside or outside the home), leading to changes in the family's economic status. Physical injuries also may lead to cognitive disabilities (e.g., in an individual with a serious head injury). Emotional and mental health issues may interfere with the parent's ability to perform his or her usual role in the home or out in the world, leading to the need to rebalance the family as activities and responsibilities become realigned.

Role of the Physician

Most medical care is provided in response to the family's initiative. The connection of primary care providers to their community often leads to knowledge of changes in the family constellation before the patient becomes symptomatic, giving the practitioner the opportunity to provide guidance. A sympathetic card following the death of a family member can express condolences and offer availability for counseling and support of the child and family as they move through the grieving process. In a similar fashion, awareness of the return of separated parents, parents returning from military service, or the arrival of grandparents into the household may allow the practitioner to express willingness to support the family during these transitions.

SUMMARY

Changes in the family structure represent nodal points that can have a significant impact on a child. Most of these events, such as the birth of a sibling or the death of a parent or grandparent, are likely to have predictable consequences, allowing the physician to anticipate the typical reactions and offer timely guidance. Nevertheless, the particular structure of a given family and its available resources become a better predictor of whether the parents (and consequently the child) will be able to navigate these rocky shoals. An understanding of the family life cycle, the developmental stage of the child, the family's emotional and economic resources, and the symptoms of childhood problems guides the physician in assessing which families are coping, and which may need monitoring and intervention. As in other areas of developmental-behavioral pediatrics, the identification of child and family counseling services facilitates timely referral when needed.

REFERENCES

American Academy of Pediatrics Committee on Psychosocial Aspects of Child and Family Health: The pediatrician and childhood bereavement. Pediatrics 105:445-447, 2000.

American Academy of Pediatrics Committee on Psychosocial Aspects of Child and Family Health: Coparent or second-parent adoption by same-sex parents. Pediatrics 109:339-340, 2002.

Bell NS, Amoroso PJ, Wegman DH, Senier L: Proposed explanations for excess injury among veterans of the Persian Gulf War and a call for greater attention from policymakers and researchers. Inj Prev 7:4-9, 2001.

Boyce WT: Coping with stressful transitions. *In* Parker S, Zuckerman B, Augustyn M (eds): Developmental and Behavioral Pediatrics: A Handbook for Primary Care, 2nd ed. Philadelphia, Lippincott Williams & Wilkins, 2005.

Carey WB, McDevitt SC: Coping with Children's Temperament. New York, Basic Books, 1995.

Carter B, McGoldrick M: The Changing Family Life Cycle. New York, Gardner Press, 1988.

Cerel J, Fristand MA, Verducci J, et al: Childhood bereavement: Psychopathology in the 2 years postparental death. J Am Acad Child Adolesc Psychiatry 45:681-690, 2006.

Perrin EC: Sexual Orientation in Child and Adolescent Health Care. New York, Kluwer/Plenum Academic Press, 2002.

Sayers SL, Farrow V, Ross J, et al: Family problems among recently returning military veterans. Presented at Session 1012—Couples and Spousal Relationships, American Psychological Association Annual Meeting, San Francisco, August 17, 2007.

Shonkoff JP, Jarman FC, Kohlenberg TM: Family transitions, crises, and adaptations. Curr Prob Pediatr 17:501-553, 1987.

Stancin T, Perrin EC: Behavioral screening. *In* Parker S, Zuckerman B, Augustyn M (eds): Developmental and Behavioral Pediatrics: A Handbook for Primary Care, 2nd ed. Philadelphia, Lippincott Williams & Wilkins, 2005.

Walsh F: Changing families in a changing world: Reconstructing family normality. *In*: Normal Family Processes: Growing Diversity and Complexity, 3rd ed. New York, Guilford Press, 2003.

INTERNET RESOURCES

Gay, lesbian, bisexual, and transgender parenting issues. Available at: http://www.gayparentingpage.com/.

Parental support for children with special health care needs and developmental disabilities: Parent to Parent-USA. Available at: http://www.p2pusa.org/.

Re-entry: Coming Home Guide. Available at: http://www.cfs.purdue.edu/mfri/pages/military/FAMILY_and_FRIENDS_1.pdf.

Resources for families with members deployed in military. Available at: http://www.cfs.purdue.edu/mfri/pages/military/deployment_support.html.

Supporting children of military parent who is deployed. Available at: http://www.cfs.purdue.edu/mfri/pages/military/Supporting_Children_of_Deployed_Parents.pdf.

RESOURCES FOR GRIEVING CHILDREN AND FAMILIES

Bibliography of books for children (grouped by age) and for professionals. Available at: http://www.childgrief.org/documents/Bibliography.pdf.

Children's Grief Education Association: Available at: http://www.childgrief.org/childgrief.htm and http://www.childgrief.org/resources.htm.

Finding a bereavement support center for children and families. The Dougy Center for Grieving Children and Families. Available at: http://www.dougy.org/default.asp?pid=3557092.

SIBLINGS

Leonard J: Twice Blessed: Everything You Need to Know about Having a Second Child—Preparing Yourself, Your Marriage, and Your Firstborn for a New Family of Four. New York, St Martin's Press, 2000.

Sears M, Sears W, Kelly CW, Adrianni R: Baby on the Way. Boston, Little, Brown Young Readers, 2001. (This is a picture book for young children.)

15 PEERS

LISE M. YOUNGBLADE, ERIC A. STORCH,
AND JOHN A. NACKASHI

Vignette

In an elite boarding school, this boy, despite upper class connections, was unpopular. He was not at all handsome, was mediocre in everything he did, and had few social graces. See what he said at age 68 in his reunion report:

Most vivid memory: "The everlasting teasing and ridicule I received at (high school)! The scars will remain until I die. Unlike Kipling I have not had 'revenge' by writing 'Stalky and Co.'"

My worst experience was: "The first 20 years of my life. Psychological counseling allowed me to join the human race at 28."

Would you follow the same career? "If my life at (high school) had been different, I might have been quite a different person. Would I have been happy? I don't know."

—Anonymous

Peer relationships provide a unique and important context for social-emotional development and adjustment, one that is complementary to parent-child relationships. Because of the relatively egalitarian nature of peer relations, children learn how to negotiate, compromise, and cooperate to maintain successful relationships. As children grow, peers provide opportunities to master skills such as perspective-taking, conflict management, loyalty, intimacy, and other social skills. Children also develop these skills with parents, but in contrast to peer relations, with parents children are dependents, receiving discipline, support, and guidance.

Not all peer experiences are equal. It is important to distinguish the terms *peer relationships* and *friendship*. In lay vernacular, they are often used interchangeably. In the professional literature, however, the terms are used to mean two different types of relationships. *Peer relationships* refers to group relations (i.e., being part of a collective of children of roughly the same age and gender). *Friendships* are dyadic, close relationships that are managed and maintained as a continuing entity. In addition, friendships involve mutual preference and choice (i.e., reciprocity), and a mutual trust, closeness, and intimacy not found among all peers. The psychological consequences for children from friendship include the consequences for more general peer relationships, such as identification and acceptance, but also include intimacy, loyalty, support, and the validation of self-worth.

Developmental research has chronicled the increasing importance and the increasing complexity of peer relationships and friendships as children grow (Bierman, 2004). First friendships generally emerge during the preschool years, evolving as children master shared pretense and cooperative play. In elementary school, children begin to become more involved in larger and more structured peer group interactions, where their friendship skills continue to develop as they learn to negotiate issues involving competition, conformity, and achievement. During preadolescence, children often form special "chumships" with same-sex peers that provide models for the skills involved in sustaining close emotional relationships, such as intimacy, loyalty, and support. In adolescence, youth may experiment with different social roles and experience a range of relationships as a way of helping them to define the person they want to be. Peer relationships and friendships during adolescence also provide support as adolescents move from dependence on their parents to autonomous functioning as adults.

Along with delineating the developmental progression and outcomes of healthy peer relationships, research also describes the outcomes children can have that result from problems with peers. The remainder of this chapter discusses dysfunctional peer experiences and offers tools and suggestions for clinicians to use as part of screening during patient visits.

PROBLEMS WITH PEER RELATIONSHIPS

Research has delineated several dimensions of peer difficulties that are of concern, including peer rejection; social withdrawal and avoidance of peer interaction; peer victimization; and lack of a close, dyadic friendship (Bierman, 2004; Cillessen and Bukowski, 2000; Deater-Deckard, 2001).

Peer Rejection

Childhood peer rejection and its role in the development of psychopathology has received more attention than any other peer-related topic, in part because of its prevalence—approximately 10% to 15% of children are rejected by their peer group. These children are actively disliked by many of their peers and are liked by few or none of them.

Peer rejection is a global term that encompasses the many behaviors used by children to exclude and hurt one another, including overt forms of control and exclusion and more subtle tactics, such as gossiping and spreading rumors. These methods, whether overt or covert, account for variance in children's maladjustment and social acceptance above and beyond the effects of aggressive behaviors. It is not simply being the recipient of aggressive acts that is linked to maladaptive outcomes, but being the recipient of coordinated efforts that keep an individual outside the boundaries of the peer group.

The short-term and long-term consequences of peer rejection are quite serious. In the short-term, these children often experience loneliness, low self-esteem, and social anxiety. Long-term consequences include poor academic performance, school dropout, juvenile delinquency, criminal behavior, and mental health problems, particularly externalizing ones, in adolescence and adulthood.

What elicits rejection? Many factors can lead to peer rejection, but the most consistently related factors, especially over the long-term, are aggressive and socially withdrawn behavior. Numerous studies have linked aggressive behavior problems in preschool, middle childhood, and adolescence to rejection from peers. Aggressive play with peers in early childhood is linked to behavioral maladjustment and difficulties with peers in middle childhood. Hostile behavior and withdrawal from social interaction in middle childhood is predictive of antisocial behavior in adolescence, extreme forms of teenage delinquency, externalizing problems in late adolescence, drug use in adulthood, and problems in other social relationships. Aggressive children are more likely to be avoided and actively targeted than nonaggressive children because the larger group seeks to isolate individuals who tend to disrupt normal peer interaction. At the same time, the experience of being rejected serves to perpetuate aggressive and externalizing problems, partly by limiting the amount and quality of the rejected child's socialization by his or her peers.

Despite clear links between aggression and rejection, not all aggressive children are rejected (Parkhurst and Asher, 1992). Approximately one third of aggressive elementary school–age children and two thirds of aggressive young adolescents are not rejected. Several factors seem to differentiate children who become rejected and children who do not. Aggressive children who are rejected tend to engage in more instrumental aggression or aggression designed to reach a specific goal; they are more likely to instigate and escalate aggressive interchanges; and they are more likely to be argumentative, disruptive, inattentive, off-task, and hyperactive.

Children's self-perceptions may be important in assessing the likelihood of negative outcomes (Patterson et al, 1990; Reinherz et al, 2000). Many rejected children describe themselves in negative terms—they say that they are less competent socially, they feel more anxious, and they expect less positive social outcomes than other children. Despite these negative self-portrayals, however, rejected children often rate themselves higher on positive indices than parents or peers, perhaps as a face-saving defense tactic. Finally, several more recent studies suggest that self-perceptions of being rejected (whether or not peer rejection is truly present) are significantly implicated in the cause of depression and suicidal ideation in childhood and adolescence.

Peer rejection, including its concomitant and long-term consequences, is an extremely difficult process to derail, in part because of its stability. Almost half of rejected children are rejected 1 year later, and 30% remain rejected after 4 years. In addition, many rejected children quickly become disliked again when put into new groups of children.

Peer Neglect, Social Withdrawal, and Peer Avoidance

Some children seem to avoid interaction with peers. In some cases, this situation refers to children who are not routinely named as liked or disliked by classmates; these *neglected* children are simply not mentioned. Neglected status is unstable, and the outcomes for these children are not much different than for average children (Newcomb et al, 1993). In large part, these children are probably not at risk; this group also may include children who simply like to spend some time alone. A smaller subgroup of these peer-neglected children may be at greater risk—those who are actively ignored. Little information is available about this subgroup of neglected children, but the clinician might want to probe for further clarification about the extent of neglect.

A group of children at risk for peer rejection and who have more serious subsequent difficulties are children who are socially withdrawn (Rubin et al, 1998). Patterns of withdrawal from social interaction in childhood seem to be stable over time and context. These children are most prone to developing feelings of loneliness and isolation and internalizing disorders, such as depression and anxiety. Although withdrawn behavior is seemingly less salient compared with aggressive, hostile behavior in early childhood, by middle childhood and through adolescence, withdrawn, internalizing behavior is strongly associated with peer rejection (Ladd, 1999; Rubin et al, 1998) (see also Chapter 41).

It is important to distinguish the quality of behavior exhibited by a child from the effect that this has on the child's peer relations. Some shy, withdrawn children experience no apparent ostracism by the peer group, whereas for others, inappropriate social withdrawal may contribute to peer rejection. Social withdrawal may indicate more serious consequences for children when it leads to or is accompanied by peer rejection than when no negative peer reactions are evident.

Peer Victimization

Peer victimization among children has been the focus of increased empiric attention over the last 3 decades (Hawker and Boulton, 2000; Nansel et al, 2001; Olweus, 1993; Storch et al, 2006). Defined as repeated exposure to negative actions on the part of one or more other individuals, 20% to 30% of youngsters are chronically victimized by peers. Although peer victimization has previously been considered an inevitable childhood occurrence, parents, school personnel, and health professionals have recognized the impact of being victimized on a range of psychosocial adjustment problems. Policy changes within schools have lagged, resulting in few improvements in the situation.

In the early 1990s and before, victimization was thought to occur primarily through physical or verbal attacks, such as hitting, pushing, cursing, or threatening. This research found that boys were victimized more frequently than girls. Such findings contradicted common knowledge about the peer experiences of girls, however, and the nature of aggressive behavior among girls and boys. More recent research has revised this conceptualization to include forms of peer maltreatment such as shunning, ignoring, and spreading rumors (Crick and Bigbee, 1998). By broadening the definition of peer victimization to include gender normative aggressive behaviors, a more balanced picture of peer experiences has been captured.

Although fewer data have been reported regarding the prospective relationships between peer victimization and adjustment, the extant findings further suggest that victimization is a distress-provoking experience. The conceptualization underlying these findings involves cognitive and behavioral components. Victimized children may internalize negative self-evaluations, resulting in greater distress and avoidance of interactions that have a high probability for victimization. Through the process of marginalization and ostracism, victimized children may have limited opportunities to build positive peer relationships that could provide physical protection and aid in coping with bullying-related distress. Cross-sectional studies have shown positive correlations between peer victimization and depressive symptoms, general anxiety, social anxiety, and externalizing symptoms. Longitudinal studies also have indicated that peer victimization predicts later symptoms of depression, social phobia, general anxiety, and internalizing and externalizing behaviors.

Lack of Friendship

The preceding sections considered peer relationships more globally from a group perspective; in this section we talk about friends—close, dyadic, mutually acknowledged relationships. Depending on the specific criteria used, approximately 10% to 20% of school-age children do not have a mutual friendship. Children without friends are not always neglected or rejected children, however. About 50% of unaccepted children have close friendships, and about 20% of average accepted children do not (Parker and Asher, 1993). Children with friends have been found to be more altruistic and to have better skills in explaining emotions. Early school adjustment has been found to be associated with having a large number of prior friendships at the time of entrance, maintaining these friendships, and developing new ones (Ladd, 1999).

Although friendship serves seemingly beneficial functions, little research is available to suggest how many friendships are desirable or sufficient, although some research has shown that the biggest difference in self-esteem is between children with no friends and children with at least one friend. In addition, it may be that quality is more important than quantity. The quality of friendships has been found to be related to social dissatisfaction or loneliness above and beyond the sheer number of friendships (Parker and Asher, 1993). One implication is that children who experience poor peer relations may be buffered against many of the associated risks and consequences if they are able to make and maintain a close friendship.

GUIDELINES FOR THE CLINICIAN

As just presented, the short-term and long-term outcomes of peer rejection, social withdrawal, friendlessness, and peer victimization are potentially quite serious. Knowing this, what are the implications for pediatricians relevant to children who present with peer problems? To aid in this discussion, Figure 15-1 presents a flow chart that may help pediatricians to structure the visit and decide on appropriate action (e.g., a referral or "wait and see"). Although extensive interviews with probes to identify the specific behavioral bases for a child's or parent's perceptions can be useful, there is no standardized, short list of questions that can be asked of either children or parents to identify quickly the nature of a child's peer relations. Certain triggers can start a conversation quickly, however, such as "tell me about your friends." Following are suggestions for gaining additional information that the pediatrician might use to determine whether or not further referral or follow-up is necessary.

The first clarifying probes might involve questions about context. Second, the pediatrician might ask about the child's perceptions of this problem. Third, the pediatrician might obtain a brief history that includes corroborating information from the parent. These are screening questions and by themselves do not diagnose a particular peer problem.

Certain behaviors and answers may raise red flags that would lead a physician to consider a referral on the spot. If a child becomes extremely distraught during the conversation, or reports feelings of profound loneliness, self-loathing, or depression, the pediatrician may want to make a mental health referral. Similarly, if the parent reports problems with multiple children, especially if corroborated by another parent or a teacher, the pediatrician may wish to make a referral for further assessment. On examination, if the physician had noted any atypical behavior, such as unusual or odd behavior, communication difficulties, or extremely poor social skills, a referral might be warranted.

The practitioner needs to decide in the course of asking the probes at what point a referral might be necessary. To the extent that there is corresponding information from the parent and the child, the pediatrician might suggest a follow-up with a school counselor. A similar referral might be based on concern from the parent. In the absence of compelling evidence for a referral, the pediatrician at least might revisit the topic at a subsequent visit. To aid the pediatrician in making these decisions,

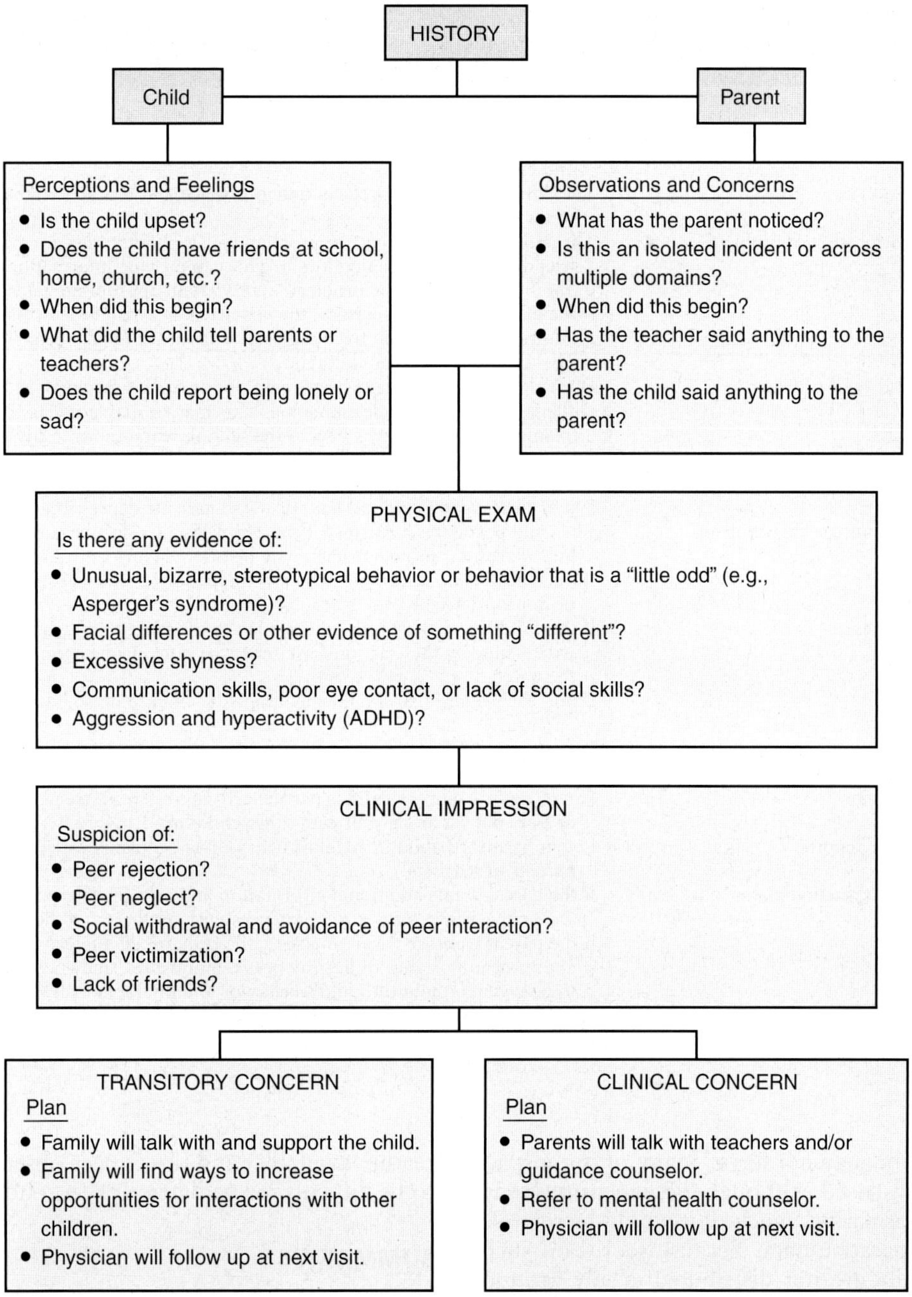

HISTORY

Child

Perceptions and Feelings
- Is the child upset?
- Does the child have friends at school, home, church, etc.?
- When did this begin?
- What did the child tell parents or teachers?
- Does the child report being lonely or sad?

Parent

Observations and Concerns
- What has the parent noticed?
- Is this an isolated incident or across multiple domains?
- When did this begin?
- Has the teacher said anything to the parent?
- Has the child said anything to the parent?

PHYSICAL EXAM

Is there any evidence of:
- Unusual, bizarre, stereotypical behavior or behavior that is a "little odd" (e.g., Asperger's syndrome)?
- Facial differences or other evidence of something "different"?
- Excessive shyness?
- Communication skills, poor eye contact, or lack of social skills?
- Aggression and hyperactivity (ADHD)?

CLINICAL IMPRESSION

Suspicion of:
- Peer rejection?
- Peer neglect?
- Social withdrawal and avoidance of peer interaction?
- Peer victimization?
- Lack of friends?

TRANSITORY CONCERN

Plan
- Family will talk with and support the child.
- Family will find ways to increase opportunities for interactions with other children.
- Physician will follow up at next visit.

CLINICAL CONCERN

Plan
- Parents will talk with teachers and/or guidance counselor.
- Refer to mental health counselor.
- Physician will follow up at next visit.

Figure 15-1. Initial screening for peer difficulties. ADHD, attention-deficit/hyperactivity disorder.

Table 15-1 provides illustrations of red flags that might lead the physician to take further action. The more red flags that occur, the more likely one would consider formal assessment or referral or both. Table 15-1 provides illustrations; it is not a diagnostic tool.

Beyond the general screening probes just described, are there tools available to assist the clinician in determining the nature and scope of the problem? The issue of detailed assessment is complicated, for two major reasons. First, problems with peers can be associated with other difficulties that require treatment, such as learning disabilities, and are part of the diagnostic picture of several mental health syndromes, including conduct disorder, anxiety disorders, autistic spectrum disorders, schizophrenic and depressive disorders, adjustment disorder, and possibly attention-deficit/hyperactivity disorder. The decision of whether or how to assess and treat peer relationship difficulties associated with these conditions would need to be made within the context of a broader mental health treatment plan, and this discussion goes beyond the scope of this chapter.

Second, many of the tools that are described are impractical for pediatricians, who often do not have easy access to school settings or other places where children's peers may be found. In addition, interpretation of some of the normed, standardized tools is facilitated by training in psychology or psychiatry, which a

Table 15-1. **Domains and Types of Red Flags for Peer Difficulties: When Follow-up or Referrals May Be Indicated**

Source	Domain	Potential Red Flags
Child	Context of problem	The problem is multicontextual (i.e., the child reports problems at school and elsewhere). The difficulty seems to occur in only one place, but it is an extremely salient place to the child.
	Clarification of problem	The child can specify what the problem is (e.g., "other kids are mean to me, my best friend doesn't like me anymore"). This can provide information to the physician about the nature of the problem, and what an appropriate referral would be. If the child cannot cite specifics, the pediatrician would at least want to seek additional information from the parent about the child's behavior and observed interactions with other children.
	History of problem	Difficulties with peers have been going on for some time. Difficulties are a recent phenomenon. This may or may not lead to further action. For example, if the child was new to the school, reassurance to the child and a "wait and see" approach might be appropriate. If it is a recent phenomenon in a relatively stable context, further probing of the child or parent or both would be suggested.
	Affect	Sad or distraught affect and flat affect can indicate depression or loneliness.
	Reasons for the problem	The child postulates a reason for the problem (e.g., "it's because I'm fat"). Depending on the reason, the pediatrician may be offered clues as to the appropriate referral. If the child has no reason for why it is happening, further probing of the parent would be appropriate.
	Actions	If the child has spoken with others, such as the parent or a teacher, the pediatrician would support these actions, ask what the outcome has been, and follow-up with the parent. If not, the pediatrician should encourage the child to do so, and to follow-up with the parent.
Parent	Corroboration	Parent corroborates the reported difficulty.
	Concern	Parent is very concerned.
	Behavior	Parent reports that the child is particularly aggressive, extremely shy or withdrawn, or does not get along well with other children.
	Other reports	Parent has heard about the child's behavior or problems with peers from other parents or teachers.
	Parent's action plan	If the parent wants additional information and asks pediatrician where to get it, reasonable suggestions are conferences with teachers and the school counselor. If the parent wants to "wait and see," the pediatrician might talk to the parent about the importance of healthy peer relationships, and encourage the parent to be vigilant about the child's behavior and interactions with other children. The pediatrician also might encourage a follow-up for further monitoring.

pediatrician may or may not have. Many of the instruments are research-based. Although these measures may provide some information, much of it would be relative and require comparative data. Because scores on such instruments usually are not distributed evenly around the midpoint of the scales, a simple examination of raw scores can be misleading. The basic implication for pediatricians is that they are in a unique position to provide a first screen for problems, but in most cases need to consider referring such cases, or developing collaborative ties with school counselors, psychologists, or others who may better be able to treat such problems.

With these caveats in mind, Table 15-2 presents a list of primary sources of information, the type of information one would get from that source, pros and cons of that type of information, and examples of available instruments. This list is not exhaustive, but is illustrative of the type of tool and information one would get from it. Generally, there are five primary sources of information: self-report from the child, parent report, teacher report, peer report, and direct observation. It is easy for pediatricians to receive information from children and parents; teacher and peer reports are expected to be less readily available; and direct peer observations are likely to be difficult for pediatricians to conduct or obtain.

SUMMARY

This chapter has presented an overview of the normative developmental progression and functions of peer relationships in childhood and adolescence. Several aspects of problematic peer relations have been discussed, including peer rejection, social withdrawal and avoidance of peer interaction, peer victimization, and lack of a close friend. Screening guidelines for pediatricians in primary care settings have been presented. Pediatricians can serve an important function in identifying children at risk for or manifesting peer difficulties. Pediatricians can respond to statements from the child or parent that may indicate peer problems. More generally, by including questions about the child's opportunities for peer interactions and about the quality of the child's friendships and peer relations in routine developmental interviews with parents, pediatricians can screen for potential problems and simultaneously increase parental awareness about this important aspect of the child's development.

Table 15-2. Sources of Information and Types of Tools Available for Peer Difficulties

Source	Type of Information	Pros	Cons	Tools Available
Child self-report	Children can provide a direct description of their perceptions of their friendships and peer relationships. For example, the practitioner might want to identify how well the child can pinpoint the nature of the difficulties, how the child feels about them (lonely, sad, angry), and how concerned the child is about the situation.	The child is the focal point. His or her perceptions and reports are likely to instigate assessment and influence treatment.	Some evidence suggests that children's self-reports of social status do not mirror the descriptions given to them by peers and teachers, and are likely to be more positive than those by others.	Pediatricians can ask screening questions about peer relationships. The Youth Self-Report of the Achenbach Child Behavior Checklist (Achenbach and Edelbrock, 2001) is a normed measure of internalizing and externalizing syndromes, but also contains social competency scales; it does not explicitly assess peer relations. Other research instruments assess the quality of friendships (Parker and Asher, 1993).
Parent report	Parents can provide anecdotal and supplemental information about their child's peer experiences.	Parents have observed their children's interactions with peers for a long time. They also have information about peers outside the school setting. In addition, parental concern is an important influence on follow-up and course of treatment.	Parents may be biased in their reports of peer relations. They may be likely to observe only friends, rather than other types of peer relationships. They may not have extensive experience with other children with which to compare their child's behavior and experience. Parents also may find it difficult to recognize or acknowledge their child's inappropriate behavior or difficulties with peers.	Pediatricians can ask screening questions about peer relationships. To the extent that the parent's report of difficulty corroborates the child's report of difficulty, practitioners may be more likely to make a referral to a school counselor, pursue additional resources for the child, and revisit the topic at the next visit. Parent perceptions of children's behavior can be assessed with the Achenbach Child Behavior Checklist (see above).
Teacher report	Teachers can provide information about children's behavior at school with peers. Teacher reports of children's social problems are an alternative means for obtaining information on peer relationships.	Teacher reports are moderately correlated with peer reports (Malik and Furman, 1993), and may be easier for pediatricians to obtain.	Physicians would need access to school settings. Some teachers are better reporters than others. Some problems are easier for teachers to identify than others (e.g., aggression may be more visible in the classroom than social withdrawal). Many of these tools are research-based, and less attention has been paid to clinical applications.	A normed, standardized tool for teachers is the Achenbach Child Behavior Checklist (Teacher's Form) (see above). Others include the Pupil Evaluation Inventory (Pekarik et al, 1976) and the Teacher-Child Rating Scale (Hightower et al, 1986). Clinicians also may interview teachers to obtain information about specific behaviors.
Peer report	Sociometric and peer behavioral assessment measures are standard techniques. For sociometric measures, children are asked to rate the likability of classmates, or are asked to nominate classmates they like or dislike. These measures yield information about social status (e.g., rejected, neglected). Behavioral ratings ask students to assess classmates' behaviors (e.g., aggressive, helpful).	Peer ratings or nominations are readily obtainable if access to the school population is available. These are the most commonly used research instruments. Much research is available to document the predictive utility of these classifications.	Practitioners would need to have ready access to school settings. Parent permission from the peers doing the ratings is required for research and may be for clinical purposes as well. Although applicable in other group settings, research documents outcomes using only classroom-based assessments of peer status.	Peer sociometrics typically ask students to list the three children they like most (or least). Status groups (e.g., rejected) are derived from these nominations. Reciprocal friendships are derived from students who nominate each other as best friends (Cillessen and Bukowski, 2000). Behavioral ratings assess classmates' perceptions of children's behaviors (e.g., the Pupil Evaluation Inventory) (see above).
Direct observation	Observations can provide detailed, precise descriptions of behavior and behavior process.	Direct observations, solely or as a supplement to other information, can provide precise descriptions of the nature and extent of a problem. The focal child's behavior is of interest, and peer responses to a child can provide an index of the child's social difficulties.	The clinician needs access to school or other settings the child is in. Observations are extremely time and resource demanding, and are best compared with observations from other involved adults (e.g., teachers) to get a complete picture.	Structured (during a task) and unstructured (during free times) observations can be made. No standard protocols exist for observations, but are based on practitioner experience, the nature of the child's difficulty, available resources, and time and individuals available.

REFERENCES

Achenbach TM, Edelbrock CS: Manual for the ASEBA School-Age Forms and Profiles. Burlington, VT, Research Center for Children, Youth, and Families; University of Vermont, 2001.

Bierman KL: Peer Rejection: Developmental Processes and Intervention Strategies. New York, Guilford, 2004.

Cillessen AHN, Bukowski WM: Recent Advances in the Measurement of Acceptance and Rejection in the Peer System. San Francisco, Jossey-Bass, 2000.

Crick NR, Bigbee MA: Relational and overt forms of peer victimization: A multi-informant approach. J Consult Clin Psychol 66:337-347, 1998.

Deater-Deckard K: Annotation: Recent research examining the role of peer relationships in the development of psychopathology. J Child Psychol Psychiatry 5:565-579, 2001.

Hawker DS, Boulton MJ: Twenty years' research on peer victimization and psychosocial adjustment: A meta-analytic review of cross-sectional studies. J Child Psychol Psychiatry 41:441-455, 2000.

Hightower AD, Work WC, Cowen EL, et al: The teacher-child rating scale: A brief objective measure of elementary children's school problem behaviors and competence. School Psychol Rev 15:393-409, 1986.

Ladd GW: Peer relationships and social competence during early and middle childhood. Annu Rev Psychol 50:333-359, 1999.

Malik NM, Furman W: Problems in children's peer relations: What can the clinician do? J Child Psychol Psychiatry 34:1303-1326, 1993.

Nansel TR, Overpeck M, Pilla RS, et al: Bullying behaviors among US youth: Prevalence and association with psychosocial adjustment. JAMA 285:2094-2100, 2001.

Newcomb AF, Bukowski WM, Patee L: Children's peer relations: A meta-analytic review of popular, rejected, neglected, controversial, and average sociometric status. Psychol Bull 113:99-128, 1993.

Olweus D: Bullying at school: What we know and what we can do. Cambridge, MA, Blackwell Publishers, 1993.

Parker JG, Asher SR: Friendship and friendship quality in middle childhood: Links with peer group acceptance and feelings of loneliness and social dissatisfaction. Dev Psychol 29:611-621, 1993.

Parkhurst JT, Asher SR: Peer rejection in middle school: Subgroup differences in behavior, loneliness, and interpersonal concerns. Dev Psychol 28:231-241, 1992.

Patterson CJ, Kupersmidt JB, Griesler PC: Children's perceptions of self and of relationships with others as a function of sociometric status. Child Dev 61:1335-1349, 1990.

Pekarik EG, Prinz RJ, Liebert DE, et al: The Pupil Evaluation Inventory. J Child Psychother 4:83-97, 1976.

Reinherz HZ, Gianconia RM, Hauf AMC, et al: General and specific childhood risk ractors for depression and drug disorders by early adulthood. J Am Acad Child Adolesc Psychiatry 39:223-231, 2000.

Rubin KH, Bukowski W, Parker JG: Peer interactions, relationships, and groups. *In* Damon W (ed): Handbook of Child Psychology, 5th ed, Vol 3. New York, Wiley, 1998, pp 619-700.

Storch EA, Masia-Warner C, Dent HC, Klein RG: Peer victimization and social anxiety in adolescence: A prospective study. Aggress Behav 31:437-452, 2006.

16 CHILDCARE

DANIEL MORAN

Vignette

At her 4-month checkup, Annie's parents brought up the question of whether it was appropriate to place her in childcare when her mother, Mirabel, returned to work the following month. They had hoped Annie's grandmother would have been able to help care for Annie, but her health is poor. The family is depending on a second income to help pay the mortgage and other expenses that have accumulated since Mirabel took maternity leave at 7 months. Mirabel admits she is distressed at the thought of leaving her child in the care of another, but is resigned to the idea and wants good advice regarding her options.

Preparing for parenthood begins for most families when they know they are pregnant. Giving birth to a child, taking the infant home from the hospital, and bonding with the infant during the first weeks of life are among the most rewarding and memorable experiences as a parent. One of many difficult decisions for a family involves the choice regarding childcare. Many parents struggle with the decision of placing the child in the care of another while one or both work. For many families, this is a financial necessity, but that does not make the decision easier. Parents question whether or not their child would be cared for appropriately, and if the decision to use childcare would have an adverse effect on their child's health, emotional well-being, or overall development.

TYPES OF NONMATERNAL CHILDCARE SETTINGS

The arrangements for childcare involve multiple factors. Childcare providers can be relatives or nonrelatives, and the settings include center-based and home-based programs in the child's own home or the home of a caregiver. The type of care being provided also varies and may include simple "babysitting," developmental interventions, or formal preacademic activities. Additionally, the nomenclature used to describe these childcare arrangements is not uniform. The terms *daycare, preschool, early childhood education, nursery school, Head Start,* and *developmental center* all can imply very different environments with a wide variation in staff education and programs offered.

Many children are exposed to a variety of childcare settings. It is common for a child to use part-time center-based childcare supplemented with nonmaternal relatives providing additional care. These variables complicate the understanding of how the quality of care and amount of time in childcare affect developmental outcomes within the context of a unique family environment.

Since 1985, the U.S. Census Bureau has been tracking childcare arrangements and providing statistics every 5 years. These data are collected from the Survey of Income and Program Participation. In the winter of 2002, the survey data indicated that for families with children younger than 5 years, approximately 62% had some form of regular childcare arrangements; 40% used relatives, and 35% used nonrelatives to provide care. Of families using nonrelatives, almost two thirds of the care was provided by organized facilities (i.e., daycare centers, preschool, or Head Start programs) (Table 16-1) (U.S. Census Bureau, 2002).

HISTORICAL PERSPECTIVE

Center-based childcare has its roots in the 19th century. These early experiences typically involved either children from socioeconomically disadvantaged families that were placed in such centers to provide enhanced stimulation and "appropriate child rearing" or a second group of children from wealthy families who sought increased instruction in the early years of life. Neither model gained wide acceptance, and both eventually faded from popular use until later in the 20th century (Caldwell, 1999).

Because of economic pressures owing to the lack of men in the labor force during World War II, women began working in the factories and other businesses, requiring them to seek other forms of childcare. Since that time, the number of children in nonmaternal childcare has steadily continued to increase. Between 1950 and 1980, the number of working women 25 to 34 years old nearly doubled. By 1998, more than 75% of all women in the same age group were in the workforce (Fullerton, 1999). Data from the U.S. Department of Labor in 2004 indicated that approximately 60% to 70% of women in the workforce had children 6 years old and younger, necessitating some form of out-of-home childcare or early childhood program (U.S. Department of Labor Bureau of Labor Statistics, 2005). The types of programs vary dramatically in terms of quality, affordability, and availability.

Table 16-1. Preschoolers (Birth to 5 Years Old) in Various Childcare Arrangements (Winter 2002)

Arrangement Type	Percent in Arrangement
In a regular arrangement	62.9
Relative care	40.2
Mother*	3.5
Father*	15.2
Sibling	2.5
Grandparent	22.7
Other relative	7.2
Nonrelative care	34.9
Organized facility	22.7
Home-based arrangement	13.8
No regular arrangement	37.2

*Reflects only the time for which the designated parent was either working or in school.
Note: Numbers of children in each type of arrangement may exceed the total because of children with multiple arrangements.
From U.S. Census Bureau, Demographics Survey Division: Survey of Income and Program Participation. 2002. Available at: http://www.sipp.census.gov/sipp.

DEBATE ON THE EFFECTS OF CHILDCARE ON CHILD DEVELOPMENTAL OUTCOMES

Against the backdrop of this dramatic increase in women entering the workforce, psychologists and others began to debate the effect nonmaternal childcare would have on a child's intellectual, emotional, and social development. Piaget, Bowlby, and others began pointing to the importance of a child's early years in shaping a child's emotional and intellectual future. Bowlby's work in the mid-20th century with institutionalized children seemed to suggest that children who were deprived of continuous access to their mothers would not have appropriate attachment and would suffer ill effects of emotional insecurity. Other researchers saw possibilities of early stimulation leading to enhanced cognitive development. These theories led to conflicting opinions on the value of nonmaternal childcare. One group advocated for the use of this form of childcare to promote better socialization, improve cognition, and enhance overall development. The opposing group suggested that the use of nonmaternal care would have deleterious effects on a child's attachment and overall emotional functioning.

In 1990, the National Academy Press published a review of the evidence available at that time regarding the effect of childcare on overall development (Hayes et al, 1990). As researchers became interested in the effects of nonmaternal childcare, data regarding these outcomes were often conflicting and confusing. Design limitations, not accounting for family differences, and variations in the childcare being studied were among the reasons why professionals, policymakers, and the public at large were confused.

NATIONAL INSTITUTE OF CHILD HEALTH AND HUMAN DEVELOPMENT STUDY

Beginning in 1991, the National Institute of Child Health and Human Development (NICHD) undertook a study to address some of the questions in this debate and to examine the relationship between children's development and their experience of childcare. The Study of Early Child Care and Youth Development is the most comprehensive study we have at this time and provides parents, pediatricians, policymakers, and other professionals with accurate research-based information about childcare and its effect on children's development. The goal of the study was to examine how differences in childcare experiences relate to children's social, emotional, intellectual, and language development, and to their physical health. It compared the development of children who were primarily in maternal care with children who spent much of their time in nonmaternal care, and detailed the association between many aspects of nonmaternal childcare (including ratings of quality, type of setting, and time spent in nonmaternal care) and children's developmental and behavioral outcomes. What is impressive about the study is that it includes significant amounts of assessment and data regarding the family environment and background. This information enables researchers, families, care providers, and policymakers to identify the net effect of childcare on various outcomes while correcting for family factors.

Study Design

Data from 1-month-old infants and their families were collected beginning in 1991. This multisite study included four phases, of which the third was concluded in 2004. The study population was diverse and included healthy children from a variety of backgrounds. Forty percent of children lived in families defined as poor or near-poor. Eighty-five percent of the children had mothers who were married or partnered. Approximately one quarter of the mothers had a high school degree or equivalent; a third had some college education. Minorities, of which half were black, constituted approximately one quarter of the children in the study group.

Childcare was defined in the study as any care provided on a regular basis by someone other than the child's mother. Children with less than 10 hours a week in nonmaternal childcare were considered to be in exclusive maternal care. Nonmaternal childcare was defined to include care from a father or other relative; care from one caregiver in the child's home; home-based, small-group childcare; and center-based childcare. The outcome variables, including cognitive/language development, social behavior, emotional development/maternal-child interaction, and health indicators, were correlated to the quality and quantity of childcare (National Institute of Child Health and Human Development Early Child Care Research Network, 2005).

Quality of childcare was evaluated on two levels. The first was what researchers described as "regulable" characteristics (i.e., adult-to-child ratio, training of caregiver, group size), and the second encompassed "process" features based on direct observation of childcare workers' positive caregiving behavior. Specifically, researchers observed for the frequency of positive physical contact, response to vocalizations, amount of positive communication with the child, encouragement of developmental progress, and lack of negative interaction. The researchers found that the more positive regulable features in a childcare setting, the more likely the settings were to have positive process features. These two aspects of childcare settings were used to define the "quality" of the childcare.

Overall, the study found that only 9% of children in childcare settings receive "a lot" of positive caregiving, 30% receive a "fair" amount positive caregiving, 53% receive some positive caregiving and 8% receive hardly any positive care giving. According to these estimates, most U.S. children are in childcare settings that would be considered somewhere between "poor" and "good." Less than 10% of the arrangements can be considered as providing very high quality childcare (i.e., optimal regulable features and frequent positive childcare experiences), and less than 10% of children are in circumstances deemed to be very low quality settings.

Outcomes of Cognitive and Language Development

School readiness and overall cognitive outcomes provide persuasive evidence to advocate for high-quality childcare. Before the NICHD study, there were numerous reports showing the positive effect on language skills for children who attended high-quality childcare centers (Roberts et al, 1989) and overall later success in school (Peisner-Feinberg and Burchinal, 1997). The positive effects of high-quality childcare on later measures of cognitive ability and school performance show persistence throughout childhood and adolescence. This evidence is often stronger for lower income families and mothers with lower levels of education (Caughy et al, 1994). The consistency of the evidence supporting early quality care and later cognitive and language success for children at risk for developmental disabilities is remarkable and fully documented in an Institute of Medicine–sponsored study (Shonkoff and Phillips, 2000).

In the NICHD study, benefits of better care were noted for all levels of income. Children who received higher quality childcare were found to have slightly better cognitive function and language development during the first 3 years of life. In childcare settings where there was more language-based stimulation, such as asking more questions and responding to vocalizations in general, the child's cognitive and language development seemed slightly better. Children who received higher quality childcare did better on standardized tests of early literacy, number skills, and other kindergarten readiness tasks. The quantity of time spent in childcare was not associated with differences in cognitive or language development.

Analyses of the data collected regarding cognitive and language development indicated that the variance in these outcomes, although related to the quality of care, is accounted for more by difference in a child's gender and family variables. It is difficult to determine whether more advantaged families, who presumably tended to select higher quality childcare, are themselves providing the environment that favors better cognitive and language development. Arguments could be made that children who spend more time in center care may have more advantages in language development because of the variety of language models, greater exposure to same-age peers, and the likely greater need to use language to have their needs met. What seems to be central for achieving optimal language functioning is an environment that includes responsive and sensitive caregiving.

Outcomes Related to Social Behavior

Before the NICHD study, large sample studies had indicated a relationship between the timing and quantity of childcare and what some may consider as indicators of maladjustment or problematic behavior. Many of the earlier studies had not taken into account selection effects that would bias the data regarding the net effect of childcare experience (Phillips et al, 1987). Families who use early childcare may differ in significant ways from families who do not and account for the findings. The lack of a comprehensive approach that included rigorous assessment of quality of childcare and enhanced understanding of family factors contributed to confusion regarding behavioral outcomes.

In studying the associations regarding childcare features and social behaviors, the researchers found that family features were more strongly predictive of children's social development and problematic behaviors than either the quality or the quantity of childcare. Children who participated in higher quality childcare tended to be more cooperative, exhibited less disobedience and aggression at 2 to 3 years of age, and displayed more positive interaction with peers at 3 years of age. Children who spent on average more than 30 hours in childcare for the first 4½ years were more likely to show problematic behaviors in kindergarten according to caregiver reports. More aggression and disobedience were noted by caregivers in children who spent more time in childcare.

Outcomes Related to Emotional Development and Maternal Interaction

The NICHD findings showed an increased risk for insecure attachment for children whose mothers showed decreased levels of sensitivity and who spent more than 10 hours in childcare. The study indicated that mothers of children younger than 3 years across all ethnic groups who spent more time in daycare showed lower levels of sensitivity in their interactions with their child. This association did not persist after 3 years of age for nonwhite families. That is, black and Hispanic mothers whose children spent more time in childcare tended to display increased levels of sensitivity to their child. Higher quality childcare was positively associated with higher levels of maternal sensitivity.

Outcomes Related to Health and Communicable Diseases

Children in the study who spent more time in childcare were slightly more likely to have an ear infection and complained more frequently of gastrointestinal symptoms. The quality of childcare did not reliably predict health outcomes. This situation may be due to minimum regulatory standards for out-of-home childcare.

Table 16-2. **Checklist for Childcare Center Evaluation**

Aspect of Childcare	Evaluation Criteria
Staff-to-child ratio and group size	
For center-based childcare	
Birth-12 mo	1:3 with groups ≤6
13-30 mo	1:4 with groups ≤8
31-35 mo	1:5 with groups ≤10
3 yr	1:7 with groups ≤14
4-5 yr	1:8 with groups ≤16
Family childcare	If there are no children <2 yr: 1 adult/6 children; when there is 1 child <2 y: 1 adult/4 children; and when there are 2 children <2 y (the maximum), no other children are recommended
Director and staff experience and training	College degrees in early childhood education Child development associate's credential Ongoing in-service training Parent's first-hand observations of care Low turnover rate
Infection control	Hand washing with soap and running water after diapering, before handling food, and when contaminated by body fluids Children wash hands after toileting and before eating Routinely cleaned facilities, toys, equipment Up-to-date immunizations of staff and children
Emergency procedures	Written policies All staff and children familiar with procedures Up-to-date parent contact lists
Injury prevention	Play equipment safe, including proper shock-absorbing materials under climbing toys Universal Back-to-Sleep practices Developmentally appropriate toys and equipment Toxins out of reach Safe administration of medicines

Adapted from Committee on Early Childhood, Adoption, and Dependent Care: Quality early education and child care from birth to kindergarten. Pediatrics 115:187-191, 2005.

Summary of the National Institute of Child Health and Human Development Study

The results of this landmark study provide a significant dataset regarding choice of daycare arrangements, advocacy for childcare financing, and future research. A clear theme that emerged from this study is that the quality of the childcare in terms of regulable factors is associated with a higher quality experience for the child, which is associated with better developmental outcomes (National Institute of Child Health and Human Development Early Child Care Research Network, 2002).

PRACTICAL ASPECTS OF CHILDCARE FOR PARENTS AND PEDIATRIC PROVIDERS

Childcare can easily cost an average of $4000 to $6000 per year and can reach more than $10,000 a year depending on the geographic location and age of the child (Schulman, 2000). Besides direct costs, there are indirect costs, such as transportation and increased medical expenditures, and many families face childcare expenses for more than one child. There is an additional burden of expenses for a working parent, such as clothing, transportation, and meals outside the home. Pediatricians and other primary care providers are in a unique position to advise families regarding their childcare options. Besides helping them determine whether or not to pursue nonmaternal childcare, pediatricians can provide key advice to families regarding how to choose an appropriate childcare setting.

The American Academy of Pediatrics (AAP) for many decades has provided strong advocacy and leadership in this area. The AAP has partnered with many other key agencies to provide checklists for families, childcare providers, and regulatory agencies regarding high-quality childcare characteristics. Zero to Three: National Center for Infants, Toddlers and Families is another source of reliable information regarding choices in childcare for professionals and parents. Publications such as *Caring for Your Baby and Young Child: Birth to Age 5* and *Caring for Our Children* from the AAP provide excellent general resources for families and professionals. In addition, the AAP and Zero to Three have publications aimed at more specific aspects of childcare, including infection control, safety measures, and aspects of policy making and advocacy. The AAP and Zero To Three programs can be reached at the following addresses:

American Academy of Pediatrics, 141 Northwest Point Boulevard, Elk Grove Village, IL 60007-1098 (www.aap.org)

Zero to Three National Center for Infants, Toddlers and Families, 2000 M Street NW, Suite 200, Washington, DC 20036 (www.zerotothree.org)

Table 16-2 summarizes the key areas to evaluate when choosing outside childcare. Adult-to-child ratio

Table 16-3. Pediatric Provider Roles in Childcare Settings

Providing advice regarding urgent health problem management
Offering guidance on managing children with special health care needs
Ensuring that each child has a medical home
Identifying authoritative sources of health information and services related to sanitation, immunization, first aid, infection control, staff health questions
Linking early childhood programs with other health professionals and services
Mediating disputes about program procedures among health professionals who give advice to the program
Training staff on health issues and identifying health training resources
Consulting on the development of health education programs for children and parents
Setting up routine health and safety surveillance
Establishing and periodically reviewing written health policies and procedures

and overall group size are key aspects in assessing the quality of care being provided. The younger the child, the smaller the ratio and overall group size should be. Childcare provider training and education give some indication about the quality of the setting. Minimal standards are post–high school training including certification in child development, early childhood education, or related fields. A college degree in one of these areas is ideal. Accreditation by national standards and license/certification by local governments should be assessed. Lastly, overall health characteristics should be examined, including infection control measures, readiness for emergencies, and injury prevention strategies.

The National Association for the Education of Young Children is an organization that has been advocating for the quality of early childhood education since 1926. More than 20 years ago, they established a voluntary system of accreditation with rigorous standards set in 10 different areas to help individual childcare centers insure quality care. Pediatricians should make families aware of this certification when counseling parents regarding out-of-home childcare. Programs seeking this highly regarded accreditation must meet standards that go well beyond state health and safety licensing requirements. Most children who are in nonmaternal childcare are in settings without this accreditation (National Association of the Education of Young Children, 2007). In addition to advising families, pediatricians can provide significant support to childcare providers. Table 16-3 outlines possible roles for pediatric providers to childcare centers.

SUMMARY

Children who experience poor quality care, whether in a childcare center or within their own home, are more likely to have significant difficulties with their overall development and performance in school. These early environments and experiences shape brain function, intelligence, and personality, and are critical to an individual's outcome. High-quality childcare, including responsive caregivers, enriched environments, and stable patterns of caregiving, are positively associated with good developmental outcomes. Pediatric providers are a key source of information and guidance to individual families and childcare center providers.

REFERENCES

Caldwell BM: Child care. *In* Levine MD, Carey WB, Crocker AC (eds): Developmental and Behavioral Pediatrics, 3rd ed. Philadelphia, WB Saunders, 1999, pp 201-208.

Caughy M, DiPietro JA, Strobino DM: Day care participation as a protective factor in the cognitive development of low income children. Child Dev 65:457-471, 1994.

Committee on Early Childhood, Adoption, and Dependent Care: Quality early education and child care from birth to kindergarten. Pediatrics 115:187-191, 2005.

Fullerton HN: Labor force participation: 75 years of change, 1950-98 and 1998-2025. Monthly Labor Review 122:3-5, 1999.

Hayes CD, Palmer JL, Zaslow MJ (eds): Who Cares for America's Children? Washington, DC, National Academy Press, 1990.

National Institute of Child Health and Human Development Early Child Care Research Network: Child care structure → process → outcome: Direct and indirect effects of child care quality on young children's development. Psychol Sci 13:199-206, 2002.

National Institute of Child Health and Human Development Early Child Care Research Network: Childcare and Child Development: Results from the NICHD Study of Early Child Care and Youth Development. New York, Guilford Press, 2005.

National Association of the Education of Young Children. 2007. Available at: http://www.naeyc.org/accreditation/.

Peisner-Feinberg E, Burchinal M: Concurrent relations between childcare quality and child outcomes: The study of cost, quality, and outcomes and child care center. Merritt-Palmer Q 43:451-477, 1997.

Phillips D, McCartney D, Scarr S, et al: Selective review of infant daycare research: A cause for concern. Zero to Three 7:18-21, 1987.

Roberts JE, Rabinowitch S, Bryant DM, Burchinal MR: Language skills of children with different preschool experiences. J Speech Hearing Res 32:773-786, 1989.

Schulman K: The High Cost of Child Care Puts Quality Care Out of Reach for Many Families. Washington, DC, Children's Defense Fund, 2000.

Shonkoff JP, Phillips DA (eds): From Neurons to Neighborhoods: The Science of Early Childhood Development. Washington, DC, National Academy Press, 2000.

U.S. Census Bureau, Demographics Survey Division: Survey of Income and Program Participation. 2002. Available at: http://www.sipp.census.gov/sipp.

U.S. Department of Labor Bureau of Labor Statistics: Women in the Labor Force: A Databook. 2005. Available at: http://www.bls.gov/cps/wlf-databook2005.htm.

17 SCHOOLS AS MILIEU

PAUL H. DWORKIN

Vignette

D.B. is a 10-year-old boy with a long-standing history of behavioral and learning problems. During the preschool years, his grandmother described him as "never sitting still, being constantly on the move, and being into everything." She also noted that D.B.'s early speech and language development "seemed slow." Since beginning elementary school, D.B. has had difficulty staying on task, completing his school work, and following the rules of the classroom and school. Results of school-based psychoeducational assessment at age 6 years included a full scale IQ of 86 (97 verbal; 78 performance) and academic delays in language arts (writing, spelling) and arithmetic. Components of his school plan have included paraprofessional support within the classroom and 3 hours per week of educational support in a resource room. He also has received community-based and school-based counseling. D.B. was begun on methylphenidate at age 6 years for attention-deficit/hyperactivity disorder.

Within recent years, D.B. has become more aggressive, often touching and hitting other children. His grandmother is worried that he has difficulty controlling his anger. He also has been reprimanded for stealing money at home and taking another student's calculator. He continues to struggle with writing and math.

D.B. has been cared for by his grandmother since infancy. D.B.'s birth history is noteworthy for maternal substance abuse, prematurity, respiratory distress, and jaundice. D.B. has mild, intermittent asthma. Despite her own chronic health problems, D.B.'s grandmother also cares for his two older sisters and periodically serves as a foster parent for children in protective custody. She acknowledges concerns with neighborhood safety and is fearful of allowing D.B. to play outside.

D.B.'s grandmother describes his inner-city school as old, in poor repair, and very crowded. She reports that teachers do not supervise students adequately, especially during lunch and recess. She is concerned with D.B.'s exposure to the large number of students with behavioral difficulties. She questions the influence of D.B.'s school on his learning and behavioral problems, and wonders whether she should request a transfer to another school, either within or beyond their school district.

The influence of where students learn on their school performance and academic achievement is a complex, controversial, politically charged issue. In the civil rights era of the 1960s and 1970s, concerns with schools in the United States focused on issues of equality and community inclusion, as expectations for racial integration and the mainstreaming of children with disabilities in the least restrictive educational environments influenced school planning and design. School boards debated the merits of such interventions as magnet schools, busing, and redistricting to promote integration, and struggled to locate and commit the resources needed to support children with special needs within the regular classroom.

In 1983, the publication of a report, *A Nation at Risk: The Imperative for Educational Reform* by the National Commission on Excellence in Education, called for a shift in emphasis of U.S. educational systems to improved academic achievement. In calling for higher standards to prepare U.S. students for the demands of the 21st century and the challenges of a global economy, the report triggered numerous reform initiatives with a focus on assessment, academic standards, and accountability. This focus culminated in the passage of the No Child Left Behind (NCLB) Act of 2001, a reauthorization of the Elementary and Secondary School Act first passed in 1965, which codified expectations for educational excellence and school accountability, while triggering an impassioned, national debate on such issues as charter schools, vouchers and parental choice, teacher qualifications and training, school finance, and valid indicators of academic achievement.

Clinicians are mindful of the extent to which a child's classroom performance is influenced by a complex interaction of child-related, family-related, and school-related factors. Despite their importance, a child's strengths and weaknesses should not be considered in isolation, but rather within the context of social and environmental circumstances. Any assessment of a child's classroom performance must consider the impact of the child's family, neighborhood, and school. Although psychosocial factors are often considered in the evaluation of a child's school functioning, characteristics of the school and classroom generally do not receive much attention. Characteristics of the specific school that a child attends seem to have a significant effect on academic achievement and classroom behavior. The school potentially can assume important roles in the prevention and the early identification of childhood maladjustment and behavioral problems. In the vignette, D.B.'s grandmother is justified in questioning the impact of his classroom and school on his performance and considering a change in school placement.

This chapter reviews school-related influences on classroom performance. School-related factors to be discussed include school resources (physical and administrative features) and characteristics of school processes. The impact of schools on disadvantaged, minority students also is emphasized. The relationships between school effectiveness and student achievement are vital considerations, whether the focus in on the performance of an individual student or on such debated public policies as the merits of student vouchers or the morning start time for beginning instruction in high schools. Yet evidence from sound, educational research is sparse. In the educational setting, teachers and students cannot be randomly assigned to different teaching methods, learning environments, and supplemental resources. Nonetheless, decades of research suggest how characteristics of schools affect learning and may inform clinical practice and advocacy.

HISTORICAL CONSIDERATIONS

The extent to which the specific school that a child attends influences classroom performance has been the subject of controversy for at least 5 decades. A survey done by Coleman and colleagues (1966) of some 645,000 students in 4000 elementary and secondary schools contributed to the belief in the 1960s that schools made very little difference. In the early 1970s, Jencks and coworkers (1972) reassessed the same data and similarly concluded that variables such as average expenditure per pupil, the number of books in the library, and the teacher-to-pupil ratio account for little of the variation among students on achievement measures. In contrast, a series of cross-sectional studies performed in the late 1970s concluded that the school a child attends can have a major impact on classroom performance, and that the type of school attended may be particularly consequential for less able students (Brookover et al, 1979; Halsey et al, 1980; Madaus et al, 1979).

The contradictory conclusions derived from such studies can be explained by methodologic differences. The earlier studies that concluded that schools exert little influence on student performance relied on limited measures of academic attainment, mainly students' verbal abilities. These surveys examined a very narrow range of school variables, primarily resources such as the number of books in the library or the number of pupils per teacher. Finally, such studies evaluated how improvements in schools would make children more alike—that is, reduce inequalities in attainment among students, rather than the more realistic goal of raising children's overall level of attainment (Rutter, 1983).

The later studies of the 1970s that suggested that schools do matter tended to overcome such methodologic deficiencies. To assess more fully the impact of schools on children, these studies examined features of schools such as process and organizational structure (see later). Researchers emphasized indicators of school effectiveness such as classroom behavior, learning attitudes, and social functioning. Despite such improvements in design, these studies were cross-sectional rather than longitudinal, and the conclusions rendered were only tentative (Rutter, 1980).

During the 1970s, a classic, well-designed, prospective study of schools within inner-city London effectively addressed methodologic limitations of earlier research and conclusively showed that "schools do indeed have an important impact ... and it does matter which school a child attends" (Rutter et al, 1979). The study involved two main stages. During the first stage, some 1500 children in one inner London borough were assessed at age 10 years (just before transferring to secondary school). Children were reassessed at age 14 years and again when leaving school to determine whether their behavior and educational progress varied according to the school attended. Results revealed large, important differences among schools in outcomes such as scores on national examinations, pupil behavior, school attendance, and delinquency rates (Rutter, 1980). Such differences were not accounted for by differences among students at the time of entry to the various schools.

The second stage of the study examined the impact of various school features on student outcome. Twelve secondary schools serving children from age 11 years onward within a large area of inner London were studied in detail. Features of schools, including physical-administrative arrangements and aspects of school processes, such as teachers' actions in lessons, were evaluated with regard to student outcome. Measures of student outcome included school behavior, school attendance, examination scores, delinquency rates, and, ultimately, occupational status. Data were gathered via a variety of strategies, including teacher interviews, pupil questionnaires, time-and-event sampled observations, and recordings made in corridors and playgrounds. In addition to showing that schools do strongly influence student outcome, results from this monumental study emphasize the greater importance of school processes compared with physical and administration features in fostering academic success and good student behavior. Subsequent research has emphasized, however, the extent to which the latter also are important in promoting students' success (Table 17-1).

PHYSICAL AND ADMINISTRATIVE FEATURES

Results from the inner London study suggest that school resources, as reflected by physical and administrative features, have a limited impact on student outcome. More recent research has emphasized, however, that characteristics of the facility do affect learning (Earthman and Lemasters, 1998).

Table 17-1. Strength of Evidence for Influence of Various School Characteristics on Student Academic Performance and Behavior

Strong Evidence for Influence
Quality of teacher-student relationship
Academic emphasis
Teachers' actions in lessons
Joint curriculum planning by school staff
General guidelines for rewards and discipline
Student and parent access to teachers, classroom, and school
Clean, tidy, attractive classrooms
Opportunity for student involvement and responsibility
Moderate Evidence for Influence
Avoidance of high student density and overcrowding
Safe, modern, well-maintained buildings
Strong, supportive teacher-student relationships
Peer group stability and achievement
Modest Evidence for Influence
Average expenditure per student
Number of books in library
Teacher-to-student ratio
Administrative autonomy (e.g., charter school)
Public or private ownership
Student instructional grouping by ability
Extent of extracurricular activities
Teacher stability

Administrative Arrangements

In the London study, whether schools were voluntary-aided (i.e., church-affiliated) or public (maintained by the local education authority) did not significantly influence student outcome. Although the greater autonomy afforded the voluntary-aided schools tended to result in slightly better outcomes, the considerable overlap in findings between the two types of schools resulted in differences that did not reach statistical significance. A more recent example is the establishment of charter schools, developed by members of the community and open to all students and receiving tax dollars based on per pupil enrollment. Such schools typically receive waivers from many legislative mandates and have greater administrative autonomy than public schools. There is little evidence to support the benefit of this model of school organization and management in meeting mandated educational standards (Miron, 2005).

Size and Space

The London study found that the size of the school and class size or overcrowding had no consistent association with student success, suggesting that it is at least possible for a school to be successful despite having fairly large classes and being overcrowded. From a practical standpoint, spacious buildings should not be regarded as a prerequisite for student success. Marginal reductions in class size from 30 to 25 students may be less worthwhile than using available funds to create much smaller remedial classes for children with special educational needs. In contrast, other research has suggested that high student density contributes to dissatisfaction, decreased social interaction, and increased student aggression (Weinstein, 1979). More recent research has shown that high student density is a significant predictor of task inattention, and overcrowding has a negative impact on student achievement in poorer school districts (Earthman and Lemasters, 1998).

Age and Condition of Buildings

Although the London study found that the age of school buildings did not seem to influence student outcome, more recent research suggests that old and obsolete buildings have a negative effect on student learning, and that safe, modern, controlled environments enhance learning (McGuffrey, 1982). Building age is likely a surrogate for such characteristics as the condition of the building, thermal control, proper lighting, acoustics, laboratory conditions, and overall aesthetics (Earthman and Lemasters, 1998). Studies suggest that students' performance is facilitated by a thermal-controlled environment, good quality lighting, attractive interior painting, avoidance of extreme unwanted noise, and properly maintained facilities (McGuffrey, 1982). Studies report higher academic achievement in newer facilities and fewer discipline problems and better attendance records (Lemasters, 1997). Factors such as better science laboratories, air-conditioned schools, pastel painted walls, less external noise, daylight in the classroom, and full-spectrum lighting with ultraviolet content correlate with measures of student performance.

Staff Provision

As previously noted, class size and the pupil-to-teacher ratio had no significant effect on student outcome within the London study. The variations among schools in pupil-to-teacher ratio (14 to 16 pupils to 1 teacher) and class size (22 to 30 students) were quite small, however. These results should not be viewed as arguing against very small classes (when feasible) or allowing large classes. Findings do suggest, however, that limited financial resources may not be best spent to improve staff provisions only modestly.

Internal Organization

In the London study, the manner in which children were grouped for teaching purposes did not influence student outcome. Whether students were placed in different tracks according to ability or taught within classes for children of differing abilities failed to affect school performance. Whether students were grouped in different grades according to age, or whether children of various ages were housed together also had no influence on outcomes.

Teachers frequently use ability grouping in the classroom with the belief that it is an effective means of promoting academic achievement. Although this is particularly common in reading, it also may be used for other subjects, such as writing, mathematics, and science. Little large-scale quantitative research has addressed this issue. Grouping may have different impacts on children of different abilities. Students of low ability may benefit from exposure to children with heterogeneous ability levels, whereas children of average ability may perform better with children of more homogeneous ability (Saleh et al, 2005).

SCHOOL PROCESSES

In contrast to the limited impact of the physical and administrative features of schools, aspects of the social organization of school life, referred to as *school processes,* have important associations with school outcome. Such processes "... create the context for teaching and learning, and seem likely to affect the nature of the school experience for both staff and pupils" (Rutter et al, 1979).

Academic Emphasis

Children's progress academically and behaviorally is favorably influenced by an appropriate emphasis on academic issues. Such an emphasis may be reflected in the frequent assignment of homework; high teacher expectations for students' academic achievement; the display of children's work on classroom walls; total teaching time per week; a high rate of students' use of the school library; and group (as opposed to individual teacher) planning of courses and lessons, with monitoring and advice provided by department heads.

Teachers' Actions in Lessons

The behavior of teachers has an important influence on student behavior and academic attainment. Pupil behavior is better in schools in which teachers spend more time on the subject matter of the lesson, as opposed to organizing or disciplining the class or distributing material. A higher proportion of teacher time spent with the whole class, as opposed to individual pupils, correlates with better outcomes in attendance, behavior, and academic achievement. Similarly, the prompt starting of lessons is found to correlate with better student behavior. In contrast, children display worse behavior in schools characterized by frequent disciplinary interventions in the classroom.

Rewards and Punishments

Academic and behavioral outcomes seem to be improved when general standards for classroom discipline are set by the school, as opposed to being left to individual teachers. High levels of corporal punishment tend to be associated with worse pupil behavior, as is teachers' use of physical punishment such as slaps. Results from the London study suggest that the establishment of general disciplinary guidelines within the school promote better pupil behavior, less delinquency, and greater success in academic achievement. Pupil behavior seems to be more favorably influenced by quiet reprimands.

Rewards and praise favorably influence outcome. Behavioral outcomes are better in schools in which teachers more often praise students' work within the classroom and publicly commend individual pupils during assemblies and other group meetings.

Pupil Conditions

As previously discussed, the extent to which schools provide a pleasant and comfortable environment for students does seem to influence student outcome. In the London study, clean and tidy, well-decorated classrooms were associated with better student behavior. Features such as the freedom to use the school buildings during breaks and the lunch period, student access to a telephone, and the availability of hot drinks were associated with greater success on examinations. A better behavioral outcome was seen when teachers expressed a willingness to see children at any time, as opposed to only at fixed times, about a problem. Similarly, better attendance and academic achievement were seen in schools in which students expressed a willingness to discuss personal problems with a staff member. In contrast, the extent of extracurricular activities did not have an effect on whether schools had good or poor outcomes.

Responsibilities and Participation

Encouraging students to assume responsibility for their actions seems to influence outcome favorably. Schools in which students are expected to assume responsibility for their own materials (e.g., books, folders, writing materials) have better outcomes for pupil attendance and behavior. Behavior and academic achievement are better among schools in which a greater proportion of pupils hold positions of responsibility, such as homework monitor, and more students actively participate in assemblies. Similarly, better student behavior is found in schools in which pupils are involved in the process of improving school effectiveness (Furtwengler, 1985). Such findings suggest the benefits of ensuring that a high proportion of students are afforded opportunities including assuming positions of responsibility and participating in group activities.

Stability of Teaching and Friendship Groups

In the London study, teacher continuity was not found to be associated with academic outcome. In contrast, schools with greater peer group stability were found to have lower rates of delinquency, as were schools in which children had met many friends outside of their class. Although such findings defy simple explanation, an undue emphasis by schools on maintaining teacher stability to promote academic success may not be justified. Subsequent research has confirmed the significant influence of peer group affiliation on academic performance (Lee et al, 1993). Peer interactions within and outside of the classroom foster a climate characterized as nonacademic or antiacademic, and the amount of time spent with peers has a significant negative impact on achievement. Regardless of their own ability level, students who affiliate with low-achieving peers have significantly lower achievement scores than students who affiliate with high-achieving peers. Despite the importance of peer group membership for educational outcomes, it is often overlooked during the assessment process. Support and counseling should consider peer group membership during the monitoring of student academic and behavioral performance.

Staff Organization

A complex interaction of external and internal factors influences educational curriculum, policies, and procedures. Examples of such external influences include familial, cultural, economic, political, and religious sources. Internal sources of influence include school boards and administrators and teachers. As previously suggested, aspects of staff organization seem to influence student outcome. The London study found that schools in which there was joint planning of courses and curriculum by the school staff, monitoring of teachers' assignments of homework, and active involvement of the senior staff in decision making had better academic and behavioral outcomes.

Many school systems have modified their organization and management procedures to create a milieu that better meets the needs of teachers, students, and families. Site-based management allows individual schools to develop their own policy and procedures for school governance and enables teachers to select professional development programs and have significant control in making school-based decisions. Middle schools have been organized in an effort to focus better on the unique developmental needs of early adolescents than the traditional junior high school. The integration of children with developmental disabilities and special needs into general classrooms with special education support services is believed to be beneficial to all students. Charter schools have been developed by members of the community to meet the needs of groups of students better. Although such schools receive public tax dollars based on per-pupil enrollment, they receive relief from many legislated mandates to enable teachers and administrators freedom in the design of curriculum and experiences. Limited research evidence suggests the importance of states exercising rigor in approving such schools to operate and in overseeing such schools in fostering academic success as measured by standardized achievement tests (Miron, 2005).

SPECIAL CONSIDERATIONS FOR DISADVANTAGED STUDENTS

Characteristics of schools attended by minority and low socioeconomic status students may be particularly important in promoting resiliency and fostering success. Generally, studies suggest that minority students from low socioeconomic status backgrounds and circumstances are exposed to greater risks and fewer resilience-promoting conditions than white students, placing such children in "double jeopardy" for poor outcomes (Borman and Rachuba, 2000). The most powerful school models for promoting the resiliency of disadvantaged children are those that actively shield children from adversity and develop strong and supportive teacher-student relationships. Studies also cite the importance of schools fostering the healthy social and personal adjustment of students, the so-called communitarian model of school organization. Such characteristics may be particularly important as families and neighborhoods become less stable and supportive (Phillips, 1997). Schools that are attentive to the psychosocial adjustment and engagement of academically at-risk students and that include initiatives to shield children actively from the risks and adversities within their homes, schools, and communities are more likely to enhance resiliency and promote academic success.

IMPLICATIONS FOR ADVOCACY

The powerful influence of schools on student performance and success has important implications for pediatric advocacy. For children experiencing school dysfunction, a child's capabilities and weaknesses should not be considered in isolation, but rather within the context of his or her environment at home and at school. Pediatricians should ensure that psychological, educational, and developmental assessments are not considered independently, but rather that findings are interpreted within the context of the setting in which the student must function. Given the limited impact of physical and administrative features on student outcomes, the pediatrician can suggest caution in attributing a student's poor performance to factors such as a large class size or old school buildings. In contrast, the pediatrician may support transfer requests when, as in the case of D.B. from the vignette, school or classroom factors may seen as contributing to performance problems.

Pediatricians can assume potentially important roles in offering support and guidance to schools, boards of education, and parent groups. Pediatricians' input can be sought in the implementation of various school policies, such as morning start times for high school students. Familiarity with the organization of schools, including the administrative, financial, power, authority, and formal and informal communication structures, should enable the pediatrician to advocate more effectively for developmentally appropriate policies. Knowledge of the importance of school process should enable the pediatrician to encourage the implementation of policies favoring appropriate academic emphasis and liberal use of rewards and discouraging the use of frequent punishments. Limited school resources may better be committed to creating small remedial classes for children with special needs, as opposed to marginally, and probably insignificantly, reducing class size for students in general.

Advocacy of pediatricians should extend to support for programs designed to prevent student maladjustment (Weissberg et al, 1983). As an influential member of the community committed to the prevention of childhood dysfunction, the pediatrician can be particularly effective in advocating for cost-effective primary and secondary prevention programs. The pediatrician's familiarity with local resources, scientific credibility, and intimate knowledge of the consequences of longstanding dysfunction can influence decisions regarding program implementation by school boards.

SUMMARY

The influence of the school environment on student performance is complex and controversial. Characteristics of the school that a child attends likely have a significant effect on academic achievement and classroom behavior. Limited research suggests that school processes, such as academic emphasis, opportunities for student involvement, and a focus on rewards rather than punishment, may be of greater importance than such physical and administrative features as the age of the school building, number of books in the library, and average expenditure per pupil. School characteristics may be particularly important in promoting the success of minority and low socioeconomic status students. Knowledge of the relationships between school effectiveness and school achievement has important implications for assessing and promoting individual student performance and public policy.

REFERENCES

Borman GD, Rachuba LT: The characteristics of schools and classrooms attended by successful minority students. Paper presented at the Annual Meeting of the American Educational Research Association, New Orleans, April 24-28, 2000.

Brookover W, Beady C, Hood P, et al: School Social Systems and Student Achievement: Schools Can Make a Difference. New York, Praeger, 1979.

Coleman JS, Campbell EQ, Hobson DJ, et al: Equality of Educational Opportunity. Washington, DC, U.S. Government Printing Office (Superintendent of Documents Catalogue No. FS 5.238:38 000), 1966.

Earthman GI, Lemasters L: Where children learn: A discussion of how a facility affects learning. Paper presented at the Annual Meeting of the Virginia Educational Facility Planners, Blacksburg, VA, February 23-24, 1998.

Furtwengler WJ: Implementing strategies for a school effectiveness program. Paper presented at the Annual Meeting of the American Association of School Administrators, Dallas, March 8-11, 1985.

Halsey AH, Health AF, Ridge GM: Origins and Destinations: Family, Class and Education in Modern Britain. Oxford, Clarendon, 1980.

Jencks C, Smith M, Acland H, et al: Inequality: A Reassessment of the Effect of Family and Schooling in America. New York, Basic Books, 1972.

Lee YE, Bryk AS, Smith JB: The organization of effective secondary schools. Rev Res Educ 19:171, 1993.

Lemasters LK: A Synthesis of Studies Pertaining to Facilities, Student Achievement, and Student Behavior. Doctoral dissertation. Blacksburg, VA, Virginia Polytechnic Institute and State University, 1997.

Madaus GF, Kellaghan T, Rakow EA, et al: The sensitivity of measures of school effectiveness. Harvard Educ Rev 49:207, 1979.

McGuffrey CW: Facilities. *In* Herbert W (ed): Improving Educational Standards and Productivity. Berkley, CA, McCutchan Publishing Corp, 1982, pp 237-288.

Miron G: Evaluating the Performance of Charter Schools in Connecticut. Kalamazoo, MI, The Evaluation Center, Western Michigan University, 2005.

National Commission on Excellence in Education: A Nation at Risk: The Imperative for Education Reform. Washington, DC, U.S. Department of Education, 1983.

Phillips M: What makes schools effective? A comparison of the relationships of communitarian climate and academic climate for mathematics achievement and attendance during middle school. Am Educ Res J 34:633, 1997.

Rutter M: School influences on children's behavior and development: The 1979 Kenneth Blackfan lecture. Children's Hospital Medical Center, Boston. Pediatrics 65:208, 1980.

Rutter M: School effects on pupil progress: Research findings and policy implications. Child Dev 54:1, 1983.

Rutter M, Maughan B, Mortimore P, et al: Fifteen Thousand Hours: Secondary Schools and Their Effects on Children. Cambridge, Harvard University Press, 1979.

Saleh M, Lazonder AW, De Jong T: Effects of within-class ability grouping on social interaction, achievement, and motivation. Instr Sci Int J Learn Cogn 33:105, 2005.

Weinstein CS: The physical environment of the school: A review of the research. Rev Educ Res 49:577, 1979.

Weissberg RP, Cowen EL, Lotyczewski BS, et al: The Primary Mental health Project: Seven consecutive years of program outcome research. J Consult Clin Psychol 51:100, 1983.

18 NEIGHBORHOOD AND COMMUNITY

LYNNE C. HUFFMAN AND PAUL H. WISE

DEFINING THE NEIGHBORHOOD

For children, the neighborhood is the relatively small environmental range and inherent relationships of home, school, and community that, together, determine the fabric of daily life. Although this sphere widens as children grow older and become more independent, this definition is intended to recognize the central importance of a child's functional environment in determining the material resources and human interaction so necessary to a child's health and social well-being.

In defining the neighborhood unit of analysis for research purposes, several options are available. These include census information and local knowledge of boundaries in cities, health districts, police districts, and school districts. Administrative data sources rely on bureaucratically defined units that vary across systems (health, education, law enforcement, social services) but tend to overlap to some extent. Such definitions of neighborhoods have primarily been limited to city or regional studies and often are used in conjunction with census data. More ethnographic accounts of neighborhoods emphasize the fact that individuals perceive boundaries differently. Some studies rely on participants' ratings of neighborhoods, and neighborhood boundaries usually are not specified. The predominance of research investigating neighborhood effects on child health has used census tract data. Tract boundaries are delineated with the advice of local communities working under Census Bureau guidelines and typically reflect prominent physical features that define neighborhoods (e.g., major streets, railroads) as well as important social and ethnic divisions.

NEIGHBORHOOD MECHANISMS OF EFFECT

The means by which neighborhood influences child health can take many forms; however, several models have been proposed. Most recently, Leventhal and Brooks-Gunn (2000) have suggested mechanisms that include the following (see also Chapter 19):

Institutional resources: the availability, accessibility, affordability, and quality of learning; social and recreational activities; childcare, schools, medical facilities, and employment opportunities present in the community.

Relationships: parental characteristics (mental health, irritability, coping skills, efficacy, and physical health); support networks available to parents; parental behavior (responsivity/warmth, harshness/control, and supervision/monitoring); and the quality and structure of the home environment.

Norms/collective efficacy: the extent to which community institutions exist to supervise and monitor the behavior of residents, particularly youths' activities (deviant and antisocial peer group behavior) and the presence of physical risk (violence and victimization and harmful substances) to children and youth. Collective efficacy includes mutual respect, institutional controls, neighborhood bonding, and perceived informal control.

Whether these mechanisms are brought into play and how they interact not only will vary according to the outcome in question but also will reflect crucial structural characteristics of neighborhoods, particularly *income and socioeconomic status* and *residential instability*. Accordingly, these dimensions are used to organize this chapter.

INCOME AND SOCIOECONOMIC STATUS: NEIGHBORHOOD POVERTY

Despite being a common focus of discussion and research, poverty has defied a single definition. In large measure, this lack of agreement reflects variation in the perceived origins of poverty and the intended use of the definition. Most often, for purposes of policy formulation and research, poverty is defined as a measure of subsistence: that level of resources that permits the maintenance of physical efficiency. Here, the measure of poverty is absolute, concerned with basics of food and shelter, and it changes only in response to changes in prices. An example of this absolute definition is the official "poverty line" for the United States, which is derived from the U.S. Department of Agriculture's estimate of food costs for a basic but nutritionally adequate diet. This figure is then multiplied by three, because studies indicated that at the time of the inception of the index several decades ago, a typical family spent approximately one third of its income on food. In 2006, the official poverty level for a family of four was $20,000 (ASPE, 2006).

In 1995, a special panel commissioned by the National Academy of Sciences recommended a different method for defining poverty (Citro and Michael, 1995). This poverty measure consisted of a budget for the three basic categories of food, clothing, and shelter (including utilities) and a small additional amount for other needs (e.g., household supplies, personal care, non–work-related transportation). Although a more refined method of determining poverty, this approach still was based on the determination of an absolute figure pegged to a set level of income or consumption. Some experts proposed changing the "absolute" measure to a "relative" one that assesses a poverty level on the basis of how a particular income relates to the general distribution of income and wealth in the rest of society (e.g., below the 10th percentile of all incomes). A different case was made for a "consumption" measure, by which spending on specific services, rather than income, is compared with a poverty threshold. Others stated that both income- and consumption-based measures are only indirect appraisals of the well-being of poor Americans, noting greater precision with measures of actual physical and emotional condition. Such "well-being" measures can track relevant indicators (e.g., health, food insecurity).

Efforts continue to identify alternative approaches for measuring the material well-being of low-income Americans. However, political and ideologic differences have made it difficult to reach agreement on reconceptualizing or reforming the measurement of poverty. Although the current federal poverty definition is widely acknowledged to have important flaws, it remains the basis for official poverty statistics and is widely used by public programs and policy deliberations to describe the level of material need in the United States.

Recent Trends in Childhood Poverty

Despite the common belief that childhood poverty has been a relatively stable phenomenon in American history, rates of childhood poverty are sensitive to economic and social trends. After 2 decades of falling poverty rates, there was a disturbing increase in the percentage of children living below the poverty line in the early 1980s, the rate climbing to more than 22% in 1983. In 1995, the portion of American children younger than 18 years and living in poverty remained more than one in five. This decreased to 17.6% in 2005 but remains the highest poverty rate among any age group in American society (U.S. Census Bureau, 2005).

The primary reasons for increases in childhood poverty are the demographic changes and decline in the earning power of the young American family. Children are more likely than in earlier periods to be raised in single-parent, female-headed households, which have a greater likelihood of being poor. In addition, real wages for young adults, particularly those with limited education, have decreased dramatically during the past 2 decades. For children, the alternative to the family for income distribution is the state. Here, too, support for children in families with insufficient earnings has deteriorated significantly. Between the mid-1970s and early 1990s, family benefits for the Aid to Families with Dependent Children (AFDC) program, the primary public mechanism dedicated to this purpose, when adjusted for inflation, declined by 40% (Brown, 1995). In 1996, however, the AFDC program was replaced by the Temporary Assistance for Needy Families (TANF) legislation; TANF was reauthorized in February 2006 under the Deficit Reduction Act of 2005. This program ended a poor child's entitlement to income support, embraced time limits for enrollment, and granted far more control over eligibility criteria, benefit levels, and oversight to individual states. Although the longer term impact of this legislation is unclear, the emphasis on state control has led to greater heterogeneity in the nature and adequacy of welfare programs across the United States.

Clinical Expression of Poverty

The clinical impact of poverty lies as much in its pervasiveness as it does in its deadening persistence. Children living in poverty experience elevated rates of developmental and medical problems and a greater likelihood that these problems will produce deleterious outcomes. This "double jeopardy" characterizes a number of disorders and represents a dual injustice; poverty distorts the promise of life by erecting biologic obstacles to health while at the same time sapping the social capacity to respond. The elements of this interaction are complex and remain poorly defined. However, several considerations are fundamental. Severe material deprivation lies at the heart of poverty's effects on child health. Even when material resources are sufficient under normal circumstances, reserves may not exist, making financial emergencies more frequent and more threatening. Stress factors are more common and found in multiplicity among poor families, and emotional supports may be inadequate for families isolated by their poverty and social alienation (Schor, 2003). Informational supports in the form of frequent access to community resources and referrals may be lacking in poor families. In addition, social support systems—a critical component of resilience—are weaker and more constrained for poor children and their families. Structural aspects of the neighborhood and the quality and breadth of school-based and non–school-based educational programs can also help determine the dimensions of the impact of poverty (Schinke, Cole, and Poulin, 2000). Together, material deprivation, heightened stress, reduced social supports, and debilitating neighborhood and school conditions can affect the full spectrum of childhood developmental needs, including stability, security, and the maintenance of a nurturing, stimulating home environment.

Childhood poverty has been linked to a variety of specific emotional, developmental, and health problems with both direct and indirect implications for child development and behavior. The influences of poverty can be viewed as elevating the likelihood of poor health by enhancing risk for poor health and reducing access to interventions that minimize the impact of elevated risk. Elevated risk can affect health by increasing the probability that an illness or traumatic event will occur and by increasing the severity with which the illness or injury affects the child. This can take the form of increased exposure or the suppression of protective factors. The effect of risk can be mediated by intervention. When there is capacity to alter the impact of risk, then disparities in access to this capacity can create inequities in outcomes. The essential element in this connection is efficacy; interventions without efficacy cannot cause differences in outcome irrespective of divergence in access. The interaction of elevated risk and reduced access is manifested in a variety of health conditions and defines, in tragic terms, the clinical expression of poverty.

Disparities in Mortality

The starkest manifestation of the impact of poverty on child health lies in its capacity to shape disparities in survival. From birth, poor children are at higher risk for death than are nonpoor children, although the dimensions of this disparity and the implications for clinical intervention vary considerably by age and cause of death.

Neonatal and Infant Mortality

Neonatal and infant mortality rates have long been recognized as sensitive indicators of social conditions. The influence of poverty on mortality during the neonatal period (<28 days) can take the form of elevated rates of low birth weight (<2500 g) or elevated rates of mortality among newborns of comparable birth weight groups (Reagan and Salsberry, 2005; Wise, 2003). The influence of poverty on birth weight distribution is modulated primarily by the health of the mother before and during pregnancy; maternal health reflects the adequacy of nutrition, age, parity, health-related behaviors (e.g., smoking, alcohol use, illicit drug use), and a range of social stresses. In addition to elevating the chance that an infant will be born at low birth weight, poverty can also increase the risk that an infant will die, even among neonates of comparable birth weights. This occurs primarily when poverty, often accompanied by inadequate health insurance coverage, affects access to tertiary care facilities. Studies show that death in the first year of life is at least 1.6 times more likely for infants of women living below the poverty level. For infants between the ages of 28 days and 1 year, the postneonatal period, the death rate doubles for infants of women living in poverty (DiLiberti, 2000). The effects of poverty in the postneonatal period (28 through 365 days of age) are expressed as increased deaths from infectious diseases, sudden infant death syndrome (SIDS), injuries, and serious sequelae of high-risk neonatal conditions. Recent efforts to educate parents about an infant's sleep position have been associated with major reductions in SIDS mortality. However, these absolute reductions have not reduced social inequalities in SIDS as these educational interventions have been more effective in relatively wealthier and better-educated populations (Pickett, Luo, and Laudale, 2005).

Mortality from Trauma

Trauma claims the life of more children than any other cause. Because the occurrence of life-threatening injury is so closely tied to the activities of daily life, the adequacy of social conditions plays an important role in shaping childhood patterns of trauma and resultant mortality. Neighborhood housing conditions can mediate trauma mortality in children, particularly those deaths not related to motor vehicle collisions (Shenassa, Stubbendick, and Brown, 2004). Poorer neighborhoods may be characterized by substandard and overcrowded housing, lack of safe recreational facilities for children, proximity of housing to busy streets, increased exposure to physical hazards, inability to purchase safety devices or to practice injury prevention measures, and limited access to health care. Other factors include fewer safe play areas, broken playground equipment, broken glass, drug activity, violence, access to firearms, limited organized sports activities or extracurricular activities, and less access to safe and affordable childcare. Primary prevention is particularly important for injury types of relatively high lethality, such as gunshot wounds, as even excellent medical care may not prevent death in many such cases (Marcin et al, 2003).

Fire

The majority of child deaths from fire are due to house fires, commonly related to parental cigarette smoking and inadequate housing and heating. In addition, demographic characteristics such as maternal education and age and number of other children in the household may influence the risk of childhood fire mortality (Scholer et al, 1998).

Motor Vehicle Casualties

Injury associated with the use of motor vehicles represents the largest contributor to traumatic mortality in childhood, affecting occupants of motor vehicles as well as pedestrians struck by motor vehicles. With some variation, particularly in some urban areas, motor vehicle occupant mortality rate is higher for children living in poverty. The reasons for this association have not been well defined. However, there appear to be significant social influences on the development of relevant health and risk-taking behaviors, including alcohol use. Pedestrian mortality is heavily influenced by social status. Because poor neighborhoods are often located in congested inner-city areas, the risk of pedestrian injury to children in this setting is likely to be elevated. The importance of the street as a play area and the lack of engineered barriers that separate children from motor vehicle thoroughfares contribute to the functional proximity of young children and moving vehicles, an association that guarantees high rates of pedestrian injury and death (Kim et al, 2007).

Homicide

Homicide is among the most important causes of death among American children. In some urban communities, homicide is the leading cause of injury-related mortality in children from birth through adolescence. The tragedy of homicide in children has defied clear understanding. However, its concentration in poor communities has been documented repeatedly (Friedman, Horwitz, and Resnick, 2005; Schnitzer and Ewigman, 2005). Child homicide can be grouped into four general categories, all of which reveal sharp social gradients:

1. neonaticide (children killed when they are neonates), when the mother is likely to be unmarried, to be adolescent, to have low socioeconomic status, and to reside with parents or other relatives;

2. infanticide (children killed during the first year of life), in which the homicide may be related to violent anger directed at the child by a caregiver in response to persistent crying or other anxiety-producing behavior;
3. in toddlers and preschool-aged children, fatal child abuse and neglect as a result of harsh punishment for the child's failure to meet unrealistic demands; and
4. among older children, community-based homicide, in which the dangers of the adult world confront the increasing independence of the preadolescent and adolescent.

In a clinical setting, family-based approaches to reducing the risk of violence against children are often useful.

Disparities in Morbidity

Preventable death may be the ultimate expression of poverty, but a variety of less severe emotional, developmental, and health problems also may affect poor children. In broad terms, children of poor families experience more days of restricted activity because of health problems and more days absent from school than do their wealthier counterparts.

Intellectual Development and Socioemotional Functioning

Poor children are at increased risk for problems of cognitive and behavioral development. Reports from the long-term follow-up studies of children in Kauai, Hawaii, revealed profound socioeconomic effects on intelligence quotient (IQ) scores (Werner and Smith, 1977). Family income and poverty status have been related to cognitive ability and academic achievement, with these relations generally strongest for the poorest families. Other contextual variables, such as residence changes, maternal relationship changes, and parent antisocial behavior and drug use, predict social maladjustment in school for disadvantaged children, including externalizing problems and peer rejection. Empiric insights have also underscored the interactive quality of social status and biologic impairments in shaping developmental outcome. In general, children of affluent families with biologic disabilities are more likely to overcome the developmental implications of their conditions than are poor children. The Kauai studies revealed that poor children with no perinatal sequelae had IQ scores similar to those of more affluent children with significant perinatal complications. The worst developmental risks are generally seen in children with perinatal insults who are also poor.

School Readiness and Achievement

Chronically poor families provide lower quality child rearing environments, and children in these families show lower cognitive performance than do other children. Any experience of poverty is associated with less favorable family situations and child outcomes than never being poor. Being poor later in childhood tends to be more detrimental than early poverty. During early childhood and adolescence, a consistent finding is that neighbors of high socioeconomic status have a positive effect on school readiness and achievement outcomes (after accounting for individual and family characteristics), especially for European Americans (Leventhal and Brooks-Gunn, 2000).

Behavioral and Emotional Problems

Living in neighborhoods marked by concentrated disadvantage significantly contributes to children's anxiety and depression (Xue et al, 2005). This connection seems to be independent of high immigrant concentration or residential instability. It also appears that collective efficacy may have a positive effect on children's mental health, at least in part through residents' use of community resources. High organizational participation may signal availability of services in the neighborhood.

Sexuality and Childbearing

Socioeconomic conditions of neighborhoods have been associated with an increased risk of adolescent and nonmarital childbearing. The proportion of families living below poverty level within a zip code is highly related to the birth rate among young teenagers in that zip code (Kirby, Coyle, and Gould, 2001). In addition, adolescent men who live in poorer neighborhoods report greater frequency of intercourse and having impregnated someone and less effective contraceptive use (Ku, Sonenstein, and Pleck, 1993). Multiple manifestations of poverty, including poverty itself, low levels of education and employment, and high levels of unemployment, may have a large impact on birth rates among young teenagers.

A study using data from the National Longitudinal Study of Adolescent Health examined the relations among neighborhood dimensions (e.g., socioeconomic characteristics, norms and opportunity structure, social disorganization) and the initiation of sex and contraceptive use at first and most recent sex (Cubbin et al, 2005). Neighborhood context (as measured by all dimensions) was modestly associated with the sexual initiation of adolescents. However, little support was found for neighborhood influence on contraceptive use, suggesting that other factors may play a more important role in shaping adolescents' contraceptive behaviors. For females, living in a neighborhood with a greater concentration of youth who were idle or black residents was associated with increased odds of sexual initiation, whereas a greater concentration of married households or Hispanic residents was associated with decreased odds of initiation. Higher initiation among males was associated with a higher concentration of poverty or idle youth, whereas lower initiation was found with a higher concentration of affluent households.

Chronic Medical Conditions

Poor children experience disproportionately high rates of serious chronic conditions. Hearing loss is more prevalent among poor children, at least in part a reflection of elevated rates of chronic otitis media and an increased likelihood that it will lead to subsequent hearing impairment and associated developmental and behavioral problems. Visual acuity is similar for poor and nonpoor children. However, poor children are less likely to have visual deficits diagnosed and corrected early, resulting in an increased rate of functional visual impairment. Reports on the prevalence of asthma among poor children are variable. However, there is evidence that the impact of asthma on poor children is greater, with higher frequency of attack, greater limitation of activity, and increased requirement for hospitalization.

Nutrition and Growth

Growth retardation, generally associated with chronic undernutrition, is more prevalent among poor children and is independently associated with poorer cognitive function (Liu, Raine, and Venables, 2003). Iron deficiency anemia, which is associated with low development scores in infancy and, later, decreased attentiveness and a higher incidence of behavioral disorders, is almost three times as prevalent among the poor as among the nonpoor in age groups 1 to 5 years and 12 to 17 years. Intake of vitamins and other essential nutrients is also far more likely to be inadequate (Skalicky et al, 2006). Although the causes are complex, poverty can exert its influence on nutrition through the misdistribution of otherwise adequate resources in the family or by the absolute inadequacy of family resources. Poverty can create profound social stress and can interrupt the provision of adequate nutrition to young children through the distortion of healthy family relationships. It can also force children into marginal caretaking situations that can complicate adequate nutrition. Yet, the most direct impact of poverty on child nutrition is the primary lack of resources to acquire adequate food. For many poor families, income available for food may represent merely the remaining portion of income once the less flexible costs of housing, utilities, and transportation are met. The absolute inadequacy of resources that leads to poor child nutrition, indeed child hunger, remains an alarming phenomenon in the United States and is one that may remain hidden from the clinician until frank clinical signs emerge.

Lead Poisoning

Lead poisoning causes a variety of significant health, developmental, and educational problems and is highly associated with poverty. The mean blood lead level of children and the percentage of children having a blood lead level of 10 mg/dL or higher increased as the percentage of the population that was black or Hispanic rose and as poverty increased. Increased crowding, older age of housing, and screening rate also were associated with higher blood lead levels. In contrast, higher blood lead levels were inversely associated with level of education, income, and home ownership (Lanphear et al, 1998). About 9 percent of children aged 1 through 5 years and enrolled in Medicaid had blood lead levels at 10 mg/dL or greater, compared with about 3 percent of the non-Medicaid population. There is also evidence that rates of elevated lead levels during pregnancy are higher in poor women. Heightened exposure in old, deteriorating housing, surrounding soils, and contaminated air is closely associated with poverty. Beyond broad measures, such as the elimination of lead from gasoline, the principal approach to combating lead poisoning is screening children for elevated lead levels. Although it is effective in identifying children with high lead burdens, screening represents a deformed public policy whereby children are used to identify lead-containing homes, rather than identifying such homes directly and eradicating lead before poisoning can occur. Lead screening is a mandatory component of the Early and Periodic Screening, Diagnosis, and Treatment component of Medicaid. However, the Government Accountability Office has reported that most children covered by Medicaid have not received such screening, and less than half of all poor and near-poor children are currently enrolled in Medicaid.

Sequelae of Low Birth Weight

The dramatic improvement in the survival of low-birth-weight newborns has been accompanied by a growing population of survivors at high risk for serious neurodevelopmental and medical problems. However, for poor children, the sequelae of low birth weight can be particularly severe. The most common medical conditions found in low-birth-weight children are asthma, upper and lower respiratory infections, and ear infections. In an examination of the long-term developmental outcome of low-birth-weight infants, those from disadvantaged backgrounds were found to fare worse than do socially advantaged children (Hogan and Park, 2000). In addition, compared with more affluent newborns of similar birth weight, poor infants have greater postneonatal mortality rates, lower IQ scores, and higher prevalence of educational difficulties. This reflects the pervasiveness of poverty and confronts the clinician with the quandary of sending a high-risk child into a suboptimal environment.

Acquired Immunodeficiency Syndrome

Acquired immunodeficiency syndrome (AIDS) in children is another problem that is intimately linked with poverty. Primarily the result of maternal transmission, infection with human immunodeficiency virus (HIV) generally implies significant morbidity and mortality risks in early childhood. Similar to high-risk neonatal survivors, children with HIV infection require a level of comprehensive and multidisciplinary services that can easily overwhelm the already inadequate local health service capacity in areas of concentrated poverty. Unlike low birth weight, however, HIV infection in a child implies the coexistence of a chronic, life-threatening illness in at least one parent. This affects profoundly the interaction among clinicians, child welfare agencies, and foster caretakers. Advances in interrupting maternal transmission and in treating infection in children have altered the risk and impact of infection. The burden remains, however, to ensure that these and all future therapeutic strides are provided equitably to all those in need.

Homelessness: An Extreme Case of Poverty

An extreme manifestation of poverty and failed societal provision is homelessness. Although precise numbers of homeless children have been difficult to establish, estimates have ranged from 200,000 to 3 million nationally. Beyond the problems inherent in measuring a population defined by a lack of residence, these estimates tend to vary owing to differences in definition, in particular the length of time a child must be without formal shelter before being considered homeless, and the political and social agenda of the group performing the count. Nevertheless, there is substantial evidence that the population of homeless children in the United States has grown since the mid-1980s. Indeed, the fastest growing component of the homeless population has been families with children; it is estimated that between 25% and 40% of the nation's homeless are families, most often headed by single women with two or three young children. Another population of homeless children is older children and adolescents labeled "runaways" or "throwaways," estimated to number almost 500,000 nationwide. Generally the product of troubled families, with high rates of physical and sexual abuse, these children are concentrated in major urban centers and often are compelled to rely on illegal and self-destructive means of subsistence including petty crime, drug trade, and prostitution.

Compared with the general population of children, homeless children have twice as many health problems, are more likely to go hungry, have higher rates of developmental delay, and possibly have higher rates of depression, anxiety, and behavior problems. School performance among homeless children is affected drastically, with seriously elevated rates of school failure and requirements for special education. Whereas overall cognitive functioning of homeless children is comparable to that of housed children, academic achievement in the areas of reading, spelling, and arithmetic are dramatically lower for homeless children (San Agustin et al, 1999). In addition to elevated risk, homeless children have drastically reduced access to comprehensive services. Immunization rates, vision and hearing assessment, and lead screening among homeless children have been shown to be seriously inadequate. Confronting the psychosocial toll of homelessness requires coordinated social service, psychological, and educational intervention, although these services are rarely available in the scope and intensity that are needed. The primary task of the clinician who cares for homeless children, like all poor children, is to provide appropriate clinical services. However, to an extent greater than for virtually all other children, the manifold risks associated with being homeless are likely to overwhelm the capacity of clinical intervention to ensure optimal outcomes. The fundamental imperative remains the establishment of decent shelter—a task that clinicians can pursue by assisting individual families with their care, by linking them to other sources of support, and by participating in the development of effective long-term solutions.

Neighborhood Violence and Danger

Violence in the lives of American children, as victims, perpetrators, and witnesses to violence, has grown to epidemic proportions. Neighborhoods that should provide a sense of familiarity and protection to children often do the opposite. Nationwide surveys have shown widespread fear among children of the potential for physical harm in their neighborhoods. The seductive lure of the drug trade and the widespread availability of guns have exposed children of the inner cities to assaults that may be unprecedented in their degree of physical and psychological violence. Children in suburban areas may also harbor significant fears of violence in their schools and on neighborhood streets.

The research literature focusing on the prevalence and impact of children's exposure to violence has grown substantially in the past few years. A large percentage of children are exposed to violence as witnesses or victims within their home in the forms of domestic abuse and television violence and on the streets and in schools in the form of assaults, attempted assaults, and physical threats (Margolin, 2005). Victimization from some form of direct violence for children between the ages of 6 and 17 years has recently been reported in the range of nearly 20% to more than 50%; and witness to violence rates, including muggings, rapes, shootings, and stabbings, has ranged from 10% to 90%, depending largely on the intensity of neighborhood poverty and drug use. Violence exposure crosses socioeconomic strata yet is more prevalent among low-income children. Exposure to violence has important physical, developmental, and emotional sequelae, including poor school functioning, emotional instability, symptoms of post-traumatic stress disorder or depression, and altered world view, and these children are more likely to become perpetrators of violence themselves (Lynch, 2003).

For all people who provide direct care to poor children, the menace of violence and intentional injury remains a source of enormous frustration. Clearly, fundamental solutions lie outside the health care system, but health professionals can play a constructive role clinically as well as be influential advocates for larger ameliorative public policies. Clinicians should explore potential at-risk situations as part of comprehensive care. This forum allows an opportunity for discussions about discipline practices, the use of verbal means of expressing anger, and strategies to address inappropriate television viewing. These discussions can also help frame a home environment that supports nonviolent resolution of conflict. The removal of guns or absolute separation of children from household guns is essential. Clinicians can also help identify young children whose environment puts them at risk for violent behavior or victimization, including those with a family history of violence, school failure, substance abuse, or gang membership. The expressed inclusion of violence prevention discussions and education within routine clinical practice may prove useful. Coordinated early referral to counseling or other supportive services may strengthen family and community-based efforts to reduce the risk of exposure to violence.

Confronting the Impact of Poverty on Child Health: Role of the Clinician

Ultimately, those who provide care to children must confront the clinical expression of poverty. Even though clinicians who care for poor children can make significant contributions through the direct provision of clinical services, the needs of poor children can never be fully met by clinical intervention alone. Rather, the role

Table 18-1. Interventions of Importance in Caring for Poor Children and Their Families

Health Services
Family planning and health services for women
Nutrition supplementation
Prevention of unintentional and intentional injuries
Comprehensive care for infants, children, and adolescents
Community-Based Services
Outreach—bridging the gap between apparent availability and actual use of services
Home visiting
Developmental and behavioral services
Strategic Activities
Community advocacy
Formulation of public policy
General Services
Economic and employment assistance
Minimum wage
Education and job training
Special Service Programs
Temporary Assistance for Needy Families (TANF)
Supplemental Food Program for Women, Infants, and Children (WIC)
Food stamps
Title V links with nonhealth services

of the clinician is defined by dual recognition of the considerable efficacy of medicine and its inherent limitations. A complete reliance on clinical services does not address the larger social forces that determine the dimensions and character of clinical need. However, the importance and relevance of clinical care should not be discounted. Alternatively, clinicians can address the needs of their patients through the linkage of clinical intervention to a spectrum of community-based services and an informed involvement in the formulation of public policies that promote the well-being of children (Table 18-1).

In a setting of poverty, the purpose of health care is to uncouple poverty from its implications for health. Although far from complete, the capacity of medical care to meet this objective is considerable. Accordingly, the primary responsibility of the clinician is the provision of high-quality health services to all children in need. This often requires the refinement of clinical practices to meet the specific needs of poor children in local communities. This, in turn, may require knowledge gained from community-based epidemiology and needs assessment activities. Nevertheless, there are specific services that hold promise for ameliorating the detrimental effects of poverty on health and development.

Lack of health insurance is a well-documented obstacle to the receipt of adequate health care. Thus, it is notable that children, especially those in low-income families and in sharp contrast to their parents, have made some gains in insurance coverage during the past decade. These improvements were driven largely by expansions in Medicaid eligibility and the establishment of the State Child Health Insurance Program (SCHIP) (Kenney, Haley, and Tebay, 2003). However, there are indications that recent improvements have reached a plateau, and some 8 million children remained uninsured in 2005, many of whom appeared eligible for Medicaid or SCHIP coverage.

Social disparities in patterns of immunization in the United States illustrate how differences in access can influence the provision of highly effective services. Children in families with incomes below the poverty level are less likely than are those with families with incomes at or above the poverty level to receive the combined series vaccination (in 2005, 79% and 84%, respectively) (Centers for Disease Control and Prevention, 2006). Several factors may account for this phenomenon, including decreased access to primary care, missed opportunities to vaccinate, and vaccination beliefs and practices among pediatric providers in poor communities that run counter to standard vaccination recommendations.

Confronting the Impact of Poverty on Child Health: Service Interventions

Health Services

Maternal Health and the Health of Women

To an important extent, inequities in the rate of poor birth outcomes are a legacy of inequities in women's health status before conception. Poor women suffer from elevated rates of a number of chronic and acute conditions, many of which affect maternal and fetal health during gestation as well as child health in subsequent years. High-quality general health care for women is essential, and clinicians who care for children should ensure that women bringing their children for services also have health care. Gynecologic and obstetric conditions noted during previous pregnancies may require significant medical management before conception. Timely access to high-quality family planning services, including counseling and reproductive health screening, helps ensure that a child is wanted and will enter a home environment that is nurturing and supportive of normal growth and development. Family planning services provide women with control over their reproductive lives and a capacity to plan for their economic responsibilities. Family planning services can reduce infant mortality rate, incidence of low birth weight, and number of stillbirths and can increase the probability that timing of birth, interval between births, and family size will serve to enhance the infant's healthy development. Despite the importance of family planning, approximately 30 million women in the United States who are at risk for unwanted pregnancy do not receive adequate health and family planning services. Almost 3 million unplanned pregnancies occur each year, with half of them being terminated by abortion. Contact with the medical system during the birth experience provides a special opportunity for clinicians to link women with appropriate reproductive and family planning services. Primary care for young children also affords ongoing contact with young mothers and a continuing clinical capacity to ensure adequate reproductive care.

Prenatal care represents a critical component of comprehensive health services for women of childbearing age. A range of services for women during the prenatal period have been shown to enhance maternal health before, during, and after delivery and represents a critical mechanism to optimize the health and early development of the newborn. Although the precise mechanisms of effect remain poorly understood, late or no prenatal care is associated with an increased incidence of low birth weight, prematurity, and death of infants of normal birth weight (Institute of Medicine, 2006). Further, there remain substantial disparities between poor and nonpoor women in the use of prenatal care services. National data reveal that approximately one in five women giving birth in the United States begins prenatal care later than the first trimester and that late initiation is heavily concentrated among poor and young women. However, recent research suggests that prenatal care should be linked to broader efforts to improve health care services to women, including improved nutrition, primary and specialty care, contraception, and treatment for smoking and illicit drug use.

Nutrition

Throughout the course of life, but particularly in pregnancy and childhood, growth and healthy development depend on adequate and balanced nutrition. For families living in poverty, limited resources can constrain both the variety and amount of necessary foods. In response, clinicians can assist such families by referrals to publicly supported nutrition programs. A primary resource is Supplemental Food Program for Women, Infants, and Children (WIC), which provides food supplements to low-income pregnant or lactating women, to infants, and to children younger than 5 years. In addition, the food stamp, school lunch, and breakfast programs and a variety of projects supported by Title V (Maternal and Child Health) have proved beneficial to enrolled families. However, these programs are often underfunded and can provide services to only a portion of all families in need. Despite repeated evaluations that document the efficacy of the WIC program, only about half of all children who meet eligibility criteria nationwide actually receive WIC services. Another important element of the effort to improve child nutrition is support for breastfeeding. Culturally sensitive, hospital-based programs that encourage breastfeeding, particularly when linked with supportive primary care involvement during the first few months after delivery, can significantly increase breastfeeding by women who are poor and possess little formal education.

Comprehensive Care

Despite the efficacy of a number of specific, isolated interventions, high-quality comprehensive care remains the foundation for ensuring optimal child health, especially for poor children who are at elevated risk for interrelated health problems. Comprehensive care strategies include the following:

Primary prevention services, which attempt to eliminate causative factors before the occurrence of illness or injury. These services include immunization, window gratings to prevent falls, and provision of contraceptives to sexually active teens.

Secondary prevention services, which address pathologic conditions that are present but not yet clearly expressed as recognized symptoms; this is particularly important in reducing the functional impact of medical problems in poor children. Such prevention often involves screening procedures, including those implemented at birth and the early detection of vision and hearing deficits as well as developmental delay.

Tertiary prevention services, which involve limiting the suffering and disability associated with a symptomatic condition, often a chronic illness. Particularly for poor children, this aspect of care generally requires a strong and continuous coordination of a range of clinical and support services.

Comprehensive care must also include a strong commitment to anticipatory guidance, school performance monitoring, and counseling. The process of providing and exchanging information about the development and social functioning of the child can enhance parents' understanding, competence, and confidence in their own perceptions and concerns. Poverty can breed isolation, but clinical guidance can play an important role in supporting parental efforts to address temperamental differences in their children (see Chapter 7), unrealistic expectations, unfounded anxieties, and the debilitating stresses of low income, crowded housing, poor education, and a climate of crime, violence, and scant hope.

It is the nature of poverty to reduce access to services as much as it is to increase need. Therefore, in poor communities, clinicians must play an enhanced role in ensuring that families receive needed care. Follow-up care takes on new significance because a variety of financial and logistical problems can undermine poor families' ability to comply with medical advice. Costs of specialty consultation or medications may be prohibitive, access to medical advice by telephone may be limited, parents may be hesitant to seek care owing to past dehumanizing interactions with the medical system, and the child's clinical status may not be known because of multiple caretakers or a chaotic social situation.

Community-Based Services

Community-based programs provide a crucial range of services and represent an important resource for clinicians caring for poor children. Such services are often targeted to children who have a specific set of conditions, whereas others attempt to enhance access to a broad range of medical and social services through intensive home visiting, follow-up care, and social supports.

Outreach

Outreach bridges the gap between the apparent availability of a service and actual use by a family in need. Parents may have a poor understanding of some of the program benefits and services available to their children.

Furthermore, even if they understand the benefits of available services, parents may not be aware of the nature or severity of their child's problem or the processes by which services can be sought. Families may also encounter poorly coordinated medical and social service systems, often with inconsistent eligibility and benefit criteria. In addition, outreach efforts can help ensure that cultural, language, and other social barriers to care are diminished and that professional staff are accountable to the community they serve.

Home Visiting

Home visiting services may be an effective means of providing services and linking families to needed resources in poor communities. Although programs vary considerably, most provide a broad range of responses to family needs. They provide information and assistance in making the home a safe and nurturing environment, address nutritional concerns, and offer social support for families isolated from relatives or community activities. Many home visiting programs focus on children with specific conditions or health care needs, providing physical therapy, home intravenous therapy, or respiratory support. Regardless of the specific need, home visiting services are most effective when they are coordinated with local clinicians and agencies and are closely integrated into a comprehensive system of care.

Developmental and Behavioral Services beyond the Health Care System

The distinctive needs of poor children can best be met by coordinated efforts that tie clinical expertise to the skills and commitment of professionals whose work extends beyond the health system to other settings where children live, work, play, and study. Teachers, daycare workers, juvenile correctional officers, foster parents, social workers, guidance counselors, and others working with children and youth with developmental and behavioral problems represent important resources for children and their families. Their insights and informed energy should be integrated into individual care plans and community-wide efforts to improve developmental outcomes. Schools offer a particularly important arena for coordinating services because school personnel are often the first to identify children in need of help and may represent a critical component of any therapeutic response. In addition, the effort to engage children with significant chronic illness in regular school settings requires a close relationship between educational and clinical personnel.

Strategic Activities

Although clinical intervention remains of critical importance to children living in poverty, the complex spectrum of risk associated with poverty cannot be addressed entirely by clinical practice alone. Clinicians may possess a special capacity to speak to the need for community-based programs and help legitimize advocacy calls for improved local services. Social networks, both formal and informal, can be important sources of support to poor families in need and can be strengthened by local professionals. This might include the collaboration of local neighborhood groups, business organizations, labor unions, religious assemblies, and a variety of other community-based institutions. At some level, clinicians must respect the need to improve public policy and recognize that the commitment to clinical intervention is inextricably tied to the struggle for social equity. This linkage will best ensure that the clinical and public commitment to optimal child development will prove both effective and just.

INCOME AND SOCIOECONOMIC STATUS: AFFLUENCE

The inclusion of affluence as a potential deterrent to healthy development is not to imply that the role of affluence might be analogous to that of poverty; it is not. Unlike poverty, affluence implies access to full societal participation that is not constrained by basic material concerns. Rather, affluence is discussed in this chapter to call attention to aspects of the affluent environment that may prove deleterious to healthy child development. There is some evidence that affluent children can report relatively low levels of happiness. In addition, there have been suggestions that parent-adolescent connections can become increasingly compromised as the demanding lives of professional parents impinge on critical "family time." A national survey by the U.S. Department of Health and Human Services has revealed that closeness to parents among adolescents tends to be inversely related to household income (America's Children, 1999).

Relations Between Affluence and Development

Among the negative outcomes in which growing up in affluence may be implicated are alcohol and drug abuse, juvenile delinquency, motor vehicle occupant injuries, suicide, cult membership, and eating disorders. Yet it remains unclear whether the primary risk is the great wealth, a rapid ascendancy into wealth, or an exclusivity of social relations that precludes peer contact with the nonwealthy. Wealth may serve as a proxy for risk; it may be associated with more potent influences, such as fame, power, lack of traditional family interactions, and intense emphasis on extraordinary achievement, that may characterize a significant proportion of wealthy families.

Aspects of Affluence with Possible Negative Effects

Aspects of the environment that may be present in a significant number of affluent families and that may be deterrents to healthy development are listed in Table 18-2. However, the suggested associations have not been subjected to repeated systematic investigation, and empiric insight into significant causal relationships remains almost entirely lacking.

Parental Absence or Neglect and Weakened Family Ties

A significant portion of affluent parents live in a style that may demand, and certainly permits, long absences from home and children. Parents who find parenthood burdensome have the means to circumvent child rearing

Table 18-2. Aspects of Affluence with Possible Negative Effects

Absence of strong, consistent parental presence and weakening of family ties
Variable and transient substitute caretakers
Unrealistic or destructive parental expectations
Overabundance of possessions with diminished need for choice and effort
Relatively easy access to cars, drugs, and alcohol

tasks in a socially sanctioned manner. Preoccupations with professional or recreational interests may eliminate protected time for parent-child involvement, nurturance, and communication. Constant professional and social demands may undermine a daily structure for family interaction and create a marked failure in the systematic transmission of family concerns, traditions, values, roles, and expressions of love based on daily events.

Isolation from Adults

Survey findings have demonstrated that youth from upper-income families are often alone at home for many hours each week. This literal isolation is associated with absence of adult supervision. Further, emotional isolation may derive from the erosion of family time together because of the demands of affluent parents' jobs and children's many after-school activities (Luthar, 2003). Feelings of high closeness to mothers were reported by approximately 75% of adolescents with family incomes of less than $15,000 but by only 65% of those with family incomes of more than $75,000 (see also Chapter 9).

Achievement Pressures and Overscheduling

Goals and standards set by affluent parents for their children may include extraordinary pressures to measure up to the success of the parents and a narrow definition of what is acceptable. Scholastics, sports, and social achievements that are good may not be good enough; they may have to be "best." The message that love and acceptance are contingent on high achievement can be particularly harmful to children with average abilities. In addition, the child's perception of parental standards may be far more stringent than the true feelings of the parents—a situation that can lead to unnecessary but real pressure on the child.

It has been speculated that overscheduling of youth of high socioeconomic status creates undue pressures and high psychopathology (e.g., anxiety and depression symptoms, substance use, delinquency) and school problems (e.g., poor grades, problematic classroom behavior). However, this hypothesis has not been supported by recent research (Luthar, Shoum, and Brown, 2006). More powerful than hours spent in activities were children's perceptions of their parents' attitudes toward achievements. Perceived parental criticism and lack of after-school supervision appear particularly detrimental. In addition, low parental expectations connote significant vulnerability for boys.

Overabundance of Possessions

Most children in wealthy families are surrounded by an abundance of possessions. This may be part of a general expression of wealth in a consumer-based society, or parents may buy expensive gifts to assuage a sense of guilt for not spending enough time with their children. Regardless, these children may have little experience with having to delay gratification or with the frustration that comes from having to do without a coveted object. This may compound the harmful effects of growing up with little contact with children from a diversity of backgrounds and social classes. Furthermore, such children may develop unrealistic expectations of the extent to which one need not adapt to life but can make the world adapt to one's whims. The expectation that familial resources will pave the way for them in life and eliminate the need for personal accomplishment may so characterize children of certain affluent families. Easy access to automobiles, drugs, and alcohol may be implicated in high rates of automobile-related injuries and substance abuse among some wealthy adolescents.

Evidence of Health and Adjustment Problems

Many children of the affluent, for whom there are unremitting demands for excellence (being average is indistinguishable from failing), develop stress-related symptoms such as insomnia, stomachaches, headaches, anxiety, and depression. Some youth come to overstate minimal health problems to have an acceptable path out of competition with others. A study of more than 800 American teens found that the most affluent youth reported the least happiness (Csikszentmihalyi and Schneider, 2000). Other research reveals that compared with inner-city, minority, low–socioeconomic status youth, affluent youth report higher levels of anxiety and depression and higher substance use, consistently indicating more frequent use of cigarettes, alcohol, marijuana, and other illegal drugs (Luthar, 2003). High–socioeconomic status youth often use substances in efforts to alleviate emotional distress or for reasons of social conformity.

The Impact of Affluence on Child Health: Role of the Clinician

Health professionals can be especially alert to the specific signals that may characterize abnormal development in affluent families. A frank discussion of these issues can be integrated into the anticipatory guidance component of primary care, and when concerns do arise, appropriate advice or referrals can be provided. Because family interactions tend to play the primary role in shaping developmental problems in affluent children, family-centered therapy is often most helpful. Clinicians can also support school and community efforts to provide organized service projects and other substitutes for the challenges of fighting for economic survival, including demanding outdoor activities in which children encounter the impartial realities of nature.

Most important perhaps is the role health professionals can play in emphasizing the critical and unique function of parenthood to those parents with the resources to leave child rearing to others. The frequently high extracurricular involvement of children of the affluent, for example, is not necessarily destructive; it is much more damaging when children believe that their parents are uninvolved and not invested in their activities and pursuits or when they believe that their failures render them unworthy in their parents' eyes. In wealthy communities, as in all others, parenting behaviors conveying acceptance and appreciation, balanced with reasonably high standards and expectations, are critical for the healthy, adaptive development of young people.

The clinician can serve as an advocate for the child, stressing the role that parents have in providing nurturance, love, and support; in setting firm and realistic limits to behavior; and in conveying to their children a clear set of traditions, ideals, and moral principles.

GEOGRAPHIC MOBILITY AND RESIDENTIAL INSTABILITY

A child's ability to thrive can be greatly enhanced by stable and familiar surroundings. Stability and familiarity breed opportunities to master developmental tasks and to develop secure relationships. Changing neighborhoods, especially frequent changes, may place the child at risk for academic, behavioral, emotional, and potentially health problems. For example, an analysis of data from the 1988 National Health Interview Survey of Child Health revealed that school-age children who moved three or more times were at increased risk for emotional or behavioral and school problems (Simpson and Fowler, 1994). However, it is difficult to know whether other family factors, such as parental job loss, could influence both geographic mobility and the risk for adverse child outcomes. The magnitude of concern increases when it is considered that nearly 40% of all school-age children have moved three or more times and that poor children are more likely to move frequently.

Geographic moves also increase the likelihood that a child does not have a specific site for health care (Fowler, Simpson, and Schoendorf, 1993). This, in turn, may place the child at risk for poor physical health and reduced receipt of health care services. In addition, delayed receipt of prior medical records often makes it difficult for new health care providers to know exactly what services, such as age-appropriate vaccinations, are needed and what physical and mental health problems deserve attention. Parents may not be familiar with the details of the physical and emotional ailments of their children, including current therapies and past evaluations. It is therefore necessary for child health care providers to create effective systems to gather prior medical record data and to be vigilant in obtaining information about children and families who have moved and are seen for the first time.

SUMMARY

For children, the neighborhood is the relatively small environmental range and inherent relationships of home, school, and community that, together, determine the fabric of daily life. The neighborhood appears to influence child health through institutional resources and collective efficacy as well as through human relationships and home environment. How these mechanisms interact depends on the health outcome in question and reflects crucial structural characteristics of neighborhoods, particularly income and socioeconomic status. Children living in poor neighborhoods experience elevated rates of developmental and medical problems and a greater likelihood that these problems will produce deleterious outcomes. Likewise, growing up in affluent families and neighborhoods may also be associated with enhanced risk for problems, including alcohol and drug abuse, juvenile delinquency, motor vehicle occupant injuries, suicide, and eating disorders. A variety of clinical and community-level interventions, both private and public in nature, may enhance a neighborhood's capacity to provide a stable and safe environment for optimal child health outcomes.

REFERENCES

America's Children. Available at: www.childstats.gov/ac1999.asp. Accessed January 4, 2007.

ASPE: http://aspe.hhs.gov/poverty/06computations.shtml, 2006.

Brown JL: Statement on Key Welfare Reform Issues: The Empirical Evidence. Medford, MA, Tufts University Center on Hunger, Poverty and Nutrition Policy, 1995.

Centers for Disease Control and Prevention: Data for 2005: National Immunization Program (2006). National Immunization Survey Data, Jan-Dec 05. Accessed January 2, 2007.

Citro CF, Michael RT (eds): Measuring Poverty: A New Approach, Washington, DC, National Academy Press, 1995.

Csikszentmihalyi M, Schneider B (eds): Becoming Adult: How Teenagers Prepare for the World of Work. New York, Basic Books, 2000.

Cubbin C, Santelli J, Brindis CD, Braveman P: Neighborhood context and sexual behaviors among adolescents: Findings from the national longitudinal study of adolescent health. Perspect Sex Reprod Health 37(3):125-134, 2005.

DiLiberti JH: The relationship between social stratification and all-cause mortality among children in the United States: 1968-1992. Pediatrics 105(1):e2, 2000.

Fowler MG, Simpson GA, Schoendorf KC: Families on the move and children's health care. Pediatrics 91(5):934-940, 1993.

Friedman SH, Horwitz SM, Resnick PJ: Child murder by mothers: a critical analysis of the current state of knowledge and a research agenda. Am J Psychiatry 162(9):1578-1587, 2005.

Hogan DP, Park JM: Family factors and social support in the developmental outcomes of very low-birth weight children. Clin Perinatol 27(2):433-459, 2000.

Institute of Medicine: Preterm Birth: Causes, Consequences, and Prevention. Washington, DC, National Academies Press, 2006.

Kenney G, Haley J, Tebay A: Children's Insurance Coverage and Service Use Improve. Snapshots of America's Families III, No. 1. Washington, DC, The Urban Institute, 2003.

Kim MH, Subramanian SV, Kawachi I, Kim CY: Association between childhood fatal injuries and socioeconomic position at individual and area levels: a multilevel study. J Epidemiol Community Health 61(2):135-140, 2007.

Kirby D, Coyle K, Gould JB: Manifestations of poverty and birthrates among young teenagers in California zip code areas. Fam Plann Perspect 33(2):63-69, 2001.

Ku L, Sonenstein FL, Pleck JH: Factors influencing first intercourse for teenage men. Public Health Rep 108(6):680-694, 1993.

Lanphear BP, Byrd RS, Auinger P, Schaffer SJ: Community characteristics associated with elevated blood lead levels in children. Pediatrics 101(2):264-271, 1998.

Leventhal T, Brooks-Gunn J: The neighborhoods they live in: The effects of neighborhood residence on child and adolescent outcomes. Psychol Bull 126(2):309-337, 2000.

Liu J, Raine A, Venables PH, et al: Malnutrition at age 3 years and lower cognitive ability at age 11 years: Independence from psychosocial adversity. Arch Pediatr Adolesc Med 157(6):593-600, 2003.

Luthar SS: The culture of affluence: Psychological costs of material wealth. Child Dev 74(6):1581-1593, 2003.

Luthar SS, Shoum KA, Brown PJ: Extracurricular involvement among affluent youth: a scapegoat for "ubiquitous achievement pressures"? Dev Psychol 42(3):583-597, 2006.

Lynch M: Consequences of children's exposure to community violence. Clin Child Fam Psychol Rev 6(4):265-274, 2003.

Marcin JP, Schembri MS, He J, Romano PS: A population-based analysis of socioeconomic status and insurance status and their relationship with pediatric trauma hospitalization and mortality rates. Am J Public Health 93(3):461-466, 2003.

Margolin G: Children's exposure to violence: Exploring developmental pathways to diverse outcomes. J Interpers Violence 20(1):72-81, 2005.

Pickett KE, Luo Y, Lauderdale DS: Widening social inequalities in risk for sudden infant death syndrome. Am J Public Health 95(11):1976-1981, 2005.

Reagan PB, Salsberry PJ: Race and ethnic differences in determinants of preterm birth in the USA: Broadening the social context. Soc Sci Med 60(10):2217-2228, 2005.

San Agustin M, Cohen P, Rubin D, et al: The Montefiore community children's project: A controlled study of cognitive and emotional problems of homeless mothers and children. J Urban Health 76(1):39-50, 1999.

Schinke SP, Cole KC, Poulin SR: Enhancing the educational achievement of at-risk youth. Prev Sci 1(1):51-60, 2000.

Schnitzer PG, Ewigman BG: Child deaths resulting from inflicted injuries: Household risk factors and perpetrator characteristics. Pediatrics 116(5):e687-693, 2005.

Scholer SJ, Hickson GB, Mitchel EF Jr, Ray WA: Predictors of mortality from fires in young children. Pediatrics 101(5):e12, 1998.

Schor EL: Family pediatrics: report of the Task Force on the Family. Pediatrics 111(6 pt 2):1541-1571, 2003.

Shenassa ED, Stubbendick A, Brown MJ: Social disparities in housing and related pediatric injury: A multilevel study. Am J Public Health 94(4):633-639, 2004.

Simpson GA, Fowler MG: Geographic mobility and children's emotional/behavioral adjustment and school functioning. Pediatrics 93(2):303-309, 1994.

Skalicky A, Meyers AF, Adams WG, et al: Child food insecurity and iron deficiency anemia in low-income infants and toddlers in the United States. Matern Child Health J 10(2):177-185, 2006.

U.S. Census Bureau: Poverty Rates by Age: 1959 to 2005. Washington, DC, Health and Human Services, 2005.

Werner E, Smith R (eds): Kauai's Children Come of Age, Honolulu, University of Hawaii Press, 1977.

Wise PH: The anatomy of a disparity in infant mortality. Annu Rev Public Health 24:341-62, 2003.

Xue Y, Leventhal T, Brooks-Gunn J, Earls FJ: Neighborhood residence and mental health problems of 5- to 11-year-olds. Arch Gen Psychiatry 62(5):554-563, 2005.

19 CULTURE AND ETHNICITY

SARA HARKNESS, CONSTANCE H. KEEFER, AND CHARLES M. SUPER

Pediatricians, like other people who serve children and their families, must increasingly deal with sociocultural differences in the context of their practice. This chapter addresses culture and ethnicity as the most general and pervasive aspect of children's environments. From this perspective, there are three challenges for pediatricians: (1) to build a broader knowledge base about cross-cultural variation in child rearing and child development; (2) to integrate this knowledge with developmental perspectives and use of standard developmental-behavioral assessment tools to make more informed clinical assessments; and (3) to develop a culturally sensitive attitude in interaction with all patients, including those from the same cultural background as the pediatrician. We first review concepts of culture and ethnicity, presenting a theoretical framework for the pediatrician to use in learning about the cultural organization of child life. Some dimensions of cross-cultural variability in the contexts of children's development from early infancy to adolescence are introduced and illustrated through three clinical cases. The chapter concludes with a discussion of culturally sensitive developmental assessment and advocacy issues in general and behavioral-developmental pediatrics.

CULTURE AND ETHNICITY

Culture and *ethnicity* are closely linked terms as used by scholars, educators, and clinicians across several fields. Anthropologists use the term *culture* to mean the way of life of a people, including both the external, socially constructed environments for living (e.g., political systems or housing patterns) and the internalized rules, expectations, and values that guide communication, thinking, and behavior. A central aspect of culture is its representation in practices of daily life. As Gottlieb (2004, pp xvi-xvii) notes:

> *Anthropologists have long promoted the notion that daily practices assumed by the members of one society as natural may be surprisingly absent elsewhere, and that such practices, seemingly unnatural in the views of outsiders, make sense when viewed in the context of a variety of cultural factors whose meanings can be discerned only after systematic analysis of the local system of cultural logic.*

The "cultural logic" to which Gottlieb refers has also been discussed in terms of "cultural models" that have motivational force because they inform members of a society about what is proper or appropriate (D'Andrade and Strauss, 1992). As LeVine (LeVine et al, 1994, p 144) wrote in applying this approach to child rearing among the Gusii people of western Kenya:

> *Thus the Gusii model of infant care can be seen as a folk system of pediatric and educational thought—embodying premises about the determinants of infant survival and early learning—or as a folk system of ethics in the parent-child relationship. It is most appropriately seen as both knowledge and morality combined in a single customary formula—moralized knowledge.*

As implied by both these authors, the "culture" of a people is not a random collection of customs, beliefs, and values but rather an organized and meaningful system, even though it may (and probably does) contain internal contradictions (Levy, 2005). Parents play a crucial role as mediators and creators of culture for their children (Harkness and Super, 1996).

Ethnicity refers to membership in a culturally defined group, usually in the context of a larger dominant society, as is the case with immigrant groups or "minorities." The internal, cognitive, and emotional dimensions are also sometimes considered under the rubric of ethnicity. As Giordano (1973, p 11) stated:

> *Ethnicity from a clinical point of view is more than distinctiveness defined by race, religion, national origin, or geography. It involves conscious and unconscious processes that fulfill the deep psychological need for security, identity, and a sense of historical continuity. It is transmitted in an emotional language within the family and is reinforced by similar units in the community.*

Ethnic categories often include several groups of varied cultural or national origin that may differ in important ways. Growing familiarity with these differences has led to a finer appreciation of the distinctive needs of particular ethnic groups in the clinical setting (McGoldrick, Giordano, and Garcia-Preto, 2005). On the other hand, societies within larger culture areas such as Asia or sub-Saharan Africa do share particular beliefs and practices, including aspects of family functioning and child rearing. At the most general level, some psychologists have argued for a distinction between "individualistic" and "collectivistic" cultures that can be drawn across a broad range of different cultural groups (Kağitçibaşi, 2007). Unfortunately, such a sweeping generalization leaves unexplained many important kinds of variability among cultural groups within each category (e.g., Asians and sub-Saharan Africans in the collectivistic category). Pediatricians, need to be careful, therefore, to avoid both the confusion inherent in keeping track of myriad different cultural groups and the oversimplification of dividing the world into two parts—essentially, ourselves versus everyone else.

Regardless of exactly how culture and ethnicity are defined, there is general recognition that they play a crucial role related to children's healthy development (Shonkoff and Phillips, 2000). Pediatricians, who have some familiarity with the ways that parents from various cultural or ethnic backgrounds (including their own) approach the universal task of raising children, are better equipped to engage in productive dialogue and decision making about the specific questions that emerge in the context of developmental-behavioral pediatrics.

THE DEVELOPMENTAL NICHE AND PARENTAL ETHNOTHEORIES

How can pediatricians become more cognizant of cultural dimensions that shape the opportunities for and challenges to the healthy development of their young patients? Given the increasing constraints on consultation time, a framework for organizing diverse pieces of information can help fill in the picture more efficiently and accurately. A useful framework for learning about children's lives from a cultural perspective is the *developmental niche* (Super and Harkness, 2002). In this approach, one takes the perspective of the child, looking outward to the environment of daily experience as it is shaped by features of the larger sociocultural setting (see Fig. 19-1). The child's developmental niche consists of three components.

Physical and Social Settings of Everyday Life

Children's environments are organized first in terms of where, with whom, and in what activities children usually spend their days. Is the infant at home alone with the mother or in a daycare center for 9 hours each day? Does the 6-year-old spend afternoons with a group of neighborhood children at the playground, does she stay home watching television with her brother, or does she help out at the family-run convenience store? What is the learning environment offered in each of these settings with regard to parental involvement, cognitive stimulation, interpersonal skills such as cooperation, and the acquisition of social roles? What are the differential patterns of risk with respect to accidental injury, physical abuse, and exposure to pathogens?

Customs of Child Care

The second subsystem involves customs of child care, that is, the caretakers' repertoire of normative strategies for child rearing. Insofar as these are part of shared cultural patterns, they are comfortable and familiar methods that do not call for careful analysis or justification—they seem "natural" and obvious to parents. Is it customary to breastfeed beyond 1 year? Do toddlers normally sleep in the same bed with their parents? Is reading a story naturally part of the bedtime routine? Do parents customarily help with homework in the evening? What are the traditional methods of discipline?

The Psychology of the Caretakers

Finally, the psychology of the caretakers forms the third component of the child's developmental niche. Of particular relevance to the pediatrician are parents' cultural belief systems or "parental ethnotheories." These culturally constructed ideas about children's behavior and development, about the family, and about parenting are influenced by the larger environments that families occupy, and they are important in parents' decision making about children's settings of daily life as well as customs of care (Harkness and Super, 1996). Although parental ethnotheories are often not explicit or developed into a coherent and internally consistent set of beliefs, when parents

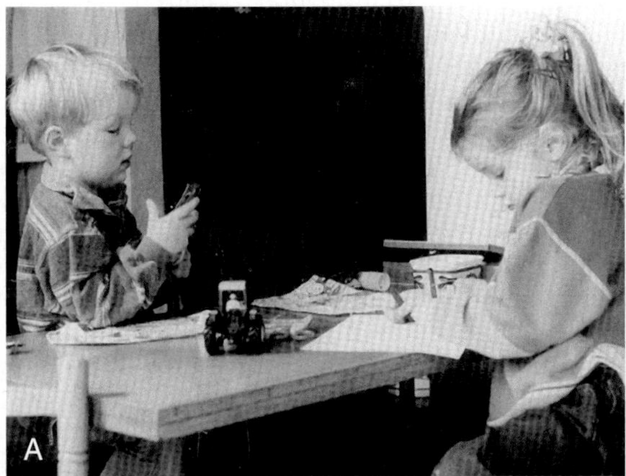

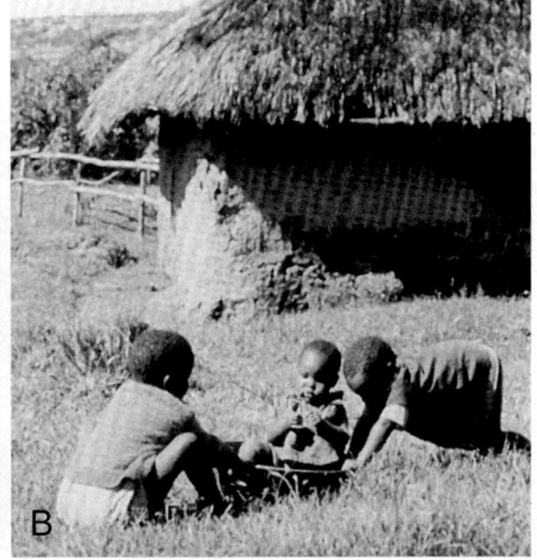

Figure 19-1. The differing developmental niches of children. *A*, In the Netherlands, a sister and brother do artwork together at their own table in the family room. *B*, In Kipsigis, Kenya, two older siblings play with baby sister, pulling her in cooking pot like a sleigh. The older children are resposible for their little sister while the mother is busy nearby.

confront choices, the culturally influenced assumptions that give meaning to the available options may be talked about more explicitly. The pediatrician can use this opportunity to help parents steer between the risks of making a choice that does not "feel right," on the one hand, and choosing a strategy that might seem "right" to begin with but is not well suited to the child's developmental or temperamental needs, on the other hand.

Parental ethnotheories form a hierarchy of beliefs that are linked indirectly although powerfully to behavior (Harkness et al, 2007). At the top of the hierarchy are the most general, implicit ideas about the nature of the child, parenting, and the family. Below this triad are ideas about specific domains, such as infant sleep or social development. These ideas are closely tied to ideas about appropriate practices and further to imagined child or family outcomes. Ideas are translated into behavior as mediated by factors such as child characteristics, situational variables, and competing cultural models and their related practices. The final results can be seen in actual parental practices or behaviors and actual child and family outcomes.

Parental ethnotheories provide a particularly helpful point of entry for the pediatrician who wishes to address a particular developmental or behavioral issue, whether it is related to sleep management in an infant or peer relations in a school-age child. In each such situation, the pediatrician may find it helpful to review three basic questions with the parent or caretaker: (1) What are the parents' expectations of the child's behavior and development at this particular point? (2) What do parents expect of themselves? What makes a "good mother" or "good father" in relation to the issue at hand? (3) What do parents expect (or hope for) from others in relation to this issue? What are the roles of other family members, friends, health care providers, or teachers? Keeping in mind these three basic questions can guide the pediatrician, in conversation with the parent, through a process of identifying the significance of a particular developmental issue and thus finding acceptable pathways to resolving it. Although such a process may seem time-consuming in the context of a busy clinical practice, it may ultimately be more efficient than the alternative of incomplete communication that leads to further office calls, lack of compliance with pediatric advice, and perhaps developmental problems.

THE CULTURAL CONTEXT OF CHILDREN'S DEVELOPMENT

Parental ethnotheories guide the settings and activities that parents organize for their children as well as their general expectations for children's development. The following examples illustrate differences that are evident at particular developmental stages.

The Postnatal Period: Care and Support of the Mother

For many middle-class American families, the postpartum period is an especially stressful time, when parents are expected—and expect themselves—to cope with the challenges of taking care of a new baby with very little support of either an informal or formal nature. Mothers just home from giving birth at the hospital may be left alone with the new baby while husbands, friends, and family are away at work, and grandparents may be unavailable or, alternatively, may be considered intrusive during the "bonding process" of the fledgling family. Exacerbating the lack of support from others may be the mother's own pressing sense of needing to "get things done" around the house. This scenario is in sharp contrast to many other cultures, both traditional and modern. Pediatricians working with immigrant families from India, for example, can expect grandparents to be in residence for several months to take care of both mother and baby. Likewise, Korean families routinely combine households during the postpartum period through moving back with grandparents or by having one or more grandparents live with them during the opening months of the baby's life (Harkness et al, 2007). In European countries, family leave policies virtually guarantee that the father will be at home for at least 2 weeks after the birth of the baby. In addition, in some countries such as the Netherlands, professionally trained postpartum care providers take care of both mother and baby for the first 10 days post partum. Family members are also expected to be closely involved in helping the new baby, and its parents, get off to a healthy beginning together. The well-known lack of contextual support in many U.S. families, coupled with mothers' own excessively high expectations of themselves, sets the stage for postpartum mood difficulties including depression and dysphoria, which in turn create risks for the development of the infant and family (Malik et al, 2007). Pediatricians can be alert to the presence or absence of external supports for the mother, as well as her own expectations of herself, as either protective or risk factors.

Infancy: Cultural Models and Developmental Agendas

According to current wisdom in the United States, infancy is a crucial period for the development of "brain architecture" essential to later success in school and in life (Shonkoff and Phillips, 2000). Parents are urged through many channels, from parenting magazines to television programs, to maximize "stimulation" of their children's cognitive and perceptual development. It is hardly an overstatement to say that a whole industry has arisen to help support parents in this endeavor (Pozniak, 2005). Although periodic warnings are sounded about the dangers of overstimulation, many middle-class parents see promotion of the child's intelligence as the central developmental agenda, starting in the opening weeks and months of the infant's life.

Cultural differences in developmental agendas are strikingly evident in comparisons with traditional agricultural societies such as those of sub-Saharan Africa, where parents have been observed to spend little time in verbal interaction with their babies while at the same time paying much more attention to the early development of motor skills such as sitting and walking (LeVine et al, 1994). Immigrant families usually carry forward these cultural models from home to the new host context, and they become evident in the pediatric context (Greenfield and Cocking, 1994; Moscardino, Nwobu, and Axia, 2006). Cultural differences in developmental agendas are not limited to such societies, however; for example, pediatric advice to mothers in the Netherlands emphasizes the importance of rest and regularity of routines, and the effects are evident in infant behavior and interaction with their mothers (Super et al, 1996). Other culturally constituted agendas for infant development focus on socioemotional intelligence (Italy) and support of physical health and well-being in the social context of the family (Spain). In another contrast, Korean middle-class mothers combine encouragement of cognitive development through early education, including reading and listening to tapes, with solicitous care for the baby as a fragile and vulnerable creature (Harkness et al, 2007).

Importantly from the perspective of the pediatrician, each of these agendas is likely to be expressed through particular caretaking practices. Thus, U.S. mothers who are concerned about cognitive development may spend a lot of time exposing their infants to various stimulating toys and equipment but be relatively unconcerned about the young baby's social contact with friends or relatives. In contrast, mothers who see the baby as needing social contact from an early age are more likely to keep the baby near others even while asleep. Likewise, cultural differences in expectations about the baby's ability to self-regulate are expressed in practices such as holding the baby while he or she falls asleep versus simply tucking the baby into bed for a nap. These practices will be best understood in the context of the ethnotheories they serve.

The Preschool Period: Getting Ready for the Transition to School

Like infancy, the preschool period has received a great deal of attention in the United States as it sets the stage for the child's later successful transition to school. Programs such as Head Start and School Readiness are premised on the observation that by comparison with many immigrant and ethnic minority groups, middle-class American children tend to start school with more developed literacy and other skills such as drawing, doing puzzles, and even playing with peers (Shonkoff and Phillips, 2000). The interesting exception to this general pattern is Asian children, who are often more advanced than their Euro-American peers at the beginning of school—a difference that preschool teachers, ironically, may also perceive as problematic (Parmar, Harkness, and Super, 2004). As with development during infancy, understanding parents' culturally shared developmental agendas for the preschool period is essential for appreciating the efforts that parents are making on behalf of their children. For example, Latino parents may emphasize the importance of being *bien educado*—"well educated" in the sense of knowing how to comport oneself competently in a variety of social situations (Delgado-Gaitan, 1994). In other cultural groups such as traditional African communities, preschool-age children are expected to begin assuming some real responsibilities for helping around the house, running errands, and taking care of younger siblings. Interestingly, when U.S. preschool children are assigned household tasks, they are generally thought of as supporting training for being "responsible" rather than for their intrinsic helpfulness (Goodnow, 1996). Each of these agendas is put into practice in the ways that parents organize their children's daily activities and interact with them. For example, Asian immigrant parents studied by Parmar, Harkness, and Super (2004) spent more time with their preschool-age children in academically related activities, although they played with their children as much as their American counterparts did; on the other hand, rural African children may spend up to half their time at home in helping activities by the age of 6 years.

Early Childhood to School Age: Temperament and Perceptions of the "Difficult Child"

Individual differences in children are recognized in all cultures, but there are sharp variations in both the developmental timing of when such differences are considered meaningful and what kinds of individual behavioral styles are seen as "difficult" for their parents and others. Parents in a rural Kipsigis community of Kenya studied by Super and Harkness in the 1970s perceived almost all babies as being the same: only babies of a particular clan were thought to be different in their social behaviors. For these parents, important differences in personality became evident around the age of 6 years, when the child was considered old enough to do tasks, such as running small errands for the family, without immediate supervision. In contrast, middle-class American parents often perceive their babies as having distinct personalities from birth onward (Harkness, Super, and van Tijen, 2000) (see also Chapter 7).

The cultural significance of individual differences in children's temperament was recognized early by Alexander Thomas and Stella Chess (1977), who found that the constellation of behavioral tendencies that defined the "difficult infant" for their urban, middle-class study population did not seem to apply to a group of Puerto Rican working-class families. The "goodness of fit" between the child's temperament and its developmental niche thus can be viewed at the level of cultural community as well as individual family. Even among middle-class families in post-industrial Western societies, there are important differences in what behavioral styles are found most challenging to parents (Super et al, 2008). For example, Italian parents were found to be very concerned about shyness but were relatively unconcerned about the child who frequently expressed negative moods or intense reactions. In contrast, Dutch parents appreciated children who would carefully evaluate new situations from a safe distance before becoming involved rather than impulsively joining in, but they found children who were too active and tended to have a short attention span to be difficult to manage. Such cultural expectations are often implicitly shared by the wider society, with policies and programs designed to match. For example, high expectations for children's quick adaptation to preschool or kindergarten in the United States are expressed in a relative absence of arrangements for children to separate more slowly from their parents, in contrast to the opposite arrangements that are routine in Sweden. Pediatricians can help parents not only to recognize the reality of constitutionally based individual differences but also to reflect on the ways that the child's developmental niche is adapted to these differences, or not, in a variety of culturally organized settings.

Middle Childhood to Adolescence: Independence and Responsibility

The cultural construct of "independence" is central for American middle-class parents' and professionals' views of child development. The infant who has trouble sleeping alone in his or her own room, the toddler who hates being strapped into a car seat, the kindergarten child who acts clingy when dropped off at school, and even the teenager who gets into arguments about coming home by a certain hour are seen as dealing with independence issues in one way or another. American parents tend to see the achievement of independence as an important goal but one that may involve internal as well as external struggles. By the time children reach school age, there is a general expectation that they will be able to handle being in new environments without their parents, in the company of peers and other adults. Indeed, the beginning of school for American children marks the start of a trend, perceived as developmentally universal, toward increasing involvement with peers and correspondingly decreasing time and involvement with family.

The ethnocentricity of this expectation has become increasingly evident in recent years as it contrasts with patterns of social development imported to the United States by various immigrant groups. Asian parents, for example, often expect their schoolchildren to spend hours after school on academic activities, whether homework or special tutoring such as is routinely offered in their home countries. Working parents from some cultures expect their children to help out at home with important responsibilities such as dinner preparation, even at the expense of homework. The notion of "responsibility" itself can also vary; for example, the Asian Indian girl who consults with her mother about decisions regarding dating is seen as behaving "responsibly," as is the Euro-American girl who makes a decision on her own to come home early from a school dance she is not enjoying (Raghavan, Harkness, and Super, in press). Pediatricians need to be aware of the varying cultural ways that parents think about their children's development of independence and responsibility, and avoid giving guidance based on their own cultural models.

CULTURE AND THE CLINICAL ASSESSMENT OF BEHAVIORAL-DEVELOPMENTAL ISSUES

Cultural differences such as those we have described manifest themselves not only in normal development but also in developmental and behavioral problems that parents and others bring to the clinical setting. In the following section, we describe and comment on three clinical cases in which cultural knowledge was needed for the assessment and management of developmental-behavioral issues.

Case 1: A Portuguese-American Toddler with Eating and Sleeping Problems

Mr. and Mrs. Gomes brought their son John, 20 months, to the developmental-behavioral clinic because of his refusal of food and inadequate weight gain and poor sleeping patterns. Mrs. Gomes (and her mother), dreading every meal and ending each one in tears, had taken to feeding John all day long, following him around with food and a spoon as he played. In addition, they had begun giving him high-calorie, milk-based supplements at bedtime. John was not and never had been allowed to feed himself. He looked thin, pale, and weak to his mother and grandmother, and that image was reinforced by neighbors and relatives. Mrs. Gomes was vulnerable to their many comments on his size, accepting them as confirmation of her inadequacy as a mother and allowing her guilt to soar. She was certain that John was anorexic, especially after hearing on the *Oprah Winfrey Show* that infants could have the disorder.

The feeding problem had been identified early: as a newborn, John had difficulty latching onto the breast, a pattern that Mrs. Gomes saw as rejection of food and, very quickly, as her failure. She stopped breastfeeding and initiated solids before 3 months of age. Sleep emerged as a problem, abruptly, within a week of the Gomes' moving from the maternal grandparents' home to their own place when John was 9 months of age. Although initially they tried to let him cry out his repeated wakenings in his own room, soon he was sleeping with them. They had lived with Mrs. Gomes' parents since John's birth, and although he was extremely attached to his grandfather, the Gomes had not realized he would notice the change. In fact, they had not anticipated any of their reactions to the separation until their first visit to the grandparents, about 2 weeks after the move, when John and all four adults burst into tears.

Developmental screening of John showed normal to superior performance in motor, language, cognitive, and social areas, but he would not leave his parents, despite his interest in going to the playroom with the psychologist. He showed great pleasure in play and initiated many contacts with the psychologist but only a few with his father and none with his mother.

A few points in the Gomes' family histories proved to be most useful in understanding and untangling the presenting problem. Mrs. Gomes' sister had been diagnosed with anorexia as a child, and Mrs. Gomes vividly remembered scenes of her mother fighting, unsuccessfully, to get food into her. Mr. Gomes and his mother, who was apparently obese, had fought with each other over his poor eating as a child, and as an adult he had been significantly overweight.

By reflecting with Mr. and Mrs. Gomes, the clinical team was able to uncover cultural and generational implications of these histories in the parents' current difficulties with John. Among their Portuguese family and community, a baby should look fat to be seen as healthy and normal, and a mother would interpret any comment about her baby's size as a reflection of her success as a good, Portuguese mother. The team acknowledged the family's trans-generational feeding and eating problems as history that was clouding the parents' current views of John and themselves but that need not repeat itself. Having clarified those implications, the team was able to propose parental behavioral changes based on developmental principles that made sense to the Gomeses on hearing them, although previously they had not been obvious; specifically, the team talked about the normal decline in children's appetite and the emergence of autonomy in the second year of life as well as the high degree of awareness that even young infants have for important people around them. The team decided to focus only on the feeding issues because they assumed that the sleep difficulties were secondary to the feeding interactions. The parents were asked to stop their involvement in John's eating and allow him total control over his intake, despite the messes and despite their fear of losing him to starvation, and the team suggested that they also discontinue the bedtime supplements. The parents were also asked to keep a record of what John ate each day.

On the return visit 2 weeks later, Mr. and Mrs. Gomes reported dramatic change in John's eating. He was now entirely self-feeding, consuming amounts that were more than adequate for the comfort of his mother and grandmother. Even more striking was Mrs. Gomes' description of a day with John: for the first time, he would approach her with toys for positive interaction, and also for the first time, she enjoyed being with him. She told the pediatrician that she had not realized she *could* play with him, having no recollection of her parents playing with her. John still insisted on sleeping with his parents, but they showed resolve in their need to be together in bed without him and he was wakening less often, probably because of the decrease in bedtime feedings. John's behavior in the clinic supported the team's optimistic appraisal of the situation. He was as pleased as before with the play, but this time he went several times to his mother's knee to show her a toy or for a cuddle before he approached his father for the same. The parents already had plans for dealing with the sleep problem, asking only for the pediatrician's approval and fine-tuning.

This case illustrates a common kind of behavioral-developmental issue for parents of toddlers in ethnic groups including not only Portuguese but also Hispanic, Italian, and some Asian (notably Indian) populations. In these cultures, it is normative for infants and young children to be hand fed by their mothers up to a much later age than would be considered appropriate in U.S. middle-class families. Feeding is often considered *the* core function and defining feature of motherhood. Because of a child's temperamental disposition or for other reasons, however, feeding practices can lead to conflicts such as the Gomes family was experiencing. The clinical response to the problem in this case, although based on developmental principles, also substituted an American middle-class cultural model of development involving increasing autonomy and separation as an alternative to the parents' previous cultural model based on interdependence. It is interesting that the parents were able to accept this different view so readily; we can speculate, however, that they were able to do so in part because the idea of autonomy was presented in relation to only one admittedly problem domain and because it was in the service of achieving the parents' primary cultural goal of getting the child to eat more (see also Chapter 58).

Case 2: An American Infant with Behavioral and Sleeping Problems

At the time that Mr. and Mrs. Pearce brought 6-month-old David to the behavioral-developmental clinic, they were desperate for relief from his constant and demanding irritability and his highly irregular sleep schedule, including nighttime sleep periods of at most 1½ hours. The problem had begun at birth with his parents' responding to his every cry, which they heard as signaling hunger. In response, they had continually increased his feedings, which now amounted to an almost unbelievable 48 ounces of milk per day in addition to a small amount of solids. David had had a few longer stretches of nighttime sleep in the past 2 months when the parents let him cry after wakening, but as they said, "He still needs us to put him to sleep" for naps, at bedtime, and after wakening at night.

Mr. Pearce was very supportive of and concerned about his wife, finding her in tears at the end of his working day. No one was getting enough sleep and he felt their lives were drifting apart. These difficulties had seriously challenged their confidence in themselves as parents. Mrs. Pearce had been given up to foster care by her mother at the age of 6 years. She had very fond memories of her foster mother, but the early break with her own mother and the death of her foster mother several years before David's birth had contributed to her vulnerability to self-doubts as a parent, thus increasing her need to respond to his every cry.

The clinical team's assessment of David showed that his development was normal in cognitive, language, and fine and gross motor development. His temperament was not extreme on most dimensions, although his diurnal schedule as reported by his parents was very irregular. It was difficult for the team to imagine him as irritable all day long. An attempt at napping during the clinic revealed behavior typical of David's difficulty falling asleep. He repeatedly raised his head from the mattress, turning it from side to side, bobbing up and down, and whimpering. The team also observed, however, that his mother constantly intervened, patting his head with every "bob."

Both parents accepted the team's observation of their overintervention with David in this brief episode in the clinic and as they described it at home. They seemed relieved to learn about the concept of overprotection that might be "no favor to the child," as Mr. Pearce later put it. They also quickly saw that their reading of most of David's cries as hunger or a need for attention, and their consequently rapid responses, had actually prevented him from developing his own skills in state regulation even though he seemed by temperament to have the capacity to do so. On the basis of this understanding, the parents accepted the team's recommendations to reduce his intake of formula and to increase solid food, to let him cry for short periods during the day if they had to attend to a task, and to keep a diary of his daily schedule.

Within a week, Mrs. Pearce reported in a telephone call that she had limited David's formula intake and that he was eating much more solid food. Along with these changes in eating, she commented that David seemed happier during the day and was even able to nap without "help" from his parents. On a return visit 2 weeks later, the positive ripple effects of the change in feeding were apparent in other areas of his behavior, such as requiring much less parental intervention for going to sleep and sustaining longer periods of nighttime sleep. Mrs. Pearce herself saw that she had overstimulated David in general—with radio playing, lights, mobiles, and a toy-filled bedroom as well as with her own attentiveness. She was thankful for the permission to pull back and since doing this was continuing to discover on her own how to tolerate his cry, how his behavior at night affected his daytime behavior, and how she and her husband could modulate their interventions, entertainment, and activities with David.

This case, like the first one, illustrates the interaction between individual family history and cultural beliefs and practices in the development of a behavioral problem. As a foster child who had suffered twice the loss of her mother, Mrs. Pearce was anxious not to fail her own child. Her attentiveness, however, was also an exaggeration of the standard mainstream American cultural model of responsive parenting. In this case, it seems that what the parents needed most was authoritative advice to counter what they had derived from a combination of personal experience and cultural images of good parenting, advice demonstrating that being a good parent might be achieved through different routes.

Case 3: Control of Female Adolescent Sexual Behavior in a Haitian Family

Dr. McHale, a Euro-American pediatrician, first met the Bernard family when they brought their children to the HMO for an introductory visit. The Bernards had emigrated from Haiti several years earlier and had three children, of whom the oldest was 16-year-old Jacqueline. Both parents were present for the initial visit, but Mr. Bernard asked and answered most questions for the children and for his wife. The pediatrician's questions about school, sports, and social activities drew short answers from the children and some intrafamily glances as the father described the close supervision of the children that either he or his wife or his brother and sister-in-law provided. The children's out-of-school social activities were limited to extended family and church.

The family's next use of the health center occurred almost a year later when Jacqueline was brought to the clinic by her father. Mr. Bernard wanted an examination to determine whether his daughter had engaged in sexual intercourse. He was angrily convinced that she had and insistent on the pediatrician's providing the proof. Jacqueline herself was sullen and uncommunicative with her father. She revealed to the pediatrician that she did have a boyfriend whom she saw secretly, but Dr. McHale's impression was that either she was withholding the full story—as she denied having intercourse—or she truly did not understand the pediatrician's vocabulary.

Dr. McHale was surprised and uncomfortable about the degree of involvement of this father in his daughter's intimate development and confused about how to relate either to his position of total control or to Jacqueline's of reticence and distrust. She explained to Jacqueline and Mr. Bernard that an examination would not provide the proof that he sought. She suggested that the family needed to find a way to manage the parents' concern for and surveillance of their daughter's social and physical maturation. In addition, she pointed out that they needed to find a way to support Jacqueline's inevitable independence and social development in this culture very different from what the parents had experienced in their own youth.

Mr. Bernard only reluctantly accepted this idea, and subsequent attempts by Dr. McHale and the child mental health consultants to work on a plan with the family failed. Several times during the next 2 years, Mr. Bernard returned with Jacqueline to request pregnancy testing or culture for sexually transmitted disease. Communication between father and daughter had not improved, and Mr. Bernard remained angry. Jacqueline was still sullen but obviously was making her own way in the local adolescent culture. Shortly before graduating from high school, Jacqueline became pregnant and soon after married her second cousin, the father of the baby.

This case illustrates, first, cultural differences in the management of adolescent sexual behavior and, second, the clash of cultures between the Haitian parental generation and the American peer culture of their children. Intergenerational disagreements concerning freedom and control, and obligations to the family, often emerge strongly during the adolescent period for acculturating families (Berry, 2007).

The most striking aspect of this case, however, is the way it illustrates the dilemma faced by the pediatrician asked to apply her expertise in a way that she finds personally and socially unacceptable. In this case, the pediatrician suggested an alternative strategy involving a change in power relationships among family members. The father, however, was apparently equally uncomfortable with this solution: he wanted help, but on his own terms. The failure in communication between the pediatrician and the father was mirrored in the failure of both parents and pediatrician to prevent the occurrence of pregnancy in the unwed adolescent daughter.

Table 19-1. Five Steps to the Development of Culturally Sensitive Attitudes, Assessment, and Intervention

1. Acquaint yourself with the child's developmental niche, including daily routines, caretaking practices, and the cultural beliefs that give these meaning for the parents.
2. Explore with parents their expectations for the child's behavior and development; their own role in protecting, managing, and nurturing the child; and the roles of other significant persons (e.g., extended family, health care providers).
3. Use standard assessments (e.g., motor, language, cognitive, social, temperament, and attachment measures) to inform your understanding of the parents' presentation of "problems" in the child's behavior and development.
4. Be aware that standard developmental assessment tools reflect the cultural biases of the population for which they were developed.
5. Use your knowledge of the parents' beliefs, practices, and goals in formulating advice for handling behavioral-developmental issues.

In thinking back on this case, Dr. McHale felt that she might have done more to reach Jacqueline herself and to learn her perspective on the situation; alternatively, perhaps Dr. McHale could have worked through Haitian community institutions such as the church. Perhaps, however, the actual outcome was not entirely culturally inappropriate: Jacqueline had finished her education, had married within the community, and could now begin a new, more independent stage of her life as a young married woman.

Cultural Themes in the Clinical Context

Cultural themes, as illustrated in these cases, can be manifested in the clinical context of pediatric care in three ways. First, behavior problems often reflect cultural themes. Parents are likely to present specific behavioral-developmental problems that are manifestations of larger cultural themes, but usually without conscious awareness of this. Second, problem domains vary cross-culturally. Particular behavioral domains—for example, sleeping, eating, language or motor development—are especially resonant with the dominant cultural themes of different societies, and this variation is reflected in the kinds of "problems" that parents report to pediatricians. Third, cultural themes relate differentially to developmental transitions, and transition points may therefore provide particular opportunities to learn about cultural themes and to consider shaping interventions appropriately. Unless the pediatrician understands the cultural aspects of the situation, even advice based on solid developmental or temperamental information is likely to fail.

A CULTURALLY SENSITIVE PRACTICE OF PEDIATRICS

Bringing cultural sensitivity, in the sense of a nonprejudiced attitude toward unfamiliar practices, to a clinical assessment of behavior and development is not sufficient. In a culturally sensitive practice, the pediatrician will approach the family and the presenting problem with general knowledge of how cultures normally organize beliefs, values, and practices into a consonant whole, with specific knowledge of both the foreign culture and his or her own, and with flexibility in the manner of negotiating information and authority during the clinical communications. Table 19-1 summarizes important steps in this process.

A Culturally Sensitive Attitude

A culturally sensitive attitude in behavioral-developmental pediatrics is both neutral and alert. Neutrality requires awareness of and perspective on one's own cultural beliefs and biases; alertness requires awareness of the possibility that any practice, problem, or response to pediatric assessment and management may have a cultural basis. This basis may be found at the level of the family culture, the ethnic community, or the dominant culture. Achieving and practicing with such a culturally neutral and alert eye requires knowledge of various cultures and ethnic groups. It can be attained through continued dialogue with patients themselves, interviews with community or religious leaders, searching the medical and social science literature on relevant ethnic groups, and even reading novels and biographic accounts by cultural insiders. A knowledgeable perspective on one's own ethnic beliefs and biases, those of the dominant contemporary American culture, and the medical system as a culture must also be attained. The sources are similar to those for knowledge of any professional issue; medical education centers and private and professional societies offer postgraduate courses for enhancing one's cultural learning, not only for knowledge but also for skill and attitude.

A culturally sensitive attitude is adaptable and clarifying, and its goal is to support parents in making effective choices in harmony with their cultural goals and beliefs. In some ways, it is antithetical to the usual medical approach because the pediatrician in this situation must listen attentively and must work to elicit the patient's own meaning, rather than impose a ready-made structure on the communication. People of differing cultures vary in intimate ways of being and thinking. Language shortcuts, slang, and even medical jargon can carry shared meanings efficiently between physician and patient of the same culture, but they cannot be used with patients of different cultures without risking the flow of mutually meaningful information (Pedersen, 1985). To avoid this, the pediatrician must often be in a receptive rather than an active mode when assessing behavioral development problems; certainty must be put aside for searching. Ballottement of the abdomen, and waiting for the informative return of the spleen, is the closest medical analogy to this sort of work. When resuming an action mode after such an attentive pause, the pediatrician should use other interactive skills, such as problem solving, rather than answer giving, in the traditional diagnostic phase; and negotiation, rather than prescription giving or unilateral decision making, in the treatment or management phase. Both of these skills require holding open several options while exploring the benefits, limitations, and possible consequences of each one. In addition, pediatric adaptability must relate not only to choices of child rearing patterns and developmental outcomes but also to differences in use of medical services and definitions of problems. Patients must play an active role in shaping appropriate care.

Because culture is an organized and meaningful system, as indicated by the niche framework, a culturally sensitive approach in pediatric practice can be systematized along the same lines. Of particular significance to the practitioner is an understanding of how cultural beliefs and goals held by parents are used to organize children's daily environments and in customary child rearing practices. In general, as we have outlined before, the beliefs of a culture will support customary practices, which, if successfully carried out, will lead to actualization of the shared values.

Many individual customs or parental practices of child rearing are based on beliefs and values that are often not made explicit by the parent. When parents have a problem with their child's behavior, discovery of their underlying beliefs is important; those beliefs often support a continued practice that may not fit that particular child's temperament, that may not be suitable to the child's developmental stage, or that may present too great a divergence from the majority culture. Reassuring or advising parents will probably fail unless their own beliefs and values are uncovered and tested. Once these are made explicit, other means of actualizing them can be sought. Taking a cultural perspective at the family level can alert one to a path of enquiry that opens up new possibilities.

Culturally Sensitive Assessment

Standardized tests normally offer the pediatrician a powerful and efficient method of assessing the nature and degree of developmental disturbance. However, variation in the cultural environments of children and their corresponding developmental differences point to the importance of considering culture and ethnicity when the pediatrician assesses behavioral development.

The application of standard tests of assessment to populations beyond the one for which norms were developed is problematic (Kazdin, 2003), and cross-cultural psychologists have been especially concerned with the possibilities for misuse and misunderstanding (Berry, Poortinga, and Pandey, 1997). The most obvious problem, that differences in experience will produce differences in norms, is not the greatest one. More serious is the fact that items in the test are usually chosen in light of cultural values and the frequency of behaviors in Euro-American children. There is little conceptual (as opposed to empiric) basis for the most popular tests, including the Bayley scales and the Denver Developmental Screening Test. What children are seen to do and the age they are seen to do it are captured in these tests, but when the tests are used on a new population, the developmental skill underlying the specific behavioral items may not be represented; in short, the construct validity may be threatened. Thus, when children of a different culture do not perform a test item, we do not know whether they have merely failed in a specific act or lack the social, representational, or motor skills that the item was designed to tap.

For example, 9-month-old infants in rural Kenya, when presented with a doll in the context of the Bayley examination, characteristically exhibit negative responses rather than the social responses (e.g., cuddling) this part of the test was designed to elicit; to the Gusii mothers, the inert doll looked too much like a dead baby (Keefer et al, 1991). It would be difficult to assess the social development of Gusii infants on the basis of their response to this item of the Bayley scale. Moreover, other potential items in the Bayley examination that would reflect culturally significant aspects of development in other ethnic groups (e.g., sharing in the African context) do not appear on these American tests at all—the test as a collection of items is biased. Thus, until the behavioral scope of such tests is widened or culture-specific adaptations are made, pediatricians should be very cautious about their application and interpretation with children of other ethnic groups (Miller, Onotera, and Deinard, 1984).

Culturally Sensitive Intervention

The pediatrician can use cultural knowledge and sensitivity, together with thoughtful use of developmental assessments, to establish a strategy of intervention relevant to the needs of both the child and the parents. In this context, understanding the issues that parents face in their own cultural environments can help the pediatrician to intervene most effectively on behalf of the child's developmental needs. The pediatrician must also be alert to issues of "goodness of fit" between the child's culturally structured home environment and the wider environments of school, peer groups, and ultimately work settings. Anthropologists have noted that parental goals are oriented to the needs of adult life as parents have experienced them in the past or imagine them to be in the future. For some cultural or ethnic groups, this orientation may not be compatible with success in middle-class American society. In situations such as this, pure cultural relativism—accepting all cultural systems as equally valid—is an inadequate response. Instead, the pediatrician faces a double challenge: first, to understand the child's home environment and development as culturally structured phenomena; and second, to help the parents and child negotiate a successful relationship with the wider world.

CULTURAL ADVOCACY ISSUES

We have suggested in this chapter that a culturally sensitive attitude in diagnosis and intervention is now an essential tool in clinical pediatrics. Children's development is shaped in part by the settings of their daily lives, the customs of care used at home, and the psychology of the caretakers, particularly parental ethnotheories. These three aspects of the developmental niche are in turn regulated by larger aspects of the culture in which the children and parents live. The broadly middle-class, Euro-American environment that forms the basis for the culture of medicine differs in important ways from the environment of many of today's pediatric patients. To hear the meaning of behaviors behind parents' depiction, to see the development underlying possibly biased standardized assessments, and to intervene in ways that will be accepted and effective, these are the challenges in creating a culturally appropriate developmental-behavioral pediatrics. To meet this challenge, the pediatrician must turn an ethnographer's eye not only toward the patient but also toward his or her own personal beliefs and those of the medical system itself. Just as the pediatrician must be an advocate for the right of the individual child to be different, he or she must also be an advocate for the right of particular cultures or subcultures to be different, even in the face of pressures from the dominant culture. Clarity and certainty, when an action is based on solid scientific data, are most useful combined with cultural knowledge and a culturally sensitive perspective that allow the rich varieties of normal human behavior and development.

SUMMARY

A culturally sensitive attitude in diagnosis and intervention is an essential tool in modern clinical pediatrics. Children's development is shaped in part by the settings of their daily lives, the customs of care used at home, and the psychology of the caretakers. These three aspects of the developmental niche are in turn regulated by larger aspects of the culture in which the children and parents live. The pediatrician must turn an ethnographer's eye not only toward the patient but also toward his or her own personal beliefs and to those of the medical system itself. To hear the meaning of behaviors underlying parents' descriptions, to see the development underlying possibly biased standardized assessments, and to intervene in ways that will be accepted and effective, these are the challenges in creating a developmental-behavioral pediatrics that allows the rich varieties of normal human behavior and development.

REFERENCES

Berry JW: Acculturation strategies and adaptation. *In* Lansford JE, Deater-Deckard K, Bornstein MH (eds): Immigrant Families in Contemporary Society. New York, Guilford Press, 2007, pp 69-82.

Berry JW, Poortinga YH, Pandey J: Handbook of Cross-Cultural Psychology, Vol. 1: Theory and Method, 2nd ed. Needham Heights, MA, Allyn & Bacon, 1997.

D'Andrade R, Strauss C: Human Motives and Cultural Models. Cambridge, Cambridge University Press, 1992.

Delgado-Gaitan C: Socializing young children in Mexican-American families: An intergenerational perspective. *In* Greenfield PM, Cocking RR (eds): Cross-Cultural Roots of Minority Child Development. Hillsdale, NJ, Erlbaum, 1994, pp 55-86.

Giordano J: Ethnicity and Mental Health: Research and Recommendations. New York, National Project on Ethnic America of the American Jewish Committee, 1973.

Goodnow J: From household practices to parents' ideas about work and interpersonal relationships. *In* Harkness S, Super CM (eds): Parents' Cultural Belief Systems: Their Origins, Expressions, and Consequences. New York, Guilford Press, 1996, pp 313-344.

Gottlieb A: The Afterlife Is Where We Come From. Chicago, University of Chicago Press, 2004.

Greenfield PM, Cocking RR: Cross-Cultural Roots of Minority Child Development. Hillsdale, NJ, Erlbaum, 1994.

Harkness S, Super CM (eds): Parents' Cultural Belief Systems: Their Origins, Expressions, and Consequences. New York, Guilford, 1996.

Harkness S, Super CM, Moscardino U, et al: Cultural models and developmental agendas: implications for arousal and self-regulation in early infancy. J Dev Processes 2:5-39, 2007.

Harkness S, Super CM, van Tijen N: Individualism and the "Western mind" reconsidered: American and Dutch parents' ethnotheories of children and family. *In* Harkness S, Raeff C, Super CM (eds): Variability in the Social Construction of the Child. New Directions for Child and Adolescent Development, No. 87. San Francisco, Jossey-Bass, 2000, pp 23-39.

Kağitçibaşi C: Family, Self, and Human Development Across Cultures: Theory and Applications, 2nd ed. Mahwah, NJ, Erlbaum, 2007.

Kazdin AE: Ethical Principles of Psychologists and Code of Conduct. Washington, DC, American Psychological Association, 2003.

Keefer CH, Dixon S, Tronick E, Brazelton TB: Cultural mediation between newborn behavior and later development: Implications for methodology in cross-cultural research. *In* Nugent JK, Lester BM, Brazelton TB (eds): The Cultural Context of Infancy, Vol. 2: Multi-Cultural and Interdisciplinary Approaches to Parent-Infant Relations. Norwood, NJ, Ablex, 1991.

LeVine RA, Dixon S, LeVine S, et al: Child Care and Culture: Lessons from Africa. New York, Cambridge University Press, 1994.

Levy R: Ethnography, comparison, and changing times. Ethos 33(4):435-458, 2005.

Malik NM, Boris NW, Heller SS, et al: Risk for maternal depression and child aggression in Early Head Start families: A test of ecological models. Infant Mental Health J 28(2):171-191, 2007.

McGoldrick M, Giordano J, Garcia-Preto N: Overview: Ethnicity and Family Therapy. New York, Guilford Press, 2005.

Miller V, Onotera RT, Deinard AS: Denver Developmental Screening Test: Cultural variations in Southeast Asian children. J Pediatr 104(3):481-482, 1984.

Moscardino U, Nwobu O, Axia G: Cultural beliefs and practices related to infant health and development among Nigerian immigrant mothers in Italy. J Reprod Infant Psychology 24(3):241-255, 2006.

Parmar P, Harkness S, Super CM: Asian and Euro-American parents' ethnotheories of play and learning: Effects on pre-school children's home routines and school behavior. Int J Behavioral Dev 28(2):97-104, 2004.

Pedersen P (ed): Handbook of Cross-Cultural Counseling and Therapy. Westport, CT, Greenwood Press, 1985.

Pozniak H: Parenting baby educators: The early learning centre: educational baby toys can really stimulate tiny minds, and the market. The Independent, October 28, 2005, p 6.

Raghavan C, Harkness S, Super CM: Asian Indian immigrant and Euro-American mothers' ethnotheories about their daughters. J Crosscultural Psychology 2009; in press.

Shonkoff JP, Phillips DA: From Neurons to Neighborhoods: The Science of Early Childhood Development. Washington, DC, National Academy Press, 2000.

Super CM, Harkness S: Culture structures the environment for development. Human Dev 45(4):270-274, 2002.

Super CM, Harkness S, van Tijen N, et al: The three R's of Dutch child rearing and the socialization of infant arousal. *In* Harkness S, Super CM (eds): Parents' Cultural Belief Systems: Their Origins, Expressions, and Consequences. New York, Guilford Press, 1996, pp 447-466.

Super CM, Axia G, Harkness S, Welles-Nyström B, Zyličz PO, Ríos Bermúdez M, Bonichini S, Parmar P, Moscardino U, Kolar V, Palacios J, McGurk H: Culture, temperament, and the "difficult child" in seven Western cultures. Eur J Dev Sci 2(1-2): 136-157, 2008.

Thomas A, Chess S: Temperament and Development. New York, Brunner/Mazel, 1977.

20 MEDIA

VICTOR C. STRASBURGER

> *"True, media violence is not likely to turn an otherwise fine child into a violent criminal. But, just as every cigarette one smokes increases a little bit the likelihood of a lung tumor someday, every violent show one watches increases just a little bit the likelihood of behaving more aggressively in some situation."*
>
> —Psychologists Brad J. Bushman and L. Rowell Huesmann (Handbook of Children and the Media, 2001, p 248)
>
> *"Parents could once easily mold their young children's upbringing by speaking and reading to children only about those things they wished their children to be exposed to, but today's parents must battle with thousands of competing images and ideas over which they have little direct control."*
>
> —Professor Joshua Meyrowitz (No Sense of Place, 1985, p 238)

Throughout the recent history of Western civilization, adults have complained about the influence of media on children and adolescents. First, it was penny novels, then comic books, then *Playboy* magazine, rapidly followed by Elvis Presley and rock 'n' roll, and now it is Paris Hilton, Britney Spears, *MySpace.com,* and other Internet sites. The fact is, there have always been objectionable media, but not every child or teen is vulnerable, nor are all media problematic. Some, in fact, are powerfully prosocial. For example, the Internet has completely revolutionized the learning and memorization of "facts" in school. Within the next decade, people will begin wearing 5-gigabyte mini-computers on their wrists, like watches, and will be able to tell you when the First Punic War was in an instant (264 BC, and Rome won). Even now, teaching about the American Civil War in school is a snap if you have access to Ken Burns' acclaimed PBS series.

So not all the media are "bad," nor are all children and teens equally affected by them; but the media remain the single most important and underrated influence on young people today. Sex, drug taking, obesity, school achievement, aggressive behavior—virtually *every* concern that a parent or a developmental expert might have about a child has some potential basis in the media (Strasburger, 2006). Adults need to think of the quality and impact of the media as an environmental health issue, which then avoids moralizing and concentrates on protecting infants, children, and teens from potential harm. At the same time, even the definition of "literacy" has changed significantly. In 1900, to be literate meant that you could read and write. In 2008, to be literate means that you can decode and understand a dizzying variety of media.

HOW CHILDREN AND TEENS USE MEDIA

Children and teens spend more time with media than they do in any other activity except for sleeping. By the time today's young people reach the age of 70 years, they will have spent 7 to 10 years of their lives watching television alone (Strasburger, 2006). More American homes have a TV set than indoor plumbing, and today's child lives in an environment with an average of four TV sets, three CD players, three radios, three VCRs or DVD players, two videogame consoles, and at least one computer. Preteens and teens can download racy videos, text message their friends, buy cigarettes and alcohol on the Internet, and leave enticing profiles on *MySpace.com.* Yet across all ages, television remains the predominant medium. Television viewing is beginning at increasingly younger ages, which has major implications in terms of early brain development (Wartella and Robb, 2007). The latest national report found that on a typical day, nearly two thirds of infants are watching television for 1½ hours (Vandewater, 2007). A 2005 Kaiser Foundation report surveyed more than 2000 third to twelfth graders nationally and found that children and teens spend an average of nearly 6.6 hours per day with a variety of different media (Fig. 20-1). Most problematically, two thirds of American teenagers have a TV set in their own bedroom, half have a VCR or DVD player, half have a video game console, and nearly one third have a computer (see Fig. 20-1). Virtually every study on the impact of media finds that children and teens with bedroom media experience more adverse effects (Strasburger, 2006). Multitasking is also common among teens (Fig. 20-2), although there are not yet good data on how this

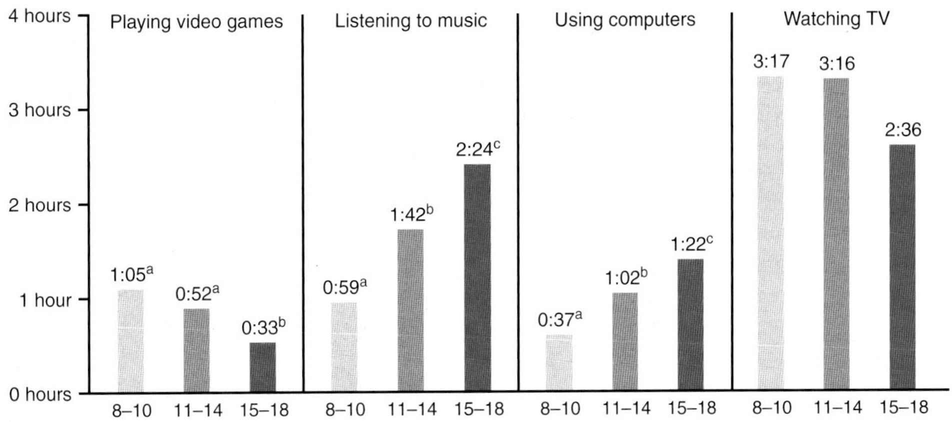

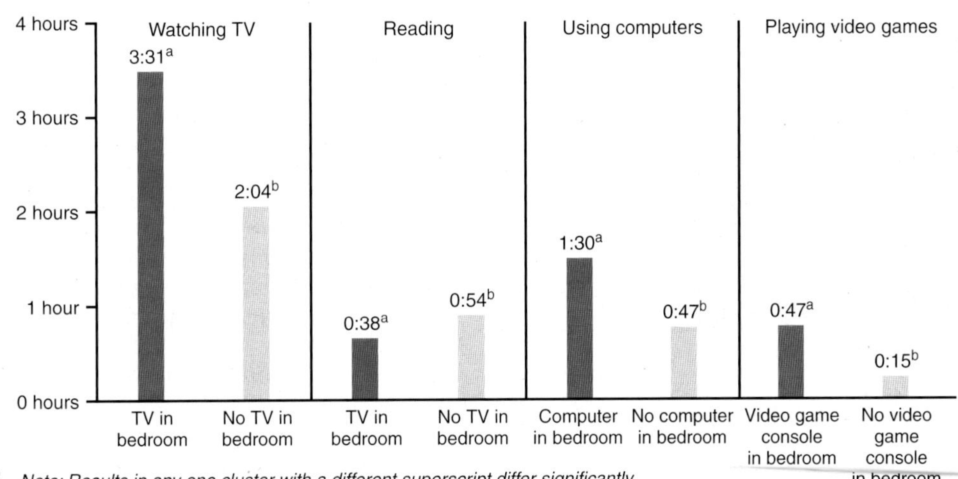

Figure 20-1. A, Even during adolescence, television remains the predominant medium for teenagers. B, The presence of a TV set in a child's or teen's bedroom increases all media use significantly and decreases reading. *(From Rideout V, Roberts DF, Foehr UG: Generation M: Media in the lives of 8-18 year-olds. Menlo Park, CA, Kaiser Family Foundation, 2005.)*

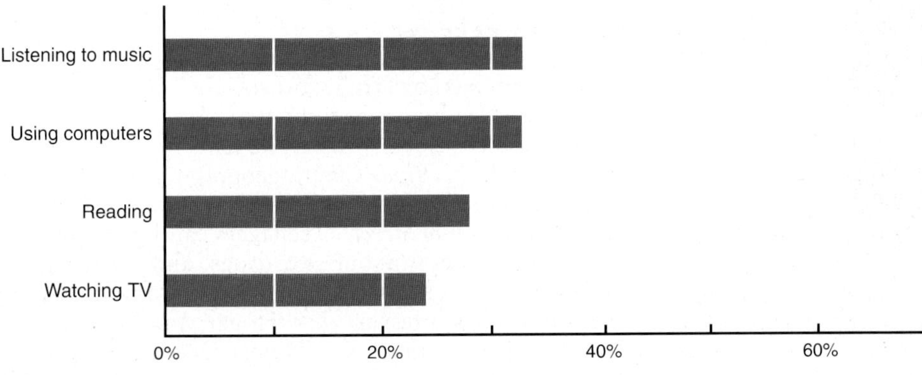

Figure 20-2. Preteens and teens frequently use several media at the same time—multitasking. At present, there is no research available on the impact that this has. *(From Rideout V, Roberts DF, Foehr UG: Generation M: Media in the lives of 8-18 year-olds. Menlo Park, CA, Kaiser Family Foundation, 2005.)*

affects their comprehension or behavior. In particular, music is frequently used as a background accompaniment to homework or talking with friends.

There are numerous theories about how television and other media affect young people. One of the most important and best-documented is the third-person effect—people think that the media affect everyone else but themselves (Strasburger, Wilson, and Jordan, 2009). For example, a sample of more than 500 teenagers nationwide thought that sexual content on television influenced teens their own age, yet less than one fourth believed that it influenced their own behavior (Fig. 20-3).

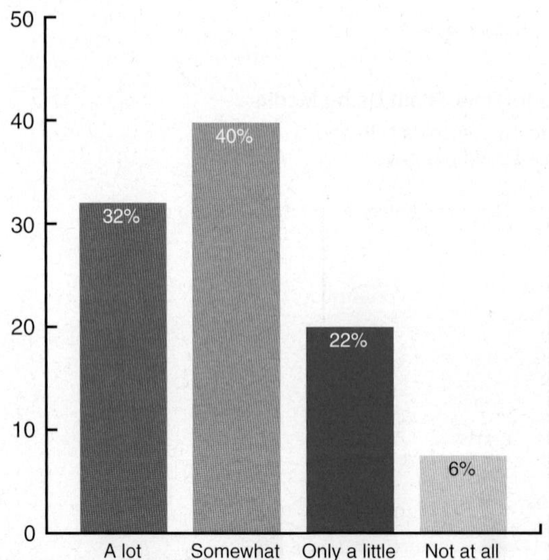

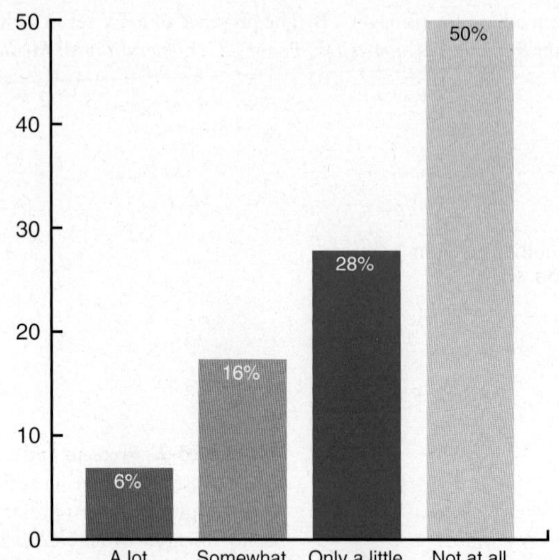

Figure 20-3. Teenagers (and adults) fervently believe that the media affect everyone else but themselves, the so-called third-person effect. *(From Kaiser Family Foundation: Teens say sex on TV influences behavior of peers [press release]. May 20, 2002.)*

Another of the most compelling theories about media influence is the super-peer theory, which states that because teens are notoriously susceptible to peer influences, the media may function as a kind of super-peer for them (Strasburger, 2006). When college students are asked to identify models of responsible and irresponsible sexual behavior, for example, they primarily cite media figures. Early-maturing girls are more likely to seek out sexual content in a variety of media and to interpret that content as approving of teen sex (Brown and Strasburger, 2007). Closely akin to the super-peer theory is the cultivation hypothesis. This says that children and teens tend to view the media world as being "real" and think that they are watching real adult behaviors. For teens, in particular, this may result in their thinking that the violence, sex, and drug taking they are viewing is *normative behavior* for people their age and older. One theory that has been thoroughly discredited is the catharsis theory, that viewers can be purged of their feelings of aggression by watching media violence, for example (Strasburger, Wilson, and Jordan, 2009).

EARLY BRAIN DEVELOPMENT

In 1999, the American Academy of Pediatrics' Committee on Public Education issued a recommendation that children younger than 2 years not be allowed to watch television (American Academy of Pediatrics, 1999). A firestorm ensued. Since then, many studies have documented the potentially negative impact of media on early brain development. The human brain is unique in being relatively immature at birth, but that allows it to develop in response to the environment in which it will function. Research shows that infants have a critical need for direct interaction with parents and other caregivers for healthy brain development and that viewing adults on television or in videos is not nearly as effective. Although educational videos for infants are now a $100 million business, there is no evidence that they are effective, and there is one study that has actually found language delays in some infants exposed to them (Zimmerman et al, 2007). Similarly, the adolescent brain is a "work in progress," and new studies show that it is not fully mature until the age of 25 years or so. Therefore, media content that is particularly relevant to teenagers—sex, drugs, and eating disorders, for example—may be very influential in their health-related decisions.

POSITIVE EFFECTS

Media can be powerfully prosocial. They can teach young children numbers and letters *(Sesame Street)*, respect for their elders *(Mister Rogers' Neighborhood)*, logical thinking *(Blues Clues)*, geography *(Where in the World is Carmen Sandiego?)*, and religious and racial tolerance *(Sesame Street)*. Teenagers can learn valuable health information about sex, drugs, and other health issues through television shows and the Internet. Numerous studies attest to this (Hogan and Strasburger, 2007). However, there *is* an almost-Orwellian aspect to media: some critics think that "mind control" is not out of the question, particularly in politics.

NEGATIVE EFFECTS

Whereas media *can* be prosocial, sadly in the United States they tend not to be. American media are among the most violent, sexually suggestive, and commercialized in the world. The average young person will view an estimated 40,000 advertisements, 20,000 acts of violence, 15,000 sexual references, and 2000 beer and wine ads annually on television alone. From a scientific standpoint, it is difficult to imagine how 6 hours a day of media immersion does *not* result in some behavioral consequences, at least in some children. However, the research is difficult to do. Where, for example, does one find a population that has not been exposed to television? In a UNESCO survey of 22 countries, 91% of the world's population of children were found to have access to a TV set. Media research is difficult social science research so that *any* reported findings are probably highly significant. Unfortunately for pediatricians and developmental-behavioral specialists, most of the research resides in the communications and psychology journals and is not easy to digest; but there is a uniformity of findings in a variety of different subject areas that is difficult to deny.

Media Violence

As early as 1952, the U.S. Senate held hearings on whether media violence was affecting young people. More than 50 years later, after more than 3500 studies—of which fewer than 30 showed no effect—the controversy should be over; yet somehow it continues. The research is *very* clear on the following effects (Anderson et al, 2003; Hogan, 2005; Strasburger, Wilson, and Jordan, 2009):

- Viewing media violence desensitizes children and teens. A variety of experiments have documented that desensitization occurs on physiologic and interpersonal levels.
- The most common aspect of American media violence is the notion of "justifiable violence" (i.e., "good guys" versus "bad guys"). This is also the most powerfully reinforcing aspect of media violence.
- For young children, media violence can be frightening and cause sleep disorders. Sleep disturbances are most commonly associated with viewing more television during the day, viewing television at bedtime, and having a TV set in the bedroom. Teens who watch 3 hours or more a day are at increased risk for sleep problems by early adulthood. Parents frequently use television and videos to try to "soothe" children before bedtime, but media tend to be exciting and stimulating. Very young children may be frightened, even by Disney videos, and certainly by inappropriate television ads for blockbuster movies. Television news can also be upsetting or frightening to young children, especially when it contains videos like those of the Virginia Tech killer.
- One fourth of all violent episodes on television involve gunplay. In movies, 40% of the top-grossing G- and PG-rated films feature at least one main character carrying a gun.
- The connection between viewing media violence and real-life aggression is nearly as strong as the link between smoking and lung cancer (Fig. 20-4). Clearly, not everyone who smokes gets lung cancer (the estimate is about 10%). Likewise, not everyone who views violence becomes violent themselves (one estimate is that 10% to 30% of real-life violence can be attributed to viewing media violence).

Several longitudinal correlational studies—which give cause and effect answers—have found that children learn their attitudes about violence at a very young age, and once learned, those attitudes are very difficult to modify.

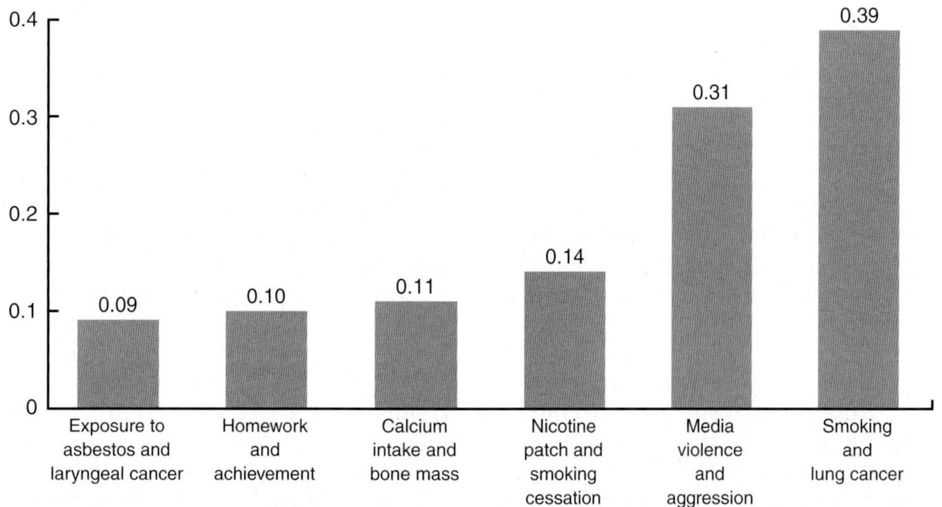

Figure 20-4. A comparison of the media violence correlation with other social risks that have been studied scientifically. *(From Strasburger VC, Wilson BJ: Children, Adolescents, and the Media. Thousand Oaks, CA, Sage, 2002.)*

The first study began in the 1960s in Upstate New York: 875 third graders were prospectively observed for 22 years. Their exposure to media violence at the age of 8 years correlated with their aggressive behavior 11 years and 22 years later, even when IQ and socioeconomic status were controlled for (Huesmann et al, 1984). Another similar study just recently concluded. In this study, a random sample of 707 children aged 1 to 10 years from two New York counties was followed for 17 years. Time spent watching television was a significant risk factor for aggressive behavior later on, especially for boys (Johnson et al, 2002). A third study from 1977 to 2003 found that viewing media violence between the ages of 6 and 9 years predicts adolescent aggressive behavior and even adult criminal behavior and spousal abuse (Huesmann et al, 2003). What seem most important in determining whether media violence will have an impact on young children are whether the child identifies with violent characters, whether the child sees television as being real, and the context of the violence (Is it condoned? Is it punished? Does it cause harm?). The correlation between media violence and aggressive behavior has been sufficiently well established in the minds of media researchers that studies are rarely done anymore.

Suicide

Several studies have demonstrated a link between media coverage of suicide, television movies about suicide, and subsequent increases in teen suicide. Even well-intentioned programs can cause an increase, and this contagion effect seems to be stronger in adolescents than in adults. The Centers for Disease Control and Prevention have issued guidelines for media reporting about suicide that encourage TV stations and newspapers not to glorify the person or to sensationalize the event.

Advertising

Children and adolescents see 40,000 ads per year on television alone. Increasingly, younger and younger children are being targeted, primarily because advertising is a $250 billion a year industry in the United States (American Academy of Pediatrics, 2006); yet a series of Federal Trade Commission (FTC) hearings in the late 1970s concluded that it is unfair and deceptive to advertise to children younger than 6 years. Several European nations either ban all advertising directed at children or severely restrict it, yet in the United States, it remains business as usual.

The impact is considerable. Tobacco manufacturers spend $30 million a day on advertising and promotion. Two large and unique longitudinal studies have found that approximately one third of all teen smoking can be attributed to tobacco advertising and promotion (Borzekowski and Strasburger, 2007). Alcohol manufacturers spend nearly $6 billion a year on advertising, and research shows that exposure to ads is a significant risk factor for teen drinking (Borzekowski and Strasburger, 2007). Prescription drug advertising is also problematic because it gives young people the mistaken impression that there is a drug to cure every problem. In particular, the makers of drugs for erectile dysfunction have come under fire for spending so much money on ads (nearly $350 million in the first 10 months of 2004 alone) that seem to portray sex as a recreational sport (Brown and Strasburger, 2007). Last but not least, advertisers spend more than $2.5 billion a year to promote fast food restaurants and another $2 billion to promote food products, most of which are unhealthy for children. Of the 40,000 ads that children see, more than half are for food, especially high-calorie snacks and sugared cereals. Several studies have documented that young children request more junk food after viewing commercials (American Academy of Pediatrics, 2006).

Sex

In modern American culture, sex is used to sell everything from shampoo to cars to beer and wine; yet when teenagers respond to the apparent cues that everyone is having sex but them, they are instructed to "just say no" and taught abstinence-only sex education. To date, abstinence-only sex education has been proved ineffective, even by multiple government studies (Trenholm et al, 2007); yet the Federal government continues to spend more than $170 million a year supporting abstinence-only sex education. In addition to the lack of evidence that it works, abstinence-only programs are competing within a media culture that is anything *but* abstinence-only. Sex on prime-time television is ubiquitous, and rarely are the risks or consequences displayed (Fig. 20-5). Music Television (MTV) rarely shows music videos anymore. Instead, MTV is filled with "reality" shows like *Next, The Real World, Flavor of Love,* and *Parental Control* that give teens inappropriate "scripts" about the opposite sex, dating, and human sexuality. The Internet is also a prime source of inappropriate sexual material for young people. Studies show that the majority of children and teens have accessed pornography online, whether inadvertently or intentionally (Fig. 20-6).

American media are unique in their reluctance to advertise birth control products and emergency contraception (Brown and Strasburger, 2007), yet erectile dysfunction drugs are advertised constantly, even during programming that children and teens may view (American Academy of Pediatrics, 2006). At least eight national, peer-reviewed studies have documented that giving teens access to birth control does *not* increase their sexual activity or decrease their age at first intercourse (Brown and Strasburger, 2007). The media represent an important access point for teens for information about contraception (and sexuality in general, for that matter). For example, the top-10 programs *ER* and *Friends* have featured story lines about emergency contraception and about condoms, respectively.

Does all of this suggestive and casual sexuality have an impact on behavior? Increasingly, the answer seems to be yes. There are now three longitudinal correlational studies (i.e., giving causal effect) that have found that children and teens exposed to more sexual content on television or in other media have a doubled risk of beginning early sexual intercourse (Brown and Strasburger, 2007). Although rock music normally does not have much behavioral impact, one study has found an association between listening to "degrading" music lyrics and

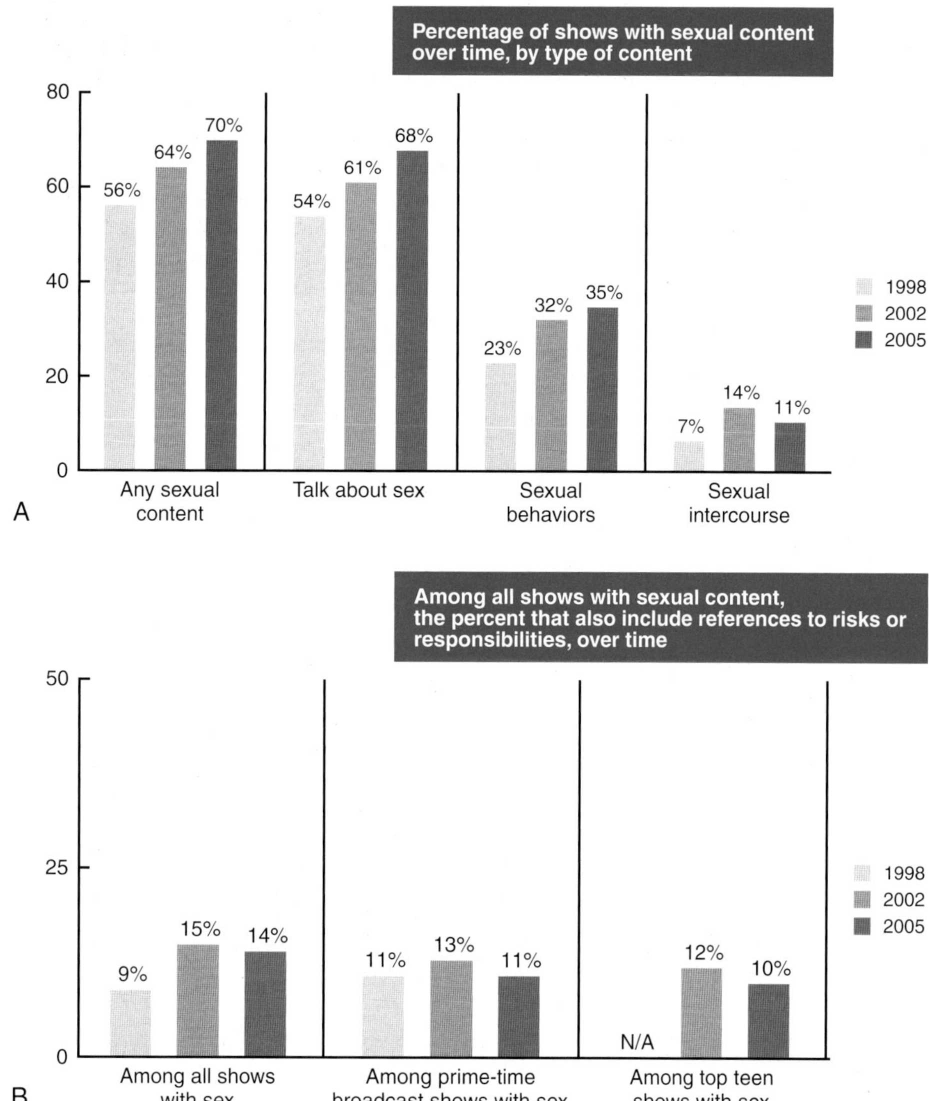

Figure 20-5. The latest in a series of content analyses of sex on prime-time television finds that the number of scenes with sexual content has nearly doubled from 1998 to 2005 to 70% (**A**). At the same time, less than 15% of shows with sexual content include references to the risks and responsibilities of having sex (**B**). *(From Kunkel D, Eyal K, Finnerty K, et al: Sex on TV 4. Menlo Park, CA, Kaiser Family Foundation, 2005.)*

earlier sexual intercourse (Martino et al, 2006). Clearly, the media make sexual activity seem like normative behavior for teens and exert super-peer pressure on them to begin sexual activity early.

Drugs

Analogous to the abstinence-only trend in American society, the "Just Say No" message of the 1980s is alive and well, too. Drug Abuse Resistance Education (DARE) is used by 80% of school districts nationwide, despite the fact that several studies have shown it to be ineffective. On the other hand, programs like Life Skills Training do work, remarkably well, but are more expensive and time-consuming than DARE. As with sex, the media are decidedly *not* anti-drug. Instead, movies and television programming are full of drug use; and more than $20 billion a year is spent on advertising tobacco, alcohol, and prescription drugs. Many beer ads use sexy

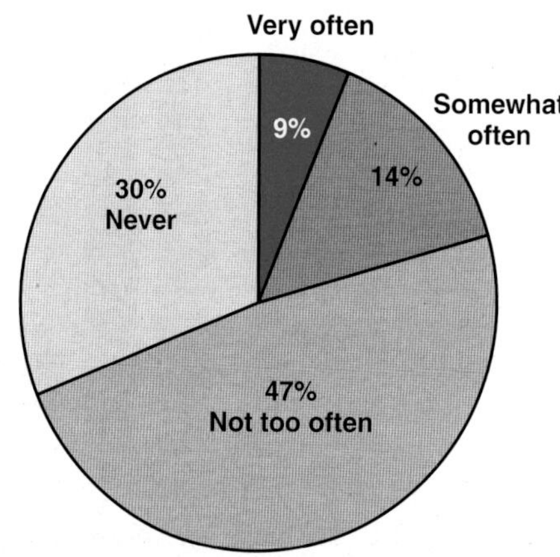

Figure 20-6. The percentage of 15- to 17-year-olds who have "accidentally" stumbled across pornography online. *(From Rideout V: Generation Rx.com: How young people use the Internet for health information. Menlo Park, CA, Kaiser Family Foundation, 2001.)*

models and adolescent humor to try to attract underage drinkers. Also featured prominently are alcohol on television and cigarette smoking in box-office hits, whereas illicit drugs are rarely seen (Fig. 20-7). On prime-time television, 71% of programs depict alcohol use, and a drinking scene is shown every 22 minutes, compared with smoking every 57 minutes and illicit drug use every 112 minutes. Children and teens who view more than 4 hours of television a day are five times more likely to start smoking than are those who watch less than 2 hours a day. A TV set in the bedroom doubles the risk. Movies are an even bigger problem, however, where cigarette smoking is making a major comeback and now ranks as perhaps the single greatest influence on whether a child or teen will begin smoking. Popular movies expose American youth to billions of smoking images (Sargent, Tanski, and Gibson, 2007), and research shows that exposure to R-rated movies doubles the risk of new smoking among teens.

The impact of advertising remains considerable as well. More than 20 studies have found that children and adolescents exposed to cigarette ads or promotions are more likely to become smokers themselves (Borzekowski and Strasburger, 2007). Several studies have found that

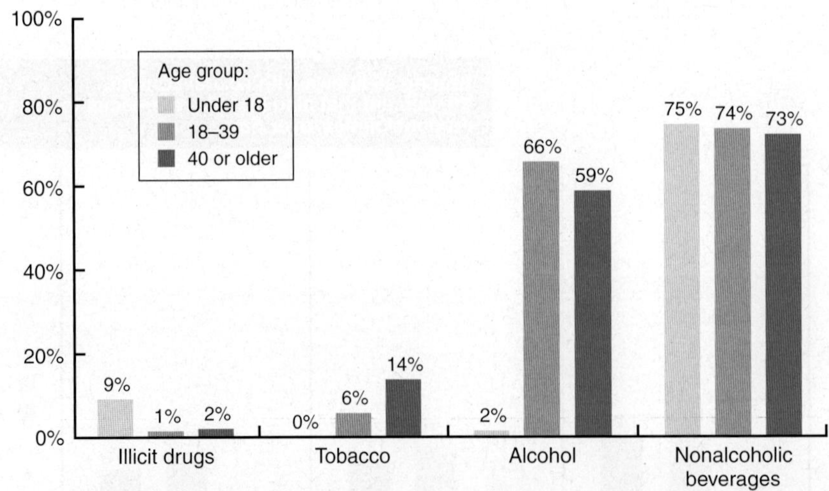

A

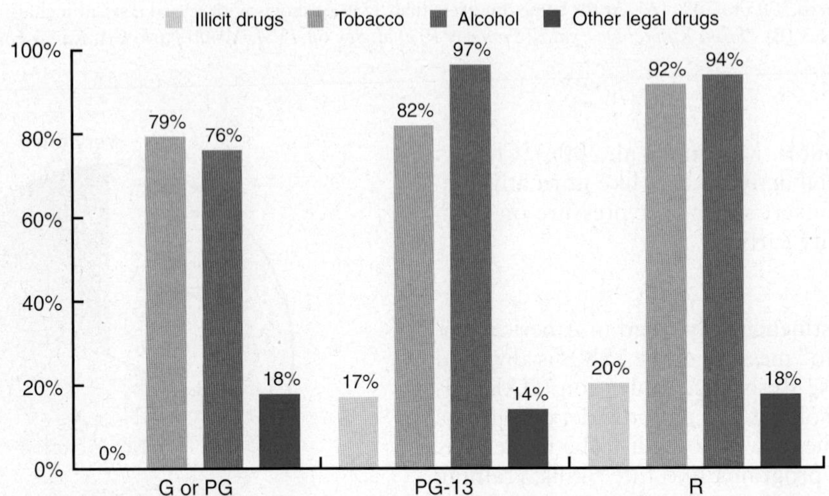

B

Figure 20-7. Drug content on television (A) and in the movies (B). Alcohol and tobacco remain the two most important drugs portrayed in mainstream media, and a G or PG rating is not protective. *(From Christenson PG, Henriksen L, Roberts DF: Substance use in popular prime-time television. Washington, DC, Office of National Drug Control Policy, 2000; and Roberts DF, Henriksen L, Christenson PG: Substance use in popular movies and music. Washington, DC, Office of National Drug Control Policy, 2000.)*

adolescent drinkers are more likely to have been exposed to alcohol advertising (Collins et al, 2007).

Obesity and Eating Disorders

Food is big business in the United States. Americans spend more money on fast food alone ($110 million) than they do on higher education, computers, or cars. Half of the nearly 40,000 ads that children and teens see annually on television are for food, especially high-calorie snacks and sugar-coated cereals (American Academy of Pediatrics, 2006; Gantz et al, 2007). Five national cross-sectional studies have found an association between television viewing and obesity (Institute of Medicine, 2006; Jordan, 2007), and one study found that children with a television set in their bedroom have a 30% increased risk of being overweight. What is not known is what the mechanism is. Media could cause poor nutritional habits through the advertising of junk food, they could displace more calorie-intensive activities, or they could increase snacking behavior.

Unfortunately, the media may also play a crucial role in the development of young girls' body self-image. For example, a large study of nearly 7000 9- to 14-year-olds found that girls who wanted to look like television or movie stars were twice as likely to have concerns about their weight, to be constant dieters, or to engage in purging behavior (Field et al, 1999). Clearly, the media "cause" an unhealthy body self-image in some young women (Brown and Strasburger, 2007); but do they cause eating disorders as well? A study of nearly 3000 Spanish 12- to 21-year-olds during a 19-month period found that those who read girls' magazines had a doubled risk for development of an eating disorder (Martinez-Gonzalez et al, 2003). A naturalistic study of the impact of introducing American television to Fiji found that 15% of teen girls reported vomiting to control their weight after American programs were introduced, compared with only 3% beforehand (Becker et al, 2002).

CONTROVERSIES

Television viewing has been associated with attentional problems in both children (Christakis et al, 2004) and adolescents (Johnson et al, 2007). Several studies have also found a relationship between television viewing and poorer academic performance (Borzekowski and Robinson, 2005), although the viewing of educational television programs by younger children is thought to be beneficial (Wartella and Robb, 2007). One study has actually found an association between early television viewing and autism (Waldman et al, 2006). Prolonged computer use and viewing violent programs have both been associated with increased social isolation. All of the controversies will require more substantial research in the future.

SOLUTIONS

Anyone concerned with child and adolescent development must learn to appreciate the impact of the media on young people. Two simple questions could elicit important information and enable interventions, if necessary (Strasburger, 2006):

1. How many hours a day does the child or teen use entertainment media?
2. Is there a TV set or Internet connection in the bedroom?

The American Academy of Pediatrics has been a leader in this public health arena since the establishment of its Task Force on Children and Television in 1983. Its recommendations include the following:

- Limit total entertainment media to no more than 1 to 2 hours per day.
- No TV sets in the bedroom.
- Severely restrict television time for children younger than 2 years.
- Co-viewing with parents.
- Work with local schools to create media education programs in the classroom.
- Work with local daycare centers to limit or to eliminate TV sets on-site.
- Work with local media outlets to increase the amount of educational programming for children and teens.

Changing the media is an altogether different proposition. Hollywood is loath to accept any outside interference, yet the entertainment community must recognize the public health implications of what they produce. More dialogue with public health organizations would be beneficial. The Federal government is equally loath to deal with media issues. For example, despite finding in the late 1970s that advertising to children younger than 6 years is inherently deceptive, the FTC refused to do anything about it because of marketplace forces (American Academy of Pediatrics, 2006). The Federal Communications Act of 1934 allows Congress to regulate what is broadcast over the public airwaves, but both cable and the Internet are impervious to regulation. A number of possibilities exist that would improve the current state of programming for children and teens:

- Mandating of media education for all kindergarteners to twelfth graders (American Academy of Pediatrics, 1999).
- Mandating of a media component for all sex and drug education programs in schools.
- Increased funding of media research.
- Specific targeting of cigarette smoking in the movies. This might entail trying to get movie sets designated as nonsmoking zones or changing the movie ratings. In May 2007, the Motion Picture Association of America (MPAA) indicated some willingness to consider doing this.
- Creation of more counteradvertising against tobacco and alcohol, not just illicit drugs.
- A ban on all tobacco advertising in all media and restriction of alcohol advertising to so-called tombstone advertising (in which the product alone is shown).

- Severe restrictions on advertising of junk foods to children and teens.
- Support for the television industry to air contraceptive ads during prime-time programming.
- Creation of a universal ratings system. The current ratings are an alphabet soup of letters and numbers that are confusing to most parents. The MPAA ratings are often inaccurate and rate more heavily for sex than for violence (Strasburger, Wilson, and Jordan, 2009). The television ratings are done by the producers themselves. The videogame ratings are also frequently inaccurate. Parents need a content-based system that will give them the maximum amount of information to make informed choices.

SUMMARY

The media are a powerful influence on the development of young people. To underestimate their influence is to miss an important opportunity to help raise healthy infants, children, and teenagers. According to the research, the media can play a major role in influencing aggressive behavior, early sexual activity, alcohol use, cigarette smoking, obesity, and unhealthy body self-image. In addition, the media's connection to eating disorders, attentional disorders, academic achievement, and autism is currently being actively investigated. Young people's exposure to media needs to be controlled by parents, and the media themselves need to be made healthier for young people.

REFERENCES

American Academy of Pediatrics: Media education. Pediatrics 104:423-426, 1999.

American Academy of Pediatrics: Children, adolescents, and advertising. Pediatrics 118:2563-2569, 2006.

Anderson C, Berkowitz L, Donnerstein E, et al: The influence of media violence on youth. Psychological Sci Public Interest 4:81-110, 2003.

Becker AE, Burwell RA, Gilman SE, et al: Eating behaviours and attitudes following prolonged exposure to television among ethnic Fijian adolescent girls. Br J Psychiatry 180:509-514, 2002.

Borzekowski DLG, and Robinson TN: The remote, the mouse, and the No. 2 pencil: The household media environment and academic achievement among third grade students. Arch Pediatr Adolesc Med 159:607-613, 2005.

Borzekowski DLG, Strasburger VC: Tobacco, alcohol, and drug exposure. *In* Calvert S, Wilson BJ (eds): Handbook of Children and the Media. Boston, Blackwell, 2007.

Brown JD, Strasburger VC: From Calvin Klein to Paris Hilton and MySpace: Adolescents, sex, and the media. Adolesc Med State Art Reviews 18:484-507, 2007.

Christakis DA, Zimmerman FJ, DiGiuseppe DL, McCarty CA: Early television exposure and subsequent attentional problems in children. Pediatrics 113:708-713, 2004.

Collins RL, Ellickson PL, McCaffrey D, Hambarsoomians K: Early adolescent exposure to alcohol advertising and its relationship to underage drinking. J Adolesc Health 40:527-534, 2007.

Field AE, Cheung L, Wolf AM, et al: Exposure to the mass media and weight concerns among girls. Pediatrics 103:e236, 1999.

Gantz W, Schwartz N, Angelini JR, Rideout V: Food for thought: Television food advertising to children in the United States. Menlo Park, CA, Kaiser Family Foundation, 2007.

Hogan MJ: Adolescents and media violence: Six crucial issues for practitioners. Adolesc Med Clin 16:249-268, 2005.

Hogan MJ, Strasburger VC: Media and prosocial behavior in children and adolescents. *In* Nucci L, Narvaez D (eds): Handbook of Moral and Character Education. Mahwah, NJ, Lawrence Erlbaum, 2007.

Huesmann LR, Eron LD, Lefkowitz MM, et al: Stability of aggression over time and generations. Dev Psychology *20*:1120-1134, 1984.

Huesmann LR, Moise-Titus J, Podolski C, et al: Longitudinal relations between children's exposure to TV violence and their aggressive and violent behavior in young adulthood: 1977-1992. Dev Psychology 39:201-221, 2003.

Institute of Medicine: Food Marketing to Children and Youth: Threat or Opportunity? Washington, DC, The National Academies Press, 2006.

Johnson JG, Cohen P, Smailes EM, et al: Television viewing and aggressive behavior during adolescence and adulthood. Science 295:2468-2472, 2002.

Johnson JG, Cohen P, Kasen S, Brook JS: Extensive television viewing and the development of attention and learning difficulties during adolescence. Arch Pediatr Adolesc Med 161:480-486, 2007.

Jordan AB: Heavy television viewing and childhood obesity. J Children Media 1:45-54, 2007.

Martinez-Gonzalez MA, Gual P, Lahortiga F, et al: Parental factors, mass media influences, and the onset of eating disorders in a prospective population-based cohort. Pediatrics 111:315-320, 2003.

Martino SC, Collins RL, Elliott MN, et al: Exposure to degrading versus nondegrading music lyrics and sexual behavior among youth. Pediatrics 118:e430-e441, 2006.

Rideout V, Roberts DF, Foehr UG: Generation M: Media in the lives of 8-18 year-olds. Menlo Park, CA, Kaiser Family Foundation, 2005. Available at: http://www.kff.org.

Sargent JD, Tanski SE, Gibson J: Exposure to movie smoking among US adolescents aged 10 to 14 years: A population estimate. Pediatrics 119:e1167-e1176, 2007.

Strasburger VC: Risky business: What primary care practitioners need to know about the influence of the media on adolescents. Prim Care 33:317-348, 2006.

Strasburger VC, Wilson BJ, Jordan A: Children, Adolescents, and the Media, 2nd ed. Thousand Oaks, CA, Sage, 2009.

Trenholm C, Devaney B, Fortson K, et al: Impacts of Four Title V, Section 510 Abstinence Education Programs: Final Report. Princeton, NJ, Mathematica Policy Research, Inc, 2007.

Vandewater EA, Rideout VJ, Wartella EA, et al: Digital childhood: Electronic media and technology use among infants, toddlers, and preschoolers. Pediatrics 119:e1006-e1015, 2007.

Waldman M, Nicholson S, Adilov N: Does television cause autism? 2006. Available at: http://www.johnson.cornell.edu/faculty/profiles/Waldman/AUTISM-WALDMAN-NICHOLSON-ADILOV.pdf. Accessed 5/14/07.

Wartella E, Robb M: Young children, new media. J Children Media 1:35-44, 2007.

Zimmerman FJ, Christakis DA: Children's television viewing and cognitive outcomes: A longitudinal analysis of national data. Arch Pediatr Adolesc Med 159:619-625, 2005.

Zimmerman FJ, Christakis DA, Meltzoff AN: Associations between media viewing and language development in children under age 2 years. J Pediatr 151:364-368, 2007.

SUGGESTED READINGS FOR PARENTS

Cantor J: "Mommy, I'm scared": How TV and movies frighten children and what we can do to protect them. San Diego, Harcourt Brace, 1998.

Christakis DA, Zimmerman FJ: The Elephant in the Living Room: Make Television Work for Your Kids. New York, Rodale Books, 2006.

Christakis DA, Zimmerman FJ: Children and television: A primer for pediatricians. Contemp Pediatr 24:31-45, 2007.

Walsh D: WHY Do They Act That Way? A Survival Guide to the Adolescent Brain for You and Your Teen. New York, Free Press, 2005.

21 DISASTERS, WAR, AND TERRORISM

Joseph F. Hagan, Jr.

Terrorism, natural disasters, and war experienced, witnessed, or described create significant trauma that now harms more individuals, including children, than since the era of World War II. War and terrorism *directly* affect wide populations and, along with natural disasters, *indirectly* reach millions more through global media. Those injured or displaced carry the tragedy of war to distant communities as refugee populations grow worldwide. Terrorists' targeting of civilians with the capacity to publicize their atrocities spreads fear widely in ways never before known. Thus, children in the 21st century have unprecedented exposure to disaster and the tragedy that ensues.

The harm of these events on the children directly involved is obvious, but the reality of the psychological impact even on children distant from disaster, war, or terrorism must be recognized. With increasing prevalence of disorders of anxiety and mood in children and adolescents as well as in adults, an understanding of children's psychological experience of community tragedy must be appreciated by professionals caring for children. Professionals must join with communities to ensure rescue, recovery, and the restoration of hope.

DISASTERS DEFINED

Natural disasters as well as the disasters of war and terrorism are traumatic events beyond normal human experience. They result in extreme physical and psychological harm (Saylor, 1993; Work Group on Disasters, American Academy of Pediatrics, 1995). Psychological experiences of children have been found to show great variance, and an American Academy of Pediatrics report noted that psychological response was influenced by both risk and protective factors (Hagan, 2005). The nature of the disaster, the level of exposure, and the extent to which a child and those around the child are personally affected are important factors. The child's individual temperament plays a vital role in determining reaction style and capacity for resiliency (see Chapter 7). Age and stage of development, prior experience, and preexisting emotional stressors as well as parental experience and response contribute to outcomes positive or negative. Recognition of this complex interactivity of protection and risk is key to understanding and assessing children's plight.

The Nature of the Traumatic Experience

Although they may be similar in terms of morbidity, mortality, and property damage, storms, earthquakes, and other natural disasters are generally less psychologically stressful than are disasters in which harm is intentionally inflicted. The increased psychopathology resulting from war and terrorist acts may be a result of deliberate acts of violence experienced, witnessed, or reported. Inhumane and intentional acts add the experience of horror to the physical experience. Acute events with little resultant disruption of the child's social environment are likely to be less psychologically damaging than are chronic traumatic events with impact on daily life and function.

Modern war is seldom waged at a Waterloo or a Gettysburg, as the battlefield of armies has expanded from field to continent. In civil conflicts, individuals in the populace become participants on the basis of race, religion, or political affiliation. Children now account for at least half of civilian casualties. Morbidity and mortality are increased by the lingering effects of war because of disrupted health and social services. The duration and chronicity of the conflict of war further potentiate the risks of harm. Serious and persisting psychological trauma results from the experience of violent events and the loss of home or parents (Wexler et al, 2006).

The seriousness of a child's personal disaster experience is proportionally predictive of response. Children may be directly or indirectly affected. Direct experiences include personal injury, injury to a family member, and loss of a family member or close relation. Threat of such loss can also be injurious. Children are indirectly affected by observing the experience of others and by media reporting.

Indirect Trauma Experiences

Modern media potentiate this effect, especially in children. Repeated images of a disastrous event suggest more sustained damage to the young child. Many children who saw the repeated images of the Twin Towers collapse assumed that not two but many buildings in New York City were attacked, representing to them an attack more horrible than the real one (Fig. 21-1). In addition, media bring distant events closer, even into the child's home. Younger children many miles from the terrorist attacks on the Pentagon and New York City felt they were at

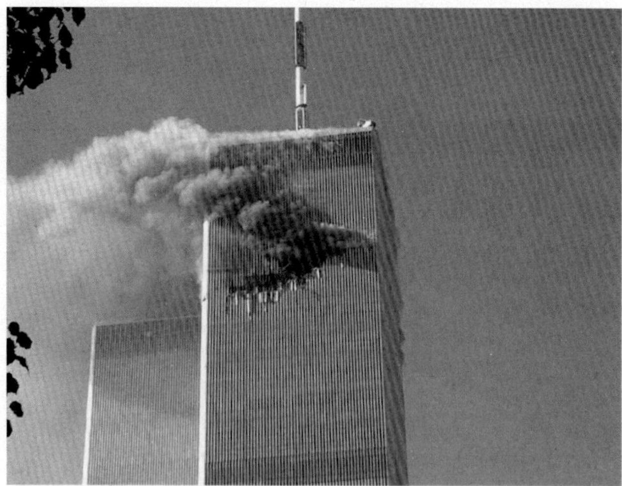

Figure 21-1. New York City, September 11, 2001: The World Trade Center North Tower after the crash of American Airlines Flight 11. (*Copyright © Larry Radar. http://larry.911photos.com.*)

proximate risk, as they did not appreciate the distance from the attacks that protected them.

In war or terrorism, the affected populations are victims of hate and threat for political rather than personal reasons. Psychological harm can occur from perceived risk of personal harm, uncertainty about one's future safety, and loss of hope. Media can serve as an inadvertent but powerful vector of the terror message. This serves the terrorist's goal to bring about abrupt change to the culture or society. Terrorist acts intend to kill a few, to maim perhaps many, but to terrorize a population.

It is apparent that such indirect exposure effect is dose responsive, and adults have control over the "dose." Communities have a role to require responsible reporting. Parents can limit psychological harm by limiting media exposure (Pine et al, 2005).

The Importance of Parents

The parental experience must be considered in measurement of the child's risk for psychological harm and in the assessment of the troubled child. Certainly, the child's survival or freedom from injury will often depend on the assistance of parents or other trusted adults. An injured or lost parent will be unable to protect the child, and a parent distracted or distressed has reduced capacity to address the child's immediate recovery needs. The importance of parents as protectors is obvious, but the child's perception of that protective role is also significant. If a parent is viewed as powerless and unable to assume or to project a protective role, the child's fearful experience is worsened.

It follows that parental composure is relevant to the child's experience. Parental anxiety will compound that of the child as well as reduce parents' sensitivity to their child's distress and impede their availability to reassure. After the September 11, 2001, attack on New York City, rates of post-traumatic stress disorder (PTSD) and depression among adults in Manhattan were doubled (Galea et al, 2002). Symptoms of PTSD declined in adults during the ensuing 3 months; but during that quarter-year, children were cared for by these affected parents and depended on them for their emotional and psychological recovery and daily needs. Delayed parental recovery is predictive of a similarly slowed return to normalcy in the child (Pine and Cohen, 2002).

CHILDREN'S RESPONSES

Adjustment to traumatic events will involve some level of behavioral reaction and symptoms. This reactivity is a normal physiologic and psychological response, mediated by survival instincts and the wish to preserve self and loved ones from harm. Quality of response is partially dependent on the type of trauma. Events involving exposure to violence or dangerous circumstances lead to a primary response of fear and later anxiety, whereas events involving loss or threat of loss of an important relationship lead to grief and dysphoria (Pine et al, 2005). Psychological responses of children to trauma can vary from mild and transient symptoms of stress and distress to acute stress reactions or acute stress disorder or to the more pervasive and prolonged consequence of PTSD. In most cases, as children are helped to cope with their distress, symptoms subside (Beauchesne et al, 2002; Work Group on Disasters, American Academy of Pediatrics, 1995). Child and adolescent mental health after the September 11, 2001, attack on New York City (Calderoni et al, 2006) and Hurricanes Katrina and Rita (Weisler et al, 2006) has been reviewed.

Stages of Response

Children's responses to disaster, terrorist acts, or war will vary over time. Immediately after the traumatic event, fright predominates with concomitant feelings of denial, disbelief, grief for loss, or relief if loved ones have not been harmed.

A few days to weeks after the traumatic event, manifestations of emotional distress predominate. Developmental regression is common in children, and common symptoms include externalizing behaviors such as hostility, irritability, and aggressive behaviors toward others and internalizing symptoms represented by depressed mood, apathy, pessimism, withdrawal, sleep disturbances, and somatization. Such signs are common, are part of the normal recovery process for children, and can be expected to last for a few weeks. Children's play and games demonstrating themes of the traumatic event are common and represent adaptive attempts at mastery. When marked distress or behavioral disorganization is noted, especially in children who experienced major loss, early referral for mental health services is indicated.

Children with adverse reactions lasting longer than 1 month are at increased risk for development of PTSD or violent and delinquent behaviors later in life (Beauchesne et al, 2002; Monson, 2002). Referral for mental health services is imperative.

Developmental Ages and Stages of Response

A child's age and stage of development determine response to the trauma experienced. Developmental stage determines a child's interpretation of events as well as the child's response to them. Interventions to assist children must be developmentally appropriate if they are to successfully alleviate distress.

The responses of younger children are marked by changes in mood, anxiety level, and internalized behavioral symptoms. They are unable to understand the event and will have difficulty distinguishing a deliberate action from an unintentional incident. They will be concerned with the consequences to themselves and their immediate family or community. The more sophisticated older children show greater comprehension of the traumatic event and of its intent and implications. They too will experience anxiety and depression. Their reactions may be complicated by anger, fear, or despair, and older children are further influenced by prior personal experience and vulnerabilities.

Infancy and Early Childhood (Birth to 4 Years)

Lacking comprehension of the traumatic event, the infant or young child's experience is one of disrupted routine and loss of loved ones and caregivers. Their perception of safety is challenged and trust is harmed. Regression and detachment can follow. Infants may show increased irritability, an exaggerated startle response, and separation anxiety. Toddlers and preschoolers typically experience behavior and skill regression. They show temper tantrums, increased dependency, and sleep disturbances and nightmares.

Middle Childhood (5 to 10 Years)

Younger school-age children will often represent their experience of trauma through play expressing trauma-related themes. Aggressive behaviors are common. Sleep disturbances, regressive behaviors, disorders of mood, and anxiety are frequently observed. With their increasing capacity for empathy, children nearing adolescence will be concerned not only for their own family's safety but also for the well-being of others.

Adolescents (11 to 21 Years)

The adolescent response is varied and highly dependent on the adolescent's experience and maturity level. In this period of complex transitions, older adolescents may have an adult range of responses. Younger adolescents, still developing emotional coping skills, will have a different spectrum of vulnerability. Whereas tasks to establish independence and to create a personal identity predominate, sudden loss can lead to regression, delay in developmental advancement, and both externalized and internalized symptoms. Self-preservation and care of family are the predominant concern of younger adolescents; their more mature friends empathically show concern for others as well. Adolescents are typically concerned with fairness, reflecting the persistence of strong concrete thinking. Volunteerism or enlistment in the armed services may be positive outcomes of this thinking; retaliation is a less positive response.

Syndromic Responses

Diagnosis and management of specific mental health conditions are discussed elsewhere in this text. Problems and disorders representing responses to natural disasters or terrorist events include the following:

- Acute stress reaction
- PTSD
- Anxiety disorders
- Depression

Whereas many children will meet DSM-IV diagnostic criteria for these disorders, far more children will be partially affected. *The Diagnostic and Statistical Manual for Primary Care (DSM-PC) Child and Adolescent Version* (Wolraich, 1996) is an important resource for understanding the symptoms of the child with behavioral and emotional health problems of significant morbidity but that do not meet the level of symptoms required for the adult diagnosis of disorder. Support and services must be available on the basis of symptomatic morbidity and not restricted by diagnosis.

MANAGEMENT—ACUTE

Preparedness

Management of the needs of families and children after disaster, terrorist act, or act of war begins with community preparedness. Emergency services in the United States are highly developed with an emphasis on rescue, triage, and attention to acute medical crises. We are less prepared for chemical events or biologic attack (Committee on Environment Health and Committee on Infectious Diseases, American Academy of Pediatrics, 2000), and there is a notable lack of hospital beds available to meet surge demands.

Availability of child-specific treatments is extremely limited in the majority of jurisdictions, including child-specific emergency response teams, child-appropriate doses or delivery systems for emergency medications, child-friendly decontamination tools and techniques, emergency department resources, pediatric intensive care beds, and pediatric ward beds (Markenson and Reynolds, 2006). Preparedness also demands pre-event consideration of how the emotional needs of affected children will be addressed. The American Academy of Pediatrics Task Force on Terrorism studied these needs after the September 11 attacks, consulted with governmental agencies, and offered recommendations (Table 21-1). The American Academy of Pediatrics continues to study the unique preparedness needs of American children (American Academy of Pediatrics, 2007).

Evacuation

Evacuation may occur before an anticipated event or in response to a sudden or unexpected event. All communities should have a plan for evacuation before a crisis. Evacuation plans will vary in their complexity and specificity on the basis of factors such as relative risk, the nature of perceived risk, population size, geography,

Table 21-1. Disaster Preparedness to Meet Children's Needs

Children are more vulnerable than adults.
Children are not little adults. Their developing minds and bodies place them at disproportionate risk based on size, minute respiration, smaller circulating blood volume, and developmental vulnerabilities.
Children have unique treatment needs.
Once children are critically ill or injured, their bodies will respond differently from adults in similar medical crises. Consequently, pediatric treatment requires special drug dosages and specially sized equipment. Children are at particular risk for hypothermia during decontamination procedures.
Children have unique mental health needs.
Just as children's developing bodies affect their response to physical trauma, children's developing minds pose unique challenges to providing quality mental health care.
Children need care from providers trained to meet their unique needs.
Because children respond differently from adults in a medical crisis, it is critical that all health care workers be able to recognize the unique signs and symptoms in children that may indicate a life-threatening situation and to respond accordingly.
Disaster planning must address and meet children's needs.
To meet the unique needs of all infants, children, adolescents, and young adults, it is critical that our community preparedness efforts involve pediatric health care experts as well as key facilities, institutions, and agencies that care for children.

Modified from the American Academy of Pediatrics Task Force on Terrorism, The Youngest Victims: Disaster Preparedness to Meet Children's Needs. Available at: http://www.aap.org/terrorism/topics/PhysiciansSheet.pdf.

proximity to safe havens, and proximity to sources of additional risk, such as a dam in the event of a flood or a nuclear power plant in the event of terrorist attack.

Plans for evacuation of a community must have clear and specific components addressing the safety of children, families, and both children and adults with special health care needs. Most existing evacuation plans rely on the ability of adults to move or to care for themselves. The New Orleans experience in Hurricane Katrina highlights the imperative of planning and planning specifically for those unable to care for themselves. The haunting photographs of unused and subsequently flooded city school buses are testimony to an inadequate and failed pre-event evacuation plan (Fig. 21-2).

Sudden abandonment of home, school, or neighborhood entails immediate loss, with the consequences of disruption, discontinuity, stress, disorganization, and losing the sense of security. Although adults might hope for return to a home undamaged, it is difficult to address the fears of children and their expectation that all is lost. The value of transitional objects to children is obvious and they should be encouraged. Contingencies should also be made for family pets, both for the safety of the pet and for the solace of the family.

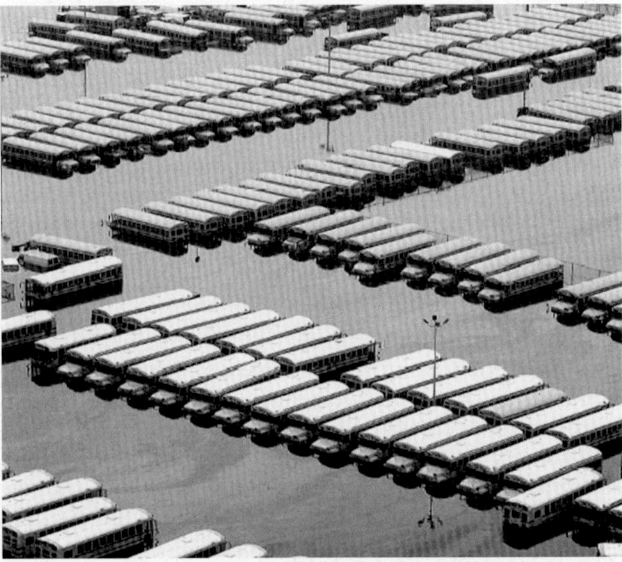

Figure 21-2. Flooded New Orleans city school buses serve as a powerful example of failed opportunities to evacuate residents from the aftermath of Hurricane Katrina. (*http://www.mackinac.org/media/images/2006/mer2006-03p1a.jpg.*)

Shelter in Place

In certain circumstances, evacuation might be impossible, as in New Orleans after the rupture of the levee, or dangerous, for example, in chemical or biologic attack. In these situations, evacuation places the evacuee, the first responder, and perhaps the accepting community at risk, and shelter must be created at the place of the event. Community leaders should include these contingencies in their disaster plan.

Shelter in place requires food, water, shelter, delivery of emergency medical services, and, if prolonged, provisions to address mental health needs. Egress out might be restricted, but access in for responders must be ensured. Inevitably, law enforcement will be involved to ensure order and to enforce boundaries; policies should be in place to ensure fairness, reasonableness, and recognition of the unique needs of children and families.

Reunification

Children will be separated from parents and caregivers in disasters. This reality must be reflected in community disaster planning if the plan is to actually work. Anna Freud's classic study of British children evacuated without their parents during the 1940 Blitz on London defined the importance of keeping families together. She found that "London children ... were on the whole much less upset by bombing than by evacuation to the country as a protection against it" (Coles, 1992).

In U.S. communities during the work or school day, parents are separated from their children, who will be at school or childcare facilities. If an evacuation order is given during these hours, parents and children are likely to be evacuated before they are reunited. A plan must exist for the rapid reunification of families.

Absent a credible system for reunification that is known by parents and trusted, evacuation will be slowed by desperate parents resisting removal as they seek to find their children. One can only speculate on the chaos of an evacuation order for Manhattan to New Jersey, with frantic parents fighting to go north or east to reclaim their children rather than west to safety. If Manhattan parents could be assured that their children would also be evacuated to New Jersey and if reunification sites and procedures were in operation, the evacuation process could flow more smoothly and have the potential for more protection of life.

Reunification of separated families did not occur smoothly after the Katrina evacuation of New Orleans. Hundreds of children were separated from families and loved ones, and reunification was finally accomplished not according to disaster planning and not by a successful governmental intervention but as a result of the unique and creative chance collaboration of a not-for-profit organization and a major television news network.

Care of Unattached Children

Pending reunification, plans must be in place for the care of unattached children. The place of detainment must be safe from the disaster and its aftermath, and personnel are to be dedicated to the care of these children. Care should be child centered to the extent possible. At a minimum, children must be kept safe from misuse or abduction. Emergency medical care and care necessitated by the disaster aftermath will be needed by some children, such as immunization for new infectious disease risks. Procedures are necessary to ensure no limitation of necessary care when parents or guardians are not available to provide consent.

MANAGEMENT—CHRONIC

Reunification and Care of Unattached Children

Parents will be lost to death, injury, or involuntary relocation. Authorities will attempt to reunite children with parents or other family. Some children will be placed in foster care. The acute problem of reunification now is a chronic condition of providing for long-term care. The emotional cost of lost love ones compounds the psychological trauma of the disaster.

Surveillance

The primary health care system in the United States has become a de facto mental health system (Heldring, 2004). Surveillance for developmental or behavioral problems is a core activity of every health encounter between professional and child. Professionals providing health and mental health care services to child survivors of disaster or terrorist act use their knowledge of the child, their awareness of the child's disaster experience, and their familiarity with common reactions to identify children struggling to adjust. Each interaction can be a therapeutic one if the provider is sensitive to the child's predicament and vigilant for signs of maladjustment. Inquiry to child or parent about child and family adjustment is appropriate.

Children distant from the disaster or terrorism event may also be affected. As previously noted, the ultimate goal of the terrorist is to scare a population and to cause the victimized community to act in a different manner. Children and parents can be helped to determine their own risk, which is often negligible. Preexisting problems with anxiety can increase this misperception of risk.

Screening

Screening for adverse reactions to disaster or terrorism is the broader action of investigating all children or adults in a community or other group who were affected by the event. Surveillance relies on knowledge and sensitivity to detect troubled victims. Screening assumes that many psychological symptoms will be private, hidden, or subtle. Screening uses some form of assessment tool, ideally one previously validated for detection of certain symptoms in similar circumstances or populations (Council on Children with Disabilities, American Academy of Pediatrics, 2006).

Screening for PTSD symptoms in Thai children after the 2004 tsunami detected prevalence rates of 13% for children living in refugee camps and 11% for children from affected villages. These rates were significant compared with the 6% prevalence in children from unaffected villages, yet this rate would hardly suggest that these children were "unaffected" (Thienkrua et al, 2006). School-based screening in New York City found high rates of disorders of mood and anxiety-related diagnoses.

Screening for the psychological sequelae to traumatic events is as essential as assessment for food and shelter needs. It is an important component of community preparedness and response. Screening needs of children are similar to those of adults, but child-specific screening techniques and tools are to be employed.

THERAPEUTIC TASKS IN HELPING CHILDREN AND ADOLESCENTS: THE RATIONALE FOR INTERVENTION OR REFERRAL

"The primary goal of healing is to integrate the traumatic loss in the child's life and minimize any long-term consequences of the event" (Gaffney, 2006). Children must establish trust and come to feel that they need not be alert for future harm. They must find sanctuary, in a physically and emotionally safe environment. With psychological safety comes the ability to trust oneself and others. Children then move beyond the trauma and its emotional burden. They become grounded as they were before the trauma. They redevelop self-care skills and seek to once again establish order in their world.

ESTABLISHING HOPE

As communities recover from a disaster, recovery includes return to a safe living environment, restoration of essential services, and gradual return to normal work pursuits for parents and school or play for children. If recovery is to be complete, the community and its people must restore hope. If they are to feel safe and free from fear, they must have hope for the future, belief in the community's ability to regrow, and trust that the likelihood of repeated disaster is low.

The alternative is to live in fear.

Communities are perhaps less safe after natural disaster or terrorist acts. The world, as perceived by American children, is perhaps less safe since 2001; but we are, for the most part, safe. Children must be afforded that sense of safety; they must be allowed hope. Do we succeed in giving this comfort?

Under threat of invasion during the Second World War, British children and their parents were exhorted in public information posters to "keep calm and carry on," a clear message of purpose and conviction. President Franklin Roosevelt told families suffering the Great Depression: "First of all, let me assert my firm belief that the only thing we have to fear is fear itself—nameless, unreasoning, unjustified terror which paralyzes needed efforts to convert retreat into advance" (Roosevelt, 1933). Children depend on trusted adults to feel safe or protected so that they might anticipate a less stress-laden future. Children living in unsafe communities or those who are victims of prejudice or racism require this trust in adults so that they too can be safe. Are contemporary parents and community and governmental leaders meeting this need? Are we teaching our children to live *with* fear, or are we, as a culture, living *in* fear?

Effective public communication about terrorism or disaster risk is essential, and it is important that planners or those governmental officials charged with keeping us safe be aware of the psychology of terrorism. Does the American public policy of a "war on terrorism" protect us or scare us, or both? Do "terror alerts" protect or terrorize? Does the attempt to communicate risk help or hurt the people warned? Risk communication must reduce anxiety if it is to minimize the risk of panic. Increasing anxiety, or terror, is the goal of the terrorist. Effective risk communication has the following characteristics (Heldring, 2004):

- The communication comes from credible and trusted authorities.
- Specific information about the risk is communicated.
- Specific information about the efforts to reduce risk are communicated.
- Actions citizens can take to reduce risk are clearly defined.
- Apprehension is acknowledged.

It is important to communicate to children that they and we are almost always safe from terrorist act, war, or natural disaster. Children must know that we will take care of them, as we take care of one another. If some feel that the world is now a more fearful place than in the past, then it is essential that we help our children live with this fear, adjust to it, feel hopeful, and plan for their futures.

CARING FOR CAREGIVERS

Personal injury or loss will also occur in caregivers. Medical professionals, providers of emergency medical services, mental health practitioners, and other members of helping professions in a disaster area are also potential victims. The caregiver's actual first response might be to ensure personal safety and the safety of family and neighbors. Proper disaster planning considers provision of emergency services if the local caregivers are lost or temporarily incapacitated. When disaster occurs, professional responders will also be affected, and personal experiences will affect one's ability to respond effectively.

Even caregivers not directly harmed by the disaster must be cognizant of self-care needs. The toll taken by fear, tension, sadness, and exhaustion must be recognized (Laraque et al, 2004).

ADVOCACY

The American Academy of Pediatrics (2007) has endorsed a number of steps to community preparedness that address the unique needs of children. Pediatricians and other health service providers for children are encouraged to serve as resources for families and advocates for community disaster-preparedness plans appropriate to the unique needs of pediatric patients. Pre-disaster planning might include the following (Hagan, 2005):

- Collaborate with other professionals who with families recognize the importance of schools in disaster preparedness.
- Help schools recognize their roles in the aftermath of disaster, especially with regard to assessment and treatment of students' mental health.
- Review evacuation and relocation plans for child and family relevance.
- Identify resources available to the community in the event of disaster.
- Identify necessary resources for children and families that are *un*available and advocate for their provision.

SUMMARY

Children and adolescents who are victims of disaster or experience the horrific trauma of war or terrorism will have predictable responses, and their caring community must address their unique needs. Comprehensive community preparedness includes provisions for children and others unable to care for themselves. Provisions must also be in place and resources exist to provide for the expected impact on the mental health of affected youth.

REFERENCES

American Academy of Pediatrics: Children & Disasters. Available at: www.aap.org/terrorism. Accessed May 20, 2007.

Beauchesne MA, Kelley BR, Patsdaughter CA, Pikard J: Attack on America: Children's reactions and parents responses. J Pediatr Health Care 16:213-221, 2002.

Calderoni ME, Alderman EM, Silver EJ, Bauman LJ: The mental health impact of 9/11 on inner-city high school students twenty miles north of ground zero. J Adolesc Health 39:57-65, 2006.

Coles R: Anna Freud: The Dream of Psychoanalysis. Reading, MA, Addison-Wesley, 1992, p 189.

Committee on Environment Health and Committee on Infectious Diseases, American Academy of Pediatrics: Chemical-biological terrorism and its impact on children: A subject review. Pediatrics 105:662-670, 2000.

Council on Children with Disabilities, Section on Developmental Behavioral Pediatrics, Bright Futures Steering Committee and Medical Home Initiatives for Children with Special Health Needs Project Advisory Committee, American Academy of Pediatrics: Identifying infants and children with developmental disorders in the medical home: An algorithm for developmental surveillance and screening. Pediatrics 118:405-420, 2006.

Gaffney DA: The aftermath of disaster: Children in crisis. J Clin Psychology 62:1001-1016, 2006.

Galea S, Ahern J, Resnick H, et al: Psychological sequelae of the September 11 terrorist attacks in New York City. N Engl J Med 346:982-987, 2002.

Hagan JF, and The Committee on Psychosocial Aspects of Child and Family Health, and the Task Force on Terrorism, American Academy of Pediatrics: Psychosocial implications of disaster or terrorism on children: A guide for the pediatrician. Pediatrics 116: 1-9, 2005.

Heldring M: Talking to the public about terrorism: promoting health and resilience. Families Systems Health 22(1):67-71, 2004.

Laraque D, Boscarino JA, Battista A, et al: Reactions in need of tri-state area pediatricians after the events of September 11: Implications for children's mental health services. Pediatrics 113:1357-1366, 2004.

Markenson D, Reynolds S, Committee on Pediatric Emergency Medicine and Task Force on Terrorism, American Academy of Pediatrics: The pediatrician disaster preparedness. Pediatrics 117: e340-e362, 2006.

Monson RB: Children in terror. J Pediatr Nurs 17:62-63, 2002.

Pine DS, Cohen JA: Trauma in children and adolescents: Risk and treatment of psychiatric sequelae. Biol Psychiatry 51:519-531, 2002.

Pine DS, Costello J, Masten A: Trauma, proximity and developmental psychopathology: The effects of war and terrorism on children. Neuropsychopharmacology 30:1781-1792, 2005.

Roosevelt FD: First Inaugural Address, 1933.

Saylor CF: Introduction: Children and Disasters: Clinical and Research Issues. *In* Saylor CF (ed): Children of Disasters. New York, Plenum, 1993, pp 1-10.

Thienkrua W, Cardozo BL, Chakkraband ML, et al, for the Thailand Post-Tsunami Mental Health Study Group: Symptoms of posttraumatic stress disorder and depression among children in tsunami-affected areas in southern Thailand. JAMA 296:549-559, 2006.

Weisler RH, Barbee JG, Townsend MH: Mental health and recovery in the golf coast after hurricanes Katrina and Rita. JAMA 296: 585-588, 2006.

Wexler ID, Branski D, Kerem E: War and children. JAMA 296: 579-581, 2006.

Wolraich ML (ed): American Academy of Pediatrics. The Classification of Child and Adolescent Mental Health Diagnoses in Primary Care: The Diagnostic and Statistical Manual for Primary Care (DSM-PC) Child and Adolescent Version. Elk Grove Village, IL, American Academy of Pediatrics, 1996.

Work Group on Disasters, American Academy of Pediatrics: Psychosocial Issues for Children and Families in Disasters: A Guide for the Primary Care Physician. Washington, DC, U.S. Department of Health and Human Services, 1995. Publication No. (SMA) 95-3022.

Part III BIOLOGICAL INFLUENCES

22 BIOMEDICAL BASIS OF DEVELOPMENT AND BEHAVIOR

Ellen Roy Elias

The past 10 years have witnessed an explosion in technologic fields and scientific understanding that is unparalleled in prior decades. These major advances encompass many fields from computer science to biomolecular techniques, from medical interventions to laboratory studies. The new and constantly improving understanding of how human embryos develop, of how the central nervous system (CNS) functions, and of the subtle molecular and metabolic changes that can cause human disease has had a significant impact on our understanding of human development and behavior. This chapter explores some of these advances and how they are important for the developmental pediatrician.

EMBRYOLOGY

The progression from a fertilized egg into a complex human with multiple organs and chemical substances (such as hormones, lipids, proteins, and ions) with billions of interconnecting cells, each containing intracellular organelles surrounded by complex cell membranes, is a miracle to contemplate. The physical changes occurring during the multiple stages in fetal life have long been understood by direct study of embryos. More recent studies have led to a clarification of many of these processes, with the understanding that some steps occur with greater complexity than what was originally thought. For example, closure of the neural tube is no longer thought to occur by a simple two-zipper process; rather, there are at least five zippers, each of which is mediated by different genes and affected by different teratogens (Van Allen et al, 1993).

The explosion of information that has emerged from the field of molecular biology has led to an immense body of knowledge about the role of developmental genes in human development. There are currently hundreds of genes that have been discovered whose normal activity is necessary for normal development and function of the brain. Important gene pathways are now known to be critical for the normal formation of all parts of the body, including the CNS.

Certain genes, for example, Sonic Hedgehog (SHH), when activated, turn on a cascade of genes downstream that are critical for normal fetal CNS development (Dorus et al, 2006; Oldak et al, 2001). Mutations in these genes can lead to major malformations; for example, mutations in SHH cause holoprosencephaly. Even more interesting is that certain post-translational modifications of gene activity can lead to malformations as severe as those caused by gene mutation. For example, binding of cholesterol to the SHH protein is essential for normal activation of the downstream cascade of genes, so that children with severe Smith-Lemli-Opitz syndrome who have an enzyme deficiency causing severe cholesterol depletion may also present with holoprosencephaly (Muenke and Beachy, 2000). See Chapters 24, 26, and 30 for more detailed information on molecular and metabolic derangements that may lead to CNS abnormalities and dysfunction.

BRAIN IMAGING

In addition to advances that have been made in embryology and developmental and molecular biology, the field of medical radiology has also seen an explosion in new techniques that allow sophisticated imaging of CNS anatomy. Computed tomography, especially with use of dye to visualize the vasculature, and magnetic resonance imaging are powerful tools that can indicate even subtle dysgenetic changes in brain structure. Computed tomographic angiography can visualize changes in blood flow to the brain caused by both congenital vascular anomalies and events such as stroke and thrombus. Magnetic resonance imaging can detect major structural abnormalities, such as agenesis of the corpus callosum, holoprosencephaly, and lissencephaly (smooth brain caused by severe neuronal migration defects), as well as more subtle findings, such as heterotopias and migrational abnormalities of neurons.

Special hardware allows magnetic resonance imaging not only to visualize anatomy but also to yield information about biochemical function with magnetic resonance spectroscopy. Positron emission tomography, the newest of the functional imaging techniques, is now being used to better understand the geography of the brain and how certain areas may malfunction in association with specific neurologic phenotypes (Hoon, Belsito, and Nagae-Poetscher, 2003).

CENTRAL NERVOUS SYSTEM INJURY

With improvements in CNS imaging and better understanding of biologic processes and their impact on brain function, we are now able to better understand how CNS injury can lead to CNS dysfunction. For example, anoxia, long known to cause brain injury and developmental disabilities, can now be understood on a biochemical level and can be imaged in a sophisticated way. This has led to different interventions to help reduce the neurologic sequelae of anoxia, such as head cooling in the neonatal intensive care unit (Gluckman et al, 2005).

With more sophistication and globalization in our society comes the risk of greater exposure to more agents that may cause brain injury. For example, the list of possible teratogens has grown astronomically during the past decade and includes a host of prescription medications, such as the anticonvulsants carbamazepine and valproate (Alsdorf and Wyszynski, 2005) and drugs such as Accutane used to treat acne, as well as illicit substances such as cocaine. Alcohol, long available and known to cause deleterious effects on the developing fetus, is still a common cause of developmental disability. An increased prevalence of infections, such as human immunodeficiency virus (HIV) infection, has also played a role in causing increased CNS morbidity.

Many of these topics are covered in greater detail in this section of the book, particularly Chapters 23, 28, and 31.

THE ROLE OF GENETICS IN DEVELOPMENTAL DISABILITIES

The developmental pediatrician cannot understand the cause behind the problems faced by patients without a basic understanding of human genetics. Simple mendelian genetics, namely, understanding of the basic mechanisms of autosomal dominant, autosomal recessive, and X-linked disorders, is extremely important. Autosomal dominant disorders are passed on from a parent to a child with a 50% chance recurrence risk with each pregnancy. Because of variable penetrance, the severity of the problems may be different (i.e., a child may have more worrisome issues than a parent), even though both the parent and the child carry the same DNA mutation. An example of a common autosomal dominant disorder with developmental implications is neurofibromatosis. A rarer autosomal dominant disorder causing macrocephaly and autism is Bannayan-Riley-Ruvalcaba syndrome, and it is associated with a high risk of malignant disease in both the child and the affected parent. Confirmation of this diagnosis with a simple blood test of the affected *PTEN* gene can have enormous implications for the family (Zhou et al, 2003).

Autosomal recessive inheritance is the genetic pattern whereby each parent caries a mutated gene on one allele. If both of these altered alleles are passed on to a child, that child will have no normal gene messages for that gene product and will be affected; there is a 25% chance of this with every pregnancy. Most metabolic disorders are inherited with this pattern. The risk of an autosomal recessive disorder increases with a family history of consanguinity (i.e., marrying a relative such as a cousin or uncle greatly increases the risk of both parents' carrying the same rare gene mutation).

X-linked inheritance is the least common of the inheritance patterns. In this situation, a gene mutation is located on one of the mother's X chromosomes. There is a 50% chance of having an affected child, if the child is male. In certain circumstances, symptoms can also be manifested in females carrying X-linked mutations, although symptoms are generally milder in the female than in the male. X-linked inheritance is seen for certain metabolic disorders and is a more common cause of retardation syndromes, for example, fragile X syndrome. Certain X-linked disorders are lethal in the male and are manifested only in females, for example, Rett syndrome.

Often, attention paid to obtaining a detailed family history and pedigree will pay off in suggesting a possible underlying diagnosis amenable to testing. Therefore, a family pedigree is an essential piece of a developmental assessment. For example, history of an affected maternal uncle can be an important clue toward the diagnosis of an X-linked disorder such as fragile X. A history of parental consanguinity raises the concern of an autosomal recessive disorder, which would have a 25% recurrence risk in future pregnancies. Even simple information such as paternal age older than 40 years, which raises the risk of a new dominant mutation, can help clinch a diagnosis. Missing a genetic diagnosis with an associated significant recurrence risk does a horrible disservice to patients and their families. Therefore, basic genetic testing should be performed in all children presenting with intellectual disability and autism, at least for the more common, diagnosable conditions (Table 22-1).

It can be daunting to consider what tests should be performed. Of all the advances that have occurred in medicine and science during the past 10 years, none has been so dramatic as the explosion of new knowledge that has occurred in the field of genetics. The incredible increase in new information now available to the developmental pediatrician can be traced to a number of factors. One factor is the Human Genome Project, completed in 2003, which was a 13-year project designed to identify all the genes in human DNA (estimated to be 20,000 to 25,000). With the completion of this major project comes the understanding of the normal DNA structure

Table 22-1. Genetic Evaluation of Children with Intellectual Disability and Autism

Chromosomes with high-resolution banding
Comparative genomic hybridization microarray
Fluorescent in situ hybridization testing, when appropriate (if a specific diagnosis is suspected on the basis of family history or phenotype)
DNA testing for fragile X syndrome
Referral to a geneticist for the following:
- Dysmorphic features
- Multiple congenital anomalies
- History of previously affected sibling or consanguinity
- Neurodegenerative course
- Suspicion of a metabolic disorder (e.g., hypoglycemia, coarse features, organomegaly)

of the human genome, allowing more accurate and timely diagnosis of genetic disorders *(www.Genomics.energy.gov)*.

Advances in molecular biology have affected the care of patients in many ways. For example, discovery of some of the genes causing the more common forms of congenital deafness, such as connexin 26, has improved the care and management of children with hearing loss. It is now possible to identify the exact cause of deafness in many cases, to provide appropriate genetic counseling to families, and to know when to screen for other associated medical problems (see Chapter 70).

New diagnostic techniques have been developed that allow greater identification of subtle DNA changes. These techniques include better karyotyping with higher resolution; fluorescent in situ hybridization (FISH), which allows detection of tiny microdeletions not visible even with high-resolution chromosome analysis; and the newest and most powerful in the genetic armamentarium, comparative genomic hybridization (CGH) microarray. CGH microarray uses computer chip technology to screen for hundreds of genes simultaneously and can detect subtle DNA rearrangements. Many geneticists are beginning to use CGH microarray instead of karyotyping, and many people in the field think that it will eventually replace chromosome analysis completely (Shaw-Smith et al, 2004).

Advances in molecular biology have made it possible to test DNA directly to look for gene mutations and changes that might not be detectible with a routine karyotype, FISH, or even microarray. This testing is now possible for many genetic disorders and can be used to confirm diagnoses causing developmental disabilities. An example of this testing is molecular testing for fragile X syndrome, looking for expansion of triplet repeats as well as methylation of the gene.

Chapters 24 and 26 expand definitions and explanations of genetic advances and illustrate how they are routinely being used to confirm diagnoses in children with developmental disabilities and behavioral disorders. Updated information on Down syndrome, the most common chromosomal abnormality seen in children, is presented in Chapter 25.

As well as advances in molecular techniques, new understanding of population genetics has led to the discovery of many genes whose alterations cause diseases affecting cognitive function and mental health. There are currently entire journals devoted to neuropsychiatric disorders such as schizophrenia, bipolar disorder, and Tourette syndrome. There has also grown a much better understanding of certain behavioral phenotypes, such as addiction (Strong, 2003).

Intense research is under way to understand what genes may be contributing to mental health disorders. Many gene loci have been associated with schizophrenia and Tourette syndrome, for example. There are also a number of genetic disorders, diagnosable with standard genetic techniques such as FISH, that have an associated psychiatric phenotype. An example is the velocardiofacial syndrome, caused by a deletion on chromosome 22q11. Schizophrenia, bipolar disorder, and depression can all be seen in patients who carry this deletion, which is passed on as a dominant trait.

A new frontier in genetics is the area of biochemical disorders and inborn errors of metabolism. This topic was not addressed in previous editions of this text, but this field has grown so enormously during the past 10 years that an entire new chapter is devoted to a discussion of those disorders for which a biochemical etiology is now known. Many of these disorders are now understood, not just on a biochemical level but on a cellular and molecular level as well. An example of this class of disorders is the group of lysosomal storage disorders. New treatments including enzyme replacement and bone marrow transplantation are now possible for some of these disorders, which were often fatal without any possible intervention in the past.

A new group of disorders are the disorders of energy metabolism, caused by abnormalities in mitochondrial function. These disorders may present with a variety of symptoms, but hypotonia and developmental delay are fairly universal. Unlike disorders associated with classic genetic patterns of inheritance, mitochondrial disorders caused by mitochondrial DNA mutations are maternally inherited. Understanding of this pattern of inheritance and how to suspect mitochondrial disorders is important for the developmental pediatrician, as these disorders are not uncommon. Mitochondrial disorders are covered in Chapter 30.

ADVANCES IN MEDICAL CARE

Pediatric care has changed significantly in several areas, particularly in the field of neonatology. The limits of viability have been pushed earlier and earlier. Although survival has improved greatly, this still may come at a cost in terms of neurologic morbidity. Chapter 27 explores this in great detail.

Major advances have also been made in other areas of pediatric care, including the ability to perform repair of complex congenital lesions affecting the heart and the increased use of transplantation for severe congenital heart disease. Transplantation has also led to increased survival for other diseases, including renal failure. Other transplants, including intestinal, liver, and lung, have led to survival in previously fatal disorders. Complex medical interventions for chronic disorders can certainly affect developmental outcome in these children, and pediatricians often find themselves caring for children with multiple, complex medical as well as developmental issues. An approach to the management of children with these complex issues can be found in Chapter 74.

Advances have been made in other areas that do not require "high-tech" surgical or medical interventions. For example, better understanding of the role of good nutrition in normal development and of how nutritional problems can affect development has been gained. Nutritional issues may even have an impact on embryologic development, such as the association between folate deficiency and neural tube defects. The important role of nutrition is discussed in Chapter 29.

SUMMARY

Advances in multiple and diverse scientific fields have led to an increased understanding of normal embryologic development, CNS form and function, and mechanisms of CNS damage. An explosion of knowledge in the field of genetics has led to in-depth understanding of multiple disease processes, in some cases down to a cellular and molecular level. This has led to discoveries of the causes of previously described diseases, descriptions of new diseases, and new approaches to management and treatment of diseases.

Although it is impossible for a developmental pediatrician to understand and to remember all of these new mechanisms and molecular tests, it is nonetheless critical for the physician evaluating and caring for children with developmental disabilities to have a basic understanding of human genetics and to know when to suspect certain problems and when to refer to a knowledgeable subspecialist.

Major advances in medical fields as diverse as neonatology, nutrition, and surgery have enabled children with complex medical issues to survive what were formerly lethal circumstances. However, children who have complex medical or genetic disorders, who have difficult deliveries, or who are born too soon may face a host of developmental challenges. These problems may persist for many years, and in fact the issue of transition to adult care providers is now necessary in many cases. During their training, adult care providers often receive little information about or exposure to the care, management, and evaluation of people with disabilities, placing pressure on the pediatrician to sort out diagnoses and management issues earlier in life.

Although it is still challenging, major advances across many fields of science and medicine have led to a greater understanding of the causes and evaluation of developmental disabilities and to improvements in management of these children.

REFERENCES

Alsdorf R, Wyszynski D: Teratogenicity of sodium valproate. Expert Opin Drug Saf 4(2):345-353, 2005.

Dorus S, Anderson JR, Vallender EJ, et al: Sonic Hedgehog, a key development gene, experienced intensified molecular evolution in primates. Hum Mol Genet 15(13):2031-2037, 2006.

Genomics.energy.gov for information on the Human Genome Project.

Gluckman PD, Wyatt JS, Azzopardi D, et al: Selective head cooling with mild systemic hypothermia after neonatal encephalopathy: Multicentre randomized trial. Lancet 365:663-670, 2005.

Hoon AH Jr, Belsito KM, Nagae-Poetscher LM: Neuroimaging in spasticity and movement disorders. J Child Neurol 18(1):S25-S39, 2003.

Muenke M, Beachy PA: Genetics of ventral forebrain development and holoprosencephaly. Curr Opin Genet Dev 10(3):262-269, 2000.

Oldak M, Grzela T, Lazarczyk M, et al: Clinical aspects of disrupted Hedgehog signaling. Int J Mol Med 8(4):445-452, 2001.

Shaw-Smith C, Redon R, Rickman L, et al: Microarray-based comparative genomic hybridization (array-CGH) detects submicroscopic chromosomal deletions and duplications in patients with learning disability/mental retardation and dysmorphic features. J Med Genet 41:241-248, 2004.

Strong C: Neuropsychiatry Reviews 4(10), December 2003.

Van Allen MI, Kalousek DK, Chernoff GF, et al: Evidence for multisite closure of the neural tube in humans. Am J Med Genet 47(5):723-743, 1993.

Zhou XP, Waite KA, Pilarski R, et al: Germline PTEN promoter mutations and deletions in Cowden/Bannayan-Riley-Ruvalcaba syndrome results in aberrant PTEN protein and dysregulation of the phosphoinositol-3-kinase/AKt pathway. Am J Hum Genet 73(2):404-411, 2003.

23 NERVOUS SYSTEM DISORDERS

KELLY KNUPP AND JULIE PARSONS

Nervous system disorders encompass abnormalities in structure or function of the brain and peripheral nervous system. They may be the results of underlying genetic conditions or injury from trauma, metabolic derangement, or infection. This chapter discusses more common nervous system disorders including seizures, head trauma, central nervous system dysgenesis, central nervous system infection, and several genetic neuromuscular disorders. For more detailed discussion of related conditions, see the separate chapters, including those on cerebral palsy (Chapter 67), inherited metabolic disorders (Chapter 30), and genetic disorders (Chapter 26).

SEIZURES

A seizure is a discrete event characterized by a change in neurologic function associated with an electrical discharge arising from neurons in the brain. Because the brain controls many functions, the clinical presentation will vary from a sudden feeling of nausea, to brief confusion, to generalized shaking associated with a loss of consciousness. Typically, a change in electrical function can be detected by electroencephalography (EEG), but not always. The electrical change can either be too deep within the brain or involve too small a portion of the cortex to be detected by EEG electrodes placed on the scalp.

Rarely is a seizure witnessed during a patient's visit. Most seizures are less than 5 minutes in duration and are frequently less than 1 minute in duration. The common feature of an event that is likely to be a seizure is a *stereotyped recurrent episode*. When this pattern is recognized, the possibility of a seizure must be considered, although this pattern is often present in other phenomena, such as syncope, headache, and cardiac arrhythmia. Therefore, ancillary testing, such as EEG and magnetic resonance imaging (MRI), can be of great benefit.

There are several types of seizures (Table 23-1); knowledge of these types will allow the practitioner to obtain a better description from families when a history is taken. The most common classification system is the International League Against Epilepsy system dividing seizures into partial seizures, arising from one part of the brain, and generalized seizures, involving the entire brain at one time. Defining of seizure type is very useful to the clinician for deciding on treatment, classifying epilepsy syndromes, and determining the cause of a seizure.

Partial seizures, also called focal seizures, can be divided into two types: simple partial and complex partial. A simple partial seizure is a seizure that involves a small part of the brain and is not associated with a change in consciousness. The seizure will clinically present as the function that the particular part of the brain represents, for example, right arm jerking arises from the left motor strip of the brain. Complex partial seizures also involve a small portion of brain but are associated with an alteration of awareness. Seizures arising from the temporal lobe provide an excellent example of this type of seizure; these typically start with an epigastric feeling followed by lip smacking, nonpurposeful or semipurposeful hand movements such as picking movements or handwringing, and confusion.

Generalized seizures involve the entire brain during the seizure but can also have a variety of presentations, such as staring spells (absence seizures), sudden fall to the ground (atonic seizures), stiffening (tonic seizure), and quick jerks (myoclonic seizure). Generalized tonic-clonic seizures are the most familiar type of seizure, but they can be either generalized in onset or focal in onset with evolution into a generalized tonic-clonic seizure. Specific details can lead to a more detailed description, which will in turn lead to better diagnosis and treatment. The use of home video has led to significant improvement in communication between patient and provider. This technology has helped clarify many episodes that were difficult to describe and thus has led to improved care for the patient.

Epilepsy means having two or more seizures separated by 24 hours in one's lifetime. It is important for this definition to be understood by both clinicians and patients because there is still a negative connotation to the diagnosis of epilepsy among the general population. Having a single seizure does not mean that one has epilepsy. In fact, 5% of children will have a seizure by the age of 20 years (Hauser et al, 1996). Only about 1% to 2% of the population has recurrent unprovoked seizures and therefore a diagnosis of epilepsy.

The most accepted epilepsy classification is that of the International League Against Epilepsy, meant to be as inclusive as possible, although it recognizes that not

Table 23-1. International League Against Epilepsy Seizure Classification

Generalized Seizures
Tonic-clonic seizures (includes variations beginning with a clonic or myoclonic phase)
Clonic seizures
Without tonic features
With tonic features
Typical absence seizures
Atypical absence seizures
Myoclonic absence seizures
Tonic seizures
Spasms
Myoclonic seizures
Massive bilateral myoclonus
Atonic seizures
Focal Seizures
Simple partial seizures
Complex partial seizures

every patient will fit nicely into a category. The classification of epilepsy relies on the seizure types that are present. The initial division is into focal onset and generalized onset. A third category that is not clearly focal or generalized recognizes that epileptiform discharges may cause encephalopathy. These categories are determined in most cases by the presenting seizure type. Another way to view pediatric epilepsy is by age. A child's brain changes over time, and the presentation of an epilepsy syndrome can and does evolve with this change. Different syndromes are more prevalent within different age groups.

Benign childhood epilepsy is a classic epilepsy syndrome characterized by focal seizures, typically occurring at night, described as focal facial twitching that spreads and evolves into a generalized tonic-clonic seizure. These patients have a characteristic EEG pattern with bilateral independent temporal central spikes. The majority of patients outgrow this epilepsy syndrome as they enter adolescence. Although it was previously thought to be "benign," more recent studies have shown that some of these children have mild learning and language difficulties related to the frequency of epileptiform discharges during sleep (Nikolai et al, 2007). Symptomatic focal epilepsies are thought to be caused be a focal area of abnormality in the brain, such as a malformation or an injury like stroke or inflammation.

Classic examples of idiopathic generalized epilepsies are benign myoclonic epilepsy in infancy, which tends to resolve quickly; and childhood absence epilepsy, which is characterized by frequent staring episodes, at times associated with eye fluttering, lip smacking, or hand automatisms. These seizures are usually brief (5 to 15 seconds) but can occur several times a day (many patients have up to 100 in a day). Owing to the frequency of absence seizures, some children present with difficulty in school because of frequent electrical disruptions. In the teenage years, juvenile myoclonic epilepsy is an emerging epilepsy syndrome. Children with this syndrome have a combination of frequent myoclonic seizures, more prevalent in the early morning hours, and less frequently occurring generalized tonic-clonic seizures. Myoclonic seizures may not initially be recognized as seizures. The clinician may have to ask specifically about this symptom.

There are generalized epilepsy syndromes grouped under epileptic encephalopathies that can have a more significant effect on development, such as infantile spasms, Lennox-Gastaut syndrome, myoclonic astatic epilepsy, and Dravet syndrome. Infantile spasms present in the first year of life and are characterized classically by clusters of sudden arm and leg extension. Clusters are usually most apparent on awaking and on going to sleep. Many children will let out a cry with each jerk as though they are uncomfortable, often inciting families to seek care. Many neurologists view this type of epilepsy as an emergency. Recent literature suggests that the longer the spasms go untreated, the worse the developmental outcome will be (Primec et al, 2006). Children whose seizures are not controlled almost universally manifest cognitive deficits. Many of these children will develop Lennox-Gastaut syndrome.

Lennox-Gastaut syndrome consists of atypical absence seizures, tonic seizures, and generalized tonic-clonic seizures in addition to a characteristic EEG pattern. These children can also have myoclonic, atonic, and partial seizures. EEG findings include slow spike and wave discharges. Most of these seizures are very difficult to control, and developmental delay is usually present. These children present in the early toddler years. Many have a history of infantile spasms preceding the development of the characteristic seizures. An underlying cause is identified in a number of these patients, including an abnormality detected on MRI, infection, hypoxia, or metabolic abnormalities.

Myoclonic astatic epilepsy of Doose is another syndrome that presents during the early preschool years. These toddlers are typically normal before the onset of seizures. Some have reported that these children may have had precocious development. These children have atonic seizures, myoclonic seizures, and staring spells. The seizures can often be difficult to control. Development seems to follow seizure control; when seizures are controlled, development improves, but when seizures are frequent, development can halt or even regress. An underlying cause is not found in these patients.

Dravet syndrome or severe myoclonic epilepsy of infancy was first described in 1982. These children initially have normal development. During the first year of life, atypical febrile seizures develop. The seizures have a prolonged duration and focality that shifts from one side of the body to the other. Around 1 year of life, myoclonic seizures become apparent, although they do not have to be present. Severe developmental delay and poor response to medication are common. A mutation has recently been found in about 80% of these patients in a sodium channel gene, *SCN1A* (Harkin et al, 2007). In a study of children developing intractable epilepsy and encephalopathy immediately after first immunization, a large number of children had a mutation in this gene (Berkovic et al, 2006).

Landau-Kleffner syndrome is another epileptic syndrome that presents in childhood and causes developmental problems. These children have infrequent seizures, but they have a loss of language characterized by verbal auditory agnosia and loss or reduction of spontaneous speech. EEG frequently demonstrates continuous epileptiform discharges (spike waves) during sleep. Treatment has been attempted with intravenous immune globulin, steroids, and high-dose diazepam with mixed results. There can be milder forms associated with varying degrees of learning difficulties.

Evaluation of the Patient

A seizure should initially be thought of as a *symptom* reflecting an alteration in the brain. The focus of evaluation should be on identification of an underlying cause of the seizure. A history should be obtained in detail to ascertain that the event was a seizure. Differential diagnosis includes breath-holding spells, syncope, night terrors, constipation, shivering, arrhythmia, and headaches. Physical examination should focus on asymmetry of neurologic function. Evidence of trauma, meningismus, papilledema, and rash is important to note.

Laboratory studies including calcium and magnesium determinations should be performed to exclude electrolyte imbalance. Calcium abnormalities can be particularly important in young children because they can indicate underlying genetic abnormality, nutrition imbalance, or endocrine abnormality. Blood count and infectious etiology should be considered in any patient with a fever. Lumbar puncture should be strongly considered in patients younger than 1 year presenting with a fever and considered in children younger than 18 months (Practice Parameter, 1996). Any patient with a fever and first-time seizure who has depressed mental status should also have a lumbar puncture.

Imaging is helpful acutely if trauma is suspected or if the child is presenting with a first seizure. Imaging available in the emergency department is typically a computed tomographic (CT) scan of the head, although MRI is becoming more readily available in some emergency departments. There are limitations to both modalities. MRI allows more detailed imaging, although acute bleeding can be difficult to appreciate. Head (CT) is often quicker, does not require children to be sedated, and visualizes intracranial blood well. However, tumors and small or early infarcts can be missed on computed tomography. Any patient with a first unprovoked seizure should ultimately undergo evaluation by MRI, regardless of the initial choice of imaging. MRI can be delayed several days if the patient has returned to baseline and does not have focal findings on neurologic examination.

EEG is frequently ordered for patients with a first seizure. If there is uncertainty that an event was a seizure, an abnormal EEG recording can provide information on recurrence risk for having more seizures. An abnormal EEG recording acutely after an event that improves over time is consistent with a seizure. Unfortunately, the correlation between seizures, epilepsy, and EEG abnormalities is not 100%. One must always consider the clinical situation when interpreting EEG results. The greatest use of EEG after a first-time seizure is in providing some additional information about the likelihood of an additional seizure. A patient with a generalized "idiopathic" seizure and an abnormal EEG recording has a likely recurrence rate around 56%. These same children with a normal EEG recording have a recurrence risk of 26% (Shinnar et al, 1990). The greatest risk factors for seizure recurrence are an abnormal EEG recording with focal findings and abnormal findings on neurologic examination.

Treatment

Treatment can be divided into two categories, acute and preventive. If a child is actively seizing, treatment is generally started 5 minutes into the seizure. The first line of treatment is a benzodiazepine. This is often followed by a loading dose of a parenteral medication, traditionally phenobarbital, phenytoin, or fosphenytoin. With the addition of new parenteral medications, these recommendations are likely to change. Formulations of benzodiazepines are available for home use, such as Diastat, a rectal administration system for diazepam. There is also literature on the intranasal and buccal use of midazolam as well as buccal lorazepam. These formulations allow families to abort a seizure in the home setting, avoiding a trip to the emergency department.

Preventive treatment is not appropriate for every child who presents with a seizure. Standard practice is to wait until a patient fulfills the definition of epilepsy (two or more seizures) before starting treatment with anticonvulsants. Several new anticonvulsants have become available during the last 2 decades (Table 23-2). There has been great debate about choice of anticonvulsants for specific syndromes, and good-quality studies for each syndrome are not available for many of the medications. Regardless of the anticonvulsant chosen, as long as the medication is well chosen for the particular type of seizure or epilepsy, the response rate to an initial drug is around 50%; the response rate to a second medication is an additional 15%. The response rate then decreases to about 5% for each additional medication alone and in combination (Kwan and Brodie, 2000). If medications are not effective, there are several alternatives: the ketogenic diet and derivatives, vagus nerve stimulator, and epilepsy surgery.

The ketogenic diet is a diet high in fat and low in protein and carbohydrate. This changes the metabolism of the brain from use of carbohydrates as a source of energy to use of ketones as an energy source. This is a very rigid diet requiring meticulous attention to all food and liquid intake, and consultation with a knowledgeable dietitian is often required. Some variations of this diet are currently being used that are better tolerated, including the Atkins diet and the low glycemic index diet.

The vagus nerve stimulator is a device that is implanted in the left upper chest wall with a wire that extends to and wraps around the vagus nerve. An electrical impulse is delivered at regular intervals to the vagus nerve. An emergency mode can be activated by a magnet swiped over the device to abort a seizure. Response rates have been reported at around 45% of children, with a more than 50% reduction in seizures and 10% with seizure freedom (Alexopoulos et al, 2006).

Table 23-2. **Anticonvulsants**

Anticonvulsant	Dosing	Seizure Type	Routine Monitoring	Typical Serum Levels
Carbamazepine	10-30 mg/kg/day	Focal seizures	CBC, electrolytes	4-12 μg/mL
Ethosuximide	15-40 mg/kg/day	Absence seizures	CBC	40-100 μg/mL
Felbamate	45-100 mg/kg/day	Broad spectrum	CBC	30-100 μg/mL
Gabapentin	30-100 mg/kg/day	Focal seizures		4-20 μg/mL
Lamotrigine	1-15 mg/kg/day (varies on the basis of additional antiepileptic drugs)	Broad spectrum; may not work for myoclonus	LFTs	5-20 μg/mL
Levetiracetam	40-100 mg/kg/day	Broad spectrum		5-50 μg/mL
Methsuximide	20 mg/kg/day	Broad spectrum	CBC	20-40 μg/mL
Oxcarbazepine	15-45 mg/kg/day	Focal seizures	Electrolytes	10-55 μg/mL
Phenobarbital	2-6 mg/kg/day	Broad spectrum	CBC	15-40 μg/mL
Phenytoin	4-8 mg/kg/day	Focal seizures	CBC, LFTs	10-20 μg/mL
Pregabalin	2-6 mg/kg/day	Focal seizures		
Primidone	5-20 mg/kg/day	Broad spectrum	CBC	4-12 μg/mL
Tiagabine	0.25-1.25 mg/kg/day	Focal seizures		5-70 μg/mL
Topiramate	5-25 mg/kg/day	Broad spectrum	Electrolytes	3-25 μg/mL
Valproic acid	20-60 mg/kg/day	Broad spectrum	CBC, LFTs	50-120 μg/mL
Vigabatrin	40-100 mg/kg/day	Focal seizures, infantile spasms	LFTs, visual fields, MRI	
Zonisamide	4-10 mg/kg/day	Broad spectrum	Electrolytes	10-30 μg/mL

CBC, complete blood count; LFTs, liver function tests; MRI, magnetic resonance imaging.

Epilepsy surgery has been employed as a method of controlling seizures for more than 50 years, but it has increased dramatically during the last 2 decades. Several types of surgeries are performed. Hemispherectomy, the removal of an entire hemisphere, is used in situations such as Sturge-Weber syndrome and hemimegancephaly. Corpus callosotomy is a surgery that separates the connections between the two hemispheres. Deeper connections through the thalamus and basal ganglia still exist. This surgery is most appropriate for patients with atonic seizures and possibly myoclonic seizures.

The majority of epilepsy surgeries are focal resections that remove the area of onset of partial seizures. Before surgery, the patient must undergo a comprehensive evaluation, including studies such as video EEG monitoring, MRI (often with specialized sequencing), neuropsychologic evaluation, single-photon emission computed tomography (with and without seizure), and positron emission tomography.

HEAD TRAUMA

Head injury is unfortunately still a common cause of injury and death in the pediatric population. In many cases, these injuries are preventable by use of helmets when bicycling, skateboarding, and skiing as well as with the use of appropriate restraints when riding in cars. In addition, proper sports equipment when playing contact sports can prevent some of these injuries. Another cause of head injury in the pediatric population is nonaccidental trauma. An estimated 37,000 children are hospitalized for traumatic brain injury a year, with 435,000 emergency department visits annually (Langlois, Rutland-Brown, and Thomas, 2004).

The Glasgow Coma Scale has been used in the emergency situation to rapidly evaluate the severity of injury and to triage patients into mild, moderate, and severe injury. The scale relies on motor, ocular, and verbal responses and must be used carefully in very young children who may not yet be verbal and able to follow commands or who are frightened and unable to cooperate with strangers. A Glasgow Coma Scale score of 13 to 15 correlates with mild head injury, a score of 9 to 12 correlates with moderate head injury, and a score of 3 to 8 is associated with severe head injury.

The mechanism of action of trauma can cause a wide variety of injuries from fracture, hemorrhage, contusion, swelling, and combinations of these. Fractures can be linear, depressed, or comminuted. Clinical signs of a basilar skull fracture are mastoid bruising (Battle sign) and periorbital bruising (raccoon sign). After a skull fracture, very young infants should be observed clinically for a growing skull fracture or leptomeningeal cyst formation. Fractures through the cribriform plate can lead to cerebrospinal fluid (CSF) rhinorrhea.

Hemorrhage can be subdural, epidural, intraparenchymal, and intraventricular. Epidural bleeding is more likely to be arterial in origin and can accumulate quickly, necessitating surgical intervention. Intraventricular hemorrhage can lead to blockage of CSF flow and require external drainage. Any blood products near the cortex can be irritating to the brain and lead to seizures.

With head injury, there may be forces causing injury opposite the site of impact, called contrecoup effects. This is related to movement of the brain within the skull that creates a second site of injury opposite the site of impact. Diffuse axonal injury can also occur and is thought to reflect shear injury deeper within the tissue related to forces of the trauma. This is most apparent in the white matter and can cause significant alteration of consciousness without significant focal injury. MRI can be very helpful in identifying this type of injury.

Children have better outcome from traumatic brain injury compared with that of adults, but many will have changes in behavior, cognition, and educational needs. The more severe the injury, the greater the sequelae of the injury. Even after mild head injury, a postconcussive syndrome has been reported (Mittenberg, Wittner, and Miller, 1997). These symptoms include headache, dizziness, fatigue, blurry vision, photophobia, memory problems, and depression.

STROKE

Stroke, although rare, happens in children as well as in adults. Stroke in the pediatric population is commonly divided into neonatal and childhood stroke. This structure is useful in thinking about etiology, in evaluation, and for ongoing research in this population. Neonatal stroke is more common, occurring in 1 in 4000 live births annually (Nelson and Lynch, 2004), whereas childhood stroke occurs in about 2 to 8 in 100,000 per year in North America (Giroud, Lemesle, and Gouyon, 1995; Kittner and Adams, 1996).

Neonatal strokes are further divided into prenatal, perinatal, and postnatal. Prenatal strokes are typically noted around 4 to 8 months postnatally with focal deficit on examination. Perinatal strokes clinically present with seizures in the first week of life due to acute injury to the cortex. Postnatal strokes present with sudden focal findings that correlate with the area of injury.

Childhood strokes can occur at any time. These are manifested with acute focal deficits that correlate with the area of injury. With strokes involving larger areas of the brain, consciousness may be impaired. The use of MRI has led to more ready identification during the past decade. Transient ischemic attack, defined as focal neurologic deficit lasting less than 24 hours, can also have findings on MRI, making some question whether this is still a useful clinical distinction.

The etiology of stroke in children is different from that of adult stroke, and there is also a difference in etiology between neonatal stroke and childhood stroke. In some cases, the cause may be obvious, such as congenital heart disease, sickle cell disease, and trauma. Patent foramen ovale is a risk factor in both adult and pediatric stroke patients. Other risk factors are vasculopathy, infection (e.g., varicella), and prothrombotic disorders. Abnormalities leading to a prothrombotic state include antiphospholipid antibodies, protein C deficiency, elevated homocystinemia, protein S deficiency, and factor V Leiden deficiency. In neonatal stroke, some antibody-mediated deficiencies can be transmitted vertically, transiently increasing the risk for stroke in the neonatal period. Moyamoya syndrome is bilateral stenosis of the internal carotid arteries causing extensive collateral circulation to occur. This produces a characteristic appearance on cerebral angiography.

As in adults, once a stroke has been identified, it is important to try to identify the cause to prevent recurrence, which is increased (up to 66%) in patients with vascular abnormalities (Fullerton et al, 2007). Evaluation should include imaging with MRI to confirm the diagnosis of stroke. If the cause of the stroke is not immediately obvious (e.g., trauma), further evaluation needs to be completed, looking for cardiac abnormalities, prothrombotic abnormalities, and infectious etiology. Angiography may be required in some patients if abnormalities in the great vessels are suspected.

Treatment of all stroke, adult and pediatric, has improved during the last decade, but this has been based almost entirely on adult studies. These treatments have employed systemic infusion of tissue-type plasminogen activator (tPA) and interventional radiology–guided intra-arterial placement of tPA directly at the site of occlusion. Both of these treatments have very specific time criteria from onset of symptoms for their use. The only randomized studies in children for stroke are in sickle cell patients. Optimal treatment of neonatal and childhood stroke requires coordination by a multidisciplinary team including a neurologist, hematologist, rehabilitation physician, and neuropsychologist.

HEADACHES

Headaches are a common pediatric complaint and can be associated with a variety of symptoms indicating the underlying illness. The differential diagnosis of a headache is vast. One must first think of headache as a symptom, not as a diagnosis. The actual number of young patients with headache is difficult to determine because children may not be able to fully articulate their symptoms, but by the age of 7 years, 37% to 50% of children have had a headache (Sillanpää, 1983; Sillanpää, Piekkala, and Kero, 1991).

Headaches are classified according to the International Headache Society classification system (Table 23-3). The most common divisions are migraine with and without aura and tension-type headache. Children have also been described to have cluster headaches, although this is less common. The headache criteria were developed primarily for the adult population, and some caveats must be considered when these same criteria are used for children. Migraine in children is generally shorter in duration and is more likely to be bitemporal than lateralized pain. There are also variants, such as brief vertigo and cyclic vomiting, that need to be considered. These are listed in the classification system. Headaches due to overuse of medications must also be considered.

Because the differential diagnosis of a headache can be vast, consideration of the chronology of a headache is useful in restricting possible causes. An acute headache is more likely to be due to infection, acute hypertension, trauma, embolism, hemorrhage, or shunt malfunction. Acute recurrent headaches are more likely to represent migraine or tension-type headaches.

Headaches that are chronically progressive are most often organic in nature. These headaches are more likely to represent tumors, infection, or increased intracranial pressure from either altered CSF flow or pseudotumor cerebri. Pseudotumor cerebri is an elevation in CSF pressure without obstruction in flow. It can be secondary to numerous causes, including antibiotic use, steroid use, obesity, hypervitaminosis, and sinus thrombosis. An ophthalmoscopic examination to evaluate for papilledema can assist in this diagnosis.

Table 23-3. Headache Classification

Migraine
Migraine without aura
Migraine with aura
Childhood periodic syndromes that are commonly precursors of migraine
Cyclic vomiting
Abdominal migraine
Benign paroxysmal vertigo of childhood
Tension-type headache
Cluster headache
Headache attributed to head or neck trauma
Headache attributed to cranial or cervical vascular disorder
Headache attributed to a substance or its withdrawal
Headache attributed to psychiatric disorder
Cranial neuralgias and central causes of facial pain

A lumbar puncture for opening pressure is the "gold standard."

Evaluation of the patient with headache includes a history that identifies the location, quality, quantity, frequency duration, timing, and associated features of the pain. A family history of headaches can be quite helpful. Many headache types have a strong familial component. It is important to ascertain medication trials, including home doses, to ensure that adequate dosing has been attempted. A detailed examination, including blood pressure, ophthalmoscopic examination, and musculoskeletal evaluation of the craniofacial and neck region, is necessary. Imaging is indicated for any first-time severe headache, for any patient with a neurologic deficit, and for change in headaches. If pseudotumor cerebri is suspected, a lumbar puncture is indicated to obtain opening pressure. Imaging should be performed before this to rule out mass lesion.

Treatment of headaches in children can be difficult because of unique qualities, such as short duration of the headaches. Treatment can be divided into abortive agents to stop an acute headache and preventive therapy. With a short duration of headache, abortive medications must be rapid acting to stop the headache before the time the headache is self-resolving. Ibuprofen and sumatriptan nasal spray are good agents for abortive therapy. Acetaminophen may also be effective. Much research needs to be done to clarify the efficacy of other agents to be used as preventive agents in children (Lewis et al, 2004).

BRAIN MALFORMATIONS

Most brain malformations can be explained by evolving anatomy of fetal brain. About 3% of neonates have major central nervous system or systemic malformations. The causes are variable, including environmental (infection, toxic) and genetic. About 60% of all central nervous system malformations are still of unknown cause (Aicardi, 1992). With improved neuroimaging such as MRI, earlier diagnoses of brain malformations are possible, and a more precise prognosis can be made in many cases.

Holoprosencephaly is a severe defect that refers to incomplete division of the forebrain (Fig. 23-1) A single large ventricular cavity results. The thalami are fused, but cerebellum and brainstem are normally formed. These defects are typically associated with severe facial and ocular abnormalities. Congenital cardiac disease and polydactyly may also be noted. Trisomy 13 and trisomy 18 can be associated, as can other genetic disorders, such as Smith-Lemli-Opitz syndrome. Mutations in the Sonic Hedgehog gene on chromosome 7 lead to holoprosencephaly. Any child with holoprosencephaly deserves a full genetic evaluation so that appropriate genetic counseling and recurrence risks can be given to the families. Severe intellectual disability, rigidity, intractable seizures, apnea, and temperature instability are common neurologic manifestations.

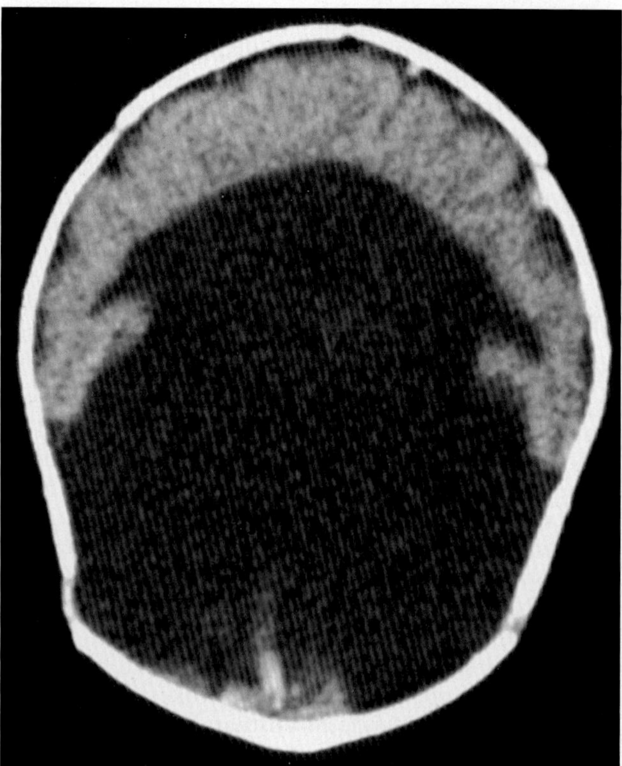

Figure 23-1. Alobar holoprosencephaly.

Septo-optic dysplasia may represent a milder form of holoprosencephaly. Agenesis of the septum pellucidum, optic nerve hypoplasia resulting in visual impairment of variable degree, and neuroendocrine disturbance including growth hormone deficiency and diabetes insipidus may result. Because of this, a full endocrinologic evaluation is warranted in these patients. Some patients may have intellectual disability, and many patients require low vision services.

Schizencephaly is characterized by unilateral or bilateral, full-thickness clefts associated with heterotopic gray matter extending from the cortical surface to the ventricular cavity (Fig. 23-2). The clefts may be open or close lipped. In close-lipped schizencephaly, the cleft walls are opposed, and CSF fluid space is absent. As a result, small clefts may be difficult to recognize. At times, unilateral open-lipped schizencephaly may be difficult to differentiate from a porencephalic cyst, which

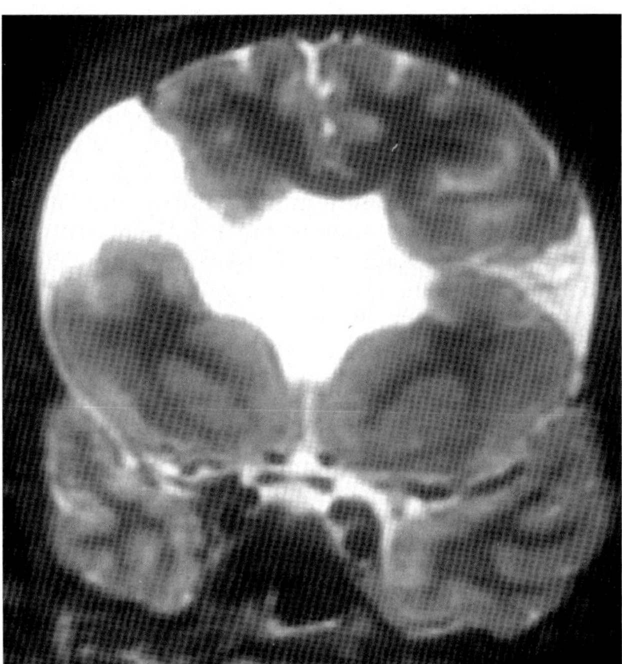

Figure 23-2. Bilateral schizencephaly: *left,* open-lipped type; *right,* closed-lipped type.

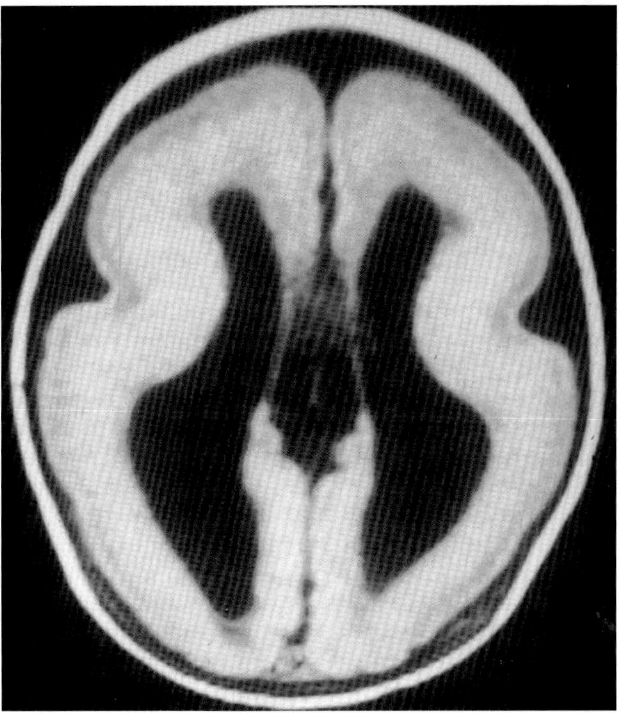

Figure 23-3. Lissencephaly.

implies cortical destruction from vascular or infectious insults. Schizencephaly accounted for 5% of all cortical malformations in a series of pediatric patients with malformations of cortical development (Leventer et al, 1999). Clinical manifestations of schizencephaly may range widely, depending on the size and extent of the clefts. Generalized or more focal motor deficits, such as hypotonia, hemiparesis, spastic quadriparesis, seizures, and variable degrees of intellectual disability or learning impairment, are noted.

Lissencephaly, meaning "smooth brain," is caused by failure of neuronal migration (Fig. 23-3). In its most severe form, a complete absence of sulcation is present. Usually only four of the usual six layers of the cortex are present. Imaging studies reveal a thickened cortex with a paucity of sulci. Enlarged lateral ventricles are noted. A small number of these cases result from a deletion of the distal portion of the short arm of chromosome 17, which is termed Miller-Dieker syndrome. In this syndrome, marked hypotonia, profound psychomotor retardation, feeding difficulties, microcephaly, and intractable seizures are characteristic.

Less severe forms of cortical migration disorders include *pachygyria* (decreased numbers of broad gyri and shallow sulci) and *polymicrogyria* (excess gyri that are too small, too crowded, and too numerous). In these cases, the general organization of the cortex may be normal with focal areas of abnormality noted. Clinical findings are variable with developmental issues ranging from learning disabilities to intellectual disabilities. A variety of bilateral or unilateral motor deficits and tone abnormalities ranging from spasticity to hypotonia with hyperreflexia may be seen.

Agenesis of the corpus callosum can be partial or complete. In isolated agenesis of the corpus callosum with no other associated brain malformations, neurologic abnormalities can include seizures, mild to moderate intellectual disability, and visual and motor incoordination. Agenesis or partial agenesis of the corpus callosum is seen in a wide variety of chromosomal, metabolic, and central nervous system malformation syndromes. Neurologic findings and developmental disabilities are understandably diverse in these cases.

NEUROMUSCULAR DISORDERS

Children with neuromuscular disorders may present with pure motor delays or more global delays, including cognitive impairment. Abnormalities causing disease may be localized to anterior horn cells in the spinal cord, peripheral nerves, or muscle fibers. Patients typically present with weakness and loss of or failure to gain motor skills. Previously, diagnostic evaluations required muscle biopsy, electromyography, or nerve conduction studies in addition to clinical history and examination. Currently, in many cases, molecular or genetic studies now confirm suspected diagnoses.

Duchenne Muscular Dystrophy

Duchenne muscular dystrophy is an X-linked recessive disorder with an incidence of 1 in 3500 male live births. Becker muscular dystrophy is less frequent, with an incidence of 1 in 30,000. Both result from mutations in the dystrophin gene. Absent dystrophin in the muscle cell membrane causes breakdown of skeletal and cardiac muscle. Boys with Duchenne muscular dystrophy typically present at 3 to 5 years of age because they are toe walkers or cannot keep up with their peers. On examination, they may have pseudohypertrophy of the calves and forearms and proximal weakness in the shoulders and particularly in the hip girdle. Most boys demonstrate a Gower maneuver (push off the floor, lock the knees, then use the hands to "climb up" the legs) as they get up from the floor and have difficulty running. Early in the course, reflexes are preserved, but as weakness of muscle groups progresses, only ankle reflexes are preserved. The majority of boys lose the ability to walk and are seated in a wheelchair by the age of 10 to 13 years. Death usually occurs in the late teens or early 20s from cardiac or respiratory dysfunction.

Medical complications of muscular dystrophy are respiratory infections and progressive respiratory failure due to weakness of the intercostal and skeletal muscles. Use of corticosteroids provides temporary improvement. Boys develop a dilated cardiomyopathy by the age of 10 years (Nigro et al, 1990), and early intervention is recommended. Carrier mothers have an estimated 10% to 15% incidence of cardiomyopathy and need to be observed as well. Progressive scoliosis typically develops in the teenage years in boys who are nonambulatory. Spinal fusion improves comfort in seating as well as pulmonary capacity. Two thirds of the boys have learning disabilities, attentional disorders, or cognitive delay. Around 2% are autistic. Early academic intervention and individual education plans are encouraged. Use of stimulant medication for attentional issues is not contraindicated in Duchenne dystrophy and can be quite helpful. Many boys will experience some depression, particularly in high school. Counseling and judicious use of antidepressants, such as selective serotonin reuptake inhibitors, typically will help the boys and their families through this period.

The diagnosis of Duchenne or Becker dystrophy at present is confirmed by laboratory studies. Creatine kinase elevation of more than 100 to 1000 times normal is noted in Duchenne dystrophy. There are very few other disorders except rhabdomyolysis that will give this marked elevation. Deletions in the dystrophin gene are present in 80% of the boys. Sequencing studies are also available to confirm a diagnosis. In most cases, muscle biopsy is no longer required.

Myotonic Dystrophy

Myotonic dystrophy, an autosomal dominantly inherited disease, is one of the more common muscle disorders. The incidence is 1/8000. A triplicate repeat of trinucleotides cytosine, guanine, and tyrosine (CTG) found on chromosome 19 causes myotonic dystrophy type 1. Affected patients have repeats numbering in the hundreds to thousands. In general, the increased size of the expansion correlates with earlier onset of symptoms and a more severe phenotype. Creatine kinase concentration may be normal to threefold increased.

Facial weakness and distal muscle weakness develop over time, but the hallmark of the disease is percussion, grip, or eyelid myotonia. Myotonia is an inability to relax contracted muscle. Grip myotonia is commonly elicited with a handshake and observing a very slow relaxation of the fingers. Myotonia is not demonstrated in infants and young children but becomes symptomatic typically around the age of 5 years.

Multiple associated features, such as early cataract formation, ptosis, male pattern baldness or hair thinning, long thin facies, high arched palate, and frontal bossing, may be noted. Cardiac arrhythmias and conduction disorders are seen in the majority of patients. Mitral valve prolapse may be present. Decreased ventilatory drive and diaphragm weakness, dysphagia, and aspiration can also cause significant morbidity. Hypogonadism and insulin resistance may develop over time. Sleep disorders and especially daytime somnolence are noted. Cognitive deficits, lack of motivation, and sometimes hostile or paranoid behavior can be seen.

Congenital myotonic dystrophy presents in the neonate as severe hypotonia, facial diplegia with poor suck and swallow, respiratory difficulty, and occasionally arthrogryposis. Intellectual disability is prominent in 50% to 60%.

Spinal Muscular Atrophy

Spinal muscular atrophy is a disorder of the anterior horn cells in the spinal cord. Spinal muscular atrophy is most commonly caused by deletions of exons 7 and 8 in the survival motor neuron gene found on chromosome 5. The inheritance pattern is autosomal recessive. There is a high carrier frequency in the United States.

There are three common forms of spinal muscular atrophy classified by age at onset and severity of functional impairment. Type 1 spinal muscular atrophy has been termed Werdnig-Hoffmann disease and is most usually fatal by 2 years of age. Children with spinal muscular atrophy type 2 can usually achieve the ability to sit but have limited walking. Patients with type 3 or Kugelberg-Welander syndrome develop weakness in teen or young adult years.

On examination, children demonstrate hypotonia, weakness with neurogenic muscle atrophy, areflexia, and hand tremor. Creatine kinase levels are normal or only mildly elevated. Cognitive and cardiac problems are not commonly seen in this disorder. Respiratory insufficiency due to weakness, early-onset scoliosis in nonambulatory children, and osteopenia are noted early in the course of the disease.

Charcot-Marie-Tooth Disease

Hereditary sensory motor neuropathy or Charcot-Marie-Tooth disease is the most common peripheral neuropathy in children. The frequency is 1/2500. There are multiple inheritance patterns in this disorder. Charcot-Marie-Tooth disease type 1A is the most common form and is a dominantly inherited disorder, usually due to a duplication of material on chromosome 17.

Clinical symptoms are progressive distal weakness and atrophy of the intrinsic muscles of the foot as well as peroneal muscles. Footdrop, steppage gait, and toe walking result. Intrinsic hand muscles may also be involved. Fine tremor is not an unusual feature. Reflexes are lost, and sensory findings such as loss of vibration, temperature sensation, and proprioception are typical. Physical examination findings also include pes cavus foot deformity and wasting of the hypothenar eminence. There is no cognitive impairment with this disorder.

INFECTIOUS DISEASES

Central nervous system infections are a common cause of hospitalizations and neurodevelopmental sequelae in children. Immunizations, improvements in perinatal care, and treatment of immunosuppressive disease have had a significant impact on reducing morbidity.

Multiple viruses are disease producing but can be difficult to isolate. Enteroviruses and arboviruses are common. Immunization status, prior travel, season of the year, and age of the patient all help determine which virus may be implicated in encephalitis. For instance, West Nile virus encephalitis would be a diagnostic consideration in the summer when mosquitoes are prevalent as the vector for transmission of this virus.

The skin, mucous membranes, lymphoid tissue, and nervous system are key components of the physical examination. Fever, headache, malaise, nuchal rigidity, nausea, decreased appetite, and rash may be noted on presentation. Altered mental status, including irritability, encephalopathy, and even coma, can be a presenting symptom of encephalitis. Patients may be aphasic or present with seizures. Focal neurologic findings may also be present. Symptoms may be very mild or life-threatening.

Laboratory studies typically show a leukocytosis with elevation in lymphocytes. An opening pressure obtained during the spinal tap will usually be elevated. CSF typically has a normal glucose concentration, a protein level that is normal to moderately elevated, and an increased white blood cell count (5 to 1000 cells per high-power field). Bacterial cultures and Gram stain should be performed in addition to cell counts, and specimens for polymerase chain reaction (PCR) analysis for enterovirus and herpes simplex virus (HSV) should be sent. Sending of serum, urine, nasal, and rectal swabs for viral studies will improve the diagnostic yield for specific viruses.

HSV infection is a treatable cause of encephalitis but may be indistinguishable from other viral encephalitides. CSF cultures for HSV have a sensitivity of less than 10%. HSV PCR of the CSF has been shown to have 98% sensitivity and 94% specificity (Aurelius, 1991; Lakeman and Whitley, 1995) and is currently the laboratory test of choice to confirm the diagnosis. Classically, HSV encephalitis is associated with hemorrhagic inflammation of the temporal lobes and is frequently bilateral.

Neonatal herpes infection is associated with considerable morbidity and mortality. Infants with seizures at the onset of therapy had greater mortality and were at higher risk for abnormal neurologic development. Early diagnosis and treatment have a positive effect on morbidity and mortality. Longer treatment (21 days) and higher doses of acyclovir (60 mg/kg/day) have improved outcomes. According to a study by Kimberlin and associates (Kimberlin, Lin, and Jacobs, 2001a, 2001b), however, there has not been much progress made in decreasing the time between diagnosis of neonatal herpes and initiation of treatment.

Enteroviruses (coxsackieviruses A and B, echoviruses, and enteroviruses 68 through 71) are a common cause of encephalitis and meningitis in the United States. Many cases are self-limited, but a large proportion of children have short-term or long-term disabilities. Enteroviral infections, in contrast to HSV infection, typically involve the entire brain. Treatment is largely supportive. Seizures resulting from viral encephalitis can be challenging to treat and may require multiple anticonvulsant medications. Close monitoring for cerebral edema, electrolyte imbalance, and respiratory complications is critical. If HSV infection is a diagnostic consideration, acyclovir should be initiated until the result of PCR analysis of CSF for HSV is negative.

Bacterial Meningitis

Bacterial meningitis is an inflammation of the membranes that surround the brain and spinal cord. About 10% of patients with bacterial meningitis die (Arditi et al, 1998), and 40% have neurologic sequelae including hearing impairment (Grimwood et al, 1995).

The etiology of bacterial meningitis is affected by the age of the patient. Group B streptococci and gram-negative enteric organisms are most common in neonates. Intrapartum antibiotic prophylactic treatment implemented by the Centers for Disease Control and Prevention in 2002 decreased the incidence of neonatal group B streptococcal disease by about two thirds (Schrag et al, 2002).

In infants and younger children, *Streptococcus pneumoniae, Neisseria meningitidis,* and *Haemophilus influenzae* type b (Hib) are the most common causes. In areas of developed countries where Hib conjugate vaccines are widely used, the incidence of *H. influenzae* meningitis has markedly decreased (Martin et al, 2004). The highest risk of *S. pneumoniae* meningitis is in children younger than 2 years. Universal use of heptavalent pneumococcal conjugate vaccine (PCV7) in infancy in the United States has reduced the incidence of invasive disease including bacterial meningitis by 90% (Black et al, 2004). Predominant causes of bacterial meningitis in older children and adolescents are *S. pneumoniae* and *N. meningitidis*.

Risk factors for bacterial meningitis in children include penetrating head injuries, CSF leaks, immunocompromised states such as human immunodeficiency virus infection, asplenia, and immunoglobulin deficiencies. Staphylococci and gram-negative organisms are responsible for infection in patients with ventriculoperitoneal shunts. In patients with cochlear implants, a more than 30-fold increase in the incidence of pneumococcal meningitis has been noted (Reefhuis et al, 2003).

Clinical features of meningitis are variable and depend on the patient's age. Fever, mental status changes, and nuchal rigidity are present in less than 50%. These findings are not specific for meningitis. Seizures are the presenting symptom in about one third of cases of bacterial meningitis and are most common in *S. pneumoniae* and *H. influenzae* type b infections (Kaplan, 1999). Petechiae and purpura are most common in meningococcal meningitis. Focal neurologic signs or papilledema raises concern about increased intracranial pressure.

Imaging should be performed before a spinal tap in these cases to avoid potential complications of herniation.

Diagnosis is confirmed by lumbar puncture. CSF findings include pleocytosis with polymorphonuclear cells predominant. If the lumbar puncture is performed early in the disease course, white blood cell counts may be normal or lymphocytes may predominate. Glucose concentration is decreased, and CSF protein concentration is typically elevated. In patients with untreated bacterial meningitis, Gram stain of CSF is positive in 80% to 90%. Positive CSF bacterial culture results decrease fairly rapidly after antibiotic therapy has been initiated. Samples for blood culture should, of course, be obtained.

Empiric therapy is determined to cover the most likely etiologic agents. In neonates, ampicillin and cefotaxime or an aminoglycoside are commonly used. Vancomycin and a third-generation cephalosporin are recommended in children older than 1 month. Duration of therapy is dependent on age, pathogen, and clinical course of disease. In children, several studies have been done to evaluate the benefit of dexamethasone as adjunctive therapy. Patients who received dexamethasone had a decrease in neurologic and audiologic sequelae compared with children who received a placebo. The benefits were greatest in patients with *H. influenzae* infection and less evident in pneumococcal meningitis (McIntyre et al, 1997).

Hearing impairment is the most common neurologic sequela of bacterial meningitis, noted in 25% to 35% of patients with *S. pneumoniae* infection and in 5% to 10% of patients with *H. influenzae* and *N. meningitidis* infections. Hypoglycorrhachia correlates with development of hearing loss as well (Fortnum, 1992; Wald et al, 1995). Learning disabilities, motor deficits, speech and language problems, and behavioral disorders are seen in approximately 10% of children after bacterial meningitis (Kooman et al, 2003).

MOVEMENT DISORDERS

Two types of movement disorders are common in pediatrics: tics and tremors.

Tremors are rhythmic, involuntary movements with a variety of amplitudes and frequencies. There are numerous causes of tremor. Resting tremors are typically found in basal ganglia disorders and therefore are not as commonly seen in the pediatric population. Action tremors do not occur at rest but are elicited with voluntary muscle contraction. Intention tremor and postural tremor are both types of action tremor. Typically, these tremors are localized to the cerebellum and its pathways. Medications such as valproic acid and sympathomimetics may cause tremor.

Essential tremor is the most common tremor type. No other neurologic abnormalities are found on examination. Arms and hands are predominantly involved. Commonly, a family history is elicited because most patients inherit this condition as an autosomal dominant disorder. The diagnosis can be made by history and examination. In patients with unilateral tremor of rapid onset or resting tremor, another diagnosis should be explored. Primidone or propranolol can be used for symptomatic treatment of tremor, but no medications are needed in the majority of patients.

Tics, including Tourette syndrome, are another common pediatric movement disorder that is often familial. Tics are repetitive, stereotypic arrhythmic movements that are mostly involuntary. Tics can be simple or complex, depending on the muscle groups involved. Forceful eye blink is a common simple motor tic, whereas touching tics are complex. Vocal tics such as sniffing and coughing are simple, whereas uttering phrases and repeating other people's words (echolalia) are complex vocal tics. Tics are frequently preceded by a premonitory urge, and tension is relieved briefly after the tic is carried out. Tics may be suppressed for several minutes voluntarily, but a "release" phenomenon typically follows suppression. Tics disappear with sleep.

Tourette syndrome is a chronic tic disorder; multiple motor and vocal tics occur during 1 year or more, following a waxing and waning course. Many children with Tourette syndrome have attentional and behavioral problems or obsessive-compulsive disorders. These comorbid conditions occur in about 50% of patients with Tourette syndrome and are present more often in boys than in girls (McMahon et al, 2002). Comorbid conditions, rather than the tics themselves, may require medical treatment.

Tics are readily diagnosed clinically. Laboratory and imaging studies are rarely indicated. On occasion, EEG may be helpful in differentiating eye flutter tics from absence seizures. Stereotypies or self-stimulation behaviors may also be confused with tic disorders.

Tics may be treated pharmacologically if they result in significant emotional distress to the child, are self-injurious or painful, or are so bothersome to others that the child requests treatment. Treatment does not usually stop tics completely. The typical waxing and waning course of tic disorders complicates treatment.

REFERENCES

Aicardi J: Malformations of the CNS. *In* Disease of the Nervous System in Childhood. London, Mac Keith Press, 1992, pp 139-181.

Alexopoulos AV, Kotagal P, Loddenkemper T, et al: Long-term results with vagus nerve stimulation in children with pharmacoresistant epilepsy. Seizure 15(7):491-503, 2006.

Arditi M, Mason EO Jr, Bradley JS, et al: Three year multicenter surveillance of pneumococcal meningitis in children: Clinical characteristics, and outcome related to penicillin susceptibility and dexamethasone use. Pediatrics 102:1087-1097, 1998.

Aurelius E, Johansson B, Skoldenberg B, et al: Rapid diagnosis of herpes simplex encephalitis by nested polymerase chain reaction assay of cerebrospinal fluid. Lancet 337:189-192, 1991.

Barth P (ed): Disorders of Neuronal Migration. London, Mac Keith Press, 2003.

Berkovic SF, Harkin L, McMahon JM, et al: De-novo mutations of the sodium channel gene SCN1A in alleged vaccine encephalopathy: A retrospective study. Lancet Neurol 5(6):488-492, 2006.

Black S, Shinefield J, Baxter R, et al: Postlicensure surveillance for pneumococcal invasive disease after use of heptavalent pneumococcal conjugate vaccine in Northern California Kaiser Permanente. Pediatr Infect Dis J 23:485-489, 2004.

Centers for Disease Control and Prevention: Diminishing racial disparities in early onset neonatal group B streptococcal disease—United States, 2000-2003. MMWR Morb Mortal Wkly Rep 53:502-505, 2004.

Chavez-Bueno S, McCracken GH Jr: Bacterial meningitis in children. Pediatr Clin North Am 52:795-810, 2005.

Fortnum HM: Hearing impairment after bacterial meningitis: A review. Arch Dis Child 67:1128-1133, 1992.

Fullerton HJ, Wu YW, Sidney S, Johnston SC: Risk of recurrent childhood arterial ischemic stroke in a population-based cohort: The importance of cerebrovascular imaging. Pediatrics 119:495-501, 2007.

Giroud M, Lemesle M, Gouyon JB, et al: Cerebrovascular disease in children under 16 years of age in the city of Dijon, France: A study of incidence and clinical features from 1985 to 1993. J Clin Epidemiol 48:1343-1348, 1995.

Grimwood K, Anderson VA, Bond L, et al: Adverse outcomes of bacterial meningitis in school age survivors. Pediatrics 95:646-656, 1995.

Harkin LA, McMahan JM, Iona X, et al: The spectrum of SCN1A-related infantile epileptic encephalopathies. Brain 130(pt 3):843-852, 2007.

Hauser WA, Annegers JF, Rocca WA: Descriptive epidemiology of epilepsy: Contributions of population-based studies form Rochester Minnesota. Mayo Clinic Proc 71:576-586, 1996.

Kaplan SI: Clinical presentations, diagnosis, and prognostic factors of bacterial meningitis. Infect Dis Clin North Am 13:579-594, 1999.

Kimberlin DW, Lin CY, Jacobs RF, et al: Natural history of neonatal herpes simplex virus infections in the acyclovir era. Pediatrics 108:223–229, 2001a.

Kimberlin DW, Lin CY, Jacobs RF, et al: Safety and efficacy of high dose intravenous acyclovir in the management of neonatal herpes simplex virus infections. Pediatrics 108:230–238, 2001b.

Kittner SJ, Adams RJ: Stroke in children and young adults. Curr Opin Neurol 9:53-56, 1996.

Koomen I, Grobbee DE, Roord JJ, et al: Hearing loss at school age in survivors of bacterial meningitis: Assessment, incidence, and prediction. Pediatrics 112:1049-1053, 2003.

Kwan P, Brodie MJ: Early identification of refractory epilepsy. N Engl J Med 342(5):314-319, 2000.

Lakeman FD, Whitley RJ: Diagnosis of herpes simplex encephalitis: Application of polymerase chain reaction to cerebrospinal fluid from brain-biopsied patients and correlation with disease. National Institute of Allergy and Infectious Diseases Collaborative Antiviral Study Group. J Infect Dis 171:857-863, 1995.

Langlois JA, Rutland-Brown W, Thomas KE: Traumatic Brain Injury in the United States: Emergency Department Visits, Hospitalizations, and Deaths. Atlanta, GA, Centers for Disease Control and Prevention, National Center for Injury Prevention and Control, 2004.

Leventer RJ, Phelan EM, Coleman LT, et al: Clinical and imaging features of cortical malformations in childhood. Neurology 53:715-722, 1999.

Lewis D, Ashwal S, Hershey A, et al: Practice parameter: Pharmacological treatment of migraine headache in children and adolescents. Neurology 63:2215-2224, 2004.

Martin M, Casellas JM, Madhi SA, et al: Impact of *Haemophilus influenzae* type b conjugate vaccine in South Africa and Argentina. Pediatr Infect Dis J 23:842-847, 2004.

McIntyre PB, Berkey CS, King SM, et al: Dexamethasone as adjunctive therapy in bacterial meningitis: A meta-analysis of randomized clinical trials since 1988. JAMA 278:925-931, 1997.

McMahon WM, Filloux FM, Ashworth JC, Jensen J: Movement disorders in children and adolescents. Neurol Clin 20:1101-1124, 2002.

Mittenberg W, Wittner MS, Miller LJ: Postconcussive syndrome occurs in children. Neuropsychology 11:447-452, 1997.

Modoni A, Silvrestri G, Pomponi MG, et al: Characterization of the pattern of cognitive impairment in myotonic dystrophy type 1. Arch Neurol 61:1943, 2004.

Nelson KB, Lynch JK: Stroke in newborn infants. Lancet Neurol 3:150-158, 2004.

Nigro G, Comi L, Politano L, Bain R: The incidence and evolution of cardiomyopathy in Duchenne muscular dystrophy. Int J Cardiol 26(3):271-277, 1990.

Nikolai J, van der Linden I, Arends JB, et al: EEG characteristics related to education impairment in children with benign childhood epilepsy with central temporal spikes. Epilepsia 48(11):2093-2100, 2007.

Practice Parameter: The neurodiagnostic evaluation of the child with a first simple febrile seizure. Pediatrics 97(5):769-772, 1996.

Primec ZR, Stare J, Neubauer D: The risk of lower mental outcome in infantile spasms increases after three weeks of hypsarythmia duration. Epilepsia 47(12):2202-2205, 2006.

Reefhuis J, Honein MA, Whitney CG, et al: Risk of bacterial meningitis in children with cochlear implants. N Engl J Med 349:435-445, 2003.

Schrag S, Gorwitz R, Fultz-Butts K, Schuchat A: Prevention of perinatal group B streptococcal disease: Revised guidelines from CDC. MMWR Morb Mortal Wkly Rep 51:1-22, 2002.

Shinnar S, Berg AT, Moshe SL, et al: Risk of seizure recurrence following a first unprovoked seizure in childhood: A prospective study. Pediatrics 85:1076-1108, 1990.

Sillanpää M: Changes in the prevalence of migraine and other headaches during the first seven school years. Headache 23:15-19, 1983.

Sillanpää M, Piekkala P, Kero P: Prevalence of headache at preschool age in an unselected child population. Cephalalgia 11:239-242, 1991.

Silva M, Licht D: Pediatric central nervous system infections and inflammatory white matter disease. Pediatr Clin North Am 52:1107-1126, 2005.

Wald ER, Kaplan SL, Mason EO Jr, et al: Dexamethasone therapy for children with bacterial meningitis. Meningitis Study Group. Pediatrics 95:21-28, 1995.

Wheless JM, Clarke DF, Carpenter D: Treatment of pediatric epilepsy: Expert opinion, 2005. J Child Neurol 20(Suppl 1):S1-S56, 2005.

24 CHROMOSOMAL DISORDERS AND FRAGILE X SYNDROME

Anne Chun-Hui Tsai, Laura Pickler,
Nicole Tartaglia, and Randi Hagerman

GENERAL FEATURES

Fifteen percent of recognized pregnancies result in a spontaneous abortion; half of those aborted fetuses are chromosomally abnormal. Six percent of stillborn infants and a similar percentage of neonatal deaths have chromosome anomalies. The fetus with a chromosome abnormality is more likely to be underdeveloped, to have malformations, or to have hydrops or demise. However, not all live-born infants are so severely affected; small or dysmorphic infants or children may also have a chromosome abnormality. Inherited chromosome problems may be suspected in couples with infertility, recurrent spontaneous abortions, and stillborn or live-born dysmorphic infants. When the diagnosis of a chromosome abnormality is made prenatally, the outcome may be difficult to predict because most available clinical findings come from observation of children diagnosed as a result of problems after birth. Chromosomal studies are indicated when there is clinical suspicion of an underlying genetic explanation for a child's physical or developmental problems. Table 24-1 summarizes specific findings that should prompt this type of evaluation.

CHROMOSOME PREPARATION AND MOLECULAR CYTOGENETICS

Karyotype

Chromosome structure is visible only during mitosis, most often achieved in the laboratory by stimulation of a blood lymphocyte culture with a mitogen for 3 days. Other tissues used for this purpose include skin, products of conception, cartilage, and bone marrow. Chorionic villi or amniocytes are used for prenatal diagnosis. Spontaneously dividing cells without a mitogen are present in bone marrow, and historically, bone marrow biopsy was done when immediate identification of a patient's chromosome constitution was necessary for appropriate management (e.g., to rule out trisomy 13 in a newborn with a complex congenital heart disease). However, this invasive test has been replaced by the fluorescent in situ hybridization (FISH) technique (see later discussion).

Cells processed for routine chromosome analysis are stained on glass slides to yield a light-and-dark band pattern across the arms of the chromosomes. This band pattern is characteristic and reproducible for each chromosome. With use of different staining techniques, different banding patterns result: G, Q, and R banding. The most commonly used is G banding. The layout of chromosomes on a sheet of paper in a predetermined order is called a karyotype. High-resolution chromosome analysis is the study of more elongated chromosomes in prometaphase. In such an analysis, the bands can be visualized in greater detail, allowing detection of smaller, more subtle chromosome rearrangements.

Fluorescent In Situ Hybridization

FISH is a powerful technique that labels a known chromosome sequence with DNA probes attached to fluorescent dyes, thus enabling visualization of specific regions of chromosomes by fluorescent microscopy. There are many different kinds of probes, including paint probes (a mixture of sequences throughout one chromosome), sequence-specific probes, centromere probes, and telomere probes. A cocktail of differently colored probes, one color for each chromosome, called multicolor FISH, or M-FISH, can detect complex rearrangements between chromosomes. FISH can detect submicroscopic structural rearrangements undetectable by classic cytogenetic techniques and can identify marker chromosomes. For pictures of FISH studies, see *www.kumc.edu/gec/prof/cytogene.html*. FISH also allows interphase cells (lymphocytes, amniocytes) to be screened for numerical abnormalities, such as trisomy 13, trisomy 18, or trisomy 21, and sex chromosome anomalies. However, because of the possible background or contamination of the signal, the abnormality must be confirmed by conventional chromosome analysis.

Comparative Genomic Hybridization and Microarray Chip

Comparative genomic hybridization (CGH) is a molecular cytogenetic method of screening for genetic changes. The alterations are classified as DNA gains and losses and reveal a characteristic pattern that includes changes at chromosomal and subchromosomal levels. Its usefulness has been well documented in cancer and more

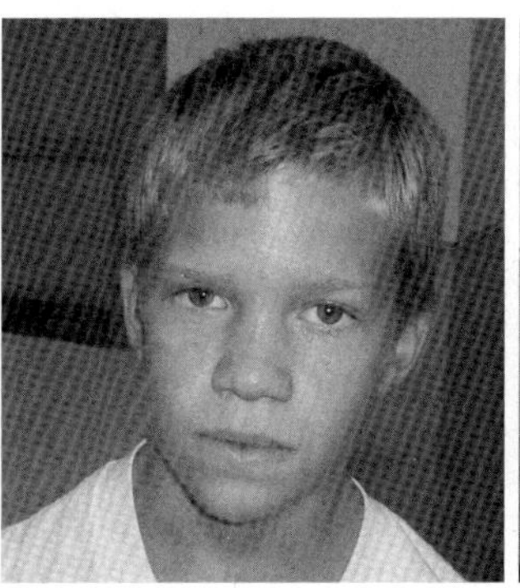
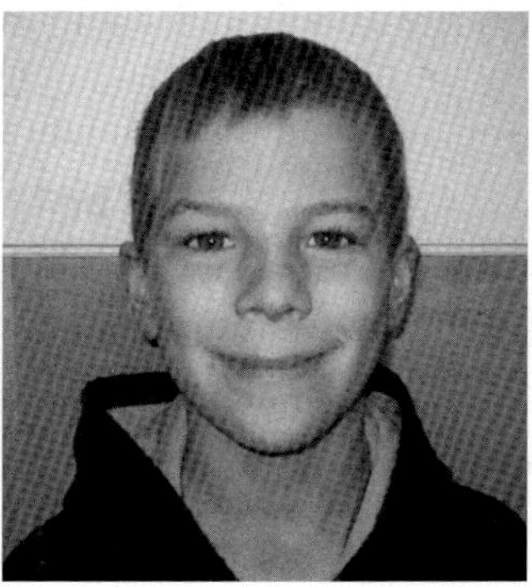
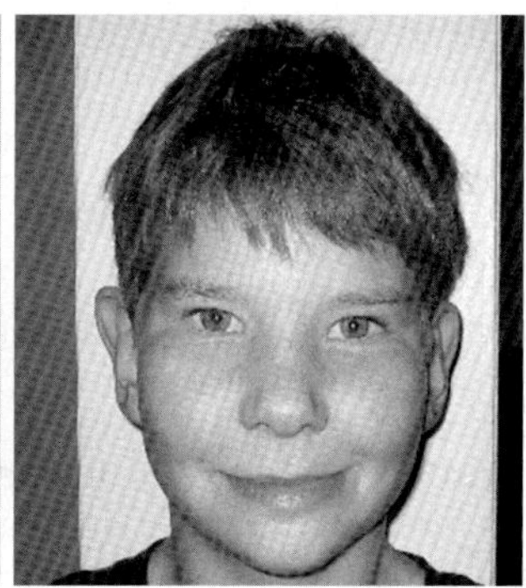

Figure 24-1. Clinical photographs of children with sex chromosomal anomalies, XXY, XYY, and XXYY syndromes.

Table 24-1. **Indications for Chromosomal Studies**
Multiple minor dysmorphic features
Major structural malformations
Increased incidence of medical problems
Microcephaly
Unexplained intellectual disability
Unexplained developmental delay
Hypotonia and severe joint laxity
Growth delay or failure to thrive
Tall or short stature
Delayed puberty or hypoplastic gonads
Multiple miscarriages

recently in detecting small chromosomal rearrangements. In the past, resolution was only around 3 to 10 Mb, not very helpful for small rearrangements. Chip technology has allowed the application of CGH on microarray technique. This technique is able to detect very small genetic imbalances anywhere in the genome. In particular, it has been used to detect interstitial and subtelomeric submicroscopic imbalances, to characterize their size at the molecular level, or to define the breakpoints of translocation. Several clinically available chip assays have been widely applied in clinical diagnosis; however, these chips are limited to all conditions that can be ascertained by FISH. Genome-wide array is the subject of current research. Results of microarray should be interpreted with caution because this technology may pick up polymorphisms that have not been previously identified.

Vignette

M. C. is a 10-year-old girl with dysmorphic features including prominent forehead, deep-set eyes, large mouth, wide-spaced teeth, digital anomalies, hypotonia, and intellectual disability (IQ of 45). Past history is significant for atrial septal defect and ventricular septal defect repair, seizure disorder, and sleep disturbance as well as self-mutilating behaviors. Family history is significant for two maternal spontaneous abortions. The differential diagnosis includes chromosomal rearrangements, telomeric rearrangements, Smith-Magenis syndrome, and 1p36 deletion. A microarray chip analysis was performed that confirmed 1p36 miscorrelations.

Chromosome Breakage Studies

Assessment of chromosome breaks and sister chromatid exchanges requires special techniques that lead to enhancement of the breaks or special staining that allows visualization of the exchanged chromatid. Two disorders are excluded by this process: Fanconi pancytopenia syndrome and Bloom syndrome. Fanconi pancytopenia syndrome is characterized by radial ray deficiencies, growth retardation, and hematologic abnormalities. Bloom syndrome is characterized by short stature, failure to thrive, and malar telangiectasias.

CHROMOSOME NOMENCLATURE

Visible under the microscope is a constriction site on the chromosome called the centromere, which separates the chromosome into two arms: p, for petite, refers to the short arm; and q, the letter following p, refers to the long arm. Each arm is further subdivided into numbered bands visible by use of different staining techniques. Centromeres are positioned at different sites on different chromosomes and are used to differentiate the chromosome structures seen during mitosis as metacentric (p arm and q arm of almost equal size), submetacentric (p arm shorter than q arm), and acrocentric (almost no p arm). The use of named chromosome arms and bands provides a universal method of chromosome description. Common symbols include del (deletion), dup (duplication), inv (inversion), ish (in situ hybridization), i (isochromosome), pat (paternal origin), mat (maternal origin), and r (ring chromosome). See the next section for definitions of these terms.

CHROMOSOME ANOMALIES

Chromosome anomalies may be numerical or structural.

Numerical anomalies can result in either aneuploidy or polyploidy. Aneuploidy is loss or gain of one or, rarely, two chromosomes, exemplified by trisomy 21 or monosomy X. Polyploidy is the addition of a complete haploid, as in 69,XXX, or 69,XYY.

Structural anomalies are rearrangements of genetic material within or between chromosomes. These may be either genetically balanced, in which there is no change in the amount of essential genetic material and the phenotype is normal, or unbalanced, with a gain or loss of essential chromosome segments. Examples include microdeletions (for further discussion, see Chapter 26);

duplication of critical regions, such as 15q11-13; and translocations or inversions.

Numerical Anomalies

Trisomy

Trisomy is the presence of three copies of a chromosome rather than the normal two copies. Trisomies for each of the autosomes except chromosome 1 have been recorded. Most trisomic embryos are lost in early pregnancy. Trisomy is the most common finding in chromosomally abnormal embryos studied after a spontaneous abortion. With rare exceptions, only autosomal trisomies 13, 18, and 21 survive to term and are seen in the population. Trisomy for sex chromosomes, such as XXX or XXY, has fewer deleterious effects on development; most of these trisomies result in term live births. The pathogenesis of trisomy is generally thought to be an error of nondisjunction. Nondisjunction is a failure of segregation of chromosomes or chromatids at cell division, which can occur during meiosis or mitosis.

Trisomy 21

Refer to Chapter 25.

Trisomy 13

The newborn incidence is approximately 1 in 5000. Most trisomy 13 fetuses spontaneously abort in the first trimester. During the second trimester, abnormalities observed on ultrasound examination include growth retardation, congenital heart lesions, midline brain and facial lesions (e.g., holoprosencephaly), and omphalocele. Newborns with trisomy 13 also have midline abnormalities (i.e., scalp cutis aplasia, brain malformations, central or unilateral facial clefts), omphalocele, and polydactyly. Almost all affected newborns have lethal cardiac anomalies. Intellectual disability in survivors is profound.

Trisomy 18

The newborn incidence is approximately 1 in 3500. Most trisomy 18 pregnancies result in spontaneous abortions or stillbirths. Abnormalities such as severe intrauterine growth retardation, congenital heart lesions, and diaphragmatic hernia are frequently detected by ultrasound examination. The newborn with trisomy 18 has a small facies with prominent occiput, small ears, overlapping fingers, and rocker-bottom heels. Almost all of these newborns have cardiac as well as other internal malformations. Newborns are more likely to be female, and they are profoundly handicapped.

Most pediatricians agree with withdrawal of life support in infants with trisomy 18 and trisomy 13. However, a small portion of parents choose to continue aggressive treatment for their children with such conditions. A support group resource, Support Organization for Trisomy 18, 13, and Related Disorders (SOFT), exists for parents and is available at *http://www.trisomy.org*.

47,XXY (Klinefelter Syndrome)

The prevalence of 47,XXY is 1 in 700 male births. There is a very large spectrum of involvement; some individuals are significantly affected by the developmental and medical features of XXY syndrome, whereas others are minimally affected. The typical clinical presentation varies with age. Approximately 5% of males diagnosed with XXY are identified by prenatal amniocentesis because XXY is associated with advanced maternal age. Another 10% are diagnosed in infancy or childhood because of speech and language delays, mild hypotonia, motor delays, academic problems, or behavioral problems. An additional 10% are diagnosed in adolescence and young adulthood by physical features (i.e., tall stature, micro-orchidism) and pubertal delays or incomplete puberty caused by testosterone deficiency, and 5% are identified during evaluation for infertility or for symptoms of hypogonadism that develop later in adult life. Studies estimate that the remaining 70% of individuals with XXY remain undiagnosed through their lifespan.

Facial features are not typically dysmorphic in XXY males (Fig. 24-1). Mild hypotonia, fifth digit clinodactyly, genu valgum, and pes planus can be present in childhood. Tall stature due to increased lower segment length begins before puberty and continues into adolescence. Adolescent and adult men may have narrowed shoulders, eunuchoid body habitus, gynecomastia (30% to 50%), and decreased muscle bulk. Progressive fibrosis of the seminiferous tubules of the testes leads to micro-orchidism and inadequate testosterone production at puberty and in adulthood, requiring testosterone supplementation. Infertility is almost universal in nonmosaic cases, although the success rate of reproductive technologies such as intracytoplasmic sperm injection in adult men with XXY is rapidly increasing. Affected adult men also have increased risks for breast cancer, osteoporosis, diabetes, hypothyroidism, and autoimmune diseases.

Early delays can be present in speech or motor development; thus, close developmental monitoring with implementation of early intervention with speech, physical, and occupational therapy is recommended when delays are identified. Expressive language is often more affected than receptive language, and prospective studies show that up to 75% of XXY children have language-based learning disabilities and reading disorders. Overall cognitive abilities are generally in the average range, although there is as extreme variability in IQ scores as seen in the general population. Prospective studies show that full-scale IQs are approximately 10 points less than those of sibling controls, often with performance IQ significantly higher than verbal IQ. A psychoeducational assessment including speech-language evaluation should be obtained in school-age children with XXY to evaluate for learning disabilities and reading disorders. Fine motor and gross motor coordination deficits and graphomotor problems are also common and benefit from occupational therapy interventions and assistive technology in the classroom.

Behavioral and emotional symptoms are not universal in XXY but can include anxiety symptoms, attention deficits (35% with attention-deficit/hyperactivity disorder [ADHD]), sensory processing problems, social withdrawal, and social immaturity relative to peers. ADHD, anxiety, and other behavioral symptoms should be assessed and treated with behavioral and psychopharmacologic interventions as indicated. In children with

XXY and social difficulties, language evaluation including pragmatic language assessment should be completed because deficits are common despite cognitive skills in the normal range. Social skills groups and other interventions for social development are also recommended. Occupational therapy strategies to improve sensory processing problems and self-regulation are also recommended as indicated. Parents should be provided with information for national support organizations, including Klinefelter Syndrome and Associates *(www.genetic.org)* and the American Association for Klinefelter Syndrome Information & Support *(www.AAKSIS.org)*.

47,XYY

The prevalence of 47,XYY is 1 per 1000 male births, although studies estimate that up to 90% of XYY males are undiagnosed. Although initially publicized as such, the diagnosis of 47,XYY is not associated with increased aggressive or criminal behaviors. Children with XYY syndrome may be diagnosed incidentally by prenatal diagnosis, or they may be identified postnatally when genetic testing is ordered for developmental delays or behavioral difficulties. The additional Y chromosome is paternally inherited; thus, there is no association with advanced maternal age. Males with 47,XYY are not dysmorphic, and the most consistent clinical feature is tall stature, with most at the 75th percentile or above. Musculoskeletal manifestations can commonly include long fingers and pes planus. Motor tics and essential tremor have been described in XYY males as well. Pubertal development and testosterone production are normal in XYY syndrome, and fertility is generally unimpaired.

Prospective studies of XYY children identified by newborn screening studies show cognitive scores within the typical range, with a slightly increased risk for language-based learning disabilities. Motor coordination deficits and graphomotor problems can also be more common. Studies that compare outcomes in prenatally versus postnatally diagnosed cases show significantly more neurodevelopmental problems in postnatally diagnosed cases, including increased developmental delays, learning disabilities, ADHD, and pervasive developmental disorder. Prenatally diagnosed cases should be monitored closely because of their risk for developmental delays, with formal developmental assessments starting at 6 to 12 months of age and prompt initiation of early intervention services when indicated. For postnatally diagnosed cases, a full developmental or psychoeducational assessment including speech-language and motor skills evaluation will guide treatment planning. XYY children can have behavioral manifestations of ADHD, including hyperactivity and impulsivity, as well as mood instability and anxiety. Assessment and treatment of ADHD and other emotional and behavioral symptoms with behavioral interventions and psychopharmacologic agents are recommended when indicated. Approximately 10% of children diagnosed with XYY have autism spectrum disorders; thus, XYY children with social deficits should be formally evaluated for autism spectrum disorders because this diagnosis has an impact on treatment and educational recommendations. Parents should also be referred to the XYY support section of Klinefelter Syndrome and Associates at *www.genetic.org*.

47,XXX

The prevalence of 47,XXX (also known as triple X, trisomy X) is 1 in 800 females. As with XYY syndrome, it is estimated that only 10% of females with XXX are identified during their lifetime. A small percentage of girls with trisomy X are diagnosed prenatally because trisomy X is associated with advanced maternal age. Postnatally diagnosed cases are most often identified by hypotonia or motor delays or speech delays in the first few years of life. The majority of 47,XXX females have no obvious physical features, although tall stature and epicanthal folds can be present. A small number may present with radioulnar synostosis, renal abnormalities, oligomenorrhea, and premature ovarian failure. Puberty and fertility are considered to be unaffected.

Prospective studies of newborns identified with trisomy X showed an increased risk for both motor and speech delays as well as later risk for language-based learning disabilities. Expressive language is typically more impaired than receptive language. Cognitive abilities are generally within the typical range, although significant learning disabilities can be present. The behavioral phenotype can include a socially inhibited temperament, although in some cases social, performance, and separation anxiety can significantly affect social and academic functioning and warrants further psychological and pharmacologic interventions. Because of the presence of attention deficits without significant hyperactivity symptoms in approximately 20% of school-age girls with trisomy X, evaluation for ADHD is recommended with standard behavioral and medication treatments. Ongoing assessment for and treatment of anxiety and other mood disorders should be continued through adolescence. Parents should be referred to support organizations, including Klinefelter Syndrome and Associates *(www.genetic.org)* and Triplo-X Syndrome *(www.triplo-X.org)*.

Monosomy

Monosomy is the presence of only one member of a chromosome pair in a karyotype. It is generally more detrimental to embryonic and fetal development than is the equivalent trisomy. Monosomy may result from nondisjunction or chromosome lag. A chromosome may lag at anaphase and be excluded from the new nucleus. In males, lag of the Y chromosome at meiosis is thought to be a common cause of X chromosome monosomy (i.e., Turner syndrome).

Turner Syndrome (45,X)

Among live-born females, 1 in 2500 has Turner syndrome. The majority of 45,X fetuses present as growth-disorganized embryos that spontaneously abort during the first trimester of pregnancy 99% of the time. These monosomies represent about 10% of early spontaneous abortions. Some 45,X fetuses are detected on ultrasound examination in the second trimester. The fetus has a cystic hygroma or a more generalized fluid collection (e.g., hydrops fetalis). Additional findings include preductal coarctation and horseshoe kidney. The majority of these fetuses are stillborn. Infants with Turner syndrome may be normal, or they may have features such as residual neck webbing from the cystic hygroma, shield chest, coarctation, and edema of the hands and feet.

The presenting features during childhood are short stature and a cardiac murmur. Treatment with growth hormone, estrogens, and androgens supervised by a pediatric endocrinologist may enable many girls with Turner syndrome to achieve normal adult heights and to develop secondary sexual characteristics. Teenagers present with primary or secondary amenorrhea or lack of secondary sex characteristics because of streak ovaries. The majority are infertile. Turner syndrome females are mentally normal but may have spatial-perceptual abnormalities that may lead to academic performance difficulties. Social relationships may be difficult during the school-age years through adulthood. Nonverbal learning disorders, psychomotor problems, and poor manual dexterity have also been described in these girls. ADHD is common enough that evaluation with standard behavioral and medication treatments is recommended. Families and educators should have normal academic expectations for girls with Turner syndrome, and prompt intervention should be initiated when a problem is suspected.

Cardiovascular disease, hyperlipidemia, hyperuricemia, type 2 diabetes, and obesity also commonly occur. Other medical problems that should be noted are development of hypertension, scoliosis, and the relatively common hearing and vision problems. Regular screening for hearing and vision problems should occur throughout life. Between 10% and 30% of women with Turner syndrome will develop hypothyroidism. Screening every year or two is prudent. An active support group is available online at *www.turnersyndrome.org*.

Many females with the Turner phenotype may have karyotypes other than 45,X. The Turner syndrome phenotype may be the result of lack of the second intact sex chromosome. Examples include X chromosome mosaicism, Xq isochromosome, and Xp deletion. However, the karyotype in spontaneously aborted fetuses and those with fetal hydrops is likely to be 45,X.

Polyploidy

Polyploidy is the state in which the chromosome count is double or triple that of a normal pregnancy. Most of these pregnancies abort by 20 weeks, making them unlikely to be seen as a live birth and subsequently ascertained by a developmental pediatrician.

Structural Anomalies

Many different types of structural chromosome anomalies exist. In clinical context, the plus sign or minus sign preceding the chromosome number indicates increased or decreased number, respectively, of that particular whole chromosome in a cell. For example, 47,XY+21 designates a male with three copies of chromosome 21. The plus sign or minus sign after the chromosome number signifies extra material or missing material, respectively, on one of the arms of the chromosome. For example, 46,XX,8q− denotes a deletion on the long arm of chromosome 8. Detailed nomenclature, such as 8q11, is required to further demonstrate a specific missing region so that genetic counseling can be provided. The following definitions illustrate use of common nomenclature. For details of current and past nomenclature convention, the reader is directed to the International System for Human Cytogenetic Nomenclature text revised in 2005. See Figure 24-2 for illustrative purposes.

Deletion (del). This refers to an absence of normal chromosomal material. It may be terminal (at the end of a chromosome) or interstitial (within a chromosome). The missing part is described by the code del, followed by the number of the chromosome involved, in parentheses, and a description of the missing region of that chromosome, also in parentheses; for

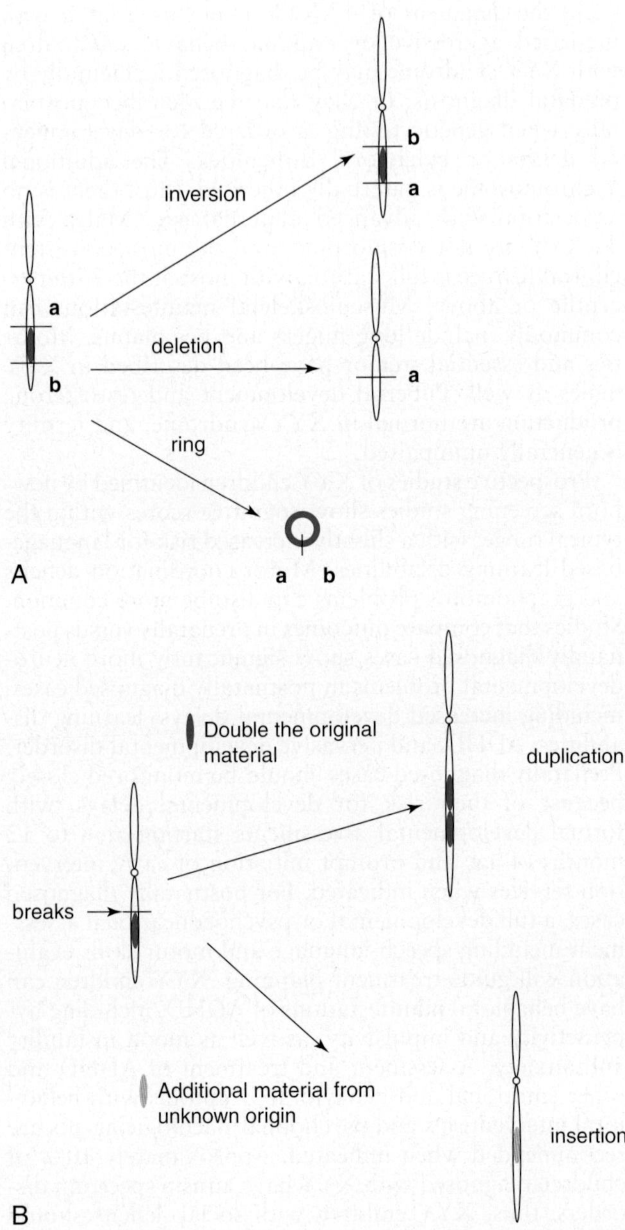

Figure 24-2. Examples of structural chromosome abnormalities: inversion, deletion, and ring (A); duplication and insertion (B).

Continued

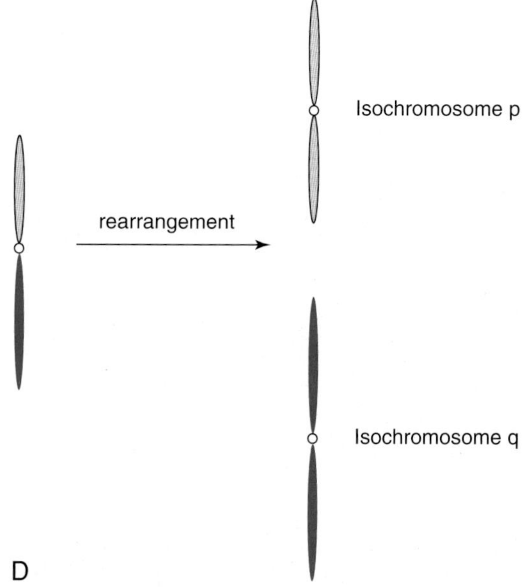

Figure 24-2. cont'd translocation (C); and isochromosome (D).

example, 46,XX,del(1)(p36.3). This chromosome nomenclature describes the loss of genetic material from band 36.3 of the short arm of chromosome 1, which results in 1p36.3 deletion syndrome. Several common deletions result in clinically recognizable conditions associated with cognitive disabilities and characteristic facial features. For example, Wolf-Hirschhorn syndrome, del(4p), results in an unusual face with "Greek helmet" appearance; cri-du-chat syndrome, del(5p), is typified by an unusual high-pitched cry and dysmorphic features.

Duplication (dup). An extra copy of a chromosomal segment can be tandem (genetic material present in the original direction) or inverted (genetic material present in the opposite direction). A well-described duplication of chromosome 22q11 causes cat-eye syndrome, resulting in iris coloboma and anal or ear anomalies.

Inversion (inv). In this aberration, a rearranged section of a chromosome is inverted. It can be paracentric (not involving the centromere) or pericentric (involving the centromere). The phenotype is usually normal. Inversion carriers may have offspring with subsequent anomalies, such as those seen in San Luis Valley syndrome, also known as recombinant 8 syndrome.

Ring chromosome (r). Deletion of the normal telomeres (and possibly of other subtelomeric sequences) leads to subsequent fusion of both ends to form a circular chromosome. Ring chromosome anomalies often cause growth retardation and cognitive disabilities.

Translocation (trans). This describes the interchromosomal rearrangement of genetic material. Translocations may be balanced (the cell has a normal content of genetic material arranged in a structurally abnormal way) or unbalanced (the cell has gained or lost genetic material as a result of chromosomal interchange). Balanced translocations may further be described as reciprocal, the exchange of genetic material between two nonhomologous chromosomes, or Robertsonian, the fusion of two acrocentric chromosomes.

Insertion (ins). Breakage within a chromosome at two points and incorporation of another piece of chromosomal material is called insertion. This requires three breakpoints and may occur between two chromosomes or within the same chromosome. The clinical presentation or phenotype depends on the origin of the inserted materials.

Isochromosome (i). One of the chromosome arms, either p or q, is duplicated and all the material from the counterpart arm is lost. This results in a mirror-image p or q arm on both sides of the centromere. Examples include maternal i(15q), which leads to Prader-Willi syndrome, and i(Xq), which causes Turner syndrome.

Mosaicism

Simply defined, mosaicism refers to the presence of two or more cell lines of different genetic or chromosomal material within one individual. Whether mosaicism is clinically relevant is dependent on the tissue involved and the percentage of abnormal genetic material present in that tissue. Mosaicism can occur in both structural and numerical chromosomal rearrangements. As a general rule, an individual with an aneuploid line in only some tissues is likely to have a phenotype less severe than but qualitatively similar to that of someone with the nonmosaic aneuploidy. Asymmetry in body distribution may result in hypoplasia or hyperplasia of the affected tissues. Mosaicism that excludes the bone marrow may give a normal karyotype in the blood. If there is a high suspicion of mosaicism based on clinical findings, a skin biopsy with use of cultured skin fibroblasts may be necessary to ascertain the abnormal karyotype. If the skin is similarly not affected, tissue sampling of other tissues may be necessary to make the diagnosis.

Mosaicism can be discussed in the context of somatic abnormalities as well as germline mosaicism, placental mosaicism, and amniotic fluid cell mosaicism. In isolated germline mosaicism, the abnormal cell lines are confined to the germ cells (egg or sperm). In this case, it is possible for mosaicism to be transmitted to offspring. In conditions in which fertility is known to be affected, germline mosaicism may result in unexpected fertility, such as in Turner syndrome or Klinefelter syndrome. Placental mosaicism and amniotic fluid cell mosaicism typically become important in prenatal diagnosis situations and may not reflect a true constitutional mosaicism of the embryo and thus should be interpreted with caution.

A mosaic state may originate in either meiosis or mitosis, which are substantially chromosome specific (not all chromosomal abnormalities have the same mechanism of origin). The zygote may have been normal or trisomic initially, followed by a postzygotic event that results either in initiation of an abnormal cell line or in "rescue" of an otherwise trisomic fetus. This is illustrated in Figure 24-3A.

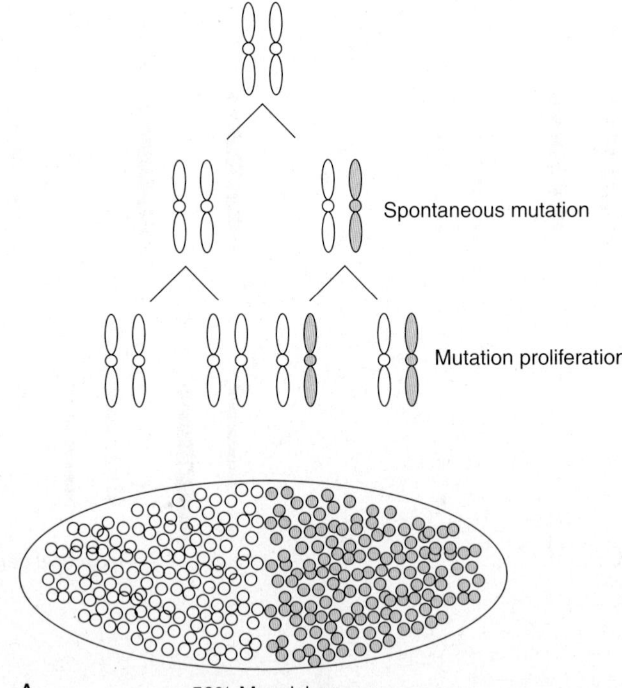

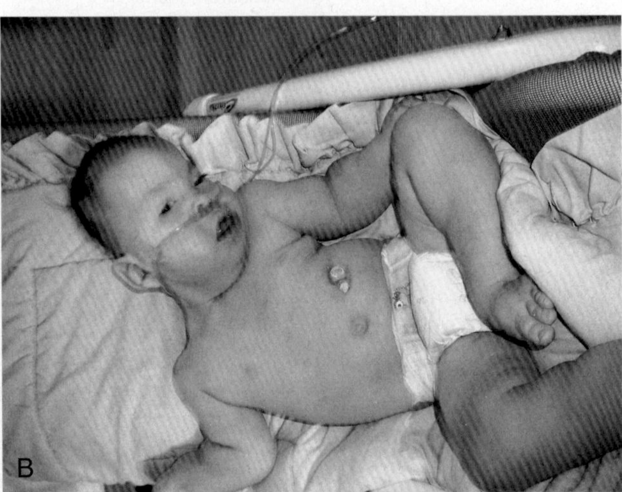

Figure 24-3. A, Mechanism of mosaic chromosomal anomalies. B, Photograph of a child with Pallister-Killian syndrome, a clinical example of mosaicism.

Trisomies 21, 13, and 18 and Turner syndrome are discussed earlier. The mosaic state of any of these conditions would generally be expected to be less severe than the full aneuploid syndrome but could range in spectrum from mild to severely affected, depending on the tissues involved. Conservative management of individuals with mosaic trisomy is the same as established medical management of the full syndrome but should be tailored to the individual. As noted before, girls with mosaic Turner syndrome may unexpectedly be fertile and should be counseled accordingly.

Mosaic trisomy 8 is much more commonly seen than a full trisomy 8 syndrome because of the early lethality of the

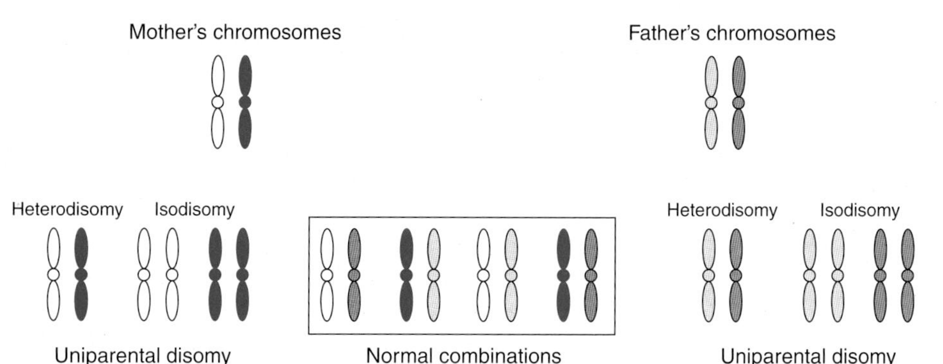

Figure 24-4. Uniparental disomy.

full trisomy 8 syndrome. Patients are dysmorphic in appearance and tend to have poor coordination. The degree of mental deficiency is variable from normal to moderate intellectual disability. Motor delays may occur. Other organ systems that may be involved include cardiac, ureteral-renal, musculoskeletal, and hematologic. On occasion, conductive deafness may occur, and auditory acuity should be suspected in patients with language delay.

Pallister-Killian syndrome (also known as Pallister mosaic syndrome, tetrasomy 12p, and Killian-Teschler-Nicola syndrome; Fig. 24-3B) is caused by true mosaicism for a small supernumerary marker chromosome 12p. In most cases, the isochromosome 12p is detected preferentially in skin fibroblasts and not in peripheral blood. This syndrome is characterized phenotypically by postnatal growth deceleration, profound intellectual disability with seizures developing in infancy, and poor speech development. Facies are dysmorphic with sparse anterior scalp hair particularly in the temporal areas during infancy, which resolves as the child ages. Streaks of hyperpigmentation or hypopigmentation of the skin may be present. Hearing and vision may be compromised and should be screened in affected individuals.

Hypermelanosis of Ito encompasses a heterogeneous group of disorders characterized by hypopigmented whorls and streaks following Blaschko's lines with associated intellectual disability, seizures, or asymmetry in other organs. According to Taibjee and colleagues (2004), only 30% to 60% of patients diagnosed clinically had a demonstrable cytogenetic abnormality. However, of those in whom an abnormality was found, 95% were either mosaic or chimeric. The exact mechanism to explain abnormal pigmentation in pigmentary mosaicism is currently unknown. A number of hypotheses have been made. Research in this area is active and ongoing.

Uniparental Disomy

Uniparental disomy (UPD) describes the situation whereby both chromosomes (or chromosomal segments) are inherited from the same parent (Fig. 24-4). The chromosomes may be identical (called isodisomy) or different (called heterodisomy). Although UPD for nearly every chromosome has been described, there are currently several more common genetic conditions associated with UPD. These include Prader-Willi syndrome (UPD 15, maternal in origin), Angelman syndrome (UPD 15, paternal in origin), Beckwith-Wiedemann syndrome (UPD 11, paternal in origin), and Russell-Silver syndrome (UPD 7, maternal in origin). These syndromes are discussed in the context of this book because of their significance for the developmental pediatrician.

Of note, Prader-Willi, Angelman, and Beckwith-Wiedemann syndromes all have other well-described alternative genetic mechanisms that result in disease, not just UPD alone. If the disease mechanism is due to UPD, the routine karyotype will be normal 46,XX or 46,XY. Typically, molecular studies are required to demonstrate UPD and must be compared with parental DNA markers. It is not enough to have normal chromosomes in structure and number; for some key genes, normal development cannot proceed without contribution from both parents.

There are four hypothetical mechanisms whereby complete UPD may occur. Errors in both meiosis and mitosis may give this result. Two separate abnormal events are required in each case to produce viable offspring. The original abnormality is usually a sporadic event, and recurrence risk for the same parents to have another child with the same error is minimal (given normal parental karyotypes). Increasing maternal age may contribute to risk because of the prevalence of meiotic errors in women of older childbearing age.

Prader-Willi and Angelman syndromes are discussed in detail in Chapter 26. Both syndromes are the result of nonfunctioning or absent genes in the PW/AS critical region on chromosome 15q11-13. Prader-Willi syndrome is due to the absence of a paternal contribution to this area. Angelman syndrome is due to absence of a maternal contribution to the same region affecting the *UBE3A* gene. The specific gene responsible for Prader-Willi syndrome has not been definitively identified at this time. Screening for either syndrome is accomplished by DNA-based methylation studies, which should be routinely used to confirm the diagnosis even in the presence of highly suggestive clinical features.

Beckwith-Wiedemann syndrome is caused by paternal UPD 11p15 approximately 20% of the time. Cardinal features of this syndrome include macroglossia, prenatal or postnatal overgrowth, and abdominal wall defects. Neonatal hypoglycemia also may be a striking early feature and is thought to contribute to subsequent developmental delay if it is poorly controlled. Most patients are cognitively normal, barring chromosomal duplication, complications of prematurity, or environmental insult such as hypoglycemia. Disruption of regulatory genes at two distinct loci (known as domains 1 and 2) is thought to cause this disorder. UPD 11p15 is highly correlated with hemihyperplasia. A subset of patients with UPD also have alterations of H19, a tumor suppressor gene. This subset of patients is at highest risk for the preferential development of Wilms and other intra-abdominal tumors. Tumor surveillance includes quarterly abdominal ultrasound examinations until 7 years of age and serum alpha-fetoprotein measurements. Inheritance is sporadic if the causal mechanism is UPD. Other genetic mechanisms producing the Beckwith-Wiedemann phenotype include methylation errors in domains 1 and 2, duplication of 11p15, *CDKN1C* gene mutations, and translocation or inversion of 11p15. Recurrence risk varies by genetic mechanism of disease.

Russell-Silver syndrome is in actuality a heterogeneous group of disorders. Approximately 10% of children with the clinical diagnosis of Russell-Silver syndrome will have a demonstrable UPD 7 defect. These cases tend to be more "classic" in their presentation, with prenatal onset of small stature, characteristic triangular facial features, clinodactyly of the fifth fingers, café au lait spots, and skeletal asymmetry. Recurrent nocturnal hypoglycemia may be seen and has been hypothesized to contribute to school difficulty. Cognition is not thought to be abnormal. Learning disabilities and attention deficit disorder appear to be increased in incidence in Russell-Silver syndrome. Autism and similar disorders like pervasive developmental disorder may also be increased. It is unclear whether these problems just appear to be increased in Russell-Silver syndrome, are innate to Russell-Silver syndrome, or are acquired through early malnutrition and hypoglycemia, both of which are preventable. In infancy and childhood, gross motor and speech delays necessitate evaluation and appropriate therapies. Key management issues with these cases involve treatment of small stature with growth hormone. In instances in which growth hormone deficiency cannot be clearly documented and growth velocity is normal, treatment with growth hormone is controversial.

Other Anomalies

Marker Chromosomes

Marker chromosomes are extra chromosomal pieces found during karyotyping that are usually derived from a structural rearrangement. They may be in the form of a ring or biosatellite chromosomes with or without centromeres. With a centromere, the structure is relatively stable; without centromeres, the marker chromosomes tend to be smaller, may exhibit mitotic instability, and may have mosaic form. Various amounts of heterochromatin or euchromatin may be present. Many markers are compatible with normal development and normal intelligence and may be inherited with no phenotypic consequence. Others, such as inverted-duplication chromosome 15 markers, can have associated phenotypic abnormalities. Identification of the marker can be achieved by FISH or microarray chip assay.

Chromosome Breakage

Chromosome breaks present as random visible lesions in metaphase chromosomes. They can lead to subsequent structural changes such as deletion and translocation.

> **Vignette**
>
> A mother brings her 2-day-old daughter to your clinic because of coloboma of iris, preauricular pits, and congenital heart defect. The mother was also noted to have preauricular pits but was physically and intellectually normal. Physical examination of the child revealed micrognathia, low-set ears, hypertelorism, down-slanting palpebral fissures, and anal stenosis. Ophthalmologic evaluation showed coloboma of choroids and retina. A karyotype of the child revealed a marker chromosome of 22 origin: supernumerary inv dup (22)(q11) chromosome. Subsequent karyotyping of the mother revealed a mosaic marker.

Minimal numbers of breaks can be identified in normal individuals; however, individuals with the group of disorders named chromosome breakage syndromes have increased breaks that are inducible by chemicals and environmental insults. Examples include Fanconi pancytopenia syndrome (covered in Chapter 26), Bloom syndrome, and ataxia-telangiectasia. Bloom syndrome is characterized by short stature, failure to thrive, and malar telangiectasia. Diagnosis can be made by observing sister chromatid changes. Ataxia-telangiectasia is characterized by progressive ataxia and telangiectasia involving eyes, conjunctiva, and other facial areas. There is a higher association of infections and malignant neoplasia. Increased breakage under normal chromosome culture can be seen, and random structural anomalies can sometimes be identified. Molecular analysis is available for these three conditions. However, because of the genetic heterogeneity, a breakage study is usually performed to further confirm the disease before specific DNA testing is offered.

Chromosome Fragile Sites

Chromosome fragile sites are gaps, and breaks can be visualized with or without modification of culture conditions. There are more than 100 fragile sites reported. The best known is a folate-sensitive fragile site at Xq27.3 that leads to fragile X syndrome (FXS), the most common inherited cause of intellectual disability and the most common single-gene mutation associated with autism. Although the name is derived from the fragile site seen on the X when cells are grown in folate-deficient media for cytogenetic analysis, the diagnosis is made today with DNA testing that reveals the trinucleotide repeat (CGG) on the 5′ untranslated portion of the fragile X mental retardation 1 gene (*FMR1*). There are normally between 5 and 44 CGG repeats in the *FMR1* gene. The protein produced from this gene, FMRP, is a regulator of translation for many other messages important for synaptic maturation and plasticity. The premutation (55 to 200 CGG repeats) is common in the general population (1 in 130 to 250 females and 1 in 800 males) and is unstable such that a female premutation carrier can pass the full mutation (>200 repeats) to her offspring, although a male premutation carrier will pass on only the premutation to all of his daughters because the sperm can only carry the premutation. The full mutation is usually methylated, so there is little or no messenger RNA (mRNA) produced from this gene and therefore little or no FMRP. It is the absence or deficiency of FMRP that causes FXS. The level of FMRP deficit correlates with IQ, such that the more FMRP present, the higher the IQ.

Although most males with FXS are intellectually disabled, approximately 15% are not and instead present with ADHD and learning disabilities. Females with FXS are usually not intellectually disabled but may present with learning disabilities, attention problems, or full ADHD in addition to having shyness and social anxiety. Math is always the most significant learning problem academically, but language deficits and visual-motor coordination problems are also common. Perseverative speech is almost universal in children with FXS, although approximately 10% are nonverbal, and selective mutism is common in the females with FXS. Approximately 30% of boys with FXS have full autism; an additional 20% meet criteria for pervasive developmental disorder not otherwise specified. Even those without autism will often have poor eye contact, hand mannerisms such as hand flapping or hand biting, and repetitive speech. All children with autism or autism spectrum disorders or intellectual disability should have fragile X DNA testing to rule out a mutation in *FMR1*; approximately 2% to 6% of children who present with autism have a fragile X mutation.

The physical features of FXS include large or prominent ears, hyperextensible finger joints, and large testicles or macro-orchidism beginning in early puberty. However, 30% of children with FXS do not have obvious physical features, so DNA testing should not be dependent on these features and is indicated in any child with developmental delay of unknown etiology. It is important to make the diagnosis as early as possible so that intervention, including speech and language therapy, occupational therapy, and special education support, can be started and appropriate genetic counseling can be given to the whole family.

Many children with FXS do well with stimulant medication for their ADHD; selective serotonin reuptake inhibitors for their anxiety; and atypical antipsychotics (such as aripiprazole) for their autism, mood instability, or aggression. Specific targeted treatments of FXS that will reverse the enhanced long-term depression that is leading to weak synaptic connections is a hope for the near future. The long-term depression in FXS occurs through up-regulation of the metabotropic glutamate receptor 5 (mGluR5) pathway that occurs in the absence of FMRP, which is normally inhibitory for this pathway. Therefore, specific treatments of FXS would include use of mGluR5 antagonists. If trials in adults with FXS are successful, these targeted treatments may be available in the future for children with FXS. In animal studies, including the fragile X knockout mouse, mGluR5 antagonists decrease seizures and help the cognitive deficits.

Clinical involvement can occur in individuals with the premutation through a different molecular mechanism called RNA toxicity. The premutation is associated with enhanced translation of the *FMR1* gene, so that two to eight times normal levels of *FMR1* mRNA are produced. This is just the opposite of FXS, in which little or no mRNA is produced. The elevated mRNA has an extended repeat length that forms a hairpin structure that binds other proteins in the neuron. This leads to dysregulation of these proteins and the eventual formation of inclusions in the nucleus of the neuron. Approximately 30% to 40% of aging men and a more limited number of women with the premutation develop tremor and ataxia, typically after the age of 50 or 60 years. This disorder may also be associated with a neuropathy in the lower extremities, autonomic problems, parkinsonian features, anxiety, mood lability, and cognitive decline. It is called the fragile X–associated tremor/ataxia syndrome (FXTAS), and it occurs exclusively in premutation carriers, not in individuals with the full mutation. Magnetic resonance imaging findings include global brain atrophy and white matter disease, especially in the middle cerebellar peduncles. Because of the occurrence of FXTAS, the family history needs to include careful questioning about neurologic problems in the grandparents or extended family members. Often, FXTAS in a grandparent is misdiagnosed as Parkinson disease or Alzheimer disease.

The premutation is also the leading cause of ovarian failure in women in the general population. Approximately 20% of women with the premutation have premature ovarian failure (stopping of menses before the age of 40 years), and an additional 20% have early menopause (menopause before the age of 45 years). Even women with the premutation who are cycling normally have an elevation of follicle-stimulating hormone compared with controls, suggesting ovarian dysfunction. This problem is also thought to be related to RNA toxicity in carriers of the premutation because it does not occur in women with the full mutation.

The premutation is thought to occasionally cause developmental issues related to RNA toxicity because some children with the premutation have problems with ADHD, shyness, social anxiety, or autism spectrum disorders. In boys who present clinically and are found to have the premutation, more than 90% have ADHD and more than 70% have autism spectrum disorders. However, in boys who are found to have the premutation through cascade testing of a family once one person is identified with FXS, only 8% have autism spectrum disorders and 38% have ADHD, although shyness and social isolation are common problems in these boys. On occasion, a child with the premutation will present with more severe problems including intellectual disability and features of FXS, and many of these individuals will have lowered FMRP, so they are truly affected with FXS (particularly in the upper end of the premutation range). In general, males can be more significantly affected by the premutation either from lowered FMRP or from elevated levels of mRNA. The problems of the premutation also respond to therapy as needed, including psychopharmacologic interventions as discussed before. For more information about involvement and treatment of individuals with the full mutation and the premutation, the families should be referred to the National Fragile X Foundation at *www.fragilex.org*.

Involvement from the fragile X gene mutation is now considered a family affair, but the pediatrician can facilitate referrals for genetic counseling, neurologic evaluations of older family members who may be affected by FXTAS, obstetric-gynecologic evaluations for those with premature ovarian failure, and counseling or psychiatric evaluations for those with emotional problems including the mothers who are carriers. Anxiety and depression are common in the carrier mothers (perhaps related to RNA toxicity), and these psychiatric problems can significantly affect the well-being of the child and the ability of the mother to nurture the child. Therefore, attention to all of the problems in the family is a necessity in this condition.

REFERENCES

Bejjani BA, Theisen AP, Ballif BC, Shaffer LG: Array-based comparative genomic hybridization in clinical diagnosis. Expert Rev Mol Diagn 5(3):421-429, 2005.

Bender BG, Harmon RJ, Linden MG: Psychosocial adaptation of 39 adolescents with sex chromosome abnormalities. Pediatrics 96:302-308, 1995.

Bojesen A, Juul S, Gravholt CH: Prenatal and postnatal prevalence of Klinefelter syndrome: A national registry study. J Clin Endocrinol Metab 18(2):622-626, 2003.

Butler MG: Imprinting disorders: Non-mendelian mechanisms affecting growth. J Pediatr Endocrinol Metab 15(Suppl 5):1279-1288, 2002.

Christoforidis A, Maniadaki I, Stanhope R: Managing children with Russell-Silver syndrome: More than just growth hormone treatment? J Pediatr Endocrinol Metab 18(7):651-652, 2005.

Chu C, Schwartz S, McPherson E: Paternal uniparental isodisomy for chromosome 14 in a patient with a normal 46,XY karyotype. Am J Med Genet 127(2):167-171, 2004.

Cohen MJ: Beckwith-Wiedemann syndrome: Historical, clinicopathological and etiopathogenetic perspectives. Pediatr Dev Pathol 8(3):287-304, 2005.

Delaval K, Wagschal A, Feil R: Epigenetic deregulation of imprinting in congenital diseases of aberrant growth. Bioessays 28(5):453-459, 2006.

Flannery DB: Pigmentary dysplasias, hypomelanosis of Ito and genetic mosaicism. Am J Med Genet 35(1):18-21, 1990.

Gardner RJM, Sutherland G (eds): Chromosome Abnormalities and Genetic Counseling. Oxford, Oxford University Press, 2004.

Graham JM Jr, Bashir AS, Stark RE, et al: Oral and written language abilities of XXY boys: Implications for anticipatory guidance. Pediatrics 81:795-806, 1988.

Jones KL (ed): Smith's Recognizable Patterns of Human Malformation. Philadelphia, Elsevier Saunders, 2006.

Liehr T, Claussen U, Starke H: Small supernumerary marker chromosomes (sSMC) in humans. Cytogenet Genome Res 107(1-2):55-67, 2004.

Mitter D, Buiting K, von Eggeling F, et al: Is there a higher incidence of maternal uniparental disomy 14 [upd(14)mat]? Detection of 10 new patients by methylation-specific PCR. Am J Med Genet 140(19):2039-2049, 2006.

Perkins RM, Hoang-Xuan TA: The Russell-Silver syndrome: A case report and brief review of the literature. Pediatr Dermatol 19(6):546-549, 2002.

Robinson A, Bender B, Linden MG: Summary of clinical findings in children and young adults with sex chromosome anomalies. *In* Evans JA, Hamerton JL (eds): Children and Young Adults with Sex Chromosome Aneuploidy Birth Defects: Original Article Series, Vol 26. New York, Wiley-Liss, for the March of Dimes Birth Defects Foundation, 1991, pp 225-228.

Schrander-Stumpel CT, Govaerts LC, Engelen JJ, et al: Mosaic tetrasomy 8p in two patients: Clinical data and review of the literature. Am J Hum Genet 50(4):377-380, 1994.

Taibjee SM, Bennett DC, Moss C: Abnormal pigmentation in hypomelanosis of Ito and pigmentary mosaicism: The role of pigmentary genes. Br J Dermatol 151(2):269-282, 2004.

Tartaglia N, Hansen R, Reynolds A, et al: ADHD and autism spectrum disorders in males with XXY, XYY, and XXYY syndromes. J Intellect Disabil Res 50(11):787, 2006.

www.genetests.org. Accessed August 10, 2006.

www.ncbi.nlm.nih.gov. Accessed August 10, 2006.

25 DOWN SYNDROME: CARE OF THE CHILD AND FAMILY

William I. Cohen (1947-2009)

Down syndrome (DS) is the most common genetic disorder causing intellectual disability. This discussion of its diagnosis and management serves the dual purpose of reminding the clinician of the important features of this condition and providing a model for the management of other developmental disabilities, combining a comprehensive understanding of the biologic disorder and an appreciation of how the parents, extended family, and community respond to the child and the child's unique needs.

DS was first described by John Langdon Down in 1865. Jérôme Lejeune discovered the presence of an extra twenty-first chromosome (trisomy 21) in individuals who fit Down's description in 1959. DS occurs in 1/733 live births or 1/150 conceptions. The higher rate for conceptions reflects the fact that one of four spontaneous abortions are fetuses with trisomies of any kind.

GENETICS

Three different chromosomal abnormalities are associated with individuals who have the phenotypic appearance of DS: trisomy 21, translocations, and mosaicism. Ninety-five percent of individuals with the physical appearance of DS have trisomy 21, which is the presence of an extra chromosome 21 as a result of nondisjunction. In nondisjunction, the chromosomes fail to pair or fail to exchange genetic material. This usually occurs at the first meiotic division, although it can occur at the second meiotic division as well. The extra chromosome is most often of maternal origin, but paternal origin occurs as well; in one study, 7% of the infants received the extra chromosomal material from their fathers. Nondisjunction occurs sporadically in individuals of all ages; however, the association of increasing maternal age and trisomy reflects a well-known age-related increase in meiosis I nondisjunction. Although trisomy 21 occurs sporadically, empirically the rate of recurrence of trisomy 21 irrespective of age is 1%. Nevertheless, for most women, the age-related risk predominates. At age 35 years, the risk is approximately 1 in 250. By age 48 years, the risk of trisomy 21 is 1 in 11.

Although there are more parents who delay childbearing into their 30s and beyond, most of the infants with DS are born to mothers younger than 35 years. Women 35 years and older account for only about 7% of births each year (and approximately 20% of infants with DS). Consequently, the other 80% are born to women younger than 35 years.

Three percent to 4% of individuals with DS have a *translocation* with the extra chromosomal material "stuck" to another chromosome. The extra 21 chromosome may be commonly attached to either chromosome 14 or chromosome 21. Fifty percent of translocations occur de novo and have a low risk of recurrence in subsequent pregnancies. However, 50% are inherited from a normal parent with a balanced translocation. These families have a high risk of recurrence in subsequent pregnancies. Therefore, parents of children with translocations are encouraged to obtain a karyotype to determine whether they are balanced carriers and therefore at risk of having a subsequent child with DS. If that were the case, the siblings of the child with DS would need to be studied to determine if they may also be carriers of a balanced translocation.

One percent to 2% of children have *mosaicism,* in which only some cells have the extra chromosome. This usually represents nondisjunction in an early postzygotic mitosis. The extent of affected tissues with an extra chromosome 21 varies with the timing of the event. Mosaicism can also occur by loss of the extra chromosome in early cell lines, so-called trisomy rescue. The greater the proportion of tissues with an extra 21 chromosome, the greater likelihood that the individual will have the characteristic DS phenotype. On the other hand, individuals with only a small proportion of cells affected may never be detected because they would be unlikely to be karyotyped.

Mosaic forms of DS tend to cause confusion for both the families and physicians, who often assume that children with mosaicism have a milder form of DS. This statement is partially correct; depending on the tissues involved, an individual who has some cell lines with an extra chromosome 21 may be indistinguishable from the typical child. However, most children with mosaicism and the full phenotypic expression of DS will show typical characteristics. On the other hand, children with subtle physical features or minimal developmental disabilities are sometimes thought by their physicians and families to have mosaic DS, even when their karyotype is consistent with trisomy 21. The confusion seems to stem from a failure to realize the enormous biologic variability of trisomy 21: from significant hypotonia with attendant delays in motor development to nearly normal muscle tone; from intellectual disability to mild variations in learning styles.

PRENATAL SCREENING AND DIAGNOSIS

In January 2007, the American College of Obstetricians and Gynecologists (ACOG) issued a practice bulletin recommending that all pregnant women be screened for DS, starting with a first-trimester blood test for free beta-human chorionic gonadotropin and pregnancy-associated plasma protein A together with an ultrasound examination for nuchal translucency. Those at risk would be offered genetic counseling and the option of chorionic villus sampling or second-trimester amniocentesis. In addition, neural tube screening with maternal serum alpha-fetoprotein determinations would be offered to women who undergo the first trimester screening. The ACOG further recommends that those women who are not screened in the first trimester obtain serum screening with alpha-fetoprotein, estriol, human chorionic gonadotropin, and inhibin A determinations. In addition, the ACOG recommends that all women, regardless of age, have access to diagnostic testing (American College of Obstetrics and Gynecology, 2007).

These recommendations elicited a strong negative reaction from the various national DS organizations, including the National Down Syndrome Congress and the National Down Syndrome Society. These advocacy groups expressed enormous consternation that these guidelines appeared to promote early identification for the purpose of termination of the pregnancy and offered to collaborate with the ACOG to provide accurate information about the lives of people with DS to families faced with these decisions.

MAKING THE DIAGNOSIS IN THE NEWBORN PERIOD

The diagnosis of DS is first suggested by a variety of physical characteristics that together indicate the consideration of this diagnosis (Table 25-1). The facial appearance of the child is often the first clue: flat profile, upslanted palpebral fissures, epicanthal folds, flat nasal bridge, small auricles (external ears), nuchal fat pad, and short head (brachycephaly). In reality, infants born vaginally often have edema of the face and eyelids, making it more difficult to detect the eye findings. On the other hand, central hypotonia, manifested as low muscle tone, may make the diagnosis easier, whereas relatively normal tone will confound the picture. A number of infants may fail to maintain their body temperature on the first day of life and require a warming bed.

The definitive diagnostic procedure is the chromosomal karyotype. In some hospital laboratories, the preliminary results may be ready within 48 hours. Ordinarily, the results may take up to 2 weeks, even longer if they are sent to a commercial laboratory. A physician or nurse in the delivery room who suspects that an infant has DS can do a great service to the family by obtaining a heparinized sample of cord blood, which can subsequently be sent to the cytogenetics laboratory if the clinical suspicion is strong enough.

Table 25-1. Diagnostic Features of Down Syndrome

Upslanting palpebral fissures	98%
Wide gap between the toes	95%
Nuchal fat pad	87%
Depressed nasal bridge	83%
Brushfield spots	75%
Brachycephaly	75%
Epicanthal folds	60%
Clinodactyly	50%
Single palmar crease	50%

INFORMING THE FAMILY

Whereas the pattern of features associated with DS and its relatively common occurrence make it easy for clinicians to suspect this condition, it can be much more challenging to decide how and when to communicate these concerns to the family. We are fortunate that much investigation has been conducted on this subject, for disabilities and congenital malformations in general and DS in particular (Holan and Cohen, 1992; Skotko, 2005). Unfortunately, most parents are dissatisfied with the way the diagnosis was communicated.

Parents want to be told by someone who has a positive attitude and is knowledgeable. However, despite its incidence, most practitioners are likely to have had limited experience with children with developmental disabilities in general or DS in particular. This may lead the physician to speak more out of personal experience than current information. Most of our opinions and beliefs reflect what we have learned in training or in the course of our years in practice. It is both unfortunate and true that physicians trained some time ago may advise families to place the child for adoption or even to institutionalize the infant. On the other hand, physicians trained more recently often have had exposure to families of individuals with DS and other developmental disabilities and have been able to appreciate the societal changes that have occurred during the last 20 years to appreciate the value of all individuals.

If you suspect DS in the newborn period, explain your concerns to the parents as soon as possible. The karyotype will confirm or deny them. Parents sense when physicians and nurses have a secret. You need *not* be certain of the diagnosis. In fact, this lack of certainty often gives families an opportunity to consider the possibility while maintaining hope. The unexpected birth of an infant with DS can rob the family of the normal child they had hoped for and imagined. The time it takes to obtain the karyotype results from the laboratory is often helpful to ease the shock and feeling of loss.

Dilemmas for the Physician in Regard to Informing the Family

None of us wishes to cause harm or distress to the families of our patients, and there is little doubt that this unexpected news can cause significant grief—an emotion experienced by both the parents and the physician. As the parents react to the discovery that their child is not who they expected, the physician cannot help feeling that he or she directly caused the parents' upset. Our intellectual certainty of the diagnosis may waver in the face of our desire to avoid the family's suffering. Some clinicians try to avoid discussion of the issue at all and seek a genetics consultation. Others cloak themselves in positive forecasts for the future of this child: "Things have never been better for children with Down syndrome." Others who suspect the diagnosis and are not certain may choose to wait for a few weeks. If we remind ourselves that we did not cause this disorder, it is possible to tell parents what we suspect and to tolerate the intense emotions that they and we are likely to encounter. As we find a way to tolerate our own sense of sadness, we are challenged to acknowledge the emotions of the parents: "It makes sense to me that you are feeling this way." Nevertheless, one must not assume that the birth of child with DS is necessarily unsuspected or, in fact, "bad news." Some parents recognize the increased likelihood of having a child with DS (associated with their age) and may choose not to have prenatal screening or diagnosis. For instance, they may have grown up with individuals with DS and have a sense of the range of possible, positive outcomes.

Here is one suggested approach to this conversation. It is mandatory that the infant be present and highly desirable for both parents to hear this information at the same time. "I have examined your baby and she is healthy. I noticed some features [which should be shown to the parents and explained with plain, nontechnical language]. These features make me think that your child may have Down syndrome. [Pause to monitor the parents' verbal and nonverbal reactions.] What do you know about Down syndrome?" This is an opportunity to provide a short description of the physical characteristics, the medical vulnerabilities (which, for example, lead to screening for cardiac problems), and the association with intellectual disability. It is most important to follow this discussion with information that will connect the family to other resources. Local DS parent groups and clinical programs as well as the national organizations have material for new parents that addresses a wide variety of concerns. They can help connect the parents with support groups as well as with families of other children with DS, which many families find most helpful. (See Internet Resources.)

MEDICAL CONDITIONS IN DOWN SYNDROME AND HEALTH CARE GUIDELINES

Health care for the child with DS combines standard well-child care protocols, as described by the American Academy of Pediatrics, with the awareness and detection of congenital abnormalities and the medical vulnerabilities that occur in greater frequency in children with DS. This has led to the development of specific screening protocols to prevent a secondary disability, which occurs when a treatable medical condition that can exacerbate a developmental problem is overlooked. For example, children with DS generally have delays in acquiring spoken language. They also are at greater risk for hearing loss. The clinician who attributes the delay in spoken language to the developmental disabilities of DS and fails to detect and then to treat or habilitate this hearing loss will further compromise language function. What follows is a systematic review of health concerns in individuals with DS.

Cardiovascular Disorders

Congenital heart disease has been estimated to occur in about 50% of infants with DS. The most commonly occurring conditions are atrioventricular septal defect, ventricular septal defect, atrial septal defect, and tetralogy of Fallot. Whereas most children with a hemodynamically significant lesion will present with cardiac signs and symptoms, in some children, an atrioventricular septal defect may be present in the absence of a murmur. These children develop early increased pulmonary vascular resistance that reduces the left-to-right intracardiac shunt, minimizes the heart murmur, and prevents symptoms of heart failure and respiratory problems. Such individuals who seem to be doing clinically well may be developing serious pulmonary vascular changes. The only reliable way to exclude serious structural congenital heart disease is by echocardiography. Therefore, a pediatric cardiologist should evaluate infants as soon as the diagnosis of DS is made.

Gastrointestinal Disorders

Congenital gastrointestinal tract malformations, such as duodenal atresia and imperforate anus, occur in approximately 5% of children with DS. Vomiting and the inability to tolerate feedings in the first 12 hours of life warrant immediate investigation. The diagnosis of intestinal obstruction may be the first clue to the diagnosis of DS. Prenatal ultrasound findings of a "double bubble" or polyhydramnios may suggest the diagnosis in utero. These conditions are rarely occult, and the obvious need for intervention makes it impossible to overlook them. Hirschsprung disease is 25 times more likely to occur in individuals with DS than in the typical child. Failure to pass meconium in the first 24 hours of life may be the first clue to this condition. Severe constipation in infancy is an indication for evaluation for Hirschsprung disease by a pediatric gastroenterologist or a pediatric surgeon because of the high mortality associated with enterocolitis in the untreated child. Chronic constipation is reported in 30% of individuals with DS. It is often successfully treated with dietary interventions, such as pear or prune juice, prunes, and Karo syrup, or over-the-counter preparations that act as stool softeners, such as Maltsupex. Some children require use of osmotic agents such as lactulose or polyethelene glycol. Failure to respond should suggest further evaluation for Hirschsprung disease or hypothyroidism. Gastroesophageal reflux occurs commonly and needs to be treated to prevent the consequences of acid reflux. Children with DS may have oral-motor dysfunction with swallowing difficulties and aspiration. An aerodigestive team (otolaryngologist, pulmonologist, and gastroenterologist) can be particularly helpful in this regard.

Celiac disease (gluten enteropathy) is reported to occur in 7% to 14% of individuals with DS. In addition to the usual symptoms of bloating, diarrhea, and failure to thrive, children with DS may have no symptoms of malabsorption. They may present with constipation, failure of linear growth, or, on occasion, behavioral abnormalities. Serologic screening with determination of immunoglobulin A tissue transglutaminase antibody and immunoglobulin A levels (to ensure that the child is not deficient in this class of immunoglobulins) will indicate those children who need a referral to a gastroenterologist to confirm the diagnosis. A biopsy is necessary before treatment is begun with a gluten-free diet. Celiac disease can occur as soon as 6 months after the exposure to gluten. Likewise, it may not be manifested for several years after the initial exposure. Clinicians must be sensitive to the various manifestations of celiac disease, both the gastrointestinal and the multiple nongastrointestinal symptoms, and re-evaluate the child accordingly (Cohen, 2006).

Ophthalmologic Difficulties

Ophthalmologic difficulties are common in children with DS, and it is important to ensure optimal visual function. Dense congenital cataracts occur more frequently in DS than in the general population. The absence of a red reflex on funduscopic examination is an indication for emergent ophthalmologic referral. Cataract extraction is critical because amblyopia (loss of vision) can occur rapidly, within 7 days in children younger than 1 year. Overall, cataracts are estimated to occur in 11% to 46% of individuals with DS, and fortunately, most of them are visually insignificant. Children with DS have an increased incidence of strabismus, nasolacrimal duct stenosis, and nystagmus. The detection of these conditions warrants timely referral. Because refractive errors occur in 50% of children with DS, they should be referred for routine ophthalmologic evaluation by 6 months of age, in the absence of obvious ocular disease.

Audiologic and Ear, Nose, and Throat Problems

Ear, nose, and throat problems are common in children with DS. Because of the characteristic midfacial hypoplasia, manifested as narrow airways, eustachian tubes, sinus ostia, and external auditory canals, children with DS are at increased risk for recurrent otitis media, nasopharyngitis or sinusitis, and the consequences of chronic serous otitis media. This is of particular significance, given the well-known difficulties in expressive language development in children with DS. The team of physicians caring for the child must ensure optimal hearing to avoid the undesirable consequence of suboptimal language development. Common upper airway abnormalities include laryngomalacia, tracheomalacia, and subglottic stenosis. Such children need an ear, nose, and throat evaluation, often including laryngobronchoscopy. Children with DS have frequent episodes of croup, and this may reflect silent reflux causing laryngeal irritation.

Sleep Abnormalities

Children and adults with DS frequently have a variety of sleep abnormalities. The anatomic features noted above, together with hypotonia, contribute to an increased incidence of obstructive sleep apnea. Even normally sized tonsils and adenoids may lead to relative obstruction, and adenoidectomy or tonsillectomy may be indicated in the presence of obvious symptoms. Some youngsters sleep sitting up and leaning forward. However, children with DS often are restless sleepers, awakening or arousing several times during the night. It is unclear whether this represents undetected airway obstruction without apnea (related to the collapse of the airway and the arousal of the child in response) or a separate, central phenomenon. In addition to the negative consequences of hypoxemia and disordered sleep on daytime wakefulness (which may lead to behavioral abnormalities such as ADHD symptoms and to learning problems), untreated obstructive sleep apnea has been associated with significant cardiac morbidity, such as pulmonary hypertension. One study of children with DS showed that 80% had abnormal sleep evaluations when abnormal arousals were included. Because parental reports of abnormal sleep do not correlate well with the results of sleep studies, clinicians should strongly consider an evaluation by a pediatric sleep center in the face of these symptoms, including full polysomnography. Although adenotonsillectomy is the first procedure performed, 50% of patients may still have obstruction after this procedure, and therefore a postoperative sleep study is needed to define the nature of the residual obstruction, which might include glossoptosis, hypopharyngeal collapse, lingual tonsillar hypertrophy, or adenoidal regrowth in the case of previous adenoidectomy. The growing awareness of sleep disorders in children with DS and the increase in sleep studies have led to the use of positive-pressure airway devices, such as continuous positive airway pressure and bilevel positive airway pressure. Although these devices are challenging to use, the efforts of pediatric sleep specialists are often able to successfully desensitize children to them (Shott, 2006).

Infectious Disease and Immunology

In addition to ear, nose, and throat infections, individuals with DS have been shown to have deficiencies of cellular and humoral immunity. Although it is rare, children with DS have been reported to have a deficiency of immunoglobulin G subclasses 2 and 4 in the face of normal total immunoglobulin G. Children with repeated serious pyogenic infections, such as pneumonia and empyema, need to have quantitative immunoglobulins measured and then to be treated accordingly (Nespoli et al, 1993; Ugazio et al, 1990). Furthermore, children with recurrent pneumonia should be evaluated for gastroesophageal reflux and aspiration. Children with DS who meet standard cardiac and pulmonary criteria for respiratory syncytial virus prophylaxis are urged to receive palivizumab to prevent infection during the winter months because their narrow airways put them at increased risk for serious morbidity. DS is associated with an increased incidence of autoimmune disorders, including thyroid abnormalities, celiac disease, juvenile-onset diabetes mellitus, juvenile rheumatoid arthritis, and alopecia areata.

Hematologic Disorders

Infants with DS often present with polycythemia, which quickly resolves. However, partial exchange transfusion may be required to treat symptomatic individuals. Erythrocytes show a persistent macrocytosis in two thirds of individuals with DS. This may be present in the face of iron deficiency anemia and give false reassurance. Thrombocytopenia occurs commonly in newborns with DS, and it is usually transient although it may be seen as part of a transient myeloproliferative disorder, which is found in 10% of infants. This condition, manifested by pancytopenia, hepatosplenomegaly, and circulating immature white blood cells, regresses spontaneously within the first 3 months of life. However, 20% to 30% of these children go on to develop leukemia. DS is the most common factor predisposing to childhood leukemia; approximately 1% of children with DS develop one of four kinds of this disorder. This is between 10 and 20 times the frequency observed in typically developing children. Fifty percent of the leukemias are lymphoid, and the other half are myeloid. Most of the myeloid leukemias are acute megakaryocytic leukemia. Both transient myeloproliferative disorder and acute megakaryocytic leukemia are associated with somatic mutations of the *GATA1* gene, which encodes hematopoietic growth factor. Acute myeloid leukemias have extremely high rates of remission and very low rates of relapse in children with DS compared with typically developing children. In one series of 33 patients younger than 4 years with DS and nonlymphocytic leukemias, all achieved a complete remission, and the group had an 80% estimated 8-year survival rate (Dixon, Kishnani, and Zimmerman, 2006). The current protocols are shorter in duration than for typically developing children and use modified doses of chemotherapeutic agents. Bone marrow transplantation has rarely been necessary, although stem cell transplantation may be indicated following recurrence.

Endocrine Disorders

In childhood and adolescence, hypothyroidism occurs frequently, in approximately 15% of the population. Most of these cases are autoimmune in nature (Hashimoto's thyroiditis). Although it is less frequent, hyperthyroidism (Graves disease) occurs as well. A population-based study of newborns with DS suggested that it is a "mild form of congenital hypothyroidism that is rarely detected by neonatal screening." Thyroid supplementation in a group of these infants led to small but statistically significant increases in motor development, length, and weight (van Trotsenburg, Vulsma, and van Rozenburg-Marres, 2005). These findings have not been replicated as yet but are suggestive of the need for sensitivity to the subtleties of thyroid disorders in children with DS. One such instance is the problem of recurrent mild elevations of thyroid-stimulating hormone in the face of free thyroxine levels at the low end of the range of normal. A number of pediatric endocrinologists empirically treat these children with thyroid replacement therapy, considering this condition to represent compensated hypothyroidism.

Musculoskeletal Conditions

The central hypotonia, combined with oral-motor immaturity and lack of coordination of suck-swallow, can interfere with the establishment of successful feeding in the newborn period. This can be particularly difficult for those mothers who wish to nurse their babies. Fortunately, lactation specialists can provide specific techniques to overcome these challenges.

Ligamentous laxity is a common finding in children with DS. Together with hypotonia, these children present as floppy and flexible. It is rare to see congenitally dislocated hips in children with DS, although hip problems do occur in adolescence. Adolescents also are prone to patellar dislocation. The most potentially serious problems caused by ligamentous laxity are related to the occiput and cervical spine. Laxity of the transverse ligaments can lead to excessive movement of C1 and C2. A small percentage of individuals with DS (estimated at 2%) will develop spinal cord compression from this excess movement. Approximately 13% of individuals with DS have more than 4.5 mm of distance between the atlas and the dens on lateral cervical spine radiographs on comparison of the neutral view with full flexion and full extension. These individuals have been described as having atlantoaxial instability and have been, in the past, considered at risk for the development of spinal cord compression. The belief that atlantoaxial instability is an asymptomatic precursor of cord compression as well as the desire to prevent any possible injury led to the recommendation that all individuals participating in Special Olympics have such studies performed. However, recent reviews of the literature have suggested that such screening may not be necessary and that individuals who are at risk for such spinal cord catastrophes either have symptoms or signs (such as neck pain, weakness in the upper extremities, gait disturbance, bladder or bowel problems, or hyperreflexia and presence of Babinski sign) or have been subjected to manipulation of the neck. This has led to the recommendation of universal precautions in administering anesthesia to children with DS, especially for ear, nose, and throat procedures.

It has been suggested that measurement of the neural canal width provides a better assessment of the likelihood of spinal cord compression. The evidence supporting the current recommendations for screening with lateral cervical spine films (flexion, extension, and neutral) is not robust; our colleagues in the United Kingdom discontinued screening 10 years ago. Until such time as the current guidelines are revised, it would be prudent, however, to continue to obtain these radiographs (including measurement of the neural canal width) between 3 and 5 years of age (the neural canal width should be greater than 14 mm). Participants in Special Olympics and therapeutic equestrian programs may need to be evaluated more frequently. Adults with DS are at greater risk for cervical spine abnormalities because of anatomic predisposition as well as the early onset of arthritic changes (Cohen, 2006). In any event, the presence of signs or symptoms warrants further neuroradiologic evaluation (magnetic resonance imaging). Symptomatic individuals must be referred for neurosurgical evaluation and treatment, which consists of fusion of C1 and C2 (Caird, Wills, and Dormans, 2006).

Neurologic and Neurodevelopmental Disorders

Epilepsy

Although seizures occur more frequently in individuals with cognitive disabilities than in the typical population, the frequency of seizures in individuals with DS ranges from 1% to 13% (Goldberg-Stern, Strawsburg, and Patterson, 2001). Half these seizures can be attributed to an underlying medical problem (such as cardiovascular disease, infection, trauma, perinatal problems, or, more rarely, moyamoya disease). Consequently, a full investigation is warranted. The other 50% are idiopathic. Of note, infantile spasms occur more frequently in children with DS. Although they are usually associated with poor neurodevelopmental outcome, timely recognition of this disorder along with rapid institution of treatment correlates with better outcomes. Children who had a delay in beginning treatment and who had a long time until the spasms stopped had a lower developmental quotient and a higher incidence of autistic features (Eisermann et al, 2003). Vigabatrin, a new anticonvulsant that is not easily available in the United States, has been associated with rapid cessation of spasms.

Autistic Disorders

These disorders are more prevalent in children and adults with DS. Whereas the incidence of autism in the general population is reported at 15 per 10,000 population, current evidence suggests that the prevalence in DS is approximately 5% to 10%. In addition to an early onset of symptoms, children with DS seem to be more likely to develop the so-called disintegrative form of autism, in which a child with adequate development of cognitive, language, and adaptive skills undergoes a dramatic regression with the emergence of typical autistic features. These children warrant a full investigation and should be considered for prolonged video electroencephalographic evaluation. The Aberrant Behavior Checklist has been shown to be useful in characterizing children with DS and autistic spectrum disorder (Capone et al, 2005).

Attention-Deficit/Hyperactivity Disorder (ADHD)

This common neuropsychiatric disorder occurs more frequently in children with DS (and cognitive disabilities in general) than in typically developing children. It is important to control for the child's developmental age in using standardized ratings. Be mindful of underlying undiagnosed medical problems, such as hyperthyroidism, hearing loss, and sleep disturbances (with or without sleep apnea), that may be responsible for the inattention or overactivity In general, children with DS respond well to current medical management with stimulant therapy, although it is wise to start with smaller than usual doses because of heightened sensitivity to psychoactive medications.

Other Neurobehavioral Disorders in Children

In addition to ADHD, children with DS commonly manifest oppositional-defiant disorder, disruptive disorder, and stereotypic movement disorder. Adolescents and adults with DS may manifest depressive disorders, obsessive-compulsive disorders, and a peculiar psychotic-like disorder. These are described in greater detail in Capone's review of the subject (Capone et al, 2006).

Alzheimer Disease

Parents of newborn infants with DS have often heard about the association of DS with Alzheimer disease, and although this is not a condition that appears in childhood, the question of the likelihood of its development may well arise. This misinformation was based on the finding of pathologic changes of Alzheimer disease in the autopsies of children with DS. None of these children had any evidence of dementia. Furthermore, studies have shown that many of the adults with behavior changes suspected of representing Alzheimer disease were found to have diagnosable, treatable conditions, such as hypothyroidism or depression (Chicoine and McGuire, 2006).

THE HEALTH CARE GUIDELINES FOR INDIVIDUALS WITH DOWN SYNDROME

A variety of screening protocols have been developed to ensure optimal health and well-being for children and adults with DS. The earliest U.S. version was proposed by Mary Coleman in 1981. The most recent version is the Health Supervision for Children with Down Syndrome, developed jointly by the Committee on Genetics of the American Academy of Pediatrics and the Down Syndrome Medical Interest Group and published in *Pediatrics* in 2001 (American Academy of Pediatrics, 2001). This protocol is designed to supplement, not replace, the standard well-child care protocols of the American Academy of Pediatrics and the American Academy of Family Physicians. Whereas previous versions reflected a consensus by clinicians, the new standard of evidence-based medicine serves as the foundation for the current revision being undertaken by the American Academy of Pediatrics and the Down Syndrome Medical Interest Group. It is expected to be released in 2009. See Tables 25-2 to 25-5 for a brief summary of the recommended screenings and consultations.

GROWTH AND DEVELOPMENT

Children with DS grow in length and height at a slower rate than do typically developing children. The mechanism is multifactorial, including metabolic and endocrine abnormalities related to the presence of extra genetic material. This growth retardation begins prenatally. Children with DS should be plotted on the DS-specific growth charts, which exist for both boys and girls from birth to 18 years of age. Growth charts for head circumference are available up to the age of 36 months (see Internet Resources). Although children with DS are likely to fall below the fifth percentile for height on the charts for

Table 25-2. Health Supervision Recommendations: Birth

Chromosomal karyotype to confirm the diagnosis
Cardiac evaluation (including echocardiography)
Objective hearing evaluation (auditory brainstem response test or evoked otoacoustic emission testing (This is routinely performed as part of Universal Newborn Hearing Screening.)
Ophthalmoscopic examination to detect dense congenital cataracts (look for red reflex)
Thyroid function testing (check state-mandated screening)
Referral for Early Intervention ("Birth to Three" developmental services)
Discussion of availability of family support
Medical genetics consultation, as indicated: discussion of future risk in subsequent pregnancies The parents of any child with translocation genotype must have a karyotype to be certain they are not balanced carriers.

Table 25-3. Health Supervision Recommendations: First Year of Life

Repeat hearing evaluation periodically at 9–12 months of age with behavioral audiometry.
Refer for eye examination by pediatric vision specialist by 6 months.
Repeat thyroid function testing (thyroid-stimulating hormone and free thyroxine) at 6 and 12 months.

Table 25-4. Health Supervision Recommendations: Ages 1 to 12 Years

Continue periodic hearing evaluations, every 6 months until pure-tone audiograms can be obtained for each ear separately. Then, assess hearing yearly.
Continue eye examinations.
Perform yearly thyroid function testing.
Recommend biannual dental care, beginning at 2 years of age.
Obtain lateral cervical spine radiographs (flexion, neutral, and extension), measuring the atlanto-dens interval and the neural canal width, between 3 and 5 years of age to look for atlantoaxial instability.
The Down Syndrome Medical Interest Group recommends screening for celiac disease at 2 years of age with immunoglobulin A tissue transglutaminase antibody and total immunoglobulin A levels.

Table 25-5. Health Supervision Recommendations: Adolescence

Continue yearly thyroid function testing.
Continue periodic vision and hearing assessments and dental care.
Refer for an adolescent medicine consultation regarding sexual health concerns.
Educational programming should focus on transition planning.

typical children, most children with DS are growth hormone sufficient. However, when children with DS cross percentile lines on the DS growth charts, they should be evaluated for endocrinopathies (such as hypothyroidism and growth hormone deficiency) as well as for celiac disease. On the other hand, school-age and adolescent children with DS have a tendency to become overweight. Therefore, growth charts for typically developing children should be used in conjunction with DS-specific growth charts because the typical charts will not accurately reflect appropriate linear growth, and the DS weight charts fail to capture the extent of the overweight problem.

Most children with DS have mild to moderate intellectual disability. They have delays in all areas of development: gross and fine motor, cognitive, language, and personal-social. There is one important exception: in general, expressive (verbal) language abilities tend to be more delayed than cognitive and receptive language skills. For this reason, it is encouraged to teach children sign language as part of a total communication approach to overcome problems in verbal expression and to improve communication in general. Learning sign language does not interfere with the subsequent development of spoken language. Adolescents and adults with DS show continued expressive language development. Nevertheless, some children do not develop any appreciable verbal expressive language. Younger children may be candidates for use of PECS (Picture Exchange Communication System), and older children without any appreciable language are candidates for augmentive communication devices.

Children with DS from 0 to 3 years of age are eligible for Early Intervention services. This federally funded program provides a range of developmental services, rendered by child development specialists, occupational therapists, physical therapists, and speech-language pathologists. The services are provided in the home.

Most new parents have no frame of reference to understand what intellectual or cognitive disability means. They may believe that the child may never walk or talk or be toilet trained. On the other hand, the frequently although inaccurately used term *developmental delay* implies that the child will eventually "catch up." Parents need to be sensitively educated to what will happen as the child grows. This understanding generally develops over time, and it can be cruel as well as incorrect to attempt to address the issue of the child's future functional abilities. The use of information such as that in Tables 25-6 and 25-7 can help orient parents to what they might expect.

After 3 years of age, local school districts are responsible for providing educational services. Individuals with disabilities are eligible for educational programming through the age of 21 years.

EDUCATION

Most children with DS are eligible for special education services under Federal laws 94-142 (passed in 1975) and 99-457 (passed in 1986). The most recent version, Individuals with Disabilities Education Act, was passed in 2004. In the not too distant past, most children with special needs were educated in special classes, sometimes, but not always, located in neighborhood schools. Within the past 20 years, following the innovative efforts of Canadian educators, individuals with special needs have been educated in inclusive settings, that is, in regular education classes alongside their age-mates. This has been accomplished by providing supportive services within the regular education setting, through a combination of assistive personnel to the pupil and support for

Table 25-6. **Developmental Milestones**

	Children with Down Syndrome		"Normal" Children	
Milestone	**Average (months)**	**Range (months)**	**Average (months)**	**Range (months)**
Smiling	2	1½-4	1	½-3
Rolling over	8	4-22	5	2-10
Sitting alone	10	6-28	7	5-9
Crawling	12	7-21	8	6-11
Creeping	15	9-27	10	7-13
Talking, words	16	9-31	10	6-14
Standing	20	11-42	11	8-16
Walking	24	12-65	13	8-18
Talking, phrases	28	18-96	21	14-32

From Pueschel SM (ed): Down Syndrome: Growing and Learning. Kansas City, Andrews, McMeel & Parker, 1978.

Table 25-7. **Self-Help Skills**

	Children with Down Syndrome		"Normal" Children	
Skill	**Average (months)**	**Range (months)**	**Average (months)**	**Range (months)**
Eating				
Finger feeding	12	8-28	8	6-16
Using spoon and fork	20	12-40	13	8-20
Toilet training				
Bowel	42	28-90	29	16-48
Bladder	48	20-95	32	18-60
Dressing				
Undressing	40	29-72	32	22-42
Putting clothes on	58	38-98	47	34-58

the instructional staff from an inclusion specialist. The spread of this form of educational programming reflects the efforts of the parents of these children who realized that their children participated in the community alongside typical children in all activities except schooling. In addition to providing role models for the children with special needs, this method of education has an enormous benefit in leveling differences between the typical children and those with special needs. If we believe that the goal of education is to prepare all individuals to function in our communities, it makes sense that we begin the process of integration earlier rather than later in the life of the individual. Nevertheless, some parents choose center-based schools for their children, believing that a self-contained special education program is a better fit for their child. Recently, some parents are seeking to identify post-secondary programs to continue their child's education after the age of 21 years, when the educational system's responsibilities cease (Fig. 25-1).

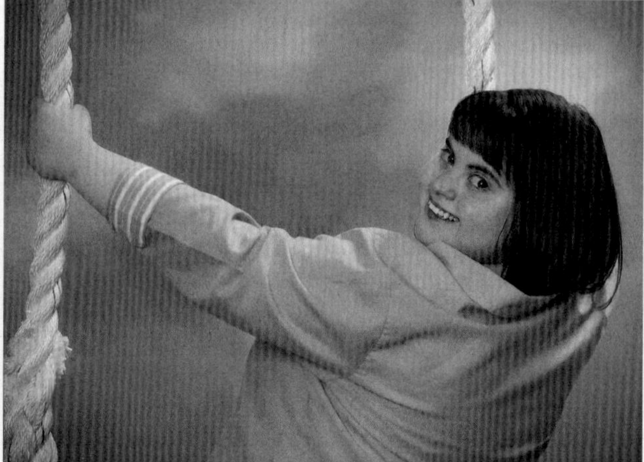

Figure 25-1. Kerry has just turned 22. She loves musical theater, singing and, dancing. She recently finished a vocational program and has just been hired to work at a department store.

ISSUES FOR ADOLESCENTS

Parents and health care providers are often challenged by the discovery that adorable little children who need love and protection grow into adolescents and young adults with mature bodies and with interests in members of the opposite sex. Failure to anticipate this inevitable progression can invite disaster. Therefore, early and frequent discussion about social-sexual training will help families recognize and advocate for appropriate educational programming within their schools. We must be mindful that the training we provide our children should focus on the kind of life we would like our children to have as adults: independent, safe from sexual exploitation and maltreatment, with companionship needs met, and aware of the rules of society (Couwenhoven, 2007). These issues are particularly important because many young people with DS have expressed the desire to develop emotional relationships. Several couples have gotten married, with the attendant media interest. These desires are natural yet remain challenging to society.

The transition process starts automatically in the educational system at 14 years of age, but it is just one of many such processes necessary. These include the transition from pediatric to adult medical care and the potential transitions to a variety of different living situations. Recently, new tools have been developed for guiding young people and their families through this journey, with use of a functional approach to strengths and interests (see Internet Resources for Transition Tool).

COMPLEMENTARY AND ALTERNATIVE THERAPIES

As is the case with other neurodevelopmental disorders such as autism, many parents of children with DS seek out a variety of complementary and alternative therapies. They learn about them from other parents and often through the Internet. These include nutritional interventions (such as multivitamin, mineral, and amino acid combinations) that are purported to enhance learning, to improve muscle tone, and to decrease medical complications. In addition, some parents may pursue chiropractic treatment, neural enhancers, facial plastic surgery, and other interventions they hope will improve the lives of their children. Attempts to scientifically document the benefits claimed have been unsuccessful. The specific aspects of these various interventions have been documented in depth on the Web site *Down Syndrome: Health Issues* (see Internet Resources). The great interest in these treatments reflects parents' hopes that their child might be spared the consequences of the cognitive disabilities so often associated with DS. Cooley (2002) has provided a compassionate guide for engaging with parents around these issues, which recognizes the different ways in which physicians and parents evaluate information in light of the discomfort traditionally trained physicians have with these interventions. In frustration, parents are more than willing to try what *might* work, and we should support their explorations as long as the interventions are safe. Finally, because many families use these treatments, we must be certain to ask what other therapies they are using for their child.

INVESTIGATION IN INTERVENTIONS TO IMPROVE COGNITION AND MEMORY

The possibility of enhancing memory and learning now appears to be more than a dream. The development of an animal model of DS (such as the Ts65dn mouse, which is trisomic for about half of the genes on human chromosome 21) has provided molecular biologists the opportunity to explore the consequences of the overexpression of genes contained on chromosome 21. Neuroscientists have demonstrated the same structural abnormalities of the hippocampus and the cholinergic pathways through the basal forebrain nuclei in these mice as are found in human brains. Further study has revealed abnormalities of synaptic function, with an increase of inhibitory control (specifically an increase in GABA A receptors), which is now believed to play a role in interfering with optimal learning and memory (Fernandez et al, 2007). Other studies of cerebellar structure reveal deficits in the granule cell layer development that may correlate with the decreased cerebellar volume found in these mice and in individuals with DS (Roper et al, 2006). The overexpression of amyloid precursor protein has been implicated in interfering with axonal function in these mice. Preliminary investigations suggest that a variety of pharmacologic interventions may ameliorate or partially correct these deficits. It is becoming apparent that these interventions would not be limited to use in infants but might be useful in children, adolescents, and even adults with DS. Although the development of specific treatments that will be safe for human subjects will likely take quite some time, these findings have galvanized the biomedical community and families alike.

CARING FOR FAMILIES OF CHILDREN WITH DOWN SYNDROME

In caring for children with DS, the tremendous societal change in attitudes toward individuals with disabilities has created a sense of positive expectation that continues to challenge what used to be minimal expectations. The celebrity of Chris Burke, who played the role of Corky on the television program *Life Goes On* (1989-1993), is but one example of the way in which thinking about DS has changed. Inclusive educational programs and participation in community activities such as scouting and camping have likewise helped develop a positive sense of expectancy.

Nevertheless, physicians who become knowledgeable about these changes must continually calibrate their response to the family. The unexpected birth of a child with DS is most often experienced as a tragedy and loss, and the physician who optimistically seeks to comfort the grieving parents with the news that "things are better now for kids with DS than ever before" is more likely to confuse or to enrage rather than comfort. Yet over time, that information will be helpful and can begin healing the wounds.

Ironically, the positive imagery from media and local and national organizations that may buoy one family's flagging spirits may inadvertently cause deep despair in another. Children with DS, like every other biologic disorder, have a spectrum of abilities and behavioral characteristics. There are indeed children who function in the severe to profound range of cognitive disability. There are children with significant neurobehavioral disorders such as ADHD and autism, which make them difficult to manage, despite expert pediatric and subspecialty care. There can be great emotional pain in having a child with a chronic condition, for which the family must anticipate future living arrangements, protection from maltreatment, and financial security. The sense of optimism that many families hold, however, appears to leave little room for these other parents to be able to openly struggle with how difficult it is to raise a child with additional special needs. Our enthusiasm can blind us to the specific experience of a given family. Parents may feel guilty about complaining, as if they should be grateful for having a child with DS. They may experience intense competitive feelings. One couple reported, "We heard about another little girl with Down syndrome who was potty trained at 4 years of age. We were devastated. Our son is 4 and is barely interested. Then we found out that it took 6 months to train her, and we were relieved. It was amazing, we were competing against this child, and, what's more, we hadn't been given the whole story."

Another couple had sought help in dealing with defiant behaviors that were very distressing to them. Sam was a charming 4-year-old who was showing behaviors appropriate for a 2½-year-old. However, on occasion, he would stare at his parents and not respond. Further investigation revealed that in the community and in his educational program, he was experiencing no difficulty whatsoever. Furthermore, they used appropriate behavioral responses. Nevertheless, they expressed enormous distress: "We know Sam will not be smart. It's clear that he is going to have to make his way in the world on the basis of his personality. And that's what really scares us. We're afraid that these misbehaviors he is having are going to really keep him from being successful." This fueled their fears for his future and their overly harsh discipline.

We best help our families by looking and listening carefully for indicators that they are experiencing distress. We must be mindful of the effect of the birth of a child with a developmental disability on the marital relationship and on siblings. The task is to make a place of DS in the family and then to put DS in its place. An overly optimistic approach may make it difficult for families to put the disorder in its place.

DOWN SYNDROME AS A MODEL FOR DEVELOPMENTAL DISABILITIES

The prevalence of DS in the population has had multiple ramifications. The last 25 years have seen a proliferation of information about DS that appears to be directly related to societal changes, such as the access to free and public education, the closing of public institutions for the care of physically and cognitively impaired people, and the advocacy of parents and organizations such as The Arc (formerly The Association for Retarded Citizens). Courageous parents failed to believe the dire predictions made for their children: they dreamed a future of unknown possibilities. The initiative for the emergence of individuals with DS from the recesses of their family's homes sprang from the passionate commitment of those parents who never doubted that their children had a future in society, their physical, developmental, and behavioral features notwithstanding. Trusting their own intuition, parents such as Marian and Frank Burke, Emily and Charles Kingsley, and Barbara and Jack Levitz, among hosts of others, challenged the conventional wisdom of the day and devised programs of supportive services that were ultimately replaced by a variety of formal educational opportunities, such as Early Intervention. Their children, Chris Burke, Jason Kingsley, and Mitchell Levitz, have now embarked on the next phase of this remarkable journey from despair to hope. They serve as role models for youngsters with DS and provide visible proof that the possibilities open to our children may not be a fantasy if we choose to maintain hope, love, and support.

Indeed, these families, with the instrumental support of local and national parent organizations, have helped spearhead the growth of a powerful partnership between consumers and the professional community of health care professionals, basic scientists, educators, therapists, and public policy advocates. The advances in inclusive education, the founding of regional DS clinics and centers, and the regional and national meetings, for parents and professionals alike, have helped fuel an explosion of both basic and applied research. The culmination of these activities has been the establishment of foundations and organizations such as the Down Syndrome Research and Treatment Foundation (in Palo Alto, California), which has sought to establish a mechanism to move quickly from the basic science of cognition and behavior to potential interventions, bypassing the usual, cumbersome, and underfunded governmental biomedical pathways (see Internet Resources).

SUMMARY

Children with DS provide a multifaceted opportunity to integrate our expertise about the medical, developmental, and emotional issues surrounding the diagnosis and management of this common condition. Our efforts to use current knowledge to minimize the impact of the medical and developmental challenges in the service of promoting maximal functional adaptation of the individual with minimal personal burden to the family make this endeavor both challenging and satisfying.

REFERENCES

American Academy of Pediatrics, Committee on Genetics: Health supervision for children with Down syndrome. Pediatrics 107(2):442-449, 2001.

American College of Obstetrics and Gynecology, Practice Bulletin No. 77: Screening for fetal chromosomal abnormalities. Obstet Gynecol 109(1):217-228, 2007.

Caird MS, Wills BP, Dormans JP: Down syndrome in children: The role of the orthopaedic surgeon. J Am Acad Orthop Surg 14:610-619, 2006.

Capone GT, Grados MA, Kaufmann WE, et al: Down syndrome and comorbid autism-spectrum disorder: Characterization using the aberrant behavior checklist. Am J Med Genet A 134:373-380, 2005.

Capone G, Goyal P, Ares W, et al: Neurobehavioral disorders in children, adolescents, and young adults with Down syndrome. Am J Med Genet C Semin Med Genet 142C:158-172, 2006.

Chicoine B, McGuire D: Mental Wellness in Adults with Down Syndrome. New York, Woodbine House, 2006.

Cohen WI: Current dilemmas in Down syndrome clinical care: Celiac disease, thyroid disorders and atlanto-axial instability. Am J Med Genet C Semin Med Genet 142C:141-148, 2006.

Cooley WC: Nonconventional therapies for Down syndrome: A review and framework for decision making. *In* Cohen WI, Nadel L, Madnick ME, (eds): Down Syndrome: Visions for the 21st Century. New York, Wiley-Liss, 2002.

Couwenhoven T: Teaching Children with Down Syndrome About Their Bodies, Boundaries, and Sexuality. Bethesda, MD, Woodbine House, 2007.

Dixon N, Kishnani PS, Zimmerman S: Clinical manifestations of hematologic and oncologic disorders in patients with Down syndrome. Am J Med Genet C Semin Med Genet 142C:149-157, 2006.

Eisermann MM, DeLaRaillère A, Dellatola G, et al: Infantile spasms in Down syndrome—effects of delayed anticonvulsive treatment. Epilepsy Res 559(12):21-27, 2003.

Fernandez F, Morishita W, Zuniga E, et al: Pharmacotherapy for cognitive impairment in the mouse model of Down syndrome. Nat Neurosci 10(4):411–413, 2007. Published online; doi:10.1038/nn1860.

Goldberg-Stern H, Strawsburg RH, Patterson B, et al: Seizure frequency and characteristics in children with Down syndrome. Brain Dev 23:375-378, 2001.

Holan JE, Cohen WI: Reflections on the informing process: Why are these people angry with me? Down Syndrome Papers and Abstracts for Professionals 15(2):4-5, 1992.

Nespoli L, Burgio GR, Ugazio AG, Maccario R: Immunological features of Down's syndrome: a review. J Intellect Disabil Res 37:543-551, 1993.

Roper RJ, Baxter LL, Saran NG, et al: Defective cerebellar response to mitogenic Hedgehog signaling in Down syndrome mice. Proc Natl Acad Sci U S A 1032:1452-1456, 2006.

Shott S: Down syndrome: Common otolaryngologic manifestations. Am J Med Genet C Semin Med Genet 142C:131-140, 2006.

Skotko B: Mothers of children with Down syndrome reflect on their postnatal support. Pediatrics 115:64-77, 2005.

Ugazio AG, Maccario R, Notarangelo LD, et al: Immunology of Down syndrome: A review. Am J Med Genet 7(Suppl):204-212, 1990.

van Trotsenburg AS, Vulsma T, van Rozenburg-Marres SL, et al: The Effect of thyroxine treatment started in the neonatal period on development and growth of two-year-old Down syndrome children: A randomized clinical trial. J Clin Endocrinol Metab 90:2204-2211, 2005.

RESOURCES FOR PARENTS AND FAMILIES

Kingsley J, Levitz M: Count Us In: Growing Up with Down Syndrome. New York, Harvest Books, 1994.

Stray-Gundersen K: Babies with Down Syndrome, 2nd ed. Bethesda, MD, Woodbine House, 1995.

RESOURCES FOR PROFESSIONALS

Down Syndrome Medical Interest Group (DSMIG US). For more information on DSMIG, contact William I. Cohen, MD, at Children's Hospital of Pittsburgh, 3705 Fifth Avenue, Pittsburgh, PA 15213, 412-692-7963; email: cohenwi@upmc.edu.

Down Syndrome Quarterly is a multidisciplinary journal that began publication in 1996. It is now published by the Down Syndrome Research Foundation in Vancouver, British Columbia. For more information, contact Jo Mills, Editor, at jo@dsrf.org, or write to *Down Syndrome Quarterly,* 1409 Sperling Avenue, Burnaby, British Columbia, Canada V5B 4J8.

Down Syndrome: Research and Practice is an international research journal for original research papers on the development, therapeutic, and educational needs of persons with Down syndrome and papers that evaluate interventions and professional practice. Available at: http://www.down-syndrome.org/research-practice/.

INTERNET RESOURCES

Down Syndrome: Health Issues. This comprehensive, award-winning site includes abundant information about Down syndrome, lists of Down syndrome clinics, and abstracts. http://www.ds-health.com/.

Growth Charts for Children with Down Syndrome. www.growthcharts.com.

Transition Planning tool. http://transition.uclid.org.

National Down Syndrome Society. http://www1.ndss.org/. Telephone: 1-800-221-4602.

National Down Syndrome Congress. http://www.ndsccenter.org/. Telephone: 1-800-232-NDSC.

Down Syndrome Research Foundation. http://www.dsrf.org.

Canadian Down Syndrome Society. http://www.cdss.ca/.

Down Syndrome Research and Treatment Foundation. http://www.dsrtf.org/.

26 GENETIC SYNDROMES AND DYSMORPHOLOGY

VIRGINIA KENT PROUD AND ELLEN ROY ELIAS

Developmental problems are characteristic of many different genetic conditions and syndromes. This chapter reviews the genetic disorders that are typical of different mechanisms of inheritance: syndromes caused by abnormalities in neighboring "contiguous" genes and disorders inherited by mendelian inheritance patterns. Autosomal dominant describes a mechanism of genetic inheritance with a 50/50 chance of occurrence in offspring that can appear sporadically with advanced paternal age. Autosomal recessive describes a mechanism of genetic inheritance with a 25% recurrence risk; it is the genetic mechanism of most metabolic disorders and some rare dysmorphic syndromes. X-linked conditions are important particularly in the context of developmental and intellectual disability. There are several hundred different X-linked forms of intellectual disability, and mapping is beginning to clarify the underlying cause of these conditions. The most common of these, fragile X syndrome, is further described in Chapter 24.

Molecular studies provide high diagnostic accuracy to confirm many of these disorders. It is often possible to predict the phenotype on the basis of specific DNA changes, known as genotype-phenotype correlation. Multifactorial conditions include those caused by multiple genes and environmental factors. Many types of developmental disabilities are due to this form of inheritance. Knowledge about an underlying genetic condition can facilitate prevention, such as preconception treatment with diet or vitamins in future pregnancies of mothers who have phenylketonuria. Finally, teratogenic mechanisms play a role in causing a significant number of developmental disabilities. Clearly, environmental factors and underlying genetic tendencies combine to affect brain formation and function from early in embryonic life throughout childhood. The natural history of these many conditions reflects a changing phenotype with age. Management of most disorders is multidisciplinary, including medical genetics, pediatrics, and developmental. A greater understanding of genetic and molecular mechanisms is beginning to allow us to better understand the etiology and management of many developmental disorders.

CHROMOSOMAL CONTIGUOUS GENE SYNDROMES

Angelman Syndrome

Angelman syndrome was initially described as "happy puppet" syndrome in 1965 in individuals with happy demeanor and awkward movements with truncal ataxia. Children with Angelman syndrome present with initial hypotonia, progressive hypertonia, and microcephaly (Fig. 26-1). Other problems include failure to thrive, mild facial dysmorphism consisting of a broad mouth and open expression with drooling, and facial hypotonia. Neurologic problems include tremor, abnormal electroencephalographic patterns, seizures, and ataxia. Angelman syndrome is a contiguous gene syndrome localized at 15q11.2-q13 due to mutation, deletion, or imprinting of the gene *UBE3A*. The incidence is between 1 in 12,000 and 1 in 20,000 live births. Because of neurologic problems and developmental delay, reproduction is limited. The mechanism for development of Angelman syndrome is based on methylation of parent-specific DNA imprints in the 15q11.2-q13 region. Specific DNA methylation testing may detect 70% to 80%, including those with a larger cytogenetic deletion or a smaller FISH deletion. As in Prader-Willi syndrome, gene imbalance in this region also occurs by uniparental disomy imprinting gene defects. In each of these mechanisms, the clinical result is due to the loss of the maternal contribution to genes expressed in the region, either maternal deletion or paternal disomy. In addition, *UBE3A* sequence analysis may detect up to 10% of individuals with a specific mutation. For an additional 10%, the mechanisms are unclear and may result from imprinting changes, for which no diagnostic testing is currently possible.

Developmental issues include neonatal hypotonia, progressive hypertonia, movement disorders with ataxia, seizures, gross motor and fine motor delay, and speech delay. Frequently, the developmental quotient is less than 50. There is often tremor, awkward gait, excessive laughter, and absent speech. Autism has been described

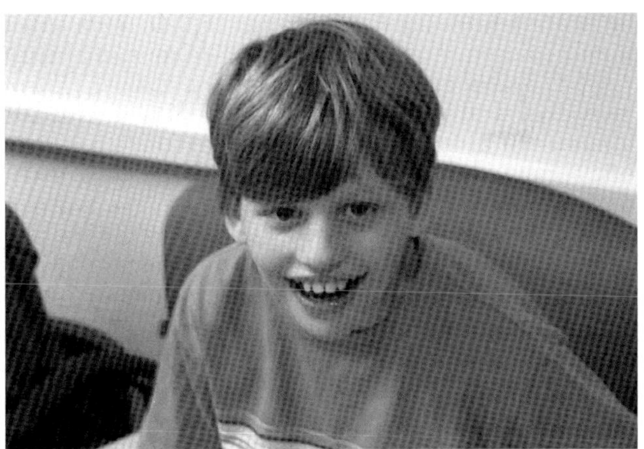

Figure 26-1. Angelman syndrome, 10-year-old boy.

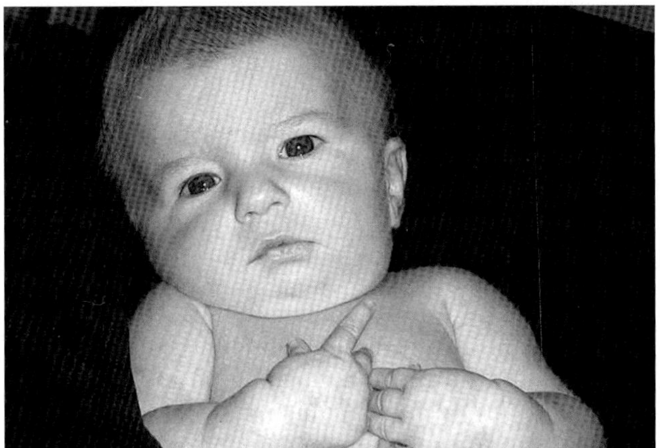

Figure 26-2. Prader-Willi syndrome, 8-week-old boy.

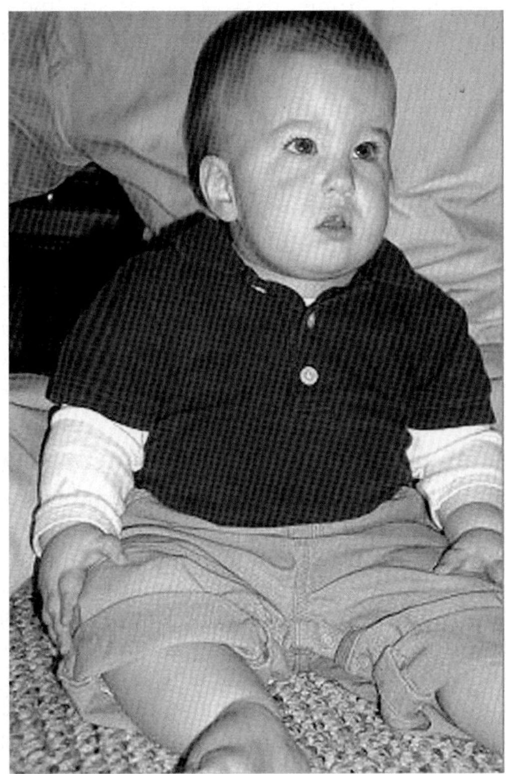

Figure 26-3. Prader-Willi syndrome, 1-year-old boy.

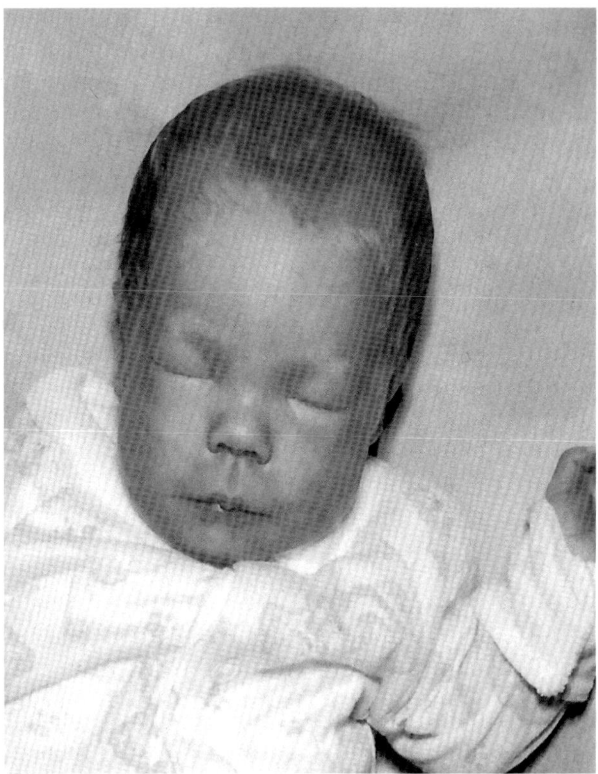

Figure 26-4. Prader-Willi syndrome, 2-week-old girl.

commonly in children with Angelman syndrome. More recent mutations in the *MECP2* gene at Xq28 (the gene for Rett syndrome) can modify imprinting of the gene *UBE3A* at 15q11 and cause clinical autism in some individuals with Angelman syndrome. This may be one of the first descriptions of two genetic syndromes in which a mutation in one gene, such as in *MECP2,* which normally would result in a different disorder called Rett syndrome, modifies the expression of another gene, namely, *UBE3A,* such that children with Angelman syndrome present with autism because of the interaction between these two genes.

Management guidelines include a multidisciplinary approach with specialists in nutrition, neurology, child development, endocrinology, and audiology. There is a support group, Angelman Syndrome Foundation, *www.angelman.org*, in addition to the American Epilepsy Society, *www.aesnet.org*.

Prader-Willi Syndrome

In 1956, Prader, Labhart, and Willi characterized the unique clinical natural history of neonatal hypotonia, failure to thrive, onset of hyperphagia at 2 to 3 years of age, developmental delay, short stature, characteristic facies with tall forehead and bitemporal narrowing, "almond-shaped" eyes, scoliosis, small hands and feet with tapered fingers, hypothalamic hypogonadism, delayed puberty, and often morbid obesity by midchildhood (Figs. 26-2 to 26-6). Prader-Willi syndrome is localized to 15q11.2, the Prader-Willi critical region, an imprinted region. The incidence of Prader-Willi

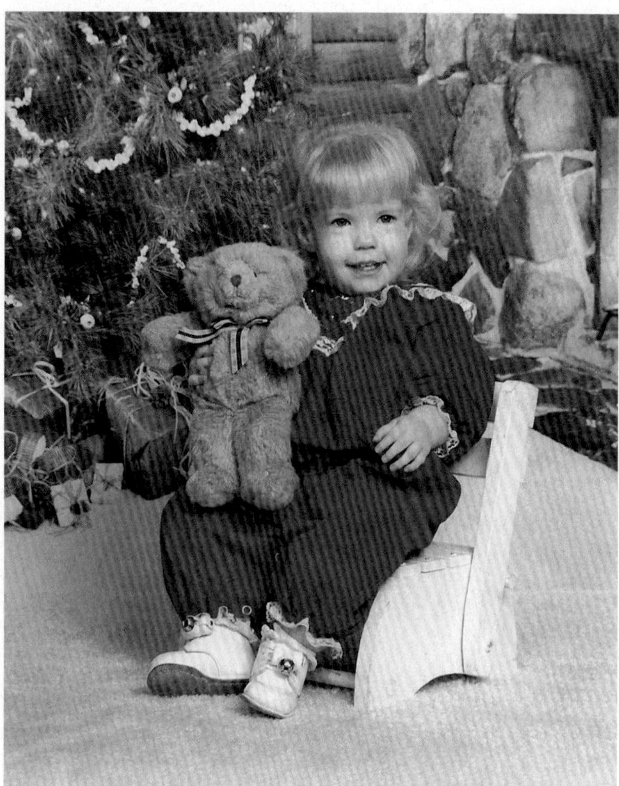

Figure 26-5. Prader-Willi syndrome, 2-year-old girl.

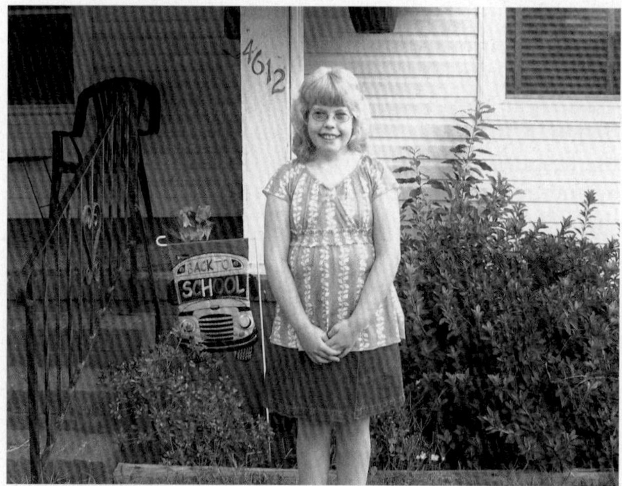

Figure 26-6. Prader-Willi syndrome, 11-year-old girl.

syndrome is between 1 in 10,000 and 1 in 25,000 births. It occurs on a sporadic nonmendelian basis, and occurrence in offspring is rare because affected individuals, both male and female, are frequently hypogonadic. There are a number of genetic mechanisms that can explain imbalance at the 15q11.2 region. Deletion of a paternal chromosome at 15q11.2 was first identified and occurs in approximately 50% of patients. For 20% of individuals, there is no visible cytogenetic deletion, but molecular deletion of the paternal 15q11.2 is identified by fluorescent in situ hybridization (FISH). With either the chromosomal or molecular FISH deletion, the recurrence to a sibling is less than 1%. An additional 25% of individuals will present with Prader-Willi syndrome due to maternal disomy at 15q11.2, frequently due to meiotic nondisjunction followed by trisomic rescue. Again, recurrence risk is less than 1%. Finally, a few individuals with Prader-Willi syndrome have an imprinting mutation that modifies the expression of the entire region. Those individuals with an imprinting gene mutation are at the highest risk of having another child, between 25% and 50% recurrence risk in a subsequent pregnancy.

Developmental issues in children with Prader-Willi syndrome focus primarily on the profound hypotonia with gross motor, fine motor, and speech delays. Additional problems occur because of the hyperphagia that generally may begin in the second year and that can be controlled with behavioral management. Temper tantrums, stubbornness, and obsessive-compulsive disorder suggest a distinctive behavioral phenotype in older children. Although the disorder Angelman syndrome is localized to the same chromosomal region and some individuals with Prader-Willi syndrome do have autism spectrum disorders, the incidence of autism spectrum disorders in Prader-Willi syndrome is much less than in Angelman syndrome.

Management guidelines were modified dramatically in 1996 because intervention with engineered human growth hormone beginning as early as 2 months of age has permitted optimization of growth and lean body mass into adulthood. In addition to modification of the food intake with close behavioral and nutritional support, growth hormone can enable normal or almost normal weight gain. It is clear that individuals with Prader-Willi syndrome have a decreased metabolic rate, so optimum calories between 3 and 4 years of age are no more than 8 to 10 kcal per centimeter of height. Other important medical issues include monitoring for osteoporosis with bone densitometry and clinical monitoring for scoliosis. Endocrine follow-up and treatment of growth, osteoporosis, and hypogonadism can significantly improve quality of life for these children. Unfortunately, there have been reports of sudden death after growth hormone treatment, so careful multidisciplinary monitoring is critical. Diabetes can occur because of the obesity and even from growth hormone treatment.

A support group, Prader-Willi Syndrome Association in America, can be found at *www.pwsausa.org*.

Williams Syndrome (Williams-Beuren Syndrome)

Williams syndrome (WBS) in children with elfin facies, neonatal hypercalcemia, and supravalvular aortic stenosis was initially described by Joseph and Parrott in 1958 and later by Williams and colleagues (1961) and Beuren and colleagues (1962), who characterized a unique facial gestalt with intellectual disability and supravalvular aortic stenosis. Clinical features include intrauterine growth restriction, microcephaly, neonatal hypercalcemia and hypercalciuria, dysmorphic facies with periorbital puffiness, stellate irides, and cardiac murmur (classically supravalvular aortic stenosis). Failure to thrive, short stature, hypotonia, joint laxity, hernias, and gastroesophageal reflux are common. Because this condition, in part, is due to an elastin arteriopathy, any arteries may have narrowing, such as renal or peripheral pulmonic vessels. In addition, other connective tissue manifestations include hoarseness of the voice, hernias, lax joints, and stretchy skin. The natural history of WBS includes in utero growth delay with microcephaly and neonatal cardiac defect with facial dysmorphism, hypercalcemia, and hypercalciuria. In infancy, failure to thrive, developmental delays, and short stature become apparent. Medical problems in childhood include hernias requiring surgery, endocrinopathies (particularly hypothyroidism and growth hormone deficiency as well as diabetes mellitus), and presentation of precocious puberty and hypertension in late childhood. By adolescence, hypertension may progress, as does high-frequency sensorineural hearing loss; and by adulthood, renal failure may become apparent.

The incidence is approximately 1 in 20,000 live births. WBS is due to a chromosomal microdeletion at 7q11.2 in the Williams-Beuren syndrome critical region. This may be a cytogenetic deletion that is visible on high-resolution banded chromosomes or detected only with a molecular FISH probe of the elastin (*ELN*) gene, found in 99% of patients with WBS. Another gene frequently deleted is *LMK1,* associated with developmental problems. WBS can be diagnosed prenatally by interphase FISH deletion of *ELN1* or *LMK1*. WBS FISH probes are included in comparative genomic hybridization (CGH) targeted arrays. As a contiguous gene syndrome, it is usually sporadic. However, autosomal dominant inheritance of isolated supravalvular aortic stenosis or "supravalvular aortic stenosis–plus" has been reported as inherited microdeletion of *ELN*. Except in these familial cases, individuals may have limited reproductive potential. There have been rare cases of siblings, but not parents, affected, more likely as a result of germline mosaicism.

Developmentally, children with WBS present in the neonatal period primarily with hypotonia and failure to thrive. Gross motor delay with walking by 2 years of age and fine motor delay become apparent in the second year. Characteristically, there is a unique, "loquacious" personality with good verbal and language skills but unique learning disabilities with visual and motor problems, hyperacusis, and strong verbal short-term memory. Although intellectual disability may be present in 75%, it is usually mild.

Management guidelines include initial cardiac evaluation together with monitoring of serum and urine calcium concentrations. It may be necessary to modify calcium intake. Periodic monitoring of thyroid and growth factors as well as ophthalmologic evaluation is indicated. Support groups include the Williams Syndrome Association at *www.williams-syndrome.org* and the Williams Syndrome Foundation at *www.wsf.org*.

Deletion 22q11.2

Deletion 22q11.2 was initially reported as DiGeorge syndrome, a multiple congenital anomaly syndrome due to abnormalities of derivatives of the third and fourth pharyngeal pouches. This contiguous gene syndrome now also includes velocardiofacial syndrome, Shprintzen syndrome, and CATCH22. DiGeorge in 1968 described a child with hypoparathyroidism and cellular immune deficiencies secondary to thymic hypoplasia. Dysmorphism in infants includes relatively wide-set eyes, flat nasal bridge, small chin, and small low-set posteriorly rotated ears. Shprintzen and colleagues in 1978 described children with speech delay, cleft palate or velopharyngeal incompetence, and congenital heart defects and adults with deep-set eyes and narrow face with a relatively long nose with prominent bridge. Clinical features of deletion 22q11.2 syndrome include growth delay, conotruncal cardiac defects (tetralogy of Fallot, interrupted aortic arch, ventricular septal defect, and truncus arteriosus), velopharyngeal incompetence and other palatal abnormalities with a characteristic facies, learning problems in 70% to 90%, hypocalcemia in 50%, and immune deficiencies in 77%. The natural history evolves from infancy, when a number of children succumb to cardiac malformations or immune deficiency complicated by calcium deficiency. It is thought that there is complete penetrance but widely variable expression even among affected family members who have the autosomal dominant deletion. The current estimate of incidence is approximately 1 in 6000 live births, with as many as 10% of cases being familial. The contiguous gene deletion at chromosome 22q11.2 may be either cytogenetic or molecular. Cytogenetic deletions of 22q11.2 at the DiGeorge syndrome critical region can also be demonstrated with a commercial FISH probe in approximately 95% of individuals. The majority are de novo, but between 7% and 10% may be inherited as an autosomal dominant trait. In approximately 3% to 5% of cases, however, individuals with the phenotype are not found to have the deletion, and additional loci, particularly at 10p13, have been described. For individuals who do not have a deletion at either locus, mutations in the gene *TBX1* have been found in research testing.

Developmental issues vary widely. Some children manifest significant developmental delay from early infancy. In others, more mild language delay may be due to eustachian tube dysfunction and chronic infections causing conductive hearing loss. Eighty percent of individuals with 22q11.2 deletion have an IQ of less than 80, with autism spectrum disorders occurring in as many as 20%. The majority of individuals will have some form of learning problems. Behavioral-psychiatric disorders, particularly bipolar disorder, attention deficit disorder, and attention-deficit/hyperactivity disorder, are common.

Management guidelines include collaboration among specialists in medical genetics, clinical pharmacology and therapeutics, child development, cardiology, and speech pathology. Cardiac evaluation with echocardiography, immune evaluation of absolute lymphocyte count with T- and B-cell subsets and humoral immune response, and measurement of ionized serum calcium to evaluate for hypoparathyroidism should occur with the initial diagnosis. Speech and language as well as feeding evaluations, renal ultrasonography, and skeletal survey looking for evidence of vertebral anomalies should also be done. Behavioral and learning problems need to be identified and treated. Support groups include The International 22q11.2 Deletion Syndrome Foundation at *www.22q.org* and the Velo-Cardio-Facial Syndrome Educational Foundation at *www.vcfsef.org*.

Smith-Magenis Syndrome

Smith-Magenis syndrome is also known as 17p deletion syndrome. This condition was first described by Smith and colleagues in 1982, and the chromosomal interstitial deletion was identified in 1986 at chromosome 17(p11.2 to p11.2). Clinical features include characteristic behavioral issues, mild to moderate intellectual disability, and developmental delay. Unique sleep disturbances are described as reverse circadian rhythm. There are distinctive facial features including a square face with broad brows, deep-set eyes, and thick, everted, tented upper lip. Many infants have failure to thrive, short stature, and hearing loss but with a normal head circumference in 80%. A characteristic hoarse voice has also been described. There is an evolution of the phenotype with age. Infants are often passive. In childhood, eye, gastrointestinal, and hearing problems become apparent. By adulthood, attenuation of the behavioral problems and a normal lifespan may be expected. Epidemiology suggests that approximately 1 in 25,000 individuals may have Smith-Magenis syndrome, and more than 100 individuals have been described worldwide. Like other contiguous gene syndromes, most of these are sporadic events, although testing of parental blood is still recommended because of the possibility of an inherited rearrangement. Children from many different ethnic groups have been described for this particular disorder. Chromosomal localization of the contiguous gene deletion on chromosome 17 at p11.2 is characteristic. Seventy percent of affected individuals have a common deletion that can be detected by high-resolution banded chromosomes. FISH with a DNA-specific probe or targeted CGH array detects approximately 95% of affected individuals. Sequencing analysis of the *RAI1* gene may identify a mutation in the remaining 5%. Some of the clinical features that have been attributed to this disorder are due to haploinsufficiency of genes in this region, and primary features have been attributed to the retinoic acid–induced gene (*RAI1*).

Developmental issues include sleep disturbances and self-injurious behaviors, which are the hallmarks of Smith-Magenis syndrome. Head banging, sensory integration issues, inattention with tantrums, and other maladaptive behaviors in the context of short stature, short fingers or brachydactyly, and mild to moderate intellectual disability frequently will suggest the diagnosis. Many children need specific therapeutic management of the sleep disturbance. Communication systems including augmentative communication and sign language may be helpful to modify the behavior. In polysomnographic studies, there has been demonstrated a decrease in rapid eye movement (REM) sleep in children with Smith-Magenis syndrome. Erratic melatonin secretion has been documented.

Management guidelines include renal ultrasonography, echocardiography, spinal radiography, immunoglobulin determinations particularly looking for evidence of immunoglobulin A deficiency, fasting lipid levels, and thyroid function. Nutritional evaluation and otolaryngologic consultation are frequently helpful. Developmental and psychological services can be most valuable in these children. A support group, Parents and Researchers Interested in Smith-Magenis Syndrome, can be found at *www.smithmagenis.org*.

Duplications in the 17p11.2 critical region have also been reported and may be expressed in children with short stature, attention deficit disorder, attention-deficit/hyperactivity disorder, and autistic-like features as well as developmental delay and intellectual disability. Many times, the duplications are discovered fortuitously in the course of evaluation for Smith-Magenis syndrome. Just as with deletion or duplication at 15q11.2, there may be additional information coming from research looking at the effect of modifying genes, and additional information about duplications in this region and association with autism may be forthcoming.

MENDELIAN GENETIC SYNDROMES AND CONDITIONS

Autosomal Dominant

Neurofibromatosis Type I

Neurofibromatosis (von Recklinghausen neurofibromatosis or NF1) was described by Crowe and associates (1956) in individuals who had at least six café au lait spots of more than 1.5 cm in diameter. Howell and Ford (1980) described an individual who was thought to have NF1 in the popular book *The Elephant Man*. It is very important to acknowledge that Joseph Merrill probably had a totally different disorder called Proteus syndrome. National Institutes of Health clinical guidelines for diagnosis of NF1 include at least two of the following: (1) six café au lait spots of more than 5 mm in diameter, (2) axillary or inguinal freckling, (3) Lisch nodules (hamartomatous tufts of pigment on the iris) in individuals older than 10 years, (4) optic glioma, (5) bony pseudarthrosis (particularly the tibia), (6) skin neurofibromas or a plexiform neurofibroma of the subcutaneous tissues, and (7) first-degree relative with neurofibromatosis.

Infants may have a few café au lait spots, but by 3 years of age, axillary and inguinal freckling becomes more common. Median age at onset of optic gliomas is 4 years, and Lisch nodules and neurofibromas may not appear until after adolescence. Scoliosis may require surgery in adolescence, and pain and paresthesias from neurofibromas become a primary problem in early adulthood. There are no current standard treatments of neurofibromatosis, but many clinical studies are under way to evaluate treatment protocols. Neurofibromatosis occurs in all populations at an incidence of approximately 1 in 3500 live births. Fifty percent of cases appear to be new mutations, but that may be difficult to determine without mutation analysis of the gene (*NF1*) at 17q11.2 that codes for neurofibrin, a tumor suppressor protein. Most disease is thought to be due to a constitutional mutation resulting in truncation of the neurofibrin protein. This protein is a critical substrate in many important signaling pathways, and deficient protein results in insufficient tumor suppressors. At this time, there is limited genotype-phenotype correlation; however, DNA testing to identify a mutation or large deletion in an affected family member can by beneficial in prenatal diagnosis, when there is a 50% recurrence risk.

Developmental manifestations show a wide variability of phenotypic expression. Twenty-five percent to 50% of patients with NF1 may have learning disabilities, and 5% to 10% have intellectual disabilities. Some neurologic and developmental problems are specifically related to the degree of central nervous system involvement with tumors; but even in individuals with no identifiable central nervous system abnormalities, there is an increased likelihood of learning problems.

The National Institutes of Health consensus management guidelines include monitoring for tumors, especially optic glioma in a young child, by ophthalmologic examination and diagnostic imaging studies. Monitoring of children for hypertension due to renal arterial dysplasia can be critical. Multidisciplinary follow-up of children by specialists in pediatrics, neurology, and orthopedics and developmental specialists is recommended. When to perform brain magnetic resonance imaging needs to depend on the neurologic examination findings and reported symptoms. Teachers, therapists, and early infant evaluation and therapy are indicated on an individual basis. Support groups include The Children's Tumor Foundation at *www.ctf.org* and Neurofibromatosis, Inc., at *www.nfinc.org*.

Marfan Syndrome

Marfan syndrome (type 1) includes a group of connective tissue disorders predominantly due to fibrillin 1 abnormalities. Marfan (1896) described the first classic patients; Boerger (1914) first noted ectopia lentis; and McKusick (1956) delineated cardiovascular complications. Fibrillin 1 is a protein found in almost every tissue. Mutations in the gene *FBN1* include cardiovascular, skeletal, and eye manifestations. Other tissues frequently involved are the skin, lungs, and dura of the central nervous system. Classic features of Marfan syndrome type 1 include dilation or dissection in the aorta at the level of the sinus of Valsalva, myopia with ectopia lentis, scoliosis with pectus excavatum or carinatum, arachnodactyly of the fingers and toes, spontaneous pneumothorax, dural ectasia, and striae or stretch marks of the skin. Other typical skeletal manifestations include disproportionate stature with an upper/lower segment ratio of less than 0.86 and a facial gestalt with a long narrow face, high arched palate, and crowded teeth. The phenotype evolves with age so that infants may have only skeletal or cardiac findings; toddlers may have a characteristic facial gestalt, myopia, and stretchy skin; and a 5-year-old may have mitral valve prolapse and lax joints. In contrast, a 14-year-old first diagnosed with a fibrillinopathy may present with only mildly disproportionate but not necessarily tall stature, spontaneous pneumothorax, pectus excavatum, mildly dilated aortic outlet, and high myopia. In adults who have not been previously recognized, fibrillinopathy may present as spontaneous ruptured thoracic aorta, dislocated lens, glaucoma, cataracts, arthritis, varicosities, and life-threatening complications in pregnancy. The incidence of type 1 fibrillinopathies is approximately 1 in 5000 to 10,000 with no ethnic, geographic, or gender preference. The gene, *FBN1,* is located at 15q11.2 and codes for the elastin protein fibrillin 1. A mutation in *FBN1* is found by sequencing in approximately 93% of individuals who have clinical findings of Marfan syndrome type 1. Marfan syndrome type 2, also called Loeys-Dietz syndrome, has recently been described to be due to mutations in transforming growth factor-beta receptor 2. Often, these patients have additional manifestations, such as craniosynostosis, hypertelorism, and congenital heart malformations. Congenital Marfan syndrome presents in the first 6 months of life. Loss of the central coding region for the protein appears to result in this more severe and potentially life-threatening form of the disorder, whereas errors in C-terminal processing primarily cause only skeletal manifestations.

Developmental issues do not usually play a major role in individuals with classic Marfan syndrome. The majority have normal intelligence with no more than the population incidence of learning disabilities, attention-deficit/hyperactivity disorder, and seizures. However, visual problems and fine motor issues due to joint laxity and arachnodactyly are often seen. It is very important to differentiate Marfan syndrome from a metabolic phenocopy, homocystinuria, which may have many similar skin and skeletal manifestations as well as dislocated lenses but is commonly found with learning disabilities, attention-deficit/hyperactivity disorder, and intellectual disability. This disorder is due to deficient conversion of homocystine by the enzyme cystathionine beta-synthetase, resulting in a buildup of methionine that may be detected on newborn screening. Importantly, homocystinuria may be treated in part with diet and vitamin therapy.

As with most genetic disorders involving proteins that affect multiple organ systems, a multidisciplinary approach is necessary for management of Marfan syndrome type 1. The American Academy of Pediatrics guidelines recommend cardiac evaluation of all individuals because early treatment with beta-blockers, losartan, and early prophylactic surgery can be lifesaving. Treatment with losartan has been shown to decrease the aortic root dilation. Recommendations for subacute bacterial endocarditis prophylaxis have recently been revised by the American Heart Association (2007). Monitoring ophthalmologically can minimize complications due to lens dislocation. Children and young adults must be monitored closely with regard to sports, eye surgery (such as Lasix surgery), and use of cardiac stimulants even in over-the-counter cold preparations.

The fibrillinopathies must be differentiated between Marfan syndrome type 1 with *FBN1* mutations and Marfan syndrome type 2 with transforming growth factor-beta 2 receptor mutations because they are different disorders with at times a similar phenotype. The support group is The National Marfan Syndrome Foundation, *www.marfan.org,* which sponsors both clinical and research studies, or The Canadian Marfan Association, *www.marfan.ca*.

Achondroplasia

Achondroplasia is one of the classic "short limb, short stature (dwarfism)" conditions. It was first described in ancient Egypt around 4500 BCE and in Ecuador around 500 BCE. The Greek derivative *achondroplasia* means "without cartilage formation." In 1994, Rousseau and colleagues described a unique mutation in the gene for fibroblast growth factor receptor 3 (*FGFR3*) as the primary cause of achondroplasia. Clinical features include short stature and rhizomelic (proximal) shortening of the arms and legs. In infancy, there are redundant skin folds over the long bones, lax hyperextensible joints, trident configuration of the fingers, bowed legs, and a thoracolumbar gibbus. Exaggerated lordosis is noted as the child begins walking by 2 to 3 years of age. Individuals with achondroplasia have absolute macrocephaly, frontal bossing with a prominent anterior fontanelle, and flat nasal bridge. There is an evolution of phenotype with fetal age, with normal growth and skeletal proportions for the first 20 weeks of intrauterine life, but disproportionate short stature often becomes apparent with bowed femurs by 30 to 33 weeks. Diagnosis may be suggested on prenatal ultrasound examination and confirmed by finding the *FGFR3* common mutation by amniocentesis. At delivery, the infant is usually well grown, although disproportionate stature can be identified with an upper to lower head to pubic bone/pubic bone to heel ratio greater than 2 (normal in a term infant is 1.65). Special growth curves for achondroplasia are helpful for monitoring stature. In the first 12 months, the gibbus in the lumbar region becomes more apparent, and in the first 2 years, low muscle tone combined with lax joints and shortened bones contribute to "apparent" gross motor delay. With the flat nasal bridge and midface hypoplasia, there is often eustachian tube dysfunction, leading to recurrent otitis media and conductive hearing loss. This can have an impact on speech development. A narrow foramen magnum can cause communicating hydrocephalus within the first year of life. Placement of a ventriculoperitoneal shunt and even foramen magnum decompression may be necessary in severe cases. By 4 years of age, like their peers, most individuals with achondroplasia have attained motor milestones, and no specific cognitive delay is expected. By 7 to 10 years of age, obesity can become a major issue complicating orthopedic deformities, especially genu valgum. By midadolescence and early teenage years, lumbar spinal stenosis and psychological issues about body image must be addressed. Limb lengthening procedures are appropriate for some teens.

The incidence of achondroplasia is between 1 in 15,000 and 1 in 40,000 live births. The *FGFR3* gene is at chromosome 4p16.3. One specific mutation occurs in 98% of affected individuals (a G380R substitution in nucleotide 1138). Hypochondroplasia, a milder variant, is due to other mutations in the *FGFR3* gene that permit better cartilage growth. Frequently, achondroplasia is sporadic and may be associated with advanced paternal age. Homozygous mutations are lethal in utero or in early infancy. Although most children with achondroplasia are cognitively normal, developmental issues may be seen. Lax joints and low muscle tone contribute to early apparent gross motor developmental delay. In addition, hydrocephalus due to narrowing at the foramen magnum may lead to more generalized delays. Short broad hands and lax joints often contribute to initial fine motor delays, and recurrent otitis media due to eustachian tube dysfunction leads to chronic hearing loss and can affect speech development. Psychological problems stemming from body image issues complicated by neurologic and musculoskeletal problems need to be addressed.

Management guidelines include prenatal genetic counseling, with chorionic villus sampling, amniocentesis, or cord blood sampling for mutation analysis if identification is made by ultrasound examination early or if one of the parents has achondroplasia. A genetic skeletal survey in the newborn period often can confirm a clinical diagnosis. Because up to 4% of individuals with achondroplasia may die in the first year of a combination of obstructive and central apnea, early computed tomography of the brain and measurement of the foramen magnum with follow-up magnetic resonance imaging and sleep study are recommended by 6 months of age or earlier, depending on clinical symptoms such as snoring, nighttime apnea, and extensor posturing. Audiologic evaluation is repeated by 6 months, and aggressive treatment of recurrent otitis media and neurosurgical, orthopedic, and pulmonary problems is performed as needed. Support groups include the Human Growth Foundation at *www.hgfound.org*, Little People of America at *www.lpaonline.org*, and The Magic Foundation at *www.magicfoundation.org*.

Autosomal Recessive

Metabolic disorders are covered extensively in Chapter 30.

Fanconi Anemia

Fanconi anemia (Fanconi pancytopenia) was first described in 1927 in Germany in a child with growth delay, mild dysmorphism, and bone marrow dysplasia. The clinical features affect heart, kidney, bone, and skin. Bone marrow failure may present with myelodysplastic syndromes, acute myelogenous leukemia, and solid tumors in infancy or aplastic anemia in adulthood. Affected individuals have an inordinate toxic reaction to chemotherapy or radiation therapy, and the chance of malignant change is approximately 25%. By 40 years of age, up to 80% of individuals may experience bone marrow failure. There are many different phenotypes due to different genes and different mutations. The in utero manifestation may resemble VACTERL association (*V*ertebral anomalies, imperforate *A*nus, *C*ardiac, *T*racheo-*E*sophageal fistula, *R*enal, and *L*imb). In early childhood, there may be short stature with myelodysplasia, hyperpigmentation, developmental delay, and characteristic facial gestalt with deep-set eyes. Adolescents or adults may present with simple myelodysplasia or malignant disease. Fanconi anemia occurs in approximately 1 in 100,000 live births with a carrier frequency for the general population in the United States, Europe, and Japan of about 1 in 300. A number of genes including *FANCA, FANCB, FANCC,* and many others have been associated with Fanconi syndrome. The gene *BRCA2* has also recently been found to be causative. Fanconi anemia is an autosomal recessive condition, and proteins produced by these genes are part of a nuclear complex involved in regulating cell cycle and DNA repair. Diagnostic testing consists of analysis of chromosomal breakage in the presence of diepoxybutane and mitomycin C in affected compared with control lymphocyte cultures. Mutation analysis of *FANCC* and sequence analysis for *FANCA, FANCC, FANCF, FANCG,* and *BRCA2* can be used for evaluating carriers and prenatal diagnosis.

Developmental issues depend on the phenotype and the time at presentation. Individuals may have normal intelligence or mild to moderate developmental delay, growth delay, and short stature.

Management guidelines must be tailored to the presenting phenotype. Lifelong monitoring for bone marrow suppression, malignant neoplasms, and ionizing radiation is required to optimize growth and nutrition and to treat associated malformations. Allogeneic hematopoietic stem cell or bone marrow transplantation has been successful. The support groups include the Fanconi Anemia Research Fund at *www.fanconi.org* and International Fanconi Anemia Registry at *www.rockefeller.edu/labheads/auerbach/clinresearch.php*.

X-Linked Disorders

There are about 400 X-linked genes causing developmental problems, intellectual disability, or autism spectrum disorder. Fragile X is the most common form of an inherited intellectual disability in girls and boys and presents with clinical phenotype due to a trinucleotide expansion, in CGG, in the *FMR1* gene. This syndrome is covered in great detail in Chapter 24. Other linked genes, such as the gene for Rett syndrome and the *UBE3A* that causes Angelman syndrome, have recently been described to modify imprinting of other genes.

Rett Syndrome

Rett syndrome ("Classic Rett syndrome") occurs in females, whereas "variant or atypical Rett syndrome" and a pattern of "neonatal encephalopathy with mental retardation" occur in males. Clinical features of the "classic form" in females include acquired microcephaly, dysfunctional handwashing movements, and seizures by 3 years of age in 90%. There is an evolution of the phenotype with normal birth parameters and development for the first 6 to 9 months, failure of developmental progress between 9 and 16 months with a potential for seizures, and progression to acquired microcephaly, dysfunctional hand movements between 2 and 3 years, and autistic-like features with loss of speech, language, and social interactions between 2 and 3 years. Between 5 and 7 years of age, there is often a latent period with plateauing or potential improvements in milestones and communication. Scoliosis, growth delay, and small cold hands and feet by adolescence provide evidence for progressive deterioration of autonomic function. Individuals with variant or atypical Rett syndrome may have behavioral and cognitive impairment without the characteristic natural history. The prevalence in females is 1 in 8000 to 10,000. The gene *MECP2* (methyl CPG binding protein 2) is found at Xq28. The protein is expressed in all tissues and is a transcriptional modifier that binds with histones in the heterochromatin and modifies imprinting of other genes. Mutations are found more frequently in the sperm, perhaps explaining why it is less common in boys. It is not clear how the protein acts in the central nervous system. Mouse models and further studies of the targets of *MECP2* protein are currently under way; 99.5% of mutations are sporadic. In males, postzygotic mosaicism may permit survival, resulting in a clinical phenotype of microcephaly, seizures, and significant cognitive delay. Diagnostic testing for *MECP2* identifies mutations in 80% of classic females. Skewed X-inactivation may lead to no clinical features in those few mothers who also have the gene.

A girl with Rett syndrome may initially have normal development, although some mothers describe developmental concerns in the first 6 months. Loss of milestones, especially speech, in a well-grown little girl particularly with failure to maintain appropriate rate of head growth needs to raise the question of Rett syndrome in spite of the lack of seizures or typical handwashing movements. The dysfunctional handwashing patterns may not become apparent for several years. Frequently, these girls can communicate by sign but have minimal expressive language.

Management includes a multifactorial team; neurologic, cognitive, and behavioral manifestations all need close monitoring. Growth and sleep disturbances with intermittent hyperpnea have been described. An electrocardiogram is indicated to evaluate for long QT, which has been found to be associated with sudden death. It is also important to be aware of the possibility of the child developing scoliosis as well as autonomic dysfunction with deficiencies in sweating and temperature control. Current studies to address genotype-phenotype correlations with new mutations are found at *www.infogenetics.org*. There is an additional gene, *CDKL5*, that has been reported to also cause an atypical form of Rett syndrome with an early-onset seizure variant. New information is currently making clear that children with Angelman syndrome may have variations in the Rett syndrome gene that contribute to the autistic features in children with Angelman syndrome (see Angelman syndrome discussion earlier). A support group, International Rett Syndrome Foundation, is found at *www.rettsyndrome.org*.

Trinucleotide Expansions

Myotonic Dystrophy, Type 1 (DM1)

Myotonic dystrophy affects muscle, brain, eye, and heart. Mild DM1 expression may begin in the mid-20s with myotonia and cataracts. Classic DM1, however, presents with distal muscle weakness and wasting, myotonia, cataracts, male pattern balding, cardiac arrhythmias, and often learning problems. There is a tendency for diabetes mellitus in adults, and women have increased miscarriages and complications of labor and delivery. The most severe form, congenital DM1, presents with profound hypotonia in the newborn period, respiratory distress requiring ventilatory support, and macrocephaly; 25% may suffer neonatal death. Survivors have developmental delay or intellectual disability. Prenatally, problems include polyhydramnios and decreased fetal movement. Infants with congenital myotonic dystrophy have a significant expansion of the trinucleotide repeat in an allele inherited from the mother. Classic DM1 presents between late childhood and early adulthood, and some mild manifestations in families are often recognized only after more severely affected individuals have been identified. Prevalence is between 1 in 8000 and 1 in 10,000 live births. The gene for DM1, dystrophia myotonica protein kinase (*DMPK*), is localized on chromosome 19q13.3. Expansion of the CTG trinucleotide repeat results in inactivation or decreased function of the enzyme. This is an autosomal dominant condition and in pedigrees can be identified with anticipation because of the unstable trinucleotide repeat generally when it is inherited through the oogenesis. More than 35 CTG repeats can result in clinical manifestations, but infants with congenital myotonic dystrophy may have more than 2000 trinucleotide repeats.

Individuals with classic DM1 may have minor intellectual deficits, but individuals with congenital myotonic dystrophy who survive may have profound facial myopathy mimicking Möbius syndrome and making it difficult to assess cognitive abilities without specialized testing. Affected infants may have significant developmental delay.

Management includes multidisciplinary evaluation and follow-up including neurology, ophthalmology, cardiology, physiatry, and genetics, providing necessary physical therapy, occupational therapy, and speech services as well as psychological services as indicated. In older individuals, abnormal swallow studies may demonstrate muscle dysfunction. Support groups are found at *www.mda.org* for the Muscular Dystrophy Association or through Muscular Dystrophy Canada at *www.muscle.ca*.

SYNDROMES WITH CANCER PREDISPOSITION

Beckwith-Wiedemann Syndrome

Beckwith-Wiedemann syndrome (or exomphalos, macroglossia, gigantism syndrome) was initially described by Wiedemann in 1964 and Beckwith in 1969. Several hundred cases have been reported of this overgrowth condition with extremely variable clinical presentation. Major findings in infants include macrosomia, hemihypertrophy, macroglossia, omphalocele or umbilical anomalies, and visceromegaly including adrenocortical cytomegaly and nephromegaly. There may be unique linear ear lobule creases and pits on the edge of the auricle. It is important to identify Beckwith-Wiedemann syndrome early because of the increased risk of embryonal tumors in infancy and childhood, especially in association with hemihypertrophy. Other clinical features may include in utero polyhydramnios, prematurity, neonatal hypoglycemia, glabellar facial nevus flammeus, other hemangiomas, cardiomegaly, structural cardiac anomalies, cardiomyopathy, diastasis recti, and advanced bone age. Tumors occur in 4% to 7% and include adrenal carcinoma, Wilms tumor, gonadoblastoma, and hepatoblastoma. Even with a classic presentation in the newborn period, there is spontaneous resolution of many of the problems, the omphalocele after surgical correction, and macroglossia with time. The chromosomal localization involves an imprinted region of critical genes located on chromosome 11p15.5. Beckwith-Wiedemann syndrome is heterogeneous; 85% of cases are sporadic, but in some there is an apparent autosomal dominant inheritance with variable expressivity. In other cases, contiguous gene duplication at 11p15 results from a defect of maternal gene expression or specific mutations in the p57 (*CDKNIC*) or in the *NSD1* gene. Microdeletions including methylation of *H19* can also cause Beckwith-Wiedemann syndrome by loss of *IGF2* imprinting, as can microdeletion of the entire *LIT1* gene. Recent data suggest a possible increase in abnormalities of imprinting in pregnancies with monozygotic twining or using assisted reproductive technology, particularly intracytoplasmic sperm injection (DeBaun et al, 2003; Maher et al, 2003). Diagnostic testing including high-resolution banded karyotype, FISH, uniparental disomy, and CGH array studies may be necessary if methylation is abnormal to characterize the underlying mechanism, which is important for counseling with regard to recurrence. Diagnostic testing by methylation studies of the 11p15.5 region can identify approximately 75% of affected individuals.

Development may be compromised by hypoxemia or profound hypoglycemia in the newborn period. In most individuals with Beckwith-Wiedemann syndrome, development is normal.

Management needs to address the airway and feeding and speech problems if there is significant macroglossia. Scoliosis may be manifested in adolescence. It is important to screen for hepatoblastoma by serum alpha-fetoprotein determinations every 3 months in the first 3 years and to screen for other embryonal tumors with a complete abdominal ultrasound examination quarterly until 8 years of age.

Whereas this overgrowth condition has been described at 11p15.5 for many years, recent information has identified abnormalities in the region in as many as 30% of individuals with the short-stature condition Russell-Silver syndrome, which may also be caused by *UPD7* (see Chapter 24).

Support groups include Beckwith-Wiedemann Children's Foundation, *www.beckwith-wiedemannsyndrome.org*, and Beckwith-Wiedemann Syndrome Family Forum, *www.beckwith-wiedemann.info*.

Costello Syndrome

Costello syndrome (fasciocutaneous skeletal syndrome) is due to a germline mutation in an *HRAS* gene that normally causes cancer when it is affected by somatic mutations. Costello syndrome was initially described by Costello (1977) with "mental subnormality and nasal papillomata." Clinical features include dysmorphic facies with epicanthal folds, depressed nasal bridge, broad mouth and coarse features, normal head circumference but short stature, developmental delay, and intellectual disability with cutis laxa and deep soft creases in the palms and soles (Figs. 26-7 to 26-9). Cardiac

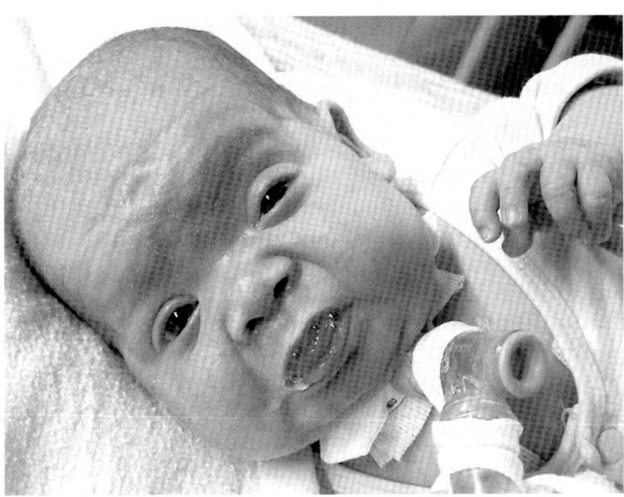

Figure 26-7. Costello syndrome, 4-month-old girl.

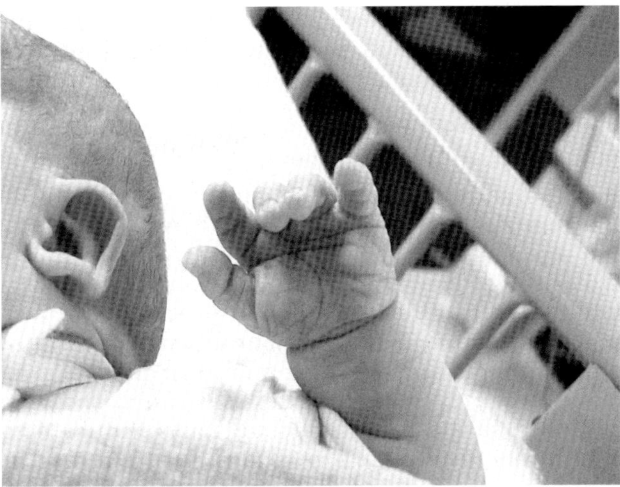

Figure 26-8. Costello syndrome, 4-month-old girl.

malformations are often complicated by dysrhythmias and hypertrophic cardiomyopathy. Benign tumors such as nasolabial, perioral, and anal papillomas are common, and malignant tumors (ganglioneuroblastoma, bladder cancer, embryonal rhabdomyosarcoma, and other malignant neoplasms) occur in up to 17% of mutation-positive cases. Individuals may present in utero with polyhydramnios, macrosomia, and occasionally cardiac arrhythmias. Infantile hypotonia and failure to thrive require gastrostomy tube placement in half of cases. In childhood, developmental delay with coarsening facial features and papillomas develop; by adolescence, short stature, intellectual disability, characteristic facies with nasolabial papillomas, and thick, coarse, darkened skin on the hands and feet are apparent. There are approximately 200 cases described worldwide with many different ethnic groups affected. The gene has been localized to chromosome 11p15.5, and two common mutations have been found in the *HRAS* gene. These two common mutations account for essentially 100% of cases. *HRAS* is expressed in the Ras/MAP kinase pathway that is also the site of germline mutations

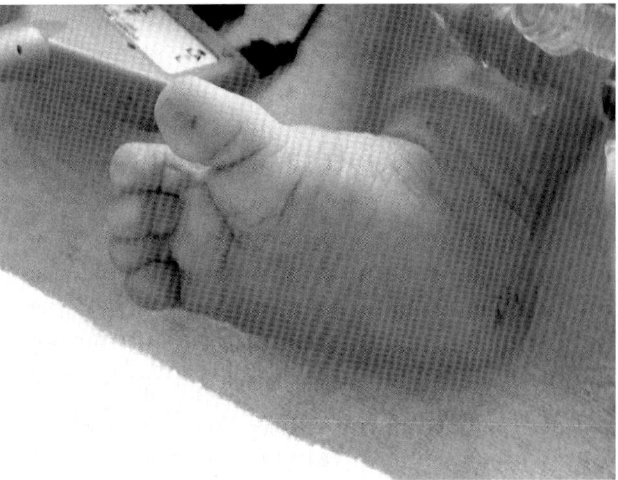

Figure 26-9. Costello syndrome, 4-month-old girl.

in two phenotypically overlapping conditions, Noonan syndrome and cardiofaciocutaneous syndrome. *HRAS* is part of the Ras signaling pathway, and mutations alter tumor suppressor functions of the pathway. Almost all cases at this time have been sporadic. Rare sibling reports are most likely due to germline mosaicism. The mechanism of rare father to son transmission of a variant Costello phenotype is unclear. Diagnostic testing is by selected mutation analysis of *HRAS*.

Developmental problems in the neonatal period include oral motor incoordination and hypotonia that frequently lead to failure to thrive. Global delay in gross and fine motor skills becomes apparent with median age of walking at 2 years and talking at 4 years. Final IQs generally are in the mild to moderate range of intellectual disability. It is notable that many infants and children with this disorder have a unique interpersonally interactive, pleasant, and engaging personality. Management includes cardiac monitoring throughout life as well as a low threshold for evaluation for malignant neoplasms. There are no clear cancer screening guidelines, but at least initial evaluation and screening, like the Beckwith-Wiedemann syndrome protocol (also due to genes localized at 11p15.5), is indicated. The Costello Syndrome Support Group is found at *www.costellokids.com*.

MULTIFACTORIAL CONDITIONS

Cleft Lip and Palate

Cleft lip with or without cleft palate is usually due to multiple genes and often unknown environmental factors. Incidence of cleft lip with or without cleft palate is 1 in 1000 live births. There are more than 500 different syndromes that may be associated with clefting. Cleft lip is more common among Asian (1.7 per 1000) and American Indian (3.6 per 1000) live births. It is less common than average in African Americans at 1 in 2500. Males are more frequently affected than are females. Cleft palate with or without cleft lip occurs in approximately 1 in 2000 births and is more common in females. Cleft palate is more likely than cleft lip to have a strongly inherited basis. Multiple genes are associated with both simple and syndromic cleft lip or cleft palate. Embryologically, the lip closes between 5 and 6 weeks and the palate by 10 weeks of gestation. Women with seizure disorders who take anticonvulsant medications have an increased risk of facial clefting, as do individuals with alcohol exposure or maternal glucose intolerance. Multifactorial recurrence for a couple with no family history and one child with cleft lip or palate is approximately 3% to 5%. This is the same as the occurrence for offspring of individuals with simple clefting. If the clefting is associated with a specific syndrome, however, the recurrence is much more difficult to predict and depends on the specific associated syndrome. For example, with autosomal dominant van der Woude syndrome, although the gene is inherited by 50% of the offspring, the specific occurrence of clefting depends on the penetrance of that gene in the family. Penetrance is calculated by comparing the number of individuals who have the gene with the members who actually have cleft lip or palate. For most multifactorial clefts in which neither parent has a cleft, the recurrence risk actually varies between 2% and 8%. Genetic testing is often unrevealing, unless there is an association with a specific condition, such as deletion 22q11.2 syndrome, Di George syndrome, needs to be considered if there appears to be a familial pattern for velopharyngeal insufficiency, especially with cardiac problems observed by history, family history, or physical examination. Testing of most children with cleft palate for deletion 22 is reasonable, and as array CGH becomes more refined and cost-effective, panels to look at syndromic or nonsyndromic clefting genes will also become more readily available.

For simple nonsyndromic clefting, developmental issues are related to speech and language complicated by palatal insufficiency and articulation. There may be additional structural malformations of the oropharynx, tongue, and lip compounded by conductive hearing loss due to eustachian tube dysfunction and chronic ear infections that compromise speech and language development.

Management is optimized by a multidisciplinary team including specialists in plastic surgery, oral surgery, dentistry, speech pathology, occupational therapy (particularly for feeding issues), genetics, and education. Support groups for children with facial clefts include Operation Smile, an international program for children with craniofacial anomalies (*www.operationsmile.org*), the Cleft Palate Foundation (*www.cleftline.org*), and the March of Dimes Birth Defects Resources at *www.marchofdimes.com*.

Congenital Heart Disease

Multiple genes have been identified for both syndromic and nonsyndromic congenital heart disease. One common gene (*VEGF*) is localized at chromosome 22q11.2/DiGeorge syndrome/deletion 22/velocardiofacial critical region. Mutations in *TBX1* in this region are also found in individuals with "conotruncal facial" syndrome with cardiac malformations. Teratogens causing congenital heart defects include maternal diabetes and alcohol. The incidence of congenital heart disease is approximately 1 in 125 live-born infants. Some children have heart defects on the basis of heart-face or heart-hand syndromes. The majority of children, however, do not have associated dysmorphic features. Genes including variations in *HRAS* or *VEGF* or *TBX1* contribute to a number of cardiac defects including hypertrophic cardiomyopathy. All children with congenital heart defects should have chromosome analysis and array CGH. Because additional loci, such as the velocardiofacial locus at chromosome 10p, are being identified, there is potential for specific array CGH for nonsyndromic or syndromic congenital heart defects.

Developmental progress is compromised by early persistent cyanosis, failure to thrive, or chronic illness. Aggressive medical and surgical management and optimization of nutrition to minimize failure to thrive will also have an impact on development. All children with congenital heart defects need to have the benefit of multidisciplinary management including specialists in pediatrics, cardiology, cardiac surgery, development, genetics, and therapies. Support groups include the March of Dimes Birth Defects Resources at *www.marchofdimes.com* and the National Organization for Rare Disorders at *www.rarediseases.org*.

CHARGE Syndrome

CHARGE syndrome (CHARGE association or Hall-Hittner syndrome) is an acronym for the combination of *c*oloboma, *h*eart anomaly, choanal *a*tresia, *r*etardation, and *g*enital and *e*ar anomalies. Clinical features include ocular coloboma that can be peripupillary, iris, retinal, macular, or nerve; choanal atresia or stenosis; cranial nerve dysfunction; and characteristic small, posteriorly rotated, cupped simple ears. It is uncommon for a child to have all manifestations of this association. The term CHARGE should be restricted to infants with at least three major malformations including choanal atresia or coloboma combined with cardinal malformations, heart, ear, and genital. Growth retardation, especially low birth weight, should not be used in the definition. The incidence of CHARGE syndrome is approximately 1 in 10,000, and gene localizations include chromosomes 8q12.1 and 7q21.1. The gene *CHD7*, chromodomain helicase DNA binding protein, at 8q21.1 is known to be associated with CHARGE syndrome, but other genes are no doubt also involved. The basic genetic mechanism, however, continues to be described as multifactorial because although the gene may be inherited in a dominant fashion, there are many other genes as well as known and unknown environmental factors that affect the expression of those genes. Diagnostic testing should include at least CGH array with high-resolution banded chromosomes, although most individuals will have normal results with these tests. Sequence analysis of *CHD7* coding region detects mutations in 60% to 65% of individuals. Large *CHD7* deletions, however, are uncommon. *CHD7* sequencing is possible and can be valuable for preconception counseling and prenatal diagnosis when the result is positive.

Most children with CHARGE association have delayed milestones and hypotonia. Development is complicated by dual sensory vision and hearing impairment as well as by vestibular dysfunction. Management in neonates requires immediate evaluation of airway, feeding, heart, and hearing. Tracheostomy or surgical correction of choanal atresia may often be necessary. Speech and language, occupational, nutrition, and physical therapies are important, and with failure to thrive, gastrostomy tube and nutrition services are critical. It is important to monitor hearing closely because children with CHARGE association can have normal IQ and be compromised by hearing and visual deficits. School and psychological services need to be provided by specialists in management of the deaf and blind. Special attention is often required for airway problems (even as older children) with anesthesia, and regular ophthalmologic and audiologic evaluations are important. Pubertal evaluation for hypogonadal hypogonadism is indicated in some children.

The support group, The CHARGE Syndrome Foundation, is at *www.chargesyndrome.org*.

Neural Tube Defects

See Chapter 74, in which particularly folic acid prevention of neural tube defects is described.

Teratogens

Fetal Alcohol Syndrome

Refer to Chapter 31.

Maternal Diabetes

There are specific effects of maternal glucose concentration and glucose intolerance that correlate with the three stages of alcohol embryopathy, depending on the timing of exposure: alcohol-related birth defects, fetal alcohol exposure, and fetal alcohol syndrome. First-trimester glucose intolerance can result in malformations, especially congenital heart defects. Maternal glucose intolerance in the second trimester can result in central nervous system, brain development, developmental, and learning issues. Third-trimester maternal glucose intolerance results in the classic infant of a gestational diabetic mother. Maternal glucose intolerance is becoming identified as a teratogen regardless of whether the mother has diabetes mellitus or is identified at 28 weeks to have gestational diabetes during gestation. Some birth defects may be due to first-trimester hypoglycemia in women with only a familial history of diabetic tendency. This can be evidently severe in infants with malformations when there is maternal obesity or genetic predisposition in a family, such as deletion 22q11.2. The Web site for the American Diabetes Association is *www.diabetes.org*.

REFERENCES

Abruzzo MA, Erickson RP: A new syndrome of cleft palate associated with coloboma, hypospadias, deafness, short stature, and radial synostosis. J Med Genet 14:76-80, 1977.

American Heart Association, Wilson S, Taubert KA, Gewitz M, et al: Prevention of infective endocarditis. Guidelines from the American Heart Association: A Guideline from the American Heart Association Rheumatic Fever, Endocarditis, and Kawasaki Disease Committee, Council on Cardiovascular Surgery and Anesthesia, and the Quality of Care and Outcomes Research Interdisciplinary Working Group. Circulation 116:1736-1754, 2007.

Angelman H: "Puppet" children: A report on three cases. Dev Med Child Neurol 7:681-688, 1965.

Beckwith JB: Macroglossia, omphalocele, adrenal cytomegaly, gigantism, and hyperplastic visceromegaly. Birth Defects Original Article Series 5(2):188, 1969.

Beuren AJ, Apitz J, Harmjanz D: Supravalvular aortic stenosis in association with mental retardation and a certain facial appearance. Circulation 26:1235-1240, 1962.

Boerger F: Ueber zwei Falle von Arachnodaktylie. Z Kinderheilk 12:161-184, 1914.

Cassidy S, Schwartz S: Prader-Willi Syndrome: Gene Tests/Gene Reviews. Seattle, University of Washington, July 12, 2006.

Costello JM: A new syndrome: Mental subnormality and nasal papillomata. Aust Paediatr J 13:114-118, 1977.

Crowe FW, Schull WJ, Neel JV: A clinical, pathological, and genetic study of multiple neurofibromatosis. Springfield, IL, Charles C Thomas Publishers, 1956.

Davenport SL, Hefner MA, Mitchell JA: The spectrum of clinical features in CHARGE syndrome. Clin Genet 29:298-310, 1986.

DeBaun MR, Niemitz EL, Feinberg AP: Association of in vitro fertilization with Beckwith-Wiedemann syndrome and epigenetic alterations of LIT1 and H19. Am J Hum Genet 72:156-160, 2003.

DiGeorge AM: Congenital absence of the thymus and its immunologic consequences: Concurrence with congenital hypoparathyroidism. Birth Defects Orig Art Ser IV:116-112, 1968.

Doyle TF, Bellugi U, Korenberg JR, et al: "Everybody in the world is my friend" hypersociability in young children with Williams syndrome. Am J Med Genet 124A:263-273, 2004.

Fanconi G: Familiäre infantile perniziosaartige Anämie. Z Kinderheilkd 117:257-280, 1972.

Howell M, Ford P: The True History of the Elephant Man. New York, Penguin, 1980.

Joseph MC, Parrott D: Severe infantile hypercalcaemia with special reference to the facies. Arch Dis Child 33:385, 1958.

Klein-Tasman BP, Mervis CB: Distinctive personality characteristics of 8, 9 and 10-year-olds with Williams syndrome. Dev Neuropsychol 23:269-290, 2003.

Loeys BL, Chen J, Neptune ER, et al: A syndrome of altered cardiovascular, craniofacial, neurocognitive and skeletal developmental abnormalities caused by mutations in TGFBR1 or TGFBR2. Nat Genet 37:275-281, 2005.

Lopez-Rangel E, Lewis M: Loud and clear evidence for gene silencing by epigenetic mechanisms in autism spectrum and related neurodevelopmental disorders. Clin Genet 69:21-22, 2006.

Maher ER, Brueton LA, Bowdin SC, et al: Beckwith-Wiedemann syndrome and assisted reproduction technology (ART). J Med Genet 40:62-64, 2003.

Marfan AB: Un cas de déformation congénitale des quatre membres, plus prononcée aux extrémités, caracterisée par l' allongement des os avec un certain degré d' aminicissement. Bulletins et memoires de la Société medicale des hôpitaux de Paris, 1896, 13:220-226, 1896.

McKusick VA: Heritable Disorders of Connective Tissue. St. Louis, CV Mosby, 1956.

Rousseau F, Bonaventure J, Legeai-Mallet L, et al: Mutations in the gene encoding fibroblast growth factor receptor-3 in achondroplasia. Nature 371:252-254, 1994.

Shprintzen RJ, Goldberg RB, Lewin ML, et al: A new syndrome involving cleft palate, cardiac anomalies, typical facies, and learning disabilities: Velo-cardio-facial syndrome. Cleft Palate J 15:56-62, 1978.

Smith ACM, McGavran L, Robinson J, et al: Interstitial deletion of (17)(p11.2p11.2) in nine patients. AJMG 24:393-414, 1986.

Smith ACM, McGavran L, Waldstein G: Deletion of the 17 short arm in two patients with facial clefts. AJHG 34(Suppl):A410, 1982.

Wiedemann HR: Complexe malformatif familial avec hernie ombilicale et macrglossie—un "syndrome nouveau." J Genet Hum 13:223-232, 1964.

Williams JCP, Barratt-Boyes BG, Lowe JB: Supravalvular aortic stenosis. Circulation 243:1311, 1961.

27 NEURODEVELOPMENTAL CONSEQUENCES OF PRETERM BIRTH: CAUSES, ASSESSMENT, AND MANAGEMENT

Mary Leppert and Marilee C. Allen

Preterm birth has become a major public health problem (Behrman and Butler, 2007). Although technologic and medical improvements in obstetric and neonatal intensive care during the 20th century dramatically improved infant survival (especially for preterm infants), preterm birth rates are rising. With no concomitant improvements in their health, neurodevelopmental, or functionaloutcomes, increasing numbers of preterm survivors strain limited health, educational, and social service resources. Multiple risk factors have been identified, but prediction of which mothers will deliver before term remains elusive. Prematurity is not a single disease, and there will be no simple solution. A paradigm shift is required that conceptualizes preterm delivery as a complex condition resulting from poorly understood mechanisms, the end result of multiple interrelated overlapping factors that vary among populations.

Immature organ systems that compromise extrauterine life are the defining characteristic of prematurity. The required physiologic, medical, and nutritional support necessary for survival can injure immature organs. Infants are born before term for a variety of reasons, including preterm labor, premature rupture of membranes, signs of fetal distress, and maternal illness. Organ injury due to factors that contribute to preterm delivery and interventions required to support extrauterine life influence the infant's health and neurodevelopment. Variations in fetal and maternal genomes account for some of the variations in the ability of a mother to sustain a pregnancy to term and of an infant's body to recover from organ injury. Continuous interactions between maternal and fetal genomes and the maternal environment and the intrauterine and extrauterine environments influence birth timing and circumstances as well as infant growth, health, neurodevelopmental, and behavioral outcomes.

Compared with children born full term, populations of children born before term have higher prevalence rates for cerebral palsy, cognitive impairment, visual impairment, strabismus, hearing loss, specific learning disabilities, attention deficit disorder, speech and language delay, executive dysfunction, working memory deficit, visual-perceptual impairment, minor neuromotor dysfunction, and fine motor difficulties (Behrman and Butler, 2007). Among children who were born before term, the proportion of survivors with cerebral palsy, cognitive impairment, school problems, specific learning disabilities, visual impairment, and multiple disabilities increases as gestational age and birth weight decrease.

Although they represent just 12% to 13% of U.S. births, preterm infants account for 64% to 75% of infant deaths, 42% to 47% of children with cerebral palsy, 27% of children with cognitive impairment, 37% of children with visual impairment, and 23% of children with hearing impairment (Alexander, 2007; Behrman and Butler, 2007; Dolk, Pattenden, and Johnson, 2001). Although infants with birth weight below 1500 g represent only 1% to 2% of U.S. births, they account for 47% of infant deaths, 22% of children with cerebral palsy, and 36% of infant hospital costs. Estimated special education costs attributed to preterm birth, beyond the cost of educating a child born full term, total $611 million per year, or $2237 per preterm survivor. The economic burden associated with preterm birth is staggering: $26.2 billion for the United States in 2005 or $51,600 per infant born before term (over the costs for a full-term infant), a conservative estimate by the Institute of Medicine (Behrman and Butler, 2007).

EPIDEMIOLOGY OF PRETERM BIRTHS

Although immaturity is the defining characteristic of prematurity, there are no reliable measures of fetal or infant maturation. The definition of prematurity has changed during the last century, from a focus on infant size (e.g., birth weight) to a more reliable indicator of immaturity, duration of pregnancy (gestational age). Preterm birth is now defined as delivery before 37 weeks of gestation (by convention, one never rounds up). Understanding the problem of prematurity requires recognition that definitions and preterm birth rates have been changing; racial, ethnic, and geographic disparities persist; and the search for etiology has widened to include studies of various genetic factors, biologic variables, environmental exposures, individual-level behaviors, and neighborhood social characteristics.

Definitions

Because of the lack of reliable indicators of gestational age or date of conception during the 19th and early 20th centuries, infants were referred to in terms of birth weight, which is easily and reliably measured. Until the 1960s, prematurity was synonymous with low birth weight (birth weight below 2500 g). Approximately one third of low-birth-weight infants are full-term infants with intrauterine growth restriction, which challenges the validity of low birth weight as a proxy for prematurity (Alexander, 2007). Although an individual infant may be both, distinguishing prematurity from intrauterine growth restriction is important in determining causes, risk factors, and health and neurodevelopmental outcomes.

Individual variation in fetal growth becomes more prominent during the third trimester. When they plotted birth weight by gestational age for their population of newborns, Battaglia and Lubchenco (1967) discovered differences in mortality and morbidity among infants who were small, appropriate, or large for gestational age. By the third trimester, many biologic and environmental factors influence fetal growth, including race or ethnicity, gender, multiple gestations, maternal drugs, environmental toxins, maternal illness, uteroplacental insufficiency, and congenital infections.

Although they are highly correlated and often thought of as interchangeable, pregnancy duration, infant size, and maturity are distinctly different concepts. There is a biologic continuum not only in birth weight for gestational age but also in degree of maturity for age or size (Allen, 2005). Just as a 12-year-old child can be tall or short for age, he or she can be more or less mature compared with other 12-year-olds. Not only may an individual infant born at 24 weeks of gestation be small, appropriate, or large for gestational age, but there is similar variation in physical and neurologic maturity for 24 weeks of gestation.

The traditional method of determining gestational age and a mother's due date (estimated date of confinement) was calculated from the first day of the mother's last menstrual period. Timing of ovulation, fertilization, and implantation has generally been unknown for the majority of women. Clinical indicators of fetal growth (e.g., fundal height) and development (e.g., detecting fetal heart tones or quickening, feeling fetal movement) could corroborate the mother's due date. The conventional definition of gestational age at birth is the time interval between the mother's last menstrual period and delivery, which includes approximately 2 weeks before conception. Wide variations in menstrual cycle timing (as much as 7 to 25 days) during a woman's childbearing years and among women account for much of the uncertainty surrounding gestational age. Even when assisted reproductive technologies precisely determine when fertilization and implantation occur, obstetricians use the traditional definition and add 2 weeks when determining gestational age.

When timing of fertilization is not known, current practice is for obstetricians to estimate gestational age by measuring the fetal size by ultrasound examination (Behrman and Butler, 2007). Because individual variation in fetal size increases with gestational age, early prenatal ultrasound examinations are more accurate than later ones, especially as late as the third trimester. Assessment of multiple measures of fetal size (e.g., crown-rump length until 12 to 14 weeks of gestation, biparietal diameter of the fetal head, femur length, sacral length, foot length, jaw size, chest circumference) improves accuracy. An early prenatal ultrasound examination provides the current clinical "gold standard" for estimating gestational age.

The major limitations of prenatal ultrasound examination for estimating gestational age are its requirement of technology and expertise, and it is most accurate when it is performed early in a pregnancy. Not all women who register for prenatal care routinely have a prenatal ultrasound examination for pregnancy dating, and prenatal care is difficult for many women at risk for preterm birth (e.g., minority or impoverished women). Postnatal assessments of gestational age are based on measurement of infant size (birth weight, length, head circumference, foot length) or degree of neurologic or physical maturity, but they are not as accurate as a prenatal ultrasound examination before 20 weeks of gestation (Allen, 2005). Comparison of different populations is problematic when method of estimating gestational age varies, especially if there is no information about methods used.

Etiologies

Preterm birth is not a disease or a syndrome but a common complex condition with multiple interrelated overlapping factors that lead to several final common pathophysiologic pathways (Behrman and Butler, 2007). Preterm birth results from multiple gene-environment interactions that involve both maternal and fetal genomes, the intrauterine environment, and the mother's body and her external environment. Among different populations, there are considerable variations in prevalence of risk factors as well as preterm birth rates. Risk factors include individual-level behavioral and psychosocial factors, neighborhood social characteristics, environmental exposures, maternal medical conditions, assisted reproductive technologies, biologic factors, and genetics. Some factors originate at or before conception. The presence of multiple risk factors is highest in women of low socioeconomic or minority status. A reflection of exposure to infection and antigens as well as maternal and fetal immune responses, inflammation appears to play an important role in one or more pathophysiologic pathways for preterm birth. Multiple gestations often result in preterm birth (i.e., 50% of twins, 90% to 100% of higher order multiples), presumably because of uterine overdistention and limitation of uteroplacental resources.

Unfortunately, differentiation of preterm births by clinical presentation raises more questions than provides answers (Alexander, 2007; Behrman and Butler, 2007). Approximately 50% of preterm infants are born after spontaneous onset of preterm labor, and another 30% to 40% are born when membranes rupture before labor (i.e., premature rupture of membranes). The proportion of infants delivered before term for maternal or fetal indications has increased to 10% to 20%, presumably because of earlier and better recognition of signs of fetal distress and maternal illness. Risk factors for spontaneous labor and premature rupture of membranes overlap (e.g., infection), as do risk factors for indicated and spontaneous preterm birth (e.g., preeclampsia, intrauterine growth restriction). The risk factors that lead to preterm labor, premature rupture of membranes, and maternal or fetal illness requiring preterm delivery are similar, but their frequency varies among different populations and by gestational age. A better understanding of specific mechanisms that lead to preterm birth would allow researchers to target prevention and treatment strategies toward more homogeneous subgroups.

Racial and Ethnic Disparities

The United States struggles with long-standing racial and ethnic disparities in preterm birth rates, infant mortality rates, distribution of gestational age at birth, and distribution of birth weight for gestational age (Alexander, 2007; Behrman and Butler, 2007). Preterm birth rates ranged from 17.8% for non-Hispanic African American, 11.9% for Hispanic, and 11.3% for non-Hispanic white mothers to 10.5% for Asian and Pacific Islander mothers in 2003. Despite decreasing preterm birth rates for African Americans and increasing preterm birth rates for white women during the last decade, African Americans continue to have higher preterm birth rates than whites do. The preterm birth rate after preterm labor decreased by 27% for African Americans while it increased by 3% for whites. Moreover, the increase in medically indicated preterm births was 32% for African Americans but as high as 55% for whites.

Race and ethnicity are classified by maternal self-report, but significant heterogeneity of each subgroup has been widely acknowledged. There is little agreement as to the extent to which racial and ethnic disparities in preterm birth rates are due to socioeconomic differences, access to care issues, racism, stress, maternal behaviors, vulnerability to infections, medical illness, exposure to environmental toxicants, or genetics.

Epidemiologic Trends in Preterm Birth and Survival

The U.S. preterm birth rate has steadily increased by 30%, from 9.7% in 1980 to 12.5% in 2004, while post-term births have decreased (Alexander, 2007; Behrman and Butler, 2007). The mean gestational age at birth decreased from 39.2 weeks in 1985-1988 to 38.8 weeks in 1995-2000. The increase was greatest in infants born at 33 to 36 weeks of gestation (8.9% of infants born from 1995 to 2000) compared with infants born before 33 weeks of gestation (2.2%) or infants born before 29 weeks of gestation (0.82%). With concomitant increases in labor induction, cesarean section (to 27.5% of births in 2003), maternal age at birth, assisted reproductive technologies, multiple gestations, and indicated preterm births as well as decreases in fetal death rates and birth rates for full-term infants with intrauterine growth restriction, the rising U.S. preterm birth rate reflects widespread medical and societal changes.

There are large geographic variations in preterm birth rates (Alexander, 2007). New England and western states have the lowest preterm birth rates (8% to 9.9%); the southeastern states and Nevada have the highest rates (>12%). Although there are widely published international comparisons of low-birth-weight birth rates, major differences in data collection and reporting make international comparisons of *preterm* birth rates problematic. Nonetheless, most developed countries report lower preterm birth rates than the United States. In 1996, when the reported U.S. preterm birth rate was 11%, it was 7.1% in Canada and 6.9% in Australia (Behrman and Butler, 2007). Differences in racial and ethnic composition of state and national populations provide only a partial explanation for these geographic differences.

Medical and technologic advances during the last few decades have dramatically lowered neonatal mortality (i.e., within 28 days from birth) and infant mortality (i.e., within 1 year from birth) rates. In the United States, dramatic decreases in gestational age–specific mortality (not changes in gestational age distribution) account for the decrease in neonatal and infant mortality rates (Alexander, 2007; Behrman and Butler, 2007). The limit of viability has been progressively lowered to 23 to 24 weeks of gestation now (with rare survival below 23 weeks of gestation). Changes in resuscitation of infants at the lower limit of viability, thereby recording them as infant deaths rather than fetal deaths, influence reported fetal and infant mortality rates. Although African American preterm infants have historically had a survival advantage (i.e., lower preterm mortality rates) over white preterm infants, this gap has narrowed. Despite their decreasing preterm birth rate, the lessening of a *preterm* infant survival advantage and the continuing high mortality for African American *full-term* infants result in higher mortality rates for all African American infants compared with all white infants.

Methodologic issues contribute to some of the disparities in birth and mortality rates (Alexander, 2007; Behrman and Butler, 2007). Countries and states have complex systems to collect and report data on births, deaths, and other indicators of public health. Persistent problems include missing data, lack of consistency in reporting (especially fetal deaths), and both systematic and random misclassifications of birth weight and gestational age data. Differing methods of calculating gestational age (e.g., from last menstrual period, best obstetric estimate, or prenatal ultrasound examinations) over time and among subgroups influence calculations of preterm birth rates, gestational age distributions, and gestational age–specific mortality rates.

Prevention and Treatment

Although medical and technologic advancements have improved infant survival, prevention of preterm birth remains problematic (Behrman and Butler, 2007).

Many randomized controlled trials of bed rest, tocolytics, antibiotics, cervical cerclage, and other strategies have failed to demonstrate consistent efficacy in reducing preterm birth rates. Inability to reliably predict which pregnant women will deliver before term is a major difficulty with randomized controlled trials of prevention strategies. Although there is evidence that intramuscular or vaginal progesterone supplementation lowers the preterm birth rate in women with a prior preterm birth (the best predictor), its routine use would have a small effect on the U.S. preterm birth rate.

Prevention of multiple gestations *is* an effective strategy for prevention of preterm births. In 2000, 12% of twins and 42% of higher order multiples were conceived with in vitro fertilization, and 21% of twins and 40% of higher order multiples were conceived with medications that promote ovulation (Reynolds et al, 2003). In vitro fertilization guidelines have been developed to limit the number of embryos transferred, and guidelines recommending ultrasound assessment after ovulation medications could further reduce multiple gestations and preterm birth rates. Fortunately, the U.S. triplet birth rate decreased from 7% in 1996 to 3.8% in 2002.

An interdisciplinary integrative research approach that evaluates multiple determinants over the lifespan (as has been done with heart disease) could provide insight into mechanisms of preterm birth pathways. Determinants include distal factors (e.g., physical and social environments) that influence a mother's predisposition and exposures as well as proximal factors (e.g., the mother's medical status and behavior). Multiple research approaches (i.e., epidemiologic, genetic, and animal studies) and integration of research findings are needed to devise effective preventive and treatment strategies for specific homogeneous subgroups of mothers at risk for preterm birth. Better assessments of gestational age, fetal and infant maturation, and mechanisms of preterm birth facilitate clinical decisions regarding maternal complications, timing of delivery, and neonatal management.

HEALTH OUTCOMES

Neonatal complications of prematurity are due to immature organ systems and organ injuries caused by conditions that contributed to preterm birth, delivery complications, or interventions required to sustain extrauterine life. The smallest and most immature infants are most vulnerable to all the complications of prematurity. The most common acute complication is respiratory distress syndrome, which can lead to chronic lung disease (also known as bronchopulmonary dysplasia). Inflammation and cytokine injury have been implicated in the pathogenesis of chronic lung disease, brain white matter injury, retinopathy of prematurity, and necrotizing enterocolitis. Preterm infants are vulnerable to infection, and antibiotics are often started at the first signs of acute or subacute deterioration. Necrotizing enterocolitis, retinopathy of prematurity, apnea and bradycardia, anemia, and brain injury (including intraventricular hemorrhage, hydrocephalus, infarction, and white matter injury) are also complications of prematurity. Feeding intolerance, gastroesophageal reflux, and concern about necrotizing enterocolitis often hinder adequate nutrition for growth and development. Although there are some randomized controlled trials, most standard treatments and interventions in the neonatal intensive care unit have not had adequate safety or efficacy studies.

During their first several years, infants born before term have higher rates of rehospitalization, surgery, respiratory infections (especially with respiratory syncytial virus), gastrointestinal problems, and reactive airway disease than do those born at term. Infants with chronic lung disease have higher risks of asthma, growth problems, and neurodevelopmental disability. Although preterm infants have a higher risk of sudden infant death syndrome than full-term infants do, this poorly understood relationship is not due to apnea of prematurity.

Although health problems are most frequent in early childhood, they persist in some children through childhood and even adolescence (Behrman and Butler, 2007). Some studies report poor growth in children born before term or with birth weights below 2500 g, but many other studies demonstrate catch-up growth into adolescence. Most adults born before term have a height and weight within 2 SD of the population mean and no significant health sequelae. Although young adults born before term have fewer risk-taking behaviors, the prevalence of smoking is similar to that of young adults born at term. Higher blood pressure has been reported in adolescents with birth weight below 1500 g than in adolescents with normal birth weight. There is a well-demonstrated association between low birth weight and cardiovascular disease in adulthood but not in adults born before term.

Visual Impairment

Retinopathy of prematurity is a vascular disorder of the retina with a multifactorial etiology, primarily due to immaturity. The retina is one of the last organs to be vascularized during fetal development, so retinopathy of prematurity is highest in the most immature and sick preterm infants. Retinopathy of prematurity occurs in up to 50% of infants with birth weight below 1000 g and in up to 90% with birth weight below 750 g (Behrman and Butler, 2007). The peak onset for threshold disease is 38 weeks postmenstrual age, and involution begins by 44 weeks postmenstrual age. Severe retinopathy of prematurity that requires laser surgery occurs in 10% of infants born before 28 weeks of gestation and in up to 40% of infants born before 26 weeks of gestation. Timely diagnosis and effective treatments have improved visual outcomes, so that only 1% to 2% of infants born before 26 to 27 weeks of gestation and 4% to 8% born at or before 24 weeks of gestation have severe visual impairment. Ophthalmologic follow-up is recommended until involution is complete and in all children with severe retinopathy of prematurity (for signs of late sequelae, including retinal detachment, cataracts, and angle-closure glaucoma).

Strabismus, amblyopia, and visual acuity problems (especially myopia) are more frequent in children born before term than in their peers born full term, with the highest risks in children with severe retinopathy of prematurity (Behrman and Butler, 2007). In a study that compared children born before 32 weeks of gestation with full-term classmates at the age of 7 years (Cooke et al, 2004), more preterm children required glasses (12% versus 4.3%) and had strabismus (13.6% versus 1.4%). As many as 24% to 31% of infants born before 26 weeks of gestation or with birth weight below 750 g require glasses, 24% develop strabismus, but only 1% to 2% have severe visual impairments (Behrman and Butler, 2007; Hack et al, 2000; Marlow et al, 2005).

Hearing Impairment

Severe hearing impairment occurs in 1.5% to 9% of children born before 26 weeks of gestation or with birth weight below 1000 g (Behrman and Butler, 2007; Doyle and Casalaz, 2001; Hack et al, 2000). Moderate to severe hearing impairment interferes with language acquisition and speech; early detection and treatment improve language and functional outcomes. Progressive hearing impairment has been reported in infants with congenital cytomegalovirus infection or persistent pulmonary hypertension. Some children born before term have difficulty with auditory processing and auditory discrimination, which influences their academic progress and behavior.

NEURODEVELOPMENTAL OUTCOMES

Antenatal Brain Development

The development of the fetal central nervous system (CNS) is a precise and timed process that is vulnerable to insult from a multitude of influences. Antenatal insults can, in turn, influence the integrity of the maternal-fetal dynamic or the timing and position of the infant at delivery. In a monograph on infantile cerebral paralysis written more than 100 years ago, Sigmund Freud stated, "It may well be possible that the same pathogenic factors that rendered intrauterine development abnormal also extend the influence to parturition; abnormal birth is the final result of an abnormal pregnancy" (Freud, 1897). Genetic, toxic, metabolic, and infectious factors can increase risk of both preterm delivery and fetal brain injury or malformation. The fetus with CNS anomalies has a higher risk of preterm birth, problems at delivery, and postnatal complications that include feeding problems, and each can further compromise neurologic development. The nature and extent of antenatal and perinatal brain injury depend on the etiology, extent, and timing of the insult. Little is known about how to promote recovery from brain injury.

Many genetic and metabolic factors influence fetal brain development. Gross structural brain malformations are seen in a number of genetic or chromosomal disorders (e.g., lissencephaly in Miller-Dieker syndrome, holoprosencephaly in trisomy 13). Other genetic disorders produce cognitive deficits without easily recognizable anatomic brain anomalies (e.g., Down syndrome). Disruption sequences and malformations (e.g., septo-optic dysplasia or DiGeorge sequence) account for a number of structural and functional brain anomalies. Metabolic abnormalities (also genetically determined) can cause serious developmental impairments after birth, but these infants are often protected in utero by maternal metabolic competence, as is the case with congenital hypothyroidism.

Antenatal exposures to infections or toxins can significantly influence fetal brain development. Maternal TORCH infections at vulnerable periods of fetal development have teratogenic effects on the fetus, with significant structural anomalies (e.g., hydrocephalus with *Toxoplasma gondii* infection, microcephaly with rubella and cytomegalovirus infection). There is evidence that maternal bacterial infections (e.g., urinary tract infections, chorioamnionitis) put the fetus at risk for neurologic impairment through inflammatory mechanisms. Fetal alcohol exposure carries a relatively high risk for cognitive, language, and learning impairments and is occasionally associated with structural brain anomalies (e.g., heterotopias). Prenatal exposure to some anticonvulsants (e.g., dilantin, valproate) and anticoagulants (e.g., warfarin, coumadin) also influences fetal brain development.

Maternal illness (e.g., chronic hypertension, preeclampsia), placental insufficiency, and cord problems (e.g., cord prolapse or knot) can lead to preterm delivery, compromised fetal brain development, or both. Thrombosis due to primary maternal clotting disorders (e.g., factor V Leiden deficiency) can compromise fetal brain structural and functional development. Preterm delivery, congenital malformations, intrauterine growth restriction, cord accidents, and obstetric problems are more common in multiple gestations.

Perinatal and Neonatal Brain Injury

Acute complications that lead to preterm delivery (e.g., maternal hemorrhage, placental abruption, cord prolapse) can acutely compromise the fetus, cause brain injury, and result in neurologic impairment. They are not good individual predictors of preterm outcomes, however, if intervention is prompt and the infant does not demonstrate signs of CNS injury on examination or neuroimaging studies. Many of the complications of prematurity (e.g., chronic lung disease, retinopathy of prematurity, necrotizing enterocolitis, sepsis, or meningitis) are associated with neurodevelopmental disability (Allen, 2002). Some may serve as a marker or proxy for severity of illness or immaturity. Measures of severity of chronic lung disease correlate with motor and cognitive outcomes (Hack et al, 2000; McGrath et al, 2000; Taylor, Klein, and Hack, 2000). Of children born before term who were on a ventilator for more than 28 days, 14% had cerebral palsy, 43% had cognitive deficits, and 4.4% had neurosensory impairment; impairments rates climbed to 80%, 100%, and 40%, respectively, for infants on a ventilator for more than 120 days (Walsh et al, 2005).

The best predictors of preterm neurodevelopmental outcome are measures of CNS structure and function (Allen, 2002). Serial head ultrasound examinations can identify CNS structural injury, especially in acutely ill preterm infants. Germinal matrix or subependymal hemorrhage (grade 1) and a small amount of intraventricular hemorrhage (grade 2) are associated with a mildly increased risk of neurodevelopmental disability (compared with preterm infants with no hemorrhage). Although intraventricular hemorrhage that dilates the ventricles (grade 3), intraparenchymal hemorrhagic infarction (formerly called grade 4 intraventricular hemorrhage), and posthemorrhagic hydrocephalus are not common, they carry a high risk of cerebral palsy and cognitive impairment. Clinical and ultrasound evidence of progressive hydrocephalus is an indication for relieving intracranial pressure by serial lumbar punctures or ventricular taps or placement of a ventriculoperitoneal or other type of shunt. As necrotic brain tissue is reabsorbed, asymmetric or irregularly shaped enlarged ventricles, porencephalic cysts that communicate with a ventricle, cysts adjacent to the ventricles (periventricular leukomalacia), or other signs of white matter injury on neuroimaging studies indicate a high risk of neurodevelopmental disability. Ventricular size on magnetic resonance imaging correlates with severity of motor and cognitive impairment in children with spastic cerebral palsy (Melham et al, 2000). Although magnetic resonance imaging has practical limitations and is not routinely obtained, qualitative analysis of magnetic resonance neuroimaging is being explored for prediction of neurodevelopmental outcome of preterm infants (Dammann and Leviton, 2006; Woodward et al, 2006).

Cerebral Palsy

Whereas the prevalence of cerebral palsy in the general population is only 0.1% to 0.2% (1 or 2/1000 live births), multiple studies demonstrate increasing prevalence of cerebral palsy with decreasing birth weight and gestational age categories (Amiel-Tison et al, 2002; Behrman and Butler, 2007; Keogh and Badawi, 2006). In a recent report from Sweden, the prevalence of cerebral palsy was only 1.1/1000 live births for children born full term but 6.7/1000 live births for children born at 32 to 36 weeks of gestation, 40.4/1000 live births for children born at 28 to 31 weeks of gestation, and as high as 76.6/1000 live births for children born before 28 weeks of gestation (Himmelmann et al, 2005). There was a similar stepwise increase when prevalence of cerebral palsy was calculated by birth weight category: from 1.2/1000 live births for birth weight above 2500 g, to 6.7/1000 for birth weight of 1500 to 2500 g, to 54/1000 for birth weight of 1000 1499 g, and to 82/1000 for birth weight below 1000 g. Dramatic improvements over time in survival of preterm infants of all gestational ages offset relatively small temporal changes in gestational age–specific rates of cerebral palsy (Behrman and Butler, 2007).

Many preterm outcome studies report the rate of cerebral palsy in *preterm survivors,* and this distinction is important in the smaller and most immature infants who have high mortality rates. Reviews of preterm outcome studies estimated that cerebral palsy developed in 7.7% of infants with birth weight below 1500 g and 10% of infants with birth weight below 1000 g (Bracewell and Marlow, 2002; Escobar, Littenberg, and Petitti, 1991). Most recent studies corroborate the observation of higher cerebral palsy rates with decreasing gestational age or birth weight categories: 11% to 12% in children born at 27 to 32 weeks of gestation, 7% to 20% in children born before 26 or 27 weeks of gestation, 6% to 6.7% in infants with birth weight below 1500 g, and 10% to 23% in infants with birth weight below 1000 g (Amiel-Tison et al, 2002; Bracewell and Marlow, 2002; Doyle and Casalaz, 2001; Hack et al, 2000; Hintz et al, 2005; Keogh and Badawi, 2006; Marlow et al, 2005; Tommiska et al, 2003).

Some of the variability in reported prevalence of cerebral palsy is due to differing definitions of cerebral palsy. Some studies focus on disabling cerebral palsy in their reports, whereas others include children with mild cerebral palsy. A large study of preterm infants born before 26 weeks of gestation in the British Isles in 1995 reported that 20% developed cerebral palsy, and it was disabling in 12% (Marlow et al, 2005). Many preterm children with mild cerebral palsy have a mild spastic diplegia (characterized by tight heel cords and toe walking) or a mild hemiplegia (characterized by marked handedness and asymmetric posture and gait). Although these children may require physical therapy services and orthotics as toddlers, most walk independently and many have minimal functional motor impairment by school age. Mild cerebral palsy is a marker, however, for increased risk of later school problems.

In studies of children with cerebral palsy, 40% to 50% were born before term and 26% were born before 32 weeks of gestation (Amiel-Tison et al, 2002; Behrman and Butler, 2007). Spastic diplegia is the predominant type of cerebral palsy in preterm children, especially in the most immature preterm children (64% to 75% of children with cerebral palsy born before 26 weeks of gestation or with birth weights below 1000 g) (Marlow et al, 2005; Tommiska et al, 2002). In preterm children born before 26 weeks of gestation who had spastic diplegia, 43% walked with an abnormal gait at 6 years, but 43% were not ambulatory (Marlow et al, 2005). The more severe form of spastic diplegia involves more proximal muscle groups and joints (knee, hip) as well as a greater need for intensive physical therapy, orthotics, and medical and surgical management of spasticity. Among preterm children with cerebral palsy, the proportion with spastic hemiplegia is low in children born before 26 weeks of gestation (3%) or 28 weeks of gestation (10%) but increases to as high as 34% for children born between 32 and 36 weeks of gestation and 15% to 30% for children with birth weight of 1500 to 2499 g (Amiel-Tison et al, 2002; Hagberg et al, 1996; Marlow et al, 2005).

Neuromotor Abnormality

Although many preterm infants demonstrate neuromotor abnormalities on examination during their first year, only a small proportion develop cerebral palsy. As early as 1972, Drillien described a constellation of abnormal neurologic findings (increased neck, trunk, and lower extremity extensor tone; increased hip adductor tone; neck and trunk hypotonia; persistent primitive reflexes) that was called transient dystonia because of resolution during infancy (Drillien, 1972). In a longitudinal study of dystonia in preterm infants, only 12% who had dystonia at 7 to 9 months developed cerebral palsy (and 83% with severe neurologic abnormalities developed cerebral palsy) (Pedersen et al, 2000). As many as

52% had normal findings on neurologic examination by 13 months and 88% had normal findings on neurologic examination by 36 months. All children who had normal examination findings at 7 to 9 months were normal at 36 months.

Several studies report that up to 35% to 50% of children born with birth weights below 1000 g have evidence of mild motor impairment or coordination problems (Behrman and Butler, 2007). At preschool age, preterm children have more problems with coordination, motor planning, and fine motor and graphomotor tasks. Most important, children with neuromotor abnormalities have a higher risk of attention deficit disorder, executive dysfunction, language delay, learning disability, and behavior problems.

Intellectual Disability and Borderline Intelligence

Mental retardation is traditionally defined as an IQ 2 SD or more below the mean (i.e., an IQ of 70 or less) accompanied by deficits in two or more areas of adaptive functioning. Many now substitute "intellectual disability" in deference to the social stigma attached to the words "mental retardation." Published follow-up studies and reviews report that children born before term have not only a higher incidence of intellectual disability but also a higher risk of borderline intelligence and learning disabilities than do children who were born full term (Aylward et al, 1989; Aylward, 2002; Behrman and Butler, 2007; Bhutta et al, 2002).

The likelihood of intellectual disability is 1.4-fold greater in children born between 32 and 36 weeks of gestation compared with children born full term, and the risk is 6.9 times greater for children born before 32 weeks of gestation (Stromme and Hagberg, 2000). Children with birth weight of 1500 to 2499 g have a 2.3 greater risk of intellectual disability than do children with birth weight of 2500 g or higher; the risk increases to 11.6 for children with birth weight below 1500 g. Nonetheless, children born before 32 weeks of gestation or with birth weight below 1500 g represent only 4% of the population of children with intellectual disability.

Although populations of children born before term demonstrate a normal range of IQ scores, the mean IQ score decreases with decreasing birth weight and gestational age categories. A meta-analysis of a large number of studies found that children born with birth weights below 2500 g had a mean IQ that was 5 to 7 points below the mean for full-term controls; a more recent meta-analysis found a weighted mean difference of 10.2 points for preterm children compared with full-term children (Aylward et al, 1989; Bhutta et al, 2002). A study of young adults with birth weights below 1500 g found a mean IQ score of 87 compared with a mean IQ score of 92 for full-term controls; 49% had IQ scores 1 SD or more below the mean compared with 33% of controls (Hack et al, 2002). Studies of children with birth weights below 1000 g report that 11% to 42% had IQ scores 2 SD or more below the mean, and 37% to 68% had scores 1 SD or more below the mean (Behrman and Butler, 2007; Doyle and Casalaz, 2001; Hack et al, 2000; Saigal, 2000; Vohr et al, 2000; Wilson-Costello et al, 2007). The impact of borderline cognition on the academic success of children must not be underestimated. Eligibility criteria for services under the Individuals with Disabilities Education Act (IDEA) in the United States vary widely among states, and many jurisdictions do not include borderline intelligence.

In the British study of 6-year-olds born before 26 weeks of gestation, 21% had IQ scores 2 SD or more below the test mean, and 46% had IQ scores 1 SD or more below the mean (Marlow, 2005). Their mean IQ score was 24 points below the mean IQ score for full-term controls (82 versus 106). Compared with IQ scores of the full-term controls (not the test norms), 41% of children born before 26 weeks of gestation had IQ scores 2 SD or more below the mean.

Academic Achievement

Academic achievement is influenced not only by a child's IQ but also by the child's language understanding, visual-perceptual abilities, graphomotor skills, attention, executive function, and ability to learn. IQ tests average a child's performance on a number of cognitive subtests, including auditory and visual memory, understanding complex language, abstract reasoning, visual perception, and visual-motor integration. Children born before term have a higher risk of difficulty in each of these areas of function. There are many definitions of specific learning disability, but most assume the child has normal intelligence and adequate exposure to teaching. Outcome studies vary in how they report school problems: some specifically test for cognitive impairments and specific learning disabilities (specific criteria also vary), some merely report grade retention or need for special education services.

No matter how school problems are measured, the smaller and more immature the infant, the higher the risk of specific learning disabilities, grade retention, and need for special education services (Behrman and Butler, 2007). The need for support services in the classroom was higher in children with birth weight below 2500 g compared with children with normal birth weight (27% versus 3.5%) (Halsey, Collin, and Anderson, 1996). Studies of children with birth weight below 800 or 1000 g report that 13% to 33% repeat a grade and approximately half require special education: 2% to 20%, special education classrooms; and 33% to 46%, special education resources in a regular classroom (Aylward, 2002; Behrman and Butler, 2007; Kirkegaard et al, 2006; Saigal, 2000; Taylor, Klein, and Hack, 2000). The prevalence of learning disabilities is 7% to 18% in full-term controls, 30% to 38% in children with birth weight of 750 to 1000 g, and 50% to 63% in children with birth weight below 750 g. Children with birth weights below 1000 g are 3 to 5 times more likely than full-term controls to fail a grade, are 2 to 6 times more likely to have learning disabilities, and require 3 to 10 times more special education resources.

Executive Dysfunction

The cognitive, metacognitive, and behavioral skills that are required to organize purposeful goals are collectively referred to as executive function. These skills or aptitudes include initiation, inhibition, organization, working memory, and impulse control and the ability to shift attention, to plan, and to reason. These executive functions affect the efficiency with which people learn, work, and socialize. Even in children with normal intelligence, executive dysfunction influences a child's capacity to learn and to function in school. A few preterm outcome studies report that children with birth weight below 1000 g have lower scores on measures of executive function compared with full-term peers, and test scores decrease with decreasing birth weight and gestational age categories (Anderson and Doyle, 2004; Harvey, O'Callaghan, and Mohay, 1999).

Attention-Deficit/Hyperactivity Disorder

The diagnosis of attention-deficit/hyperactivity disorder (ADHD) is somewhat subjective, and unrecognized cognitive impairments and learning disabilities make it difficult to assess the effect of preterm birth on child behavior. Although it is not a universal finding, a number of studies report a 2- to 6-fold increase in ADHD symptoms in school-age children with birth weight below 1000 or 1500 g compared with full-term controls (Aylward, 2002, 2005; Behrman and Butler, 2007; Bhutta et al, 2002; Saigal et al, 2001). Another study found that children with ADHD were 3.1 times more likely than children without ADHD to have been born with birth weight below 2500 g (Mick et al, 2002).

The cumulative effect of slightly lower cognitive potential, more difficulty with executive function, increased likelihood of learning disability, and ADHD behaviors can have profound academic consequences. Academic achievement for these children may require tutoring, coaching of study strategies and organizational skills, behavior modification, and classroom modification. Pharmacologic intervention for attention deficits requires weighing of academic and social benefits against the child's health status, nutrition, and growth.

Adolescent and Adult Functioning

Limited data have been published on the functional abilities of adolescents and young adults born before term in the 1970s and early 1980s (Behrman and Butler, 2007; Grunau, Whitfield, and Fay, 2004; Hack et al, 2002, 2004; Saigal et al, 2006). Although they were more likely than full-term controls to repeat one or more grades, to require special education, or to leave school early, 74% to 82% graduated from high school and 30% to 32% matriculated into colleges (but they were less likely than controls to enter 4-year colleges). Teenagers and young adults who were born before term do not perceive themselves as different from their peers on most measures of behavior and emotion. Some teenagers born before term rated themselves lower in scholastic, athletic, romantic, and job competency than their full-term peers, but they also reported fewer problems with delinquency, marijuana, or alcohol. Their parents reported that they have more difficulty with behavior, social acceptance, athletics, social skills, attention, and scholastic competency than parents of full-term controls described. Young women born before term and their parents reported more difficulty with withdrawn behaviors, anxiety and depression, fewer friends, poorer family relationships, and less sexual activity than full-term controls.

In a study of teenagers with birth weight below 1000 g who were high-school graduates, they rated themselves lower in measures of job competency and viewed themselves as needing more help from others in finding and securing employment (Grunau, Whitfield, and Fay, 2004). Another study of 22- to 25-year-olds found no differences between those with birth weight below 1000 g and controls in terms of employment, living independently, or marriage/cohabitation (Saigal et al, 2006).

Many contributory and confounding factors, including health status, socioeconomic status, cognitive deficits, academic history, and difficulties with attention and executive function, vary among these various studies of young adult outcomes.

Furthermore, it is not yet possible to know adult outcomes for preterm infants born in the last decade and treated with antenatal or postnatal steroids, surfactant, and technologic advances.

NEURODEVELOPMENTAL SUPPORT AND FOLLOW-UP

Neurodevelopmental Support in the Neonatal Intensive Care Unit

Preterm infants in a neonatal intensive care unit (NICU) are exposed to multiple medical procedures and overwhelming sensory stimuli, and these influence neuromaturation just as the intrauterine environment influences fetal neuromaturation. Strategies for providing support for preterm neuromaturation include minimizing procedures, pain management, decreasing sensory input overload, involving parents in their infant's care, encouraging mothers to provide breast milk, modifying nursing routines according to the infant's needs, paying careful attention to how an infant is positioned and supported, and facilitating non-nutritive sucking (Aucott et al, 2002; Behrman and Butler, 2007). As long as they are contingent on infant responses, interaction with the infant and gentle stimulation can be beneficial. This requires recognition of signs of stress and distress. Kangaroo care, which involves skin-to-skin contact as the naked infant is positioned upright on a parent's chest, originated in South America but has been adopted in many NICUs in the United States. Als' Neonatal Individualized Developmental Care and Assessment Program (Als, 1998) is a highly organized comprehensive system for supporting preterm infants in the NICU that has generated widespread interest. There are limited data on short-term benefits for each of these intervention strategies, but further research is needed to assess long-term outcomes.

After Discharge from the Neonatal Intensive Care Unit

The American Academy of Pediatrics Council on Children with Disabilities (2006) has recently updated its policy statement to include an algorithm for developmental surveillance and screening to identify and to refer infants with atypical development. This is most germane to infants born before term because of their high incidence of major impairments and minor morbidities. Specific high-risk neonatal follow-up clinics monitor high-risk NICU infants, identify early signs of neurodevelopmental disability, provide comprehensive evaluations, and refer them for appropriate community services. Ideally, their comprehensive assessments use a multidisciplinary model, with participation by specialists in developmental pediatrics, physical and occupational therapy, nursing, social work, and clinical neuropsychology.

In the NICU developmental follow-up clinic, assessment of infant milestone achievement and serial neurodevelopmental examinations identify developmental delays and impairments. Children who develop cerebral palsy demonstrate persistent neuromotor abnormalities on examination and motor delay; the more severe the cerebral palsy, the earlier the motor delay and the more severe the neuromotor abnormalities. Severe cerebral palsy can be identified during the first year, but follow-up to 2 years may be necessary to diagnose mild cerebral palsy.

Cognitive abilities are difficult to assess early in infancy and in infants with motor impairment. Early language abilities that progress along a typical timeline are reassuring for cognitive abilities, and language acquisition progresses rapidly between 12 and 36 months. Language delays, including failure to acquire appropriate vocabulary or to use phrases, are early markers of three very different developmental disorders: hearing impairment, cognitive impairment, and communication disorders. Each has a very different prognosis and requires specific interventions. The identification of early language delay and its cause allows early diagnosis and early, appropriate interventions.

The high-prevalence/low-severity disorders, including fine motor difficulties, graphomotor disorders, learning disabilities, and attention deficits, require follow-up to preschool and school age. Fine motor problems become most apparent by 3 to 5 years as the child has difficulty with buttons, snaps, or tying shoes. Graphomotor disorders become more apparent in kindergarten and early elementary school, as do learning disabilities, while written language disabilities may not be appreciated until middle school, when efficiency becomes an issue.

The Individuals with Disabilities Education Act (IDEA) has evolved to include service provision within their community for children from birth through their educational years. Part C services are for children from birth to 3 years, and part B provides services for children from 3 years until enrollment in a formal education setting. Intervention programs under IDEA are the mainstay of services for children born before term, but eligibility for services varies tremendously from jurisdiction to jurisdiction. There is not universal agreement as to whether one should correct for degree of prematurity when evaluating developmental delay in children born before term and, if so, for how long (Allen, 2002). Correction is most important in the most preterm infants and during the first year. For a 6-month-old who was born at 23 weeks of gestation, most will expect the child's abilities to be at a 2-month level (the age corrected for degree of prematurity), not at the 6-month level. Arithmetically, correction for degree of prematurity can influence developmental scores up to the age of 8 years (Rickards et al, 1989).

SUMMARY

Prematurity is an important but complex public health problem that will not be easily solved. Preterm birth results from multiple causal pathways with multiple interrelated biologic, psychosocial, and environmental risk factors that vary in frequency among different populations. Despite medical and technologic advancements that have led to dramatic improvements in preterm survival and lowering of the limits of viability, there have been no concomitant improvements in sequelae, and the preterm birth rate is rising, not falling.

Children born before term have higher rates of health sequelae, developmental disabilities, and functional impairments than do children born full term. Despite this, most preterm survivors do not have major disabilities and are functional as adults. The more immature the infant, the higher the risk of disability and impairment, and the more severe the sequelae tend to be. An inherent limitation of neonatal follow-up literature is an obligatory time lag: there is no way to know how the preterm survivors we are now caring for in our NICUs will do during childhood or as adults.

Costs incurred by providing high-risk obstetric care, neonatal intensive care, and developmental and educational support during childhood would be better spent preventing preterm births. This requires a focused multidisciplinary research approach, with sustained, stable funding, to better understand mechanisms of preterm birth and how various genetic, psychosocial, and environmental risk factors influence these mechanisms. Until prevention of preterm birth is feasible, effective treatment strategies need to be developed to prevent injury to the brain and other organs and to support ongoing neuromaturation and recovery from injury.

REFERENCES

Alexander GR: Prematurity at birth: Determinants, consequences, and geographic variation. Appendix B. In Behrman RE, Butler AS, (eds): Preterm Birth: Causes, Consequences, and Prevention. Institute of Medicine Committee on Understanding Premature Birth and Assuring Healthy Outcomes, Washington, DC, National Academies Press, 2007.

Allen MC: Preterm outcomes research: A critical component of neonatal intensive care. Ment Retard Dev Disabil Res Rev 8(4):221-233, 2002.

Allen MC: Assessment of gestational age and neuromaturation. Ment Retard Dev Disabil Res Rev 11(1):21-33, 2005.

Als H: Developmental care in the newborn intensive care unit. Curr Opin Pediatr 10:138-142, 1998.

American Academy of Pediatrics, Policy Statement: Identifying infants and young children with developmental disorders in the medical home: An algorithm for developmental screening and surveillance. Pediatrics 118:405-420, 2006.

Amiel-Tison C, Allen MC, Lebrun F, Rogowski J: Macropremies: Underprivileged newborns. Ment Retard Dev Disabil Res Rev 8(4):281-292, 2002.

Anderson PJ, Doyle LW; Victorian Infant Collaborative Study Group: Executive functioning in school-aged children who were born very preterm or with extremely low birth weight in the 1990s. Pediatrics 114:50-57, 2004.

Aucott S, Donohue PK, Atkins E, Allen MC: Neurodevelopmental care in the NICU. Ment Retard Dev Disabil Res Rev 8(4):298-308, 2002.

Aylward GP: Cognitive and neuropsychological outcomes: More than IQ scores. Ment Retard Dev Disabil Res Rev 8:234-240, 2002.

Aylward GP: Neurodevelopmental outcomes of infants born prematurely. Dev Behav Pediatr 26:427-440, 2005.

Aylward GP, Pfeiffer SI, Wright A, Overhauls SJ: Outcome studies of low birth weight infants published in the last decade: A metaanalysis. J Pediatr 115:515-521, 1989.

Battaglia FC, Lubchenco LO: A practical classification of newborn infants by weight and gestational age. J Pediatr 71(2):159-163, 1967.

Behrman RE, Butler AS (eds): Preterm Birth: Causes, Consequences, and PreventionInstitute of Medicine Committee on Understanding Premature Birth and Assuring Healthy Outcomes. Washington, DC, National Academies Press, 2007.

Bhutta AT, Cleves MA, Casey PH, et al: Cognitive and behavioral outcomes of school-aged children who were born preterm: A meta-analysis. JAMA 288(6):728-737, 2002.

Bracewell M, Marlow N: Patterns of motor disability in very preterm children. Ment Retard Dev Disabil Res Rev 8(4):241-248, 2002.

Cooke RW, Foulder-Hughes L, Newsham D, Clarke D: Ophthalmic impairment at 7 years of age in children born very preterm. Arch Dis Child Fetal Neonatal Ed 89:F249-F253, 2004.

Dammann O, Leviton A: Neuroimaging and the prediction of outcomes in preterm infants [editorial]. N Engl J Med 355(7):727-729, 2006.

Dolk H, Pattenden S, Johnson A: Cerebral palsy, low birthweight and socio-economic deprivation: Inequalities in a major cause of childhood disability. Paediatr Perinat Epidemiol 15(4):359-363, 2001.

Doyle LW, Casalaz D: Outcomes at 14 years of extremely low birthweight infants: A regional study. Arch Dis Child Fetal Neonatal Ed 85:F159-F164, 2001.

Drillien CM: Abnormal neurologic signs in the first year of life in low-birth weight infants: Possible prognostic significance. Dev Med Child Neurol 14:575-584, 1972.

Escobar GJ, Littenberg B, Petitti DB: Outcome among surviving very low birthweight infants: A meta-analysis. Arch Dis Child 66:204-211, 1991.

Freud S: Infantile cerebral paralysis. In Russin LA, trans: Nothnagels Handbuch. Vienna, 1897. Florida, University of Miami Press, 1968.

Grunau RE, Whitfield MF, Fay TB: Psychosocial and academic characteristics of extremely low birth weight (800 g) adolescents who are free of major impairment compared with term-born control subjects. Pediatrics 114(6):e725-e732, 2004.

Hack M, Wilson-Costello D, Friedman H, et al: Neurodevelopment and predictors of outcomes of children with birth weights of less than 1000 g: 1992-1995. Arch Pediatr Adolesc Med 154(7):725-731, 2000.

Hack M, Flannery DJ, Schluchter M, et al: Outcomes in young adulthood for very-low-birth weight infants. N Engl J Med 346(3):149-157, 2002.

Hack M, Youngstrom EA, Cartar L, et al: Behavioral outcomes and evidence of psychopathology among very low birth weight infants at age 20 years. Pediatrics 114:932-940, 2004.

Hagberg B, Hagberg G, Olow I, Wendt L: The changing panorama of cerebral palsy in Sweden. VII. Prevalence and origin in the birth year period 1987-90. Acta Paediatr 85(8):954-960, 1996.

Halsey CL, Collin MF, Anderson CL: Extremely low-birth-weight children and their peers: A comparison of school-age outcomes. Arch Pediatr Adolesc Med 150:790-794, 1996.

Harvey JM, O'Callaghan MJ, Mohay H: Executive function of children with extremely low birthweight: A case control study. Dev Med Child Neurol 41:292-297, 1999.

Himmelmann K, Hagberg G, Beckung E, et al: The changing panorama of cerebral palsy in Sweden. IX. Prevalence and origin in the birth-year period 1995-1998. Acta Paediatr 94(3):287-294, 2005.

Hintz SR, Kendrick DE, Vohr BR, et al: National Institute of Child Health and Human Development Neonatal Research Network: Changes in neurodevelopmental outcomes at 18 to 22 months' corrected age among infants of less than 25 weeks' gestational age born in 1993-1999. Pediatrics 115(6):1645-1651, 2005.

Keogh JM, Badawi N: The origins of cerebral palsy. Curr Opin Neurol 19:129-134, 2006.

Kirkegaard I, Obel C, Hedegaard M, Henriksen TB: Gestational age and birth weight in relation to school performance of 10-year-old children: A follow-up study of children born after 32 completed weeks. Pediatrics 118:1600-1606, 2006.

Marlow N, Wolke D, Bracewell MA, Samara M: Neurologic and developmental disability at six years of age after extremely preterm birth. N Engl J Med 352(1):9-19, 2005.

McGrath MM, Sullivan MC, Lester BM, Oh W: Longitudinal neurologic follow-up in neonatal intensive care unit survivors with various neonatal morbidities. Pediatrics 106(6):1397-1405, 2000.

Melham ER, Hoon AH, Ferrucci JT, et al: Periventricular leukomalacia: Relationship between lateral ventricular volume on brain MR images and severity of cognitive and motor impairment. Radiology 214:199-204, 2000.

Mick E, Biederman J, Prince J, et al: Impact of low birth weight on attention-deficit hyperactivity disorder. J Dev Behav Pediatr 23(1):16-22, 2002.

Pedersen SJ, Sommerfelt F, Markestad T: Early motor development of premature infants with birthweight less than 2000 grams. Acta Paediatr 89:1456-1461, 2000.

Reynolds AJ, Martin JA, Jeng G, Macaluso M: Trends in multiple births conceived using assisted reproductive technology, United States 1997-2000. Pediatrics 111:1159-1162, 2003.

Rickards AL, Kitchen WH, Doyle LW, Kelly EA: Correction of developmental and intelligence test scores for premature births. Aust Paediatr J 25(3):127-129, 1989.

Saigal S: Follow up of very low birthweight babies to adolescence. Semin Neonatol 5:107-118, 2000.

Saigal S, Stoskopf BL, Streiner DL, Burrows E: Physical growth and current health status of infants who were of extremely low birth weight and controls at adolescence. Pediatrics 108(2):407-415, 2001.

Saigal S, Stoskopj B, Streiner D, et al: Transition of extremely low-birth-weight infants from adolescence to young adulthood. JAMA 295:667-675, 2006.

Stromme P, Hagberg G: Aetiology in severe and mild retardation: A population-based study of Norwegian children. Dev Med Child Neurol 42:76-86, 2000.

Taylor HG, Klein N, Hack M: School-age consequences of birth weight less than 750 g: A review and update. Dev Neuropsychol 17:189-321, 2000.

Tommiska V, Heinonen K, Kero P, et al: A national two-year follow up study of extremely low birthweight infants born in 1996-1997. Arch Dis Child Fetal Neonatal Ed 88:F29-F35, 2003.

Vohr BR, Wright LL, Dusick AM, et al: Neurodevelopmental and functional outcomes of extremely low birth weight infants in the National Institute of Child Health and Human Development Neonatal Research Network, 1993-1994. Pediatrics 105(6):1216-1226, 2000.

Walsh MC, Morris BH, Wrage LA, et al: Extremely low birthweight neonates with protracted ventilation: Mortality and 18-month neurodevelopmental outcomes. J Pediatr 146:798-804, 2005.

Wilson-Costello D, Freidman H, Minich N, et al: Improved neurodevelopmental outcomes for extremely low birth weight infants in 2000-2002. Pediatrics 119(1):37-45, 2007.

Woodward LJ, Anderson PJ, Austin NC, et al: Neonatal MRI to predict neurodevelopmental outcomes in preterm infants. N Engl J Med 355:685-694, 2006.

28 HUMAN IMMUNODEFICIENCY VIRUS INFECTION IN CHILDREN

Sharon Nichols and John Farley

EPIDEMIOLOGY

More than 2 decades have passed since the clinical syndrome now known as acquired immune deficiency syndrome (AIDS) was first described and ultimately demonstrated to be caused by the human immunodeficiency virus type 1 (HIV-1) retrovirus. The syndrome was described in children in urban areas of the United States in the early 1980s, with abnormalities in child development a hallmark of the disease. Presently worldwide, at least 1500 infants are born each day with perinatally transmitted HIV infection (World Health Organization, 2006). Whereas interventions to prevent mother-to-child transmission have resulted in a dramatic reduction in the number of infected infants in developed country settings, the challenge of the massive program development required has limited the impact of efficacious interventions in resource-limited settings.

Through 2005, more than 9000 cases of children in the United States with AIDS were reported to the U.S. Centers for Disease Control and Prevention. The most common risk factor is mother-to-child transmission (92.9%), and the second is receipt of contaminated blood or blood products (6.6%) (Centers for Disease Control and Prevention, 2005). Less commonly, cases in children have also been ascribed to sexual abuse, mucous membrane exposure to blood, and exposures such as to contaminated needles in the health care setting. Black non-Hispanic and Hispanic children are affected disproportionately in the United States. Among women of childbearing age, injection drug use is a common risk factor for HIV infection but remains second to heterosexual transmission. HIV-infected women are less likely to receive prenatal care than are women in the general population, and HIV-affected families in the United States are more likely to be poor. Thus, perinatally infected children may have multiple risk factors for developmental and behavioral problems. An increasing number of adolescents acquire HIV infection sexually or through injection drug use. Because of major improvements in the care of children with perinatally acquired HIV disease in the United States (Gortmaker et al, 2001), most will survive through adolescence. Thus, additional behavioral issues common to adolescents with chronic illness, such as maintaining adherence to therapy, are a growing challenge.

COURSE OF ILLNESS AND LABORATORY MONITORING

Perinatal HIV transmission may occur in utero, close to or during delivery, or post partum through breastfeeding. In the absence of treatment, the tempo of disease progression in children is considerably more rapid than in adults; up to 25% develop an infectious or neurologic complication in the first year of life (Duliege et al, 1992). It is hypothesized that children infected in utero may be at the highest risk for rapid disease progression. With the use of potent antiretroviral therapy known as highly active antiretroviral therapy (HAART), optimal obstetric care, and avoidance of breastfeeding, the risk of perinatal transmission can be reduced to below 2% (Madger et al, 2005). The cornerstone of prevention of perinatal transmission is universal counseling and voluntary HIV testing for all pregnant women, which should be advocated by all health care providers.

Although HIV pathogenesis is not as well characterized in children, it is likely to be similar to that in adults. After infection, dendritic cells transport HIV virions to regional lymph nodes within 48 hours of exposure. There, $CD4^+$ T-lymphocyte cells become infected. HIV in the blood increases rapidly during the first weeks of infection in adults, then declines dramatically, reaching a stable set-point within 6 months. Cell-mediated responses rather than antibodies are likely to be the key immune activities leading to viral suppression. Perinatally infected infants reach peak viremia at 1 to 2 months of life but unlike adults have only minimal declines in plasma virus during the next several months (Shearer et al, 1997). This may be related to the failure of infants to mount an effective immune response or transmission of a virus that has mutated to escape the maternal immune response. After infection, ongoing HIV replication results in generalized immune activation with higher levels of programmed cell death and T-cell turnover. The ability of the thymus to generate new T cells may be impaired. As the $CD4^+$ T-lymphocyte absolute count is higher in children than in adults, standards for mild, moderate, and severe $CD4^+$ T-lymphocyte suppression vary by age (Table 28-1). Ultimately, the germinal center organization of lymph nodes is lost. In children in particular, significant B-lymphocyte dysfunction with

Table 28-1. **Categories of Immune Suppression among HIV-Infected Children Based on Age-Specific CD4+ Cell Counts and Percentage**

	<12 Months		1-5 Years		6-12 Years	
Immune Category	No./mm³ (%)		No./mm³ (%)		No./mm³ (%)	
Category 1: no suppression	>1500	(>25)	>1000	(>25)	>500	(>25)
Category 2: moderate suppression	750-1499	(15-24)	500-999	(15-24)	200-499	(15-24)
Category 3: severe suppression	<750	(<15)	<500	(<15)	<200	(<15)

Centers for Disease Control and Prevention: 1994 revised classification system for human immunodeficiency virus infection in children <13 years of age. MMWR Morb Mortal Wkly Rep 43(RR-12):1-19, 1994.

impaired humoral immunity also occurs. With time, the immune system becomes unable to respond to infectious pathogens. Opportunistic infections or other serious complications occur, and the child meets the AIDS case definition (Centers for Disease Control and Prevention, 1994). The use of HAART has resulted in fewer children experiencing severe immunosuppression. Thus, in the United States, the most common complications are now bacterial pneumonia, herpes zoster, dermatophyte infections, and oral candidiasis. Bacteremia, *Pneumocystic jerovici (carinii)* pneumonia, *Mycobacterium avium* complex infection, lymphoid interstitial pneumonitis, and disseminated fungal infection are now uncommon (Gona et al, 2006).

Virologic testing is used to determine the infection status of infants born to HIV-infected mothers; definitive testing is possible by 4 months of age among non-breastfed infants. HIV RNA assays (viral load measurement) assess the magnitude of HIV plasma viremia and are used for the clinical monitoring of HIV-infected children to determine if antiretroviral therapy is recommended and to evaluate response to antiretroviral therapy. The severity of HIV disease and risk of disease progression are determined by age, presence or history of HIV-related or AIDS-defining illnesses, level of CD4+ cell immunosuppression (see Table 28-1), and magnitude of HIV plasma viremia (Working Group on Antiretroviral Therapy, 2006).

PSYCHOSOCIAL ISSUES

Despite advances in treatment of HIV in children, the psychosocial issues associated with the disease continue to be tremendous. In the United States and other countries where HAART is widely used, HIV is now treated as a chronic illness more than as a terminal one. Although this is obviously a welcome change, the treatment of chronic illnesses carries a different and significant burden for patients and their providers. This is particularly true for adolescents, who may focus on the short-term problems associated with treatment side effects over the long-term importance of viral control. Issues of treatment adherence are especially significant for this population and are discussed in detail later.

The use of HAART has succeeded in preventing many of the physical complications of HIV in children and in other members of their families. However, these children and their families continue to face significant psychosocial and emotional issues. Families affected by the disease are also disproportionately affected by poverty, and managing the complicated health care tasks required to treat HIV infection adds to their level of stress. Substance abuse in the family or by the infected adolescent can interfere with treatment adherence and raise the risk of the adolescent's infecting other youth. Children are affected by emotional issues related to HIV infection, such as the fear of death, the loss and change of caregivers, the anxiety over medical procedures and pain, and the secrecy and isolation that are sometimes still associated with the disease. Owing to the continued stigma associated with HIV infection, the family may be reluctant to avail itself of support from family, friends, or school personnel because of concerns about disclosure of the diagnosis. This may be particularly true for immigrant families, who have different cultural attitudes toward HIV infection and medical care as well as the added stress of adjusting to a new culture. Medical providers who are aware of the presence of HIV infection in the family are in an excellent position to guide the family toward counseling and social work resources and to discuss issues of diagnosis disclosure. Support groups, educational materials, and provision of access to Internet resources can increase the family's ability to cope. Making such resources available to the family is of course particularly critical to assist the child and family with bereavement issues at times of loss of a caregiver or in preparation for the child's own death, should that become likely.

For families of perinatally infected children, disclosure of the child's HIV diagnosis to him or her as well as revealing the parent's HIV status is often a difficult issue. Parents may be reluctant to discuss the child's diagnosis because of concerns about inadvertent disclosure to others by the child as well as the desire to protect the child emotionally. In 1999, the American Academy of Pediatrics recommended diagnosis disclosure to children perinatally infected with HIV, 25% to 90% of whom were unaware of their HIV status at that time (American Academy of Pediatrics, Committee on Pediatric AIDS, 1999). Guidelines for this process and for determining the child's developmental appropriateness for disclosure are discussed by Gerson and colleagues (2001).

As perinatally infected children survive into adolescence, they join those infected at that time in facing decisions about disclosure of their diagnosis to sexual partners. An accurate understanding of their HIV disease is also important at that time for them to take on health care tasks for their own survival. In a study of

40 HIV-infected youth aged 13 to 24 years, Wiener and Battles (2006) found that they rated disclosure to dating partners as their most difficult disclosure challenge, but those who did disclose experienced greater feelings of self-competence with peers. In their sample, youth who had disclosed their diagnosis more in general were also more likely to disclose to romantic partners. This suggests that working with children and families on disclosure issues before the child begins sexual activity may increase the likelihood that the youth will later reveal his or her HIV status to potential sexual partners. Providers in adolescent medicine should offer support to the youth, and to the partner as well when appropriate, through the process of diagnosis disclosure. It is important for providers to be aware of the laws of their state regarding notification of sexual or needle-sharing partners of their patients' HIV status.

Adolescents who are infected with HIV through high-risk behaviors have additional psychosocial issues and stresses that present challenges to their health care providers. In a study of risk-infected adolescents in a southern urban U.S. environment, Kadivar and associates (2006) found relatively high rates of running away and unstable housing, parental and youth substance abuse, parental abandonment or neglect, sexual abuse or assault, other sexually transmitted diseases, depression, and involvement with the juvenile justice system. These youth may also struggle with issues of sexual identity and disclosure of sexual preference to their families. Identifying youth infected in adolescence with HIV and involving them in consistent care are difficult but critical. Providers should bear in mind that HIV infection may not be at the top of the list of stresses faced by these young people, and connecting them with social work, housing resources, and mental health and substance abuse treatment may be an important step in enabling them to focus on their health and long-term survival.

HIV INFECTION AND CHILD DEVELOPMENT

Growth

Growth, nutrition, and metabolism, requisite for normal child development, are affected by HIV disease. Causes can include decreased oral intake (due to anorexia, food aversion or refusal, barriers to food access or preparation, altered taste, early satiety, or neurologic dysfunction), increased nutrient losses (due to vomiting, diarrhea, or malabsorption), increased nutrient requirements (due to fever, secondary infection, or end-organ complications), and metabolic or endocrine dysregulation (due to cytokine production or endocrine deficiencies) (Chantry and Moye, 2006). Thus, growth failure or failure to thrive is common. In addition to poor growth in infancy and childhood, teens are at risk for delayed puberty and adrenarche, with increased risk associated with degree of immunosuppression (Buchacz et al, 2003).

Behavioral and Emotional Issues

Mental health and behavioral issues have been a key issue of concern for caregivers and providers of children with HIV infection. Studies of perinatally infected youth suggest a relatively high rate of psychiatric disorders in this population. For example, the large Pediatric AIDS Clinical Trials Group 219C cohort study found an incidence of psychiatric hospitalization of 6.17 cases per 1000 person-years among children younger than 15 years compared with the reported incidence of 1.7 per 1000 person-years in the general pediatric population. The majority of patients were admitted for depression or behavioral disorders (Gaughan et al, 2004). Mellins and colleagues (2006) found that 55% of a sample of 47 perinatally infected youth aged 9 to 16 years met criteria for a psychiatric diagnosis, primarily anxiety, attention-deficit/hyperactivity, conduct, and oppositional defiant disorders. Although relatively high rates of attention-deficit/hyperactivity disorder have been observed in younger children with HIV infection, studies that have used a well-matched control group of children exposed to HIV in utero but not infected have found comparable rates of attention-deficit/hyperactivity disorder in that group (Chiriboga et al, 2005; Mellins et al, 2003). These studies suggest that other variables, such as environmental, maternal, and genetic factors, as well as the stresses of living with a potentially terminal illness, stigma, and family loss and disruption may contribute to or be responsible for the high rates of some psychiatric disorders in perinatally infected children and adolescents. Nevertheless, pediatricians who treat this group of children should be aware of the high rate of conditions that indicate the need for psychotherapeutic intervention.

Neurodevelopment

HIV infection in childhood, particularly when the virus is perinatally acquired, can have devastating effects on central nervous system functioning. Encephalopathy was recognized early in the epidemic as a significant aspect of HIV disease that is particularly common in children (Mitchell, 2001), especially infants (Tardieu et al, 2000). Although opportunistic infections of the brain due to immunodeficiency are less common in children than in adults, the virus itself can enter the central nervous system. There, it is thought to affect central nervous system functioning indirectly, primarily by infection of microglia and macrophages and resulting release of neurotoxic products rather than by infection of neurons themselves. Significant nervous system side effects, such as peripheral neuropathy, fatigue, and depression, can also be associated with medications used to treat HIV infection.

Before antiretroviral medications were developed and came into wide use, it was not uncommon for infants with perinatally acquired HIV infection to develop a severe, progressive HIV encephalopathy (PHE). This was characterized by a prominent motor component, with bilateral pyramidal tract signs and eventual spastic diplegia; loss of developmental milestones; decreased emotional expressiveness; and, in some cases, focal neurologic signs. Neuroimaging revealed poor brain growth and resulting microcephaly and calcification of the basal ganglia. Belman and colleagues (1988) noted three common disease courses: a rapidly progressive encephalopathy leading to death, a subacute but nonetheless steadily progressing course, and a static or plateau profile with continued attainment of milestones but at a slower rate than in typical development. Children who survived infancy could develop progressive encephalopathy at a later point; however, static encephalopathy was more common in this group. Children infected later in development, generally through contaminated blood products or clotting factor at that time, showed a clinical course more similar to that of adults, with a long asymptomatic period and eventual impairments in motor speed, executive functions such as cognitive flexibility, and visual processing (Cohen et al, 1991). Studies comparing school-age hemophilic children and adolescents with and without HIV infection found that among those with HIV infection, decreased cognitive functioning was related to greater immune dysfunction (Loveland et al, 2000) but was subtle in the early stages (Sirois and Hill, 1993).

The introduction of zidovudine led to the first reports of the arrest and reversal of the deficits associated with PHE by treatment with antiretroviral medications (Brouwers et al, 1990). However, impaired cognitive and motor functioning continued to be a significant risk for children with perinatal HIV infection (Chase et al, 2000) and to predict later disease progression (Pearson et al, 2000). In addition to decreased global cognitive functioning, deficits in specific areas were observed, such as language and expressive behavior (Wolters et al, 1995). Since the advent of HAART, PHE has continued to decrease in frequency (Chiriboga et al, 2005; Shanbhag et al, 2005). Chiriboga and colleagues reported a decline in the rate of PHE from 31% in 1992 to less than 2% in 2000 in their cohort of perinatally infected children.

Despite the decrease in progressive encephalopathy, however, studies of neurodevelopment in the age of HAART suggest that cognitive problems may still be a significant concern for children with perinatally acquired HIV infection, particularly those with immune impairment (Jeremy et al, 2005). The Women and Infants Transmission Study followed a relatively large sample of children of mothers with HIV infection from birth and administered regular neurodevelopmental evaluations. The investigators compared the developmental status of 117 study participants who were born with HIV infection with that of 422 who were HIV exposed but uninfected (Smith et al, 2006). The children were evaluated at the ages of 3 and 7 years by use of the McCarthy Scales of Children's Abilities, a measure of general cognitive ability that also yields standardized domain scores in the areas of verbal, perceptual-performance, quantitative, memory, and motor abilities. Children who were HIV infected were further divided into two groups, those who experienced a class C (AIDS-defining) event during the course of the study (HIV/C; N = 33) and those who did not (N = 84). The groups were similar in the rates of other factors that present risks to neurodevelopment, including prematurity and prenatal exposure to drugs and alcohol. The investigators found that after adjustment for other health and environmental variables, the HIV-infected children who had an early class C event had significant impairment compared with the other two groups in all domains at both time points. Children who had HIV infection but did not experience an early AIDS-defining illness were similar to uninfected children, with both groups receiving test scores in the average range. The rate of change between the two time points did not differ between the groups. Thus, the HIV-infected children who experienced early, significant illness displayed global impairment but continued to develop, albeit at a consistently lower level than for the children in the other groups.

In summary, the current literature suggests that in the age of HAART, neurodevelopmental problems in children with perinatally acquired HIV infection are relatively subtle, compared with matched controls, until significant immunocompromise has occurred, at which time progressive encephalopathy can still occur. Mild global impairment has been well documented; more specific deficits can occur in a variety of areas but have been most commonly observed in language and fine motor skills. More severe motor impairments, including spastic diplegia, and global cognitive decline are seen with progressive encephalopathy. In examining a child with HIV infection, particularly one with well-controlled disease, the pediatrician should bear in mind that the child may be subject to numerous other developmental risks that are common in this population. These include low socioeconomic status, educational disadvantage, family disruption and loss of caregivers, parental and environmental substance abuse, coinfection with cytomegalovirus and other congenital infections (possibly with associated hearing deficits), side effects of medications, prenatal exposure to drugs and alcohol, and birth risks such as prematurity and low birth weight. Studies are currently being conducted to determine if prenatal exposure to antiretrovirals places the child at risk for developmental problems. Fatigue and depression due to HIV infection or antiretrovirals can have an impact on concentration, psychomotor speed, and other aspects of cognitive functioning. Referral for neuropsychological testing, neurologic evaluations, and neuroimaging can help disambiguate whether the child's cognitive impairments are related to HIV infection and thus indicate a need for treatment changes. It can also clarify whether interventions are needed.

Regardless of the cause of a perinatally infected child's cognitive impairment, the pediatrician must be aware of the possibility of significant service needs. Referrals for early intervention services, including occupational, physical, and speech therapy, are frequently necessary for infants and preschool children affected by HIV infection. As they get older, a disproportionate number of the children qualify for special education services. Chiriboga and associates (2005) noted that children in their study who had arrested PHE and significant improvement of cognitive symptoms nevertheless had a high rate of placement in special education (71%). Even children in that study who had never been diagnosed with PHE had a 24% rate of special education placement. The American Academy of Pediatrics (2000) made the point that pediatricians should be familiar with federal and state special education laws to assist families and make appropriate referrals for HIV-infected children with special education needs. For example, the federal Individuals with Disabilities Education Act provides access to educational and other services for children with developmental disabilities and health impairments if their condition has the potential to interfere with school attendance and performance. Other regulations that are relevant for children with special health care needs include Section 504 of the Rehabilitation Act of 1973. By providing referrals for developmental evaluations and for early intervention and special education programs as soon as the need is suspected, the pediatrician may be able to prevent HIV-infected children from falling behind their peers and being at risk for school failure and dropping out of school. As more and more perinatally infected children survive into adolescence, the need for vocational planning and preparation for independence becomes critical and should receive an early focus by the treatment team.

Although the stigma associated with HIV infection is less than in the past, it still exists, and communication with schools can be a sensitive topic for HIV-infected children and their caregivers. Families have the right to choose whether the child's HIV status is disclosed to the school, and pediatricians need to determine whether disclosure has occurred before any contact with schools occurs. Families may choose to disclose only to the school nurse or certain personnel to facilitate administration of medications at school when necessary. In a survey of 92 school-age children with HIV infection, Cohen and associates (1997) found that 53% of families had not informed the school of the child's HIV status; in those cases in which disclosure had occurred, the school nurse was most frequently the person who was informed. Pediatricians may find themselves in a position in which they are able to provide education to school staff and decrease their concerns about having an HIV-positive child in their classroom, thus facilitating a more normalized educational experience for the child.

MEDICAL MANAGEMENT

In addition to prophylaxis to prevent some opportunistic infections among severely immunosuppressed children, antiretroviral therapy is the mainstay of medical management. As of September 2006, there were 22 antiretroviral drugs approved for use in HIV-infected adults and adolescents in the United States. Thirteen of these had an approved pediatric treatment indication. These drugs fall into several major classes: nucleoside analogue or nucleotide analogue reverse transcriptase inhibitors, non-nucleoside reverse transcriptase inhibitors, protease inhibitors, and fusion inhibitors. Per current U.S. guidelines, "Aggressive combination therapy with at least three drugs from at least two classes of drugs (HAART) is recommended for initial treatment of infected infants, children, and adolescents because it provides the best opportunity to preserve immune function and delay disease progression" (Working Group on Antiretroviral Therapy, 2006). For patients initiating HAART, the goal of therapy is optimal viral suppression (a sustained viral load measurement below the threshold of detection). In the absence of optimal viral suppression, the patient is at risk for acquisition of resistance mutations, which may limit future treatment options. The medical indications for initiation of HAART therapy remain a topic of discussion among experts. A consideration in the choice of the initial antiretroviral regimen is the potential for side effects and limitations in subsequent treatment options should resistance develop. However, there are also a number of important behavioral and developmental factors. These include an understanding of the barriers to adherence, particularly the complexity of dosing schedule, food requirements, and palatability problems. There are several types of distinct adverse drug effects that may be most common with certain antiretroviral drugs or drug classes (Table 28-2). Some of these adverse effects result in appearance changes that may present challenges with adjustment and willingness of the child to adhere to treatment. Serious psychiatric adverse experiences, notably depression, have been reported in patients treated with the non-nucleoside reverse transcriptase inhibitor efavirenz.

Psychiatric or behavioral comorbidity has been noted among HIV-infected children in the United States. The pediatrician may be required to consider the use of psychotropic medications for a patient who is already being treated with HAART. It is important to appreciate that a number of antiretroviral agents as well as some psychotropic medications use the cytochrome P-450 enzyme system for metabolism. The cytochrome P-450 system consists of several isozymes, six of which mediate

Table 28-2. **Distinct Adverse Drug Effects Most Common with Certain Antiretroviral Drugs or Drug Classes**

Antiretroviral Drug or Drug Class	Most Common Adverse Effects
Zidovudine	Hematologic adverse events associated with drug-induced bone marrow suppression
Nucleoside reverse transcriptase inhibitors	Mitochondrial dysfunction, including lactic acidosis, hepatic toxicity, pancreatitis, and peripheral neuropathy
Stavudine and the protease inhibitor drugs and to a lesser degree certain other nucleoside reverse transcriptase inhibitors	Lipodystrophy and metabolic abnormalities including fat maldistribution and body habitus changes, hyperlipidemia, hyperglycemia, insulin resistance, and diabetes mellitus; osteopenia, osteoporosis, and osteonecrosis also reported
Non-nucleoside reverse transcriptase inhibitors and the nucleoside reverse transcriptase inhibitor abacavir	Allergic reactions such as rashes and hypersensitivity reactions

Working Group on Antiretroviral Therapy and Medical Management of HIV-Infected Children: Guidelines for the Use of Antiretroviral Agents in Pediatric HIV Infection. 2006. Available at: http://www.aidsinfo.nih.gov/guidelines.

most drug metabolism (1A2, 2C9/10, 2C19, 2D6, 2E1, 3A). Cytochrome P-450 isozymes can be inhibited or induced by certain drugs, and other drugs being administered concomitantly may be affected by these changes (substrates). This may result in drug toxicity or subtherapeutic plasma levels requiring dose adjustment. Medications used to treat attention deficit disorder, including methylphenidate hydrochloride and dextroamphetamine sulfate, do not use the cytochrome P-450 system for metabolism; amoxetine hydrochloride uses the cytochrome P-450 2D6 isozyme. Whereas concomitant administration of amoxetine hydrochloride and antiretroviral agents has not been formally studied, there is no contraindication listed (Eli Lilly, 2005). Fusion inhibitors and nucleoside reverse transcriptase inhibitors generally do not affect cytochrome P-450 activity. The non-nucleoside reverse transcriptase inhibitors nevirapine and efavirenz are generally cytochrome P-450 inducers; delavirdine is an inhibitor of isozyme 3A. Protease inhibitors are generally cytochrome P-450 inhibitors to varying degrees. Some psychotropic medications, particularly benzodiazepines, selective serotonin reuptake inhibitors, and some newer antidepressants, should be used with caution or not coadministered with these agents (University of Liverpool, 2006). As information is often updated and new agents are approved, consultation with a pharmacist is recommended for all patients receiving HAART who are also psychotropic medication treatment candidates.

ADHERENCE TO THERAPY

Nonadherence is well established as a major cause of clinical failure of HAART, and intermittent nonadherence is a particular problem. Studies in adults have demonstrated that more than 95% adherence to HAART is necessary for durable suppression of viral load (Miller and Hayes, 2000). In the presence of selective pressure by antiretroviral agents, high rates of viral replication and viral mutation lead to the development of drug resistance. Mutations conferring resistance against one antiretroviral agent often confer cross-resistance to other agents. Thus, poor adherence can render a whole class of antiretrovirals ineffective.

A person with a chronic illness must adhere to a medical regimen even though there is no cure, often in the absence of visible symptoms. While our understanding of HIV therapy is evolving, lifelong treatment is likely to be required. Pediatric chronic illness presents many unique adherence challenges. Caregivers are responsible for the adherence of children and so have a profound impact on adherence. Children living in families in which the adult caregiver is ill, is subject to significant stress, lacks effective organizational skills, lacks social support, or is not motivated to administer medications will have a high risk of nonadherence. Use of outreach staff to provide additional support for families with such challenges may enhance adherence. Adherence of children to complex medical regimens is influenced by the parent's or caregiver's knowledge of the illness, understanding of the therapeutic recommendations, and duration of treatment (Parrish, 1986). Providers need to emphasize caregiver education and realize that adherence will likely decrease over time without intervention.

Children's understanding of and reactions to illness change during development through a series of systematic stages that correspond to cognitive abilities (Peterson, 1989). The child's level of cognitive, motor, social, emotional, and psychological functioning affects the course and management of the disease. Their ability to perceive their own illness, to approach medical treatment, and to respond to interventions is influenced by their developmental level. It is important for care providers to be certain that a child's understanding of his or her illness and adherence interventions are periodically updated to keep pace with cognitive and emotional development.

Although it is a crucial component of good clinical care, assessment of adherence to HAART in HIV-infected children and youth is challenging and labor-intensive. Caregiver interview or self-report is considered especially subject to bias, as parents may inflate their adherence report to satisfy clinicians. However, it can be used to identify some poor adherers, and good adherence assessed by self-report is associated with good clinical outcomes (VanDyke et al, 2002; Williams et al, 2006). The pill count method to estimate adherence involves a comparison between the amount of medication remaining in the child's bottle and the amount that should be remaining based on the amount and dosage of the initial prescription and the length of time since the patient began using the bottle. This method does provide a measure of adherence over time but is subject to bias due to "pill dumping" (i.e., the parent may not leave all unused pills in the bottle in an effort to falsely increase the apparent level of adherence and please the clinician), and determination of the date when the patient commenced use of the current bottle can be a challenge. The chances of pill dumping bias or reporting bias are minimized by use of pharmacy medication refill records (i.e., comparing refill data from the pharmacy with the estimated refill requirement if all doses were administered). The method generally overestimates adherence because the availability of medication in the home does not necessarily mean the medication was actually administered. Pharmacy refill records and pill counts provide a general assessment of the number of doses taken but fail to yield any information about patterns of poor adherence. Electronic monitoring of adherence offers a more detailed assessment, demonstrating problems with dosing intervals in addition to missed doses. The Medication Event Monitoring System (Aprex/Aardex Corp., Menlo Park, CA) uses a microprocessor in the medication container cap to record the date and time of each vial opening. Electronic monitoring is considered by many to be the "gold standard" for adherence assessment.

Child and parent (or other caregiver) characteristics associated with adherence and strategies to improve adherence have been reported. In a large sample of HIV-infected children in the United States assessing adherence by self-report, factors associated with nonadherence included increasing age in years, female child, detectable HIV viral load, occurrence of recent stressful life events, repeating a grade in school, self-assessment of adherence by the child, and diagnosis of depression or anxiety. Factors associated with improved adherence included having an adult other than the biologic parent as the primary caregiver, use of a buddy system to remember to take medications, higher caregiver education level, previous adherence assessments, and taking antipsychotic medications (Williams et al, 2006). A number of other caregiver self-report studies report that poor palatability and unpleasant or inconvenient formulations remain major barriers to excellent adherence in children. Antiretroviral therapy regimens requiring less frequent administration have been associated with better adherence in HIV-infected adults and children. Thus, providers should choose the least complex and most palatable regimen possible. As an alternative to liquid formulations, some of which are notorious for palatability problems, a procedure for teaching young children to swallow pills was first described in 1984 and is now commonly employed by pediatric HIV care providers (Dahlquist and Blount, 1984). If palatability problems are anticipated, delaying initiation of the regimen while pill-swallowing training is attempted should be considered. Care providers should work with families to plan how adherence will be incorporated in the daily "routine." Whenever possible, medication dosing should be "cued" to another regular event, such as mealtimes or washing up at bedtime. Adherence aids such as pill boxes with a compartment for doses for each day and time or an alarm device should be encouraged. A prospective randomized trial of an intensive home-based nursing intervention has been described showing that nursing intervention is associated with improved adherence to HAART and better virologic outcome (Berrien et al, 2004). This suggests that interventions to enhance caregiver knowledge and self-efficacy, to overcome child-related barriers to adherence, and to provide social support are effective for some caregivers.

SUMMARY

Although advances in medical management have reduced the likelihood of many of the more severe sequelae of HIV infection in children and youth, significant behavioral and developmental challenges remain. Although HIV-affected families in the United States are disproportionately affected by poverty and substance abuse, all HIV-infected children commonly face emotional and psychosocial issues such as fear of death, death or change of parent or caregiver, anxiety, secrecy, and isolation. Physical development may be affected by the disease or its treatment. Although antiretroviral treatment has decreased the incidence of progressive encephalopathy, subtle neurodevelopmental problems are common and often require service referral. A high rate of psychiatric and behavioral disorders has been reported, and drug interactions between some antiretroviral agents and some psychotropic medications need to be considered. Poor adherence to antiretroviral therapy must be addressed because it is the major cause of treatment failure and may limit future therapeutic options.

REFERENCES

American Academy of Pediatrics, Committee on Pediatric AIDS: Disclosure of illness status to children and adolescents with HIV infection. Pediatrics 103:164-166, 1999.

American Academy of Pediatrics, Committee on Pediatric AIDS: Education of children with human immunodeficiency virus infection. Pediatrics 105:1358-1360, 2000.

Bagenda D, Nassali A, Kalyesubula I, et al: Health, neurologic, and cognitive status of HIV-infected, long-surviving, and antiretroviral-naive Ugandan children. Pediatrics 117:729-740, 2006.

Belman AL, Diamond G, Dickson D, et al: Pediatric acquired immunodeficiency syndrome: Neurologic syndromes. Am J Dis Child 142:29-35, 1988.

Berrien VM, Salazar JC, Reynolds E, et al: Adherence to antiretroviral therapy in HIV-infected pediatric patients improves with home-based intensive nursing intervention. AIDS Patient Care STDS. 18:355-363, 2004.

Brouwers P, Moss H, Wolters P, et al: Effect of continuous-infusion zidovudine therapy on neuropsychologic functioning in children with symptomatic human immunodeficiency virus infection. J Pediatr 117:980-985, 1990.

Buchacz K, Rogol AD, Lindsey JC, et al: Delayed onset of pubertal development in children and adolescents with perinatally acquired HIV infection. J Acquir Immune Defic Syndr 33:56-65, 2003.

Centers for Disease Control and Prevention: 1994 revised classification system for human immunodeficiency virus infection in children <13 years of age. MMWR Morb Mortal Wkly Rep 43(RR-12):1-19, 1994.

Centers for Disease Control and Prevention: HIV/AIDS Surveillance Report. 2005. Available at: http://www.cdc.gov/hiv/topics/surveillance/resources/reports. Accessed December 1, 2006.

Chantry CJ, Moye J: Growth, nutrition, and metabolism. *In* Zeichner SL, Read JS (eds): Handbook of Pediatric HIV Care. Cambridge, Cambridge University Press, 2006, pp 273-308.

Chase C, Ware J, Hittelman J, et al: Early cognitive and motor development among infants born to women infected with human immunodeficiency virus. Pediatrics 106:e25, 2000.

Chiriboga CA, Fleishman S, Champion S, et al: Incidence and prevalence of HIV encephalopathy in children with HIV infection receiving highly active anti-retroviral therapy (HAART). J Pediatr 146:402-407, 2005.

Cohen J, Reddington C, Jacobs D, et al: School related issues among HIV-infected children. Pediatrics 100:1-5, 1997.

Cohen SE, Mundy T, Karassik B, et al: Neuropsychological functioning in human immunodeficiency virus type 1 seropositive children infected through neonatal blood transfusion. Pediatrics 88:58-68, 1991.

Dahlquist LM, Blount RL: Teach a six-year-old girl to swallow pills. J Behav Ther Exp Psychiatry 15:171-173, 1984.

Duliege AM, Messiah A, Blanche S, et al: Natural history of human immunodeficiency virus type 1 infection in children: Prognostic value of laboratory tests on the bimodal progression of disease. Pediatr Infect Dis J 11:630-635, 1992.

Eli Lilly and Company: Amoxetine hydrochloride [package insert]. 2005. Available at: http://www.pdr.net/druginformation. Accessed January 15, 2007.

Gaughan DM, Hughes MD, Oleske JM, et al: Psychiatric hospitalizations among children and youth with HIV infection. Pediatrics 113:e544-551, 2004.

Gerson AC, Joyner M, Fosarelli P, et al: Disclosure of HIV diagnosis to children: When, where, why, and how. J Pediatr Health Care 15:161-167, 2001.

Gona P, Van Dyke RB, Williams PL, et al: Incidence of opportunistic and other infections in HIV-infected children in the HAART era. JAMA 296(3):292-300, 2006.

Gortmaker SL, Hughes M, Cervia, J, et al: Effect of combination therapy including protease inhibitors on mortality among children and adolescents infected with HIV-1. N Engl J Med 345:1522-1528, 2001.

Jeremy RJ, Kim S, Nozyce M, et al: Neuropsychological functioning and viral load in stable antiretroviral therapy–experienced HIV-infected children. Pediatrics 115:380-387, 2005.

Kadivar H, Garvie PA, Sinnock C, et al: Psychosocial profile of HIV-infected adolescents in a Southern US urban cohort. AIDS Care 18:544-549, 2006.

Loveland KA, Stehbens JA, Mahoney EM, et al: Declining immune function in children and adolescents with hemophilia and HIV infection: Effects on neuropsychological performance. J Pediatr Psychol 25:309-322, 2000.

Madger LS, Mofenson L, Paul ME, et al: Risk factors for in-utero and intrapartum transmission of HIV. J Acquir Immune Defic Syndr 33(1):87-95, 2005.

Mellins CA, Brackis-Cott E, Dolezal C, et al: Psychiatric disorders in youth with perinatally acquired human immunodeficiency virus infection. Pediatr Infect Dis J 25:432-437, 2006.

Mellins CA, Smith R, O'Driscoll P, et al: High rates of behavioral problems in perinatally HIV-infected children are not linked to HIV disease. Pediatrics 111:384-393, 2003.

Miller LD, Hayes RD: Adherence to combination antiretroviral therapy: Synthesis of the literature and clinical implications. AIDS Read 10:177-185, 2000.

Mitchell W: Neurological and developmental effects of HIV and AIDS in children and adolescents. Ment Retard Dev Disabil Res Rev 7:211-216, 2001.

Parrish J: Parent compliance with medical and behavioral recommendations. *In* Krasnegor N, Arasteh J, Cataldo M (eds): Child Health Behavior. New York, Wiley, 1986, pp 453-501.

Pearson DA, McGrath NM, Nozyce M, et al: Predicting HIV disease progression in children using measures of neuropsychological and neurological functioning. Pediatrics 106:e76, 2000.

Peterson L: Coping by children undergoing stressful medical procedures: Some conceptual, methodological, and therapeutic issues. J Consult Clin Psychol 57:380-387, 1989.

Shanbhag MC, Rutstein RM, Zaoutis T, et al: Neurocognitive functioning in pediatric human immunodeficiency virus infection. Arch Pediatr Adolesc Med 159:651-656, 2005.

Shearer WT, Quinn TC, LaRussa P, et al: Viral load and disease progression in infants infected with human immunodeficiency virus type 1. N Engl J Med 336:1337-1342, 1997.

Sirois PA, Hill SD: Developmental change associated with human immunodeficiency virus infection in school-age children with hemophilia. Dev Neuropsychol 9:177-197, 1993.

Smith R, Malee K, Leighty R, et al: Effects of perinatal HIV infection and associated risk factors on cognitive development among young children. Pediatrics 117:851-862, 2006.

Tardieu M, Le Chenadec J, Persoz A, et al: HIV-1–related encephalopathy in infants compared with children and adults. Neurology 54:1089-1095, 2000.

University of Liverpool, HIV Pharmacology Group: NNRTI Drug Interactions, Protease Inhibitor Drug Interactions. 2006. Available at: www.hiv-druginteractions.org. Accessed January 1, 2007.

Van Dyke RB, Lee S, Johnson GM, et al: Reported adherence as a determinant of response to highly active antiretroviral therapy in HIV-infected children. Pediatrics 109:e61, 2002.

Wiener LS, Battles HB: Untangling the web: A close look at diagnosis disclosure among HIV-infected adolescents. J Adolesc Health 38:307-309, 2006.

Williams P, Storm D, Montepiedra G, et al: Predictors of adherence to antiretroviral medications in children and adolescents with HIV infection. Pediatrics 118:e1745-1757, 2006.

Wolters P, Brouwers P, Moss H: Pediatric HIV disease: Effect on cognition, learning, and behavior. Sch Psychol Q 10:305-328, 1995.

Working Group on Antiretroviral Therapy and Medical Management of HIV-Infected Children: Guidelines for the Use of Antiretroviral Agents in Pediatric HIV Infection. 2006. Available at: http://www.aidsinfo.nih.gov/guidelines. Accessed December 1, 2006.

World Health Organization: Antiretroviral therapy of HIV infection in infants and children in resource-limited settings: Towards universal access, recommendations for a public health approach. 2006. Available at: http://www.who.int/hiv/pub/guidelines. Accessed December 1, 2006.

29 NUTRITION ASSESSMENT AND SUPPORT

Marilyn Stevenson and Nancy F. Krebs

The nutrient requirements of children are influenced by their growth rate and body composition and the composition of new growth. These factors vary with age and are especially important during early postnatal life. Growth rates are higher in early infancy than at any other time, including the adolescent growth spurt. Growth rates decline rapidly starting in the second month of postnatal life.

Nutrient requirements also depend on body composition. In the adult, the brain, which accounts for only 2% of body weight, contributes approximately 20% to the total basal energy expenditure. In contrast, in a full-term neonate, the brain accounts for 10% of body weight and more than 40% of total basal energy expenditure. Thus, in the young infant, total basal energy expenditure and the energy requirement of the brain are relatively high.

Composition of new tissue also influences nutrient requirements. For example, fat accounts for about 40% of weight gain between birth and 4 months but for less than 5% between 24 and 36 months. The corresponding figures for protein are 11% and 21%; for water, 45% and 68%. The high rate of fat deposition in early infancy has implications not only for energy requirements but also for the optimal composition of infant feedings. The high fat content of human milk (and thus of modern infant formulas) efficiently supports fat deposition. Because of the high nutrient requirements for growth and the body composition, the infant is especially vulnerable to undernutrition. Slowed physical growth rate is an early and prominent sign of undernutrition in the young infant. The limited fat stores of the very young infant mean that energy reserves are quite limited. The relatively large size and continued growth of the brain render the central nervous system especially vulnerable to the effects of malnutrition in early postnatal life.

Children are also particularly vulnerable to the effects of malnutrition during periods of rapid growth and development. Such vulnerability is common in infants who are born prematurely, in young children with chronic diseases that interfere with absorption or growth, and in those with delayed or altered development that affects feeding skills and behaviors. Neuromuscular dysfunction, cognitive delays, seizures, impaired vision, medications, disordered hunger and satiety cues, perioral sensitivity, and behavioral problems are all risk factors for malnutrition in young children with disabilities.

GROWTH ASSESSMENT

Growth assessment typically and most readily includes weight, length (or height for children older than 2 years), and head circumference measurements. These are plotted on National Center for Health Statistics growth references *(www.cdc.gov/growthcharts),* which are based on cross-sectional samples of infants and children in the United States (Kuczmarski et al, 2000). Detailed guidelines for procedures to obtain accurate anthropometric measures are available through the Centers for Disease Control and Prevention Web site, *http://www.cdc.gov/nchs/data/nhanes/nhanes_03_04/BM.pdf.*

Because the growth patterns of children with special needs are often abnormal compared with usual references, often falling below the 5th percentiles for weight and height, particular care must be given to the assessment of patterns of growth and rates of growth. A steady pattern of growth well below the 5th percentile may be less cause for concern than a deceleration of growth from the 75th to 25th percentiles. Although the term *growth* is often used nonspecifically, distinction is appropriately made between weight gain and linear growth, both of which are interrelated but not equally responsive to nutritional deprivation or manipulation. Weight represents the composite of energy reserves (i.e., fat) and lean body mass and body water. Linear growth reflects musculoskeletal growth and is governed by many non-nutritional factors, including endocrinologic and genetic influences, making it somewhat less modifiable by nutritional intake.

Proportionality of weight to length or height is another indicator of nutritional adequacy. Body composition may be altered by the underlying condition. This includes especially muscle mass, which is often abnormal if a child is nonambulatory or hypotonic. Although extremes of undernutrition may have an impact on muscle bulk, disuse will generally have a more profound impact. Thus, in such cases, total weight must be considered in the context of body composition. Similarly, microcephaly can contribute to low total weight, especially in an infant or young child, when the size of the head is relatively large compared with the rest of the body. Brain growth, represented by head circumference, may also be primarily influenced by non-nutritional factors. Use of the weight for length (or body mass index graphs for children older than 2 years) gives an indication of whether the child is gaining in weight proportional to linear growth. "Ideal" weight for length is the weight at the 50th percentile (median) for a given length on the weight/length chart. Normal weight range for a given length is considered to be within 10% (above and below) of the median.

Head circumference should be measured, plotted on age- and sex-adjusted references, and compared with weight and length or height for age percentiles. An exceptionally large head, as with hydrocephalus, may contribute disproportionately to weight and give false interpretation to adequate weight gain or weight-to-length assessment. Alternatively, microcephaly will also affect total weight, and weight status should be interpreted accordingly. As noted, muscle mass is often disproportionately low in children with special needs (e.g., those with Down syndrome or untreated Prader-Willi syndrome). Children with conditions such as cerebral palsy or fetal alcohol syndrome often have low fat stores, reflecting relative inadequacy of energy intake or an inherent lean body habitus. Assessment of body composition by measurement of skin fold thickness (with skin calipers) to estimate subcutaneous fat stores and arm circumference to estimate muscle body mass may be very useful in interpreting body weight and adequacy of energy and fat stores.

Adjustment for prematurity is typically made for the first 24 months of corrected age and gives a more accurate perspective of absolute weight and length measurements. For example, an infant born at 28 weeks of gestation would be plotted at an adjusted age 3 months less than chronologic age. Use of the weight-for-length reference is another way to assess proportionality of weight and length that is independent of age norms.

Disease- or condition-specific growth charts have little practical value in monitoring growth. Data for these charts have often inevitably come from a small sample size or from a population receiving poor nutritional or medical intervention. Specialty growth charts may be useful in comparing children to others with the same syndrome and in identifying expected patterns of growth for the condition. They are best used in conjunction with the National Center for Health Statistics growth charts for monitoring growth and proportionality.

Because determination of ideal weight is dependent on length or height measurement, obtaining accurate measurement is important yet often difficult in special populations. Alternative methods to use of a length board or stadiometer include the knee-height caliper, which measures the length from heel to knee and applies a formula to estimate height (Table 29-1), and upper arm length or tibia length measurement formulas (Bell and Davies, 2006; Stevenson, 1995).

ENERGY AND NUTRIENT REQUIREMENTS

Children with developmental disabilities exhibit a wide range of mental and physical deficits; therefore, determination of the nutritional requirements of children with special needs is not standardized, even within groups of children with the same condition. This necessitates an empiric approach for each child, guided by knowledge of nutritional needs of normal children and by the limited data available for selected subgroups of children with special needs.

The energy needs of children with cerebral palsy have been studied. Both resting energy expenditure and total energy expenditure have been found to be lower than in control groups. Resting energy expenditure is primarily determined by lean body mass, and these findings are consistent with a lower lean body mass in the subjects (Stallings et al, 1996). Guidelines for estimation of calorie needs of children older than 5 years with cerebral palsy, Down syndrome, spina bifida, and Prader-Willi syndrome have been published (Ekvall, 1993) (Table 29-2). These guidelines are useful as a starting point, but because of variability in severity, activity level, and associated illness within these populations, calorie goals must always be individually estimated and monitored. This ideally involves assessing current energy intake and making adjustments, upward or downward, to the current regimen on the basis of growth (weight and linear) at regular assessment intervals.

Protein requirements are usually assumed to be the same as published Dietary Reference Intakes for age and are based on ideal weight (Otten, Hellwig, and Meyers,

Table 29-1. Estimation of Stature from Knee Height in Children Ages 6 to 18 Years

White boys	Stature in cm = (knee height × 2.2) + 40.54
White girls	Stature in cm = (knee height × 2.15) + 43.21
Black boys	Stature in cm = (knee height × 2.18) + 39.6
Black girls	Stature in cm = (knee height × 2.02) + 46.59

Modified from Stevenson RD: Use of segmental measures to estimate stature in children with cerebral palsy. Arch Pediatr Adolesc Med 149:658-662, 1995.

Table 29-2. Estimation of Energy Needs of Children Older than 5 Years with Special Health Care Needs

Condition	Energy Needs (kcal/cm)
Cerebral palsy or motor dysfunction	
Mild, ambulatory	14
Severe, nonambulatory	11
Down syndrome	
Girls	14
Boys	16
Prader-Willi syndrome	
Growth maintenance	10-11
Weight loss	8.5
Spina bifida	
Weight maintenance	9-11
Weight loss	7

Modified from Ekvall S: Pediatric Nutrition in Chronic Diseases and Development. New York, Oxford University Press, 1993.

2006). Obtaining adequate protein may be difficult if energy needs are very low. Pediatric enteral feeding products may not supply enough protein if calorie intake is less than 50 calories per kilogram, in which case modular protein additives may need to be added. High-quality dietary protein may be lacking in oral diets for children who have difficulty chewing meat, who avoid dairy, or who have a limited variety of foods in their diet.

Fluid requirements are based on body weight. Many children with oral motor dysfunction have difficulty handling liquids because of the rapid transit through the oral cavity. They may have increased losses associated with drooling; cognitive deficits may contribute to inability to communicate thirst. When calorically dense enteral formulas are used to meet energy needs with a relatively small volume, fluid intake may be suboptimal if additional free water is not provided. It is thus not unusual for children with special needs to fail to meet fluid needs, which may, in turn, predispose to constipation and chronic mild dehydration.

Vitamin and mineral needs have also not been established specifically for this population. The Recommended Dietary Allowance or, in some cases, Adequate Intakes for vitamins and minerals are used to estimate an appropriate level of intake for an individual (Otten, Hellwig, and Meyers, 2006). On the other hand, intakes should not routinely exceed the published tolerable upper intake limits (Otten, Hellwig, and Meyers, 2006). The risks for inadequate nutrient intake are generally more likely to be attributed to inadequate dietary intake than to increased nutrient needs. A complete children's multivitamin-mineral tablet (i.e., a product that includes both vitamins and minerals) may be given daily if dietary intake from an entire food group is missing or energy requirements are very low. Several case reports have been published of specific micronutrient deficiencies occurring in the context of extremely limited variety, based on either limited child preferences or perceived intolerance to multiple foods (see vignette). Increased intakes for calcium and vitamin D are indicated for the nonambulatory, non–weight-bearing child to optimize bone mineralization. This is especially important during early adolescence when bone mineralization is maximal. Although more empiric than evidence based, typical recommended intakes are at least 150% of the Adequate Intakes for these nutrients. Calcium is not included in significant amounts in vitamin-mineral supplements and should be given in addition to any vitamin preparations. Fluoride supplementation should be considered for children fully dependent on ready-to-feed formula and without additional intake of fluoridated water.

Vignette: Micronutrient Deficiency

A 9-year-old boy with autism was transferred from an outside hospital with a presumptive diagnosis of Henoch-Schönlein purpura. The patient presented to the outside hospital with a chief complaint of acute refusal to walk, swollen knees, and "rash." Initial diet history on admission was "normal for age." Further inquiry revealed that he ate only one food at a time; food for approximately the past 6 months had been soft pretzels with cheese. Before that, he ate corn chips as primary food. The history was negative for consumption of fortified liquid supplements or a multivitamin-mineral supplement. Past medical history was otherwise unremarkable except for developmental delays and seizure disorder; before the onset of these symptoms, the patient was described as ambulatory and active. Medication included only phenytoin.

Vital signs were within normal limits (no hypertension).

Physical Examination

In general, this was an agitated, uncooperative, prepubertal boy who appeared well nourished.

Skin: nonpalpable purpuric lesions on feet and ankles, with extension up to knees; no petechiae; no lesions on buttocks.

Head, eyes, ears, nose, and throat: no bleeding gums or oral lesions; no epistaxis; eyes without icterus or injection; neck supple and without adenopathy; lungs clear; cardiovascular examination unremarkable.

Abdomen: nontender and without organomegaly.

Extremities: 2-3+ pitting edema in feet and ankles, with extension up to knees.

Rectal examination findings normal; stool heme negative.

Neurologic examination grossly intact but difficult to perform owing to poor cooperation.

Laboratory Studies

Complete blood count with slightly low hemoglobin and hematocrit values, normocytic mean cell volume; normal platelet count; erythrocyte sedimentation rate, 15; urinalysis, negative; prothrombin time, prolonged at 15; blood urea nitrogen and creatinine concentrations normal.

Discussion

Although examination findings are not entirely inconsistent with Henoch-Schönlein purpura, the history did not indicate the typical progression of macular rash starting on distal aspects of lower extremities and buttocks. The absence of hypertension, palpable lesions, signs or symptoms of bowel ischemia, and laboratory findings suggestive of systemic inflammation (no elevated erythrocyte sedimentation rate, thrombocytosis, or leukocytosis) does not support

(Continued)

Vignette: Micronutrient Deficiency—cont'd

Henoch-Schönlein purpura as the diagnosis. The extremely limited diet, which indicated no intake of fruits and vegetables, and the findings of extensive ecchymoses along with prolonged prothrombin time raised the possibility of vitamin K and vitamin C deficiencies. The patient received parenteral vitamin K on admission, with normalization of prothrombin time, but without improvement in other symptoms. Plasma ascorbic acid level was determined; the result was below the lower limit of normal, consistent with a diagnosis of scurvy.

This case illustrates the importance of recognition of the potential of nutritional deficiencies to cause skin findings. The history of an extremely limited diet without fortified products or micronutrient supplements in a developmentally delayed child should have brought the possibility of a nutrient deficiency to mind, especially when several diagnostic criteria were not met for a more common diagnosis. Similar case reports have been published (Duggan, Westra, and Rosenberg, 2007).

In young children with special needs who are not receiving fortified formulas, dietary preferences may not include good sources of iron or zinc, two trace minerals for which requirements are relatively high in infancy and early childhood, when growth is relatively rapid and when postnatal brain development is still active. Iron is essential for normal erythropoiesis and for normal brain development. The bone marrow and red blood cell production is prioritized, however, over other tissues, including the brain. Iron deficiency has been associated with both cognitive and motor deficits. When these occur in early childhood, they appear to be only partially reversible with iron therapy, presumably because of the impact of the insult during a "critical window" of brain development. Iron deficiency anemia represents severe deficiency. Mild to moderate deficiency, reflected by depleted stores, is associated with adverse neurodevelopmental consequences (American Academy of Pediatrics, 2004b).

Zinc is essential for normal growth, immune function, and neurocognitive development. Unlike iron, stores of zinc are limited, and mild to moderate deficiency can occur relatively quickly with limited absolute intake or intake from dietary sources that have limited bioavailability, such as foods containing absorption inhibitors like phytate, which is found in grains and legumes. The effects of mild zinc deficiency are well documented and include growth faltering (both linear and weight gain), anorexia, and impaired immune function. Neurodevelopmental delays have also been documented, particularly related to motor development. More severe deficiency is associated with these signs as well as a characteristic acral-orificial dermatitis and diarrhea.

Flesh foods, especially red meats, are excellent natural and highly bioavailable sources of these two minerals. However, for a variety of reasons, including the texture and need for coordinated chewing, taste preferences, and tradition, meats often are not routinely consumed by young children with special needs. Although infant cereals are typically highly fortified with iron, once a young child transitions to ready-to-eat cereal, this dietary source is often not replaced by comparably fortified foods. Food fortification with zinc is more limited than for iron, so young children who do not consume commercial fortified enteral formulas may have marginal zinc intakes if their diets do not contain meats. If iron status was adequately supported during the latter part of infancy, iron stores may be maintained with the amounts typically contained in a multivitamin supplement. With iron deficiency, however, a period of therapeutic supplementation with iron alone will be necessary to replete stores and to attain normal iron status. Infant liquid multivitamin drops do not contain zinc, nor do many of the chewable preparations for children older than 2 years. There is no commercially available liquid zinc supplement comparable to liquid iron supplements; a liquid zinc supplement can be obtained by prescription from compounding pharmacies.

Benefits of megadoses (>10-fold Recommended Dietary Allowance levels) of vitamins for children with Down syndrome, autism, and other conditions have not been supported by evidence from controlled trials.

DIETARY ASSESSMENT

Assessment of an infant's intake should most importantly determine whether the infant is breastfed (or receiving human milk) or formula fed. This is a critical distinction because of the differences in feeding and nutritional issues between these two feeding modes. Although many infants will receive a mixture of feedings, the following discussion highlights issues assuming full intake from either human milk or formula.

The benefits of breastfeeding to infant health and development are without question, but this requires clinicians to be aware of physiologic issues that are inherent with breastfeeding. A general resource for breastfeeding management, including for infants with special needs, has been published by the American Academy of Pediatrics (American Academy of Pediatrics, 2006). If the infant has feeding difficulties (e.g., due to prematurity, developmental delays, or congenital anomalies), maternal milk supply can easily and quickly become diminished. In such circumstances, a good milk supply can be maintained with pumping. The demands on the mother of pumping, however, must also be recognized, and support will be important for sustained success. Early recognition of potentially inadequate milk supply due to poor infant feeding is critical for avoidance of growth faltering. Fortification of expressed human milk may be beneficial for infants with special needs (e.g., those born prematurely or those for whom adequate volume is a challenge). Human milk fortifiers designed for premature infants are available while the infant is in the nursery but are not routinely available after discharge. Expressed milk can be fortified with standard powdered infant formula to increase the calorie (and nutrient) density.

Adequacy of milk intake by a breastfed infant will usually be assessed first and foremost by adequacy of growth. The composition of human milk is quite consistent, and only in rare circumstances will a deficiency of milk nutrient composition or energy density be a cause of growth faltering. During the first several months of life, milk volume and intake are much more susceptible to shortfall due to either maternal or infant causes or an interaction between them.

For formula-fed infants, assessment should establish that the formula is a standard commercial infant formula. Alternative home-prepared mixtures or plant-based "milks" (e.g., rice, soy, hemp) have been associated with cases of severe malnutrition. Assessment should also confirm appropriate preparation of the formula, typically to 20 kcal per ounce of energy density. Formulas should contain a minimum level of iron fortification, that is, at least 4 mg iron per liter. Although daily intake is somewhat easier to quantify for bottle-fed infants, adequacy of a given intake is again determined by adequacy of infant growth.

Complementary foods should be started by approximately 6 months of age, and assessment should include consideration of both quantity and quality. Human milk is low in iron, and complementary foods (or supplements) are essential to meet the infant's iron needs once the infant's stores at birth are depleted. Strategies to meet iron requirements for term breastfed infants include use of iron-fortified infant cereal, pureed meats, or iron supplements, starting by approximately 6 months. For preterm or low-birth-weight infants, iron depletion occurs earlier, typically before 6 months. For these infants, a daily iron supplement of 2 mg/kg/day is recommended from 1 month of age. By approximately 6 months, the breastfed infant also needs a source of zinc in addition to that provided in human milk. Because many infant cereals are not zinc fortified, pureed meats are the best dietary source of zinc. Infants' digestive tracts are essentially mature by 6 months, and meats can thus be safely introduced as an early complementary food at this age and provide an excellent source of highly bioavailable zinc and iron. Pureed fruits and vegetables are often among the first complementary foods introduced. They offer variety and exposure to different tastes. The nutrients they provide, however, are usually not limited in the milk of healthy, well-nourished lactating mothers. For formula-fed infants, the specific choices of complementary foods are less important because the fortification of the formula will continue to provide relatively generous amounts of all nutrients. Gradual introduction of a variety of foods, starting at approximately 6 months, is appropriate.

Developmental cues that indicate readiness for non-liquid foods include regression of tongue-thrusting reflex and other primitive reflexes, ability to sit upright with minimal support, reaching for objects and bringing to mouth, ability to bring hands to midline, and absence of choking with non-liquid foods. If development is significantly delayed, expectations for complementary feeding should be adjusted accordingly. For breastfed infants, this may indicate need for micronutrient supplements, especially iron and possibly zinc, to replace the intake of these essential nutrients that would otherwise have been derived from foods. For formula-fed infants, there is no nutritional necessity for complementary foods, and introduction can be delayed until the infant achieves the appropriate developmental milestones. If progression to complementary foods is significantly delayed, referral to a pediatric occupational therapist or speech-language therapist may be helpful to specifically work on oral motor function and feeding skills (American Academy of Pediatrics, 2004a).

For older children, dietary assessment should include a basic review of food groups included in the child's usual diet. Growth may be progressing along normal growth channels, masking concern for nutrient deficiencies from limited food choices. Overconsumption of milk is a classic example. Consumption of more than 32 ounces per day for a young child is associated with iron deficiency anemia because of displacement by the milk of iron-fortified foods or meats. Autistic children often exhibit limited dietary choices and may benefit from a pediatric feeding specialist (e.g., pediatric dietitian, occupational therapist, or speech therapist). Although vitamin-mineral supplements may be offered to cover nutritional inadequacies, the usual pediatric vitamin-mineral supplements may not be well accepted in this population because of the taste or texture of the supplements. Thus, if a routine screening indicates a highly restricted diet, whether it is due to the child's preferences or to real or perceived intolerance, with absence of one or more food groups and without use of fortified products or nutrient supplements, the risk of nutritional deficiencies should be considered.

Commonly used medications in children with disabilities, including anticonvulsants, laxatives, steroids, stimulants, and antipsychotic medications, may have nutritional implications. Some affect appetite, and others can interfere with nutrient absorption or utilization (Table 29-3).

PHYSICAL EXAMINATION

Components of the physical examination that are most reflective of and responsive to nutritional status are general appearance, skin, hair, and mucosal surfaces. General appearance includes amount of subcutaneous fat (e.g., wasting, which reflects inadequate energy intake; or normal to generous fat, which reflects adequate or excessive energy intake). As discussed before under growth assessment, distinguishing between subcutaneous fat and muscle mass can be used to assess energy needs. Skin fold measurements, if available and appropriately obtained, can help characterize these body composition differences. Evidence of micronutrient deficiencies should particularly be considered in the presence of skin findings, including detectable pallor, bruising, petechiae, and rashes that are unusual in character or severity. Abnormal hair texture, easy pluckability, or visible change in pigmentation may represent nutritional deficits, including inadequate or poor-quality protein intake. Edema, generalized or limited to lower extremities, may suggest hypoalbuminemia of nutritional origin or congestive heart failure secondary to micronutrient deficiency.

The neurologic examination provides an opportunity to assess developmental level. Loss of deep tendon reflexes is associated with micronutrient deficiencies, notably vitamin E deficiency, which may occur with fat malabsorption, or vitamin B_{12} deficiency, which may be seen in vegans without supplementation or in the breastfed infant of an unsupplemented vegan mother.

An overview of examination findings associated with specific micronutrient deficiencies is provided in Table 29-4. Obviously, the physical examination is also important for identification of other underlying pathologic processes that may affect growth or nutritional needs.

BIOCHEMICAL ASSESSMENT

Laboratory testing is often less informative than the history and examination but can certainly be used to screen for gross deficiencies or metabolic abnormalities or to offer confirmatory data. Biochemical screening is typically limited to a complete blood count, but as noted before, anemia due to iron deficiency reflects severe deficiency and thus is a late diagnosis. If the child presents in a vulnerable age range (e.g., older infant or toddler) for iron deficiency or a dietary pattern suggests inadequate intake, a better assessment is provided by obtaining a serum ferritin concentration and transferrin saturation (and derived iron-binding capacity) in addition to the complete blood count. Because ferritin is elevated as part of the acute-phase response, interpretation is enhanced by obtaining a concurrent marker of inflammation (e.g., a C-reactive protein level or erythrocyte sedimentation rate). Without evidence of hepatic dysfunction, edema, or moderate to severe protein-energy malnutrition, serum albumin concentration is unlikely to be low or informative. Prealbumin is another circulating protein that has a shorter half-life than albumin and reflects more acute changes in nutritional status, but in an outpatient assessment, it typically provides little additional information beyond that available from the history, anthropometry, and examination. Both albumin and prealbumin are also depressed with acute inflammation. Specific circulating levels can be obtained for most vitamins, or, in some cases, intermediary metabolites

Table 29-3. Potential Nutrient-Drug Interactions for Drugs Commonly Prescribed for Children with Developmental Delays

Medication	Interaction	Recommendation
Anticonvulsants	Decreased absorption or altered metabolism:	Supplemental vitamin D, folate
Phenytoin	vitamins D, B_6, B_{12}, folate	Consider supplemental vitamin B_6 or B_{12}
Phenobarbital	Constipation	High-fiber diet
		More fluid
Laxatives	Decreased absorption of fat-soluble vitamins	Take before bed, not with meals
Mineral oil		
Steroids	Decreased absorption or increased excretion of calcium, phosphorus	Supplemental calcium, vitamin D
	Increased weight gain, stunting	Calorie-controlled diet
Stimulants	Reduced appetite	Take after meals
	Poor weight gain, stunting	High-calorie diet
Antipsychotics	Increased weight	Adjust calorie content of diet
	Decreased weight	

Table 29-4. Summary Table of Micronutrient Deficiency Findings in History or Examination

	Rash or Skin Findings	Mouth Lesions	Neurologic Symptoms	Anemia	Other
Vitamin C	X (purpura)	X	X	X	
Thiamin			X		
Riboflavin		X			
Niacin	X		X		
Folate		X		X	
Vitamin B_{12}		X	X	X	
Vitamin B_6		X	X	X	
Vitamin A	X				Corneal dryness and thickening, blindness
Vitamin D					Rickets, epiphyseal widening
Vitamin E			X	X	
Vitamin K	X (purpura)			X	
Iron			X	X	
Zinc	X		X		Growth impairment, anorexia, delayed puberty
Calcium			Tetany		Bone mineral depletion
Phosphorus					Impaired muscle function, including cardiorespiratory arrest

reflect nutrient deficiencies. Such tests are not routinely obtained but rather as indicated from other findings in the nutrition assessment.

In the evaluation of potential underlying disease to explain poor growth, first-line screening tests may include a comprehensive metabolic panel, including electrolyte and mineral values, glucose concentration, renal function tests, and liver function profile. Thyroid function testing should be reserved for cases with linear growth plateauing, short stature, or findings on history or examination suggestive of thyroid dysfunction. Urinalysis and stool microscopy for fat malabsorption are also useful screening tests. Second-tier tests for growth faltering, which should be guided by other findings or risk, include serologic testing for celiac disease (tissue transglutaminase), gastrointestinal imaging (e.g., upper gastrointestinal series), serum amino acids, and urine organic acids to screen for inborn errors of metabolism.

INTERVENTIONS

Poor weight gain often can be improved with increasing the calorie density of infant formula, offering energy-dense foods and beverages, and enhancing the calorie content of low-energy foods by addition of fats. This includes providing whole milk to drink and setting limits on consumption of water, juice, and sports drinks. Flavored instant breakfast powder added to whole milk or milk mixed with cream supplies additional calories and nutrients. Flavored liquid pediatric nutritional supplements (e.g., PediaSure) are expensive but are often available through the local Special Supplemental Nutrition Program for Women, Infants, and Children (WIC) or some insurance carriers; private label versions are sold at most major retailers. These drinks contain milk protein but are lactose free and are broadly fortified with micronutrients. Protein- and micronutrient-fortified high-calorie juice beverages are available from pharmaceutical sources and are useful for children who refuse the creamy texture and flavor of milk.

When children exhibit signs of food refusal to certain textures, fatigue with eating, inability to advance diet to age-appropriate foods, coughing or choking with eating or drinking, or prolonged time required to eat, a referral for evaluation by an occupational or speech therapist with expertise in child feeding may provide helpful insights into the processes underlying the child's feeding challenges. An upright modified barium swallow study may also be helpful to evaluate for aspiration and to identify textures that can be managed safely by the child.

Tube feedings, either by nasogastric or gastrostomy device, should be considered when attempts to maximize the diet orally have failed to produce steady weight gain, when unreasonable amounts of time (more than 45 minutes per meal) are required for oral feeding, when inadequate hydration leads to severe constipation, or when oral feedings are not safe because of risk of aspiration. Ideally, tube feedings should not replace all oral feeding when aspiration is absent, but they may be used to augment inadequate dietary intake or to provide liquids that may be unsafe or difficult to consume in adequate amounts. The feeding tube also offers a convenient way to administer medications to the child. When oral intake is desired in addition to tube feedings, it is imperative to balance the impact of provision of substantial energy needs through the tube on the child's physiologic regulation of energy intake. It is unreasonable to expect that a child's oral intake will substantially increase if nutritional needs are largely being met by the tube feedings. Once growth has been normalized or improved, a trial of reduced formula intake can be initiated, with monitoring of weight status while the child is given opportunity to adjust oral intake to meet needs (see also later).

The choice of enteral feeding products depends on the child's age and the specific feeding issues. Initially, the tube-fed infant is given infant formula. A premature transitional formula should be given if the infant was born before 36 weeks. Specialized formulas such as those made from hydrolyzed casein with medium-chain triglycerides and elemental or metabolic formulas may be prescribed to meet special needs. There is no need to add baby foods to the feeding tubes of infants who are receiving a standard formula in amounts adequate to achieve normal growth.

A tube-fed child older than 12 months or larger than 10 kg should receive a pediatric enteral feeding product. These products are designed to meet the usual energy, protein, vitamin, and mineral requirements for the child up to 10 years of age. The protein source is typically intact milk protein, but these formulas are lactose free. Products differ in the balance of casein and whey proteins, which may have an impact on tolerance. The whey fraction of milk protein stays liquid in an acidic environment, and there is some evidence that whey-predominant formulas have a faster rate of gastric emptying (Khoshoo et al, 1996). The protein in many pediatric enteral formulas is predominantly casein, which tends to coagulate in the stomach, thereby delaying gastric emptying. In some children, this may be associated with feeding intolerance, with more episodes of vomiting, gagging, and retching. Optimizing the gastric emptying rate by choosing a whey-predominant formula for developmentally impaired children, who may have an element of gastrointestinal dysmotility, may lead to improved success in feeding.

Constipation and diarrhea are common problems in tube-fed children; managing hydration and fiber content of tube feedings can help normalize stooling patterns. The free water content of most intact protein formulas is about 85%. Additional water may be necessary if energy needs and formula volumes are low. Most pediatric enteral feeding products are available with and without fiber. The insoluble fiber such as cellulose provides bulk and promotes peristalsis. The soluble fiber–containing formulas act as prebiotics, stimulating the growth of beneficial bacteria, and may help improve water and electrolyte absorption and slow transit time.

Blending table foods such as meat, fruit, vegetable, and cereal with milk, juice, and water is an alternative to pre-prepared pediatric enteral tube feeding products. This method may be more economical for the uninsured, but sanitation in the food preparation and storage process must be ensured, and analysis of the recipe for nutritional adequacy by a pediatric dietitian is recommended.

Specialty pediatric enteral formulas that contain partially hydrolyzed proteins (casein or whey), peptides, and free amino acids as a nitrogen source are available for infants or children with allergies or protein sensitivity. Some of these formulas also contain a fat blend with a mixture of long- and medium-chain triglycerides, which are helpful in the management of malabsorption. Pediatric physician nutrition specialists or gastroenterologists as well as pediatric dietitians are useful resources to recommend enteral formula products. A list of pediatric formulas and their features is provided in Table 29-5.

Bolus feedings should be given when possible. For the child who is fed both orally and with tube, feeding regimens include having the child eat at regular mealtime intervals, following each meal with an enteral feeding. The child who eats orally may be allowed to eat and drink throughout the day as desired and then be given enteral feedings overnight by feeding pump to supplement intake to achieve calorie and fluid goals. When enteral tube feedings are the sole source of nutrition, a bolus feeding schedule should be developed to provide bolus volumes as tolerated and timed throughout the day to be convenient to caretakers and school schedules. Daytime boluses may also be supplemented with nocturnal pump feedings if the child is unable to meet enteral feeding goals by day.

For feeding intolerance, especially gastroesophageal reflux symptoms in infants, continuous feedings may need to be provided. For the convenience of the child and caregivers, it is best to try to deliver the highest rate of feeding tolerated to decrease the total hours of feeding time required to meet fluid and nutritional needs.

On occasion, a child who is tube fed will not be able to tolerate the volume of formula needed for adequate growth, and provision of a formula with increased calorie density becomes necessary. The usual calorie density of pediatric enteral formulas is 1 kcal/mL (30 kilocalories per ounce). At this time, there is only one pediatric ready-to-feed formula available as 1.5 kcal/mL. A few formulas come as a powder and thus may be concentrated to a higher calorie density by adjusting the amount of powder and water. Providing a high-calorie adult formula of 1.5 to 2 calories/mL may be an option for an older child. Another option is to add calories from a carbohydrate or fat-carbohydrate modular supplement to the formula. Any of these choices alters the nutrient profile and potential tolerance of the feedings. Those

Table 29-5. Pediatric Tube Feeding and Oral Formula Selection

Typical Use	Features	Formula Examples
Standard pediatric tube or oral feeding	Intact cow milk protein	PediaSure* Resource Just for Kids† Nutren Junior†
Standard pediatric tube feeding	Blenderized foods from chicken, fruits, and vegetables; contains some milk protein Not flavored for oral intake	Compleat Pediatric†
Constipation	Intact cow milk protein 5-6 g fiber per 1000 mL	PediaSure with Fiber* Resource Just for Kids with Fiber† Nutren Junior with Fiber†
Delayed gastric emptying	Intact cow milk protein 50% whey protein	Nutren Junior Nutren Junior with Fiber
Gastroesophageal reflux	Intact cow milk protein 50% whey protein	Nutren Junior Nutren Junior with Fiber
Impaired gut function	Semi-elemental Peptide-based proteins	Peptamen Junior† Vital jr*
Malabsorption	Elemental 100% free amino acids Contains medium-chain triglycerides Powdered products—calorie density may be manipulated	Elecare* Vivonex Pediatric†
Protein allergy	Elemental Contains 100% free amino acids	Neocate Junior‡ Elecare
Poor weight gain	Intact milk protein 1.5 kcal/mL (45 kcal/oz)	Resource Just for Kids 1.5,† Resource Just for Kids 1.5 with Fiber†
Poor milk acceptance	Clear liquid oral supplement Fruit flavored, fat-free, intact milk protein Fortified with vitamins and minerals; not intended as sole source of nutrition	Enlive* Boost Breeze†

All formulas are lactose free, meet 100% Dietary Reference Intakes for most nutrients in approximately 1000 mL, are intended for children ages 1 to 10, and provide 30 kcal/oz (1 kcal/mL) unless otherwise indicated.
*Ross Products Division, Abbott Laboratories, Columbus, OH.
†Nestle Nutrition, Glendale, CA.
‡Nutricia North America, Gaithersburg, MD.

formulas concentrated to 1.5 calories/mL provide additional protein loads. Use of carbohydrate may precipitate osmotic diarrhea, and carbohydrate or carbohydrate-fat supplements do not add additional vitamins or minerals for those who need them. See Table 29-6 for a list of commonly used formula additives.

Weaning from tube feedings may be the eventual outcome for some children as development of oral skills progresses and safety of oral feedings is demonstrated on an upright modified barium swallow study. The child should be medically stable, with the underlying condition that led to the tube corrected or stabilized. Weaning should be attempted only when the child's nutritional status is optimal, as some loss of weight may be inevitable during the weaning process. A weight loss of up to 10% may be tolerated if the child is at an ideal weight for age and length when the weaning process is initiated. Regular monitoring of oral progress, weight, and energy and fluid intake by a pediatric dietitian or physician is necessary during the weaning process. Guidelines for transitioning from tube feedings to oral feedings are provided in Table 29-7.

Some programs transition the child from tube to oral feeding by use of an intensive, behaviorally based program that lasts only a few weeks. This approach is highly structured, providing firm, consistent introduction of foods without regard to the child's initial response. These programs may be successful with some children. The child must be at a sufficiently high developmental level to respond to behavior modification techniques, and the parents must be able to attend and to comply with the rigorous training and follow-up.

SUMMARY

Children with special health care needs require adequate and appropriate nutritional intake to achieve optimal growth and development. Although the principles of nutrition assessment are the same as for normal healthy children, including assessment of dietary intake, growth, physical examination, and laboratory biomarkers, the interpretation is more complex because of differences in growth potential, body composition, activity levels, and associated medical conditions. Similarly, the options for nutrition support are more complex if developmental or gastrointestinal conditions dictate special routes or quality of feedings. In all cases, the child must be examined and treated as an individual, with sufficient monitoring to promptly identify either inadequate or excessive growth and to make appropriate adjustments to quantity or quality of the nutritional intake. This population is vulnerable to manipulations of nutritional intake for which the practitioner should be aware. Regular attention to nutritional needs and nutrition status in clinical practice can make it possible that every child with special needs will grow and develop to his or her own potential.

Table 29-6. Formula Additives

Typical Use	Features	Examples
Calorie booster	Powdered carbohydrate from glucose polymers 23 kcal/tablespoon	Polycose*
Calorie booster	Emulsified fat, mixes well, contains essential fatty acids 4.5 kcal/mL	Microlipid†
Calorie booster	Powdered fat and carbohydrate 42 kcal/tablespoon	Duocal‡
Protein booster	Powdered whey protein Lactose free 6 g protein/scoop	Resource Beneprotein†
Fiber booster	Powdered soluble fiber from guar gum 3 g fiber/tablespoon	Resource Benefiber†

*Ross Products Division, Abbott Laboratories, Columbus, OH.
†Nestle Nutrition, Glendale, CA.
‡Nutricia North America, Gaithersburg, MD.

Table 29-7. Guidelines for Transition from Tube Feeding to Oral Feeding

To prepare for the physiologic feelings of hunger and satiety, the feeding schedule should be adjusted to deliver daytime boluses, simulating quantity and timing of daytime meal and snack schedules.
The child should then be offered regular meals and snacks by mouth, followed by the supplemental enteral feedings.
The calories given by tube may be decreased by approximately 25%. This amount has been suggested to be adequate to invoke enough hunger to promote increased oral intake without allowing excessive weight loss as oral intake increases (Blackman and Nelson, 1985).
Feedings may be continually decreased as oral intake improves.
Continue to meet water needs by tube if needed. Fluids are often the last consistency to be safely or easily consumed.
When the child can meet at least 75% of the energy needs by mouth, tube feedings may be discontinued and weight monitored.
The unused feeding tube should remain in place for several months to allow enough time to document consistent physical growth, especially during periods of acute illness.

REFERENCES

American Academy of Pediatrics, Committee on Nutrition: Complementary feeding. *In* Kleinman RE (ed): Pediatric Nutrition Handbook, 5th ed. Elk Grove Village, IL, American Academy of Pediatrics, 2004a, pp 103–115.

American Academy of Pediatrics, Committee on Nutrition: Iron deficiency. *In* Kleinman RE (ed): Pediatric Nutrition Handbook, 5th ed. Elk Grove Village, IL, American Academy of Pediatrics, 2004b, pp 299–312.

American Academy of Pediatrics: American College of Obstetricians and Gynecologists: Breastfeeding Handbook for Physicians. Elk Grove Village, IL, American Academy of Pediatrics; Washington, DC, American College of Obstetricians and Gynecologists, 2006.

Bell KL, Davies PS: Prediction of height from knee height in children with cerebral palsy and non-disabled children. Ann Hum Biol 33:493-499, 2006.

Blackman JA, Nelson CL: Reinstituting oral feedings in children fed by gastrostomy tube. Clin Pediatr (Phila) 24:434-438, 1985.

Duggan CP, Westra SJ, Rosenberg AE: Case records of the Massachusetts General Hospital. Case 23-2007. A 9-year-old boy with bone pain, rash, and gingival hypertrophy. N Engl J Med 357:392-400, 2007.

Ekvall S: Pediatric Nutrition in Chronic Diseases and Development. New York, Oxford University Press, 1993.

Khoshoo V, Zembo M, King A, et al: Incidence of gastroesophageal reflux with whey- and casein-based formulas in infants and in children with severe neurological impairment. J Pediatr Gastroenterol Nutr 22:48-55, 1996.

Kuczmarski RJ, Ogden CL, Grummer-Strawn LM, et al: CDC growth charts: United States. Adv Data 314:1-27, 2000.

Otten JJ, Hellwig JP, Meyers LD (eds): Dietary Reference Intakes: The Essential Guide to Nutrient Requirements. Washington, DC, National Academies Press, 2006.

Stallings VA, Zemel BS, Davies JC, et al: Energy expenditure of children and adolescents with severe disabilities: a cerebral palsy model. Am J Clin Nutr 64:627-634, 1996.

Stevenson RD: Use of segmental measures to estimate stature in children with cerebral palsy. Arch Pediatr Adolesc Med 149:658-662, 1995.

30 INBORN ERRORS OF METABOLISM

JEFFREY M. CHINSKY AND ROBERT D. STEINER

In the past, inborn errors of metabolism referred to pathologic conditions caused by the inherited deficiencies of enzymes of intermediary metabolism that produced the accumulation of toxic intermediates or deficiency of products, with resulting disease manifestations. Therefore, several dozen disease conditions became identified, and diagnostic and treatment options were incorporated into medical practice, often requiring the assistance of a subspecialist in the field, usually the clinical geneticist or clinical biochemical geneticist and neurologist. As knowledge of the molecular biology of disease has rapidly expanded, the term is now applied to hundreds of pathologic conditions, many of which are defined by the enzymatic deficiency or gene mutation, rather than by the metabolites present in excess, that leads to diagnosis. It is beyond the scope of this chapter to develop an encyclopedic resource for the practitioner on this topic. For that purpose, the reader is referred to the list of references at the end of the chapter. Rather, the focus of this chapter is to provide the developmental-behavioral pediatric practitioner an operating structure in which to consider inborn errors of metabolism as causes of developmental delay or behavioral abnormalities. The reported incidence of identification of an inborn error of metabolism in a patient with developmental delay or intellectual disability is about 1% (Moeschler and Shevell, 2006). This small percentage represents a large heterogeneous collection of disorders, and therefore, by its nature, the approach has to be one of broad screening with use of historical and clinical clues to help guide the process.

Classically, most inborn errors of metabolism have been defined by their acute or episodic presentations, often in infancy, of an extreme illness, usually with overt changes in neurologic or other organ function, or by easily noted physical abnormalities. Classic forms of these disorders were associated with marked deficiencies or absences of defined enzymes. Screening for these disorders consisted of either examination of blood or urine for known abnormally accumulated substances or abnormal deficiencies or direct enzymatic testing. However, nonclassic forms of all of these disorders may be manifested outside of the typical neonatal period, often as a result of some varying amount of residual enzymatic activity in the patient. In addition, variant phenotypic expression of disorders may occur in patients with mutations both identical to and distinct from those described for classic inborn errors of metabolism. Therefore, nonclassic or variant-type inborn errors of metabolism may be manifested at any age and may not show all or even any of the features usually associated with the classic descriptions of these disorders. The practitioner must maintain an index of suspicion in the approach to diagnosis of any of these disorders, especially when the patient is out of infancy. It is not always clear what environmental or combination of circumstances lead to manifestations of illness in these patients. Many anecdotal associations have helped focus laboratory testing, but approaches to screening by necessity must be broad. Often, a tiered approach rather than the "shotgun" approach is more useful. Watchful waiting for the development of additional manifestations that direct diagnostic testing is a part of the work-up of most of these patients with atypical presentations. Explaining the need for patience to the parents is a necessary part of the counseling session of most patients with unexplained developmental delays or behavioral abnormalities undergoing metabolic disease evaluation.

GENERAL APPROACH

The general diagnostic approach to the evaluation of patients with behavioral or developmental abnormalities is discussed in several other chapters of this book. Usually, before these patients reach the clinical biochemical geneticist or metabolic disease specialist, they have already undergone fairly comprehensive etiologic evaluations. Neuroimaging has often already been performed, as have screening karyotypes and other studies discussed elsewhere in the text. Additional key items must therefore be kept in mind in considering inborn errors of metabolism to identify possible avenues for further investigation. A list of clinical or laboratory findings that may be apparent after the initial (or later) consultation is provided in Table 30-1. Throughout this text, whenever associations have been reported, these are noted by the finding followed by the disorder in parentheses. However, these associations are still few and in some cases anecdotal associations. Often, after consultation with the clinical biochemical geneticist or metabolic disease specialist, the practitioner will want to review any positive (or pertinent negative) findings described by the specialist or listed on laboratory results, and texts are available for that purpose, some of which are listed at the end of this chapter. The tables provided in this chapter are meant to be a starting guide for clinical and laboratory evaluation.

Table 30-1. Initial Clinical or Laboratory Findings Suggestive of Inborn Errors of Metabolism

Intermittent or recurrent unexplained illness	Spinal gibbus-type formation
Developmental delays	Marfanoid appearance
Regression or loss of psychomotor skills	Digital anomalies (syndactyly, arachnodactyly)
Intermittent or new-onset behavioral or psychiatric abnormalities	Imaging abnormalities
Failure-to-thrive (growth or weight gain)	Dysostosis multiplex
Neurologic abnormalities	Punctate calcifications ("stippled epiphyses")
Hypotonia	Abnormal laboratory values
Dystonia or disorders of movement	Acidosis (elevated anion gap)
Dysmetrias and ataxia	Persistent metabolic acidosis (normal or elevated gap)
Seizures, especially recalcitrant, difficult to control	Respiratory alkalosis
Unexplained lethargy or coma	Hypoglycemia
Somatic abnormalities	Elevated or low-absent urine ketones
Coarse facies, macrocephaly, prominent eyebrows	Urine reducing substances (in absence of glucosuria)
Hepatomegaly or hepatosplenomegaly	Hyperammonemia
Hair (brittle, sparse, alopecia)	Low blood urea nitrogen (especially with appearance of dehydration)
Skin abnormalities (dermatitis, buttock dimpling, angiokeratomas)	Lactic acidosis
Ophthalmologic abnormalities	Hyperuricemia
Corneal or lenticular opacities	Low uric acid
Retinal abnormalities	Low cholesterol
Abnormalities of extraocular movements	Unexplained abnormalities on magnetic resonance imaging or computed tomography of the head
Unexplained deafness (sensorineural hearing loss)	Basal ganglia abnormalities
Skeletal abnormalities	Cerebral calcifications
Unexplained contractures, clawed extremities	Leukodystrophy, abnormal white matter, delayed myelination

Modified from Moeschler JB, Shevell M; American Academy of Pediatrics Committee on Genetics: Clinical genetic evaluation of the child with mental retardation or developmental delays. Pediatrics 117:2304-2316, 2006.

As with all consultations, the initial approach in evaluation of the patient with developmental delay or intellectual disability or behavioral abnormalities for inborn errors of metabolism must focus on a comprehensive history, both of the patient and of the immediate and extended family. Because most of the inborn errors of metabolism are rare, autosomal recessive disorders, parental consanguinity increases the likelihood of one of these being present. This information may not be provided with general questioning. More specific questioning about the possibilities of cousin relationships, ancestry of branches of the family from neighboring or the same small towns or villages, and the like sometimes is the only way to elicit such information. Family history of stillbirths or of infant or childhood deaths needs to be explored because many of these may at first be incorrectly ascribed to common illnesses ("pneumonia," "severe dehydration from gastroenteritis," unknown meningitis or encephalitis, "sepsis" without a defined organism) when instead they may have been due to an undiagnosed inborn error of metabolism. Death of male infants may suggest a family history of the X-linked urea cycle defect ornithine transcarbamylase deficiency. Undiagnosed neonatal or infantile deaths as well as unexplained acute or chronic illnesses may suggest a need for one type or another work-up for inborn error of metabolism. History of conditions such as apparent life-threatening episodes and near-miss sudden infant death syndrome should lead to more extensive questioning, often sending the parents of your patient back to their own families for further information. Family history not only of intellectual disability but also of behavioral or psychiatric disorders may provide clues to the identification of familial risk for a specific inborn error of metabolism. This should include consideration of poor school performances (including special education classes) in family members. Similarly, dietary histories in family members (apparent meat or protein avoidance, vegetarianism, unexplained food "allergies" without typical urticarial or anaphylaxis history, history of food avoidance due to association with headaches, and the like) may prompt further evaluations for inborn error of metabolism.

The pregnancy history may be revealing. A prior history of nonimmune hydrops fetalis may suggest a number of inborn errors of metabolism including lysosomal storage disorders, congenital defects of glycosylation, a type of glycogen storage disease (IV), some mitochondrial or respiratory chain disorders, neonatal hemochromatosis, several glucose pathway enzyme deficiencies (glucose-6-phosphate dehydrogenase, pyruvate kinase, glucose phosphate isomerase) affecting red blood cell stability, and others. Maternal HELLP (hemolysis, elevated liver enzymes, and low platelets) syndrome and acute fatty liver of pregnancy may be associated with fetal fatty acid oxidation disorders, such as long-chain 3-hydroxyacyl-CoA dehydrogenase deficiency. Even prolonged hyperemesis of pregnancy may be the clue needed to consider the possibility of these disorders in the fetus or family. Widespread newborn screening for hyperphenylalaninemia (phenylketonuria) has now been in place for more than 40 years. However, many of the treated female patients have long discontinued the diet and are becoming pregnant without the consultation of a specialist and institution of dietary restriction of phenylalanine intake in a timely fashion. The syndrome identified in infants of untreated mothers with phenylketonuria includes intrauterine growth restriction or small for gestational age, microcephaly, congenital heart disease (10%), and developmental delay or intellectual disability. Even if the

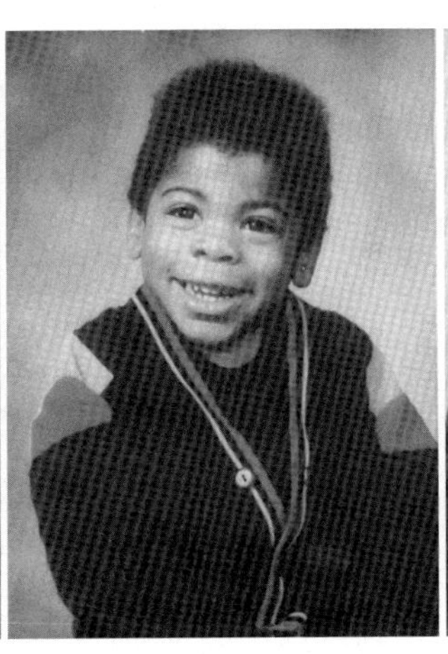
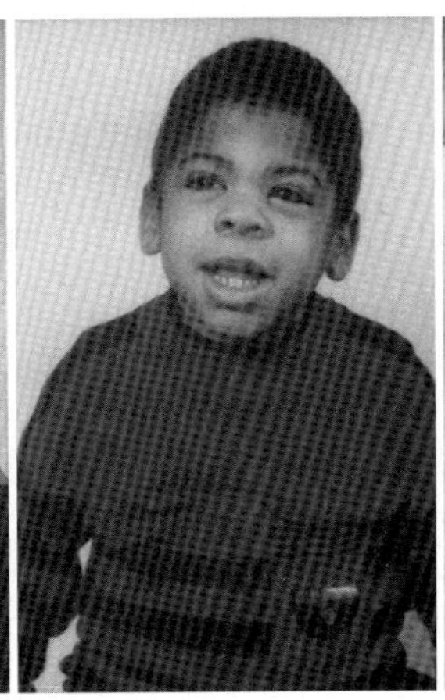
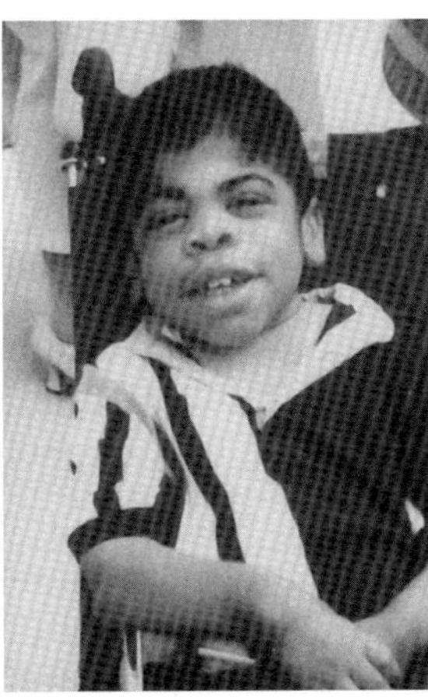

Figure 30-1. **Mild progression of classic features of Hunter syndrome (MPS II).** The patient had minimal evidence of MPS II at initial evaluation for developmental delay. Photographs at ages 3 to 6 years demonstrate progression to classic coarse facial features, accompanied by organomegaly and dysostosis multiplex, observed at 10 years of age *(right)*.

mother claims to have been "treated" during pregnancy, the timing of institution of effective treatment (optimal levels of phenylalanine achieved before conception or before the end of the first trimester) is paramount in determining the likelihood of these consequences. These infants usually do not themselves have phenylketonuria. Instead, they suffer the consequences of the fetal environment (hyperphenylalaninemia) provided by the mother. For best outcomes, women with phenylketonuria should be receiving effective dietary restriction before conception.

In reviewing the patient's own medical history, careful attention must be paid to any emergency department visits or hospitalizations for what may have been considered typical childhood illnesses, especially vomiting, diarrhea, and other forms of gastroenteritis. Any type of prior neurologic acute presentation, unless there is a specific etiologic diagnosis (e.g., culture- or laboratory-proven meningitis or encephalitis), should be suspect. Abnormal laboratory results (i.e., hypoglycemia, mild metabolic acidosis, mild hyperammonemia) are often "excused" in patients who are the products of intrauterine growth restriction or have had a prolonged course of poor oral intake due to vomiting. If laboratory tests were obtained, review may suggest the possibility of an inborn error of metabolism previously not considered (see Tables 30-1 and 30-3). The ability to review previous clinical and laboratory data becomes extremely important, and records from previous illness should be actively sought. In addition, the historical review should ensure that optimal nutrition has been offered in the patient's diet. The combination of breastfeeding with no supplementation may expose the infant to the variances of maternal diet (e.g., strict vegetarianism, which could lead to vitamin B_{12} deficiency in the child). Similarly, inadequate dietary intakes of certain vitamins, minerals, and even major food groups (i.e., very low protein) may exaggerate normal metabolic responses or unmask latent inborn errors of metabolism.

An attempt should be made to determine if the patient had an "expanded" newborn screen, currently referring to the analysis of newborn screening blood spots by tandem mass spectroscopy (MS/MS) for many plasma amino acids and acylcarnitines. Newborn screening in the United States is not standardized nationally, so not all states use this powerful technique to screen for 25 to 50 inborn errors of metabolism. Some states and developed countries currently screen for as few as five disorders. Although newborn screening is expanding, it is set up as a screening rather than as a diagnostic test. There will always be patients with conditions that are included in newborn screening who are not identified by newborn screening for various reasons including insufficient oral intake, inadequate follow-up, missed testing, sample mix-up, and physiologic false-negatives. Therefore, a history of a negative newborn screen makes certain disorders less likely but does not necessarily exclude those disorders. Importantly, not all inborn errors of metabolism are uniformly detected on such screening regimens, even when they are subsequently known to be present (e.g., biotinidase deficiency, certain urea cycle defects, homocystinuria, intermittent maple syrup urine disease). If there is an item in the history that suggests screening for any of these disorders, do so even though it often involves repeating tests included in the "expanded" newborn screens.

The patient's physical and neurologic examination history may suggest clues that were not previously present or emphasized. A clear history of developmental regression (loss of psychomotor skills not associated with an acute event) may suggest a number of lysosomal storage or similar disorders. Children who demonstrate neurologic or developmental delays or regression may have associated physical findings (hepatosplenomegaly, macrocephaly, ophthalmologic or skeletal changes) that may help guide selection of screening and diagnostic tests (Fig. 30-1; see Tables 30-4 and 30-7). Neurologic or developmental regression may also be present in nonclassically defined forms and contexts. A middle-school or high-school child whose grades deteriorate in association with behavioral changes may have metachromatic leukodystrophy, adrenoleukodystrophy, or Niemann-Pick type C, among others, although the first impulse is to rule out drug use and other social and behavioral reasons for the change. This change in school performance may occur even before notable changes on either brain imaging or physical examination. Strokelike episodes are associated with a number of inborn errors of metabolism, often with resultant dystonia, dyskinetic conditions, and developmental delays that may initially be manifested with the episode, then appear to improve, then appear to become more permanent or progressive. It may take several years before the involvement of basal ganglia secondary to "metabolic strokes" associated with a variety of organic acidemias (e.g., methylmalonic and propionic acidemias) is noted on neuroimaging studies (Fig. 30-2). Many individuals with inborn errors of metabolism have history of periods of waxing and waning developmental progression. Others, such as with glutaric aciduria type I, may have apparent normal development for many months before a devastating illness with metabolic crises or strokelike event leaves them with a dystonic or dyskinetic condition, sometimes with associated developmental delay. However, many individuals with developmental delay associated with inborn errors of metabolism present no differently from most children with otherwise undiagnosed developmental delay or intellectual disability—there is simply slower than normal but continuing progression of attainment of milestones, however small the positive gains, up until a certain point. This point of apparent termination is sometimes due to physical limitations (muscle contractures, neurologic complications such as dystonias), but many times these individuals enter adulthood with apparent delays for which no further intellectual accomplishments appear to be attained. Again, for that reason, it is important to look for associations or patterns that may provide clues for appropriate avenues of investigation: motor delays in the absence of other neurologic abnormalities (some organic acidemias, mitochondrial abnormalities), speech delays in the absence of other delays (3-methylglutaconic aciduria, verbal apraxias associated with galactosemia), speech delays with later behavioral abnormalities with little initial effect on motor milestones (Sanfilippo [MPS III] and Hunter [MPS II] syndromes, succinic semialdehyde dehydrogenase deficiency), motor delays with hypotonia (mitochondrial disorders), developmental delays with self-injurious behavior (Lesch-Nyhan syndrome), or apparent sleep disorder (MPS III). There are a large number of such associations that may be gleaned through a thorough history. Similarly, a thorough physical examination may reveal hepatomegaly, hepatosplenomegaly, macrocephaly, ophthalmologic abnormalities, or other clues

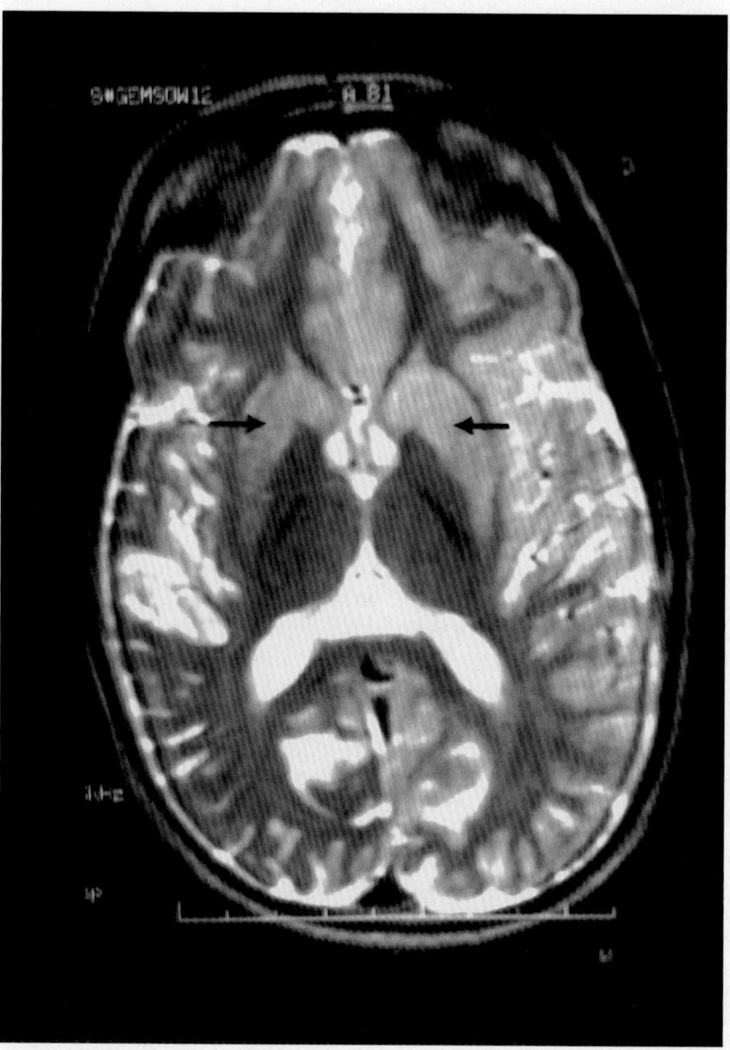

Figure 30-2. Abnormal basal ganglia T2 signals of magnetic resonance imaging of the brain in a patient with propionic acidemia. Note increased signals of putamen and caudate regions *(arrows)* but not of adjacent basal ganglia (globus pallidus) or thalamus. These were not observed until 6 years of age, 3 years after first prolonged coma-producing episode at 3½ years of age with resultant hemiplegic choreoathetosis that resolved in the subsequent 9 months. They are not evident on a routine computed tomographic scan of the head. There are also diffuse increased signals in the subcortical white matter.

to help guide diagnostic testing. A formal ophthalmologic consultation is appropriate to determine if any other physical clues are present (specific retinal, lenticular, or corneal abnormalities). A summary of many of these associations can be found in Table 30-4 and more complete coverage in the referenced texts. Importantly, keep in mind that many of these abnormalities may not yet be present at the time of initial referral for developmental delay. For example, as shown in Figure 30-1, it took several years for this patient with Hunter syndrome (MPS II) to develop recognizable features associated with the condition (such as coarse facies or skeletal abnormalities). In this case, initial mild hepatomegaly, associated with continuing mild developmental delay, led to early diagnosis of MPS II. Considering that enzyme replacement therapy for this and several other lysosomal disorders is now available, it is important to identify these disorders as early as possible.

LABORATORY EVALUATION

It is recommended that all patients with unexplained developmental delays undergo complete genetics evaluation, which should include comprehensive dysmorphologic, ophthalmologic, and neurologic examinations as well as brain imaging studies. Laboratory tests should include both cytogenetic and submicroscopic examinations (fluorescent in situ hybridization and molecular) as well as both screening and targeted testing for inborn errors of metabolism. Because inborn errors of metabolism represent a large diverse collection of conditions due to errors in any one of many interacting metabolic pathways, selection of discriminating or diagnostic tests for any individual inborn error of metabolism is daunting. For that reason, consideration of an initial set of screening tests is mandated (Table 30-2), some of which may have already been performed as part of a routine medical evaluation for illness. In review of past laboratory results, ensure that thyroid function tests were previously performed. As stated, a tiered approach is best, based on diagnostic clues gleaned from the complete history, physical examination, and reported initial laboratory values.

Patients with inborn errors of metabolism and developmental delays may be divided among those who have presented with an acute clinical deterioration, those with a more indolent course but in which developmental delay or neurologic abnormalities become more manifest, and those with physical or somatic features known to be associated with certain groups of conditions, such as lysosomal storage disorders. For those patients presenting with acute illness leading to an emergency department or hospital visit, evaluation of the parameters usually "routinely" obtained may suggest one or more of the conditions listed in Table 30-3 and focus subsequent evaluations. The initial laboratory tests that should be included are listed in Table 30-2; these will help determine if likely errors in amino acid, fatty acid, or carbohydrate metabolism or mitochondrial function are present. This includes determination of serum glucose, bicarbonate (including determination of anion gap when acidosis is present), and blood urea nitrogen (very low in illness expected to demonstrate higher levels due to "dehydration" is suggestive of urea cycle defect) concentrations; serum transaminases and liver function tests; direct or indirect bilirubin levels; plasma ammonia and lactate levels; and urine analysis (be sure it includes ketones and some way of differentiating

Table 30-2. Screening Laboratory Investigations for Inborn Errors of Metabolism as Causes of Developmental Delay or Behavioral Abnormalities

Blood Tests	*Consider "Second-Tier" Testing (see text for details)*
Review from history	Plasma acylcarnitine profile (first or second tier)
Complete metabolic panel	Simultaneous plasma lactate and pyruvate (very few reliable analyses available for pyruvate, special handling required)
Glucose (note time related to last meal or symptoms)	Urine for quantitative amino acids (if plasma levels are low, renal Fanconi syndrome, failure-to-thrive)
Electrolytes, bicarbonate, anion gap, blood urea nitrogen, creatinine	Carnitine levels (plasma and urine, total, free versus esterified)—especially with hypotonia
Liver function tests (aspartate aminotransferase, alanine aminotransferase, albumin)	Serum transferrin electrophoresis (congenital disorders of glycosylation screen)
Bilirubin (including direct fraction)	Plasma or serum very-long-chain fatty acids (more severe neurologic deficits, seizures) (include phytanic acid and plasmalogens, if available)
Complete blood count	Urine for mucopolysaccharides, oligosaccharides (including sialylated species), individual white blood cell enzymatic tests as indicated for possible lysosomal storage disorder
Plasma quantitative amino acids	Serum uric acid
Plasma ammonia (if not done previously)	Urine uric acid/creatinine ratios
Lactate (especially with persistent metabolic acidosis, mild or moderate)	Serum or plasma cholesterol
Creatine kinase (especially with hypotonia or weakness)	Plasma sterols by gas chromatography–mass spectrometry (7-dehydrocholesterol and others)
Plasma acylcarnitine profile (first tier if no prior newborn tandem mass spectroscopy screen)	Urine purine and pyrimidine panels
Simultaneous plasma lactate and pyruvate (first tier if prior persistent high lactate)	Plasma and urine creatine and guanidinoacetate levels
Urine Tests	Plasma copper and ceruloplasmin—severe seizures, movement disorder, or neurologic course, psychiatric disturbances
Urine for organic acid analysis	Cerebrospinal fluid amino acids, lactate and pyruvate, neurotransmitters
Urine analysis (including ketones and reducing substances)	
Metabolic screens (differing availability and types): ferric chloride, dinitrophenylhydrazine, Acetest, reducing substances, mucopolysaccharide screen, others	

Table 30-3. **Typical Laboratory Patterns in Classes of Inborn Errors of Metabolism**

	Laboratory Findings*			
Type of Disorder†	**Hyperammonemia**	**Acidosis (Anion Gap)**	**Ketones**	**Hypoglycemia**
Urea cycle defect	++	– (pH > 7.45)‡	–	–
Organic acidemia				
Amino or organic acids	+	++	high	+
Fatty acid oxidation	+/–	+/–	low-absent§	++
Mitochondrial disorder	–	+	+/–	+/–
Carbohydrate disorder	–	+	+	+
Peroxisomal disorder	–	–	–	–
Lysosomal storage (MPS, SPHL)	–	–	–	–

*Usually present and marked (++), usually absent (–), may be present (+), variable finding (+/–).
†Organic acidemias are divided into those derived from errors in metabolism of amino acids and fatty acid oxidation disorders; lysosomal storage refers to mucopolysaccharidoses (MPS) and sphingolipidoses (SPHL).
‡Respiratory alkalosis in clinical settings of shocklike appearance in which metabolic acidosis would otherwise be expected is a marker of hyperammonemia.
§Low level or absence of ketones associated with hypoglycemia is usually either excessive insulin function or a fatty acid oxidation or ketogenesis disorder.

non–glucose reducing substances from glucose). Some fatty acid oxidation defects and organic acidemias may first be suspected in infants with mild delays by the presence of low but persistent direct bilirubinemia reflecting ongoing metabolic liver involvement (e.g., long-chain 3-hydroxyacyl-CoA dehydrogenase deficiency). If appropriate, subsequent screens for these disorders by obtaining plasma for amino acids, acylcarnitine profile, and carnitine levels and urine for organic acids are indicated at that time of acute presentation. If these were not initially obtained, one may do so at the first follow-up visit or initial consultation with the developmental-behavioral pediatrician. However, detection of certain identifying metabolites or patterns for specific disorders may be limited because of the decrease in these levels during "well" or acutely recovered periods. For example, certain fatty acid oxidation disorders may be missed by urine organic acid analysis when urine is collected when the patient is well but identified by more sensitive plasma acylcarnitine profiles (whose screening potential for organic acidurias, however, is less broad).

A complete blood count may be useful because some organic acidemias and other inborn errors of metabolism depress bone marrow function. One may want to further evaluate hypoglycemia, looking for carbohydrate disorders (e.g., glycogen storage diseases, fructose metabolism disorders, galactosemia), by checking for elevations in cholesterol, triglyceride, uric acid, and lactate concentrations and the presence of urine reducing substances. Most of these disorders are not associated with developmental delay unless there have been complications of prolonged hypoglycemia and acidosis. However, many organic acidurias (fatty acid and amino acid inborn errors of metabolism) are associated with developmental delays, and screenings based on hypoglycemia should include testing for these disorders (Table 30-4). Mitochondrial or other myopathies may be screened by checking creatine kinase concentration and simultaneous pyruvate with lactate levels, but results of screening tests for mitochondrial disorders can be negative. Analysis of urine amino acids and phosphate (compared with serum phosphate) may be useful to determine if an associated renal Fanconi syndrome (glucosuria, phosphaturia, aminoaciduria, renal tubular acidosis) is present. Renal tubular acidosis not due to inborn errors of metabolism is in the differential diagnosis of causes of metabolic acidosis. In addition, renal tubular dysfunction is associated with some inborn errors of metabolism usually associated with liver disease as well as others (e.g., tyrosinemia, galactosemia, hereditary fructose intolerance, cystinosis; see Table 30-4). Analysis of urine amino acids may also help sort out some of the abnormalities that may or may not be evident on the plasma amino acid and urine organic acid analyses.

If cerebrospinal fluid (CSF) is obtained, quantitative amino acids or other diagnostic compounds may help identify causes of new-onset severe seizures, for example, in nonketotic hyperglycinemia (elevated CSF glycine compared with plasma glycine levels) or disorders of neurotransmitters (i.e., creatine disorders). When CSF is obtained in this setting, it should be tested for the usual parameters plus amino acids and lactate, and some CSF should be frozen at −80°C for later evaluation for neurotransmitters. Difficult-to-control seizure disorders with more severe neurologic findings may also be an indication to screen for peroxisomal and certain other rare disorders. History of skeletal punctate calcifications or stippled epiphyses and certain dysmorphic facial features (i.e., elongated forehead) may suggest peroxisomal disorders. These may be screened by obtaining plasma for very-long-chain fatty acids (optimally with red blood cell plasmalogens and plasma phytanic acid). Disorders of copper metabolism (Menkes syndrome with low serum copper and ceruloplasmin levels) and uric acid metabolism (very high serum urate levels in Lesch-Nyhan syndrome, very low levels in molybdenum cofactor deficiency and related disorders) may be considered. It is recommended to all emergency department practitioners and hospitalists who are likely to be the first to evaluate these patients with acute presentations that frozen plasma and CSF samples be saved for consideration of future diagnostic evaluations for inborn errors of metabolism. Importantly, many of the disorders have successful treatment regimens (dietary restrictions, vitamin

Table 30-4. **Inborn Errors of Metabolism Suggested by Clinical and Laboratory Features Associated with Developmental Delay***

Behavioral or Psychiatric Symptoms

Sanfilippo (MPS III) syndrome
Hunter (MPS II) syndrome
Urea cycle defects (any) (especially ornithine transcarbamylase deficiency in girls)
Adrenoleukodystrophy
Metachromatic leukodystrophy
Homocystinuria
- Cobalamin disorders
- Methylene tetrahydrofolate reductase deficiency

Hurler-Scheie/Scheie (MPS I) syndrome
Wilson disease
Late-onset GM_2 gangliosidosis
Late-onset neuronal ceroid lipofuscinosis
Purine disorders
- Lesch-Nyhan disease (self-mutilation)

Porphyrias
Disorders of creatine
Niemann-Pick type C
Mitochondrial disorders (e.g., MELAS)

Speech Disorders (as Presenting Sign)

Galactosemia (verbal dyspraxias)
3-Methylglutaconyl-CoA hydratase deficiency
Ethylmalonic aciduria
D-Glyceric aciduria

Sensorineural Deafness

Peroxisomal disorders
Mitochondrial disorders
Canavan disease
Biotinidase deficiency
Phosphoribosylpyrophosphate synthetase (purine) abnormality
Mucopolysaccharidoses (I, II, IV)
Mannosidosis

Renal Abnormalities

Polycystic kidneys
- Zellweger syndrome (peroxisomal)
- Congenital disorders of glycosylation
- Glutaric aciduria II
- Smith-Lemli-Opitz syndrome
- Carnitine palmitoyltransferase II deficiency

Renal Fanconi syndrome
- Cystinosis
- Galactosemia
- Tyrosinemia type I (intellectual disability rare)
- Hereditary fructose intolerance
- Lowe syndrome
- Mitochondrial disorders (rare)
- Glycogen storage disease I (intellectual disability rare)
- Lysinuric protein intolerance
- Wilson disease

Unusual odors
- Musty or mousy: phenylketonuria
- Maple syrup: maple syrup urine disease
- Sweaty feet: isovaleric acidemia; glutaric acidemia type II
- Cabbage: tyrosinemia
- Acrid: glutaric acidemia type II
- Fishy: trimethylaminuria, tyrosinemia
- Swimming pool: hawkinsinuria
- Cat urine: β-methylcrotonylglycinuria
- Treatments of inborn errors of metabolism
  - Carnitine for organic acidurias
  - Phenylacetate for disorders of the urea cycle

Skeletal Abnormalities

Dysostosis multiplex
- Hurler disease (all MPS I forms)
- Hunter disease (MPS II)
- Sanfilippo disease (MPS III)
- Maroteaux-Lamy (MPS VI; intellectual disability rare)
- Sly disease (MPS VII)
- I-cell disease (mucolipidosis II)
- Multiple sulfatase deficiency
- GM_1 gangliosidosis
- Galactosialidosis

Generalized
- Morquio syndrome (MPS IV)

Scoliosis
- Homocystinuria
- Congenital disorders of glycosylation
- Morquio syndrome (MPS IV)

Gibbus formation (spine)
- Mucopolysaccharidoses

Chondrodysplasia punctata
- Peroxisomal disorders
- β-Glucuronidase deficiency

Eye Abnormalities

Lens dislocation
- Homocystinuria
- Molybdenum cofactor deficiency
- Sulfite oxidase deficiency
- Marfan syndrome (rare with intellectual disability)

Upward gaze abnormality
- Niemann-Pick type C
- Mitochondrial disorders (Kearns-Sayre, Leigh syndromes)

Macular cherry-red spot
- GM_2 gangliosidosis (Tay-Sachs, Sandhoff diseases)
- Niemann-Pick disease
- GM_1 gangliosidosis
- Krabbe disease
- Galactosialidosis
- Sialidosis
- Mucolipidoses
- Multiple sulfatase deficiency
- Farber disease
- Cytochrome *c* oxidase deficiency

Corneal opacities
- Cystinosis (lysosomal transport defect)
- Mucopolysaccharidosis (MPS) syndromes
  - Hurler (MPS I)
  - Morquio (MPS IV)
  - Maroteaux-Lamy (MPS VI)
  - Sly (MPS VII)
- Mucolipidoses (I-cell disease, mucolipidosis III)
- Oligosaccharidoses
  - Galactosialidosis
  - Mannosidosis
- Sphingolipidoses
  - GM_1 gangliosidosis
  - Fabry disease (intellectual disability rare)
- Multiple sulfatase deficiency

Lenticular opacities (cataracts)
- Galactosemia
- Homocystinuria
- Peroxisomal disorders
- Smith-Lemli-Opitz syndrome
- Mitochondrial disorders
- Lowe syndrome
- Mevalonic aciduria
- Hyperornithinemia
- Multiple sulfatase deficiency
- Lysinuric protein intolerance
- Fabry disease (intellectual disability rare)

Retinitis pigmentosa
- Peroxisomal disorders
- Congenital disorders of glycosylation
- Mitochondrial disorders
- Mevalonic acidemia
- Long-chain 3-hydroxyacyl-CoA dehydrogenase deficiency
- Hunter (MPS II) syndrome

(Continued)

Table 30-4. Inborn Errors of Metabolism Suggested by Clinical and Laboratory Features Associated with Developmental Delay—cont'd

Skeletal Abnormalities—cont'd

- Sjögren-Larsson syndrome
- Abetalipoproteinemia

Brain Imaging Abnormalities

Leukodystrophies
- Krabbe disease
- Metachromatic leukodystrophy
- Adrenoleukodystrophy
- Canavan disease (includes U fibers)
- Salla disease (includes U fibers)
- L-2-Hydroxyglutaric aciduria (U fibers)
- Multiple neurologic syndromes

Subdural effusions
- Glutaric aciduria type I
- D-2-Hydroxyglutaric aciduria
- Dihydropyrimidine dehydrogenase deficiency
- Pyruvate carboxylase deficiency
- Menkes disease

Basal ganglia abnormalities
- Organic acidemias (especially propionic, methylmalonic, and glutaric acidemias)
- Mitochondrial disorders, including Leigh disease, pyruvate carboxylase and pyruvate dehydrogenase deficiencies
- GM_1 gangliosidosis
- Krabbe disease
- Molybdenum cofactor deficiency
- Tetrahydrobiopterin defects
- Renal tubular acidosis (calcifications)
  - Carbonic anhydrase II deficiency
  - *SLC4A4 (NBC1)* defects

Cerebral calcifications (includes basal ganglia calcifications)
- Adrenoleukodystrophy
- GM_2 gangliosidosis
- Krabbe disease
- L-2-Hydroxyglutaric aciduria
- Mitochondrial disorders
  - Leigh syndrome
- Folate disorders
- Biopterin disorders
- Biotinidase deficiency

Macrocephaly

- Glutaric aciduria type I
- Hurler disease (MPS I)
- Krabbe disease
- Canavan disease
- Tay-Sachs disease
- Mannosidosis
- Multiple acyl-CoA dehydrogenase deficiency (glutaric aciduria type II)
- L-2-Hydroxyglutaric aciduria
- D-2-Hydroxyglutaric aciduria
- 4-Hydroxybutyric aciduria
- 3-Hydroxy-3-methylglutaric-CoA lyase deficiency
- Multiple sulfatase deficiency
- Neonatal adrenoleukodystrophy (peroxisomal disorder)
- Pyruvate carboxylase deficiency

Hair Abnormalities

Alopecia
- Biotinidase deficiency
- Holocarboxylase synthase deficiency
- Methylmalonic and propionic acidemias
- Acrodermatitis enteropathica
  - Zinc deficiency
- Congenital erythropoietic porphyria

Pili torti: Menkes disease

Trichorrhexis nodosa
- Menkes disease
- Argininosuccinic aciduria
- Argininemia
- Lysinuric protein intolerance

Skin Abnormalities

Angiokeratomas
- Fabry disease (intellectual disability rare)
- GM_1 gangliosidosis
- Schindler disease
- Galactosialidosis
- Sialidosis
- Fucosidosis
- Mannosidosis

Ichthyosis
- Steroid sulfatase deficiency
- Multiple sulfatase deficiency
- Congenital disorders of glycosylation (type 1f)
- Refsum disease
- Sjögren-Larsson syndrome
- Gaucher disease
- Krabbe disease

Nodules
- Farber disease
- Congenital disorders of glycosylation
- Hunter syndrome (MPS II)

Thickened or dimpled skin
- Congenital disorders of glycosylation (abnormal fat pads, dimpling)

Thickened
- GM_2 gangliosidosis
- Sly disease (MPS VII)
- I-cell disease (mucolipidosis II)
- Sialidosis
- Galactosialidosis

Inverted nipples
- Congenital disorders of glycosylation
- Menkes disease
- Biopterin synthesis disorders
- Molybdenum cofactor deficiency
- Isolated cases of citrullinemia, methylmalonic and propionic acidemias, pyruvate carboxylase deficiency, very-long-chain acyl-CoA dehydrogenase deficiency

Hematologic Abnormalities

Hemolytic anemias
- Pyroglutamic aciduria (5-oxoprolinuria)
- Pyrimidine disorders
- Purine disorders
- Glycolytic disorders
- Wilson disease

Megaloblastic anemias
- Abnormalities of cobalamin (vitamin B_{12}) and deficiencies
  - CblC, CblD, CblF
  - Methylmalonic acidemia and homocystinuria
  - Transcobalamin II deficiency
- Abnormalities of folate and deficiencies
- Mevalonic aciduria
- Orotic aciduria (pyrimidine disorders)
- Pearson syndrome

Leukopenia
- Organic acidurias (especially methylmalonic, isovaleric, and propionic acidurias)
- Folate abnormalities
- 3-Oxothiolase deficiency
- Transcobalamin II deficiency
- Mitochondrial disorders (Pearson syndrome)

Elevated Creatine Kinase

- Disorders of fatty acid oxidation
- Mitochondrial disorders
- Carnitine palmitoyltransferase II deficiency
- Glycogen storage diseases (type III, type V, phosphofructokinase deficiencies)—intellectual disability rare
- D-Hydroxyglutaric aciduria

Table 30-4. Inborn Errors of Metabolism Suggested by Clinical and Laboratory Features Associated with Developmental Delay—cont'd

Elevated Creatine Kinase—cont'd	*Hypouricemia*
3-Oxothiolase deficiency Mevalonic aciduria Myoadenylate deaminase deficiency	Molybdenum cofactor deficiency Xanthine oxidase deficiency Phosphoribosylpyrophosphate synthetase deficiency Purine nucleoside phosphorylase deficiency Wilson disease Cystinosis or other Fanconi syndrome
Hyperammonemia	*Leigh Syndrome*
Urea cycle defects Organic acidurias (especially methylmalonic, propionic, and isovaleric acidurias and glutaric aciduria type II) Fatty acid oxidation defects Multiple carboxylase deficiency (biotinidase and holocarboxylase synthase deficiencies) Pyruvate dehydrogenase complex deficiency	Pyruvate dehydrogenase complex deficiency Pyruvate carboxylase deficiency Mitochondrial disorders (includes electron transport defects) Fumarase deficiency 3-Methylglutaconic aciduria Biotinidase deficiency Sulfite oxidase deficiency

*This table represents a starting point for consideration of focused screenings for inborn errors of metabolism. It is derived from multiple references listed at the end of the chapter, primarily in the summary tables found in Fernandes et al (2000), Gilbert-Barness and Barness (2000), Hoffmann et al (2002), Nyhan, Barshop, and Ozand (2005), and Wappner and Hainline (2006), to which the reader is referred for more comprehensive listings. It is not meant to be all-inclusive.

or cofactor supplementations, drugs used as alternative pathways for excretion of toxic metabolites). Earlier identification of an inborn error of metabolism leads to lower likelihood of repetitive central nervous system (CNS) insults from such "metabolic decompensations," with less effect on ultimate developmental outcome.

Acute or new-onset "behavioral" or "psychiatric" patterns should also be evaluated with suspicion for inborn errors of metabolism (see Table 30-4). Intermittent irritability, fatigue, complaint of headaches, and changes in behavior, especially after periods of no food intake (on arising in the morning, skipping meals) or after high protein intake (after dinner), should always make one suspicious. Plasma ammonia levels are not routinely obtained in pediatric emergency departments, and this habit has to change. The presence of intermittent hyperammonemia or hypoglycemia should always be determined in these types of patients. The presence of low ketone levels in association with hypoglycemia should be an indicator to screen for disorders of fatty acid oxidation and ketone metabolism (urine for organic acids, plasma carnitine levels, and acylcarnitine profiles). Initial laboratory results suggesting a respiratory alkalosis (pH >7.5) in a clinical setting of lethargy, coma, or suspected shocklike illness with expected metabolic acidosis being absent should be evaluated with an immediate test for hyperammonemia. These states may be due to deficiencies in the enzymes of the urea cycle themselves or secondary inhibitions from the metabolites of many organic acidurias (see Table 30-3). Both hyperammonemia and, to a lesser extent, ketoacidosis may be manifested solely with unexplained vomiting, which at any time may lead to more serious mental status changes. Ammonia levels therefore need to be obtained more frequently with these types of presentations and during the subsequent treatment courses of these presentations.

Many diseases with "classic" infantile presentations of acute mental status changes (vomiting, lethargy, seizures) leading to apnea or coma have been noted to be associated in some cases with a more subclinical chronic presentation with no history of acute metabolic-type collapse. For example, maple syrup urine disease (branched-chain α-ketoaciduria), a disorder of the catabolism of the branched-chain amino acids leucine, isoleucine, and valine, typically is described by this infantile presentation at 1 to 2 weeks of life. However, a number of patients have been referred for evaluation of developmental delay, often with mild to moderate ataxia or dysmetria and no history of emergency department presentation. These patients demonstrate plasma and urine abnormalities (very high urine ketone levels, with or without metabolic acidosis, and elevated plasma branched-chain amino acids) that are no different from those of patients who present with more classic infantile signs and symptoms. They may be referred to as intermediate, chronic, or subacute types. Similarly, some patients present only intermittently with signs and symptoms associated with severe laboratory abnormalities but between episodes demonstrate no laboratory abnormalities (intermittent type). Many organic acidemias fall into these three categories. For that reason, initial or previous serum chemistries and urine analyses should always be considered to start the investigative process of developmental delay.

Physical or somatic findings may suggest other laboratory investigations, especially in more chronic-type presentations. For example, organomegaly, corneal clouding, radiographic bone abnormalities suggesting dysostosis multiplex, and coarse features, associated or not with developmental delays, may suggest lysosomal storage disorders, some of which may be screened by urinary tests for mucopolysaccharides and oligosaccharides. Ultimate diagnosis depends on specific enzymatic testing, usually routinely performed on white blood cell pellets. However, a common mistake is to request the wrong enzyme test. Always request the test by naming the disease entity that you are considering, not just the enzymatic assay that you may have just researched. Other physical findings that may assist the

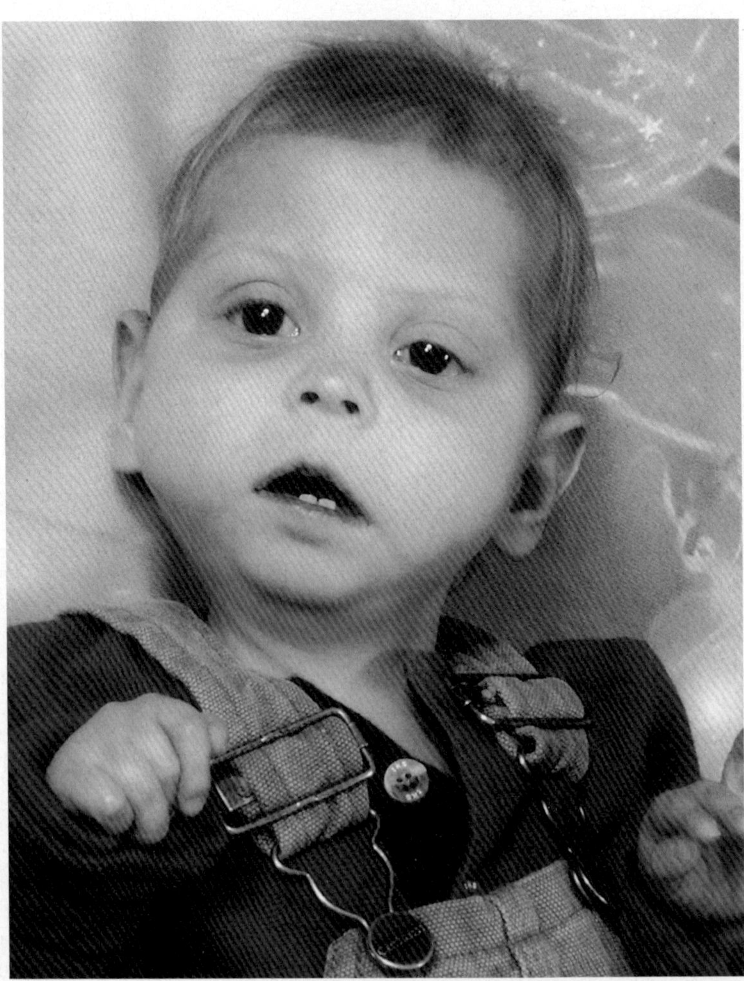

Figure 30-3. Smith-Lemli-Opitz syndrome at 1 year of age. Marked developmental delay with microcephaly, narrow frontal area, broad nasal tip with anteverted nares, prominent glabella with elongated philtrum, tented upper lip (Cupid's bow or carp-shaped), and micrognathia. Associated abnormalities included cleft palate, ambiguous genitalia, 2,3 toe syndactyly, cholestatic liver disease, and renal dysplasia with hypertension. (Courtesy of E. Elias, MD.)

investigation include alopecia or dermatitis (biotinidase or holocarboxylase synthase deficiency—screen by urine organic acids), abnormal hair (Menkes disease with pili torti—screen by serum copper and ceruloplasmin; argininosuccinic acid lyase deficiency, a urea cycle defect—screen by plasma amino acids), ectopic lens (homocystinuria, sulfite oxidase deficiency), inverted nipples (congenital disorders of glycosylation), macrocephaly (glutaric aciduria type I, Canavan disease, Tay-Sachs disease, a few other lysosomal storage disorders, among others), cataracts and other ophthalmologic findings, and dysmorphic features (high forehead of Zellweger syndrome or the facies and 2,3 syndactyly of Smith-Lemli-Opitz syndrome; Fig. 30-3). Many of these associations may be found in Table 30-4, and its references have more extensive listings. Discussions with specialists in clinical biochemical genetics early in the investigative process should also help guide selection of many of the second-tier laboratory evaluations.

HYPERAMMONEMIA AND DISORDERS AFFECTING THE UREA CYCLE

Ammonia is produced as a natural byproduct of ongoing catabolism of amino acids. During times of decreased calorie intake, the breakdown of the carbon skeletons from amino acids is begun by removal of their amino group in a series of transamination reactions that ultimately shuttle the amino group into the urea cycle. This prevents the accumulation of ammonia, a compound toxic to many cells, which may produce cerebral edema and neuronal damage. The efficient functioning of the urea cycle in the liver produces urea, the excretory form of these nitrogen-containing amino groups, and prevents these harmful effects of tissue accumulation of ammonia, the free form of these amino groups. The clinical manifestations of hyperammonemia may include vomiting, poor feeding, irritability, headache, confusion, listlessness, and hyperpnea, which may lead rapidly to lethargy, coma, seizures, and respiratory arrest. Hyperammonemia appears to have a direct stimulatory effect on the respiratory centers of the brain, leading to a respiratory alkalosis. This laboratory result contrasts with what is usually expected in a sick child appearing in shock (i.e., metabolic acidosis). Reported "normal" laboratory values should always be considered suspicious in a child appearing very sick, whose pH, bicarbonate, and blood urea nitrogen levels should otherwise be anything but normal value.

In infants especially, persistent or recurrent vomiting of unknown etiology should always lead to consideration of hyperammonemia because this can rapidly progress to a critical illness without treatment. In older children and adults, developmental delay and neurologic abnormalities

Table 30-5. Urea Cycle Disorders

Carbamyl phosphate synthetase deficiency (carbamyl phosphate synthetase commits the ammonium moiety to the functioning urea cycle)
N-Acetylglutamate synthetase deficiency (*N*-acetylglutamate synthetase provides cofactor for carbamyl phosphate synthetase)
Ornithine transcarbamylase deficiency (ornithine transcarbamylase begins the urea cycle by reacting carbamyl phosphate with ornithine to produce citrulline)
Argininosuccinic acid synthetase deficiency (citrulline reacts with added aspartic acid to produce argininosuccinic acid)
Argininosuccinic acid lyase deficiency (argininosuccinic acid degraded to arginine and fumarate)
Arginase deficiency (produces urea for excretion and ornithine to be recycled to ornithine transcarbamylase, completing the cycle)

on examination may be evident from both clinically apparent and subclinical episodes of hyperammonemia in the past. For many of these past episodes, the plasma ammonia may not have been measured and therefore wide suspicion is important. Both acute behavioral and psychiatric manifestations have been described, and children and adults have described the difference when they have their "ammonia headaches" compared with migraines and other discomforting episodes. Obtaining a measure of plasma ammonia needs to be a priority in any child in whom mental status changes, defined very broadly, are evident. There are both acute and chronic forms of all of the disorders that affect the urea cycle, and clinical suspicion is paramount. The urea cycle may not be functioning adequately because of either mutations in the genes encoding the enzymes of the urea cycle (primary urea cycle disorders) or the toxic accumulation of products of other inborn errors of metabolism (notably the organic acidemias) that directly negatively affect the functioning of these enzymes. The degree of hyperammonemia at times may be just as high in these conditions as in the primary urea cycle disorders. Screening is accomplished by measurement of plasma ammonia levels, plasma amino acids, and urine for organic acids (including orotic acid). Quantitation of amino acids in the urine may also be helpful.

Several inherited disorders of the urea cycle (urea cycle disorders) are due to insufficiency or total absence of one of the six enzymatic activities contributing to the complete urea cycle (Table 30-5).

They are all autosomal recessive genetic disorders except for ornithine transcarbamylase (OTC) deficiency, an X-linked disorder. OTC deficiency should be suspected when family history reveals male newborn or infant deaths. Because of the random nature of X-inactivation, many girls carrying an OTC mutation have clinical symptoms. Some are severely affected with presentation in early infancy; others have symptoms including headaches, intermittent ataxia or encephalopathy, behavioral and psychiatric abnormalities, or developmental delays. Teenage girls often learn to avoid high protein–containing meals, and therefore dietary preferences can provide helpful clues as well. Several older male children have also been identified, not having the devastating infantile illness, by mutations producing partial enzymatic activity. OTC deficiency is therefore *not* only a neonatal disease. Approximately 60% of the diagnoses of OTC deficiency are now made in patients older than 1 month (Smith et al, 2005). OTC deficiency screening is accomplished by analysis of urine for organic acids (being sure to include orotic acid, an accumulated byproduct) and plasma amino acids (usually demonstrating low citrulline, the product of the enzymatic reaction, and increases in glutamine and alanine from hyperammonemia). The amino acid abnormalities and orotic acid elevation can be subtle in late-onset cases, so the index of suspicion should remain high, and consultation with a clinical biochemical geneticist or metabolic disease specialist may be helpful in suspected cases without clear laboratory evidence. DNA testing for mutations is clinically available at several laboratories.

Each of the urea cycle disorders will have its own pattern of amino acids and urea cycle compounds on plasma amino acid screen, and interpretation from biochemical genetics laboratories is usually provided. However, at the time of clinical decompensation, urea cycle disorders should be suspected in the face of a respiratory alkalosis and low blood urea nitrogen concentration for clinical illness (problematically reported as normal range), and an ammonia level should be immediately determined. Initial treatment involves intravenous fluids containing high glucose concentration (D10 at twice maintenance to start), cessation of all protein feeds until studies sort out the diagnosis, and use of compounds for alternative pathways of excretion of the amino moieties (e.g., sodium phenylacetate and sodium benzoate) as well as urea cycle intermediates (usually arginine if the diagnosis is unknown, citrulline if the diagnosis is known to be carbamyl phosphate synthetase or OTC deficiencies). Chronic treatment of these disorders includes protein restriction, sodium phenylbutyrate and benzoate (for alternative pathways of ammonia excretion), and either citrulline or arginine (which now becomes an essential amino acid).

Urine organic acid analysis should always be performed because many inherited disorders of amino acid catabolism and fatty acid oxidation produce byproducts that interfere with the functioning of the urea cycle. Notably, propionic and methylmalonic acidemias produce hyperammonemia accompanied by marked metabolic acidosis, not respiratory alkalosis, and fatty acid oxidation disorders may have normal bicarbonate and blood urea nitrogen levels on serum chemistries (see Table 30-3). Mental status changes as well as developmental delays may be due to intermittent hyperammonemias from a number of these and other conditions. Lysinuric protein intolerance is due to mutations affecting genes involved in dibasic amino acid transport. Urine amino acid analysis will demonstrate increases in the excretion of cystine, ornithine, lysine, or arginine, with resultant decreases observed in plasma amino acids. This disorder often presents in later infancy or childhood with growth delays, hypotonia, and hepatomegaly but variable developmental abnormalities, depending on the history of hyperammonemic episodes. A helpful screen is serum ferritin, often elevated in this condition, as are lactate dehydrogenase and thyroxine-binding globulin.

Hyperammonemia-hyperornithinemia-homocitrullinemia syndrome may present with variable developmental delays, irritability, myoclonic spasms, hemiparesis or paraparesis, seizures, and numerous other neurologic findings at any age. Intermittent episodes of hyperammonemia often lead to typical symptoms and signs of vomiting, lethargy, ataxia, or coma, and cortical atrophy on computed tomography or magnetic resonance imaging of the head may be evidence of subclinical attacks. Postprandial hyperammonemia may be interspersed with normal levels of ammonia. Plasma and urine amino acids are useful screens, demonstrating hyperornithinemia, orotic aciduria, and homocitrullinuria. Elevated levels of ornithine may be present in other disorders with developmental delay, such as ornithine aminotransferase deficiency with gyrate atrophy of the choroid and retina and renal Fanconi syndrome, but these do not have episodes of hyperammonemia. Nonetheless, their presence may be suspected from the pattern on plasma and urine amino acid analysis.

DISORDERS OF AMINO ACIDS AND ORGANIC ACID METABOLISM

Organic Acidurias

Many of the conditions referred to as organic acidemias or acidurias are the result of inherited deficiencies of the enzymatic steps catalyzing the breakdown of the branched-chain amino acids leucine, isoleucine, and valine. Description of all of the large number of disorders is beyond the scope of this book. However, most organic acid disorders will produce metabolites detected by urine organic acid analysis. The most familiar of the branched-chain amino acid disorders are maple syrup urine disease (branched-chain ketoaciduria, more accurately referred to as maple syrup disease because not only the urine may have this odor), isovaleric acidemia, propionic acidemia, and methylmalonic acidemia. These conditions are manifested with episodic illness, often clinically devastating, with prominent ketoacidosis, often reflected by an increased anion gap. They may be accompanied by hyperammonemia or hypoglycemia (see Table 30-3). Other disorders of amino acid metabolism to suspect with this type of presentation include glutaric acidurias types I and II, multiple carboxylase deficiency, and 3-hydroxy-3-methylglutaric (HMG) acidemia (HMG-CoA lyase deficiency). Both HMG-CoA lyase deficiency and glutaric aciduria type II may be distinguished by absence of ketosis in the face of profound acidosis and hypoglycemia (see later). A variety of clinical subtypes of disorders of amino acid metabolism have been observed with classic neonatal or infantile presentations of vomiting, listlessness, lethargy, seizures, ophthalmoplegias, apnea, coma, and death if untreated; intermittent episodes of clinical collapse but with normal periods (and normal laboratory values) between collapse; and intermediate forms presenting with developmental delays and varying findings of ataxia or dysmetria but no history of such devastating clinical episodes.

Screening of plasma amino acid and plasma carnitine levels and urine organic acid analyses will often identify the disorders. Plasma acylcarnitine profiles may help detect if not confirm the disorders in the absence of direct enzymatic testing. They all require amino acid–specific restricted diets and often vitamin supplementation because many of these enzymes use vitamin cofactors whose dietary supplementation may help augment activities in mutations causing residual rather than complete absence of activities. These vitamins include thiamine, cobalamin, biotin, riboflavin, folate, and others. Several of these conditions are manifested by hypotonia, in part because of carnitine deficiency, a compound used to replace coenzyme A attached to many of the acyl moieties (carboxylic acid derivatives) generated during branched-chain amino acid catabolism. The acylcarnitine compounds are then excreted in the urine, depleting the body of free carnitine required for transport of long-chain fatty acids into mitochondria for oxidation, ultimately leading to production of ketone bodies required as energy substrates. Many of these disorders may be detected by newborn screening with MS/MS (where available), but the absence of their "positivity" on such screens does *not* rule them out in a child presenting at a later age. On occasion, metabolites of drugs (e.g., valproic acid) may produce organic acid results that may overlap those seen in some of these disorders. The biochemical geneticist and metabolic disease specialist should be helpful in sorting these out. Many of these disorders demonstrate abnormalities on computed tomography or magnetic resonance imaging of the head, including abnormal basal ganglia signals and cerebral atrophy, which may take years to appear (see Fig. 30-2).

Biotinidase and Multiple Carboxylase Deficiencies

Biotinidase deficiency and holocarboxylase synthase deficiency (multiple carboxylase deficiency) produce deficiencies in carboxylating enzymatic activities requiring the cofactor biotin, usually provided in normal diets. Dietary biotin requires biotinidase to free biotin into a usable form for attachment to other enzyme proteins (carboxylases) through the subsequent action of holocarboxylase synthase. Lack of either enzymatic activity will cause patients to demonstrate intermittent clinical signs and symptoms similar to those seen with inherited disorders of the individual carboxylating enzyme step (propionyl-CoA carboxylase, 3-methylcrotonyl carboxylase, pyruvate carboxylase). Deficiencies of either biotinidase or holocarboxylase synthetase may present with alopecia and dermatitis (probably related to fatty acyl-CoA carboxylase deficiency), ataxia, and lactic acidosis. The metabolic acidosis due to lactic acidosis is often difficult to treat with dietary bicarbonate and citrate supplements, but it responds quickly to high doses of biotin (usually 10 mg daily).

Newborn screening by enzymatic measurement of biotinidase is very sensitive for biotinidase deficiency, but newborn MS/MS for amino acids and acylcarnitines can miss these disorders because the metabolites of branched-chain amino acid metabolism may not have accumulated to detectable levels usually associated with clinical symptoms and acidosis. This cause of developmental delay and intellectual disability is preventable if supplemental biotin is provided early in life.

Glutaric Acidurias

Disorders of lysine catabolism produce a group of organic acidurias that have a common presentation complex of ataxia, seizures, myoclonus, extrapyramidal symptoms (dyskinesias), "metabolic stroke," and macrocephaly. The best known is glutaric aciduria type I (deficiency of glutaryl-CoA dehydrogenase), which often remains unsuspected until a devastating strokelike illness leaves the infant or child with neurologic consequences, often with dystonia as a prominent feature. Alternatively, the child may present with "atypical" cerebral palsy, with dystonic or dyskinetic features but no clinical history of an episode associated with likely brain injury. There may be history of hypotonia and unusual movements or posturing of extremities during routine illnesses or after immunizations. Infants generally demonstrate overt macrocephaly or increasing rate of head growth during 3 to 6 months of age, before any strokelike or metabolic episode. Brain imaging (computed tomography or magnetic resonance imaging) may reveal prefrontal collections (prefrontal hygromas) of CSF, often misinterpreted as evidence of chronic subdural bleeding. The diagnostic metabolites may be picked up by MS/MS during newborn screening, but identification or necessary follow-up of asymptomatic neonates may be missed. Diets restricted for lysine and tryptophan, supplemented with riboflavin and carnitine (if deficiency is documented), and careful education of families and primary care physicians to promote early administration of intravenous fluids containing glucose with any significant illness may prevent neurologic sequelae if they are instituted before the first acute clinical episode with overt neurologic deterioration. It is unclear if there is any reversal of symptoms if treatment is started after the acute severe clinical episode.

Screening of plasma amino acids and urine organic acids and plasma acylcarnitine profiles should identify glutaric aciduria type I. Other biochemically related disorders that should also be identified with the testing described include the L-2- and D-2-hydroxyglutaric acidurias, 2-oxoadipic aciduria, and glutaric aciduria type II (now termed multiple acyl-CoA dehydrogenase deficiency). L-2 Hydroxyglutaric aciduria is among the few causes of leukodystrophy that demonstrates involvement of the subcortical U fibers (see Table 30-4). Multiple acyl-CoA dehydrogenase deficiency (glutaric aciduria type II) is a condition of multiple enzymatic deficiencies that depend on flavin cofactors. Interruption of the normal flavoprotein-dependent transfer of electrons from these reactions into the electron transport system of the mitochondria produces the multiple deficiencies observed, including that of glutaric acid metabolism and fatty acid oxidation (see later).

Hyperphenylalaninemias

Several inborn errors of metabolism have historically been categorized as aminoacidopathies or disorders of amino acid metabolism, many of which were associated with intellectual disability that appeared preventable or were ameliorated by dietary restriction of the offending amino acid. The classic disorder is phenylketonuria (PKU), a long-standing component of successful newborn screening in preventing intellectual disability. However, certain children with PKU are still missed on newborn screening as a result of sample mix-up, reporting error, follow-up deficiency, and other reasons, and any child with unexplained intellectual disability, especially with acquired microcephaly, should have plasma amino acid screening (and other tests) to look for this and other disorders. It has long been established that hyperphenylalaninemia has toxic effects associated with the developing brain, both during infantile growth (children with PKU) and during gestation (infants of mothers with PKU). Aside from intellectual disability, the manifestations of children with PKU include pigment "abnormalities" (typically, but not always, blue eyes and fair skin), eczematous rash, and neurologic sequelae including seizures, variable microcephaly, and hyperactivity. These result from the absence of the enzyme phenylalanine hydroxylase, with subsequent inability to convert phenylalanine to tyrosine. Therefore, amino acid testing will show elevated levels of phenylalanine and variable decreased levels of tyrosine. These are easily detected on newborn screens including MS/MS, which is rapidly replacing the previous bacteriologic methods of identifying hyperphenylalaninemia. As with all newborn screens, the lack of reporting of a positive newborn screen in any individual patient with developmental delay does not preclude the possibility of this diagnosis. Often, these individuals may have a musty (mousy) odor and a history of unexplained infantile vomiting illnesses, irritability, and a mild rash ascribed as atopic (eczema) that does not respond well to topical therapies. Of note, the phenylalanine hydroxylase enzyme has a cofactor, tetrahydrobiopterin, that is also necessary in the formation of several neurotransmitters. All patients with hyperphenylalaninemia need to be screened for this cofactor defect. Without testing for tetrahydrobiopterin defects, this cofactor defect can become evident when dietary restriction of phenylalanine does not prevent clinical sequelae in children identified by newborn screens with elevated phenylalanine. PKU (or hyperphenylalaninemia) responds to diet restricted for phenylalanine intake, careful monitoring of amino acid levels, and supplementation with tyrosine, which becomes an essential amino acid in this disorder. Cofactor defects require more specialized treatment.

There are individuals with so-called benign hyperphenylalaninemia, caused by milder deficiencies of phenylalanine hydroxylase, as well as transient hyperphenylalaninemias of infancy, with no apparent clinical sequelae. However, it can be difficult to determine early on, when treatment is most effective, whether these infants have potential for development of sequelae similar to classic PKU. Many should therefore be started on treatment, with subsequent follow-up studies suggesting when dietary restriction can be relaxed. However, at a later age, especially during reproductive years, these women should be retested. As described earlier in this chapter, hyperphenylalaninemia during pregnancy may result in intrauterine growth restriction, microcephaly, intellectual disability, and congenital heart disease. This syndrome, termed maternal PKU, is preventable if the mothers are prescribed restricted diets for phenylalanine, with resultant declines of their plasma phenylalanine levels documented and maintained before conception and throughout pregnancy. Note that these infants usually do not have PKU and will not show elevations of their plasma phenylalanine levels after several days of age. Therefore, maternal history is important in the evaluation of children with unexplained developmental delay. A mother may be unaware of her past history of PKU because dietary treatment of PKU, which is now recommended to be lifelong, was discontinued as early as 6 years of age in some centers in previous years. Plasma amino acid testing of the mother may be indicated if it is warranted by clinical suspicion.

Homocystinurias and Disorders of Methionine and Cysteine

Homocystinuria can be produced by a number of inherited disorders of metabolism. It is a multisystemic condition that may affect the skeleton, eye, vascular system, and CNS. The basis of much of the findings is the increased thrombosis, thromboembolic events, and resultant strokes, both subclinical and overt, in a variety of organs as well as the connective tissue disorder caused by the abnormal accumulation of homocysteine. Many individuals have easily identified findings, including a marfanoid skeletal habitus (but with osteoporosis) and ectopia lentis (often a downward dislocation of the lens noted by iridodonesis, a shimmering appearance to the iris), but these may only be evident well into the childhood or teenage years. Vascular disease with increased tendency toward major complications including pulmonary embolism and strokes is noted in both childhood and adult ages. Intellectual disability and behavioral problems are common but may be variable in degree. Considering that individuals are normal at birth, these adverse outcomes can often be ameliorated if not totally prevented with appropriate therapy. Newborn screening programs employing MS/MS will often identify these individuals by detection of elevated plasma methionine, but it is the homocystine in urine and plasma, which usually accumulates weeks to months after birth, that leads to diagnostic confirmation and appropriate treatment. The absence of activity of cystathionine β-synthase, an enzyme often responsive to vitamin B_6 (pyridoxine), is found in many but not all patients. The condition may also be due to disruption of several vitamin B_{12}–dependent pathways (often termed remethylation defects) that are identified by production of homocystinuria and homocystinemia but with low or normal levels of plasma methionine (i.e., deficiency of methylene tetrahydrofolate reductase). Clinical forms of methylmalonic aciduria with homocystinuria (cblC and cblD subtypes of methylmalonic acidemia) are well established on the basis of common cobalamin (vitamin B_{12})–associated pathways. Additional forms (cblE and cblG subtypes) may be manifested with elevations of homocysteine but not methylmalonic acidemia. All four of these cobalamin disorder subtypes may be manifested with developmental delay and associated megaloblastic anemia. Cystathionine β-synthase deficiency homocystinuria is treated with pyridoxine, dietary restriction of methionine, and often betaine, a product used to provide alternative pathways of excretion for homocysteine. The cobalamin disorders are treated with vitamin B_{12}, variable diet restriction, carnitine, folate, and betaine.

Developmental delay is usually present early in life in children with homocystinuria, but there is a heterogeneous pattern of symptoms. Some individuals are not referred for evaluation until behavior and psychiatric abnormalities become paramount. Rage attacks, psychomotor seizures, depression, schizophrenia, and personality disorders have all been anecdotally reported with the condition. By then, the other features of the condition (ophthalmologic and skeletal) are usually evident. Seizures are common but have not been reported in the majority of pediatric patients before strokes. Because many of the children present early for developmental delays without signs of regression, screening plasma amino acid analyses and urine amino acid and organic acid studies should identify this condition if the samples are handled properly. On occasion, urine organic acid screens will report the presence of cystathionine, a compound related to the homocysteine metabolic pathway. In the absence of elevated homocysteine, this is thought to be a benign condition even though there are anecdotal reports of its association with intellectual disability. Similarly, persistent elevated plasma methionine is unlikely to have etiologic significance if the laboratory findings of homocystinuria, tyrosinemia type I, or other more common and easily identifiable inborn errors of metabolism causing hypermethioninemia are not present. Some of these elevations normalize with time. It often is helpful to specifically obtain a "total" blood homocysteine level to avoid artifactual but expected absences of homocysteine observed in plasma amino acid analyses.

Elevations of 5-oxoproline are occasionally observed in urine organic acid screens. This may reflect rare disorders affecting glutathione, a tripeptide of glutamate, cysteine, and glycine, or related pathways. However, patients with urea cycle defects (OTC deficiency), homocystinuria, and severe liver dysfunction and toxicities of any etiology may also present with 5-oxoproline in the urine.

Tyrosinemias

Several inborn errors of metabolism result in elevations of plasma tyrosine. Classically, only tyrosinemia type II is variably associated with intellectual disability, although the chronic debilitating symptoms associated with untreated tyrosinemia type I may impede the normal attainment of motor milestones, especially in late infancy or early childhood. Both may be detected by screening plasma amino acid and urine organic acid analyses. Tyrosinemia type II (tyrosine aminotransferase deficiency), also known as oculocutaneous tyrosinemia, is associated with the development of irritative dermatitis of the palms and soles and eventual keratitis of the cornea (dendritic type ulcers). Both symptom complexes respond to dietary restrictions of tyrosine and phenylalanine, from which it is derived. Intellectual disability of varying degrees has been associated with this condition in about 50% of cases reported, but it remains unclear whether the hypertyrosinemia causes the intellectual disability. It is unclear if dietary restriction prevents intellectual disability in tyrosinemia type II as it does in PKU, but it is prudent to start all diagnosed patients on this therapeutic regimen. It clearly improves the skin and eye findings, preventing more permanent ophthalmologic problems. Varying degrees of abnormal behaviors, hyperactivity, language delays, seizures (uncommonly), and microcephaly and one case of self-mutilation tendencies have been anecdotally reported.

Tyrosinemia type III is due to the deficiency of the next enzyme of the pathway, 4-hydroxyphenylpyruvate dioxygenase. It is unclear if it is an actual disease condition, but it has been mainly described in children being screened for causes of developmental delay or intellectual disability. There are no reported abnormalities of liver, eye, or skin, but the persistent abnormally high levels of tyrosine from infancy distinguish it from those detected on newborn screens that eventually are labeled transient hypertyrosinemia of the newborn, thought to be more an infant liver maturation process. No data exist for the therapeutic effects of tyrosine- and phenylalanine-restricted diets, but it appears prudent to initiate these as early as possible.

Tyrosinemia type I, the hepatorenal form, is due to deficiency of an enzyme several steps removed from direct catabolism of tyrosine, fumarylacetoacetase (or fumarylacetoacetate hydrolase). The diagnosis is confirmed by documentation of an abnormal metabolite, succinylacetone, in blood and urine, although it is often not detected in plasma amino acid screens. Tyrosinemia type I is associated with variable but progressive liver dysfunction, often leading to cirrhosis and renal tubular dysfunction (vitamin D–resistant rickets due to hypophosphatemia); intermittent neurologic symptoms resembling acute intermittent porphyria may produce hyponatremic seizures, posturing and seizures, and hypertension with mental status changes. At times, there has been a cabbage-like odor associated with patients. Dietary restriction of tyrosine and phenylalanine provides variable amelioration, but the progressive nature of the condition usually persists. Long-term outcomes in untreated tyrosinemia are usually associated with hepatocellular carcinoma or liver failure, both requiring hepatic transplantation. Recently, the introduction of 2(2-nitro-4-trifluoromethylbenzoyl)-1, 3-cyclohexanedione (NTBC) to the therapeutic regimen has dramatically altered the course of the observed hepatic and renal symptoms.

FATTY ACID OXIDATION DISORDERS

The term *organic acidurias* historically referred to disorders of both amino acid metabolism and fatty acid oxidation. The fatty acid oxidation disorders are now considered a separate category because of similarities in presentation and laboratory findings, overlapping but different from the disorders of amino acids (see Table 30-3). Any patient with episodes of hypoglycemia associated with low levels or absence of ketones should be screened for these disorders by blood acylcarnitine profiles. However, some patients with fatty acid oxidation defects may excrete ketones even during crises, especially as neonates. Patterns in urine organic acid analyses and carnitine levels of blood and urine may be helpful, but plasma acylcarnitine profiles often provide diagnostic confirmation. Many of these disorders may be detected by MS/MS-based screening programs, but beware false-negatives or lack of testing and follow-up in any individual patient. Transport of long-chain fatty acids into mitochondria for fatty acid oxidation is provided by carnitine, whose deficiency may be due to primary disorders or secondarily to its attachment to the excess various acyl moieties generated from the carbon skeletons of long-, medium-, or short-chain fatty acids and subsequent urinary excretion in these fatty acid oxidation disorders. Multiple enzymes with specific chain length requirements (very long, long, medium, and short) have been identified, as have disorders due to their deficiencies. The field continues to expand, but the current listing of disorders includes those listed in Table 30-6.

A detailed discussion of these disorders is beyond the scope of this text (for review, see listed references). They all may present with lower than expected levels of acetoacetate and β-hydroxybutyrate, the circulating blood ketone bodies. Their accumulating intermediates or deficient substrate production for vital ongoing metabolic processes may variably affect the CNS, muscle, and heart tissues, producing symptoms suggestive of fatty acid oxidation disorders. Episodes of vomiting with variable mental status changes (listlessness or lethargy progressing to coma), hypoketotic hypoglycemia, variable acidosis and hyperammonemia, apparent life-threatening episodes, seizures, hepatomegaly or variable liver test abnormalities (direct bilirubinemia, mild elevations in aspartate aminotransferase and alanine aminotransferase), chronic muscle weakness (variable creatine kinase elevations), cardiomyopathy, failure-to-thrive, and a range of chronic CNS findings from hypotonia to spastic diplegia, developmental delays, peripheral neuropathies, and retinal changes have all been described. Much of the CNS disease may be related to clinical or

Table 30-6. Fatty Acid Oxidation Disorders

Carnitine transporter defect
Carnitine translocase deficiency
Carnitine palmitoyltransferase I and II deficiencies
Short-chain acyl-CoA dehydrogenase deficiency
Short-chain 3-hydroxyacyl-CoA dehydrogenase deficiency
Medium-chain acyl-CoA dehydrogenase deficiency
Long-chain L-3-hydroxyacyl-CoA dehydrogenase deficiency
Trifunctional protein deficiency (one form of long-chain 3-hydroxyacyl-CoA dehydrogenase deficiency)
Very-long-chain acyl-CoA dehydrogenase deficiency
Multiple acyl-CoA dehydrogenase deficiency
- Glutaric aciduria type II
- Ethylmalonic-adipic aciduria

3-Hydroxy-3-methylglutaryl-CoA lyase deficiency (last step in both leucine and fatty acid oxidation metabolism)

subclinical decompensations associated with otherwise typical childhood illnesses leading to lack of adequate caloric intake. Identification of these disorders early will usually prevent these sequelae, but a large percentage (up to 40% before routine screening) presented with initial episodes associated with infantile death, usually in the context of an otherwise expected benign viral-like illness. In children presenting with unexplained developmental delays, especially with hypotonia, routine screening with plasma carnitine levels and acylcarnitine profiles and urine organic acid analysis should identify these disorders as well as other potentially serious organic acidurias. The most important therapeutic regimen involves avoidance of fasting or prolonged periods without calorie intake. Modified fat diets and carnitine and vitamin therapies are tailored to the individual disorders identified.

CENTRAL NERVOUS SYSTEM DISORDERS ASSOCIATED WITH AMINOACIDOPATHIES AND NEUROTRANSMITTERS

Several inborn errors of metabolism appear to directly affect neurotransmitter function. Glycine cleavage deficiency, an enzymatic activity isolated from both liver and brain, results in nonketotic hyperglycinemia. It usually presents with severe neonatal neurologic devastation, often in the form of unremitting seizures, in which elevations of glycine in the CSF are noted, irrespective of the presence of similar elevations in the plasma. However, the variably elevated plasma glycine level may be the first clue to this diagnosis. It is the increased ratio of CSF to plasma glycine (>0.09; normal, <0.04) that is important for the diagnosis, and thus CSF for quantitative amino acid analysis must be obtained at the same time as plasma amino acids. The patients are usually normal at birth but by 2 days of age may demonstrate hiccupping (thought potentially to be a seizure equivalent), with eventual myoclonic or severe tonic-clonic seizures, and a characteristic burst suppression electroencephalographic pattern. Hypotonia progresses to spasticity, and many die within weeks to months. Profound psychomotor retardation is the norm for surviving patients with classic nonketotic hyperglycinemia. In contrast, there are transient, atypical, and late-onset forms of apparent nonketotic hyperglycinemia. Transient forms may appear just as severe as classic forms, but they appear to improve by 2 months of age, with declines in CSF glycine concentration. Many but not all have no neurologic sequelae in subsequent years, but this form has been reported in only a handful of patients, whereas hundreds have been diagnosed with classic nonketotic hyperglycinemia. In contrast, late-onset forms may be manifested in normal neonates or infants who then develop severe unremitting seizures with characteristic electroencephalographic or other neurologic signs and symptoms that may be variable, presenting at any age. CSF analysis for amino acids is often not performed in later onset neurologic disease unless severe symptoms are present, and therefore it is unclear if glycine cleavage defects represent rare or more common causes of these types of presentations. For all three types of glycine cleavage deficiency conditions, therapies involving benzoate (to promote renal clearance and to lower body glycine levels) and dextromethorphan (NMDA antagonist) have been tried on the basis of glycine excitatory neurotransmitter effects on the CNS *N*-methyl-D-aspartate (NMDA), receptor with variable results. The anticonvulsant valproate should probably be avoided in these conditions because of some evidence that it inhibits the activity of this enzyme complex, leading to elevations of glycine. Treatment of classic nonketotic hyperglycinemia has not been proved to ameliorate the profound psychomotor retardation, and in the opinion of several clinical biochemical geneticists, classic nonketotic hyperglycinemia remains a lethal condition.

Tyrosine hydroxylase deficiency, the first step in the pathway of catecholamine biosynthesis (levodopa, dopamine, norepinephrine), has been identified in very few patients. However, their pattern of presentation is similar, with dystonias, hypokinesias, or rigidity during infancy or early childhood. The diagnostic test to keep in mind is measurement of catecholamines in CSF. Urine catecholamine measurements are not particularly useful. Many of the enzymes of the catecholamine (as well as serotonin) neurotransmitter pathway are biopterin or pyridoxine cofactor dependent. Although diagnosis of pathway enzymatic deficiencies depends on CSF analysis for specific patterns of accumulated intermediates, initial amino acid and organic acid analyses of plasma and urine occasionally suggest the elevation of these intermediates. Suggestive clinical presentations include infants with extrapyramidal movement disorders, hypotonia, and oculogyric crises (aromatic L–amino acid decarboxylase deficiency); boys with borderline intellectual disability with behavioral abnormalities (violent or aggressive) and stereotypic hand movements (monoamine oxidase A deficiency); and later childhood- or teenage-onset dystonias (guanosine triphosphate cyclohydrolase I deficiency—first step in biopterin cofactor synthesis, may have hyperphenylalaninemia). Both pyridoxine- and folinic acid–responsive seizures may be the result of enzymatic deficiencies of either these or other neurotransmitter pathways.

Defects of sulfite oxidase metabolism (in the metabolic pathway of cysteine), due to either the enzyme deficiency itself or molybdenum cofactor defect, have also been associated with refractory seizures and severe psychomotor retardation. Some individuals with these disorders have dislocated lens. Molybdenum cofactor deficiency is associated with extremely low serum uric acid levels. It produces a combined deficiency of xanthine oxidase and sulfite oxidase, whose products may be identified on plasma and urine amino acid and organic acid analyses. It is usually identified in infants with severe, refractory seizures whose first metabolic screens are negative. It is not clear how variable this condition may be. Few patients with late onset have been clearly identified. Specialized testing for urine *S*-sulfocysteine is diagnostic in many cases.

An increasing number of children with developmental delay (mild to moderate, especially language) and acting out behavior are being identified with succinic semialdehyde dehydrogenase deficiency. This enzyme is in the pathway of glutamic acid metabolism in the brain involved in the formation and regulation of levels of gamma-aminobutyric acid, a known neurotransmitter. The etiology of vitamin B_6 (pyridoxine)–responsive seizures is thought to reside in the upstream portion of this pathway and is a separate condition. Succinic semialdehyde dehydrogenase deficiency is identified by the presence of 4-hydroxybutyric acid on urine organic acid analysis, but this metabolite may be missed even by experienced laboratories. This compound is thought to accumulate in the CNS and to cause neuroexcitatory abnormalities as well as the enzymatic deficiency affecting the normal regulation of gamma-aminobutyric acid levels. More than 150 individuals have been described with this condition, which is variably manifested during childhood with intellectual delays, seizures, hypotonia, ataxia, and variable aggressive behaviors or autistic features. For that reason, any child presenting to the developmental pediatrician with some subset of these findings should have urine analysis of organic acids, keeping this condition as well as numerous other organic acidurias in mind. Although the anticonvulsant vigabatrin has been postulated to have a potential therapeutic effect in this disorder by decreasing the upstream substrate of this reaction, its toxic side effects have limited clinical studies, and no results of its clear efficacy are available at present.

There are several disorders of ornithine metabolism that may be manifested with developmental delays. Hyperammonemia-hyperornithinemia-homocitrullinemia syndrome is discussed earlier. Disorders of creatine metabolism may first be suggested by urinary screening tests. One of these, guanidinoacetate methyltransferase deficiency, is manifested with elevations of ornithine but low arginine levels in plasma accompanied by low levels of creatine in brain proton magnetic resonance spectroscopy patterns. Patients usually demonstrate developmental delays, hypotonia, seizures, and extrapyramidal movements. Many of the patients presenting with later onset have absence of speech or autistic behavior accompanying the intellectual disability. Some have striking behavioral patterns. When magnetic resonance imaging of the brain is ordered in a child with developmental delay, seizures, intellectual disability, or other related concerns, consideration should be given to adding such magnetic resonance spectroscopy studies to detect these and other disorders of inborn errors of metabolism.

PURINE AND PYRIMIDINE DISORDERS

The association of intellectual disability and self-injurious behaviors in boys with Lesch-Nyhan syndrome, an X-linked disorder of the purine salvage pathway (hypoxanthine-guanine phosphoribosyltransferase [HGPRT] deficiency), has long been known. These infants are typically normal for 3 to 4 months, and then motor delays associated with hyperreflexia, spasticity, and choreoathetoid movements become apparent during months to years. Compulsive, self-destructive behaviors involving self-biting are characteristic. Although many have intellectual disability, several do not, but the dysarthrias may be confusing. Hyperuricemia may be manifested in infancy as urinary crystals in the diaper, gout, or renal disease at older ages. Some do not have hyperuricemia until after puberty. Allopurinol therapy is available to prevent urate stones, but it does not alter the neurologic disease. Urine purine and pyrimidine metabolite testing in specialized laboratories is diagnostic. Enzyme (HGPRT) testing is available.

Isolated xanthine oxidase deficiency is thought to be benign, but if it is associated with sulfite oxidase deficiency through molybdenum cofactor deficiency, a syndrome of refractory seizures and ultimate severe intellectual disability is often present (discussed earlier). Very low levels (undetectable) of plasma uric acid are noted, and urine screens demonstrate sulfur-containing metabolites. It is unclear if therapies involving low purine diets, molybdenum, and experimental drugs are helpful.

Patients with seizures, developmental delay, ataxia, and autistic features identified by hypouricosuria may have 5′-nucleotidase superactivity, one of several rare disorders of pyrimidine metabolism. A similar one with additional varying neurologic features is uridine monophosphate synthase deficiency, producing massive orotic aciduria (found on urine organic acid testing) and megaloblastic anemia, unresponsive to vitamin B_6, vitamin B_{12}, and folate. Orotic acid crystals in diapers may have been reported. Both of these are reported to respond to uridine supplementation.

Elevated urinary excretion of uracil and thymine may be observed in patients with seizures, intellectual disability, hypertonia or hyperreflexia, microcephaly, or autistic features who have dihydropyrimidine dehydrogenase deficiency. Not all patients with this deficiency exhibit neurologic findings. Similarly, abnormal pyrimidine products (urinary dihydrouracil and dihydrothymine) may be seen in a similar albeit rarer disorder, dihydropyrimidinase deficiency. Recent recommendations for screening of children with autistic features include as a third tier serum and urine uric acid. If increased levels are noted, enzymatic testing for HGPRT (decreased) and phosphoribosylpyrophosphate synthetase superactivity (increased) can be performed; if decreased levels are noted, a purine and pyrimidine panel (uracil excretion, xanthine, hypoxanthine) can be performed to look for these types of disorders.

PEROXISOMAL DISORDERS

Disorders of peroxisomal function have many overlapping features, usually associated with several of the following: psychomotor retardation; hypotonia or severe weakness; intractable seizures; cataracts, retinal degeneration, or any impairment of vision or sensorineural hearing; dysmorphic facial features; findings on computed tomography or magnetic resonance imaging of the head consistent with neuronal migration defects, heterotopias, and leukodystrophy; liver function abnormalities; and calcific stippling of epiphyses. A clinical pearl is that peroxisomal disorders should be considered in any child with both hearing and visual deficits. In the past, attempts at distinguishing individual clinical disorders were made, but current

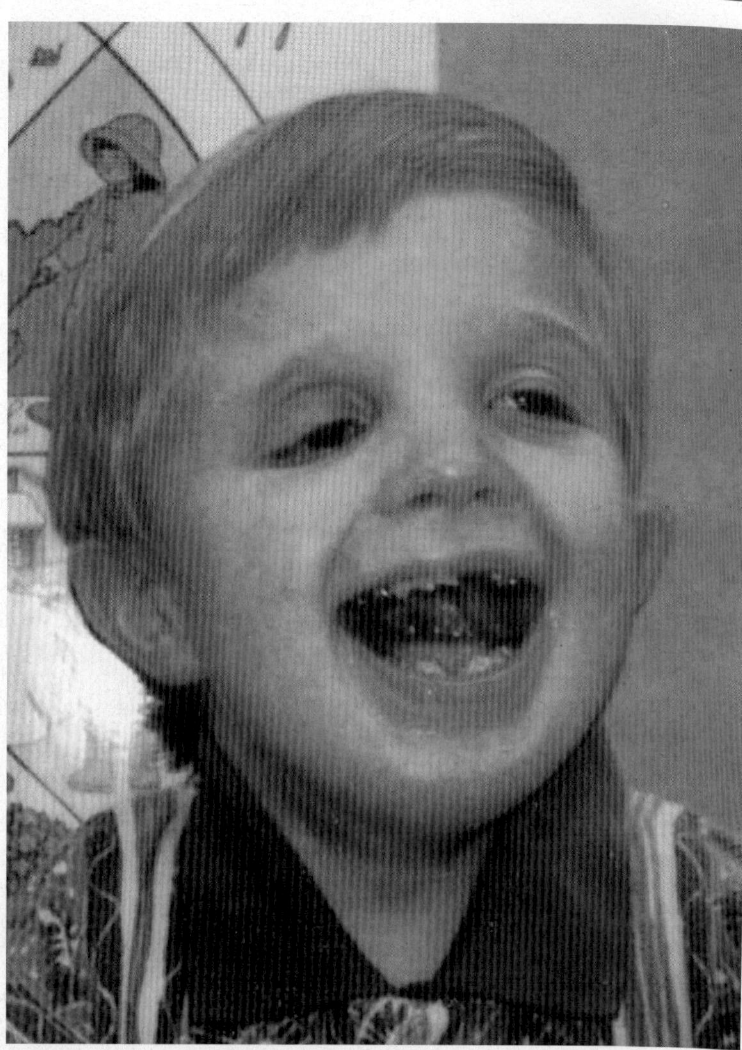

Figure 30-4. Infantile Refsum disease (peroxisomal). Facial dysmorphisms, although mild, are apparent, including brachycephaly, deep-set orbits, and downslanting palpebral fissures. These brachycephalic patients with epicanthal folds and round facies may be mistaken for Down syndrome on initial evaluation but have normal karyotype. Screening for very-long-chain fatty acids helps identify a peroxisomal disorder in a child with dysmorphic features and developmental delay.

molecular assessments suggest that this is not always clear-cut. Several had very distinguishing features in classic cases. For example, Zellweger syndrome (hepatocerebrorenal syndrome) was considered for rare hypotonic infants with intractable seizures, characteristic facial features (high prominent forehead, cataracts or other ophthalmologic abnormalities, hypoplastic superior orbital ridges, depressed nasal bridge with epicanthal folds), cystic disease of kidney, hepatomegaly, findings on computed tomography or magnetic resonance imaging of the head of abnormal neuronal migration, and epiphyseal stippling. This is a disorder of peroxisomal biogenesis; liver electron microscopy shows absent or markedly abnormal peroxisomes, and enzymatic tests show multiple peroxisomal enzymatic deficiencies. Confirmation of abnormalities in plasma very-long-chain fatty acid analysis identified these children with peroxisomal dysfunction and decreased erythrocyte plasmalogens; elevated plasma pipecolic acid and bile acid intermediates were noted. Although it was initially described as a disorder causing infantile death at a few months of age, several other children were noted with similar features, and it has now become apparent that defects of individual peroxisomal enzymes and function or additional peroxisomal biogenesis syndromes exist. These include neonatal adrenoleukodystrophy, infantile Refsum disease (particularly with pigmentary degeneration of the retina, sensorineural deafness, and anosmia; Fig. 30-4), rhizomelic chondrodysplasia punctata (severe rhizomelic shortening of proximal limbs), hyperpipecolic aciduria, and a long list of peroxisomal enzymatic deficiency syndromes. Genomic analysis will ultimately help differentiate these categories. Although urine organic acids may show abnormalities, analysis of very-long-chain fatty acids (plasma or serum increased ratio of C26:C22) is diagnostic in most cases. More specific testing for diagnostic confirmation and specific diagnosis, such as for decreased plasmalogens (whole blood or erythrocytes), increased phytanic and pipecolic acids (plasma), and other studies, may then be directed by specialists who observe these children. Because less severe forms of these peroxisomal disorders are being identified outside of infancy (see Fig. 30-4), it is important for the specialist in developmental pediatrics to keep these screening tests in mind.

A different presentation needs to be kept in mind for the peroxisomal disorders causing adrenoleukodystrophy and related disorders (adrenomyeloneuropathies).

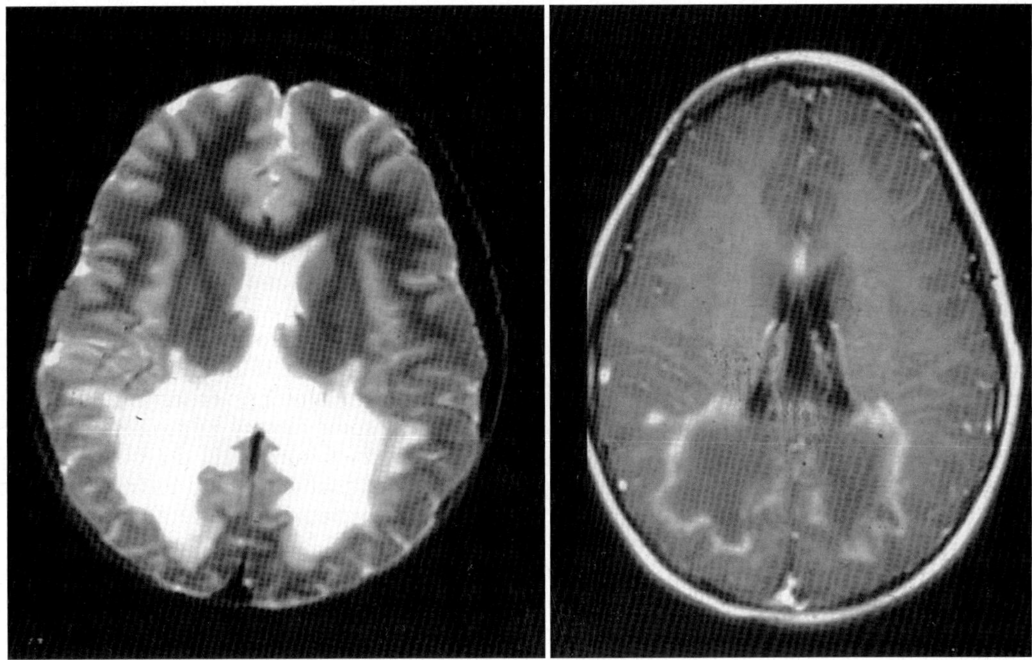

Figure 30-5. **Adrenoleukodystrophy.** Magnetic resonance images of a patient with X-linked adrenoleukodystrophy *(left)* demonstrate abnormal signals reflecting parieto-occipital areas of demyelination, which will progress in a caudal-rostral fashion with time. Magnetic resonance imaging with contrast material *(right)* demonstrates classic enhancement at the periphery of the demyelinated zone in the occipital region. *(Courtesy of G. Raymond, MD.)*

Adrenoleukodystrophy is an X-linked progressive demyelinating disorder variably associated with adrenal dysfunction. Affected children may often first present with behavioral or school performance abnormalities that progress to overt neurologic abnormalities. Loss of vision and hearing may be manifested first by language or speech problems or difficulties with assigned tasks. Classically, onset is in childhood, beginning at 3 to 10 years of age, but later onsets have been noted. Screening for abnormalities of very-long-chain fatty acids allows early identification. There is a characteristic caudal to rostral pattern of demyelination of cerebral white matter noted on computed tomography or magnetic resonance imaging (Fig. 30-5), but this may not be evident at the time of initial presentation for behavioral or school performance issues. Some patients may present with findings solely referable to adrenal dysfunction (Addison disease). Those patients with prolonged variable periods of apparent lack of neurologic involvement represent the adrenomyeloneuropathy group, who may begin to show neurologic compromise at any time, including later adulthood. Those with adrenomyeloneuropathy typically do not exhibit brain dysfunction but rather show spinal cord dysfunction. A high index of suspicion for this disorder is needed, even in female patients, because there has been clinical expression observed in female heterozygotes for this X-linked disorder. Currently, there are no definitively proven effective therapeutic measures available for adrenoleukodystrophy, although the efficacy of Lorenzo's oil (glyceryl trioleate and glyceryl trierucate 4:1) is debated. Bone marrow stem cell transplantation may prevent deterioration in boys who begin to show CNS involvement, but it is not indicated presymptomatically. However, supportive measures are extremely helpful, and the treatments for the adrenal dysfunction are clinically effective. Therefore, early identification of individuals with this disorder through judicious use of the screening laboratory tests is highly recommended. It is hoped that effective therapy will be demonstrated sometime soon.

DISORDERS OF CARBOHYDRATES

Glycogen Storage Diseases

If well treated, both early and in an effective prospective manner, most patients with listed forms of glycogen storage disease (I-IX) should not have significant problems with intellectual development. Most forms are manifested with signs and symptoms of liver or muscle dysfunction, including hypoglycemia and varying hepatomegaly, muscle weakness, and hypotonia. Some forms (glycogen storage disease I and Fanconi-Bickel syndrome [GLUT-2 defect]) may exhibit an associated renal Fanconi–type picture, often first identified by aminoaciduria during work-ups for failure-to-thrive and rickets-like picture. When developmental delay or intellectual disability is noted in glycogen storage diseases, it usually is the result of severe hypoglycemic episodes. Glycogen storage disease II, Pompe disease, is a lysosomal disorder due to acid maltase (α-glucosidase) deficiency, with progressive hypotonia, weakness, macroglossia, hepatomegaly, and cardiomegaly. Enzyme replacement therapy is now available for this disorder, and early identification is extremely important in attempts to prevent the relentless development of the cardiomyopathy and subsequent cardiac and respiratory failure.

Galactosemia

Classic galactosemia has been associated with apparent delays in speech, language, and other intellectual functions. Galactosemia classically is manifested in the newborn period with a clinical picture of neonatal hepatitis that may include hypoglycemia, acidosis, hyperbilirubinemia, and renal Fanconi syndrome and that may be associated with a concurrent systemic infection with *Escherichia coli*. Cataracts or lenticular opacities may be noted. Symptoms develop from the inability to properly metabolize galactose, derived from the intake of milk sugar, lactose (disaccharide glucose-galactose). Newborn screening programs have been successful at decreasing the mortality of this disorder in developed countries, but false-negative results on newborn screening have been noted, and affected neonates are often becoming ill as the results of newborn screening are being reported. Classic galactosemia, manifesting within the first 2 weeks of life, is due to deficiency of galactose-1-phosphate uridyltransferase. The excess galactose and metabolites accumulating in blood and urine is easily detected with appropriate testing. Testing of urine for reducing substances (i.e., Clinitest) is an effective screening test, provided the child had remained on oral intake of lactose-containing feeds (breast milk or formulas). The presence of reducing sugar in urine is rapidly lost when intravenous fluids containing glucose are used instead, even for as little as 24 hours. Similarly, numerous formulas no longer contain lactose, and intake of these also will produce a negative urine screen for reducing substances. The clinical illness is rapidly reversed by the removal of the offending source of galactose (lactose-containing formulas or breast milk). For various reasons, some of them delineated before, some children go undiagnosed until they present with later-recognized complications, including developmental abnormalities. These include reports of mild intellectual deficits, delayed speech development and especially verbal dyspraxias, and some difficulties in visual perceptions, spatial orientation, and performance of visual-motor tasks. Of note, girls generally have ovarian dysfunction associated with hypogonadism, delayed puberty, and infertility. Importantly, despite treatments with galactose elimination diets, even starting in the first few days of infancy, these complications of ovarian dysfunction (near 100%) and abnormalities in speech-language function (about 70%) are observed. Erythrocyte tests of galactose 1-phosphate levels and galactose-1-phosphate uridyltransferase activities should identify these individuals when they present during the childhood years. More extensive intellectual disability may be due to the medical complications of the infantile illness (i.e., meningitis or hypoglycemic seizures). A number of variants with decreased activity but not absence of this enzyme have been identified, and current studies suggest that most are not associated with these long-term sequelae.

Other variants of galactosemia exist, with deficiencies in either uridine diphosphate galactose 4-epimerase or galactokinase. Both enzymes may be assayed in red blood cell samples. Cataracts are the only major abnormality observed in galactokinase-deficient patients. Complete deficiency of epimerase has been associated in a few patients with symptoms, signs, and outcomes similar to those of classic galactosemia, including impaired psychomotor development. Many more patients, however, exist with forms ascribed to partial deficiency or nonsystemic forms (isolated red blood cell deficiency with normal liver activity). Most of these patients are neurologically normal. At least one patient with red blood cell epimerase deficiency has been described with no systemic signs of illness, including negative urine reducing substances and normal urinary galactitol excretion pattern, who nonetheless demonstrated language delays during the second to third years of life and is now thought to have some autistic features. Development of optimal treatment for severe epimerase-deficient patients is difficult; some dietary galactose is probably necessary because of the nature of the defect, interacting metabolic replacement pathways, and endogenous production of galactose unaffected by diet.

Disorders of Fructose Metabolism

Hereditary fructose intolerance, due to deficiency of aldolase B (fructose-1-phosphate aldolase) in the glycolytic-gluconeogenic pathway, is not usually associated with psychomotor retardation. However, the patient's inability to handle sucrose may produce behavioral abnormalities, especially in school-age children being introduced to fruits or candies. Severe metabolic illness can result from fructose ingestion, with concurrent hypoglycemia and liver and kidney dysfunction. It is a difficult diagnosis to prove, in the past often involving a potentially dangerous intravenous fructose tolerance test and subsequent tissue (liver, renal, intestinal mucosa) enzymatic analysis. However approximately two thirds of the cases have a small number of known genomic mutations, and these alleles are amenable to clinical screening. Fructose-1,6-diphosphatase deficiency is manifested similarly to glycogen storage disease type I, and although multiple metabolic derangements exist (hypoglycemia, lactic acidosis, apparent liver dysfunction), outcomes usually are not associated with developmental abnormalities if diagnosis is made early and the episodes are treated appropriately and aggressively.

Congenital Disorders of Glycosylation

Most patients with congenital disorders of glycosylation (CDG) have psychomotor retardation, and other systems, especially the liver, are affected. Details of clinical disorders are being identified in association with specific deficiencies in the enzymatic steps involved in the addition of sugar moieties to a variety of important intermediates of structural carbohydrates and glycoproteins. A large group involve phosphomannomutase deficiency, CDG type Ia, with infantile hypotonia, abnormal eye movements, eventual psychomotor retardation but no regressions, variable seizures or strokelike episodes, failure-to-thrive with feeding abnormalities, hepatomegaly, later skeletal or heart abnormalities, and varying striking dysmorphic features (including inverted nipples, dimpled skin, or focal sites of lipoatrophy or dystrophy). The appearance of fat pad accumulations, especially near or over the buttocks, in infants should alert clinicians to screen for this disorder. Inverted nipples are associated with this as well as anecdotally with rare cases of several other inborn errors of metabolism (see Table 30-4). Progressive muscle atrophy and weakness may be observed in those who survive to the second decade of life. Several liver function abnormalities (elevated transaminases, low serum albumin, low serum antithrombin III—etiology for strokelike episodes) may be observed, especially in type Ib, and low thyroglobulin (thyroxine-binding globulin) may be observed during evaluations for possible hypothyroidism. Screening tests involve isoelectric focusing of serum transferrin, now widely clinically available. The inherited defect prevents the normal glycosylation of this and other serum proteins, readily observed as underglycosylated forms on electrophoretic analysis.

Most of the developing long list of subtypes of CDG are manifested with psychomotor retardation and may be identified by abnormal glycosylation patterns of transferrin. At least one group, type Ib, is associated with congenital hepatic dysfunction with fibrosis and protein-losing enteropathy but demonstrates normal mental development. This type, however, may be at risk for thrombotic strokes due to a relative hypercoagulability state, and the complications of subclinical or overt strokes may be confused with later developmental delay erroneously thought secondary to the cumulative effects or complications of the associated systemic disease (protein-losing enteropathy, diarrhea, vomiting, failure-to-thrive, villous atrophy). For all of the CDG groups, there are ongoing studies to determine if alternative carbohydrate moiety supplementations, oral or intravenous, will have therapeutic effects. The complications of type Ib have been reported to respond to multiple daily doses of oral D-mannose. The other forms of CDG to date have eluded attempts at treatment. It has been recommended that all patients being evaluated with any form of psychomotor retardation have a serum transferrin isoelectric focusing (often now listed as CDG screen) or similar screen performed.

MITOCHONDRIAL DISORDERS

Many inborn errors of metabolism may be manifested with metabolic acidosis including lactic acidosis as a secondary complication of poor tissue perfusion and cellular dysfunction. One group, however, has been related directly to disorders of pyruvate metabolism (defects in pyruvate dehydrogenase complex or pyruvate carboxylase) and demonstrated elevations of plasma lactate and alanine as a consequence of the conversion of presumed excess intracellular pyruvate. The use of a lactate/pyruvate ratio to help identify these patients became more widespread, but clinical significance could be attached only when the plasma lactic acid was high, and it became clear that sampling artifacts abound. As more patients with chronic lactic acidosis have been identified, several have been ascribed to defects in the mitochondrial electron transport chain. Mutations in the genes encoding these enzymes may reside in either nuclear or mitochondrial DNA. As more of these disorders have been identified, it has become apparent that not all patients have chronic lactic acidosis, many do not have abnormal pyruvate/lactate ratios, and often the only mechanism for laboratory diagnosis is proper handling and assay of muscle biopsy tissue for the enzymes of interest. Some enzymes may be assayed from fibroblast cultures (those of pyruvate metabolism and tricarboxylic acid cycle), but defects of the electron transport system are particularly difficult to demonstrate unless testing is performed in highly specialized laboratories, and even there, tissue-specific difference of expression of electron transport chain enzymes can lead to the need for testing of other tissues. Most important, because there is clinical overlap with many other inborn errors of metabolism (e.g., organic acidurias), comprehensive testing to rule these out first must be performed by the appropriate screening tests. Of note, the lactic acidosis may not be clear from plasma sampling, and CSF studies for lactate, pyruvate, and amino acids are often required for complete screening.

Mitochondrial disorders generally demonstrate multisystem involvement because of the presence of mitochondria in all cells. However, sometimes only single-organ systems appear clinically affected. Signs and symptoms referable to the skeletal and cardiac muscle systems should always be suspect. Children with developmental delay or intellectual disability and hypotonia of unknown etiology in which extensive work-up has ruled out other inborn errors of metabolism and genetic syndrome causes often fall into this category. Other CNS signs may include seizures, ophthalmoplegias, ataxia (which may be intermittent rather than chronic), strokelike episodes, and cranial nerve dysfunction. Blindness with a variety of ophthalmoscopic abnormalities and sensorineural deafness may be present. Other organs may show symptoms manifesting as feeding disorders, intermittent vomiting episodes, failure-to-thrive, severe constipation or chronic abdominal pain, liver or kidney disease, diabetes, thyroid dysfunction, and respiratory dysfunction. Clinical presentations may be of acute severe metabolic illness with severe acidosis, with or without hypoglycemia, and severe CNS depression or a more indolent, chronic type of picture with poor growth and development. One group of these disorders became known as Leigh syndrome (subacute necrotizing encephalomyelopathy), usually demonstrating a progressive encephalopathy with typical brain imaging abnormalities, including multiple symmetric foci of necrosis (spongy degeneration) observed particularly in the basal ganglia, thalamus, and brainstem but also in the cerebellum, spinal cord, and even optic nerve. Often these lesions are not first manifested on computed tomography of the head but require magnetic resonance imaging of the brain and associated studies. Many of these children, perhaps up to 80%, demonstrate the clinical appearance of the disorder by 2 years of age and die within the subsequent 2 years. However, an ever-increasing number of individuals have been identified with all forms of variation of this presentation despite having similar genetic basis of disease. Leigh syndrome is now known to be caused by several different mitochondrial disorders. Similarly, Alpers disease (progressive infantile poliodystrophy) is probably a group of disorders affecting individual mitochondrial enzymatic activities (e.g., pyruvate metabolism, electron transport chain). It often is diagnosed by specific testing after identification of progressive gray matter degeneration and cirrhosis of the liver. Comprehensive family history can be extremely valuable, especially if a pattern of inheritance suggesting maternal transmission of clinical symptoms (mitochondrial inheritance) is evident. Both nuclear and mitochondrial DNA mutations may affect the functioning of these mitochondrial enzymes, and therefore pedigree patterns of autosomal recessive, X-linked, and maternal inheritance have been described.

Because of the varied presentations, a high level of clinical suspicion needs to be maintained, especially in children with all forms of developmental delay associated with either ataxia and dystonic or extrapyramidal cerebral palsy or hypotonia of unknown causes. These are often difficult diagnoses to make, and involvement of a specialist in the field early during the investigation is recommended. Aside from Leigh syndrome, some other more common categories of these disorders include the following: mitochondrial encephalopathy, lactic acidosis, and strokelike episodes (MELAS); myoclonic epilepsy and ragged red fiber (MERRF) disease; chronic progressive external ophthalmoplegia disease (CPEO); neuropathy, ataxia, and retinitis pigmentosa; Kearns-Sayre syndrome (likely to be a subset of adult CPEO with progressive external ophthalmoplegia, ptosis, pigmentary retinopathy, heart block, ataxia, and sensorineural deafness); Pearson syndrome (anemia or pancytopenia, hepatic dysfunction, exocrine pancreatic insufficiency); Leber's hereditary optic neuropathy; and many others. An increasing number of mitochondrial DNA mutations are becoming amenable to screening, but they still represent only a handful of the numerous causes of these diseases. Aside from these described clinical presentations, suspicion may be raised by the following: persistent, or intermittent, elevated plasma lactic acid; elevated CSF lactate, pyruvate, and alanine and other amino acids; elevated tricarboxylic acid intermediates; lactate or 3-methylglutaconic acid on urine organic acid analysis; muscle biopsy demonstrating ragged red fibers (peripheral accumulation of mitochondria); brain magnetic resonance spectroscopy with elevated lactate; or abnormally appearing mitochondria on histologic or electron microscopic examination.

LYSOSOMAL STORAGE DISORDERS

A large number of syndromes are due to inherited defects in the enzymatic activities located in the lysosome, present in cells to provide ongoing turnover of a number of cellular compounds. Groupings of this disorder include the mucopolysaccharidoses (MPS), with abnormal accumulation of glycosaminoglycans; sphingolipidoses, mucolipidoses, and disorders of other lipid-type substances; oligosaccharidoses; and glycogen storage disease (Pompe disease, glycogen storage disease type II, previously described in the text under disorders of carbohydrate metabolism). Clinical features are referable to the sites of abnormal accumulations affecting otherwise normal function or physical structure. Some combination of CNS effects, including developmental delay and intellectual disability but notably regression in milestone achievements, coarse facies, skeletal abnormalities (including the specific radiographic findings of dysostosis multiplex for MPS disorders), corneal and lenticular opacities, variable retinal abnormalities (including cherry-red spot on macula), deafness, hepatosplenomegaly, cardiac valvular disease, dermatologic findings (such as angiokeratomas), macrocephaly, pancytopenia, bone marrow foam cells or lipid-laden macrophages or reticuloepithelial cells in other organs, and other findings help clinically classify the dozens of disorders in this group of inborn errors of metabolism. For example, the mucopolysaccharidoses can be clinically subdivided into the presence or absence of several main clinical features including intellectual disability, corneal clouding, organomegaly, coarse facies, and dysostosis multiplex, but wide clinical variability exists for each of these defining clinical "distinguishing" features (Table 30-7). Most important, all of these types of storage disorders should be considered when developmental regression is indicated on clinical history. Not only CNS but somatic features may variably progress quickly or slowly, with intermittent periods of stability of changing features, after identification of the patient. Enzymatic testing is available for nearly all of the disorders, often through leukocyte preparations easily sent to specialty laboratories. The availability of clinical screening tests for accumulated compounds in urine (glycosaminoglycans, oligosaccharides) offers a place to start with testing for some of these disorders, but these urine tests lack sensitivity and specificity. Of note, MPS III disorders are well known to be variably missed by these urine tests because they may not accumulate massive amounts of the diagnostic metabolites. Specific enzymatic testing should be sought as soon as some clinical defining features (subtle hepatosplenomegaly, dysostosis multiplex) are evident in a child with any form of developmental delay. Consultation with a clinical biochemical geneticist or metabolic disease specialist early in arranging appropriate studies can save time and expense in the laboratory investigation.

The onset of developmental regression in the presence or absence of organomegaly necessitates evaluation for lysosomal storage disorders. The absence of organomegaly may help guide selection of enzymatic assays to be performed—testing first for Tay-Sachs disease (GM_2 gangliosidosis), some forms of Krabbe disease, and metachromatic leukodystrophy compared with other sphingolipidoses with organomegaly presenting similarly (e.g., Niemann-Pick diseases, Gaucher disease, GM_1 gangliosidoses, mucopolysaccharidoses). Coarse facies, especially early, and complaints referable to musculoskeletal joint dysfunction or spinal abnormalities (e.g., gibbus formation) should suggest mucopolysaccharidoses, in which early skeletal studies for dysostosis multiplex, even before overt clinical symptoms, can be extremely helpful (see Table 30-7). Investigation for characteristic ophthalmologic findings (corneal abnormalities, retinitis pigmentosa, optic atrophy, cherry-red macula) is extremely important. Obviously, brain imaging can be extremely helpful, especially if early findings of leukodystrophy are evident (Fig. 30-6; see also Fig. 30-5).

Table 30-7. **Characteristics of Mucopolysaccharidoses**

		Clinical and Laboratory Features†					
Syndrome	**Accumulated Compound***	**Intellectual Disability**	**Organomegaly**	**Corneal Clouding**	**Coarse Facies**	**Dysostosis Multiplex**	**Enzyme Defect**
Hurler (MPS IH)	DS, HS	+	+	+	+	+	α-L-Iduronidase
Scheie (MPS IS)	DS, HS	–	–	+	+/–	+	α-L-Iduronidase
Hurler-Scheie (MPS IHS)	DS, HS	+/–	+	+	+/–	+	α-L-Iduronidase
Hunter (MPS II)	DS, HS	+/–	+	–	+	+	Iduronate sulfatase
Sanfilippo types							
A (MPS IIIA)	HS	+	+/–	–	+/–	+/–	Heparin *N*-sulfatase
B (MPS IIIB)	HS	+	+/–	–	+/–	+/–	α-*N*-Acetylglucosaminidase
C (MPS IIIC)	HS	+	+/–	–	+/–	+/–	Acetyl-CoA: α-D-glucosaminide-*N*-acetyltransferase
D (MPS IIID)	HS	+	+/–	–	+/–	+/–	N-Acetyl-α-D-glucosaminide-6-sulfatase
Morquio types							
A (MPS IVA)	KS	–	–	+/–	–	‡	Galactose-6-sulfatase
B (MPS IVB)	KS	+/–	+/–	+/–	+/–	‡	β-Galactosidase
Maroteaux-Lamy (MPS VI)	DS	–	+	+	+	+	Arylsulfatase B (acetylgalactosamine-4-sulfatase)
Sly (MPS VII)	DS, HS, CS	+	+	+	+	+	β-Glucuronidase
MPS IX	Hyaluronan	+	–	–	–	§	Hyaluronidase

*Accumulated compounds: DS, dermatan sulfate; HS, heparan sulfate; KS, keratan sulfate; CS, chondroitin 4-sulfate and chondroitin-6 sulfate.
†Typically present (+), typically absent (–); variably present (+/–), usually mild if present.
‡Marked generalized skeletal abnormalities are observed in Morquio type A, but they are not dysostosis multiplex.
§Other skeletal findings, especially joints.
Modified primarily from Nyhan WL, Barshop BA, Ozand PT: Atlas of Metabolic Diseases, 2nd ed. New York, Oxford University Press, 2005, p 502.

Table 30-8. **Lysosomal Storage Disorders with Somatic and CNS Involvement**

MPS I, II, III, and VII
Gaucher disease (glucosylceramide β-glucosidase or glucocerebrosidase)
Niemann-Pick disease (sphingomyelinase)
GM_1 gangliosidosis (β-galactosidase)
Farber disease (ceramidase) (nodule formation over joints, vocal cords)
Multiple sulfatase deficiency (arylsulfatases A, B, C) (MPS features with ichthyosis)
Galactosialidosis (β-galactosidase and α-neuraminidase)
Mannosidosis (α- or β-mannosidase)
Fucosidosis (α-fucosidase)
Sialidosis type II (sialidase or α-neuraminidase)
Aspartylglucosaminuria (aspartylglucosaminidase)
Mucolipidoses II (I-cell disease) and III (*N*-acetylglucosaminophosphotransferase)
Niemann-Pick type C—lipid storage disorder (intracellular cholesterol esterification)

Although rare, disorders of sialic acid metabolism (Salla disease) may be indicated by the uncommon finding of U fiber involvement on magnetic resonance imaging that demonstrates diffuse white matter involvement. This rare finding is also observed in two unrelated leukodystrophic disorders, Canavan disease (deficiency of neuronal aspartoacylase activity, described later in text), and L-2-hydroxyglutaric aciduria (previously described).

Some of the lysosomal storage diseases to consider if developmental delay or intellectual disability is associated with somatic tissue involvement (organomegaly, coarse facies, and others) are listed in Table 30-8.

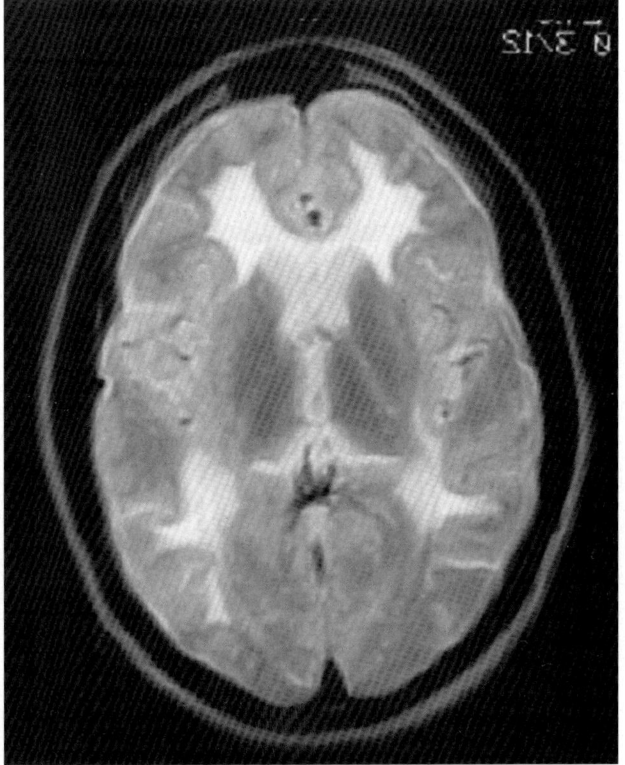

Figure 30-6. Metachromatic leukodystrophy. Magnetic resonance imaging in patient with juvenile metachromatic leukodystrophy demonstrates diffuse areas of demyelination. *(Courtesy of S. Naidu, MD.)*

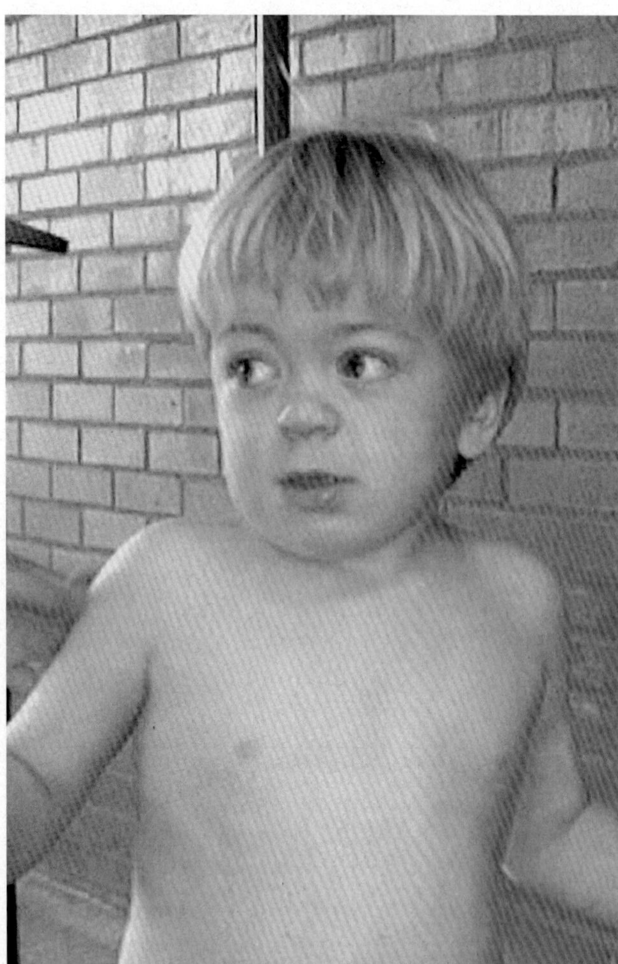

Figure 30-7. Hunter syndrome (MPS II). This child with very mild facial features was identified early by organomegaly and gibbus formation.

Table 30-9. Initial Presentations Primarily of CNS Disease in Lysosomal Storage Disorders

MPS III
GM2 gangliosidosis (Tay-Sachs and Sandhoff diseases) (hexosaminidase A or B)
Krabbe disease (β-galactocerebrosidase)
Metachromatic leukodystrophy (arylsulfatase A)
Sialidosis type I (α-neuraminidase)
Schindler disease (α-*N*-acetylgalactosaminidase)
Neuronal ceroid lipofuscinosis (multiple types, most with retinal dysfunction)
Gaucher disease type III (glucocerebrosidase) (may have early horizontal gaze palsy)

In contrast, initial presentations primarily of CNS disease (without organomegaly) are listed in Table 30-9.

Several lysosomal sphingolipidoses and lipid storage disorders do not appear to be associated with CNS abnormalities, including the most common presentation of Gaucher disease, type I (glucocerebrosidase deficiency), which is usually associated with organomegaly and bone marrow involvement; Fabry disease (α-galactosidase A deficiency), an X-linked disorder that may be manifested with painful acroparesthesias or hypohidrosis in childhood, corneal whirl pattern, angiokeratomas, and eventual vascular disease (leading to ischemia and infarction) affecting the kidney, heart, and brain in adulthood; Wolman disease (lysosomal acid lipase deficiency) with hepatosplenomegaly, calcification of the adrenal glands, infantile vomiting and diarrhea or steatorrhea, abdominal distention, and severe failure-to-thrive; cholesterol ester storage disorder (also lysosomal lipase deficiency), a milder disorder in childhood but with hepatosplenomegaly, hypercholesterolemia, and liver dysfunction in adulthood; and several mucopolysaccharidoses (see Table 30-7), including some forms of MPS I (α-L-iduronidase deficiency but residual activity, Scheie syndrome), MPS IV (Morquio A syndrome, *N*-acetylgalactosamine-6-sulfatase deficiency; and Morquio B syndrome, β-galactosidase deficiency), and MPS VI (Maroteaux-Lamy syndrome, *N*-acetylgalactosamine-4-sulfatase deficiency).

Of importance to keep in mind during initial evaluation of developmental or behavioral disorders is that all of these disorders may have variable expressions with respect to timing and severity of classically described findings. Any male child with developmental delays with even hints of organomegaly or coarse features should be considered for testing for Hunter syndrome (X-linked MPS II) (Fig. 30-7; see also Fig. 30-1). Behavioral features may suggest testing not only for MPS II but also for MPS III (Sanfilippo syndromes, especially type B) (Fig. 30-8; see also Fig. 30-7). Early gibbus formation or other skeletal abnormality (especially dysostosis multiplex) or even associated symptoms of apparent "stiff joints" should lead to consideration of testing for these as well as for MPS I (Scheie, Hurler-Scheie variants) (Fig. 30-9). Urinary glycosaminoglycan analysis may be obtained through spot tests, which are quick but have suffered from both false-positives and false-negatives. It is often a good initial screening test, but under specific clinical circumstances, it may be prudent to advance directly to enzyme testing for MPS I, II, or IIIB. Because dysostosis multiplex may be seen in other forms of lysosomal storage disorders, urine testing for oligosaccharides as well as for mucopolysaccharides adds a broader differential to initial testing. Recent advances in enzyme replacement therapy for some of the mucopolysaccharidoses and sphingolipidoses support the earlier use of diagnostic tests for the work-up of these potentially treatable disorders.

OTHER DISORDERS TO CONSIDER

Canavan Disease

This disorder is due to the absence of aspartoacylase activity, resulting in urinary excretion of *N*-acetylaspartic acid, now available as a screening test for the disorder (request specifically as part of urine organic acid analysis). Although infants appear normal at birth, hypotonia and developing macrocephaly are usually apparent within a few months, with worsening rather than maturing neurologic functions. Imaging studies of the brain demonstrate diffuse symmetric white matter

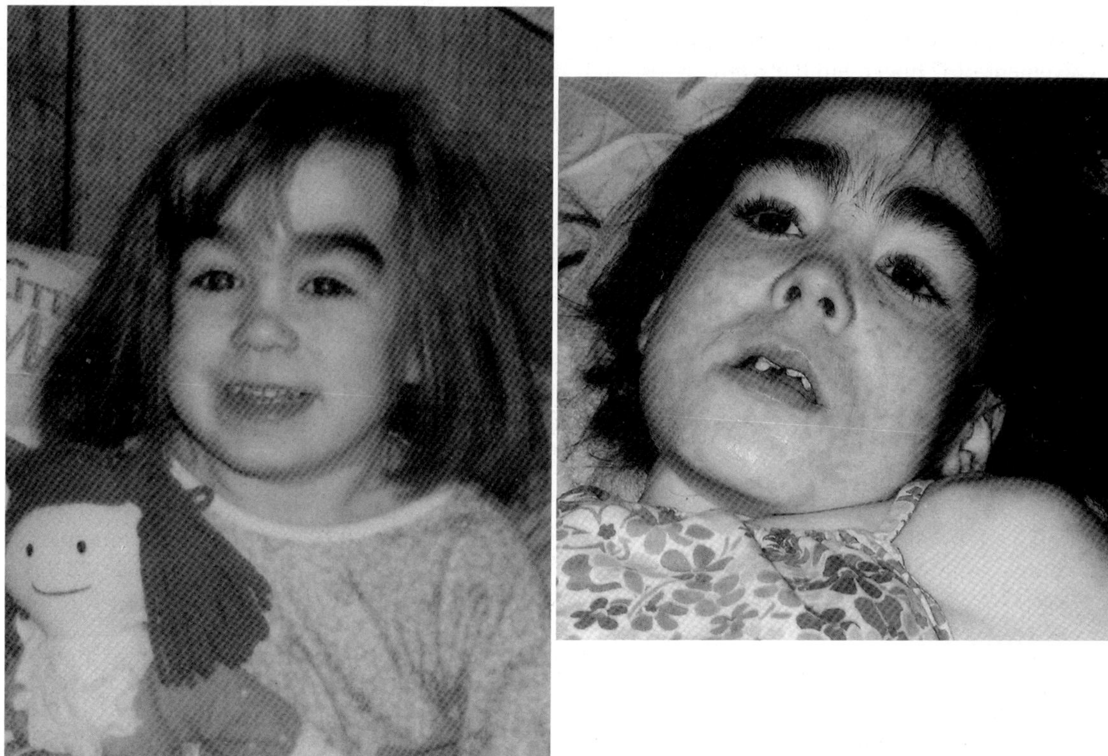

Figure 30-8. **Sanfilippo B (MPS IIIB).** The patient always had prominent eyebrows, thought initially to be more a familial trait. She was evaluated for developmental delay at 3 years of age, presenting with mild hepatomegaly *(left)*. The somewhat more evident facial coarsening developed only at a much later age, when frank hepatomegaly and dysostosis multiplex were apparent *(right)*.

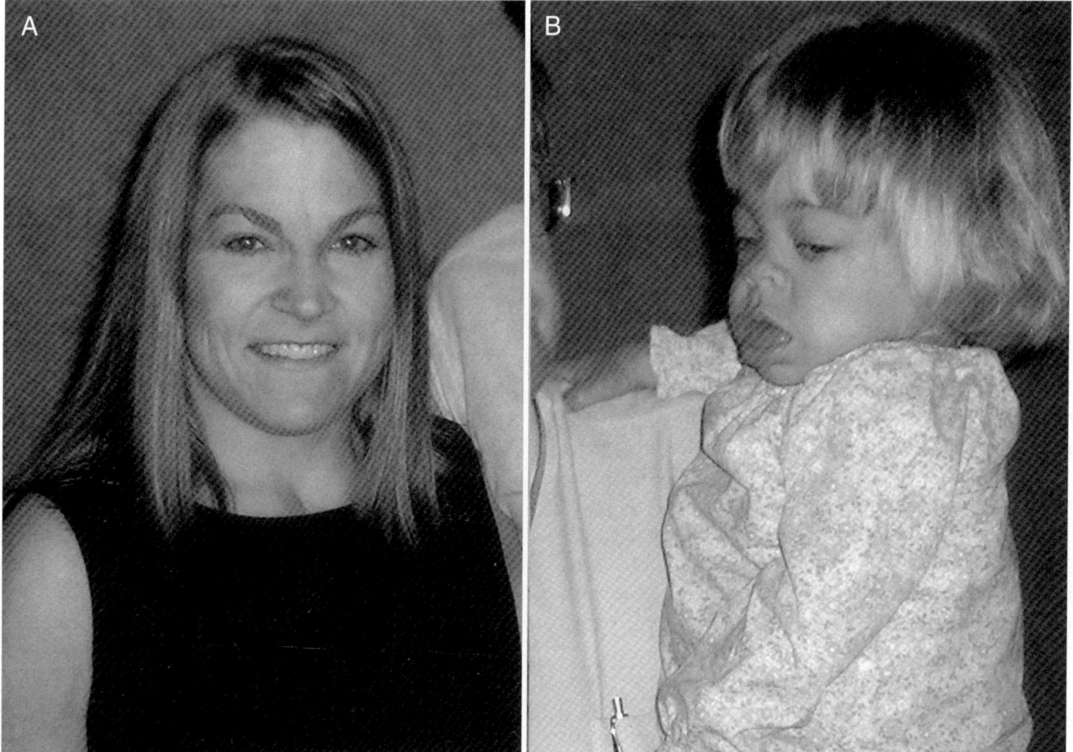

Figure 30-9. **Two forms of MPS I: α-iduronidase deficiency. A,** An adult woman with Hurler-Scheie or Scheie variant α-iduronidase deficiency. No evident dysmorphism with no apparent effect on CNS functioning until adulthood; she was initially evaluated as a child for joint stiffness limiting movements. **B,** Classic Hurler disease. Note marked facial coarsening and extremity contractures at 3 years of age. The patient was initially evaluated for gibbus deformity.

changes resembling classic lysosomal storage disease leukodystrophies, but with the less common observation of involvement of U fibers. Similar to the lysosomal storage disorders, there are both infantile and juvenile presentations, and computed tomography or magnetic resonance imaging changes may not be observed in all cases at the time of initial evaluation. Its symptoms and signs may be very aggressive after birth or more gradual, demonstrating a regressive pattern. Similar to Tay-Sachs disease, Canavan disease is most common among those of Ashkenazi Jewish descent, but it may be observed in all ethnicities. Rather than macular cherry-red spot, ophthalmologic examination may reveal signs of optic atrophy and retinal pigmentation.

Smith-Lemli-Opitz Syndrome

An autosomal recessive disorder of cholesterol metabolism, Smith-Lemli-Opitz syndrome may be suspected in children with overt dysmorphic features and multiple congenital anomalies in which screening cholesterol levels are low (see Fig. 30-3). However, because the serum cholesterol level may be in the normal range, measurement of the more specific plasma level of its precursor, 7-dehydrocholesterol, is indicated for consideration of this disorder. This is performed by ordering laboratory testing for plasma sterols by gas chromatography–mass spectrometry, which will identify patterns suggesting not only Smith-Lemli-Opitz syndrome but also other disorders of cholesterol metabolism (desmosterolosis, lathosterolosis).

The dysmorphic and somatic features of Smith-Lemli-Opitz syndrome are often striking and may include microcephaly, narrow forehead, ptosis, ophthalmologic findings including cataracts, abnormally positioned ears, broad anteverted nares, micrognathia with varied palatal defects (high arched palate, cleft uvula, abnormal alveolar ridges), syndactyly (especially digits 2 and 3 of the lower extremities), postaxial polydactyly of either upper or lower extremities and other limb anomalies, varied cardiac and genitourinary abnormalities (ambiguous genitalia, male-female sex reversal, cryptorchidism, inguinal hernia, renal cysts), increased frequency of gastrointestinal anomalies (pyloric stenosis, gastroesophageal reflux disease, Hirschsprung disease, malrotation), adrenal abnormalities (both glucocorticoid and mineralocorticoid deficiencies), and multiple others at varying frequency. Intellectual disability is the norm among survivors. A variety of imaging abnormalities of the brain have been observed, and any patient with findings consistent with holoprosencephaly sequence should be tested for this disorder. Mutations in the gene encoding 7-dehydrocholesterol reductase have been identified. This syndrome has variable clinical expression, ranging from prenatal and neonatal deaths to subclinical cases identified in family members of a propositus.

Current therapeutic approaches include supplementation of diets with cholesterol and rarely bile salts, with modest results. Behavioral abnormalities with autistic features may be present in patients with Smith-Lemli-Opitz syndrome, who may have mild to severe dysmorphic and somatic features. Of note is that these autistic behavioral abnormalities may be ameliorated with supplemental cholesterol in some patients. For that reason, even patients with no obvious or only mild dysmorphic features but with autistic behavioral features should be screened for errors in cholesterol metabolism.

SUMMARY

Evaluation of developmental delay is usually both a process of recognizing distinct clues for laboratory testing and a process of elimination of a wide range of metabolic disorders with overlapping features and extensive variations in presentations. Table 30-1 lists findings suggestive of inborn errors of metabolism. Tables 30-2 and 30-4 may be useful guides for work-up considerations. An excellent summary table is described in Cleary and Green (2005).

From the history, decide which children have had what might be considered intermittent acute neurologic or metabolic collapses by presentations to hospitals—many organic acidemias (amino acid and organic acid disorders), fatty acid oxidation and mitochondrial disorders, and urea cycle defects may be manifested this way. Check plasma amino acid, ammonia, and lactate concentrations and urine organic acid levels and consider others from Table 30-2.

Hypotonia and weakness are present in innumerable conditions. However, remember to check creatine kinase, lactate, plasma amino acid, and urine organic acid levels and to request acylcarnitine profile and possibly carnitine studies as part of the initial screens.

Multisystem disorders to keep in mind are Smith-Lemli-Opitz syndrome (plasma sterol testing), peroxisomal disorders (very-long-chain fatty acids), congenital disorders of glycosylation (transferrin isoform studies), and mitochondrial disorders.

With more severe neurologic states (i.e., severe seizures, associated deafness and eye findings), consider peroxisomal disorders (plasma very-long-chain fatty acids), mitochondrial disorders (lactate and pyruvate, urine organic acids), serum ceruloplasmin (Menkes syndrome) and uric acid (low in molybdenum cofactor and sulfite oxidase defects; high in Lesch-Nyhan defect [self-mutilation]) determinations, CSF studies (lactate, pyruvate, amino acids, neurotransmitters), and magnetic resonance spectroscopy.

Any organomegaly, facial coarseness, and joint or spine abnormalities (i.e., gibbus deformation), even slight, should suggest screening for mucopolysaccharidoses. In a male patient, consider the X-linked Hunter syndrome enzymatic testing directly.

Abnormal behavior, acting out, difficulties at night with sleep, and the like should lead one to consider enzyme testing for: MPS III (Sanfilippo B syndrome), if the child is male, test for MPS II (Hunter syndrome), succinic semialdehyde dehydrogenase deficiency (urine organic acids), partial urea cycle defects (plasma amino acids, ammonia, and urine for orotic acid), later onset metachromatic leukodystrophy (arylsulfatase A), and X-linked adrenoleukodystrophy (very-long-chain fatty acids). Consider also screens for creatine disorders (urine and magnetic resonance spectroscopy) and homocystinuria (cofactor forms).

With macrocephaly, check head imaging results for leukodystrophic changes or subdural effusions (e.g., prefrontal hygromas) and consider glutaric aciduria type I (urine organic acids or acylcarnitine profile), Canavan disease (urine *N*-acetylaspartate), and various sphingolipidoses and mucopolysaccharidoses (individual white blood cell enzymatic tests).

Consider plasma sterol testing in children with 2,3 syndactyly of toes, especially with hypotonia, dysmorphic facies, or other congenital anomalies (Smith-Lemli-Opitz syndrome).

With facial dysmorphism, not only Smith-Lemli-Opitz syndrome (plasma sterols) but peroxisomal disorders (plasma very-long-chain fatty acids), congenital disorders of glycosylation (plasma transferrin isoforms), and storage disorders (mucopolysaccharidosis screens and enzymatic testing) should be considered.

Any odd urine odor or persistent or intermittent metabolic acidosis should be checked with urine organic acid analysis.

The evaluation of patients with autism spectrum disorders for inborn errors of metabolism remains loosely defined, with only occasional individual diagnoses made. Some groups of disorders to keep in mind after initial first-tier studies have been performed include those of cholesterol metabolism (Smith-Lemli-Opitz syndrome), purine and pyrimidine metabolism, sulfation defects, gamma-aminobutyric acid metabolism (succinic semialdehyde dehydrogenase), and creatine metabolism.

Several texts have very helpful tables listing clinical associations with inborn errors of metabolism, including those of Nyhan, Barshop, and Ozand (2005), Hoffman and colleagues (2002), Fernandes, Saudubray, and van den Berghe (2000), and Gilbert-Barness and Barness (2000). Some of the information from these and other sources is presented in Table 30-4.

REFERENCES

Clarke JTR: A Clinical Guide to Inherited Metabolic Diseases. New York, Cambridge University Press, 1996.

Cleary MA, Green A: Developmental delay: When to suspect and how to investigate for an inborn error of metabolism. Arch Dis Child 90:1128-1132, 2005.

Fernandes J, Saudubray JM, van den Berghe G: Inborn Metabolic Diseases: Diagnosis and Treatment, 3rd ed. New York, Springer-Verlag, 2000.

Gilbert-Barness E, Barness L: Metabolic Diseases: Foundations of Clinical Management, Genetics, and Pathology. Natick, MA, Eaton Publishing, 2000.

Hoffmann GF, Nyhan WL, Zschocke J, et al: Inherited Metabolic Diseases. Philadelphia, Lippincott Williams & Wilkins, 2002.

Leonard JV, Morris AAM: Diagnosis and early management of inborn errors of metabolism presenting around the time of birth. Acta Paediatr 95:6-14, 2006.

Moeschler JB, Shevell M; American Academy of Pediatrics Committee on Genetics: Clinical genetic evaluation of the child with mental retardation or developmental delays. Pediatrics 117:2304-2316, 2006.

Nyhan WL, Barshop BA, Ozand PT: Atlas of Metabolic Diseases. 2nd ed. New York, Oxford University Press, 2005.

Schaefer GB, Lutz RE: Diagnostic yield in the clinical genetic evaluation of autism spectrum disorders. Genet Med 8:549-556, 2006.

Scriver CR, Beaudet AL, Sly WS, Valle D (eds): The Metabolic and Molecular Bases of Inherited Disease, 8th ed. New York, McGraw-Hill, 2001.

Smith W, Kishnani PS, Lee B, et al: Urea cycle disorders: Clinical presentation outside the newborn period. Crit Care Clin 21:S9-S17, 2005.

Wappner RA, Hainline BE: Introduction to inborn errors of metabolism. *In* McMillan JA (ed. in chief): Oski's Pediatrics: Principles and Practice, 4th ed. Philadelphia, Lippincott Williams and Wilkins, 2006, pp. 2145-2150.

Winter SC, Buist NRM: Clinical treatment guide to inborn errors of metabolism 1998. J Rare Dis 4:18-46, 1998.

31 TOXINS

Fred M. Henretig

Theories and practical advice on child development rightly point to the importance of the environment, but usually only to the psychosocial part. Not to be forgotten are the various elements of the physical or nonhuman surroundings: natural conditions and disasters, housing, diet, medicines, and physical dangers such as toxins in the air, water, food, and elsewhere. This chapter reviews the hazards for development and behavior of prenatal toxins such as alcohol, breast milk contaminants such as cocaine, and postnatal environmental toxic exposures, especially lead, mercury, polychlorinated biphenyls, and pesaticides.

The causes of most developmental disorders, including attention deficit disorder and autism, are poorly understood, but exposures to a number of environmental toxins have been suggested by both epidemiologic and experimental evidence. The most concerning of these agents are lead, mercury, polychlorinated biphenyls, and pesticides. In July 2000, an expert committee of the U.S. National Academy of Sciences concluded that 3% of all childhood developmental disorders in America are the direct consequence of toxic environmental exposures and that an additional 25% are likely to be the result of an interaction between such exposure and individual susceptibility (National Academy of Sciences, 2000).

This chapter reviews toxic influences on the central nervous system (CNS) with special reference to those environmental toxins that are significant, direct causes of functional brain damage in children. Many severe intoxications are capable of causing impaired or inadequate substrate delivery to the brain, for example, secondary to profound respiratory depression with consequent hypoxia (e.g., alcohols, barbiturates, opioids, other sedative-hypnotics), circulatory failure and shock (calcium channel antagonists, beta-adrenergic blockers), hypoglycemia (ethanol, sulfonylureas), or status epilepticus (lead, tricyclic antidepressants, camphor, isoniazid), with resulting neurologic sequelae. In addition, innumerable specific neurotoxins have been described in the toxicology and neurology literature; the focus here is on prenatal and postnatal exposure to those drugs and environmental pollutants with specific pathologic and epidemiologic predilection for cognitive or behavioral effects in young children. Additional discussions of potentially toxic influences on development and behavior are contained elsewhere in this text in the chapters concerning prenatal health, diet and nutrition, and adolescent substance abuse.

GENERAL PRINCIPLES OF PEDIATRIC NEUROLOGIC TOXICITY

The interaction between various exogenous toxins and the CNS is predictably complex. This is particularly true when the prolonged developmental sequence for brain architecture and function is considered. The neurotoxic effects of exposure to a particular xenobiotic may vary greatly, depending on total dose, acuity, and timing of exposure. These principles may be better conceptualized after a brief review of human neurovascular and brain ontogeny.

The CNS tends to be protected from some toxic influences by the blood-brain barrier. Highly polar compounds tend to be excluded, whereas lipid-soluble, nonpolar compounds tend to cross the barrier easily. The integrity of the barrier varies with age, and the immature brain allows many more substances through. Thus, inorganic lead poisoning can cause severe encephalopathy in young children but primarily a peripheral neuropathy in adults. The anatomic substrate of the blood-brain barrier is not yet fully understood, but three major concepts include (1) the function of glial cells wrapped around capillary endothelium, (2) the unique properties of the capillary endothelium of the brain, particularly the finding of zonulae occludentes, or structures joining the endothelial cells together into tight junctions, and (3) the extracellular basement membrane between endothelial cells and glia and neurons.

Not all areas of the brain are equally affected by a given toxin, even when it does cross the blood-brain barrier. Variation can result from different vascular patterns and unique sensitivities of different cell types caused by differing neurochemistry. Thus, a considerable degree of selectivity occurs in the neuropathologic effects of any given potential neurotoxin.

An additional consideration is the rapid prenatal and postnatal developmental changes in brain structure, which may be adversely influenced by toxins. The development of the brain begins as early as 3 weeks of gestation, when the neural plate is formed from the ectoderm. The neural plate then undergoes axial fusion, developing into the neural tube, with closure occurring by simultaneous cranial and caudal progression. After neurulation, subsequent sequential developments are neuronal proliferation, migration, differentiation, synaptogenesis, apoptosis, and myelination. These begin after the gestational age of 28 days and continue into postnatal life, with active glial and synapse evolution until about 3 years of age. All of these processes may be affected by environmental toxic exposures (Mendola et al, 2002; Schmid and Rotenberg, 2005). At birth, all large neuronal cell bodies are in place in the cerebral cortex and basal ganglia. However, synaptic connections are relatively sparse. During the first 2 years of life, there is tremendous growth of these connections, such that by the age of 2 years, synaptic density is almost twice that of adulthood. During the next few preschool-age years, these synapses are "pruned" selectively, presumably on the basis of sensory and motor stimulation. This process may be altered in the presence of even subtle toxic influences that affect neurotransmitter function as well as more overt neuronal damage from global insults such as hypoxia and hypoglycemia. Alteration of dendritic architecture may result in difficulties with fine neurocognitive function, such as memory, attention, and problem solving skills. Such a paradigm has been invoked, with experimental evidence in animal models, for the effects of low-level lead toxicity on intellectual function (Goldstein, 1992).

Unique Pediatric Vulnerabilities to Environmental Toxins

Children may be relatively more vulnerable to many toxic agents than adults are for several reasons beyond the prolonged neurologic developmental sequence, including greater relative exposure, immature metabolism, and longer lifespan for chronic toxic effects, including carcinogenesis, to be manifested. They have higher body surface to mass ratios, higher metabolic rates, and higher minute ventilation for body size than adults do. Thus, for an inhalational exposure, they are breathing more toxin per kilogram of body weight per minute than an adult counterpart exposed to the same degree of air contamination (i.e., a higher dose). They "live closer to the ground," with many toxins being heavier than air and thus more concentrated in a child's breathing zone than would be the case for an adult. For ingested toxins, through food or water, the same body size and metabolic considerations mean that children will ingest relatively higher doses of toxin from contaminated food or water. Children also tend to have more hand-to-mouth activity than adults do, so if their hands become contaminated, the risk of toxin ingestion also increases proportionally. Children have immature metabolic pathways, especially in early infancy. This might mitigate, or exacerbate, certain toxic exposures. For example, some environmental toxic compounds, such as polyaromatic hydrocarbons, are believed to require activation by pathways that are undeveloped in infancy (Landrigan and Garg, 2002), and so infants with this exposure may suffer less adverse consequence than an older child or adult with a comparable exposure. On the other hand, some toxins are detoxified by intact metabolic pathways (e.g., organophosphate pesticides) and thus may be relatively more toxic to young children. Last, many toxic effects require years or decades to become manifested fully. This is particularly true for suspected carcinogens and agents linked to neurodegenerative diseases.

Specific Hazards in the Prenatal and Perinatal Periods

Many drugs and toxins (e.g., alcohol) exert overt adverse effects on the developing structure and function of the CNS with high-dose exposure in utero. Many such agents at lower doses may cause milder effects on postnatal cognitive function without overt structural abnormality (e.g., fetal alcohol effects), and comparable subtle effects may result from maternal exposure to several other substances. Additional perinatal concerns related to drug toxicity include the effects of maternal medications used during parturition and lactation and of those given directly to the newborn (Fine, 2006). Another important mechanism by which prenatal toxicity can have an impact on postnatal behavior is passive addiction of the fetus to drugs used by the mother.

PRENATAL TOXIC EXPOSURE AND IMPACT ON POSTNATAL COGNITION AND BEHAVIOR

Prenatal Exposures

The impact of a given prenatal drug or toxin exposure on the subsequent postnatal health of the exposed child is a complex process. An important distinction is the clinical severity of the exposure on the mother and its chronicity. Acute toxic overdoses in pregnancy are uncommon but do occur, often as a result of depression related to the woman's having become pregnant or in the desire to abort. The consequences of a single overdose of most agents on the fetus is usually related to the impact on maternal cardiorespiratory and metabolic status, and if the pregnant woman remains stable from these standpoints, the fetus is not commonly adversely affected.

Chronic exposures to certain therapeutic agents, drugs of abuse, and environmental toxins, however, are more regularly associated with recognizable teratogenic and neurocognitive postnatal effects on the fetus. Teratogenicity implies that a subtoxic or therapeutic exposure in the mother may cause structural or functional abnormalities in the fetus. Numerous teratogens are now known or suspected; among the more important are androgens and progestins, several anticonvulsants (carbamazepine, phenytoin, valproic acid), antineoplastic agents (cyclophosphamide, chlorambucil, methotrexate), coumadin, ethanol, iodine, lead, methylmercury, polychlorinated biphenyls, ionizing radiation, retinoids, nicotine (smoking), tetracycline, thalidomide, and trimethoprim.

Substance abuse during pregnancy constitutes an important and unfortunately common form of chronic prenatal toxin exposure. The consequence of prenatal substance abuse on the subsequent behavior and development of the exposed child during infancy and childhood is a complex process that involves considerable overlap of prenatal and postnatal influences (Fine, 2006). Many mothers who are chemically dependent, for example, are also of low socioeconomic status, are malnourished, use multiple agents including alcohol and cigarettes, have underlying medical problems (some of which may be secondary to their substance abuse), and may suffer significant emotional disorders and social problems. All these factors may independently have an impact on prenatal CNS microstructure and function as well as on the subsequent postnatal maternal-child interaction and therefore complicate the interpretation of the specific effect of the individual substance, if any, on postnatal behavior and cognition. It is difficult to control for all such factors in clinical studies; in addition, these studies tend to rely on interviewer or questionnaire ascertainment of exposure, which may not be accurate. Such factors may account in part for the disparities noted between studies on the incidence of significant adverse effects on children born to mothers who admit to recreational use of drugs such as alcohol, cocaine, opiates, and marijuana. Although in comparison to controls, there may be a statistically significant increase in the observed rate of the studied adverse effect (e.g., congenital anomalies) or lower average performance scores on standardized testing (e.g., intelligence, behavioral effects), many exposed children will appear to have outcome measures similar to those in the control group. However, very subtle manifestations may have occurred in exposed children yet are difficult to detect and to quantify. Animal studies are more readily controlled than human epidemiologic research but less useful for observing subtle alterations in behavior and development; even these, as well as in vitro studies, are subject to confounding factors secondary to the occurrence of undernutrition or absence of specific nutritional factors, such as vitamins, that might attenuate the effect of putative toxins in vivo.

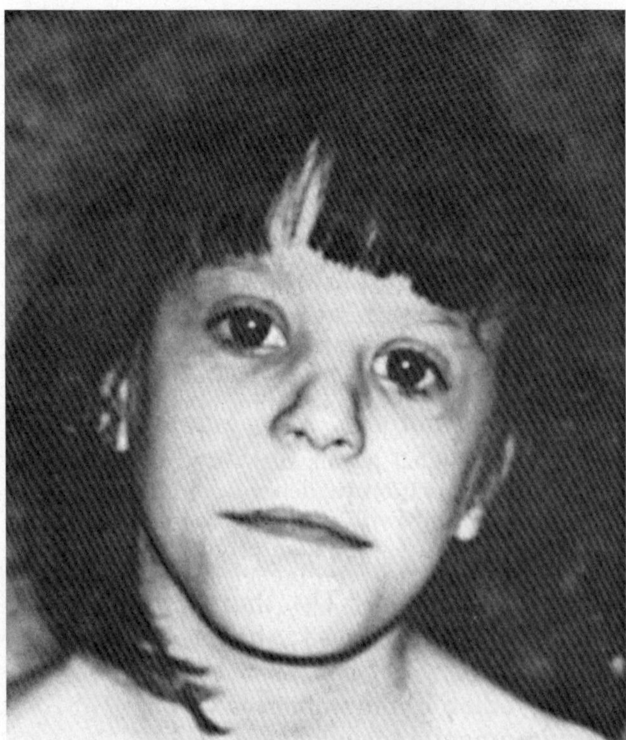

Figure 31-1. Fetal alcohol syndrome. This 8-year-old girl was born to a chronically alcoholic woman. She is mildly retarded and growth deficient with facial features typical of fetal alcohol syndrome (short palpebral fissures, flat nasal bridge with epicanthal folds, long smooth philtrum with thin upper lip). *(From Graham JM Jr: Manual for the Assessment of Fetal Alcohol Effects. Seattle, University of Washington Press, 1982.)*

Alcohol

Chronic, heavy alcohol consumption during pregnancy may result in a constellation of congenital anomalies termed the fetal alcohol syndrome (Stratton et al, 1996). Alcohol's toxic effects are likely due to several mechanisms, including interference with neuronal migration, impaired development and function of neurotransmitter receptors, and actual neuronal necrosis (apoptosis). Major features of fetal alcohol syndrome include intrauterine growth restriction, intellectual disability, and facial dysmorphogenesis (microcephaly, short palpebral fissures, epicanthal folds, maxillary hypoplasia, cleft palate, hypoplastic philtrum, and micrognathia; Fig. 31-1). Fetal alcohol syndrome is usually associated with the consumption of 2 to 3 ounces of ethanol per day (e.g., four to six standard "drinks" of hard liquor or its equivalent) or binge drinking (five or more drinks on one occasion). It is estimated that 4% of women who drink to this degree during pregnancy will give birth to children with fetal alcohol syndrome (Fine, 2006).

In the absence of frank growth retardation or congenital anomalies (e.g., fetal alcohol syndrome), several studies have found children born to women who drink heavily during pregnancy at increased risk for developmental deficits (American Academy of Pediatrics, 1993). Various terms have been applied to these milder syndromes of fetal alcohol effects, including partial fetal alcohol syndrome and alcohol-related neurodevelopmental disorder (Mendola et al, 2002; Stratton et al, 1996). These have included milder anomalies and attention-deficit/hyperactivity disorder, fine motor impairment, clumsiness, and subtle speech disorders. The spectrum of disorder probably represents the degree of ethanol exposure and its timing, with the full fetal alcohol syndrome representing teratogenic effects resulting from exposure that was heavier and earlier in pregnancy. It has been difficult to define a precise threshold for toxicity because of the many confounding factors already mentioned. In addition, alcohol consumption has often been characterized as average number of drinks per day, without always distinguishing binge drinking (which is more likely to result in higher blood alcohol levels) from daily "social drinking" (e.g., a glass of wine with dinner, which is less likely to result in toxic blood levels). Current dogma proscribing any ingestion of alcohol during pregnancy may be counterproductive, raising unnecessary guilt in otherwise healthy mothers who drink sparingly, and fails to focus on the real problem of chronic alcoholism with its attendant comorbidity on the fetus produced by malnutrition, smoking, medical illness, and so on. Nevertheless, the American Academy of Pediatrics (1993) recommends that pregnant women and those planning a pregnancy should abstain from alcohol entirely.

Cigarettes

Cigarette smoke contains the toxins nicotine and carbon monoxide as well as numerous other potentially toxic compounds (e.g., aromatic hydrocarbons). Prenatal exposure to cigarette smoking is believed to result in decreased birth weight, probably because of the vasoconstrictive effect of nicotine on uterine blood flow, and the effect of carbon monoxide on decreasing fetal hemoglobin oxygen-carrying capacity (Byrd and Howard, 1995). Other effects may result from additional toxins, decreased maternal calorie intake, or both. Postnatal effects on behavior and development ascribed to prenatal cigarette exposure include cognitive deficits, decreased attention span, hyperactivity, and increased aggression. Maternal cigarette smoking has been specifically associated with several measures of impaired cognition, after control for several covariates in a low-risk population, including impaired visuospatial function, lower language and reading scores, and reduced overall intelligence (Mendola et al, 2002).

Cocaine

Maternal cocaine use is highly related to numerous catastrophic complications of gestation and the perinatal period (Volpe, 1992). Major CNS anomalies, intracranial hemorrhages, abruptio placentae, and decreased birth weight and head circumference are seen, presumably secondary to the peripheral vasoconstrictive and central monoaminergic effects of this potent drug. Less drastic postnatal effects have also been observed in infants with prenatal exposure. In the neonatal period, some such infants have increased tremulousness, poor feeding, irritability, abnormal sleep pattern, and, occasionally, seizures. Older cocaine-exposed infants do not regularly exhibit persistent cognitive deficits on standard tests (e.g., Bayley Scales of Infant Development) in comparison to appropriate control infants. However, there is some evidence for the association of prenatal cocaine exposure with deficits in fine and gross motor development and negative impact on school-age behaviors (Bada et al, 2007; Mendola et al, 2002).

Marijuana

In general, light to moderate use of marijuana during pregnancy has not been clearly associated with subsequent cognitive deficits. One study found an exposure of one or more "joints" per day, but not lesser use, during the third trimester of pregnancy to be associated with a 10-point deficit on Bayley Scales of Infant Development at the age of 9 months. This effect was no longer apparent at 19 months of age (Richardson et al, 1995). Other evidence has suggested some deficits in executive functions, including visuospatial analysis and attention, despite the absence of significant changes in IQ (Mendola et al, 2002).

Opiates

The most profound effect of prenatal opiate exposure is the neonatal withdrawal syndrome (see the section on neonatal withdrawal syndrome). Long-term studies of cognitive function in older children born to heroin-addicted or methadone-maintained mothers are inconsistent in their findings. Postnatal environmental influences seem to be important in the intellectual outcome. For example, heroin-exposed children tend to show cognitive deficits, whereas children born to mothers provided comprehensive prenatal care in a methadone maintenance clinic do not. Similar differences are noted in comparing infants born to heroin-addicted mothers who are subsequently raised at home with their birth parents versus those who are adopted (Ornoy, 2003). However, some deficits in attention and behavioral issues remained, even in the adopted children.

Polychlorinated Biphenyls

Polychlorinated biphenyls (PCBs) and related compounds (polychlorinated dibenzofurans and polychlorinated dibenzodioxins, or dioxins) are a large group of chemicals that were used widely in industry from the 1930s to 1970s as insulators and lubricants in electrical equipment. They have been banned in the United States and most Western countries since the 1970s, but they have persisted in the environment, particularly as oils that pollute water supplies, which are then consumed by aquatic organisms and become concentrated increasingly in animal tissue as they progress up the food chain. Being fat-soluble chemicals, they tend to occur in greatest concentration in beef, dairy products, and fish that are relatively high in fat (Schmid and Rotenberg, 2005).

The adverse effects of PCBs were first recognized after high-dose prenatal exposures resulted in epidemics of severe toxicity, in this case occurring in Japan in 1968 and Taiwan in 1979 from contaminated cooking oil. Children exposed in utero were noted to have a variety of developmental defects, including reduced birth weight, deformed nails, gingival hypertrophy, and subsequent IQ deficits bordering on intellectual disability. Later studies found that more subtle but pervasive effects were associated in childhood with prenatal PCB exposure at background exposure levels in populations from Michigan, North Carolina, and Europe. These included memory and attention deficits, decreased verbal abilities, and adverse behavioral and emotional effects. Elevated maternal PCB levels are associated with decreased maternal thyroid function, which may in part explain the associated negative effects of PCBs on infant neurocognitive development (Stein et al, 2002).

Obstetric Anesthesia

A number of drugs are considered for administration to women during labor, including analgesics, anxiolytics, and labor-inducing and, conversely, tocolytic agents. Many of these are associated with potential neonatal behavioral effects (Hoyer, 2002).

A popular drug for maternal analgesia during labor has been meperidine. However, the slow placental transfer and subsequent metabolism of this compound by the fetus allow considerable accumulation. Thus, infants born between 1 and 4 hours after meperidine administration to the mother are likely to experience significant CNS depression. This eventuality can be managed with supportive care and naloxone, 0.01 to 0.1 mg/kg, administered intramuscularly or intravenously (start with 0.01 mg/kg; if no effect, use 0.1 mg/kg).

Both systemic analgesics and regional anesthetic agents have also been shown to have significant effects on newborn behavior. Decreased motor maturity and increased irritability have been noted at 3 days of age after regional anesthesia alone. Systemic agents have been found to affect some variables such as habituation and orientation on the Brazelton Neonatal Behavioral Assessment Scale throughout the first month of life. These effects may represent increased pharmacologic action resulting from immaturity of the neonatal blood-brain barrier or metabolic pathways, or both, or they may represent a contribution from interference with normal maternal-infant bonding caused by the combined effects on mother and infant. Anxiolytic agents such as lorazepam may contribute to a "floppy infant syndrome," which fortunately resolves spontaneously without recognized sequelae.

Oxytocin is used to induce or to augment labor. Its use is rarely associated with uterine tetany and resultant compromised placental blood flow with consequent fetal distress. Tocolytic agents such as magnesium may result in depressed infantile neurologic function and reflexes.

Neonatal Withdrawal Syndrome

A large number of drugs used habitually by pregnant women, including, most notably, opiates as well as alcohol, barbiturates, benzodiazepines, and several other miscellaneous sedative-hypnotic agents, can cause the neonatal withdrawal syndrome. Many women who are addicted to opiates are polydrug abusers, which complicates the diagnosis of and therapy for the clinical withdrawal state in their newborns.

Opiates

Classic features of neonatal opioid withdrawal include wakefulness, jitteriness, irritability that is inconsolable, tremor, hypertonicity and hyperreflexia, vomiting, diarrhea, poor feeding, and failure-to-thrive. Severe cases can be rarely accompanied by seizures. Most infants of heroin-addicted women display symptoms early, 65% in the first 24 hours of life. Withdrawal in infants born to mothers taking methadone is manifested slightly later, usually on the second or third day of life, and the duration of the symptoms tends to be longer. Although methadone withdrawal is generally less severe, these infants are more likely to exhibit disturbed feeding patterns and failure to gain weight. Both heroin- and methadone-addicted infants show lower than average gains in development on follow-up testing, although the consensus among researchers is that these differences are probably related more to covariables, such as poverty and malnutrition, than to drug effects per se. Management of acute neonatal opioid withdrawal includes swaddling, hypercalorie diets, and, for severe cases, pharmacologic treatment. Breastfed neonates may be less likely to require pharmacologic treatment than are those who were bottle fed. The American Academy of Pediatrics recommended tincture of opium as first-line pharmacotherapy for neonates with opiate withdrawal, and phenobarbital for neonatal sedative-hypnotic withdrawal, in its 1998 statement (American Academy of Pediatrics, 1998). Many authorities currently use oral morphine sulfate or methadone interchangeably with tincture of opium. Phenobarbital can be helpful as an adjunct in severe cases or in situations in which opioid addiction is complicated by barbiturate or sedative-hypnotic abuse.

Other Drugs

Neonatal withdrawal from short- and long-acting barbiturates, benzodiazepines, tricyclic antidepressants, other sedative-hypnotics, and alcohol is also well described. These syndromes share features of opiate withdrawal and, in particular, can be associated with seizures. Onset varies with the pharmacologic characteristics of the agents (e.g., early for alcohol and short-acting barbiturates; later for phenobarbital). Most such infants can be successfully managed with phenobarbital and supportive care.

Substances in Breast Milk

An additional precaution for the perinatal period is that of illicit drugs or prescribed medications, taken by nursing mothers, that might pass through breast milk. This topic has been summarized by the American Academy of Pediatrics (2001). General considerations for prescription medications include the necessity of using the medication at all, the possibility of safer alternatives, and the timing of dosing in relation to nursing so that drug transfer is minimized (e.g., just after breastfeeding or just before the infant's longest sleep period).

One area of particular concern to this discussion is that of subtle developmental effects linked to alcohol exposure of breastfed infants. Postnatal exposure to alcohol through breastfeeding was associated with significantly lowered scores on the Psychomotor Development Index of the Bayley scales in infants at 1 year of age, even at levels of one drink daily (Little et al, 1989). Although the amounts of alcohol estimated to be ingested through breastfeeding are small, the authors suggested that repetitive doses of alcohol can accumulate in the infant during breastfeeding, as had been shown for other drugs such as caffeine. However, a more recent effort to replicate this finding, in a population from Avon County, England, found no such association when infants were tested at 18 months of age (Little et al, 2002).

The epidemic of illicit cocaine abuse has been the focus of great concern in regard to teratogenic and perinatal morbidity. Altered sensorium and seizures have also been observed in infants ingesting cocaine in the perinatal period from breastfeeding (both through milk and from direct contact with cocaine used as a local anesthetic for sore nipples) as well as from environmental acquisition through passive inhalation of "crack" smoke, ingestion of crack, or both.

Breast milk has also been found to contain PCBs, and breastfed infants are exposed to a considerable fraction of their total lifetime dose within the first few months of life. Nevertheless, the potential negative impact of PCB exposure through breast milk is considered less consequential than the numerous proven advantages, and breastfeeding in this context is still recommended without qualification. Pregnant and breastfeeding mothers can take some reasonable steps to limit PCB exposure to their infants by minimizing consumption of high-fat animal tissues, particularly cheeses and processed meats. Some authors have suggested that women avoid significant weight loss while lactating, as fat breakdown liberates PCBs (Schmid and Rotenberg, 2005).

HAZARDS IN INFANCY AND CHILDHOOD

This section highlights significant toxicologic causes of acquired cognitive and behavioral dysfunction in older infants and children. In addition, adverse cognitive effects of some commonly prescribed therapeutic drugs are discussed.

Lead

Extent of Problem

Lead poisoning, currently defined by the Centers for Disease Control and Prevention (CDC) as blood lead levels in excess of 10 μg/dL, still affects more than 300,000 American children aged 1 to 5 years despite decades of prevention efforts (CDC, 2002). Although recent surveys have found a significant decline in average U.S. lead levels, presumably because of decreased environmental contamination by airborne lead derived from leaded gasoline and decreased use of lead solder in canned foods, pockets of excessive lead contamination still persist among inner-city, impoverished, minority children. For example, children enrolled in Medicaid have an incidence of lead poisoning three times higher than that of those not enrolled. In addition, refugee, immigrant, and foreign-born adopted children remain at especially great risk. Children from "lower risk" groups who reside in older homes with deteriorated paint may also be found to have elevated lead levels. Thus, the number of potential victims of lead-induced effects is still considerable.

Lead sources are numerous, including automobile exhaust emissions, industrial waste, and widespread contamination from deterioration of surfaces painted with lead-based paint (Fig. 31-2). Additional sources include battery casings burned as fuel, dirt and dust in contaminated areas that rest on children's hands and toys, occasional food or water contamination (especially if improperly glazed ceramic cups or plates are used), and lead dust and particles on parental clothing from occupational exposure. Children are more efficient than adults at absorbing ingested lead; this process is further enhanced by concomitant nutritional deficiency, particularly low-iron, high-fat diets, which often coexist with lead paint exposure in low-income families.

Hazards for Development and Behavior

Lead is a typical heavy metal poison, with wide-ranging toxicity on multiple organ systems. Its principal toxic effects relate to its affinity for biologic electron donor ligands (especially sulfhydryl groups), which allows it to bind to and then have an impact on numerous enzymatic, structural, and receptor proteins, and its chemical similarity to calcium, leading to interference with many calcium-mediated pathways, particularly in mitochondria and second-messenger systems regulating cellular energy metabolism. Lead may have an impact on the heme synthesis pathway, leading to microcytic anemia, and injure the kidneys, but its most dramatic manifestation in children is neurotoxicity, particularly acute encephalopathy (Fig. 31-3). Typically, a 1- to 3-year-old child presents with stupor or coma and seizures, which are often protracted. The illness can be heralded by days of nausea, vomiting, and irritability or listlessness. The pathologic features of acute encephalopathy involve both a vascular lesion, with capillary leak and increased intracranial pressure, and direct neuronal damage, particularly in the thalamus, hypothalamus, and basal ganglia. Current government-mandated screening and lead abatement programs have resulted in a marked decline in the incidence of lead encephalopathy, but it is still observed rarely. Management considerations for lead encephalopathy include appropriate intensive care with optimal cardiorespiratory support, seizure and intracranial pressure control, close monitoring of fluid provision and urine output to avoid fluid overload but to maintain urine flow, and specific chelation therapy with use of calcium disodium edetate and dimercaprol, as detailed elsewhere (Henretig, 2006). However, the

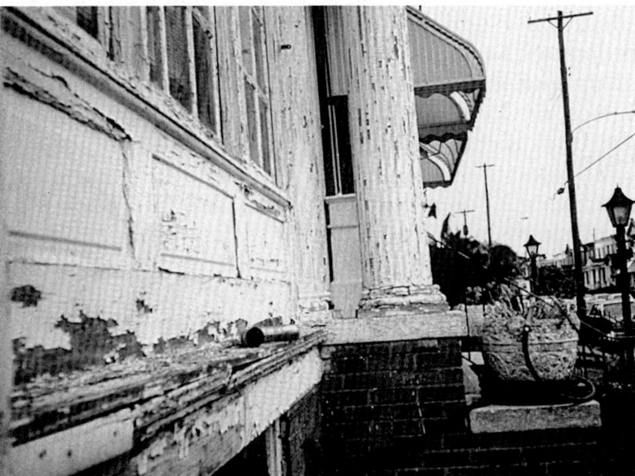

Figure 31-2. A typical inner-city row house with peeling lead paint. *(Courtesy of Carla Campbell, MD, and Philadelphia Department of Public Health, Philadelphia, PA.)*

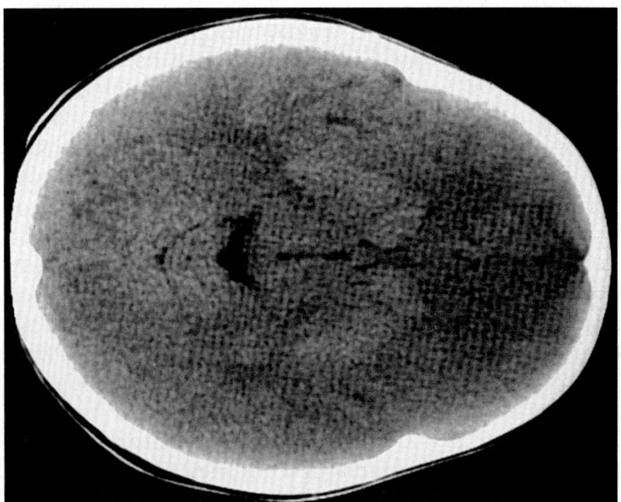

Figure 31-3. Computed tomography scan of the head of a child with acute lead encephalopathy, demonstrating cerebral edema. *(Courtesy of Eric Faerber, MD, and the Department of Radiology, St. Christopher's Hospital for Children, Philadelphia, PA.)*

greatest public health concern surrounding childhood lead exposure is related to subencephalopathic effects on the CNS. Numerous studies have attempted to elucidate and to quantify cognitive and behavioral deficits in children with "low" lead levels (generally in the 40- to 80-μg/dL range, but recent studies have extended this to levels as low as 10 μg/dL) who were overtly asymptomatic. Many of the early studies were retrospective, and many were poorly controlled. In addition, it is difficult to control for some confounding variables such as innate hyperactivity or learning disability, poor parental supervision, nutritional deficiency, inadequate intellectual stimulation, and low parental intelligence quotient (IQ). Thus, despite the considerable public health consequences of defining asymptomatic lead poisoning as a significant disease with the capacity for intellectual impairment, it has been difficult to demonstrate such causality with precision.

The first large, well-controlled study that addressed most methodologic criticisms compared the neuropsychological performance of 58 first- and second-grade children in whom the dentin of shed primary teeth showed a high lead content with that of 100 control children with low dentin lead levels (Needleman et al, 1979). There was a 4-point deficit in the Wechsler Intelligence Scale for Children (Revised) full-scale IQ in the high-lead group (106.6 versus 102.1). In addition, more than 2000 children with known dentin lead levels were evaluated blindly by teacher ratings of classroom behavior. The occurrence of nonadaptive behaviors such as distractibility and impulsiveness was significantly associated in a stepwise dose-related fashion with dentin lead content.

Studies have attempted to extend the potential lower limits of both lead burden and critical age by using a longitudinal design, enrolling children at birth or even prenatally. A prospective study of 249 Boston children from birth to 2 years of age found an inverse relationship between prenatal lead exposure and development, with an estimated difference of 4.8 points on the mental scale of the Bayley Scales of Infant Development between the low- and high-exposure groups (Bellinger et al, 1987). Another study from Cincinnati also found an inverse relationship between prenatal and neonatal blood lead levels and mental scale scores, resulting in a 16- to 22-point mental developmental scale deficit at 6 months of age (Dietrich et al, 1987). Postnatal lead exposure was related to effects on development in a longitudinal cohort study from the lead smelter community of Port Pirie in South Australia (McMichael et al, 1988). This study of 537 children found that the blood lead level at each age, particularly at 2 and 3 years, and the integrated average level were inversely related to development, with an estimated deficit of 7.2 points. Of note, an 11-year follow-up of the 1979 Boston study found that impaired academic status and neurobehavioral function was still related to the lead content of teeth shed 11 years earlier (Needleman et al, 1990). Measures of cognitive status that correlated with lead burden included failure to graduate high school, frequency of reading disability, and lower high-school class rank. Finally, a more recent study evaluated IQ in patients 6 months to 5 years old and found that blood lead levels were inversely correlated with IQ scores at 3 and 5 years of age and that the magnitude of this decrement was 4.6 points for each 10 μg/dL increase in blood lead level. Of particular concern, this effect was even greater for children in the lowest (1-10 μg/dL) range (Canfield et al, 2003).

Although there may always be some slight doubt about the causal relationship between low lead exposure and cognitive effects, the studies of the past decade meet many if not most of the usual criteria for relating causality to epidemiologic associations: temporal relationship, strong statistical association, dose-response gradient, control for confounding variables, consistent findings across studies, and biologic plausibility. The cumulative weight of these prospective studies adds to the conviction that occult lead poisoning is a significant cause of cognitive deficits.

Pediatric Management

Current recommendations for prevention and screening of children at risk have been summarized (CDC, 2002). Children with a high priority for annual screening include those aged 1 to 3 years (up to 6 years if not previously screened) who live in high-risk, inner-city communities; siblings or playmates of children with known lead poisoning; children who live in or near older homes, especially if they are undergoing renovation; and any child with additional specific exposure risks based on cultural or family occupational criteria (see Table 31-2).Additional at-risk groups who are seen for common pediatric problems include children with acute accidental ingestions and those presenting with foreign bodies in the ears, nose, or throat. Intervention should include prompt termination of lead exposure, although this is often difficult to enforce. It is extremely important to remove children from exposure during active lead removal programs.

The overall treatment of lead poisoning is detailed elsewhere (American Academy of Pediatrics, 1995; CDC, 2002; Henretig, 2006) but briefly summarized here. All at-risk children should be screened (Table 31-1), and those with elevated lead levels should have close monitoring and follow-up (Table 31-2) and be provided educational and environmental interventions as appropriate (Table 31-3). Treatment of asymptomatic patients with lead levels greater than 45 μg/dL is generally agreed on by most authorities; however, the value of chelation therapy to modify the possible neurobehavioral toxicity is unproved. The oral chelating agent succimer (2,3-dimercaptosuccinic acid) has been used increasingly, with an exceptional safety profile, and this agent is currently the drug of choice for asymptomatic patients with lead levels of 45 to 69 μg/dL. The National Institutes Health sponsored a prospective, placebo-controlled study of succimer chelation therapy in asymptomatic children with blood lead levels of 20 to 44 μg/dL that found only modest efficacy of succimer in reducing blood lead levels when they were tested 1 year after therapy initiation. Furthermore, cognition, neuropsychiatric function, and behavior were not benefited by treatment when they were studied at 3 years after enrollment (Rogan et al, 2001) or at 7 years (Dietrich et al,

Table 31-1. Clinical Manifestations of Lead Poisoning in Children

Clinical Findings	Usual Blood Lead Levels (µg/dL)
Severe	>70-100
Neurologic: encephalopathy (coma, altered sensorium, seizures, bizarre behavior, ataxia, apathy, incoordination, loss of developmental skills; papilledema, cranial nerve palsy, signs of increased intracranial pressure)	
Gastrointestinal: persistent vomiting	
Hematologic: pallor (anemia)	
Mild-Moderate	50-70
Neurologic: hyperirritable behavior, intermittent lethargy, decreased interest in play, "difficult" child	
Gastrointestinal: intermittent vomiting, abdominal pain, anorexia	
Asymptomatic	0-49
Neurologic: impaired cognition, behavior; impaired fine motor coordination	
Miscellaneous: impaired hearing, growth	

Modified from Henretig FM: Lead. *In* Flomenbaum NE, Goldfrank LR, Hoffman RS, et al (eds): Goldfrank's Toxicologic Emergencies. New York, McGraw-Hill, 2006, pp 1308-1324.

2004). Currently, the American Academy of Pediatrics and the CDC recommend aggressive environmental remediation and optimization of nutritional status (Table 31-3), without routine chelation therapy, for such children (CDC, 2002).

Mercury

Another heavy metal with the potential for significant neurotoxicity and widespread human exposure is mercury. Severe elemental mercury and inorganic mercury salt poisoning (responsible for pink disease, or acrodynia, from mercurous chloride teething lotions or diaper powder) has become rare. However, a more insidious concern is that of chronic exposure to organic mercurials, particularly methylmercury, resulting from contamination of the food chain. Large outbreaks have occurred in Minamata Bay, Japan, from eating fish contaminated by factory waste discharged into the bay and in Iraq from contaminated bread baked from grain treated with methylmercury as a fungicide (Schmid and Rotenberg, 2005). Severe CNS effects occurred in both instances, with a particular susceptibility noted in the fetuses of poisoned pregnant women (almost 30% of children born during the height of the Minamata Bay epidemic had moderate or severe developmental disabilities).

Recent concern has centered, as for lead, on more subtle neurocognitive effects that may be attributed to chronic low-level mercury exposure through fish or other food consumption (Mendola et al, 2002; Schmid and Rotenberg, 2005). For example, a large study in the Faroe Islands identified deficits in pediatric cognitive function, particularly language, memory, and attention, occurring at levels of prenatal mercury exposure that were less than 3% of the toxic threshold suggested by the Iraq outbreak (Grandjean et al, 1997). This and other similar studies have concluded that excessive mercury exposure, defined as more than 0.1 µg/kg/day by the U.S. Environmental Protection Agency, through seafood consumption should be avoided by women of childbearing age and young children. The U.S. Food and Drug Administration now recommends that at-risk populations (women who are or may become pregnant, nursing mothers, and young children) avoid the largest

Table 31-2. Management Guidelines for Pediatric Lead Exposure

Screen

Screen children at 1, 2, and 3 years of age (up to age 6 years if not tested previously), if
- The child lives in or regularly visits a home built before 1950
- The child lives in or regularly visits a home built before 1978 undergoing remodeling or renovation (or has been within 6 months)
- The local health department considers the child's community to be high risk
- The child is at risk by virtue of
  - Low-income family, receipt of poverty assistance
  - Personal, family, or playmate history of lead poisoning
  - Parental occupational, industrial, hobby exposures
  - Proximity to major roadway
  - Hot tap water for consumption
  - Cultural exposures (folk remedies, cosmetics, ceramic food containers, trips, residence outside United States, international adoptees)
  - Parents are migrant farm workers
  - History of pica for paint chips, dirt, foreign bodies, and the like
  - History of iron deficiency
  - Development disability

Follow-up

Venous Blood Lead Level (µg/dL)	Management Overview
<9	Retest in 6 months; parental education (see Table 31-3)
10-14	Retest in 3 months; education; refer to health department for case management
15-19	Retest in 6 weeks; refer to health department for case management; education; environmental investigation and control
20-44	Retest in 1-2 weeks; refer to health department for case management; clinical evaluation; education; environmental investigation and control
45-69	Within 48 hours: retest; clinical evaluation; chelation therapy with oral succimer or intravenous calcium disodium edetate; refer to health department for case management; education; environmental investigation and control
≥70	Emergently hospitalize child and retest; immediate chelation therapy, typically with intramuscular dimercaprol and intravenous calcium disodium edetate; refer to health department for case management; education; environmental investigation and control

Modified from Centers for Disease Control and Prevention: Managing Elevated Blood Lead Levels Among Young Children: Recommendations from the Advisory Committee on Childhood Lead Poisoning Prevention. Atlanta, GA, Centers for Disease Control and Prevention, 2002.

Table 31-3. Educational and Environmental Interventions for Reducing Childhood Lead Exposure

Notify local health department.
Home lead paint abatement: use professional contractors, if possible; use plastic sheeting, low dust-generating paint removal; replace lead-painted windows; floor treatment; final cleanup with high-efficiency particle air vacuum, wet mopping.
Avoid or restrict access to the most hazardous areas of the home and yard.
Dust control: wet mopping, sponging with high-phosphate detergent; frequent hand, toy, pacifier washing.
Reduce soil lead exposure by planting grass and shrubs around the house.
Use only cold, flushed tap water for consumption.
Optimize nutrition: avoid fasting; iron- and calcium-sufficient diet; iron and calcium supplementation as necessary.
Avoid food storage in open cans.
Avoid imported ceramic containers for food and beverage use.
Evaluate parental occupations and hobbies and any other possible "exotic" sources of lead exposure beyond that due to lead paint chips or dust.

Modified from Henretig FM. Lead. *In* Flomenbaum NE, Goldfrank LR, Hoffman RS, et al (eds): Goldfrank's Toxicologic Emergencies. New York, McGraw-Hill, 2006, pp 1308-1324.

predator fish, such as shark, swordfish, tilefish, and king mackerel, which contain mercury at nearly 1 ppm. Most other popular seafood, such as canned (non-albacore) tuna, salmon, pollock, cod, catfish, flatfish, shrimp, scallops, clams, and crabs, do not require express consumption advice beyond a general limit of approximately 2 pounds per week. Albacore tuna is a special case; the Food and Drug Administration recommends a limit of 6 ounces per week for at-risk persons, although some consumer groups think that is still too high (Sue, 2006). Up-to-date recommendations for appropriate limits on fish consumption are available at Internet Web sites of the U.S. Environmental Protection Agency and the U.S. Food and Drug Administration (e.g., *http://www.epa.gov/mercury/advisories.htm*).

Another, more controversial source of organic mercury is thimerosal, the bacteriostatic agent used for years in many vaccines and other biologicals. Thimerosal is a compound with an ethylmercury moiety. Although it is a potentially neurotoxic organic mercury, ethylmercury is not identical to methylmercury, and its neurotoxicity is believed to be comparatively less. Still, concern arose that the amount contained in many childhood vaccines would result in a cumulative dose for some infants that slightly exceeded the recommended maximum daily doses (of methylmercury) averaged over time. In particular, it has been suggested that such low-level mercury exposure might be associated causally with autism. In response to these concerns, the American Academy of Pediatrics in 1999 called for thimerosal to be removed from childhood vaccines, and since 2001, except for influenza vaccine, all U.S. vaccines contain none or only trace amounts. Subsequently, a number of carefully performed studies have tried to validate the association between thimerosal-containing vaccines and autism or other neurodevelopmental disorders and found none (Sue, 2006). The diagnosis of methylmercury poisoning is difficult to confirm by laboratory testing. Blood levels may be elevated (>1-2 μg/dL). Hair levels of mercury have been used in research studies but are subject to external contamination and are not currently recommended for routine clinical use. Treatment is not regularly effective, although some animal studies have shown succimer to be promising (Sue, 2006). Of note, despite the overwhelming volume of research negating the purported relationship of thimerosal to autism, parents of children with this disorder may understandably search desperately for treatment options, and many have turned to unorthodox medical practitioners, including some who advocate chelation therapy in uncontrolled therapeutic "trials." To address this situation, the National Institute of Mental Health announced in September 2006 that it would inaugurate a controlled trial of chelation therapy for children with autism (*www.nimh.nih.gov/press/autism.irp.trials.cfm*).

Other Metals

Aluminum, arsenic, thallium, and manganese are additional, rare causes of neurotoxicity that more typically is manifested as overt encephalopathy, along with varying associated features, rather than by subtle developmental effects. These uncommon metal poisonings are reviewed in detail along with specific recommendations for management in reference toxicology texts.

Pesticides

The term *pesticide* denotes a broad group of heterogeneous compounds that are used to prevent, to repel, or to kill pests, especially insects but also rodents, nematodes, fungi, and unwanted plants (e.g., herbicides). In this discussion, the focus is primarily on the organophosphorus insecticides, which as a group have significant mammalian toxicity in acute overdose and also have raised concern for subtle neurocognitive effects in children from background, low-level chronic exposure.

The organophosphates are acetylcholinesterase inhibitors, thereby disrupting normal cholinergic neurotransmitter function. In overt poisonings, they cause an acute toxidrome that is well recognized and characterized by profound CNS disturbances, ranging from lethargy to coma or seizures, and cholinergic symptoms including bronchospasm, bronchorrhea, and several additional muscarinic effects often recalled by the mnemonic SLUDGE (salivation, lacrimation, urination, defecation, gastrointestinal cramping, and emesis). Such patients may have life-threatening illness and are typically treated with atropine and pralidoxime for the acute overdose (Osterhoudt et al, 2006).

These agents are used widely in the home, in the home garden, and for agricultural applications and as such are accessible to children through dermal, oral, and inhalational routes. A national survey of human exposure to multiple environmental pollutant chemicals in 1999-2000, by the CDC, found that children aged 6 to 11 years had urine organophosphate metabolite levels that were twice as high as those of adults aged 20 to 59 years. Although concern for chronic, low-level pesticide exposure is significant (e.g., the U.S. Congress passed the 1996 Food Quality Protection Act to restrict access of young children to pesticides), the evidence for adverse health effects in this context is sparse. One interesting study from Mexico compared two agricultural communities, one using pesticide-based agriculture, the other not. Several measures of neurocognitive function, such as coordination and human-figure drawing, were performed better by children in the non–pesticide-using group. However, pesticide levels were not reported for individual tested children (Weiss et al, 2004).

Inhalational Toxins

Both the accidental or intentional acute exposure to carbon monoxide and the chronic inhalation abuse of various solvents have been associated with CNS syndromes. Chapter 45 provides a more detailed discussion of adolescent substance abuse.

Carbon Monoxide

Exposure to carbon monoxide fumes is the most common cause of death from poisoning in the United States, accounting for 3500 to 4000 fatalities per year. Many cases are secondary to smoke inhalation from house fires, although a clinically important and more challenging group to recognize includes individuals with subtle neuropsychiatric or systemic afebrile "flulike" symptoms, or both, resulting from faulty furnaces, automobile exhaust, improperly vented water heaters, kerosene heaters, and so on. One study in the Children's Hospital of Philadelphia emergency department found a surprisingly high incidence (nearly 30%) of carbon monoxide exposure during the winter months in just such a group of 46 patients (Baker et al, 1988).

Toxicity of carbon monoxide is mediated primarily by cellular hypoxia. It decreases oxygen delivery by binding to hemoglobin to form carboxyhemoglobin and by shifting the oxyhemoglobin dissociation curve to the left; it can also bind to mitochondrial cytochrome oxidase and inhibit cellular respiration as well. As such, carbon monoxide poisoning especially affects organs most susceptible to hypoxia: the heart and brain. In acute, severe exposures, patients may have coma, convulsions, cardiovascular collapse, and respiratory failure. Many survivors (up to 40%) of severe carbon monoxide poisoning have neuropsychiatric sequelae. The effects of severe but nonlethal carbon monoxide exposure on pregnant women can also be manifested as fetal demise or cerebral palsy in the infant. Prolonged low-dose exposure through cigarette smoking (which can produce carboxyhemoglobin levels of 5% to 15%) in pregnancy has been associated with lower birth weights and increased neonatal mortality rates. The mainstays for treatment of acute carbon monoxide poisoning are immediate removal from exposure, provision of appropriate supportive care and 100% oxygen, and consideration, if feasible, of the use of hyperbaric oxygen therapy for selected patients, especially those who are pregnant (Fine, 2006).

Solvents

The general background for intentional inhalant abuse is discussed in Chapter 45. Several organic solvents have been associated with CNS sequelae, particularly toluene (glue sniffing) and gasoline. The neuropathic effects of toluene include ataxia, tremors, emotional lability, and cognitive effects. Gasoline abuse leads to an encephalopathy characterized by ataxia, tremor, chorea, and myoclonus; there can also be an organic psychosis with hallucinations, paranoia, and violence. The neurologic sequelae of chronic gasoline inhalation are believed to result from tetraethyl lead toxicity, and the diagnosis can be confirmed by finding elevated blood lead levels. The treatment of organic lead toxicity in this context is primarily supportive, with sedation as indicated. For those patients with significantly elevated blood lead levels, one might consider a trial of chelation therapy as described before for inorganic lead encephalopathy, but it has not been found to be particularly efficacious.

SUMMARY

Children are uniquely vulnerable to toxic influences because of relatively increased exposure, immaturity of physiologic processes, and the prolonged developmental timeline of the human nervous system. A number of environmental toxic hazards are well substantiated, and many more are under investigation. Unfortunately, much of the data supporting such associations is derived from human epidemiologic studies or from animal models. Each of these is somewhat difficult to extrapolate to individual clinical encounters. Nevertheless, pediatricians must strive to stay current with environmental research and be able to apply that scholarship and reasonable interpersonal judgment to counsel families on the potential consequences of clinical exposures, to mitigate guilt and anxiety that are unreasonable, and to provide or to refer for appropriate therapy when such is available.

REFERENCES

Alpert JJ, Zuckerman BZ: Alcohol use during pregnancy: WHAT is the risk? Pediatr Rev 12:375-379, 1991.

American Academy of Pediatrics, Committee on Substance Abuse and Committee on Children with Disabilities: Fetal alcohol syndrome and fetal alcohol effects. Pediatrics 91:1004-1006, 1993.

American Academy of Pediatrics, Committee on Drugs: Treatment guidelines for lead exposure in children. Pediatrics 96:155-160, 1995.

American Academy of Pediatrics, Committee on Drugs: Neonatal drug withdrawal. Pediatrics 101:1079-1088, 1998.

American Academy of Pediatrics, Committee on Drugs: The transfer of drugs and other chemicals into human milk. Pediatrics 108:776-789, 2001.

Bada HS, Das A, Bauer CR, et al: Impact of prenatal cocaine exposure on child behavior problems through school age. Pediatrics 119:e348-e359, 2007.

Baker MD, Henretig FM, Ludwig S: Carboxyhemoglobin levels in children with nonspecific flu-like symptoms. J Pediatr 113:501, 1988.

Bellinger D, Leviton A, Waternaux C, et al: Longitudinal analyses of prenatal and postnatal lead exposure and early cognitive development. N Engl J Med 316:1037, 1987.

Byrd RS, Howard CR: Children's passive and prenatal exposure to cigarette smoke. Pediatr Ann 24:640-645, 1995.

Canfield RI, Henderson CR, Cory-Slechta DA: Intellectual impairment in children with blood lead concentrations below 10 μg per deciliter. N Engl J Med 348:1517-1526, 2003.

Centers for Disease Control and Prevention: Managing Elevated Blood Lead Levels Among Young Children: Recommendations from the Advisory Committee on Childhood Lead Poisoning Prevention. Atlanta, GA, Centers for Disease Control and Prevention, 2002.

Dietrich KN, Krafft KM, Bornschein RL, et al: Low-level fetal lead exposure effect on neurobehavioral development in early infancy. Pediatrics 80:721, 1987.

Dietrich KN, Ware JH, Salganik M, et al: Effect of chelation therapy on the neuropsychological and behavioral development of lead-exposed children after school entry. Pediatrics 114:19-26, 2004.

Fine JS: Reproductive and perinatal principles. *In* Flomenbaum NE, Goldfrank LR, Hoffman RS, et al (eds): Goldfrank's Toxicologic Emergencies. New York, McGraw-Hill, 2006, pp 465-486.

Goldstein GW: Neurologic concepts of lead poisoning in children. Pediatr Ann 21:384-388, 1992.

Grandjean P, Weihe P, White R, et al: Cognitive deficit in 7-year-old children with prenatal exposure to methylmercury. Neurotoxicol Teratol 19:417-428, 1997.

Henretig FM: Lead. *In* Flomenbaum NE, Goldfrank LR, Hoffman RS, et al (eds): Goldfrank's Toxicologic Emergencies. New York, McGraw-Hill, 2006, pp 1308-1324.

Hoyer A: Effects on the fetus of maternal drugs during labor. Pediatr Rev 23:256-257, 2002.

Landrigan PJ, Garg A: Chronic effects of toxic environmental exposures on children's health. Clin Toxicol 40:449-456, 2002.

Little RE, Anderson KW, Ervin CH, et al: Maternal alcohol use during breastfeeding and infant mental and motor development at one year. N Engl J Med 321:425, 1989.

Little RE, Northstone K, Golding J, et al: Alcohol, breastfeeding and development at 18 months. Pediatrics 109:e72, 2002.

McMichael AJ, Baghurst PA, Wigg NR, et al: Port Pirie Cohort Study: Environmental exposure to lead and children's abilities at the age of four years. N Engl J Med 319:468, 1988.

Mendola P, Selevan SG, Gutter S, Rice D: Environmental factors associated with a spectrum of neurodevelopmental deficits. Ment Retard Dev Disabil Res Rev 8:188-197, 2002.

National Academy of Sciences: Scientific Frontiers in Developmental Toxicology and Risk Assessment. Washington, DC, National Academy Press, 2000.

Needleman HL, Gunnoe C, Leviton A, et al: Deficits in psychologic and classroom performance of children with elevated dentine lead levels. N Engl J Med 300:689, 1979.

Needleman HL, Schell A, Bellinger D, et al: The long-term effects of exposure to low doses of lead in childhood—an 11-year follow-up report. N Engl J Med 322:83, 1990.

Ornoy A: The impact of intrauterine exposure versus postnatal environment in neurodevelopmental toxicity: Long-term neurobehavioral studies in children at risk for developmental disorders. Toxicol Lett 140-141:171-181, 2003.

Osterhoudt K, Shannon M, Burns Ewald M, Henretig F: Toxicologic emergencies. *In* Fleisher GR, Ludwig S, Henretig FM (eds): Textbook of Pediatric Emergency Medicine, 5th ed. Philadelphia, Lippincott Williams & Wilkins, 2006.

Richardson GA, Day NL, Goldschmidt L: Prenatal alcohol, marijuana, and tobacco use: Infant mental and motor development. Neurotoxicol Teratol 17:479-487, 1995.

Rogan W, Dietrich K, Ware J, et al: The effect of chelation therapy with succimer on neuropsychological development in children exposed to lead. N Engl J Med 344:1421-1426, 2001.

Schmid C, Rotenberg JS: Neurodevelopmental toxicology. Neurol Clin 23:321-336, 2005.

Stein J, Schettler T, Wallinga D, Valenti M: In harm's way: Toxic threats to child development. J Dev Behav Pediatr 23:S13-S22, 2002.

Stratton K, Howe C, Battaglia FC (eds): Fetal Alcohol Syndrome: Diagnosis, Epidemiology, Prevention and Treatment. Committee to Study Fetal Alcohol Syndrome, Institute of Medicine. Washington, DC, National Academy Press, 1996.

Sue Y-J: Mercury. *In* Flomenbaum NE, Goldfrank LR, Hoffman RS, et al (eds): Goldfrank's Toxicologic Emergencies. New York, McGraw-Hill, 2006, pp 1334-1344.

Volpe JJ: Effect of cocaine on the fetus. N Engl J Med 327:399-407, 1992.

Weiss B, Amler S, Amler RW: Pesticides. Pediatrics 113:1030-1036, 2004.

Part IV GENERAL PHYSICAL ILLNESS—DEVELOPMENTAL-BEHAVIORAL ASPECTS

32 ACUTE MINOR ILLNESS

William B. Carey

Vignette

After breakfast, Sally Smith calls her friend Martha to see how her 2-year-old son Michael is doing with his ear infection. Martha is trying to get some sleep following a difficult night combating Michael's fever. Sally reassures her that the fever is only a symptom and not the disease itself, but the doctor has repeatedly impressed on Martha the importance of keeping the fever down. He has told her about the harmful effects of the fever itself and about the likelihood of continuing rise with possible seizures and brain damage if it is not reduced promptly. She has sponge-bathed him and given him antipyretics intermittently throughout the night because the doctor told her that a good parent should do that. The boy cried throughout the sponging. Martha was exhausted and fell asleep at about 4 AM. She feels guilty and inadequate.

The minor illnesses and injuries of childhood occupy about half the time of the average primary care physician, and yet they tend to be regarded as having little or no relevance to the child's development and behavior. This chapter points out the considerable interactions that these universal experiences do have with the child's developmental-behavioral status.

Acute minor illness is defined here as ordinary, brief health problems, such as the common respiratory and gastrointestinal infections and the familiar instances of physical trauma experienced by all children. These are the usual minor complaints that account for almost all the visits to primary health care clinicians because of illness. There is reason to believe that the assumption of their unimportance is incorrect and is attributable to insufficient attention and research. A comprehensive critical review of the meager literature more than 35 years ago summarized available data and called for further investigation (Carey and Sibinga, 1972). This chapter draws primarily on that review as to content and organization. Only a little additional material has been published since then (Crocetti et al, 2001; Cunningham, 1989; Richtsmeier and Hatcher, 1994; Schmitt, 1980; Sibinga and Carey, 1976). The recommendations are based more on a pooling of the experience of many pediatricians rather than on extensive formal research findings.

STRESSES IN THE CHILD AND PARENTS

The child with an acute minor illness experiences the discomfort of the illness and its treatment, the emotional reactions to and fantasies about the illness (such as feelings of guilt, fear, anger, sadness, and apathy), the loss of normal social contacts at school and elsewhere outside the home, the restrictions (such as bed rest and diet), the decreased or altered sensory input, and a change in the relationship with the parents, who may become either more indulgent or more hostile (Freud, 1952).

The parents endure stresses of two sorts: those that arise from the illness itself and its management, such as more responsibility and expense, interference with employment, and less sleep and recreation; and the extraneous factors that complicate the parents' reaction to the illness, such as the parents' personal problems, preexisting physical or behavioral difficulties in the child, and situational pressures, such as unemployment or marital discord (see also Chapter 10 regarding various forms of family dysfunction). Another unrelated factor may be the vulnerable child syndrome, in which some parents continue to be inappropriately overconcerned about their children's health long after they have completely recovered from an early health crisis (see Chapter 34). The Family and Medical Leave Act passed by the U.S. Congress in 1993 allows parents leave for the care of

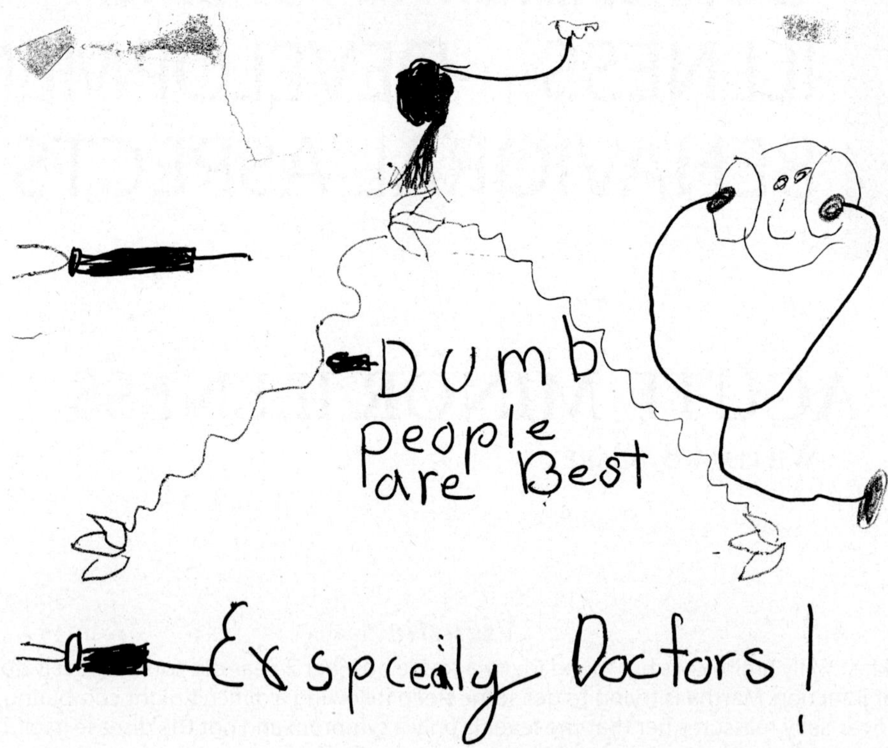

Figure 32-1. A young child's conflicting feelings about her doctor.

their children's major illnesses, such as hospitalizations, but makes no provision for more common and equally disruptive minor illnesses (Heymann et al, 1996).

Effects of Stressors

The effect of acute minor illness on children's behavior, although well known to parents and clinicians, has scarcely been studied. Various possible behavioral reactions, such as dependency, withdrawal, irritability, rebelliousness, and feelings of inferiority, have been reported, but a comprehensive, systematic delineation of these reactions and their determinants and consequences is still awaited. The child's temperament influences his or her experience of the illness and reactions to it (Fig. 32-1), which are likely to affect the clinical manifestations and outcome (see Chapter 7).

The parents may also suffer from fears and anxieties, anger, guilt, fatigue, depression, distortions, and misconceptions. They are expected to master these feelings and to adjust sufficiently to meet their child's needs. Ineffective responses may consist of inappropriate feelings or lack of understanding (such as too much or too little anxiety, persistent misconceptions about the illness or its treatment, or an excessive sense of personal injury) or inability to muster appropriate behavior to deal with the illness (such as difficulty in carrying out a reasonable share of the treatment process in conjunction with the physician, as evidenced by noncompliance with the treatment plan).

It seems likely that minor illness and its management account for only a small portion of the more chronic behavioral variations and problems in children, yet these effects are real and must be acknowledged and dealt with. Any experienced pediatrician can think of striking examples of unfavorable outcomes, such as the child who is treated by the parents for years as a semi-invalid because a physician had felt compelled to reveal and to stress the existence of a functional heart murmur without considering or assessing the impact of this information on the child and the parents, or the child who is made to feel guilty or inadequate because of recurrent respiratory or urinary infections.

On the other hand, as Parmelee (1997) has observed, it is possible that childhood illnesses "not only aid the process of the development of social competence and a healthy personality, but they may be necessary for this process. In turn, social competence and a healthy personality provide us the greatest capacity for coping with illness." The recurring experience of minor illnesses furnishes children with a multitude of opportunities to broaden their knowledge of themselves, of their caregivers, and of the relationships between them. Positive outcomes can include enhanced social competence and self-assurance.

NURTURING SICK CHILDREN AND SUPPORTING PARENTS

A useful way to describe principles of management of minor illness is in terms of the three components: the illness itself, the child, and the parents—how the needs of each are sometimes not met, why this happens, what the consequences may be, and finally how to avoid these complications. Even the best trained, most compassionate physician makes occasional lapses of good judgment in these matters; the objective is to keep "pediatric pathogenesis" to a minimum (Carey and Sibinga, 1972).

Treat the Illness

Treatment of illness can go awry in three main ways. Probably the most common error we physicians make in the management of minor illness is in overdiagnosis and overtreatment. For example, unnecessary antibiotics are frequently prescribed for viral upper respiratory infections. Insignificant findings, such as a functional heart murmur or tibial torsion, may be overinterpreted, made into a "pseudo-disease," and managed with greater attention than they deserve. Fostering fever phobia in parents continues to be a common error in primary care (Crocetti et al, 2001; Schmitt, 1980). Physicians apparently err in this direction for two principal reasons: problems within the physician himself or herself, such as insufficient training or excessive anxiety; and pressures from the parents, such as their common urging that something decisive be done about recurrent respiratory infections (see Chapter 10 concerning exaggeration of illness by parents, including Munchausen syndrome by proxy). Possible consequences of overmanagement include generating fear that the child is sicker than he or she really is, producing harm from unnecessary procedures (Sibinga and Carey, 1976), and promoting excessive dependence on the physician and his or her treatment.

Undermanagement and mismanagement and their causes and consequences are sufficiently well known to require no further elaboration here.

Obviously, the primary role of the pediatrician or other clinician is to treat the illness. This means the use of appropriate diagnostic and therapeutic measures with avoidance of the pitfalls already mentioned. In particular, non-illnesses or pseudo-diseases should not be diagnosed or treated. Also, reasonable steps should be taken to help the parents and the child prevent recurrences or spread of the illness. Risk-taking behaviors that predispose to illness and injury should be discouraged.

Nurture the Sick Child

Undoubtedly the most common problem in the medical management of the sick child is that the illness itself is treated but the person with the problem is neglected. The clinician may be inadequately sensitive and attentive to the emotional needs of the sick child. The cause is usually a narrowness of interest or a deficiency of empathy. This preoccupation with the illness itself makes it more likely that the experience will be more frightening and stressful for the child than it needs to be.

On the other hand, overattention to the child's feelings, as with our own children or those of our friends or colleagues, with whom we are too closely involved emotionally, may mean that sound professional judgment and proper diagnosis and treatment are in jeopardy (Carey and Sibinga, 1968).

Third, inappropriate handling of the child—with dishonesty or belittling of his or her concerns for whatever reason—must invariably make the illness experience more hazardous for the child.

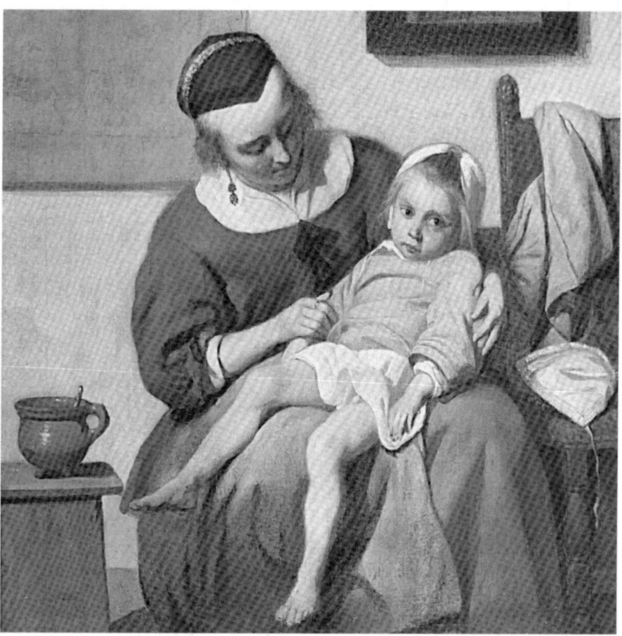

Figure 32-2. Acute minor illnesses can have significant behavioral impact. *(Gabriel Metsu: The Sick Child. With permission from the Rijksmuseum–Stichting Museum, Amsterdam.)*

Nurturing the sick child means that the physician can reduce the stress of the illness by keeping the discomfort, trauma, and restrictions of the management to a minimum; that he or she can promote the child's adjustment to the illness by listening to the child's concerns and responding to them honestly and supportively; and, at times, that the illness experience can even be an opportunity for psychological growth (Fig. 32-2). By learning about the illness and his or her ability to tolerate discomfort and to overcome a problem with the help of the family and physician, the child can gain in self-confidence and avoid developing a sense of physical inferiority or personal inadequacy (Parmelee, 1997).

Support the Parents

Although it may be difficult to define what support for the parents should consist of, there is little problem in identifying unsupportive patterns in the physician-parent relationship. These errors in management are attributable to a variety of professional and personal failings in the physician.

Two common errors are overdomination and oversubmissiveness. The playing of too dominant a role by the physician in the care of minor illness stifles self-reliance in parents, as when the physician attempts to dictate every detail of the management and leaves nothing to the parents' own resources. Too much submission to the parents' wishes results in abdication of the physician's proper advisory status. Pleasing parents is a reasonable objective but not when it goes, for example, to the extent of allowing parents to change the physician's mind about use of an antibiotic.

Neglect of the parents entails not giving sufficient attention to their feelings, their need for information, or their help in handling the illness. Insufficient empathy for the parents and being excessively busy are two common sources of this problem. Neglected parents become confused and helpless and are likely to turn elsewhere for assistance.

Inappropriate handling of the parents, such as giving them misinformation about the illness or its management, or doing anything that needlessly upsets them, is, of course, likely to leave them with feelings of incompetence and perhaps with an unwarranted attachment to the physician through fear or misguided gratitude. The vignette at the beginning of the chapter is an example of this phenomenon.

Probably the best way to be supportive to parents with a sick child is to determine their needs and expectations, to help them deal with the illness and the sick child, to be available in case of further need, and to promote their general self-confidence in handling illness. Following the general guidelines for establishing and maintaining the therapeutic alliance (see Chapters 75 and 86), this process includes listening to the parents' concerns, supplying needed information, helping them use their own ideas and resources as much as possible, giving suggestions about altering potentially dangerous remedies, and providing reassurance. Ineffective but harmless home remedies need not be routinely disapproved. If the parents' fears are disproportionate to the situation, their basis deserves some investigation.

Well-supported, self-reliant parents are more likely to manage well the illness and the child, to relieve the physician of needless repetition of instructions, and to face other aspects of child rearing with greater confidence.

SUMMARY

The average American pediatrician spends about half of his or her time dealing with minor illnesses, yet problems in development and behavior related to minor illness and its management have been largely ignored. There can be little doubt that the child's developmental and behavioral status affect the experience of and reaction to the illness. The extent of the impact of acute minor illnesses on the child's development and behavior is certainly considerable but demands greater clarification. The discussion deals both with the dangers of "pediatric pathogenesis" and with the great opportunities for promotion of the child's progress and mental health through skillful handling of these events. It remains a major area for expansion of knowledge through research and for enhancement of professional skills.

REFERENCES

Carey WB, Sibinga MS: Should pediatricians provide medical care for their friends' children? Pediatrics 42:106, 1968.

Carey WB, Sibinga MS: Avoiding pediatric pathogenesis in the management of acute minor illness. Pediatrics 49:553, 1972.

Crocetti M, Moghbeli N, Serwint J: Fever phobia revisited: Have parental misconceptions about fever changed in 20 years? Pediatrics 107:1241, 2001.

Cunningham AS: Beware overtreating children. Am J Dis Child 143:786, 1989.

Freud A: The role of bodily illness in the mental life of children. Psychoanalytic Study Child 7:69, 1952.

Heymann SJ, Earle A, Egleston B: Parental availability for the care of sick children. Pediatrics 98:226, 1996.

Parmelee AH Jr: Illness and the development of social competence. J Dev Behav Pediatr 18:120, 1997.

Richtsmeier AJ, Hatcher JW: Parental anxiety and minor illness. J Dev Behav Pediatr 15:14, 1994.

Schmitt BD: Fever phobia: Misconceptions of parents about fevers. Am J Dis Child 134:176, 1980.

Sibinga MS, Carey WB: Dealing with unnecessary medical trauma to children. Pediatrics 57:800, 1976.

33 HOSPITALIZATION, SURGERY, AND MEDICAL AND DENTAL PROCEDURES

ELLEN C. PERRIN AND DEBORAH SHIPMAN

In 2000, children and adolescents 1 to 17 years old accounted for 5% of hospital stays in the United States. More and more hospitalizations of children are the result of trauma or are associated with the management of a chronic physical illness. Children with acute illnesses are often cared for outside the hospital, and many elective surgical procedures are performed in day-surgery units. These changes have come about largely as a result of efforts to contain escalating health care costs but also in part because of the recognition among health care professionals and parents that hospitalization itself is associated with extra stresses to children and their families that may be avoided by alternative methods of care.

In addition to hospitalization, children and adolescents experience stress from outpatient medical procedures and surgery and even routine visits to the dentist. All of these represent an underlying loss of control and an alteration in the rhythms of a child's everyday life. Even routine venipuncture at the time of a yearly health maintenance visit can cause anxiety in children. Outpatient or day surgery has become the norm for many routine surgical procedures, including such common procedures as placement of myringotomy tubes and dental surgery. The increased number of these types of procedures has led to an increased recognition of the needs of children before, during, and after these traumatic events. The need for parental involvement has been increasingly recognized as vital in preparing a child for and supporting the child through medical procedures.

Major changes in hospital structure, design, and policies have created an environment that is increasingly supportive to children and families and have radically altered the experience of hospitalization during the past half-century (Thompson, 1986). A great deal of literature has become available for parents and for children to prepare them for hospitalization, and many medical centers provide tours and preparation programs for children anticipating surgery and hospitalization. Wards and patient rooms are designed more appropriately, and play space, appropriate recreation, and Child Life programming are often available. Hospital policies generally allow and even encourage siblings and friends to visit and one or both parents to room-in with children (in a few states, such policies are formally legislated).

SOURCES OF STRESS

General

In their interaction with the world of medicine, young children often have difficulty understanding what is happening to them. When they are ill, they do not understand what part they have had in causing or controlling the illness or why hospitalization and the associated painful procedures are necessary. Young children cannot comprehend the reasons for such traumatic impositions as separation from their parents, being forced to live temporarily in a strange and sterile environment, having to endure painful procedures (sometimes even with the assistance of their parents), and the pain and discomfort that may be associated with the condition itself. Children up to school age may confuse their condition and their hospitalization with some form of immanent justice (e.g., retribution for a rule they have disobeyed or for unacceptable thoughts or activities).

As children get older, their ideas about the causation of illness become more sophisticated, but they do not understand the complexity of the mechanisms of disease and health until well into adolescence (Perrin and Gerrity, 1981). Their limited understanding of illness and its management results in complicated distortions and bizarre notions of their own ability to affect the onset and outcome of the illness (Schonfeld, 1996). Because health care professionals do not necessarily predict accurately how and what children understand about their illness and its treatment, it is helpful to review with children their conceptions and misconceptions to avoid maladaptive responses (Perrin and Perrin, 1983). No matter what else is occurring related to medical care, children experience, both in reality and in their fantasy, a frightening loss of control. In that children have a greater belief than do adults in the effectiveness of powerful others (usually adults) in determining their health and well-being, they are especially vulnerable to the ineffectiveness of their own actions and wishes.

Medical Procedures and Dental Visits

Children undergo numerous injections and venipunctures early in life. Studies have examined the various parental factors and coping strategies for children undergoing these procedures. Parents can help their children most effectively after they examine their own previous experiences and fears. They can help their child have a less stressful experience if they are psychologically available to them.

Each child will have a unique perspective that is based on temperament, previous experience, and age. Temperamental factors affect both the children's reactions to painful experiences and the ease with which their parents can prepare them for the procedure. Children's cognitive ability affects not only their experience and memory of painful procedures but also their parents' and caregivers' perception of their response to painful procedures. In a study examining the response of children with autism to a needlestick procedure, parents consistently underreported both their child's historical pain sensitivity and their child's pain response during the procedure (Nader et al, 2004).

Statistics from the Centers for Disease Control and Prevention show that in 1991, approximately 20 million children underwent invasive procedures. Children have high levels of anxiety while awaiting medical procedures, and this can affect later interactions with health care professionals and dysfunction in health-seeking behaviors (Zelikovsky et al, 2000). Evidence-based medicine supports the use of cognitive-behavioral techniques for reducing anxiety before and during medical interventions, and these techniques have implications for children's ability to function after the interventions (Melnyk, 2000). The American Academy of Pediatric Dentistry has developed guidelines for the use of "behavior guidance" techniques, which they define as "a continuum of interaction involving the dentist, the patient, and the parent directed toward communication and education." Behavior guidance is considered important not only to facilitate dental examination and procedures but to increase compliance with recommended oral health practices outside of the office setting.

Surgery

The effects of anesthesia and surgery on children's development have been studied extensively. These medical procedures can affect children's cognitive, emotional, and behavioral development. A high level of "preoperative anxiety" is one of the most important factors in predicting the development of such disorders as enuresis, sleep disturbances, and changes in mood (Calda et al, 2004). Higher levels of anxiety before surgery have direct physiologic effects that cause poor wound healing and susceptibility to infection (McCann and Zeev, 2001). Children who experience greater levels of anxiety before surgery are at risk for increased pain and general poor cooperation with medical staff (Kain et al, 2006). The level of parental anxiety also contributes to outcomes and is equally important to address before surgery (Melnyk and Feinstein, 2001). An examination of risk factors that predict higher stress levels should be undertaken to identify children at greatest risk and to tailor preoperative procedures appropriately.

Table 33-1. **Sources of Anxiety Related to Hospitalization**

Separation from parents, siblings, friends
New adults and children
Disruption of usual routines
Unfamiliar food, bed, clothes, rules
Interruption of schoolwork
Painful and frightening procedures
Guilt, shame
Poor understanding of the experience
Loss of control; enforced dependency
Worry about body integrity, death
Loss of privacy
Parental anxiety

Hospitalization

Admission to a hospital is disruptive and bewildering; even after multiple admissions, children report anxiety about and discomfort from the process of entering this strange and frightening world (Table 33-1). The child who is admitted to a hospital is separated from the usual surroundings and routines of his or her everyday life: the support and care of parents, everyday interactions with siblings, school life, and social and sports activities with friends. These interruptions are frequently unplanned, are usually unpleasant, and interfere with children's efforts to maintain autonomy and control. In addition, they generally occur when the child is already anxious and uncomfortable or in pain related to the illness or trauma that precipitated the hospitalization. Even for the few children with severe chronic illnesses who spend many days in the hospital, their smoother adjustment to hospital life and routines comes at a cost in disruption of normal social and emotional development.

At the time of hospitalization, children encounter new routines and new adult caretakers and meet other children with a variety of medical problems. They are automatically thrown into a bizarre and unfamiliar environment in which even the most basic functions, such as eating and sleeping, are different from their normal pattern and are under someone else's control. They are introduced to a variety of new technologic equipment and all of the flashing lights and beeps that go with these devices. They may undergo a number of procedures that begin during the process of being admitted to the hospital; these are at the least unfamiliar and often accompanied by discomfort or pain. Almost every child is subjected to poking and pricking, physical restraints, dietary changes, restriction in activity, and perhaps isolation.

EFFECTS ON CHILDREN

Most children who are hospitalized with current hospital procedures are able to cope effectively without any lasting effects on their behavior (Vernon and Thompson, 1993). Children in the most vulnerable age groups, those in whom the preexisting nurturing relationships are tenuous, and those for whom the detrimental or frightening effects of the illness or trauma are overwhelming may cope poorly and require extra attention.

Table 33-2. Common Behavioral Symptoms after Hospitalization or Surgery

Regression (thumb sucking, bed-wetting, baby talk)	Sleep disturbances
Conflicts about eating	Aggressiveness, acting out
Increased dependency	Fear of physicians and nurses
School phobia	Depression
Decreased attentiveness; academic failure	Encopresis

There has been extensive investigation of the psychological impact of hospitalization. The initial work focused primarily on the effects of the separation from parents that accompanied a hospital stay (Douglas, 1975) and began to explore children's fears about their body integrity when faced with surgery or extended illness (Davenport and Werry, 1970). Through the 1970s, there were many further elaborations of the vulnerability of children to the many unique stresses of hospitalization and descriptions of the character, extent, and longevity of the behavioral evidence of children's subsequent distress (Gabriel and Danilowicz, 1978; Quinton and Rutter, 1976; Vernon et al, 1975). Since the late 1970s, a large number of interventions have been designed to prevent or to ameliorate children's distress. Most evaluations have concluded that such programs are beneficial, as evidenced by less maladaptive behavior after hospitalization, more rapid physiologic signs of recovery, and growth in both knowledge and understanding (Watson and Visram, 2003).

Emotional difficulties are greatest among children between 6 months and 6 years of age and increase markedly if hospitalization is long or recurs frequently. Parents and teachers of children recently hospitalized report behavior problems suggestive of difficulties with separation, fearfulness, and regression (Table 33-2) (Thompson and Vernon, 1993). The number of children who demonstrate behavior problems in this period is greater among children with two or more admissions or who stayed in the hospital more than 2 weeks than among those with a single or a shorter admission. Because children with chronic illnesses are likely to be admitted to hospitals more frequently and to stay longer than generally healthy children, it is possible that these findings are confounded with the known increased prevalence of behavior problems in children with chronic illnesses (Perrin et al, 1993). Davenport and Werry (1970) found no effects of hospitalization 2 weeks after hospital stays of less than 48 hours. There is a direct relationship between difficulties with adjustment after discharge and the amount of visiting the child is allowed (and therefore the amount of separation the child experiences while in the hospital). Studies comparing inpatient treatment with day surgery or outpatient care have demonstrated that although medical outcome was equivalent, hospitalized children displayed higher levels of overall psychological upset than did the group treated on an outpatient basis (Scaife and Campbell, 1988).

Children's prior experience with illness and hospitalization (their own, their peers', or family members') informs their reactions to hospitalization and procedures. It is often helpful to understand children's recent experiences or memories to help them separate their current experience from other experiences. Children's intelligence and temperamental style also contribute to their ability to manage and to cope with the stresses and threats they confront in hospitalization. Parents can often be helpful in anticipating children's usual reactions to new circumstances, painful or threatening procedures, and separations. Commercially available books and videotapes may guide parents in their support of their children (Perrin and Starr, 2000).

Parents' attitudes toward the child's illness or condition, and their own experiences with hospitalization and illness, may also profoundly influence their child's reaction to hospitalization and the child's ability to cope with it. Parents for whom the illness or trauma and hospitalization generate an apparently excessive amount of anxiety may be helped by learning specific stress management techniques (e.g., hypnosis, deep relaxation, meditation) that may also be helpful for their children. Numerous studies have confirmed that parents can be taught to help their children manage painful procedures by using these techniques (Powers et al, 2005). It is important to provide parents with opportunities to get information about their children, to be able to express their concerns and fears to the clinicians working with their children, and, in some cases, to share their emotional reactions and concerns in a caring and safe support group environment. Support groups in the context of children's hospital wards might include such topics as dealing with terminal illness, guilt, financial concerns, working with siblings, and strategies for coping with the subsequent physical and emotional needs of the index child and the rest of the family. Many children's hospitals have created libraries geared to providing information about childhood illness and chronic health issues for children, adolescents, and parents.

EFFECTS OF CHILDREN'S ILLNESSES, PAIN, AND PROCEDURES ON CLINICIANS

It is challenging for nurses, residents, and senior physicians to watch children bewildered, confused, and in pain. Health care providers must understand their own feelings about illness and death as well as about the necessity for painful procedures to be effective in providing support to children. It is helpful for all members of the health care team to be involved collaboratively with parents in important decisions about the care provided to children and families. Conflicts among members of the professional team regarding the division of labor, control of decision making, and responsibility for communication can seriously undermine children's care. Clinicians may identify powerfully with children, or with their parents, and find that such identification interferes with their ability to make dispassionate clinical decisions and to enforce hospital regulations. Past family and personal history with illness, hospitalization, and death may color their ability to deal directly with

Table 33-3. **Opportunities Related to Hospitalization**

Parents and children have the opportunity to
Demonstrate and receive nurturing by parents, siblings, friends
Increase knowledge and skills about the child's illness and its care
Increase participation in care
Foster communication with health care professionals
Develop or enlarge social networks
Increase available support
Improve understanding of general mechanisms of health and illness
Improve confidence and sense of mastery
Health care professionals have the opportunity to
Develop an alliance with the child
Observe the child for an extended time (play, interactions with peers, family members, adults)
Assess family's strengths and needs
Observe pattern of the illness, response to medications
Provide education, modeling
Obtain consultations
Encourage self-care and increase participation and confidence

the powerful affective responses certain children and families may evoke in them. Neither excessive identification nor artificial distancing from children and families is optimally helpful to their patients.

Professionals may have the greatest difficulty in maintaining open communication with children and parents when the child's condition and needed procedures are particularly painful for them. Silence may be interpreted by the child as abandonment or anger as the result of his or her condition and thus may compound the intrinsic difficulty of the circumstance. The death of a child in the hospital is one of the most stressful personal and professional experiences faced by health care providers. It may trigger a grief response similar to that following a personal loss. It is important for health care professionals to have permission and support to discuss these experiences and to have their personal needs met at these times. It is often helpful to encourage some introspection about their own history of losses and a discussion of the impact of their patient's death on their personal and professional lives. Such social institutions as funerals and memorial services can be as helpful to health care providers as they are to families. In some hospital settings, teams of professionals organize support systems to ensure that the expertise and skills of members of multiple related disciplines are available to address these issues. Such support systems often include representatives from the clergy, Child Life, nursing, psychiatry, psychology, and social work (see Chapter 36).

OPPORTUNITIES FOR PREVENTION AND INTERVENTION

Hospitalization is an opportunity for a child's "medical home" to play an important role in the provision of coordinated care. The medical home provider should partner with parents to ensure that the child's medical needs and the child's and family's emotional needs are met. The role of the medical home provider includes preparing families for hospitalization, communicating with providers in the hospital, and helping families interpret medical information and communicate with hospital personnel. Children and families can sometimes grow through an illness or a hospitalization (Parmelee, 1993; Solnit, 1960) as outlined in Table 33-3. Illness and hospitalization provide opportunities for parents and siblings to care for and nurture the child. The experience provides opportunities for children to increase their understanding of their illness and its care, to increase participation in their own care, and to communicate with health care providers, their parents, and other children about the illness. Hospitalization may be a time when both parents and children can expand their social network, meeting children and families with medical concerns similar to their own. It also provides an opportunity for parents to learn more about their child's illness, gaining both information and skills; to increase their ability to observe their child; and to increase their sense of competence in their ability to care for the child.

Children's involvement in decision making about their medical care has been shown to enhance self-esteem and overall well-being. Children who are prepared for surgery and are supported through their hospitalization recover more quickly and have few emotional problems related to the surgery. Presurgery programs should inform the child of the nature of the medical intervention, preview the hospital experience, and allow time for the child to process the information in a safe environment (home). Children of different ages will have different needs in terms of information and different ways in which they express their fears and concerns. Many pediatric hospitals and clinics have developed preadmission preparation programs, and they are available to parents through the Internet and in the form of written materials. More general age-appropriate materials can also be helpful in normalizing the experience of medical care and allowing children time to "practice" and accept the future intervention.

It is important that hospital staff be prepared to support parents in their demanding role as children's primary caretakers, both during the hospital stay and afterward. They should encourage participation in resource groups for parents and for older children and should refer parents to the increasing body of literature written for parents and children about surgery, hospitalization, and medical procedures. Decreasing maternal anxiety and facilitating maternal involvement in care can decrease negative behavioral responses of children after hospitalization (Melnyk, 2000). One-to-one parent and family-to-family supports are unique in increasing parents' feeling of competence and improving coping and problem solving skills. Siblings should be given age-appropriate information about their brother's or sister's illness (Kleiber et al, 1995) and encouraged to visit and stay in touch with the hospitalized child. The hospital should recognize the importance of family visitation, including siblings, and liberal visitation policies should be established.

Hospitalization also provides special opportunities for health care professionals. The extended period in the hospital allows them to develop or to strengthen

Table 33-4. Factors Affecting Consequences of Hospitalization

Child's age and development
Whether it is a first or recurrent hospitalization
Length of separation
Prior preparation about hospitals, procedures
Child's temperament, personality, and coping style
Characteristics of illness or injury
Family's response to illness or injury
Family cohesiveness and communication
Procedures or surgery required
Amount of pain and discomfort
Responsiveness of hospital environment
Consistency of hospital personnel

their alliance with the child and to observe his or her play and interactions with other children, with family members, and with caregiving adults. It allows them to observe the family's strengths and its ongoing needs, the pattern of the child's illness and its response to medications, and the child's response to pain. Pediatricians and other health care professionals can also use the hospital environment to obtain consultations, to provide education about the illness and its care, to model appropriate care, and to encourage increased participation in the management of the illness on the part of both the child and the parents, improving compliance with medical recommendations in the future.

MINIMIZING STRESSES

Currently accepted cognitive-behavioral techniques for reducing anxiety before and during medical procedures include such techniques as relaxation through the use of breathing exercises, hypnosis, and distraction with visual imagery or external stimuli such as videos and television. Parents play a broad role in the development of children's coping skills, and they are integral to a child's ability to use learned coping techniques. Parents should take advantage of myriad print and Web site materials that are now available concerning medical care. These materials can provide information, normalize the experience for children, and help children develop coping strategies with the help of their parents. For parents, these materials provide a new level of understanding and empathy for their children. In addition, clinical personnel should be aware of and trained in these techniques so that they may coach children and parents when necessary. Many pediatric hospitals have been proactive in encouraging parents to take part in preparing their children for medical procedures and for coping with pain during and after procedures. For children who routinely undergo invasive medical procedures, ongoing training (e.g., in yoga or relaxation and meditation techniques) can be beneficial.

Current recommendations from the American Dental Society stress the importance of predicting the child's reaction by taking into account developmental level, attitudes toward dental care, and temperament. There is an emphasis on communication with the child and individualized techniques. Communication with parents as to expected procedures is also an important influence on the future behavior of the child. Studies have shown that maternal "dental anxiety" contributes to the child's overall experience of dental care. Parents should share in the decision making process about behavior guidance and treatment. Last, when children are not able to control their fear reaction or become hysterical during treatment, the dentist should decide on the medical necessity of the procedure, consult with parents, and opt to discontinue treatment when appropriate. Further communication with the child and parents and use of alternative behavior guidance techniques may allow needed (but not life-threatening) treatment in the future.

A number of variables affect the balance of positive and negative outcomes from a child's hospitalization (Table 33-4). What a child and family experience and learn from a hospital stay is strongly influenced by hospital procedures (Table 33-5) and by its health care professionals (Plank, 1971).

Numerous studies have demonstrated unequivocally that systematic preparation for hospitalization or surgery not only reduces children's psychological distress during and after a hospitalization but also results in more adaptive physiologic responses (Melamed and Ridley-Johnson, 1988). Prepared children have been documented to be more cooperative with procedures, to have less resistance to anesthetic induction, to have lower heart rate and blood pressure, to require fewer

Table 33-5. Minimization of Stress

Before Hospitalization
Outpatient procedures, evaluation, and treatment whenever possible
Involvement of parents in decisions about procedures and hospitalizations
Television, school, and community programs about illness and hospitals
Prehospitalization tours
Specific information about planned procedures and hospitalizations
Parents present as much as possible
During Hospitalization
Rooming-in for parents
Encourage visiting for siblings, peers, extended family
Child Life program (recreation and therapeutic play)
Limited number of nurses and other caregivers
Child's choice of clothes, food, activities
Maximal mobility
Pain control
Procedures
Limited number
Preparation of child
Child's choice of when, where, and with whom
Limited waiting time
Parents accompany and support child
Hospital Structure
Rooming-in facilities
Play space
Waiting space near operating and recovery rooms
Comfortable accommodations for parents
Cheerful, child-oriented decor
Single- and double-bed rooms

medications during the recovery period, and to take less time to first voiding and adequate fluid intake after a surgical procedure than children who were not formally prepared before their surgery.

The number of hospital admissions should be kept to a minimum, and their length should be limited as much as possible. It is advisable to avoid hospitalization between the ages of 6 months and 4 years. Health professionals should encourage education about health, illness, and hospitals through television and in schools and should facilitate children's hospital tours and meetings with other children and their families who are or who have recently been in the hospital. All children should participate in an organized program preparing them for the experiences associated with planned surgical or diagnostic procedures (inpatient or outpatient) and hospital stays. Parents should participate in all aspects of planning for and care of children hospitalized or having outpatient procedures.

The factor under the most direct control of health care professionals is the nature of the hospital environment itself and the manner in which surgery and other procedures are carried out. Every pediatric hospital should have a playroom with opportunities for recreation and developmentally appropriate activities to help children deal effectively with their illness, trauma, medical care, and hospitalization. Play provides opportunities for children to re-create a familiar experience that can comfort them and make the hospital setting less threatening. Pediatric hospital units should have a trained staff of Child Life professionals who participate in decisions about the manner and scheduling of children's procedures and who are integrally involved in preparing children and parents for hospitalization, surgery, and procedures. These professionals provide individualized services to children that focus on the child's strengths, present developmentally appropriate information to children, and establish therapeutic relationships with children and parents (Neff, 2000).

School programs for children of all ages should be integrated into the larger Child Life program to facilitate learning from the child's experiences with illness and hospitalization as well as from prescribed curricula. At one pediatric hospital, a "school room" staffed by teachers is available to hospitalized school-age children, and bedside teaching is available as well. Children who keep up with assignments and learning during hospitalization have a less difficult time reentering school after hospitalization. To the greatest extent possible, children should stay connected to their classmates and teachers. Friends may be able to visit, and children can use e-mail, phone calls, or letters to stay in touch. Teachers can help by initiating class projects that provide pictures and cards for hospitalized students. This allows children to maintain all important social contacts during prolonged hospitalizations or stays at home. Psychologists, social workers, and psychiatrists are often helpful as members of the overall health care team.

Nurses should be assigned in such a way as to minimize the number of different adults caring for a child. Parents should be encouraged to stay with their child as much as possible, and liberal visiting hours should allow friends, teachers, and siblings to visit frequently.

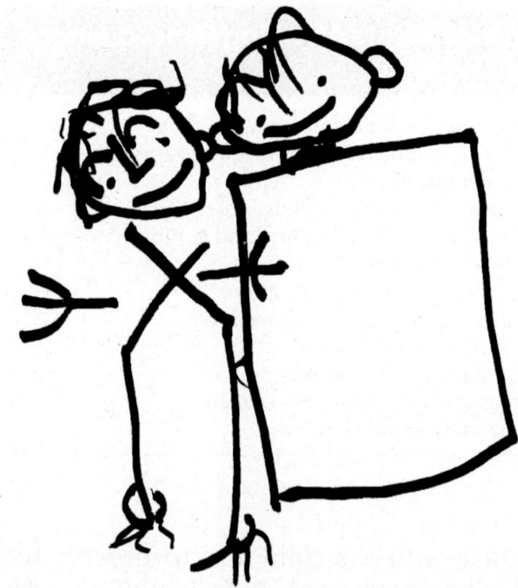

Figure 33-1. A 4-year-old child's expression of feeling about the importance of parental presence in the hospital.

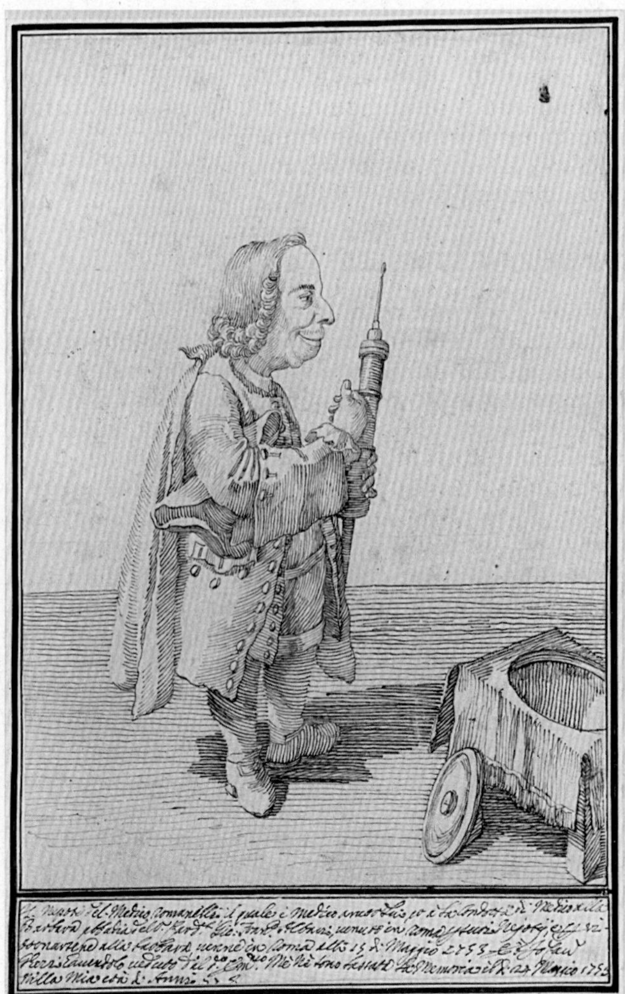

Figure 33-2. Health care professionals can control the nature of the hospital environment to minimize frightening experiences such as this. *(Ghezzi, Pierleone: Doctor Holding an Enema Syringe Caricature. Philadelphia Museum of Art: Purchased with funds from the SmithKline Beecham [formerly Beckman] Corporation for the Ars Medica Collection.)*

Pediatric hospitals can be constructed in such a way that children have opportunities both for being alone or with their family or close friends and for group activities with their peers. This means that rooms with one or two beds and space for parents to stay are preferable to larger wards. Parents should be encouraged to participate in decision making and care as active members of the health care team (Fig. 33-1).

Procedures, even minor ones such as drawing blood, initiation of intravenous therapy, and radiographic studies, are best limited to those that are absolutely necessary for the child's care. Children should be honestly and appropriately informed about procedures, and whenever possible, they should be performed at a time, with people, and in a place of the child's choice. Parents should be present whenever possible. Maintaining the child's mobility and autonomy and limiting pain and discomfort are important ways to safeguard the child's security and well-being (Fig. 33-2).

The professionals caring for children in the hospital should be prepared to explain to children and their parents the mechanisms involved in their illness or injury, the plans for its care, and the expected outcomes of treatment. They should facilitate and encourage children's taking the maximum possible control of necessary procedures and other aspects of managing their illness both during the hospitalization and after discharge.

SUMMARY

A child's developmental-behavioral status can both influence and be influenced by medical care experiences, including medical procedures, dental care, surgery, and hospitalizations. Physicians should be aware of the stresses involved in these experiences and the effects they may have on children. Many opportunities for minimizing the stresses on children and their families can make the experiences as positive as possible. Health care clinicians should also be cognizant of the personal impact that these experiences may have on them. Health care professionals helping parents and children to cope with these intrusions should refer to the extensive materials available through many children's hospital Web sites, the Institute for Family-Centered Care, and many others available commercially.

REFERENCES

Calda J, Pais-Ribeiro J, Carneiro S: General anesthesia, surgery and hospitalization in children and their effects upon cognitive, academic, emotional and sociobehavioral development—a review. Paediatr Anaesth 14:910-915, 2004.

Davenport H, Werry J: The effect of general anesthesia, surgery, and hospitalization upon the behavior of children. Am J Orthopsychiatry 40:806-824, 1970.

Douglas J: Early hospital admissions and later disturbances of behavior and learning. Dev Med Child Neurol 17:456-480, 1975.

Gabriel HP, Danilowicz D: Post-operative responses in "prepared" children after cardiac surgery. Br Heart J 40:1046-1051, 1978.

Kain Z, Mayes L, Caldwell-Andrews A, et al: Preoperative anxiety, postoperative pain, and behavioral recovery in young children undergoing surgery. Pediatrics 118:651-658, 2006.

Kleiber C, Montgomery LA, Craft-Rosenberg M: Information needs of the siblings of critically ill children. Child Health Care 24:47-60, 1995.

McCann E, Zeev N: The management of preoperative anxiety in children: An update. Anesth Analg 93:98-105, 2001.

Melamed B, Ridley-Johnson R: Psychological preparation of families for hospitalization. J Dev Behav Pediatr 9:96-102, 1988.

Melnyk B: Intervention studies involving parents of hospitalized young children: An analysis of the past and future recommendations. J Pediatr Nurs 15:4-13, 2000.

Melnyk B, Feinstein F: Mediating functions of maternal anxiety and participation in care on young children's posthospital adjustment. Res Nurs Health 24:18-26, 2001.

Nader R, Oberlander T, Chambers C, Craig K: Expression of pain in children with autism. Clin J Pain 20:88-97, 2004.

Neff J; American Academy of Pediatrics, Committee on Hospital Care: Child life services. Pediatrics 106:1156-1159, 2000.

Parmelee AH Jr: Children's illnesses and normal behavioral development: The role of caregivers. Zero to Three 13:4-10, 1993.

Perrin EC, Gerrity PS: There's a demon in your belly: Children's understanding of illness. Pediatrics 67:841-849, 1981.

Perrin EC, Newacheck P, Pless IB, et al: Issues involved in the definition and classification of chronic health conditions. Pediatrics 91:787-793, 1993.

Perrin EC, Perrin JM: Clinicians' assessments of children's understanding of illness. Am J Dis Child 137:874-878, 1983.

Perrin EC, Starr S: Addressing common pediatric concerns through children's books. Pediatr Rev 21:130-138, 2002.

Plank E: Working with Children in Hospitals. Cleveland, Case Western Reserve University Press, 1971.

Powers S, Jones S, Jones B: Behavioral and cognitive-behavioral interventions with pediatric populations. Clin Child Psychol Psychiatry 10:65-77, 2005.

Quinton D, Rutter M: Early hospital admissions and later disturbances of behavior. Dev Med Child Neurol 18:447-459, 1976.

Scaife J, Campbell I: A comparison of the outcome of day care and inpatient treatment of pediatric surgical cases. J Child Psychol Psychiatry 29:185-198, 1988.

Schonfeld DJ: The child's cognitive understanding of illness. *In* Lewis M (ed): Child and Adolescent Psychiatry: A Comprehensive Textbook. Baltimore, Williams & Wilkins, 1996, pp. 943-947.

Solnit AJ: Hospitalization: An aid to physical and psychological health in childhood. Am J Dis Child 99:155-163, 1960.

Thompson R: Where we stand: Twenty years of research on pediatric hospitalization and health care. Child Health Care 14:200-210, 1986.

Thompson RH, Vernon DT: Research on children's behavior after hospitalization. J Dev Behav Pediatr 14:28-35, 1993.

Vernon D, Foley J, Sipowicz R, Shulman J: The Psychological Responses of Children to Hospitalization and Illness. Springfield, IL, Charles C Thomas, 1975.

Vernon DT, Thompson RH: Research on the effect of experimental interventions on children's behavior after hospitalization. J Dev Behav Pediatr 14:36-44, 1993.

Watson A, Visram A: Children's preoperative anxiety and postoperative behaviour. Paediatr Anaesth 13:188-204, 2003.

Zelikovsky N, Rodrigue J, Gidycz C, Davis M: Cognitive behavioral and behavioral interventions help young children cope during a voiding cystourethrogram. J Pediatr Psychol 25:535-543, 2000.

RESOURCES FOR CHILDREN AND FAMILIES

Many books describing hospitalization, medical procedures, trauma, and acute illness are available for children of all ages.

Institute for Family-Centered Care. Available at: www.familycenteredcare.org. 7900 Wisconsin Ave, Suite 405, Bethesda, MD 20814; (301) 652-0281; institute@iffcc.org.

MEDLINEplus has an illustrated online medical encyclopedia that allows parents and children to look up all kinds of procedures so that they will know what to expect.

PBS: Talking with kids about health. Available at: www.pbs.org/parents/talkingwithkids/health/.

Starbright World is a free online community that connects kids living with chronic and serious illness and offers illness-related computer games to teach kids through play. Available at: www.starbright.org/projects/sbw/index.html.

Sesame Solutions: Health provides health-related games, stories, and activities for kids, starring Sesame Street characters plus advice for parents on communication. Available at: sesameworkshop.org/parents/solutions/health.

The Dougy Center for Grieving Children provides age-appropriate information and resources for children who have experienced the death of a parent or sibling. Available at: www.dougy.org/.

Band-Aides and Blackboards is a gathering place for kids who are growing up with medical problems where they can tell their story and read about other kids in similar circumstances. Available at: www.lehman.cuny.edu/faculty/jfleitas/bandaides.

KidsHealth offers health games and information for kids plus relevant advice for parents. Available at: www.kidshealth.org/index.html.

34 EARLY HEALTH CRISES AND VULNERABLE CHILDREN

Brian W. C. Forsyth

Vignette

The mother of a newborn infant asks if the baby's glucose test could be repeated before hospital discharge "just to be sure he's okay." The pediatrician starts to reassure her that repeating the test is not necessary because the glucose concentration was found to be normal shortly after birth and is no longer a concern now that the baby is older. The mother, however, appears quite anxious about her healthy newborn, so the pediatrician decides on a different approach and instead asks her about her pregnancy and whether she had had any problems. She relates a story that includes a threatened abortion and prolonged bed rest, and when asked whether there was ever a time that she thought "he might not make it," she becomes tearful and talks about an earlier miscarriage. This conversation allows the pediatrician to acknowledge her fears, to express empathy, and to talk about the fact that when someone has been as fearful about her child as she has, such fears can persist, despite her baby's being so healthy. He comments that it will be important for them to continue to discuss this as her child grows, leaving this as an opening so that at future clinic visits he can relate again to this conversation and address the fears and parental behaviors that can result in the vulnerable child syndrome.

Green and Solnit (1964) first coined the phrase "the vulnerable child syndrome" in a paper describing children with severe behavioral and learning problems, all of whom had a history of experiencing a serious illness or accident early in life. Although these children had recovered fully from the early life-threatening events, their parents continued to view them as abnormally susceptible to illness or death. These continuing parental fears, and the resulting abnormal interactions between the parents and their children, were considered responsible for the children's abnormal psychological development. Although this concept had been described previously in the literature, this landmark paper with its use of the term *vulnerable child* brought focus to a psychodynamic process in which the major etiologic factor is the parents' perceptions of vulnerability rather than other factors that might make the child truly vulnerable for adverse outcomes.

Presently, the term *vulnerable child syndrome* is reserved for children who demonstrate all aspects of the syndrome as described by Green and Solnit (Table 34-1). The term *vulnerable child* is commonly used to refer to instances in which parents perceive their children to be abnormally susceptible to illness or death, although the children do not necessarily exhibit the consequences of the parents' abnormal perceptions.

There is a spectrum of vulnerability, with the vulnerable child syndrome representing the extreme end of the spectrum. Both the etiology of vulnerability and the resulting sequelae may be varied; less severe experiences than a near-death experience, such as problems with crying behavior in early infancy, may cause parents to view their child as abnormally vulnerable (Forsyth and Canny, 1991). Similarly, the expression of the disorder might be different; for example, a child who is viewed by parents as vulnerable might be brought to the physician more frequently for minor medical complaints but might not necessarily demonstrate the psychological or behavioral consequences described in the vulnerable child syndrome.

PREVELANCE OF VULNERABILITY

The true prevalence of perceived vulnerability is difficult to ascertain because it is dependent on the way in which vulnerability is defined. In a community-based study of 1095 children aged 4 to 8 years who were being seen by health care providers, 10% of parents viewed their children as vulnerable with use of the Child Vulnerability Scale (Forsyth et al, 1996). Twenty-one percent of all mothers reported that they had prior fears that their child might die. However, with use of the definitions employed in the study, only 1.8% of children had all three features of the vulnerable child syndrome: (1) prior fears that the child might die, (2) continuing perceptions of vulnerability, and (3) behavior problems (as defined by the Child Behavior Checklist). In another study conducted in medical clinics, 27% of children were described by their parents as vulnerable (i.e., "uniquely threatened by an episode of illness"), although for 40% of these, there was no medical basis for concern (Levy, 1980).

Table 34-1. Diagnostic Criteria for the Vulnerable Child Syndrome

An event early in the child's life that the parent considered to be life-threatening
The parent's continuing unrealistic belief that the child is especially susceptible to illness or death
The presence of a behavioral or learning problem in the child

From Forsyth BWC: Vulnerable children. *In* Parker SJ, Zuckerman BS, Augustyn MC (eds): Developmental and Behavioral Pediatrics, 2nd ed. Philadelphia, Lippincott Williams & Wilkins, 2005.

ETIOLOGY OF VULNERABILITY

A number of different types of events and illnesses have been described in the literature as contributing to increased parental perceptions of vulnerability (Table 34-2). Examples include complications of pregnancy (Burger et al, 1993), premature birth (Perrin, 1989), neonatal jaundice (Kemper et al, 1989), hospitalization for infectious illnesses, and problems of feeding and crying behavior in early infancy (Forsyth and Canny, 1991). Some of these are truly life-threatening events, whereas others are minor problems that are medically insignificant; it is the parents' understanding and beliefs about the problem that are most important in contributing to perceptions of vulnerability, rather than the reality of the diagnosis as understood by the physician (Carey, 1969). A particular example of this has been referred to in the literature as nondisease to describe such entities as innocent cardiac murmurs (Bergman and Stamm, 1967) and sickle cell trait (Hampton et al, 1974), which to the physician are of little consequence but which parents may view with concern and, as a result, treat their child differently.

In general, the earlier in a child's life that an event occurs, the more likely it is to contribute to the parents' perceptions that the child is vulnerable. In some instances, the event that initiates the parents' fears for a child may not be related to a condition of the child but may have occurred before the child's birth, for example, an earlier miscarriage or the experience of the death of a previous child. Also, a crisis that occurred around the time of a mother's pregnancy, such as an illness or death of a close relative, might contribute to irrational fears of death. The newborn period is a time when parents are likely to be particularly anxious about their child's well-being, and medical care that is insensitive to their understanding and concerns might contribute to long-standing perceptions of vulnerability.

In a review of published research related to the vulnerable child syndrome, Thomasgard and Metz (1995) identified a number of other parental factors that have been associated with vulnerability; for example, perceptions of vulnerability are more prevalent among women who are unmarried, are younger, are less educated, and have lower family incomes. Psychological factors that can contribute to a parent's tendency to view a child as vulnerable include a lack of support and a lack of emotional warmth in relationships; maternal depression, particularly in the postpartum period; and a lack of sense of competence in being a parent and feeling less in control of one's life (Estroff et al, 1994). In a follow-up study of premature infants, maternal anxiety measured at the time of discharge from the newborn intensive care unit was the one factor in a multivariate analysis that was later associated with increased perceptions of vulnerability when the children were aged 1 year (Allen et al, 2004).

Table 34-2. Antecedents of the Vulnerable Child

Preexisting
Death of a relative or previous child early in life
Prior miscarriage or stillbirth
Pregnancy Related
Pregnancy complications (e.g., vaginal bleeding)
Abnormal screening results (e.g., abnormal α-fetoprotein)
Delivery complications
Newborn Period
Prematurity
Neonatal illness or complications
Congenital abnormalities
Hyperbilirubinemia
False-positive results of screening (e.g., phenylketonuria)
Early Childhood
Excessive crying, colic, spitting up
Any serious illness
Admission to hospital for such things as "to rule out sepsis"
Self-limited infectious illnesses (e.g., croup, gastroenteritis)

From Forsyth BWC: Vulnerable children. *In* Parker SJ, Zuckerman BS, Augustyn MC (eds): Developmental and Behavioral Pediatrics, 2nd ed. Philadelphia, Lippincott Williams & Wilkins, 2005.

Green and Solnit, in their original description of the vulnerable child syndrome, also identified as a predisposing factor a mother's "displacement of unacceptable feelings toward the child or of unacceptable thoughts and reactions associated with the birth of the child." It is important, however, to emphasize that the vulnerable child syndrome is a result of the parent's view of the child as somehow defective and is not due to a lack of emotional bonding between the parent and child.

CLINICAL PRESENTATION OF THE VULNERABLE CHILD

The vulnerable child may present with a number of different types of problems divided by Green and Solnit (1964) into the following major categories.

Difficulties with Separation

An example of this is a parent's reluctance to leave the child in the care of a babysitter. The parent's sense of the child's being vulnerable and the resulting abnormality in interactions with the child lead to a decrease in the child's sense of autonomy and independence. Parents may complain of the child's sleep problems, although this may in part be because the child is sleeping in the parents' bed or the parents are regularly checking on the sleeping child to make sure that the child is still alive.

Symptoms of Infantilization

In some cases, the parents are unable to set appropriate disciplinary limits for the child and are overindulgent and excessively protective of the child. The child may become disobedient and argumentative and may refuse to eat.

Often the child's episodes of negative behavior disintegrate into physical fighting, with hitting and biting, and the parent is unable to handle the behavior appropriately. Most description of children's behavior in the vulnerable child syndrome come from clinical reports, although there has been some research that has examined child behavior. In a follow-up study of premature infants, Allen and colleagues (2004) assessed children when they were 1 year old and demonstrated that increased parental perceptions of vulnerability were associated with an increase in abnormal adaptive behaviors even in those children who had no medical sequelae of prematurity, such as cerebral palsy or growth delay. Importantly, however, there was no association between parental perceptions of vulnerability and either motor development or mental development as measured by the Bayley scale, except in those cases in which there was true medical vulnerability.

Overconcern with Minor Medical Problems

A parent who perceives his or her child to be vulnerable is often a frequent visitor to the clinician for what the clinician considers to be only minor medical problems. There is often excessive focus on such things as the regularity of the child's bowel movements and complaints that the child has a sickly appearance or has circles under the eyes. The child may have psychosomatic problems, such as recurrent abdominal pain or headaches, and may have frequent absences from school. Sometimes Munchausen by proxy syndrome must be considered.

School Underachievement

Even though school underachievement was initially described by Green and Solnit, it is usually not the major presenting problem in the vulnerable child syndrome. The child's school performance may suffer because of distractible, hyperactive behavior in the classroom. The parents' earlier reluctance to separate from the child and the unspoken fear that the child is unsafe out of the parents' presence may be transferred to the child, and the resulting preoccupation and anxiety can interfere with the child's abilities to concentrate and to learn.

MAKING THE DIAGNOSIS

Whenever a clinician sees a child with one or more of the aforementioned problems, the possible etiologic role of an earlier event and abnormal parental perceptions of vulnerability should be considered (Fig. 34-1). To make the diagnosis, the clinician must obtain a history that not only identifies the initiating event but also captures the quality of the parents' fears of the risk to the child and provides insight into the abnormal interaction between the parent and child. In addition, history taking that is sensitive to the fears of the parent helps initiate the therapeutic process by conveying to the parent a sense of understanding and empathy.

Often it is necessary to obtain again the child's medical history, beginning from the mother's pregnancy and including a history of family illnesses or death. Because parents are truly concerned about their child, they usually welcome the suggestion that a full review of everything that has gone on in the past may shed some light on the child's present problems. Whenever the parent reports a prior problem or concern, no matter how minor it was, the details of what the physician said at that time and what the parents understood and feared might be helpful in making the diagnosis. Empathic comments such as "That must have been very frightening to you" and questions such as "Did you at any time fear that he might not make it?" often allow the parents to express their real concerns. If, on the other hand, the event was truly of little concern to the parents, they usually say so. Attention should also be paid to issues of separation, both early in the child's life and when the child starts daycare or school. Questions should be asked about the parents' level of worry when they are separated from their child and how comfortable they are leaving the child with a babysitter.

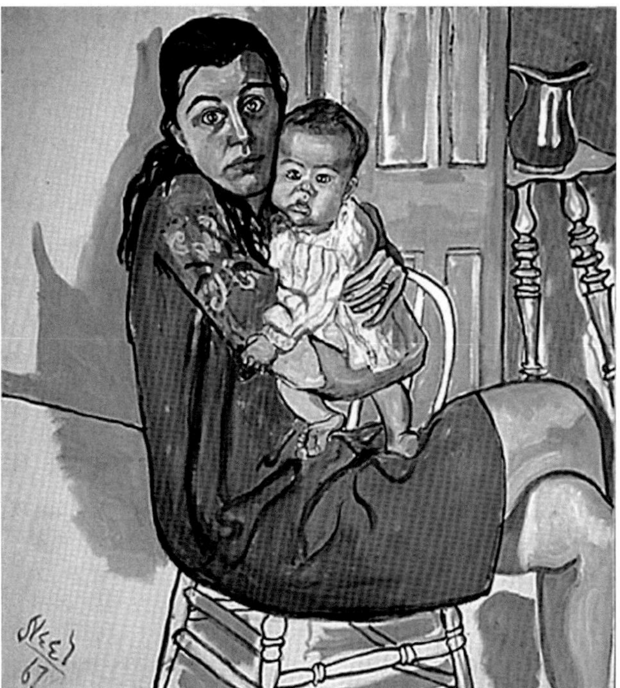

Figure 34-1. **Picture of mother and child.** It is the parents' understanding and beliefs about the problem that are most important in contributing to perceptions of vulnerability, rather than the reality of the diagnosis. *(© 1998 Estate of Alice Neel.)*

Although it is unlikely to be useful in a clinical setting, the Child Vulnerability Scale was developed to be used in research to measure parents' perceptions of their children's vulnerability (Forsyth et al, 1996). Both the clinical history and the Vulnerable Child Scale have been helpful in identifying factors that contribute to vulnerability.

MANAGEMENT

Suggestions for the prevention and management of the vulnerable child syndrome are summarized in Table 34-3.

Prevention

Unfortunately, one of the consequences of present-day advances in technology and the increase in screening for hereditary and congenital disorders is that there is also

Table 34-3. Prevention and Management of the Vulnerable Child Syndrome

Prevention at the Time of the Health Crisis
Understand and discuss parents' beliefs about even minor problems.
Do not use terms, such as allergy and colitis, that suggest a diagnostic entity when there is no real evidence supporting it.
Recognize when parents are particularly anxious about an event and specifically deal with their fears.
Management
After a thorough evaluation, provide a clear statement of the child's physical health.
Help the parents understand the link between the present problem and their past anxieties about their child's health.
Support and advise parents about interacting with their child in an appropriate manner.
Make a referral for a psychiatric evaluation and treatment if necessary.

an increase in false-positive results (Filly, 2000; Getz and Kirkengen, 2003). Whereas a result that is later shown to be falsely positive may have significant implications for parents and the way they view their child, the pediatrician often is unaware of the results of screening tests that are done prenatally, and questions may need to be asked specifically about these when a history of the mother's pregnancy is reviewed. In discussing a false-positive screening test result, there needs to be exploration of the parent's beliefs and understanding and an explanation of the different natures of the two tests (screening versus confirmatory) and conclusive statements that leave no doubt about the correct diagnosis.

Because a parent's understanding of the severity and implications of an illness or event might be very different from reality, it is important that even in minor illnesses the clinician take time to understand parents' beliefs and to discuss them appropriately. Clinicians need to be aware of the implications of the "medicalization" of symptoms that may be concerning to parents but are often within the normal physiologic spectrum. An example of this might be "infantile reflux" and how it is treated. In a study conducted in the United States, 67% of infants between the ages of 4 and 6 months were reported by their parents to have reflux, and 16% of these had been treated with a change of the infant's formula (Nelson et al, 1997). In contrast, a study done in Thailand reported a prevalence of reflux of only 8.4% at 4 months of age, and all of these had been managed with parental reassurance (Osatakul et al, 2002). Whereas ethnicity might explain some of these differences, it is more likely that the approach to the symptom and its management account for the major differences.

Another example is the infant with colic, for which changing of infant formulas is also prevalent (Polack, 1999). Suggesting that the infant is allergic to the formula and requires a "special formula" implies to the parents that the child has a medical problem that requires a specific treatment. In a follow-up study of children reported to have problems of feeding and crying behavior in early infancy, those who had received a formula change were twice as likely to be perceived as vulnerable at age 3½ years compared with those whose problem had been managed without a formula change (Forsyth and Canny, 1991). This would suggest that the clinician's approach to managing a problem of this type can have long-lasting consequences. In this example, if the clinician describes colic as a self-limited condition affecting normal infants, the risk for the parents to perceive their child as vulnerable may be diminished. Some parents may wish to change the formula, but even so, a statement by the clinician ahead of time that the infant can go back to the regular formula within a few weeks serves to emphasize to the parents that this is a self-limited condition without long-lasting effects (see also Chapter 57).

When discharging a child from the hospital after an acute illness, the clinician should review the diagnosis with the parents, emphasize that recovery is or will be complete, and point out that the child is no more vulnerable to illness than other children are. When a parent is particularly anxious after an illness or other event that could later contribute to perceptions of vulnerability, it may be helpful to ask further questions, such as, "Has this brought to mind other things that you've experienced before?" and "Is there anything that you are particularly worried about?" Such questions enable the clinician to deal specifically with the parents' fears and to point out the erroneous links they may have made between two unrelated events. It might also be helpful to question the parents at a later date about an event. Having parents relate their understanding of what went on might help the clinician identify any erroneous beliefs.

Approach to Management

Whenever it is recognized that parental perceptions of vulnerability are affecting or may affect a child's behavior or development, an approach that might be helpful includes the following.

1. The clinician should take an in-depth history and perform a conspicuously meticulous physical examination before giving the parents a clear statement that the child is physically healthy. There should be no equivocal comments, such as "He doesn't look too bad." Conducting laboratory tests just to prove to the parents that there is nothing physically wrong can have the opposite effect of suggesting to them that the clinician is continuing to look for something wrong but has not yet found it.
2. The clinician needs to help the parents understand and accept the notion that the child is considered special by the family and that this derives from their response to earlier events. It is helpful to explain this process as a recognized entity and not something that is particularly unique to them—that parents who experience the level of anxiety that they have continue to be fearful for their child and that this has an effect on the way they interact with their child, sometimes with a deleterious effect on the child.
3. The parents need to be supported in dealing with the child in a more appropriate manner. Advice should be given on setting consistent limits and discontinuing infantilizing behaviors. Issues of overprotection and problems of separation may need to be examined, and parents may need to be advised on how to respond

differently to somatic complaints. In instances when a child probably does have an underlying abnormality (e.g., cerebral palsy after premature birth) but the parents have exaggerated perceptions of their child's vulnerability, the primary care clinician should help the parents distinguish between those issues that are of real concern and those that relate to their past experiences and anxieties. In doing this, the clinician often needs to give parents very specific explanations and advice on how to respond to their child in various circumstances.

4. Although many of these problems can be managed by a primary care clinician, a referral for psychiatric evaluation and therapy may be necessary in some instances. Whether the focus of treatment is primarily on the child or the parents, the importance of the parental perceptions of vulnerability in sustaining the problem needs to remain a central part of the therapy.

In most instances, the time taken by a clinician to establish a diagnosis of vulnerable child syndrome does not necessarily have to be long, particularly if the possibility of the diagnosis is entertained from the beginning and the history is obtained in a systematic fashion, searching for etiologic factors and developing an understanding of the parents' perceptions of the child's vulnerability.

RESILIENCY

Even though the focus of this chapter is primarily on the adverse psychological effects of early health crises, the concept of resiliency in children is in some respects the other side of the coin from vulnerability and also needs to be considered. The vulnerable child syndrome does not develop in all children who experience a serious life-threatening event, and after an acute, self-limited event most parents continue to have relatively normal perceptions of their children. As noted previously in describing a large community-based study, only 1.8% of children were defined as having the vulnerable child syndrome, although 21% of the mothers had reported that they at some time had feared that their child might die (Forsyth et al, 1996). The term *resiliency* is most often used to describe the protective process that results in more positive outcomes for individuals who are at risk because of either adverse social factors (e.g., poverty) or psychological factors (e.g., maternal depression). There is also a body of literature that describes resiliency among children with chronic illnesses or conditions, children who thrive and do well psychologically despite their handicaps.

Resiliency is not just the result of one or even multiple factors but a process with many contributing factors. For any individual, the sense of resiliency may change over time and may be influenced by developmental changes (Rutter, 1993). Both preceding and succeeding circumstances may be important. There may, at times, be a turning point in a person's life when the individual becomes more resilient and less vulnerable, with a resulting change in that person's path in life. From the Kauai Longitudinal Study in which 698 infants were studied into adulthood, Werner (1989) and colleagues identified three different areas that contribute to the development of resiliency: (1) individual factors, such as temperament (high activity, sociability, and attention span), cognitive skills, and internal locus of control; (2) familial factors, such as the concern of parents for the well-being of their children, despite their own experience of stresses such as poverty and marital discord; and (3) external support factors, such as the presence of another caring adult in the life of a child. For children with chronic illness, a number of familial factors that contribute to resiliency have been described. These include the development of good communication within families, the engagement in active coping efforts, the ability to attribute a positive meaning to the situation, and the ability to balance the illness with other family needs (Patterson and Blum, 1996).

There has been little examination of what factors might decrease parental perceptions of vulnerability after an acute, self-limited problem early in a child's life and protect the child from possible adverse psychological consequences. However, it is likely that some of the same individual and familial factors that contribute to the development of resiliency for children with chronic illnesses might also protect children who experience an acute health crisis from being perceived as vulnerable. Also, for the child perceived as vulnerable by his or her parents, there is the potential that intervening factors later in development might play a role in contributing to a sense of resiliency rather than vulnerability.

SUMMARY

There has been a substantial increase in our understanding of the vulnerable child syndrome in the decades that have passed since it was first described. The results of research have illustrated how different types of problems in early infancy, some of which appear quite minor and of little consequence, can affect parents' perceptions of their children's vulnerability for years after an event. Almost certainly, the earlier an event happens in a child's life, the more likely it is to affect the parents' developing view of their child; thus, it is most important that clinicians recognize and address early on incidents that could potentially have long-lasting consequences. Similarly, when a child presents with symptoms such as behavior problems or repeated complaints of minor medical problems, the possibility of the vulnerable child syndrome should be considered and explored. A clinician's role in helping parents develop a more realistic view of their child can potentially have an important effect on promoting a child's healthy development.

REFERENCES

Allen EC, Manuel JC, Legault C, et al: Perception of child vulnerability among mothers of former premature infants. Pediatrics 113:267-273, 2004.

Bergman AB, Stamm SJ: The morbidity of cardiac non-disease in school-children. N Engl J Med 276:1008-1013, 1967.

Burger J, Horwitz SM, Forsyth BWC, et al: Psychological sequelae of medical complications during pregnancy. Pediatrics 91:566-571, 1993.

Carey WB: Psychologic sequelae of early infancy health crises. Clin Pediatr 8:459-463, 1969.

Estroff DB, Yando R, Burke K, Synder D: Perceptions of preschoolers' vulnerability by mothers who had delivered preterm. J Pediatr Psychol 19:709-721, 1994.

Filly RA: Obstetric sonography: The best way to terrify a pregnant woman. J Ultrasound Med 19:1-5, 2000.

Forsyth BWC, Canny PF: Perceptions of vulnerability 3½ years after problems of feeding and crying behavior in early infancy. Pediatrics 88:757-763, 1991.

Forsyth BWC, Horwitz SM, Leventhal JM, Burger J: The Child Vulnerability Scale: An instrument to measure parental perceptions of child vulnerability. J Pediatr Psychol 21:89-101, 1996.

Getz L, Kirkengen AL: Ultrasound screening in pregnancy: Advancing technology, soft markers for fetal chromosomal aberrations, and unacknowledged ethical dilemmas. Soc Sci Med 56:2045-2057, 2003.

Green M, Solnit AJ: Reactions to the threatened loss of a child: A vulnerable child syndrome. Pediatrics 34:58-66, 1964.

Hampton ML, Anderson J, Lavizzo BS, Bergman AB: Sickle cell "nondisease": A potentially serious public health problem. Am J Dis Child 128:58-61, 1974.

Kemper K, Forsyth B, McCarthy P: Jaundice, terminating breastfeeding and the vulnerable child. Pediatrics 84:773-778, 1989.

Levy JC: Vulnerable children: Parent's perspectives and the use of medical care. Pediatrics 65:956-963, 1980.

Nelson SP, Chen EH, Syniar G, Christoffel KK: Prevalence of symptoms of gastroesophageal reflux during infancy: A pediatric practice-based survey. Arch Pediatr Adolesc Med 151:569-572, 1997.

Osatakul S, Sriplung H, Puetpaiboon A, et al: Prevalence and the natural course of gastroesophageal reflux symptoms: A 1-year cohort study of Thai infants. J Pediatr Gastroenterol Nutr 34:63-67, 2002.

Patterson J, Blum RW: Risk and resilience among children and youth with disabilities. Arch Pediatr Adolesc Med 150:692-698, 1996.

Perrin E, West P, Culley B: Is my child normal yet? Correlates of vulnerability. Pediatrics 83:355-363, 1989.

Polack FP, Khan N, Maisels MJ: Changing partners: The dance of infant formula changes. Clin Pediatr 38:703-708, 1999.

Rutter M: Resilience: Some conceptual considerations. J Adolesc Health 14:626-631, 1993.

Thomasgard M, Metz WP: The vulnerable child syndrome revisited. J Dev Behav Pediatr 16:47-53, 1995.

Werner EE: High risk children in young adulthood: A longitudinal study from birth to 32 years. Am J Orthopsychiatry 59:72-81, 1989.

35 CHRONIC HEALTH CONDITIONS

Ute Thyen and James M. Perrin

Vignette

Sandra Suarez is an 8-year-old girl with type 1 insulin-dependent diabetes mellitus. Diagnosed at 4 years of age after an episode of bed-wetting and polyuria, she currently receives multiple insulin injections each day and tests her blood sugar three times a day. Her after-school activities include soccer three afternoons a week, with the other days at a more sedentary after-school program. Although she's proficient at self-injection, as is her mother, her father still has difficulties with needles. Both parents have faced limitations in their jobs—Sandra's mother has turned down promotions because they would have required moving, and her father now works part-time to be available if Sandra has any crises related to her condition. John, Sandra's 6-year-old brother, is in first grade and has had problems with daydreaming and not staying on task. Sandra's primary care physician, while evaluating John's needs, is working with the endocrinology group at the nearby medical center to make sure the family knows about the diabetes and is getting some family therapy to help with adjustment to Sandra's condition and planning ahead for likely changes with adolescence (Fig. 35-1).

CHRONIC HEALTH CONDITIONS: A DEFINITION

Chronic illnesses in childhood include a wide variety of health conditions: rare chromosomal disorders, rheumatoid arthritis, epilepsy, asthma, juvenile diabetes, and malignant neoplasms, among others. Children and their families face a bewildering number of conditions—most rare, some described in only a handful of cases. Among chronic *physical* conditions, only asthma and recurrent otitis media occur more often than 1 per 100 children. All neurologic diseases (including seizure disorder but excluding autism) taken together approach a prevalence of 1 per 100 children. Other physical conditions are relatively to extremely rare. Mental health conditions, including attention-deficit/hyperactivity disorder (ADHD), depression, and anxiety, in contrast, occur with relatively high frequency. Many children also experience serious chronic health problems of unknown etiology without a clear diagnosis. The experience of child health professionals with chronic conditions differs substantially from that in adult medicine, where a much higher percentage of patients have a smaller number of relatively common chronic illnesses, such as coronary artery disease, malignant neoplasms, adult-onset diabetes, and degenerative arthritis.

Although the treatment and outcomes of and clinical services for different chronic conditions vary substantially, children with chronic conditions and their families share many common tasks: adaptation to life with a chronic condition, mastering of variations in usual developmental transitions, and adjustment to the economic and psychosocial impact of a chronic condition. Studies of the developmental and behavioral implications of chronic conditions in childhood have examined individual conditions, but taken together, this work documents the common consequences and service needs of children with a diverse group of conditions, and clinical care should address these common needs.

General definitions of chronic conditions typically address two main criteria: duration of illness, usually at least 3 to 12 months or the likelihood of permanence (e.g., leukemia, diabetes); and severity, as indicated by limitations in age-appropriate activities, need for long or recurrent hospitalizations, or need for care beyond that generally experienced by healthy children with occasional acute, self-limiting illnesses. This definition of a chronic condition focuses on the consequences of the conditions more than on the specific diagnosis, and recent work has led to measures of chronic conditions based on this notion (Bethell et al, 2002; Stein and Silver, 2002).

The use of a general definition of chronic conditions allows attention to common behavioral and developmental characteristics of all children with these conditions, including characteristics that may influence behavior and development: duration, age at onset, interference with age-appropriate activities, visibility, expected survival, course (stable versus progressive), level of certainty (episodic versus predictable), mobility, physiologic and sensory impact, impact on cognition and communication,

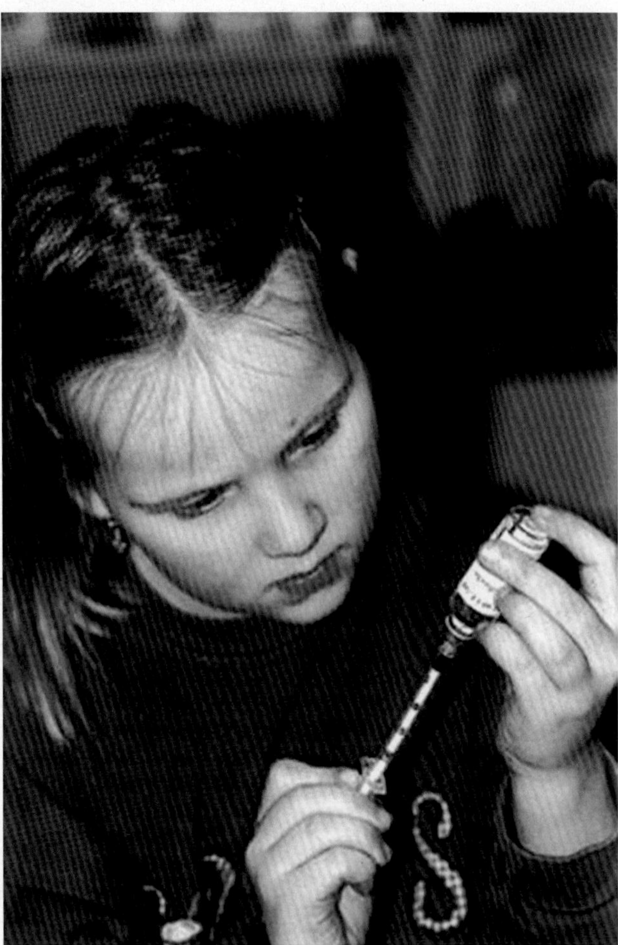

Figure 35-1. Eight-year-old Sandra developed diabetes type 1. She initally learns how to calculate the required dose and draw up insulin and to self-inject the insulin in the subcutaneous tissue of her thighs or abdominal wall. Later she received pens for easier self-administration. Because of recurrent hypoglycemia at night, an insulin pump may be an option for her.

and psychological and social impact (Perrin et al, 1993b). These dimensions, which may fluctuate over time, characterize a child's condition more effectively than does diagnosis alone and help frame the impact of the condition on social and psychological growth.

The term *condition* includes both illnesses (diseases) and disabilities. Examples of chronic illnesses are asthma, Crohn disease, diabetes, and epilepsy. Disabilities include cerebral palsy, loss of limb function, vision or hearing impairment, and intellectual disability. Illness and disability may coexist in the same child and may have different manifestations at changing stages of the illness or the child's growth and development. Children and adolescents with chronic conditions may have no clinical evidence of illness or disability at the time of assessment, for example, symptom-free infants who test positive for human immunodeficiency virus infection, apparently healthy children receiving continued replacement therapy or medications, or children during a symptom-free phase of a relapsing condition. The World Health Organization has introduced conceptually helpful terminology, the International Classification of Functioning, Disability, and Health (ICF), to classify chronic health conditions

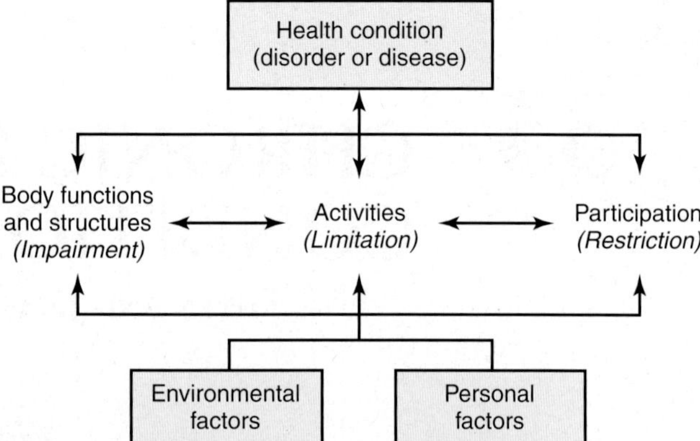

Figure 35-2. The International Classification of Functioning, Disability, and Health (World Health Organization).

on the levels of body structures and functions, activities and limitations, and participation and restrictions in the context of a variety of facilitating or limiting environmental factors (Fig. 35-2). As a part of the World Health Organization Family of International Classifications, the ICF complements the International Classification of Diseases (World Health Organization, 2001).

The manifestations of disability and chronic conditions in childhood and adolescence differ in nature, intensity, and impact from those in adults, mainly because of the impact on developmental tasks and behavior. The ICF-CY (for children and youth), developed partly to respond to these differences, provides a conceptual framework to describe levels of activities and participation among children and youth, with attention to environmental factors that other definitions address less directly (Lollar and Simeonsson, 2005).

EPIDEMIOLOGY OF CHRONIC CONDITIONS IN CHILDHOOD

The chronic health conditions of children and youth reflect both a large group of individually rare conditions and the growing epidemics during the past 2 to 3 decades of three major groups of more common conditions: asthma, obesity, and mental health diagnoses. Rates of disability due to a chronic condition have grown fourfold among children and youth in the United States since 1960. Much of the early growth in prevalence of chronic conditions—from around 1960 to 1980—reflected improvements in survival of children with conditions that had previously had fatal outcomes for most or all children during childhood (Gortmaker and Sappenfield, 1984). These conditions include many childhood cancers, most congenital heart disease, spina bifida, and cystic fibrosis—all of which children now mainly survive well into adulthood, although at times with significant physical and psychological morbidity or with secondary conditions. Children who have had leukemia, for example, have risks for development of second cancers as adults. What had been for families (and clinicians) preparation for short lifespans became instead developing strategies for coping with a long-term health condition.

Chronic conditions such as arthritis, cancer, heart disease, and hemoglobinopathies currently appear to have stable rates, with little evidence for growth or decline in incidence. They account for a substantial portion of all chronic conditions among children and youth, although the substantial growth in obesity, asthma, and mental health conditions accounts for more. A few other conditions have had a small marginal impact on these rates (e.g., exposure to toxic substances in utero and human immunodeficiency virus 1 infections). Other factors have also contributed to higher rates of childhood chronic conditions. Whereas the overall numbers of children surviving prematurity or low birth weight have increased during the past 3 decades, the incidence of major sequelae has not. Infants of extremely low birth weight have substantial risk of visual and hearing defects, chronic lung disease, cerebral palsy, or intellectual disability, but this increase among children who previously would not have survived has been offset by the benefits of modern neonatology for quantitatively larger groups of infants with low birth weight or gestational age of more than 32 weeks who are much more likely to survive with no impairment than in years past. New genetic interventions may eradicate some diseases; those relatively rare conditions that continue to have high mortality rates will likely undergo technologic breakthroughs. Newly emerging public health threats include infectious diseases, such as tuberculosis and human immunodeficiency virus infection, and new viral diseases, such as avian influenza, that easily spread with increased mobility worldwide and currently affect predominantly children in Asia and Africa but may be expected to create problems also in the Western Hemisphere.

Rising rates of chronic conditions related to social and environmental exposures are to be expected. Complex living situations, experience of trauma, and family instability may contribute to an increase of mental health disorders. Physical disorders often occur in combination with developmental problems in growing numbers of young people.

Since 1980, however, much of the growth in chronic conditions reflects epidemics of more common conditions, specifically, obesity, asthma, and mental health conditions (especially ADHD, depression, and autism spectrum disorders). Current population estimates (0-18 years) are as follows: obesity, approximately 11,250,000 (Ogden et al, 2002); asthma, 5,250,000 (Mannino et al, 2002); and ADHD, 4,000,000. In contrast, current population estimates for those earlier conditions that have experienced great improvements in survival include the following: cystic fibrosis, 22,500; spina bifida, 60,000; sickle cell anemia, 37,500; and hemophilia, 7500. Although these latter conditions have had generally stable rates in the population since 1980, rates of obesity, asthma, and ADHD have more than doubled since the early 1980s (see also Chapter 54).

Prevalence figures using a generic, consequences-based approach (National Survey of Children with Special Health Care Needs) estimate that 12.8% (95th percent confidence interval, 12.6-13.0) of U.S. children and youth 0 to 18 years of age have a chronic condition (van Dyck et al, 2004). The wide geographic variation (e.g., 15.5% in Maine to 11.0% in Utah) indicates impacts of culture and access to health care. Mental health and developmental problems are reported at high rates in the 2003 National Survey of Children's Health. The most commonly diagnosed problems among children 6 to 17 years of age were learning disabilities (11.5%), ADHD (8.8%), and behavioral problems (6.3%); among preschoolers, speech problems (5.8%) and developmental delay (3.2%) were most common. One in 200 children was diagnosed with autism. Rates of parental concerns about emotional, developmental, or behavioral problems were even higher; for example, 41% of parents had concerns about learning difficulties and 36% about depression or anxiety. Children with developmental disabilities had lower self-esteem, had more depression and anxiety, had more problems with learning, missed more school, and were less involved in sports and other community activities. Their families experienced more difficulty in the areas of childcare, employment, parent-child relationships, and caregiver burden.

Boys have higher rates of chronic physical conditions than do girls, some because of an X-linked inheritance pattern (e.g., hemophilia, Duchenne muscular dystrophy); in others, because male gender is an independent risk factor for adverse outcomes (sequelae of prematurity, childhood accidents and injuries); and in others, for unknown reasons. Poor children also have higher rates of chronic conditions and often more severe illness (partially attributable to barriers to care) and higher rates of long-term conditions resulting from low birth weight or prematurity or secondary to childhood injury. Specifically, poor children are more likely to develop severe asthma, they run twice the risk of ketoacidosis if they are diabetic, they have higher rates of severe iron deficiency anemia, and they have two to three times the risk for development of permanent complications from bacterial meningitis.

IMPACT OF CHRONIC ILLNESS ON DEVELOPMENT AND BEHAVIOR (Table 35-1)

Psychosocial Factors Affecting Chronic Conditions

Most chronic conditions result from a combination of predisposing constitutional factors, influenced by psychological and environmental factors. The etiology of most diseases is biologic (e.g., inborn errors of metabolism or chromosomal abnormalities), although some conditions reflect primarily environmental factors (e.g., lead poisoning) and others mostly social (e.g., head injury secondary to preventable accidents). Thus, social and psychological factors influence the causation of some chronic conditions.

Social and psychological factors also affect the course and severity of chronic illness. Poor children especially lack access to health care, coordination of care, and information and other resources to cope with the illness. Among families with children with special health care needs, low-income and uninsured children are at much higher risk to encounter unmet health needs compared with higher income and insured children (van Dyck et al, 2004).

Social and community factors can influence the child's or family's ability to normalize life with a chronic illness or disability, providing both facilitators and barriers,

Table 35-1. Factors That Influence Development and Behavior among Children with Chronic Health Conditions

Illness or Condition Characteristics (Other Than Specific Diagnosis)
Severity (physiologic or sensory impact)
Duration
Age at onset
Interference with age-appropriate activities
Expected survival
Course (stable versus progressive)
Certainty (predictable versus uncertain)
Impact on mobility
Impact on cognition and communication
Pain
Child Factors
Gender
Intelligence and communication skills
Temperament
Coping skills and patterns
Family Factors
Family functioning
Parental mental health
Household structure (number of adults and children)
Socioeconomic status
Social Factors
Cultural attitudes
Access to health care
Community resources
Geography
School and daycare systems

and thus affect outcomes of chronic conditions, personal aspirations, and preparation for work and independent living. State or federal legislation such as the Americans with Disabilities Act, ensuring access and equal opportunities for people with disabilities, helps overcome barriers and restrictions. However, in terms of environmental barriers, personal and public attitudes may be just as limiting as physical barriers.

Chronic conditions act as a chronic stressor for the child and family. Family members may experience multiple and conflicting emotions and use a wide range of cognitive and behavioral strategies that have both problem-solving and emotion-regulating functions in the process of coping. *Coping* describes a dynamic process in which emotions and appraisal of the stress continually affect and influence each other and change the relationship between the individual and the environment. *Adjustment,* different from coping, describes the outcomes of coping at a specific point in time. Most children and adolescents adhere to certain patterns of coping strategies, dependent on prior experience, learning, beliefs, culture, and environmental influences, although mechanisms change over time and at different stages of development. Although coping mechanisms have had less study in children than in adults, age, gender, and situation appear to predict coping strategy, which is also highly variable among children. Children and adults make use of a wide variety of coping patterns. Although problem-focused coping strategies have been associated with more positive emotions in response to stress, different coping strategies may be adaptive, depending on the situational circumstances and options available. Clinicians should observe and support the child's preferred coping style rather than change it. A very limited number of coping strategies in an individual should alert the clinician that the coping repertoire may be restricted and adaptive mechanisms poor. Changing clinical practice patterns that pay more attention to self-help activities, strategies to aid empowerment, sharing of responsibility, and listening to children as they understand their illness and try to cope with it may benefit children (Perrin et al, 1993a) (see also Chapter 7).

Effects of Chronic Conditions on Development

Adjustment to chronic illness often involves transitions different from those experienced by other children and families as well as common transitions made more difficult by the presence of a chronic condition. The age at onset of the condition and the stage of the child's development affect coping and adjustment. Many children with a stable congenital condition, such as a limb deficiency, spina bifida or cerebral palsy, or hearing or vision impairment, experience their condition not as an illness at all but as being different from others. The impact of a chronic condition will also vary with the specific impact it has on mastering of developmental tasks and whether limitations can be overcome by supportive environments, specific training programs, therapies, or technologic aids. Development is a continuous process in all areas, such as psychomotor, emotional, and social milestones, but certain ages have characteristic developmental tasks. The more pervasive a chronic health condition is, affecting more than one area of functioning, the greater is the challenge for successful coping and adaptation. Cognitive impairment and mental health conditions generally pose a greater risk for maladjustment compared with conditions without these features.

Conditions with a progressive course or limited life expectancy (e.g., muscular dystrophy) create significant issues in family adaptation and anticipation of an early loss. Conditions with unstable or unpredictable courses are a constant source of stress and may tax individuals' and families' ability to cope. Conditions requiring frequent or prolonged hospitalizations or isolation at home create a serious challenge to early parent-infant bonding in young children and to schooling and acquisition of knowledge, socializing with peers, and participation in community life in older children.

In infancy, illness may affect basic growth, cause failure to thrive, and bring about excessive fatigue. The child may be less responsive than other children or may have physical characteristics that interfere with normal nurturing responses of parents. In blind children, for example, normal responsive smiling does not develop, and parents may perceive this phenomenon as indicating an unresponsive, unrewarding infant. Infants with hearing disability show delay in language acquisition, difficulties in communication, and higher rates of behavior problems. Extensive medical or surgical care during this period often makes the child special and vulnerable in the eyes of parents, and the sense of vulnerability may persist for years, even when medical and surgical care ceases.

As toddlers, children should become more independent and explore their environment vigorously. Chronic illness may slow the development of early independence, diminish the child's resilience, and delay the acquisition of normal developmental milestones. It may limit the child's developing sense of competence and task mastery. For school-age children, frequent absences resulting from illness interfere with learning and usual socialization. Children with visible conditions may feel different or may be subject to teasing. Normal separation from family in early school years may become more difficult because of needs for additional care by parents or increased time at home rather than in school.

Adolescents must develop a new sense of identity, work on their individual identities, develop increasingly adult forms of sexuality, and maintain their educational and vocational development. Many chronic illnesses force continuing dependence on caregivers for medical care or other in-home treatments. Attempts to develop independence in adolescence may lead to rebellion and denial, such as the teenager with diabetes who stops monitoring glucose concentration or diet or who changes insulin dosages whimsically. Sexual development may be affected by disease directly (as with myelomeningocele) or by fears of sexual inadequacy (as in cystic fibrosis). Much of the health care for children and adolescents with chronic illness emphasizes the specific condition they have, neglecting other necessary elements of health supervision and prevention. Teenagers with chronic conditions may require more careful preparation and counseling about sexuality than do other children. Chronic illness may affect competitiveness in athletic activities, although health professionals and parents just as commonly underestimate the athletic capabilities of teenagers with chronic illness. Like children without illness, those who are less active in athletics should find other activities that allow them to excel and enhance their self-esteem.

Chronic illness may hamper the development of appropriate individual identity. The development of an appropriate identity emphasizes being a child or adolescent rather than having a disease. Parents, professionals, and adolescents themselves often generalize from the disease to the whole person, labeling the youngster a diabetic or a leukemic, rather than a child or teenager with diabetes. All involved should be encouraged to use "people first" rather than "disease first" language.

Health-Related Quality of Life in Youth with Chronic Conditions

Health-related quality of life has emerged as a major outcome in studies of the effects of growing up with a chronic condition on individuals and families. The World Health Organization defines health as not only a physical status but also a subjective representation of function and well-being—how a person feels, psychologically and physically, how she or he manages with other persons and copes with everyday life. This perceived health is known as health-related quality of life (HRQOL) and describes a multidimensional construct covering physical, emotional, mental, social, and behavioral components of well-being, as perceived by the individual. Health status (including physical, emotional, and social functioning) and quality of life represent distinct but overlapping concepts (Smith et al, 1999). Health status may be defined as objective description of functional and structural abilities (body structures and functions in the ICF terminology) and generally uses measures such as the amount or frequency of performing a typical task or daily activity. Quality of life represents the subjective appraisal of one's health status at a given time. Although one would expect some correlation of health status and HRQOL, it can be relatively weak. Given people's potential to cope with and to adapt to adversity, the impact of impairment changes greatly over time, and subjective HRQOL may be very good indeed despite ill health. In people affected by chronic conditions and disabilities, the conceptual distinction appears to be of great importance: a limited range of activities does not necessarily imply dissatisfaction with one's personal life and well-being.

Development of instruments to measure health-related quality of life in children and adolescents creates more difficulties compared with that in adults:

1. dimensions relevant to HRQOL may be different from dimensions found to be relevant for adults and must be developed with use of qualitative research methods to identify meaningful items and domains;
2. each age requires developmentally and psychometrically sound instruments; and
3. parent proxy instruments may be required for some populations, such as very young children or those with mental disabilities, although the equivalence of self-report and proxy measures remains unclear in these populations (White-Koning et al, 2005).

Major progress has been achieved in the development of generic instruments for children and adolescents, although few are available in more than one language (Eiser and Morse, 2001). Whereas generic instruments allow comparisons of children and adolescents with and without chronic conditions and different groups of children with chronic conditions, they may not adequately reflect the specific impact of a condition. Some developers of generic instruments have therefore provided scales or modules for certain conditions, such as asthma, diabetes, and rheumatoid arthritis.

Studies report impaired HRQOL in comparison with apparently healthy children in children with asthma (Sawyer et al, 2001) or epilepsy (Sabaz et al, 2001). The effect of reduced HRQOL has been described across various conditions by use of generic instruments (Varni et al, 2001). Different conditions may affect different domains. For example, children with rheumatoid arthritis are much more likely to report reduced HRQOL in the physical dimension than are children with conditions without much pain. Children with congenital impairments report limitations less in the physical domain than in social domains. Studies on HRQOL in parents of children with chronic conditions often demonstrate greater decrease in HRQOL compared with the effects documented in children.

Behavioral Impact of Chronic Conditions

Chronic conditions in children increase the risk of associated psychological and behavioral problems. Most larger, community-based studies indicate an approximate doubling of these rates among children with chronic conditions compared with apparently healthy controls. (For a comprehensive review, see Thompson and Gustafson, 1996.) Meta-analyses of behavioral or developmental issues in children with chronic conditions support higher levels of total adjustment problems, with increased rates of both internalizing and externalizing difficulties, and lower self-esteem (Bennett, 1994; Lavigne and Faier-Routman, 1992). Nonetheless, behavioral and psychological differences between apparently healthy children and those with chronic conditions, albeit significant, are generally small, and most children and adolescents with chronic conditions have scores on scales of behavior, mood, or social adaptation within the normal ranges. Of interest is the finding of little variation among different chronic conditions in rates of psychological or behavioral problems. This approximate doubling of risk appears to affect all children with chronic conditions, regardless of the specific diagnosis. The main exception to this finding is that children with chronic conditions affecting the central nervous system directly or indirectly have much higher risk of maladjustment.

Both cognitive impairment and mental health problems may result from the illness directly (e.g., hydrocephalus, brain malformations, head injuries, epilepsy, or encephalitis) or indirectly through the effect of treatments (e.g., neurotoxic medications or radiation therapy in childhood leukemia; adrenergics or steroids for asthma; anticonvulsant medications). For example, the iatrogenic effects of treatment of leukemia have been associated with a mean decline of 10 intelligence quotient points, with attention, concentration, short-term memory, processing speed, sequencing ability, and visual-motor coordination being most affected. The side effects of phenobarbital for seizure prophylaxis in young children include slowing of cognitive development and, at times, severe behavioral problems.

The mechanisms of increased risk for adjustment problems have not been carefully studied. The increased risk of children with neurologic conditions points to the importance of some condition characteristics or at least the particular impact of central nervous system disease on behavior. Theoretical considerations drawing on knowledge of family development and parent-child interaction indicate parent and family adjustment as a powerful mediator of the effect of chronic stress on the child. Maternal self-esteem and depression are highly correlated with child psychological status in many studies, as is high perceived stress in the child and family environment. Psychological difficulties presumably follow from the demands that a chronic condition places on a child and family beyond the complexities of normal development and psychological growth. Surprisingly, disease severity does not seem to have an impact on child adjustment (Perrin et al, 1989). Although it might be expected that children with the most severe illnesses would have the highest risk of problems in adjustment, few studies have found any association of severity and adjustment. Indeed, some early studies found that children with less severe forms of a condition had greater problems with psychological adjustment than did those with more severe forms. These earlier findings do not appear to be supported in more recent studies. Overall, the level of intellectual functioning appears to have an impact on adjustment, with children with lower levels expressing more behavior problems and poorer social functioning. Higher levels of intellectual functioning may protect children with chronic conditions from maladjustment. Whether a condition is congenital or acquired later in childhood or adolescence and the longitudinal effects of course and duration of the condition on behavior have not been well studied.

Chronic Conditions: Implications for Education and Work

Attending school is important for children's academic, social, and emotional development and for their future success, yet children with chronic conditions miss a substantial number of school days each year for several reasons: exacerbations of the condition; acute illnesses not related to the chronic condition but likely to have a more protracted course in a child with compromised health status; hospitalizations for treatments; physician or hospital appointments; psychological problems secondary to peer reactions, lack of confidence, or poor academic achievement resulting in school avoidance; and perceptions of vulnerability in parents and inappropriate health beliefs. Inadequate school policies or nursing care may exclude children who must take medicine, are incontinent or need respiratory therapy, or require parents to come to school. Children with mobility impairments may face barriers to schools or classrooms. Special education placements are commonly used, despite the fact that most children with mobility problems have no special learning problems that require special education programs. Especially with mental health conditions, such as ADHD, schools play critical roles, partly in testing children and more in helping them with their social and educational performance. Whether a child with ADHD succeeds depends greatly on the services available and the attitude of the school toward behaviors associated with ADHD (Ustun, 2007).

Children who must be at home for extended periods may receive home teaching, especially if the absence is at least for 2 or more consecutive weeks. Yet the child with asthma who has frequent brief absences may find such home services unavailable. Even when it is available, home teaching typically consists of only a few hours per week and is a poor substitute for the full range of classroom teaching. Furthermore, home teaching cannot replace peer interactions and the socialization that accompanies them. Helping a child maintain active contact with classmates by having them deliver homework and books is one important way of helping to maintain integration.

Psychosocial problems in children and adolescents may persist into young adulthood. Young men who had chronic physical conditions in childhood or adolescence had significantly higher risks for depression and anxiety, use of mental health specialists, poor educational qualifications, and periods of unemployment. Those with cardiac or respiratory disorders had the highest risks for psychological distress and absence of educational qualifications, those with neurologic and musculoskeletal disorders had the highest rates of social isolation, and those with visual or auditory problems had longer spells of unemployment. In contrast, women with a history of childhood chronic conditions had an elevated risk only for having seen a mental health specialist (Pless et al, 1993). Compared with apparently healthy adults, young adults with a history of chronic physical conditions in childhood are more likely to develop nonspecific psychosomatic complaints (i.e., headaches, back and shoulder pain, dizziness, or palpitations) unrelated to their chronic condition or an overt somatization disorder (Kokkonen and Kokkonen, 1995). The effects of cultural attitudes, which may stigmatize certain diseases, and societal levels of acceptance and tolerance may affect how young people with a chronic condition perceive their quality of life and well-being.

Effects of Chronic Conditions on the Family

For many families, a key transition takes place at discharge from the hospital, when major responsibility for the child's care transfers from hospital staff to family. Other unusual transitions may include repeated hospitalizations. More typical transitions in a child's life include starting school, development of autonomy in preadolescence, and initiation of sexual relationships in adolescence, all potentially changed by the presence of a chronic condition. Many parents perceive their child with a chronic condition as vulnerable and respond with varying degrees of protection, often reflecting a realistic need of the child but sometimes restricting the child's individual development by overprotection. With many conditions, children rely on additional support from their parents to deal with daily medications or treatments, threatening development of autonomy and self-efficiency in adolescents in particular. In general, psychological factors may affect adjustment to the illness and adherence to treatment regimens, perceptions of vulnerability in patients and parents, and susceptibility to secondary mental health problems in both the child and the family.

Each stage of family development is characterized by a set of tasks, for which the family develops its own coping strategies. Societal, historical, cultural, and geographic factors all influence family development and form the context for family beliefs, myths, taboos, expectations, role models, and patterns of adaptation. Developmentally stable (maintenance) periods are interspersed by developmentally less stable (transitional) periods. Normative transitions include the birth of a child, school entry, and onset of adolescence. Unexpected transitions include disruptive life events, such as catastrophic or chronic illness in a family member, and loss and separation.

Families whose child is born with or develops a chronic condition pass through a relatively predictable sequence of emotional reactions, similar to those that follow separation and loss: shock (inability to express feelings, to communicate, or to share feelings); disbelief (denial, wishful thinking); grieving and anger (blaming behavior, lack of control, inappropriate criticism, depression, helplessness, withdrawal behaviors); stabilizing period (demystification, use of cognitive control behavior, adapting to day-to-day routine); and maturation and acceptance (emotional adjustment, feelings of personal development and growth). The different stages are not mutually exclusive, crises may cause setbacks, and different family members typically go through different stages at different times.

Modern medical treatments and advanced technology such as dialysis, intravenous feeding, parenteral or enteral alimentation, and mechanical ventilation offer great opportunities and many choices for children and adolescents with chronic conditions, both prolonging life and improving quality of life. Technologic advances have allowed the transfer of care for children assisted by technology from hospitals to families and communities, and care at home became an accepted alternative. Emerging parent advocacy for their children demanded care at home, pointing to the devastating effects of prolonged hospital admissions and parent-child separation. Families now provide care for most childhood chronic conditions, relying on hospitals only for acute, life-threatening complications of disease or for review by subspecialists. Providing that care typically requires a broad array of multidisciplinary services that vary substantially according to the health condition and the needs of the child and families (Figs. 35-3 to 35-5). Families' experiences with care at home, in particular having substantial hours of nursing in the home, have been ambivalent. Families appreciate having their child home and receiving qualified nursing care. Yet, family privacy, control of parenting and care issues, and independence are in jeopardy. For many families, there may be no guarantee that the services provided at a community level or the hours allotted will be determined with the child's or the family's needs in mind. The training and expertise of nurses may not be sufficient to meet the child's special health care needs (Perrin et al, 1993c).

The resilient family effectively uses resources within and outside the family system to prevent breakdown and to promote adaptation to a chronic condition (Rolland and Walsh, 2006). Parents of children with chronic illness must monitor the child's health, check equipment, administer medications, provide physical therapy, or carry children with mobility impairments, all tasks beyond the normal ones of parenting. Whereas severity appears to show little association with adjustment in children and youth, the impact on parents does show an increase with severity, reflecting the workload of supporting a child with a severe chronic condition (Thyen et al, 2003). Parents often report feelings of fatigue, depression, and social isolation. The extra burdens of care particularly affect family cohesion, along with less opportunity for social, recreational, and cultural activities in families with a child with a chronic health condition. Overt family dysfunction or family breakdown as a result of a child's chronic illness is uncommon, although families may pay a high price in terms of opportunities, social relationships, career choice, and personal growth to cope with the burden of care. Parents of children with

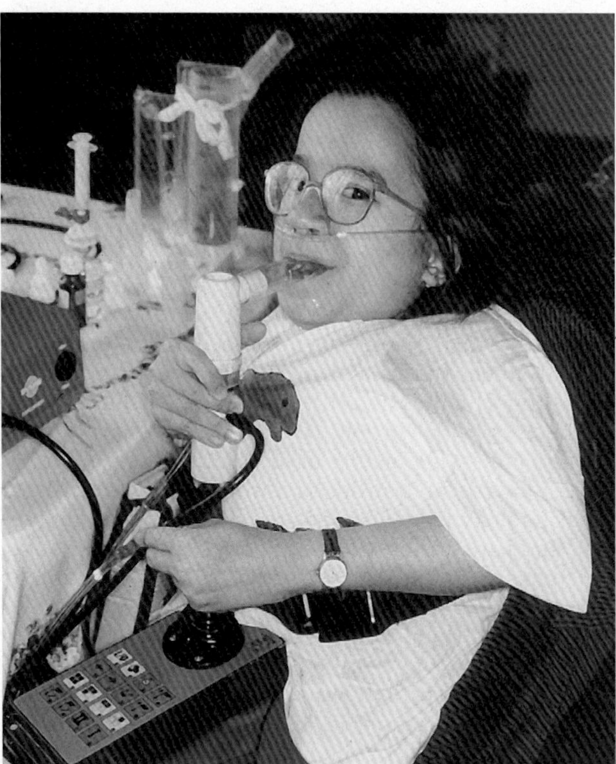

Figure 35-3. Michelle is a 19-year-old woman with osteogenesis imperfecta, restrictive lung disease, cardiomyopathy, intermittent obstructive bowel disease, and frequent fractures. Michelle depends on continuous oxygen, regular respiratory therapy, frequent use of medications per nebulizer, continuous positive-pressure airway ventilation at night, and intravenous fluids during episodes of intestinal obstruction. She depends on help in all activities of daily living, with her mother being the main caregiver. She recently finished high school with good reports. She enjoys reading and writing on her personal computer. She is mobile with her electric wheelchair.

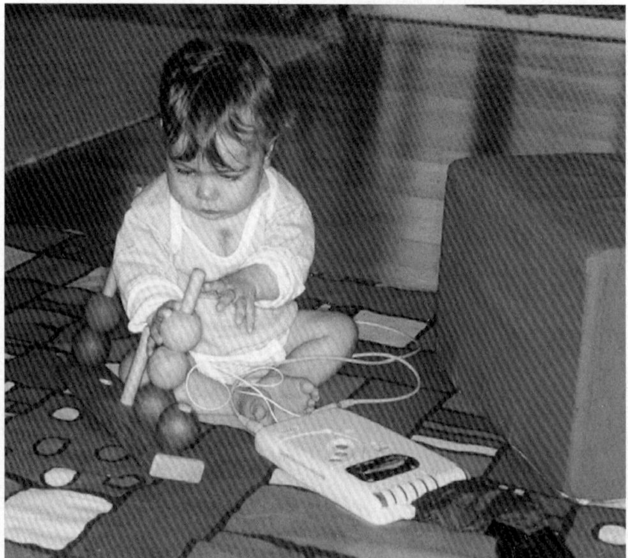

Figure 35-4. One-year-old Finn is on a cardiac monitor. He has complex congenital heart disease (transposition of the great arteries, double inlet left ventricle, mitral valve stenosis and insufficiency, high-grade stenosis of the pulmonary arteries). His first cardiac surgery was at age 4 weeks, and his second operation was at age 10 months after signs of progressive heart failure and congestive liver disease developed. He awaits a third major operation at age 18 months. He has failure to thrive and short stature; however, his cognitive and motor development are somewhat slow but still age appropriate. He is the youngest of three children, and hospitalizations at the cardiac surgery center 300 miles from home are a logistic problem, but the family receives social support from grandparents and neighbors.

chronic conditions in community-based studies have increased rates of mental health problems, particularly higher rates of depression, but no significant increase in single parenthood, social isolation, alcohol problems, or family dysfunction. In contrast, studies of clinical populations indicate more marital discord, dysfunctional family patterns, and overt psychiatric disturbances in families, probably reflecting selection biases in these populations. In families of children with chronic arthritis as an example, mothers experienced more depressed mood than did fathers but also reported a greater sense of mastery over time. Depressed mood was related to greater functional disability and psychosocial problems in their children and lack of family support. Parental mood and strain also appear to predict child adjustment over time.

Among two-parent families, mothers are significantly less likely to work outside the home if they have a child with a chronic condition. Participation in the workforce outside the home may, however, be a protective factor for mental and social well-being of mothers (Thyen et al, 1999). Chronic illness in children has major financial costs as well; the relatively small number of children with severe physical conditions consume at least a third of all child health expenditures. Parents face sizable out-of-pocket expenses, not only for uncompensated health care costs but also for adaptations to the home, transportation, and extra child care. Lost income because of a parent's quitting a job due to the child's chronic condition and curtailed career opportunities further increases financial burden (Kuhlthau and Perrin, 2001).

The multiple demands on the family often leave less parental time for siblings. The few studies of adjustment to a sibling's chronic condition present a mixed picture. Some children find the experience of helping to nurture a sibling with chronic illness one that helps them develop their own skills, enhances their maturity, and improves their resilience. Others find the parental neglect such a problem that they become depressed, develop aggressive and acting out behavior, do poorly in school, and are otherwise diminished in their own psychological health. The correlates of adjustment of siblings are not well understood, although parental mental health and the family environment are likely to play major mediating roles.

Families benefit from and contribute to the network of relationships and resources in the community. Effective social support helps families cope better with chronic stress. Self-help and advocacy groups have helped many parents access information, recruit tangible support, and foster a sense of worth and importance of the work they accomplish. In integrating complex medical, educational, social, and emotional needs of this population, the focus shifts from provider as "expert" to family-provider partnerships and from the child as the target of treatment to

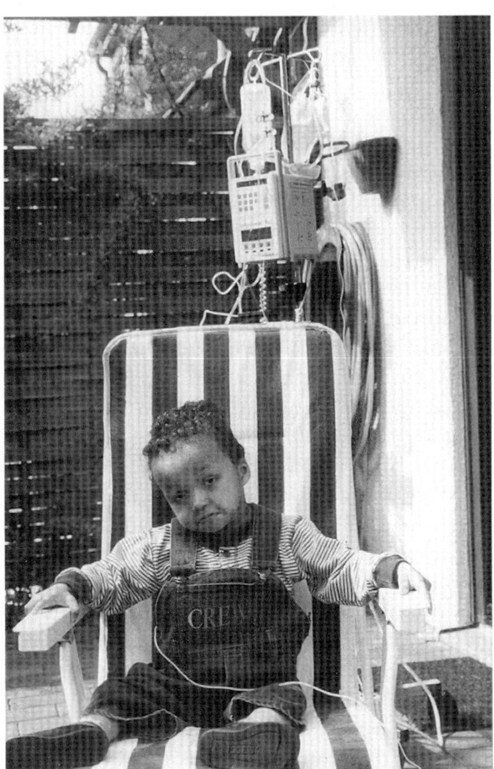

Figure 35-5. Two-year-old Leon has prune-belly syndrome with severe obstructive uropathy and inability to have normal bowel movements. The picture shows him with his infusion set for total parenteral nutrition. He depends on parenteral nutrition on a continuous basis (20 to 24 hours/day) through a Broviac catheter, frequent intermittent catheterization, nebulizer for intermittent obstructive airway disease, care of his gastrostomy and colostomy, and frequent intravenous administration of antibiotics. He lived in a hospital for the first 1½ years of his life; his mother was single with multiple social problems and was unable to take him home; he lives with foster parents and has made excellent progress developmentally. He walks independently and talks in two-word sentences. He receives intensive early intervention services. However, his health is still fragile, and he is frequently hospitalized briefly because of some complications in his management.

interventions that include the social context of the individual child, especially the family. Rising consumerism, supplementary education and information by nonmedical organizations, self-help and parent support groups, and access to the World Wide Web have considerably helped families access information and other families for mutual support.

MANAGEMENT BY CLINICIANS (Table 35-2)

Coordination of Care and the Medical Home

Children without chronic conditions usually receive all their care close to home from a community-based pediatrician, family physician, or nurse practitioner. Children with chronic conditions receive their care from a multitude of different providers, including the primary care clinician, hospital-based subspecialists, home health agencies, specialized therapists, and sometimes alternative sources of care. Their care may be spread over different sites, sometimes at considerable distance from home, contributing to fragmentation of care. Families with children with chronic conditions may benefit from efforts to coordinate care.

Table 35-2. Areas of Pediatric Evaluation and Intervention

Medical Care
Health maintenance and preventive care
Acute illness care
Chronic illness care, collaborating with subspecialty health providers
Identification of Behavioral and Developmental Consequences
Periodic assessment
Monitoring and referral
Assessment of Family Strengths
Knowledge
Social support
Coping skills
Psychological status
Education about Illness
Developmentally appropriate
Ongoing
Decision making
Planning for Education
Medication and treatment
Emergency plans
Implications of condition for participation in classes and outside activities
Special evaluation or placements

The concept of a medical home has been advocated for all children, but especially those with special health care needs (Medical Home Initiatives for Children with Special Needs Project Advisory Committee, 2002), to avoid fragmented care and overuse and underuse, to promote interagency cooperation, to alleviate stress for families, and ultimately to improve outcomes such as health status, health-related quality of life, and participation in school and community. The characteristics of the medical home include development of registries of patients with chronic health conditions, implementation of practice standards for their care, access to educational materials for children and families, and partnership with families in decision making. The complexity of services needed often calls for collaborative teams within a practice to carry out medical home responsibilities (Perrin, 2006).

Access to specialist services is crucial, in particular during the initial diagnostic phase and later for continued update and monitoring of treatments as well as for having access to first-hand information on new treatment options. Pediatricians can help families manage care by ensuring access to state-of-the-art medical and surgical care and other specialized therapies or programs. Such services are often organized specifically for individual conditions and are highly efficient in providing specific treatments. Primary care providers must closely cooperate with specialists, ensure exchange of information, and act as facilitator to access specialized services. Families must have good information to help them make sense of medical advice that is often conflicting.

Case management activities have a long history in human services, in which staff from public or voluntary private agencies have helped families, often from economically deprived backgrounds, to determine needs and to gain access to services. As a process, case management is an orderly, planned provision of services intended to facilitate a client's functioning at as normal a level as possible and as economically as possible. The experience with care at home has changed the use and definitions of case management as it applies to children and families (Perrin and Bloom, 1994). The newer and more adequate term *care coordination* places less emphasis on access and management and more on aspects of communication, service delivery, and family support, with the understanding that the professional responsible for coordination works with the family to develop an agenda or a list of short-term and long-term goals and priorities of each family member in close cooperation with the family.

Not all families need care coordination. Family members usually develop increasing competence to direct the management of the child's needs and services provided. Care coordination services may particularly help during the year after the onset of the child's condition, at the time of discharge from the hospital, or during difficult transitional periods (e.g., during school entry). The medical home can help ensure coordination of care, often collaborating with other professionals: nurses, social workers, and educators.

The functions of care coordination include teaching families about their child's care, developing a care plan and revising it periodically according to the child's and family's needs, helping the family to access necessary services, communicating effectively with all care providers including home health services and social and educational services, and helping to resolve conflicts among service providers. Social and emotional support for the family is an important part of the care coordinator's work.

Decision Making

The past 30 years have seen tremendous expansion of the role of the family in caring for children with chronic conditions and in decision making about their child's care. From an approach that often excluded parents from involvement in decision making (Massie and Massie, 1976), parents now assume major responsibilities in these areas, partly following the increased use of home rather than hospital care and partly reflecting major growth in consumerism in health care (Perrin et al, 1993c). Work done by Family Voices and Brandeis University allowed the first systematic characterization by parent leadership of the issues faced by parents in raising children with chronic conditions, much also documented in the National Survey of Children with Special Health Care Needs. That work documented needs for several types of services (specialty medical services and mental and home health care). Providing families resources to take care of their children with chronic conditions and involving them in key decisions have led to increased parent satisfaction and increased adherence to mutually agreed on treatment plans. Building on the experience of parent involvement in educational planning through Individual Educational Plans, health care programs increasingly use Family Service Plans, in which parents and professionals together plan for a child's care.

Children with chronic conditions should always receive developmentally appropriate information about their condition and have their questions answered (Joffe et al, 2006). Children and adolescents are able to participate in decision making and to give informed consent at a much earlier age than legal age. Providing ongoing information to the child requires additional developmental knowledge and competency on the part of the professionals, who also often need to advise parents about how to talk to their child. As children progress from childhood to young adulthood, they should take increasing responsibility for self-management of their chronic condition, as part of the usual process of developing independence and autonomy and achieving transition to young adulthood. Application of developmental concepts along with knowledge about how children understand illness and how they use strengths, resources, and skills to cope will help clinicians care effectively for children and adolescents with chronic conditions.

Increasing effort goes to educating children about their chronic illnesses; however, few curricular materials have been developed that take into account developmental changes in children's concepts of illness. Structured educational programs are available for the more prevalent conditions, such as asthma, diabetes, obesity, and epilepsy. There is at least some evidence that these programs enhance knowledge and understanding, self-management skills, and autonomy and lead to less hospitalization and emergency care. Long-term outcomes in terms of better health status and improved health-related quality of life have been insufficiently studied. Most programs require parents' participation and are standardized for school-age children and for adolescents; very few address issues of siblings. Access to such programs varies greatly and may not be included in the child's insurance benefits.

Prevention and Management of Developmental and Behavioral Problems

The special needs of families with children who have long-term illnesses require that a wide range of services be available to these families. Pediatricians can help families manage care by ensuring access not only to medical and surgical care but also to a broader array that includes preventive mental health services, appropriate home nursing and educational services, planning and monitoring of educational placement, social services, and, at times, other specialized therapies. Furthermore, the pediatric view should include parents and siblings as well as the child with the condition. Modern medical treatments and advanced technology offer great opportunities and many choices for children and adolescents with chronic conditions, both prolonging life and improving quality of life. Families must have good information to help them make sense of medical advice that is often conflicting.

Clinicians working with children with chronic illness should ensure that these children receive all the usual aspects of preventive care and health supervision, including efforts to identify, prevent, and manage mental health conditions in the child. Additional pediatric responsibilities include identification of behavioral and developmental consequences of chronic illness for the child; assessment of family strengths and coping skills and identification of family problems, including those of sibling adjustment; education of the child and family about illness; and help in planning an appropriate educational setting for the child. Given the high cost of many chronic conditions, physicians should also know how to refer families to sources of support, both private and public (Bauman et al, 1997) (see Part V).

Identification of Behavioral-Developmental Consequences

Most children with severe long-term illness are psychologically healthy and without developmental problems. Yet the clinician must be vigilant in developmental and behavioral assessment of children with chronic illnesses and assess both the level at which a child is functioning and the need for referral. Primary care providers apparently recognize adjustment problems in some of their patients with chronic conditions. However, only about half of children with a serious chronic condition and a behavioral or emotional problem receive mental health services (Weiland et al, 1992).

Assessment of Family Strengths

Pediatricians should help families increase the support available to them, become more knowledgeable about their child's health needs, and strengthen their skills both in coping and in nurturing their child. Pediatricians should be particularly sensitive to maternal depression and marital dysfunction, knowing how to identify these problems and where to refer parents when necessary. Although most families need only anticipatory guidance, parent counseling, and empathy, at times a mental health referral is in order (Sabbeth and Stein, 1990).

Education about Illness

Education about illness must take into account the child's developmental level. Explanation of illness and its treatment should be targeted to the child's (and parents') abilities. Education must be a continuing process as the child develops more cognitive sophistication. Periodic review of the child's understanding of illness helps inform the physician of areas needing attention. Pediatricians can help explain the often confusing information that families receive from multiple providers. To do so, they must themselves communicate effectively with specialists and remain current with the main issues of the specific health condition.

Clinicians need to help children and their families make adequate and autonomous decisions. For adults, the principles of informed consent guide clinicians to inform the patient and to respect the patient's decisions. For children and adolescents, the process to achieve informed consent is far more complex. Informed consent requires autonomy and full ability to make judgments, of which children are capable to a limited extent, and should be replaced by a collaborative principle of combined parental permission, child assent, and physician agreement.

Education of children and families seems necessary but is not sufficient to enhance their self-care skills. Relatively little is known about the exact context of information that families need. Does the child with asthma need to learn about lung physiology, chest anatomy, and the mechanisms of actions of medications and why he or she develops certain kinds of symptoms, where medicines are kept, or how to use them? Much experimentation must continue in this area, and it should take into account the developmental status of the child.

Planning for Education

School is the main workplace of children. Pediatricians should help families work with schools to ensure the best placement for the child. Some children require special education services because of the effect of the illness on their cognitive abilities. Most children with chronic illness can participate in regular education programs, at times requiring modification of the school environment or the school day. Many require planning for dispensing of medication or for emergency care, and school staff need information about the illness and its consequences for the child's participation in school. Pediatricians should see that adequate transfer of information occurs and that satisfactory planning occurs for the child.

SUMMARY

Chronic illness and disabilities both affect and are affected by the development and behavior of children. Although only a minority of children have major chronic health conditions, the complexity of the diagnosis and management of these children and their families calls for extensive pediatric involvement with much interdisciplinary collaboration and coordination of care. Special pediatric roles other than that of providing medical care include identification of developmental-behavioral concerns, assessment of family strengths, education about illness, and planning for education.

References

Bauman LJ, Drotar D, Leventhal JM, et al: A review of psychosocial interventions for children with chronic health conditions. Pediatrics 100(2 Pt 1):51-244, 1997.

Bennett DS: Depression among children with chronic medical problems: A meta-analysis. J Pediatr Psychol 19(2):149-169, 1994.

Bethell CD, Read D, Stein RE, et al: Identifying children with special health care needs: Development and evaluation of a short screening instrument. Ambul Pediatr 2(1):38-48, 2002.

Eiser C, Morse R: Quality-of-life measures in chronic diseases of childhood. Health Technol Assess 5(4):1-157, 2001.

Gortmaker SL, Sappenfield W: Chronic childhood disorders: Prevalence and impact. Pediatr Clin North Am 31(1):3-18, 1984.

Joffe S, Fernandez CV, Pentz RD, et al: Involving children with cancer in decision-making about research participation. J Pediatr 149(6):862-868, 2006.

Kokkonen J, Kokkonen ER: Psychological and somatic symptoms in young adults with chronic physical diseases. Psychother Psychosom 64(2):94-101, 1995.

Kuhlthau KA, Perrin JM: Child health status and parental employment. Arch Pediatr Adolesc Med 155(12):1346-1350, 2001.

Lavigne JV, Faier-Routman J: Psychological adjustment to pediatric physical disorders: A meta-analytic review. J Pediatr Psychol 17(2):133-157, 1992.

Lollar DJ, Simeonsson RJ: Diagnosis to function: Classification for children and youths. J Dev Behav Pediatr 26(4):323-330, 2005.

Mannino DM, Homa DM, Akinbami LJ, et al: Surveillance for asthma—United States, 1980-1999. MMWR Surveill Summ 51(1):1-13, 2002.

Massie R, Massie S: Journey. New York, Knopf, 1976.

Medical Home Initiatives for Children with Special Needs Project Advisory Committee: American Academy of Pediatrics. Pediatrics 110(1 Pt 1):184-186, 2002.

Ogden CL, Flegal KM, Carroll MD, et al: Prevalence and trends in overweight among US children and adolescents, 1999-2000. JAMA 288(14):1728-1732, 2002.

Perrin EC, Ayoub CC, Willett JB: In the eyes of the beholder: Family and maternal influences on perceptions of adjustment of children with a chronic illness. J Dev Behav Pediatr 14(2):94-105, 1993a.

Perrin EC, Newacheck P, Pless IB, et al: Issues involved in the definition and classification of chronic health conditions. Pediatrics 91(4):787-793, 1993b.

Perrin JM: The changing contours of pediatric practice. Ambul Pediatr 6(6):303-304, 2006.

Perrin JM, Bloom SR: Coordination of care for households with children with special health needs. *In* Wallace HM, Nelson RP, Sweeney PJ (eds): Maternal and Child Health Practices. Oakland, CA, Third Party Publishing, 1994, pp 711-718.

Perrin JM, MacLean WE Jr, Perrin EC: Parental perceptions of health status and psychologic adjustment of children with asthma. Pediatrics 83(1):26-30, 1989.

Perrin JM, Shayne MW, Bloom SR: Home and Community Care for Chronically Ill Children. New York, Oxford University Press, 1993c.

Pless IB, Power C, Peckham CS: Long-term psychosocial sequelae of chronic physical disorders in childhood. Pediatrics 91(6):1131-1136, 1993.

Rolland JS, Walsh F: Facilitating family resilience with childhood illness and disability. Curr Opin Pediatr 18(5):527-538, 2006.

Sabaz M, Cairns DR, Lawson JA, et al: The health-related quality of life of children with refractory epilepsy: A comparison of those with and without intellectual disability. Epilepsia 42(5):621-628, 2001.

Sabbeth B, Stein RE: Mental health referral: A weak link in comprehensive care of children with chronic physical illness. J Dev Behav Pediatr 11(2):73-78, 1990.

Sawyer MG, Spurrier N, Kennedy D, et al: The relationship between the quality of life of children with asthma and family functioning. J Asthma 38(3):279-284, 2001.

Smith KW, Avis NE, Assmann SF: Distinguishing between quality of life and health status in quality of life research: A meta-analysis. Qual Life Res 8(5):447-459, 1999.

Stein RE, Silver EJ: Comparing different definitions of chronic conditions in a national data set. Ambul Pediatr 2(1):63-70, 2002.

Thompson RJ, Gustafson KE: Adaptation to Childhood Chronic Illness. Washington, DC, American Psychological Association, 1996.

Thyen U, Kuhlthau K, Perrin JM: Employment, child care, and mental health of mothers caring for children assisted by technology. Pediatrics 103(6 Pt 1):1235-1242, 1999.

Thyen U, Sperner J, Morfeld M, et al: Unmet health care needs and impact on families with children with disabilities in Germany. Ambul Pediatr 3(2):74-81, 2003.

Ustun TB: Using the international classification of functioning, disease and health in attention-deficit/hyperactivity disorder: Separating the disease from its epiphenomena. Ambul Pediatr 7(1 Suppl):132-139, 2007.

van Dyck PC, Kogan MD, McPherson MG, et al: Prevalence and characteristics of children with special health care needs. Arch Pediatr Adolesc Med 158(9):884-890, 2004.

Varni JW, Seid M, Kurtin PS: PedsQL 4.0: Reliability and validity of the Pediatric Quality of Life Inventory version 4.0 generic core scales in healthy and patient populations. Med Care 39(8):800-812, 2001.

Weiland SK, Pless IB, Roghmann KJ: Chronic illness and mental health problems in pediatric practice: Results from a survey of primary care providers. Pediatrics 89(3):445-449, 1992.

White-Koning M, Arnaud C, Bourdet-Loubere S, et al: Subjective quality of life in children with intellectual impairment—how can it be assessed? Dev Med Child Neurol 47(4):281-285, 2005.

World Health Organization: International Classification of Functioning, Disability, and Health. Geneva, Switzerland, World Health Organization, 2001.

36 PALLIATIVE AND END OF LIFE CARE FOR CHILDREN AND FAMILIES

LINDA S. GUDAS AND GERALD P. KOOCHER

This chapter is intended as a guide to integrating concepts of palliative and end of life care into the practices of pediatricians, family physicians, and other health care professionals working with children and families confronting loss and death. The following pages summarize important treatment approaches in different sites of care. The development of normal children's views of death are reviewed and linked to the care of seriously ill children. Family-centered care and the role of the health care team are discussed. The need for further educational services and research is briefly mentioned.

Advances in medical care have allowed children with serious, complex, and rare conditions to live longer, necessitating consideration of four aspects of pediatric palliative care. The first involves care of a child with an acute, acquired, life-threatening illness (e.g., metastasized cancer). The second aspect, also an acute condition, involves managing sudden, severely traumatic injuries (e.g., the child involved in a car crash or man-made or natural disaster). The third and more frequent circumstance involves the care of a child with a chronic, life-shortening condition (e.g., cystic fibrosis or AIDS), when numerous medical crises and an unpredictable course create uncertainty of quality and duration of life. Finally, a perinatal or neonatal death may occur (e.g., the delivery of a child with a prenatal diagnosis of a fatal condition). In such situations, a family must prepare for both a birth and the death of their infant. Any of these courses can form the basis for a host of psychological stressors, whether from the trauma of the news of a serious accident or from the emotional accommodation to uncertainties among children and families facing progressive life-limiting conditions (often described as a Damocles syndrome) (Koocher and O'Malley, 1981). In all four aspects of care, families struggle with whether they should anticipate the child's death and accommodate to the impending loss or suppress their anxieties about possible or probable death while hoping for the best. The coping styles and pace of adaptation will often vary among family members. Reactions of parents, siblings, and loved ones represent major challenges to health care workers and cause for preventive mental health in pediatrics to specifically address the needs of these children.

INCIDENCE OF DEATH

Approximately 55,000 children younger than 19 years die every year in this country (Institute of Medicine, 2003). The majority of child deaths occur during the first year of life (around 50%), and of those deaths, most occur during the neonatal period. After the first year of life, unintentional injuries or accidents constitute the most frequent cause of death, with more than half of those occurring between the ages of 15 and 19 years. Cancer is the most frequent illness cause of all child death, with sudden infant death syndrome (SIDS) leading the infancy period. The majority of children and adolescents die or are pronounced dead in institutions; of those, approximately 56% occur in inpatient settings (intensive care units, delivery rooms, long-term care facilities) and 16% in outpatient settings (emergency departments, disaster sites, accident sites) (Institute of Medicine, 2003; Knapp et al., 2005). In addition to these deaths, thousands more children live for years with debilitating conditions. Such statistics become a concern considering the well-documented lack of professional training in as well as the availability of services for pediatric palliative care.

DEFINITIONS

Palliative care has historically represented comfort care provided in hospital or hospice to individuals at the end stage of life when medical problems no longer respond to curative measures. Whereas control of pain and prevention of suffering remain primary goals of palliative care, such services can best be viewed as a continuum of care from the time of diagnosis (when care will benefit the child who survives as well as the child who dies) to the end of life (when some curative or life-prolonging measures, such as organ transplants or blood transfusions, may still benefit the ill child). Pediatric palliative care, then, involves a multidisciplinary approach that seeks to prevent or to relieve physical and emotional distress produced by life-threatening or life-limiting disorders and that enhances the life of children and families living under these conditions. The goal focuses on achieving optimal quality and normality of life (Hutchinson et al, 2003;

Institute of Medicine, 2003). Such care includes active interventions, accessible in multiple settings (schools, hospitals, home), and regards healing and palliation as parallel, nonconflicting processes (Browning and Solomon, 2005; Himelstein et al, 2004). Good palliative care addresses cultural and religious differences, specifically in regard to meaning and significance of illness, death, expression of suffering and grief, and value of life. It involves inclusion of the child and family in treatment and decision making in a supportive manner and places the dignity of the child as paramount.

End of life or terminal care involves the process of helping the child and family to prepare for an anticipated death (e.g., discussing life supports) and to manage the end stage of fatal conditions (e.g., removal of a breathing tube) (Institute of Medicine, 2003). As a part of palliative care, end of life care promotes culturally sensitive communications that assist children and their families in understanding diagnosis, prognosis, and treatment options. Consistent with the philosophy of palliative care, end of life care can occur concurrently with curative or healing measures. Because some children experience and recover from multiple medical crises, end of life care should become a continuous part of the health care plan from beginning to end of treatment. The Institute of Medicine (2003) emphasizes that one cannot reliably predict which children will die and which will live through such episodes even after initial treatments have failed. This component of uncertainty reiterates the need for continuing review of treatment goals with the child, brothers and sisters, parents, and extended family members. Himelstein and colleagues (2004) identify four steps for the health care provider to consider in end of life or advanced care planning: (1) identify and include the decision makers, (2) determine the patient's and family's understanding of the illness and prognosis, (3) establish goals of care, and (4) share decisions about the use of lifesaving measures and interventions.

Bereavement care, a component of pediatric palliative care, is the supportive process of grief work necessary to help children and families cope after experiencing loss through death. Chapter 37 discusses such care in detail, but remember that grieving constitutes an ongoing, continuous process throughout the course of any life-threatening condition (Milstein, 2005). Health care providers should vigilantly strive to help children and families address losses as they occur at various milestones and transitions in the progression of their illness. For example, even at the initial diagnosis, children and families struggle with the concept that their lives will never "be like before," and anticipatory grief begins. For example, parents experiencing a high-risk pregnancy fear daily for the life of their unborn child. Families and children who struggle over time with the uncertainties of survival under a "Damoclean threat" (Koocher and O'Malley, 1981) experience a chronic sorrow. Grief, then, begins well before the time of death. Professionals must also remain cognizant of their own feelings of loss while caring for (and caring about) those they cannot cure. Physicians especially must come to terms with their orientation as healers while often facing helplessness and impotence in managing end-stage disease. Caregivers also grieve.

DEVELOPMENTAL CONSIDERATIONS OF ILLNESS AND DEATH

To understand a child's reaction to life-threatening conditions and death, professionals delivering pediatric palliative care must be mindful of important developmental differences in children's ability to conceptualize the nature and consequences of their illnesses and to make sense of and to master the concept and reality of death. Developmental studies have documented acquisition of the universality and irrevocability of death concepts as well as highlighting children's own awareness of their potential death (Koocher, 1973). Age is only one variable; emotional, social, and cognitive development each plays its own role in shaping the child's response. Personal experience with loss, separation, and illness may also facilitate comprehension of concepts of illness and death.

Infants lack the ability to recognize that their health circumstances differ from others and make little connection of causality with respect to the disease process and the treatment program. Nor can infants and toddlers understand all dimensions of death, especially its permanence. However, even very young children demonstrate the beginnings of concepts of separation and loss, as in games such as "all gone" and "peek-a-boo." Primitive protest, despair, separation anxiety, and detachment often occur at withdrawal of nurturing caretakers and can be perceived as akin to abandonment. Very young children also respond in reaction to observing distress in others. Emotional expression in the infant links directly to impulse and sensation. Behavioral manifestations of loss may include lethargy, irritability, or failure-to-thrive in extreme cases. Toddlers have better capacities to understand parental separation but can show regressive behavior, such as loss of toilet training or excessive clinging, especially under traumatic situations (e.g., car accidents or natural disasters). As the infant becomes a toddler, speech and language development makes it possible to communicate directly about the disease and treatment process. During these early years, the presence of a parent or, at minimum, the primary nurse during examinations or procedures can enhance the young child's coping abilities and compliance by providing the reassuring voice of a caretaker.

During the preschool period, egocentricism and magical thinking, which accompany preoperational thought, dominate concerns about causes of illness-related events and death. The child does not show well-established cause and effect reasoning in the illness-treatment process and can still think of death as a consequence of a specific thought or action rather than as a biologic process. For example, a young child might believe he became ill as a punishment for acting mean toward his siblings. Preschoolers' constructions of reality originate with their physically observable world, limited by their own experiences. They understand death as a changed state (Himelstein et al, 2004) and consider death as akin to sleep, moving away, or other known experiences of the living. Regression, longing, self-blame, sadness, and anger may accompany loss.

With the beginning of concrete operational thought at around the age of 6 or 7 years, the child can clearly differentiate between self and others, becomes capable of perspective taking, and thereby begins to recognize the irreversibility and permanence of death. A beginning understanding of biologic processes of the human body fosters a more realistic understanding of illness or trauma. School-age children may have many questions about their condition, although they might not always have the vocabulary or feel permission to ask them. Mood and reactivity become more stable, but fantasies and fears become more important to overall emotional reactivity and adaptation. The middle-school–age child tends to experience more anxiety, more overt symptoms of depression, and more somatic complaints than do younger children (Gudas, 1993), and contact with the child's primary care physician may provide great reassurance. A visit to the pediatrician can often prove helpful for healthy surviving siblings as well, especially for the child with somatic symptoms, and particularly when the ill sibling's death follows medical illness. In the preadolescent years, mastery and competency-based activities help form adaptive mechanisms in the face of emotional stress. Intellectual problem solving becomes useful as a defense mechanism. Responses to death and loss may be manifested in school or learning problems. Thus, collaboration with the child's school may provide important diagnostic information and opportunities to mobilize intervention and support. Information gathered from the media, peers, and parents can form lasting impressions, a relevant concern in helping children cope with the aftermath of disasters or accidents.

At the time of adolescence, with its accompanying abstract reasoning and formal operational thought, a more complete comprehension of death becomes possible. Death and end of life become concepts rather than events. Teenagers become aware of the complex physiologic systems of the body in relationship to both life and death. Responses to loss may revolve around multisystem syndromes (e.g., eating disorders, conversion reactions) as well as symptoms limited to the more immediate perceptions, as with younger children (e.g., stomachaches). The teenage years, marked by feelings of omnipotence, self-absorption, and narcissism, place teens at risk for denial of a life-threatening condition and lack of adherence to a treatment plan. The diagnosis of a life-altering illness additionally halts their move toward independence and development of a distinct sense of identity. Resentment, mood swings, rage, and risk-taking behaviors can emerge as the adolescent seeks answers to questions of values, safety, and fairness. Alternatively, the adolescent may seek philosophical explanations or spiritual meanings (e.g., How will I be remembered?). With the onset of hypothetical thinking and metacognition, alternatives that might not have occurred to the younger child become more prevalent (e.g., What will happen if the treatments don't work?). A future orientation becomes meaningful, and the long-range consequences of illness and treatment take on salience for the first time (e.g., Death means one is at peace and feels no pain.). Older children with serious conditions react most severely to perceived threats to their competence, expressing fears of falling behind in school or reacting with marked depression and anxiety to mobility losses. An ill teenager suffers intense concern with the loss of peer interaction and school activities because these become the primary delineators of evolving self-esteem in adolescence. All adolescents may demonstrate fascination with dramatic or sensational death (e.g., suicides, car crashes, disasters). Death of a peer can feel especially traumatic, particularly if that peer carried a similar health condition (e.g., cystic fibrosis). Consultation with the adolescent's pediatrician, who has known the teenager over time, could prove valuable in determining emotional risk factors and the need for psychological intervention.

Those professionals delivering palliative care must understand how children's ability to understand illness and death varies dramatically as a function of the child's developmental level. Such awareness is relevant in dealing with the ill child as well as with siblings and friends. Readers will find a more extensive review of children's developmental responses to death, dying, and grief in Gudas (1993), Koocher (1981), and Gudas and Koocher (2004).

UNDERSTANDING THE SERIOUSLY ILL AND DYING CHILD'S RESPONSE TO DEATH

The practice of withholding information about the diagnosis and prognosis from the dying child and family was generally abandoned many years ago, as clinicians learned that "protecting" children from the seriousness of their condition does not alleviate the child's or the family's concerns. However, whereas advances have occurred in informing children and families of their right to accurate and truthful medical knowledge, little has been done to equip health care providers with the knowledge or skills to effectively do so (Browning and Solomon, 2005). In a recent survey of 446 pediatric hospital staff members and community physicians, Contro and associates (2004) discovered that 71% of the residents, 40% of the attending physicians, and 43% of the nurses felt inexperienced, inadequate, and distressed in communicating with families and patients about issues of palliative care. In the same study (Contro et al, 2004), 68% of the family members interviewed (66 family members of 44 deceased children) reported distress caused by uncaring delivery of bad news and careless remarks by providers, resulting in lasting pain and complication of their and their child's grief. The professional literature repeatedly documents the need to educate all health care professionals working and communicating with gravely ill children on developmentally sensitive discussions of death and dying (Bagatell et al, 2002; Institute of Medicine, 2003).

Reviews of professional opinion and research data have consistently stressed that children as young as 5 or 6 years have a very real understanding of their illness, and still younger children show definite reactions to increased parental stress and other effects of a terminal illness on themselves and their families. Despite the recognition by children of their serious illness, conceptualizations of death and loss do not really differ from the general developmental trends already noted. The predominant modes of response tend to reflect age-related concerns about separation, pain, and disruption of usual life activities. Even among healthy children, substantial elements of anxiety exist with regard to death (Koocher, 1981). It should come as no surprise, therefore, to find a variety of adverse psychological symptoms and behavioral problems among dying children and members of their families.

In situations of loss and terminal illness, clinicians and researchers have begun to document observation of a process of potential reactions that occur, and often recur, over time. Ztalin (1995), for example, refers to two phases of patient response to or understanding of terminal illness. The first phase involves reacting and questioning, which includes the influence of family and social networks, issues of cause and control, illness severity, and beliefs about world view. The second phase involves assimilation, in which the patient and family attempt to place the illness within the context of their lives. In response to loss and death, Rando (1993) refers to a schema that divides such responses into three phases (avoidance, confrontation, and accommodation), each of which is characterized by a major response set toward the loss. Researchers studying children's reactions to loss and grief increasingly refer to psychological tasks rather than to predictable stages that children should master to cope effectively.

The crucial point, however, is to recognize the great variability in human response and the nonlinear progression of emotional responsiveness and conceptualization in terms of reactions rather than lock-step stages. For example, in thinking about adolescents diagnosed with AIDS or cancer, a significant, direct, and continuing expression of anger may well be seen. The adolescent is also much less likely to reach a stage or phase of acceptance of death. Case management must therefore be focused on individual patient responses and needs. Clinicians should not fall into the conceptual trap of pondering why a patient has not yet reached a certain stage or task at an expected juncture or feel concerned that a patient has regressed if he or she seems to engage in reworking reactions seen at previous points in time.

Another factor impinging on children's emotional reactivity and ability to cope with a serious medical condition involves their awareness and understanding of what is happening to them physiologically. For example, pediatric patients certainly know when they feel energetic or lethargic. An ill child who feels weak might more likely acknowledge a poor prognosis than the alert, active child; yet neither child might truly come to an acceptance of his or her fate. Primary care providers can better assess concerns paramount to the child by determining what the child has been told and by whom and what questions the child wants to ask about his or her condition.

KEY PSYCHOLOGICAL ISSUES FOR THE CRITICALLY ILL CHILD AND FAMILY

Children confronting terminal illnesses or facing an uncertain but potentially fatal outcome stand at substantial risk for emotional problems as a function of stress. Depending on the trajectory of the disease process, even children who were asymptomatic before becoming ill will predictably experience increased anxiety, sleep and appetite changes, social isolation, emotional withdrawal, depression, apathy, and marked ambivalence toward adults providing their primary care. These reactions are best regarded as responses to acute or chronic stress rather than as evidence of psychopathology. Children or families with preexisting emotional disorders will often experience an exacerbation of symptoms. When children feel that the outcome they will confront (i.e., death) is independent of their own behavior, the accompanying emotional stress and feelings of helplessness and hopelessness are dramatic.

Separation

The infant or toddler in an unfamiliar setting with strangers as caretakers (as when hospitalized) seeks parental reassurance and comfort and finds separation even more anxiety producing than does the healthy child. Arranging for parents to sleep in the hospital room with their child and to become integrally involved in the child's care is vital at this age. At times, the parents' heightened anxiety or withdrawal resulting from anticipatory grief can cause them to defer basic care of their child to the nursing staff. Alternatively, when the parents cannot detach from the responsibility of caring for the child, they may need permission to be relieved of such care. The primary health care team should assist the parents in openly discussing their emotional reactions to help them address their personal and family needs and to provide for the child's ongoing physical care and comfort.

By approximately 3 years of age, the preschooler can increasingly understand and tolerate parental absences. The presence of a life-threatening illness and the need for prolonged hospitalizations, however, can lead to regressive behavior and an increased need for parental reassurance. The preschool-age child can perceive death as a type of separation or parting from others. Fears and fantasies about illness and dying can be confused with concern about separation. The adolescent typically is concerned about potential family withdrawal related to anticipatory grief, censoring of medical information, and social withdrawal of peers due to their friends' anxieties about serious illness. Acceptance by peers is paramount to the adolescent's sense of identity and self-esteem. Isolation from normal peer activities poses difficulties for many adolescents.

Parents' presence and active involvement in the child's care remain essential throughout the childhood and adolescent years. This involvement includes the option to be present during medical procedures. Most health care facilities are aware of the comfort this provides the child and family and currently allow parental participation in basic treatments and procedures, such as dressing changes and insertion of intravenous lines. However, controversy remains, both in clinical settings and in the literature (Groopman, 2006; Knapp et al, 2005), as to whether parents should be exposed to such lifesaving procedures as intubation and resuscitation, particularly when the child is unconscious. Does the presence of parents provide comfort, help them come to terms with the child's condition, and allow them to feel that they have done everything they could? Or will parental presence disrupt or contribute to increased psychological trauma? The primary nurse and pediatrician (not actively involved in the procedure) can become invaluable liaisons between the staff and the parents in determining appropriateness and observing parental reaction.

Pain Management

Treatment of life-threatening illness requires many painful and noxious procedures and treatments. In addition to facilitating the parents' physical presence, comforting and reassuring, the treatment team can use other strategies to deal with the anxious anticipation of adverse procedures as well as the management of pain.

Every child needs preparation for procedures in clear, understandable language. An explanation of the procedure, commensurate with the child's age and ability to comprehend, helps the child anticipate what will transpire and provides an increased sense of control. Play therapy techniques, such as providing children with a stuffed toy animal and asking them to insert an intravenous line with use of actual equipment, offer an opportunity to address emotional concerns and to use mastery as a coping strategy before the actual procedure. The young child who complains of pain during a procedure can learn distraction techniques, such as deep breathing, squeezing a parent's arm when the pain intensifies, or the use of visual imagery techniques. Allowing the child to maintain some control can also help decrease fear and helplessness. For example, the clinician can suggest that it is okay to scream or cry during a procedure, as long as the child remains relatively motionless. Deep muscle relaxation and hypnosis can also prove useful with school-age children and adolescents, both as an aid in reducing anxiety and as a strategy to control chronic pain (such as "phantom pain" after amputation or pain from an invasive procedure). Consultation with a mental health provider, who can help the child better understand the psychological consequences of his or her pain and who can provide skilled behavioral techniques, is appropriate.

Vignette

Jill, 4 years of age, had severe distress reactions in response to venipuncture. Play therapy sessions were introduced and included elaborate preparations for drawing blood from her plush toy animal, Snoopy. She was also provided a party blower noisemaker for Snoopy to use during the procedure. After a few consultations, Jill was able to tolerate venipuncture herself, using a party blower, without overt signs of distress. The intervention allowed Jill to express herself, to gain some mastery over her feelings of anxiety, and to learn a distraction technique.

Control

The diagnosis of a life-threatening condition creates an emotional crisis in the family. The loss of control implicit in the diagnosis is one of the most devastating aspects of the crisis. Parents can experience the loss of ability to protect their child from harm and to positively influence their child's future. Their feelings of loss of control can generate intensification of concern and caretaking behavior, thus helping regain a sense of mastery when they feel helpless. Often, however, the staff can experience this behavior as overprotective and infantilizing.

Vignette

A 10-year-old girl was put on life support after an anoxic brain injury. Her parents did not leave her side for several days. They eventually asked the nurse if she thought they might "miss something" if they went home for a brief time to attend to their other children. The mother also expressed a fear that her daughter might need her while she was away. The parents were told, "She is not responsive and won't know if you are not here. You don't need to stay all the time." These parents could have been better reassured by such words as, "We don't know how much she knows is going on. We will be with her and remind her that you will return soon. We will call you if we observe anything new."

The preadolescent child, who seeks achievement in many areas, can experience the loss of control to plan his or her life. The child might displace anger onto schedules or hospitalizations that interfere with afterschool activities. For example, a 9-year-old child can become furious that chest physical therapy for progressive symptoms of cystic fibrosis interrupts play dates with friends. Anger about the diagnosis may not appear directly. The preadolescent child might attempt to regain control by testing parental limits. The parents might, in turn, curtail discipline out of guilt or concern for their sick child. Rather than making the child feel special, however, this behavior can make the child feel more out of control.

Loss of control has a heightened impact during adolescence. Adolescents strive for autonomy and increasing independence from parents. When hospitalizations or disease symptoms impede such developmental progress by virtue of decisions made by medical personnel that affect the adolescent's health and daily life, patients often feel bombarded. The hospital experience can foster passivity and regressive dependence that inhibit the adolescent's growing sense of mastery over the environment. The ability to experience competence through school, social experiences, and planning for the future is also seriously disrupted when treatments or symptoms make it difficult to keep up.

Another adolescent task involves development of mastery over one's changing body. The physical changes accompanying serious illnesses directly challenge body image integrity. For instance, alopecia, a frequent side effect of chemotherapy, becomes a visible, inescapable reminder to the patient of the disease as well as a possible source of embarrassment and decline in self-esteem. Comfort and confidence in sexual attractiveness are also severely challenged by the effects of both the disease and its treatment.

With children and adolescents, the loss of control accompanying a hospitalization adds stress. The patient's daily schedule is disrupted, and familiar people and activities are absent. Some patients might feel uncomfortable at some particular time of the day, coinciding with a missed special activity or lonely late-evening hours. Simple measures, such as permitting patients to wear their own clothes in the hospital or allowing some choices in time for procedures (e.g., Shall we do this now or after lunch?), can increase the child's sense of control.

Trust and Honest Communication

Seriously ill children have many fears and apprehensions about their condition. They often sense the tendency of parents, loved ones, and medical personnel to withhold or to minimize information. Such tendencies can leave children with confusing or misleading information about treatments, procedures, or course of care.

Vignette

Susan, aged 9 years, complained of feeling treated like a baby during a hospitalization. Her physician would compliment her pajama choices or ask about her stuffed toy animals but did not talk with her about discussions and decisions made about her care, which she knew were being decided in the hallway with residents. Susan commented to her psychologist, "I want to know if I need to have another lumbar puncture and when I can go home. I don't care if he likes my teddy bear!"

Open communication with children provides an opportunity to dispel unnecessary worries and to concentrate on the adjustment required for the realities of treatment. Children have the right to timely and accurate information necessary to understand their care goals and options and to participate in their care in a developmentally appropriate manner (Browning and Solomon, 2005). Only through such discussions can the hopes, wishes, and preferences of the child be addressed. A child who can ask questions and receive honest answers about the illness and treatment will feel more a part of the medical regimen, trust his or her caretakers, and feel less anxious. Although such communication may initially be difficult for the clinician, the ultimate gains in adherence and security from such discussions will prove invaluable. Parents and health care providers may benefit from a consultation with a mental health provider to assist them in addressing issues in a developmentally sensitive way and in determining what and how much the child understands.

Vignette

Joey, aged 6 years, was dying of an aggressive, inoperable brain tumor. With the help of Joey's psychologist, his parents and neurologist explained to Joey that all the medicines and radiation could not stop the tumor from growing. He could go home, where his parents and the visiting nurses would take care of him, making sure he gets his medicine if any part of him hurts. He was told that when his tumor got too big, his body would stop working and he would die. His parents explained that he would go to heaven to live with God and his Auntie Helen and that someday the whole family would be together again. Later that day, the psychologist went back to see Joey in his hospital room and said to Joey, "We talked about some hard things this morning." Joey retorted, "I hate Auntie Helen!" The therapist, responding to both the family's belief system and to Joey's statement and its underlying concern, replied, "Lots of boys and girls have died and gone to heaven, so you won't have to hang out with Auntie Helen. But I bet you're upset about dying, too." The management of this situation respected family beliefs and allowed Joey, his parents, and the medical team to truthfully discuss Joey's prognosis and gave Joey permission to communicate with others about his end of life.

FAMILY-CENTERED MANAGEMENT OF PALLIATIVE CARE

Viewing family-based intervention as an absolute necessity will foster optimal adaptation and support of the patient. The costs of chronic illness to the patient's family are substantial in both emotional and financial terms. The course of the illness will likely tax the adaptive capacities of the parents, both as individuals and as a couple. Brothers and sisters will also likely experience an extra burden of stress. If the patient does die, a family of grief-stricken survivors remains. The practitioner who overlooks the family as a part of the "patient care" locus will ultimately compromise care for the ill family member.

Professionals must remain aware that the typical or normal behavior in the family of a child with terminal or life-threatening illness differs from the behavior of the same family before the diagnosis. Professionals immersed in the process of treating such families or who have known the families for many years can easily overlook this truism. For example, competent, articulate parents talking retrospectively of the day they first learned of their child's diagnosis frequently report, "After the doctor told us our child had leukemia, she said some other things.... I don't remember what they were." The "other things" may have dealt with treatments about to begin; but the parents, overwhelmed by the threat of a potentially terminal illness, often feel too stunned to absorb the information. Such predictable reactions routinely occur under these circumstances, and the health care team can implement measures to assist such parents. Communication between specialists and the primary care physician should include information important for the parents to absorb (e.g., imminent treatments, side effects of medications). Parents may feel more comfortable communicating with their pediatrician's office for clarification or reassurance. Follow-up phone calls to the family by the physician or nurse can routinely assess the parents' level of functioning and ability to absorb information accurately. Writing down information or providing written resources allows the parents to have concrete reminders. The Institute of Medicine offers helpful suggestions to present difficult news to families, including having someone present trained to respond to the family's needs and ready to stay with the family, having both parents present, asking if the parents would like to have anyone else present, and providing a tape of the conversation for them to review as needed (Institute of Medicine, 2003).

In coping with life-threatening illness, family members must confront the problem of managing their own emotions as well as the practical aspects of daily living. Learning to deal with chronic stress, disruption, and uncertainty makes the ability to cope a continually trying task. Koocher and O'Malley (1981) summarize the burdens of coping as balancing the needs of the patient in the home with those of healthy siblings, fostering the patient's normal social and emotional development while coping with long-term uncertainty, and dealing with unresolved anticipatory grief should the child survive.

Increased marital stress and financial strain are predictable phenomena. The quality of the marital relationship before diagnosis serves as an important predictor of the adequacy of marital coping with the crisis. A decreased sense of parental competence can further impair coping. The survival of a marriage can be linked to survival of the patient, but professional counseling and parent support groups can play important roles in helping to manage parental and marital stress (Koocher and O'Malley, 1981).

The relationship of sisters and brothers to their parents also changes if they experience decreased attention and support. Siblings may feel angry at both the ill child and the parents who have failed to protect them from the consequences of the illness. Increased stress in the home and the resulting changes that occur (loss of family time, changes in routine) may feel as distressing to the brothers and sisters as the condition of their sibling. Such a response is particularly common when the sibling is newly born and little time has passed for emotional attachment. School and peer relationships can also suffer. In other instances, brothers and sisters can plunge into academic pursuits as a means of escaping stresses at home or to prove their competence in an effort to combat family feelings of hopelessness. Peer relationships can be interrupted for practical reasons, such as school absences to visit the ill child or to retreat into the family. Sisters and brothers can also feel alienated from friends who do not understand their irritability and preoccupation. Development of somatic complaints as a means of garnering parental attention or to identify with the ill child has also been observed.

Open communication between the patient's primary care provider and the siblings, including family counseling sessions, constitutes one beneficial approach. Siblings may have many questions and fantasies that necessitate clarification but that the parents alone may not be able to answer. Parents' efforts to spend "special time" with their healthy children, to provide consistency, to continue important family routines, and to aid their children in maintaining as normal a life as possible also become important. By knowing something of the family's premorbid interactions and individual coping skills, the primary care provider can help evaluate and understand children's reactions and advise and assist the family in responding to their needs.

The family's pediatrician stands in a unique position to assist the parents, ill child, and siblings. In addition, the pediatrician can facilitate transfer of information about the family within and across sites of care to other health care providers involved in the palliative care of the child. Such support, anticipatory guidance, and sharing of information have been associated with positive long-term bereavement adjustment (American Academy of Pediatrics, Committee on Psychosocial Aspects of Child and Family Health, 2000; Knapp et al, 2005).

MANAGING PEDIATRIC PALLIATIVE CARE IN DIFFERENT SITES

Seriously ill children receive care in a variety of settings. The psychological issues and needs of pediatric patients and their families can differ, depending on the locus of care. Practitioners should be sensitive to and capable of recognizing the distinctions. The important point for health care professionals to remember is that individual family members must be viewed in the context of the current treatment circumstances and the personal meanings of those events. A family who manages well under one set of circumstances can have very different reactions during subsequent conditions. The distinction might well be based on an attribution or perception not evident to the physician managing the case. This phenomenon underscores the importance of a team approach to care that includes mental health professionals.

Emergency Department

Whereas the actual death of a child in the emergency department is an uncommon occurrence, the emergency department physician and health care team must prepare to treat and to manage the life-threatening illnesses and conditions likely to enter their doors and that cause children to die. As previously noted, injuries and accidents constitute the number one cause of death in children; SIDS leads the cause of death in the infancy period. Inevitably, these children arrive urgently to the emergency department for triage and care. In addition, the child with a life-threatening illness or condition may come to an emergency department in a medical crisis. The mother in premature labor or with a high-risk pregnancy may also present to an emergency department staff.

Several characteristics distinguish the emergency department from other sites at which children may die:

1. Staff must prepare to respond to the emotional, medical, cultural, procedural, and legal aspects of caring for a seriously ill patient while simultaneously

supporting a family in the acute process of grief (Knapp et al, 2005).
2. More than one family member may be affected (as in a disaster or accident or an imperiled newborn and mother).
3. Parents of the child may be unavailable at the time.
4. Medicolegal procedures may be complicated and emotionally difficult, as in trauma cases or SIDS, when overwhelmed parents facing the imminent death of their child must endure an investigation as to the cause of the child's condition.
5. Often no prior established relationship exists between the emergency department staff and the child and family (Knapp and Mulligan-Smith, 2005).

The importance of the trusted and familiar family physician to communicate with and to guide the family through the trauma of an emergency department experience, even if such communication is initially by telephone contact, is evident. In addition, the primary care physician, aware of the family's cultural and religious beliefs, can assist the family and staff in making decisions about further necessary care that accommodate the family's values and customs. Such decisions include additional invasive procedures, postmortem care of the body, organ donation, and autopsy if the child dies.

Clearly, similarities in needs exist between children and families in palliative care and those who die in the emergency department. Most applicable are attention to pain relief, facility design, timely provision of accurate and understandable language, provision of immediate and long-term bereavement support, identification of community-based resources, and family involvement in decision making (Knapp et al, 2005).

Outpatient Clinics and Offices

Outpatient care for the child with a life-threatening condition is generally more reassuring than care in other sites. Children spend more time in the company of familiar caretakers in the pediatrician's office or a hospital clinic where they have received care over time. A degree of normality associated with sleeping in one's own bed and returning to the familiar family home can prove supportive and reassuring. However, the stresses on family members can be great in some instances. Arranging for care of siblings, missing time at work, managing household chores, and other such disruptions can be quite stressful, depending on the frequency and duration of the stay and the treatment required.

As life-limiting and life-threatening conditions progress, outpatient treatments and visits increase. We know that even young children have an awareness of their medical conditions and that children seem to know innately when they are dying. We also know of the increased sense of isolation dying children tend to experience. Pediatric health care providers who work with cancer patients well know how anxiety levels in children with leukemia often increase in parallel with increases in the frequency of outpatient clinic visits. This finding is opposite of what is found in youngsters with chronic non–life-threatening illnesses. Even children who have previously coped relatively well become acutely sensitive to changes in frequency of visits, treatments, and procedures. Encouraging the child to ask questions about his or her condition not only will alleviate some anxiety but will empower the child to become active in his or her care. Effective communication between the child and the managing clinicians in the outpatient setting will also begin to build a healthy rapport that will continue throughout the child's palliative care. If the child has not yet established a relationship with a mental health provider, such developments create a crucial time for introducing supportive therapy.

Inpatient Settings

During an inpatient stay, a child requires more reassurance and emotional support for a longer period than during outpatient visits. Many hospitals now provide rooming-in opportunities and encourage parents or other family members to participate in caring for their child. However, in some settings or circumstances (e.g., intensive care units), such involvement by family members may be limited. Some hospital stays can be seen as "routine" therapeutic admissions; others can generate anxiety, realistic or not, that the illness has worsened. Even children who otherwise seem to be coping well through a prolonged illness can experience specific problems (such as conditioned reflex vomiting), anxiety linked to painful procedures, depressive reactions to progressive loss of physical capacities, or family inhibitions (Koocher and O'Malley, 1981). Although seemingly a paradoxical reaction to the cessation of a noxious experience, hospitalizations and stressful treatment regimens can become imbued with some protective value.

For children with complex medical problems that require inpatient, home, and community-based services from many different professionals, organizations, and settings that may be separated geographically, institutionally, and even culturally from one another, the burden of coordination of services can be overwhelming (Institute of Medicine, 2003). For the families of the hospitalized child with a life-threatening illness, continuity of care is paramount to feeling confidence in and trustful of the quality of care their family member receives. Without continuity, parents often feel they must "start from scratch" with each hospital admission. Heller and Solomon (2005) interviewed 36 bereaved parents of children with life-threatening conditions who died after receiving care at three geographically dispersed teaching hospitals. Three types of continuities emerged as key in ensuring that the parents felt confident their child would receive the best possible care:

1. informational continuity—information on prior events is available to all care providers and used to give care appropriate to their child's current circumstances;
2. relational continuity—the importance of providers' knowing the patient as a person, allowing predictability and coherence in care; and
3. management continuity—types of care from different providers complement one another in a coherent way, that is, a shared management plan. In the absence of continuous, caring relationships with staff, parents reported frustration, hypervigilance and mistrust about the quality of care their child received.

This study demonstrates that the presence of one or more professionals who remain present throughout the child's course of hospitalization mitigates parents' anxieties and concerns.

Because the focus of care in hospital settings is on cure, the child with life-threatening or terminal illness stands in a unique position compared with those children who will return to a healthy life. By not forgetting the curative aspect of palliative care, the maintenance of a sense of normality and optimal quality of life for the hospitalized child becomes critical. Continuity of daily life activities becomes a key issue. Socialization, through visits, phone calls, and letters from friends and schoolmates, is encouraged. Making the hospital a familiar setting by bringing in personal articles from home promotes continuity and familiarity, a gesture especially helpful for the young child. Ensuring that the patient continues as an active, responsible person who makes choices should be the central priority. This active stance is best introduced to patients as a way of helping them cope with disease and hospitalization. Choices can include activity room programming, academic tutoring, developing a support network by introducing newly diagnosed patients to each other and to "veterans," allowing patients to participate in decisions concerning medical procedures, and soliciting and responding to feedback from the child. These components create an atmosphere in which the child can maintain a sense of dignity and control and should have a positive effect on the child's ability to cope with his or her illness.

Location of End of Life Care

Patients in the terminal stages of disease receive care in a variety of settings. The medical team should discuss location of terminal care with the family and patient at appropriate points in the course of the child's illness, at a time when the family can plan and have questions thoroughly explored. Mental health and social service clinicians are important consultants for planning at this stage to help the family reach a decision that is personally, financially, and practically reasonable for them. The family needs to be reassured that the entire medical team will support them in whatever decision they reach and that the hospital team will work closely with the home care or hospice team to provide continuity of care. Some families may benefit from meeting a home care or hospice nurse who can answer questions of the child and family and discuss the eligibility criteria for accepting children as patients.

Currently, the majority of children who die do so in the hospital. Allowing the child to die at home, in hospice care, or in a continuing care facility is an alternative that warrants consideration by all individuals involved in the child's care. Parents and families often feel reassured and more useful when they are able to care for their child at home (Hutchinson et al, 2003). However, some other parents may feel insecure and tense in dealing with the side effects of treatments, administering medications, or other aspects of home care. Transition to the home may also leave the family with a feeling of isolation or abandonment from the hospital providers who have become trusted caretakers (Milstein, 2005). Home and community-based care settings also carry with them potential concerns, such as provider anxiety and burnout or depletion of financial resources. More than one family member should be prepared to provide skilled care for the ill child to allow sharing of both the physical and emotional responsibility.

At some point, home care may prove to be insufficient or too complex for the family alone. The child's pediatrician may stand in a pivotal and nonthreatening role to help the family make the decision that additional care may be indicated. Parents can be reassured that those professionals skilled in palliative care will work alongside others so that some of the professional team remains familiar to the family and so it does not seem that the referring team has given up on them (Hutchinson et al, 2003). If hospice proves a viable option, issues related to competence, reliability, and trust are salient for the family. By definition, hospice care implies that the family has acknowledged the terminal nature of the illness and that the family unit agrees they can no longer care for their child by themselves. With the affirmation of the child's pediatrician, the parents can be reassured that they are neither "giving up on" nor "letting go of" their child; nor by choosing hospice are they "giving over" the care of their child. Instead, families can be helped to see that by providing a program of highly qualified and compassionate services, they are actively planning for a meaningful experience for the remainder of their child's life.

THE ROLE OF THE INTERDISCIPLINARY TEAM

Throughout the patient's treatment, the family and child establish a network of medical providers whom they come to know and trust. A typical pediatric palliative care team will include the inpatient physician or intensivist, primary nurse, mental health professional, outpatient pediatrician and nurse, and visiting nurse. A palliative care specialist, medical specialists, physical therapists, occupational therapists, nutritionists, and hospice nurses and workers may also join the team. Open, frequent communication among team members ensures a uniform approach and underscores the consistent availability of the staff to the patient and family. Liaison with school counselors, teachers, clergy, or other community members can also prove helpful in providing additional support. The designation of an overall team coordinator experienced in palliative care issues, who takes responsibility for gathering data and presenting the synthesized information to the family, is crucial for clear communication. This prevents overly anxious parents from "splitting" team members, which can lead to confusing or distorted information.

The primary care physician is often the person the family wants to become this team coordinator, for the family relies on their pediatrician (and the office staff) to be the reliable and consistent professional to transition with them through the diagnosis, treatment, death, and bereavement process of their child and to then be available to continue to treat the surviving siblings. Numerous studies report that the presence of such a continuous advocate, reviewer of services, and manager of

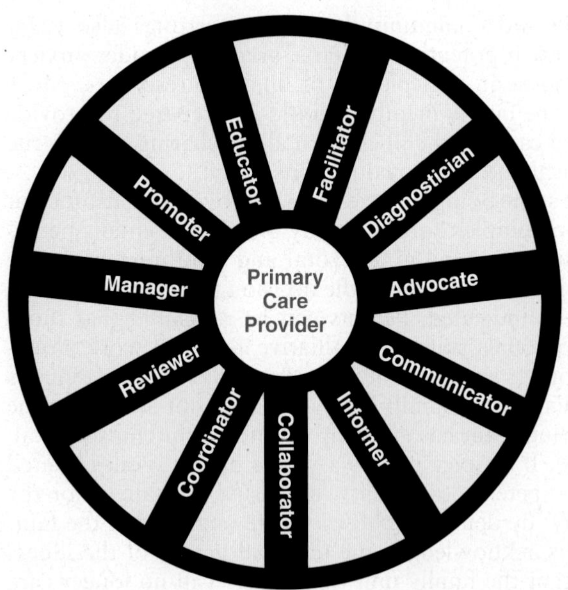

Figure 36-1. Role of the primary care provider in pediatric palliative care.

transmission of information helps minimize symptoms of traumatic stress and emotional suffering. Whether the child dies within a short time or survives for years or even decades before an early death, ill children, parents, and siblings want to share and hear difficult news with the key team member who has known them over time. Although this responsibility may seem burdensome and time-consuming, many of these services require simply "being there" over time. The multiple roles the primary care provider can fulfill have been discussed throughout this chapter and are illustrated in Figure 36-1.

The mental health professional can offer support to the patient, family, and medical staff by consulting with them on the assessment of the patient's developmental level, the meaning of psychological and psychogenic symptoms, and the care and management of the patient. Indirect consultation can lead to direct patient contact or can allow improved care without such referral. The mental health clinician can also facilitate creation of a forum to discuss team members' emotional reactions to providing care to patients with life-threatening conditions.

The mental health provider can best serve the patient and family by conducting an initial evaluation at the time of diagnosis. At this juncture, the psychological consultant can assess the family's functioning and interactional style and make recommendations for managing predictable stresses. The early intervention can help manage predictable reactions and decrease family tension by helping the family facilitate clear communication and mutual support. This initial assessment also permits early intervention when one or more family members seem at risk. If mental health services are routinely introduced early on and integrated as part of the standard care of the patient, no stigma is associated with the service. Families should not feel singled out as being "crazy" or in need of psychological intervention. Patients additionally benefit by virtue of the fact that all caregivers interact closely and more efficiently.

In responding to the needs of end of life care with a child and family, the medical and mental health professionals can help families set reasonable (i.e., concrete, realistic, and focused) goals over which they have control, even as they face diminished physical control. For example, alleviation of pain is a goal of the child, family, and health care providers and can be obtained only through working in collaboration.

EDUCATIONAL AND RESEARCH NEEDS IN PEDIATRIC PALLIATIVE CARE

There is a significant lack of formal education in pediatric palliative care in medical schools and residency programs (Bagatell et al, 2002; Browning and Solomon, 2005; Contro et al, 2004; Institute of Medicine, 2003; Knapp et al, 2005). Among those training programs that do offer formal education in death and dying, a significant lack of standards exists. Consequently, many physicians delivering pediatric care report feeling unprepared to deal with end of life and bereavement care for children, with much of their experience occurring on a trial and error basis (Bagatell et al, 2002; Institute of Medicine, 2003). In addition, the health care system in the United States has failed to meet the needs of children requiring end of life and bereavement care (Browning and Solomon, 2005; Institute of Medicine, 2003), notably owing to lack of funding and reimbursement of time and services from insurance companies. Whereas integration of formal training of pediatric palliative care into the curriculum of medical schools or offering specific fellowship programs for pediatric care specialists may seem a Herculean task, we must begin to more effectively relieve the physical and emotional pain of these children and families. Bagatell and colleagues (2002), for example, designed and implemented a low-cost, six-session seminar for pediatric residents at the University of Arizona. This program included sessions involving symptom management and discussion of end of life care with families and issues arising at the time of death. Pre- and post-testing of the residents suggested an increase in skill acquisition and comfort level in managing children dealing with end of life issues. Health care providers and family members are increasingly seeking information on informative Web sites (Table 36-1).

Research needs in pediatric palliative care include protocols and procedures for implementation in the hospital as well as curriculum designs in medical schools to prepare physicians to provide expert care on a pediatric palliative care team. Such programs must remain sensitive to developmental differences in children, cultural and religious differences, ethical and legal issues, and management of symptoms at different stages of illness. Clinical research is necessary to learn more about the experiences of children and families to identify risk factors, to facilitate communication, to improve quality of life, and to coordinate care. Such research is problematic, for many reasons, however. Prospective studies, observing the child at diagnosis and continuing with the family into bereavement, are desperately needed to determine appropriate timing and approaches to care.

Table 36-1. **Web Sites**

Site	Information
www.aahpm.org American Academy of Hospice and Palliative Medicine	Training guidelines for fellowships in palliative care Educational programs Book resources Board membership
www.eperc.mcw.edu End of Life/Palliative Education Resource Center (EPERC)	Educational materials Conferences Self-study program Resources
www.ippcweb.org Initiative for Pediatric Palliative Care	Research Assessment Curriculum modules Educational development
www.chionline.org Children's Hospice International	All inclusive programs for children and families How to develop programs Raising standards
www.depts.washington.edu/healthtr Adolescent Health Transition Project	Time lines for transition of care Health history form for transfer of care Information for teens

The length of such research and the ethical and practical issues of working with an ill child are of concern. Retrospective studies raise significant risks of retraumatization of families as well as validity and reliability issues in assessing children and families whose level of functioning varies over the course of the illness and who are actively grieving.

SUMMARY

Many professionals are fearful of working with children who will die and with their families. Most often, these practitioners cite their own helplessness or sense of inadequacy in the face of death as a basis for their apprehension. The ill children and their families also have fears but desperately need and want skilled support of professionals who can provide encouragement and advice about how to cope with their stress and uncertainty. Clinicians who participate in the final days of a child's life will forever be indelibly etched into the family's memories of that event and incorporated into the meaning of the child's death for the family. The impact pediatric providers can have on offering positive experiences for these children and their families is immeasurable. The emotional rewards of working with families during this difficult time are substantial.

REFERENCES

American Academy of Pediatrics, Committee on Psychosocial Aspects of Child and Family Health: The pediatrician and childhood bereavement. Pediatrics 105(2):445-447, 2000.

Bagatell R, Meyer R, Herron S, et al: When children die: A seminar for pediatric residents. Pediatrics 110(2):348-353, 2002.

Browning DM, Solomon MZ: The initiative for pediatric palliative care: An interdisciplinary educational approach for healthcare professionals. J Pediatr Nurs 20(5):326-334, 2005.

Contro NA, Larson J, Scofield S, et al: Hospital staff and family perspectives regarding quality of pediatric palliative care. Pediatrics 114(5):1248-1252, 2004.

Groopman J: Being there. The New Yorker, April 3, 2006:34-39.

Gudas L: Concepts of death and loss in childhood and adolescence: A developmental perspective. *In* Saylor CE (ed): Children and Disasters. New York, Plenum Press, 1993, p 67-84.

Gudas LS, Koocher GP: Grief and bereavement. *In* Behrman RE, Kliegman, RM, Jenson HB (eds): Nelson Textbook of Pediatrics, 17th ed. Philadelphia, WB Saunders, 2004, pp 117-120.

Heller KS, Solomon MZ: Continuity of care and caring: What matters to parents of children with life-threatening conditions. J Pediatr Nurs 20(5):335-346, 2005.

Himelstein BP, Hilden JM, Boldt AM, Weissman D: Pediatric palliative care. N Engl J Med 350(17):1752-1762, 2004.

Hutchinson F, King N, Hain RD: Terminal care in paediatrics: Where we are now. Postgrad Med J 79:566-568, 2003.

Institute of Medicine; Field MJ, Behrman RE (eds): When Children Die: Improving Palliative and End-of-life Care for Children and their Families. Washington, DC, National Academies Press, 2003.

Knapp J, Mulligan-Smith D; Committee on Pediatric Emergency Medicine: Death of a child in the emergency department. Pediatrics 115(5):1432-1437, 2005.

Koocher GP: Childhood, death and cognitive development. Dev Psychol 9(3):369-375, 1973.

Koocher GP: Development of the death concept in children. *In* Bibace R, Walsh ME (eds): The Development of Concepts Related to Health: Future Directions in Developmental Psychology. San Francisco, Jossey-Bass, 1981, pp 85-99.

Koocher GP, O'Malley JE: The Damocles Syndrome: Psychosocial Consequences of Surviving Cancer. New York, McGraw-Hill, 1981.

Milstein J: A paradigm of integrative care: Healing with curing throughout life, "being with" and "doing to." J Perinatol 25:563-568, 2005.

Rando T: Treatment of Complicated Mourning. Champaign, IL, Research Press, 1993.

Ztalin DM: Life themes: A method to understanding terminal illness. Omega 31:185, 1995.

37 AFTER THE DEATH OF A CHILD: HELPING BEREAVED PARENTS AND BROTHERS AND SISTERS

WILLIAM LORD COLEMAN AND
JULIUS BENJAMIN RICHMOND (1916-2008)

"Bereaved parents live two lives simultaneously, one with their child and one without their child. They live both lives every day."

—William Lord Coleman

"Bereaved parents, at some point, must integrate the death of their child into their lives and continue to live. There is never closure."

—Julius Benjamin Richmond

Vignette

A pediatrician read of the death (drowning in a lake) of a 5-year-old boy (Joel) in his practice. He felt uncomfortable and confused whether he should contact the family. He decided to wait until Joel's sister's next office visit (in 1 month) and then "say something."

Joel's mother and 10-year-old sister Kathy sat silently in the examination room. Kathy had her arm around her mother. Their eyes seemed to search his face: Does he know? Will he say something? He greeted them, then sat silently, uncertain what to do or say, as if waiting for them to mention Joel's death first.

After a short silence, he said softly, "I'm very sorry about Joel's passing." They mumbled "Thank you." Tears filled their eyes. After a respectful pause, he asked, "How are you getting by?" The mother had taken an indefinite leave of absence from work. The father was working longer hours "to keep busy and distracted." Kathy had many excused absences from school, her grades were dropping, and she had quit the soccer team. After the memorial service and interment of Joel's ashes, the family had received only occasional calls and letters. "Everyone seems to have disappeared . . . as if everything was normal again, like Joel had never died."

The pediatrician was deeply moved and was worried about the impact on Kathy and that she might be assuming the role of "caretaker." Painfully aware this was not a routine well-child visit, he told them he would reschedule it. He wanted to help, but at this moment he did not know what to do. In parting, he determined to find support for the family and to address Kathy's situation. He scheduled a "family visit" (mother, father, Kathy) at 5:00 PM for the following week.

The death of a child* is the most devastating and life-defining event parents can ever experience. It defies the natural order: parents should not bury their children. The child will never be again, and the death leaves an emptiness never filled. The loss destroys the parents' hopes of loving and developing a healthy, happy child to be a positive and productive member of society. When a child dies, something in the parents and siblings dies too, expectations and hopes of a future together. The grief and yearning are unimaginable to others because

Both authors lost their sons, Dale K. Richmond (1950-1971) and Justin L. Coleman (1976-2003). This chapter is dedicated to them and to all lost children everywhere.

* *Child* includes a fetus, infant, child, adolescent, and grown adult. The child may be a biologic child, stepchild, adopted child, foster child, grandchild, or of any relationship. *Pediatrician* includes all who care and advocate for children and their families. *Parent* includes all who love, protect, and care and provide for children—biologic parents, grandparents, stepparents, adoptive parents, foster parents, and siblings.

the experience is so removed from any life event that they may have known (Finkbeiner, 1996; Rando, 1986).

Grief is often described in metaphors: Grief is a wave. It rushes in from the ocean, without warning, monstrous, silent or roaring, crushing the grief stricken. Eventually the wave recedes, leaving them in a strange calm to crawl, to stand, to walk, and then to continue on. Over time, the waves gradually become ripples quietly tugging on their ankles, barely noticeable but always felt. The monstrous waves return intermittently, and again the ripples return. They are always there.

Brothers and sisters, "the forgotten mourners," are deeply affected both by their parents' grief and by their own special loss. The circle of grief is wide. For every child who dies, approximately 10 people are deeply affected.

Grief also affects those who have "lost" children other than by certain known death: through relinquishing their children for adoption; by kidnapping, running away, or leaving home and never returning; by severely incapacitating injuries, mental illness, or substance abuse; and even by being imprisoned for life.

The goal of this chapter is to help pediatricians learn of

- grief and bereavement and their impact on parents and brothers and sisters;
- supportive measures, including resources and referrals, for the bereaved in the office or clinic; and
- supportive measures at the bedside for the grief stricken when the child dies.

GRIEF AND BEREAVEMENT: THEIR IMPACT ON PARENTS AND BROTHERS AND SISTERS

Parents and siblings grieve in their own ways: each at his or her own level of suffering, for his or her own duration, privately or publicly, silently or openly, and alone or with others. The parents' ways of grieving strongly influence the child's expression of grief. The child's and parents' individual temperaments and their "fit" must be considered (Carey and McDevitt, 1995). Children also perceive death by their developmental levels (Lewis and Schonfeld, 2002).

Various factors influence the ways in which parents and siblings grieve (Table 37-1). Appreciation of these factors enables pediatricians to be more understanding and comforting (Wessel, 2003).

First, pediatricians can better understand grief reactions by seeing grief as falling into two general "stages" (Maciejewski et al, 2007). These stages do not fit the five stages (denial, anger, bargaining, depression, acceptance) faced by those experiencing their own approaching deaths (Kubler-Ross, 1969). The initial stage of grief is profound sorrow and despair. The later stage is acceptance and yearning. The stages are both circular and sequential: at times, each stage circling back around to affect the other; at other times, progressing. The bereaved always experience the recurrent waves and ripples, but over time, the ripples become more present than the waves.

Normal grief reactions affect the physical, emotional, psychological, and social-behavioral health and function of the bereaved (Table 37-2). Anger, sadness, and denial are primal survival tools that pediatricians should

Table 37-1. Factors Influencing Expressions of Grief

Parents and Siblings	Parents	Brothers and Sisters
The manner of death	Parent–dead child relationship, including "unfinished business"	Developmental status
Family cohesion	"Special meaning" of child	Individual temperament
Mutual support	Age of child	How parents grieve
Responses of friends, extended family	Individual temperament	Surviving sibling–child relationships
Physical and mental health	Quality of marriage	Surviving siblings' relationships
Access to resources	Parent's ability to show affection	Responses at school (teachers, peers)
Cultural: religious beliefs, traditions	Career demands	
	Responses of colleagues	

Table 37-2. Normal Grief Reactions (A Selective List): What Pediatricians Should Monitor and Care For

Physical	Emotional-Psychological	Behavioral-Social
Lethargy	Disbelief; why?; if only; what if?	Restlessness, sighing
Sleep disturbances	Sadness, depression, even suicidal ideation	Screaming
Tightness in the chest	Crying, keening (anguished wailing)	Calling out to lost child
Other somatic complaints	Helplessness, guilt, anxiety	Avoiding activities outside of home
Weight gain or loss	Feel "I'm going crazy," "Am I normal?"	Withdrawal from friends and acquaintances
	Feel like "damaged goods"	Avoiding or treasuring reminders of child (his or her room, clothing, photos, music)
	"Emotional coma," "walking dead"	Disorganization, indecision
	Afraid to be alone; loneliness	Memory and concentration loss
	Thinking endlessly about the child and circumstances of death	Marriage strained, broken, strengthened

acknowledge and validate. Pediatricians should be vigilant and thorough in detecting these symptoms, explaining them as normal reactions, monitoring them, and treating or referring as necessary (Zisook and Zisook, 2005). They must be especially sensitive to when parent and sibling grief becomes depression (Heneghan et al, 2004); Park et al, 2007). Some parents may even feel suicidal, wanting to "join" the dead child (Li et al, 2005). Delayed grief reactions occur sometime after the death, such as close to the death anniversary or birthday (anniversary reactions).

Relationships among parents and siblings can be strained. Marriages can be strained also. Family relationships and marriages can also be strengthened.

The death and family grief may recall a personal event and stir strong emotions in the pediatrician. A bit of pediatrician self-disclosure can be supportive, but not too much (McDaniel et al, 2007; Redinbaugh et al, 2003).

SUPPORTIVE MEASURES, INCLUDING RESOURCES AND REFERRALS, FOR THE BEREAVED IN THE OFFICE OR CLINIC

A Child's Death, the Family's Grief, and the Role of the Pediatrician

Pediatricians experience the death of children more than all other physicians. Although trained in "how to deliver bad news" (Fallowfield and Jenkins, 2004), most pediatricians are not comfortable and knowledgeable helping the grief-stricken family at the time of the child's last breath, during the time immediately after the death, or after the family has left the hospital (Vazirani et al, 2000). The family context, however, is the domain of pediatricians. Pediatricians know the child and parents better than any professional does (American Academy of Pediatrics, 2003). Pediatricians will feel more comfortable in giving initial help if they remember that just because they encounter or discover the family's grief, they do not necessarily have to assume long-term personal care or responsibility for the family. However, as pediatricians, they are endowed with clinical and moral obligations to care for children and their families, and they are expected to make referrals and to find resources for the family and to monitor their well-being. Pediatricians help the bereaved by showing they care. Parents look to pediatricians for advice and support for medical and mental health problems (Kahn et al, 1999).

Caring for the Family and Remembering the Child

Primary care pediatricians usually are not present when a child dies. This includes developmental-behavioral pediatricians and other outpatient or clinic-based subspecialists. Hospital-based pediatricians (residents, hospitalists, emergency medicine, intensive care, and chronic illnesses specialists), however, are more likely at the bedside with the family when the child dies. The primary care pediatrician's care for parents and siblings may begin before the death in anticipated, expected deaths and certainly after the death when the family leaves the hospital, when they are enveloped by profound grief. Grief lasts longer than a 2-hour memorial service. The end of a child's life is the beginning of the family's bereavement, the rest of their life without their child. Pediatricians, with their long-term and trusted relationships with families, are uniquely positioned and privileged to help families heal.

The most healing and restoring measures are the continued caring and presence of extended family and friends, keeping the child's memory alive and not letting the child slip into oblivion, never again hearing the child's name. This is the parents' worst fear. On learning of the child's death, the pediatrician might consider contacting a relative or family friend, even the family's minister, rabbi, priest, or imam. The purpose is to organize a group of friends who will prepare hot dinners to deliver to the family nightly for a few weeks and/or arrange other supportive measures.

There is a medical adage: "For patients, it is more important to know how much the physician cares than to care how much the physician knows." At this time, this is never more true. The pediatrician can schedule supportive office visits to inquire about the family's well-being, to remember the dead child (stories, photographs), to let the family share feelings, and to monitor their health and well-being. The pediatrician should encourage the family to have "family meetings" at home as they have in the office or clinic (Coleman, 2001). When a child dies by suicide or neglect, family members may be hesitant to speak for fear of being judged or hesitant to share their feelings of being stigmatized.

In deaths of older teens or adults who have been living in the adult world, parents normally do not know as much about their adult lives. Stories from adult friends are deeply appreciated because they yield hitherto unknown information, understanding, and appreciation of the lost adult children (filling in the blank parts of a "life portrait"). Pediatricians can suggest that parents locate and contact these adult friends (Table 37-3).

The pediatrician should remember the three *A*'s, three key interventions:

- Acknowledgment (of the family's journey of feelings from the grief to the hope to live again).
- Anticipatory guidance (to inform the family of the normal grief reactions, the "stages," and how to appreciate their own signs of healing).

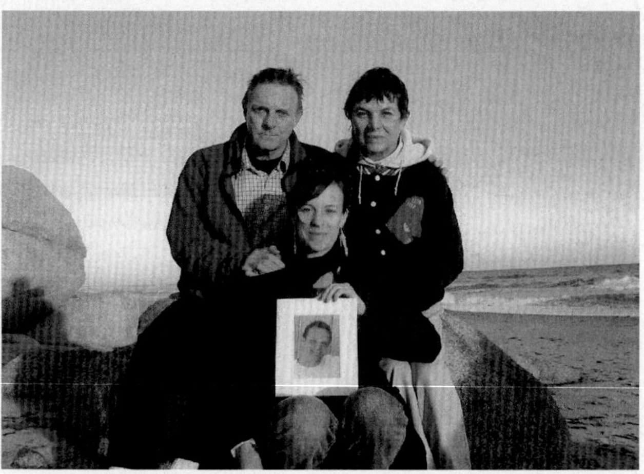

Figure 37-1. Justin L. Coleman with his family.

- Availability (to be there for the family and to observe the brothers and sisters).

A variety of supportive measures are listed in Table 37-4.

Finding Resources and Referrals

Most pediatricians, including some developmental-behavioral subspecialists, do not have the expertise or time for extended grief counseling. They may see the family for one or two visits or maybe none; but, for *all* families, they should suggest and encourage referrals and resources (Table 37- 5). Families (even individuals within the family) seek out resources only when they are ready. Some never reach out, preferring to heal individually or within their family. Whatever their choice, when families return for subsequent office visits, pediatricians must always remember the dead child by name.

Finding Sources of Solace

Pediatricians can respectfully inquire about the family's possible religious support and beliefs regardless of the pediatrician's own personal beliefs. Faith and religion and spirituality can be very helpful to those who seek it and want it. Faith and religion are universal sources of solace and give the bereaved the strength to endure, the hope to go on, the courage to recognize their own confusion and uncertainty, and a knowledge and acceptance of their own weaknesses and mortality (Koenig et al, 2001). Other sources of solace are art, music, nature, and literature (e.g., "grief literature").

Special places, offering remembrances, solitude, peace, and quietness also give solace. These places have special meaning or hold memories of past good times with the child and might include a gravesite, memorial bench, park, walking trail, school, athletic field, garden, memorial stone, lake or seaside, a tree with a ribbon tied to a branch, or the child's bedroom.

Table 37-3. What Helps: What Physicians, Family, and Friends Can Do

Know that every bereaved person grieves in his or her own way.
Know the two general, recurring stages of grief: profound sadness/emptiness and acceptance/yearning.
Put aside your feelings of discomfort or sadness to console the family.
Contact the family as soon as possible (phone message, letter; try not to e-mail). Do not expect a reply (at least not soon).
Always call the dead child or teenager by his or her name.
Keep communications brief (verbal and written); e.g., "I'm sorry for your loss, for the death of __________."
Attend the funeral or memorial service, if possible.
Offer to be of help or available to do anything (e.g., running errands).
Organize friends to bring the family cooked dinners for a month.
Introduce a friend or acquaintance who has lost a child to the newly bereaved family when the time seems right.
Suggest or give the family books on grief and loss.
Visit with the family and share stories or feelings; just be there.
Send letters, make phone calls on important dates—the dead child's birthday and the death anniversary.
Always remember the dead child and his or her family.
Help the family find resources (see Table 37-5).

Table 37-4. Supportive Measures by the Pediatrician in the Office or Clinic

Keep a special calendar to remember the death anniversary dates of children in the practice.
Write a personal letter of remembrance to parents and brothers and sisters on the death anniversary.
Keep a photograph of the dead child in a sibling's medical chart (paper and electronic, if possible) to share at the family's visits.
Always call the lost child by name; if appropriate, hugs are welcome.
Encourage family members to keep personal journals.
Inquire about the well-being of every family member, even if that person is not present.
Facilitate an office family meeting to help them share and support each other.
Encourage home family meetings—especially when sharing at home is difficult.
Refer the family or individuals to the appropriate specialist when they are ready.
When the family or individuals are ready, suggest local grief support (hospital, church, temple) or the nearest chapter of The Compassionate Friends (see Table 37-5).
When office grief counseling ends, schedule future, later visits; encourage visits as necessary.
Remember and use the three A's: Acknowledgement, Anticipatory (guidance), Availability.

Table 37-5. Referrals and Resources

Referrals	
Counseling professionals knowledgeable in grief and bereavement (not just "normal grief"), family dynamics, and child development	
Psychologists, clergy, social workers, counselors, family therapists, marriage psychiatrists, and developmental-behavioral pediatricians	
Physicians knowledgeable in treating depression and medication (parents and siblings)	
Resources	
The Compassionate Friends is a national support organization with more than 600 local chapters. It offers pamphlets, books, and videos and sponsors an annual 2-day meeting. It also supports the annual International Candle Lighting. On the second Sunday of each December, parents gather at 7:00 PM (local time) to light candles in remembrance.	www.compassionatefriends.org National office (toll free) 877-969-0010
Improving driver training requirements, advocating for stricter penalties for those who sell alcohol to minors	www.allstate.com\teen
The National Suicide Prevention Lifeline	1-800-273-TALK www.suicidepreventionlifeline.org
Grief Watch	www.griefwatch.com
Crisis, Grief, and Healing	www.webhealing.com (links to hundreds of online resources)
Connect for Kids	www.connectforkids.org
Organ donation	www.organdonor.gov
Mothers Against Drunk Driving (MADD)	www.madd.org
Gun safety	www.kidsandguns.org

Another Pediatrician Role: Helping the Family Appreciate Their Healing

Acute grief reactions slowly yield to lifelong bereavement, but often the parents and brothers and sisters are not aware of the signs of healing and so cannot appreciate their beginning to live again. Pediatricians can help each member measure his or her own healing and that of others by inquiring about certain behaviors and by encouraging family meetings at home (Table 37-6).

Brothers and Sisters: The Forgotten Mourners

Surviving brothers and sisters are the "forgotten mourners" because parents usually receive the majority of the attention and support. Siblings often have to "delay" and "mute" their grieving. They may feel "ignored" as they put aside their own grief and loss to participate in supportive activities at home (support parents, cook meals, clean house, answer phone). The nature of their prior sibling relationship can affect their mood even years later (Waldinger et al, 2007). Brothers and sisters may suffer even more as every day they experience their parents' grief in the most intimate, unavoidable, and unmitigated way (DeVita-Raeburn, 2004). The pediatrician's support for brothers and sisters is essential and invaluable (Table 37-7).

Finally, pediatricians will do well to remember to avoid a variety of intentional, hurtful remarks and actions for themselves to teach others to avoid them too (Table 37-8).

SUPPORTIVE MEASURES AT THE BEDSIDE WHEN THE CHILD DIES

Every parent who has lost a child will always remember how she or he first heard about or witnessed the worst life event imaginable. Some children die slowly (weeks, months, years), and others die acutely (instantly, hours, days). The family's grief begins before the child dies. During a slow death (e.g., chronic illness, severe injury), parents often experience fluctuating levels of concern, have anticipatory grief (which can "buffer" or lessen the acute grief reaction at the actual death), and at times may even wish for the child to die to end the suffering of all, especially the child. Parents, in turn, feel horrified that they could think such thoughts and ask themselves, How could I? They may then respond with a defense reaction formation, becoming very protective and caring and asking lots of questions of the pediatrician who is also facing his or her own emotions (Baider and Wein, 2001). As death nears, parents feel increasing remorse and sadness and a resurgence of love for the child. At the death, with the last hope extinguished, parents may feel guilt and relief. Now the wave of grief begins to crush them.

In acute death, immediately before their child dies, parents feel indescribable anxiety and confusion (Knapp and Mulligan, 2005). Parents ask, Why my child? He was such a good child, why has God done this to him? When children die suddenly (e.g., motor vehicle crashes, suicide, war, acute illness), parents may displace their anger onto the pediatrician, regardless of the pediatrician's behavior. This is more likely if the pediatrician fails to

Table 37-6. **Signs That the Parent or Sibling Is Healing (Never Cured)**
In their journals, members will note changes over time.
Does not think of child as often and is not overwhelmed by thoughts
Can reach out and comfort others
Can attend social events (and is invited) and can be in the spirit of the event
Shares stories; gives photos, books, clothing to relatives and friends
Laughs again (and without guilt)
Can mention child's name and tell stories without crying or sadness
Asks others about their children

Table 37-7. **Issues Affecting Brothers and Sisters and Clinical Implications for the Pediatrician**
Sibling's grief overshadowed by parents' grief
Sibling's "survival guilt" ("I should have died"; "I was always the bad kid"; "I was mean to her")
Brothers and sisters need assurance that the death is not their fault.
Parents may fill their loss by another pregnancy; may take attention from siblings.
Parents may withdraw emotionally or displace feelings and expectations of the dead child onto the sibling.
Discussion (in office and later at home) helps brothers and sisters understand and accept the death, make adjustments, and improve their functioning.
Siblings and parents each may want or need time alone and time together with the pediatrician during office visits.
A physical examination might assure a sibling of his or her good health if the child died of a medical illness.
Years later, if they become parents and their own parents die, siblings' grief may re-emerge.
"Unfinished business" between brothers and sisters and the dead child will require discussion.
Pediatricians should encourage siblings' questions and expressions of grief, guilt, anger, confusion, resentment, hope, and healing.

Table 37-8. **What Might Hurt (Even with Good Intentions)**
"She's no longer in pain."
"It's God's will. He is in a better place."
"I know just how you feel."
"You can have more children."
"You'll get over it."
"You must feel terrible."
"At least you have other children."
"My son lost his puppy and he was so sad."
"My son's in jail but I love him."
"Life is not fair."
Trying to talk the bereaved out of their feelings
"Hurrying" the bereaved through their grief, e.g., resuming prior activities, attending social events (life as usual)
Friends, even relatives, avoiding talk about the lost child and the family's grief
Professional and workplace colleagues avoiding talk about the lost child and the family's grief
Discussing trivial matters at a grief-related event
Comparing (unfavorably) the child and siblings
Discussing one's children (achievements, activities, or problems) for too long

Table 37-9. The Dying and the Dead Child: The Bedside Pediatrician's Roles

Take charge initially.
Page a more experienced team member (known to the family), if appropriate.
Always call and refer to the child by his or her name.
Respect and protect the family's need for privacy, praying, crying, and being silent.
Be present or available only enough to comfort; if unsure, ask them what would help.
Offer to get a phone or to make calls, or ask if they might want a camera.
Suggest that the family cut a lock of hair and remove personal items.
Answer sensitive questions in a comforting way. (Did she suffer? Could he hear me when I told him that I loved him?)
Be patient. The family may not hear or remember anything that is said at this time.
Be aware of and respect different cultural, religious, and individual values.
The pediatrician should consider the possibility of organ donation and then call the organ donation team as quickly as possible so they can speak to the parents. Organs are "viable" only 6 to 10 hours after death (see Table 37-5).

show sympathy or consideration, even if it is out of her or his own helplessness or sense of blame or failure (Seecharan et al, 2004). Pediatricians also may hesitate to speak or to reach out because they mistakenly fear that their attempts might trigger a torrent of grief and tears, making the bereaved even sadder, in turn making pediatricians even more uncomfortable. Sometimes their attempts are so awkward that they unintentionally, out of their own discomfort, hurt or offend the bereaved, making the situation even worse.

At this time, pediatricians *must* put aside their feelings of discomfort and recognize and attend to the needs of the family. The presence of the silent pediatrician can be very comforting to the family. A simple "I am sorry" or a touch on the shoulder or a hug, if appropriate, means much to the family. Affirming their feelings is very supportive, for example, "I am so sorry for your unspeakable loss." Parents will always remember and be comforted by these acts of kindness.

If the parents are not present at the time of death, the pediatrician phoning the parents must be both comforting and direct, answer their questions honestly and briefly, and promise to "explain more" when they arrive. The pediatrician should ask them to get to the hospital quickly but safely and might urge them to have a friend drive or to take a taxi.

During the time surrounding death (the minutes and hours before and after death), pediatricians can be immensely supportive and helpful (Bagatell et al, 2002) as they quickly assume key responsibilities (Table 37-9).

SUMMARY

Approximately 60,000 children aged 0 to 19 years die each year in America. Pediatric residents and hospital-based subspecialists are invariably at the bedside when the child dies. However, the majority of pediatricians (primary care, developmental-behavioral, and other outpatient specialists) see the parents and brothers and sisters after the child has died and they have left the hospital.

Pediatricians play essential roles, whether in helping the grief-stricken family at the bedside when the child dies or in helping the bereaved family (parents, brothers and sisters, and others) through office visits in the weeks, months, and years after the death. Pediatricians also help family members find supportive resources, and they make appropriate and timely referrals. Even parents who lose their only child also need and benefit from the pediatrician's initial support and guidance.

This chapter briefly describes the grief process, its impact on parents and brothers and sisters, and various supportive measures by pediatricians, whether at the bedside or later in the office or the clinic.

REFERENCES

American Academy of Pediatrics, Task Force on the Family: Family pediatrics. Pediatrics 111:1541-1571, 2003.

Bagatell R, Meyer R, Heron S, et al: When children die: A seminar series for pediatric residents. Pediatrics 110:348-353, 2002.

Baider L, Wein S: Reality and fugues in physicians facing death: Confrontation, coping, and adaptation at the bedside. Crit Rev Oncol Hematol 40:97-103, 2001.

Carey WB, McDevitt SC: Coping with Children's Temperament: A Guide for Professionals. New York, Basic Books, 1995.

Coleman WL: Family-Focused Behavioral Pediatrics. Philadelphia, Lippincott Williams & Wilkins, 2001, pp. 240-243.

DeVita-Raeburn E: The Empty Room: Surviving the Loss of a Brother or Sister at Any Age. New York, Scribner, 2004.

Fallowfield L, Jenkins V: Communicating sad, bad, and difficult news in medicine. Lancet 363:312-319, 2004.

Finkbeiner A: After the Death of a Child: Living with Loss through the Years. Baltimore, Johns Hopkins University Press, 1996.

Heneghan AM, Mercer M, DeLeone NL: Will mothers discuss parenting stress and depressive symptoms with their child's pediatrician? Pediatrics 113:460-467, 2004.

Kahn RS, Wise PH, Finkelstein JA, et al: The scope of unmet maternal health needs in pediatric settings. Pediatrics 103:576-581, 1999.

Knapp J, Mulligan D: Death of a child in the E.D. Pediatrics 115(5):1432-1437, 2005.

Koenig H, McCullough M, Larson D: Handbook of Religion and Health. New York, Oxford Press, 2001.

Kubler-Ross E: On Death and Dying: What the Dying Have to Teach Doctors, Nurses, Clergy, and Their Own Families. New York, Touchstone, 1969.

Lewis M, Schonfeld D: Dying and death in childhood and adolescence. *In* Lewis M (eds): Child and Adolescent Psychiatry, 3rd ed. Philadelphia, Lippincott Williams & Wilkins, 2002, pp. 1239-1245.

Li J, Laursen TM, Precht DH, et al: Hospitalization for mental illness among parents after the death of a child. N Engl J Med 352:1190-1196, 2005.

Maciejewski PK, Zhang B, Block SD, Prigerson HG: An empirical examination of the stage theory of grief. JAMA 297:716-723, 2007.

McDaniel S, Beckman H, Morse D, et al: Physician self-disclosure in primary care visits: Enough about you, what about me? Arch Intern Med 167:1321-1326, 2007.

Park ER, Storfer-Isser A, Kelleher KJ, et al: In the moment: Attitudinal measure of pediatrician management of maternal depression. Ambul Pediatr 7:239-246, 2007.

Rando T (ed): Parental Loss of a Child. Champaign, IL, Research Press, 1986.

Redinbaugh EM, Sullivan AM, Block AM, et al: Doctor's emotional reactions to recent death of a patient: Cross sectional study of hospital doctors. BMJ 327:185-191, 2003.

Rochelle B, Meyer R, Herron S, et al: When children die: A seminar series for pediatric residents. Pediatrics 110:348-353, 2002.

Seecharan GA, Andresen EM, Norris K, et al: Parents' assessment of quality of care and grief following a child's death. Arch Pediatr Adolesc Med 158:515-520, 2004.

Vazirani RM, Slavin SJ, Feldman JD: Longitudinal study of pediatric house officers' attitudes toward death and dying. Crit Care Med 28:3740-3745, 2000.

Waldinger RJ, Vaillant GE, Orav EJ: Childhood sibling relationships as a predictor of major depression in adulthood: A 30-year prospective study. Am J Psychiatry 164:949-954, 2007.

Wessel MA: The primary pediatrician's role when a death occurs in a family in one's practice. Pediatr Rev 24:183-185, 2003.

Zisook S, Zisook SA: Death, Dying and Bereavement. Philadelphia, Williams & Wilkins, 2005.

READINGS FOR PARENTS

Grollman EA: Living When a Loved One Has Died. Boston, Beacon Press, 1995. A guide through the grief to healing, remembering, and living again.

Hancock B: Riding with the Blue Moth. Champagne IL, Sports Publishing LLC, 2005. A father's account of his son's death, the impact on the family, and his cross-country solo bicycle ride to honor his son.

Hickman M: Healing After Loss: Daily Meditations for Working Through Grief. New York, Perennial Press, 2002. These 365 one-page meditations (each a relevant quote and words of comfort and guidance) can be read over and over.

Part V OUTCOMES—BEHAVIORAL AND EMOTIONAL

SECTION A Social Relationships

38 THE SPECTRUM OF SOCIAL COGNITION

Robin L. Hansen and Gordon L. Ulrey

Vignette

Miya, a 6½-year-old girl, was referred by her parents because she is having problems in school. Her teacher has said that she finds her difficult to manage in the classroom because she is frequently out of her seat, disturbing her classmates, and is often argumentative when asked to resume work. The teacher also notes that Miya has difficulty making and maintaining friendships and increasingly asks to be allowed to "help" in the classroom rather than going to recess with her classmates. She reports that Miya seems anxious when she is in unstructured situations but does better in structured activities. Her parents are also concerned about problems with peers. She rarely gets invited to birthday parties, and few classmates came to her last birthday party although her parents made sure that the entire class was invited. The parents report that she plays much better with her 3-year-old neighbor and 12-year-old cousin than with children her own age. They have few behavior problems at home, where she is an only child. When tested by the school psychologist, Miya's cognitive ability, both verbally and nonverbally, was at a high level (IQ 135), as were her achievement skills in reading, writing, and written language.

This vignette illustrates several common concerns related to social behaviors about which pediatricians, other primary physicians, psychologists, and other mental health professionals are frequently asked. Although Miya is intellectually gifted, there is a large discrepancy between her cognitive abilities and her social functioning. She is struggling with her social interactions with peers and having difficulties in school meeting classroom expectations.

Our objective in this chapter is to provide a model for understanding social cognitive abilities that will facilitate both assessment and treatment of children with weaknesses akin to Miya's. Although we know sociability when we see it, we have difficulty clinically defining it, measuring it, and thus assessing it. We conceptualize sociability as composed of social cognitive abilities as well as the tendency to affiliate with others. Some children have age-appropriate social cognitive skills and prefer to be alone, whereas others want to interact with others but lack the skills to initiate or to maintain relationships. In this chapter, we focus on social cognitive abilities (see Chapter 41 for discussion of social withdrawal).

A rich and varied literature investigating components of social behavior, including developmental, genetic, cultural, and environmental aspects, has recently been enriched by research on the neurologic circuitry serving these abilities. Understanding of the neural basis helps us understand how social cognitive processes mediate social behaviors in ways that are distinct from, although complementary to, intellectual abilities. Studies of the autism spectrum disorders have provided the most compelling evidence of the importance of social cognitive skills to regulate social behaviors (Hobson et al, 2006). Of course, not all children with social cognitive deficits should be diagnosed with autism spectrum disorders.

COMPONENTS OF SOCIAL COGNITION

Adolphs defines social cognition as "our abilities to recognize, manipulate and behave with respect to socially relevant information, including the ability to construct representations of relations between the self and others and to use those representations flexibly to guide social behavior" (Adolphs, 2001). Studies of social cognition have suggested that there is overlap with intellectual cognitive domains, but although complementary, these are distinct processes with separate but interconnected neural systems (Adolphs, 2003; Amodio and Frith, 2006). Like intellectual cognitive processes, social cognitive processing skills exist on a spectrum that we recognize clinically, but which has not yet been as well documented or measured in psychometrically sound or clinically accessible ways.

Computer models of artificial intelligence illustrate the distinct aspects of intellectual and social cognition. Pinker describes intelligence as "the ability to attain goals in the face of obstacles by means of decisions based on rational (truth-obeying) rules" but also states, "In our daily lives we all predict and explain other people's behavior from what we think they know and what we think they want" (Pinker, 1997). Interpretations of the behaviors and emotions of others are often described as intuition or common sense. Problems encountered in developing "thinking machines" or artificial intelligence systems are related to their reliance on explicit knowledge along with the inability of this system to use knowledge that is implicit in the other things it knows (Pinker, 1997). The shortcomings of a computational theory of mind illustrate the importance of a child's development of both causal and inferential processing to interpret social information. The development of social cognitive skills is essential for learning to understand the thoughts, intentions, and emotions of self and others. The development of the ability to follow the "rules" of social play, to show empathy, and to regulate one's own responses to unstructured or ambiguous social environments reflects a child's developing social cognitive abilities.

Joint attention is a very early component of social cognition important to understanding how young children engage caregivers, emerging midway through the first year of life. The child will look at an object and communicate an interest in showing it to or sharing it with another person. Similarly, the child will show interest in an object that another is showing or communicating about. The child focuses attention on an object and the person conjointly, communicating by gesture, eye contact, and facial expression.

The maturation of social reciprocity during early childhood requires developing empathy. Developmental research suggests that most children demonstrate some understanding of how others feel during the second year of life and that this ability is tied to other social cognitive skills (Emde, 1998; Gallese, 2005). The construct of "theory of mind" refers to the ability to make inferences about what another person believes or feels (Amodio and Frith, 2006). Baron-Cohen uses the concept of "mindblindness" to describe the difficulties individuals with autism spectrum disorders have in perceiving and comprehending the thoughts, feelings, or intentions of others, which is a major contributor to the social difficulties experienced by individuals with Asperger syndrome or high functioning autism, despite their relatively intact intellectual cognitive skills (Baron-Cohen, 1995).

Children who are seen as highly sociable have skills that help them understand or even anticipate how peers or caregivers feel and their intentions—they are good "mind readers." The social cognitive capacity for developing empathy is critical for developing peer friendships. Children with less developed empathy have greater difficulty establishing friendships and may be seen by caregivers or teachers as self-centered and difficult to engage. Failure to appreciate or to take into account the needs or interests of others often reflects poorly developed empathy.

The effective use of communicating and comprehending social meaning through language is another important construct of social cognition. The pragmatics of language relate to how well a child understands a situation's context when communicating. Children with pragmatic language disorder have difficulty with both self-expression and interpretation of the meaning and intentions others are trying to communicate. The ambiguities of teasing and joking are difficult for children with poor pragmatic language skills to understand and will affect their sociability. Children on the autism spectrum often have unusual prosody (rhythm) of their spoken language that sometimes seems flat or scripted or may have exaggerated but atypical inflexion patterns. Less pronounced difficulty with both pragmatics and prosody affects children's sociability. Reponses to verbal commands or requests may be overly literal; children may not understand that the way something is said changes the meaning. A child's sense of humor should be in synchrony with peers when social abilities are well developed. Children who fail to understand social nuances, particularly changes in timing or tone of voice related to humor, may have a very high level of intellectual cognition but a mismatch in their social cognitive skills.

The construct of central coherence has also been useful for understanding differences in the ability to perceive faces or other body language behavior and to infer social meaning in interactions with others (Happe and Frith, 2006). Central coherence relates to social cognition in regard to the ability to integrate and to make sense of a wide range of social information. All the components of social cognition require interpretation and inference to comprehend the intentions or feelings of others. Children with weak central coherence often focus on specific or isolated details and are less able to see a gestalt of more complete configurations; they have trouble seeing the forest for the trees.

THE NEURAL BASIS OF SOCIAL COGNITION

Research on the neural correlates of social cognition in children is expanding rapidly.

Changes in function and structure underlie normative brain development in this area. Moreover, important differences in processing of information related to social behaviors have been demonstrated in children and adults with autism spectrum disorders that have increased our knowledge related to the neural circuitry involved in social cognitive processing (Pennington et al, 2006).

Neural structures that have been primarily investigated in the development of social cognitive skills include the higher order visual cortices in the temporal lobe, medial frontal cortex, amygdala, hippocampus, basal ganglia, and fusiform gyrus. These regions function as a complex interconnected neural network (Amodio and Frith, 2006; Pelphrey et al, 2004a, 2004b). Many components of social cognition seem to have distinct neural systems or structures within the broader social cognitive framework. Mirror neurons, a particular class of visuomotor neurons distributed in the superior temporal sulcus, discharge both when one is doing an action and when one is observing an action. This neural system plays a functional role in mediating imitation as well as in interpreting the actions of others and is postulated to be linked to the evolution and understanding of speech in humans (Rizzolatti and Craighero, 2004). The role of the mirror neuron system in social perception relates primarily to the development of self-other awareness, the initial stages of evaluating the social communicative intentions of others by analysis of eye gaze direction, facial expression, body movements, and other types of biologic movement (Hurley and Charter, 2005; Pennington et al, 2006).

Imitative learning is critical for both intellectual cognition and social cognition. A child's ability to understand actions of others is essential for development of reciprocity in play. The perception of social cues, including gestures, language pragmatics, and prosody as well as mood or intention, requires neurocognitive processing of mirror neurons. Whereas changes in vocal intonations or rhythm change the meaning of oral communication, nonverbal cues such as posture, facial expressions, or other gestures express information also critical for interpreting social intention. The ability to "read" and to use body language is widely accepted as an important aspect of social cognition. The development of these skills is also interdependent on mirror neuron processing and related neural circuits.

Specific areas of the brain are involved in face recognition. Studies of face recognition reveal that skills vary from individuals who "never forget a face" to individuals who are unable to recognize even familiar faces or are unable to easily interpret emotional state from facial expressions. Eye contact and recognition of emotions in facial expression have been investigated for both cultural influences and influences on early attachment behaviors. Imaging studies have found that the fusiform gyrus is important in the neural circuitry of face recognition (Adolphs, 2001; Pelphrey et al, 2004a). Recognition of emotions in facial expression has been investigated for the influences of both culture and early experiences (Pollak and Sinha, 2002).

DEVELOPMENTAL COURSE

The components of social cognition emerge throughout development. Recognition of the emergence, or lack thereof, of these social cognitive skills during appropriate developmental stages is important for early identification of children with social cognitive deficits.

Infancy

Infants have been described as "prewired" to be social beings (Gopnik et al, 1999). We now have research that helps us begin to understand how this "wiring" may be constructed. Rogers reviews the literature on infant imitation of facial movements that provides evidence for a specific neural network. Possibly the motor neuron system, present at birth, is capable of perception-action couplings, which appear to be a starting state for the development of self-other representations (Rogers, 2006). This predisposition emphasizes the importance of behaviors that facilitate engaging with others, such as eye contact and social smiling, and the feedback provided by reciprocal synchronized parental responses, particularly as the infant's repertoire of volitional behaviors expands. Eye contact, social smiling, reaching, and emerging joint attention skills have all been identified as behaviors that reflect social cognitive skills in infancy. The emergence of the social smile at 2 to 3 months heralds what Emde and colleagues have termed "an awakening of sociability" with enhanced capacity for eye-to-eye social contact and reciprocity (Emde, 1998). Midway through the first year, infants should begin to use social referencing, monitoring the emotional expressions of others to modulate emotion as well as behaviors, and the emergence of joint attention skills should be observed.

Toddler/Preschool

Socialization demands increase during this phase, and many children for whom there were no concerns in infancy related to social development may now struggle with social difficulties. Children in the toddler/preschool age not only learn how to communicate their thoughts to others, but they also develop skills for expressing intention and emotions to them. A critical social cognitive skill that also develops is the ability to infer or to predict another's thoughts as well as other children's intentions and feelings. From these abilities emerge the capacity for empathy and response behaviors of soothing and helping (Emde, 1998). These social cognitive communication skills emerge as children develop an understanding of social rules in different settings and relationships. Children learn to process social information, which requires self regulating and monitoring and the ability to modify one's own behaviors in relation to social perception and understanding of the expression of intention by others.

Preschoolers develop the ability to construct narratives that reflect their social cognitive development and serve to organize and communicate their social-emotional experiences as their language skills expand. This helps them deal with emotionally unexpected situations or conflicts. These narratives are also reflected in their social, imaginative play with peers. Reciprocity in play requires children to observe and to recognize feelings and beliefs of others, which they can match with their own.

School Age

Social cognitive abilities in school-age children are largely reflected in their ability to function in increasingly socially ambiguous situations. Children with well-established social cognitive skills are able to function successfully and flexibly in both structured (classroom, clubs) and unstructured (recess, lunch period) situations. The major difference between the classroom and playground is the degree of externally imposed structure and routine of each day. The playground represents a much more ambiguous social environment than the classroom. Children who play cooperatively on the playground must negotiate and agree on rules of interaction, which are both implicit and explicit. The children must be able to interpret the intent of other children in a fluid manner (social mirroring). Children with more developed social cognitive abilities have more skills for "navigating" social ambiguities. The concept of "street smarts" is often used to describe children and adolescents who are skilled at coping with or thriving in unstructured social environments. The complementary but distinct relationship between intellectual cognition and social cognition is clear in observing children who do and do not adapt well to ambiguous social situations.

Adolescence

The demand for social reciprocity among adolescents increases and becomes even more complex. The ambiguities of social group affiliations and emerging sexual identity of adolescents often are stressful, even for adolescents with solid social cognitive skills. In addition, the need to establish social reciprocity and to be accepted by peers of both sexes is a major developmental task for this age group. Adolescents are also increasingly subjected to social testing or teasing from both sexes. Interpretation of humor, kidding around, and being criticized "playfully" all require social cognitive skills to interpret the subtle meaning based in context, gestures, tone of voice, and timing during these complex social engagements.

DIAGNOSTIC CONSIDERATIONS

In assessing children with social difficulties, it is critical to consider characteristics of social cognitive skills as well as environmental, cultural, and familial factors that have an impact on socialization. Although it is well understood that environmental factors play a major role in the development of language, intellectual, and social behaviors, we also know that abnormal brain functions (developmental or acquired) may interfere with the basic skills of language, cognition, and social functioning in spite of optimal opportunities in the environment for learning. It is important to identify children with disorders of social cognition or mental health and other neurodevelopmental disorders, including genetic disorders such as sex chromosome disorders, and to assess the degree to which impairments in intellectual cognition contribute to social difficulties (Tartaglia et al, 2007). Children with delays in intellectual cognitive development generally have social cognitive skills appropriate to their intellectual level. Children with acquired brain injury also have behavioral and social difficulties (Yeates et al, 2004).

Environmental and cultural issues contribute to social difficulties as well and must be assessed in every child with social difficulties. Both the *Diagnostic Classification of Mental Health and Developmental Disorders of Infancy and Early Childhood,* revised edition (DC:0-3R), and the *Diagnostic and Statistical Manual for Primary Care* (DSM-PC) emphasize the importance of environmental and parent-child relationship issues in assessing children with behavioral concerns and provide frameworks for considering their impact. DC:0-3R uses a five-axis classification system, similar to the *Diagnostic and Statistical Manual of Mental Disorders,* fourth edition, text revision (DSM-IV-TR), specifically emphasizing direct assessment of parent-child relationships, psychosocial stressors, and emotional and social functioning in addition to clinical disorders and medical-developmental disorders (American Psychiatric Association, 2000). Along with the DSM-IV-TR, these diagnostic classification models should be familiar to health care professionals working with children (American Psychiatric Association, 2000). These systems delineate the criteria for diagnosis of disorders that may be present in children with social difficulties and that are important in the differential diagnosis of children with social cognitive deficits. The range of disorders that need to be carefully considered include regulatory disorders of sensory processing, disorders of attachment, autism spectrum disorders, nonverbal learning disorders, social anxiety disorders, disruptive behavior disorders such as attention-deficit/hyperactivity disorder, oppositional defiant disorder, conduct disorder, post-traumatic stress disorder, and mood disorders.

Research from the International Consortium for the Study of Social and Emotional Development, reviewed by Rubin (2002), illustrates the importance of including cultural and gender-specific factors in assessing children with social difficulties. Differences in cultural expectations regarding eye contact with strangers and speaking outside the home to unfamiliar adults are examples of cultural expectations that will affect children's social success in situations that have expectations different from those in their home. Issues of second language acquisition related to social abilities also need to be assessed. Stressors in the caregiving environment, such as interpersonal, financial, medical, and mental health disturbances, can affect children's social behaviors and need to be considered as well.

ASSESSMENT AND INTERVENTION

The clinical assessment of children with social problems requires an appreciation of the range of behaviors associated across the spectrum of social cognition and abilities. Tables 38-1 to 38-4 list observable social behaviors across the developmental periods from infancy to adolescence that reflect social cognitive processes. The higher levels of social behaviors are indicators of appropriately developing social cognitive skills. The skills reflecting lower social behaviors are those most commonly observed that suggest some compromise or deficits in social cognition. There are also parent report, teacher report, and self-report measures for children that provide more extensive or collateral information when behavior difficulties are reported that can help differentiate underlying problems. Table 38-5 lists screening

Table 38-1. Spectrum of Social Skills: Infancy

High Sociability	Low Sociability
Seeks caregiver's contact	Indifferent to caregiver contact
Seeks eye contact	Avoidance of or brief eye contact
Reciprocal smile	Random smiles or object and activity related
Reaches for caregiver	Few gestures for social contact, hand flapping
Vocalizes with caregiver	Few vocalizations, little reciprocity of vocalizations
Reacts to absence of caregiver	Little response to caregiver absence
Soothed by caregiver	Unresponsive to soothing
Joint attention emerging	No evidence of joint attention

Table 38-2. Spectrum of Social Skills: Toddler/Preschool

High Sociability	Low Sociability
Joint attention	Isolated attention
Stranger recognition	Indiscriminant response
Easy to engage	Difficult to engage in social interactions
Imitation of language and actions	Little imitation
Emerging symbolic play	No pretend play, scripted imitation
Adaptive to change	Difficulty with transitions, new situations
Uses language for social initiation	Jargon, echolalic speech
Well-regulated activity	Poorly regulated activity
Imaginative role play with peers	Difficulty with unstructured peer play

Table 38-3. Spectrum of Social Skills: School Age

High Sociability	Low Sociability
Enjoys peer play	Prefers play with older or younger peers or adults
Shares toys	Difficulty sharing, destroys own toys
Chosen for teams and games	Dislikes recess, gets teased
Has favorite friend	Friend changes frequently or has trouble
Peer group of friends	Withdraws from group play, activities Prefers to be alone or withdrawn
Talks with peers and adults easily	Refuses to speak in school and in unfamiliar groups or is inappropriately intrusive, loud
Variety in play patterns	Scripted, repetitious play or rigid with rules
Able to shift activities, groups easily	Prefers classroom to recess, resists change
Responds to others' distress	Ignores crying, distress in peers or parents
Able to joke with peers	Misses jokes, very literal interpretation
Uses a variety of gestures socially	Few or inappropriate gestures in social interactions
Understands personal space	Intrusive in other's personal space

Table 38-4. Spectrum of Social Skills: Adolescence

High Sociability	Low Sociability
Highly engaged with peers	Prefers solitary activities
Has close, trusted friends same age	Prefers solitary fantasy play, fantasy fiction; younger or older peers
Good reciprocal conversations	Little social conversation with peers
Speech patterns adjusted to peers and adults	Little adjustment; overly formal or pedantic
Appreciates humor	Confused with jargon, joking; literal
Tolerates changes, new situations	Difficulty with change, unpredictable activities without clear rules
Concern for others' feelings, ideas	Little response to others' distress, ideas
Initiates and receives calls from peers	Few calls or social activities with peers
Wide range of school, leisure activities	Activities restricted in range, solitary (e.g., excessive electronic games or science fiction)

Table 38-5. Screening Tools for Children with Social and Behavioral Difficulties

Infant/Toddler Symptom Checklist: 7-30 months (DeGangi et al, 1995)
Modified Checklist for Autism in Toddlers (M-CHAT) (Robins et al, 2001)
Social Competence and Behavior Evaluation, Preschool Edition (LaFreniere and Dumas, 1995)
Social Communication Questionnaire: 48 months and older (Rutter et al, 2003)
Social Responsiveness Scale: 4-18 years; parent, teacher/caregiver forms (Constantino and Gruber, 2005)
Behavior Assessment System for Children–2: 2-5 years, parent, teacher forms; 6-11 years, parent, teacher forms; 12-21 years, parent, teacher, and self-report forms (Reynolds and Kamphaus, 2004a, 2004b, 2004c)
Adaptive Behavior Assessment System II: 0-5 years, 5-21 years; parent, teacher/care provider, self-report forms (Harrison and Oskland, 2004
ASEBA Child Behavior Checklist: 1½-5 years, 6-18 years; parent, teacher report forms (Achenbach, 1997; Achenbach and Rescorla, 2000, 2001)
Short Sensory Profile (Dunn, 1999)
What I Think and Feel (Revised Children's Manifest Anxiety Scale) (Reynolds and Richmond, 1998)

tools that can be clinically useful in assessing children with social difficulties. Few specifically measure social cognitive processing per se, but they are helpful in systematic collection of information with standardized norms for comparison across a range of behaviors and contexts. They must be used in conjunction with additional clinical information that provides a more comprehensive context for interpretation.

Behavioral concerns common in children with social cognitive difficulties, along with treatment recommendations, are presented in a developmental context, reflecting the emergence of social cognitive abilities and changing expectations for social behaviors at different developmental stages.

Infancy

Infants who have difficulty with emotional regulation or do not show behaviors that reflect the development of increasingly complex social interactions with their caregivers should be further evaluated. It is important to separate temperamental traits that reflect behavioral styles of reactivity affecting the infant's ability to respond to caregivers and different environmental contexts from underlying early social cognitive abilities, if possible. Helping parents to understand the range of temperament traits as well as the range of sociability in typically developing infants is important, as is providing information about ways to accommodate their child's temperament and to promote sociability (see Chapter 7). Prospective studies of infants at risk for autism because of an older sibling with autism have demonstrated by 12 to 18 months of age fewer gestures and delays in both receptive and expressive language, decreased eye contact, decreased response to name, and differences in responsiveness to people and objects (Bryson et al, 2007; Cassel et al, 2007; Mitchell et al, 2006). Infants with these characteristics need to be closely observed and referred for early intervention services focused on improving social and language skills. It is important to assess and to facilitate parent-child interactions for infants showing minimal engagement cues or poorly regulated affect. Pediatricians and other health care professionals can help support parents who have interactive styles that are either underresponsive or overresponsive to their child's cues. Helping parents understand their child's temperament traits as well as their own parenting style in relationship to their child's temperament can be extremely helpful when these seem to be a component of the child's reported difficulties. Recognition of early signs of poorly attuned parent-child interactions or disturbed regulatory function is critical for health professionals and can be facilitated by knowledge of social cognitive behaviors of infants that reflect early levels of social ability.

Toddler/Preschool

Children who fail to appreciate the needs of others frequently will have social difficulties related to poorly developed empathy. Children with poorly developed empathy are more likely to be isolated from peers, who experience the child as not following the implicit rules of taking turns or sharing and may complain that he or she is "unfair." The child who will engage only when his or her own interests are involved will have difficulty sustaining relationships. Children who behave with less empathy than expected for their age require thoughtful assessment. There are important environmental, psychological, and social cognitive factors that have an impact on developing empathy. Failure to engage in reciprocal social interactions with peers is frequently an indicator of poorly developed social cognitive skills. Knowledge of a child's cultural background and expectations and opportunities to form peer relationships is also necessary to determine the extent to which a child should be expected to engage with peers. Whereas limited exposure or opportunity to develop social play may relate to isolated nuclear families or limited exposure to similar-aged peers, it should resolve with appropriate opportunities provided (e.g., daycare, school). Concerns that children prefer to play with older or younger children may also reflect social cognitive difficulties. Parents may report to the primary care clinician that their child gets along very well with adults but never is invited for play dates or birthday parties. The expectations and demands for social reciprocity are different, depending on how close the other person is to being a same-aged peer. The younger playmate is more likely to tolerate less reciprocity because of allowing the older child to control the interaction. In contrast, play with older children often is controlled by them. However, when play is with a peer, there is much less acceptance of behaviors that show little mutual understanding of intent or social rules.

Daycare and preschool may both increase concerns about social difficulties as well as provide opportunities for greater development of age-appropriate social skills through structured and unstructured play with peers and adults outside the family. Additional observations can also be made of children's social behaviors that may help clarify the primary difficulties if there is an experienced daycare provider or teacher. Young children with social cognitive difficulties will need perceptive, experienced teachers who can help children navigate peer play in structured and unstructured activities, provide explicit input about the feelings and intentions of other children if needed, and help the parents learn these skills without necessarily categorizing the behaviors as pathologic. Use of explicit modeling of social reciprocity in play and age-appropriate social stories may be helpful (Gray, 1994, 2000).

School Age

When children present with behaviors that suggest an attention disorder or hyperactive behaviors, the child's individual differences in neurocognitive skills, which mediate social-emotional functioning, must be considered. Deficits in working memory and executive function are often associated with social behavior problems and illustrate the interdependence between social and intellectual cognition. Children who primarily have difficulties with peers for social cognitive reasons rather than for other attentional or emotional factors often show patterns of behavior such as difficulties with social ambiguities. They may function very differently in structured (classroom, clubs) versus unstructured (recess, lunch) social encounters.

Just as we provide treatment to support or to facilitate learning to read or to improve language skills, children with low social cognitive skills need explicit interventions. Parents need support to understand the importance of providing more structure to support the development of social skills through direct instruction and input, particularly around ambiguous social encounters. For example, before an unstructured social encounter (recess, lunch, play dates), the child can be coached about expected behaviors and responses to anticipated behaviors of others. The child can review brief lists of tips related to social rules and rehearse through role play with parents or other adults. Use of social stories can be very helpful for children to internalize a variety of age-appropriate "social scripts" that can provide a scaffold for their social encounters (Gray, 1994, 2000). Many schools and therapists provide interventions for children with social cognitive deficits, often called social skills groups (Winner, 2000).

Adolescents

Adolescents with poor social cognitive skills are vulnerable to feelings of isolation and abandonment that can be dramatic. At a stage in life when separation from parents and affiliation with peers is essential, the sense of existential angst associated with being unaccepted by peers can compromise the regulation of mood and increase social anxiety and isolation.

Indicators of struggles with social skills in adolescence often include behaviors such as preference for solitary activities, preoccupation with fantasy play or fiction, and preference for exclusive play with younger peers or adults. This play may include peers but is not socially interactive in a flexible manner, such as strong preferences for electronic games, science fiction, or role-playing games. Games or activities that minimize or eliminate the social ambiguities are preferred because feedback is limited to text on computers without other social cues, such as tone of voice, timing, or body language involved. Role playing is also appealing because there is a prescribed interaction that is known or expected, minimizing both ambiguity and demands for reciprocity. Why would a shy, socially anxious adolescent choose to be on stage? Acting a role defines social expectations and eliminates the need for interpretation of intention or feelings of others.

The overfocused interests that often develop in adolescents with social difficulties are a coping mechanism to deal with the social ambiguities of adolescence. As long as they are discussing something about which they are very knowledgeable, there is less need to interpret social behaviors of others.

When adolescents are observed to be socially isolated or choosing activities that minimize or eliminate peer interactions, clinicians should obtain more information about social-emotional functioning. The adolescent with low sociability needs more structured peer activities. Social coaching, social role playing, and supportive social groups offer opportunities to expand their social abilities (Winner, 2000). Helping the adolescent understand how structured social encounters (school programs, clubs, church) differ from unstructured activities (parties, dates) can increase their awareness and improve their preparation for these encounters. Parents may need support to limit time with electronic games and to increase structured social activities. Social skills groups are very helpful in providing the opportunity to discuss and to role play social situations and to get explicit feedback from peers in a supportive, structured group setting.

SUMMARY

When behaviors associated with social difficulties are reported, it is helpful to consider the effect to which social cognitive skills are a factor. When a history seems to eliminate cultural, environmental, trauma, or health factors, the child's behavior associated with social cognitive abilities should be considered. Most children will not meet the criteria for a neurodevelopmental disorder, such as an autism spectrum disorder. However, consideration of skills in the social cognitive spectrum can be useful. Interventions for social functioning problems often relate to an increase in structured activities, such as clubs and organized activities with same-aged peers. The child also may benefit from more direct, explicit teaching when the skills have not developed. Appreciation of the spectrum of social cognitive abilities, similar to the wide variation of intellectual or physical abilities distributed normally in individuals, and of the complementary but distinct neural circuits that underlie these skills is important to health care professionals caring for children and families.

REFERENCES

Achenbach TM: Manual for ASEBA School-Age Forms & Profiles. Burlington, VT, University of Vermont, Research Center for Children, Youth, & Families, 1997.

Achenbach TM, Rescorla LA: Manual for ASEBA Preschool Forms & Profiles. Burlington, VT, University of Vermont, Research Center for Children, Youth, & Families, 2000.

Achenbach TM, Rescorla LA: Manual for ASEBA School-Age Forms & Profiles. Burlington, VT, University of Vermont, Research Center for Children, Youth, & Families, 2001.

Adolphs R: The neurobiology of social cognition. Curr Opin Neurobiol 11(2):231-239, 2001.

Adolphs R: Investigating the cognitive neuroscience of social behavior. Neuropsychologia 41(2):119-126, 2003.

American Psychiatric Association: Diagnostic and Statistical Manual of Mental Disorders, 4th ed, text revision. Washington, DC, American Psychiatric Association, 2000.

Amodio DM, Frith CD: Meeting of minds: The medial frontal cortex and social cognition. Nat Rev Neurosci 7(4):268-277, 2006.

Baron-Cohen S: Mindblindness—An Essay on Autism and Theory of Mind. Cambridge, MA, MIT Press, 1995, pp 1–7.

Bryson SE, Zwaigenbaum L, Brian J, et al: A prospective case series of high-risk infants who developed autism. J Autism Dev Disord 37(1):12-24, 2007.

Cassel TD, Messinger DS, Ibanez LV, et al: Early social and emotional communication in the infant siblings of children with autism spectrum disorders: An examination of the broad phenotype. J Autism Dev Disord 37(1):122-132, 2007.

Constantino J, Gruber C: Social Responsiveness Scale (SRS). Los Angeles, Western Psychological Services, 2005.

DC:0-3R: Diagnostic Classification of Mental Health and Developmental Disorders of Infancy and Early Childhood, revised edition. Washington, DC, Zero To Three Press, 2005.

DeGangi G, Poisson S, Sickel R, Wiener A: Infant/Toddler Symptom Checklist—A Screening Tool for Parents. Tucson, AZ, Therapy Skill Builders, 1995, pp 1-58.

Diagnostic and Statistical Manual for Primary Care (DSM-PC), Child and Adolescent Version; Wolraich ML, Felice ME, Drotar D (eds). Elk Grove Village, IL, American Academy of Pediatrics, 1996.

Dunn W: Manual for Sensory Profile. San Antonio, TX, Harcourt Assessment Company, The Psychological Corporation, 1999.

Emde R: Early emotional development: New modes of thinking for research and intervention. *In* Warhol JG (ed): New Perspectives in Early Emotional Development. Johnson & Johnson Pediatric Institute, 1998, 29-45.

Gallese V: "Being like me": Self-other identity, mirror neurons, and empathy. *In* Hurley S, Chater N (eds): Perspectives on Imitation: From Neuroscience to Social Science, Vol. 1. Mechanisms of Imitation and Imitation in Animals. Cambridge, MA, MIT Press, 2005, pp 101-118.

Gopnik A, Meltzoff AN, Kuhl PK: Ancient questions and a young science. *In* The Scientist in the Crib—Minds, Brains, and How Children Learn. New York, Morrow, 1999, pp 1–22.

Gray, C: The Original Social Story Book. Arlington, TX, Future Horizons, 1994.

Gray, C: The New Social Story Book. Arlington, TX, Future Horizons, 2000.

Happe F, Frith U: The weak coherence account: Detail-focused cognitive style in autism spectrum disorders. J Autism Dev Disord 36(1):5-25, 2006.

Harrison P, Oskland T: Adaptive Behavior Assessment System, Second Edition. San Antonio, TX, Pearson Education Inc, 2004.

Hobson PR, Chidambi G, Lee A, Meyer J: Foundations for self-awareness: An exploration through autism. Monogr Soc Res Child Dev 71(2) 1-28:128-154, 2006.

Hurley S, Charter N: Introduction: The importance of imitation. *In* Perspectives on Imitation: From Neuroscience to Social Science, Vol. 2. Imitation, Human Development, and Culture. Cambridge, MA, MIT Press, 2005, pp 1-52.

LaFreniere P, Dumas J: Social Competence and Behavior Evaluation, Preschool Edition. Los Angeles, Western Psychological Services, 1995.

Mitchell S, Brian J, Zwaigenbaum L, et al: Early language and communication development of infants later diagnosed with autism spectrum disorder. J Dev Behav Pediatr 27(2 Suppl):S69-S78, 2006.

Pelphrey KA, Adolphs R, Morris JP: Neuroanatomical substrates of social cognition dysfunction in autism. Ment Retard Dev Disabil Res Rev 10(4):259-271, 2004a.

Pelphrey KA, Morris JP, McCarthy G: Grasping the intentions of others: The perceived intentionality of an action influences activity in the superior temporal sulcus during social perception. J Cogn Neurosci 16(10):1706-1716, 2004b.

Pennington B, Williams J, Rogers S: Conclusions. *In* Rogers SJ, Williams JHG (eds): Imitation and the Social Mind. New York, Guilford Press, 2006, pp 431-453.

Pinker S: Thinking machines. *In* How the Mind Works. New York, Norton, 1997, pp 59-148.

Pollak SD, Sinha P: Effects of early experience on children's recognition of facial displays of emotion. Dev Psychol 38(5):784-791, 2002.

Reynolds CR, Kamphaus R: Manual for BASC-2, 6-11 ages Forms & Profiles. Circle Pines, MN, AGS Publishing, 2004a.

Reynolds CR, Kamphaus R: Manual for BASC-2, Preschool Forms & Profiles. Circle Pines, MN, AGS Publishing, 2004b.

Reynolds CR, Kamphaus R: Manual for BASC-2, 12-21 ages Forms & Profiles. Circle Pines, MN, AGS Publishing, 2004c.

Reynolds CR, Richmond BO: Revised Children's Manifest Anxiety Scale (RCMAS): What I Think and Feel. Los Angeles, Western Psychological Services, 1998.

Rizzolatti G, Craighero L: The mirror-neuron system. Annu Rev Neurosci 27:169-192, 2004.

Robins DL, Fein D, Barton ML, Green JA: The Modified Checklist for Autism in Toddlers: An initial study investigating the early detection of autism and pervasive developmental disorders. J Autism Dev Disord 31(2):131-144, 2001.

Rogers S: Studies of imitation in early infancy: Finding and theories. *In* Rogers SJ, Williams JHG (eds): Imitation and the Social Mind. New York, Guilford Press, 2006, pp 3-26.

Rubin KH: "Brokering" emotion dysregulation: The moderating role of parenting in the relation between child temperament and children's peer interactions. *In* Zuckerman BS, Lieberman AF, Fox NA (eds): Emotional Regulation and Developmental Health: Infancy and Early Childhood. New Brunswick, NJ, Johnson & Johnson, 2002, pp 81-99.

Rutter M, Bailey A, Berument S, et al: Social Communication Questionnaire (SCQ). Los Angeles, Western Psychological Services, 2003.

Tartaglia N, Hansen R, Hagerman R: Advances in genetics. *In* Odom SL: Handbook of Developmental Disabilities. New York, Guilford Press, 2007, pp 98-128.

Winner MG: Inside out: What makes a person with social cognitive deficits tick? 2000. Available at: www.socialthinking.com.

Yeates KO, Swift E, Taylor HG, et al: Short- and long-term social outcomes following pediatric traumatic brain injury. J Int Neuropsychol Soc 10(3):412-426, 2004.

39 OPPOSITIONAL BEHAVIOR/ NONCOMPLIANCE

WILLIAM J. BARBARESI

Vignette

The parents of 3-year-old Joseph report that they "can't get him to do anything." When asked to pick up his toys, Joseph either ignores the request or whines. His parents respond by loudly repeating the request. Joseph, in turn, loudly refuses or starts to have a tantrum. On some days, his parents find it "easier to just pick up the toys ourselves" to "preserve the peace." Joseph also has a difficult time making transitions, particularly from play activities to less interesting activities, such as meals. At other times, Joseph's parents find that they can "yell loud enough" to get Joseph to comply. Joseph's parents feel that the majority of their interactions with Joseph involve unsuccessful and unpleasant attempts to "get him to obey."

DEFINING OPPOSITIONALITY/NONCOMPLIANCE

Oppositionality/noncompliance refers to "the refusal to initiate or complete a request made by another person" or the failure to follow a rule that is in effect, even if it is not specifically stated at the time of the noncompliant behavior (Forehand and McMahon, 1981). In this chapter, the terms *oppositional behavior* and *noncompliance* are used interchangeably. Researchers have described four "categories" of noncompliant behavior (Stifter et al, 1999):

1. Defiance: failure to follow directions, accompanied by behaviors such as whining or aggressive behavior;
2. Passive noncompliance: ignoring adult commands while maintaining a neutral affect;
3. Self-assertion: verbal refusal to comply with an adult request while maintaining neutral affect; and
4. Avoidance: actively moving away from an adult in response to an adult command.

Oppositional behaviors may occur only in certain situations (home, school, daycare) or only in response to certain adult authority figures (parents, teachers) or peers (Hoffenaar and Hoeksma, 2002). Oppositionality has both behavioral and emotional aspects (Hoffenaar and Hoeksma, 2002). In addition to the easily observable behaviors associated with oppositionality, oppositional children may respond to threats to their autonomy with anger and show a lack of fear in response to discipline. This pattern of behavior contrasts with the guilt or shame that nonoppositional children typically show when they are disciplined (Hoffenaar and Hoeksma, 2002). Oppositional and noncompliant behaviors are often developmentally appropriate, particularly among toddlers and preschool-age children.

Oppositional behavior occurs on a continuum, with normal toddler and preschooler resistance at one end and clearly deviant behaviors consistent with a diagnosable "disorder" at the other end (Hoffenaar and Hoeksma, 2002). A certain degree of oppositionality in toddlers may be viewed as a mechanism by which toddlers begin to assert their independence and individuality. Thus, oppositional behavior may facilitate the toddler's emotional maturation from totally dependent on to more independent of her or his parents.

Oppositional and noncompliant behaviors represent some of the most common concerns among parents of children from toddlers through adolescents and are the most frequently reported behavior problems in primary care pediatric practice (MacDonald, 2003). Disruptive behavior problems also constitute the most common reason that preschool-age children are brought to mental health clinics (Keenan and Wakschlag, 2002).

In addition to the "normal" oppositionality that is seen in all age groups, oppositional behavior may present significant challenges to parents while not rising to the level of a diagnosable disorder (Wolraich, 1997). Oppositional behavior may be observed as a complicating behavior problem among children with other developmental and behavioral disorders, such as autistic disorder and intellectual disability. At the extreme end of the spectrum of oppositional/noncompliant behavior, children may have symptoms sufficient to warrant a formal diagnosis of oppositional defiant disorder. Finally, children may manifest oppositional defiant disorder as a comorbid condition with other conditions, such as attention-deficit/hyperactivity disorder.

In this chapter, the focus is on oppositional and noncompliant behaviors, not on "diagnosable disorders" of oppositionality/noncompliance. However, the majority of the literature on oppositionality focuses on the severe end of this behavioral spectrum, including primarily children with oppositional defiant disorder and conduct disorder as defined in the *Diagnostic and Statistical Manual of Mental Disorders,* fourth edition, text revision (Burke et al, 2002; Loeber et al, 2000).

RISK FACTORS FOR THE DEVELOPMENT OF OPPOSITIONALITY/NONCOMPLIANCE

Most of the information about risk factors for the development of oppositional and noncompliant behavior comes from studies of children with frank disorders including oppositional defiant disorder and conduct disorder (Burke et al, 2002; Loeber et al, 2000). Whereas this limits the utility of this information for understanding oppositional behavior in children with symptoms that do not warrant a diagnosis of a disorder, it does provide some information about factors that contribute to the development and maintenance of oppositional behavior.

Environmental Risk Factors

Socioeconomic disadvantage has clearly been associated with the development of more severe forms of disruptive behavior (Burke et al, 2002). Specific risk factors include parental unemployment, residing in public housing, and high neighborhood crime rates (Burke et al, 2002). Children who are physically or sexually abused or neglected are clearly more likely to develop significant disruptive behaviors than are children who have not been abused (Burke et al, 2002). It has also been shown that family socioeconomic disadvantages reduce the likelihood that children's oppositional behavior will improve in response to parent management training (Kazdin, 1997). Adopted children are at risk for oppositional behavior disorders, particularly with pre-adoption risk factors such as abuse or neglect, later age at adoption, and pre-adoption placement in multiple foster homes (Simmel et al, 2001). A history of physical or sexual abuse is associated with diagnosed oppositional behavior disorders (Ford et al, 2000). Children living in poverty have been found to have a decrease in oppositional behavior disorders when their families move out of poverty (Costello et al, 2003). Exposure to parental separation during childhood is associated with increased risk for oppositional behavior disorders during adolescence (Fergusson et al, 1994).

Genetic and Biologic Risk Factors

Twin studies and familial aggregation studies have provided support for a genetic contribution to the more severe end of the oppositional behavior spectrum, although it is difficult to separate genetic and environmental influences on oppositionality, even with these research approaches (Burke et al, 2002). Parent ratings of oppositional behavior of monozygotic twins are concordant to a degree that is comparable to ratings of reading ability (Simonoff et al, 1998). Underarousal of the autonomic nervous system, reflected in lower baseline heart rates, and lower salivary cortisol levels have been associated with oppositional defiant disorder (Burke et al, 2002). Young children with significant oppositional behaviors have been found to manifest autonomic underarousal, similar to responses seen in adolescents and adults with significant antisocial behaviors (Crowell et al, 2006). Young children with callous or unemotional traits, based on parent and teacher ratings, appear to be at particularly high risk for severe oppositional and disruptive behaviors (Christian et al, 1997).

Temperament

The concept of temperament is reviewed in detail in Chapter 7. In brief, temperament refers to the "how" of a child's behavior, or "behavioral style," rather than to the motivation behind a particular behavior (Chess and Thomas, 1986). In the original Thomas and Chess longitudinal study of temperament, 10% of children manifested a constellation of "difficult" temperamental traits including irregularity, negative responses to or withdrawal from novel stimuli, slow or poor adaptability to change, and intense, often negative mood (Chess and Thomas, 1986). Thomas and Chess stressed the importance of "goodness of fit" between parenting style and a child's unique set of temperamental traits. These concepts are useful in describing the evolution of oppositional behavior. Young children with difficult temperaments may manifest intense, negative responses to parental commands, particularly if they involve compliance in emotionally charged contexts, such as bedtime or mealtime. The reaction of the difficult child may prompt some parents to remove the demand on the child, thus reinforcing the child's negative response and contributing to the development of noncompliance. Alternatively, parents may respond with increasingly coercive attempts to elicit compliance, thereby inadvertently reinforcing the child's initial, negative, noncompliant response. Although temperament serves as a useful conceptual framework for understanding oppositionality in young children, there is limited empiric support for a causal relationship between innate temperament and oppositionality (Stifter et al, 1999). Recently, however, it has been found that infants who showed poor ability to regulate their emotional response to frustrating experiences were more likely to manifest oppositionality as toddlers (Stifter et al, 1999). Similarly, children with significant problems with anxiety have been found to have oppositional behaviors; if a child becomes anxious when demands are placed on him or her, the likelihood of noncompliance may increase (Garland and Garland, 2001).

Parenting

Poor parenting has been shown to be associated with disruptive child behavior, including oppositionality (Burke et al, 2002). However, the effects of poor or ineffective parenting are often confounded by the presence of parental psychopathology, making it difficult to disentangle the relative importance of these factors

(Burke et al, 2002). Nevertheless, certain parenting behaviors do seem to be associated with the development of disruptive and oppositional behaviors; these include lack of parental involvement, lack of parental warmth, harsh and inconsistent discipline, and physically aggressive punishment (Beauchaine et al, 2005; Burke et al, 2002). Mothers of teenagers with oppositional behavior disorders manifest higher rates of conflict behaviors in interactions with their children than do other mothers of teenagers without oppositional behavior disorders (Fletcher et al, 1996). These parenting behaviors would clearly fit the description of aversive responses to child behavior, as described later, and may contribute to the development of oppositionality in this manner.

THE NEGATIVE REINFORCEMENT TRAP: PARENTAL REINFORCEMENT AND THE DEVELOPMENT OF NONCOMPLIANCE

Parent-child interaction patterns have long been assumed to play an important role in the development of noncompliant behavior (Forehand and McMahon, 1981). Parents often place demands on their young children, and many such demands may be described as aversive to the child (e.g., "It's time to go to bed." or "Stop playing and pick up your toys."). In response to this aversive event, the child may manifest a coercive response (e.g., whining, yelling, or a tantrum). Under certain circumstances, an optimal parental response might include a single and simple repetition of the requirement, followed by a compassionate remark about how challenging the request may be from the child's perspective, and then firm limit setting on escalating behavior. However, parents may respond to the child's coercive response by removing the original aversive event, thereby negatively reinforcing the child's noncompliant behavior. Alternatively, the parent may respond by in turn presenting another aversive event (e.g., yelling, repeating the original command), to which the child may respond by escalating his or her original coercive response (e.g., kicking, screaming). Ultimately, the child may respond by compliance with the original request, but if this occurs only in response to a more aversive parental demand, the child learns to respond only to the parent's more aversive approach of yelling, screaming, and repeating commands (Fig. 39-1). Parents may also inadvertently reinforce coercive, noncompliant behavior by positive reinforcement. For example, when told that it is time to stop playing, the child may whine and cry. In an effort to elicit compliance, the parent may talk to the child, comfort the child, or attempt to explain the reason for the request, thereby positively reinforcing the child's noncompliant response. If such parent-child interactions are repeated many times, a lasting and indeed worsening pattern of oppositionality and noncompliance may evolve (Forehand and McMahon, 1981).

DEVELOPMENTAL COURSE OF OPPOSITIONAL/ NONCOMPLIANT BEHAVIOR

Manifestations of oppositionality and noncompliance change with the child's developmental stage (Figs. 39-2 and 39-3). For example, infants may run away from their parents or ignore parental requests. Toddlers may respond to parental requests by having frank tantrums, particularly at key points during the day, such as bedtime or mealtimes. School-age children may procrastinate or engage in arguments over parental requests to complete basic household chores. Adolescents are likely to manifest oppositionality in more worrisome situations, such as failure to adhere to curfews and breaking family or societal rules about proscribed behaviors, such as alcohol use.

Research on risk factors for severe forms of oppositional behavior offers insight into factors that increase the likelihood that normative oppositionality in the toddler and young child may progress to functionally significant oppositional behavior or frank oppositional behavior disorders. Nevertheless, as with our understanding of risk factors for oppositionality, most of the research on progression of oppositional behaviors comes from literature on frank disorders (oppositional defiant disorder and conduct disorder). It has clearly been established that more severe disruptive behavior disorders (conduct disorder) are almost always preceded by oppositional behavior disorders, leading some researchers to characterize oppositional defiant disorder as a "subsyndromal form of conduct disorder" (Biederman et al, 1996). It has been shown that young, preschool-age children with significant oppositional behavior disorders are likely to continue to exhibit oppositional behavior disorders over time (Lavigne et al, 2001). Factors such

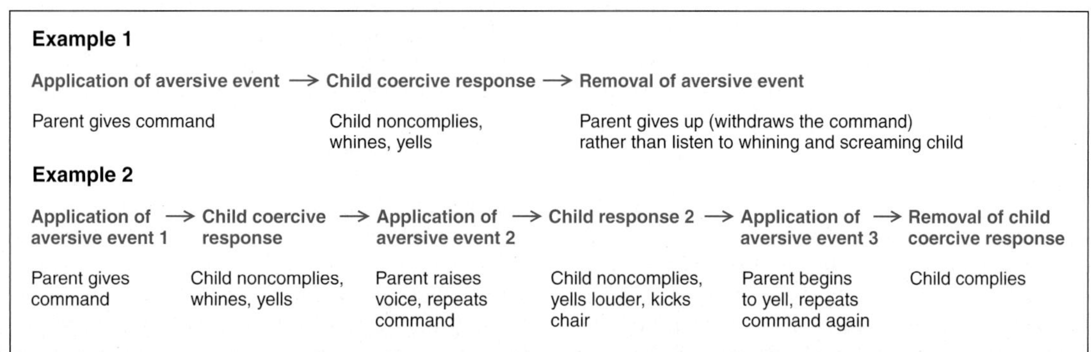

Figure 39-1. Negative reinforcement and the development of oppositional behavior. *(From Forehand RL, McMahon RJ: Helping the Noncompliant Child: A Clinician's Guide to Parent Training. New York, Guilford, 1981.)*

V65.49 Aggressive/Oppositional Variation	
Oppositionality Mild opposition with mild negative impact is a normal developmental variation. Mild opposition may occur several times a day for a short period. Mild negative impact occurs when no one is hurt, no property is damaged, and parents do not significantly alter their plans.	**Infancy** The infant sometimes flails, pushes away, shakes head, gestures refusal, and dawdles. These behaviors may not be considered aggressive intentions, but the only way the infant can show frustration or a need for control in a response to stress, e.g., separation from parents, intrusive interactions (physical or sexual), overstimulation, loss of family member, change in caregivers. **Early Childhood** The child's negative behavior includes saying "no" as well as all of the above behaviors but with increased sophistication and purposefulness. The child engages in brief arguments, uses bad language, purposely does the opposite of what is asked, and procrastinates. **Middle Childhood** The child's oppositional behaviors include all of the above behaviors, elaborately defying doing chores, making up excuses, using bad language, displaying negative attitudes, and using gestures that indicate refusal. **Adolescence** The adolescent's oppositional behaviors include engaging in more abstract verbal arguments, demanding reasons for requests, and often giving excuses.

Figure 39-2. DSM-PC oppositional behavior variant. *(From Diagnostic and Statistical Manual for Primary Care [DSM-PC], Child and Adolescent Version; Wolraich ML, Felice ME, Drotar D [eds]. Elk Grove Village, IL, American Academy of Pediatrics, 1996.)*

V71.02 Aggressive/Oppositional Problem	
Oppositionality The child will display some of the symptoms listed for oppositional defiant disorder. The frequency of the opposition occurs enough to be bothersome to parents or supervising adults, but not often enough to be considered a disorder.	**Infancy** The infant screams a lot, runs away from parents a lot, and ignores requests. **Early Childhood** The child ignores requests frequently enough to be a problem, dawdles frequently enough to be a problem, argues back while doing chores, throws tantrums when asked to do some things, messes up the house on purpose, has a negative attitude many days, and runs away from parents on several occasions. **Middle Childhood** The child intermittently tries to annoy others, such as turning up the radio on purpose, making up excuses, begins to ask for reasons why when given commands, and argues for longer times. These behaviors occur frequently enough to be bothersome to the family. **Adolescence** The adolescent argues back often, frequently has a negative attitude, sometimes makes obscene gestures, and argues and procrastinates in more intense and sophisticated ways.

Figure 39-3. DSM-PC oppositional behavior problem. *(From Diagnostic and Statistical Manual for Primary Care [DSM-PC], Child and Adolescent Version; Wolraich ML, Felice ME, Drotar D [eds]. Elk Grove Village, IL, American Academy of Pediatrics, 1996.)*

as parental substance abuse and low socioeconomic status appear to increase the likelihood that oppositional behaviors will progress over time (Loeber et al, 1995). However, many children with significant oppositional behaviors do not progress to more serious behavior disorders over time (Lahey et al, 1992).

EPIDEMIOLOGY

It may be neither possible nor necessary to precisely define the "prevalence" of oppositional behaviors, particularly if one is referring to the "normative" oppositionality that occurs in all children. It is more important to recognize that behavior problems are identified as one of the most common problems encountered in pediatric practice, with oppositional behaviors among the most common behavior problems (MacDonald, 2003). To the extent that difficult temperament profiles contribute to the development of troubling levels of oppositionality, it may be expected that approximately 10% of children manifest functionally significant levels of oppositionality (Chess and Thomas, 1986).

At the more severe end of the spectrum, oppositional defiant disorder is among the most frequent of the behavioral disorders diagnosed by pediatricians (Williams et al, 2004). Prevalence estimates of frank oppositional behavior disorders range from 1% to approximately 10% (Dick et al, 2005; Maughan et al, 2004). Oppositional behavior disorders have been found to be common in every country and ethnic group in which they have been studied (Arcia and Fernandez, 2003; Bird et al, 2001; Gau et al, 2005; Harada et al, 2004; Srinath

Table 39-1. **Guide to Obtaining History of Noncompliant Behavior**

Setting	Description	Frequency	Duration	Parent Response	Child Response
Bedtime					
Mealtime					
Bath time					
On phone					
Visitors at home					
Visiting others					
Car					
Public places (e.g., stores)					
School					
Siblings					
Peers					
Other parent/relative					
Disciplinary procedures					
Other					

From Forehand RL, McMahon RJ: Helping the Noncompliant Child: A Clinician's Guide to Parent Training. New York, Guilford, 1981

et al, 2005). Oppositionality is most accurately viewed as a component of normal child development and a common behavior disorder in all cultures, races, and ethnic groups. Whereas frank disorders of oppositionality are more common in boys, oppositional behavior may be equally common among both genders (Lahey et al, 2000).

ASSESSMENT OF OPPOSITIONAL/ NONCOMPLIANT BEHAVIOR

An assessment of oppositional behavior depends on understanding basic behavior principles. First, clinicians must distinguish between negative and positive reinforcement of a child's noncompliant or oppositional behavior (Forehand and McMahon, 1981). Negative reinforcement refers to the withdrawal of an aversive event in response to a noncompliant or oppositional behavior (e.g., removing a parental request for compliance when a child resists the parental request). In contrast, positive reinforcement occurs when a pleasant consequence occurs in response to a behavior (e.g., parental attention or soothing in response to a noncompliant behavior). Both negative and positive reinforcement may contribute to the development of oppositional/noncompliant behaviors, as described earlier. These concepts should be kept in mind when inquiring about a child's oppositional/noncompliant behavior.

Oppositional and noncompliant behaviors can be understood only in the context of parent-child interaction. It is therefore essential to inquire not only about the nature, timing, and frequency of problem behaviors but also about the antecedents and the consequences (including parental response) to these behaviors. For most clinicians, this information may be most efficiently obtained through a careful interview. This should begin with open-ended questions about problem behaviors. Subsequently, the interview should focus on common situations in which oppositional and noncompliant behaviors typically occur (Table 39-1). During the interview, the clinician will obtain additional, important information by gauging the parents' perceptions about the severity and origins of the child's behavior as well as the parents' ability to understand the ways in which their parenting may contribute to the problem behaviors. For example, it may become apparent that the child manifested consistently negative and resistant responses to parental demands at an early age, suggesting a difficult temperament. Parents may also demonstrate varying degrees of insight into the extent to which their responses may sustain or even worsen their child's oppositional behavior. For some families, the negative interactions surrounding a child's oppositionality may constitute the predominant parent-child interaction in the family system. Finally, the interview will allow the clinician to assess the parent's approach to parenting. This should include information about the method, timing, and consistency of discipline techniques employed by the child's parents or guardians.

It is also important to identify risk factors that increase the likelihood of both the development and maintenance of oppositional behaviors (see earlier). This task will be inherently easier for clinicians who have a long-term relationship with a child and his or her family.

Several tools are available to the clinician in collecting information that will assist in identifying the origins, severity, and functional impact of oppositional behaviors (Burns and Patterson, 2000; Conners et al, 1998; Lengua et al, 2001). It may be useful to assess parents' stress level in response to their child's challenging behavior (Abidin, 1995). However, there is no single scale or group of scales that can take the place of a careful clinical interview, particularly if the goal is to understand the behavior of the child without regard to a particular diagnostic framework.

PREVENTION AND TREATMENT

Parents and their oppositional/noncompliant children often seem locked in a negative, stressful, and unproductive relationship that is not satisfying for either the parent or the child. In clinical practice, such parent-child relationships often seem to literally be defined and dominated by this cycle of negative interaction. Parents often describe their management of their child's behavior as an effort to "survive the crisis of the moment," even when they seem to recognize that the strategies that allow them to end a negative child behavior may increase the likelihood that the behavior will recur. More often, parents who are locked in such negative interaction cycles with their children do not recognize the factors that initiated and sustain the child's negative, oppositional behaviors. Knowledgeable primary care clinicians may be able to prevent the development of more severe forms of oppositional behavior by providing sound advice and guidance on positive parenting approaches that help parents avoid the negative reinforcement trap and positive reinforcement trap described before. For the developmental and behavioral clinician, it is likely that parents and children will be evaluated at a point when oppositional behavior problems are more firmly established.

In the vignette at the beginning of this chapter, the parent's of 3-year-old Joseph may not have recognized their son's temperamentally determined difficulty with transitions. This trait may have increased the likelihood that Joseph would not respond to parental requests, in turn leading his parents to adopt more forceful yet less effective management strategies ("yelling loud enough"). Joseph and his parents were thus locked in a typical negative reinforcement trap. At times, Joseph's parents lacked the energy to enforce their requests, thereby compounding Joseph's noncompliance by inadvertent, positive reinforcement. If Joseph's parents had understood their son's temperamentally determined difficulty with transitions, they may have been able to adopt management approaches that would not have led to the negative interactions that eventually dominated their interactions with Joseph.

Parent management training is an empirically supported psychosocial treatment for children with oppositional behavior problems (Brestan and Eyberg, 1998; Webster-Stratton, 2005). A number of different parent management training programs have been developed. Two such programs with long track records and research support are those developed by Forehand and Webster-Stratton (Forehand and McMahon, 1981; Webster-Stratton, 2005). These and other effective parent management approaches have several key features in common. The interventions are based on an understanding of the need to reverse the negative parent-child interactions that perpetuate oppositional behaviors. Specific instruction in more appropriate parenting techniques, including limit setting and discipline, are not introduced until after parents have been taught to re-establish positive interactions with their children. Parent management approaches have been demonstrated to decrease oppositional behaviors both immediately after the intervention and in follow-up studies lasting up to several years (Forehand and McMahon, 1981; Reid et al, 2004; Webster-Stratton, 2005). Perhaps most important, parent management training has been found to interrupt the progression of disruptive behavior patterns in young children (Reid et al, 2004). Following is a description of the basic steps included in effective parent management interventions (Forehand and McMahon, 1981; Webster-Stratton, 2005).

Re-establishing Positive Parent-Child Interactions

Whereas parents of oppositional children are typically anxious to learn limit setting and discipline approaches that will end their child's problem behaviors, this is *not* the initial goal of parent management training. Parents are instead given explicit, guided instruction and practice in positive, play-based interactions with their children. This intervention includes attending to and subsequently rewarding desirable child behaviors as part of the play interaction as well as ignoring undesirable behaviors. The goal of this stage of the intervention is to replace negative parental attention and reinforcement of undesirable behaviors (the positive and negative reinforcement traps) with positive parental attention and reward for desirable behaviors.

Limit Setting and Giving Directions

Key skills taught to parents during this phase of intervention include identifying important household rules, providing clear and concise directions, using limited "warnings" as reminders to comply with requests, and avoiding coercive, negative interactions with the child. The goal of this stage of intervention is to increase the child's compliance with a more appropriate, well-defined set of rules for appropriate behavior.

Effective Discipline

This stage of the intervention teaches parents to employ time-out as a discipline strategy. In addition to the basic steps involved in implementing a time-out, parents are taught ways to avoid engaging in power struggles during the time-out, how to follow through with children who refuse to enter or stay in time-out, and how to implement time-out outside the home. The goal of this stage of the intervention is to replace coercive, ineffective discipline with a more effective, noncoercive approach.

Generalizing to Other Settings

By definition, parent management training focuses on improving the parent-child interaction to improve child behavior in the context of the family environment. For young, preschool-age children, this may be the only objective of the intervention. However, many children with oppositional behaviors are school aged. For these older children, oppositional behaviors may lead to significant functional impairment in the school setting and with peers. Interventions that focus exclusively on parent management have not been shown to improve oppositional behaviors in school or with peers (Webster-Stratton et al, 2004). For this reason, Webster-Stratton and colleagues have added intervention modules that help parents equip their children with skills that improve behavior in learning environments and teacher training that is analogous to parent management training approaches (Webster-Stratton et al, 2004; Webster-Stratton, 2005).

Factors That Affect Response to Parent Management Training

Whereas parent management training benefits many children with oppositional and disruptive behaviors, approximately 30% to 50% of children either fail to show significant improvement or fail to sustain improvement over time (Webster-Stratton, 2005). This failure has led researchers to attempt to identify factors that are associated with decreased likelihood of response to parent management training. Unfortunately, these are the same factors that are associated with initial risk for oppositional behavior problems and include marital discord, socioeconomic disadvantage, maternal depression, and parental substance abuse (Forehand and McMahon, 1981; Webster-Stratton, 2005). Clinicians should be aware of the need for careful, longitudinal monitoring of children with these risk factors.

PHARMACOLOGIC TREATMENT OF OPPOSITIONAL BEHAVIOR

There is some evidence to suggest that oppositional behaviors may diminish in response to psychopharmacologic treatment in certain, limited circumstances. In particular, children with attention-deficit/hyperactivity disorder and significant oppositionality may show short-term improvement in oppositional behavior when they are treated with psychostimulants (Farmer et al, 2002). However, there is *no empiric support* for psychopharmacologic treatment of oppositional behavior in general (Farmer et al, 2002).

SUMMARY

Oppositional behaviors are among the most common problems encountered in pediatric practice. Oppositional behaviors may be more likely to develop in children with a constellation of difficult temperamental traits, particularly if the child is socioeconomically disadvantaged or if the family is characterized by marital discord, maternal depression, or parental substance abuse. However, functionally significant oppositional behaviors may occur as a feature of normal development and in families that do not have any of these risk factors. Coercive parent-child interactions play a central role in the initiation and progression of oppositional behaviors. Effective, empirically supported interventions for oppositional behavior problems are based on systematic parent management training. Further research is needed to develop clinically useful instruments to assess oppositional behaviors, particularly for children who have functionally significant problems but do not meet criteria for a diagnosable disorder.

REFERENCES

Abidin RR: Parenting Stress Index, 3rd ed. Professional Manual. Odessa, FL, Psychological Assessment Resources, Inc, 1995.

American Psychiatric Association: Diagnostic and Statistical Manual of Mental Disorders, 4th ed, text revision. Washington, DC, American Psychiatric Association, 2000.

Arcia E, Fernandez MC: Presenting problems and assigned diagnoses among young Latino children with disruptive behaviors. J Atten Disord 6(4):177-185, 2003.

Beauchaine TP, Webster-Stratton C, Reid MJ: Mediators, moderators, and predictors of 1-year outcomes among children treated for early-onset conduct problems: A latent growth curve analysis. J Consult Clin Psychol 73(3):371-388, 2005.

Biederman J, Faraone SV, Milberger S, et al: Is childhood oppositional defiant disorder a precursor to adolescent conduct disorder? Findings from a four-year follow-up study of children with ADHD. J Am Acad Child Adolesc Psychiatry 35(9):1193-1204, 1996.

Bird HR, Canino GJ, Davies M, et al: Prevalence and correlates of antisocial behaviors among three ethnic groups. J Abnorm Child Psychol 29(6):465-478, 2001.

Brestan EV, Eyberg SM: Effective psychosocial treatments of conduct-disordered children and adolescents: 29 years, 82 studies, and 5,272 kids. J Clin Child Psychol 27(2):180-189, 1998.

Burke J, Loeber R, Birmaher B: Oppositional defiant disorder and conduct disorder: A review of the past 10 years, part II. J Am Acad Child Adolesc Psychiatry 41(11):1275-1293, 2002.

Burns GL, Patterson DR: Factor structure of the Eyberg Child Behavior Inventory: A parent rating scale of oppositional defiant behavior toward adults, inattentive behavior, and conduct problem behavior. J Clin Child Psychol 29(4):569-577, 2000.

Chess S, Thomas A: Temperament in Clinical Practice. New York, Guilford, 1986.

Christian RE, Frick PJ, Hill NL, et al: Psychopathy and conduct problems in children: II. Implications for subtyping children with conduct problems. J Am Acad Child Adolesc Psychiatry 36(2):233-241, 1997.

Conners CK, Sitarenios G, Parker JD, Epstein JN: The revised Conners' Parent Rating Scale (CPRS-R): Factor structure, reliability, and criterion validity. J Abnorm Child Psychol 26(4):257-268, 1998.

Costello EJ, Compton SN, Keeler G, Angold A: Relationships between poverty and psychopathology: A natural experiment. JAMA 290(15):2023-2029, 2003.

Crowell SE, Beauchaine TP, Gatzke-Kopp L, et al: Autonomic correlates of attention-deficit/hyperactivity disorder and oppositional defiant disorder in preschool children. J Abnorm Psychol 115(1):174-178, 2006.

Dick DM, Viken RJ, Kaprio J, et al: Understanding the covariation among childhood externalizing symptoms: Genetic and environmental influences on conduct disorder, attention deficit hyperactivity disorder, and oppositional defiant disorder symptoms. J Abnorm Child Psychol 33:219-229, 2005.

Farmer EM, Compton SN, Bums BJ, Robertson E: Review of the evidence base for treatment of childhood psychopathology: Externalizing disorders. J Consult Clin Psychol 70(6):1267-1302, 2002.

Fergusson DM, Horwood LJ, Lynskey MT: Parental separation, adolescent psychopathology, and problem behaviors. J Am Acad Child Adolesc Psychiatry 33(8):1122-1131; discussion 1131-1133, 1994.

Fletcher KE, Fischer M, Barkley RA, Smallish L: A sequential analysis of the mother-adolescent interactions of ADHD, ADHD/ODD, and normal teenagers during neutral and conflict discussions. J Abnorm Child Psychol 24(3):271-297, 1996.

Ford JD, Racusin R, Ellis CG, et al: Child maltreatment, other trauma exposure, and posttraumatic symptomatology among children with oppositional defiant and attention deficit hyperactivity disorders. Child Maltreat 5(3):205-217, 2000.

Forehand RL, McMahon RJ: Helping the Noncompliant Child: A Clinician's Guide to Parent Training. New York, Guilford, 1981.

Garland EJ, Garland OM: Correlation between anxiety and oppositionality in a children's mood and anxiety disorder clinic. Can J Psychiatry 46(10):953-958, 2001.

Gau SS, Chong MY, Chen TH, Cheng AT: A 3-year panel study of mental disorders among adolescents in Taiwan. Am J Psychiatry 162(7):1344-1350, 2005.

Harada Y, Saitoh K, Iida J, et al: The reliability and validity of the Oppositional Defiant Behavior Inventory. Eur Child Adolesc Psychiatry 13(3):185-190, 2004.

Hoffenaar PJ, Hoeksma JB: The structure of oppositionality: Response dispositions and situational aspects. J Child Psychol Psychiatry 43(3):375-385, 2002.

Kazdin AE: Parent management training: Evidence, outcomes, and issues. J Am Acad Child Adolesc Psychiatry 36(10):1349-1356, 1997.

Keenan K, Wakschlag LS: Can a valid diagnosis of disruptive behavior disorder be made in preschool children? Am J Psychiatry 159(3):351-358, 2002.

Lahey BB, Loeber R, Quay HC, et al: Oppositional defiant and conduct disorders: Issues to be resolved for DSM-IV. J Am Acad Child Adolesc Psychiatry 31(3):539-546, 1992.

Lahey BB, Schwab-Stone M, Goodman SH, et al: Age and gender differences in oppositional behavior and conduct problems: A cross-sectional household study of middle childhood and adolescence. J Abnorm Psychol 109(3):488-503, 2000.

Lavigne JV, Cicchetti C, Gibbons RD, et al: Oppositional defiant disorder with onset in preschool years: Longitudinal stability and pathways to other disorders. J Am Acad Child Adolesc Psychiatry 40(12):1393-1400, 2001.

Lengua LJ, Sadowski CA, Friedrich WN, Fisher J: Rationally and empirically derived dimensions of children's symptomatology: Expert ratings and confirmatory factor analyses of the CBCL. J Consult Clin Psychol 69(4):683-698, 2001.

Loeber R, Green SM, Keenan K, Lahey BB: Which boys will fare worse? Early predictors of the onset of conduct disorder in a six-year longitudinal study. J Am Acad Child Adolesc Psychiatry 34(4):499-509, 1995.

Loeber R, Burke JD, Lahey BB, et al. Oppositional defiant and conduct disorder: A review of the past 10 years, part I. J Am Acad Child Adolesc Psychiatry 39(12):1468-1484, 2000.

MacDonald EK: Principles of behavioral assessment and management. Pediatr Clin North Am 50(4):801-816, 2003.

Maughan B, Rowe R, Messer J, et al: Conduct disorder and oppositional defiant disorder in a national sample: Developmental epidemiology. J Child Psychol Psychiatry 45:609-621, 2004.

Reid MJ, Webster-Stratton C, Baydar N: Halting the development of conduct problems in head start children: The effects of parent training. J Clin Child Adolesc Psychol 33:279-291, 2004.

Simmel C, Brooks D, Barth RP, Hinshaw SP: Externalizing symptomatology among adoptive youth: Prevalence and preadoption risk factors. J Abnorm Child Psychol 29(1):57-69, 2001.

Simonoff E, Pickles A, Meyer J, et al: Genetic and environmental influences on subtypes of conduct disorder behavior in boys. J Abnorm Child Psychol 26(6):495-509, 1998.

Srinath S, Girimaji SC, Gururaj G, et al: Epidemiological study of child and adolescent psychiatric disorders in urban and rural areas of Bangalore, India. Indian J Med Res 122(1):67-79, 2005.

Stifter CA, Spinrad TL, Braungart-Rieker JM: Toward a developmental model of child compliance: The role of emotion regulation in infancy. Child Dev 70(1):21-32, 1999.

Webster-Stratton C: The incredible years: A training series for the prevention and treatment of conduct problems in young children. *In* Hibbs ED, Jensen PS (eds): Psychosocial Treatments for Child and Adolescent Disorders: Empirically Based Strategies for Clinical Practice. Washington, DC, American Psychological Association, 2005.

Webster-Stratton C, Reid MJ, Hammond M: Treating children with early-onset conduct problems: Intervention outcomes for parent, child, and teacher training. J Clin Child Adolesc Psychol 33:105-124, 2004.

Williams J, Klinepeter K, Palmes G, et al: Diagnosis and treatment of behavioral health disorders in pediatric practice. Pediatrics 114(3):601-606, 2004.

Wolraich ML: Diagnostic and Statistical Manual for Primary Care (DSM-PC) Child and Adolescent Version: Design, intent, and hopes for the future. J Dev Behav Pediatr 18(3):171-172, 1997.

40 AGGRESSION, VIOLENCE, AND DELINQUENCY

STEPHEN S. LEFF, CALLISTA TULLENERS,
AND JILL C. POSNER

Vignette

A 10-year-old girl comes to the office for an evaluation for abdominal pain. This is her third visit in 2 weeks for the same complaint. She has no fever, vomiting, diarrhea, constipation, or other constitutional complaints. Her mother is becoming increasingly concerned because her daughter has missed 8 days of school. The child's physical examination findings are normal with the exception of mild, periumbilical tenderness without rebound or guarding. On further questioning at this third visit, the girl reluctantly reveals that a classmate has been spreading rumors about her and she feels like "all her friends are turning on her."

BACKGROUND

Helping children and adolescents recognize and appropriately respond to conflict situations is often left to parents, school systems, or psychotherapists. However, there are many things that pediatric health care providers can do to understand the scope of the problem, to assess a child's behavioral tendencies, to monitor a child's behavioral progress, and to work collaboratively with parents and schools.

Low-level aggressive behavior (such as hitting, pushing, or threatening others) is present as early as preschool and is a constant source of frustration and concern for many children as they become older. In fact, a nationwide study indicated that 29.9% of sixth to tenth graders reported moderate or severe involvement with bullying, with 13% being involved as the bully, 10.6% being involved as the victim, and 6.3% being involved as both a bully and a victim (Nansel et al, 2001). In addition to those youth involved as a bully, as a victim, or as both a bully and a victim, many students frequently witness these low-level conflicts when they occur at school. These individuals have been termed bystanders because they do not actively try to resolve the conflict but passively support the aggressor or bully by not intervening. Thus, low-level aggression and victimization occur frequently among school children and are important issues to address for all students, not just for the aggressors or victims.

In the first part of the chapter, we define aggression and then distinguish it from several related constructs. Then we discuss some of the current subtypes of aggression and provide information on the etiology and theoretical premises of the development of aggression. In the second part of the chapter, we focus on the pediatrician's role in curtailing the problem of youth violence. Finally, in the last part of the chapter, we discuss practical issues including straightforward techniques that pediatric health care providers can use with children and families around problems of aggression and also tips on recognizing when referral to a mental health specialist may be indicated.

DEFINITIONAL ISSUES

Table 40-1 includes definitions for terms that are used in this chapter. Aggression is behavior that is intended to harm or to hurt another individual. Physical or overt aggression includes dominant actions such as hitting, pushing, and shoving. Relational or social aggression includes socially manipulative behaviors, such as starting rumors, ignoring others on purpose, threatening to withdraw friendships, and using social exclusion to harm one's social standing (Crick and Grotpeter, 1995). The term *bullying* is often used interchangeably with *aggression,* even though the research has clearly differentiated these two terms. Bullying is a form of aggression in that it is intended to harm or to hurt another individual either physically or socially and meets two additional criteria (see Rigby, 2002). First, the behavior must occur within the context of an imbalance of power, either physically, such that one child is stronger or larger than the victim, or psychologically, such that the bully has higher social standing than the victim. Second, the bullying behavior must occur repeatedly over time. Thus, when two children of equal strength or status become involved in an occasional conflict or fight, the term *bullying* is not appropriate. However, if the tallest child in the class

Table 40-1. **Definitions**

Term	Definition
Aggression	Behavior that is intended to harm or to hurt another individual
Physical or overt aggression	Physical acts that are intended to harm or to hurt the physical body, such as hitting or pushing
Relational or social aggression	Socially manipulative acts that harm or hurt another's feelings or social standing, such as gossiping or using social exclusion
Bullying	Aggression that occurs within an imbalance of power and that occurs repeatedly
Violence	Serious acts of delinquency
Delinquency	Serious physical aggression and criminal behavior

repeatedly makes fun of the shortest child in the class, then bullying may be the appropriate characterization. The definition of bullying is broad enough to encompass both physical and relational forms of aggression.

The term *violence* is often used to refer to serious actions of delinquency. For instance, violence is often thought of as extremely serious physically aggressive behavior (such as assault, robbery, or rape), criminal behaviors, and delinquent actions (including fire setting, property destruction, and the like). It is imperative that educators, school-based mental health professionals, and primary care physicians work together to focus on the low-level day-to-day forms of aggression and bullying that occur frequently in the elementary and middle schools across the nation so that they do not build to the more serious forms of violence and delinquency in the high-school settings (see Leff et al, 2001).

EPIDEMIOLOGY OF AGGRESSION AND ASSOCIATED PROBLEMS

In the past, aggressive behaviors were largely conceptualized as being physical, direct, and overt in nature (e.g., hitting, pushing, or kicking), and therefore boys were viewed as being considerably more aggressive than girls. However, the gender gap is lessened when one considers the way in which children typically aggress toward others, boys in a physical and overt manner, and girls in a social, indirect, and often covert manner affecting one's social standing (see Crick and Grotpeter, 1995).

Both forms of aggression have been associated with a number of comorbidities. Physical aggression is associated with academic deficits, social problem solving difficulties, emotional arousal deficits, peer relationship problems, and, for some children, extension of physically aggressive behavior into adolescence and adulthood (Loeber et al, 1993). Relational aggression is associated with internalizing problems (such as loneliness, depression, and anxiety), peer relationship difficulties, and problem solving deficits (Crick and Grotpeter, 1995). Thus, children who engage in low-level aggressive behaviors (either physical or relational) during the elementary and school-age years are likely to experience a number of comorbid difficulties that can cause significant impairment as they become older. Similarly, being the victim of these types of aggressive actions also has negative repercussions. For example, victims often experience internalizing symptoms (somatic complaints, such as headaches and stomachaches), have strained peer relationships, and are often unhappy at school (Kochenderfer and Ladd, 1996).

SUBTYPES OF AGGRESSION

In this chapter, we briefly review three common conceptualizations to categorize children's aggression.

Reactive Versus Proactive Aggression

Reactive aggression is impulsive and a reaction to a situation (e.g., the child pushes another child because he was pushed himself). Proactive aggression is planned to accomplish a specific goal (e.g., a child pushes another so that she can be the first in line). Children who exhibit reactive aggression tend to have many impulsive behavior problems, have difficulty regulating their emotional arousal, demonstrate social skills and problem solving deficits, and are typically more disliked than those children who exhibit high levels of proactive aggressive behavior. Proactive aggressive children expect that the aggressive action will benefit them in some way and possess relatively high levels of self-confidence compared with reactive aggressive youth.

Physical Versus Nonphysical Forms of Aggression

For many years, the study of aggression focused on physical or overt behaviors related to dominance. However, physical, overt aggression does not fully recognize the sometimes subtle and indirect manner that girls often display when they are angry at their peers. This form of aggression, called relational, social, or indirect aggression, is exhibited with the intention of damaging another child's social standing within the peer group. Interventionists are now beginning to broaden the scope of treatment to include techniques that may be helpful in decreasing both physical and nonphysical forms of aggression (Leff et al, 2007).

DSM-IV: Oppositional Defiant Disorder and Conduct Disorder

The *Diagnostic and Statistical Manual of Mental Disorders,* fourth edition (DSM-IV), classifies youth's aggressive and noncompliance behaviors into two distinct diagnostic categories, oppositional defiant disorder and conduct disorder (DSM-IV, 1994). Oppositional defiant disorder consists of a pattern of noncompliant and defiant behavior toward authority figures. To meet the diagnostic criteria of oppositional defiant disorder, youth must exhibit at least four of eight noncompliant and argumentative behaviors (e.g., arguing with adults, actively defying requests, blaming others for one's actions) for at least a 6-month period. This pattern of behavior is usually seen before the age of 8 years. Prevalence rates vary between 2% and 15%, depending on the study and sampling technique used. See Chapter 39 for a more extensive discussion of oppositional defiant disorder.

Conduct disorder is a more serious diagnostic category than oppositional defiant disorder and consists of a pattern of behavior in which the rights of others and major societal rules and norms are frequently violated. In general, conduct disorder is associated with alcohol and drug use, early sexual behavior, and persistent recklessness and risk-taking behaviors. Prevalence rates for conduct disorder range from 1% to 10%. Conduct disorder is differentiated from oppositional defiant disorder because it often involves serious aggression toward people or animals, destruction of others' property or belongings, and deceit or theft. There are both child-onset and adolescent-onset subtypes of conduct disorder.

ETIOLOGY OF AGGRESSION AND VIOLENCE

Research examining the etiology of aggression and violence has primarily focused on the physical forms of aggression. Most researchers believe that aggression and violence are multidetermined, complex phenomena that are first expressed relatively early in the child's life. Further, research has clearly demonstrated that aggression is often quite stable over time, especially if early preventive treatments are not undertaken. In this section of the chapter, we briefly review several of the theoretical premises for the etiology of aggression. These models are not mutually exclusive. Many theorists posit that they should be integrated for best understanding the complexity of aggression and violence.

Biologic/Psychobiology

Prior research suggests that one may inherit a biologic vulnerability or underlying temperament to exhibit aggression, which has been called a diathesis. It is thought that aggressive behavior most likely results from the interaction between a diathesis (this biologic predisposition toward being aggressive) and an environmental or psychosocial stressor that influences one to act in an aggressive manner (diathesis-stress model). Aggressive behavior is complex and multidetermined.

A number of genetic and pharmacologic studies have increased our knowledge of the role of neurotransmitters, hormones, and enzymes that may influence aggressive behavior. Here we review a few recent findings about neurotransmission and neuroanatomy. Studies have found that high levels of dopamine or low levels of serotonin may be associated with aggressive behavior in both humans and animals (Nelson and Chiavegatto, 2001). The frontal lobes are posited to suppress or to inhibit signals from lower brain regions, such as the amygdala, which has been associated with emotional arousal, excitement, fear, and aggression. The orbital frontal region of the brain is thought to be involved in the modulation of aggressive behavior. Lesions of the frontal lobe may increase the risk of aggressive and violent behaviors (Grafman et al, 1996).

Social Learning

Social learning theories suggest that children learn to exhibit aggressive behaviors because they observe others acting aggressively and can see how these behaviors are reinforced over time (Bandura, 1973). Social learning theories emphasize the importance of the social context and posit that individuals can learn by observing others' actions and whether these individuals are positively or negatively reinforced when exhibiting aggressive behaviors. Research by Bandura has also suggested that young children imitate adults' aggressive actions that they witness in contrived social settings. Thus, aggressive behavior is thought to occur because it has been either modeled or reinforced over time.

Social Information Processing

Social information processing models of aggression and development suggest that the way in which a child processes a series of social cues has an impact on how the child will eventually behave in the social situation (Crick and Dodge, 1994). For instance, physically aggressive children are thought to have deficits in a number of these sequential social cognitive dimensions, including encoding of environmental cues, interpretation of intentionality, generation of social goals, generation of behavioral alternatives, evaluation of these alternatives, and, finally, enacting of the behavior. Social information processing models help explain both the development and maintenance of aggressive behaviors and also suggest approaches to prevention and treatment of aggression.

Developmental/Ecologic

Developmental/ecologic theories of aggression suggest that behavioral sequences become entrenched because of the series of interactions an individual has with others in his or her social environment (Bronfenbrenner, 1986). The child's behavior is believed to be influenced greatly by his or her biology; interactions with parents and siblings, peers, diverse school personnel, and caregivers; and the larger community and cultural context in which he or she resides. Each of these interactions influences children as they mature and in many cases are thought to play a role in the development and maintenance of aggression.

Integration of Theories

Many researchers use a diathesis-stress framework for understanding the integration of theories and the interplay between nature and nurture in the influence of aggression. A diathesis-stress model suggests that aggressive behavior occurs when a predisposed child (a child with a genetic or psychological vulnerability) is in a stressful or provoking situation or environment. Thus, the biologic and social information processing theories suggest the importance of different types of biologic and psychological vulnerabilities, whereas the social learning and developmental/ecologic (and also social information processing) theories focus more heavily on the influence of environmental stressors in the expression of aggression.

UNIQUE ROLE OF PEDIATRIC HEALTH CARE PROVIDERS

Youth violence has emerged as a major public health concern in the United States because of its high prevalence and associated morbidity and mortality. Health

Table 40-2. Potential Roles for Pediatric Health Care Providers in Regard to Violence and Aggression

Anticipatory guidance and prevention
Screening for aggression, victimization, and related issues
Assessment of children who are aggressors, victims, or both or frequent witnesses and bystanders
Referral for mental health services
Office-based counseling
Research
Collaboration with school and community efforts

care providers, pediatricians in particular, are uniquely poised to address violence prevention at the clinical level. Practical ways for pediatric health care providers to partake in violence prevention have been proposed (Table 40-2), and research to learn more about the success and implementation of such efforts is currently under way.

Pediatric health care can capitalize on the physician-patient relationship, inherent in the primary care pediatric setting, to champion prevention of youth violence (Rivara and Farrington, 1995). Pediatric health care providers develop relationships not only with the individual patient but also with his or her family throughout all phases of childhood development. Often, the pediatric health care provider's reach extends beyond the walls of the office as many are well integrated into the communities that they serve. Moreover, pediatric health care providers are adept at offering preventive care services and are knowledgeable about activities such as screening, treatment, and advocacy. Therefore, pediatric health care providers are situated on the front lines to recognize and to respond to the problems associated with youth violence.

The American Academy of Pediatrics and national experts who have called for health professionals to take a more active role in youth violence prevention recommend educating families about youth violence, counseling patients directly, enhancing parents' behavioral management skills, discussing discipline practices and parent-child communication, advocating for gun safety, and referring patients or families to community programs (Barkin et al, 1999). Further, pediatricians should provide initial screening for a child's involvement in frequent peer conflicts at school either as an aggressor, as a victim, or as both an aggressor and a victim. Asking screening questions to understand the child's friendships, problem solving skills, and communication and relationships with his or her parents is extremely helpful. After the identification of significant challenges in these areas through screening, further assessment, appropriate treatment by the pediatric health care provider, or referral to a mental health specialist should take place.

Anticipatory guidance in the form of patient education and parent education and training is an additional means for pediatric health care providers to address youth violence that has been found to avert later problems (Task Force on Violence, 1999). Specific components of anticipatory guidance include advising parenting classes, offering counseling or support, advocating for gun safety, and discouraging corporal punishment and discussing alternative forms of discipline. Encouragement of "nurturing and nonviolent behaviors" is another recommendation. Pediatric health care providers can also become involved in violence-related research through practice-based research projects (Task Force on Violence, 1999).

Pediatric health care providers can assist in integrating treatment care plans relating to violence prevention and behavioral management across important life contexts, including the home, school, and community. As such, pediatric health care professionals play an essential role in coordinating and organizing services for many youth and their families.

Pediatric health care providers encounter barriers as they assume these roles in addressing youth violence. These barriers include limited training in prevention programming, relatively short office visits, and substantial reimbursement challenges for many patients. The following section offers practical suggestions related to assessment, advocacy, treatment, and referral.

SCREENING, ASSESSMENT, AND REFERRAL

We recommend that pediatric health care providers screen for and assess four primary dimensions: involvement in low-level peer conflicts at school and social skills functioning, ability to make and to maintain friendships, problem solving abilities, and communication and connection with parental and adult figures.

Involvement in Peer Conflicts at School and Social Skills Functioning

Screening questions, detailed in Table 40-3, will help the pediatric care provider understand whether children become involved in frequent peer conflicts at school, what role they may play in these conflicts (e.g., aggressor, victim, or both), the settings in which they typically occur, how the conflicts usually develop, and whether there is a school staff member or other responsible adult aware of and assisting with these issues. If the child and parent report relatively frequent peer conflicts (e.g., happening several times a month), if the child or adult is concerned by the conflicts, or if there are no adults who can support the child within the school setting, it is recommended that the provider conduct further assessment of the peer conflicts.

Several teacher and parent report measures allow pediatric health care providers to quickly and efficiently assess how well a child is interacting with his or her classmates. Two teacher report measures, the Behavioral Assessment Scale for Children (Reynolds and Kamphaus, 1992) and the Teacher Report Form (Achenbach, 1991), are commonly used to assess how children are functioning across a number of different externalizing and internalizing behaviors. Each has demonstrated strong psychometric properties in numerous studies and has been found to be moderately to highly associated with other indices, such as peer report measures and behavioral observations. Briefer teacher report measures, such as the Children's Social Behavior Questionnaire (Crick, 1996), have shown much promise in providing a quick

Table 40-3. Questions for Youth

Conflicts

Do you frequently become involved in conflicts at school or within other settings?
Can you describe the conflict, argument, or fight and also whether it is physical (e.g., hitting or pushing) or nonphysical (e.g., gossiping, social exclusion, verbal taunts)?
What is your role in the conflict (e.g., aggressor, victim, or bystander)?
Where at school (or elsewhere) do these conflicts typically occur?
Do you have conflicts during the lunch recess period at school? If yes, please describe.
How does the conflict typically start?
How often do you become involved in these types of conflicts?
Are any adults at school aware of these conflicts?
How concerned are you by these conflicts?

Friendships

Is it easy for you to make and to keep friends?
Do you have a lot of friends? If so, please tell me about some of your friends.
Do you have a best friend? If so, can you tell me about him or her?
What activities or things do you like to do with your friends?
Are your friends nice to other children and youth?

Problem Solving

How can you tell when there is about to be a problem or conflict at school?
If you become involved in a conflict, argument, or fight with another child your age, do you usually think that it was the other person's fault?
What do you do to try to resolve conflicts, arguments, or fights when you are involved?
What do you do to try to resolve conflicts, arguments, or fights when they happen to other children?

Communication with Parents and Adult Figures

If you become involved in a conflict, fight, or argument, is there anyone you can talk to about it at home, at school, or within your neighborhood? Is it helpful when you talk with this individual?

and efficient index of the child's level of physically aggressive, relationally aggressive, and prosocial behaviors. The advantages of using teacher reports are that they are easy to administer and to score, they do not require the health care provider to interfere with valuable class time or the teacher to interrupt clinical care, and they are consistent with typical referral practices as teachers often refer students who are having externalizing behavior problems (Leff et al, 1999).

Parents are often unfamiliar with their child's behavior in school settings in which conflicts typically occur (e.g., playground, lunchroom, hallways) and thus may not be sensitive reporters for subtle peer relationship difficulties. Parent report measures have utility in providing information about the child's behavioral functioning in the home and community. The parent version of the Behavior Assessment System for Children and the Child Behavior Checklist have demonstrated strong psychometric properties across numerous studies. The parent version of the Children's Social Behavior Questionnaire is easily administered, scored, and interpreted. Finally, the Social Skills Rating System (Gresham and Elliot, 1990) has been used across a number of studies to assess children's social skills. This measure has parent, teacher, and self-report versions and provides a good understanding about the type and severity of children's social skills difficulties.

On the primary assessment tools mentioned (Behavior Assessment System for Children, teacher and parent versions; Teacher Report Form; Child Behavior Checklist), a standardized total score can be generated for externalizing behaviors or more specifically related to the aggression subscales of these instruments. If this standardized score is at or above the 90th percentile, this may suggest that follow-up treatment or referral to a mental health specialist is needed.

Screening for Peer Relationships and Friendships

How one is treated by one's friends and what one learns in the context of early peer relationships can have a considerable impact on one's use of aggressive behaviors. Rejection by one's peers has been clearly associated with aggressive and nonaggressive behavior problems at the preschool, middle-school, and high-school levels; patterns of prosocial play behaviors with peers in early childhood have been associated with positive behavioral functioning as youth reach adolescence (see Deater-Deckard, 2001). Further, research has demonstrated that having a best friend can serve as a powerful buffer against a host of negative outcomes and that the protective effects of positive friendships can even extend to lessening the effects of a challenging home situation. As such, it is recommended that pediatric health care providers screen for the child's or youth's ability to develop and to maintain close friendships and assess whether the child has at least one prosocial best friend. In Table 40-3, we include several questions to help pediatric health care providers quickly and efficiently determine the quantity and quality of the child's friendships, whether the child has a prosocial best friend, and whether the child experiences difficulties during the lunch recess period as conflicts and social exclusion often occur in this unstructured and sometimes less supervised social context (Leff et al, 2004).

Problem Solving Abilities

There are few well-validated and brief assessment tools of social problem solving skills, even though many aggression prevention programs teach children a series of problem solving steps following the social information processing model (Crick and Dodge, 1994) described earlier. It is possible to briefly screen for a child's flexibility in using problem solving skills in the context of challenging social situations by asking questions about how the child would interpret and think through different social situations. The child's responses to these questions help the pediatric health care provider to determine whether an appropriate treatment is providing problem solving strategies to the child and parent within a primary care setting (see Chapter 86) or whether referral of the child to a mental health specialist is needed for intensive social skill and problem solving training (see Chapter 89). In addition, several questions related to the child's empathic behaviors and perspective taking skills are also instructive for treatment planning (see Table 40-3).

Parent-Child Communication

It is extremely important for a pediatric health care provider to screen for and to assess how well a child and parent are communicating about the child's social relationships, school behaviors, and overall psychosocial adjustment. A youth who shows high levels of aggression, peer rejection, or social withdrawal is more at risk if he or she does not have an adult to confide in. Although there are few well-validated and brief assessment tools in this area, several specific screening questions can be asked by pediatric health care providers in the context of an office visit as outlined in Table 40-3. These questions will provide a deep understanding for the pediatric health care provider about the child's home and school context and can be helpful in the referral and treatment recommendation process.

TREATMENT STRATEGIES

In this last section, we discuss some straightforward techniques that pediatric health care providers can use to address low-level conflicts and peer relationship struggles with their patients and families in the context of the office visit. These techniques are likely to be warranted when the screening questions provided in Table 40-3 indicate that a child has difficulties with conflicts (as an aggressor, victim, or both), social skills and friendships, and problem solving challenges. It is recommended that pediatric health care providers refer the child and family to a mental health specialist if these techniques cannot be implemented or if brief interventions do *not* help to alleviate the low-level aggression and peer relationship difficulties. We discuss strategies within each of the following four areas and summarize the recommendations in Table 40-4.

Table 40-4. Tips Related to Intervention Strategies

Strategies for Addressing Peer Victimization at School

Establish a "go-to" or point person at school.
Avoid bullying hot spots at school (e.g., less well supervised areas of the playground).
Stay close to good friends when unable to avoid bullying hot spots.
Participate in structured and supervised activities during school recess.
Make good decisions about which activities or groups of friends to join.
Inform school personnel if a child is being bullied, especially through nonphysical means that they may not be aware of.

Promoting Friendships

Have short structured outings or play dates within a structured and fun setting.
Be a good friend to others.
Set specific goals related to the development and maintenance of prosocial friendships.

Promoting Problem Solving, Perspective Taking, and Empathy Skills for Aggressors

Promote problem solving strategies by helping the child slow down and think through potential social conflict situations and by asking the child the following questions:
- What led to the problem?
- What did the child do to contribute to the problem?
- What did the other child do to contribute to the problem?
- What were the child's choices in the situation?
- What are the consequences associated with each potential choice?

Use modeling and role playing to help children learn problem solving strategies (having parents reflect on the strategies used to stay calm and think through tough interpersonal situations).
Help parents learn to reinforce appropriate problem solving steps.
Assist the child in building empathy and perspective taking skills by asking questions when reading stories or discussing the child's day. Sample questions include the following:
- How do you think he or she felt in this situation? How could you tell this by looking at his or her face and body?
- How would you have felt in this situation?

Promote empathy and perspective taking by discussing the benefits of sharing and compromising.

Promoting Positive Parent-Child Communication

Create a special time each evening to play a fun game or to talk about the child's day.
Use floor-time techniques for short child-directed, positive-oriented play sessions.

Strategies for Addressing Peer Victimization at School

Pediatric health care providers can help children who are frequently victims of peer aggression or bullying. First, it is suggested that they talk to their patients and their families about bullying "hot spots" at school. Typically, these are unstructured school settings, such as unsupervised areas on the playground during recess, in the lunchroom, in the hallways, and during transition times (Leff et al, 2004). If the child recognizes the areas in which he or she or others are most likely to be victimized, the child can take certain actions to become prepared within these settings. It is helpful to remind children and families that there is power in numbers. As such, it is strongly recommended that when the child is unable to avoid a bullying hot spot, he or she should try to stay close to a good friend or to other children who are not frequently bullied.

The pediatric health care provider can also advise the child and parent to establish a "go-to" person at school who can talk with the child if he or she is concerned by any peer relationship issues that may arise. This key individual can often be helpful in the case of nonphysical forms of bullying, which may not be readily apparent or even understood by various school personnel. Thus, the key individual, if supportive and properly educated about the difficulties associated with relational and verbal forms of aggression, can often be helpful in alerting other school personnel to the occurrence of the more subtle form of victimization. A number of different school staff could serve as the go-to person, including the school counselor, the school psychologist, a teacher, or a playground or lunchroom supervisor. The go-to person needs to be an approachable adult who is willing to collaborate with the youth, parent, and pediatric health care provider if necessary to help ensure a safe and productive school experience for the youth.

There are also several playground-related strategies that children can employ to lower the chances that they will be the target of peer aggression. First, it is recommended that children participate in structured and organized activities during the school recess period if possible. Research has demonstrated that children play more cooperatively and prosocially when they are given the opportunity to participate in structured activities during recess (Leff et al, 2004). Second, pediatric health care providers can educate children and parents about basic peer group entry techniques that can be extremely helpful when employed on the playground during recess. These include helping children learn to be discriminating in terms of deciding which activities and groups to try to join and in which to participate. For instance, an activity that includes many of their friends is a much better one to try to join than a similar activity that includes children who are known to bully or bother others. Further, pediatric health care providers can highlight the importance of waiting for the right moment to try to enter a group, such as when there is a natural break in the activity (e.g., the ball goes out of bounds in basketball, or when girls switch positions in a jump-rope game), and that a positive-oriented comment about the game or the children playing the game (e.g., That looks like fun, do you need another person to play?) is often better received than a disruptive or negative comment.

Strategies for Promoting Friendships

There are several ways in which pediatric health care providers can advise parents on how to promote positive interactions between their child and the child's classmates or peers, whether their child is an aggressor or victim. One strategy is for the parent to set up a short, highly structured play date for their child and another peer. Essentially, the parent helps to promote their child's friendships by maximizing the likelihood of a successful play date in this manner. Another simple but effective strategy is to encourage the child to be friendly to others, as research has demonstrated that being friendly and interested in others' activities is associated with the development of friendships and prosocial actions.

Promoting Problem Solving, Empathy, and Perspective Taking Skills for Aggressors

Pediatric health care providers can help parents learn how to work with their children who are aggressive to build problem solving skills. The parent can ask the child a series of questions designed to help him or her slow down and think through the different problem solving steps as opposed to reacting impulsively in challenging social situations. It is important that parents emphasize that when a conflict occurs, often both parties contribute to the situation in some manner. The types of questions we recommend include asking the child what the antecedents to the problem were and what the child or others may have done to contribute to the problem. Next, it is important that parents explore with children what their choices are in potential conflict situations and whether they think about the consequences of each choice before deciding on how to react in the situation. Also, problematic social situations provide a strong opportunity for parents to model staying calm and thinking through situations thoroughly by considering all alternatives, as opposed to reacting to the situation emotionally or impulsively.

There are also many different ways that parents can help their children become empathic and consider another child's perspective. For instance, when reading a story with their child, a parent can ask the child how he or she thinks the main character would be feeling and how he or she would have felt in a similar situation. Further, this type of coaching can be extremely useful by having children take on the perspective of "the victim" in potential conflict situations. Parents can encourage their children's use of "I" statements to help build empathy. For instance, the child would learn to say "I feel upset when you bump into me on the playground during recess." Finally, parents can also promote empathy and perspective taking skills by reinforcing times in which the child shares or compromises in his or her peer relationships.

Promoting Positive Parent-Child Communication

Strategies that pediatric health care providers can recommend for parents to improve communication with their children can be helpful for all children and their parents, regardless of whether the child is an aggressor, a victim, or a bystander of aggression. One strategy is to have parents and children set aside a short period of uninterrupted time, such as 10 or 15 minutes several times a week, when they can play a fun game together, talk about their days, or do other mutually enjoyable activities together. Another variation on this strategy is to use the special time for "floor time" (Greenspan and Wieder, 2006). Floor time is a technique in which children direct the play with the adult for short periods, while the adult pays positive attention to the child's actions, comments on the child's actions, and follows along as appropriate. The important part of this technique is that the parent allows the child to exhibit creativity and excitement while providing an opportunity for positive praise and parent-child communication.

SUMMARY

Pediatric health care providers are in a unique role in the prevention of youth violence. Pediatric health care providers can become involved in the prevention of violence through many activities, including advocacy, anticipatory guidance, practice-based research projects, and coordination of care services for their patients. This chapter focuses on their role in the screening for and assessment of low-level aggression and related comorbidities. Pediatric health care providers are uniquely situated to direct screening, assessment, and follow-up treatment or referral to a mental health specialist to help their patients better navigate peer-related challenges associated with being the aggressor or victim of low-level conflicts at school. Specifically, screening questions can be used to determine whether a child is struggling with peer aggression or victimization, social skills development and friendship making skills, problem solving and perspective taking abilities, and communication between the child and parent. A number of straightforward treatment strategies exist that will help equip pediatric health care providers with more of the knowledge and strategies to successfully provide short-term follow-up treatment in this important area.

REFERENCES

Achenbach TM: Integrative Guide for the 1991 CBCL/4-18, YSR, and TRF Profiles. Burlington, VT, University of Vermont, Department of Psychiatry, 1991.

Bandura A: Aggression: A Social Learning Analysis. Englewood Cliffs, NJ, Prentice-Hall, 1973.

Barkin S, Ryan G, Gelberg L: What pediatricians can do to further youth violence prevention—a qualitative study. Inj Prev 5:53-58, 1999.

Bronfenbrenner U: Ecology of the family as a context for human development: Research perspectives. Dev Psychol 22:723-742, 1986.

Crick NR: The role of overt aggression, relational aggression, and prosocial behavior in the prediction of children's future social adjustment. Child Dev 67:2317-2327, 1996.

Crick NR, Dodge KA: A review and reformulation of social information-processing mechanisms in children's social adjustment. Psychol Bull 115:74-101, 1994.

Crick NR, Grotpeter JK: Relational aggression, gender, and social psychological adjustment. Child Dev 66:710-722, 1995.

Deater-Deckard K: Annotation: Recent research examining the role of peer relationships in the development of psychopathology. J Child Psychol Psychiatry 42:565-579, 2001.

Diagnostic and Statistical Manual of Mental Disorders, 4th ed. Washington, DC, American Psychiatric Association, 1994.

Grafman J, Schwab K, Warden D, et al: Frontal lobe injuries, violence, and aggression: A report of the Vietnam head injury study. Neurology 46:1231-1238, 1996.

Greenspan SI, Wieder S: Engaging Autism: Using the Floortime Approach to Help Children Relate, Communicate, and Think. Cambridge, ME, Da Capo Press, 2006.

Gresham FM, Elliot SN: The Social Skills Rating System. Circle Pines, MN, American Guidance Service, 1990.

Kochenderfer BJ, Ladd GW: Peer victimization: Cause or consequence of school maladjustment. Child Dev 67:1305-1317, 1996.

Leff SS, Angelucci J, Goldstein AB, et al: Using a participatory action research model to create a school-based intervention program for relationally aggressive girls: The Friend to Friend Program. *In* Zins J, Elias M, Maher C eds: Handbook of Prevention and Intervention in Peer Harassment, Victimization, and Bullying. New York, Haworth, 2007, pp 199-218.

Leff SS, Costigan TE, Power TJ: Using participatory-action research to develop a playground-based prevention program. J School Psychol 42:3-21, 2004.

Leff SS, Kupersmidt J, Patterson CJ, Power TJ: Factors influencing teacher predictions of peer bullying and victimization. School Psychol Rev 28:505-517, 1999.

Leff SS, Power TJ, Manz PH, et al: School-based aggression prevention programs for young children: Current status and implications for violence prevention. School Psychol Rev 30:343-360, 2001.

Loeber R, Wung P, Keenan K, et al: Developmental pathways in disruptive child behavior. Dev Psychopathol 5:101-132, 1993.

Nansel TR, Overpeck M, Pilla RS, et al: Bullying behaviors among US youth: Prevalence and association with psychological adjustment. JAMA 285:2094-2100, 2001.

Nelson RJ, Chiavegatto S: Molecular basis of aggression. Trends Neurosci 24:713-719, 2001.

Reynolds CR, Kamphaus RW: The Behavior Assessment System for Children, Teacher Rating Scales (BASC-TRS). Circle Pines, MN, American Guidance Service, 1992.

Rigby K: Bullying in childhood. *In* Smith PK, Hart CH eds: Blackwell Handbook of Childhood Social Development. Oxford, Blackwell, 2002.

Rivara FP, Farrington DP: Prevention of violence: Role of the pediatrician. Arch Pediatr Adolesc Med 149:421-429, 1995.

Task Force on Violence: The role of the pediatrician in youth violence prevention in clinical practice and at the community level. Pediatrics 103:173-181, 1999.

41 SOCIAL WITHDRAWAL AND ISOLATION

RAYMOND H. STARR, JR.,
AND HOWARD DUBOWITZ

Vignette

John was a difficult child from birth. As an infant, he was upset easily by new situations and people, cried a lot, and was difficult to soothe. Caring for him was frustrating and upsetting for his parents. Initially, their reactions were caring; however, gradually, they changed, first to increasing anger at John and finally to neglecting John's needs. John's father lost his job shortly after John was born, adding the stress of income loss to the frustration of having a difficult child. John developed an insecure attachment, crying uncontrollably when his mother picked him up at daycare and increasingly withdrawing from new people and situations. As he entered preschool, he avoided playing with peers, preferring solitary activities. As he got older, John had difficulty learning how to behave in peer or adult-child social situations. He became anxious. In childhood, he was rejected and unpopular. His parents tried mightily to get him to engage in social activities. As John approached adolescence, he developed a negative perception of his abilities to socialize with others, a frame of mind that led to further withdrawal. Over time, his internalizing difficulties broadened into major depression.

Social withdrawal and isolation are rooted in infancy and may have an impact on development and well-being that is lifelong. This chapter discusses social withdrawal and isolation from the framework of developmental psychopathology. This view considers the multiple influences that, over time, may interact, perhaps leading to psychopathology.

Social withdrawal and isolation are characteristic of a number of disorders, and differential diagnosis presents a challenge. Table 41-1 lists conditions in which social withdrawal and isolation may co-occur, including autism, hearing or language difficulties, anxiety, and depression. This chapter focuses on assessment, treatment, and prevention of cases in which the primary presenting problem is social withdrawal and isolation. This is not a simple task. For example, children with social withdrawal and isolation often develop into adolescents and adults who have anxiety and depressive disorders. The material in this chapter must be considered in conjunction with the descriptions provided in other relevant entries in this volume, that is, normal differences in temperament and behavioral adjustment (see Chapter 7) and social cognitive ability and inability (see Chapter 38).

The developmental psychopathology approach relies on two principles (Vasey and Dadds, 2001). The first consists of three elements: multidetermination, multifinality, and equifinality (Vasey and Dadds, 2001). In multidetermination, factors interact, producing unique outcomes. Multifinality states that a factor can lead to differing outcomes in multiple contexts. For example, identical twins can become very different adults on the basis of their distinctive profiles and the reaction of others toward them. Similarly, equifinality emphasizes the multiple pathways leading to a single, specific outcome. Thus, a socially withdrawn adult may have experienced trauma or may simply prefer solitary activity. Second, developmental adaptations can be shaped by risk and protective factors that have negative (exacerbating) or positive (buffering) effects. In addition, all of these events must be considered in relation to the developing child. For example, behavior problems can differ by the child's age and sex.

DEFINING SOCIAL WITHDRAWAL AND ISOLATION

Children's interests in and ability to affiliate with others vary. Social withdrawal and isolation range from normal behavior patterns to problematic, deviant ones. Social withdrawal and isolation incorporate a broad and complex range of behaviors (Rubin et al, 2003). Some people prefer to be quiet rather than talkative, to be alone rather than in groups, or to occupy themselves with objects rather than with people. These preferences

Table 41-1. **Possible Causes of Social Withdrawal and Isolation**

	Definition	Possible Causes
Social withdrawal	Limitations in social interaction based on voluntary or internal factors	Normal temperamental variation Cultural or language differences from dominant group Autism spectrum disorder Hearing loss Language or learning disorder Hypothyroidism Chronic illness Anxiety Depression Selective mutism
Isolation	Limitations in social interactions based on external factors	Low-density population area Limited transportation for social events Cultural differences in beliefs or values about frequency and nature of social interactions Restrictive parenting style

are often variations within the normal range. Others may have experienced discomfort or abuse and shun social contacts and the resulting painful consequences. The many and varied forms of social withdrawal and isolation in childhood have different causes, correlates, and consequences; manifestations that vary by context and age; and implications for treatment and prevention. When social withdrawal and isolation reach the clinical level, that is when they cause significant suffering or limit functioning, these difficult behaviors are classified as internalizing problems. Internalizing problems involve emotional and behavioral overcontrol encompassing anxiety disorders, depression, and phobias. These are contrasted to externalizing problems that involve undercontrol, including aggression, attention-deficit/hyperactivity disorder, conduct disorders, and oppositional defiant behavior. Internalizing and externalizing problems do not represent end points of a continuum and they frequently co-occur.

Labels that refer to this condition often are used interchangeably. For example, many people perceive "socially withdrawn," "isolated," "shy," and "inhibited" as equivalent when these behaviors are more properly seen as related albeit different constructs (Rubin et al, 2003). Thus, although both social withdrawal and isolation involve limited social interaction, social withdrawal can be seen as more voluntary and isolation as more of a consequence of external factors (Rubin and Coplan, 2004). Table 41-1 lists potential causes of both social withdrawal and isolation.

Rubin and Coplan (2004) describe a number of subtypes of what they call "solitude": "active isolation" occurs when others avoid interaction or play with a child; "social (passive) withdrawal" occurs when a child isolates himself or herself from others. Within the latter, "anxious solitude" is characterized by a conflict between approach and avoidance that creates anxiety. In contrast, anxiety is not present in children with low social approach motivation.

In spite of these efforts, the field lacks definitional clarity and agreement. Thus, the closely related construct of shyness is described as mild to debilitating inhibition or discomfort in interpersonal settings that interferes in a person's personal or career objectives. Like social withdrawal and isolation, shyness has physiologic, cognitive, affective, and behavioral manifestations. The critical nature of definitional distinctions is discussed later when cross-cultural issues are considered.

EPIDEMIOLOGY

Exact estimates of the proportion of children with social withdrawal and isolation are not available. What data are available describe clinical disorders or major risk factors. However, anxiety disorders are one of the most common forms of adult psychopathology. Approximately 7% of adults experience clinical levels of social phobia in a given year (National Institute of Mental Health, 2006). Similarly, anxiety disorders are among the most common reasons for mental health treatment referrals in children, with generalized anxiety disorder having a lifetime prevalence rate of slightly less than 4% (Vasey and Dadds, 2001) and social phobia being present in 1% to 2% of children (Crozier and Alden, 2001). In addition, there are high rates of comorbidity for various anxiety disorders. A lack of close friends in adolescence is a predictor of low self-esteem in adults. If we consider a chronic lack of a close friend to be a proxy for social withdrawal and isolation, then significant numbers of adolescents are at risk for problems. For example, 15% of fifth graders have no close friend. Overall, studies have found incidence rates of anxiety disorders ranging from 10% to 17%, with higher rates among girls and younger children (Vasey and Dadds, 2001).

A child's age and gender are associated with social withdrawal and isolation and related behavior problems (Rubin and Coplan, 2004). As is discussed later, children withdrawn in early childhood tend to exhibit a negative behavioral trajectory with age. They are increasingly rejected by their peers, form negative self-concepts, and become more isolated and depressed in the absence of appropriate interventions. In addition, boys who exhibit social withdrawal and isolation in early childhood are more at risk for later behavior problems than are girls. This may be a result of shy and withdrawn behaviors being considered less appropriate for boys. Indeed, parents view social

Table 41-2. **Factors Contributing to the Development of Social Withdrawal and Isolation**

Life Stages	Infancy	Toddler-Preschool	School Age	Adolescence
Child factors	Dysregulated behavior Easy arousal Difficulty in calming	Behavioral inhibition Poor peer relationships Insecurity in social situations Immaturity	Isolation Anxiety Poor self-esteem Awareness of social differences and deficits	Loneliness Unpopular Withdrawn Peer victimization Internalizing disorders
Parental responses	Insecurity about parenting Avoidance of child	Anxiety Excessive vigilance Overinvolvement and overprotection	Negative parental perceptions Negative parental care Coercive parenting	
Additional contributions	High social stress Limited social support for parents Limited parent knowledge about child development Maltreatment	Low sociability among parents Beliefs in strong responses to inappropriate behavior Limited out-of-home experiences	No friends Friends who are also withdrawn or isolated Peer rejection	

withdrawal and isolation in boys less favorably. Whereas outcomes of social withdrawal and isolation differ by gender, the prevalence does not appear to differ by gender.

THEORY

The study of social withdrawal and isolation has a long history and has been considered by many different theorists. Psychoanalyst Sullivan considered the presence of a close peer ("chum") in adolescence a critical element in typical social and personality development. Developmental theorists such as Werner and Bronfenbrenner emphasized the contexts of development in which multiple, nested, and interacting contexts in combination with individual characteristics must all be considered to fully understand development.

The developmental psychopathology approach exemplifies a holistic or multifactorial view. Attachment theory focuses on early parent-infant relationships as a model for all other relationships. Family systems theory emphasizes family dynamics. Biologically oriented models also incorporate interactions across contexts (Vasey and Dadds, 2001). Finally, learning theory emphasizes how environmental events shape behavior (Vasey and Dadds, 2001).

Rubin and colleagues (2003) emphasize understanding the interactions among these processes at different ages. Multiple feedback loops are established between child, maternal, and contextual factors. In the absence of intervention, these interactions can escalate into maladaptive child behaviors.

The cycle of social withdrawal and isolation often begins in the neonatal period and is characterized by dysregulated behavior (an easily aroused and difficult-to-calm child) and a mother who, while concerned for her infant, is vigilant and overly solicitous. This combination can lead to a wary, behaviorally inhibited toddler, particularly in the case of an insecure-resistant or avoidant mother-child attachment in which the mother remains anxious, vigilant, and overly involved. When this happens, her behaviorally inhibited child can reinforce these maternal behaviors, resulting in an escalating spiral.

Peer relationships become increasingly important in preschool. The child's social inhibition often correlates with a growing fear of peer interactions. In turn, these behaviors may be reinforced by peers who escalate their victimization of the vulnerable child. Teachers may observe precursors of social withdrawal and isolation: immaturity, high anxiety, and insecurity in social contexts. Mothers may become overprotective and overcontrolling rather than allowing "children to be children." In addition, mothers of inhibited children may see the child's behaviors as internally rather than externally controlled.

The preschool child's withdrawal may be exacerbated by unsupportive parental and peer behaviors. The withdrawn child often experiences a lack of success in peer relations and by early elementary school becomes yet more withdrawn, isolated, anxious, and inhibited. Increasing cognitive maturity in later elementary school allows children to be able to compare social behaviors and to be aware of their deficient social interactions. Still further isolation and withdrawal may result from negative self-esteem, negative peer behaviors and perceptions, and negative maternal care and perceptions. The child's social behavior becomes increasingly aberrant. The child turns into a teenager who is lonely, withdrawn, unpopular, likely to suffer peer victimization, and perhaps depressed. All of these factors may interact and combine to aggravate relationship difficulties and internalizing behavior problems.

Finally, external factors help shape the cycle of social withdrawal and isolation. As suggested by ecologic models, societal values, demography, and living conditions all are important. Similarly, stressors and social support shape parental responses to and attitudes about their child's behaviors. Finally, parental attitudes and knowledge about child development are an important influence.

ETIOLOGY

This section reviews research on the causes and correlates of social withdrawal and isolation. A wide range of research is reviewed to outline the factors that should be considered in diagnosis of and intervention with children at risk for development of these internalizing disorders or who already exhibit behavior problems. Table 41-2 summarizes the child factors, parental responses, and general environmental conditions associated with social withdrawal and isolation. Whereas these factors are discussed in roughly chronologic order, it is important to consider their possible presence and influence over a wide age range.

Temperament

Temperament refers to a constitutionally based pattern of emotional responses to social and environmental stimuli (see Chapter 7). It includes response rapidity, intensity, and predictability as well as overall mood and motivation. It is a major theme in considering infant and child development and also plays an important part in adolescent and adult personality (Vasey and Dadds, 2001). Social withdrawal and isolation have been important constituents of temperament since Thomas, Chess, and Birch (1969) developed the construct. Indeed, one of their three typologies, the "slow to warm up child," resembles the prototypical infant with social withdrawal and isolation.

There are many different approaches to describing temperament. All view it as biologically based, observable soon after birth, and representing stable, relatively long lasting behavioral dispositions that respond to stimuli in a consistent manner. However, manifestations of temperament can vary over time. Crying by an 8-month-old child separated by a barrier from a desired toy is an adaptive response. The same behavior by a 2-year-old would be maladaptive; trying to overcome the barrier would be adaptive.

One model described by Fox and colleagues (2005) provides the basis for the present discussion. Temperament has two interacting dimensions: (1) intensity and latency of reactions to stimuli and (2) self-regulation, the ability to control reactions to stimuli. The ability to self-regulate has an impact on the consequences of high reactivity to stimuli (e.g., crying). Low self-regulation and high reactivity, particularly when parental responses are inappropriate, can initiate a negative trajectory with child behaviors worsening over time. In the absence of helpful intervention, the rate of acceleration is likely to increase.

The ability to regulate attention and emotion begins to develop in infancy and is physiologically based (Calkins and Fox, 2002). Infants presented with upsetting stimuli learn a number of strategies to avoid emotional distress, such as redirecting their attention to other objects or people. Emotions as well as cognitions begin to be regulated in infancy. Of particular importance are the development of the ability to control negative affect by soliciting help and support from others and the acquisition of self-soothing abilities.

Deficits in emotion regulation are biologically based (Fox et al, 2005). Much of the research in this area has been concerned with behavioral inhibition, a pattern of avoidance and negative response to unfamiliar people and stimuli. Behaviorally inhibited individuals show several patterns of central nervous system activation. These include increased asymmetric frontal lobe electroencephalographic activation, with the right frontal lobe being more reactive, and increased limbic system and amygdala activation. Similarly, new events and people cause greater heart rate acceleration and increased cortisol secretion.

Behavioral research supports these biologically based findings (Fox et al, 2005). For example, infants who displayed negative responses to new situations at 4 months of age tended to have greater right frontal lobe activation at 9 months, and those who had these reactions at both time points were found to be socially withdrawn 4-year-olds. These and other findings support the model of Rubin and coworkers (2003). Consistently inhibited toddlers are fearful in infancy, show greater distress on separation from their mothers, and may have mothers who are overinvolved with their play or decisions. Similarly, preschoolers with higher right frontal lobe electroencephalographic activation were rated by their mothers as having more internalizing problems.

Behavioral inhibition and its correlated temperamental aspects represent relatively stable traits that in the absence of intervening experiences last over time. Temporal patterns for behavioral inhibition parallel the stability of other characteristics such as intelligence. That is, correlations between ages increase with the age of the individual at the measurement points.

To summarize, temperament, an inborn, biologically based response pattern, has important developmental consequences. It is correlated with behavioral inhibition, inhibited responding to new people and events. Behavioral inhibition can be measured in several ways, is relatively stable over time, and has significant consequences for social relationships.

Parent-Child Relationships and Attachment

Research on the parental correlates of social withdrawal and isolation has concentrated on three areas: parental belief systems, parenting behaviors, and attachment. Parental beliefs and behaviors interact with child biologic characteristics (i.e., genetics, temperament, behavioral inhibition, and age and sex). For example, infant shyness is predicted by low sociability among biologic as well as adoptive mothers (Daniels and Plomin, 1985). Beliefs and behaviors also are interrelated; mothers of socially withdrawn children are more likely than are those of outgoing children to believe that social skills should be directly taught and that inappropriate behaviors should be responded to strongly, even coercively.

It is difficult to separate elements that contribute to social withdrawal and isolation. For example, child age, maternal beliefs about the nature of social competence, attitudes about responses to inappropriate child social behavior, and extent of perceived social support interact in determining the maternal coercive behavior. In addition, an insecure attachment relationship, an adverse life context, and low social support predict coercive parenting tactics. However, increased social support can moderate these influences (Rubin et al, 1989).

Parental behaviors are important in originating and maintaining social withdrawal and isolation (Crozier and Alden, 2001). First, parents may use overcontrol and coercion to manage their child's behavioral inhibition. This occurs not only in task-oriented settings, where parental control might be expected, but also during unstructured, free play, where there are no such demands. Parental behaviors may actually inhibit development by limiting the child's chances to learn through play in novel environments.

The second set of correlated behaviors includes overly solicitous, protective, and intrusive parenting (Rubin and Coplan, 2004). That is, parents of shy, behaviorally inhibited children limit their child's exposure to social situations in which they might experience upset. As a result, these children do not learn to manage such encounters and withdraw even more. Parents thus reinforce their child's biologically based behavioral predispositions.

Parental factors may reinforce and maintain social withdrawal. Parents are aware of the child's inhibited response patterns, seek to help the child cope with the inhibitions by being overly protective and solicitous, and thus limit exposure to new events and people, exacerbating the inhibition. Thus, socially reticent 4-year-olds are more likely to be reticent 3 years later (Crozier and Alden, 2001).

These interactions of child characteristics, parental beliefs, and parental behaviors parallel the development of attachment, the prototypical relationship template. Relationships through life are based on this template. Securely attached infants learn to trust others and develop positive self-esteem by feeling worthy of others' trust. Additional skills that develop from this framework include reciprocity in social relations and empathy. Children with deviant attachments are more likely to develop inappropriate forms of these skills. Thus, temperamentally overreactive infants with unresponsive or insensitive parents tend to develop insecure-ambivalent attachments (Crozier and Alden, 2001). They are ambivalent, seeking and then avoiding contact, and at greater risk of becoming behaviorally inhibited toddlers.

Peer Relationships

Peer relationships become increasingly important as toddlers become preschoolers. These relationships provide opportunities to learn reciprocity, to cooperate in pursuing common goals, to help form accurate self-perceptions, and to foster emotional security. Along with attachment bonds, they form templates for future relationships (Rubin et al, 2005). Insecure parent-child attachment relates to both peer relationships and the presence of externalizing and internalizing problems. Two factors are key (Rubin et al, 2005): having at least one friend and being accepted by peers. For example, children victimized by peers who lacked a close friend were more likely to have externalizing and internalizing behavior problems. However, when best friends have behavior problems, young teens are more likely also to display such problems, suggesting that the influence of a close friend need not be positive.

Considering this, it is surprising that socially isolated and withdrawn children neither lack close friends nor have unstable friendships (Rubin et al, 2005). Most children report that they have a close friend. It is the nature of this friendship, not its presence or absence, that is important. Withdrawn children's friendships lack support, intimacy, and validation. Behavior problems are found in children who both lack friends and are shy and withdrawn or have a close friend who also has similar, negative behaviors.

In summary, peer relationships and friendships maintain and reinforce early behavior patterns. They provide a context for the development of key aspects of behavior, and in turn, the presence, absence, and consequences of friendships have lifelong implications. The roles of peers and friendships are not revolutionary. Rather, they are evolutionary, enhancing, inhibiting, and modifying existing behavioral tendencies.

CHILD MALTREATMENT AS AN INTEGRATIVE EXAMPLE

Child abuse and neglect serve as an example of the many factors related to social withdrawal and isolation. Both social withdrawal and isolation and maltreatment are complex, multiply determined phenomena. Environmental factors, child temperament, and parental knowledge and behaviors all play a role in the occurrence and the developmental sequelae of both abuse and neglect. As is the situation for social withdrawal and anxiety, combinations of multiple elements rather than any single, isolated factor are important. Between 60% and 95% of maltreated children have insecure, problematic attachment relationships (Cicchetti and Toth, 2005), which in turn are correlated with behavioral inhibition, social withdrawal, and, in adults, depression. In addition, both adults and peers rate maltreated children as more socially withdrawn and ostracized by their peers. Finally, maltreated children and adults are more anxious and depressed.

Adults maltreated in childhood are at greater risk for internalizing problems. Equifinality is illustrated by the fact that many aspects of maltreatment may play a role in this outcome. For example, abuse is often seen as related to parental overcontrol and neglect to undercontrol. Yet, both are linked with internalizing behavior problems as a function of the child's feeling unable to modify either set of circumstances. Multifinality is also a factor. Bolger and Patterson (2001) noted that whereas both neglect and sexual abuse independently correlate with internalizing disorders, their co-occurrence is an even stronger predictor. In addition, rates of problems were highest when both types of maltreatment were accompanied by poverty.

CULTURE: AN ADDITIONAL CONSIDERATION

Cultural differences in the presence, acceptability, and appropriateness of social withdrawal and isolation exemplify the complexities of dealing with children who are socially withdrawn and isolated in clinical settings. For example, attitudes toward social withdrawal and isolation vary widely across societies (Rubin and Coplan, 2004). Behaviorally reserved and shy children are viewed positively in China; they are seen as more socially competent, more accepted by peers, and more successful in school than is the case in Western countries. Researchers are beginning to understand cultural differences (Cheah and Rubin, 2003). For example, reserved, shy behavior

Table 41-3. **Assessment Options for Social Withdrawal and Isolation**

Techniques	Specific Techniques or Instruments	Comments
Parent interview	Questions: How is she or he doing at home? at school? with friends? What would you like your child to be doing socially? History of interventions for social withdrawal and isolation, including apparent reasons for success or failure of approaches Assessment of child's temperament and behavioral style (see Chapter 78) Parental beliefs and attitudes Formal interviews, such as Kiddie Schedule for Affective Disorders and Schizophrenia–Present and Lifetime Versions	Observe parental comfort or anxiety with child's sociability If concerned, obtain history of parents' sociability as youth and current level of anxiety or depression
Child interview	Questions: Who are your friends? Where do you play with them? What do you like to do? What do other people think of you and your friends? How does your friend make you feel?	Presence of friends may not be as informative as nature of friendship Withdrawn children do not get support and validation from friends
Informal observation	General appearance of the child Social behavior with other children in waiting room Parent-child interactions during initial wait and during stress Ability of child to converse with adults	Children older than 3 years should be able to converse briefly
Standardized checklists or questionnaires	Child Behavior Checklist, including Teacher Report Form and Youth Self-Report Strengths and Difficulties Questionnaire Social Anxiety Scale for Children–Revised Social Phobia and Anxiety Inventory for Children Anxiety Disorders Association forms	May not yield definitive diagnosis, but rather inventory of behavior problems
Other sources	Daycare provider or teacher Coaches, tutors, other adults	These sources can provide narrative information or complete standardized checklists or questionnaires

appears superficially similar to social withdrawal, although in reality they differ significantly. Chinese mothers view social withdrawal negatively but value reserved behavior in children. Indeed, they view and respond to withdrawal more negatively than do American mothers. This difference may reflect the need to foster different values and characteristics in collectivist compared with more individualistic cultures. Thus, whereas all cultures value social competence, the nature of that competence varies. Caution is warranted in generalizing from studies of European-American groups to children and families from different cultures (Rubin et al, 2003).

ASSESSMENT

Assessment aims to determine whether a behavior problem is present and to decide on a course of remedial action. If a problem is suspected, a first issue is whether the exhibited behavior is within the range considered to be "normal." This requires knowledge of normal behavior and also the thoughts and feelings of the child and those in the child's environment about the acceptability of the behavior. The possible ramifications of the behavior should be assessed in clarifying the child's functioning, in different contexts (home, school, with peers).

Social withdrawal and isolation can be assessed in varied ways. Table 41-3 summarizes assessment options. Parent and child interviewing, informal observation, completion of standard forms, and unstructured direct observation can be integrated into routine practice. Additional input from a daycare provider or teacher can be valuable. The following recommendations are based on examination of the developmental precursors and correlates of social withdrawal and isolation. Authors differ in which assessment approaches are best.

Informal Assessment

Informal assessments are an important part of every clinical visit. A major component is observing and asking about beliefs, behaviors, and interactions. One key question is whether the child appears to be socially withdrawn or isolated. A second question is how that might be impeding his or her functioning—at home, with friends, at school. It is also important to ascertain how the child feels about his or her situation. Then, there is the question of what may be contributing to the behavior problem. Fourth, determine what interventions have been tried, including how the parent responds to the child. The possible role of different cultural beliefs and practices should be considered. The important factors vary somewhat by age of the child.

In *infancy,* key foci include child temperament, parental history, parenting beliefs, and parent-infant interaction. Examples include observing how the parents perceive their infant, how they soothe their upset child, and their level of anxiety and asking what concerns they may have. The family history could include mental health problems such as anxiety disorders. Such issues can be raised in an initial visit within a context of "getting to know you." Pediatricians also need to be aware of normal stranger anxiety, which develops around 9 months of age, producing selective social withdrawal without impairing relationships with familiar adults and children.

The focus changes with *toddlers* to issues of attachment and the child's initial social relationships with adults and peers. A child's recall of a previous pediatric visit may evoke fear and withdrawal. It is always useful to ascertain how the child usually behaves, in a variety of settings. Parents should be encouraged to seek input from daycare and preschool providers and teachers about their child's social interactions and their responses.

Direct interviewing of the child is useful in assessing how a child engages the larger social environment and becomes appropriate in the *preschool and middle childhood years*. One can ask children about friendships, what they like to do with friends, their feelings, and whether anyone bothers them. Other issues, such as changes in family structure and function, life events, and parental monitoring of child activities, can be addressed.

Peer relations and extrafamilial activities become more important in *adolescence*. Issues include solitary and group activities, computer use, and parent-teen communication patterns.

To conclude, these factors should be looked at over time. Are things getting better for the child, or worse? What do parents and teens see as problem areas? Do they agree on areas where things seem to be going well or poorly? What is being done to resolve these situations? Input from childcare and educational professionals can be valuable.

Formal Evaluation

Questionnaires and checklists, although commonly used, have problems. First, self-reports of internalizing problems lack validity before middle childhood. Thus, reports are obtained from others, typically parents and teachers. Whereas self-reports become increasingly valid with age, correlations between adolescent, parent, and teacher reports remain low. These respondent appraisal differences are due to the difficulty of observing internal emotional states that underlie social withdrawal and isolation and reporting individuals' differing perspectives on the child. Additional factors are important. For example, attachment organization is related to informant disagreement. Greater adolescent-parent disagreement about internalizing and externalizing problems was present among insecurely attached teens. Clinicians should consider reports from multiple individuals and be open in interpreting discrepant views. For example, whereas clinicians rely more on parental than on teen problem reports in diagnosis and treatment planning, this may not be a good idea. Indeed, agreement may not be a key factor. Instead discrepant reports can be viewed as a consequence of different perspectives on experiences; parents do not necessarily know their teen's inner life.

Formal assessments include screening and diagnostic instruments. The most commonly used comprehensive screening measures have been developed by Achenbach (Achenbach and McConaughy, 1997). Forms include the Child Behavior Checklist (forms for 1.5-5 and 6-18 years), the Teacher Report Form (6-18 years), and the Youth Self-Report (11-18 years). All are easily completed in about 15 minutes. Norms and scoring procedures are available for such scales as total, internalizing, and externalizing behavior problems; withdrawn or depressed; and social problems. Child Behavior Checklist results can be used in various ways, ranging from using responses as the basis for further interviewing to informing referral decisions.

Other screening instruments merit consideration. For example, the Strengths and Difficulties Questionnaire (Goodman and Scott, 1999) has psychometric properties comparable to the Child Behavior Checklist, is short (25 items), and has multiple forms (parents and teachers of 3- and 4- to 16-year-olds; a self-report form for 11- to 16-year-olds). Whereas its usefulness in the diagnosis of social withdrawal and isolation has not been evaluated, other characteristics make it worth considering as a screen. Still other screening measures have a narrower focus on anxiety disorders. These include the Social Anxiety Scale for Children–Revised and the Social Phobia and Anxiety Inventory for Children (Crozier and Alden, 2001). The Social Anxiety Scale for Children–Revised has subscales for Social Avoidance in General, Social Avoidance in New Situations, and Fear of Negative Evaluation; the Social Phobia and Anxiety Inventory for Children examines Assertiveness/General Conversation, Traditional Social Encounters, and Public Performance. Finally, the Anxiety Disorders Association of America (2007) has simple measures that screen for anxiety disorders. There are separate forms for parents and adolescents. If social withdrawal and isolation are suspected, more formal assessments can be performed.

More formal interviews have been designed specifically for diagnosis, treatment planning, and outcome evaluation. These include the Anxiety Disorders Interview Schedule for Children and the Kiddie Schedule for Affective Disorders and Schizophrenia–Present and Lifetime Versions (Crozier and Alden, 2001).

Summary

Assessment of behavioral disorders is a complex task. The clinical examination and interview, careful observation, and multiple informants, especially childcare and educational professionals, remain the mainstays of practice. When significant problems seem apparent, the clinician may pursue further observation and interviewing along with screening measures in deciding on a course of action. Others may opt to refer the child to a mental health professional for further evaluation.

TREATMENT

Pediatricians can offer basic guidance in helping parents respond to social withdrawal and isolation. If appropriate, they can be reassured that their child's behavior is not necessarily problematic, especially if the child appears content. They can be encouraged to accept it as within a normal range, albeit difficult for some in a culture that usually values assertive behavior. Parents can encourage children to the extent that they can participate socially in at least some settings without emotional upset. However, parents should be advised of the risks of aggressively pushing children to socialize; sensitivity and gentle encouragement to engage in situations in which the child could realistically experience successful interactions are needed. Gradual introduction of the child to difficult or stressful situations may help desensitize the child, allay anxiety, and build coping skills. Specific guidance may be needed, depending on contributors to the problem. For example, parents may need to intervene if their child is being bullied at school. Further actions may include evaluation and possible treatment of the child, treatment of parental anxiety disorders, or both.

Whereas social withdrawal and isolation are the result of multiple factors, most interventions have emphasized increasing the amount and quality of social interactions in diagnosed children. Social skills training has a history of successful use in moderately withdrawn children. They are directly instructed in using and practicing a standard set of target skills for interacting with others. Other common approaches are based on social learning theory and involve modeling, reinforcement, and direct coaching about appropriate social responses. Although interventions have typically been implemented by adults including teachers and parents, use of peers as change agents has become common. In that context, competent peers act as role models and alleviate anxiety through positive reinforcement of targeted social behaviors.

Existing treatment approaches have problems. First, many people know how they should behave but cannot take appropriate actions. Such difficulties are compounded in social withdrawal and isolation by limited abilities and opportunities to control social fears and anxiety (Rubin et al, 1996). Second, treatments are based on adult protocols and are not designed with the needs of children in mind (Hudson et al, 2002). Consider temperament and physiologic factors. Greater reactivity to new people and situations can lead to increased avoidance, which in turn creates a stronger reaction in threatening situations. The ability to learn to identify situations as nonthreatening and to respond adaptively to similar future situations is thus limited by a lack of opportunity to habituate to such circumstances. Avoidant behaviors are reinforced.

The few controlled studies of treatment efficacy have evaluated cognitive-behavior therapies (Crozier and Alden, 2001). In general, studies of social withdrawal and isolation–related disorders link individual and group therapy to decreased symptom levels. Some research suggests that therapy is more effective when parents are involved and when the children are older. This finding suggests that greater cognitive maturity enhances treatment effectiveness. Finally, results of some studies suggest that cognitive-behavior therapy can have long-lasting effects, particularly in preventing more severe pathologic processes, such as substance abuse and depression.

Social Effectiveness Training for Children (Crozier and Alden, 2001) is one promising cognitive-behavioral intervention. It includes both group (social skills training, peer generalization) and individual (direct exposure to anxiety-arousing situations) components. Weekly social skills training sessions emphasize conversational skills, listening, and interpersonal assertiveness. Peer generalization activities provide direct practice in pleasant social situations. Direct exposure activities are individualized to meet each child's anxieties.

The age of the child is a key factor in deciding on appropriate treatment (Crozier and Alden, 2001). As noted, cognitive-behavior therapy is most appropriate with older children. Similarly, parental involvement works better from infancy through middle childhood. Parents can learn to assess temperament and respond appropriately to their child's needs. This also aids secure attachment formation. Parents should be screened for the presence of psychopathology, and if it is present, appropriate treatment should be initiated before or with child problem-oriented training. For example, treatment for anxiety disorders in late middle childhood was less effective when parents had untreated anxiety problems (Hudson et al, 2002). As children get older, peers become more important, and interventions such as Social Effectiveness Training for Children provide appropriate experiences (Table 41-4).

Psychopharmacologic treatment is commonly used (Crozier and Alden, 2001). Limited data suggest that it can be effective in the short term, but questions remain about long-term safety and efficacy. Selective serotonin reuptake inhibitors are highly effective. Whereas monoamine oxidase inhibitors are very effective, dietary interactions limit their practicality. In all, few studies have compared the efficacy of differing drug classes or the effectiveness of psychopharmacologic and behavioral treatment approaches.

PREVENTION

Prevention efforts have focused on ameliorating factors that place children at risk for social withdrawal and isolation (Vasey and Dadds, 2001). These include child characteristics and both proximal and distal environmental influences on development. With regard to the child, it is worth considering genetics (the genetic basis

Table 41-4. Treatment Options for Social Withdrawal and Isolation as a Function of Age

Age	Treatment options
Infancy	Attention to the infant's needs Close physical contact and support Limited environmental stimulation Social support for family
Toddler-preschool	Gentle encouragement to interact Social stories Opportunities to rehearse before social situations
School age	Practice before stressful situations Modeling Peers as change agents Direct coaching Relaxation Social skills groups Behavior management and cognitive-behavior therapy Multiple approaches, such as Social Effectiveness Training for Children
Adolescence	Social skills training Peer generalization Interpersonal assertiveness Direct exposure to arousing situations Cognitive-behavior therapy Psychopharmacology for anxiety or depression

of anxiety disorders), temperament (i.e., behavioral inhibition), coping style (e.g., avoidant), and cognitive style (e.g., pessimistic). Proximal environmental influences include parental psychopathology, inappropriate modeling, learning, and parental overprotection. More distal influences include social class and its correlates (e.g., housing), negative life events, other stressors, and neighborhood characteristics.

In spite of the prevalence of social withdrawal and isolation and related disorders, prevention has received little attention (Vasey and Dadds, 2001). Child-oriented strategies include direct and vicarious modeling, acquiring anxiety management skills (e.g., relaxation training, positive imagery), rehearsal and role play, and positive reinforcement of appropriate social skills. Environmentally targeted efforts include reducing parental anxiety; modeling appropriate behaviors; and using caregiving behaviors appropriate to the child's anxiety profile, age, and other characteristics. Recommended prevention strategies vary for children of different ages and risk factor constellations (Vasey and Dadds, 2001). Thus, parent skills training can be used prenatally when there is a genetic history of anxiety disorders, in infancy when insecure attachments may develop, in childhood when a parent is overcontrolling or overly critical, and in adolescence to help a parent cope with excess anxiety. Psychotherapy may be useful at any age when parental psychopathology is present. Coping skills training can be helpful with older children and adolescents who are having problems starting school, are transitioning into new schools, or are subject to high stress levels (e.g., divorce or trauma).

Research suggests that these and other strategies are useful and have potentially important implications (Hudson et al, 2002). For example, prevention can work, even with very young children, when it incorporates parental involvement. Older children and adolescents may have behavior problems that are more resistant to change and may also find it more difficult to form a therapeutic relationship. Other benefits include reduced anxiety soon after program onset and transfer of learned skills to other situations; the long-lasting nature of these improvements may alter the trajectory of behavior problem development. In part, program effectiveness appears to be related to situations being seen as less threatening and anxiety provoking as well as to decreased environmental support for withdrawal and isolation.

SUMMARY

Social withdrawal and isolation are not rare. It is an issue pediatricians and other primary care clinicians may observe or hear about from concerned parents. Children naturally manifest a broad spectrum of behavior. An initial question is whether the social withdrawal and isolation are within the "normal" range or are causing emotional harm or impairing a child's functioning. Social withdrawal and isolation may be a relatively isolated phenomenon or part of other conditions, such as depression, that should be considered. In addition, as illustrated by the vignette at the beginning of this chapter, social withdrawal and isolation may lead to an array of mental health and social problems (i.e., multifinality). In considering the etiology of social withdrawal and isolation, it is evident that there may be several contributors, including a child's temperament, the parent-child relationship, peer influences (i.e., equifinality), and aspects of the social environment, such as levels of support. The chapter offers strategies for assessment of social withdrawal and isolation. Some of these can reasonably be performed in pediatric primary care; others warrant a mental health evaluation. An important principle is to obtain information from multiple sources, including childcare and educational professionals, and from the child. Interventions need to be tailored to the individual child and family. These include practical steps that can reasonably be part of pediatric care. Clearly, some children need referrals to mental health professionals. Pediatric providers have a distinct opportunity to try to prevent social withdrawal and isolation and its deleterious effects in at-risk children.

REFERENCES

Achenbach TM, McConaughy SH: Empirically Based Assessment of Child and Adolescent Psychopathology: Practical Application, 2nd ed. Thousand Oaks, CA, Sage, 1997.

Anxiety Disorders Association of America: Self Tests. Available at: http://www.adaa.org/GettingHelp/SelfHelpTests.asp. Accessed April 29, 2007.

Bolger KE, Patterson CJ: Pathways from child maltreatment to internalizing problems: Perceptions of control as mediators and moderators. Dev Psychopathol 13:913-940, 2001.

Calkins SD, Fox NA: Self-regulatory processes in early personality development: A multilevel approach to the study of childhood social withdrawal and aggression. Dev Psychopathol 14:477-498, 2002.

Cheah CSL, Rubin KH: A cross-cultural examination of maternal beliefs regarding maladaptive behaviors in preschoolers. Int J Behav Dev 28:83-94, 2003.

Cicchetti D, Toth SL: Child maltreatment. Annu Rev Clin Psychol 1:409-438, 2005.

Crozier WR, Alden LE (eds): International Handbook of Social Anxiety: Concepts, Research, and Interventions Relating to the Self and Shyness. Chichester, England, Wiley, 2001.

Daniels D, Plomin R: Origins of individual differences in infant shyness. Dev Psychol 21:118-121, 1985.

Fox NA, Henderson HA, Marshall PJ, et al: Behavioral inhibition: Linking biology and behavior within a developmental framework. Annu Rev Psychol 56:235-262, 2005.

Goodman R, Scott S: Comparing the Strengths and Difficulties Questionnaire and the Child Behavior Checklist: Is small beautiful? J Abnorm Child Psychol 27:17-24, 1999.

Hudson JL, Kendall PC, Coles ME, et al: The other side of the coin: Using intervention research in child anxiety disorders to inform developmental psychopathology. Dev Psychopathol 14:819-841, 2002.

National Institutes of Mental Health: The Numbers Count: Mental Disorders in America. 2006. Available at: http://www.nimh.nih.gov/publicat/numbers.cfm#Social.

Rubin KH, Burgess K, Kennedy AE, Stewart S: Social withdrawal in childhood. *In* Mash E, Barkley R (eds): Child Psychopathology, 2nd ed. New York, Guilford, 2003, pp 372-406.

Rubin KH, Coplan R, Chen X, et al: Peer relationships in childhood. *In* Bornstein M, Lamb M (eds): Developmental Psychology: An Advanced Handbook, 5th ed. Hillsdale, NJ, Erlbaum, 2005, pp 469-512.

Rubin KH, Coplan RJ: Paying attention to and not neglecting social withdrawal and isolation. Merrill-Palmer Quarterly 50:506-534, 2004.

Rubin KH, Mills RSL: Maternal beliefs about adaptive and maladaptive social behaviors in normal, aggressive, and withdrawn preschoolers. J Abnorm Child Psychol 18:419-435, 1990.

Rubin KH, Mills RSL, Krasnor L: Maternal beliefs and children's social competence. *In* Schneider B, Attilli G, Nadel-Brulfert J, Weissberg R (eds): Social Competence in Developmental Perspective. New York, Kluwer, 1989, pp 313-331.

Rubin KH, Rose-Krasnor L, Bigras M, et al: Predicting parental behavior: The influences of setting conditions, psychosocial factors, and parental beliefs, 1996. Available at: http://www.rubin-lab.umd.edu/pubs/Downloadable%20pdfs/kenneth_rubin/parent-child%20relationships%20and%20parenting/QUEBEC96.pdf.

Thomas A, Chess S, Birch HG: Temperament and Behavior Disorders in Children. New York, New York University, 1969.

Vasey MW, Dadds MR (eds): The Developmental Psychopathology of Anxiety. New York, Oxford University Press, 2001.

42 ADJUSTMENT AND ADJUSTMENT DISORDERS

Robert Needlman

Vignette

Jim, a 12-year-old boy in seventh grade, is brought to his primary care physician's office because of fighting in school. He has been suspended twice in the last 3 months, most recently for swearing at a teacher. Previously a B-C student, his grades are dropping because he refuses to complete homework. He claims that school is stupid and that nobody there likes him. Although once an avid soccer player, now, after school, he spends his afternoons in his room playing video games. He usually responds to family members with irritation. His mother feels he is "sad," although he seemed excited during a recent trip to an amusement park. On detailed questioning, his mother realizes that Jim's current problems developed after his father lost his factory job 5 months ago, forcing the family to move to a smaller apartment in a poorer part of town.

Cases like Jim's raise a number of questions. Assuming that his maladaptive behaviors and emotions are a response to his father's recent job loss, how are the event and the child's behavior actually linked? Why has this child not been able to cope more effectively? What diagnoses does his current status suggest? How can the clinician differentiate a temporary downswing from an adjustment disorder from an incipient emotional disorder? What interventions are likely to help? What is the prognosis?

This chapter discusses adjustment and adjustment disorders. Adjustment is a broad concept dealing with how a child responds to stress. Stress refers to internal or external factors that challenge a child's well-being (see Chapter 50). Coping is a concept that encompasses responses to stress, focusing on the moment-to-moment responses. Adjustment refers to the child's reactions to stress over weeks and months. At this most general level, a certain circularity is unavoidable: adjustment is an adaptive response to stress, whereas stress is anything that requires the child to make an adjustment. Stressors can be physiologic in nature (i.e., illness or injury) or psychosocial (loss and threatened loss of security, relationships, or stature). Research into the psychobiology of stress is beginning to draw connections between the physiologic and psychological dimensions of stress and adjustment (Susman, 2006).

Children cope with stress every day; a child wakes up and cannot find a clean shirt to put on; he gets teased on the bus; he struggles on a math test; he does not get a part in the school play. The classic children's book *Alexander and the Terrible, Horrible, No Good, Very Bad Day* by Judith Viorst portrays the universal experience of disappointment and frustration. Children cope in various ways. They encourage and console themselves; they seek distractions; they complain to friends or family members. If their distress rises to the point of being noticed, it may alert a support system including siblings, parents, and teachers. If these corrective processes fail, the child may come to medical attention.

The question then arises, Why have this child and this child's supporter system been unable to adjust? Table 42-1 summarizes possible causes. The stress may be too large. Multiple stressors may be acting together. The child's internal coping skills may be weak, or the coping style may be maladaptive (Newcorn and Strain, 1992). The support systems may be inadequate, perhaps because the people who might be supportive are distracted by their own problems. These problems may in turn reflect deficiencies in their own support systems. For example, a mother loses access to psychiatric care after her own health insurance is cut; as a result, her anxiety disorder goes untreated, and she is unable to respond appropriately to her child's anxious behavior. The child's adjustment disorder may therefore reflect problems at multiple levels, from individual to family to society.

CONCEPTS OF STRESS AND ADJUSTMENT

Stress Response Systems

At the individual level, moderate to severe stress activates two major neuroendocrine systems (Bauer et al, 2002). The sympathetic-adrenal-medullary system provides a rapid, short-lived response transmitted through the sympathetic nervous system and mediated by serum catecholamines. Sympathetic-adrenal-medullary system activation is characterized by increased heart rate, blood pressure, and muscle tension and redistribution of blood flow to striated muscle, the well-known fight-or-flight response. The hypothalamic-pituitary axis provides a longer term response. Serum cortisol rises approximately

Table 42-1. Possible Causes of Poor Adjustment to Stress

Cause	Examples
Nature of stress	Extremely severe stress Multiple stressors Unfamiliar stress
Child factors	Temperamental differences, such as limited adaptability, inhibition, difficult child Early or chronic stress Other psychiatric conditions, including attention-deficit/hyperactivity disorder, anxiety, and depression Chronic medical conditions
Family factors	Weak social support Multiple stressors Distraction by other issues Other conditions, including mental or physical health disorders and substance abuse
Environmental and cultural factors	Mismatch of child or family style with cultural norms and expectations Immigration War, famine

20 to 30 minutes after a stressor, followed somewhat later by increases in blood glucose concentration fueled by protein catabolism, decreased immune responsiveness, and emotional distress. The balance between these two systems influences the effects of a particular stressor on the individual's physical and emotional health (Bauer et al, 2002).

Sympathetic nervous system responses are counterbalanced by activation of the parasympathetic nervous system, the main fibers of which travel along the vagus nerve. Vagal outputs regulate heart rate, and vagal tone can be gauged by measuring variability of heart rate in response to respiration, a value termed respiratory sinus arrhythmia. Higher vagal tone has been associated with greater ability to withstand stress and to self-regulate emotional responses to stressors (Porges, 1995). Lower vagal tone, by contrast, may be associated with poorer response to social stress in infancy and may render children more vulnerable to the corrosive effects of later stress. Vagal tone can be measured in infants and suggests that the ability to handle stress early on is the product of genetics or the intrauterine environment. As the child grows, additional experiences may alter vagal tone. In a longitudinal study, school-age children with lower vagal tone showed more behavior problems in the presence of parental problem drinking (El-Sheikh, 2005).

Individual differences in physiologic response to stressors have been conceptualized as a core feature of temperament (Boyce et al, 1992). Many features of the response to stress appear to be enduring individual traits (see Chapter 7 for a discussion of temperament and the contribution of Chess and Thomas). For example, Kagan has demonstrated a high level of continuity between behavioral inhibition in infancy and social inhibition during preschool. Children with the highest levels of inhibition showed unusually sustained heart rate elevations when presented with unexpected objects during infancy. High and sustained heart rates in response to novelty predicted both internalizing and externalizing behavior problems in early childhood (Kagan, 1997).

Long-Term Effects of Stress

Stressors can be conceptualized as internal or external factors that threaten to disrupt an organism's physical or psychological homeostasis. In children, homeostasis includes physical growth and psychological development as well as current well-being. Repeated adaptation to persistent stressors requires ongoing adjustments in arousal, a process that has been termed *allostasis*. Exposure to highly arousing or challenging environments imposes a high degree of allostatic load, which may result in either physical or psychological morbidity both during childhood and into adulthood. Early stressful experiences have been linked to long-term morbidity including depression and suicide but also heart disease, hepatitis, and cancer, among others (Bauer and Boyce, 2004). The model that emerges is complex, with vulnerability to stress stemming from genetic influences, early prenatal and postnatal physiologic stressors, and early and continuing psychosocial adversity. In turn, forced adaptation to early and persistent stressors (allostasis) may induce long-standing changes in reactivity that render the child more vulnerable to stress.

The mechanisms linking early adversity with later morbidity are complex, including continuity of high-risk social and physical environments as well as enduring endocrine and neurologic changes. Susman argues that prenatal and early neonatal stress predisposes vulnerable children to psychophysiologic hypoarousal, which in turn makes them prone to early and persistent antisocial behavior (Susman, 2006). Early exposure to severe stress, such as experienced by victims of physical or sexual abuse, has been associated with exaggerated cortisol and catecholamines in response to subsequent stressors (Bauer and Boyce, 2004).

Chronic stress has been tied to immunologic dysfunction, including numerical and functional changes in lymphocytes, decreased antibody responses to various antigens, abnormal cytokine levels, and corresponding increases in respiratory infections. Notably, these effects show great individual variation. That is, they appear in children who are stress sensitive (as determined prospectively by various measures, such as vagal tone) but to a much lesser extent in others (Boyce and Jemerin, 1990).

Resilience

The converse of stress vulnerability is resilience. Like vulnerability, resilience in children can be traced to both psychological and social conditions. For example, Werner's longitudinal study of children growing up in poverty on the island of Kauai found that children who thrived tended to be physically attractive, temperamentally easy, and intelligent and also to have at least one adult mentor (Werner, 1992). Positive child temperament and positive social environments may have interactive as well as additive effects. Among preschool children rated by their teachers as temperamentally easy, externalizing problems were infrequent, regardless of the level of family conflict reported by parents, evidence of a protective effect. Internalizing problems in temperamentally easy children were actually *lower* in families with *higher* conflict, an unexpected interaction. By contrast, as expected, preschoolers rated as temperamentally difficult living in high-conflict families showed the highest levels of both internalizing and externalizing problems (Tschann et al, 1996).

Ecologic and Cultural Perspectives

Resilience, like stress, occurs at multiple levels of organization. For example, a neighborhood might organize itself into a block watch to increase the security of children walking to school, thereby reducing the stress of bullying. The municipal government might install better lighting or assign additional police protection. In turn, the federal government might allocate funds to support local initiatives.

Culture influences what experiences are stressful and how those stresses are expressed as illness. Cultural psychiatrists argue that mental health and illness must be understood with reference to specific societies and cultures. They point out, for example, that there are mental illnesses such as *ataque de nervios* in Puerto Rico and neurasthenia in China that do not fit within the *Diagnostic and Statistical Manual of Mental Disorders* (DSM-IV) framework, whereas diagnoses such as personality disorders and eating disorders arise exclusively in the industrialized West (Lewis-Fernandez and Kleinman, 1995).

Of particular relevance to adjustment disorders is the observation that in contrast to "psychologized presentations of psychiatric disorder," such as sadness as a principal symptom of depression, "decades of cross-cultural research indicate that the majority of humanity displays somatic symptomatology" (Lewis-Fernandez and Kleinman, 1995). Conversely, symptoms that in the industrialized West are understood to be manifestations of organic dysfunction may in other cultures be considered evidence of spiritual derangement. In *The Spirit Catches You and You Fall Down,* Anne Fadiman describes how a young child's seizure disorder is understood differently by her Cambodian family than by her American physicians. In this carefully documented account, the failure to adequately bridge the cultural divide results in mutual frustration and a tragic outcome (Fadiman, 1997).

Cultures have not only characteristic responses to stress but also characteristic approaches to adjustment. Some cultures promote discussion of problems; others encourage sublimation or meditation. Children are inducted into the cultural norms implicitly through social learning and explicitly through direct education.

Changes in culture brought about by immigration can also be a source of adjustment disorder (McGoldrick and Giordano, 1996). Changes in the cultural milieu bring potential conflicts for individuals because of differences in the expression of stress or the approach to coping in the immigrant versus mainstream cultures. Moreover, immigrants who have recently been traumatized by war and life as refugees suffer a double burden of stress. On the other hand, social support in the receiving country can reduce psychological morbidity among recently immigrated adolescents (Schweitzer et al, 2006).

ADJUSTMENT DISORDERS

Adjustment, in the sense of psychological well-being in the face of adversity, encompasses everything from coping with developmentally necessary challenges to responses to extreme trauma. In contrast to this broad concept, the diagnosis of adjustment disorders attempts to designate a group of psychiatric diagnoses that occupy an intermediate ground between reactions that are merely concerning and those severe enough to merit other major psychiatric diagnoses. Although fraught with theoretical and practical difficulties, the diagnosis of adjustment disorders remains important for its frequency and its association with sometimes serious outcomes (Greenberg et al, 1995; Kovacs et al, 1995; Newcorn and Strain, 1992; Portzky et al, 2005).

Diagnostic Challenges

As defined in the DSM-IV (American Psychiatric Association, 2000), the diagnosis of adjustment disorder requires four features: (1) emotional or behavioral symptoms that arise within 3 months of the onset of an identified stressor; (2) the symptoms are greater than would be expected in response to the stressor or are severe enough to interfere with normal functioning; (3) the symptoms do not meet the criteria for another Axis I diagnosis; and (4) the symptoms resolve within 6 months after the cessation of the stressor. In addition, DSM-IV excludes bereavement. The International Classification of Diseases (ICD-10) criteria are similar, except they allow that adjustment disorders may continue for more than 6 months after the stressor ends.

An obvious difficulty with the DSM-IV diagnosis is that although it calls for the existence of "symptoms," it does not specify their precise nature or number. In this respect, adjustment disorder differs significantly from many other DSM-IV diagnoses, for example, major depression. A rough indication of the kinds of symptoms that compose adjustment disorder is apparent from the six subtypes: adjustment disorder with depressed mood; adjustment disorder with anxiety; adjustment disorder with mixed anxiety and depressed mood; adjustment disorder with disturbance of conduct; adjustment disorder with mixed disturbance of emotions and conduct; and adjustment disorder unspecified. Although the diagnostic guidelines do not specify particular symptoms under each of these headings, presumably the symptoms are similar to those included in the corresponding major psychiatric diagnoses. This similarity raises the question of how the adjustment disorders are differentiated from their corresponding Axis I diagnoses. Presumably in adjustment disorder, the symptoms are fewer in number or lesser in magnitude, because otherwise the Axis I diagnosis would supersede the diagnosis of adjustment disorder. Thus, for example, an adolescent might experience symptoms including sadness, tearfulness, and anhedonia; if the symptoms were sufficient to merit the diagnosis of major depression, that would be the diagnosis, rather than adjustment disorder with depressed mood.

Adjustment disorder *can* be diagnosed in addition to an Axis I diagnosis, as long as the adjustment disorder cannot be accounted for by the other diagnosis. For example, a child with dysthymia could merit an additional diagnosis of adjustment disorder with anxiety if the anxiety symptoms arose in response to an identified stressor. Adjustment disorders share some characteristics with acute stress disorder and post-traumatic stress disorder. However, in adjustment disorder, the stressors are typically less extreme, and core features of post-traumatic stress disorder, such as nightmares and behavioral avoidance, are absent.

By definition, adjustment disorders are time limited. When symptoms persist well beyond the original stressor, the diagnosis must change (American Psychiatric Association, 2000). However, there is no sure way to distinguish ahead of time between cases of adjustment disorder that are destined to resolve and those that mark the beginning of more chronic psychiatric conditions (Andreasen and Hoenk, 1982). Therefore, it is unclear whether the adjustment disorder *turns into* another Axis I disorder (usually with the "not otherwise specified" modifier) or whether the condition was that disorder all along. Moreover, the time frame of 6 months is arbitrary and constant regardless of the age of the child.

The 6-month time limit begins after the inciting stressor ends. If the stressor persists over time, then the adjustment disorder can be prolonged indefinitely, becoming chronic adjustment disorder. An example of a time-limited stressor might be the breakup of an adolescent romance; examples of persisting stressors include a chronic medical illness such as sickle cell disease, the multiple ongoing stresses subsumed under the heading of poverty, and a parent's chronic psychiatric illness. Often, children are exposed to a mixture of acute and chronic stressors that change over time, and it may be difficult to define a precise beginning and end. The existence of apparently stress-related responses that begin later than 3 months after the stressor and last longer than 6 months suggests a degree of arbitrariness in the DSM-IV timing criteria (Newcorn and Strain, 1992).

The diagnosis of adjustment disorder relies on a presumed connection between a stressor and subsequent symptoms; however, both stressors and symptoms are common and therefore may arise together by coincidence. In diagnosis of adjustment disorder, therefore, special care should be taken to consider alternative explanations, including potentially treatable medical conditions, such as hyperthyroidism and hypothyroidism, whose symptoms can mimic those of psychological distress. Given all of the difficulties enumerated, it is not surprising that the reliability of the diagnosis is relatively low compared with other DSM-IV diagnoses (Newcorn and Strain, 1992).

Prevalence and Symptoms

The prevalence of adjustment disorder in a community-wide sample of children has been estimated at between 4% and 8%. The generalizability of the finding may be limited, as the data come from Puerto Rico more than 25 years ago (Bird et al, 1988). Adjustment disorder represents between 25% and 65% of psychiatric diagnoses among children and adolescents seen in outpatient settings. In another survey, 16% of psychiatric outpatients younger than 18 years had diagnoses of adjustment disorder. Boys and girls are diagnosed with equal frequency (Newcorn and Strain, 1992).

A review of psychiatric inpatients from Iowa, in the 1970s, included 199 adolescents with transient situational disturbance, the precursor of adjustment disorder. Altogether, 77% had behavioral symptoms, including drug use (37%), truancy or suspensions (36%), chronic rule violations (34%), and low academic performance (33%); less commonly, the adolescents showed temper outbursts (30%), thefts (17%), and persistent lying (13%). Depressive symptoms were seen in 64%, including dysphoric mood (41%), suicidal thoughts or attempts (29% and 25%, respectively), sleep difficulties (22%), appetite changes (19%), guilt (21%), diminished concentration (11%), and anhedonia (10%). The adolescents presented with an average of 3.8 symptoms apiece. The nature and number of symptoms suggest that adjustment disorder is not a benign condition. Events precipitating the admissions commonly included school problems (60%), parental rejection (27%), alcohol or drug use (26%), parents separated or divorced (25%), and girlfriend or boyfriend problems (20%) (Andreasen and Wasek, 1980).

In a 1995 study in a suburban psychiatric hospital in New Jersey, adjustment disorder was diagnosed in 7% of adults and 34% of children 18 years and younger who were admitted emergently (Greenberg et al, 1995). Among the 54 adolescents with adjustment disorder, 89% had presented with suicidality. The most common admitting diagnosis was adjustment disorder with depressed mood (50%) followed by adjustment disorder with mixed disturbance of emotions and conduct (41%); 6% also were diagnosed with substance use disorders. By the time of discharge, 39% of the adolescents had their adjustment disorder diagnosis changed, most often to conduct disorder or oppositional defiant disorder (Greenberg et al, 1995).

In a 2004 study of 302 Finnish adolescents seen in a psychiatric outpatient clinic, 89 (30%) were diagnosed with adjustment disorder, of whom 25% reported suicide attempts, threats, or ideation. Suicidal adolescents with adjustment disorder were more likely to have had previous psychiatric care or foster placement and to have dysphoric moods (Pelkonen et al, 2005). Suicide may develop rapidly in adolescents with adjustment disorders with prominent symptoms of depression (Portzky et al, 2005).

Adjustment Disorders and Medical Illness

Adjustment disorders are common among children and adolescents with chronic medical conditions. A review of studies of survivors of childhood cancer, for example, found frequent behavioral and emotional difficulties, including problems of depression, anxiety, stressed peer relations, and poor school and work performance. Nonetheless, the majority of cancer survivors are psychologically well (Stuber, 1996). Notably, the most stressful aspect of cancer for many children is not the threat of death but rather the trauma of repeated medical interventions (see Chapter 50).

Adjustment disorders were diagnosed in 33% of a cohort of 74 children with recently diagnosed insulin-dependent diabetes, with an additional 3% diagnosed with major depression and other Axis I disorders (Kovacs et al, 1985). Typical adjustment disorder symptoms included depressed mood, feelings of friendlessness, irritability, social withdrawal, and general anxiety. High family income and preexisting marital harmony were associated with lower risk of adjustment disorder; that is, they appeared to confer resilience. Recovery from the adjustment disorder occurred for most of the children within the first 3 months and was nearly universal by 9 months after diagnosis.

Asthma is another chronic illness with a well-documented connection to adjustment problems. Recurrent, potentially life-threatening illness may undermine psychological well-being directly and by interfering with normal parenting. At the same time, emotional upset is a common asthma trigger, and behavior problems are associated with poor medication compliance. Educational interventions aimed at improving child and family adjustment, as well as knowledge about asthma itself, have been shown to reduce the asthma severity (Davis and Wasserman, 1992).

Adjustment Disorders and Psychosocial Stressors

As noted, adjustment disorders arise in response to common problems in school, at home, and with peers, particularly boyfriend or girlfriend problems. Increasingly, bullying is recognized as a major source of stress and potential cause of adjustment disorders. Family stressors, such as divorce or the death of a sibling, result in adjustment disorders in many but not all children. Other stressors, such as sexual abuse or parental alcoholism, may surface only after much patient investigation, if at all. The risk increases when there is a convergence of temperamental and social (i.e., parenting) risks (Lengua et al, 2000).

An underappreciated risk factor is family relocation, as described in the Vignette at the beginning of the chapter. A family move can mean losing friends and facing unfamiliar peers at school and in the neighborhood. In a 1993 analysis of a national dataset, children who had moved frequently were 1.8 times more likely to have four or more behavior problems on a standardized measure, even after controlling for income, sex, single parenting, parent education, race, and other potentially confounding factors. Developmental delays, educational problems, and grade retention were also associated with frequent moves (Wood et al, 1993).

For many school-age children and adolescents, self-esteem is linked to achievement, whether academic, athletic, or artistic. Highly competitive children may be especially vulnerable to development of emotional problems in response to disappointing performance. A case report of adjustment disorder in a college basketball player illustrates the point (Shell and Ferrante, 1996). Learning disabilities, particularly dyslexia, have been associated with behavior disorders, both internalizing and externalizing. Treatment of emotional problems associated with learning disabilities should be considered at the same time as planning for special education.

Prognosis

The prognosis for children diagnosed with adjustment disorder has been characterized as a "glass half full." In a 5-year follow-up of 52 adolescents, 23 (44%) were completely well at follow-up; another 14% were well but had had significant problems during the follow-up interval (Andreasen and Hoenk, 1982). Among younger children with adjustment disorder, the prognosis may be worse, with only 26% reported completely well at 4-year follow-up. Prognosis depends on the nature of the stressor, individual child characteristics, and family and social supports (Kovacs et al, 1995; Lengua et al, 2000; Stuber, 1996). For example, the death of a parent or suicide of a peer may be more likely to evoke symptoms of depression compared with receiving a diagnosis of a serious medical illness (Kovacs et al, 1995).

In a longitudinal study of 30 psychiatrically referred children aged 8 to 13 years with adjustment disorder, the disorder resolved during a period of 8 to 9 months in all cases. Many of the children also had comorbid psychiatric conditions. Compared with a matched control group who had psychiatric disease but no adjustment disorder, children with adjustment disorder had similar rates of psychiatric disturbance during the 7 to 8 years following the diagnosis of adjustment disorder. In other words, in this group of psychiatrically involved children, the presence of adjustment disorder did not affect the long-term prognosis (Kovacs et al, 1994). In contrast, in the study of children with newly diagnosed insulin-dependent diabetes mellitus, discussed before, about 8% of the children received psychiatric diagnoses within 5 years of the original diagnosis of insulin-dependent diabetes mellitus. Children who developed adjustment disorder had a much higher rate of long-term morbidity; 48% of children with adjustment disorder developed a new psychiatric disorder within 5 years compared with 16% of children who did not have adjustment disorder (Kovacs et al, 1995).

Newcorn and Strain (1992) reviewed immediate and long-term responses to common stressors of loss of a parent or sibling, divorce, and serious physical illness. In general, variability is the rule. Many children show initial adjustment problems, mainly symptoms of depression, anxiety, and a drop-off in school performance. Most children recover from these early disturbances, but many also go on to experience long-standing problems with low self-esteem, sleep, school performance, concentration, and peer relations. The risk for development of persisting problems is increased in children who have preexisting problems, such as hyperactivity, anxiety, and aggressiveness.

Prevention and Treatment

Little has been written that explicitly addresses the prevention of adjustment disorders in children and adolescents. However, a number of principles can be gleaned from the literature. Primary prevention entails building resiliency, within children, families, and larger systems. Pediatric preventive initiatives aimed at promoting physical and psychological well-being may play a role in the prevention of adjustment problems (see Chapter 86). A promising candidate for such intervention might be language development. Young children use language to self-regulate their emotions and behavior, and language delays are associated with preschool behavior problems. Primary care interventions that promote early reading aloud have been associated with increased child language competence in high-risk populations (Mendelsohn, 2002). Specifically to encourage adjustment to stress, children can be taught a vocabulary to describe their stress and their reaction to it. They then have tools for engaging their social support network. They can also read or be read stories that highlight successful adjustment to comparable stresses and resilient characters.

Preventive guidance might be especially important for children with temperamental traits that may make them more vulnerable to the effects of stress, for example, children judged to be low in adaptability, "slow to warm up," or "difficult." Similarly, children in families with medical or social histories that suggest exposure to higher allostatic load might benefit from training in relaxation, self-hypnosis, meditation, or other self-regulation strategies, even before a particular stressor comes to the fore (see Chapter 46).

Secondary prevention would target children known to be at risk for the development of adjustment disorder. A limited body of research has evaluated specific strategies. For example, a randomized prospective trial of 332 children, aged 4 to 16 years with chronic medical issues, investigated the role of nurse home visiting. The intervention sought to raise family well-being and parental competence and to lower parental stress. The nurse visitors forged relationships with families, showing emotional support and providing information individualized to the needs of the family. Concerns about the child's behavior or school functioning, parenting, and family relationships were common. Parent ratings of behavior problems did not change in response to the intervention, but parent-rated psychosocial adjustment was better in the intervention group, as was child-reported positive self-concept (Pless et al, 1994).

Tertiary prevention would be aimed at ameliorating the effects of identified adjustment disorders, speeding the resolution of symptoms, and reducing the incidence of later psychiatric diagnoses. Nonpharmacologic approaches that support self-control and enhanced coping strategies might be useful (see Chapters 46 and 50) and would include relaxation–mental imagery, cognitive-behavioral therapy, creative expression, family counseling, and parent guidance. Where adjustment disorders are linked to stressors in the school, interventions to ameliorate the stressors might prove effective, such as working with teachers to eliminate bullying or to support positive peer interactions. Similarly, when stressors are identified at home, parent guidance (or, for example, marital therapy) may prove the most effective. In cases in which impairment is severe, pharmacologic treatments might provide rapid relief. The choice of medication would presumably follow from treatments for related internalizing and externalizing disorders. However, studies evaluating specific therapies in children diagnosed with adjustment disorders are lacking.

REFERENCES

American Psychiatric Association: Diagnostic and Statistical Manual of Mental Disorders, 4th ed, text revision. Washington, DC, American Psychiatric Association, 2000.

Andreasen NC, Hoenk PR: The predictive value of adjustment disorders: A follow-up study. Am J Psychiatry 139(5):584-590, 1982.

Andreasen NC, Wasek P: Adjustment disorders in adolescents and adults. Arch Gen Psychiatry 37(10):1166-1170, 1980.

Bauer AM, Boyce WT: Prophecies of childhood: How children's social environments and biological propensities affect the health of populations. Int J Behav Med 11(3):164-175, 2004.

Bauer AM, Quas JA, Boyce WT: Associations between physiological reactivity and children's behavior: Advantages of a multisystem approach. J Dev Behav Pediatr 23(2):102-113, 2002.

Bird HR, Canino G, Rubio-Stipec M, et al: Estimates of the prevalence of childhood maladjustment in a community survey in Puerto Rico. The use of combined measures. Arch Gen Psychiatry 45(12):1120-1126, 1988.

Boyce WT, Barr RG, Zeltzer LK: Temperament and the psychobiology of childhood stress. Pediatrics 90(3 pt 2):483-486, 1992.

Boyce WT, Jemerin JM: Psychobiological differences in childhood stress response. I. Patterns of illness and susceptibility. J Dev Behav Pediatr 11(2):86-94, 1990.

Davis JK, Wasserman E: Behavioral aspects of asthma in children. Clin Pediatr (Phila) 31(11):678-681, 1992.

El-Sheikh M: Does poor vagal tone exacerbate child maladjustment in the context of parental problem drinking? A longitudinal examination. J Abnorm Psychol 114(4):735-741, 2005.

Fadiman A: The Spirit Catches You and You Fall Down: A Hmong Child, Her American Doctors, and the Collision of Two Cultures. New York, Farrar, Straus, and Giroux, 1997.

Greenberg WM, Rosenfeld DN, Ortega EA: Adjustment disorder as an admission diagnosis. Am J Psychiatry 152(3):459-461, 1995.

Kagan J: Temperament and the reactions to unfamiliarity. Child Dev 68(1):139-143, 1997.

Kovacs M, Feinberg TL, Paulauskas S, et al: Initial coping responses and psychosocial characteristics of children with insulin-dependent diabetes mellitus. J Pediatr 106(5):827-834, 1985.

Kovacs M, Gatsonis C, Pollock M, Parrone PL: A controlled prospective study of DSM-III adjustment disorder in childhood. Short-term prognosis and long-term predictive validity. Arch Gen Psychiatry 51(7):535-541, 1994.

Kovacs M, Ho V, Pollock MH: Criterion and predictive validity of the diagnosis of adjustment disorder: A prospective study of youths with new-onset insulin-dependent diabetes mellitus. Am J Psychiatry 152(4):523-528, 1995.

Lengua LJ, Wolchik SA, Sandler IN, West SG: The additive and interactive effects of parenting and temperament in predicting adjustment problems of children of divorce. J Clin Child Psychol 29(2):232-244, 2000.

Lewis-Fernandez R, Kleinman A: Cultural psychiatry. Theoretical, clinical, and research issues. Psychiatr Clin North Am 18(3):433-448, 1995.

McGoldrick M, Giordano J: Overview: Ethnicity and family therapy. *In* McGoldrick M, Giordano J, Pearce JK (eds): Ethnicity and Family Therapy, 2 ed. New York, Guilford, 1996, pp 1-27.

Mendelsohn AL: Promoting language and literacy through reading aloud: The role of the pediatrician. Curr Probl Pediatr Adolesc Health Care 32(6):188-202, 2002.

Newcorn JH, Strain J: Adjustment disorder in children and adolescents. J Am Acad Child Adolesc Psychiatry 31(2):318-326, 1992.

Pelkonen M, Marttunen M, Henriksson M, Lonnqvist J: Suicidality in adjustment disorder—clinical characteristics of adolescent outpatients. Eur Child Adolesc Psychiatry 14(3):174-180, 2005.

Pless IB, Feeley N, Gottlieb L, et al: A randomized trial of a nursing intervention to promote the adjustment of children with chronic physical disorders. Pediatrics 94(1):70-75, 1994.

Porges SW: Cardiac vagal tone: A physiological index of stress. Neurosci Biobehav Rev 19(2):225-233, 1995.

Portzky G, Audenaert K, van Heeringen K: Adjustment disorder and the course of the suicidal process in adolescents. J Affect Disord 87(2-3):265-270, 2005.

Schweitzer R, Melville F, Steel Z, Lacherez P: Trauma, post-migration living difficulties, and social support as predictors of psychological adjustment in resettled Sudanese refugees. Aust N Z J Psychiatry 40(2):179-187, 2006.

Shell D, Ferrante AP: Recognition of adjustment disorder in college athletes: A vignette. Clin J Sport Med 6(1):60-62, 1996.

Stuber ML: Psychiatric sequelae in seriously ill children and their families. Psychiatr Clin North Am 19(3):481-493, 1996.

Susman EJ: Psychobiology of persistent antisocial behavior: Stress, early vulnerabilities and the attenuation hypothesis. Neurosci Biobehav Rev 30(3):376-389, 2006.

Tschann JM, Kaiser P, Chesney MA, et al: Resilience and vulnerability among preschool children: Family functioning, temperament, and behavior problems. J Am Acad Child Adolesc Psychiatry 35(2):184-192, 1996.

Werner EE: The children of Kauai: Resiliency and recovery in adolescence and adulthood. J Adolesc Health 13(4):262-268, 1992.

Wood D, Halfon N, Scarlata D, et al: Impact of family relocation on children's growth, development, school function, and behavior. JAMA 270(11):1334-1338, 1993.

43 SEXUALITY: ITS DEVELOPMENT AND DIRECTION

Jennifer B. Hillman and
Michael G. Spigarelli

Vignette

Jodi is a 9-year-old girl who presents to the primary care provider with a chief complaint of a "hormonal problem." Jodi's parents are concerned because they think she is acting "like a boy." They are searching for a medical explanation and a "fix" for her behavior. They recall that as an infant, she used to touch herself "down there" during diaper changes. As a preschooler, she used to straddle the couch and "rub herself," leading them to scold and punish her repeatedly to stop this "obscene" behavior. When she was younger, she preferred to play with her brother's trucks, trains, or balls over baby dolls. They also caught her "playing doctor" with friends from school on several occasions. More recently, they have noticed she likes to play soccer, football, and video games with the boys in the neighborhood. She has even started to dress like a boy with baseball hats, sports T-shirts, tennis shoes, and baggy jeans. Jodi's father is really concerned that she has some kind of hormonal imbalance that makes her act like a boy. He remembers his sister acting in a similar way and she grew up to be a "spinster." Her mother thinks Jodi has taken being a "tomboy" to an extreme. They are asking for testing, a diagnosis, and treatment.

This vignette illustrates myriad concerns about the development of sexuality. In this chapter, we address the issues of normal sexual development, sexual identity, gender identity, gender expression, and sexual orientation. We also describe specific circumstances that may affect the sexuality of children, including puberty and the timing of puberty, sexual orientation, mental and physical disabilities, chronic medical conditions, abuse, and psychiatric conditions.

Sexuality, by definition, refers to sexual behaviors in all sexual organisms. For humans, sexuality encompasses the expression of sexual sensation and related intimacy between human beings and the expression of sexual identity. Sexuality is the way in which one interacts with others, taking into account gender, relationships, and cultural norms. The idea that sexuality is either normal or abnormal is based on cultural beliefs within the society in which the individual lives that help determine "normal" or "abnormal." Sexuality and its related topics are difficult concepts for children and adults to comprehend. Moreover, discussion of these issues with children and adolescents is often an extremely sensitive area for both parents and medical providers.

Human sexuality is shaped throughout the life of an individual, beginning at birth and ending with death, on the basis of physiologic, psychological, social, political, cultural, familial, spiritual, and religious factors in an individual's environment. Every individual develops a unique sexual identity because of the individual life experiences that shape sexuality. This concept is difficult for most adults to fully comprehend, particularly when the adult view of one's own sexuality was developed in a dominant culture different from the one in which the child is being raised. This can lead to the delivery of mixed messages for children, from both their parents and their culture, as well as for their parents, from both the primary and the new culture, regarding "normal" sexual development because of variations in the interpretation of cultural norms that leads to further differentiation in sexuality.

To help frame the discussion of human sexuality, it is necessary to define some of the typical terms that are used. *Gender* is simply the distinction between being either male or female. Typically, this information is discovered during the prenatal period with ultrasound examination or within seconds of a child's birth. *Gender identity* refers to the awareness of being male or female. It is believed that gender identity develops around the second or third year of life. *Gender role* is one's outward expression of maleness or femaleness. This is thought to be an ongoing process. Individuals with incongruent gender role and gender identity are typically referred to as being *transgendered*. An individual's pattern of sexual arousal toward other individuals is considered the *sexual orientation*. *Sexual identity* refers to an individual's personal assessment of sexual orientation as heterosexual, homosexual, bisexual, or asexual. There can be discordance between sexual identity and sexual orientation. For example, a married woman may desire to have sex with women. She would be considered bisexual by sexual orientation. However, she may consider herself to be heterosexual by sexual identity. Sexual identity and orientation begin to develop during pre-adolescence and can vary over time for some individuals.

NORMAL DEVELOPMENT OF SEXUALITY

The development of human sexuality is an ongoing process, with each phase building on the previous experience. From infancy through adulthood and well into the geriatric stages of life, sexuality is in evolution. It is important for medical providers to be knowledgeable about, comfortable with, and aware of human sexuality in all stages of life. Table 43-1 summarizes normal sexual behaviors based on the child's age.

Infancy

The prenatal and infancy period has a large impact on the development of human sexuality. By the time of birth, gender has been determined, and familial and cultural ideas about the child's gender begin to be expressed. Gender roles in infancy are largely being determined for the children by parents, caretakers, and family members. For example, a female infant's parents may choose to dress their daughter only in pink clothing. Conversely, parents may dress their male and female twins in the same clothing regardless of the child's gender. There is no intrinsically correct way to dress a male or female infant. In addition, there are no studies showing that color or type of clothing has an impact on maleness or femaleness. Choice of clothing color and type is simply an expression of gender role determined by the parents and family members and will ultimately be part of sexuality and its development.

During infancy, there are a few other key events that may have an impact on sexuality. For male infants, circumcision is typically done within days of birth. The decision about circumcision is typically based on parental cultural and religious beliefs. Female infants may have vaginal discharge or bleeding in the neonatal period due to exposure to maternal hormones in utero. By 6 months of age, many infants will begin to explore their genitals during diaper changes or bathing. In addition, male infants frequently have erections. Parental response to circumcision, self-exploration, and self-stimulation has an impact in shaping sexuality. All of these expressions of sexuality are part of the normal developmental process. Infants should not be punished or ridiculed for expression of human sexuality, and parents should receive adequate information to allow them to feel empowered as parents.

Toddlers and Preschoolers

Friedrich and colleagues (1991) demonstrated that there is a peak in outward expression of sexual behaviors between the ages of 3 and 5 years. Toddlers become increasingly aware of their gender and gender identity as girl or boy (Calderone, 1985). Genital touching may increase during this period, particularly when the child is upset or tired. Friedrich and colleagues (1991) surveyed Midwestern parents of 2- to 12-year-old children about frequency of sexual behaviors. They found that 64.1% and 54.4% of parents of male and female children aged 2 to 6 years, respectively, endorsed touching of sex parts at home. In addition, this age group had the highest frequency of the following commonly reported sexual behaviors: tries to look at people undressing, shows genitals to adults, masturbates with the hand, touches breasts, kisses nonfamily children and adults, undresses in front of others, touches genitals at home, scratches crotch, and identifies with boy or girl toys. A similar

Table 43-1. Common Sexual Behaviors of Children and Adolescents

Age	Sexual Behaviors
Infancy (birth through 1 year)	Exploration of genital area during diaper changes Erections in boys Masturbation
Toddlers and preschoolers (ages 1 to 4 years)	Masturbation Touching mother's breasts or other body parts Taking clothes off Showing genitals to other children or adults
School-age to early adolescence (ages 5 to 11 years)	Masturbation (public displays decrease) Sex play between peers, such as playing "house" or "doctor," in which children explore sexuality through looking at and touching of genitals Asking questions and talking about sex Dressing up as the opposite sex as dramatic play
Adolescence	Continued masturbation, increasingly private Exploration of sexual intimacy with the same or opposite sex Awareness and questioning of sexual orientation Initiation of sexual intercourse

follow-up study was conducted by Friedrich and colleagues in 1998. The findings of this study were similar to those of the initial study in that the most common sexual behaviors observed by female caregivers among children aged 2 to 5 years were standing too close to people, touching genitals in public places, touching mother's or other women's breasts, touching genitals when at home, and trying to look at people when they are nude or undressing. Touching of genitals in public places was more commonly reported among caretakers of male children.

Gustafsson and coworkers (1995) studied the sexual behaviors of Swedish preschool-age children at daycare centers. Surveys of the daycare providers revealed that searching for body contact, responding to adult-initiated body contact, watching genitals of other children, and reacting to sexual words were not uncommon. Another epidemiologic study of British preschool children found that touching of one's own genitalia, attempting to touch a woman's breasts, showing of one's own genitalia, looking at another child's genitalia, and rubbing one's own genitalia were relatively common observances by daycare staff. Less commonly observed behaviors included putting a finger into another's vagina or anus, a mouth to another's genitalia or anus, or a penis into a vagina; asking for genitalia to be touched; and putting a mouth on a doll's genitalia (Davies et al, 2000). These behaviors should raise the question of exposure to adult sexual practices or sexual abuse.

Observation of sexual behaviors in children may lead to concern for sexual abuse among parents and pediatricians. Knowledge of normal expression of sexual behaviors is critical to help differentiate between sexual abuse and normal sexual behaviors. Providers should put into context the frequency of sexual behaviors, the quality or type of sexual expression, and the general context of the family's outward expression of sexuality. If self-exploration is increasingly problematic for families, providers should encourage parents to redirect children when they are touching themselves in public settings and to be more tolerant within the home. Further evaluation for suspected sexual abuse may also be warranted.

Toddlers and preschoolers become increasingly curious about sexuality at the time that they are developing verbal and cognitive language skills. Children this age will begin to ask questions about sexuality. The American Academy of Pediatrics recommends that proper terminology be used for all anatomic parts (American Academy of Pediatrics, 2001a). The use of nicknames for genitals can lead to confusion and embarrassment later in life. Parents and caregivers should take advantage of teachable moments, such as the birth of a sibling or a new cousin, to explain how babies are brought into the world.

Preschoolers may engage in forms of dramatic play that involves dressing up in costumes or attire typically worn by the opposite sex, playing "nurse" or "doctor," and acting out roles as mommy and daddy. Although there are no published data on the frequency of these behaviors, experts agree that these behaviors are commonplace. Finch (1967) stated that "some sex play between children is nearly universal." He went on to say that sex play is a means to satisfy children's curiosity about their own bodies and those of others. These childhood explorations are typically transient and innocent.

Parents may become concerned and alarmed by witnessing these behaviors. This type of play is developmentally appropriate and important. It is a way for children to learn about the adult world and to try out different roles in a nonthreatening manner. Punishment for dressing as the opposite sex can have an impact on healthy sexual development. Likewise, harsh threats, such as those to harm genitalia or other severe forms of punishments for failure to curtail sex play, are traumatic to the child. Burch (1952) went so far as to say that "sudden scolding or a terrifying scene will do more harm than good." Other experts have suggested that "making a scene" may teach children that sexual behavior elicits a response from parents, and they may tend to use their sexuality to gain attention. The key is for children to be allowed to explore their world in a safe environment that is consistent with socially acceptable practices.

School-Age Children

Sigmund Freud termed the period between 6 and 11 years the latency period because of his belief that innate sexual wishes are thought to be relatively quiet. School-age children are typically involved in same-sex relationships, and playgroups tend to include children of the same gender. However, researchers have found that self-stimulation still occurs in both male and female children. It appears that rather than being latent, as Freud suggested, at this stage of development, these behaviors exist but have become more private and discrete, which in part explains the need for privacy while dressing and bathing. In addition, children are increasingly interested in what it means to be male or female as well as their gender role and identity.

School-age children are beginning the process of acquiring a foundation on which they will build in the years ahead for many domains, including sexuality. Therefore, it is increasingly important for parents to have ongoing discussions about sexuality and touching. School-age children should know the difference between appropriate and inappropriate touch. They should also be able to talk about their body parts without feeling embarrassed or believing they are either naughty or dirty. Open discussion about sexual issues, beginning early in a child's life, sets the stage for future communication, which will become particularly important during the teen years.

The early stages of puberty may be seen in school-age children. For girls, breast development may begin as early as the age of 8 years; the average age of thelarche is approximately 11 years. The onset of puberty in boys is, on average, later than in girls; the first sign, testicular enlargement, occurs on average around 11.5 years of age. Testicular enlargement may begin as early at 9.5 years (Marshall and Tanner, 1969). Discussions between parents and pediatricians, and parents and children, about the timing and progression of puberty are very important. Parents should be made aware of the timing of the changes that occur to allow children to feel the most comfortable with these changes.

The onset of puberty brings a sense of urgency for parents to discuss "the birds and the bees." It is not uncommon for parents to implore the pediatrician's assistance in explaining sexual intercourse and reproduction to their child. The discussion about sex and conception should begin when the child first starts to ask questions and should be ongoing, with as much or as little information as the parent thinks the child can handle and understand. As the child progresses through puberty, discussions about sexual relationships and intercourse will likely become more personal and individualized.

Pre-Teens

The majority of pre-teens have entered puberty. Nearly half of pre-teen girls have reached menarche. Along with menarche may come associated problems: menstrual cramps, menstrual migraines, unpredictable bleeding, nausea, and abdominal bloating. Pre-teen boys may experience nocturnal emissions or "wet dreams." These changes are all part of normal sexual and pubertal development.

Pre-teens should understand what sexual intercourse entails. Both boys and girls should be provided information and knowledge about how sexually transmitted infections are acquired and prevented. Both boys and girls should have knowledge about how pregnancy can be achieved and prevented. In addition, they should have a clear understanding of what constitutes sexual abuse. Although most public and parochial school systems have organized sexual education programs, the curriculum varies considerably. Parents and physicians should assess the pre-adolescent's knowledge of sexuality and related issues. It is during these years that a portion of every physician office visit should be set aside for a private discussion between pre-teen and provider. This fosters the development of a positive relationship between patient and provider while sending the clear message that children deserve the respect to be allowed to discuss personal and potentially embarrassing issues with their health care provider.

Adolescence

The teenage years are a period of transition, both mentally and physically, from childhood into adulthood. Although neither the natural history nor the precise origin of sexual orientation is fully understood, it is thought that sexual orientation is established by the conclusion of childhood. It is during adolescence that this awareness of sexual identity leads to the further exploration of sexual orientation. These aspects of sexuality may be very evident to some teenagers, their parents, and their health care providers. For others, there may be only a glimpse of insight into these issues, and the extent of these changes will be experienced only in adulthood. It is common for adolescents to experiment with their sexual identity and sexual relationships. Retrospective questionnaires reveal that a fair number of homosexual adults reported having had relationships and sexual encounters with persons of the opposite sex as adolescents. Likewise, an equal percentage of adults who consider themselves heterosexual report having had sexual activity with the same sex during adolescence (Frankowski, 2004).

Issues related to sexual identity and orientation can be a source of anxiety and insecurity for the questioning or sexually aware adolescent. Young homosexual adolescents have unique health risks, including social stigma; potential isolation from peers, friends, and family members; depression; and suicide. Health care providers and parents should not assume an adolescent's sexual orientation and should ask gender-neutral questions when talking to teenagers about sexuality. This careful approach promotes a safe and healthy environment in which the questioning teen may feel comfortable discussing concerns about sexual orientation. See the section on sexual identity and orientation for more information.

Data from the Youth Risk Behavior Survey from 2003 reveal that 46.7% of high-school students reported ever having had sexual intercourse, and 34.3% of students nationwide reported having had sexual intercourse in the 3 months preceding the survey (Grunbaum et al, 2004). The prevalence of sexual activity among girls aged 15 years is reported to be 24%, with an increase to 62% by the age of 18 years (Abma and Sonenstein, 2001). Data from the Youth Risk Behavior Survey revealed that approximately 60% of male twelfth-grade students had ever had sexual intercourse. In addition, 4.2% of girls and 10.4% of boys reported having had sexual intercourse before the age of 13 years (Abma and Sonenstein, 2001). See the later section on sexual intercourse for more details.

The initiation of sexual intercourse brings with it many issues related to human sexuality. Prevention, detection, and provision of appropriate medical care for those at risk or soon to be at risk for pregnancy and sexually transmitted diseases (STDs) are the most pressing for pediatricians and adolescents. Parental conflict about the timing of initiation of sexual activity may also develop. Physicians caring for adolescents should provide confidential care that includes time alone with the adolescent during all visits and discussion of sexual intercourse and contraception and education about sexually transmitted infections, including human immunodeficiency virus (HIV) infection. Potentially sensitive questions, such as those about sexuality and gender, should be asked only while alone with the adolescent patient; asking them with a parent or guardian present may force adolescents to lie to protect themselves and then force them to lie in the future to not lose the respect of their health care provider.

Counseling about Normal Development

The vignette about Jodi at the beginning of the chapter illustrates several typical sexual behaviors at different stages of Jodi's development. All of Jodi's behaviors are normal expressions of sexuality that parents may or may not notice during a child's development. Touching of one's genitals, masturbation, choice of toys, and playing doctor are part of normal behavior, as are her choice of clothing and desire to be athletic. Providers presented with this or a similar scenario should reassure the parents and encourage them to allow their child to express himself or herself. They should feel comfortable in their ability to reinforce that the behaviors are normal and therefore there is no need for any additional evaluation for an underlying medical cause.

SPECIFIC ISSUES RELATED TO THE DEVELOPMENT OF CHILD AND ADOLESCENT SEXUALITY

Gratification Behavior and Masturbation

Vignette

At 5 months of age, Cindy was first noted to have episodes of stiffening of her body and arching of her back alternating with moaning and groaning. These episodes lasted anywhere from 5 to 20 minutes and occurred nearly every day, with more episodes happening when Cindy was particularly tired. Sometimes her face reddened and she appeared dazed. As she grew older, the spells tended to increase in frequency and duration. When she was nearly 2 years old, her parents sought evaluation by a pediatric neurologist for epilepsy. Careful dissection of the history revealed that Cindy was responsive during the episodes, sometimes able to carry on conversations while rocking and stiffening rhythmically. In addition, home videotaping of the episodes revealed rhythmic pelvic rocking and flexion throughout episodes, distractibility and extinction of the behavior by parental interruptions, facial flushing, and diaphoresis.

The word *masturbation* is derived from the Latin *manus*, meaning "hand," and *stupratio,* meaning "defilement" (Nechay et al, 2004). This historically suggests that this practice was considered impure. The modern meaning of the term implies stimulation of the genitals often resulting in orgasm (Leung and Robson, 1993). Currently, masturbation is generally accepted as a normal part of human sexuality and development. This behavior can be referred to as gratification behavior, gratification disorder, infantile masturbation, and self-stimulation behavior.

Although Still described masturbation in infants and children in the 1900s (1909), the true incidence and onset of this behavior are not known. Leung and Robson (1993) report gratification behavior typically beginning at 2 months, with a peak at 4 years of age. Meizner (1987) observed in utero masturbation by ultrasound examination. Estimates on the frequency of masturbation are fraught with uncertainty, particularly given the nearly universal belief by parents that their child would never masturbate. In that light, a lower bound prevalence estimate of masturbation at some time in life was estimated to be 90% of boys and 50% to 60% of girls (Leung and Robson, 1993).

The medical literature on childhood self-stimulation behavior remains sparse, with fewer than 20 case reports typically describing infants and children presenting with bizarre attacks or "episodes" that have resulted in extensive medical evaluations. Gratification behavior has been mistaken for seizures (Fleisher and Morrison, 1990; Livingston et al, 1975; Wulff and Ostergaard, 1992; Yang et al, 2005), abdominal pain (Couper and Huynh, 2002; Fleisher and Morrison, 1990), and other movement disorders like dystonia and dyskinesia (Mink and Neil, 1995). Masturbatory behavior often involves posturing and stiffening, jerking movements, elevations in heart rate and blood pressure, and unusual vocalizations (grunting), which leads to suspicions of epilepsy or colicky abdominal pain. Nechay and colleagues (2004) retrospectively reviewed the existing case reports of children diagnosed with gratification disorder or infantile masturbation. The majority of the patients were referred for evaluation of epilepsy, and more than half of the cases developed symptoms before the age of 1 year. Nine cases used home video to confirm a diagnosis of gratification disorder. In a more recent review of 12 cases of masturbation in infancy and childhood, Yang and associates (2005) suggested practical points for management of this behavior (Table 43-2).

Gratification behavior may alert parents or providers to the possibility of sexual abuse. Wells' study of parental report of behaviors did not find "masturbating more" to be a statistically significant behavior associated with sexual abuse or alleged sexual abuse (Wells et al, 1995). Other characteristics of masturbatory behavior, such as the frequency, the ability to redirect the child, and the child's demeanor during the behavior, may be helpful in discriminating between normal sexual behavior and that concerning for sexual abuse. The behaviors found to be associated with increased risk of sexual abuse, described in a study of children's sexual behaviors in preschool settings as reported by daycare staff, were the most rarely reported sexual behaviors: attempting to insert or inserting a penis or finger into another child's genitalia, attempting to have oral contact with another child's genitalia, putting the mouth on a doll's genital area, and asking to be touched in the genital area (Davies et al, 2000).

Table 43-2. **Evaluation and Management of Masturbatory Behavior That Is Suggestive of Seizure Disorder, Abdominal Pain, or Movement Disorder**

Videotape the event or behavior in question.
Assist parents in changing their view of the child's behavior as a disease or problem.
Scolding or threatening of the child for the behavior is not appropriate.
Redirect or distract the child.
Suggest a milestone or time frame for the child to end the behavior, at least in public.
For parents offended by the term *masturbation,* substitute the term *gratification behavior*.

Adapted with permission from Yang ML, Fullwood E, Goldstein J, Mink JW: Masturbation in infancy and early childhood presenting as a movement disorder: 12 cases and a review of the literature. Pediatrics 116:1427, 2005.

Case Resolution

The vignette demonstrates that masturbation can involve much more than overt stimulation of the genitals. It can be a full-body experience that includes elevation of the heart rate, sweating, and vocalizations. Often, masturbation may be thought to represent seizures, apneic events, or behavior problems. Observation of the child either directly or with the use of videotape can help clinicians and parents determine the pattern and source of the episodes. Masturbation itself should be considered a normal and appropriate part of all stages of development. Rather than trying to avoid discussions or to suppress the behavior, a more open and informed discussion will benefit caregivers, medical providers, and, most important, the child in question.

Initiation of Sexual Intercourse and Related Practices

Vignette

Stacey is a 17-year-old girl who presents to her primary care provider's office for her annual soccer physical. She is an outstanding athlete, with college aspiration and the interest of various recruiters who are impressed with her academic and athletic abilities. When her mother is asked to leave the room for a brief confidential discussion, her mother states emphatically, "Don't worry, we are best friends and she tells me everything." Her mother announces that "she is *not* having sex" as she leaves the room. In private, Stacey confides in you that she has been sexually active (vaginal intercourse) with her boyfriend for the past 6 months and that they use condoms when they can buy them privately and without embarrassment, but that can be difficult. She notes that she was extremely worried 2 months ago when her period was late, so worried that she failed her first examination in AP English. Her period did come; she and her boyfriend were still worried, so they tried a few home pregnancy tests, which were all negative, prompting them to agree not to have sex again. This pledge lasted less than 1 week, and at present she is concerned because she is due to have a period in the next few days.

Studies indicate that a significant proportion of adolescents engage in noncoital sexual activities that include kissing, touching of breasts and genitals, and oral sex. Typically, these behaviors precede the onset of sexual intercourse. Schofield (1965) described five stages of dating and petting that occurred in a relatively predictable sequence among the 15- to 19-year-old heterosexual British youths he studied. Stage 1 involved limited heterosexual contact, kissing, and dating without kissing. Stage 2 progressed to kissing and stimulation of breasts while still clothed. Stage 3 included stimulation of breasts under clothes and genital stimulation or apposition. Sexual intercourse with a single partner defined stage 4. Sexual intercourse with more that one partner was considered stage 5. Other researchers have found a similar developmental sequence to the initiation of sexual intercourse. A study by Halpern-Felscher and coworkers (2005) evaluated adolescent perceptions, attitudes, and behaviors about oral versus vaginal sex. This study of ninth-grade adolescents revealed a higher percentage of students who reported having ever had oral sex versus vaginal sex, 19.6% and 13.5%, respectively. Among 15- to 19-year-old teenagers in the National Survey of Family Growth from 2002, 55.2% of boys and 54.3% of girls engaged in oral sex. Interestingly, interview findings revealed that teens engaging only in oral sex considered themselves "virgins" and did not feel exposed to the risks associated with sexual intercourse (Centers for Disease Control and Prevention, 2005). It is important to ask about all forms of sexual contact during the confidential visit with adolescents. This information is vital for your assessment of high-risk behavior and helps guide your discussion of education about prevention of STDs, contraception, and healthy relationships.

Nearly half of all high-school students have ever had sexual intercourse, and approximately one third of students nationwide are currently sexually active (defined as "had sex in the 3 months prior to being surveyed") (Grunbaum et al, 2004). The overall percentage of students who have ever had sexual intercourse decreased from 1990 through 2001 (Grunbaum et al, 2002). In the United States, boys typically initiate sexual intercourse before girls do; the average age at first intercourse is 16 to 17 years in boys and 17 to 18 years in girls (Seidman and Rieder, 1994). According to data from the National Survey of Family Growth looking at premarital sexual intercourse among 15- to 19-year-old white and black girls from 1970 through 1988, black girls appear to initiate sexual intercourse earlier than white girls do. Among black girls, lower socioeconomic status is associated with earlier first intercourse (Centers for Disease Control and Prevention, 1991). Data from the National Survey of Adolescent Males (1988-1991) looking at the relation of sexual activity to age and race among adolescent men aged 15 to 19 years revealed that black men initiate sexual intercourse earlier than white men do (Seidman and Rieder, 1994). On the basis of data from the Youth Risk Behavior Survey, this racial disparity between age and initiation of sexual intercourse is decreasing (Grunbaum et al, 2002, 2004). Epidemiologic studies reveal that once adolescents are sexually experienced, they do not generally plan intercourse. They tend to have multiple serial sexual relationships and report having sexual intercourse relatively infrequently (Seidman and Rieder, 1994). It needs to be stated that one act of sexual intercourse can potentially lead to the development of pregnancy as well as acquisition of STDs, and therefore the frequency or relative infrequency should not affect clinical care.

Initiation of sexual activity before 13 years of age is strongly associated with an increased number of lifetime partners, less consistent use of condoms, teen pregnancy, and increased prevalence of sexually transmitted infections (Coker et al, 1994; Greenberg et al, 1992). The timing of initiation of sexual intercourse is influenced by an array of factors; the most influential factors are the social influences of parents, siblings, sexual partners, and friends. Coker and colleagues analyzed data from 1991 to determine correlates and consequences of early initiation of sexual behavior. The following factors were consistently associated with early age at first sexual intercourse among all race categories and both genders: carrying a weapon to school, getting into physical fights in the previous year, beginning to smoke cigarettes, and first alcohol use before the age of 13 years (Coker et al,1994).

In addition to the concern for pregnancy and STDs, other important issues that are associated with sexual activity should be discussed with teens. Adolescents frequently report sexual pressure and violence; studies indicate that as many as 33% of sexually active 15- to 17-year-olds were involved "in a relationship where they felt things were moving too fast sexually," 29% reported feeling pressure to have sex, and 24% had "done something sexual they didn't really want to do." With respect to being pressured into engaging in sexual acts that they did not want to do, 21% of teens surveyed by the Kaiser Family Foundation reported having oral sex to "avoid having sexual intercourse." Abusive relationships, particularly those that involve physical violence, have been reported in as many as 9% of ninth- to twelfth-grade students surveyed, who were physically forced to have sexual intercourse during some point in their past.

Summary

Stacey's case illustrates a typical adolescent presenting for a sports physical. The key is to provide time to confidentially ask about sexuality and sexual experiences. Once you are aware of the adolescent's sexual debut or pending debut, you have the opportunity to counsel her about contraception, sexually transmitted infections, and other risk factors. As she has placed trust in you by providing this information, she is seeking help, guidance, and testing or treatment. Given her current concerns about pregnancy, a urine pregnancy test should be performed in the office, with the results provided as rapidly as possible, as she will likely not fully hear anything you have to offer until she knows the results. Once the pregnancy test results are obtained, the urine can be sent for STD screening.

This very typical scenario brings up many preventive medicine topics, including STD screening, pregnancy prevention, risk behavior identification, and reassurance that you are there to provide. If you are unwilling to provide these services, she deserves to be referred to a provider who is comfortable providing these services. A brief discussion about relationship safety and healthy sexuality is also very helpful for the adolescent's developing sexuality. Most offices providing care for adolescents have free condoms available for distribution, and we recommend this. Regarding the adolescent's mother and the confidentiality of the adolescent, we always encourage adolescents to have ongoing discussions and openness with their parent or guardian about sex and relationships. If the adolescent refuses to discuss sexual relationships with a parent, it is critical to maintain confidentiality and to provide ongoing support for the adolescent.

Sexual Orientation and Homosexuality

Vignette

Juan, a 9-year-old boy, is brought in by his parents because they are very concerned that he likes to dress up in female clothing. It is not unusual for Juan to be found dressed up in his mother's gowns and high-heeled shoes. His mother and father have been uncomfortable with his behavior for years. His mother recalls that when Juan was 3 years old, he liked to play with typical girls' toys like dolls and dress-up clothes. More recently, he is involved in skateboarding but also takes dance classes, although his parents have refused his request to sign up for ballet and tap classes. Juan denies any desire to be or to become a girl, and he typically hangs out with male friends. He is unsure of sexual attraction or orientation but plans to marry and have children someday.

Sexual identity is how individuals describe themselves as heterosexual, homosexual, bisexual, asexual, or uncertain. Sexual orientation involves the patterns of sexual thoughts, fantasies, and attractions toward other individuals. The word *homosexual* has been used since 1869 (Friedman and Downey, 1994) to describe individuals who have the potential to have sexual attraction to those of the same sex. Before 1973, homosexuality was considered a psychiatric diagnosis and was included in the *Diagnostic and Statistical Manual of Mental Disorders*. Although stigmatization toward individuals with homosexual orientation remains, there has been much progress in understanding of human sexual orientation in the last few decades.

Alfred Kinsey conducted interviews of men and women in the United States of sexuality and sexual behaviors in the 1950s. Based on his studies, he estimated that 8% of men and 4% of women were exclusively homosexual for a period of at least 3 years during adulthood. Thirty-seven percent of men and 20% of women reported at least one homosexual experience resulting in orgasm (Kinsey et al, 1948, 1953). Critics have stated that Kinsey's studies were not representative of the general population and his research techniques were not valid. In the late 1980s, Fay and colleagues reported that at least 20% of men had at least one sexual experience with another man resulting in orgasm and only 3% of the adult male population reported having occasional or more often homosexual contact in the preceding year (Fay et al, 1989). According to the National Survey of Men conducted in 1991, 2.3% of men aged 20 to 39 years had had sex with someone of the same gender in the preceding 10 years; 1.1% had had such activity exclusively (Billy et al, 1993). Data on the prevalence of homosexuality among women is sparse, but estimates are generally lower than those for men.

Data on sexual orientation and behaviors among adolescents reveal that homosexual experiences are not uncommon during the adolescent years. Kinsey reported that in the period from puberty to 20 years of age,

28% of boys and 17% of girls had one or more homosexual experiences (Kinsey et al, 1948, 1953). In 1973, Sorenson reported that 17% of boys and 6% of girls between the ages of 16 and 19 years reported at least one homosexual experience. Remafedi and colleagues (1992) surveyed Minnesota high-school students in seventh through twelfth grades about sexual orientation. They found that 88.2% of students were "mostly or totally heterosexual"; 10.7% of students were "unsure" of their sexual orientation; 0.7% were bisexual; and 0.4% were mostly or totally homosexual. In addition, the prevalence of students describing themselves as homosexual increased with age. The proportion of boys and girls engaging in homosexual activity as adolescents who go on to identify as homosexual adults is not known.

Further understanding of what it means to be a homosexual male or female in the United States continues to be the subject of research. Homosexual youth are two to three times more likely to attempt suicide than are their heterosexual counterparts (Gibson, 1989). The National Gay and Lesbian Task Force found that 45% of gay men and 20% of lesbians surveyed were victims of verbal and physical assaults in school (Kourany, 1987). Garofalo and associates (1998) surveyed adolescent high-school students in Massachusetts as part of the 1995 Youth Risk Behavior Survey of health risk behaviors and sexual orientation. They found more than 30 statistically significant health risk behaviors positively associated with self-reported gay, lesbian, or bisexual orientation, including weapon carrying, fighting, multiple substance abuse, and sexual risk behaviors. In addition, non-heterosexual youth were found to be at higher risk for dropping out of school, being kicked out of their homes, and turning to life on the streets for survival (Garofalo et al, 1998). Risks of HIV infection are also higher among homosexuals, with higher seroprevalence rates in descending order among black adolescents, "mixed race or other" adolescents, Hispanic adolescents, and Asian and white adolescents (Valleroy et al, 2000). It is safe to say that homosexual adolescents have unique sociologic, psychological, and medical risks.

The medical care of the homosexual youth is the same as that of their heterosexual counterparts and should be provided with particular attention to the risks associated with being homosexual. Health care providers should discuss sexual identity, orientation, and behaviors with all adolescent patients so that appropriate risk assessment can be made. If providers do not feel comfortable discussing these issues in a nonjudgmental way, they should refer the patient to someone who is capable of providing this type of care. During discussions about sexual orientation, it is important for providers to ask questions in a gender-neutral manner. For example, use "Have you been in a romantic relationship before?" in place of "Do you have a boyfriend?" (Table 43-3).

Research is beginning to demonstrate a relationship between sexual orientation and biologic factors such as brain morphology and ability to detect pheromones. These observations provide supporting evidence that sexual orientation is not a choice but an intrinsic characteristic of each individual. The first study that purportedly described this observable biologic difference (LeVay, 1991) demonstrated that an area of the anterior hypothalamus (INAH3) is smaller in both heterosexual women and homosexual men. Another study, by Savic and colleagues (2005), evaluated sexual orientation dimorphisms seen with two putative human pheromones. These observational studies describe associational data and as such cannot address causality. They underscore the concept that more research is necessary.

Table 43-3. **Special Considerations for Non-Heterosexual (Gay, Lesbian, or Bisexual) Adolescents**

Refer adolescents if you have personal barriers to providing appropriate care.
Assure the patient that his or her confidentiality will be protected.
Help the adolescent work through his or her feelings. Be hesitant to define sexual orientation at this age on the basis of same-sex feelings and sexual experiences.
Identify risky behaviors (e.g., unprotected sexual intercourse, substance abuse).
Ask about mental health and refer if necessary.
Offer support and advice for adolescents in dealing with potential conflict with family and friends.
Encourage transition to adult care when appropriate.

Adapted with permission from Frankowski BL: Sexual orientation and adolescents. Pediatrics 113:1827, 2004.

Summary: How to Handle This Boy and His Parents?

Juan's situation demonstrates several important complex issues, such as gender identity and orientation, coupled with his parents' fears about his gender and sexual orientation. The parents' concern has been leading them to prohibit certain behaviors and desires, which can contribute to ongoing issues throughout pre-adolescence and adolescence. Care should be taken to reassure the parents that Juan's behaviors are typical for his age and will continue to be expressed (even in spite of parental demands to the contrary). Certainly, some of the underlying concern involves the possibility that Juan will ultimately describe himself as homosexual or transgender. This "fear" should be addressed, with a discussion that neither homosexual nor transgender orientation is a choice for anyone involved (individual, parent, teacher, neighbor, or other individual) and attempts to change this orientation will not work and can only be detrimental to the child. Given the parental concerns and the apparent need for reassurance, this child should be seen relatively frequently.

Sexuality of Children with Disabilities and Chronic Disease

Vignette

Molly is nearly 25 years old and has cerebral palsy. She only recently made her first appointment with an adult primary care physician. She has delayed transitioning her care for as long as possible because she has felt so connected to her pediatrician. This time, her mother waits in the waiting room while Molly enters the examination room alone. Several minutes are devoted to collecting the medical history of cerebral palsy and scoliosis and the list of orthopedic surgeries and medications. Before the examination, the internist asks more personal questions about substance use, educational and career plans, romantic interests, previous history of intimacy, and plans to initiate sexual intercourse. Molly bursts into tears. When she is able to express why she had cried, she responds, "No one has ever cared about me enough to ask me about my sexuality. Everyone treats me like a child."

Regarding sexuality, adolescents with developmental delay, disability, and chronic medical conditions are no different from their nondiseased or nondisabled counterparts. Historically, children with disabilities have been thought of and treated as asexual individuals. It is no longer acceptable to ignore sexuality and its related issues in caring for children and adolescents with any type of chronic illness or developmental delay. Moreover, these children experience differences in their social exposures and relationships that may further complicate their sexual development, making it critical for the medical provider to discuss issues of sexuality routinely and openly.

In addition, most children with congenital defects and developmental delay eventually progress through puberty. Children with neurodevelopmental disabilities are 20 times more likely than their counterparts to experience early pubertal changes (Siddiqi et al, 1999). More specifically, children with cerebral palsy typically begin puberty earlier and complete puberty later than do typically developing children (Worley et al, 2002). Among girls with spina bifida, the incidence of precocious puberty approaches 20% (Elias and Sadeghi-Nejad, 1994). Divergence from the norm in terms of the timing of puberty can further affect developing sexuality, especially in youth with disabilities who are already singled out as different.

Suris and colleagues (1996) compared the sexual behaviors of adolescents with chronic disease and disability with those of adolescents without chronic disease and disability. Overall, there was no difference among male and female adolescents with and without chronic conditions reporting ever having had sexual intercourse. Both male and female adolescents with visible conditions were more likely than controls to report ever having a sexually transmitted disease. Cheng and Udry (2002) used data from the National Longitudinal Study of Adolescent Health 1994-1995 to evaluate sexual behaviors of adolescents with physical disabilities in the United States. They found that male and female adolescents with physical disabilities were as likely to be sexually active as the nondisabled. Specifically, by the age of 16 years, 37% of nondisabled boys with average pubertal development had initiated sexual intercourse; 48%, 44%, and 39% of boys with minimal, mild, and more severe disabilities had initiated sexual intercourse. Among girls, a similar trend was observed, with 34% of nondisabled girls of average pubertal development ever having had sex. Among the disabled, 52%, 36%, and 42% of girls with minimal, mild, and more severe disabilities had initiated sexual intercourse (Cheng and Udry, 2002).

Children with disabilities have a right to the same education about sexuality as their peers. According to the American Academy of Pediatrics (1996), an underlying premise of sexuality education is that sexuality is a source of pleasure and a basis for bonding and human relationships. Other stated goals of sexuality education include giving children a sense of being attractive members of their respective genders with the expectation of satisfying adult relationships; teaching children to be assertive in protecting the privacy of their own bodies and reporting violations to trusted adults; and conveying information about conception, contraception, and STDs (American Academy of Pediatrics, 1996). Instructing students with disabilities may require alterations in the delivery of the curriculum so that a particular child can understand the material. Use of anatomically correct dolls, role playing, and repetition of material may be useful in some situations (Table 43-4).

Gynecologic care of adolescents with disabilities should be no different from that provided to adolescent girls without disabilities. Adolescents with disabilities may experience many of the common gynecologic symptoms of adolescence: anovulatory cycles with irregular menstrual bleeding, vaginal discharge and pruritus, and concern for STDs. Consideration of the underlying disability and associated medical issues is important in sorting out and treating gynecologic concerns. Inspection of the genitalia as part of routine examination of children and adolescents is important to document normal anatomy. Rarely is a pelvic examination indicated in an adolescent who is not sexually active (Quint, 1999). If a pelvic examination is necessary, girls with and without disabilities should be informed of the procedures and instruments to be used. Those with disabilities may tolerate the procedure better if they are offered the presence of a trusted caregiver, modification of the position during examination (frog-leg position versus stirrups), and use of distraction techniques.

Table 43-4. **Major Objectives of Sexuality Education for Children with Disabilities**
Teach children how to express physical affection in a manner appropriate for the child's apparent age, not developmental or chronologic age.
Discourage inappropriate displays of affection in the community (e.g., hugging strangers).
Express clear expectations of behavior that conforms with family and societal standards for privacy and modesty.
Teach children the difference between acceptable behaviors in a private setting and those acceptable in public (e.g., masturbation).
Teach children about the right to refuse to be touched at any time and to convey any history of having been inappropriately touched to a trusted adult.
Discuss pleasure and affection when educating children about sex.

Adapted with permission from the American Academy of Pediatrics, Committee on Children with Disabilities: Sexuality education of children and adolescents with developmental disabilities. Pediatrics 97:275, 1996.

In 1993, the National Center on Abuse and Neglect reported that children with disabilities have 2.2 times greater risk of sexual abuse during childhood compared with those without disability (Crosse et al, 1993). Subsequent studies have found similar results (American Academy of Pediatrics, 2001b; Suris et al, 1996). Furthermore, child abuse may result in disabilities, which can in turn result in further sexual and physical abuse, setting up a vicious circle (Jaudes and Diamond, 1985). One proposed explanation of this increased risk related to the relative social isolation of children with disabilities, leaving fewer opportunities for the child or adolescent to develop close and trusting relationships with which to share concerns about alleged abuse. In addition, cognitive deficits may affect the child's ability to understand what constitutes sexual abuse. Other factors that further confound this issue include daily dependence on family members and caregivers for intimate care, increased exposure to a large number of caregivers, and inappropriate social skills (Murphy, 2005).

Summary: How to Counsel the Young Woman with Disabilities: Intimacy, Prevention of Unwanted Pregnancy, and STDs

Molly's situation is a far too common scenario in which the complexities of medical care are coupled with a pervasive discomfort among primary care providers and pediatric subspecialists discussing sexuality and sexual activity. This attitude undervalues the individual and not only promotes unsafe practices but prevents appropriate preventive medical and prenatal care. It is incumbent on all those who provide care to pre-adolescent individuals, irrespective of condition or health status, to provide appropriate, confidential, and comprehensive care including pubertal development, healthy sexual development, and intimacy counseling as well as the prevention of sexual abuse, STDs, and undesired pregnancy. It cannot be overstated that all individuals deserve the best care as described throughout the chapter.

SUMMARY

Sexuality is an intrinsically necessary and normal component of human development with an understandable direction to the path it takes in every individual. As normal as sexuality and sexual development is, the discussion or even mere acknowledgement of its existence remains exceedingly uncommon in public and medical realms. As care providers, we have the obligation to promote healthy development and reduction in predictable risks for each and every one of our patients. Certainly, sexuality can be an extremely sensitive subject of discussion with children and adolescents for both parents and care providers. This initial sensitivity can be reduced with adequate factual knowledge, openness, and a desire to provide the best care possible. The discussion of sexuality is not and should not be seen as an isolated question or series of questions but rather as a process. This process, when it is done well, is done continuously throughout development with the necessary provision of privacy between medical care provider and child or adolescent. In this manner, as individuals develop their sexual identity, they are surrounded by and supported by their parents and health care providers and have adequate time to ask questions and to seek advice before they are forced to make potentially life-threatening decisions.

REFERENCES

Abma JC, Sonenstein FL: Sexual activity and contraceptive practices among teenagers in the United States, 1988 and 1995. Vital Health Stat 23(21):1, 2001.

Adams PF, Marano MA: Current estimates from the National Health Interview Survey, 1994. Vital Health Stat 10(193):1, 1995.

Alexander B, Schrauben S: Outside the margins: Youth who are different and their special health care needs. Prim Care 33:285, 2006.

American Academy of Pediatrics: Committee on Children with Disabilities: Sexuality education of children and adolescents with developmental disabilities. Pediatrics 97:275, 1996.

American Academy of Pediatrics, Committee on Psychosocial Aspects of Child and Family Health and Committee on Adolescence: Sexuality education for children and adolescents. Pediatrics 108:498, 2001a.

American Academy of Pediatrics, Committee on Child Abuse and Neglect and Committee on Children with Disabilities: Assessment of maltreatment of children with disabilities. Pediatrics 108:508, 2001b.

Benson V, Marano MA: Current estimates from the National Health Interview Survey, 1992. Vital Health Stat 10(189):1, 1994a.

Benson V, Marano MA: Current estimates from the National Health Interview Survey, 1993. Vital Health Stat 10(190):1, 1994b.

Billy JO, Tanfer K, Grady WR, et al: The sexual behavior of men in the United States. Fam Plann Perspect 25:52, 1993.

Brown B, Brown JD: Adolescent sexuality. Prim Care 33:373, 2006.

Burch B: Sex and the young child. Parents Magazine 27:36, 1952.

Calderone MS: Adolescent sexuality: Elements and genesis. Pediatrics 76:699, 1985.

Centers for Disease Control and Prevention: Premarital sexual experience among adolescent women—United States, 1970-1988. MMWR Morb Mortal Wkly Rep 39:929, 1991.

Centers for Disease Control and Prevention: Sexual behavior and selected health measures: Men and women 15-44 years of ago, United States, 2002. Adv Data 362:1, 2005.

Cheng MM, Udry JR: Sexual behaviors of physically disabled adolescents in the United States. J Adolesc Health 31:48, 2002.

Coker AL, Richter DL, Valois RF, et al: Correlates and consequences of early initiation of sexual intercourse. J Sch Health 64:372, 1994.

Cotton S, Mills L, Succop PA, et al: Adolescent girls' perception of the timing of their sexual initiation: "Too young" or "just right. J Adolesc Health 34:453-458, 2004.

Couper RT, Huynh H: Female masturbation masquerading as abdominal pain. J Paediatr Child Health 38:199, 2002.

Crosse SB, Kaye E, Ratnofsky AC: Report on the Maltreatment of Children with Disabilities. Washington, DC, National Center on Child Abuse and Neglect, Administration for Children and Families, U.S. Department of Health and Human Services, 1993.

Davies SL, Glaser D, Kossoff R: Children's sexual play and behavior in preschool settings: Staff's perceptions, reports, and responses. Child Abuse Neglect 24:1329, 2000.

Duncan P, Dixon BA, Carlson J: Childhood and adolescent sexuality. Pediatr Clin North Am 50:765, 2003.

Earl DT, Blackwelder RB: Management of chronic medical conditions in children and adolescents. Prim Care 25:253, 1998.

Elias ER, Sadeghi-Nejad A: Precocious puberty in girls with myelodysplasia. Pediatrics 93:521, 1994.

Fay RE, Turner CF, Klassen AD, et al: Prevalence and patterns of same-gender sexual contact among men. Science 243:338, 1989.

Finch SM: Sexual activity of children with other children and adults. Clin Pediatr (Phila) 6:1, 1967.

Fleischer DR, Morrison A: Masturbation mimicking abdominal pain or seizures in young girls. J Pediatr 116:810, 1990.

Frankowski BL: American Academy of Pediatrics Committee on Adolescence: Sexual orientation and adolescents. Pediatrics 113:1827, 2004.

Friedman RC, Downey JI: Homosexuality. N Engl J Med 331:923, 1994.

Friedrich WN, Grambsch P, Broughton D, et al: Normative sexual behavior in children. Pediatrics 88:456, 1991.

Friedrich WN, Fisher J, Broughton D, et al: Normative sexual behavior in children: A contemporary sample. Pediatrics 101:9, 1998.

Garofalo R, Wolf RC, Kessel S, et al: The association between health risk behaviors and sexual orientation among a school-based sample of adolescents. Pediatrics 101:895, 1998.

Gibson R: Report of the Secretary's Task Force on Youth Suicide: Prevention and Intervention in Youth Suicide. Rockville, MD, U.S. Department of Health and Human Services, 1989.

Greenberg J, Magder L, Aral S: Age at first coitus: A marker for risky sexual behavior in women. Sex Transm Dis 19:331, 1992.

Grunbaum JA, Kann L, Kinchen SA, et al: Youth risk behavior surveillance—United States 2001. MMWR Morb Mortal Wkly Rep 51:1, 2002.

Grunbaum JA, Kann L, Kinchen SA, et al: Youth risk behavior surveillance—United States 2003. MMWR Surveill Summ 53:1, 2004.

Gustafsson PA, Larsson I, Lundin B: Preschoolers' sexual behavior at daycare centers: An epidemiological study. Child Abuse Neglect 19:569, 1995.

Halpern-Felscher BL, Cornell JL, Kropp RY, et al: Oral versus vaginal sex among adolescents: Perceptions, attitudes, and behavior. Pediatrics 115:845, 2005.

Jaudes PK, Diamond LJ: The handicapped child and child abuse. Child Abuse Neglect 9:341, 1985.

Kaiser Family Foundation, National Survey of Adolescents and Young Adults: Sexual Health Knowledge, Attitudes and Behaviors. Menlo Park, CA, Henry Kaiser Family Foundation, May 2003.

Kinsey AC, Pomeroy WB, Martin CE: Sexual Behavior in the Human Male. Philadelphia, WB Saunders, 1948.

Kinsey AC, Pomeroy WB, Martin CE: Sexual Behavior in the Human Female. Philadelphia, WB Saunders, 1953.

Kourany R: Suicide among homosexual adolescents. J Homosex 13: 111-117, 1987.

Leung AK, Robson WL: Childhood masturbation. Clin Pediatr (Phila) 32:238, 1993.

LeVay S: A difference in hypothalamic structure between heterosexual and homosexual men. Science 253:1034-1037, 1991.

Livingston S, Berman W, Pauli LL: Masturbation simulating epilepsy. Clin Pediatr (Phila) 14:232, 1975.

Marshall WA, Tanner JM: Variations in pattern of pubertal changes in girls. Arch Dis Child 44:291, 1969.

Meizner I: Sonographic observation of in utero fetal "masturbation." J Ultrasound Med 6:111, 1987.

Mink JW, Neil JJ: Masturbation mimicking paroxysmal dystonia or dyskinesia in a young girl. Mov Disord 10:518, 1995.

Murphy NA: Sexuality in children and adolescents with disabilities. Dev Med Child Neurol 47:640, 2005.

Murphy NA, Elias ER: Sexuality of children and adolescents with developmental disabilities. Pediatrics 118:399, 2006.

Nechay A, Ross LM, Stephenson JB, et al: Gratification disorder ("infantile masturbation"): A review. Arch Dis Child 89:225, 2004.

Newacheck PW, Taylor WR: Childhood chronic illness: Prevalence, severity, and impact. Am J Public Health 82:364, 1992.

Pathela A, Hajat A, Schillinger A, et al: Discordance between sexual behavior and self-reported sexual identity: A population-based survey of New York City men. Ann Intern Med 145:416, 2006.

Prater CD, Zylstra RG: Medical care of adults with mental retardation. Am Fam Physician 73:2175, 2006.

Quint EH: Gynecologic health care for adolescents with developmental disabilities. Adolesc Med 10:221, 1999.

Remafedi G: Male homosexuality: The adolescent's perspective. Pediatrics 79:326, 1987.

Remafedi G, Resnick M, Blum R, et al: Demography of sexual orientation in adolescents. Pediatrics 89:714, 1992.

Rosenthal SL, Von Ranson KM, Cotton S, et al: Sexual initiation: Predictors and developmental trends. Sex Transm Dis 28:527, 2001.

Savic I, Berglund H, Lindstrom P: Brain response to putative pheromones in homosexual men. Proc Natl Acad Sci USA 102:7356-7361, 2005.

Schofield M: The Sexual Behavior of Young People. Boston, Little, Brown, 1965.

Seidman SN, Rieder RO: A review of sexual behavior in the United States. Am J Psychiatry 151:330, 1994.

Siddiqi SU, Van Dyke DC, Donohoue P, et al: Premature sexual development in individuals with neurodevelopmental disabilities. Dev Med Child Neurol 41:392, 1999.

Sorenson RC: Adolescent Sexuality in Contemporary America. New York, World Publishing, 1973.

Suris J, Resnick MD, Cassuto N, et al: Sexual behavior of adolescents with chronic disease and disability. J Adolesc Health 19:124, 1996.

Valleroy LA, MacKellar DA, Karon JM, et al: HIV prevalence and associated risks in young men who have sex with men. Young Men's Survey Study Group. JAMA 284:198-204, 2000.

Wells RD, McCann J, Adams J, et al: Emotional, behavioral, and physical symptoms reported by parents of sexually abused, nonabused, and allegedly abused prepubescent females. Child Abuse Neglect 19:155, 1995.

Woodard LJ: Sexuality and disability. Clin Fam Pract 6:941, 2004.

Worley G, Houlihan CM, Herman-Giddens ME, et al: Secondary sexual characteristics in children with cerebral palsy and moderate to severe motor impairment: A cross-sectional survey. Pediatrics 110:897, 2002.

Wulff CH, Ostergaard JR, Storm K: Epileptic fits or infantile masturbation? Seizure 1:199, 1992.

Yang ML, Fullwood E, Goldstein J, Mink JW: Masturbation in infancy and early childhood presenting as a movement disorder: 12 cases and a review of the literature. Pediatrics 116:1427, 2005.

SECTION B

Self-Relations, Self-Esteem, Self-Care, and Self-Control

44 SELF-CONCEPT

CAROL S. DWECK AND ALLISON MASTER

Common sense is typically the only guide parents and many professionals use in child rearing. Yet, common sense is not the gold standard in pediatric medicine. Drugs and medical procedures, no matter how much they are touted in advance or how sensible they seem, are not used to treat millions of children without extensive testing. Why should it be any different for child rearing? To address this concern, there has recently been a loud call for evidence-based child rearing practices, ones that withstand the rigors of scientific testing before they are recommended for widespread use with children. Researchers are responding to this call and have begun to build such a body of knowledge.

This chapter translates research on self-concept into recommendations for clinicians and parents, showing how parents and others can interact with children in ways that build self-esteem. We emphasize that parents can support the development of self-esteem in their children by teaching them that their abilities and talents are not simply inborn qualities that automatically produce success or failure but rather can be developed through effort and practice. We present research findings that fly in the face of common sense, demonstrating, for example, that praising children's abilities, far from building motivation and lasting confidence, sets them up for fear of failure and for the risk of underachievement. Most important, we describe what forms of praise and feedback are best for fostering the qualities we value in our children and the qualities they value in themselves.

We begin by describing three different scenarios in which the pediatrician or other health care clinician is asked to counsel a family about issues of self-concept and self-esteem. Notice that these examples come from different domains of functioning.

Vignette

The Brilliant but Unmotivated Child

Allen is an intellectually brilliant child of 13. He had taught himself to read at 3 and was inventing math tricks at 4, and when his parents had him tested, his IQ score was off the charts. His unusual abilities earned him a place at *the* elite private school in his city. He is popular there. Recently he stopped doing his homework and studying for tests. He says the work is beneath him, and he takes every opportunity to tell his parents how intellectually superior he is to the other students. His parents are distraught as they see his grades plummeting, and they take him to the pediatrician for evaluation. What should the pediatrician tell them?

Vignette

The Talented but Low-Confidence Child

Janie has always been fascinated with drawing. When she was little, she took her crayons with her everywhere she went and produced little works of art. As her artwork began to get attention, her parents encouraged her and delighted in her success but did not put pressure on her. Now, at 16, Janie just entered a nationwide art competition. Her confidence was shaky as she submitted her painting, and it sank even lower as she waited for the results to be announced. She asked herself and her parents, "Have I humiliated myself going up against the most talented young artists in the whole country?" Her parents called her pediatrician, asking him how they should handle it if she loses. The wise pediatrician knew that they would also have to think about what to tell her if she won. When the prizes are announced, much to her amazement, Janie takes top honors. What would the pediatrician have recommended that her parents say to her?

Vignette

The Promising Child Who Failed

Nine-year-old Elizabeth just completed her first gymnastics meet. Lanky, flexible, and energetic, she is just right for gymnastics, and she loves it. Of course, she was a little nervous about competing, but she felt confident of doing well. She had even thought about the perfect place in her room to hang the ribbon she would win. In the first event, the floor exercises, Elizabeth went first. Although she did a nice job, the scoring changed after her performance and she lost. Elizabeth also did well in the other events, but not well enough to win. By the end of the evening, she had received no ribbons and was devastated. The parents, after a turbulent night of mourning the loss, call the pediatrician in the morning for advice on how to handle the situation. What is the right thing for them to do? Should they tell Elizabeth that *they* think she was the best? that she was robbed of a ribbon that was rightfully hers? that gymnastics is not all that important? that she has the ability and will surely win next time? or that she did not really deserve to win quite yet?

DEFINITIONS

Self-concept refers to *beliefs* children have about themselves. In this chapter, we focus on children's beliefs about whether their talents and abilities are fixed or can be developed. *Self-esteem* refers to children's *feelings* about themselves—whether they feel good about their competencies and feel that they are worthy people. We will see that some self-concepts make it easier for children to feel good about themselves and to maintain these feelings even in the face of setbacks. One measure of self-esteem is how children speak about themselves. However, more important, we can infer that a child has high self-esteem when she or he is actively engaged in activities, is eager for challenges, and demonstrates resilience in the face of setbacks. We infer that children have low self-esteem when, regardless of whether they declare that they are bright or capable, they are reluctant to try new activities or withdraw after failure and disappointment. These indices of self-esteem—motivation, confidence, and willingness to continue after setbacks—may be at odds with what children declare about themselves. In addition, they may not be consistent across all domains of functioning but rather may differ within a child as we consider that child's behavior during academic pursuits, athletic competitions, musical performances, or social encounters.

PRAISING ABILITIES AND TALENTS CAN BACKFIRE

As the self-esteem movement was reaching its peak, parents and teachers went out of their way to ensure children's success and to protect them from failures. In fact, we polled parents and found that 85% of our sample agreed that you *must* praise your children's ability to make them feel good about themselves and help them succeed (Mueller and Dweck, 1998). Children who are vulnerable and have fragile motivation—those who are afraid of hard tasks and who give up in the face of difficulty—are overconcerned with their abilities (Dweck, 1999). When they confront a challenging task, these children worry about how smart they look. When they hit a setback, they worry that a deficiency has been exposed, and they become discouraged or defensive. These signs of poor self-esteem are often true not only of children who have poor skills but of many very bright and high-achieving children.

Praising children's ability, far from boosting their confidence, can make them preoccupied with their ability. It tells them that we adults judge their underlying ability from their performance. It conveys to them that their competence is what we adults care about most and value them for, and it makes them fear that if they do not succeed and look smart, we will not value them any longer. These findings were demonstrated in an illustrative series of experiments with late grade-school students (Mueller and Dweck, 1998). Children were given problems from a nonverbal IQ test. After the first set of 10 problems, on which all children generally did well, they received one of three forms of praise:

- One third of the children were praised for their intelligence: "Wow, that's a really good score. You must be smart at this!"
- One third were praised for their effort: "Wow, that's a really good score. You must have worked really hard!"
- One third were simply praised for their performance: "Wow, that's a really good score."

The prediction was that the second group was more likely than the first to remain engaged and confident in the face of difficulty. The group that was simply praised for their performance would fall somewhere in between the other two groups on our measures.

What happened? After the 10 initial problems and the praise, the children had to choose another task for later: Did they want a hard task that they could learn something from, or did they want an easy task that they were sure to do well on (and thus continue to look smart). The majority of the intelligence-praised children wanted to do the easier task and not jeopardize the intelligence praise they had gotten. The overwhelming majority (in one study 90%) of the effort-praised children wanted to try the hard task that they could learn something from. When the emphasis was on effort, children had no fear of making mistakes.

Next, all the children received a series of 10 really hard problems, ones designed for older children. Afterward, when asked why they thought they had trouble with them, how much they were enjoying the task, and whether they wanted to take some problems home to work on, the children who had been praised for their intelligence said they thought they were having trouble because they were not good at the task or were not smart enough. So the very children who were told they were smart when they succeeded thought they were *not* smart when they met with difficulty. In contrast, the students who had been praised for their effort thought that the hard problems just called for more effort or a new strategy. The fact that they had been praised for the *process* they had engaged in allowed them to remain focused on the process when they most needed it.

When the students rated the problems for enjoyment, those who had been praised for their intelligence showed a sharp decline in enjoyment after the hard problems. They were unable to sustain that enjoyment when the problems became more challenging. In truth, how could they enjoy problems that were making them feel stupid? In contrast, the children who had been praised for their effort showed no decline in their enjoyment. A number of them said they liked the hard ones the best. In other words, when they were focused on effort and learning, the hard problems were a welcome challenge, not an unwelcome threat.

The children were offered a chance to take some problems home with them and asked how much they would like to do so. After the hard problems, the intelligence-praised children had a greatly reduced desire to have anything further to do with the problems. "Thanks, but I already have these at home," one boy claimed. These children felt that they lacked ability and that further effort would be both futile and aversive. In contrast, the effort-praised children still showed a strong desire to take problems home to work on further.

To find out how the difficulty would affect children's performance, the children got a third set of 10 problems to work on. These problems were equal in difficulty to the first set, meaning that they were somewhat challenging but that most children could do well on them, as they had on the first set of problems. Yet, the group that had been praised for their intelligence now did significantly worse than they had originally and did the worst of the three groups. The intelligence praise followed by difficulty had undermined their ability to perform well on this IQ test. In contrast, the group that had been praised for effort did significantly better than they had originally. They had clearly benefited from their sustained engagement, perhaps even teaching themselves better strategies as they struggled with the difficult problems. They now performed the best of the three groups. The effort praise and their continued focus on *process* had raised their IQ scores!

Finally, to see how defensive children would be about their less-than-perfect performance, the children were asked to write (anonymously) to children in another school about the task we had given them and we left a space for them to report their scores. Almost 40% of the children who had been praised for their intelligence *lied* about their scores—and always in the same direction. Only about 12% or 13% of the children in other groups did this. This finding suggests that when you have been praised for your intelligence, your performance becomes an index of your worth. Thus, a poor score is shameful and needs to be hidden. When your performance simply speaks to your current skill level on a new task that you are striving to master, a poor score on a very hard task is nothing to be ashamed of.

These results were surprisingly strong, and they have been replicated over and over. Praise for intelligence does not build lasting confidence and does not give children the motivation to persevere in the face of difficulty. This does not mean that children do not enjoy intelligence praise. They do indeed. In fact, they often display self-satisfied smiles as they receive the praise. However, those smiles are short-lived and disappear completely when these children begin working on the more challenging problems. In short, praise for intelligence appeared to trap children in the desire to look smart without effort and to be so worried about their ability that they could not cope constructively with setbacks.

What is more, these effects are found in ethnically and racially diverse samples and in rural as well as in urban contexts. Although we focused on intelligence in these studies, the same principle holds for praising musical or artistic talent, or athletic prowess, or any ability.

ADULTS SEND MESSAGES AND CHILDREN HEAR THEM

Children are exquisitely attuned to the messages that we adults send. Children want to feel competent and they want to feel valued and loved. The praise we offer children gives them this information about how they should think of themselves. The intelligence praise tells them that to feel competent and to be valued, they have to be smart. As soon as they pick up this message, they reject tasks that could jeopardize this image of themselves as smart. The effort praise, on the other hand, tells them that competence is about working hard and that hard work is what adults respect.

Children as young as 4 years have these reactions (Cimpian et al, 2007). Beneficial effects are not limited to effort praise but are similar for different *kinds* of process feedback (Kamins and Dweck, 1999). After all, praise for effort is not always appropriate. Praise for children's strategies is just as effective. So, as long as adults put the emphasis on some part of children's *process*—their effort, their concentration, the approach they used, the choices they made, the patience they showed, the learning they engaged in—children are likely to remain engaged, learning oriented, and resilient in the face of challenges. The lesson is that parents should praise their children for what they put into a task, not for what the task reveals about their children's talents or abilities. Table 44-1 differentiates process praise from person praise.

Criticism should also be directed at the process (Kamins and Dweck, 1999). Constructive or process criticism is feedback that helps children understand what they can do differently to produce better results on their next try. It helps them realize, for example, that more studying, different study strategies, more background skills, or more help from the teacher is necessary for them to do better in the future. Criticizing children's abilities ("I guess you're not a math person." "You have your father's tin ear.") or simply criticizing their performance does not provide this kind of useful information, nor does glossing over or excusing their errors!

Table 44-1. **Differentiation of Process Praise and Person Praise**

Process Praise	**Person Praise**
Appreciation of effort	Appreciation of talent
Understanding what the child did to achieve success	Attributing success to a child's innate abilities
Clarity on why a performance was noteworthy	General praise of the performance and child

SELF-CONCEPT

Children's beliefs about intelligence and talent form the basis for much of their motivation (Aronson et al, 2002; Butler, 2000; Cury et al, 2006; Dweck, 1999, 2006; Dweck and Leggett, 1988; Ommundsen, 2003; Robins and Pals, 2002; Trzesniewski and Robins, 2003). That is why person and process praise and criticism are so powerful—they tell children not only about what adults value but also about the very nature of intelligence and other types of talent.

Children and adults can think of their intelligence (or any personal attribute) as a fixed trait—you only have a certain amount and that's that. We call this an entity theory of intelligence because, here, intelligence is conceived of as a fixed *thing*. We have also called this a fixed mindset, and we use this term here for simplicity. Alternatively, children and adults can think of their intelligence as a quality that can be developed over time through their efforts. We have called this an incremental theory of intelligence because, here, intelligence is conceived of as something that can be *increased*. We have also called this a growth mindset, and we will do so here.

Alfred Binet, the inventor of the IQ test, had a radical growth mindset (Binet, 1909/1973). He believed that children's basic capacity to learn could be transformed through education, and he spent most of his career devising educational programs that would accomplish just this (Siegler, 1992). An increasing number of psychologists are pointing out the malleable nature of important parts of intelligence, and neuroscientists are finding that the brain remains more plastic as we age than was previously believed (see Chapter 8).

These mindsets are an important part of children's self-concepts. Children who believe in fixed intelligence are more vulnerable than those who believe in expandable intelligence (see Dweck, 1999). In fact, many of the harmful effects of person praise may come from the fact that it communicates to children that intelligence is a stable underlying trait that can be read from their performance (Mueller and Dweck, 1998). Many of the beneficial effects of process praise may come from the fact that it suggests that intellectual competence can be enhanced through hard work. Let us see how this works.

First, children who believe that intelligence is fixed are chronically worried about how smart they are. If they have only a certain amount of this precious attribute, then they need to believe that they have a noteworthy amount. Many studies have shown that students with a fixed mindset will pass up opportunities to learn important new things when there is a risk of making errors or exposing deficiencies (Blackwell et al, 2007; Hong et al, 1999). Instead, they choose easier tasks at which they are sure they can succeed. In their minds, it is better to safeguard their self-concept than to learn. We have even shown that students with a fixed mindset will shy away from learning things that are critical to their future academic success (Hong et al, 1999). In this sense, they choose to protect their self-concept in the present at the cost of their success in the future.

For children with a growth mindset, learning is a priority. Because they believe that they can develop their intellectual skills, they look for opportunities to do so. For them, it is a waste of time to display their abilities when they could be increasing them. This does not mean that these children do not care about doing well in school or getting high scores on tests; it simply means that they put a premium on learning whenever possible and see high scores as evidence of learning rather than as evidence of superior inborn ability. In a number of studies, it has been shown that these students are the ones who end up getting better grades in school, especially when schoolwork becomes challenging (Blackwell et al, 2007; Grant and Dweck, 2003).

Conversely, students with the fixed mindset do not believe in the power of effort (Blackwell et al, 2007; Hong et al, 1999). They believe that if they have ability, they should not need effort to succeed, and that if they need effort to succeed, then they do not have ability. They (erroneously!) believe that geniuses have made their great contributions without exerting much effort, when in fact research shows that geniuses are often the people who worked harder than anyone else (Ericsson, 1996). This critical belief puts fixed-mindset students in a real bind. They want to succeed to look and feel smart, but they cannot work hard at it or they will feel dumb. It also means that as the work becomes more difficult in school, these are often the students who stop working—think about Allen in our opening example. Every exertion of effort undermines the idea that they are intelligent or gifted.

In contrast, students in a growth mindset believe wholeheartedly in effort. For them, it is what turns on and powers their ability and what allows them to increase their ability over time. It is what allowed geniuses to flower and to make their great discoveries or contributions. This means that within a growth mindset, there is no conflict about exerting effort—it fosters rather than undermines ability, and it is highly effective.

Children in a fixed mindset have negative reactions to setbacks, just like the children who received intelligence praise in the studies we described earlier. Those in a fixed mindset view the setbacks as revealing a lack of ability, and they respond to the setback by becoming discouraged or defensive (Blackwell et al, 2007; Hong et al, 1999).

They might withdraw their effort from this task or school subject. To save face, they might blame others (like the teacher) for their disappointing performance, or they might say that they were not really interested in the task or school subject, even if it was something they were enthusiastic about shortly before. Students in a fixed mindset have even told us that to perform better in the future, they would seriously consider cheating (Blackwell et al, 2007). If they believe they lack ability permanently, and they do not believe in effort, there are very few constructive paths open to them.

Children in a growth mindset are certainly very disappointed when they do not do as well as they expected, but their reactions are utterly different. They do not see these setbacks as indictments of their underlying ability. They see them as a reflection of the effort or strategy they used and they believe that the remedy lies in applying more effort or using different learning, study, or test-taking strategies in the future. In one study, with pre-med college students, we found that students in a growth mindset bounced back from an initial poor grade in a critical course. They did this by studying more effectively. Students in a fixed mindset usually did not recover from an initial poor grade (Grant and Dweck, 2003).

As we noted before, students in a growth mindset often end up doing better than their fixed-mindset counterparts, even when they begin with equal ability or past accomplishments (Blackwell et al, 2007; Grant and Dweck, 2003; Trzesniewski and Robins, 2003). In one study (Blackwell et al, 2007, Study 1), we observed adolescents for 2 years as they entered seventh grade and made the transition to junior high school. This is a particularly vulnerable time for many students. The schoolwork often becomes substantially more difficult, the grading becomes more stringent, and the educational environment often becomes less personal and nurturing. In addition, many students have the sense that the grades they earn are now a more important index of how they will do in the future. It is in these more challenging environments that students' mindsets make the most difference.

Early in their first semester, we assessed whether students had entered junior high school with a fixed or growth mindset. We did this by asking them to agree or to disagree with fixed-mindset or growth-mindset statements like the following:

Your intelligence is something very basic about you that you cannot really change. (fixed mindset)

Everyone, no matter who they are, can substantially increase their intelligence. (growth mindset)

Students who, overall, agreed with the first type of statement were classified as holding a fixed mindset, whereas those who overall agreed with the second type of statement were classified as holding a growth mindset. Interestingly, both groups of students—the students who held a fixed mindset and those who held a growth mindset—had entered junior high with equivalent achievement test scores. The safer, less threatening environment of grade school did not push the two groups apart. However, from the very first semester of junior high, the two groups diverged in their grades, and this difference increased steadily during the next 2 years.

MINDSETS AND SELF-ESTEEM

The fixed and growth mindsets we have been describing not only are an important part of children's self-concepts but also have important implications for children's self-esteem (Niiya et al, 2004; Nussbaum and Dweck, 2008; Robins and Pals, 2002; Trzesniewski and Robins, 2003). Fixed and growth mindsets play a role both in how stable students' self-esteem is and in how students repair their self-esteem after a failure.

On conventional measures of self-esteem, children with the fixed and growth mindsets often do not differ. However, when students are observed over challenging periods of their lives, such as the transition to junior high school or their college years in a top university, the two groups diverge (Robins and Pals, 2002; Trzesniewski and Robins, 2003). The students with a growth mindset gain self-esteem. As they meet and master the challenges, their confidence in themselves grows. In contrast, those with a fixed mindset lose self-esteem. The fact of continually hitting challenges and having to apply effort erodes their self-confidence. Table 44-2 includes some questions that a clinician could ask children to assess their mindset and the answers typical of children with fixed versus growth mindsets.

In general, then, the fixed mindset makes self-esteem more fragile and unstable because mistakes and challenges can easily undermine children's confidence in

Table 44-2. **Clinical Indicators of Mindset**

Indicator	Growth Mindset	Fixed Mindset
What does the individual think it takes to succeed?	Effort, practice	Intelligence, talent
What does the individual think makes a genius?	Hard work	Innate ability
What is the individual's typical response to new challenges?	Yes, please	No, thank you
How does the individual respond to setbacks?	The individual looks for new approaches and strategies.	The individual blames others, becomes defensive, or gives up.
What might you see if the individual experiences failure?	The individual tries again with a new approach.	The individual lies about performance, makes excuses.
What might you expect if you know the test is very difficult?	Sustained effort at studying	Cheating, procrastination

themselves. Mindsets make a difference for how students *repair* their self-esteem when it is injured (Nussbaum and Dweck, 2008). Suppose a student has had an important failure, one that was caused by and has revealed a skill deficit. Students can try to repair the deficit that led to the failure; or they may try to salvage their self-esteem by blaming the teacher or the test, by making excuses (illness, fatigue), or by finding people who did even worse than they did. In a series of studies (Nussbaum and Dweck, 2008), we looked at how students in different mindsets repair their self-esteem. In these studies, students were given a very hard test to work on and then received feedback that they had done poorly on their initial attempt. At this point, most students, regardless of their mindset, showed a drop in their confidence in their abilities.

Our participants were then shown a set of icons on a computer screen. These icons represented other students who had taken the same test in the past, and the icons were labeled with the scores these past students had earned. If the participants clicked an icon, they would see a description of the strategies that that student had used to try to do well on the task. Obviously, clicking on the icons of students who had done well on the test would yield better and more useful strategy information than clicking on the icons of students who had done poorly. What did our participants do?

Those in a fixed mindset consistently chose to examine the strategies of students who had performed worse than they had. Rather than try to seek information that would help them learn and improve, these students wanted to feel better than someone else. Interestingly, it worked! After looking at a variety of bad strategies, these students now said that they felt really good about their abilities. However, it was in some sense false self-esteem because they clearly had not repaired their skill deficit and were not in a better position to do well the next time.

In contrast, those in a growth mindset consistently chose to look at the strategies of students who had performed substantially better than they had. This worked too, and after examining a host of these good strategies, they now felt very good about their abilities. In this case, they had not only repaired their confidence but had done what they could to be better prepared the next time around.

This and other research suggests that those in a fixed mindset often suffer from false, easily deflated confidence (Niiya et al, 2004). Students in a fixed mindset given easy and hard problems spend time dwelling on the easy problems and avoiding hard problems. Ironically, they may end up with an even higher opinion of their abilities than students in the growth mindset, who had to grapple with the hard problems. However, when required to focus on hard problems, their confidence plummets well below that of students with a growth mindset. Coming face to face with the true level of their skills is deflating.

Students in a fixed mindset are more likely to engage in "self-handicapping," meaning that they do things that put their performance in jeopardy but at the same time give them an esteem-saving reason for a poor showing. In a fixed mindset, short-term ego needs are often more important than longer term growth or even success.

In summary, a belief in fixed ability makes children's self-esteem fragile because, in this framework, so many things—inevitable things like mistakes or effort—call that ability into question. A belief in fixed ability also makes self-esteem repair a defensive process instead of a learning process because fixed ability cannot be repaired. In contrast, a belief in expandable ability makes children's self-esteem more hardy and resilient because setbacks give them motivation to enhance or to repair their abilities.

Teaching a Growth Mindset

The good news is that the growth mindset can be taught. Mindsets are beliefs, and beliefs can be changed. Teaching a growth mindset changes students' motivation and performance in school (Aronson et al, 2002; Blackwell et al, 2007; Good et al, 2004). In these studies, students were taught about the brain and, in that context, learned that their brains formed new connections every time they learned something new and that, in this way, they became smarter over time. They were also taught how to apply this to their schoolwork. At the end of the workshops, their motivation and school performance were compared with those of the control groups. The control groups had also received noteworthy workshops, such as workshops teaching useful study skills.

In all cases, the students who had received the growth-mindset workshops showed significantly better grades or achievement test scores than did students in the control groups. In addition, teachers' reports and students' reports suggested that those in the growth-mindset workshops now had enhanced motivation to learn, better study habits, and more resilience in the face of setbacks. Here is an example of what one math teacher said about a formerly turned-off boy: "L., who never puts in any extra effort and doesn't turn in homework on time, actually stayed up late working for hours to finish an assignment early so I could review it and give him a chance to revise it. He earned a B+ on the assignment (he had been getting C's and lower)."

In all of these workshops, students seemed fascinated by the brain and by the idea that they could do things to help their brains to work better and to grow new connections over time. This idea made them excited about learning because it was something they were now doing for themselves rather than to please others. Many students said things like this: "My favorite thing from Brainology [the workshop] is the neurons part where when you learn something there are connections and they keep growing and growing. I always picture that when I'm in school!" Teachers said things like this about their students: "They have offered to practice, study, take notes, or pay attention more to ensure that connections will be made" (see Dweck, 2006).

Clinical Implications

Let us return to the idea that parents' feedback sends messages and go back to the three children from the beginning of the chapter. We should now have a better idea of how pediatricians should tell their parents to respond to them and why.

First, let us revisit Allen, the brilliant 13-year-old who retired from hard work at school, all the while touting his superior intellect. Many parents would respond to this situation by reassuring Allen of his exceptional intelligence and agreeing with him that he was smarter than his fellow students. They would see this as boosting his confidence and motivating him to work harder in school. They might also try to monitor him better, checking up on his homework and urging him to study before upcoming tests. They might deprive him of privileges until his homework was finished or until he put in a respectable amount of study time.

However, given what we know now, this hardly seems like the best course of action. Allen was most likely in a fixed mindset. His prodigy status was his claim to fame, something that made him special, better than others, and made his parents proud. Now, however, he entered a school with lots of smart students, and the work was hard enough that he could not just coast along on sheer brains as he could before. He was frightened. What if he was someone who had to work hard for accomplishments like the ordinary kids? Would he lose his special status and the respect and love of his parents?

His parents' insistence on his brilliance would simply play into these fears. Instead, his parents need to change his (and their) thinking, putting the emphasis on learning and skill development rather than on innate brilliance. They need to communicate that true genius and great contributions come from hard work and that even Thomas Edison, Mozart, Darwin, the Curies, and Cezanne all put in many years of obsessive labor before they made their great contributions. Actually, there are virtually no examples of great contributions without great effort. At the same time, the parents need to put this philosophy into action, praising real effort, challenge seeking, and commitment when they see it and *not* praising easy A's or effortless success. They need to convey that simply doing things that come quickly and easily is meaningless.

In the same vein, the parents of Janie, the winner of the art contest, are in danger of falling into the praise-for-talent trap. Their daughter's shaky confidence followed by her huge success might present an irresistible opportunity to assure her of her talent. Instead, they need to use the occasion to emphasize how her love of art, hard work, perseverance, and courage had paid off. There may also be hard periods ahead if Janie gets into the big-time art world, in which many talented people vie for success. A fixed mindset, with its fragile confidence and defensive reactions, will not serve her well. Instead, that emphasis on hard work, perseverance, and courage is what will more likely see her through.

What about Elizabeth, the aspiring gymnast whose early hopes were crushed at her first meet? Telling her that *they* thought she was the best is telling her a lie. It will undermine their credibility, such that they will not be reliable sources of feedback for her in the future. Telling her she was robbed of a ribbon is teaching her to be a poor sport when she loses. Telling her that gymnastics is not important teaches her to devalue activities after a setback. Telling her that her ability will bring her success next time is telling her that inherent ability is the only factor that matters—but if it did not bring her success this time, why should it bring her success next time? Telling her she did not yet deserve to win may seem harsh, but put in a more caring way, it is true and it is helpful. Elizabeth's parents can point out that she is a relative newcomer and that there were many girls in the competition who had worked longer and harder than she had. She could do gymnastics, if she wanted, just for fun, but if she also wanted to win in the future, she would have to put in a lot of time and effort to develop her skills. Rather than filling their child with defensive rationalizations, they will be giving her a plan for future success.

Mindsets also operate in the social realm. Children who believe their social skills can be developed fare better in the face of social setbacks and rejections. They are more likely to remain positive about themselves and are less likely to respond defensively to a rejection (Erdley et al, 1997). Parents can help their children to navigate the complex social world by helping them develop an openness to learning in this arena as well.

A Note on Culture and Diversity

Research on praise and the growth-mindset workshops has been conducted on diverse samples of white, Asian, black, and Hispanic students, and the same general results have been obtained with each group (Aronson et al, 2002; Blackwell et al, 2007; Good et al, 2004; Mueller and Dweck, 1998; Robins and Pals, 2002). In addition, research has been conducted across Europe (Cury et al, 2006) and Asia (Hong et al, 1999), with similar findings. Although there is greater emphasis on effort in some Asian cultures than in the United States, the fixed and growth mindsets appear to operate in similar ways across cultures (Grant and Dweck, 2001).

The growth mindset is particularly critical for groups that have been stereotyped as having low ability, such as blacks in various academic areas or female students in math. Studies have shown that the achievement gap between blacks and whites or between female and male students is largest for students in a fixed mindset and is greatly reduced for students in a growth mindset (Dar-Nimrod and Heine, 2006; Good et al, 2004). This is because students in a fixed mindset are more likely to fall prey to stereotypes (which are, in essence, beliefs about fixed ability) and to have these stereotypes undermine their performance. Students in a growth mindset, who believe that their ability can be developed, can remain motivated and effective even in the face of stereotypes.

Children with Physical Deformities and Disabilities

Many children have physical deformities, cognitive impairments, and other disabilities that differentiate them from their classmates. They face an additional set of challenges as they develop their self-concept and self-esteem. They often recognize the differences between themselves and others. They are unfortunately subject to explicit and subtle forms of prejudice and to the expectations that

Table 44-3. Recommendations

Praise and criticism
Praise effort and improvement, not ability.
Do not praise easy successes.
Give honest, constructive critiques.
Convey that
Abilities can be developed.
Effort and learning make the brain grow stronger.
Success is about progress, not easy perfection.
Show children that
Challenges are fun.
Mistakes are interesting and helpful.

one disability, such as cerebral palsy, implies a cognitive impairment, such as intellectual disability. Parents may themselves have ambivalent feelings about their children with disabilities as they attempt to deal with their own grief and guilt. Physical appearance, difficult temperaments, slow language development, and cognitive impairments may all challenge parents to provide consistent affection, engagement, and support to their children.

Specific research on how to support these children to develop confidence, motivation, and resilience is required. From what we have learned in studies of children developing typically, it is highly likely that the best course of action will be to acknowledge the deformities or disabilities as outside the child's control, neither denying the impact of the condition on the child and his or her functioning nor attributing any special characteristics to the child on the basis of the condition. At the same time, parents, teachers, and other important adults in the child's life can support the development of a growth mindset, encouraging the child to put out effort to develop skills, strengths, and assets in the domains in which effort and practice will improve skills.

SUMMARY

Although much remains to be discovered about how best to nurture a child's self-concept, researchers have begun to replace conventional wisdom with empiric evidence. This chapter has presented some of that evidence that leads to the recommendations summarized in Table 44-3. Praising children's effort rather than their intelligence or talents and teaching children that abilities can be developed can unlock their motivation to learn and foster resilience in the face of obstacles. These methods shape a positive and adaptive self-concept, allow children to maintain their self-esteem, and help them develop their abilities to the fullest.

REFERENCES

Aronson J, Fried C, Good C: Reducing the effects of stereotype threat on African American college students by shaping theories of intelligence. J Exp Soc Psychol 38:113-125, 2002.

Binet A: Les idées modernes sur les enfants [Modern Ideas on Children]. Paris, Flamarion, 1909/1973.

Blackwell LS, Dweck CS, Trzesniewski K: Implicit theories of intelligence predict achievement across an adolescent transition: A longitudinal study and an intervention. Child Dev 78:246-263, 2007.

Butler R: Making judgments about ability: The role of implicit theories of ability in moderating inferences from temporal and social comparison information. J Pers Soc Psychol 78:965-978, 2000.

Cimpian A, Arce H, Markman EM, Dweck CS: Subtle linguistic cues affect children's motivation. Psychol Sci 18:314-316, 2007.

Cury F, Elliot AJ, Da Fonseca D, Moller AC: The social-cognitive model of achievement motivation and the 2 × 2 achievement goal framework. J Pers Soc Psychol 90:666-679, 2006.

Dar-Nimrod I, Heine SJ: Exposure to scientific theories affects women's math performance. Science 314:435, 2006.

Dweck CS: Self-Theories: Their Role in Motivation, Personality, and Development. Philadelphia, Psychology Press, 1999.

Dweck CS: Mindset. New York, Random House, 2006.

Dweck CS, Leggett EL: A social-cognitive approach to motivation and personality. Psychol Rev 95:256-273, 1988.

Dweck CS, Mangels J, Good C: Motivational effects on attention, cognition, and performance. *In* Dai DY, Sternberg RJ (eds): Motivation, Emotion, and Cognition: Integrated Perspectives on Intellectual Functioning. Mahwah, NJ, Erlbaum, 2004, pp 41-56.

Ehrlinger J, Dweck CS: Attention and overconfidence: The role of implicit theories. Unpublished manuscript. Palo Alto, CA, Stanford University, 2007.

Erdley C, Cain K, Loomis C, et al: The relations among children's social goals, implicit personality theories and response to social failure. Dev Psychol 33:263-272, 1997.

Ericsson KA (ed): The Road to Excellence: The Acquisition of Expert Performance in the Arts and Sciences, Sports, and Games. Mahwah, NJ, Erlbaum, 1996.

Good C, Dweck CS, Rattan A: An incremental theory decreases vulnerability to stereotypes about math ability in college females. Unpublished data. New York, Columbia University, 2004.

Grant H, Dweck CS: Cross-cultural response to failure: Considering outcome attributions within different goals. *In* Salili F, Chiu C, Hong Y (eds): Student Motivation: The Culture and Context of Learning. New York, Plenum, 2001, pp 203-219.

Grant H, Dweck CS: Clarifying achievement goals and their impact. J Pers Soc Psychol 85:541-553, 2003.

Hong YY, Chiu C, Dweck CS, et al: Implicit theories, attributions, and coping: A meaning system approach. J Pers Soc Psychol 77:588-599, 1999.

Jourden FJ, Bandura A, Banfield JT: The impact of conceptions of ability on self-regulatory factors and motor skill acquisition. J Sport Exerc Psychol 13:213-226, 1991.

Kamins M, Dweck CS: Person vs. process praise and criticism: Implications for contingent self-worth and coping. Dev Psychol 35:835-847, 1999.

Martocchio JJ: Effects of conceptions of ability on anxiety, self-efficacy, and learning in training. J Appl Psychol 79:819-825, 1994.

Mueller CM, Dweck CS: Intelligence praise can undermine motivation and performance. J Pers Soc Psychol 75:33-52, 1998.

Niiya Y, Crocker J, Bartmess EN: From vulnerability to resilience: Learning orientations buffer contingent self-esteem from failure. Psychol Sci 15:801-805, 2004.

Nussbaum AD, Dweck CS: Defensiveness versus remediation: Self-theories and modes of self-esteem maintenance. Pers Soc Psychol Bull 34:599-612, 2008.

Ommundsen Y: Pupils' affective responses in physical education classes: The association of implicit theories of the nature of ability and achievement goals. Eur Phys Educ Rev 7:219-242, 2001.

Ommundsen Y: Implicit theories of ability and self-regulation strategies in physical education classes. Educ Psychol 23:141-157, 2003.

Rhodewalt F: Conceptions of ability, achievement goals, and individual differences in self-handicapping behavior: On the application of implicit theories. J Personality 62:67-85, 1994.

Robins RW, Pals JL: Implicit self-theories in the academic domain: Implications for goal orientation, attributions, affect, and self-esteem change. Self Identity 1:313-336, 2002.

Sarrazin P, Biddle S, Famose JP, et al: Goal orientation and conceptions of the nature of sport ability in children: A social cognitive approach. Br J Soc Psychol 35:399-414, 1996.

Siegler RS: The other Alfred Binet. Dev Psychol 28:179-190, 1992.

Steele CM, Aronson J: Stereotype threat and the intellectual test performance of African-Americans. J Pers Soc Psychol 68:797-811, 1995.

Sternberg RJ: Intelligence, competence, and expertise. *In* Elliot A, Dweck CS (eds): The Handbook of Competence and Motivation. New York, Guilford Press, 2005, 15-30.

Trzesniewski K, Robins R: Integrating self-esteem into a process model of academic achievement. Symposium paper presented at the Biennial Meeting of the Society for Research in Child Development, Tampa, FL, April 2003.

Wood R, Bandura A: Impact of conceptions of ability on self-regulatory mechanisms and complex decision making. J Pers Soc Psychol 56: 407-415, 1989.

45 SUBSTANCE USE, ABUSE, AND DEPENDENCE AND OTHER RISK-TAKING BEHAVIORS

John R. Knight

Misuse of psychoactive substances is one of our nation's greatest public health problems and one of great relevance to pediatricians. Treatment of medical problems related to use of tobacco, alcohol, and other drugs places a considerable drain on time and other health care resources. Even more important is the cost in human pain and suffering to individual users and their family members. Physicians can make a difference by screening all adolescents for use of alcohol and drugs and intervening early before serious harm results. This chapter presents an overview of the problem and describes practical methods for screening, assessment, office intervention, and referral to treatment. Because this problem often affects families, the chapter ends with a discussion of substance misuse by parents.

ADOLESCENT DEVELOPMENT

Adolescence describes the psychosocial changes that occur as individuals leave childhood and develop into independent, contributing members of adult society. To accomplish this, a number of behavioral strategies may be employed, including experimentation, exploration, risk taking, limit testing, and questioning of established rules and authority. Whereas these strategies are often functional, they can lead to serious injury and illness when they are combined with alcohol or drug use. Simple warnings about risks associated with substance use may be insufficient. All too often, warnings elicit the classic response "Don't worry, that can never happen to me." On the more positive side, research has shown that adolescence is not a tumultuous period of emotional lability and suicidality (Offer and Schonert-Reichl, 1992). In fact, it is a very positive period when interpersonal relationships are transformed and new cognitive abilities emerge. In social relationships, there is movement from predominant family influence (preconformist), to peer influence (conformist), to independent thinking (postconformist) (Petersen and Leffert, 1995). Cognitively, the development of formal operations leads to the ability to think in the abstract (Piaget and Inhelder, 1958). Propositional logic, that is, the formation of hypotheses and consideration of many possible solutions, emerges. Adolescents also develop metacognition, or the ability to think about the thought process itself. These new abilities are essential for the establishment of therapeutic physician-patient relationships and for counseling interventions, such as cognitive-behavioral therapy and motivational enhancement.

RISK AND PROBLEM BEHAVIORS

Problem behavior theory and social cognitive theory provide a conceptual framework for understanding risk behaviors during adolescence. Problem behavior theory defines *risk behavior* as anything that can interfere with successful psychosocial development and *problem behavior* as risk behaviors that elicit either formal or informal social responses designed to control them (Jessor and Jessor, 1977). These may cluster to form a "risk behavior syndrome" when they serve a common social or psychological developmental function (e.g., affirming individuation from parents, helping to achieve adult status, gaining acceptance from peers). These behaviors may help the adolescent cope with failure, boredom, social anxiety, unhappiness, rejection, social isolation, low self-esteem, or lack of self-efficacy. Adolescents who are poor students may use drugs as a way of achieving social status among their peers.

Social cognitive theory posits a "triadic reciprocal causation," in which behavior, personal determinants, and environmental influences all interact to determine behavior (Bandura, 1977). According to this theory, individuals learn how to behave through a process of modeling and reinforcement, imitating behaviors observed in others that are perceived to have positive consequences. Therefore, exposure to successful, high-status role models who use drugs will likely influence adolescents. Health risk and problem behaviors are both purposeful and functional. Peer influences may suggest to adolescents that drug use and sexual behaviors are necessary if one is to become popular, cool, sexy, grown-up, sophisticated, macho, or tough.

EPIDEMIOLOGY

According to the Monitoring the Future study, three of every four students have begun to drink by the end of high school, half have gotten drunk at least once, half have tried an illicit drug, and one in four has tried an illicit drug other than marijuana (Johnston et al, 2006). Rises in usage of specific drugs can be predicted by two factors: an increase in the perceived availability of the drug and a decrease in the perceived risk of harm associated with use of the drug. Misuse of alcohol and drugs is found among all demographic subgroups, with higher risk of drinking associated with being male, white, and from middle to upper socioeconomic status families. Usage among Latino adolescents has been increasing during recent years. Compared with previous years, the 2005 Monitoring the Future data also indicate that illicit drug use is declining slightly, but misuse of prescription drugs (including narcotic analgesics, stimulants, and tranquilizers) is rising (Johnston et al, 2006).

Tobacco

Positive developments regarding tobacco use in recent years include decreased acceptability of cigarette smoking in public places and a widespread perception that tobacco use is hazardous to health. There has also been an increase in the number of laws restricting tobacco use and better enforcement of laws prohibiting sale of tobacco products to minors. Despite these advances, prevalence of tobacco use among high-school students has remained essentially unchanged, with nearly a quarter (23%) of high-school seniors reporting current smoking (Johnston et al, 2006). This makes cigarettes the drug most commonly used on a daily basis among high-school students. Some consider tobacco to be a "gateway" drug for youth, and cigarette smokers are more likely to be heavy drinkers and to use illicit drugs (Epps et al, 1995).

Alcohol

The majority of adolescents report drinking (Eaton et al, 2006). The average first-time drinker is 12 to 13 years old. The prevalence of binge drinking, defined as having five or more drinks in a row, is reported at 25% among ninth to twelfth graders in the United States (Eaton et al, 2006). Whereas heavy episodic drinking is slightly more prevalent among boys than among girls, in recent years girls have been catching up. Drinking often occurs in cars or at parties from which young people drive home. Accidents are the leading cause of death among young people in the United States, and 39% of motor vehicle fatalities are alcohol related (National Highway Traffic Safety Administration, 2006). Although most teenagers report they are aware that driving after drinking is dangerous, 28.5% have accepted a ride during the past 30 days from a driver who had been drinking, and almost half of the students who drink have taken this risk (Eaton et al, 2006).

Illicit Drugs

Half of twelfth graders have tried some kind of illicit drug. The most commonly used substances are marijuana, volatile inhalants, amphetamines, and narcotics other than heroin. Thirty-eight percent of high school students have tried marijuana and 20% have used it within the past month (Eaton et al, 2006). Frequent marijuana use is particularly problematic for students because it can result in decreased attention, memory, and motivation and lead to a downward spiral of worsening academic performance and increased use (Jacobsen et al, 2004). The potency of this drug has increased almost sixfold during the past 30 years, making it more hazardous than that smoked during the 1960s by present-day parents of teenage children. Inhalants are a class of drugs whose use is particularly prevalent among younger adolescents (Johnston et al, 2006). These are defined as fumes or gases that produce euphoria when they are inhaled and include solvents, glues, aerosols, and butane. These chemicals are found in many common household products and thus are readily available to young people. Inhalants may be brought into school as small bottles of typewriter correction fluid. This is the only class of drug whose use is highest among eighth graders, the youngest group surveyed; 17% of eighth graders have tried some form of inhalant (Johnston et al, 2006).

Prescription Drugs

Medications that have clinical utility in some situations, such as the opioids, anxiolytics, and psychostimulants, also have potential for abuse and dependence. Among high-school seniors, lifetime misuse of opioid analgesics (e.g., oxycodone, hydrocodone) is 12.8%; sedatives (barbiturates), 10.5%; tranquilizers (e.g., clonazepam), 9.9%; and amphetamines (e.g., Dexedrine, mixed salt amphetamine), 13.1%. During the past 2 decades, an increase in the number of children being treated with stimulant medications (Safer et al, 1996) has been associated with an increase in the diversion, sale, and abuse of stimulants. Methylphenidate spansules can be ground up and then self-administered by nasal insufflation ("snorting") or injection. Like cocaine, this can potentially lead to sudden cardiac arrhythmia and death. Many youth misuse stimulant medications as "study pills" rather than to get high (Wilens et al, 2006). Children with attention-deficit/hyperactivity disorder (ADHD) are at increased risk for development of substance use disorders as they become adolescents and adults. However, appropriate treatment of ADHD with stimulant medications appears to be protective (Wilens et al, 2003). Because there is significant co-occurrence of ADHD and substance abuse, clinicians should regularly assess patients with ADHD for substance use and recommend adult supervision of stimulant medication storage and administration when treating high-risk youth. Because some teenagers consider drug use "cool" and appealing, over-the-counter stimulant medications (e.g., "stay-awake" pills or "diet pills") may also be misused.

RISK FACTORS

Genetic, familial, social, environmental, and characterologic factors have been found to influence the development and manifestation of substance use problems. Genetic predictors, found in both twin and adoption studies, suggest that alcohol use disorders are at least mildly inheritable, particularly from fathers to sons (Murray and Clifford, 1983). Parental use of alcohol or drugs or permissive attitudes about substance use have also been implicated in youth substance abuse (Patton, 1995). Socially, having substance-abusing friends is associated with increased likelihood of initiation of substance use (Freeland and Campbell, 1973). Peer influences do not predict the development of substance use problems or disorders (Patton, 1995). In fact, adolescents who use for social reasons are more likely to stop than are those who use for psychological reasons (Kandel and Raveis, 1989). Environmental risk factors for substance use disorders include deprivation and low socioeconomic status (Dusenbury and Botvin, 1992). Personality characteristics associated with substance abuse problems include low assertiveness, low self-esteem, low self-efficacy, low self-confidence, low social confidence, and external locus of control (Dusenbury and Botvin, 1992). Substance users also tend to have lower religiosity, higher identification with counterculture, higher impulsivity, higher anxiety, and stronger need for peer approval (Newcomb and Felix-Ortiz, 1992). However, the most powerful predictor of substance use disorders is younger age at first use. Those who begin drinking during the preteen years are four times more likely to develop alcohol dependence later in life compared with those who do not begin until college (Hingson et al, 2006).

ASSOCIATED PROBLEMS

Significant comorbidity exists between substance abuse and depression, bipolar disorder, ADHD, and antisocial behavior disorders (Bukstein et al, 1989). The use of alcohol and drugs is also associated with violence, weapon carrying, truancy, juvenile delinquency, and early sexual experimentation (DuRant et al, 1997, 1999). This last association is an important factor in the present epidemic of human immunodeficiency virus (HIV) infection and acquired immune deficiency syndrome (AIDS). Use of drugs increases the risk for HIV exposure by impairing judgment, increasing the likelihood of participating in sexual behavior, and reducing the likelihood of condom use (Friedman et al, 1993).

STAGES OF USE

According to the *Diagnostic and Statistical Manual for Primary Care, Child and Adolescent Version* (DSM-PC), substance use occurs on a continuum from the "developmental variation" of experimentation, through "substance use problems," to the disorders of abuse and dependence (Wolraich et al, 1996). A developmental model of substance use progression is described here and illustrated in Figure 45-1.

Abstinence is the stage at which adolescents have not yet begun to use any psychoactive substances. An initial trial of tobacco, alcohol, or other drugs defines the stage of *experimental use*. It is characterized by use of substances that are usually obtained from and used with friends. At this stage, intoxicants produce a mild euphoria with a return to baseline mood and feeling. The teenager thus experiences a good feeling without serious adverse consequences. However, experimentation can still be a hazardous activity for teens. They have insufficient experience to know their own limits or safe "doses" of alcohol and drugs. Urged on by their peers, they may rapidly consume toxic quantities without realizing the potential danger. They may put themselves and others at risk by participating in hazardous activities like operation of a motor vehicle.

Nonproblematic use is characterized by the intermittent, continuing use of alcohol or drugs in the absence of negative consequences. In adult drinkers, this may be referred to as social drinking. This term is misleading if

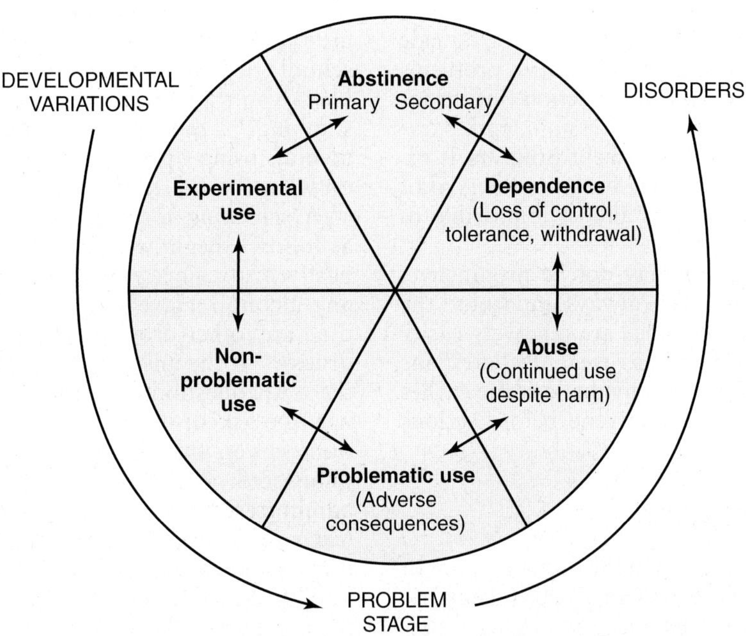

Figure 45-1. Adolescent drug and alcohol use: a developmental view.

it is applied to teenage drinking, however, as the typical "social" pattern is episodic heavy drinking. In addition to alcohol, most nonproblematic users tend to use marijuana and prescription drugs.

Problematic use is said to occur when adverse consequences develop as a result of use, even though the individual may not acknowledge that there is any causal link. Substance-related problems can include school failure, detentions, suspensions, problems with parent or peer relationships, motor vehicle accidents, other injuries, emergency department visits, physical or sexual assaults, and legal problems, among others. These are often accompanied by significant changes in dress, behavior, and peer group. At the problematic use stage, alcohol- or drug-induced euphoria may or may not be followed by return to baseline mood and feeling. There may be associated anxiety, discomfort, and guilt feelings and changes in both quantitative and qualitative aspects of their use (i.e., increased amounts, increased frequency, and increase in variety of substances used). At this stage, some individuals are still able to cut back or stop their use with limited intervention. Others progress to the disorders of abuse and dependence, which require more intensive intervention and treatment.

Substance abuse is a maladaptive pattern of substance use that causes impairment in social or school functioning, recurrent physical risk or legal problems, and continued use despite harm occurring during a 12-month period, with no diagnosis of dependence (American Psychiatric Association, 1994). *Substance dependence* is a disorder characterized by a maladaptive pattern of compulsive use, negative consequences, loss of control over use, preoccupation with use, and tolerance or withdrawal. *Tolerance* is the need to use more and more to get the usual effect. *Withdrawal* is feeling ill when substance use is stopped or a blocking agent is administered (e.g., naloxone). Tolerance and withdrawal symptoms can be physiologic, psychological, or both. Dependence is synonymous with *addiction,* characterized by constant use of substances when available, solitary use, disrupted family ties, and loss of outside supports. Significant medical and psychiatric problems may develop, including hepatic dysfunction, infectious diseases, overdoses, blackouts, depression, and paranoia. Referral to an intensive treatment program is often required. *Secondary abstinence* becomes the goal of treatment, as control over use is almost impossible to re-establish once it is lost.

All of these stages may or may not be progressive. Whereas appropriate diagnosis is always important, the disorders of abuse and dependence are relatively easier to recognize and more difficult to treat. Pediatricians should therefore try to identify individuals at the earlier stage of problematic use and intervene before serious harm results.

SCREENING AND ASSESSMENT

Screening for substance abuse should occur as part of routine adolescent medical care (Kulig, 2005). Pediatric clinicians should consider substance use when adolescents present with behavioral problems, school failure, or emotional distress. The most effective method of screening is a confidential history, taken without parents present in the room. Teenagers will reliably report use of alcohol and drugs if they are assured of confidentiality (Brener et al, 2002). They should be told that "anything you tell me will be kept confidential unless I think there is a risk to your safety, or someone else's safety. Should that happen, I will let you know, and you and I together will figure out how to tell your parents. I will not give information about you to someone else behind your back." The interview should begin with general questions about health and then progress to psychosocial functioning. The HEADS FIRST mnemonic (see Chapter 6) summarizes the areas that should be covered in all adolescent interviews.

Some clinicians may prefer to use a questionnaire for screening purposes, such as the Problem Oriented Screening Instrument for Teenagers (POSIT) (Rahdert, 1991). This is a 139-item yes or no questionnaire developed by the National Institute on Drug Abuse, written at a sixth-grade reading level, which includes 10 scales: alcohol and drug use, physical health, mental health, family relations, peer relations, educational status, vocational status, social skills, leisure/recreation, and aggressive behavior/delinquency. The POSIT has been found to have good reliability among adolescents in a medical office setting (Knight et al, 2001).

On beginning a substance use history, a "transitional" strategy in information gathering works best (Adger and Werner, 1996). Begin with questions about use of legitimate substances (i.e., prescribed and over-the-counter medications). Then progress to asking about those substance that are socially tolerated (tobacco, alcohol), to those that are socially disapproved of (marijuana), to those that are frankly illegal and socially proscribed (cocaine, heroin). With younger adolescents, a second transitional strategy involves moving from a general statement about use, to a question about use among school peers, to a question about friends' use, to a question about personal use. "I know that kids your age are often curious about cigarettes. Has anyone in your school tried smoking? How about any of your friends? Have you thought about it at all? Have you ever tried smoking?" The style of the interview should be nonjudgmental, using open-ended questions and concentrating on what the *effects* have been of alcohol or drug use.

A screening for substance abuse can be structured as follows. Begin with three *use* questions. "During the past year (or since your last clinic visit), have you drunk any alcohol? Have you smoked marijuana? Have you used any other drug to get high (including prescription drugs)?" If the answer to all three questions is no, only the CAR question from the CRAFFT screen (Fig. 45-2) need be asked; if the answer to any of the three questions is yes, the entire CRAFFT screen should be administered. The CRAFFT screen consists of six orally administered yes or no questions that are easy to score (each yes answer = 1). Key words in the test's six items form its mnemonic (CRAFFT).

The last CRAFFT question may be broken into several parts: "Have you gotten into any trouble recently?" and if the answer is yes, "Were you using

C	Have you ever ridden in a CAR driven by someone (including yourself) who was "high" or had been using alcohol or drugs?
R	Do you use alcohol or drugs to RELAX, change your mood, feel better about yourself, or fit in?
A	Do you ever use alcohol or drugs while you are by yourself ALONE?
F	Do your FAMILY or FRIENDS ever tell you that you should cut down on your drinking or drug use?
F	Do you ever FORGET things you did while using alcohol or drugs?
T	Have you ever gotten into TROUBLE while you were using alcohol or drugs?

Figure 45-2. CRAFFT questions. Two or more yes answers suggest a serious problem. *(Reprinted with permission, Children's Hospital Boston, 2007. All rights reserved. From Knight J, Shrier L, Bravender T, et al: A new brief screen for adolescent substance abuse. Arch Pediatr Adolesc Med 153:591-596, 1999; Knight JR, Sherritt L, Shrier LA, et al: Validity of the CRAFFT substance abuse screening test among adolescent clinic patients. Arch Pediatr Adolesc Med 156:607-614, 2002.)*

alcohol or drugs at the time?" and if the answer is yes again, "Do you think there could be a link between your alcohol or drug use and getting into that trouble?" Adolescents may not have yet made this association. Asking these questions in serial fashion elicits more information and also begins the process of intervention by increasing the adolescent's awareness of problems. A CRAFFT total score of 2 or higher has a sensitivity of 80% and a specificity of 86% for identifying substance abuse or dependence (Knight et al, 2002). A positive CRAFFT test result indicates a need for additional assessment.

The assessment interview with the adolescent should include a thorough alcohol and drug use history, including age at first use, current pattern of use (quantity and frequency), and impact on physical and emotional health, school, and family and negative consequences from use (e.g., legal problems). The assessment should also include a screening for co-occurring mental disorders, parent or sibling alcohol and drug use, and other risk behaviors such as illegal activities and sexual promiscuity (American Academy of Pediatrics, 1998). A parent interview may be included as part of a substance use assessment, although parents typically underestimate the severity of use of their teenage children (Fisher et al, 2006).

A complete physical examination should be performed, including a full set of vital signs. When performing the eye examination, be sure to note pupil size. Nasal mucosa should be examined for inflammation or erosion characteristic of drug insufflation (snorting). Liver and spleen should be carefully palpated. A skin examination may reveal needle marks, although this finding is quite uncommon in adolescents presenting for regular medical care. Abnormal breath sounds (e.g., wheezing) may be found in patients who are smoking tobacco, marijuana, cocaine, or heroin. Urine and serum toxicologic examinations are of limited usefulness and are generally less sensitive than a good history. Except in a true emergency, laboratory testing should not be performed without the knowledge and consent of the patient (American Academy of Pediatrics, 1996). Pediatric clinicians should avoid performing drug screens at the request of parents or legal authorities. They may order drug tests as an adjunct to outpatient treatment when the results will be available only to the patient and treatment team. Clinicians must be familiar with sensitivity and specificity (threshold values) for specific drugs and the different methods of testing. Urine specimens must be collected by direct observation or according to the Mandatory Guidelines for Federal Drug Testing Programs *(http://www.drugfreeworkplace.com)*. Urine specific gravity and creatinine level must always be determined because urine concentration directly affects the validity of the test. All positive screen results must be confirmed by gas chromatography and mass spectrometry. In general, serum half-lives of drugs of abuse are brief, and urine testing reflects drug use only within the last 48 hours. A notable exception is marijuana, whose active ingredient, Δ^9-tetrahydrocannabinol (THC), and its carboxylic acid metabolite may be detected in the urine for several weeks after discontinuation of daily use (Woolf and Shannon, 1995). Therefore, when drug testing for THC is being done as part of a treatment program, serial urine specimens must be sent out for *quantitative* THC and creatinine determinations. Abstinence is supported by a finding of serial decreases in the THC: creatinine ratio.

Adolescent patients may present with symptoms of acute or pathologic intoxication. Table 45-1 lists the signs and symptoms of intoxication or withdrawal and treatment options for common drugs of abuse. After the assessment, pediatric clinicians must make an initial determination of problem severity and need for treatment (Fig. 45-3).

Individuals who are experimental users or regular users do not necessarily need to be referred to mental health specialists. They are amenable to brief office interventions as described later. On the other hand, teenagers who seem likely to have a diagnosis of abuse or dependence should be referred to specialized treatment as soon as possible. Clinicians should also refer those who have signs or symptoms of a co-occurring mental disorder, such as major depression, bipolar disorder,

Table 45-1. Medical Management of Drug Intoxication and Withdrawal

Names and Preparations	Intoxication: Signs and Symptoms	Intoxication: Treatment	Withdrawal: Signs and Symptoms	Withdrawal: Treatment
Alcohol				
Beer Wine Hard liquor	*Mild-moderate:* ↓ level of consciousness, poor coordination, ataxia, nystagmus, conjunctival injection, slurred speech, orthostatic hypotension	Observation and supportive care, protect airway, position on side to avoid aspiration	*Mild-moderate:* restlessness, agitation, coarse tremor, ↑ sensitivity to sensory input, nausea, vomiting, anorexia, autonomic hyperactivity (tachycardia, hypertension, hyperthermia), anxiety or depression, headache, insomnia	Thiamine, 100 mg PO or IM daily Folate, 1 mg PO daily Multivitamins, 1 daily Benzodiazepine taper over 3-7 days (chlordiazepoxide, 25-50 mg q6h × 24 hr, then 25 mg q6h × 48 hr; or diazepam, clonazepam, oxazepam)
	Severe: respiratory depression, stupor, coma, death *Chronic:* pancreatitis and cirrhosis are rare in adolescents.	Ventilatory support, intensive care	*Severe:* seizures, hallucinations, delirium, death	Seizures: benzodiazepines (lorazepam, 0.1-0.2 mg/kg/dose IV or PR, repeat 0.05 mg/kg every 5 minutes if needed; usual maximum dose = 4 mg, but larger doses may be needed) Hallucinations: haloperidol
	Pathologic: belligerent, excited, combative, psychotic state (even after small amount in susceptible person)	Physical restraint Low-dose benzodiazepine (lorazepam, 1-5 mg PO as needed) or haloperidol, 1-5 mg q4-8h IM or 1-15 mg/dose PO		
Miscellaneous information: Alcohol is highly addictive, and withdrawal from it is associated with serious, potentially lethal side effects that begin 6 to 24 hours after the last drink. Alcohol dependence is rare in adolescents, however, but alcohol-related deaths are not. Adolescents tend to be binge drinkers and are at high risk for alcohol-related accidents and acute alcohol poisoning.				
Cannabis				
Marijuana *Pot, herb, grass, weed, reefer, dope, buds, sinsemilla, Thai sticks* THC capsules Hashish Hashish oil	*Acute:* euphoria, sensory stimulation, pupillary constriction, conjunctival injection, photophobia, nystagmus, diplopia, ↑appetite, autonomic dysfunction (tachycardia, hypertension, orthostatic hypotension), temporary bronchodilation	Reassurance and observation		
	Chronic: gynecomastia, reactive airway disease, ↓sperm count, weight gain, lethargy, amotivational syndrome	Discontinuation of use, symptomatic treatment and care (bronchodilators for wheezing)	*Chronic users:* mild irritability, agitation, insomnia, electroencephalographic changes	Reassurance Symptoms disappear in 3-4 days
	Pathologic: panic, delirium, psychosis, flashbacks	Psychosis: neuroleptic medication		
Miscellaneous information: Cannabis derivatives have low potential for causing physiologic withdrawal symptoms. These drugs are commonly used by adolescents, however, and are associated with adverse psychological effects, including tolerance and withdrawal. The potency of marijuana has greatly increased during the past 25 years.				

Hallucinogens				
Phencyclidine (PCP) *Angel dust, super grass, peace weed* Ketamine *Special K* Lysergic acid diethylamide (LSD) *Acid, blotters, orange sunshine, blue heaven, microdot, sugar cubes* Mescaline *Mesc* Peyote *Buttons, cactus* Psilocybin *Magic mushrooms, 'shrooms* Jimson weed *Locoweed* Nightshade	Acute: perceptual (visual, auditory) distortion and hallucinations, nystagmus, feelings of depersonalization, mild nausea, tremors, tachycardia, hypertension, hyperreflexia *Chronic:* flashbacks	Reassurance and observation For anticholinergics (i.e., Jimson weed, nightshade), symptoms are more severe and may require gastric lavage, benzodiazepine sedation, and hospitalization. Discontinuation of use	Psychological	Reassurance
	Pathologic: panic, paranoia, psychosis	Psychosis: close observation in a quiet room Benzodiazepines (lorazepam, 1-5 mg PO) Use of neuroleptic medication is controversial.		
Miscellaneous information: PCP may be sprinkled on marijuana and smoked. Exposure can thus occur without the user's knowledge.				
Inhalants				
Nitrous oxide *Laughing gas, whippets* Amyl nitrite *Poppers, snappers* Butyl nitrate *Rush, bullet, climax*	*Acute:* euphoria, disorientation, sedation, conjunctival injection; acute toxicity to central nervous system, liver, kidneys Nitrates: sudden hypoxemia, hypotension	Symptomatic medical treatments	Psychological Physiologic—unknown	Reassurance, support
Chlorohydrocarbons Aerosol spray cans Hydrocarbons Gasoline, glue, solvents, white-out (typewriter correction fluid)	*Chronic:* peripheral nerve, central nervous system, liver, and kidney damage Leaded gasoline (not in United States): plumbism	Discontinuation of use, supportive therapies (e.g., dialysis) Plumbism: chelation therapy		
	Pathologic: cardiac arrhythmia and arrest	Resuscitation, hospitalization		
Miscellaneous information: Nitrous oxide is sometimes sold at rock concerts inside balloons. Nitrate compounds have been most popular among gay men, allegedly to enhance sexual experiences. The volatile hydrocarbon compounds are favored by younger adolescents and popular in some Latin American countries, on Native American reservations, and in Latino communities within the United States.				
Stimulants				
Cocaine *Coke, snow, flake, blow, nose candy* Crack *Freebase, rocks* Amphetamines *Speed, black beauties*	*Acute:* exhilaration, euphoria, restlessness, irritability, insomnia, pupillary dilation, tachycardia, arrhythmia, chest pain, hypertension, anorexia, hyperpyrexia, hyperreflexia	Reassurance and observation Symptomatic care Agitation: high-dose benzodiazepines (diazepam, 10-25 mg) Tachycardia, hypertension (controversial; see below) Hyperthermia: external cooling		

(Continued)

Table 45-1 Medical Management of Drug Intoxication and Withdrawal—cont'd

Names and Preparations	Intoxication: Signs and Symptoms	Intoxication: Treatment	Withdrawal: Signs and Symptoms	Withdrawal: Treatment
Methamphetamine *Crank, crystal meth, ice* Methylphenidate (Ritalin) Pemoline (Cylert) Prescription diet pills Didrex, Tenuate, Ionamin, Sanorex, and others "Legal speed": over-the-counter diet or stay-awake pills	*Chronic:* (if snorting: inflamed nasal mucosa, septal erosion or perforation) confusion, sensory hallucinations, paranoia, depression *Pathologic:* sudden cardiac arrest, hypertensive crisis, seizures	Discontinuation of use, symptomatic treatment and care Psychosis: neuroleptic medication Resuscitation, hospitalization Hypertensive crisis: beta-blockers, phentolamine, nitroprusside Seizures: IV lorazepam (see alcohol section above) or phenytoin, 15-20 mg/kg slow IV push with cardiac monitor	*Chronic users:* severe depression with suicidal or homicidal ideation, exhaustion, prolonged sleep, voracious appetite	Close observation, reassurance Symptoms disappear in 3-4 days
Miscellaneous information: Whereas use of cocaine and crack has declined somewhat in recent years, amphetamines have become more popular. Methamphetamine is more commonly available in California, the West, and the Southwest. With the increased public awareness of ADHD and the popularity of stimulant medications to treat it, Ritalin has now become a drug of abuse among some adolescents. It can be ground up and "snorted" and has been implicated in several reports of sudden cardiac arrest and death. So-called legal speed, over-the-counter preparations that are available in pharmacies and through mail order houses, can cause toxic effects similar to those of more potent stimulants when taken in high doses.				
Depressants				
Benzodiazepines Valium, *V's,* Librium, Serax, Klonopin, Tranxene, Xanax, Halcion, Rohypnol, *ruffies* Barbiturates Nembutal, Seconal, Amytal, Tuinal, *downers, barbs, blue devils, red devils, yellows, yellow jackets* Methaqualone Quaaludes, *ludes, sopors*	*Mild-moderate:* central nervous system sedation, pupillary constriction, disorientation, slurred speech, staggering gait *Severe:* respiratory depression, hypothermia, coma, death *Pathologic:* paradoxical disinhibition, hyperexcitability	Observation and supportive care, protect airway, position on side to avoid aspiration Acute overdose: gastric lavage Supportive: ventilator, warming blanket, ICU care Symptoms pass in a matter of hours Physical restraint, low-dose benzodiazepine rarely needed	*Mild-moderate:* restlessness, anxiety, agitation, tremor, abdominal cramps, nausea, vomiting, hyperreflexia, hypertension, headache, insomnia *Severe:* seizures, delirium, hyperpyrexia, hallucinations, death	Gradual reduction of the drug of dependence, *or* Phenobarbital substitution (calculate phenobarbital equivalent of daily dose, or give 3-4 mg/kg/day ÷ q8h) with gradual taper, *or* Change short-acting benzodiazepine to longer acting benzodiazepine and then taper Seizures: lorazepam Hallucinations: haloperidol (see alcohol section above for doses)
Miscellaneous information: These compounds are all similar to alcohol in effect and highly addictive. Withdrawal symptoms are severe and may begin 12 to 16 hours after the last dose or may be delayed for up to a week.				

Narcotics				
Heroin *Smack, horse, junk, brown sugar, big H, mud* Opium Prescription narcotics Morphine, meperidine fentanyl, oxycodone (OxyContin, *OCs*), hydrocodone (Vicodin), codeine, propoxyphene (Darvon), and others	*Acute:* euphoria, pupillary constriction, depression of respirations and gag reflex, bradycardia, hypotension, constipation	Airway protection, judicious use of naloxone at repeated intervals		*Acute detoxification:* Methadone (PO) Children: 0.7 mg/kg/day ÷ q4-6h Adult: 30-40 mg/day in 3-4 divided doses, with 5 mg/day taper Clonidine (PO) Children: 5-7 μg/kg/day ÷ q6-12h (maximum dose = 0.9 mg/day) Adult: 0.1 mg test dose, check postural blood pressure; if stable, 0.1-0.2 mg PO q4-6h *Long-term treatment:* Long-term therapeutic support Methadone maintenance (specialized clinics only) or buprenorphine induction and maintenance (can be prescribed by physicians who complete 8 hours of training and acquire DEA waiver)
	Chronic: complications of IV use include hepatitis B, HIV/AIDS, subacute bacterial endocarditis, brain abscesses	Discontinuation of use, targeted medical care for infectious complications	*Chronic users:* restlessness, lacrimation, yawning, pupillary dilation, rhinorrhea, sniffing, sneezing, sweating, flushing, tachycardia, hypertension, muscle cramps, abdominal cramps, nausea, vomiting, diarrhea	
	Pathologic: acute overdose may cause respiratory arrest and death	Intubation and ventilation Naloxone (IV, IM, SC, ETT): Children < 20 kg: 0.1 mg/kg/dose q2-3h Children > 20 kg: 2-5 mg/dose		
Miscellaneous information: Individuals who abuse narcotics seldom seek treatment for intoxication. They are more often found semicomatose and brought to the hospital by friends or emergency medical services for treatment. In treating an overdose, remember that naloxone has a shorter duration of action than most narcotic drugs do, and doses therefore need to be repeated at fairly frequent intervals. These patients require lengthy periods of observation (12 to 24 hours) in the hospital.				
Designer Drugs				
Fentanyl analogues Synthetic heroin, *China White* Meperidine analogues *MPPP, MPTP*	Similar to narcotics (above)	Similar to narcotics (above)	Similar to narcotics (above)	Similar to narcotics (above)
Amphetamine analogues *MDMA, Ecstasy, Adam, EVE, STP, PMA, TMA, DOM, DOB, and others*	Similar to amphetamines (above)	Similar to amphetamines (above)	Similar to amphetamines (above)	Similar to amphetamines (above)
Miscellaneous information: More popular on the West Coast, designer drugs can be both stronger and cheaper than the parent compound. Quality is not controlled during illicit manufacturing, posing great danger to users. For example, MPTP, a contaminant of the meperidine analogue MPPP, causes irreversible Parkinson disease.				

ADHD, attention-deficit/hyperactivity disorder; DEA, Drug Enforcement Administration; ETT, via endotracheal tube; ICU, intensive care unit; SC, subcutaneous injection; THC, tetrahydrocannibinol.

References:
Barone MA (ed): The Harriet Lane Handbook, 14th ed. St. Louis, Mosby, 1996.
Chang G, Kosten TR: Emergency management of acute drug intoxication. *In* Lowinson JH, Ruiz P, Millman RB (eds): Substance Abuse: A Comprehensive Textbook. Baltimore, Williams & Wilkins, 1992.
Schonberg SK (ed): Guidelines for the Treatment of Alcohol- and Other Drug-Abusing Adolescents. Treatment Improvement Protocol Series 4. Rockville, MD, U.S. Department of Health and Human Services, Public Health Service, Substance Abuse and Mental Health Services Administration, Center for Substance Abuse Treatment, 1993. DHHS publication 93-2010.
Wesson D (ed): Detoxification from Alcohol and Other Drugs. Treatment Improvement Protocol Series 19. Rockville, MD, U.S. Department of Health and Human Services, Public Health Service, Substance Abuse and Mental Health Services Administration, Center for Substance Abuse Treatment, 1995. DHHS publication (SMA) 95-3046.

Acknowledgment: Michael Shannon, MD, MPH (Toxicology Program), and Brigid Vaughan, MD (Department of Psychiatry), at Children's Hospital, Boston, assisted with preparation of this table.

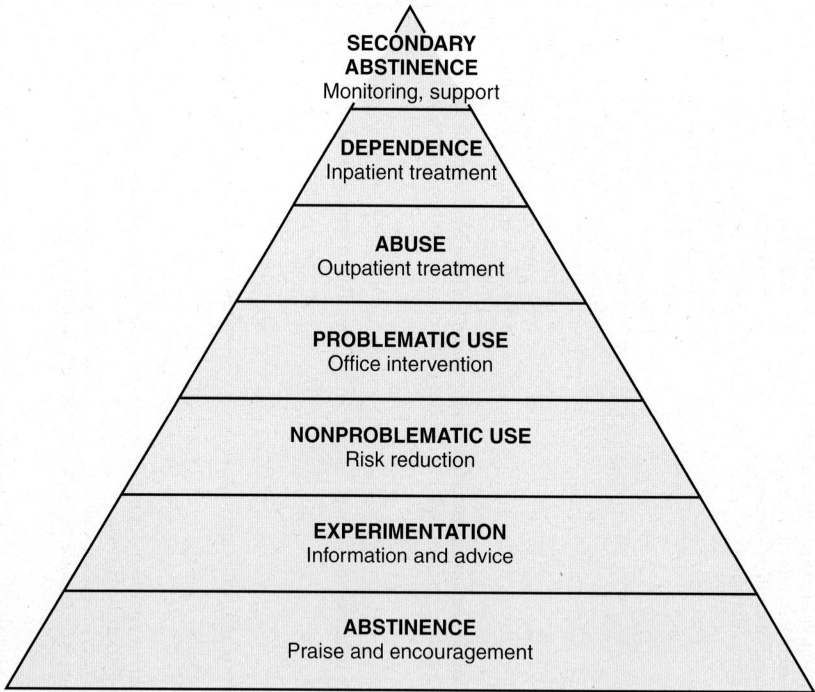

Figure 45-3. The substance use intervention pyramid.

bulimia, or ADHD. In all cases, the most important assessment has to do with the immediate safety of the patient. If it is at all in jeopardy, immediate admission to a hospital should be arranged.

BRIEF OFFICE INTERVENTION

Brief interventions involve less time than is associated with formal treatment programs, can be delivered by nonspecialists, emphasize self-help and self-management, reach large numbers of patients, and are considerably less expensive than conventional treatment (Heather, 1989). To be effective, an intervention for substance use must be appropriate to the stage of use. For abstinence, practitioners should offer praise and encouragement. Make a statement such as "I think it's great that you have decided to stay away from trying cigarettes, alcohol, or other drugs. That's a very intelligent choice. I'm really proud of you. I also want you to know that I understand how tempting it can be for teens to try them, and so I still plan to ask you about this again on your next visit. If things ever change, I hope you'll trust me enough to talk with me about it. My only concern is for your health." For the stages of experimentation and nonproblematic use, the intervention should be aimed at reducing risk, such as that associated with driving after drinking or riding with an intoxicated driver. One approach, the Contract for Life *(http://www.sadd.org/contract.htm)*, is an agreement between teens and their parents. The teen promises not to drive after drinking or to accept an unsafe ride; the parents promise to provide safe transportation any time, day or night, if their teenager calls and to defer a discussion of the circumstances until later. Adolescents who have progressed to the stages of problematic use or abuse may be amenable to outpatient counseling based on cognitive-behavioral therapy of motivational enhancement (Kadden et al, 1994; Miller and Rollnick, 2002). Those with dependence likely will require more intensive treatment, including detoxification, residential rehabilitation, or day hospital programs.

A useful model for understanding behavior change is illustrated in Figure 45-4 (Prochaska et al, 1994). *Precontemplation* is a precursor to the process of change. The individual at this stage has not yet begun to consider change as an option. His or her problems are attributed to misfortune, misunderstanding, or other external forces. Defensive thinking is prominent and may be manifested as denial, minimization, projection, rationalization, justification, or blaming of others. *Contemplation* is heralded by consideration on the part of the individual that he or she may indeed have a problem. The pros and cons of changing behavior are being weighed. Individuals are ambivalent about changing problem behaviors. *Determination* is characterized by making a clear decision to change. At this stage, the mind has changed but the behavior has not. A quit date may be set or a plan made to get help. *Action* is defined by evidence of actual change in behavior. It takes a while for the individual to feel comfortable with the new behavior. He or she may struggle with urges to resume the use of alcohol or drugs. When the new behavior becomes learned enough to be automatic, the individual is said to be in *maintenance,* which may lead to either a permanent exit *(termination)* from the change cycle or *relapse* and entry into another cycle. Relapse is part of the early recovery process, and patients should not be stigmatized or abandoned when one occurs. The relapse should be viewed as a learning experience. Supports and treatments should be reviewed and increased.

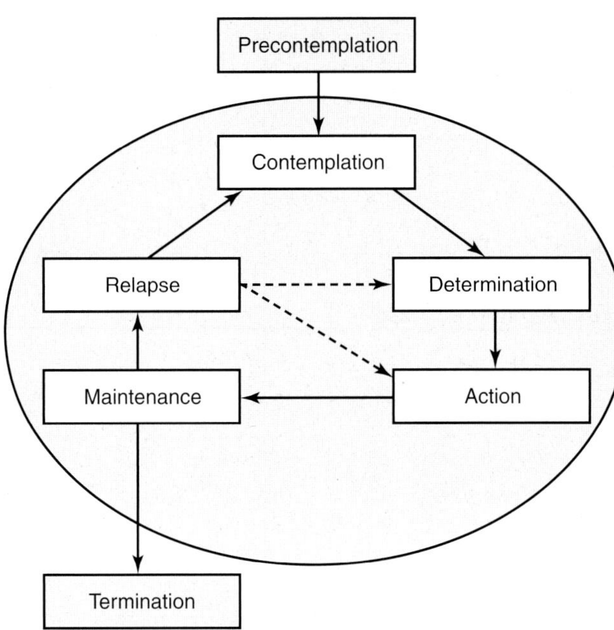

Figure 45-4. Stages of change. *(From Prochaska JO, DiClemente CC: Transtheoretical therapy: Toward a more integrative model of change. Psychotherapy 19:276-288, 1982; Prochaska JO, Velicer WF, Rossi JS, et al: Stages of change and decisional balance for 12 problem behaviors. Health Psychol 13:39-46, 1994; Prochaska JO: Strong and weak principles for progressing from precontemplation to action on the basis of twelve problem behaviors. Health Psychol 13:47-51, 1994.)*

According to stages of change theory, the goal of any single patient encounter is to facilitate movement of the patient from any one stage to the next (Miller and Rollnick, 2002). For individuals at the precontemplation stage, the clinician should try to raise doubt and increase the awareness of risks and problems. This may be done by skillful questioning ("Have you ever considered that you might not have gotten suspended from school if you hadn't been smoking pot?") or by simple delivery of information ("Are you aware that car accidents, particularly those caused by drinking, are the number one cause of death for young people your age?"). For those in contemplation, the clinician should acknowledge the ambivalence ("So it sounds like part of you wants to stop and part of you wants to keep on drinking."), try to evoke reasons to change, and then tip the balance in favor of change. Once determination is reached, the goal of the intervention is to help the adolescent find the best course of action. This is done by listing treatment options, making an appropriate referral, and following up. During maintenance, the clinician should offer positive reinforcement and discuss relapse prevention strategies. The content of an effective brief intervention statement is summarized in the FRAMES mnemonic, illustrated in Figure 45-5 (Miller and Sanchez, 1994).

The clinician should begin with feedback concerning problem or risk behavior by listing the facts, stated in the patient's own words. Facts are less likely to lead to arguments than interpretations or diagnoses are. Emphasize that the patient is the one who is responsible for changing his or her behavior. Advice should be clear, with an emphasis on stopping alcohol and drug use completely. When the teenager is unwilling to stop, a menu of options including cutting down and risk reduction should be offered. Further choices involve options for formal treatment, including referral to counseling, 12-step support groups, and intensive treatment programs. The clinician must project an attitude of empathy and faith in the patient's ability to make the necessary change (self-efficacy). Clinicians should avoid attempts to pressure the patient, as this may only lead to increased resistance to change. It is better to try to elicit self-motivational statements from the adolescent ("How might you imagine your life could improve if you gave up using drugs?") and then summarize and support those statements that favor change. Most important of all, the clinician must establish and maintain a supportive relationship with the adolescent. The relationship needs to be firm, consistent, and nonrejecting. A written behavior change contract is a useful adjunct to office intervention. One example is the Change Plan Worksheet illustrated in Figure 45-6 (Miller et al, 1994). In the example shown, the young person has contracted to stop using alcohol and drugs and to enter a formal treatment program if unable to follow through.

F	**FEEDBACK** on personal risk or impairment
R	Emphasis on personal **RESPONSIBILITY** for change
A	Clear **ADVICE** to change
M	A **MENU** of alternative change options
E	Therapist **EMPATHY**
S	Facilitation of client **SELF-EFFICACY** or optimism

Figure 45-5. The FRAMES mnemonic. *(From Miller WR, Zweben A, DiClemente CC, Rychtarik RG: Motivational Enhancement Therapy Manual: A Clinical Research Guide for Therapists Treating Individuals with Alcohol Abuse and Dependence. Rockville, MD, National Institute on Alcohol Abuse and Alcoholism, 1994.)*

TREATMENT

Pediatric clinicians should be familiar with treatment resources in their own communities. Programs vary in both intensity and philosophy, but complete abstinence from alcohol and drugs is the primary goal. In general, treatment programs fall into one of the following categories: detoxification, replacement therapy, residential treatment, and outpatient treatment.

Detoxification programs are relatively short-term inpatient programs whose goal is the medical management of physiologic withdrawal symptoms (outpatient detoxification is now more widely available). Traditionally, these programs have concentrated on alcohol dependence because alcohol withdrawal symptoms can be life-threatening. Detoxification is also appropriate for individuals who are addicted to sedatives, barbiturates, heroin, and other opioids. Many teenagers do not require detoxification because physiologic dependence is less common in this age group. In those cases in which it is necessary, detoxification should be viewed as a first step in treatment and always followed by long-term counseling and support.

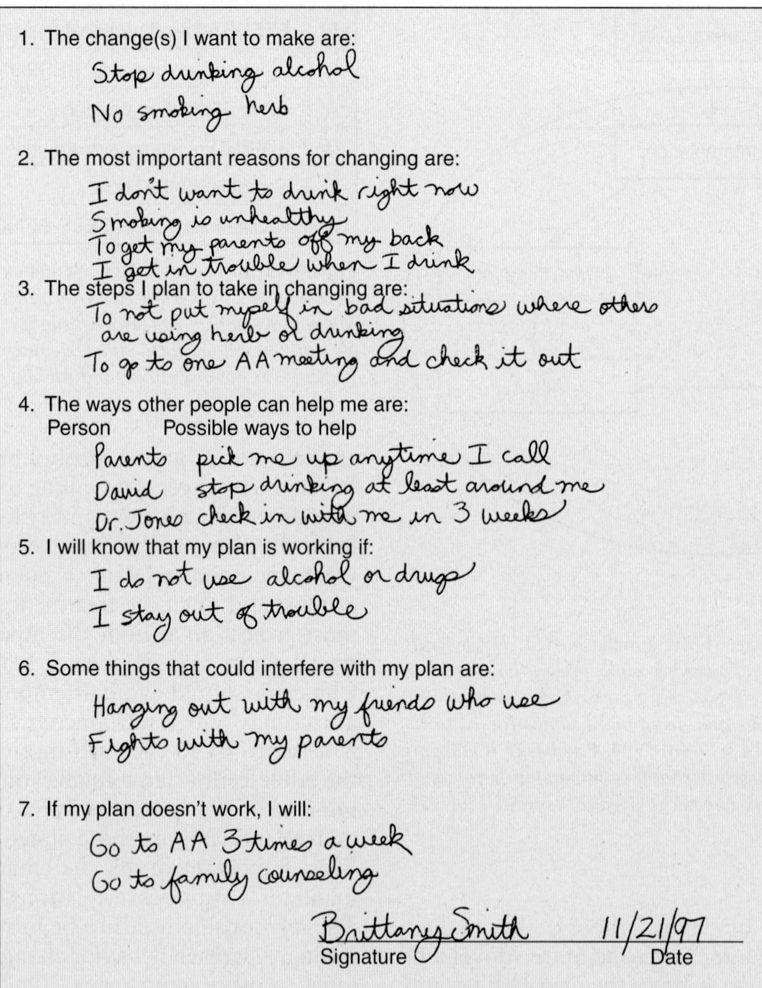

1. The change(s) I want to make are:
   Stop drinking alcohol
   No smoking herb
2. The most important reasons for changing are:
   I don't want to drink right now
   Smoking is unhealthy
   To get my parents off my back
   I get in trouble when I drink
3. The steps I plan to take in changing are:
   To not put myself in bad situations where others are using herb or drinking
   To go to one AA meeting and check it out
4. The ways other people can help me are:

Person	Possible ways to help
Parents	pick me up anytime I call
David	stop drinking at least around me
Dr. Jones	check in with me in 3 weeks

5. I will know that my plan is working if:
   I do not use alcohol or drugs
   I stay out of trouble
6. Some things that could interfere with my plan are:
   Hanging out with my friends who use
   Fights with my parents
7. If my plan doesn't work, I will:
   Go to AA 3 times a week
   Go to family counseling

Brittany Smith 11/21/97
Signature Date

Figure 45-6. Change plan worksheet.

Replacement therapy, such as methadone or buprenorphine maintenance, may be the treatment of choice for narcotics (i.e., oxycodone, heroin) addiction. Methadone is a synthetic opioid drug and full mu-receptor opioid agonist that in therapeutic doses does not produce euphoria and also blocks the euphoric effect of other narcotics. Buprenorphine is a partial mu-receptor opioid agonist that works in similar fashion to methadone but has a more favorable side effect profile (e.g., less drowsiness) and can be prescribed by physicians who receive 8 hours of training and obtain a special waiver from the Drug Enforcement Administration (information available online at *http://www.buprenorphine.samhsa.gov/*).

Methadone can be dispensed only in specially licensed clinics, which has limited its usefulness. Replacement therapy is most effective when it is combined with outpatient counseling, group therapy, educational and vocational assistance, and psychosocial support.

Residential treatment programs saw a rapid rise in popularity during the 1970s and 1980s. They were intensive, highly structured, month-long programs run by medical providers, counselors, psychologists, and family therapists. In recent years, many of these programs were closed as managed care entities became reluctant to fund this relatively expensive form of treatment. These programs tend to be long term (6 to 12 months), highly structured, founded on self-help or 12-step principles, and often staffed by recovering addicts. A present-day example of this type of treatment is Phoenix House. Other residential programs are designed to remove the adolescent substance abuser from his or her environment (e.g., wilderness programs) but have not been scientifically evaluated. All of these residential treatment programs are best reserved for those teenagers for whom outpatient treatment has failed or who have a high degree of antisocial behavior associated with their substance use.

Outpatient treatment is a useful first option. Most adolescents who receive substance abuse treatment receive it in an outpatient setting. Treatment settings can vary from structured hospital-based day treatment to varying combinations of individual counseling, family therapy, group therapy, cognitive-behavioral therapy, hypnosis, biofeedback, acupuncture, random drug testing, and self-help groups. Teenagers should be referred to programs that specialize in people their own age. Group therapy is a component of virtually all treatment programs, and adolescents do not relate well to groups of older adults. For those adolescents at the problematic use–abuse end of the spectrum, simple outpatient counseling by a mental health professional specially trained in adolescent substance use may be sufficient.

C	Have you ever felt you should **CUT DOWN** on your drinking?
A	Have people **ANNOYED** you by criticizing your drinking?
G	Do you ever feel bad or **GUILTY** about your drinking?
E	Do you ever have a drink first thing in the morning **(EYE-OPENER)** to steady your nerves or get rid of a hangover?

Figure 45-7. The CAGE questions. A positive screen is two or more yes answers. *(From Bush B, Shaw S, Cleary P, et al: Screening for alcohol abuse using the CAGE questionnaire. Am J Med 82:231-235, 1987; Ewing JA: Detecting alcoholism: The CAGE questionnaire. JAMA 252:1905-1907, 1984.)*

Referral to 12-step support groups, like Alcoholics Anonymous or Narcotics Anonymous, may also be useful. Clinicians can obtain a "meeting list" from one or both of these fellowships and should become familiar with its use. Contact can be made with recovering volunteers by calling the number listed in the telephone directory. These volunteers are usually happy to recommend specific meetings in the local area that are appropriate for young people and may often volunteer to bring the patient to a meeting and introduce the individual to the group. Twelve-step groups are developmentally challenging for adolescents and will often not work without an interested recovering person who acts as initial liaison or "temporary sponsor." Participation in 12-step fellowships is associated with improved abstinence after treatment (Kelly et al, 2002).

The clinician must continue to support adolescents who are in treatment. Follow-up visits should be scheduled at regular intervals. Find out what the components of treatment are or what goes on in 12-step groups. Then check with the adolescent at each visit to see how things are going and offer encouragement and support. "So tell me, have you joined an AA group? Have you found a sponsor yet? Which of the 12 steps are you working on now?" Never hesitate to tell a recovering adolescent how proud you are of him or her. The process of recovery is a difficult one for all individuals and poses special challenges (e.g., changing friends, accepting that they have a "chronic" disease) during the teenage years.

Family members should be encouraged to participate in treatment with their child. They may need to receive counseling themselves and may also benefit from self-help groups like Al-Anon. Whereas parents should not become overly restrictive, they must be encouraged to adopt a firm, yet reasonable, stance. In the most severe cases, they may need the support of the clinician in taking a very difficult position (i.e., informing a teenager who continues to use that he or she must either go into treatment or find another place to live). On occasion, clinicians will encounter parents who are either unwilling or unable to assist in treatment. For example, they may refuse to eliminate alcohol or other drugs from the house, often because they have a substance use problem of their own.

SUBSTANCE-ABUSING PARENTS

It has been estimated that there are 11 million children and adolescents in the United States who have an alcoholic parent, or one of every eight children (MacDonald and Blume, 1986). Clinicians should routinely ask about parental use of alcohol and drugs during office visits. Particular vigilance is called for when seeing children in the medical clinic with chronic vague complaints or when they present to school function clinics or mental health programs. Children of alcoholics have long been known to be at risk for serious medical problems, such as fetal alcohol syndrome and fetal alcohol effect (Jones et al, 1973). Having an alcoholic parent is associated with higher health care costs and a host of medical problems including sleep disturbance, gastrointestinal problems, musculoskeletal complaints, vascular and migraine headaches, chronic fatigue, decreased appetite, and other problems (Emshoff and Price, 1997). Having an alcoholic parent also places a child at higher risk for becoming a substance abuser later in life (Smart and Fejer, 1972). It is also associated with mental health problems such as ADHD, anxiety disorder, depression, and conduct disorder (Earls et al, 1988). School problems are also common among children of alcoholics. They are more likely to have language-based learning difficulties, poor attention, behavioral problems, suspensions, truancy, absenteeism, and grade retention; and yet they are less likely to receive special educational services than are other children with special needs (Emshoff and Price, 1997). Within the family, parental abuse of alcohol is associated with increased family violence, separation and divorce, parental absence, poverty, and child abuse and neglect (Johnson and Leff, 1997). In addition, children of drug-addicted parents are susceptible to special problems, which include passive exposure to smoked drugs and chemicals used to manufacture drugs and the more severe problem of congenital HIV infection and AIDS. Children of drug abusers also are exposed to chaos within the home, often due to illegal activity surrounding the acquisition, sale, and use of illicit substances. Despite all these risks, studies have been inconsistent in identifying personality characteristics of children from substance-abusing families (Johnson and Leff, 1997). Clinicians should avoid labeling them and always consider relative strengths and weaknesses within the child and the home.

The CAGE questions, shown in Figure 45-7, are a useful screening tool. A yes answer to two or more questions is highly predictive of a diagnosis of alcohol abuse or dependence (Bush et al, 1987). The pediatric clinician should explain a positive result, share his or her concern, and suggest that the parent go for a formal substance abuse evaluation. If a child is at significant risk, clinicians must insist on an evaluation. Figure 45-8 lists the essential components of an intervention with parents.

F Give parents a listing of the **FACTS** that have led to your concern.

R Explain that you are legally **REQUIRED TO REPORT**.

A Have **ANOTHER PERSON** present. There is strength in numbers, and this will help avoid later confusion about exactly what was said or recommended.

M The intervention should be a series of **MONOLOGUE**s, not a discussion or debate. If interrupted, ask the parents to please let you finish; you will then be happy to listen to them without interrupting.

E Referring the parents for formal EVALUATION is the goal of the intervention. Avoid giving a diagnosis of substance use or abuse, which will lead to arguments.

R If the individual is acutely intoxicated, arrange for a RIDE. Do not allow him or her to drive. Insist that you receive a REPORT BACK from the evaluation. This will let you know it has been done and help you better care for the child.

Figure 45-8. Principles of effective intervention with parents. *(From Wilson CR, Knight JR: When parents have a drinking problem. Contemp Pediatr 18:67-79, 2001.)*

After such an intervention, clinicians should not avoid future contact with the parent. Remember that parents so affected are sick people rather than bad people. When at all possible, this view should be communicated to the children. They should be told that their parent's disease is not their fault, and its "cure" is not their responsibility. Individual and family counseling is needed, and a referral to child-centered support groups (i.e., Alateen, Alatot) may be helpful.

SUMMARY

Substance use and misuse is a leading cause of morbidity and mortality for adolescents in the United States. Pediatric clinicians should routinely screen all teenagers and view use of alcohol and drugs on a spectrum from the high-prevalence, low-severity phenomenon of experimentation through the low-prevalence, high-severity disorders of abuse and dependence. For low-severity cases, brief office interventions are appropriate. Once a teenager has progressed to abuse or dependence, referral to specialty treatment is needed. Clinicians should be familiar with treatment resources in the local community and provide follow-up during the process of recovery. More research is needed on what constitutes effective treatment. All health care providers should also be aware that children may be affected by substance use and misuse on the part of their parents. Questions about parental use of alcohol and drugs should be part of a family screening. When problems are identified, clinicians should refer parents to adult mental health professionals for formal evaluation and treatment and insist on being a part of continuing family health care.

REFERENCES

Adger H, Werner MJ: The pediatrician. Am J Addict 5(4):s20-s29, 1996.

American Academy of Pediatrics: Testing for drugs of abuse in children and adolescents. Pediatrics 98(2):305-307, 1996.

American Academy of Pediatrics: Tobacco, alcohol, and other drugs: The role of the pediatrician in prevention and management of substance abuse. Pediatrics 101(1):125-128, 1998.

American Psychiatric Association: Diagnostic and Statistical Manual of Mental Disorders, 4th ed. Washington, DC, American Psychiatric Association, 1994.

Bandura A: Social Learning Theory. Englewood Cliffs, NJ, Prentice-Hall, 1977.

Brener ND, Kann L, McManus T, et al: Reliability of the 1999 youth risk behavior survey questionnaire. J Adolesc Health 31(4):336-342, 2002.

Bukstein OG, Brent DA, Kaminer Y: Comorbidity of substance abuse and other psychiatric disorders in adolescents. Am J Psychiatry 146(9):1131-1141, 1989.

Bush B, Shaw S, Cleary P, et al: Screening for alcohol abuse using the CAGE questionnaire. Am J Med 82:231-235, 1987.

Durant RH, Knight J, Goodman E: Factors associated with aggressive and delinquent behaviors among patients attending an adolescent medicine clinic. J Adolesc Health 21(5):303-308, 1997.

DuRant RH, Smith JA, Kreiter SR, Krowchuk DP: The relationship between early age of onset of initial substance use and engaging in multiple health risk behaviors among young adolescents. Arch Pediatr Adolesc Med 153(3):286-291, 1999.

Dusenbury L, Botvin GJ: Substance abuse prevention: Competence enhancement and the development of positive life options. J Addict Dis 11(3):29-45, 1992.

Earls F, Reich W, Jung KG, Cloninger CR: Psychopathology in children of alcoholic and antisocial parents. Alcohol Clin Exp Res 12(4):481-487, 1988.

Eaton DK, Kann L, Kinchen S, et al: Youth risk behavior surveillance—United States, 2005. MMWR Surveill Summ 55(5):1-108, 2006.

Emshoff J, Price A: Prevention and intervention options for children of alcoholics. Monograph presented at meeting on Core Competencies for Involvement of Health Care Professionals in the Care of Children and Adolescents in Families Affected by Substance Abuse. Washington, DC, Office of National Drug Control Policy, 1997.

Epps RP, Manley MW, Glynn TJ: Tobacco use among adolescents. Pediatr Clin North Am 42(2):389-402, 1995.

Fisher SL, Bucholz KK, Reich W, et al: Teenagers are right—parents do not know much: An analysis of adolescent-parent agreement on reports of adolescent substance use, abuse, and dependence. Alcohol Clin Exp Res 30(10):1699-1710, 2006.

Freeland JB, Campbell RS: The social context of first marijuana use. Int J Addict 8:317-334, 1973.

Friedman LS, Strunin L, Hingson R: A survey of attitudes, knowledge, and behavior related to HIV testing of adolescents and young adults enrolled in alcohol and drug treatment. J Adolesc Health 14(6):442-445, 1993.

Heather N: Psychology and brief interventions. Br J Addict 84(4): 357-370, 1989.

Hingson RW, Heeren T, Winter MR: Age at drinking onset and alcohol dependence: Age at onset, duration, and severity. Arch Pediatr Adolesc Med 160(7):739-746, 2006.

Jacobsen LK, Mencl WE, Westerveld M, Pugh KR: Impact of cannabis use on brain function in adolescents. Ann N Y Acad Sci 1021: 384-390, 2004.

Jessor R, Jessor SL: Problem Behavior and Psychosocial Development. New York, Academic Press, 1977.

Johnson JL, Leff M: Overview of the Research on Children of Substance Abusers. Core Competencies for Involvement of Health Care Professionals in the Care of Children and Adolescents in Families Affected by Substance Abuse, Executive Office of National Drug Control Policy, Washington, DC, 1997.

Johnston LD, O'Malley PM, Bachman JG, Schulenberg JE: Monitoring the Future National Results on Adolescent Drug Use: Overview of Key Findings, 2005. Bethesda, MD, National Institute on Drug Abuse, 2006. NIH Publication 06-5882.

Jones KL, Smith DW, Ulleland CN, Streissguth P: Pattern of malformation in offspring of chronic alcoholic mothers. Lancet 1:1267-1271, 1973.

Kadden R, Carroll K, Donovan D, et al: Cognitive-Behavioral Coping Skills Therapy Manual: A Clinical Research Guide for Therapists Treating Individuals with Alcohol Abuse and Dependence. Rockville, MD, National Institute on Alcohol Abuse and Alcoholism, 1994.

Kandel D, Raveis V: Cessation of illicit drug use in young adulthood. Arch Gen Psychiatry 46(2):109-116, 1989.

Kelly JF, Myers MG, Brown SA: Do adolescents affiliate with 12-step groups? A multivariate process model of effects. J Stud Alcohol 63(3):293-304, 2002.

Knight JR, Goodman E, Pulerwitz T, DuRant RH: Reliability of the Problem Oriented Screening Instrument for Teenagers (POSIT) in an adolescent medical clinic population. J Adolesc Health 29(2):125-130, 2001.

Knight JR, Sherritt L, Shrier LA, et al: Validity of the CRAFFT substance abuse screening test among adolescent clinic patients. Arch Pediatr Adolesc Med 156:607-614, 2002.

Kulig JW: Tobacco, alcohol, and other drugs: The role of the pediatrician in prevention, identification, and management of substance abuse. Pediatrics 115(3):816-821, 2005.

MacDonald D, Blume S: Children of alcoholics. Am J Dis Child 140(8):750-754, 1986.

Miller W, Sanchez V: Motivating young adults for treatment and lifestyle change. *In* Howard G, Nathan P (eds): Issues in Alcohol Use and Misuse by Young Adults. Notre Dame, IN, University of Notre Dame Press, 1994, pp 51-81.

Miller WR, Rollnick S: Motivational Interviewing: Preparing People for Change, 2nd ed. New York, Guilford, 2002.

Miller WR, Zweben A, DiClemente CC, Rychtarik RG: Motivational Enhancement Therapy Manual: A Clinical Research Guide for Therapists Treating Individuals with Alcohol Abuse and Dependence. Rockville, MD, National Institute on Alcohol Abuse and Alcoholism, 1994.

Murray RM, Clifford CA, Gurling HMD: Twin and adoption studies: How good is the evidence for a genetic role? *In* Galanter M (ed): Recent Developments in Alcoholism, Vol. I. New York, Plenum, 1983, pp 25-48.

OSC1: Traffic Safety Facts: 2005 Data. Washington, DC, National Center for Statistics and Analysis, 2006. Available at: http://www-nrd.nhtsa.dot.gov/pdf/nrd-30/NCSA/TSF2005/AlcoholTSF05.pdf. Accessed October 18, 2004.

Newcomb MD, Felix-Ortiz M: Multiple protective and risk factors for drug use and abuse: Cross-sectional and prospective findings. J Pers Soc Psychol 63(2):280-296, 1992.

Offer D, Schonert-Reichl K: Debunking the myths of adolescence: Findings from recent research. J Am Acad Child Adolesc Psychiatry 31(6):1003-1013, 1992.

Patton L: Adolescent substance abuse: Risk factors and protective factors. Pediatr Clin North Am 42(2):283-293, 1995.

Petersen A, Leffert N: Developmental issues influencing guidelines for adolescent health research: A review. J Adolesc Health 17:298-305, 1995.

Piaget J, Inhelder B: The Growth of Logical Thinking from Childhood to Adolescence. New York, Basic Books, 1958.

Prochaska JO, Velicer WF, Rossi JS, et al: Stages of change and decisional balance for 12 problem behaviors. Health Psychol 13(1):39-46, 1994.

Rahdert ER (ed): The Adolescent Assessment/Referral System Manual. Rockville, MD, U.S. Department of Health and Human Services, Public Health Service, Alcohol, Drug Abuse, and Mental Health Administration, 1991.

Safer DJ, Zito JM, Fine EM: Increased methylphenidate usage for attention deficit disorder in the 1990s. Pediatrics 98(6):1084-1088, 1996.

Smart R, Fejer D: Drug abuse among adolescents and their parents: Closing the generation gap in mood modification. J Abnorm Psychiatry 79:153-160, 1972.

Wilens TE, Faraone SV, Biederman J, Gunawardene S: Does stimulant therapy of attention-deficit/hyperactivity disorder beget later substance abuse? A meta-analytic review of the literature. Pediatrics 111(1):179-185, 2003.

Wilens TE, Gignac M, Swezey A, et al: Characteristics of adolescents and young adults with ADHD who divert or misuse their prescribed medications. J Am Acad Child Adolesc Psychiatry 45(4):408-414, 2006.

Wolraich ML, Felice ME, Drotar D (eds): The Classification of Child and Adolescent Mental Diagnoses in Primary Care (DSM-PC). Elk Grove Village, IL, American Academy of Pediatrics, 1996.

Woolf AD, Shannon MW: Clinical toxicology for the pediatrician. Pediatr Clin North Am 42(2):317-333, 1995.

46 SELF-CONTROL AND SELF-REGULATION: NORMAL DEVELOPMENT TO CLINICAL CONDITIONS

KAREN OLNESS

Vignettes

Ben, age 32 months, hears his mother say that there is ice cream for dessert. He immediately says, "I want ice cream." He is told that he may have ice cream after he finishes his spaghetti. He jumps off his chair and throws himself on the floor, shouting that he wants ice cream now.

Sarah, age 9 years, is seated at the dinner table with her parents and siblings. Family conversation is animated and cheerful. Sarah is glum. After poking at her food for a few minutes, she leaves the table, saying she has to study for her math test. An 11-year-old brother says, "What are you worried about? It's only a fourth-grade math test." Sarah begins to cry and runs to her room.

David, age 44 years, is 5 feet 10 inches tall and has weighed more than 260 pounds for the past 20 years. His cholesterol level is 250 mg. His family physician has helped him develop a plan to lose weight, which includes exercise and careful attention to food choices. David finished a low-fat dinner and followed this with a 2-mile walk. Now he is watching television and thinks that a dish of ice cream would really taste good. He heads for the freezer.

These vignettes are typical American scenes, but there are daily challenges to self-regulation in every culture, every school, every work, and every social situation. The behavior of 32-month-old Ben is "normal" for his developmental stage. The frustration of his parents' reasonable requirement that he finish dinner before eating dessert overwhelms his ability to regulate his emotions. Sarah is manifesting test anxiety, a common problem among children and adolescents. She may be well prepared for the test, but she is unable to control her fears that the exam is too difficult for her. The challenge to David's self-control is one that is familiar to a majority of Americans, whether the temptation is chips or cookies or ice cream or beer.

The extent to which self-control and self-regulation are developed throughout childhood and adolescence predicts much of life's success and happiness. Humans must learn to regulate motor, physiologic, thinking, and emotional responses. How they accomplish self-control affects day-to-day activities such as eating, toileting, speaking, sleeping, and dressing in early years and more complex activities such as driving, negotiating interpersonal conflict, participating in sports, playing a musical instrument, working, taking personal responsibility for health, and parenting as life proceeds. The ability to control impulses and to modulate responses relates to how well individuals cope with both expected and unexpected events (see Chapter 50), how they master new tasks, and their social competency (see Chapter 38). Whereas most professionals think about self-control and self-regulation in terms of emotional regulation, there are relationships among all types of self-regulation. Success or failure in achieving control of motor or physiologic responses may affect emotional regulation and vice versa.

Good self-control in adults is associated with skills in executive functions, which in turn favorably affects outcomes in many areas of life. Executive functions are self-regulatory or control functions that organize and direct all cognitive, behavioral, and emotional activity. Executive functions include the ability to select relevant task goals, to plan and organize the means to solve complex problems, to inhibit potent or practiced responses when appropriate, to shift problem solving strategies flexibly, and to monitor and evaluate one's own behavior. High executive function is associated with success in many areas of life. The loss of executive function, as well as the loss of important motor functions, affects many humans in their seventh and eighth decades, leading to the requirement for assistance by others. Adolescents who never develop normal executive function may require assistance throughout their lives.

Self-efficacy, the perception that one can accomplish specific goals or tasks, is also highly relevant to self-control and self-regulation. For example, adolescents who are successful in diabetes self-management also have high self-efficacy (Ianotti et al, 2006). A child or adolescent who perceives that he or she is not in control or unable to cope with a specific problem may become anxious or depressed. Paradoxically, some children with unrealistic self-confidence, leading to risk-taking behaviors, may demonstrate poor self-control in both home and school.

NORMAL DEVELOPMENT OF SELF-CONTROL AND SELF-REGULATION

Many of the antecedents of normal self-regulation are present during brain development in the human fetus. The bulk of neurons are produced prenatally, and pruning occurs postnatally. Normal neuron cell migration occurs between 5 to 6 and 25 to 26 weeks of gestation, and errors in this migration will result in brain abnormalities, which can adversely affect many functions.

After birth, the most obvious self-control process begins in motor areas. Myelination of long tracts occurs rapidly in the first year of life as control of motor development proceeds from head to feet. A normal infant develops control of arms before legs and gradually demonstrates accuracy in reaching, grasping, transferring, and manipulating. By a year of age, the infant has control of the fine pincer grasp, and this is about the time that infants have sufficient control of legs to begin to walk. The sequence of gross motor and fine motor development has been well documented, and delays in expected motor control can be easily recognized through careful observation and neurologic examinations (Brazelton, 1973).

Essential to self-control of thinking, including information processing and memory, is normal brain development. By 1 year, myelination of all regions of the corpus callosum is under way, and this is essential for increased speed of information processing as the child matures. Studies of the electrophysiologic organization of the central nervous system indicate that there is relative immaturity during the first 2 to 4 months after birth. Maturation is evident with increased regularity in sleep-wake cycles, and the infant manifests increasing self-regulation of behavior. Both axons and dendrites develop well into the second year and lead to formation of synapses and synthesis of neurotransmitters. As this occurs, the toddler manifests increasing self-modulation.

A normal toddler manifests increasing self-control of motor, language, and cognitive skills. Normal control tasks of toddlers include bowel and bladder control, use of utensils to eat, undressing and dressing, and ability to interact positively with peers and to begin sharing and taking turns. Gradually, the toddler abandons tantrums as a means of coping with frustration and becomes more adept at explaining his or her frustrations. Yet noncompliance with adult requests remains frequent in preschoolers as they struggle for autonomy. Normal children are most likely to develop self-control and self-reliance if parents are authoritative and firm but also warm, encouraging, and rational (Sturner and Howard, 1997).

As a normal child moves into preschool and early school years, he or she acquires increasing control of motor skills, often learning and enjoying many physical activities, including riding a tricycle, riding a bicycle, and playing jump rope, T ball, soccer, and games such as hide-and-seek. He or she increases drawing skills and coloring skills and learns to read. As the child experiences successes, he or she is motivated to develop further skills.

A normal child will be motivated to improve self-control throughout grade school, especially in areas of special interest. At this time, many children develop skills in computer games or sports or chess. However, the child does not yet have abstract reasoning ability and, in spite of skills in many areas, should not be given responsibilities that require abstract reasoning.

Young adolescents often have problems of self-control over the new domains in their lives and make poor judgments with respect to use of drugs and sexual behavior. Their brains are not yet mature. Adult levels of synapses in the middle frontal gyrus (i.e., prefrontal cortex) are not reached until middle to late adolescence. This development is associated with development of abstract reasoning ability and increased executive function as well as abilities in multitasking. Most normal adolescents, after the age of 16 years, will improve their self-control, including their judgment and decision making. Some adolescents, depending on the extent of early brain injury from many possible causes, may never develop normal self-control or executive functions.

The neural basis of self-control and self-regulation relies heavily on the prefrontal cortex. The prefrontal cortex is located anterior to the motor cortices in the frontal lobe of the brain. It begins to develop in late infancy and continues to develop throughout adolescence. This region of the brain plays a fundamental role in internally guided behavior through working memory and executive control operations. The different subregions may have separate functions related to executive control (Wagner et al, 2001). The dorsolateral prefrontal cortex is implicated in attention and working memory. The ventromedial prefrontal cortex, with connections to and from the amygdala, is implicated in controlling emotions, such as fear. The orbitofrontal cortex is implicated in sensory integration and decision making.

There are several studies indicating that stressors can cause working memory deficits through increased catecholamine levels (Arnsten and Li, 2005). Chapter 50 provides definitions of stress, the physiologic correlates, and the nature of coping. In situations of high stress, interventions to reduce stress and to encourage coping (see Chapter 50) or adjustment (see Chapter 42) can be anticipated to improve prefrontal cortical function and subsequent self-control and self-regulation.

CAUSES OF ABNORMALITIES IN SELF-CONTROL AND SELF-REGULATION

Table 46-1 summarizes many different causes of delays or deficits in the development of self-control and self-regulation. Events that occur in the fetal and neonatal periods may be predictors of later problems in self-control and self-regulation. Infants who are born before term may have neurodevelopmental disabilities that reduce self-regulation capacities. Many small premature infants manifest irregular state development, which is later associated with poor performance on motor skills and cognitive tests at school age. Their early problems with state regulation and later motor and cognitive difficulties may be the result of subtle or obvious neural injuries and also the result of long-term stress during their neonatal period. Problems with state regulation are also true for full-term infants who are small for gestational age. Infants born with genetic diseases such as Down syndrome or fragile X disease or those with conditions such as fetal alcohol syndrome have abnormal neural function and cognitive impairment that interferes with self-control, which makes it unlikely that most will be able to support themselves independently as adults.

Infants born with normal motor and cognitive potential may experience brain injuries from infectious diseases, malnutrition, metabolic diseases, or head injuries, which lead to abnormalities in their self-control abilities (Olness, 2003). They may later experience stressful life events that impair self-regulatory abilities. Examples include divorce of parents, deaths of family members, natural or manmade disasters, life-threatening or chronic illness, and child abuse. Post-traumatic stress may occur after any of these events, and symptoms may include deficits in self-control and self-regulation (Schwarz and Perry, 1994). Young infants who lack a mother or mother surrogate may have difficulties in forming secure attachments, and this also is associated with later problems in self-control and self-regulation (Ainsworth, 1979).

Table 46-1. Causes of Delays and Deficits in Self-Control and Self-Regulation

Cause	Examples
Early life experience	Prematurity Small for gestational age
Abnormal neural functions and cognitive impairment	Genetic disorders Neurologic disorders
Acquired brain injury	Infections Trauma
Temperamental differences	Difficult temperament
Stressful events	Divorce Lack of a maternal figure
Motor or speech impairments	Cerebral palsy
Perceived incompetence	Enuresis and encopresis
Limited parental guidance	

Table 46-2. Problems of Self-Regulation (School Age)

Persistent temper tantrums beyond 6 years	Thumb sucking	Conditioned fears, e.g., weather	Disruptive behavior
Performance anxiety, e.g., piano recital, dance recital, examination anxiety	Eating disorders	Dyshidrosis	Aggression
Nocturnal enuresis	Substance abuse	Trichotillomania	Bullying
Encopresis	Sleep problems	Simple tics	Socially inappropriate behavior
Nail biting	Attention-deficit/hyperactivity disorder	Habit cough	Oppositional behavior

There is much data to document that infants and children have intrinsic temperamental qualities that will also affect their coping styles and adaptation (Thomas and Chess, 1977). Some have low sensory thresholds, which make them less able than other children of the same age to self-regulate, for example, when they have night wakings or when they are in a new, noisy environment. There are also data that document the negative effects of environmental stressors on autonomic regulation (Gunnar and Vazquez, 2006).

Children with motor or speech impairments or disfigurements may, in spite of normal cognitive abilities, have problems in self-control and self-regulation because they perceive themselves as inadequate or incompetent. Some children at school age who are otherwise normal may have problems such as enuresis or encopresis that cause them to lose confidence because of lack of control in these specific areas. Sometimes such problems have a biologic basis, such as constipation (both enuresis and encopresis) or hyperthyroidism (enuresis), which should be identified and treated. All problems of self-control and self-regulation deserve careful diagnostic evaluations.

Tables 46-2 and 46-3 list many examples of poor self-control and self-regulation during school age and adolescence.

IMPORTANT ADDITIONAL CONTRIBUTIONS TO SELF-CONTROL

Children develop health-related lifestyles early in life. These depend on parental guidance, cultural norms, and school environments. Many children lack self-control with respect to healthy lifestyles, including issues of diet, exercise, and sleep hygiene. There is increasing public interest in imposing personal responsibility for health on American adults (Steinbrook, 2006), many of whom did not receive sufficient direction with respect to matters such as diet, exercise, and smoking when they were children.

In North America, each large city contains dozens of enclaves representing different cultures and different cultural norms, including those relating to self-regulation.

Table 46-3. Problems of Self-Regulation (Adolescent)

Substance abuse	Habit disorders, e.g., nail biting	Difficulty in completing tasks	Self-injury
Eating disorders	Trichotillomania	Dyshidrosis	Absence from school
Sleep disorders	Self-management of a chronic illness, e.g., diabetes	Antisocial behaviors	Inappropriate expressions of sexuality
Attention-deficit/hyperactivity disorder	Difficulty in organizing schedule	Compliance with medical regimens	Enuresis or encopresis
Performance anxiety	Careless driving	Aggression	Tantrums

Although Americans are said to be individualistic, many are not because they have lived in cultural environments that value extended family more than the individual. Control and regulation are provided within the extended family, and there are fewer opportunities for individual decisions. Acquisition of self-control is also influenced by the religious environment in which one develops and the extent to which religious guidelines are reinforced by the family and local community.

DIAGNOSTIC EVALUATIONS

In making assessments of problems in self-control, it is helpful to ask questions about the problem, how it is perceived, and where it is causing the greatest difficulty (Table 46-4) in addition to usual questions about health history. The reason for asking about how parents respond to worry or anxiety is to emphasize to the child that his or her parents do worry sometimes and do recognize their personal responses to worry or to determine if the child's response to anxiety is similar. It is also important to have parents describe what things the child does well, because the child may not realize that parents do have some positive thoughts about him or her.

Motivational interviewing techniques are useful in exploring problems related to self-regulation (Erickson et al, 2005). Motivational interviewing is conducted in a way that supports autonomy and shows respect for views of the child or adolescent. Motivational interviewing explores how a child or adolescent feels about changing behavior indicative of poor self-control and perceptions about how life might be different when a behavior is changed. For example, it is helpful to ask a child with enuresis what will be different when all of his or her beds are dry. If the child does not have a clear idea about the benefits of having dry beds, he or she may need some time before embarking on a treatment program.

In evaluating problems of self-regulation, it is essential to evaluate the parents (or guardians) and home environment. What are the parents' beliefs and philosophies about raising children? What are the culture and ethnic background of the family? Did the parents have similar problems? Do they continue to have these problems? What is the educational level of the parents? Do the parents have learning disabilities? What have been major family stressors? Questionnaires in advance of the visit may provide some of this information. It may also be important to see parents only during an initial visit and to see the child with parents during the second visit. Sometimes it is helpful to request films of the child's behavior at home or to ask to review photo albums about the child and family.

Depending on the problem, decisions should be made about additional testing, including physical examinations and laboratory, radiologic, or psychometric assessments. It is important to rule out causes such as metabolic diseases, attention-deficit/hyperactivity disorder, learning disabilities, or an event in the fetal or perinatal period that may have compromised cognitive function years previously. It may be appropriate to request permission to speak with the child's teacher and to obtain information about any psychometric testing done in school as well as information about academic performance.

Table 46-4. Questions Related to Problems in Control

What is the self-regulatory limitation?
Where does it cause the most difficulty (e.g., in home or in school)?
Does this child have identified learning disabilities?
How does this child learn?
Are there problems in controlling impulses?
Are there problems in controlling anger?
What are the things the child enjoys doing most?
What things does the child do well?
Does the child have a chronic illness, such as asthma or sickle cell disease?
What is the child's expectation with respect to outcomes related to the problem?
What is the parents' physiologic response to worry or anxiety?
How do family members respond to the child's problem?
Are there family members who have or who had similar problems?
What does the child believe is the cause of the problem?
What does the family believe is the cause of the problem?
Describe the child's personality as an infant.
Describe the child's personality as a toddler.
What is the cultural background of the family?

TREATMENT

If a biologic basis is identified for a self-regulation problem, efforts should be made to treat it. For example, if a child with onset enuresis has hyperthyroidism, the condition can be treated. If a child with disruptive behavior in school is found to have myotonic dystrophy, the basic problem cannot be treated. However, it is often helpful for families to have more precise explanations for problems in self-control, even if the basic problem cannot be treated. Such information may assist their plans with respect to how much continuing guidance a child may need when adulthood is reached, whether a legal guardianship should be established, and what financial issues need to be addressed.

If evaluation has determined that the child has a learning disability that contributes to the self-regulation problem or complicates treatment, this factor must be considered by physicians, therapists, and teachers. An example might be a child with test anxiety who has a math disability, making it unlikely that he or she can perform well in math tests in spite of efforts to reduce the anxiety. If a self-regulation issue relates to the developmental stage of the child (e.g., temper tantrums in a 2-year-old or toilet training problems in a 30-month-old child), parents should be provided with explanations about normal development and provided with strategies to facilitate mastery in their young children.

Some problems of self-regulation may be treated successfully by providing the child or adolescent an opportunity to learn self-hypnosis with or without biofeedback (Table 46-5). For some conditions, such as performance anxiety or nocturnal enuresis, training

Table 46-5. Applications of Hypnosis and Biofeedback in Pediatrics

Domain	Examples	Domain	Examples
Habit problems	Thumb sucking Simple tics Habit cough Nocturnal enuresis Nail biting	Pain management	Acute (procedures in office or emergency department) Chronic (sickle cell disease, recurrent headaches, hemophilia)
Performance anxiety	Sports performance Music performance Examinations	Anxiety associated with chronic disease	Malignant neoplasms Sickle cell disease Hemophilia Tourette syndrome Diabetes Rheumatoid arthritis Cystic fibrosis Cyclic vomiting syndrome
Control of conditions involving autonomic dysregulation	Conditioned hyperventilation Conditioned dysphagia Raynaud phenomenon Reflex sympathetic dystrophy	Other	Insomnia Warts Conditioned hives Problems with pill swallowing

in hypnosis may be the primary treatment. For other conditions, especially chronic illnesses such as cancer, diabetes, cystic fibrosis, or asthma, training in hypnosis is a helpful adjunct.

Hypnotherapy is a strategy for teaching a child to focus attention on specific mental images for therapeutic purposes (Olness and Kohen, 1996). It usually involves some degree of relaxation. All hypnosis is, in fact, self-hypnosis, and successful therapy depends on the child's willingness to continue practice at home. The self-hypnosis coach or teacher must choose methods that are consistent with the child's interests, learning styles, and mental imagery preferences. The addition of biofeedback often increases the child's interest in the process.

Biofeedback provides visual or auditory evidence of physiologic changes, such as increased peripheral temperature, reduced heart rate, decreased galvanic skin resistance, and relaxed muscle tone. This feedback is transformed into computer images that appeal to a child. Examples include a balloon that moves as the child stabilizes pulse rate variability, a bear that smiles as galvanic skin resistance is reduced, and a race car that moves as skin temperature is increased. Children then understand that they change a body response when they change their thinking.

It is important that child health professionals take basic training in hypnosis and biofeedback with children before using these methods in the office or hospital setting (see organizations providing training in Table 46-6).

Guidelines for Teaching Self-Hypnosis

1. Emphasize your role as a coach or teacher. You teach the child or adolescent how to practice. The child decides if and when he or she will continue practice.
2. Communicate in a way that increases the child's sense of being in control. Consider the child's preferences carefully and give him or her choices in the training process.
3. Take time to help the child understand something about the mechanism of the problem (e.g., making a diagram about how pain is understood in the brain).
4. Therapeutic suggestions must be consistent with the child's wishes and previous explanations.
5. Allow the child to use his or her personal preferred mental imagery, which might be visual or auditory or kinesthetic or olfactory.
6. Help parents to understand that the child is the learner and must control the practice.
7. Help the child to think about a future without the problem.
8. Provide the child with some system to record progress in his or her practice and achievement of his or her goals.
9. Offer the child a way to communicate with you if he or she has questions or forgets some part of the practice. This could be by phone or e-mail.

There are fringe benefits for children who develop the type of self-regulation ability described in this

Table 46-6. Organizations That Provide Hypnotherapy or Biofeedback Training

Society for Developmental and Behavioral Pediatrics
Annual workshop on hypnosis with children (www.sdbp.org)
6728 Old McLean Village Drive
McLean, VA 22101

American Society of Clinical Hypnosis (www.asch.net)
140 N. Bloomingdale Road
Bloomingdale, Illinois 60108-1017

Society for Clinical and Experimental Hypnosis
E-mail: sceh@mspp.edu
Massachusetts School of Professional Psychology
221 Rivermoor Street
Boston, MA 02132

University of Minnesota Department of Continuing Medical Education
UMHC Box 203
Room 3-110 Owre Hall
University of Minnesota Medical School
Minneapolis, MN 55455

American Society of Applied Psychophysiology and Biofeedback
Frank Andrasik (e-mail:fandrasik@ihmc.us)
University of West Florida
40 South Alcaniz Street
Pensacola, FL 32502

Vignette

Andrea is a 9-year-old girl who had migraine headaches diagnosed when she was 7 years old. Her mother also has migraine headaches, which began in childhood. The migraine episodes gradually increased in frequency to two or three each month. Each episode lasted 8 to 24 hours, and if they began in school, she had to leave the classroom. Symptoms included a right temple area headache with nausea, vomiting, runny nose, cold hands, and cold feet. At the age of 8 years, she was evaluated by a child neurologist who ordered a head computed tomography scan, which was normal. He prescribed ibuprofen for acute migraine episodes and cyproheptadine (Periactin) for prevention. Ibuprofen gave partial relief of discomfort. Andrea tried to continue normal activities but usually had to give up and then slept for several hours. She would feel weak for a day or two after each migraine episode ended.

She was referred to a behavioral pediatrician to learn self-hypnosis with biofeedback for prevention of migraine episodes. One of her favorite activities was bicycle riding with friends. She was taught a self-hypnosis induction involving bike riding. The pediatrician monitored her peripheral temperature and noted that her temperature increased 3 degrees while she imagined riding her bike with friends. He emphasized that she achieved this change simply by changing her thinking. He asked her to practice the 10-minute self-hypnosis exercise twice daily for a month. When Andrea returned 2 weeks later for a follow-up visit, she had had no migraine episodes. The pediatrician taught her some pain management methods to use with self-hypnosis in the event that she should have a migraine episode. At the third visit, she said that a migraine episode started but she immediately sat down and practiced her self-hypnosis and pain control. The episode ended a few minutes later. The pediatrician asked her to continue practice once daily and to let him know her progress by e-mail. During a 1-year follow-up, she had only two mild migraine episodes, which she stated that she controlled herself.

vignette. They have increased confidence in other areas, and they can apply their skills in self-hypnosis over a lifetime. Thomson (2005) has written a book for child health professionals and families that is based on strategies of hypnosis and includes 32 stories about animals with various self-regulation difficulties ranging from fears of storms to performance anxiety to enuresis. These creative stories have a general appeal, and each emphasizes confidence and coping.

For children who experience anxiety and pain from chronic illnesses, Culbert (2005) has developed a comfort kit that is useful in the office or hospital setting. It includes booklets for children and adolescents, families, and child health professionals. It emphasizes self-regulation skills and self-control. In the kit are distractors such as bubbles, a pinwheel, and stickers. There is also a massage pen, a comfort ruler, a squeeze ball, and a stress card that measures temperature. It includes breathing exercises and emphasizes that the child can "take charge of comfort."

RETURNING TO THE VIGNETTES

Ben, Age 32 Months

Ben's behavior represents typical challenges for a 32-month-old child (and his caretakers) in learning to defer gratification. Assuming that his parents understand his developmental stage and have established a time-out place, Ben's behavior would best be handled with few words, calmness by the family, and maybe a brief timeout for him. Although this approach is generally effective over time as normal brain development continues and parents are consistent, it might not be the right approach for a child with developmental delay or disability.

Sarah, Age 9 Years

Test anxiety and other types of performance anxiety are not unusual among grade-school children. If this is a frequent problem for Sarah, the parents should request help. The pediatrician or family physician might ask Sarah about the math class, the types of math problems, homework, and her sleep habits. The pediatrician should also assess her school performance in the present and previous years, whether there might be a math disability, and how Sarah and other family members cope with stress.

Training in self-hypnosis is a reasonable first approach to helping a child cope with uncomplicated test anxiety. If Sarah has good math ability, it is important, at this juncture, to give her a self-regulation tool that will increase her sense of competency. If she is found to have a math disability, arrangements must be made with her teacher to give her more time for exams, and Sarah may also need a tutor. Offering self-hypnosis may also be a helpful adjunct.

David, Age 45 Years

David's issues in yielding to food temptation are probably known to most Americans, in an environment where food is abundant and cheap. At an intellectual level, he and many of his peers understand why they should eat "healthy" and exercise more. Yet it is difficult to imagine denying one's self food items associated with rewards or special occasions from one's early childhood memories. David's physician might explore with David his willingness to change and also rule out depression. If depression is present, this needs treatment. The physician might use techniques from motivational interviewing described before.

PSYCHOTHERAPY

Problems of self-regulation and self-control are often associated with problems of anxiety or depression, personality disorders, or other psychiatric diagnoses.

Children may be referred to child psychologists or child psychiatrists who will provide a diagnostic assessment. Depending on their evaluation, they may offer a number of interventions, including medications, behavior modification, counseling, hypnosis, and biofeedback. An example would be an adolescent with performance anxiety related to obsessive-compulsive disorder who might respond to a combination of medications and counseling. Leora Kuttner, a child psychologist, has produced two teaching videotapes for child health professionals who work with children who have cancer. These tapes demonstrate nonpharmacologic interventions to reduce pain and anxiety and also provide evidence for the positive long-term effects of such interventions (Kuttner, 1999).

WHEN THE CAPACITY FOR SELF-REGULATION IS LIMITED

There are children who, in spite of therapeutic efforts, may not succeed in developing skills in self-regulation. This may relate to intellectual disability, learning disabilities, or severe mental illness. In these situations, it is important that child health professionals provide guidance and support to parents, who may need to continue close care and supervision of a child throughout their lifetimes. Child health professionals should learn about community resources for such children, including respite time for parents. Examples include children with severe memory impairment who cannot remember the sequence of tasks taught to them and children with Prader-Willi syndrome who require frequent monitoring by parents into adulthood. In spite of cognitive handicaps, it is helpful to identify some skill area for each impaired child and to give positive feedback related to that area as well as further opportunities to develop the talent.

SUMMARY

Excellent physical and mental self-regulation in the human requires smooth, interactive functioning of metabolic, endocrine, neural, cardiovascular, and musculoskeletal pathways. When there are limitations in any of these pathways, the capacity to self-regulate may be inhibited. Some of these inhibiting factors are eliminated as the child matures; some may be treated. Others lead to permanent limitations or handicaps. The capacity to self-regulate motor, sensory, cognitive, and emotional responses is essential to successful lives. Impediments to development of effective self-regulation and self-control in the child can lead to family problems, school problems, and eventual problems in the adult world. It is important to recognize problems of self-regulation, to evaluate causes, and to intervene as early as possible when these problems are recognized. Hypnosis and biofeedback may be useful treatments for problems in self-control and self-regulation.

REFERENCES

Ainsworth M: Infant-mother attachment. Am Psychol 34:932-937, 1979.

Arnsten AFT, Li BM: Neurobiology of executive functions: Catecholamine influences on prefrontal cortical function. Biol Psychiatry 57:1377-1384, 2005.

Brazelton TB: Neonatal Behavioral Assessment Scale. Philadelphia, JB Lippincott, 1973.

Culbert T: Comfort Kit for Kids and Families. Minneapolis–St. Paul, MN, Children's Hospitals and Clinics, 2005.

Erickson SJ, Gerstle M, Feldstein SW: Brief interventions and motivational interviewing with children, adolescents, and their parents in pediatric health care settings. Arch Pediatr Adolesc Med 159:1173-1180, 2005.

Gunnar MR, Vazquez DM: Stress neurobiology and developmental psychopathology. *In* Cicchetti D, Cohen DJ (eds): Developmental Psychopathology, 2nd ed. New York, Wiley, 2006.

Iannotti RJ, Schneider S, Nansel TR, et al: Self-efficacy, outcome expectations, and diabetes self-management in adolescents with type 1 diabetes. J Dev Behav Pediatr 27:98-105, 2006.

Kuttner L: No Fears, No Tears: 13 Years Later. Vancouver, Canada, Canadian Cancer Society, 1999.

Olness K: The global epidemic of cognitive impairment. J Dev Behav Pediatr 24:120-130, 2003.

Olness K, Kohen DP: Hypnosis and Hypnotherapy with Children. New York, Guilford, 1996.

Schwarz ED, Perry BD: The post-traumatic response in children and adolescents. Psychiatr Clin North Am 17:311-327, 1994.

Steinbrook R: Imposing personal responsibility for health. N Engl J Med 355:753-756, 2006.

Sturner RA, Howard BJ: Preschool development. Part 2: Psychosocial/behavioral development. Pediatr Rev 18:327-336, 1997.

Thomas A, Chess S: Temperament and Development. New York, Brunner & Mazel, 1977.

Thomson L: Harry the Hypno-potamus: Metaphorical Tales for the Treatment of Children. London, Crown House Publishing, 2005.

Wagner AD, Maril A, Bjork RA, Schacter DL: Prefrontal contributions to executive control: fMRI evidence for functional distinctions within lateral prefrontal cortex. Neuroimage 14:1337-1347, 2001.

SECTION C **Internal Status: Feelings and Thoughts**

47 MAJOR DISTURBANCES OF EMOTION AND MOOD

AMY CHEUNG AND PETER JENSEN

Vignette

Jenna was a previously bright and competent young adolescent who earned As and Bs in all of her subjects. When she turned 15 years old and entered the 10th grade, she began to fail tests and courses. Her mother became concerned that she was spending increasing time in her room and did not want to get out of bed in the morning. However, her mother's efforts to get her out led to many family fights. Jenna also became more irritable, frequently starting fights with her younger sister.

Her parents sought counsel from the primary care physician, who referred the family to a mental health professional. The psychiatrist elicited that Jenna could no longer focus on school work and had lost interest in hanging out with her friends. She admitted she was sad most of the time and cried for no reason. She could not fall asleep at night because her mind was racing with worries about her school work and problems with her friends. Even after sleeping for more than 10 hours, she still felt tired all day long. She started having thoughts that life is not worth living and thought about taking some pills to "sleep and never wake up" but had no explicit plans to kill herself.

The psychiatrist diagnosed Jenna with depression and prescribed one of the selective serotonin reuptake inhibitors. During the course of the next 4 months, Jenna's symptoms improved. Her school work also improved and she finished the school year, failing only one subject. Because she was feeling so much better, she decided to have a trial off her medication while she was at camp for the summer. The following fall, she complained of feeling stressed about the school year. She began to have trouble with her sleep again. Two months into the school year, Jenna was diagnosed with a recurrence of her depression. She began treatment once again with the same selective serotonin reuptake inhibitor.

Mood and anxiety disorders in children and adolescents have received increasing recognition during the past few decades as a serious public health issue that poses a significant burden on children, adolescents, and their families. With this increased recognition, effective treatments have been developed in parallel. However, there remains a significant gap between what evidence is available and what is incorporated into daily practice. Epidemiologic data show that many of these youth go unidentified and untreated until adulthood (Chang et al, 1988; Kramer and Garralda, 1998). Because of many barriers to access, including the shortage of mental health providers, pediatric settings have become the de facto mental health clinics for children and adolescents (Regier et al, 1993). Therefore, pediatric professionals need to become skilled in the identification and management of commonly presenting mental health disorders in children and adolescents, particularly anxiety and depressive disorders.

Mood disorders, including depression and bipolar disorder, can affect up to 10% of children and adolescents before adulthood (American Academy of Child and Adolescent Psychiatry, 2007c; Cheung and Dewa, 2006). Mood disorders occur more commonly in adolescents than in children. Even though most pediatric primary care providers believe it is their responsibility to recognize depression in their patients, many struggle with the diagnosis and management (Olson et al, 2001). In fact, only 17% routinely inquire about depressive symptoms in their patients, a rate much lower than for other areas, such as sexual activity and birth control (Halpern-Felsher et al, 2000; Middleman et al, 1995). Many primary care physicians are reluctant to prescribe medications for depression. Therefore, pediatric providers require further support for the identification and management of mood disorders in their patients.

Anxiety disorders are more common in children than in adolescents. Anxiety disorders are receiving increasing attention because of their frequent presentation in school-age children. Consequently, research addressing anxiety disorders has now moved beyond pediatric and mental health clinics and into school-based settings.

Furthermore, universal prevention programs have been developed for children at risk for anxiety disorders (Bernstein et al, 2005).

In this chapter, we review the most common mood and anxiety disorders presenting in pediatric settings. These include depressive disorders, bipolar disorder, social phobia, separation anxiety disorder, and generalized anxiety disorder. We draw on the existing literature as well as expert opinion on the identification and management of these disorders. For depressive disorders, we also draw primarily from the recently completed Guidelines for Adolescent Depression in Primary Care (GLAD-PC). Finally, we address the issue of suicide in children and adolescents. Because suicide rarely occurs in children younger than 13 years, the focus of this review is on suicidal ideation in children and suicidality (including attempts and ideation) and completed suicide in adolescents.

MAJOR DEPRESSION

Depressive disorders are among the most common mental disorders affecting children and adolescents. Several studies have been conducted to assess prevalence of these disorders in community-dwelling children and adolescents, with depression prevalence estimates ranging from 1% to 3% in prepubertal children and from 3% to 9% in adolescents (Fleming et al, 1989). Before the onset of puberty, the gender ratio is generally 1:1 or equal. After puberty, girls have been shown to be at higher risk for depression (Fleming et al, 1989). The gender ratio is generally maintained throughout adulthood, with women having a twofold to threefold higher risk for development of depression (Kornstein, 2001). The lifetime prevalence rate of depression in adolescents has been estimated to be as high as 20% to 25% (American Academy of Child and Adolescent Psychiatry, 1998). The prevalence of another persistent form of depression, dysthymic disorder, is approximately 3% in adolescents. The prevalence of other depressive disorders (i.e., adjustment disorder, psychotic depression, bipolar depression) has not been well documented or studied (Lewinsohn et al, 1993).

The etiology of depression has been examined in numerous studies, and no necessary or sufficient causes have been identified. However, the numerous risk factors that have been linked to depression fall into three categories: biologic, psychological, and social-environmental (Waslick et al, 2002). Among the biologic correlates, the most significant and well studied factor is genetics or heredity of depression. Numerous studies have shown higher rates of depression in adult relatives of depressed children and adolescents (Weissman et al, 1997). Furthermore, the increased rates appear to be specific to depression alone and not to all types of psychiatric disorders. Rates of depression have been found to be higher in offspring of parents with mood disorders as well as in twins of patients with depressive disorders (Weissman et al, 1997). The high rates of depression within families may not be explained by genetics alone. Other possible risk factors, such as the impact of living with a family member with a mood disorder, have been implicated and need to be further explored. For example, emerging evidence shows that treatment of maternal depression can improve outcomes in offsprings (Weissman et al, 2006).

In terms of psychological correlates, cognitive factors have been the most studied. In fact, altering cognition forms the basis of cognitive-behavioral therapy in both youth and adults with depression. Social and environmental factors, including poverty and social economic status, have been associated with increased risk of emotional disturbances such as depression (Costello et al, 1996). Other environmental issues, such as peer relationships and parenting capacities, have also been connected or associated with the development of depression. (For an in-depth review, refer to Waslick et al, 2002.)

Although depression may occur at any age, the risk for development of depression increases significantly with puberty. The long-term sequelae of depression in children and adolescents have not been fully studied. However, high recurrence rates, up to 60%, have been reported. Moreover, depressed patients have higher rates of impaired functioning, substance abuse, suicide attempts, and psychiatric hospitalizations (Weissman et al, 1999).

The most significant sequela of depression is suicide. Psychological autopsy studies of patients who have committed suicide have found a high association with psychiatric disorders, with more than 50% of children and adolescents who committed suicide having a diagnosis of depression (Brent et al, 1993). A longitudinal follow-up study of depressed adolescents found that there was an 8% rate for completed suicide in this population, much higher than that in the general population (Weissman et al, 1999).

Assessment and Diagnosis

The assessment of children and adolescents with depressive disorders should include an interview with the patient alone as well as interviews with families or parents (Zuckerbrot and Jensen, 2006). Further collateral history, with permission from the families or patients, may also be gathered from other sources, such as schools and other adults involved in the life of the child or adolescent. To help identify and evaluate depression, clinicians can use self-report instruments such as the Beck Depression Inventory (Beck and Steer, 1987) and the Kutcher Adolescent Depression Scale (Brooks et al, 2003). The use of these instruments alone for the confirmation of diagnosis is not recommended, but they can aid in the diagnosis when they are accompanied by an in-depth clinical interview.

The diagnostic criteria for major depressive disorder are shown in Table 47-1. Children and adolescents may meet criteria for a number of different depressive disorders, including dysthymic disorder or adjustment disorder with depressive symptoms. Dysthymic disorder features most of the symptoms of depression, but they are less severe and are present for at least 1 year. Adjustment disorder with depressive features may be indistinguishable from major depression on the basis of symptoms. However, there is a clear stressor that preceded the development of the depressive symptoms. Other disorders in the differential diagnosis include bereavement and

Table 47-1. Diagnostic Criteria for Major Depressive Episode (DSM-IV-TR)

A. Five (or more) of the following symptoms have been present during the same 2-week period and represent a change from previous functioning; at least one of the symptoms is either (1) or (2).
 (1) depressed mood most of the day, nearly every day, as indicated by either subjective report (e.g., feels sad or empty) or observation made by others (e.g., appears tearful)
 (2) markedly diminished interest or pleasure in all, or almost all, activities most of the day, nearly every day (as indicated by either subjective account or observation made by others)
 (3) significant weight loss when not dieting or weight gain
 (4) insomnia or hypersomnia nearly every day
 (5) psychomotor agitation or retardation nearly every day
 (6) fatigue or loss of energy nearly every day
 (7) feelings of worthlessness or excessive or inappropriate guilt
 (8) diminished ability to think or concentrate, or indecisiveness, nearly every day
 (9) recurrent thoughts of death (not just fear of dying), recurrent suicidal ideation without a specific plan, or a suicide attempt, or a specific plan for committing suicide

B. The symptoms do not meet criteria for a Mixed Episode.

C. The symptoms cause clinically significant distress or impairment in social, occupational, or other important areas of functioning.

D. The symptoms are not due to the direct physiological effects of a substance (e.g., a drug of abuse, a medication) or a general medical condition (e.g., hypothyroidism).

E. The symptoms are not better accounted for by Bereavement, that is, after a loss of a loved one, the symptoms persist for longer than 2 months or are characterized by marked functional impairment, morbid preoccupation with worthlessness, suicidal ideation, psychotic symptoms, or psychomotor retardation.

From American Psychiatric Association: Diagnostic and Statistical Manual of Mental Disorders, 4th ed, text revision. Washington, DC, American Psychiatric Association, 2000.

depressive disorder secondary to a medical condition or to substance use. Postpartum depression may also occur in adolescents after pregnancy. Adolescents who present with depressive symptoms may also have a cycling mood disorder, such as bipolar disorder or cyclothymia.

The presentation of depression in children and adolescents may vary compared with adults presenting with depression. In particular, children with depression often present with somatic complaints and have a withdrawn and sad appearance. Older children or adolescents are more likely to present with irritability than with a sad mood. Teenagers may also present with reactivity of mood, that is, their mood can seem normal at times, with periods of tearfulness, sadness, or irritability. Reactivity of mood frequently confuses clinicians and parents who are caring for an adolescent. Finally, adolescents are also more likely to present with hypersomnia and hyperphagia compared with adults with depression.

One other factor complicating the diagnosis of depression in adolescents is the nature of adolescence itself, as teens may often experience moodiness, irritability, and withdrawal from parental figures. Therefore, clinicians as well as parents and other caregivers of adolescents need to be aware of the differences in clinical presentation between normal adolescence and depressive disorders.

Table 47-2. Cognitive-Behavioral Therapy and Interpersonal Therapy for Adolescents

Therapy	Key Components
Cognitive-behavioral therapy	Thoughts influence behaviors and feelings, and vice versa. Treatment targets patient's thoughts and behaviors to improve his or her mood. Essential elements of cognitive-behavioral therapy include increasing pleasurable activities (behavioral activation), reducing negative thoughts (cognitive restructuring), and improving assertiveness and problem solving skills to reduce feelings of hopelessness.
Interpersonal therapy for adolescents	Interpersonal problems may cause or exacerbate depression and that depression, in turn, may exacerbate interpersonal problems. Treatment targets patient's interpersonal problems to improve both interpersonal functioning and his or her mood. Essential elements of interpersonal therapy include identifying an interpersonal problem area, improving interpersonal problem solving skills, and modifying communication patterns.

From Columbia Treatment Guidelines: Depressive Disorders (Version 2). New York, Columbia University, Department of Child and Adolescent Psychiatry, 2002.

A final consideration in the assessment and diagnosis of depressive disorders is the impact of comorbid conditions. The most common comorbidities are anxiety disorders, behavioral disorders, substance abuse or dependence, eating disorders, and learning disabilities. Patients with comorbidities are generally more difficult to treat and, even with symptom reduction, their functioning may remain poor.

Management

After the diagnosis of depression is made, the initial management should include both psychoeducation and safety planning with patients and families. First, families and patients need to understand that depression is a frequently chronic and recurrent condition. The aims of psychoeducation are also to improve adherence with treatment and to reduce the risk of relapse or recurrence. Peer support for parents or caregivers and for patients may also be helpful. Safety planning is another critical component of psychoeducation, given the high association between suicidality and completed suicide with depressive disorders. Patients as well as their parents and caregivers should be educated that the disorder is associated with a risk of suicide (see Antidepressants and Suicidality in this chapter).

Psychotherapy

Two forms of psychotherapy have been shown to be efficacious in depression: interpersonal therapy for adolescents (IPT-A) and cognitive-behavioral therapy (CBT). The core components of IPT-A and CBT are shown in Table 47-2 and discussed in Chapter 89. Interpersonal therapy was first developed for the treatment of adult depression and was modified for adolescents by Mufson and colleagues (1999). Several studies have demonstrated the effectiveness of IPT-A in resolving depressive symptoms in adolescents, with use of both group and individual treatment formats. Furthermore, recent trials have been completed in "real-world" settings, such as school-based clinics, with good outcomes (Mufson et al, 2004). Numerous studies have also demonstrated the efficacy of CBT in group and individual formats for prevention and for treatment of depression in children and adolescents (Compton et al, 2004).

Only one federally funded, randomized controlled trial in adolescent depression examined and compared the effectiveness of CBT in combination with antidepressant medication versus medication alone or CBT alone (March et al, 2004). This study, the Treatment for Adolescents with Depression Study (TADS), found that those youth treated with CBT alone did not fare any better than those treated with placebo. However, those treated with CBT along with antidepressant medication (fluoxetine) showed the highest response and remission rates along with better functioning. Overall findings suggested that psychotherapy or antidepressant medication alone might be started as the initial treatment for youth with mild or moderate depression with no complicating factors, such as psychosis or other comorbid illnesses. If no response is seen within 4 to 6 weeks, combination therapy with antidepressant medication or psychotherapy should be tried. If both options are available, the emerging evidence from TADS indicates that it may be advisable for clinicians to begin combination therapy with psychotherapy and antidepressant medication in outpatients who are diagnosed with major depressive disorder.

Importantly, given the controversy about the emergence of suicidality in youth treated with antidepressants, Bridge and colleagues examined suicidality rates in depressed adolescents enrolled in a psychotherapy trial but not treated with antidepressants. Rates for new-onset or worsening suicidality among depressed youth treated with psychotherapy only were similar to those treated with antidepressants in the medication trials (Bridge et al, 2005).

Antidepressants

Treatment trials involving tricyclic antidepressants for depression in children and adolescents showed no benefit from treatment. Furthermore, studies indicated that these medications were associated with risk of mortality due to overdose and cardiac toxicity. Therefore, tricyclic antidepressants are no longer used in the treatment of depression, although they may still be useful in the management of other disorders in children and adolescents.

With the emergence and increasing availability of the selective serotonin reuptake inhibitors (SSRIs) and their more favorable side effect profile (compared with the tricyclic antidepressants), SSRI prescription rates have grown tremendously during the past decade in the pediatric population. Rates of use have grown much more quickly than the evidence base supporting pediatric use, however. Currently, there are eight high-quality randomized controlled trials examining the efficacy of antidepressant medications in children and adolescents with depression. The age of the population studied ranged from 7 to 17 years. Three trials with fluoxetine all demonstrated efficacy compared with placebo. In contrast, three trials with paroxetine were all found to be negative on the basis of the primary outcome measures. Studies of three other agents, citalopram, escitalopram, and sertraline, showed statistically significant improvement among those treated with medication versus placebo in some outcomes but not in others (Bridge et al, 2007; Cheung et al, 2006). In the trials with venlafaxine, the medication was less efficacious in children compared with adolescents, and the emergence of side effects was also higher for the younger age group.

In view of these somewhat discrepant findings, the generally accepted conclusion currently is that antidepressant treatment (principally fluoxetine) may be effective in youth with moderate to severe depression. Close monitoring is needed to watch for clinical improvement as well as the possible emergence of adverse events.

The common starting dose for these medications and common side effects are shown in Table 47-3 and in Chapter 90. Clinicians should use standardized forms to record their clinical assessments, to evaluate side effects, and to document their follow-up visits with patients. (See page 471 for a discussion of the association of antidepressant use and suicidality.)

Antipsychotics

In depressed patients who also present with psychotic symptoms, antipsychotics have been used along with antidepressant medications. The most commonly used class of antipsychotics is the atypicals, which include risperidone, olanzapine, and quetiapine. However, no studies on psychotic depression have been conducted in the pediatric population. Therefore, the dosages used for children and adolescents are generally comparable to those used in adults. For readers interested in learning more about the use of atypical antipsychotics in youth,

Table 47-3. Dosing and Adverse Effects of Selective Serotonin Reuptake Inhibitors

Medication	Starting Dose	Effective Dose	Maximum Dosage	Not to Be Used with	Common Adverse Effects
Citalopram	10 mg/od	20 mg	60 mg	MAOIs	Headaches, gastrointestinal upset, insomnia
Fluoxetine	10 mg/od	20 mg	60 mg	MAOIs	Headaches, gastrointestinal upset, insomnia, agitation, anxiety
Fluvoxamine	50 mg/od	150 mg	300 mg	MAOIs	Headaches, gastrointestinal upset, drowsiness
Paroxetine	10 mg/od	20 mg	60 mg	MAOIs	Headaches, gastrointestinal upset, insomnia, agitation, anxiety
Sertraline	25 mg/od	100 mg	200 mg	MAOIs	Headaches, gastrointestinal upset, insomnia
Escitalopram	5 mg/od	10 mg	20 mg	MAOIs	Headaches, gastrointestinal upset, insomnia

MAOIs, monoamine oxidase inhibitors.

refer to a full review by Pappadopulos and colleagues (2003) and to Chapter 90.

BIPOLAR DISORDER

Bipolar disorder is less prevalent than major depression in the pediatric population. The prevalence of bipolar disorder in adolescents aged 14 to 18 years has been estimated at 0.95%, with the majority of these adolescents reporting symptoms of hypomania, a less severe form of mania, rather than full-blown mania (American Academy of Child and Adolescent Psychiatry, 2007a). Much less is known about the prevalence in children. From surveys of adult bipolar patients, approximately 17% report symptom onset before the age of 10 years (American Academy of Child and Adolescent Psychiatry, 2007a). Although the prevalence of bipolar disorder in adults is equal for men and women, gender differences among children and adolescents with bipolar disorder is not known (American Academy of Child and Adolescent Psychiatry, 2007a).

Attention-deficit/hyperactivity disorder (ADHD) may precede or coexist in more than 60% of children or adolescents with bipolar disorder (Carlson et al, 2000). However, although there is suggestion that these disorders represent different spectrums of the same disease process, only 1.3% of children diagnosed with ADHD between the ages of 6 and 12 years go on to develop bipolar disorder as young adults (Carlson et al, 2000).

Several factors have been associated with the development of bipolar disorder. Genetics, as with other mood disorders, play a significant role. Individuals with a first-degree relative with bipolar disorder are four to six times more likely to develop the disorder themselves (American Academy of Child and Adolescent Psychiatry, 2007a).

Assessment and Diagnosis

An assessment for bipolar disorder should include an evaluation for the symptoms of mania or hypomania and depression as well as an assessment of any functional impairment. To gather this information, clinicians should interview both the patient and the family or caregiver. To further aid in the assessment, the use of rating scales may be helpful. Commonly used instruments include the Child Behavior Checklist and the Young Mania Rating Scale (American Academy of Child and Adolescent Psychiatry, 2007a). However, these instruments cannot be used alone for the diagnosis of bipolar disorder but rather should be a component of the diagnostic assessment.

Table 47-4 shows the diagnostic criteria for bipolar disorder. The diagnostic criteria do not distinguish between adults and children and adolescents. Furthermore, although the *Diagnostic and Statistical Manual of Mental Disorders,* fourth edition (DSM-IV), states that individuals may be diagnosed with bipolar disorder with an episode of mania without depression, clinically, patients with bipolar disorder generally present with initial episodes of depression and then subsequent episodes of mania. Patients also generally experience periods of depression or mania with stretches of normal mood in between.

The significant overlap between ADHD and bipolar disorder symptoms makes it difficult to distinguish between these conditions. Differences in presentation that can help in deciding whether symptoms are related to bipolar disorder or ADHD include the earlier onset of ADHD symptoms (before the age of 7 years) and the persistent nature of the symptoms (no symptom-free periods). The presentation of prepubertal bipolar disorder has only further blurred the line between these two disorders in the pediatric population. For example, prepubertal children with bipolar disorder frequently present with continuous symptoms of mania or hypomania that do not remit (American Academy of Child and Adolescent Psychiatry, 2007a). This is different from the typical presentation of bipolar disorder in older adolescents and adults. The diagnosis of bipolar disorder or manic episode in older adolescents closely resembles that of adult patients with bipolar disorder.

A final critical issue in diagnosis is that many symptoms of bipolar disorder, such as mood dysregulation, poor attention, excessive activity, and increased self-esteem, depend on the developmental age of the child. Therefore, any assessment must take into account what is "normal" developmentally for a given patient. For example, the attention span of a 5-year-old is much less than that of a 10-year-old, and self-control over emotions such as tears and anger is expected to gradually increase throughout childhood and adolescence. Clinicians who do not have a good understanding of developmental issues may mistakenly label normal behavior as symptoms of bipolar disorder.

Management

Treatments of bipolar disorder in the pediatric population have not been systematically evaluated, but common mood stabilizers used to treat adults with bipolar disorder are also used clinically in children as young as preschoolers. A list of common mood stabilizers and their side effects are noted in Table 47-5. Each of these medications is described in detail here.

Table 47-4. Diagnostic Criteria for Bipolar Disorder (Manic Episode) (DSM-IV-TR)

A. Abnormally and persistently elevated, expansive, or irritable mood, lasting at least 1 week.
B. Three (or more) of the following symptoms:
 (1) inflated self-esteem or grandiosity
 (2) decreased need for sleep
 (3) more talkative or pressure to keep talking
 (4) racing thoughts
 (5) distractibility
 (6) increase in goal-directed activity
 (7) excessive involvement in pleasurable activities that have a high potential for painful consequences
C. Impaired occupational, social, or relationship functioning; hospitalization; psychosis.
D. Not due to a substance or medical condition.

From American Psychiatric Association: Diagnostic and Statistical Manual of Mental Disorders, 4th ed, text revision. Washington, DC, American Psychiatric Association, 2000.

Table 47-5. Dosing and Adverse Effects of Mood Stabilizers

Medication	Starting Dose	Effective Dose	Maximum Dosage	Possible Interactions	Common Adverse Effects
Lithium	150 mg/od	Based on serum levels*	Based on serum levels*	Nonsteroidal anti-inflammatory drugs	Acne, gastrointestinal upset, fatigue, cognitive slowing, tremor, hypothyroidism
Valproic acid	250 mg/od	Based on serum levels*	Based on serum levels*	Carbamazepine, lamotrigine	Gastrointestinal upset, irregular menstrual periods, weight gain
Carbamazepine	100 mg/od	Based on serum levels*	Based on serum levels*	Valproic acid, lamotrigine	Headaches, gastrointestinal upset, drowsiness
Risperidone	0.5 mg/od	2-4 mg	6 mg	None	Weight gain, elevated cholesterol, elevated glucose, drowsiness, muscle stiffness, elevated prolactin
Olanzapine	1.25 mg/od	5 mg	15 mg	None	Weight gain, elevated cholesterol, elevated glucose, drowsiness

*Serum levels (12 hours after dose): lithium, range 0.5-1.0 mEq/L; valproic acid, range 50-100 μg/mL; carbamazepine, range 4-12 μg/mL.

Lithium

There are several small randomized controlled trials looking at children and adolescents with bipolar disorder and the efficacy of lithium (American Academy of Child and Adolescent Psychiatry, 2007a). These findings suggest some benefit with lithium in this population. Several naturalistic studies also support the efficacy of lithium. For example, Strober and colleagues (1990) conducted an open study of children who responded to lithium but who were nonadherent with continued treatment. Those who were nonadherent relapsed much quicker than did those who continued with lithium (American Academy of Child and Adolescent Psychiatry, 2007a).

Anticonvulsants

Anticonvulsants have been widely used and well studied in children with epilepsy. However, the evidence for bipolar disorder has been limited to case reports or small case series. Emerging evidence suggests that anticonvulsants may be helpful in managing this disorder in the pediatric population (American Academy of Child and Adolescent Psychiatry, 2007a).

The common side effects of anticonvulsants are shown in Table 47-5. One noted association is the development of polycystic ovary syndrome in postpubertal girls. Polycystic ovary syndrome is characterized by obesity, hydroid androgynism (which can present as alopecia, acne, and increased facial hair), hyperinsulinemia, and lipid abnormalities. The link between valproic acid and polycystic ovary syndrome was first described in epileptic patients. However, patients with epilepsy may already be at increased risk for endocrine disorders, and the increased occurrence of polycystic ovary syndrome may not be associated with the medication alone. Furthermore, these patients have had extended exposure to anticonvulsants compared with those with bipolar disorder.

Atypical Antipsychotics

Both risperidone and olanzapine have been used in open trials for adolescents with bipolar disorder. Barzman and colleagues in 2006 conducted a controlled trial comparing valproate with quetiapine. Both valproate and quetiapine were found to be effective (Barzman et al, 2006). The use of atypical antipsychotics in this population requires further research, given the risk of hyperglycemia (diabetes), elevated lipids, and substantial weight gain.

Selective Serotonin Reuptake Inhibitors

There are no randomized controlled trials examining the efficacy of antidepressants in bipolar disorder. The American Academy of Child and Adolescent Psychiatry (2007a) conducted a systematic chart review that found the use of SSRIs improved the symptoms of bipolar depression but also increased the risk for manic relapse.

ANXIETY DISORDERS

Anxiety disorders commonly present in childhood and adolescence. In contrast to mood disorders, onset of anxiety occurs earlier in childhood, often preceding the onset of mood disorders. In this section, we review four commonly presenting anxiety disorders: social phobia, separation anxiety disorder, panic disorder, and generalized anxiety disorder. We also briefly review post-traumatic stress disorder. Obsessive-compulsive disorder is described in Chapter 48.

The etiology of anxiety disorders is manifold. Stresses and traumatic life events, such as forced separations, can increase the risk of anxiety disorders (Beidel and Turner, 2005). Furthermore, these disorders also run in families, although no specific gene has been isolated (American Academy of Child and Adolescent Psychiatry, 2007b). Other factors, such as attachment style and parent-child interactions, also increase the risk of anxiety disorders in children and adolescents with temperamental vulnerability (American Academy of Child and Adolescent Psychiatry, 2007b).

Social Phobia

Social phobia (SP) is a common disorder in children and adolescents. SP affects up to 2% of children and adolescents with a peak age at onset between 11 and 12 years (Beidel et al, 2004). These patients present with excessive fears about being in public spaces or social situations and fears of speaking in front of others. The diagnostic criteria for SP are shown in Table 47-6. SP

Table 47-6. Diagnostic Criteria for Social Phobia, Separation Anxiety Disorder, and Generalized Anxiety Disorder (DSM-IV-TR)

Diagnostic Criteria for Social Phobia

A. A marked and persistent fear of one or more social or performance situations in which the person is exposed to unfamiliar people or to possible scrutiny by others. The individual fears that he or she will act in a way (or show anxiety symptoms) that will be humiliating or embarrassing.
B. Exposure to the feared social situation almost invariably provokes anxiety, which may take the form of a situationally bound or situationally predisposed Panic Attack.
C. The person recognizes that the fear is excessive or unreasonable.
D. The feared social or performance situations are avoided or else are endured with intense anxiety or distress.
E. The avoidance, anxious anticipation, or distress in the feared social or performance situation(s) interferes significantly with the person's normal routine, occupational (academic) functioning, or social activities or relationships, or there is marked distress about having the phobia.
F. In individuals under age 18, the duration is at least 6 months.
G. The fear or avoidance is not due to the direct physiological effects of a substance, or a general medical condition, and is not better accounted for by another mental disorder.
H. If a general medical condition or other mental disorder is present, the fear in Criterion A is unrelated to it.

Diagnostic Criteria for Separation Anxiety Disorder

A. Developmentally inappropriate and excessive anxiety concerning separation from home or from those to whom the individual is attached, as evidenced by three (or more) of the following:
(1) recurrent excessive distress when separation from home or major attachment figures occurs or is anticipated
(2) persistent and excessive worry about losing, or about possible harm befalling, major attachment figures
(3) persistent and excessive worry that an untoward event will lead to separation from a major attachment figure (e.g., getting lost or being kidnapped)
(4) persistent reluctance or refusal to go to school or elsewhere because of fear of separation
(5) persistently and excessively fearful or reluctant to be alone or without major attachment figures at home or without significant adults in other settings
(6) persistent reluctance or refusal to go to sleep without being near a major attachment figure or to sleep away from home
(7) repeated nightmares involving the theme of separation
(8) repeated complaints of physical symptoms (such as headaches, stomachaches, nausea, or vomiting) when separation from major attachment figures occurs or is anticipated
B. The duration of the disturbance is at least 4 weeks.
C. The onset is before age 18 years.
D. The disturbance causes clinically significant distress or impairment in social, academic (occupational), or other important areas of functioning.
E. The disturbance does not occur exclusively during the course of a Pervasive Developmental Disorder, Schizophrenia, or other Psychotic Disorder and, in adolescents and adults, is not better accounted for by a Panic Disorder with Agoraphobia.
Specify if:
Early Onset: if onset occurs before age 6 years

Diagnostic Criteria for Generalized Anxiety Disorder

A. Excessive anxiety and worry (apprehensive expectation), occurring more days than not for at least 6 months, about a number of events or activities.
B. The person finds it difficult to control the worry.
C. The anxiety and worry are associated with three (or more) of the following six symptoms:
(1) restlessness or feeling keyed up
(2) being easily fatigued
(3) difficulty concentrating
(4) irritability
(5) muscle tension
(6) sleep disturbance
D. The focus of anxiety and worry is not confined to features of another Axis I disorder.
E. The anxiety, worry, or physical symptoms cause clinically significant stress or impairment in social, occupational, or other important areas of functioning.
F. The disturbance is not due to the direct physiological effects of a substance (e.g., a drug of abuse or a medication) or a general medical condition (e.g., hyperthyroidism) and does not occur exclusively during a Mood Disorder, a Psychotic Disorder, or a Pervasive Developmental Disorder.

From American Psychiatric Association: Diagnostic and Statistical Manual of Mental Disorders, 4th ed, text revision. Washington, DC, American Psychiatric Association, 2000.

affects both genders equally before puberty; but after puberty, girls are more likely to be affected (Bernstein et al, 1996).

Separation Anxiety Disorder

Although it can occur throughout childhood and adolescence, separation anxiety disorder (SAD) most commonly affects children aged 5 to 7 years with a peak age at onset between 7 and 9 years. The key symptom of SAD is worry about separation from a caregiver and fear of harm to either the caregiver or the child during the period of separation (see Table 47-6). School refusal is a common feature of SAD. Estimates of SAD in the general population range from 3% to 5% (Bernstein et al, 1996). Although this number is high, recovery for SAD is one of highest among anxiety disorders. Studies have suggested that SAD is more common among girls than among boys (Bernstein et al, 1996).

Generalized Anxiety Disorder

Previously known as overanxious disorder, generalized anxiety disorder (GAD) has gained increased recognition as a common presenting disorder in childhood. The peak age at onset is between 10 and 13 years. The principal symptom of GAD is worry, and in children, somatic complaints, such as stomachaches, may also be present (see Table 47-6). The prevalence rate of GAD is estimated at 1% to 2% in children (Costello et al, 1996) and 4% in adolescents (Whitaker et al, 1990). Some evidence suggests that no gender differences exist in children and adolescents with GAD (American Academy of Child and Adolescent Psychiatry, 2007b). GAD persists in only a minority of children and adolescents in long-term follow-up, but almost half of these patients go on to develop other types of anxiety disorders.

Panic Disorder

Panic disorder (PD) is rarely reported in children and occurs in less than 1% of adolescents (American Academy of Child and Adolescent Psychiatry, 2007b; Whitaker et al, 1990). Children and adolescents with PD have recurrent panic attacks. These patients may endorse a number of symptoms during the attacks, including diaphoresis, nausea, shortness of breath, and palpitations (Table 47-7). Along with physical symptoms, a patient may also have cognitive symptoms, such as thoughts they he or she may be dying or "going crazy." According to the DSM-IV diagnostic criteria, these symptoms must peak within 10 minutes. Panic attacks may occur without a trigger or occur in the context of certain stressor situations, such as crowded places (e.g., malls).

Post-Traumatic Stress Disorder

Post-traumatic stress disorder (PTSD) remains one of the most understudied anxiety disorders. The symptoms of PTSD develop in response to an exposure to a traumatic event. Depending on the type of trauma, the rate of development of PTSD in the pediatric population can vary from 5% (hurricane) to 100% (school bus hijacking) (Beidel and Turner, 2005). The clinical features of PTSD include several distinct components (Table 47-8). The most common cluster of symptoms of PTSD that patients experience after exposure to a traumatic event is the re-experience of the event. This can occur in the form of dreams, flashbacks, or thoughts. These re-experiences may occur after a trigger associated with the trauma (e.g., a smell) or spontaneously. A second cluster of symptoms is avoidance. Patients will avoid any places, situations, or people that are associated with the trauma. Finally, patients will experience symptoms of hyperarousal, including sleep disturbance, irritability, poor concentration, and exaggerated startle response. Unfortunately, there is little known about the natural history of this disorder. There is a suggestion that girls may be more likely to develop PTSD after exposure to trauma (Beidel and Turner, 2005).

Table 47-7. DSM-IV Criteria for Panic Attack and Panic Disorder Without Agoraphobia

Panic Attack

A discrete period of intense fear or discomfort, in which four (or more) of the following symptoms developed abruptly and reached a peak within 10 minutes:
(1) palpitations, pounding heart, or accelerated heart rate
(2) sweating
(3) trembling or shaking
(4) sensations of shortness of breath or smothering
(5) feeling of choking
(6) chest pain or discomfort
(7) nausea or abdominal distress
(8) feeling dizzy, unsteady, lightheaded, or faint
(9) derealization (feeling of unreality) or depersonalization (being detached from oneself)
(10) fear of losing control or going crazy
(11) fear of dying
(12) paresthesias (numbing or tingling sensations)
(13) chills or hot flushes

Panic Disorder

A. Both (1) and (2):
(1) recurrent unexpected Panic Attacks
(2) at least one of the attacks followed by 1 month (or more) of one (or more) of the following:
(a) persistent concern about having additional attacks
(b) worry about the implications of the attack or its consequences (e.g., losing control, having a heart attack, "going crazy")
(c) a significant change in behavior related to the attacks

B. Absence of Agoraphobia.

C. The Panic Attacks are not due to the direct physiological effects of a substance (e.g., a drug of abuse, a medication) or a general medical condition (e.g., hyperthyroidism).

D. The Panic Attacks are not better accounted for by another mental disorder, such as Social Phobia (e.g., occurring on exposure to feared social situations), Specific Phobia (e.g., on exposure to a specific phobic situation), Obsessive-Compulsive Disorder (e.g., on exposure to dirt in someone with an obsession about contamination), Post-traumatic Stress Disorder (e.g., in response to stimuli associated with a severe stressor), or Separation Anxiety Disorder (e.g., in response to being away from home or close relatives).

From American Psychiatric Association: Diagnostic and Statistical Manual of Mental Disorders, 4th ed. Washington, DC, American Psychiatric Association, 1994.

Management

Treatment of GAD, SAD, and SP includes both psychotherapy and medications (see Chapter 89). In general, CBT, in either group or individual format, has been shown to be effective in treating anxiety in children and adolescents (American Academy of Child and Adolescent Psychiatry, 2007b). In children with anxiety disorders, parent management is also helpful either alone or in conjunction with therapy for the child (American Academy of Child and Adolescent Psychiatry, 2007b). CBT has also been shown to be efficacious when it is delivered in other settings, such as school-based interventions (Compton et al, 2004). Therefore, CBT is recommended for first-line treatment of these disorders in children. Other components that have been shown to be effective in conjunction with group or individual CBT include parental involvement and early intervention for those with subsyndromal or mild symptoms. Therapies based on cognitive-behavioral theories have also been developed for the treatment of PD and shown to have positive effects (American Academy of Child and Adolescent Psychiatry, 2007b). Psychotherapeutic treatments of PTSD have included components of CBT, exposure, and psychoeducation. These have generally been shown to be effective (Beidel and Turner, 2005).

Antidepressants

Although no medications have been approved by the Food and Drug Administration for use in children or adolescents for GAD, SAD, PD, PTSD, or SP, SSRIs have been used clinically in children and adolescents with these disorders. There is increasing evidence from controlled trials indicating improved clinical outcomes in children and adolescents treated with fluoxetine (GAD, SAD, SP), fluvoxamine (GAD, SAD, SP), paroxetine (SP), sertraline (GAD), and venlafaxine (GAD) (see Chapter 90 for a general discussion of antidepressants and page 471 for a discussion of antidepressants and suicidality). Although previously thought to be effective, anxiolytics such as benzodiazepines and tricyclic antidepressants such as imipramine are no longer recommended. The evidence for the use of pharmacologic treatment for PD and PTSD remains limited (Masi et al, 2006).

SUICIDE IN CHILDREN AND ADOLESCENTS

Completed suicide and suicidality, which includes ideation, gestures, and attempts, is a serious consequence of psychiatric disorders. Although it rarely occurs in children younger than 13 years, completed suicide is a leading cause of death in adolescents. Every year, more than 2000 adolescents in the United States commit suicide. Among those who do complete suicide, 90% or more

Table 47-8. DSM-IV Criteria for Post-Traumatic Stress Disorder

A. The person has been exposed to a traumatic event in which both of the following were present:
  (1) the person experienced, witnessed, or was confronted with an event or events that involved actual or threatened death or serious injury, or a threat to the physical integrity of self or others.
  (2) the person's response involved intense fear, helplessness, or horror. **Note:** In children, this may be expressed instead by disorganized or agitated behavior.

B. The traumatic event is persistently reexperienced in one (or more) of the following ways:
  (1) recurrent and intrusive distressing recollections of the event, including images, thoughts, or perceptions. **Note:** In young children, repetitive play may occur in which themes or aspects of the trauma are expressed.
  (2) recurrent distressing dreams of the event. **Note:** In children, there may be frightening dreams without recognizable content.
  (3) acting or feeling as if the traumatic event were recurring (includes a sense of reliving the experience, illusions, hallucinations, and dissociative flashback episodes, including those that occur on awakening or when intoxicated). **Note:** In young children, trauma-specific reenactment may occur.
  (4) intense psychological distress at exposure to internal or external cues that symbolize or resemble an aspect of the traumatic event
  (5) physiological reactivity on exposure to internal or external cues that symbolize or resemble an aspect of the traumatic event

C. Persistent avoidance of stimuli associated with the trauma and numbing of general responsiveness (not present before the trauma), as indicated by three (or more) of the following:
  (1) efforts to avoid thoughts, feelings, or conversations associated with the trauma
  (2) efforts to avoid activities, places, or people that arouse recollections of the trauma
  (3) inability to recall an important aspect of the trauma
  (4) markedly diminished interest or participation in significant activities
  (5) feeling of detachment or estrangement from others
  (6) restricted range of affect (e.g., unable to have loving feelings)
  (7) sense of a foreshortened future (e.g., does not expect to have a career, marriage, children, or normal life span)

D. Persistent symptoms of increased arousal (not present before the trauma), as indicated by two (or more) of the following:
  (1) difficulty falling or staying asleep
  (2) irritability or outbursts of anger
  (3) difficulty concentrating
  (4) hypervigilance
  (5) exaggerated startle response

E. Duration of the disturbance (symptoms in Criteria B, C, and D) is more than 1 month.

F. The disturbance causes clinically significant distress or impairment in social, occupational, or other important areas of functioning.

Specify if:
Acute: if duration of symptoms is less than 3 months
Chronic: if duration of symptoms is 3 months or more
Specify if:
With Delayed Onset: if onset of symptoms is at least 6 months after the stressor

From American Psychiatric Association: Diagnostic and Statistical Manual of Mental Disorders, 4th ed. Washington, DC, American Psychiatric Association, 1994.

have at least one psychiatric diagnosis and more than 50% had a diagnosis of a mood disorder, such as major depressive disorder or bipolar disorder. Suicidality is also a common occurrence. In recent surveys of high-school students in the United States, up to 20% had serious thoughts about suicide in the previous 12 months (Morbidity and Mortality Weekly Report, 2002). Suicidality occurs more frequently in girls. Girls are three times more likely to attempt suicide. However, boys are five times more likely to complete suicide. Other subpopulations, such as Native Americans and bisexual or homosexual youth, are at greater risk of completing suicide.

In terms of method of suicide, firearms are the leading cause of death for boys and girls who complete suicide. More than 90% of suicide attempts involving a firearm are lethal. The presence of a firearm in the home regardless of storage method is associated with a higher risk of adolescent suicide. Therefore, many organizations, including the American Academy of Pediatrics and the Canadian Pediatric Society, endorse the removal of firearms from homes with children and adolescents.

Finally, distinction should be made between patients who have suicidality and those who self-harm (i.e., cutting or burning). This latter group generally does not have an intent to die. These youth require therapeutic interventions different from those for youth with suicidality. The rate of self-harm in adolescents can be as high as 17%. Because of these differences, the following sections focus on the prevention and management of suicide and suicidality in teenagers and not self-harm behaviors.

Table 47-9. Factors to Consider in Deciding Whether to Hospitalize an Adolescent

Strong indicators for hospitalization
- Abnormal mental state (psychotic, manic)
- Persistent wish to die
- Highly lethal method (access to guns, tall buildings)

Factors that favor hospitalization but that are not in themselves sufficient
- Prior attempt
- Male sex
- Family history of suicide
- Inadequate care or supervision at home
- Age 16 years or older

Contraindications to hospitalization
- No Factor 1 categories and: prepubertal or only small overdose or superficial cutting

Reprinted in part from Shaffer D, Greenberg T: Suicide and suicidal behaviors in children and adolescents. *In* Shaffer D, Waslick B (eds): The Many Faces of Depression in Children and Adolescents. Washington, DC, American Psychiatric Publishing, 2002, p 151.

Management

Key management strategies for adolescents who present with suicidality include addressing underlying psychiatric disorders and keeping the adolescents safe during treatment until their suicidality resolves. Whether an adolescent who presents with suicidality is hospitalized will depend on a number of factors. Table 47-9 is a list of considerations that should be given to the hospitalization of adolescents who present with suicidality.

Safety Planning

If a clinician decides that a patient does not require hospitalization, a treatment plan for the related psychiatric disorders must be established as well as a safety plan for emergency communication in case of worsening suicidality or the emergence of new crises. The safety plan should include a list of emergency contacts that the patients can use if their suicidality worsens or if an acute crisis arises (Table 47-10). The clinician should ensure that the information on the list is accurate and current. Previously, safety planning frequently included a contract with the adolescent to not make any attempts. However, no research shows that contracting

Table 47-10. Example of a Safety Plan: GLAD-PC Toolkit Safety Plan

1. Encourage adolescents and parents to make their homes safe. In teens ages 10 to 19, the most common method of suicide is by firearm, followed closely by suffocation (mostly hanging) and poisoning. All guns and other weapons should be removed from the house, or at least locked up. Other potentially harmful items such as ropes, cords, sharp knives, alcohol and other drugs, and poisons should also be removed.
2. Ask about suicide. Providers and parents should ask regularly about thoughts of suicide. Providers should remind parents that making these inquiries will not promote the idea of suicide.
3. Watch for suicidal behavior. Behaviors to watch for in children and teens include
   - expressing self-destructive thoughts
   - drawing morbid or death-related pictures
   - using death as a theme during play in young children
   - listening to music that centers around death
   - playing video games that have a self-destructive theme
   - reading books or other publications that focus on death
   - watching television programs that center around death
   - visiting Internet sites that contain death-related content
   - giving away possessions
4. Watch for signs of drinking. If a child has depression, feels suicidal, and drinks a lot of alcohol, the person is more likely to take his or her life. Parents are usually unaware that their child is drinking. If your child is drinking, you need to discuss this with your child and the clinician.
5. Develop a suicide emergency plan. Work with patients and parents to decide how do proceed if a child feels suicidal. It is important to be specific and provide adolescents with accurate names, phone numbers, and addresses.

www.gladpc.org. Ways to Help Prevent Suicide in Depressed Adolescents. Adapted from materials prepared by Families for Depression Awareness (www.familyaware.org).

with adolescents decreases the rate of suicide or suicide attempts.

Diagnosis and Treatment of Underlying Disorders

Once immediate safety has been established for the patient, the clinician should consider the treatment and management of any underlying psychiatric disorders, such as depression or anxiety. The use of SSRIs has been shown to be effective in the treatment of depressive and anxiety disorders in adolescents. However, worsening suicidality or new-onset suicidality occurs in a small number of adolescents who are treated with antidepressant medications (Table 47-11).

Dialectical behavioral therapy is the only psychotherapeutic technique that has been shown to be effective in reducing the number of suicide attempts in adults (see Chapter 89). Currently, no therapy for children or adolescents has been shown to be effective in decreasing suicidality. One study (March et al, 2004) demonstrated that patients with depressive disorders who are randomized to cognitive-behavioral therapy with or without concurrent treatment with antidepressants had a lower rate of worsening or new-onset suicidality compared to those on placebo or medication alone.

Antidepressants and Suicidality

In 2004, the Food and Drug Administration, after receiving reports of increased suicidality in children and adolescents treated with antidepressants, conducted an independent review of all clinical trials data of newer classes of antidepressants (fluoxetine, fluvoxamine, paroxetine, sertraline, citalopram, venlafaxine, mirtazapine, bupropion, nefazodone). The results of the analysis showed a twofold increase in the risk of worsening or new-onset suicidality in children and adolescents treated with antidepressants versus those treated with placebo. Table 47-11 shows the relative risk of suicidality in adolescents treated with antidepressants compared with those taking placebo. On the basis of the clinical trials evidence, the Food and Drug Administration issued a Black Box warning on both currently available antidepressants and any new antidepressants developed for use in the pediatric population. Recommendations from the Food and Drug Administration included weekly face-to-face meetings for the first 4 weeks at the initiation of medication and after any dose changes. The value of this follow-up schedule is not supported by research evidence. This monitoring schedule was later removed from the Black Box warning, and clinicians are now advised to monitor closely for the emergence of adverse effects.

Non–trial-based data provide contradictory evidence. First, postmortem studies examining toxicology reports of youth who completed suicide found that very few had antidepressants in their systems at the time of their suicide (Leon et al, 2006). Second, two epidemiologic studies showed decreased rates of completed suicides in youth in areas with higher rates of antidepressant prescription (Olfson et al, 2003). Finally, a recent meta-analysis showed that adolescents with depression were more likely to benefit from treatment with antidepressants than to be harmed by them; the number needed to treat was 10, and the number needed to harm was 112 (Bridge et al, 2007).

Numerous professional organizations including the American Academy of Pediatrics and the American Academy of Child and Adolescent Psychiatry have issued guidelines that continue to endorse the use of antidepressants in children who present with serious psychiatric disorders, such as depression and anxiety. Recommendations do not mandate strict adherence to any specific follow-up schedule but instead recommend close observation and follow-up of patients based on the clinical judgment of the treating clinician. Families are also advised to monitor closely for worsening of mood symptoms, worsening or new onset of suicidality, or other behavioral side effects in children and adolescents who are treated with antidepressant medication.

Table 47-11. **Risk of Suicidality with Antidepressants**

Antidepressant	Risk of Suicidality with Antidepressant Compared with Placebo*
Bupropion	NE
Citalopram	1.37
Fluoxetine	1.52
Fluvoxamine	5.52
Mirtazapine	1.58
Nefazodone	NE
Paroxetine	2.65†
Sertraline	1.48
Venlafaxine	4.97†

*Risk ratios comparing rates of suicidality in patients treated with antidepressants versus those taking placebo.

†Results considered statistically significant (if 95% confidence interval does not cross over 1).

NE, no events occurred in either the antidepressant or placebo groups.

Prevention

Prevention of suicide has often been endorsed by clinicians and policy makers alike. Given that most adolescents who commit suicide have at some point been diagnosed with an underlying psychiatric disorder, screening directly or indirectly for untreated psychiatric disorders would be a useful first step. Numerous screening instruments have been developed for use in the pediatric population. One example is the Columbia TeenScreen Program, which is used in school settings in many states in the United States to assess for psychiatric disorders and suicidality in adolescents. Educational programs for parents, teenagers, and other adult caregivers of teenagers are essential to help increase the identification of those who are at

Table 47-12. Risk Factors for Suicide in Adolescents

History of major depressive disorder or other forms of mood disorders
Previous suicide attempts
Family history of psychiatric disorders or suicidal behaviors
Access to lethal means (i.e., handgun)

risk for suicide. Education for clinicians, particularly primary care providers, and teachers is also essential because they have frequent contact with children and adolescents. Research studies show that only one of five primary care providers ask about suicidality in their adolescent patients routinely. Because one of the more significant precipitating factors for suicide is a stressful life event, adolescents may also benefit from interventions that help them develop increased coping skills for stress, such as problem solving and relaxation strategies. Furthermore, crisis services may also be helpful for those who are unable to cope with stressful life events.

Clinicians evaluating adolescents and their families should assess for risk factors associated with suicide and suicidality (Table 47-12) and also should advise parents and families on limiting access to lethal means within their homes. Substance use is highly associated with both suicidality and completed suicide. Of significance is that intoxication with a substance frequently increases impulsivity in adolescents, and this commonly leads to suicide attempts or completed suicide. Other precipitants include psychosocial problems, such as conflicts with family members or parents, breakup of a romantic relationship, academic difficulties, and legal problems. The availability of or access to the means for suicide is also a significant risk factor for completed suicide in adolescents. In adult research, smaller packaging of medications frequently used for suicide attempts, such as acetaminophen and acetylsalicylic acid, has been shown to decrease the rates of suicide by those methods.

Finally, suicide in teens may emerge in clusters or on the basis of "contagion." This contagion effect may be linked to the social desirability of suicide. Frequently, when adolescents commit suicide, they are glorified post mortem, leading to a social desirability for others to follow suit. Therefore, guidelines have been developed to minimize the effect of reporting on individual suicides. However, only limited research has been conducted to examine the effectiveness of these guidelines.

Conclusion

Suicide remains one of the leading causes of death in adolescents, and suicidality, which includes thoughts, gestures, and attempts, is common in both children and teens. Clinicians must educate themselves as well as families and patients to develop effective interventions that are tailored to address the risk factors in each individual patient. Furthermore, research is needed to address the lack of effective psychotherapeutic treatments for those with suicidality.

SUMMARY

Mood and anxiety disorders commonly present in children and adolescents and can lead to significant burden on patients and families if they are unrecognized and untreated. Our understanding of these disorders in children and adolescents has greatly improved during the past few decades and is reflected in the recent changes in the diagnostic criteria for these disorders.

Accompanying these changes in our understanding are the advances in treatment. Although these treatments are generally safe, all treatments have risks and benefits, and clinicians must weigh these for each individual patient. Furthermore, patients and families need to be fully informed and become active participants in the management plan.

Finally, although the diagnostic criteria and treatments of mood and anxiety disorders in children and adolescents are similar to those used in adults, clinicians must understand the developmental issues that can influence diagnosis and management in this age group to effectively manage these disorders.

REFERENCES

Aalto-Setala T, Marttunen M, Tuulio-Henriksson A, et al: Depressive symptoms in adolescence as predictors of early adulthood depressive disorders and maladjustment. Am J Psychiatry 159:1235-1237, 2002.

American Academy of Child and Adolescent Psychiatry: Practice parameters for the assessment and treatment of children and adolescents with depressive disorder. J Am Acad Child Adolesc Psychiatry 37:1234-1238, 1998.

American Academy of Child and Adolescent Psychiatry: Practice parameters for the assessment and treatment of children and adolescents with bipolar disorder. J Am Acad Child Adolesc Psychiatry 46:107-125, 2007a.

American Academy of Child and Adolescent Psychiatry: Practice parameters for the assessment and treatment of children and adolescents with anxiety disorder. J Am Acad Child Adolesc Psychiatry 46:267-283, 2007b.

American Academy of Child and Adolescent Psychiatry: Practice parameters for the assessment and treatment of children and adolescents with depressive disorder. J Am Acad Child Adolesc Psychiatry 46:1503-1526, 2007c.

Barzman DH, DelBello MP, Adler CM, et al: The efficacy and tolerability of quetiapine versus divalproex for the treatment of impulsivity and reactive aggression in adolescents with co-occuring bipolar disorder and disruptive behavior disorder(s). J Child Adolesc Psychopharmacol 16:665-670, 2006.

Beck AT, Steer RA: Manual for the Beck Depression Inventory. San Antonio, TX, The Psychological Corp, 1987.

Beidel DC, Turner SM: Childhood Anxiety Disorders. New York, Routledge, 2005.

Beidel DC, Morris TL, Turner MW: Social phobia. *In* Morris TL, March JS (eds): Anxiety Disorders in Children and Adolescents. New York, Guilford Press, 2004, pp 141-163.

Bernstein GA, Borchardt CM, Perwien AR: Anxiety disorders in children and adolescents: A review of the past 10 years. J Am Acad Child Adolesc Psychiatry 35:1110-1119, 1996.

Bernstein GA, Layne AE, Egan EA, et al: School-based interventions for anxious children. J Am Acad Child Adolesc Psychiatry 44:1118-1127, 2005.

Brent DA, Perper JA, Moritz G, et al: Psychiatric risk factors for adolescent suicide: A case-control study. J Am Acad Child Adolesc Psychiatry 32:521-529, 1993.

Bridge JA, Barbe RP, Birmaher B, et al: Emergent suicidality in a clinical psychotherapy trial for adolescent depression. Am J Psychiatry 162:2173-2175, 2005.

Bridge JA, Iyengar Salary CB, et al: Clinical response and risk for reported suicidal ideation and suicide attempts in pediatric antidepressant treatment. JAMA 297:1683-1696, 2007.

Brooks SJ, Krulewicz SP, Kutcher S: The Kutcher Adolescent Depression Scale: Assessment of its evaluative properties over the course of an 8-week pediatric pharmacotherapy trial. J Child Adolesc Psychopharmacol 13:337-349, 2003.

Carlson GA, Bromet EF, Sievers SB: Phenomenology and outcome of subjects with early- and adult-onset psychotic mania. Am J Psychiatry 157:213-219, 2000.

Chang G, Warner V, Weissman MM: Physicians' recognition of psychiatric disorders in children and adolescents. Am J Dis Child 142:736-739, 1988.

Cheung A, Dewa C: Canadian Community Health Survey: Major depressive disorder and suicidality in adolescents. Healthcare Policy 2:76-89, 2006.

Cheung A, Dewa C: Mental health service use among youth with major depressive disorder and suicidality. Can J Psychiatry 52:228-232, 2007.

Cheung A, Emslie G, Mayes T: Safety and efficacy of SSRIs in youth depression. J Child Psychol Psychiatry 46:735-754, 2005.

Compton SN, March JS, Brent D, et al: Cognitive-behavioral psychotherapy for anxiety and depressive disorders in children and adolescents: An evidence-based medicine review. J Am Acad Child Adolesc Psychiatry 43:930-959, 2004.

Costello EJ, Angold A, Burns BJ, et al: The Great Smoky Mountains Study of Youth: Goals, design, methods, and the prevalence of DSM-III-R disorders. Arch Gen Psychiatry 53:1129-1136, 1996.

Fergusson DM, Woodward LJ: Mental health, educational, and social role outcomes of adolescents with depression. Arch Gen Psychiatry 59:225-231, 2002.

Fleming JE, Offord DR, Boyle MH: Prevalence of childhood and adolescent depression in the community. Ontario Child Health Study. Br J Psychiatry 155:647-654, 1989.

Halpern-Felsher BL, Ozer EM, Millstein SG, et al: Preventive services in a health maintenance organization: How well do pediatricians screen and educate adolescent patients? Arch Pediatr Adolesc Med 154:173-179, 2000.

Kessler RC, Avenevoli S, Ries Merikangas K: Mood disorders in children and adolescents: An epidemiologic perspective. Biol Psychiatry 15:1002-1014, 2001.

Kornstein SG: The evaluation and management of depression in women across the life span. J Clin Psychiatry 62(Suppl 24):11-17, 2001.

Kramer T, Garralda ME: Psychiatric disorders in adolescents in primary care. Br J Psychiatry 173:508-513, 1998.

Leon AC, Marzuk PM, Tardiff K, et al: Antidepressants and youth suicide in New York City, 1999-2002. J Am Acad Child Adolesc Psychiatry 45:1054-1058, 2006.

Lewinsohn PM, Hops H, Roberts RE, et al: Adolescent psychopathology, I: Prevalence and incidence of depression and other DSM-III-R disorders in high school students. J Abnorm Psychol 102: 133-144, 1993.

March J, Silva S, Petrycki S, et al: Fluoxetine, cognitive-behavioral therapy, and their combination for adolescents with depression: Treatment for Adolescents with Depression Study (TADS) randomized controlled trial. JAMA 292:807-820, 2004.

Masi G, Pari C, Millepiedi S: Pharmacological treatment options for panic disorder in children and adolescents. Expert Opin Pharmacother 7:545-554, 2006.

Middleman AB, Binns HJ, Durant RH: Factors affecting pediatric residents' intentions to screen for high risk behaviors. J Adolesc Health 17:106-112, 1995.

Morbidity and Mortality Weekly Report: Youth risk behavior surveillance. CDC 51:ss-4, 2002

Mufson L, Dorta KP, Wickramaratne P, et al: A randomized effectiveness trial of interpersonal psychotherapy for depressed adolescents. Arch Gen Psychiatry 61:577-584, 2004.

Mufson L, Weissman MM, Moreau D, Garfinkel R: Efficacy of interpersonal psychotherapy for depressed adolescents. Arch Gen Psychiatry 56:573-579, 1999.

Olfson M, Shaffer D, Marcus SC, Greenberg T: Relationship between antidepressant medication treatment and suicide in adolescents. Arch Gen Psychiatry 60:978-982, 2003.

Olson AL, Kelleher KJ, Kemper KJ, et al: Primary care pediatricians' roles and perceived responsibilities in the identification and management of depression in children and adolescents. Ambul Pediatr 1:91-98, 2001.

Pappadopulos E, Macintyre JC, Crismon ML, et al: Treatment recommendations for the use of antipsychotics for aggressive youth (TRAAY). Part II. J Am Acad Child Adolesc Psychiatry 42:145-161, 2003.

Regier DA, Narrow WE, Rae DS, et al: The de facto mental and addictive disorders service system: Epidemiologic catchment area prospective 1-year prevalence rates of disorders and services. Arch Gen Psychiatry 50:85-94, 1993.

Rushton JL, Forcier M, Schectman RM: Epidemiology of depressive symptoms in the National Longitudinal Study of Adolescent Health. J Am Acad Child Adolesc Psychiatry 41:199-205, 2002.

Shaffer D, Greenberg T: Suicide and suicidal behaviors in children and adolescents. *In* Shaffer D, Waslick B (eds): The Many Faces of Depression in Children and Adolescents. Washington, DC, American Psychiatric Publishing, 2002, p 151.

Strober M, Morrell W, Lampert C, et al: Relapse following discontinuation of lithium maintenance therapy in adolescents with bipolar I illness: A naturalistic study. Am J Psychiatry 147:457-461, 1990.

Swedo SE, Leonared HL, Garvey M, et al: Pediatric autoimmune neuropsychiatric disorders associated with streptococcal infections: Clinical description of the first 50 cases. Am J Psychiatry 155:264-271, 1998.

Waslick B, Kandel R, Kakouros A: Depression in children and adolescents. *In* Shaffer D, Waslick B (eds): The Many Faces of Depression in Children and Adolescents. Washington, DC, American Psychiatric Publishing, 2002, p 19.

Weissman MM, Warner V, Wickramaratne P, et al: Offspring of depressed parents: 10 years later. Arch Gen Psychiatry 54:932-940, 1997.

Weissman MM, Wolk S, Goldstein RB, et al: Depressed adolescents grown up. JAMA 281:1707-1713, 1999.

Weissman MM, Pilowsky DJ, Wickramaratne PJ, et al: Remissions in maternal depression and child psychopathology: a STAR*D-child report. JAMA 295:1389-1398, 2006.

Whitaker A Johnson J, Shaffer D, et al: Uncommon troubles in young people. Arch Gen Psychiatry 47:487-494, 1990.

Zuckerbrot RA, Jensen PS: Improving recognition of adolescent depression in primary care. Arch Pediatr Med 160:694-704, 2006.

48 SCHIZOPHRENIA, PHOBIAS, AND OBSESSIVE-COMPULSIVE DISORDER

ANTONIO Y. HARDAN AND ANDREW R. GILBERT

Vignette

Melinda, a 14-year-old girl living with her biologic parents, was referred by her pediatrician for a psychiatric evaluation and treatment of unusual behaviors. Melinda had been doing well until about 6 months before the visit, when her parents noticed a decline in her academic functioning. Her grades dropped progressively from straight As to mostly Cs and Ds. Family members noticed a change in her personality. She became irritable with a low level of tolerance for frustration and an increasing level of social isolation. What triggered the psychiatric evaluation was a phone call from school describing bizarre behaviors. The teacher reported that Melinda had become afraid that someone was trying to hurt her. She began talking to herself loudly, making statements about the devil being after her, and accusing her peers of plotting to kidnap her. The parents stated that they have not seen these behaviors but admitted being relatively absent from home recently because of working long hours and being away with travel. Medical, personal, and developmental histories were unremarkable except for the presence of a paternal uncle who was receiving treatment for schizophrenia. During the interview, the adolescent was difficult to engage and had made limited eye contact. At times, she began talking to herself and appeared to be laughing for no apparent reason. Her affect was irritable, and she refused to answer some questions. She acknowledged feeling paranoid and talked about aliens trying to poison and hurt her. She also admitted to hearing voices that made negative comments about her and at times provided a critical commentary on her actions. She denied any command auditory hallucinations demanding her to perform an act. The primary care physician called for an urgent visit with a child psychiatrist. At that visit, Melinda was initiated on 0.5 mg of risperidone for 2 weeks, then 1 mg afterward. During the following few months, her symptoms improved progressively with a decrease in paranoid delusions and hallucinations; she appeared much improved at the 6-month follow-up with no psychotic thinking noted.

Most primary care providers and developmental-behavioral pediatricians are very comfortable identifying, assessing, and treating some mental health and behavioral disorders, such as attention-deficit/hyperactivity disorders. However, for the most part, pediatricians generally refer children with major psychiatric disorders, such as schizophrenia and obsessive-compulsive disorder (OCD), to mental health professionals because such mental health practitioners have specific knowledge, skills, and experience to treat these children. Nonetheless, primary care providers and developmental-behavioral pediatricians need to be aware of the manifestations and early signs of these severe conditions so that an appropriate referral is made. In addition, primary care clinicians must be prepared to provide a medical home for children with these disorders. The provision of a medical home requires at least broad understanding of the clinical issues, functional implications, and psychosocial impact of these conditions.

A division of psychiatric disorders into two major categories—disorders of mood and disorders of thought—was introduced by Emil Kraepelin. This chapter describes major psychiatric disorders outside the realm of mood disorders. We now know that these conditions may have an affective component even though the primary symptoms relate to thought and thought disorders. We also know that these disorders result in impaired functioning at home and in school, with family and peers. Psychotic and two specific anxiety disorders, phobias and OCD, are described here. Mood disorders are developed in Chapter 47. This overview takes a developmental approach, which we consider essential in the understanding of these disorders. We also hope that the discussion will facilitate communication and collaboration between child psychiatrist and pediatric health care providers.

CHILDHOOD PSYCHOSES

Childhood psychoses are thought disorders characterized by psychotic symptoms or a loss of contact with reality, including changes in the usual patterns of thinking, perceiving, believing, and behaving. The term *thought disorders,* also known as formal thought disorders, is used to describe a pattern of disordered language use, which is presumed to reflect disordered thinking. Like the adult versions, childhood psychoses are frequently accompanied by delusions and hallucinations. Delusions are fixed, firm, and false beliefs that are maintained by the believer despite overwhelming contradictory evidence. Hallucinations are false perceptions of one or another of the five senses: sight, hearing, taste, touch, or smell.

A disturbance of thinking is usually considered a symptom of psychotic mental illness, although it occasionally appears in other conditions. They include schizophrenia with childhood onset, schizophreniform disorder, schizoaffective disorder, delusional disorder, shared psychotic disorder, brief psychotic disorder, psychotic disorder due to a general medical condition, substance-induced psychotic disorder, and psychotic disorder not otherwise specified. Although much more common in adulthood, thought disorders can have their onset as early as 5 years of age (Masi et al, 2006).

SCHIZOPHRENIA WITH CHILDHOOD ONSET

Clinical Description

Clinical Features

The onset of schizophrenia is typically in late teens to mid-30s, but the disorder can occur in childhood, with no reports of onset before 5 years of age. Schizophrenia is defined as a chronic deterioration (at least 6 months) from previous level of functioning, accompanied by psychotic features, but with no evidence of toxic or organic etiology, and in the absence of prominent affective (either depressive or manic) symptoms. Psychotic symptoms may include delusions (e.g., thought broadcasting, thought insertion, being controlled by someone, ideas of reference, or persecutory delusions) or hallucinations (frequently auditory hallucinations, such as voices commenting on a person's behavior or two voices having a conversation). Affect is often blunted or inappropriate, and speech is digressive, vague, circumstantial, or incoherent (Masi et al, 2006; Schothorst et al, 2006). Although not definitive, evidence points to continuity between children at risk for schizophrenia, early-onset schizophrenia, and adult-onset schizophrenia (Remschmidt and Theisen, 2005).

Developmental Aspects

Symptoms of schizophrenia are sometimes difficult to identify in children. Children may experience hallucination, delusions, and thought disorder typical of schizophrenia. However, their limited cognitive and language development and difficulties separating reality from fantasy make it difficult to apply diagnostic criteria. In addition, delusions and hallucinations are usually less complex in children. Interestingly, this pattern of symptoms is usually observed in adult individuals with developmental disorders who develop psychotic symptoms.

As symptoms of psychosis emerge, children with schizophrenia experience a deterioration of their level of functioning, or never achieve the expected level of functioning (American Psychiatric Association, 2000). Blunted affect and inappropriate laughter are almost universally present in children with schizophrenia. Auditory and visual hallucinations are frequently reported. Children might hear several voices making an ongoing critical commentary or even command hallucinations telling them to hurt themselves or others. Visual hallucinations are relatively more common in children than in adults with schizophrenia. They are often frightening, and children report seeing skeletons, scary individuals, and the devil. Delusions are observed in more than half of all children with psychosis, have various themes including persecutory and religious themes, and increase in frequency with age (Masi et al, 2006; Remschmidt and Theisen, 2005).

Differential Diagnosis

Schizophrenia must be differentiated from other forms of psychosis (Table 48-1). Acute psychotic presentation can be associated with various causes of organic brain syndrome, including infection, autoimmune phenomena (e.g., lupus, multiple sclerosis), structural lesions, medications (e.g., steroids), illicit drugs (e.g., PCP), and metabolic disorders (e.g., Wilson disease or porphyria).

Table 48-1. **Differential Diagnosis of Schizophrenia**

Disorders	Clinical Characteristics
Schizophreniform disorder	Duration of psychotic symptoms of more than a month but less than 6 months
Schizoaffective disorder	Coexistence of mood and psychotic symptoms
Delusional disorder	Believable delusions
Brief psychotic disorder	Psychotic symptoms of short duration (<1 month)
Psychotic disorder due to a general medical condition	Existence of a medical condition justifying the psychotic symptoms
Substance-induced psychotic disorder	Evidence from the history, physical examination, or laboratory findings of recreational substance or prescription use
Psychotic disorder, not otherwise specified	Not enough information available
Obsessive-compulsive disorder	Presence of insight

In many of these disorders, psychosis is accompanied by symptoms of delirium or dementia. Delirium is an acute and relatively sudden decline (developing during hours to days) in attention-focus, perception, and cognition, commonly associated with a disturbance of consciousness. In contrast, dementia is characterized by a progressive decline (developing during months to years) in cognitive function due to damage or disease in the brain beyond what might be expected from normal aging.

Bipolar disorder can be accompanied by psychosis in either the depressive or manic phase. In the depressive phase, psychoses generally are related to mood, such as in the case of nihilistic or somatic delusions or self-deprecatory auditory hallucinations. Psychosis during mania is exacerbated by sleep disturbances and tends to be grandiose or paranoid in nature. The course and associated symptoms, even more than the nature of the psychotic symptoms, determine whether the disorder is classified as schizophrenia or psychosis related to an affective disorder. In schizophrenia, dysphoria occurs secondary to psychotic disintegration, whereas in depression, the psychotic symptoms have onset coincident with the affective symptoms. In schizoaffective illness, the affective component remits, but the thought disorder persists. Schizophrenia can be differentiated from autism and pervasive development disorders insofar as the pervasive developmental disorders have an earlier age at onset and are frequently associated with seizures, intellectual disability, and an almost complete lack of appropriate language or social interactions. Patients with autism do not experience hallucinations or delusions. Schizophrenia may also need to be distinguished from schizotypal personality disorder, which may be thought of as a forme fruste of schizophrenia. Patients with schizotypal personality disorder may be circumstantial without being incoherent, and they may have odd beliefs or magical thinking (e.g., belief of clairvoyance or telepathy and, in children, bizarre fantasies or preoccupations) without truly experiencing psychosis.

Epidemiology

The prevalence of childhood-onset schizophrenia is not known, but it is thought to be relatively rare, less than 5 in 10,000 (Remschmidt and Theisen, 2005; Schothorst et al, 2006). Prevalence rates appear to be greater among boys, at least in clinically referred cases. In adolescence, the prevalence is estimated to be 50 times greater than in younger children, with probable rates of 1 to 2 per 1000. In contrast, rates are much higher in adults, reaching 1 to 1.5 percent.

Etiology: Neurobiology and Risk Factors

The risk for development of schizophrenia in the children of a schizophrenic parent is about 10%, or about 10-fold the prevalence in the general population. The risk is increased even more if the parent had an especially early age at onset, there was evidence of perinatal distress at birth, and the perinatal stress is accompanied by an enlarged third ventricle and an increased ventricle-to-brain ratio. In addition, there is some evidence that schizotypal traits (e.g., a tendency to prefer one's own company or engaging in fantasy or magical thinking and idiosyncratic speech) represe nt a precursor of schizophrenia and are found to be much more common in the families of patients with schizophrenia.

Onset of puberty seems to precipitate early-onset schizophrenia in girls. Precursors of early-onset schizophrenia include movement disorders, poor sensory-motor integration, and impaired coordination. Neuropsychiatric difficulties, including fine motor problems and visual tracking difficulties, are commonly noted. Imaging studies have shown decreased cerebral volume, increased size of the lateral ventricles, and relative sparing of white matter. Interestingly, longitudinal studies have pointed to an increase in ventricular volume over time.

Treatment

The first critical step in the pediatric management of early-onset schizophrenia is its identification. Psychosis and bizarre behavior are not difficult to recognize. Adolescent patients who refuse to go to school and seem guarded about their reasons for refusing school attendance may have paranoid ideation. Schizophrenia is best managed by a child psychiatrist; however, the families of such patients require pediatric support, and the potential medical complications of neuroleptic treatment should be monitored closely (Masi et al, 2006).

Because of the rarity of this condition among youth, little is known about the optimal treatment of such patients in childhood and adolescence. Initial studies have examined the use of typical antipsychotics, such as haloperidol, but the side effect profile of these medications, including extrapyramidal symptoms and tardive dyskinesia, has limited their use. Studies have examined second-generation antipsychotics and have evaluated their efficacy and safety. Clozapine appears to be the most effective medication, with two well-designed studies reporting its superiority over haloperidol (Kumra et al, 1996) and olanzapine (Kumra et al, 2008). Clozapine was superior for relief of both negative and positive symptoms but has the serious side effect of blood dyscrasia, necessitating careful monitoring for development of this condition. However, clozapine has no extrapyramidal side effects and presumably has a much lower risk of tardive dyskinesia.

The advent of second-generation antipsychotics, such as clozapine, risperidone, olanzapine, quetiapine, ziprasidone, and aripiprazole, has increased the hope of a better treatment of early-onset schizophrenia (Masi et al, 2006). However, the benefits observed from these medications remain limited, and the prognosis is frequently guarded. Taking into consideration the poor response observed, psychosocial interventions remain essential. Psychoeducation and family support are critical to optimize the functioning of the patient and to prevent relapse. Environmental manipulations, especially in school, are frequently required to alleviate the social skills deficits, attentional disturbances, and academic difficulties frequently observed in early-onset schizophrenia.

Prognosis and Course

Little is known of the course of pediatric schizophrenia, except the prognosis is relatively poor and the condition chronic. A disturbing trend in early-onset schizophrenia is the continued loss in intelligence quotient over time (Jacobsen and Rapoport, 1998). Patients with prominent negative symptoms (e.g., flat affect, withdrawn) have a particularly poor response to treatment and a refractory prognosis. Suicide is a real risk, especially among young adult men with a previously high level of functioning who have a chronic and relapsing course. In such patients, comorbid depression and hopelessness have been observed to be associated with suicide.

DELUSIONAL DISORDER AND SHARED PSYCHOTIC DISORDER

Delusional disorder is a thought disorder that is characterized by holding on to non-bizarre delusions, that is, beliefs about events that occur in real life and hence are possible (e.g., being followed). There are seven types based on the predominant content of the delusions, allowing clinicians to specify the theme of delusions. The types include erotomanic, grandiose, persecutory, jealous, and mixed. The mean age at onset is about 40 years, but the range for the age at onset runs from 18 years to the 90s. Other psychotic symptoms are usually not present. This disorder is not usually observed in children and adolescents, but youth could be involved as part of a shared psychotic disorder also known as induced delusional disorder, folie à deux, or folie à famille (Zillessen et al, 1996). It is a characterized by an individual's or individuals' developing a delusion in the context of a close relationship with another person who has an already established delusion. The common themes of these delusions are paranoid and involve a parent, the primary patient, and a spouse as well as children, the secondary patients, in a complex psychosocial situation. A recently published case report described a 12-year-old boy who was hospitalized after his father developed a delusional disorder, paranoid type, and led to the development of a folie à famille that included the mother (Wehmeier et al, 2003). Treatment of individuals with delusional disorder and shared psychotic disorder includes a combination of pharmacotherapy and psychotherapy and requires, at times, hospitalization of the primary patient. Whereas the prognosis of delusional disorder is guarded, long-term outcome of children with shared psychotic disorder is good, especially if the primary patient is well-treated.

BRIEF PSYCHOTIC DISORDER

Epidemiologic information on brief psychotic disorder in adults and in children is limited. Reliable estimates of prevalence and even the average age at onset are not available. Although rigorous studies are lacking, it is generally believed by clinicians that this disorder is rare, and it is more common in young patients than in older individuals. Brief psychotic disorder is characterized by the existence of brief psychotic symptoms lasting for at least one day and less than a month. It can occur shortly after, and probably related to, stressful events; postpartum onset is identified as one of the traumatic incidents described especially in teenage girls. Chapter 49 describes such a case in a young man with intellectual disability. The treatment of brief psychotic disorder is challenging, and acutely psychotic patients might require a brief hospitalization. Psychopharmacologic interventions are an essential component of the management of these individuals, and typical and atypical antipsychotics are the main medications used. Psychotherapy is supportive and includes a considerable psychoeducational aspect.

OTHER PSYCHOTIC DISORDERS

Whereas schizophrenia is the most common psychotic disorder, there are, however, several other psychotic disorders that could be observed in children and adolescents. This group includes schizophreniform disorder, schizoaffective disorder, psychotic disorder not otherwise specified, psychotic disorder due to a general medical condition, and substance-induced psychotic disorder.

The symptoms of schizophreniform disorder are similar to those of schizophrenia except that the symptoms last at least 1 month but less than 6 months (American Psychiatric Association, 2000). Schizoaffective disorder is characterized by the presence of symptoms for both schizophrenia and a mood disorder. However, during the illness, delusions and hallucinations must have been present for at least 2 weeks in the absence of prominent mood symptoms (American Psychiatric Association, 2000). Psychotic disorder, not otherwise specified, is a category applied to individuals with psychotic symptoms such as delusions, hallucinations, and disorganized speech and behaviors that do no meet the diagnostic criteria for a specific disorder. It is often used when not enough information is available to allow a comprehensive assessment and accurate diagnosis.

Whereas no clear causes can be identified for most psychotic symptoms, the evaluation process should include a consideration of the possibility that the psychosis is caused by a general medical condition or is induced by a substance. In fact, in an effort to highlight the importance of bearing in mind these conditions, the *Diagnostic and Statistical Manual of Mental Disorders*, fourth edition, text revision (DSM-IV-TR), has listed psychotic disorder due to a general medical condition and substance-induced psychotic disorder. These disorders describe situations in which a general disease process, such as brain tumor, or ingested compounds, such as a prescribed medication or a recreational substance, can precipitate psychotic symptoms. The early diagnosis of such conditions is crucial in providing the appropriate treatment.

SPECIFIC PHOBIA AND SOCIAL PHOBIA

A phobia is defined as an irrational fear that produces avoidant behavior of the feared subject, activity, or situation. Phobic reactions can be very disruptive to a child's academic and social functioning and can potentially lead to grave consequences.

In addition to agoraphobia, two other phobias are included in the DSM-IV-TR: specific phobia and social phobia (American Psychiatric Association, 2000).

Specific Phobia

Phobic disorders are related to avoidance precipitated by certain triggers, such as animals, situations, or places. Fears are common among children. Among children aged 7 and 11 years, the prevalence of specific phobias is approximately 2.4% and 0.9%, respectively (Anderson et al, 1987; Silverman and Moreno, 2005), with a marked female preponderance. It is thought that parental history of anxiety disorder (particularly phobias), anxious temperament, and traumatic occurrences (e.g., a dog bite, leading to dog phobia) all play a role in the genesis of phobic disorders.

Many phobic disorders never come to medical attention because those suffering from the disorder can simply alter their life to avoid contact with the precipitant for their phobic reactions. However, children with simple phobia that leads to school avoidance often are referred for treatment of "school refusal." The differentiation between a fear and phobia is in the degree of anxiety in response to exposure, the extent of the avoidant behavior, and the concomitant functional impairment. School phobia may result in the avoidance of school, but the fear is not related to separation, as in the case of separation anxiety disorder. Behavioral interventions have a well-documented efficacy in the treatment of phobias. Such interventions include desensitization through graduated imagined or real exposure.

Social Phobia

Social phobia (SP), also known as social anxiety disorder, is a common anxiety disorder related to excessive embarrassment and extreme shyness in novel social situations. What differentiates SP from more common shyness is that children and adolescents with SP frequently avoid situations that they believe to be potentially scrutinizing, such as most social and performance situations (American Psychiatric Association, 2000). Thus, significant functional impairment characterizes SP.

Clinical Description

Clinical Features

Diagnostic criteria for SP include a persistence of symptoms, characterized by avoidance of novel and public social situations, for at least 6 months, that are severe enough to interfere with social adaptation, and these symptoms must be established across multiple situations (American Psychiatric Association, 2000). One extreme manifestation of SP in younger children is selective mutism, in which children do not speak in one or more major social situations when speaking is expected, despite speaking in other situations. In selective mutism, patients do not speak for at least 1 month (not limited to the first month of school) (Leonard and Topol, 1993).

SP frequently emerges during childhood, with a mean age at onset of approximately 15 years. Parental or school concerns are the usual cues to the presence of SP. Children and adolescents with SP will frequently describe fears related to reading, speaking, eating, or writing in public. These symptoms can occur in multiple contexts, usually associated with typical age-appropriate social environments and situations, such as classrooms, birthday parties, school dances, sporting events, social clubs, public bathrooms, and informal social gatherings (Beidel et al, 1999; Hoffman et al, 1999). Children and adolescents frequently experience somatic symptoms, such as racing heart, sweating, blushing, lightheadedness, and gastrointestinal distress, when they are confronted with a potentially anxiety-provoking situation (Beidel et al, 1991).

Diagnosis

A clinical diagnosis should include the following: psychiatric interview with the child; interview with parents, including complete developmental and family history; and review of systems. There are several psychometrically sound measures that can assist with diagnosis, including the clinician-rated Liebowitz Social Anxiety Scale for Children and Adolescents and the self-report Social Phobia and Anxiety Inventory for Children (Beidel et al, 1996; Storch et al, 2004).

Comorbidity

SP in childhood and adolescence is associated with significant comorbidity. SP is frequently accompanied by other anxiety and mood disorders, such as generalized anxiety disorder, specific phobia, and depression (Albano et al, 1996; Beidel et al, 1999; Coyle, 2001).

Developmental Considerations

Although SP is frequently diagnosed during adolescence, children as young as 8 years have been diagnosed with the disorder. Younger children may express a phenotype characterized by greater frequency and severity of tantrums and clingy behaviors, whereas older adolescents may express more avoidant behavior related to peers and social situations (Beidel and Turner, 1998).

Differential Diagnosis

The main differential diagnoses include other conditions, such as mood and anxiety disorders, that interfere with social relationships. In depression, there may be social withdrawal, but this is often antedated by satisfactory social relationships. Schizoid disorder of childhood is characterized by a lack of interest in social relationships with strangers, whereas socially phobic children both desire and fear contact with same-age peers who are not well known to them. Schizotypal children have evidence of thought disorder, such as loosening of associations and magical thinking. Children with autism and pervasive developmental disorders have disordered social relationships but usually show other stigmata of these disorders, such as impaired language development, repetitive and stereotyped patterns of behavior and interests, and difficulty in forming and sustaining social bonds.

Epidemiology

SP is estimated to occur in approximately 1% of children and adolescents. Because of the substantially higher lifetime prevalence of SP in adulthood (13.3%), SP may be underdiagnosed in childhood and adolescence, mislabeled as "shyness," and this may be due to methodologic factors (Costello et al, 2004; Kessler et al, 1994).

Etiology

There is evidence suggesting that shyness and behavioral inhibition may both constitute risk factors for the development of SP (Hayward et al, 1998). Although causality cannot be confirmed, studies suggest that classic conditioning experiences, social learning through modeling, and anxious and controlling parenting styles may all contribute to the risk for development of SP. Furthermore, twin studies suggest that shyness, behavioral inhibition, and SP may be heritable (Chavira and Stein, 2005).

Treatment

Cognitive-behavioral therapy (CBT) has been found to be effective in the treatment of children and adolescents with SP (see Chapter 89). Both family-based and group CBT have also been found to be effective (Mancini et al, 2005). Similarly, pharmacologic agents have been found to be beneficial. Both placebo-controlled and open-label studies support the efficacy of selective serotonin reuptake inhibitors in the treatment of SP (see Chapter 90). The selective serotonin reuptake inhibitors appear to reduce the severity of symptoms of SP and are generally well tolerated (Mancini et al, 2005).

Prognosis

Untreated SP may lead to significant impairment, including underachievement in academics and work as well as difficulties with relationships (Schneier et al, 1994; Stein, 1996; Van Ameringen et al, 2003). SP tends to be chronic, with approximately only 27% of patients achieving spontaneous remission.

OBSESSIVE-COMPULSIVE DISORDER

OCD is a disabling neuropsychiatric condition characterized by obsessions (recurrent, intrusive thoughts, ideas, or images) and compulsions (repetitive, ritualistic behaviors). For patients with OCD, obsessions lead to substantial anxiety and emotional discomfort, and compulsions are carried out to neutralize the anxiety. Pediatric patients with OCD, in general, are not comfortable with their obsessions (ego-dystonic) and are interested in eliminating them. For a diagnosis of OCD, the symptoms must cause significant impairment in terms of time (approximately more than 1 hour a day), distress, and interference in functioning (American Psychiatric Association, 1994).

Clinical Description

Clinical Presentation

Common obsessions include contamination fears (dirt, germs, or illness), aggressive/harm obsessions (excessive worries about danger or catastrophic events, such as death or illness happening to self or loved ones), separation, hoarding and saving, symmetry/ordering, and doing things "just right." Intrusive sexual thoughts and religious obsessions are more common in adolescence than in childhood. Common compulsions are washing, checking, repetitive counting, arranging, touching, and hoarding. At least four symptom dimensions (contamination/washing, symmetry/ordering, hoarding, obsessive/with or without checking) have been found to be temporally stable throughout childhood and adulthood as well as familial (Delorme et al, 2006; Hasler et al, 2007; Mataix-Cols et al, 2005).

Diagnosis

A clinical diagnosis should include the following: psychiatric interview with the child; interview with parents, including complete developmental and family history; symptom rating and monitoring of severity over time with use of the Children's Yale-Brown Obsessive Compulsive Scale; review of systems, with special attention to neurologic and infectious disease signs, symptoms, and history. OCD symptoms secondary to a recent group A beta-hemolytic streptococcal infection should always be ruled out.

Comorbidity

Studies suggest that approximately 80% of children and adolescents with OCD have at least one comorbid psychiatric disorder (American Psychiatric Association, 2000). Common comorbid conditions, as described before, include the following: major depression and other mood disorders; other anxiety disorders; OCD spectrum disorders; tic disorders; disruptive behavioral disorders, particularly attention-deficit/hyperactivity disorder and oppositional defiant disorder; speech/developmental disabilities; eating disorders; pervasive developmental disorders.

Developmental Aspects

It can be difficult to separate the symptoms of OCD from developmentally normal childhood rituals. Superstitious and magical thinking ("step on a crack, break your mother's back") are part of normal development, frequently appearing around the ages of 5 to 8 years. In general, these normal thoughts and behaviors do not lead to the substantial functional impairment or avoidance behaviors characteristic of OCD and other anxiety disorders. Interestingly, there are few differences between OCD in childhood and adulthood; indeed, the DSM-IV criteria are the same, although it is noted that children may have less insight and their symptoms may be more ego-syntonic.

Although pediatric OCD patients may have less insight than adult patients do, recent factor analytic studies suggest that symptoms of OCD remain temporally stable throughout childhood and adulthood. The following characteristics of the disorder and findings from research studies may support a neurodevelopmental versus acquired degenerative etiopathogenic theory of OCD: frequent childhood onset; similar presentation in childhood and adulthood may suggest that the risk emerges during development; similarity with normal childhood rituals; high comorbidity with Tourette disorder, which is characterized as a neurodevelopmental disorder; early-onset OCD is more likely to have a family history; and presence of neurologic soft sign abnormalities observed at illness onset with absence of deterioration with illness progression (Rosenberg and Keshavan, 1998).

Differential Diagnosis

Normal developmental rituals can be difficult to distinguish from OCD symptoms in children and adolescents (Table 48-2). The most important factor in ruling out normal rituals from OCD is the level of discomfort and dysfunction that accompanies the thoughts and behaviors. Tourette and tic disorders are frequently comorbid with OCD; although tics may neutralize anxiety, they are different from compulsions in that they are not triggered by an obsession (Cohen and Leckman, 1994). Pediatric autoimmune neuropsychiatric disorders associated with streptococcal infections (PANDAS) may represent a subtype of pediatric OCD; however, PANDAS appear to have a temporal relationship with the onset of streptococcal infections, have a more sudden and severe onset, and are frequently associated with tics and abnormal choreiform-like movements (Snider and Swedo, 2004). OCD spectrum disorders, including trichotillomania, onychophagia (nail biting), chronic skin picking, other impulse control disorders, and body dysmorphic disorder, are often comorbid with OCD but can also be confused with compulsions (Geller, 2006). Like tics, many impulse control disorders, such as nail biting and hair pulling, are anxiety neutralizing but do not have an obsession attached to them. Body dysmorphic disorder can be very much like OCD; however, the obsessions and compulsions of the patient with body dysmorphic disorder are focused on or driven by a specific body region (e.g., nose, teeth, hair). Similar to body dysmorphic disorder, eating disorders such as anorexia and bulimia can involve OCD-like symptoms, including obsessional thoughts and ritualistic behaviors. The focus of eating disorders, however, is on body image and involves specific eating-related rituals, such as purging and restricting.

Although primary psychotic disorders are rare in childhood, early-onset psychosis and prodromal schizophrenia can be characterized by delusions similar to obsessions. The rule of thumb in distinguishing delusions from obsessions is the level of insight present in the individual. Furthermore, the delusions and behaviors associated with a primary psychosis are more likely to be bizarre and accompanied by negative symptoms, such as a blunted affect and isolative behavior. Rumination within depressions may appear to be similar to obsessions; however, ruminations tend to be characterized by worries about mundane events and conditions in the individual's life (such as school, friends, and family), whereas obsessions tend to be characterized by specific dimensions, such as contamination, symmetry, and hoarding. Repetitive rituals and restricted interests characteristic of pervasive developmental disorders, such as Asperger disorder, can appear similar to obsessions and compulsions. In general, children and adolescents with pervasive developmental disorders suggest that they enjoy their repetitive thoughts and ritualistic behaviors (ego-syntonic), in contrast to children with ego-dystonic OCD symptoms.

Table 48-2. **Differential Diagnosis of Obsessive-Compulsive Disorder**

Differential Diagnosis	Clinical Characteristics
Normal developmental rituals	Transient
Tourette and tic disorders	Association with tics
PANDAS*	History of streptococcal infection
Trichotillomania and onychophagia	Presence of tissue damage
Body dysmorphic disorder	Focus on body parts
Early-onset psychosis and prodromal schizophrenia	Presence of hallucinations and delusions
Pervasive developmental disorders, such as Asperger disorder	Early history of social deficits

*Pediatric autoimmune neuropsychiatric disorders associated with streptococcal infections.

Epidemiology

Estimated prevalence rates of OCD in the pediatric population are between 0.5% and 4%. Studies suggest a bimodal distribution of inci- dence, with one peak in childhood and another in adulthood. The mean age at onset of pediatric OCD is approximately 10.3 years, and the mean age at assessment is approximately 13.2 years. OCD may occur in children as early as 3 years of age. Boys tend to have an earlier age at onset than do girls. The male-to-female ratio is 7:1 for cases with onset before 10 years and 1:1.5 for onset after puberty; the average male-to-female ratio in pediatric OCD is 3:2. Mild subclinical obsessions and compulsions are common in the general population (4% to 19%). Approximately one third to one half of adult OCD cases have a childhood onset (Flament et al, 1988; Leonard et al, 2005).

Etiology

The causes of OCD remain to be fully elucidated; however, there are several hypotheses about its etiology and pathogenesis (Rauch and Jenike, 1993). Because of the effectiveness of serotonin reuptake inhibitors in treating OCD, serotonergic abnormalities are potentially involved in the development and expression of the disorder. OCD is associated with several basal ganglia illnesses, including tic disorders, Huntington chorea, and Sydenham chorea; basal ganglia abnormalities in OCD are also supported by neuroimaging studies. Recent evidence suggests that severe pediatric OCD symptoms in conjunction with tics and a sudden onset of symptoms may be associated with group A beta-hemolytic streptococcal infections. A potential subtype of OCD, pediatric autoimmune neuropsychiatric disorders associated with streptococcal infections (PANDAS), has been described and may be related to an autoimmune response, similar to what is seen in Sydenham chorea.

OCD is also highly familial (Nestadt et al, 2000; Pauls et al, 1995). OCD and subclinical obsessive-compulsive symptoms are present in 18% to 30% of first-degree relatives. Relative risk in family members of affected children is approximately 25% (double that found in relatives of adult-onset cases). Studies suggest that genetic and nongenetic factors are about equally important in risk for development of OCD.

Treatment

Psychotherapy

Behavioral therapy/cognitive-behavioral therapy (BT/CBT), involving graded exposure to anxiety-provoking stimuli and ritualizing prevention, is recommended as a first-line intervention (O'Kearney et al, 2006). Augmentation of BT/CBT with medication may lead to better outcomes compared with medication alone (O'Kearney et al, 2006; Pediatric OCD Treatment Study Team, 2004). Family therapy and behavioral family intervention are important and effective approaches that target the affective and cognitive aspects of the parent-child relationship as well as the role of the OCD in the family context (Leonard et al, 2005).

Pharmacotherapy

First-line agents include selective serotonin reuptake inhibitors (fluoxetine, sertraline, fluvoxamine, paroxetine, citalopram, and escitalopram) and the tricyclic antidepressant clomipramine. Clomipramine, fluoxetine, sertraline, and fluvoxamine are approved by the Food and Drug Administration for the treatment of OCD in childhood and adolescence. It is generally recommended that maintenance therapy continue for at least 1 to 2 years after improvement is observed. Relapses are common, and long-term treatment is advised after two relapses.

Combination Therapy

Expert consensus guidelines for children and adolescents with OCD recommend starting treatment with either CBT or with the combination of CBT and pharmacotherapy (O'Kearney et al, 2006; Pediatric OCD Treatment Study Team, 2004). The decision to use combination therapy depends on several factors, including the severity of the OCD and any comorbid conditions, such as mood disorders, that may benefit from pharmacotherapy.

Prognosis and Course

OCD is chronic and at times a very disabling condition. Pooled mean persistence rates are 41% for full OCD and 60% for full or subthreshold OCD. Age at onset (earlier), duration of illness (longer), and inpatient status predicted an increased persistence. Comorbid psychiatric conditions and poor initial treatment response are also poor prognostic factors. Comorbid tic or mood disorders have been associated with increased OCD severity (Leonard et al, 2005).

SUMMARY

The dissemination of information on early-onset schizophrenia and severe anxiety disorders to primary care providers is a critical step in optimizing treatment outcomes of children and adolescents suffering from these conditions. Knowledge about the most commonly observed signs and symptoms will help clinicians in the early identification of these disorders, leading to adequate referral and initiation of appropriate interventions.

There is mounting evidence supporting the crucial role of early intervention in preventing poor outcome in psychiatric disorders in general and in children and adolescents in particular (Cornblatt, 2002; Killackey and Yung, 2007). Whereas clinical methods of identification should be implemented, future research promises the possible identification of biologic markers that might help not only in the early treatment but in the identification of children and adolescents who are at high risk for development of specific disorders (Diwadkar et al, 2006; Gothelf et al, 2007). These markers will help in the development of neurobiologically homogeneous groups in light of the emerging evidence indicating the existence of shared pathophysiologic mechanisms among different disorders. For example, neuregulin 1, a gene on chromosome 8p12, appears to play a role in influencing susceptibility to bipolar disorder and schizophrenia, and it might predispose to the development of mood-incongruent psychotic features in individuals with manic symptoms (Green et al, 2005). The examination of symptoms across the Kraepelinian divide and the identification of biologic markers are new approaches that will allow a better characterization of behavioral syndromes and will be instrumental in the development of preventive and therapeutic strategies to childhood-onset psychiatric disorders.

REFERENCES

Albano AM, Chorpita B, Barolo D: Childhood anxiety disorders. *In* Mash EJ, Barkley RA (eds): Child Psychopathology. New York, Guilford, 1996, pp 196-241.

American Psychiatric Association: Diagnostic and Statistical Manual of Mental Disorders, 4th ed. Washington, DC, American Psychiatric Association, 1994.

American Psychiatric Association: Diagnostic and Statistical Manual of Mental Disorders, 4th ed, text revision. Washington, DC, American Psychiatric Association, 2000.

Anderson JC, Williams S, McGee R, Silva PA: DSM-III disorders in preadolescent children. Prevalence in a large sample from the general population. Arch Gen Psychiatry 44:69-76, 1987.

Beidel D, Christ MG, Long PJ: Somatic complaints in anxious children. Abnorm Child Psychol 19:659-670, 1991.

Beidel DC, Turner SM: Shy Children, Phobic Adults: Nature and Treatment of Social Phobia. Washington, DC, American Psychological Association, 1998.

Beidel DC, Turner SM, Fink CM: Assessment of childhood social phobia: Construct, convergent and discriminative validity of the Social Phobia and Anxiety Inventory for Children. Psychol Assess 8:235-240, 1996.

Beidel D, Turner SM, Morris T: Psychopathology of childhood social phobia. J Am Acad Child Adolesc Psychiatry 38:643-650, 1999.

Chavira DA, Stein MB: Childhood social anxiety disorder: From understanding to treatment. Child Adolesc Psychiatr Clin North Am 14:797-818, 2005.

Cohen DJ, Leckman JF: Developmental psychopathology and neurobiology of Tourette's syndrome. J Am Acad Child Adolesc Psychiatry 33:2-15, 1994.

Cornblatt BA: The New York high risk project to the Hillside recognition and prevention (RAP) program. Am J Med Genet 114:956-966, 2002.

Costello EJ, Egger HL, Angold A: Developmental epidemiology of anxiety disorders. *In* Ollendick TH, March JS (eds): Phobic and Anxiety Disorders in Children and Adolescents. New York, Oxford University Press, 2004, pp 61-91.

Coyle JT: Drug treatment of anxiety disorder in children. N Engl J Med 344:1226-1227, 2001.

Delorme R, Bille A, Betancur C: Exploratory analysis of obsessive compulsive symptom dimensions in children and adolescents: A prospective follow-up study. BMC Psychiatry 6:10, 2006.

Diwadkar VA, Montrose DM, Dworakowski D, et al: Genetically predisposed offspring with schizotypal features: An ultra high-risk group for schizophrenia? Prog Neuropsychopharmacol Biol Psychiatry 30:230-238, 2006.

Flament MR, Whitaker A, Rapoport JL: An epidemiological study of obsessive-compulsive disorder in adolescence. J Am Acad Child Adolesc Psychiatry 27:764-771, 1988.

Geller DA: Obsessive-compulsive and spectrum disorders in children and adolescents. Psychiatr Clin North Am 29:353-370, 2006.

Gothelf D, Feinstein C, Thompson T, et al: Risk factors for the emergence of psychotic disorders in adolescents with 22q11.2 deletion syndrome. Am J Psychiatry 164:663-669, 2007.

Green EK, Raybould R, Macgregor S, et al: Operation of the schizophrenia susceptibility gene, neuregulin 1, across traditional diagnostic boundaries to increase risk for bipolar disorder. Arch Gen Psychiatry 62:642-648, 2005.

Hasler G, Pinto A, Greenberg BD, et al; OCD Collaborative Genetics Study: Familiality of factor analysis–derived YBOCS dimensions in OCD-affected sibling pairs from the OCD Collaborative Genetics Study. Biol Psychiatry 61:617-625, 2007.

Hayward C, Killen JD, Draemer HC: Linking self-reported childhood behavioral inhibition to adolescent social phobia. J Am Acad Child Adolesc Psychiatry 37:1308-1316, 1998.

Hoffman S, Albano AM, Heimberg R: Subtypes of social phobia in adolescents. Depress Anxiety 9:15-18, 1999.

Jacobsen LK, Rapoport JL: Research update: Childhood-onset schizophrenia: Implications of clinical and neurobiological research. J Child Psychol Psychiatry 39:101-113, 1998.

Kessler RC, McGonage KA, Zhao S: Lifetime and 12-month prevalence of DSM-III-R psychiatric disorders in the United States. Results from the National Comorbidity Survey. Arch Gen Psychiatry 51:8-19, 1994.

Killackey E, Yung AR: Effectiveness of early intervention in psychosis. Curr Opin Psychiatry 20:121-125, 2007.

Kumra S, Frazier JA, Jacobsen LK, et al: Childhood-onset schizophrenia. A double-blind clozapine-haloperidol comparison. Arch Gen Psychiatry 53:1090-1097, 1996.

Kumra S, Kranzler H, Gerbino-Rosen G. et al: Clozapine and "high-dose" olanzapine in refractory early-onset schizophrenia: A 12-week randomized and double-blind comparison. Biol Psychiatry 63:524-529, 2008.

Leonard HL, Ale CM, Freeman JB, et al: Obsessive-compulsive disorder. Child Adolesc Psychiatr Clin North Am 14:727-743, 2005.

Leonard HL, Topol DA: Elective mutism. Child Adolesc Psychiatr Clin North Am 2:697-707, 1993.

Mancini C, Van Ameringen M, Bennett M: Emerging treatments for child and adolescent social phobias: A review. J Child Adolesc Psychopharmacol 15:589-607, 2005.

Masi G, Mucci M, Pari C: Children with schizophrenia: Clinical picture and pharmacological treatment. CNS Drugs 20:841-866, 2006.

Mataix-Cols D, do Rosario-Campos MC, Leckman JF: A multidimensional model of obsessive-compulsive disorder. Am J Psychiatry 162:228-238, 2005.

Nestadt G, Samuels J, Bienvenu JO: A family study of obsessive-compulsive disorder. Arch Gen Psychiatry 57:358-363, 2000.

O'Kearney RT, Anstey KJ, von Sanden C: Behavioural and cognitive behavioural therapy for obsessive compulsive disorder in children and adolescents. Cochrane Database Syst Rev 4:CD004856, 2006.

Pauls D, Alsobrook JH, Goodman W: A family study of obsessive-compulsive disorder. Am J Psychiatry 152:76-84, 1995.

Pediatric OCD Treatment Study Team: Cognitive-behavior therapy, sertraline, and their combination for children and adolescents with obsessive-compulsive disorder. JAMA 292:1969-1976, 2004.

Rauch SL, Jenike MA: Neurobiological models of obsessive-compulsive disorder. Psychosomatics 34:20-32, 1993.

Remschmidt H, Theisen FM: Schizophrenia and related disorders in children and adolescents. J Neural Transm Suppl 69:121-141, 2005.

Rosenberg DR, Keshavan MS: Towards a neurodevelopmental model of obsessive-compulsive disorder. Biol Psychiatry 43:623-640, 1998.

Schneier FR, Heckelman LR, Garfinkle R: Functional impairment in social phobia. J Clin Psychiatry 55:322-331, 1994.

Schothorst PF, Emck C, van Engeland H: Characteristics of early psychosis. Compr Psychiatry 47:438-442, 2006.

Silverman WK, Moreno J: Specific phobia. Child Adolesc Psychiatr Clin North Am 14:819-843, 2005.

Snider L, Swedo SE: PANDAS: Current status and directions for research. Mol Psychiatry 9:900-907, 2004.

Stein MB: How shy is too shy? Lancet 347:1131-1132, 1996.

Storch EA, Masia-Warner C, Dent HC: Psychometric evaluation of the Social Anxiety Scale for Adolescents and the Social Phobia and Anxiety Inventory for Children: Construct validity and normative data. J Anxiety Disord 18:665-679, 2004.

Van Ameringen M, Mancini C, Farvolden P: The impact of anxiety disorders on educational achievement. J Anxiety Disord 17:561-571, 2003.

Wehmeier PM, Barth N, Remschmidt H: Induced delusional disorder: A review of the concept and an unusual case of folie à famille. Psychopathology 36:37-45, 2003.

Zillessen KE, Trott GE, Warnke A: Induced delusional disorder in childhood and adolescence. Z Kinder Jugendpsychiatr Psychother 24:117-126, 1996.

49 BEHAVIORAL CHALLENGES AND MENTAL DISORDERS IN CHILDREN AND ADOLESCENTS WITH INTELLECTUAL DISABILITY

LUDWIK S. SZYMANSKI

Vignette

A young man, 17 years of age, with moderate cognitive impairment due to the fragile X syndrome was referred to a child and adolescent psychiatrist because of aggressive behavior. He attended a special education class and had been doing very well at school until a week before the referral, when he attacked his gym teacher. The history clarified that he became embarrassed because she demanded that he jump rope, an activity that is very difficult for him. When she prompted him physically, he pushed her away. This push was interpreted as aggression. Male teachers were called, who restrained him on the floor. After that, he started to believe that the teachers restrained him to rape him and that music broadcast at the school had coded messages to that effect. The mental health team made a diagnosis of a brief psychotic disorder. He was treated with antipsychotic medication and supportive therapy. Within 2 months, he recovered completely.

Behavioral problems are one of the most frequent impediments to the progress and community integration of children and adolescents who have intellectual disability (ID). Whereas externalizing behaviors, especially disruptive ones, are the usual reason for referral for mental health consultation, less obvious symptoms such as depression, anxiety, and lack of motivation may impair adaptation as well. Thus, consideration of an individual's observable behaviors as well as emotional well-being should be an integral part of any medical care.

Terms such as *behavioral disorders, challenging behaviors, emotional disorders,* and *mental disorders* have been used in these instances, although only mental disorder is clearly defined. The *Diagnostic and Statistical Manual of Mental Disorders*, fourth edition, text revision (DSM-IV-TR), conceptualizes *mental disorder* as "a clinically significant behavioral or psychological syndrome or pattern that occurs in an individual and that is associated with present distress (e.g., a painful symptom) or disability (i.e., impairment in one or more important aspects of functioning) or with a significantly increased risk of suffering death, pain, disability, or an important loss of freedom" (American Psychiatric Association, 2000, DSM-IV-TR, p. xxxi). Thus, any behavioral problem serious enough to require treatment might be included here. The term *behavioral disorder* is sometimes used for problems thought to be a reaction to an environmental situation that do not meet criteria for a formal psychiatric diagnosis. For example, a child with ID, placed without appropriate educational supports in a classroom where the program is too difficult, may resort to disruptive behaviors that are not evident in other settings. However, this is an artificial distinction and not particularly helpful.

EPIDEMIOLOGY

It is now generally agreed that the prevalence of mental disorders in people with ID is higher than that in the comparable population without such disability, even as high as 64% (Bregman, 1991). All types of mental disorders have been described, and there is no evidence of occurrence of disorders unique to this population. In a more recent study of a population-based cohort, 42% of the children with severe ID and 33% of those with mild ID had psychiatric diagnosis (Strømme and Diseth, 2000). Interestingly, only one third of them were seen previously by a child psychiatrist. It is postulated that the increased prevalence of psychiatric disorders in this population is related to several factors, including neuropathology, impaired cognitive and language skills, and the person's repeated experiences of failure (Dykens, 2000). It is now also recognized that certain syndromes underlying ID may be associated with certain behavioral phenotypes (patterns of behavior and psychopathology), and this topic is discussed in more details in Chapters 24, 25, and 26.

DIAGNOSTIC CONSIDERATIONS

Children and adolescents who have ID often have other disabilities as well. Both the primary and associated disorders may contribute to their behavioral difficulties. Thus, the assessment should not be limited to providing a formal "psychiatric label" and coding but should be comprehensive, based on biopsychosocial principles. The most recent classification manual of the American Association on Intellectual and Developmental Disability (2002; previous name: American Association on Mental Retardation) specifies a multidimensional approach to ID. The dimensions are intellectual abilities, adaptive behavior, participation, interaction and social roles, health (physical and mental), and context (environments and culture). This schema is a useful guide for mental health assessment. The diagnostic assessment should include description of the clinical presentation justifying the diagnosis, the patient's strengths and liabilities, and comprehensive recommendations. A "generic" diagnosis, such as "aggression," is usually not sufficient. Aggressive behavior is a symptom that might be associated with depression, psychosis, or personality disorder as well as with environmental factors, such as inappropriate educational placement and inappropriate care. Each of these different potential causes would require different interventions (Szymanski et al, 1998). For instance, an aggressive youngster with ID who is in a behavioral program because of "attention getting" may actually have an underlying psychotic disorder; another youth with superficially similar symptoms and treated with an antipsychotic drug might not have a psychotic illness but may be reacting to an inappropriate educational placement.

Table 49-1. **Commons Reasons for Requesting Mental Health Evaluation**

Complaints	Comments
Disruptive behaviors	By and large, a most common reason May include range of behaviors from irritability, impulsivity, overactivity, and temper tantrums to aggression Depends also on degree of caregiver's tolerance
Aggressive behaviors	May range from swearing ("verbal aggression") to dangerous physical attacks
Self-destructive and stereotypic behaviors	Range from self-stimulatory (e.g., rocking, hand flapping, light gazing) to life-threatening (head banging, eye hitting, self-biting)
Depressed mood	May include withdrawal, sad expression, passivity, noncompliance, sleeping and eating problems, anhedonia
Social adaptation problems	Manifestations depend on age May include lack of interest in others, withdrawal, lack of eye contact, inappropriate behavior toward others, not respecting interpersonal boundaries, not understanding rules of game
Developmental delay	Caregivers are concerned that a delay in acquiring a developmental skill or in academic learning is due to emotional factors.
Bizarreness	Hallucinations, delusions May include any of the above behaviors if manifested to an extreme degree
Second opinion	Caregivers unsatisfied with an earlier diagnosis of ID sometimes search for one more acceptable to them, such as Asperger disorder.

PSYCHIATRIC DIAGNOSTIC ASSESSMENT

Reasons for Referral

Individuals with ID may be referred for psychiatric consultation for a variety of reasons. These vary, depending on age, developmental level, perceptions of the caregivers, and underlying etiology (and its behavioral phenotype). It is important to understand the reasons for referral at this time (especially if the problem has existed for some time). Some of the common referral complaints are summarized in Table 49-1.

History

The clinical assessment is done in the context of the total clinical picture, including developmental levels in various domains, associated disabilities, and psychosocial factors. Detailed history is essential, beyond the standard chief concern, history of present concern, and the like. Multiple informants (such as parents, teachers, and therapists) might provide better description of the problem than would a single observer, such as in what situations the problems in question do and do not occur and their response to various management techniques (Table 49-2).

The patient should have a recent, comprehensive medical review. It should rule out comorbid medical disorders, especially disorders known to have increased prevalence in an ID-associated syndrome that the patient might have. In children and adolescents who do not have communicative language, a pain or discomfort from an undiagnosed medical condition is a frequent cause of a behavioral change.

Clinical Interview

The clinical interview with the patient is essential. It includes not just verbal interview but observation of a child's behavior and interaction with parents and peers in the waiting room, where one may in fact obtain more information than through an "interrogation" of a frightened child in the examining room (Table 49-3). The clinician should avoid starting with a barrage of questions or superficial reassurances but should spend some time in a low-key, supportive interaction, trying to establish a relationship with the patient. The level and quality of a child's communication patterns should be assessed, such as by watching how the child communicates with the parents. With verbal children, an interview conducted in a supportive, friendly manner, with some directiveness

Table 49-2. Outline of History Taking

Chief concerns	Problems: when they started, significant events around time at onset, detailed and concrete description of behavioral manifestations, in what situations they do and do not occur
Caregivers' expectations of this referral	Overt and hidden "agenda," reasons for referral at this time (e.g., recent behavior change, reduced caregiver's tolerance)
Management of the problems so far	Behavioral-environmental and medical: detailed descriptions, consistency, adverse effects, length of treatment, results; include alternative therapies and remedies
Past history	Developmental and health, genetic history Etiology of disability and diagnostic evaluations Educational and habilitative history; services received, their appropriateness, progress
Environmental-psychosocial history	Family: composition, living situation, supports and services, significant environmental events and changes
Child's personal characteristics	Strengths, skills (communication, self-care, social, academic, others), attention span, mood, self-control, unusual behaviors Understanding of own disability, motivation for independence Interpersonal: relationship to significant persons, expression of affection, empathy, trust, separation anxiety, peer relationships Sexuality: awareness, related behaviors
Family and caregivers	Understanding of and attitudes toward child's disability, appropriateness of expectations, management of the child (appropriateness, consistency), ability to advocate for the child Effects of child's disability on family's functioning
Psychiatric "review of systems"	Mood: appropriateness, cyclicity, dysfunctional moods (depression, anxiety, agitation) Delusions, hallucinations, fears or phobias, obsessions and compulsions; stereotypic, self-stimulatory, self-injurious behaviors History of regression, loss of skills
Suggestions of past abuse	History of overt abuse, suggestive symptoms: regression, preoccupation with sexuality, vigilance, flashbacks, frightening dreams, re-enactment of traumatic event; avoidance of certain stimuli, places, persons

and structure, in concrete language understandable to the child, may yield significant information. The best opening gambit is to focus on the child's strengths and successes rather than on presenting problems. Nonverbal techniques, such as observation of the child's play, are also helpful. The parents should be asked whether the child's behavior during the interview was representative of the behavior in other settings.

Rating Instruments and Other Materials

Rating scales, such as Conners Rating Scales (parents' and teachers' versions), Reiss Screen, and the Aberrant Behavior Checklist, may supplement the clinical observations (Reiss, 1994). Other instruments with which the clinician is familiar can be used, and they may be helpful for screening purposes. An important caution is that the rating scales may not have been normed on individuals with ID, and therefore interpretation of the results may be difficult.

If possible, the parents should be asked to bring past and recent home videos of the child. They may provide valuable information about behavioral change over time and the child's behavior in natural environments.

Table 49-3. Outline of Observation and Interview of the Patient

General appearance	Phenotypic features, grooming
Behavior	Attention span, distractibility, impulsivity, self-stimulatory/self-injurious behaviors, stereotypies, unusual preoccupations
Play	Spontaneity, imagination, perseveration, use of play materials, predominant themes, age appropriateness
Mood and affect	Nonverbal expression of mood, predominant mood, appropriateness, variability
Interpersonal interaction	Relatedness to others, eye contact, referential looking, expression of affection, seeking affection, verbal and nonverbal patterns of relating, interaction with peers, separation anxiety
Language skills	Verbal and nonverbal communication, prosody, intelligibility, complexity of language, stereotypies Ability to express self and to communicate, ability for interactive conversation
Interview	Orientation, understanding of the purpose of the visit, understanding of own disability, preoccupations, unusual features (e.g., delusions, obsessions, flight of ideas)

Use of Diagnostic Categories

In most cases, the diagnosis can be made by use of the standard diagnostic schema of the DSM-IV-TR. Certain modifications might be necessary, depending on the patient's level of development and communication skills in particular (just as with young children without ID). There have been attempts to develop criteria for diagnosis of mental disorders comorbid with ID. The Royal College of Psychiatrists in England published a manual applicable to adults. In the United States, the National Association for the Dually Diagnosed is currently developing a similar manual (primarily for adults). In any case, the diagnostician should consider whether there is an issue of dangerousness (to self and others) and of abuse.

DIAGNOSIS OF SPECIFIC MENTAL DISORDERS

In the following section, some of the main categories of mental disorders are briefly reviewed. The focus is on adaptation of the DSM-IV diagnostic criteria to persons who have an ID.

Pervasive Developmental Disorders

Currently, in the DSM-IV-TR, the pervasive developmental disorder category includes autistic disorder, Asperger disorder, pervasive developmental disorder not otherwise specified, Rett disorder, and childhood disintegrative disorder. The less specific term *autism spectrum disorders* is frequently used, which is usually meant to refer to the first three disorders in the pervasive developmental disorder category. The diagnosis of autistic disorder requires qualitative impairment in social interaction (such as in eye contact, peer relationships, sharing emotions); qualitative impairment in interpersonal communication; and restricted, repetitive, and stereotyped patterns of behavior (such as preoccupation with restricted patterns of interest, nonfunctional routines, motor mannerisms). Stereotypic behaviors of children with significant ID are often seen as signs of an autism spectrum disorder, and many are referred for psychiatric consultation with the question of whether the child has autistic disorder or ID. However, 75% to 80% of children with autistic disorder have comorbid ID. Thus, these diagnoses are not mutually exclusive. Therefore, the more accurate diagnostic question is whether the child has an autism spectrum disorder comorbid with ID. Children with significant ID alone usually are able to develop social interaction, although their patterns of relating and social communication are immature for their chronologic age, and prolonged observation may be required to recognize it. Pervasive developmental disorders are discussed in detail in Chapter 69.

Psychotic Disorders

The prevalence of schizophrenia (in adults with ID) is thought to be 1% to 3% (Reiss, 1994). Schizophrenia and other psychotic disorders may be difficult to diagnose accurately in individuals who have significant ID because in the absence of language, recognition of hallucinations, delusions, and thought disorder may not be possible. In such patients, the less specific diagnosis of undifferentiated schizophrenia or psychotic disorder not otherwise specified might have to be made on the basis of behavioral changes compared with premorbid behavior. In particular, the appearance of symptoms of social or affective withdrawal, bizarre behaviors not seen before, and deterioration in the level of functioning may suggest such a diagnosis. On the other hand, psychosis should not be diagnosed in a person with significant ID merely on the basis of self-stimulatory or aggressive behavior. In children and adolescents who have 22q11.2 deletion syndrome (which may also be associated with ID), there is an increased prevalence of psychosis and psychotic symptoms (26.7%) as well as autism spectrum disorders (50%) (Vorstman et al, 2006).

Mood Disorders

It is now well accepted that all forms of mood disorders can be seen in individuals with ID. There have even been reports of depression in persons with Down syndrome, who are usually consi-dered happy and social (Szymanski and Biederman, 1984). Suicide of individuals with ID has been described. The diagnosis of depression in this population is often missed. Individuals who are depressed are often ignored because they may be quiet and may not disturb their caregivers. The clinical manifestations of the disorder may be modified by a person's level of cognitive skills, language, and experiences. As with psychoses, verbal productions cannot be used to assess the affective state if the individual has limited or no language. However, most of the diagnostic criteria for mood disorders in the DSM-IV-TR can be satisfied on the basis of observations made by others (such as caregivers). These include observations of vegetative signs (sleeping and eating disorders), psychomotor retardation, agitation or aggressive behaviors, withdrawal, anhedonia, tearfulness, irritability, and general appearance of sadness. The individual may be described as refusing to engage in previously preferred activities. As opposed to those who have dementia, although they may appear as having regressed in skills, they can still perform them if they try. Individuals with ID who have even limited language skills can provide quite good information about their feelings and mood, although they are likely to use concrete and simple descriptions, such as stating that they feel sick or not well rather than depressed (American Academy of Child and Adolescent Psychiatry, 1999). They might also act aggressively (Reiss and Rojahn, 1993), such as individuals with psychomotor retardation who are forced to participate in required activities. Symptoms of manic episodes will be likewise modified in this population (American Academy of Child and Adolescent Psychiatry, 1999). For example, whereas they will not engage in indiscriminate shopping, sexual adventures, or business investments, they may appear silly or agitated, shout, try to engage in activities that they clearly cannot perform, vocalize constantly, or engage in public masturbation.

Stereotypic Movement Disorder and Self-Injurious Behaviors

As defined by the DSM-IV-TR, this disorder is characterized by nonfunctional motor behaviors, such as persistent rocking, hand shaking, and self-biting, that are repetitive, are driven, and result in significant functional impairment. A specifier "with self-injurious behavior" is added if the behavior (such as self-hitting, head banging) results in an injury requiring medical care. Serious damage may result from these behaviors, such as retinal detachment and blindness. Often the individual may switch from one type of behavior to another. Stereotypic behaviors occur in up to one third of persons who have ID, and severe self-injurious behavior occurs in 2% (Reiss, 1994). Self-injurious behavior is more common when the retardation is severe and in certain ID-associated syndromes, such as Lesch-Nyhan and Cornelia de Lange. The causes of these behaviors are still a matter of controversy. Psychophysiologic mechanisms, such as disorders in endogenous opioid and serotonin systems, have been postulated. The true cause is probably multidetermined, with both neurobiologic and environmental factors playing a role. Environmental factors (e.g., the secondary gain of attracting the caregivers' attention) may maintain such behavior. In some nonverbal individuals, the self-injurious behavior may be related to pain from a medical condition. Thus, these behaviors might be related to different factors, and therefore comprehensive diagnostic assessment is a prerequisite for treatment (Harris, 2006). The treatment is also multifocal, depending on causative factors that are involved. It may include behavioral modification (such as rewards for positive behavior and teaching replacement behaviors), milieu manipulation (e.g., proper education or work placement, reduction of unnecessary stimulation), and teaching of alternative communication skills (if needed). Psychotropic drugs (antipsychotics and selective serotonin reuptake inhibitors) may have an important role. In any case, combination of measures rather than a single intervention are needed (Harris 2006).

Post-traumatic Stress Disorder

The possibility of post-traumatic stress disorder should be kept in mind in any assessment of persons who have ID and otherwise unexplained history of behavior change. This disorder is frequently unnoticed (Ryan, 1994) because the patients might be unable to report it. Symptoms such as distressing flashbacks, dreams, avoidance of places and activities related to the trauma, and hypervigilance may be seen as well as behavioral changes similar to those seen in abused children (mood changes, irritability, sleep disorder, sexualized behaviors).

TREATMENT

Treatment Planning

Clinicians should resist the temptations and pressure to immediately "prescribe something to take the edge off" challenging behaviors before the total clinical picture and potentially explanatory factors involved are understood. The first step is, of course, assessment of immediate safety of the patient and others and, if necessary, implementation of measures to ensure safety, which may include close supervision, medication, and hospitalization. The general principles of treatment planning are delineated in Table 49-4.

Table 49-4. Treatment Planning

Ensure safety	Assess dangerousness to self and others; if necessary, ensure safety through close supervision, supports, medication, or hospitalization, as needed.
Prerequisite: diagnostic assessment	Comprehensive understanding of the problems
Coordinated treatment planning	Mental health treatment must be coordinated with comprehensive treatment in all relevant areas, including habitation and education. Team collaboration of all involved care providers is essential.
Environmental supports	Environmental management issues and needs that contribute to the problem must be addressed, including appropriate health, education, habilitation, and housing.
Least intrusive measures	The least intrusive measures, with the best risk-to-benefit ratio and the least chance of adverse effects, should be employed first.
Multimodal treatment	Several treatment modalities may have to be employed as appropriate: supportive/cognitive psychotherapy, medications, behavioral treatment, milieu management.
Goal-oriented treatment	Specific ultimate and intermediate treatment goals and priorities should be developed.
Patient's and caregivers' collaboration	Caregivers and the patient, as much as possible, should participate in development of the treatment plan, understand it, and collaborate in its implementation.
Follow-up	Mechanisms for comprehensive follow-up of treatment progress and side effects should be developed, including collection of reliable behavioral data from caregivers, patient reassessments, and laboratory testing.
Evidence-based treatment	Initial and continuation treatments should be based on evidence of effectiveness. Ineffective ones should be discontinued.
Legal and ethical issues	Human rights and legal issues in the particular jurisdiction should be respected (e.g., obtaining valid informed consents).

Specific Treatment Measures

Psychotherapies

Recently, there has been considerable discussion on the utility of psychotherapy for individuals with ID. On the basis of meta-analysis of published studies, some researchers have concluded that various forms of psychotherapy, including group and individual, are moderately effective (Prout and Nowak-Drabik, 2003), whereas others contested these conclusions (Sturmey, 2005). One has to keep in mind that there is also a dearth of scientific studies on effectiveness of psychotherapy in general. Part of the problem is that it is difficult to define precisely psychotherapy and to implement it in a standardized manner. Furthermore, psychotherapy is not an impersonal, technical procedure but an interpersonal process in which personal factors play a major role, and these are difficult to define and to quantify. However, defined broadly as a "treatment procedure performed by a trained mental health professional, through application of psychologically based verbal and nonverbal means... and with definite goals of improving the patient's coping abilities and/or ameliorating psychopathological symptoms" (Szymanski, 1980), psychotherapy with individuals who have ID may be very effective. The prerequisite is that the therapist be well trained and experienced with this population. Communication measures appropriate for the patient and structured approaches are important. The patient should have some degree of language (including speech, sign language, even computer typing) that will permit effective communication with the therapist. Group therapy may be very effective because it provides peer support and social opportunities.

Psychotherapy is further discussed in Chapter 89.

Psychotropic Drugs

The use of these drugs is described in detail in Chapter 90. In using these drugs, physicians must follow the same principles of evidence-based treatment as they would with patients who do not have ID. They should be used in a lowest effective dose and follow-up data should prove their effectiveness. A "Christmas tree" treatment model should be avoided (adding one drug after another if the previous one is not effective, rather than discontinuing the ineffective one), unless a combination is clearly proved to be effective. These drugs should be prescribed (as any other drug is) by a physician who is thoroughly familiar with them. They should be a part of a comprehensive treatment program, not a substitute for it. Various treatment modalities, such as psychotherapy, milieu therapy, and behavior modification, have a synergistic effect with the medications. As much as possible, these drugs should be used for their designated action in specific disorders. For example, antipsychotics should be used primarily for treatment of psychotic disorder and not as a nonspecific "major tranquilizer." Whereas they are often prescribed "for aggression," there is really no specific anti-aggression drug. Aggressive behavior may be caused by psychosis, depression, a painful condition, anger, or reaction to environmental conditions, each of which requires quite different interventions. High doses of an antipsychotic drug might suppress any aggressive behavior but at the cost of side effects and suppression of the person's general functioning.

Another caveat in the use of drugs in this population concerns side effects (American Academy of Child and Adolescent Psychiatry, 1999). Children and adolescents who do not have verbal skills may have considerable difficulty in reporting side effects. They should be monitored carefully, according to predetermined criteria and baseline data. Some side effects may mimic original symptoms; for example, akathisia resulting from a too rapid withdrawal of an antipsychotic, particularly a first-generation one, may look like an increase in preexisting agitation, especially if the patient cannot describe how he or she feels. The involuntary movements of tardive dyskinesia may be difficult to differentiate from preexisting stereotypies. Videotaping of the patient's behavior before the drug is started may help in this differentiation.

A useful summary of precautions necessary with the use of psychotropic medications in persons who have ID has been issued by the Health Care Financing Administration (reviewed in American Academy of Child and Adolescent Psychiatry, 1999). Other useful resources are Reiss and Aman (1998), Rush and Frances (2000), and Harris (2006).

Psychotropic drugs are further discussed in Chapter 90, milieu therapy in Chapter 89, and behavior modification in Chapter 87.

PREVENTION OF EMOTIONAL MALADJUSTMENT

The Primary Care Clinician's Role

Pediatricians and other primary care clinicians have an excellent opportunity to provide the family of a child with ID with support and guidance, which is important in preventing a child's emotional and behavioral problems. Most parents understand that primary care clinicians cannot cure most cases of ID, but they want from them explanations of the child's problems, support, guidance, and education as to what they can do for the child. The not uncommon statement of the physician, "There is nothing you can do," is particularly destructive because it conveys an attitude of helplessness and hopelessness.

What the family needs, first of all, is to learn from the clinician to regard the child as an individual who has human worth like every other child. The physician who inquires about and points out the child's personal characteristics and strengths (rather than focusing on the impairments only), who talks to the child and responds with understanding to parental questions, conveys the message of respect and individualization. Providing the parents with up-to-date information about the child's condition, referring them for a second opinion to a specialized clinic and for support to a parents' group, advising on services, and giving "permission" to set limits and proper expectations for the child are all important. The pediatrician can teach the family to provide the child with appropriate stimulation, to set the necessary limits, to promote the child's independence, and to focus on the child's strengths rather than disabilities. All of this will help the child develop a positive self-image.

The pediatric clinician should also be able to provide early identification of behavioral problems that are related to environmental situations or to normal developmental crises. It is important to help the parents to learn to give the child attention when he or she behaves appropriately, rather than to focus only on measures to be taken after the child misbehaves.

Use of Psychiatric Consultation

If there is a suspicion of a more pervasive, functionally limiting, behavioral or emotional disturbance, referral for child psychiatric consultation is indicated. One should avoid the common tendency to refer only patients who are disturbing to others while neglecting those who are otherwise disturbed. Choice of a consultant is important; many child psychiatrists have little experience and training in developmental disabilities. Psychiatrists associated with specialized developmental disabilities clinics are usually familiar with this population. The success of a consultation depends to a considerable degree on good communication between the pediatrician and the child psychiatrist. A clear statement of the reasons for consultation is necessary, as are developmental and medical history and careful assessment for possible medical conditions that might be related to the behavioral symptoms. The child should not be referred for "medication review" but for a comprehensive psychiatric assessment. Conversely, prompt and preferably detailed feedback by the consultant is important. The psychiatrists are expected to synthesize the available information about the child into a comprehensive assessment rather than to limit themselves to prescribing medication or making psychological interpretations only.

SUMMARY

Behavioral problems are one of the most frequent factors, if not the most frequent one, preventing children and adolescents who have ID from functioning according to their abilities. They are at increased risk for mental disorders. The prevalence of psychopathology in this population has been reported to be as high as 64%. The diagnostic process is similar to the evaluation of children who do not have ID, but it may have to be modified according to the child's developmental level, particularly in the area of communication skills. Also, the treatment measures are the same as with children and adolescents without ID. Comprehensive diagnostic assessment is a prerequisite to treatment. Referral for child psychiatric consultation is indicated if the child's disturbance is pervasive, there is a potential for danger to the child or others, and first-line treatment by a nonpsychiatrist has not been successful.

REFERENCES

American Academy of Child and Adolescent Psychiatry: Practice parameters for the assessment and treatment of children, adolescents, and adults with mental retardation and comorbid mental disorders. J Am Acad Child Adolesc Psychiatry 33(Suppl):12, 1999.

American Association on Mental Retardation: Mental Retardation: Definition, Classification, and Systems of Supports, 10th ed. Washington, DC, American Association on Mental Retardation, 2002.

American Psychiatric Association: Diagnostic and Statistical Manual of Mental Disorders, 4th ed, text revision. Washington, DC, American Psychiatric Association, 2000.

Bregman J: Current developments in the understanding of intellectual disability. Part II: Psychopathology. J Am Acad Child Adolesc Psychiatry 30:861, 1991.

Dykens EM: Annotation: Psychopathology in children with intellectual disability. J Child Psychol Psychiatry 41:407-417, 2000.

Harris JC: Intellectual Disability. Oxford, UK, Oxford University Press, 2006.

Prout HT, Nowak-Drabik KM: Psychotherapy with persons who have mental retardation. An evaluation of effectiveness. Am J Ment Retard 108:82-93, 2003.

Reiss S: Handbook of Challenging Behavior: Mental Health Aspects of Intellectual Disability. Worthington, OH, IDS Publishing, 1994.

Reiss S, Aman MG: Psychotropic Medications and Developmental Disabilities: The International Consensus Textbook. Columbus, OH, Ohio State University, 1998.

Reiss S, Rojahn J: Joint occurrence of depression and aggression in children and adults with mental retardation. J Intellect Disabil Res 37:287-294, 1993.

Rush AJ, Frances A (eds): The Expert Consensus Guideline Series. Treatment of Psychiatric and Behavioral Problems in Mental Retardation. Am J Ment Retard 105(special issue 3):159-228, 2000.

Ryan R: Posttraumatic stress disorder in persons with developmental disabilities. Community Ment Health J 30:45-54, 1994.

Strømme P, Diseth TH: Prevalence of psychiatric diagnoses in children with mental retardation: Data from a population-based study. Dev Med Child Neurol 42:266-270, 2000.

Sturmey P: Against psychotherapy with people who have mental retardation. Ment Retard 43:55-57, 2005.

Szymanski LS: Individual psychotherapy with retarded person. *In* Szymanski LS, Tanguay PE (eds): Emotional Disorders of Mentally Retarded Persons. Baltimore, University Park Press, 1980, pp 131-147.

Szymanski LS, Biederman J: Depression and anorexia nervosa of persons with Down's syndrome. Am J Ment Defic 89:246, 1984.

Szymanski LS, King B, Goldberg B, et al: Diagnosis of mental disorders in people with intellectual disability. *In* Reiss S, Aman MG (eds): Psychotropic Medications and Developmental Disabilities: The International Consensus Handbook. Columbus, OH, Ohio State University, 1998, pp 3-17.

Vorstman JAS, Morcus MEJ, Duijff SN, et al: The 22q11.2 deletion in children: High rate of autistic disorders and early onset of psychotic symptoms. J Am Acad Child Adolesc Psychiatry 45:1104-1113, 2006.

SECTION D **Coping/Problem Solving**

50 COPING STRATEGIES

OLLE JANE Z. SAHLER AND JOHN E. CARR

Vignette

The mother of a 5-year-old diagnosed with acute lymphoblastic leukemia seeks help because her son has received considerable attention to help him cope with his illness, including music therapy to help with procedural pain. Now she realizes that she needs a strategy to help her cope because his behavior is "terrible." Appropriate in a case such as this one is the paradigm of problem solving skills training: **I**dentify the problem, **D**etermine options, **E**valuate and choose the best, **A**ct, and **S**ee if it worked.

The mother reports that when her son is receiving high-dose steroids every 3 weeks, he has uncontrollable tantrums, hits his 2-year-old sister, and sleeps poorly. Reducing the dose is not possible.

I. She identifies poor sleeping as the main issue because she believes he would be less irritable if he slept more. However, since he became ill, he sleeps in the parents' room on a cot. The boy wakes up and stays awake for hours when they try to go to bed.

D. As options, she lists (1) giving him sleeping medication, (2) parents going to sleep at his bedtime, and (3) returning him to his own room. She really wants to return her son to his own bed. Past attempts have resulted in all-night screaming episodes.

E. She thinks she will be more successful if she makes the change during a non-steroid week. She remembers that he has told her he is scared. She develops a plan to take him to the store to purchase a "very special" night-light for his own room. She also recognizes that her concern about the nighttime battle makes her feel anxious and is probably making him more hyper.

When steroids have been discontinued for 2 days and he is entering the 12 days of his cycle when his behavior is most manageable, she discusses his sleeping in his room after having a bath and reading stories beginning the following night.

A. She and her son shop for the night-light. The next evening, she gives him a leisurely bath. He then plugs in the light, has a story, and goes to sleep at 8 pm.

S. He wakes up at 11 pm when his parents are getting ready to go to bed and wants to sleep on the cot. She holds firm with the plan, and although the scene repeats for the next 2 nights, on the third night he stays in his room.

STRESS, ADAPTATION, AND ILLNESS

Many illnesses result from the body's attempts to adapt to "stress." Derived from physics, stress originally referred to forces causing structural or systemic strain. Applied to medicine, stress refers to any challenge to the integrity of the organism and includes the complex *interaction of biologic, behavioral, cognitive, sociocultural, and environmental changes that can disrupt homeostasis*. Any such challenge will strain the body's systems and set into motion an array of adaptive and defensive mechanisms within each of these systems. Disease and dysfunction typically result from the body's failed adaptive responses and occasionally from successful adaptive responses (e.g., autoimmune disorders).

THE STRESS RESPONSE

The stress response involves a complex set of physiologic, cognitive, and behavioral reactions that physiologist Walter Cannon called the fight-or-flight response. Hans Selye distinguished between "eustress," *the optimal degree of arousal* required to perform or to learn well, and "distress" or unhealthy stress, arousal that impedes performance, generally in instances of high stress (Yerkes-Dodson law). Two corollaries apply: (1) learning is relatively difficult; and (2) performing well-learned tasks or behaviors is relatively easy and therefore the typical response (Carr et al, 2007). A terminally ill teenage girl who is usually noncommunicative is unlikely to discuss her impending death with the health care team, even though they feel a discussion will be of benefit.

In the *acute stress response*, energy is mobilized from storage sites while further storage is temporarily halted; muscles are fueled for fight or flight. Noncritical functions are put on hold (e.g., digestion and reproduction). To achieve this state, sympathetic neural pathways, originating in the hypothalamus, trigger release of epinephrine at synapses and from the adrenal medulla. Concurrently, norepinephrine is released at all other sympathetic synapses. Once the stress ceases, parasympathetic pathways originating in the hypothalamus activate cholinergic neurons in the same end organs. This reaction rapidly dissipates the state of arousal.

In the *chronic stress response*, the hypothalamus secretes corticotropin-releasing hormone. The anterior pituitary secretes adrenocorticotropic hormone, which is transported to the adrenal cortex and stimulates glucocorticoid secretion into the circulatory system. The person momentarily feels aroused, on edge, or even anxious. With chronic stress, the stress response is continuously triggered. Over time, the body's adaptive systems begin to break down.

LEARNING, COGNITION, AND THE STRESS RESPONSE

Lazarus and Folkman (1984) proposed that the impact of a stressor is mediated by the individual's ability to accurately *appraise* the stressor. The stress response is also influenced by the individual's *vulnerabilities*. A patient can be vulnerable genetically (sickle cell anemia), cognitively (depression, defeatist beliefs), behaviorally (substance abuse), or socioculturally (poor, undernourished, denied health care or economic opportunities). *Coping skills* (see later) reflect the individual's adaptive abilities in the form of behavioral skills, cognitive strategies, and sense of efficacy based on past successes as well as motivated effort. *Social support* refers to the validation, support, and assurance of assistance that the individual can count on from others. Other *resources* include material, financial, educational, intellectual, cognitive, health, creative, and social skills and benefits the individual can call on.

The *conditioning* of physical symptoms to psychosocial triggers and reinforcers begins with the stress response. During the lifespan of the individual, the homeostatic process of adapting to stress involves learning complex interactions among biologic, behavioral, sociocultural, cognitive, and environmental experiences. The biologic symptoms become conditioned to beliefs, emotions, behaviors, and events, all of which then acquire the ability to trigger, to reinforce, and to maintain these symptoms (Carr and Kappes, 2007). The intensity and duration of a stressor may be perceived differently by various individuals as a result of life experiences, beliefs, and memories. One person's severe stressor may only be another person's mild challenge.

PSYCHOLOGICAL CONSEQUENCES

Chronic stress, which induces continued emotional arousal, can result in chronic *anticipatory anxiety*, a learned sensitivity to fear-inducing situations. Similarly, continuous exposure to loss or failed coping can lead to depression and *learned helplessness*. Emotional responses to stressful situations can become conditioned to specific cognitions (e.g., memories, self-statements). The cognitions then serve as cues for activating these same emotional states (e.g., "Every time I try to study for a math test I feel stupid and know I'll fail, so why study?").

Responses to stress are idiosyncratic, that is, influenced by personal experiences that define the nature and intensity of any stressor condition and the individual's self-efficacy or self-confidence in his or her ability to cope. Thus, the stress response can be moderated by interventions that modify predisposing vulnerabilities (biologic, cognitive, behavioral, sociocultural), stress appraisal abilities (cognitive), coping skills, and social support. Stress is a naturally and continuously occurring phenomenon; learning to manage stress is a more realistic goal than trying to eliminate it.

WHAT IS COPING?

Webster's dictionary defines coping as "overcoming problems and difficulties." A related definition that helps describe how this overcoming might be accomplished is "shaping or conforming, especially conforming to the shape of another." Thus, coping can be thought of as altering some part of oneself to maintain homeostasis, balance, or equilibrium between excessive demands and inadequate resources (Lazarus and Folkman, 1984). Coping can be adaptive when the alterations (modifications, pliability) allow the individual to fit better with environmental conditions, resulting in stress-related growth or at least maintenance of the integrity of the individual. Coping can also be maladaptive, resulting in a poorer environmental fit or injury to or even destruction of the individual.

Helping professionals often want to assist children and their families in coping with stress. However, prescribing instruction in "empirically supported" coping strategies will not resolve the adaptive crises of every child for several reasons (Somerfield and McCrae, 2000): (1) some people are near their adaptive capacity; (2) not all stresses can be dealt with by an individual or the family and must be addressed by social or organizational-level coping strategies; and (3) temperament (see Chapter 7) and personality differences influence how effectively new coping strategies can be adopted. Temperament or personality style, which is not easily changed, may be a stumbling block to successful adaptation (e.g., a person who is anxious will find it difficult to relax, a person who is highly dependent will find it very difficult to make decisions about next steps). Fortunately, *learned optimism* (versus learned helplessness as described earlier) is possible (Shatte et al, 1999).

Vulnerability (Diathesis-Stress Interaction)

A diathesis is a "constitutional" predisposition toward a behavior, cognition, abnormality, or disease. A child may have a predisposition toward anxious behavior or depressive thoughts just as he or she may have a predisposition toward allergies or coronary artery disease.

A tendency exists within a certain environment, social milieu, or level of cognitive development that may provide the precipitate circumstances that allow the predisposition to become manifested (Burke and Elliott, 1999). A child may be predisposed to anxiety, but it is not until the child is faced with the challenge of repeated stress from chronic asthma or painful procedures, as part of the treatment for cancer, for example, that the anxiety becomes manifested. The response of the parents (e.g., the parent who has an air filter installed in the heating system, or the parent who provides information, support, and distraction during the painful procedure) can moderate the extent to which the predisposition is expressed.

Resiliency

Resiliency is the ability to cope with (face, overcome, be strengthened by) adversity. Initially, children and young people are naturally resilient because they have little experience with the negative consequences of certain situations or activities and believe they have some (magical) control over what happens (egocentrism). Resiliency comes from what the child has (external resources) and who the child is and what the child can do (internal resources). It is possible to build resiliency by increasing either external or internal resources. External resources include people who are trustworthy, structures and boundaries that provide safety, role models, and encouragement to be autonomous. Internal resources include the ability to see themselves as lovable and appealing, to do kind things for others, to be proud of themselves, to communicate effectively, to solve problems, to manage feelings and impulses, to be empathetic, and to establish trusting relationships. Parents help children build resiliency by providing a safe and nurturing environment, spending time with the child, and allowing the child to make mistakes and to learn constructively from them.

COPING STYLE AND STRATEGIES

Coping skill can be conceptualized as a combination of coping style and range of implementable coping strategies. Coping style is a mixture of attributional style (perceived source of stress, locus of control, optimistic or pessimistic outlook on finding a solution) and personality characteristics, such as risk tolerance, sense of self-efficacy, and introversion or extroversion. Coping strategies reflect the repertoire of responses to the stress that the individual has available and can use successfully. Whereas personality is relatively fixed, coping strategies can be taught explicitly or through modeling.

Coping strategies can be divided into three major categories: active coping, passive coping, and avoidance. Table 50-1 provides examples of active and passive coping. An approach like music therapy, discussed later, combines active and passive coping.

Avoidance can be understood as denial: it is as if the person has decided that there is no stressor, and therefore there is no need to change behavior, perception, or emotional response. In this situation, the only way the individual can deal with it is to "forget" it or distract oneself from trying to deal with it. Avoidance can also result from a sense that although the situation is indeed stressful, it can never be changed. Avoidance and denial strategies may be appropriate stop-gap measures, such as when the stress is so acute that to acknowledge it immediately would be overwhelming (e.g., initially disbelieving that someone has died: "Who died? I can't believe it. I just saw him."). They can also be the best response when the infraction is small or inadvertent. Problems arise, however, when the acute response becomes fixed despite all evidence to the contrary or when a person's actions are essential to the resolution of a problem (e.g., "I don't have to check the medicine bottle. I know Johnny wouldn't skip his meds.").

Table 50-1. **Examples of Active and Passive Coping**

Active Coping	Passive Coping
Gathering information	Distraction by others
Securing social support	
Prioritizing tasks	
Turning to religion	
Requesting and accepting help from family and friends	
Active distraction	
Biofeedback	
Problem solving	

THE ROLE OF THE FAMILY

The first training ground for all behavior is the home. Children inherit physiologic, somatic, and personality characteristics from their parents and live in the same milieu with the same resources. Children are great mimics, and in watching their parents respond to stress by crying, getting angry, withdrawing, or developing somatic symptoms, they perceive it as "the" way to handle similar situations in their own lives. Frequently, parents, discontent with their own coping style, see it in their child and become determined to make their child change. "Do as I say, not as I do" has been a parental mantra for centuries. The family can be a change agent but only by changing itself.

Most of the time, under usual circumstances, what we have learned to do (typically, unconsciously) through modeling of our parents or other adults in the environment is sufficient to function satisfactorily and even very well. Thus, adults and children faced with a dilemma ("Should I tell someone my friend has an eating disorder, takes drugs, drinks and drives . . .?") will find a sounding board (family member, friend, teacher, clergyperson) to help them decide what to do. A person who has set too high a goal ("This garden party has to be perfect.") will find an alternative site when it starts to rain or change appraisal ("Rain on your wedding day is good luck.") The range of possible solutions to given situations is determined by culture, resources (e.g., economic constraints), and personality.

Under unusually stressful circumstances or uncommon situations, like the diagnosis of cancer in a child, the usual repertoire of the family may be insufficient to deal with the extraordinary challenges presented by the illness. For example, if this is the first person to ever have a serious illness in the family, there may be no precedent for how to deal with the tertiary care medical establishment. The "elders" most often looked to for advice may have little to offer. Under these circumstances, it becomes essential for families to learn new skills.

WHY CHANGE COPING STYLE OR LEARN NEW STRATEGIES?

The easiest time to help facilitate behavior change for coping is when the stress is incapacitating. For example, parents may not be able to insist that their child with school refusal stay at school a full day until they have used up all their sick leave and are in jeopardy of losing income. At this point, they begin to react to the child's persistent complaints of pain by finding adaptive strategies so that the child and they can cope more appropriately (i.e., the child goes to school and the parents to work).

The area of nonpharmacologic management of procedural and illness-related pain (e.g., sickle cell crisis) is the focus of much ongoing clinical and research activity on coping. The use of anesthesia and conscious sedation has gained tremendous popularity, but these agents are not without undesirable side effects, including respiratory depression, arrest, and even death. A wide variety of interventions, including music therapy, biofeedback and psychological and educational preparation (describing the procedure in simple terms, demonstrating the instruments to be used on dolls, and showing an actual child undergoing the procedure), have been examined (Mahajan et al, 1998). Studies by Kazak and coworkers (1996) and by Schiff and coworkers (2001) have shown that combined sedative and distraction techniques or other multimodal interventions are effective in reducing the distress of painful procedures. Interestingly, a study of procedural distress in children with cancer found that behavioral indicators and self-report (cognitive) measures showed desirable changes in response to coping strategies training even though physiologic parameters (heart rate, blood pressure) were not significantly different between groups (Walco et al, 2005).

MUSIC THERAPY AS DISTRACTION

According to the American Music Therapy Association (2005), music therapy is the evidence-based clinical use of music interventions to accomplish individualized (nonmusical) goals within a therapeutic relationship by a credentialed professional who has completed an approved music therapy program. Music therapy is neither learning how to play an instrument nor passive listening. Music therapy is the use of *patient-chosen* music-based modalities such as listening, drumming, lyric writing or analysis, or composition for a specified end, such as calming anxiety, dissipating anger, feeling loss, or relieving depressive or sad feelings.

In the pediatric literature, music therapy has often been used for its distractive qualities. However, it is not pure distraction. In our work with children receiving Botox injections to relieve cerebral palsy–induced contractures (Sahler et al, 2004), the music provided by the therapist is chosen by the child or, if the child is not verbal, by the parents. The therapist engages the child through eye contact and seeks to have the child participate in the music making to the extent possible, whether it is banging on a drum, mouthing the words, or singing. If quiet and calm are desired, the therapist plays softly and slowly. At the time of injection, the therapist and child (and parents and often health care givers as well) join in the song, singing loudly. It is possible that the loud singing actually takes the place of wailing or crying.

In our satisfaction surveys, we have found that the parents appreciate the opportunity to have something constructive to do (sing along) and that the entire team feels more relaxed and is likely to play musical games with the child. An interesting side effect is that other practitioners and patients have found that Botox injection days are no longer filled with disruptive screaming that frightens other children. The treatment offers an alternative way to express discomfort that is more socially and personally (especially for older children) acceptable, and it can engage the entire team, thus fundamentally changing the procedure room milieu.

BIOFEEDBACK

Biofeedback is a type of applied psychophysiology. Olson (1995) offers the following comprehensive definition:

> *As a process, applied biofeedback is (1) a group of therapeutic procedures that (2) utilizes electronic or electromechanical instruments (3) to accurately measure, process, and "feed back" to persons (4) information with reinforcing properties (5) about their neuromuscular and autonomic activity, both normal and abnormal, (6) in the form of analogue or binary, auditory and/or visual feedback signals. (7) Best achieved with a competent biofeedback professional, (8) the objectives are to help persons develop greater awareness and voluntary control over their physiological processes that are otherwise outside awareness and/or under less voluntary control, (9) by first controlling the external signal, (10) and then with internal psychophysiological cues.*

Chapter 46 discusses biofeedback in the context of self-control and self-regulation.

Biofeedback can involve measurement of physiologic parameters such as, among others, heart rate, respiratory rate, skin conductance, blood pressure, and brain wave activity. See Chapter 46 for details. A commonly used physiologic measure to monitor degree of relaxation is finger temperature (thermal biofeedback). As an individual enters into the relaxed state, the temperature of the fingers increases. By using a sensor attached to a transducer that feeds a graphic representation on the computer screen, the patient can watch variations in finger temperature in response to different thoughts, imaginings, or breathing patterns.

Initially, patients typically experience "performance anxiety." ("This should be easy. . . . Why is my temperature going *down*?") Most will then report deciding that they "don't care," at which point they begin to relax and their temperature begins to rise. The most important part of the exercise is review of the "report screen," which graphs the rise and fall of temperature over time, and they are asked to recall what they were thinking about or what changes in breathing they tried. This review of their conscious efforts to relax is the distinguishing factor of biofeedback from other types of relaxation exercises, such as self-hypnosis and guided imagery. With practice, patients are able to move into the relaxed state within a few seconds, and temperature rises during a 10-minute period increase from a degree or less to as much as 10 to 12 degrees. Direct visualization of the benefits of entering into the relaxed state can be used to abort chronic pain episodes by having the patient learn to move into relaxation as soon as the symptom begins. The basic principles of the fight-or-flight response provide explanations for why abdominal pain (decreased splanchnic perfusion) and headache (increased perfusion accompanied by throbbing) would be ameliorated by relaxation. If the patient is motivated to get better, straightforward reliance on biofeedback is often sufficient. If the patient is deriving significant secondary gain from the symptom, formal psychotherapy or pharmacotherapy may be required as well.

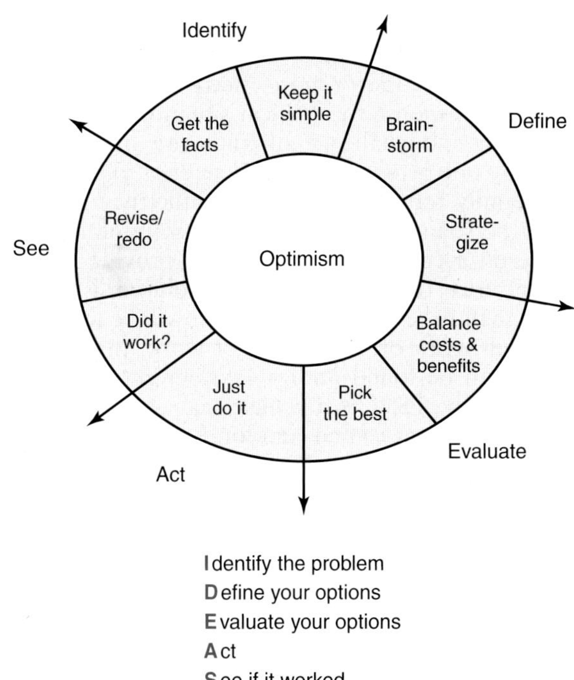

Figure 50-1. The Bright IDEAS system for problem solving.

PROBLEM SOLVING SKILLS TRAINING

Problem solving therapy is a form of cognitive-behavioral therapy that has been shown to be especially useful in the treatment of such disorders as depression and anxiety (D'Zurilla and Nezu, 1999). The premise of problem solving therapy is that individuals can be instructed in problem solving skills as a method of coping with stress and emotional distress. As originally conceptualized, problem solving is a five-stage process:

1. problem orientation (the cognitive and motivational set with which the individual approaches problems in general);
2. problem definition and formulation (delineation of a problem into concrete and specific terms and the identification of specific goals);
3. generation of alternatives (production of an exhaustive listing of possible solutions without regard to their consequences);
4. decision making (selection of the optimal solution); and
5. solution implementation and verification (monitoring and evaluation of the actual solution outcome after its implementation).

Problem solving skills training (PSST) is a term that we have chosen when applying the problem solving therapy approach to individuals who are distressed but do not manifest psychopathology or clinical levels of emotional distress. We have used PSST with the mothers of newly diagnosed cancer patients to help them cope with the everyday as well as the extraordinary stresses this diagnosis carries, especially during the first weeks and months after diagnosis, when response to surgery or induction therapy may be still unknown (Sahler et al, 2002, 2005). To make the overall objectives of the PSST program easily understood and remembered, the acronym Bright IDEAS and the logo of a lighted bulb are used. The letters **I** (Identify the problem), **D** (Determine the options), **E** (Evaluate options and choose the best), **A** (Act), and **S** (See if it worked) signify the five essential steps of problem solving (Fig. 50-1). Each week, participants are given a "homework" assignment to identify and solve a problem of specific interest to them. Their problem solving effort is reviewed at the following session. With PSST, as in the vignette that opened the chapter, mothers experience a noticeable sense of increased self-efficacy and enhanced well-being. By using their own "real-life" problems, we are able to show immediate relevance as well as immediate success. Our intervention consists of eight 1-hour individual sessions. Other researchers have provided interventions as 1-day events or three or four 2-hour sessions to individuals, families, or groups.

The steps of problem solving have been tested in a wide educational and sociodemographic range of mothers, from geographically disbursed white and black Americans, to newly immigrated monolingual Spanish-speaking mothers, to sophisticated urban Israeli and nomadic Arab mothers in the Middle East. The approach is generic, but the solutions are idiosyncratic and reflect the sociocultural background of the mother. The solutions usually come from the experience of the mother and her family. What is "new" is applying a systematic approach to trying solutions that have a reasonably high likelihood of being successful or, if they are not, understanding that alternative solutions can be generated until the "right" solution is found. Under extreme stress, however, people tend to revert to more primitive forms of coping and become easily susceptible to despair, rather than using their most sophisticated coping skills. PSST is a framework for more effective reasoning.

Thus, in response to identical situations, open communication and challenge of authority might be espoused by one person, whereas deference to the wishes of the family for privacy and self-sufficiency might be another person's solution; yet a third solution might be reliance on a community network to provide physical and emotional resources. The exact solution is less important than believing that a solution will be found and that it will work or, if it does not work, that another solution can be found until a satisfactory result is attained. Finally, PSST is a vehicle that can be used for both problem-focused and emotion-focused coping. The goal, as with all coping strategies, is to increase sense of mastery and to relieve perceived stress.

Although our work has been confined to mothers of newly diagnosed childhood cancer patients, Varni, Katz, and coworkers (Katz and Varni, 1993; Varni et al, 1993, 1994) were among the first to use problem solving–based social skills training with children, focusing primarily on social group and school reentry problems as children were being discharged from the hospital after surgery or chemotherapy. Issues addressed included What do you tell someone who asks you why you have no hair? and What should you do if someone picks on you because you take medicine that makes you fat? Each child determines the best solution for him- or herself following the Bright IDEAS model. Children as young as 7 years can participate successfully. Rehearsal of responses with the therapist or a parent adds significantly to the child's confidence and self-efficacy.

SUMMARY

Coping is the action taken by a person confronted with a stressor to return to a state of homeostasis. Coping skill is the marriage of style and strategy. Most coping is active and requires the individual to participate in altering either the situation or his or her perception of it. Avoidance is sometimes the most appropriate solution. Children learn how to cope with the stresses in their environment from the people who are in that environment. Coping strategies can also be taught formally. Cognitive understanding of autonomic and automatic physiologic responses is brought under conscious control through the mechanism of "feeding back" information about physiologic state. The skills to formally appraise a problem, to generate multiple solutions, to choose the best for that particular individual, and then to determine if the solution was successful or requires refinement have the power to reduce such potentially devastating states as depression and anxiety.

REFERENCES

American Music Therapy Association: What is music therapy? 2005. Available at: http://www.musictherapy.org/faqs.html#WHAT_IS_MUSIC_THERAPY.

Burke P, Elliott M: Depression in pediatric chronic illness: A diathesis-stress model. Psychosomatics 40:5-17, 1999.

Carr JE, Kappes BM: Stress, adaption, and illness. *In* Sahler OJZ, Carr JE (eds): The Behavioral Sciences and Health Care, 2nd ed. Göttingen, Germany, Hogrefe & Huber, 2007, pp 55-62.

Carr JE, Sawchuk CN, Nunes J: Learning processes. *In* Sahler OJZ, Carr JE (eds): The Behavioral Sciences and Health Care, 2nd ed. Göttingen, Germany, Hogrefe & Huber, 2007, pp 63-72.

D'Zurilla TJ, Nezu AM: Problem-Solving Therapy: A Social Competence Approach to Clinical Intervention, 2nd ed. New York, Springer, 1999.

Katz ER, Varni JW: Social support and social cognitive problem solving in children. Cancer 71:3314-3319, 1993.

Kazak AE, Penati B, Boyer BA, et al: A randomized controlled prospective outcome study of a psychological and pharmacological intervention protocol for procedural distress in pediatric leukemia. J Pediatr Psychol 21:615-631, 1996.

Lazarus R, Folkman S: Stress, Appraisal and Coping. New York, Springer, 1984.

Mahajan L, Wyllie R, Steffen R, et al: The effects of a psychological preparation program on anxiety in children and adolescents undergoing gastrointestinal endoscopy. J Pediatr Gastroenterol Nutr 27:161-165, 1998.

Olson RP: Definitions of biofeedback and applied psychophysiology. *In* Schwartz MS (ed): Biofeedback: A Practitioner's Guide, 2nd ed. New York, Guilford, 1995, pp 27-31.

Sahler OJ, Fairclough DL, Phipps S, et al: Using problem-solving skills training to reduce negative affectivity in mothers of children with newly diagnosed cancer: Report of a multisite randomized trial. J Consult Clin Psychol 73:272-283, 2005.

Sahler OJZ, Hunter BC, Oliva R, et al: Music therapy as procedural support during botulinum toxin injections. Abstract. Pediatr Res 55:87A, 2004.

Sahler OJ, Varni JW, Fairclough DL, et al: Problem-solving skills training for mothers of children with newly diagnosed cancer: A randomized trial. J Dev Behav Pediatr 23:77-86, 2002.

Schiff WB, Holtz KD, Peterson N, Rakusan T: Effect of an intervention to reduce procedural pain and distress for children with HIV infection. J Pediatr Psychol 26:417-427, 2001.

Shatte AJ, Reivich K, Gillham JE, Seligman MEP: Learned optimism in children. *In* Snyder CR (ed): Coping: The Psychology of What Works. New York, Oxford University Press, 1999, pp 165-181.

Somerfield MR, McCrae RR: Stress and coping research: Methodological challenges, theoretical advances, and clinical applications. Am Psychol 55:620-625, 2000.

Varni JW, Katz ER, Colegrove R Jr, Dolgin M: The impact of social skills training on the adjustment of children with newly diagnosed cancer. J Pediatr Psychol 18:751-767, 1993.

Varni JW, Katz ER, Colegrove R Jr, Dolgin M: Perceived social support and adjustment of children with newly diagnosed cancer. J Dev Behav Pediatr 15:20-26, 1994.

Walco GA, Conte PM, Labay LE, et al: Procedural distress in children with cancer: Self-report, behavioral observations, and physiological parameters. Clin J Pain 21:484-490, 2005.

Part VI

OUTCOMES—SCHOOL FUNCTION AND OTHER TASK PERFORMANCE

51 SCHOOL ACHIEVEMENT AND UNDERACHIEVEMENT

LYNN MOWBRAY WEGNER

Vignette

Alice, an 8-year-old third-grade student in an upper middle class public school, gets along very well with all the other children in her class and her teacher. Alice's parents are concerned about her classroom achievement. Her teacher had Alice's older sister as a student and she also wonders at the difference in the two girls with respect to their academic attainment. Alice's sister consistently mastered every classroom task with little effort and good humor. Alice has a similar sunny disposition, but her performance usually falls in the lower range of mid-average. Alice's parents, both attorneys, requested a conference, and the three adults could not find a logical reason for this discrepancy between the two siblings. "Why don't you discuss this with Alice's pediatrician and see if there might be a medical reason for Alice's apparent underachievement?" suggested the teacher.

On the first day of kindergarten, all children are potential Rhodes scholars! Even if the child has been attending daycare and preschool for several years, the first day of "real school" is a milestone in every family. The family anticipates sharing the child's care and nurture with teachers and other school personnel. This care becomes a combined responsibility. The child must navigate the transition between the primary influence of the home and a larger world with different expectations, and each setting contributes uniquely and importantly to the child's educational experience. Educating children is important at many levels: to the child, the family, and society.

In the medical home, pediatricians providing health maintenance for children are often consulted before school entry to help parents decide the "best" school setting or "when" it is best for the child to enter formal schooling. Later, if children do not perform at levels expected by their families or teachers, pediatricians again often are consulted for recommendations about further formal assessment and school placement. Sometimes, children perform below parental expectations, and sometimes their achievement clearly exceeds stated thresholds. Pediatricians who provide medical care for children are expected to be child development experts. Moreover, parents expect the pediatrician to be able to apply this knowledge to the acquisition of academic skills from the early primary through the secondary school years. School achievement is not merely "being smart enough." Achievement is very dependent on a complex and interwoven system reflecting societal, familial, and child elements (e.g., cognition, temperament, language, memory, attention, visual-spatial, fine and gross motor). These factors contribute to the child's ability to acquire information and new skills in the school setting. The proficient pediatrician will consider the matrix of societal, familial, and individual elements when trying to discern the factors affecting a particular child's academic achievement profile.

The three areas (Fig. 51-1) are discussed individually and then considered as elements in "school achievement." This discussion examines the factors affecting children to attain academic achievement commensurate with their cognitive level or those affecting children who

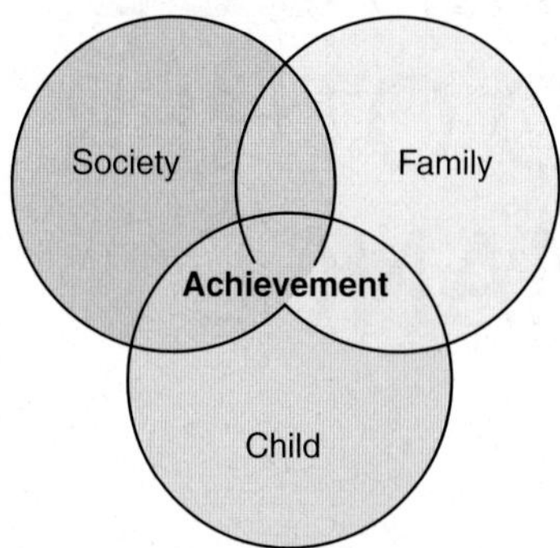

Figure 51-1. Academic achievement: Interplay of individual profile, family factors, and community characteristics.

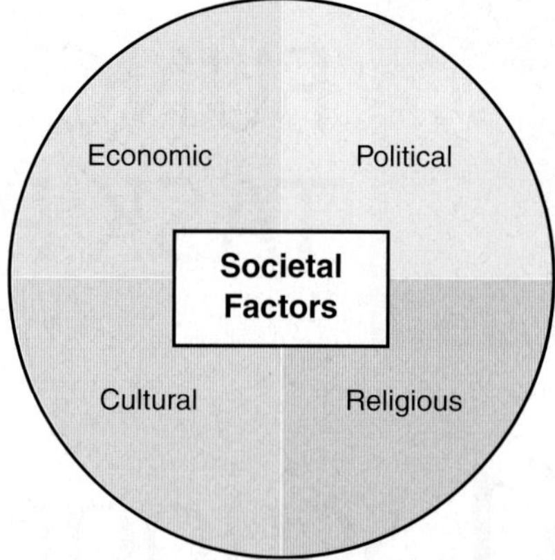

Figure 51-2. Societal factors that influence educational systems.

do not "make the grade." Finally, suggestions are offered to help direct the pediatrician's surveillance efforts to avoid unexpected academic struggles.

SOCIETAL FACTORS

Within each community, there are economic, political, cultural, and even religious influences on the educational system offered (Fig. 51-2). Whereas there are national federal mandates, control of local schools often is left to local officials with state oversight. This can create pockets of inequality as more affluent communities may be able to provide, and expect, more diversity of resources and experiences for their children. Communities with larger tax bases can support larger school budgets. Teacher salaries may be greater, schools may be better maintained, and "perishable goods" such as books, computers and software, and CD-ROMS may be more easily updated. Innovative programs may be explored as school personnel are able to attend professional trainings to learn about these offerings. Conversely, communities with fewer economic resources may not be able to attract teachers with advanced skills, more experience, or professional choices. There may be inadequate or outdated textbooks, fewer supplemental classes, and less ability to address individual student differences as completely.

Often interwoven with the economic forces are political agendas. Although a community may need a larger budget for school use, local politicians may be reluctant to promote tax increases. Their personal professional agendas may directly compete with school needs. Overarching local concerns may be a higher influence on curriculum because certain topics may be considered inappropriate. Restricting books in the school libraries is one example of this. Curriculum control is sometimes used as a means of inserting political influence in school policies.

Cultural and frequently associated religious influences can be subtle when the school is located in a geographic region populated by a preponderance of families from a particular ethnic group with specific cultural heritage and religious beliefs. If the majority believe a certain way, there is an assumption the schools will follow suit. If, however, there are many religions represented in the families, more strident and vocal groups may exert undue influence, and dissention from the others may follow. The dictum "separation of church and state" is sometimes difficult to follow when community political leaders represent a majority religious group in the community.

School administrators reflect these larger societal factors as well as their personal values and beliefs. Whereas school system administrators must follow federal and state mandates, most district systems are given significant leeway to permit local mores to set local standards (e.g., sex education, traditional man-woman marriage versus same-gender marriage/union, evolution versus creationism). These local school officials may respond to influential local groups and individuals with strong opinions about curriculum, policy, and procedures. These administrators also have their individual perspectives about how things should be run, and they often have the ability to make school policies fit their perspectives.

Teachers also bring their professional training and individual values to the classroom. The variability of teacher preparation is staggering. Some teachers have master's degrees from extremely strong education programs; other teachers may have only a few education courses taken while they receive on-the-job training. The length of the teaching career is variable also. The teacher's personal beliefs are brought to the classroom every day.

It is clear that the educational experience being offered to each child is complex and reflects many factors beyond the control of the child and family. Some of these factors are readily apparent: an aging school facility can be seen from the curb. Other equally important factors are much more subtle and may not be discerned until a problem arises. For example, a child who refuses to pray or to say the Pledge of Allegiance because of religious reasons may uncover pervasive community values. Both apparent and subtle factors are important.

FAMILY FACTORS

Families are the first communities of which children are members. It is safe to say that at this time (early 21st century), there are no "typical" families (see Chapter 9). Children may live with birth parents, adoptive parents, grandparents, other relatives, single parents, parents who are married but do not live together, same-sex parents, or foster parents, or they may be truly raised by paid caretakers while their actual parents are frequently absent. These arrangements may be variably

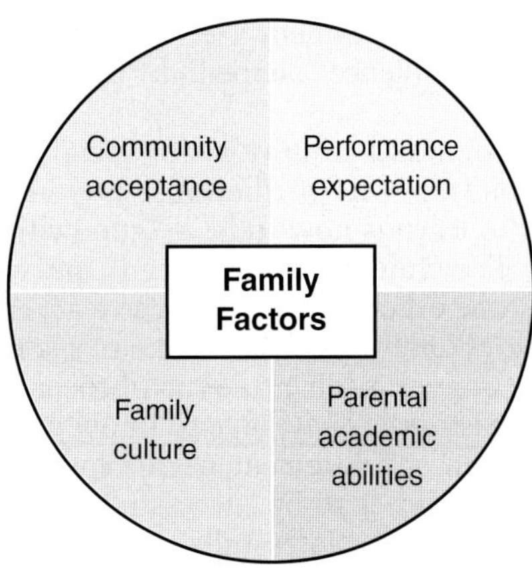

Figure 51-3. Family factors that influence student educational achievement.

accepted by the community, and this acceptance may affect the child's functioning in the family. Community acceptance also may affect the child's ability to function as an "equal" citizen in the school community (Fig. 51-3).

Families also have culture. The family culture sometimes is consistent with the larger community, and sometimes there is lack of congruity. If the family values are at odds with the larger community, conflicts can arise, and these may interfere with the child's successful academic achievement. For example, a family with strict religious adherence (e.g., Passover, Yom Kippur, Ramadan) may require school absences not synchronous with the established attendance schedule. The child may miss tests, field trips, or special opportunities. Depending on the school and community acceptance, these absences may be excused and the child allowed to make up the missed time, or the child may be penalized. There are laws prohibiting discrimination on the basis of religion, but discrimination can be subtle.

This "subtle" discrimination may also occur when the family does not meet community expectations. Biracial children may experience this. Children whose parents have unpredictable work schedules may not consistently come for school open houses or teacher conferences. This may be perceived by school personnel or other parents as "lack of interest" in school matters. Parents who have legitimate but out of the ordinary occupations (e.g., bartenders, entertainment industry) may have their parenting skills regarded more severely than those of more "traditional" parents. Children who live with relatives and are not cared for by a parent whose career precludes daily contact with the child may overhear adults make assumptions about the parents' affection and concern for the child. Children with parents in prison are often innocent victims of hostility directed at their absent parent with secondary judgments of the child's character.

Sometimes, the culture of the family excludes the community. If the family perceives the larger community as being "hostile" or alien to its values, the child may receive the message that only the family, or those of whom the family approves, are "safe" and acceptable. In this manner, the child may reject acceptance from the school community. Reinforcement is accepted only from the family. The family standards of achievement are those only accepted.

Family standards as the sole reference point for the child's academic performance may create false impressions. If the child is perceived as having more capability than he or she is able to demonstrate, the child may receive the message "You are lazy. You are not working hard enough. You could do better work if you tried harder. You are capable of better performance in your school work." Conversely, if the family has diminished expectations (e.g., "Girls in this family are not good at math."), a child with weak academic performance may not be offered a careful assessment of why his or her performance is weak.

The child's parents or primary caretakers can have a tremendous impact on successful daily school functioning. Parental disorganization and problems with time management and scheduling can upset the most conscientious student. If the child has a primary developmental condition, such as attention deficit disorder, weak parental organizational skills compound problems with getting to school on time, completing homework assignments and returning them to school, locating materials for extra projects, and even getting to bed on time so the child has adequate rest. A parent with substance abuse habits can undermine the child's sense of security and regularity. Not only can parental mental illness make the child genetically vulnerable to similar conditions, but poor emotional regulation clearly can affect daily routines and habits supporting successful school participation.

Parental learning disabilities can have a significant impact on the child's ability to master academic tasks. Not only is there an inherited pattern to some learning disabilities (Williams and O'Donovan, 2006), but many children rely on their parents to provide additional explanation and help in the evenings with homework assignments. The child whose parent struggles with basic reading, math, and written expression skills will not have the advantage of this additional home support. Many adults have significant shame about their weak basic academic skills and may try to hide this information from their children by "being too busy" to help them or telling them "You are just being lazy by asking for my help."

Finally, much has been written about socioeconomic status and the impact on child health and development. Magnetic resonance imaging studies of normal brain development in children between 6 and 18 years of age and neuropsychological testing of children in low-income families (<$35,000/year) showed significantly weaker performance on cognitive and achievement tasks emphasizing integrative skills (e.g., reading comprehension, written expression) (Waber et al, 2007). The authors of that study interpreted these results to suggest that lower economic family conditions do not provide rich and stimulating experiences enhancing cognition and accompanying complex academic tasks.

THE CHILD

Children are products of their families and the larger community, but foremost, each has a unique profile of strengths and weaknesses (Fig. 51-4). Whereas

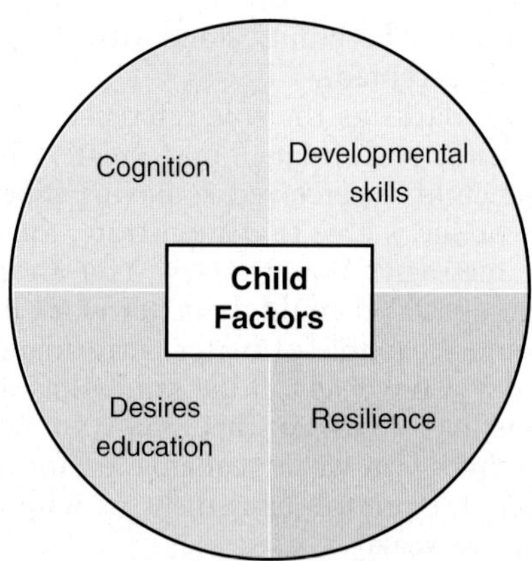

Figure 51-4. Individual characteristics of the child that affect academic performance.

community and familial responses may mitigate and enhance this profile, there are independent qualities strongly predictive of academic success. Success here is loosely described as "successful attainment of skills commensurate with the child's cognitive profile."

If the universal descriptor of "academic achievement" is successfully passing all grades, then cognition is the best predictor of academic success (Sattler, 1992). Standardized measures of intelligence correlate most closely with academic success (Lezak et al, 2004). These tests were developed with the primary intention of identifying those children who were most likely, all other factors aside, of successfully completing a formal educational program (i.e., "school"). Children with "full-scale" intelligence scale scores in the "average" range or higher (i.e., IQs > standard score 85) stand a better chance of being able to acquire the academic skills requisite to fluid reading speed and acceptable comprehension, math calculation and understanding, and expression of their ideas in written form.

If "intelligence" is closely examined, there are developmental skills clearly identifiable as contributing to this measured intelligence. Receptive and expressive language, selective attention, immediate and long-term recall, working memory, visual-spatial skills, and fluid processing all are potential domains of individual strength on which to build (see Chapter 55).

These areas also can be individual weaknesses that may be addressed for either remediation or bypass. What is important is that intelligence is perceived not as a composite but rather as a synergistic amalgam. Every child has an individual strength:weakness profile, and those children who are successful in school are taught to recognize their individual areas of strength to use when their weaker areas are emphasized during the school day.

Another important characteristic of academically successful children is resilience (see Chapter 50). Strongly resilient children do not buckle when they fail, either absolutely or relatively. This resilience may reflect their basal level of academic skills or their personal motivation to succeed in school. Some children are extremely motivated to learn and are not dissuaded by "failure." These children persevere in the face of academic struggles. They may possess a strong self-concept as part of their inherent temperament (see Chapter 7), or they have had their resilience "shaped" by the parenting style in their homes.

The classroom is a laboratory for social skills and interaction abilities. One of the most important skills a child needs to learn is how to be a "good citizen" in the classroom. The child must have needs met and respect the needs of the other students and the teacher. Children vary in their abilities to share, to take turns, to start and to maintain conversations, to control their bodies, and to request assistance. They have to know when to listen and when to talk. Children enter school with potentially very different abilities to be successful group members. Some children have successfully attended daycare or preschool and have demonstrated this ability. Other children have had home training that has made them ready to adapt to the classroom setting.

Another important characteristic of children who succeed in school is their personal belief that education is important to their present and future well-being. Young children have these feelings imparted to them by their families, who articulate the importance of education to them. As they become older, the personal acceptance of these beliefs is essential to help maintain the motivation to attend school and to give the best effort to assignments. This personal "ownership" of education's value becomes an integral part of the child's resilience to school struggles. If the child does not receive ongoing support from the family with respect to the value of education, even a mild setback can lead the child to reject school as important to him or her.

THE PEDIATRICIAN'S ROLE IN ANTICIPATORY CARE

The pediatrician can play a central role and be a significant agent in helping children to achieve school success from early childhood experiences in daycare or preschool through post-secondary education (Levine, 2002). Table 51-1 shows the various points for medical monitoring and intervention.

Genetic Elements

Certain genetic disorders have identified cognitive patterns clearly affecting a child's ability to master new information. Many of these conditions (e.g., trisomy 21, fragile X and other "expansion disorders") have variable expression in the child, and early intervention can frequently be associated with relatively optimal school performance. Careful family history can alert the clinician to assess the infant for any physical features suggesting particular inheritance or supplemental newborn screening. Prompt referral as soon as physical signs are identified can result in appropriate referral for supportive developmental interventions and family advocacy. Malformations may suggest syndromes with subsequent developmental and cognitive effects (e.g., velocardiofacial syndrome).

Prenatal Factors

Maternal and paternal age at conception, maternal habits such as alcohol use and cigarette smoking, maternal hypertension during pregnancy, and other indicators

Table 51-1. Topics Related to School Achievement: What May Be Discussed at Anticipatory Care Visits

Age	Considerations
Infant	Genetic elements
	Cognitive
	Fragile X
	Trisomy 21
	Malformations
	Velocardiofacial
	Prenatal factors
	Parent age at conception
	Alcohol or tobacco use
	Hypertension during pregnancy
	Birth and perinatal events
	Intraventricular hemorrhage
	Secondary visual impairments
	Central nervous system infections
Birth–3 years	Child
	Formal developmental screening
	Months 9, 18, and 30 or 36
	New concerns by family or physician
	Regular developmental surveillance
	Parent
	Maternal postpartum depression
	Referral to mental health programs
	Surveillance of family "wellness"
	Parental literacy
	Referral to adult literacy groups
3 years–kindergarten entry	Child
	Continue formal developmental screening
	Continue developmental surveillance
	Interaction with same-age children
	Independent play
	Sustained interest
	Interactive conversations with adults
	Variety of activities
	Parent
	Discussion about early education
	Family ambitions
	Community pressures
	Mistaken ideas
Kindergarten entry	Parent
	Community expectations
	Family history
	Child's characteristics
	Parents' personal school experiences
Early elementary years (grades 1-3)	Child
	Factors affecting standardized test performance
	Personal characteristics
	Physical
	Sensory deficits
	Medical conditions
	Motor skills
	Neuropsychological
	Attention
	Memory
	Reasoning
	Language
	Comprehension
	Temperament
	Stress and frustration management
	Emotional
	Previously diagnosed mental health conditions
	School
	Resources
	Facility conditions
	Student-teacher temperament synchrony
	Home
	Learning atmosphere
	Educational support
	Daily routine
	Parent and child expectations
	Peers
	Acceptance in social group
	Peer attitudes toward achievement
	Parent
	Review and explain testing reports
Later elementary years	Child—continue developmental surveillance
	Independence
	Initiates parental involvement
	Turns in assignments
	Asks specific questions to facilitate learning
	Cognitive changes
	Reading at appropriate grade level
	Understanding peer humor
	Peer influence
	Social hierarchies
	Attitudes toward academic achievement
	Differences in physical development
	Strengths and weaknesses identification
	Observation in the examination room
	Noting examples of stronger functioning by parents
	Parent
	Encouragement toward independence
Middle school	Child and school
	Chronic illness
	Educational and cognitive aspects
	Current research
	Effects of treatment
	Use of offered accommodations
	School personnel support
	Peer acceptance
	Parent
	Emphasize need for autonomy and individuation
	Contact school
	Suggest classroom modifications
High school	Adolescent
	Identification of personal areas of strength
	Facilitate communication between child and parent
	Parent
	Unresolved need for success
Post-secondary education/vocational training	Young adult
	If previously received supplemental services: apprenticeships

of possible fetal hypoxemia (including maternal iron deficiency anemia) and suboptimal fetal growth have been associated with developmental conditions later associated with school and behavior struggles.

Birth and Perinatal Events

Significant adverse events during delivery and prolonged neonatal complications, such as intraventricular hemorrhage with subsequent hydrocephalus, secondary visual and hearing impairments, central nervous system infections, and other significant congenital abnormalities, potentially may affect cognition and educational attainment in later childhood.

Birth Through Three Years

Between birth and 3 years of age, expert opinion recommends regular developmental surveillance as well as formal developmental screening with standardized instruments at 9 months, 18 months, and 30 or 36 months of age.

Identifying Infants and Young Children with Developmental Disorders in the Medical Home: An Algorithm for Developmental Surveillance and Screening

Formal screening also may properly be offered at any other time if the child's family or the pediatrician has new concerns. All U.S. states have early intervention services for young children, and pediatricians may make referral for formal developmental testing at any time before 36 months of age (*www.cdc.gov/ncbddd/child/devtool.htm*).

During these early years, formal screening for maternal postpartum depression, surveillance for indicators of family "wellness," and careful but clear addressing of parental literacy are important to help develop a strong and supportive family home in which the child can grow and be nurtured. Referral to local mental health programs and adult literacy groups can begin interventions benefiting everyone in the family.

Three Years Through Kindergarten Entry

Developmental support for children in this age range is usually provided through the public school systems. Whereas referrals certainly can be made after 36 months of age, it can be more difficult to obtain formal standardized assessment of the child's cognitive, language, and motor skills if the family's economic resources are limited. It is for this reason that referral for formal assessment before 3 years is emphasized. Nonetheless, children with identified developmental delays may enter the school system–sponsored structured preschool programs. For this reason, continued developmental surveillance and screening with a standardized instrument is optimal care for children in this age group.

As part of the developmental surveillance, asking the parent how the child interacts with other same-age children in paired situations as well as in larger group settings is important. As the child becomes older, there should be more independent play, more sustained interest in a preferred activity, and increasing length of interactive conversations with adults.

Asking the parents if the child freely participates in many different types of activities—coloring, assembling puzzles, imaginative play, riding a scooter or tricycle, listening to books being read aloud, and reciting nursery rhymes—can point to areas of further discussion if the child routinely avoids certain areas.

Pediatricians are often asked about the "best" preschools for their patients. Many parents mistakenly believe that young children need to be taught to read and to count before they enter kindergarten. The wise pediatrician will ask the parents what they think is important about attending preschool. That query can open a discussion about family ambitions, community pressures, and possibly mistaken ideas about early education. A thoughtful conversation often can help the parents decide for themselves the best preschool setting for their child.

Kindergarten Entry

The kindergarten physical examination appointment is often a well-attended visit because many school systems demand a school form completed by a physician. The pediatrician can be very helpful in providing some common-sense anticipatory suggestions. Regular bedtimes, breakfast in the morning, time for exercise after school, and time and place for homework completion should be emphasized. With respect to parenting, maybe the most important suggestion is to develop the habit of praising the child's efforts and not the outcome. This is very important as reading and written expression often require repeated attempts to master a subskill, and children may become tired and want to give up their attempts. They need to know that their parents appreciate and value the hard work they are showing as they work to master these skills.

Parents may quickly perceive that the kindergarten their child is attending is much different from the experience they had as 5-year-olds. Adults inspecting kindergarten curriculum may have the sense "We aren't in Kansas anymore, Toto!" As elementary curricula seem to move more quickly and encourage the acquisition of more complex skills at a younger and younger level, skills that were once the purview of first grade are now expected by the end of the kindergarten year. Some parents, sensing the intensity of the kindergarten curriculum, want the pediatrician's advice about not having the child enter kindergarten when the fifth birthday is reached. Other parents may allow matriculation but then want to retain the child for a second year of kindergarten for "maturing" purposes. Again, the community expectations, the family's history, and the child's characteristics all must be considered. This is another excellent time for a thoughtful explication of the parents' personal school experiences and an emphasis on their decision making rather than taking the pediatrician's expert opinion.

Early Elementary Years

Grades 1 through 3 are the foundation for skills used throughout the remainder of the child's school years. Learning to read, to do arithmetic functions, and to express ideas in written form may be the first tasks in which a child shows struggles. Parents want to know if early problems with classroom learning suggest more serious cognitive or processing problems, and this can be difficult to discern. Teachers are loathe to separate children in these early grades as being "deficient" and may try a variety of informal interventions before requesting formal psychoeducational testing either to identify or to describe a "learning disability." If the teacher does not communicate concerns about the child's progress to the parents, many parents assume the child is meeting expectations. The news that the child is being referred to the school's student support team for further assessment either can come as a shock to the family or can be welcomed that "finally something is being done." Many parents do not understand the testing process, the results from standardized testing, and what appropriate interventions should be offered if the child is found to meet criteria for a learning disability. The pediatrician can be helpful by offering to review the test report and explaining the standard scores in the context of a normally distributed curve. Seeing the information displayed in this graphic manner sometimes makes the numbers more understandable. There also are books explaining psychological tests to nonpsychologists (Wodrich, 1997).

For the typical nonstruggling student, the third grade is usually the first formal testing experienced, when children are given the high-stakes educational achievement testing mandated by No Child Left Behind legislation. Learning disabilities aside, Table 51-2 illustrates many factors potentially affecting the child's ability to learn classroom material and also to demonstrate this acceptable mastery on these tests. These factors should be considered throughout the academic course through college entry.

When children do not pass these examinations, additional testing will identify neuropsychological factors; however, the environmental and temperamental contributors are best assessed through interviews, observations, and checklists. By reviewing the medical record, the pediatrician can find much of this other information and can be a valuable member of the assessment team.

Table 51-2. Factors Affecting Standardized Test Performance

Personal Characteristics

- Physical
  - Sensory deficits affecting acquisition of tested material (vision, hearing)
  - Medical conditions, acute and chronic (Brown, 1999)
  - Fine motor and gross motor: precision, strength, and speed
- Neuropsychological factors
  - Attention
  - Memory: short-term, working, and long-term retrieval
  - Reasoning ability, possibly reflecting fluid processing, working memory, and processing speed (WISC Book)
  - Visual-spatial skills
- Language
  - Comprehension (both aural and reading) affected by receptive skills and prior exposure to the "language" of the test (Leonard, 1998)
- Personal experience
  - Past exposure to material covered on the test
- Temperament
  - Perceived stress of the testing and internal coping style
  - Past temperamental factors affecting learning
  - Persistence
  - Frustration management
  - Coping with both failure and success
- Emotional factors
  - Previously diagnosed mental health conditions: attention deficit disorder; depression
  - Anxiety-related disorders
  - Bipolar disorder

Environmental Factors

- School
  - Resources available for teaching and learning content: teacher qualifications; current resources for content (books, computers, consultants)
  - Physical building conditions
  - Temperament synchrony between the student and teacher
- Home
  - Availability for supplemental learning opportunities provided in the home
  - Support for consistent and complete homework mastery
  - Predictable daily routine, including meals, physical exercise, and adequate sleep
  - "Good fit" between parents' and child's expectations for school performance
- Peers
  - Child's acceptance by peers in the social group
  - Peer attitudes toward school and academic achievement

Later Elementary School Years

As the child progresses in school, the demands increase. Not only does the complexity of the material increase, with resulting emphasis on more adept integration of all the neuropsychological elements described in Table 51-2, but there is an expectation the student will function more independently. This can create problems for the child in several ways.

First, if the parents are not also emphasizing more independent management of school homework and projects, the student is not practicing independence out of the classroom. This can be seen in children not remembering to have parents sign forms brought home, not turning in completed homework although the parent made sure it was in the book-bag, or needing the parent's presence as they do their assignments. Second, teachers in later grades may function more as "consultant" rather than as teacher. That is, they may present the content in a lecture but then expect the students to ask specific questions about what they do not understand. There certainly are independent learners who can proceed and handle assignments with only minimal questioning of the teacher. Some children, however, cannot articulate what it is they do not understand; they need for the content to be presented in a slightly different manner. This may be misperceived as being overly dependent on the teacher for help, and the teacher may refuse to help them. Asking if the child shows independence at home can help resolve this confusion.

Older elementary children are expected to be transitioning into more conceptual and higher order language use and understanding. Their reading material is less about concrete and tangible topics. This change in language use and understanding is developmental and may begin as early as 9 years and yet in other students may not be mastered until later middle school. An informal sign that the child is not understanding more conceptual language is the complaint that appropriate grade-level books are "boring." When they are reading for pleasure, they may choose books at a lower level than they are capable of reading. Similarly, they may not understand the humor of same-age peers, although they used to easily tell jokes and understand them.

Peer relations also become increasingly more important as children approach the middle school years (see Chapter 15). The complex social hierarchies can take a significant amount of emotional energy, and some students will become internally distracted in the classroom as they mull over an unkind remark casually made in the lunchroom by a former close friend. Peer attitudes toward academic achievement also can be a significant factor in a student's willingness to actively participate in classroom discussions or enrichment after-school programs. Concerns about their physical development in comparison with peers also can significantly affect a child's social interactions in the classroom. As more students are retained because of failure to pass high-stakes testing, there will be more "old for grade" students, and the discrepancies between physical size and development will likely increase.

Finally, identification of the gifted student should not be forgotten (see Chapter 52). As everyone has a personal profile of strengths and weaknesses, there may be students who clearly excel and are identified early in their school years as intellectually bright. There are other students, however, who quietly do their work and may show one area of significant talent. These children should not be ignored as just showing a "splinter strength." It is possible they may fall in the designation of "academically gifted and learning disabled." That is, they will show superior scores on standardized intelligence testing, but their academic achievement testing falls in the average range of standard scores. If no one probes for more careful and formal scrutiny, the child will be passed along as average. This is a situation in which the pediatrician can make a significant contribution by noting examples of stronger functioning described by the parents or observed in the examination room. The pediatrician then can be the professional requesting further assessment by the school.

Middle School

The middle-school years can be a maelstrom for children, parents, and school personnel. All the issues described for the late elementary school-age child are present and made even more dramatic by the physical and cognitive changes experienced by young adolescents. Puberty encompasses the physical and sexual changes; adolescence demonstrates the enduring psychosocial and learning/cognitive transitions between childhood and adult life. The content demands of middle-school subjects increase also, and concomitantly supports offered in the elementary schools seem to fade. More is expected in the ability to organize their assignments, to maintain prolonged focused attention, to understand increasingly more conceptual and higher order language, and quickly to shift topics as they transition between classes and people with whom they interact. This appears to be true for both those students who have identification as "specifically learning disabled" and those who receive support through "other health impaired" identification. At the same time support is changed, the typical young and mid-adolescent does not want to appear different from peers and may refuse any offered supplemental services. The needs do not abate, but the intervention certainly changes. Parents may seek help from the pediatrician to advocate for the school to continue to honor accommodations offered in elementary school as they are clearly needed for the student to make academic progress. When contact is made with the school for this purpose, a successful strategy is to focus on the eventual goal of school attendance through the twelfth grade and high-school graduation. Asking how this student will successfully manage the content of middle-school courses and develop the skills requisite for successful mastery of high-school demands can help focus the discussion more on strengths of the middle-school teachers to enhance development and less on what will or will not be offered. If the pediatrician makes suggestions about classroom modifications (preferential seating, copies of class notes, after-school assistance in how to stage long-term projects), the process may be viewed as less adversarial.

Another manner in which the pediatrician can be helpful to both school personnel and the child is to act as a resource for information about the educational and cognitive aspects of chronic illnesses. Although most laypeople understand that central nervous system disorders (e.g., seizure disorders, past history of meningitis or head trauma with prolonged loss of consciousness, congenital brain malformations) could have a clear impact on learning, they may not understand other conditions and the relationship to cognition. This might include midline heart defects, sickle cell anemia, insulin-dependent diabetes, and asthma. Discussions about chronic health conditions might include review of current research about cognition and the condition, effects of treatment, need for hospitalization, and reduced endurance once the child is in the classroom.

Pediatricians also may be drawn into a discussion with the student to encourage the use of offered accommodations. Whereas parents may have many directives about what they want their child to do, the pediatrician may be viewed as more neutral, and thus recommendations made may be taken more seriously by the student. An especially important aspect to this discussion is to acknowledge humiliation protection and how the student may accept the support and avoid as much as possible teasing by peers.

High School

High school may begin in either the ninth or tenth grade, but high school is clearly different from all other school experiences, as parents and teachers remind the students that high-school grades "count." These are the courses and grades the colleges, technical schools, and specialized vocational programs will use to determine eligibility after the senior year. If you ask middle-class ninth-grade students what they plan to do after high school, most will give an answer including further education. It is important to try to ensure that all students leaving high school have solid reading and reading comprehension, practical math skills, and the ability to express their ideas clearly in written form. If a student's parents did not have a strong educational background, they may not have an accurate understanding of their child's ability level relative to that expected by a graduating senior. The pediatrician may have to be the strong advocate for ensuring that the student is offered assistance to graduate with as much of the basic skills as possible. Adults concerned with adolescents must remember that this age also includes first work experiences, social distractions and preoccupations, excessive media consumption, and risks of tobacco or alcohol and other substances for abuse.

On the other end of the spectrum are those students whose parents bought infant clothing for them with the logo of an Ivy League college and who are determined their child will matriculate into a "top" college. This can be a very difficult situation if the student does not have the academic or personal profile consistent with this demanding institution or if the student does not follow his or her parents' wishes. Sometimes, the decision about college can uncover the parents' unresolved needs for success and how these needs are being channeled through the child. The pediatrician can be helpful here by emphasizing in the child's early adolescent years the need for autonomy and individuation from the parents. Encouraging the adolescent to identify personal areas of strength and to pursue these for a sense of mastery and accomplishment will provide a buffer for any academic setbacks. It is a rare child who completely ignores his or her parents' suggestions, as the family messages can be incredibly powerful, but emotionally healthy children may choose a path in which they know they can find success rather than temporarily appease the parent. In this situation, the pediatrician can use skills as both a child and parent advocate to help facilitate communication between the child and parent and meaningfully contribute to an acceptable resolution to the differing needs of each.

Planning for Post-Secondary Education or Vocational Training

Ideally, these plans were being developed at the beginning of high school. Certain factors can prevent the best plan's being followed. An intervening serious health condition may change the student's plans from going to college in another state to attending a local and less stressful community college. Family disruption through the death of a parent or divorce may change the financial support available to the student, and the student may realistically have to defer formal training or education to be self-supporting. Emotional and mental health conditions can change the academic trajectory of a promising student.

Most high schools have guidance counselors to advise students, but the services that these overextended professionals can offer are usually limited to developing the letters of recommendation for the student. If a student is not planning to attend a post-secondary technical or academic program, and if the student ever received supplemental school services as either learning disabled or "other health impaired," it is very important to see if that student would be eligible for vocational rehabilitation consultation. Whereas these resources can be variable in the completeness of services offered, they should know about training centers and other community programs for individuals who do not have the educational background to enter a more advanced technical school. Apprenticeships can be another avenue for more specialized training, and this can be invaluable for students who are not reading at a high-school level and who learn best through on-the-job training.

For all students, the pediatrician can be a strong ally in communicating with teachers and other school personnel, making suggestions about improving time management and organizational skills, developing appropriate medication plans when indicated, facilitating family dialogue, and making evidence-based suggestions about diet, sleep, and exercise. The final years of secondary school can be tumultuous for students and parents. The pediatrician can be the voice of calm for them all.

SUMMARY

School performance is a multifaceted marker of a child's development, and pediatricians can make significant contributions to helping the child be as successful as he or she is capable. Knowledge of the community characteristics, the family background, and the child's individual physical, developmental, and emotional strengths and weaknesses places the pediatrician in a position to help guide the child through preschool programs all the way to high-school graduation. Actively soliciting information at all appointments about school performance and showing a genuine interest in mastery of educational tasks demonstrate the pediatrician's desire to be a partner with the child and family in their common goal of helping the child manage the academic challenges as the child develops physically, emotionally, and socially.

REFERENCES

American Academy of Pediatrics: Identifying infants and young children with developmental disorders in the medical home: An algorithm for developmental surveillance and screening. Pediatrics 118:405-420, 2006.

Brown RT (ed): Cognitive Aspects of Chronic Illness in Children. New York, Guilford, 1999.

Leonard LB: Children with Specific Language Impairment. Cambridge, Mass, MIT Press, 1998.

Levine MD: Educational Care. Cambridge, MA, Educator Publishing Service, 2002.

Lezak MD, Howieson DB, Loring DW, Hannay HJ: Neuropsychological Assessment, 4th ed. New York, Oxford University Press, 2004.

Sattler JM: Assessment of Children, Revised and Updated, 3d ed. San Diego, Jerome M. Sattler, Publisher, 1992.

Waber DP, De Moor C, Forbes PW, et al: The NIH MRI study of normal brain development: Performance of a population based sample of healthy children aged 6 to 18 years on a neuropsychological battery. J Int Neuropsychol Soc 13:729, 2007.

Wehman P: Life Beyond the Classroom: Transition Strategies for Young People with Disabilities, 3rd ed. Baltimore, MD, Paul Brookes, 2001.

Williams J, O'Donovan MC: The genetics of developmental dyslexia. Eur J Hum Genet 14:681, 2006.

Wodrich DL: Children's Psychological Testing: A Guide for Nonpsychologists. Baltimore, MD, Paul Brookes, 1997.

52 THE GIFTED CHILD

MARY C. KRAL

Children who are gifted compose 5% to 20% of the general school-age population, depending on how "gifted" is defined or the criteria used to identify students who are gifted (Pfeiffer and Stocking, 2000). Primary care physicians may be the first line of professionals consulted by parents of gifted children. *Is my preschooler gifted? How can I nurture my child's talents? What is the best educational setting for my gifted child? Why is my child not achieving at a level consistent with his or her high ability?* Primary care physicians are frequently placed in the position of assisting parents with answers to these questions and directing them to appropriate resources and educational opportunities. The following summary of the current research on identification of, appropriate educational programming for, and special challenges faced by children who are gifted is provided as a resource for the primary care provider.

DEFINITIONS OF GIFTEDNESS

"Gifted" means different things to different people in different contexts and cultures. Some equate gifted with high intelligence, others with high academic achievement. Still others highlight the domain-specific mastery characteristic, for example, of musically or artistically gifted individuals. What constitutes giftedness in terms of cognitive abilities, talents, personality traits, or environmental contributions is the source of ongoing investigation and public debate. Researchers and educators alike differ in how they define giftedness, and the empiric literature is characterized by the absence of a common vocabulary or universally defined terms, making comparisons across studies difficult. Within the realm of education, there is no federal definition recognized by all states—a child who qualifies for gifted programs in one state may not be eligible for similar programs in a different state.

Historically, gifted has been equated with high intellectual functioning. In the early 20th century, Lewis Terman defined gifted as an intelligence quotient (IQ) at or above 150 on the Stanford-Binet Intelligence Scale (Terman et al, 1926). Subsequently, the 98th percentile (IQ = 130) has commonly been used as the cutoff for giftedness. More recently, some school districts recognize students with IQs of 120 or above as eligible to receive gifted programming.

The problem with viewing exceptionally high IQ as synonymous with giftedness is that a fixed proportion of the population is always selected (e.g., top 3% to 5%; Renzulli, 2005). Research suggests that heritability accounts for most of the variance in IQ among children in middle and upper socioeconomic classes. However, for children from low-resource backgrounds or minority groups, environment—not genes—makes a bigger difference (Turkheimer et al, 2003). As such, use of an IQ cutoff as the criterion for gifted will underidentify children from low-resource backgrounds. An additional problem with use of intelligence test scores to define giftedness is the limited predictive utility of these scores. IQ correlates only modestly with academic achievement, and noncognitive factors also account for a significant proportion of variance in academic attainment, including but not limited to motivation, interest, self-efficacy, and self-regulation skills. In addition, intelligence test scores are poor predictors of real-world functioning, such as job performance (Neisser et al, 1996). Finally, IQ scores do not capture the range of cognitive abilities. Therefore, classifications that emphasize IQ for placement will miss those children with "uneven giftedness" (e.g., nonverbal intelligence > verbal intelligence). For all of these reasons, IQ cutoff criteria frequently result in underidentification of gifted children.

Modern-day conceptualizations of giftedness recognize that general intellectual ability is an important component of giftedness but reject the notion that intelligence is a unitary construct. For example, Howard Gardner's (1999) "multiple intelligences" highlights the multifactorial nature of giftedness by defining eight domain-specific intelligences: linguistic, logical-mathematical, musical, bodily-kinesthetic, spatial, interpersonal, intrapersonal, and naturalistic. Similarly, Robert Sternberg suggests that intelligence is not a fixed entity but a flexible and dynamic one, a form of developing expertise involving noncognitive and cognitive components. Specifically, Sternberg's WICS model (2005) asserts that gifted individuals possess a *s*ynthesis of *w*isdom (balancing intrapersonal, interpersonal, short- and long-term goals), *i*ntelligence (ability to adapt to one's environment and to learn from experience), and *c*reativity (applying and balancing innovative, analytical, and practical abilities). Joseph Renzulli (1978, 2005) also emphasizes the confluence of multiple factors in defining giftedness. In his three-ring model, Renzulli suggests that creative-productive people possess an interaction among three basic traits: (1) above-average ability, defined as high general intellectual functioning or well above average domain-specific performance, such as general verbal ability; (2) high levels of task commitment, defined as perseverance, hard work, intrinsic motivation, and self-efficacy; and (3) high levels of creativity, or original, unconventional, ingenious thinking. These three rings interact against a background of personality and environmental variables (e.g., educational opportunities) to give rise to gifted products. The multiple factors that give rise to gifted behaviors require special attention from parents, primary care providers, and educators.

DEVELOPMENTAL ASPECTS OF GIFTEDNESS

Cognitive Development

The term *giftedness* often sparks the nature-nurture debate. Those assuming the nature side of the argument emphasize the inborn, heritable ability and intrinsic drive of the gifted child (e.g., high IQ), whereas those assuming the nurture side of the argument suggest that giftedness is the product of hard work or deliberate practice (Bloom, 1985). According to modern-day theorists, as detailed previously, high ability is a necessary but not sufficient component of giftedness. Opportunity also plays a large role in the development of giftedness, including family support, societal and cultural values, educational opportunities, and resources.

When considering their cognitive development, Winner (1997) suggests that gifted children are qualitatively different from children of average ability. Specifically, gifted children excel at higher order reasoning, independent solution of abstract problems, and transfer of skills to novel situations. Gifted children also are characterized by an intrinsic drive to master specific domains of interest. Signs of giftedness may emerge early in development, including early onset of language, excellent memory, intense curiosity, long attention span when engaged in activities of high interest, metacognitive awareness of problem solving strategies, and efficient use of learning strategies. Many children who are gifted acquire reading skills before entering kindergarten, demonstrate facility with numbers, and excel at abstract problem solving. Although many gifted children demonstrate evenly developed intellectual functioning, many evidence domain-specific gifts in language or nonverbal/quantitative reasoning. Finally, gifted children may evidence uneven development that is characterized by acquisition of cognitive skills in advance of social and emotional development.

Social-Emotional Development

In a review of the research, Neihart and colleagues (2002) reported that most gifted children are socially and emotionally well adjusted. Contrary to myths promoted by the media, rates of suicide or school violence are not higher among students who are gifted. Rather, Neihart and colleagues report low rates of delinquency among students who are gifted compared with average students. In the National Education Longitudinal Study from the National Center for Educational Statistics, students placed in gifted programs reported higher self-perceptions of their social relationships and emotional development and tended to have fewer serious school behavior problems compared with students enrolled in regular educational programming (Sayler and Brookshire, 1993). Similarly, Bain and Bell (2004) reported that the majority of gifted elementary and middle-school students reported high self-concepts compared with a high-achieving group of students and had a stronger tendency to attribute social success to ability and effort (internal locus of control) rather than to luck or task difficulty.

A number of steps have been suggested for the promotion of healthy social and emotional development among children who are gifted. First, the role of the family cannot be understated. Three family characteristics have been shown to facilitate social and emotional resilience among gifted youth: parents who have high expectations of their gifted children and model high achievement, parents who give their children more independence, and parents who provide stimulation and nurturance (Winner, 2000). Second, schools that set high expectations for achievement and provide appropriate, individualized educational programming also promote social and emotional adjustment among gifted students. Reis and Renzulli (2004) suggest that appropriate educational programming for gifted students should include (1) accelerative learning experiences targeting areas of academic strength along with supports in areas of identified weakness (i.e., learning disabilities or attention-deficit/hyperactivity disorder), (2) mentoring that teaches students how to cope with the pressures and social stress associated with high academic ability and early presentation of career information, and (3) integration of social-emotional curriculum approaches to help gifted children support one another, including social opportunities with peers of similar abilities, interests, and motivation.

APPROACHES TO EDUCATING THE GIFTED CHILD

During the past 50 years, research and educational programming focused on gifted students have grown. At the federal level, although specific legislation recognizes the unique educational needs of students who are identified as gifted and talented (e.g., the Jacob Javits Gifted and Talented Students Education Act, recently reauthorized in 2001 as part of the No Child Left Behind Act), the federal government does not mandate services for gifted students. Gifted and talented programming is not part of the Individuals with Disabilities Education Act. Rather, the majority of programs and services that students receive are determined by state laws and policies and funded at the state and local level. State laws that define gifted and talented programming and teacher training requirements, along with available funding for gifted education, vary widely. Most states and school districts use the following definition (U.S. Department of Education, 1993) :

> *Children and youth with outstanding talent perform or show the potential for performing at remarkably high levels of accomplishment when compared with others of their age, experience, or environment. These children and youth exhibit high capability in intellectual, creative, and/or artistic areas, possess an unusual leadership capacity, or excel in specific academic fields. They require services or activities not ordinarily provided by the schools. Outstanding talents are present in children and youth from all cultural groups, across all economic strata, and in all areas of human endeavor. (p. 26)*

Most leaders in the field agree that cognitive ability tests should constitute part but not all of the identification process. They agree that other indicators of potential also should be used in the identification process and should be given equal consideration in selecting those students eligible for special services. Most agree that the selection process should take into consideration multiple variables, and in the final analysis, the informed judgment of educators should prevail over strict cutoff scores on psychometric instruments. Despite these ideals, in this era of high-stakes testing, identification of students eligible for special programs typically relies on test scores (i.e., intelligence test cutoffs or performance on academic achievement tests).

Curriculum Alternatives

In general, research suggests that gifted students require a differentiated curriculum that addresses their learning needs to maintain academic interest and high levels of achievement. The following is a brief introduction to the various curriculum alternatives for gifted education. Empiric support for the effectiveness of each of the following programs is limited. There are three main approaches to gifted education: ability grouping, acceleration, and enrichment.

Ability grouping refers to the practice of using test scores or other measures of achievement to assign students to groups within the classroom. This practice may involve part-time assignment to both regular and special classes or full-time grouping with students of similar abilities within the classroom. Magnet schools are a good example of ability grouping for students who are gifted and talented or students with special interest areas (e.g., science and math or the arts). Research suggests that gifted students who receive a differentiated curriculum through flexible grouping practices evidence higher academic achievement at all grade levels compared with those students who do not receive a differentiated curriculum (Kulik and Kulik, 1992).

Acceleration is an educational procedure that is based on the assumption that gifted students learn at an accelerated rate and generally master advanced-level academic material. Acceleration is a placement, not an educational program. Accelerative procedures may include early entrance into kindergarten, grade advancement, early entry into college, and dual enrollment in high school and college. Curriculum compacting is another example of accelerative programming, whereby a number of courses are "compressed" into one or students are exempt from instruction in an area in which they demonstrate mastery. Opponents of acceleration suggest that this form of educational programming is detrimental to the social, emotional, or physical development of gifted students, and acceleration practices are not commonly used by most school districts. However, in a review of the research, Gross and van Vliet (2005) reported positive outcomes for exceptionally gifted students who were permitted radical acceleration (i.e., early entry into college), including sustained interest and involvement in academic activities, high levels of academic success, and transition into high-status careers. Moreover, there was no evidence for social or emotional maladjustment when exceptionally gifted students participated in well-planned acceleration procedures. Positive outcomes for students who participate in radical acceleration procedures were associated with high achievement motivation, persistence, effective study skills, and involvement in educational decision making.

Enrichment refers to additional or new curricular material not delivered in regular education or instructional strategies that supplement what is taught in the regular education classroom (e.g., pull-out programs). Advanced Placement (AP) courses, part-time college courses, and summer programs are examples of enrichment programs. Gifted students report an increase in social self-concept when they participate in summer enrichment programs (Rinn, 2006). However, pull-out programs have been criticized for not providing appropriate educational programming throughout the school day or across all subject areas.

CHALLENGES FACED BY SOME GIFTED CHILDREN

The Underachieving Gifted Child

The gifted child who does not evidence ability-consistent academic achievement represents one of the most frustrating dilemmas for primary care providers and parents alike. Gifted underachievement, most commonly defined as a severe and persistent discrepancy between a student's academic performance and actual ability, represents a significant problem for some children. In a review of the research on gifted underachievement during the last 5 decades, Reis and colleagues (2005) reported that the beginning stages of academic underachievement among gifted students occur in elementary school, perhaps because of an unchallenging curriculum. Subsequently, underachievement appears to be periodic and episodic, occurring in some years and not others and in some classes but not others. Eventually, increasing episodes of underachievement will result in a more chronic pattern for some students.

Gifted underachievement is often a complex problem involving multiple factors (Reis and McCoach, 2000, 2002):

- Curriculum factors: Gifted underachievers report that they are bored or unchallenged by the regular education curriculum. In general, research suggests that when given an appropriately stimulating academic environment, gifted students perform at more advanced levels than their peers.
- Peer factors: Underachieving gifted students report that the influence of peers is the single strongest force undermining their achievement. Specifically, some gifted students succumb to the pressure to be like their peers, hiding their abilities in an attempt to be accepted by their typically developing peers (Winner, 2000).
- Family factors: Parenting styles may interact with the behaviors of some underachievers, yet no clear pattern exists about the types of parental behaviors that may influence or cause underachievement (Reis et al, 2005). Such family characteristics as inconsistent parenting styles (Rimm, 1995), parents with less positive affect, parental disinterest toward education, overly strict or overly lenient parenting, and family conflict have been correlated with gifted underachievement.
- Child factors: Depression, anxiety, perfectionism, rebellion, low motivation, low self-regulation, or low self-efficacy can lead to academic underachievement among gifted students. Academic underachievement may be symptomatic of more serious cognitive or emotional issues, such as an unrecognized dual diagnosis (e.g., attention-deficit/hyperactivity disorder, learning disability, or depression).

Solutions

Research documenting the effectiveness of specific interventions for gifted underachievement has been inconclusive. However, the growing literature on gifted underachievement suggests that a focus on strengths and interests is critical to reversing the pattern of underachievement (Baum et al, 1995; Dole, 2000; Reis et al, 2005). In addition, interventions that target family, child, peer, and academic factors are recommended. Specifically, psychological interventions that target family dynamics (e.g., increased positive parent-child interactions, increased parental interest and investment in their child's education, and use of reward systems) and characteristics of the student (e.g., cognitive and emotional obstacles, such as low self-efficacy) are recommended. Academic interventions should include curricular changes that tap areas of giftedness and high interest and establish clear academic goals and objectives with rewards for attainment of these goals. There is some evidence that more rigorous academic challenge may actually have a positive impact on underachievement. Peer groups that support achievement can be an important part of preventing and reversing underachievement. In this regard, busier adolescents who are involved in clubs, extracurricular activities, sports, and religious activities are less likely to underachieve in school. Regular patterns of work and practice also seem to help talented students develop an achievement model in their own lives. For example, scheduled time for extracurricular activities and regular time for homework and reading can help develop positive self-regulation strategies. Finally, the coordinated efforts of caring adults, such as a mental health provider, coach, or teacher, can help ensure that these areas are effectively targeted (Baum et al, 1995; Callahan and Kyburg, 2005).

The Socially Isolated Gifted Child

Among those gifted students who experience social or emotional difficulties, social isolation may result from a number of factors. Early investigations reported that the gifted adolescent who feels lonely may be experiencing stress and depression in reaction to the burdens of "success" (Kaiser and Berndt, 1985). Cornell (1990) reported that compared with popular students of average ability, unpopular high-ability students are characterized by lower reported levels of social self-concept and academic self-efficacy. Finally, Pfeiffer and Stocking (2000) have suggested that some gifted students become socially or emotionally maladjusted because of difficulties identifying a peer group with similar abilities; disparity between the instructional environment and the capabilities of the gifted child; or unrealistic expectations on the part of parents or teachers that can lead to defiant behavior, depression/hopelessness, academic underachievement, or substance abuse.

Some gifted children may be the target of peer bullying. Peterson and Ray (2006) conducted a national survey of 432 eighth-grade students identified as gifted to determine the prevalence rates of bullying among gifted students. The prevalence of being bullied at some time during kindergarten through the eighth grade was 67%. Name-calling was the most prevalent type of bullying across all grades and was rated as the worst type of bullying, followed by teasing about appearance and teasing about intelligence and grades. Students reported that the greatest emotional impact of bullying occurred in the fifth grade, although emotional distress related to being bullied persisted between the fifth and eighth grades. Boys were more likely than girls to be targets or instigators of bullying, to think violent thoughts, or to engage in violent behaviors at school. Many victims told no one and suffered in silence. The authors concluded that bullying of gifted children and adolescents occurs fairly universally and at higher rates than in some reports of the prevalence of bullying in the general school-age population. As such, for the gifted child, peer bullying may contribute to difficulties incorporating intelligence and academic accomplishments comfortably into an identity.

Solutions

In addition to supporting and encouraging accelerative learning experiences, Neihart and colleagues (2002) suggest that educational programming for gifted students should address social and emotional development. In this regard, educational programming for gifted students should (1) ensure time to learn with others of similar abilities, interests, and motivation; (2) supply opportunities to explore areas of interest with a variety of peers; (3) provide mentoring or coaching to cope with stress, criticism, and the social demands associated with high achievement; (4) present career information early; and (5) develop approaches to help gifted students support one another (e.g., group interventions that provide direct instruction in conflict resolution, decision making, and leadership). Because teasing and peer bullying occur fairly universally, primary care providers and educators should be attuned to the peak incidence of teasing about appearance and intelligence in the middle-school years and proactively work toward prevention of bullying by building a positive, safe school culture (Peterson and Ray, 2006). The most effective interventions are comprehensive, involving the entire school, rather than simply targeting the victim. An excellent resource on the subject is available through the American Psychological Association and includes prevention strategies from kindergarten through high school, school-wide education programs, and guidelines for anti-bullying policies (Orpinas and Horne, 2005).

The Perfectionistic Gifted Child

Perfectionism, holding excessively high standards for performance, afflicts some students who are gifted. Research suggests that although adaptive levels of perfectionism can fuel persistence and productivity for some gifted students, excessive levels of perfectionism can lead to immobilizing anxiety, avoidance behaviors, and failure (Schuler, 2002). Dixon and coworkers (2004) studied perfectionistic tendencies in a group of gifted high-school students. By use of cluster analysis of the Multidimensional Perfectionism Scale, personality measures, and indicators of psychiatric symptoms, four typologies were yielded (Table 52-1). Those adolescents with maladaptive types of perfectionism also reported high levels of self-doubt, excessive concern about making mistakes, excessively critical parents, poor self-image, and inadequate coping strategies. Dixon and colleagues suggest that maladaptive perfectionism may become more differentiated in adolescence.

Solutions

Knowledge about the various types of perfectionism among gifted students can help primary care providers, parents, and educators understand the barriers to their success (Dixon et al, 2004). Important components of intervention include assisting the child in setting high yet realistic goals, encouraging effort rather than placing undue emphasis on cognitive ability, and valuing the lessons learned from mistakes (Schuler, 2002). When excessively high standards lead to a crippling fear of failure and subsequent underachievement, psychological interventions are indicated. Mental health professionals may assist in the identification of possible obsessive-compulsive tendencies or depression and provide effective remediation of maladaptive perfectionism.

The At-Risk Gifted Child

According to the National Research Center on the Gifted and Talented, gifted children from low-resource families or minority groups are underidentified and underrepresented in gifted and talented educational programs. Moreover, a majority of gifted and talented students who drop out of school are from lower socioeconomic backgrounds or had reduced access to educational opportunities or technology (e.g., computers). For many students from low-resource or minority groups, the

Table 52-1. A Typology of Perfectionism in Gifted Adolescents

Perfectionism Type	Perfectionism Profile	Adjustment Profile
Mixed-adaptive	This type is well organized and has few doubts about his or her ability to complete tasks; sets high personal standards but does not overreact or respond negatively to mistakes. Parents have high expectations but are not excessively critical.	This type reports few psychiatric symptoms but a strong sense of mastery coping and superior adjustment, perceptions of personal security, and academic competence.
Pervasive	This type is well organized but has strong doubts about his or her ability to complete tasks; sets high personal standards but overreacts and responds negatively to mistakes. Parents have high expectations and are excessively critical.	This type reports more psychiatric symptoms (somatic complaints, obsessive-compulsive tendencies, depression, anxiety), a poorer self-image, a lower sense of personal security, and a pattern of dysfunctional coping.
Nonperfectionist	This type is confident in his or her ability to complete tasks but shows little preference for organization, order, or neatness; does not set very high personal standards and does not respond negatively to mistakes. Parents do not have high expectations and are not excessively critical.	This type is substantially similar to the mixed-adaptive type on measures of psychiatric symptoms, personal security, and coping, although the nonperfectionist reports less academic competence and a weaker superior adjustment compared with the mixed-adaptive type.
Mixed-maladaptive	This type is overly concerned about mistakes and doubts his or her ability to complete tasks successfully; sets relatively lower personal standards and shows relatively little preference for organization, order, or neatness. Parents set very high standards and are excessively critical.	This type reports more psychiatric symptoms (somatic complaints, obsessive-compulsive tendencies, interpersonal sensitivity), a poorer self-image, a lower sense of personal security, and a pattern of dysfunctional coping.

Adapted permission from Dixon FA, Lapsley DK, Hanchon TA: An empirical typology of perfectionism in gifted adolescents. Gifted Child Q 48:95-106, 2004.

cultivation of giftedness is complicated by limited "educational capital," including reduced financial means and restricted access to cultural, health, and educational resources, in addition to psychological and social pressures and racial and ethnic discrimination (Borland and Wright, 1994; Gordan and Bridgall, 2005).

In a review of the literature, Neihart (2006) suggested that many gifted students from low-resource families or minority groups experience an "affiliation/achievement conflict" when they perceive that the expression of their giftedness would be in conflict with or not valued by members of their cultural group. Withdrawal from academic pursuits is a common reaction to the cognitive dissonance that occurs when a student first becomes aware of this conflict, usually during adolescence. For example, gifted African American students may experience peer pressure to underachieve for fear of acting "white" (Ford, 1994). Peer influence and pressure in working-class families to marry young and to secure a job represent additional pressures faced by gifted children from low-resource families or minority groups. Underachievement in at-risk populations should therefore be viewed as a sociocultural phenomenon (Ford, 1994; Grantham, 2004; Neihart, 2006).

In a review of the literature, Moore and colleagues (2005) reported that "noncognitive" factors more effectively predict persistence among academically gifted African American students than do achievement and performance variables (e.g., tests and grades). These noncognitive factors include self-confidence, realistic self-appraisal, understanding of and ability to cope with racism, preference for long-range goals over more immediate short-term goals, support of academic pursuits from others, successful leadership experience, community service, and knowledge acquired in a field. Similarly, in a 3-year study of 35 economically disadvantaged, ethnically diverse, academically gifted high-school students, Reis and associates (2005) reported that the presence of at least one supportive adult, peer support, and involvement in productive after-school or summer activities distinguished those students who excelled academically.

Solutions

Mentoring or coaching has been promoted as one strategy to cultivate academic giftedness among students from low-resource families or minority groups. Callahan and Kyburg (2005) suggest that the greater a gifted student's distance from that expected in terms of the typical professional (e.g., African Americans in mainstream science), the greater the need for role models who are closely matched to the student in terms of attitude, values, lifestyle, background experience, race, and gender. Neihart (2006) suggests that gifted students from low-income families or minority groups must master "code switching," a process of deliberately changing behaviors to accommodate the expectations of different environments. As such, at-risk gifted students need "cultural brokers" or caring adults who understand gender, class, racial, or ethnic factors and can identify these factors in a variety of contexts, mediate potential conflict, and build bridges. Finally, coaching may provide direct instruction in the social skills necessary for leadership in a variety of cultural contexts, including authority, self-control, and conflict resolution. For instance, in some ethnic cultures, behaviors that are encouraged in accelerated educational programs (e.g., questioning authority, critical thinking) are discouraged at home because they are perceived as disrespectful of authority.

Family and peers represent important moderators of academic success among gifted students from low-income or minority groups. Ford (1994) recommends building strong family-school-community relations for these students to nurture resilience. Even among low-income families, conditions favoring high achievement are the same as those described in the general population: supportive families that value education and work, favorable educational and financial resources, positive and encouraging parenting practices, and higher degree of stimulation (Robinson et al, 2002). Peer group networks also may provide a forum for open discussions about the hidden and overt expectations regarding class, race, and achievement, including explicit labeling of the unfairness some at-risk gifted students encounter (Neihart, 2006).

Finally, the curriculum must enable access to gifted and talented programming and academic resources for members of low-resource and minority groups (Swanson, 2006). Academic enrichment that incorporates a multicultural curriculum to integrate ethnic identity and cultivation of academic giftedness is recommended (Ford, 1994). Neihart (2006) describes optimal academic settings for at-risk gifted students as "welcoming learning environments" that address identity and learning goals concurrently and normalize the conflicts that some at-risk gifted students experience.

The Twice Exceptional Gifted Child

Children who are gifted and also possess a second exceptionality are frequently misunderstood and often do not receive appropriate educational programming that addresses the range of their needs. For example, education personnel are less likely to refer students with learning disabilities (Minner et al, 1987) or emotional-behavioral disorders (Minner, 1989) for gifted and talented programs. However, the unidentified second exceptionality often impedes the academic success of the student who also is gifted. Because gifted students who are underachieving may suffer from undiagnosed learning disabilities or attention-deficit/hyperactivity disorder, it is important to exclude the possibility that a dual diagnosis is responsible for the student's underachievement (see also Chapter 51).

Solutions

Careful, professional evaluation, including comprehensive psychological or neuropsychological evaluation, may assist the primary care provider with accurate diagnosis. Intervention should include a differentiated curriculum that provides both enrichment and instructional supports. For example, a 504 Accommodation Plan may be required to help the gifted student with attention-deficit/hyperactivity disorder compensate for everyday behaviors associated with executive dysfunction (e.g., poor organizational skills, limited task initiation or persistence, deficits in working memory). In addition, several key components that foster resilience among twice exceptional students have been highlighted: early identification of both exceptionalities, educational programming that targets strengths and weaknesses (i.e., enrichment and remediation), direct instruction in compensatory strategies, and provision of accommodations at an early age to promote academic success. Twice exceptional students also may benefit from psychological interventions that address their unique emotional needs, assist in the development of awareness about their strengths and weaknesses, and promote realistic goal setting. Finally, supportive adults and extracurricular activities that showcase the gifted child's strengths promote resilience among twice exceptional students (Baum, 1990; Dole, 2000).

THE ROLE OF THE PRIMARY CARE PROVIDER

Identification

The primary care provider is in an ideal position to first identify potential giftedness early in development when children present with precocious language/vocabulary development or exceptional problem solving skills. The primary care provider also may recognize the signs of unidentified gifted students (e.g., gifted underachievers) as the child advances in school. Referral for a comprehensive psychoeducational or neuropsychological evaluation may assist with accurate identification of high ability and possible comorbid conditions, such as learning disabilities or attention-deficit/hyperactivity disorder. Finally, the primary care provider may be the first-line professional to learn about the social or emotional maladjustment of the gifted child and refer families for effective psychological or psychiatric intervention.

Parenting

The primary care provider also is in an ideal position to encourage appropriate parent-child interactions, to promote developmentally appropriate expectations for behavior, and to educate families about the unique social, emotional, and academic needs of the gifted child. Parents may feel pressure to provide enriched experiences and may feel the burden of time and financial investment. The primary care provider can alleviate these pressures by educating the family about normal child development, linking the families to resources such as the National Research Center on the Gifted and Talented, and recommending appropriate educational programming. Research suggests that family dynamics make a stronger contribution to the achievement outcomes of gifted children than demographic variables. Specifically, parents who set high and clear expectations promote higher achievement in their children. Strong extended family relations also tend to promote emotional health, social competence, and self-efficacy. Finally, an authoritative parenting style, characterized by both flexibility and firmness, contributes to greater academic achievement in children who are gifted (Neihart, 2006). The primary care provider may coach parents from diverse backgrounds about these key components of effective parenting (Table 52-2).

Table 52-2. What Gifted Students Desire from Their Parents

According to their survey of hundreds of children identified as gifted and talented, Galbraith and Delisle suggest that the following are the top 10 things gifted students wish their parents would or would not do:

1. Be supportive and encouraging; be there for us; be on our side.
2. Don't expect too much of us; don't expect perfection.
3. Don't pressure us, be too demanding, or push too hard.
4. Help us with our schoolwork/homework.
5. Help us to develop our talents.
6. Be understanding.
7. Don't expect straight As.
8. Allow us some independence; give us space; trust us, because chances are we know what we're doing.
9. Talk to us; listen to us.
10. Let us try alternative education or special programs.

Adapted with permission from Galbraith J, Delisle J: The Gifted Kids' Survival Guide: A Teen Handbook. Minneapolis, Free Spirit Publishing, 2004.

Educational Programming

The primary care provider should become familiar with state and local definitions guiding the provision of gifted programming. Definitions may be obtained from state departments of education or the National Association for Gifted Children. Because identification of students eligible for gifted educational programming may vary from school district to school district, the primary care provider also may consult with district school psychologists about identification procedures and gifted programming specific to a given school. Research clearly indicates that gifted students require accelerated learning experiences to maintain interest and high achievement. Therefore, in addition to educational programming, the primary care provider may become familiar with extracurricular opportunities, such as summer programs and weekend college courses.

SUMMARY

Current conceptualizations of giftedness highlight the cognitive and noncognitive components necessary for gifted products, including, for example, high intellectual ability, creativity, persistence and motivation, and self-efficacy. Although children who are gifted represent a heterogeneous group from diverse backgrounds, those factors that promote healthy cognitive, social, and emotional development are largely the same and include supportive families that set high expectations for academic achievement; individualized, accelerative educational programs that address areas of strength and weakness; and opportunities to interact with peers who have similar abilities, interests, and motivation. The primary care physician is in an ideal position to guide parents of gifted children by first recognizing the signs of gifted behavior early in development and referring for comprehensive psychoeducational or neuropsychological evaluation when indicated. The primary care physician also may provide families with guidance on developmentally appropriate expectations for behavior and effective parenting strategies. Finally, the primary care physician may be the first to identify potential social or emotional problems among children who are gifted and direct families to appropriate psychological interventions or mentoring.

REFERENCES

Bain SK, Bell SM: Social self-concept, social attributions, and peer relationships in fourth, fifth, and sixth graders who are gifted compared to high achievers. Gifted Child Q 48:166-178, 2004.

Baum S: Gifted but Learning Disabled: A Puzzling Paradox. Reston, VA, Council for Exceptional Children, 1990. ERIC Digest No. E479.

Baum SM, Renzulli JS, Hébert TP: Reversing underachievement: Creative productivity as a systematic intervention. Gifted Child Q 39:224-235, 1995.

Bloom B: Developing Talent in Young People. New York, Ballantine, 1985.

Borland JH, Wright L: Identifying young, potentially gifted, economically disadvantaged students. Gifted Child Q 38:164-171, 1994.

Callahan CM, Kyburg RM: Talented and gifted youth. *In* DuBois DL, Karcher MJ (eds): Handbook of Youth Mentoring. Thousand Oaks, CA, Sage, 2005, pp 424-439.

Cornell DG: High ability students who are unpopular with their peers. Gifted Child Q 34:155-160, 1990.

Dixon FA, Lapsley DK, Hanchon TA: An empirical typology of perfectionism in gifted adolescents. Gifted Child Q 48:95-106, 2004.

Dole S: The implications of the risk and resilience literature for gifted students with learning disabilities. Roeper Rev 23:91-96, 2000.

Ford D: Nurturing resilience in gifted black youth. Roeper Rev 17: 80-85, 1994.

Gardner H: Intelligence Reframed: Multiple Intelligences for the 21st Century. New York, Basic Books, 1999.

Gordon EW, Bridgall BL: Nurturing talent in gifted students of color. *In* Sternberg RJ, Davidson JE (eds): Conceptions of Giftedness, 2nd ed. New York, Cambridge University Press, 2005, pp 120-146.

Grantham TC: Multicultural mentoring to increase black male representation in gifted programs. Gifted Child Q 48:232-245, 2004.

Gross MUM, van Vliet HE: Radical acceleration and early entry to college: A review of the research. Gifted Child Q 49:154-171, 2005.

Kaiser CF, Berndt DJ: Predictors of loneliness in the gifted adolescent. Gifted Child Q 29:74-77, 1985.

Kulik JA, Kulik CC: Meta-analytic findings on grouping programs. Gifted Child Q 36:73-77, 1992.

McCoach DB, Kehle TJ, Bray MA, Siegle D: Best practices in the identification of gifted students with learning disabilities. Psych Schools 38:403-411, 2001.

Minner S: Initial referral recommendations of teachers toward gifted students with behavioral problems. Roeper Rev 12:78-80, 1989.

Minner S, Prater G, Bloodworth H, Walker S: Referral and placement recommendations of teachers toward gifted handicapped children. Roeper Rev 9:247-249, 1987.

Moore JL, Ford DY, Milner R: Recruitment is not enough: Retaining African American students in gifted education. Gifted Child Q 49:51-67, 2005.

Neihart M: Dimensions of underachievement, difficult contexts, and perceptions of self. Roeper Rev 28:196-202, 2006.

Neihart M, Reis S, Robinson N, Moon SM (eds): The social and emotional development of gifted children. What do we know? Waco, TX, Prufrock Press, 2002.

Neisser U, Boodoo G, Bouchard TJ, et al: Intelligence: Knowns and unknowns. Am Psychologist 51:77-101, 1996.

Orpinas P, Horne AM: Bullying Prevention: Creating a Positive School Climate and Developing Social Competence. Washington, DC, American Psychological Association, 2005.

Peterson JS, Ray KE: Bullying and the gifted: Victims, perpetrators, prevalence, and effects. Gifted Child Q 50:148-168, 2006.

Pfeiffer SI, Stocking VB: Vulnerabilities of academically gifted students. Special Services Schools 16:83-93, 2000.

Reis SM, Colbert RD: Hébert TP: Understanding resilience in diverse, talented students in an urban high school. Roeper Rev 27:110-120, 2005.

Reis SM, McCoach DB: The underachievement of gifted students: What do we know and where do we go? Gifted Child Q 44:152-170, 2000.

Reis SM, McCoach DB: Underachievement in gifted and talented students with special needs. Exceptionality 10:113-125, 2002.

Reis SM, Renzulli JS: Current research into the social and emotional development of gifted and talented students: Good news and future possibilities. Psychol Schools 41:119-130, 2004.

Renzulli JS: What makes giftedness? Reexamining a definition. Phi Delta Kappan 60:180-184, 1978.

Renzulli JS: The three-ring conception of giftedness. *In* Sternberg RJ, Davidson JE (eds): Conceptions of Giftedness, 2nd ed. New York, Cambridge University Press, 2005, pp 246-279.

Rimm S: Why Bright Kids Get Poor Grades and What You Can Do About It. New York, Crown Trade Paperbacks, 1995.

Rinn AN: Effects of a summer program on the social self-concepts of gifted adolescents. J Secondary Gifted Educ 17:65-75, 2006.

Robinson NM, Lanzi RG, Weinberg RA, et al: Family factors associated with high academic competence in former Head Start children at third grade. Gifted Child Q 46:278-290, 2002.

Sayler MF, Brookshire WK: Social, emotional, and behavioral adjustment of accelerated students in gifted classes, and regular students in eighth grades. Gifted Child Q 37:150-154, 1993.

Schuler PA: Perfectionism and the gifted adolescent. J Secondary Gifted Educ 12:183-196, 2002.

Sternberg RJ: The WICS model of giftedness. *In* Sternberg RJ, Davidson JE (eds): Conceptions of Giftedness, 2nd ed. New York, Cambridge University Press, 2005, pp 327-342.

Swanson JD: Breaking through assumptions about low-income, minority gifted students. Gifted Child Q 50:11-25, 2006.

Terman LM, Baldwin BT, Bronson E, et al: Genetic Studies of Genius: Mental and Physical Traits of a Thousand Gifted Children, 2nd ed. Stanford, Stanford University Press, 1926.

Turkheimer E, Haley A, Waldron M, et al: Socioeconomic status modifies heritability of IQ in young children. Psychol Sci 14:623-628, 2003.

U.S. Department of Education: National excellence: A case for developing America's talent. Washington, DC, Author, 1993.

Winner E: Exceptionally high intelligence and schooling. Am Psychologist 52:1071-1081, 1997.

Winner E: The origins and ends of giftedness. Am Psychologist 55:159-169, 2000.

RESOURCES FOR PROFESSIONALS

Essential Readings in Gifted Education (Sally M. Reis, series editor; Thousand Oaks, CA, Sage Publications) is a collection of seminal articles published in *Gifted Child Quarterly,* a lead journal in the field of gifted and talented research.

National Research Center on the Gifted and Talented (NRC/GT) is a collaborative effort between several academic institutions and state departments of education in an effort to plan and to conduct research about giftedness. The NRC/GT can be accessed on the Internet at *www.gifted.uconn.edu/nrcgt.html.*

RESOURCES FOR PARENTS AND GIFTED CHILDREN

National Association for Gifted Children (NAGC) is a national advocacy group of parents, educators, and affiliate groups who have joined together in an effort to promote appropriate gifted education. The NAGC has affiliates in nearly every state and publishes a quarterly magazine, *Parenting for High Potential.* The NAGC Web site (*www.nagc.org*) provides information about national and state policies on gifted education, including state definitions, funding, and policies about acceleration. The Web site also includes information about national conventions, parent and teacher resources, and publications.

Judy Galbraith's *The Gifted Kids' Survival Guide for Ages 10 and Under* and Judy Galbraith and James R. Delisle's *The Gifted Kids' Survival Guide: A Teen Handbook* (Minneapolis, Free Spirit Publishing) offer guides to the myriad issues faced by children and adolescents who are gifted, including identification of appropriately challenging educational programs and the social and emotional aspects of being gifted. These guides also include extensive lists of resources (books and Web sites) for parents and children.

53 ADAPTATION AND MALADAPTATION TO SCHOOL

TERRILL BRAVENDER

In the 21st century, the United States is an information-driven, highly technologic society, and education is the key to success. The U.S. Department of Labor estimates that 12 of the 20 fast-growing jobs will require at least a bachelor's degree, and an additional five will require other specialized training. The importance of education is also reflected in current unemployment statistics. In the second quarter of 2006, the unemployment rate was 7.0% among those who have not completed high school, 4.3% among high-school graduates, 3.7% for those with some college, and 2.1% for those with a college degree or higher (Bureau of Labor Statistics, 2006). For those who are employed, the differences in salaries are even more pronounced. In 2004, the median income was $22,000 per year for full-time workers with less than a high-school diploma, $31,000 for those with a high-school diploma, and $51,000 for those with a bachelor's degree (Internet Staff and Population Division). In addition, there are positive associations between income and health, and the level of education, independent of income, also plays an important role in determining overall health status.

Adaptation to school is complex, and problems in this area can result from a broad range of influences. Such problems may occur in conjunction with diagnoses covered in other chapters, such as attention deficit disorder, specific learning disabilities, and psychiatric diagnoses such as anxiety or depression, but these comorbid diagnoses do not have to be present. The term *maladaptation to school* refers to a spectrum of behaviors that run from school disengagement to school avoidance and ultimately to school dropout. When school-related behavior problems do arise, parents may look to a variety of health care providers for impartial evaluation and guidance. The clinician's primary role is to identify or to exclude medical, developmental, psychological, or other issues that may have an impact on behavior in school, although *excluding* a problem may be as important as *identifying* a problem. Even when a specific problem is not identified, parents will often look to a trusted clinician for help. The provider's role then is to act as an impartial advocate for the child and to assist the family in developing appropriate school attendance and behavior strategies. Throughout the evaluation, it is useful to remember that there are many influences on school adaptation, including issues that are related not only to the child but also to the school itself, peers, and the family. Too often, a frustrated parent focuses solely on the child without also examining these other domains.

EVALUATION

The evaluation should begin by eliciting the specifics of the school problems, not just "he hates going to school." One should assess whether these are new or persistent problems, whether the problems encompass all subjects or just specific classes or teachers, and whether the child is disruptive only at school or also at home. Routine questions about past and current medical history as well as a medication history may be important. Family history is an important component of the assessment and should include questions about other family members' school experiences and parental expectations about school and school attendance. Attention should also be paid to histories of mental illness, incarceration, substance abuse, and discipline practices. Assessments of the home environment may be revealing. Appropriate sleep and media use are important determinants of school engagement and attendance, and these should be explored thoroughly. Additional home environment assessments should include who lives in the home (permanently and transiently), how available the parents are to their children, and what sorts of family routines are established. A succinct dietary history should be obtained. If previous developmental or educational testing has been performed, the parents should be asked to provide copies of the evaluations for inclusion in the medical record. A directed physical examination is important, with particular care paid to the child's growth and developmental parameters. The child's mood, affect, and behavior in the office should be assessed to help screen for depression, severe anxiety, or hyperactivity. Routine hearing and vision screening should be performed.

A variety of physical, developmental, and behavioral issues may have an impact on adaptation to school and are summarized in Table 53-1. Although hidden medical diagnoses having an impact on school engagement are fairly rare, one must keep a broad differential diagnosis in mind. Some issues may be apparent, with the school-engagement effects hidden (such as with chronic

Table 53-1. Differential Diagnosis of Issues Related to School Behavior

Physical Issues	*Behavioral Issues*
Chronic illness	Oppositional defiant disorder
History of prematurity	Conduct disorder
Recurrent or persistent otitis media	Depressive disorders
Hearing or vision loss	Anxiety disorders
Medication side effects	School avoidance or school phobia
Seizure disorder	Substance abuse (in patient)
Lead poisoning	Sleep disturbances
Iron deficiency anemia	Excessive media use
Hypothyroidism	***Family Issues***
Somatization disorders	Chronic illness in family member
Developmental Issues	Substance abuse (in family member)
Learning disabilities	Physical or sexual abuse
Intellectual disability	Exposure to violence in home
Attention deficit disorder	***School Issues***
	Poor fit for student's temperament

illnesses or medication side effects), whereas others may truly be hidden medical diagnoses (such as absence seizures or thyroid disorders). Between 10% and 20% of school-age children have some sort of chronic illness (Boekaerts and Roder, 1999). Any chronic illness, from the severe (such as cancer) to the more benign (such as allergic rhinitis), may affect school performance, and children with lower school performance are at greater risk for disengagement. Up to one third of aggressive and disruptive students may have at least one chronic medical, nonpsychiatric illness (Rappaport et al, 2006). Asthma clearly has an impact on children's school attendance and performance and is the most common chronic illness of childhood. Other chronic health issues that should be considered include prematurity, chronic hearing loss, visual impairment, absence seizures, lead exposure, iron deficiency anemia, thyroid disease, and somatization disorders. Being overweight has been linked to poor school performance but is likely to be a marker for other issues, such as comorbid chronic health problems or lower socioeconomic status.

Behavioral and emotional disorders can dramatically affect school performance. Although both girls and boys may experience any of these disorders, boys are more likely to present with externalizing problems, such as oppositional defiant disorder or conduct disorder, whereas girls are more likely to present with internalizing disorders such as depression or anxiety, both of which are associated with school refusal. Adolescent substance use can clearly affect school engagement and attendance in dramatic ways, but which comes first, the school problems or the substance use, is less clear. In some instances, school problems and a lack of school connectedness may actually precede academic problems (Fothergill and Ensminger, 2006). The answer to which comes first is likely to depend on the individual. Adolescents who are less engaged with school are more likely to start using alcohol or drugs, and those who use these substances are more likely to have worsened school engagement and attendance. Substance use by parents may also affect school connection. Whereas the effect of prenatal exposure to alcohol or drugs is well known, ongoing substance abuse by parents can have long-term effects on their children's physical health, social and emotional development, and school performance (Conners et al, 2004), which in turn are likely to have an impact on school engagement. Traumatic events, such as prior or ongoing sexual or physical abuse, may affect school performance. Traumatic experiences and post-traumatic stress disorder are not uncommon in children and adolescents; one population-based study noted that approximately 40% of participants had experienced at least one *Diagnostic and Statistical Manual of Metal Disorders* trauma by the age of 18 years (Giaconia et al, 1995). In this study, about 14% of those with trauma histories developed post-traumatic stress disorder and were more likely to exhibit academic failure in addition to other psychological and physical health problems. Simply being exposed to violence in the home, even when it is not directed at the children, is associated with worsened school performance (Hurt et al, 2001). Finally, children who must serve as caregivers for chronically ill parents or other family members are at greater risk for school disengagement (Siskowski, 2006).

SCHOOL DISENGAGEMENT

Vignette

Jordan is a bright 15-year-old boy in ninth grade who presents to his pediatrician after his parents found marijuana in his bedroom. He has not done well in school this year, failing three classes and barely passing the remainder. Previously social and outgoing, he has recently been spending most of his time at home alone in his room. His parents became concerned, but their work demands had recently increased, and they had little time to investigate. He had a successful middle-school experience, making good grades in advanced classes and participating on the school football and lacrosse teams. Unfortunately, most of Jordan's friends have gone to different high schools. He was unable to join the football team this past fall because his parents were not available to provide transportation. When lacrosse season started in the spring, he felt that the transportation situation had not changed, so he told his parents he was not interested in playing. In a conference with Jordan and his parents, Jordan agreed to cease using marijuana if he were able to join the lacrosse team at his high school. His parents agreed that they would assist in finding appropriate transportation to and from practices as long as his grades improved and he remained drug free.

There has been significant interest recently in the importance of children's sense of connection to school. Referred to varyingly as positive orientation to school, school attachment, school bonding, and, more recently, school connectedness, it has been studied by use of different methods and definitions. Despite these differences, some common themes have emerged. A student who feels a sense of belonging, likes school, has good friends, is invested in current and future academic progress, and participates in extracurricular activities can be considered to have a high level of connectedness. Schools that provide fair and effective discipline and that have teachers who are perceived as caring and supportive also promote school connectedness among their students. Each of these individual domains has demonstrated relevance to grades, school participation, liking, and belonging. All of these factors are highly associated with student outcomes (Libbey, 2004).

School disengagement can be manifested as either disruption or withdrawal. When a child exhibits disruptive behaviors, school disengagement must be differentiated from oppositional and defiant behaviors, premeditated aggressiveness, and impulsivity associated with attention deficit disorder. These externalizing behaviors may be associated with school disengagement, but they also may be misdiagnosed in a child who is simply not connected to his or her school, and the management approaches are likely to be quite different. Students whose disengagement is manifested as withdrawal may be labeled as having depression or the primarily inattentive type of attention deficit disorder. Again, although these issues may be associated with academic disengagement, making the proper diagnosis will aid in development of appropriate interventions.

The need to feel like one belongs in school and is cared for in school is important not only for students' academic performance and school behavior but also for their emotional and physical well-being. Students who are disengaged are at greater risk for a variety of other behavioral health problems and also view themselves as less healthy than those students who are more connected to their schools. Indeed, this concept of school connectedness has emerged as an important intervention area for protecting adolescents from harm (Resnick et al, 1997). School connectedness is influenced by students' perception of caring teachers as well as by high performance expectations. School policies designed to influence adolescent behaviors (such as locker searches, drug testing, and punitive threats) have been found to have much less effect on adolescent behaviors than does the promotion of school connectedness. School connectedness is not simply an inherent attribute; it can be promoted through systematic interventions. Interventions designed to promote school bonding and implemented in elementary school can have enduring effects in reducing risky adolescent health behaviors in high school (Hawkins et al, 1999). Other programs designed to promote school connectedness have emphasized self-discipline (rather than external, punitive controls) and have been able to significantly reduce incidents of fighting and acting out in class while still maintaining classroom decorum (Freiberg, 1989; McNeeley et al, 2002). Interestingly, the more intensely the self-discipline measures were implemented, the better the students' behavior.

School connectedness is mediated by a number of variables that can be divided into system variables and individual-level variables and are summarized in Table 53-2.

System Variables

Teachers who are empathetic, are consistent, encourage self-management for discipline issues, and allow students to make decisions can improve their classroom management and thus improve students' feelings of connectedness. Harsh discipline, such as "zero tolerance" policies for alcohol infractions, have been shown to decrease connectedness. These policies usually mandate expulsion for first offenses and are designed to improve school safety. However, students who attend such schools are likely to report feeling less safe than those students who attend schools with more moderate discipline policies. Smaller schools seem to promote more connectedness than larger schools do, yet classroom size does not show such consistent effects. One explanation for this finding is that classroom sizes are rarely large enough to inhibit development of coherent social units. When schools become too large, though, it may become difficult for teachers to know all of the students and provide a warm, caring atmosphere for so many people. School connectedness is higher in schools that are racially or ethnically segregated and lowest in schools that are integrated (McNeeley et al, 2002). It has been noted that when schools are integrated, friendships tend to self-segregate within individual racial and ethnic groups. When friendship patterns are segregated in this manner, students of all racial and ethnic groups feel less connected to school. Further compounding the problem is that minority students may disproportionately

Table 53-2. Factors Influencing School Connectedness

	Positively Influence	**Negatively Influence**
System variables	Empathetic teachers Consistent discipline Student self-management for discipline Students involved in decision making Smaller schools	Harsh discipline "Zero tolerance" for minor infractions Difficult classroom management Larger schools
Individual variables	Higher grades Extracurricular activities Younger students Male students Nonminority students	Lower grades Skipping school Older students Female students Minority students

be assigned to lower-track classes together, thus exacerbating the segregated friendship patterns. Whereas some have advocated segregation of schools by race and gender to enhance educational experiences for girls and minorities, there is a potential danger in the fact that an unequal distribution of resources typically follows school segregation. Further, the National Longitudinal Study of Adolescent Health has demonstrated that some schools that are highly integrated also have high levels of school connectedness. What differentiates these particular schools is an area ripe for future research.

Individual Characteristics

Students who participate in extracurricular activities, such as sports, clubs, or performing arts groups, feel more connected to their schools, as do those who get higher grades. Lack of school connectedness is associated with higher rates of skipping school. Female students and members of minority groups demonstrate lower levels of school connectedness. Interestingly, students' school connectedness decreases as they get older, and there seems to be a significant drop-off between elementary and middle school. This is clearly a critical period for intervention and prevention efforts.

Despite the best efforts of schools and students, there occasionally is simply a poor fit between a particular student and teacher. A child's individual temperament may play a role in this and should be further investigated, as discussed in detail in Chapter 7.

Management

The goals of management include preventing further disengagement (which can progress to truancy and dropout) and promoting improved school connectedness. Specific interventions should be tailored to any underlying issues identified and to each specific situation. It is crucial that any underlying comorbid conditions (such as attention deficit disorder or depression) be treated appropriately. General intervention guidelines are as follows.

Behavioral Interventions

For disruptive students, behavioral contracts between teachers, parents, and the student can be effective. Positive reinforcement and consistency are essential for success. Children who are too disruptive to the other students may need to be placed in a special classroom with more structure.

Developing Strengths

A lack of connectedness to school can significantly affect children's self-esteem, further alienating them from participating in academic work and extracurricular activities. These children should be encouraged to develop specialties in areas of strength or interest and encouraged to apply these areas of special strength to the school environment.

Educational Services

These services are important, particularly for students with diagnosed learning disabilities. Special education focused on skill development as well as language, occupational, and physical therapy may be indicated.

Counseling

Individual counseling should be focused on a student's gaining insight into the relationship between his or her behavior and possible underlying emotional difficulties. It may also assist with the underlying anxiety about school participation that often accompanies school disengagement.

Social Skills Training

Some students are disengaged because of social skills difficulties, and those with attention deficit disorder may also benefit. Social skills training should take place in a group setting with children of similar age, and such programs are available in many communities and even within some schools.

SCHOOL AVOIDANCE

Vignette

Maggie, a 9-year-old healthy girl, presented to her pediatrician for abdominal pain and dizziness. She had been seen by other members of the medical practice twice in the past month for similar problems, and her mother had taken her to a local urgent care for evaluation the week before. Maggie indicated that pain was located near her bellybutton but could not describe it any further. She had no history of vomiting, diarrhea, or constipation and had no ill contacts. The pain tended to start soon after awakening and tended to resolve by the time they sought medical attention. The pain did not bother her on the weekends. Further history revealed that Maggie's parents had recently separated, and Maggie and her mother had moved to a new apartment in a different school district. When asked about school, Maggie stated that she wanted to go to school but that she couldn't because her stomach hurt too much. She has missed so much school that her teacher has begun sending schoolwork home, and Maggie's mother wonders if she should hire a tutor to teach Maggie at home.

School avoidance behaviors include school refusal (also referred to as school avoidance or school phobia) and truancy. Both are manifested by a child's resistance or refusal to attend school, but the two terms are often used to highlight differences in what is driving the behavior. The literature includes various interpretations and often overlapping meanings of these terms, so appropriate definition of these terms is important. This chapter uses *school avoidance* to describe all behaviors involving repeated missing of school that is not due to physical illnesses, including simple truancy. The term *school refusal* is used in place of school phobia and is differentiated from truancy, which implies a more volitional behavior.

School Refusal

School refusal may be distinguished from truancy by the following features:

1. Severe difficulty in consistently attending school, often resulting in prolonged absences.
2. Severe emotional distress when faced with having to go to school. This may be manifested by fearfulness, temper tantrums, or complaints of physical illness without an obvious organic cause.
3. The child remains at home during school hours with full knowledge of his or her parents.
4. The child does not exhibit significant antisocial behaviors, such as delinquency, substance abuse, disruptiveness, or risky sexual activity (Berg et al, 1969).

School refusal affects boys and girls equally, and children of all levels of socioeconomic status are equally affected. Although school avoidance may occur in isolation, there are high rates of comorbid psychiatric diagnoses. Anxiety disorders are quite common, as is depression, whereas conduct and oppositional defiant disorders are uncommon. There are three peak ages at onset of school avoidance behaviors:

1. At school entry (ages 5 to 6), which is often related to separation anxiety.
2. At entry into middle school (ages 11 to 13), which is the typical age for complex school avoidance presentations that involve anxiety and affective dysregulation.
3. High school (ages 14 and older) is more associated with truancy, and school avoidance at this age is more likely to be associated with serious psychiatric illnesses.

Typically, children will begin complaining of vague problems about school or sometimes will not even mention school but will complain of physical symptoms. These physical complaints may include abdominal pain, headaches, dizziness, or nausea for which no physical cause can be found. These vague complaints related to going to school may then progress to complete refusal to attend school or to remain at school despite the best efforts of parents and school staff. Most children will state that they want to go to school but are unable to do so because of their symptoms. The child's symptoms are usually present on mornings before school and quickly disappear if the child is allowed to remain at home. Some parents may find it difficult to accept that the origins of the child's physical complaints are rooted in psychological distress. Parental anxiety that there may be a hidden, serious medical condition will only serve to increase the child's anxiety and worsen the problem. This emphasizes the importance that a full medical examination be conducted to rule out any organic cause of the symptoms (Elliott, 1999). Some children may actually have a physical illness (such as gastritis) that is related to school avoidance. Treatment of such medical problems is important, but in many cases, simply treating the medical problem may not actually affect school attendance.

Further evaluation should begin by differentiating school avoidance behavior from truancy. Although it is possible for children to exhibit both behaviors, it is unusual for these problems to occur at a similar time in the same child. Next, it is important to assess the child's general functioning at home and at school as well as to assess for anxiety and depression. The family's reaction to the school refusal as well as how the school is reacting to the absences is important. On occasion, a specific incident at school or at home will be noted as a precipitant of the behavior. This incident may not seem significant to the clinician or parents (such as being scolded at school), but it may be enough in a sensitive child to start the school avoidance process. More often, though, if the child does not exhibit an anxiety disorder or depression, the etiology is related to ongoing family or peer conflict or academic difficulties. Once begun, the process may become self-perpetuating because the more time the child spends away from school, the more anxious he or she may become about attending again.

Management

Interventions should be tailored to each child. A variety of behavioral, psychodynamic, cognitive, or pharmacologic approaches may used separately or in combination. This author's bias is toward use of a strict behavioral approach that is mainly exposure based, but it should also include interventions designed to teach relaxation and self-calming techniques to affected children. In most situations, an immediate return to school should be emphasized to help reduce the reinforcement of being home. If a child does develop a physical illness requiring school absence, the home should be made as unentertaining as possible. The child must remain in bed and may not watch television, read books, play games, or interact with a parent. The reason given to the child is that if he or she is too sick to go to school, he or she is too sick for these other activities.

In conjunction with behavioral interventions, the school day may need to be modified, particularly during the initial exposure phase. Any modifications (such as shortening the school day) should be written in a contract and agreed on by teachers, school administrators, clinicians, and parents. Modifications may also include minimizing exposure to particularly stressful areas and should emphasize those aspects of school that the child finds to be positive. Once the contract is in place, the student should not be allowed to negotiate the terms. Homebound tutoring, online class work, and home schooling should be avoided because these convey the message that staying home is an appropriate alternative. If home schooling does become necessary, it should be conducted only in a time-limited manner, with a contract written that includes a date for school re-entry (Freemon, 2003).

Other specific interventions for various clinical situations are as follows.

1. If a child is fearful of school for a good reason, such as being bullied, or has legitimate fears of being harmed, these fears need to be taken seriously and

addressed appropriately. Schools are required to provide safe learning environments for all children, and if a child is bullied or threatened, it becomes a problem that the school legally must address.

2. Somatic symptoms should not be minimized or dismissed. Just because a child has school avoidance does not mean that the child cannot develop organic causes of abdominal pain. Similarly, even if an organic cause of pain cannot be identified, it does not mean that the child is not experiencing pain. The child should be told that you believe the pain is real, and even though there is no medication that will help, the parents and treatment team are going to help him or her learn to cope with what he or she is feeling so that the child can get back to school.
3. On re-entering school, socially challenging and less structured areas such as the bus stop, physical education class, and the lunchroom may need to be avoided until the child's confidence is re-established.
4. Children who have a significant anxiety component may benefit from psychotropic medications. Selective serotonin reuptake inhibitors may be considered. In addition, a low dose of a benzodiazepine may be helpful for the anticipatory anxiety that may occur on initially re-entering school.
5. Concerns about explaining their absences to other students may worsen school avoidance. Rehearsing what to say when these inevitable questions arise can alleviate some of this anxiety.
6. Recruiting a friend or dependable peer to accompany the child or even just to check in with the child throughout the day may be helpful.
7. Allowing the child to have a cell phone is a bit tricky. Most schools have strict limits on cell phone use, but cell phone communication may be able to be worked into a behavioral contract. A child may be allowed to telephone the parents once or twice daily at specific times to check in, but if the cell phone is abused by the child making increasingly frequent calls, the privilege will be lost.
8. Social skills groups may be helpful for some children with social cognitive deficits.
9. Children with neurodevelopmental dysfunctions will benefit from a variety of enhanced learning opportunities, bypass strategies, and appropriate behavioral and medication treatments.
10. Children with chronic illnesses may present special challenges. These children often exhibit a rate of absenteeism that is out of proportion to what would be directly attributable to the specific chronic illness. Special considerations should be taken to ensure that their medical appointments and medication regimens do not interfere with school attendance, disrupt the school experience, or call special attention to them.

Truancy

Intentional, unauthorized absence from school, or truancy, is a problem that affects most school districts in the United States. The prevalence of truancy is difficult to assess across different schools because of variations in reporting, so most estimates are based on students' self-reports. As might be expected, the numbers of students skipping school increase as students get older. One recent study found that nationwide, almost 11% of eighth graders and 16% of tenth graders reported skipping at least 1 day of school in the past 4 weeks (Henry, 2007). Although the No Child Left Behind Act requires schools and districts to report attendance rates, differences in state definitions mean that there remain no aggregate national data on truancy. The consequences of chronic truancy may be significant; skipping school has been associated with poor academic performance, school dropout, teen pregnancy, and social maladjustment. The effects of truancy also persist into adulthood and are associated with job instability, violence, marital problems, criminal behaviors, and incarceration. Although a main predictor of school truancy in adolescents is parental educational level, other predictors may help guide interventions. These predictors include adolescent substance abuse, having unsupervised time after school, and school disengagement. School disengagement variables include feeling unsafe in school, feeling unlikely to graduate from high school, and feeling unlikely to attend college.

Truant students may face direct legal consequences due to poor attendance. Many schools will automatically fail students who miss a particular number of classes. If the school files a truancy petition, the child or parent may face legal sanctions. Compulsory education laws often hold parents responsible for their children's school attendance, particularly for younger children. Parents and their truant children may face fines or orders for parents to attend school with their children or to attend parenting classes. In extreme and fortunately unusual cases, parents may face social services investigations or loss of custody of their children and even be sentenced to jail (Smink and Heilbrunn, 2005).

Management

Truancy interventions are similar to those involved with school dropout because chronic truancy is a path that often leads to dropout. Whereas individual behavioral management certainly plays a role (particularly involving behavioral contracts developed by parents, school personnel, and other care providers), the most important interventions are programmatic in nature. Truancy reduction programs vary as much as the schools and districts that they serve. These programs may involve school attendance review boards, alternative schools, distance learning initiatives, individual case managers, and even the court system in conjunction with social services. Although many of these programs have shown short-term success in reducing truancy rates, the long-term effects of these programs are unknown. Unfortunately, despite such ongoing efforts at decreasing truancy and its eventual outcome of school dropout, dropout rates in the United States have not changed in the past 2 decades.

SCHOOL DROPOUT

Vignette

Bobby is a 17-year-old with a long history of attention deficit disorder and academic difficulties. His high school recently instituted a 2-year foreign language requirement for graduation. Bobby has failed first-year Spanish three times and is now refusing to take it yet again in his senior year. "Why should I bother?" he asks. "There's no way I can graduate now, anyway, since I have to have 2 full years." Instead of starting twelfth grade, he has been working at an automobile repair shop near his house. Bobby says that the owner thinks Bobby would make a good mechanic, but there is no way for him to get the training he needs without a high-school diploma.

Before the American Civil War, most elementary education was offered in "common schools," which, although publicly operated, were not necessarily publicly funded, and parents often paid some form of tuition. In the period after the mid-19th century, the majority of the United States offered publicly funded primary school education, usually serving children through the age of 14 or 15 years. The "high-school movement" of the early 20th century dramatically improved access to secondary schooling, and the number of publicly funded high schools increased dramatically between 1910 and 1940 (Goldin, 1999). The first compulsory education law in the United States was passed by Massachusetts in 1852. Mississippi was the last state in the country to establish compulsory education laws in 1918. Although the ages at which students are required by law to attend school vary by state, children are required to begin school at the age of 5, 6, or 7 years and must attend through the age of 16, 17, or 18 years. There are movements currently, in many states that do not already require it, to extend compulsory education to the age of 18 years. Despite the legal requirement to attend school, dropout is, unfortunately, a frequent outcome of school maladaptation. There are numerous negative consequences to school dropout, including higher rates of unemployment, lower wages when employed, and lower general health status regardless of income.

Data on dropout rates must be reviewed with caution, realizing that differently defined rates are often reported. The *event dropout rate* refers to the percentage of students who left high school between the beginning of one school year and the beginning of the next without earning a high-school diploma or its equivalent, such as a Graduate Equivalency Degree (GED). In 1972, the high-school event dropout rate was 6.1%. This rate slowly trended downward until 1990, when it was 4.7%. Despite small year-to-year fluctuations, this rate has been essentially unchanged since that time, and the event dropout rate in the 2004 was also 4.7%. This means that almost 1 of every 20 high-school students who started high school in 2003 was no longer in school at the end of the academic year and translates to 486,000 dropouts. There are wide variations in dropout rates from state to state, ranging from 1.9% in Wisconsin to 10.5% in Arizona. The *freshman graduation rate* estimates the proportion of public high-school freshmen who graduate with a regular diploma 4 years after starting ninth grade. Nationally, approximately 75% of freshman graduate on time. The state-specific rates vary widely from a low of 57% in Nevada to a high of 88% in Nebraska. The *status completion rate* refers to the percentage of individuals in a given age range who are no longer in high school and who have completed a degree. In 2004, approximately 80.5% of 18- to 24-year-olds in the United States held a high-school diploma, and 6.3% had passed the GED examination, giving a total status completion rate of 86.8%. The converse of this is, of course, the school dropout problem, the *status dropout rate*. This rate reflects the cumulative number of dropouts within a given population. Nationally, in 2004, there were approximately 3.8 million individuals aged 16 to 24 years who were classified as high-school dropouts, representing 10.3% of this age group (Laird et al, 2007).

Those who drop out of school are at risk for a number of adverse consequences. Dropouts are more likely to be unemployed, and those who are working are likely to be underemployed. In 2003, the median income (including full-time and part-time workers) for high-school dropouts older than 18 years was $12,184, whereas the median for those who had either a high-school diploma or GED was $20,431. Dropouts are more likely to be in prison and even on death row. The U.S. Department of Justice reports that approximately 75% of state prison inmates and 59% of federal prison inmates did not complete high school. More than half of death row inmates are high-school dropouts. It has been estimated that even just a 1% increase in average education levels would save approximately $1.4 billion in incarceration costs and would reduce arrest rates by 11% (Center for Mental Health in Schools, 2000).

Management

Prevention efforts are critical, particularly given that individual-level interventions have shown little benefit. An examination of the reasons that youth drop out of school can help guide such programs. These reasons are summarized in Table 53-3. The most common reason, given by more than half of dropouts, is that they simply did not like school. Other more concrete reasons include failing school, being suspended, job conflicts, and having friends who also dropped out of school (U.S. Department of Education, 1990). These reasons should be viewed as the final outcome of a long process of disengagement from school. Academic failure, disengagement from extracurricular activities, and high numbers of school absences are all interrelated, and such problems may begin to be manifested as early as first grade (Kemp, 2006). Thus, ideal interventions should be seen as prevention efforts focused on these longer term disengagement issues. Unfortunately, programs that focus on individuals at risk are

Table 53-3. Youth Reported Reasons for Dropping Out of School

	Percentage Endorsing Reason	
	Male	**Female**
School related		
Did not like school	58	44
Was failing school	46	33
Could not get along with teachers	52	17
Could not keep up with school work	38	25
Felt I didn't belong	32	14
Could not get along with students	18	22
Was suspended too often	19	13
Was expelled	18	9
Did not feel safe at school	12	13
Job related		
Had to get a job	15	16
Could not work and go to school at the same time	20	8
Family related		
Was pregnant	—	31
Got married	3	24
Became a parent	5	23
Had to support a family	5	14
Wanted to have a family	5	14
Had to care for family member	5	12
Peer related		
Friends dropped out	17	11

likely to be less efficacious than systematic approaches that emphasize flexible approaches to academics and school structure. For example, schools should be able to have the autonomy and flexibility to offer different curricula to students with different strengths, such as vocational and technical training as well as traditional academic subjects. Students who have difficulty succeeding in these traditional academic areas would then have the opportunity to receive training and find success earlier in their education. Many of these at-risk students may eventually receive such training, but only after having to experience failure and potentially dropping out of a traditional school. Success earlier in schooling may also improve self-esteem as well as the perception that these students have about education. Unfortunately, given many of the current policies in place that require frequent testing and strict academic benchmarks, few schools have the autonomy to provide needed vocational and technical training for their most at-risk students.

In the case noted in the vignette, Bobby was fortunate enough to be able to enroll in a local community college's vocational high-school program. He was able to pursue his certified mechanics program while accumulating credit toward a high-school diploma. He graduated on time, just after his 18th birthday. Bobby earned a mechanics certificate a year later and decided to pursue a specialized apprentice program. He now is working as a mechanic for a professional auto racing team.

SUMMARY

Adaptation to school is an important predictor of academic success. Students who experience maladaptation to school are at risk for school avoidance, truancy, and, eventually, dropout. Recent research into adaptation, often referred to as school connectedness, has found that a feeling of connection to school not only is indicative of academic success but also predicts fewer risky behaviors and less truancy. Despite the many efforts aimed at dropout prevention, dropout rates in the United States have not changed during the past 2 decades. Regular screening for school adaptation and attendance is an important component of clinical interactions, and prevention of school dropout is critical. Although screening and management often focus on individual students, prevention efforts should be focused on system variables, with particular attention paid to promoting school connectedness and offering alternative pathways to school completion, such as vocational education.

REFERENCES

Berg I, Nichols K, Pritchard C: School phobia—its classification and relationship to dependency. J Child Psychol Psychiatry 10:123-141, 1969.

Boekaerts M, Roder I: Stress, coping, and adjustment in children with a chronic disease: A review of the literature. Diabil Rehabil 21(7):311-337, 1999.

Bureau of Labor Statistics: Labor Force Statistics from the Current Population Survey. 2006. Available at: ftp://ftp.bls.gov/pub/suppl/empsit.cpseed3.txt. Accessed August 25, 2006.

Center for Mental Health in Schools: An Introductory Packet on Dropout Prevention. School Mental Health Project, Department of Psychology, UCLA, 2000. Available at: http://smhp.psych.ucla.edu/qf/transition_tt/dropout.pdf. Accessed June 1, 2007.

Conners NA, Bradley RH, Mansell LW, et al: Children of mothers with serious substance abuse problems: An accumulation of risks. Am J Drug Alcohol Abuse 30(1):85-100, 2004.

Elliott JG: School refusal: Issues of conceptualisation, assessment, and treatment. Practitioner review. J Child Psychol Psychiatry 40(7):1001-1012, 1999.

Fothergill KE, Ensminger ME: Childhood and adolescent antecedents of drug and alcohol problems: A longitudinal study. Drug Alcohol Depend 82(1):61-76, 2006.

Freemon WP: School refusal in children and adolescents. Am Fam Physician 68(8):1555-1560, 2003.

Freiberg HJ: Turning around at-risk schools through consistency management. J Negro Educ 58:372-382, 1989.

Giaconia RM, Reinhertz HZ, Silverman AB, et al: Traumas and posttraumatic stress disorder in a community population of older adolescents. J Am Acad Child Adolesc Psychiatry 34(10):1369-1380, 1995.

Goldin C: A Brief History of Education in the United States. Cambridge, MA, National Bureau of Economic Research, 1999.

Hawkins J, Catalano R, Kosterman R, et al: Preventing adolescent health-risk behaviors by strengthening protection during childhood. Arch Pediatr Adolescent Med 153(3):226-234, 1999.

Henry KL: Who's skipping school: Characteristics of truants in 8th and 10th grade. J School Health 77(1):29-35, 2007.

Hurt H, Malmud E, Brodsky NL, Giannetta J: Exposure to violence: Psychological and academic correlates in child witnesses. Arch Pediatr Adolesc Med 155(12):1351-1356, 2001.

Internet Staff and Population Division: Educational Attainment in the United States: 2004. U.S. Census Bureau, Population Division, Education and Social Stratification Branch. Available at: http://www.census.gov/population/www/socdemo/education/cps2004.html. Accessed August 25, 2006.

Kemp SE: Dropout policies and trends for students with and without disabilities. Adolescence 41(162):235-250, 2006.

Laird J, DeBell M, Chapman C: Dropout Rates in the United States: 2004. Washington, DC, U.S. Department of Education, National Center for Education Statistics, 2007. NCES 2007–024.

Libbey HP: Measuring student relationships to school: Attachment, bonding, connectedness, and engagement. J School Health 74(7):274-283, 2004.

McNeeley CA, Nonnemaker JM, Blum RW: Promoting school connectedness: Evidence from the National Longitudinal Study of Adolescent Health. J School Health 72(4):138-146, 2002.

Rappaport N, Flaherty LT, Hauser ST: Beyond psychopathology: Assessing seriously disruptive students in school settings. J Pediatr 149(2):252-256, 2006.

Resnick MD, Bearman PS, Blum RW, et al: Protecting adolescents from harm. Findings from the National Longitudinal Study on Adolescent Health. JAMA 278(10):823-832, 1997.

Siskowski C: Young caregivers: Effect of family health situations on school performance. J School Nursing 22(3):163-169, 2006.

Smink J, Heilbrunn JZ: Legal and Economic Implications of Truancy. Clemson, SC, Clemson University, 2005.

U.S. Department of Education: National Education Longitudinal Study of 1988, First Follow-up Study. Washington, DC, National Center for Education Statistics, 1990.

54 ATTENTION AND DEFICITS OF ATTENTION

Lisa Albers Prock and Leonard Rappaport

Attention is an elusive concept. Research psychologists often split attention into several apparently distinct subcomponents or abilities. These components are assessed by careful experimental procedures. However, they do not necessarily correlate with a child's typical approach to schoolwork and homework in the real world. Developmental-behavioral pediatricians, psychiatrists, and clinical psychologists often lump the subcomponents into a superordinate category. Implicitly, they emphasize the ability to concentrate over time in the face of distraction. They evaluate children's ability to attend primarily by asking teachers and parents to rate the child on a variety of global behaviors. However, individuals demonstrate varying degrees of attention as a function of the specific task or stimuli, situation-specific needs and expectations, and their level of motivation. At any age, from preschool through adulthood, individuals may present with a complex and variable capacity to regulate attention to function in a variety of settings. Intrinsic and extrinsic factors may affect an individual's ability "to attend" at any moment in time.

An important controversy is whether variations in attention (and a related construct, activity level) represent a continuum of normal behavior or whether attentional weaknesses represent a neurologically based behavioral disorder. Critics of the "disorder model" cite multiple weaknesses in the theoretical construct of disorders of attention and argue that performance one or two standard deviations from the average does not necessarily imply a physiologic basis for a disorder (Carey, 2002) (see also Chapter 7). Similar issues also can be found in classifications of other behaviorally defined disorders that do not have specific known causes or diagnostic tests that identify disease.

Some children and adults have severe, persistent, and pervasive difficulties in sustaining attention, and these difficulties adversely alter academic and social functioning. Under these circumstances, the diagnosis of attention-deficit/hyperactivity disorder (ADHD) may be appropriate. The diagnosis is based on clinical features without corroborating neurologic or laboratory findings. The diagnosis implies that other neurologic, medical, and psychosocial explanations for attentional weaknesses have been considered. A difficulty in establishing the diagnosis of ADHD is that it may coexist with other diagnoses, including learning disorders, tics, seizures, lead intoxication, and child abuse. However, the diagnosis of ADHD implies that some conditions, such as seizure disorder, lead poisoning, and parent-child conflict, have been ruled out or appropriately addressed. There are many analogies in medicine. For example, fever is a continuum. It exists in many different conditions. Treatment with antipyretics normalizes body temperature without treating the cause of the fever.

Personal characteristics that have been associated with attentional deficits can also be viewed as strengths in settings other than the traditional school. For example, distractibility may be a disadvantage in the classroom but an advantage for a soldier in the field. Partial completion of multiple tasks may bring poor grades in school but good income for a salesman. A high energy level may be quite problematic for the child during a long and sedentary school day but can be a wonderful asset on the playing field after school.

In this chapter, we adopt the nomenclature of clinicians working in the field, with the knowledge that this may change as we gain more knowledge over time. Throughout this chapter, following the *Diagnostic and Statistical Manual for Primary Care,* we use the term *attentional problems* to describe individuals presenting with attentional weakness. We reserve ADHD for children and adults who have severe and persistent problems and have met specific clinical criteria for research purposes (Diagnostic and Statistical Manual of Mental Disorders, 4th ed, text revision, 2000). These criteria require pervasive challenges, with modulation of one's attention, activity, and behaviors leading to maladaptive behaviors and functional limitations that are inconsistent with an individual's developmental level and environmental expectations.

NEUROSCIENCE AND NEUROPSYCHOLOGY OF ATTENTION AND ATTENTION DISORDERS

Neuroimaging

Observations from the fields of neuroscience, neuropsychology, and clinical medicine have contributed to our evolving understanding of the concept of attention and disorders of attention. Recent studies have examined the structure and function of neurologic structures associated with attention regulation through modern structural and functional neuroimaging. These studies provide a picture of an integrated network subserving attention.

Neuroscientists and neuropsychologists consider multiple process components as composing attention (Casey and Durston, 2006; Mirsky, 1996): focus (identification of a stimulus in the environment); encoding/processing of the detected information; appropriately sustained attention (including screening out of nonrelevant environmental stimuli); appropriate shifting of attention; inhibition of involuntary shifting of attention (distractibility); and orchestration of a response to the incoming information. There are anatomic correlates to these components identified in studies of children and adults with no attentional issues.

- *Focusing* on a particular stimulus requires input from the superior temporal and inferior parietal cortices as well as striatal input as mediated via the the basal ganglia.
- *Encoding* of information to which one is attending requires the function of the hippocampus and the amygdala.
- *Sustaining attention* appears to be served by rostral midbrain structures, including the pontine reticular activation formation and thalamic nuclei.
- *Shifting attention* from one stimulus to another, either voluntarily or involuntarily, requires prefrontal cortex activity.

At the same time, specific brain lesions have been correlated with attentional problems associated with the diagnosis of ADHD, providing additional information about the complex networks required for attention. Dysfunction in the frontal-subcortical pathways is the most commonly invoked theory for ADHD. This theory is supported by the finding that deficits associated with ADHD are similar to the impaired functions of adults with frontal lobe damage. Another structure implicated in ADHD is the locus ceruleus, a small nucleus of norepinephrine neuronal cell bodies that originate in the midline pontine tegmentum and then arborize throughout the brain, including the cerebral cortex. The role of locus ceruleus neuron activation appears to be in supporting attention to the environment and screening out irrelevant details while supporting focus on the relevant stimuli (Pliska, 1996).

More than 60 studies have found individual and group differences in the size of numerous brain regions between patients with and without ADHD symptoms. Consistent with neuroanatomic and neurochemical findings, volumetric structural magnetic resonance imaging studies comparing individuals diagnosed with ADHD and controls suggest an important role of frontostriatal circuitry, frontal cortex, and basal ganglia (caudate, putamen, globus pallidus). Another group difference is intracortical connections through the corpus callosum. Finally, differences in the cerebellum have also been reported. The findings of association between structural differences and the behavioral profile of ADHD do not determine whether local structural changes are the cause of or secondary to ADHD symptoms. In addition, group differences are not of sufficient magnitude to allow use of structural imaging in diagnosis.

Functional neuroimaging studies (positron emission tomography and functional magnetic resonance imaging) have supported the importance of frontostriatal pathways in attention. A single-photon emission computed tomographic study has found differences in dopamine transporter density in adults with ADHD in comparison to adults without ADHD (Dougherty et al, 1999). However, similar to structural imaging studies, functional imaging studies do not consistently agree on the locus or lateralization of brain findings in individuals diagnosed with ADHD as opposed to those without ADHD. Functional studies have the same logical limitation as structural studies do, leaving unanswered whether correlations between activations and symptoms are a cause or effect of the attentional problems.

Developmental changes have also been seen in response to inhibition and other aspects of attention. These changes are associated with differences in the number and identity of areas of activation on functional imaging. In addition, adults with ADHD demonstrate a prominent decrease in metabolism in premotor cortex, superior frontal cortex, striatum, and thalamus compared with adults without ADHD. The magnitude of the differences changes from childhood to adulthood.

Neurochemistry

Evidence from studies examining brain structure (neuroimaging), brain function (neuropsychology, functional imaging studies), and responses to medications (psychopharmacology) suggest the importance of dopamine- and norepinephrine-mediated frontostriatal pathways in the pathophysiology of ADHD. Psychostimulants commonly used to treat symptoms of ADHD have been found to influence both dopaminergic and noradrenergic systems. Nearly all medications effective in treating the symptoms of individuals diagnosed with ADHD have been demonstrated to directly or indirectly increase dopamine activity in frontostriatal pathways. Neuropharmacologic studies support the concept of ADHD as a disorder of hypodopaminergic function or dopamine insensitivity.

DEVELOPMENTAL TRAJECTORY OF ATTENTION SKILLS

Any individual's ability to regulate her or his level of attention, activity, and impulses evolves from infancy through adulthood. Both neurologic maturation and real-life experiences have an impact on the rate of change and the precision of these skills. In addition, level of motivation and intelligence also alter one's ability to selectively attend to a specific environmental stimulus. As a result, a child's attention regulatory skills must be evaluated within the context of the child's chronologic and developmental age. With increasing neuromaturation, one's ability to inhibit or to override routine or reflexive behaviors in favor of more controlled or situation-appropriate and adaptive behaviors generally improves. In some situations (e.g., inhibition tasks), young children may use more brain regions than do adults to perform similar tasks.

Studies of children beginning in infancy have described three core components integral to demonstration of one's level of attention in any situation: (1) alerting/arousal, (2) inhibition, and (3) attentional control. The developmental information integrates with neural functions to provide a picture of this complex function.

Alerting/Arousal

To demonstrate attention to any specific environmental stimulus, an individual must maintain alertness to detect salient stimuli in the environment. A child's ability to disengage, shift, and re-engage attention typically develops throughout infancy. For example, even at 3 months of age, parents report being able to distract an upset child with exposure to a novel stimulus; but as interest and attention wane, a child's distress returns, suggesting that distress reduction may be the result of shifting of attention, not reduction in the noxious stimulus.

Regions of the right frontal and parietal cortices and the norepinephrine system appear to be critical in maintaining focus on a particular object or person (Posner and Rothbart, 2005). Studies of individuals with epilepsy have demonstrated that midline structures are also necessary for arousal. This model also suggests that alertness (focus on one specific item) leads to "quieting" of other brain activities by the release of norepinephrine, resulting in an increased signal-to-noise ratio in specific brain areas.

Inhibition

A child's ability to inhibit inappropriate behaviors (response inhibition) typically increases with age. One common task thought to measure response inhibition in the clinical setting is the go/no-go paradigm, in which children are asked to respond to every stimulus except one (e.g., respond to all letters except Z). A child's ability to refrain from responding to the no-go stimulus is used as a measure of response inhibition. During the preschool and school-age years, response inhibition tends to improve for most children.

Neuroimaging studies using the go/no-go paradigm have demonstrated signal increases in several brain regions (ventral prefrontal cortex, inferior frontal cortex, and anterior cingulate gyrus) with development; children show reduced brain activity on this task compared with adults, although the brain activation in these same regions increases when inhibition is required (Casey et al, 2001; Vaidya, 2005). In children far more than in adults, basal ganglia structures also appear to be involved in response inhibition. Children diagnosed with ADHD who behaviorally show a high rate of errors of commission, or false alarms, demonstrate significantly lower activity than do control children in their basal ganglia region activity during performance of a go/no-go task (Durston, 2003). However, when children diagnosed with ADHD took stimulant medication to address symptoms of inattention and impulsivity, their basal ganglia activity more closely resembled that of control children as their behavioral performance improved (Vaidya, 2005).

Attentional Control

In the real world, children (and adults) are expected to selectively focus on relevant tasks while simultaneously suppressing information that is irrelevant or misleading at that time. One task used to study this component of attention is the Stroop paradigm. In this task, participants are asked to identify the color of ink in which a word is written. The task requires inhibition of word reading because reading the word is a more automatic response than saying the color (e.g., saying *red* when the word *blue* is printed in red ink requires inhibition of reading *blue*). Neuroimaging studies implicate that the anterior cingulate cortex is particularly important for detecting and resolving this attentional conflict.

Shifting attention is measured by tasks such as the Wisconsin Card Sorting Task. This task requires participants to change the sorting rule they are using as a result of the positive and negative feedback they receive on the basis of their responses. Typically, healthy children learn to shift their behavior and their implicit categories when the rules change. Adults adjust more quickly than do children. Adults with dorsolateral prefrontal cortex lesions have impaired performance on these tasks. In addition, adults with frontal lobe lesions perform this task quite similarly to a typically developing 3-year-old child.

ATTENTION-DEFICIT/HYPERACTIVITY DISORDER AS A DIAGNOSIS

The core features required for diagnosis of ADHD have been revised during the past half-century with each iteration of the *Diagnostic and Statistical Manual of Mental Disorders* (Tables 54-1 and 54-2). ADHD is currently diagnosed on the basis of the presence of behavioral symptoms of inattention or hyperactivity-impulsivity. These domains are dissociable but frequently co-occur. To ensure that the core symptoms are pervasive, clinical diagnostic criteria must be observed in *at least two settings*. To ensure that the symptoms are profoundly disruptive, diagnostic criteria currently require that an individual is *functionally impaired*. To ensure that the symptoms are persistent, the criteria require that they have been present for at least 6 months and began before the age of 7 years. Finally, the *Diagnostic and Statistical Manual of Mental Disorders*, fourth edition, text revision (DSM-IV-TR), requires that the symptoms are *not attributable to another primary disorder* (DSM-IV-TR, 2000).

Most researchers and clinicians follow the framework outlined in the DSM-IV-TR (2000) in making the diagnosis of ADHD (see Table 54-1). Four specific subtypes of ADHD are outlined in the DSM-IV-TR:

1. ADHD, combined type (accounting for 85% of those with ADHD)
2. ADHD, predominantly inattentive type
3. ADHD, predominantly hyperactive-impulsive type
4. ADHD, not otherwise specified

Table 54-1. Diagnostic Criteria for Attention-Deficit/Hyperactivity Disorder

A. Either 1 or 2 (or both):

(1) *inattention:* six (or more) of the following symptoms of inattention have persisted for at least 6 months to a degree that is maladaptive and inconsistent with developmental level:

- (a) often fails to give close attention to details or makes careless mistakes in schoolwork, work, or other activities
- (b) often has difficulty sustaining attention in tasks or play activities
- (c) often does not seem to listen when spoken to directly
- (d) often does not follow through on instructions and fails to finish schoolwork, chores, or duties in the workplace (not due to oppositional behavior or failure to understand instructions)
- (e) often has difficulty organizing tasks and activities
- (f) often avoids, dislikes, or is reluctant to engage in tasks that require sustained mental effort (such as schoolwork or homework)
- (g) often loses things necessary for tasks or activities (e.g., toys, school assignments, pencils, books, or tools)
- (h) is often easily distracted by extraneous stimuli
- (i) is often forgetful in daily activities

(2) *hyperactivity-impulsivity:* six (or more) of the following symptoms of hyperactivity-impulsivity have persisted for least 6 months to a degree that is maladaptive and inconsistent with developmental level:

Hyperactivity

- (a) often fidgets with hands or feet or squirms in seat
- (b) often leaves seat in classroom or in other situations in which remaining seated is expected
- (c) often runs about or climbs excessively in situations in which it is inappropriate (in adolescents or adults, may be limited to subjective feelings of restlessness)
- (d) often has difficulty playing or engaging in leisure activities quietly
- (e) is often "on the go" or often acts as if "driven by a motor"
- (f) often talks excessively

Impulsivity

- (g) often blurts out answers before the question has been completed
- (h) often has difficulty awaiting turn
- (i) often interrupts or intrudes on others (e.g., butts into conversation or games)

B. Some hyperactive-impulsive or inattentive symptoms that caused impairment were present before age 7 years.

C. Some impairment from symptoms is present in two or more settings (e.g., school or work and at home).

D. Clear evidence of clinically significant impairment in social, academic, or occupational functioning.

E. Symptoms do not occur exclusively during the course of pervasive developmental disorder, schizophrenia, or other psychotic disorder and are not better accounted for by another mental disorder (e.g., mood disorder, anxiety disorder, dissociative disorder, or personality disorder).

Based on the Diagnostic and Statistical Manual of Mental Disorders, 4th edition, text revision. Washington, DC, American Psychiatric Association, 2000.

Table 54-2. Evolution of Diagnosis of Attention-Deficit/Hyperactivity Disorder

Year	Citation	Comments
1902	George Still published in *Lancet*	Initial clinical description of 43 children with "moral impulse control" difficulties related to neurologically based difficulties with sustaining attention
1930s	Clinical use of "minimal brain damage" and then "minimal brain dysfunction"	Attribution of behavioral symptoms to "brain insults," including infections, toxin, head trauma; use of stimulants began in 1930s
1960s	"Hyperkinetic reaction of childhood" enters the DSM-II (1968)	Increased used of stimulants prescribed to address symptoms
1970s		Central role of "attention" and focus on subtypes related to presence or absence of impulsivity/activity and modulation of arousal, impulsive responses
1980	DSM-III (1980) "hyperkinetic syndrome" changed to "attention deficit disorder ± hyperactivity" in DSM-III-R (1987)	Consideration of core features of "primary inattention" to environment versus "failure to inhibit appropriate response"; changed from ADD (attention deficit disorder) to ADHD (attention-deficit/hyperactivity disorder) on the basis of field trials using behavioral rating scales
1990s	DSM-IV (1994) evidence-based redefinition of ADHD criteria	Emphasizing pervasiveness and impairment caused by symptoms
	National Institute of Mental Health (NIMH) conference to review state of ADHD diagnosis and treatment (1998)	NIMH conference reviews ADHD diagnostic trends and practices, suggesting both inappropriate and inadequate diagnosis of ADHD
2000s	American Academy of Pediatrics practice guidelines for primary care providers (2001)	American Academy of Pediatrics guidelines emphasize assessment in two or more settings with standardized questionnaires and consideration of comorbidities

Key components of the DSM-based diagnosis of all ADHD subtypes include the following:

- symptoms of inattention or symptoms of hyperactivity-impulsivity, often operationally defined by a symptoms checklist;
- onset of symptoms in childhood (before 7 years of age) and duration greater than 6 months; and
- functional impairments in two or more settings; not primarily attributable to other disorders (including pervasive developmental disorders, anxiety disorders, thought disorders).

The criteria do not specifically prevent individuals with underlying developmental or emotional disorders, such as an autism spectrum disorder or an anxiety disorder, from being diagnosed with ADHD. The criteria encourage clinicians to avoid use of ADHD as a primary diagnosis if a child's inattention or distractibility may be understood to reflect another disorder that responds to another type of intervention.

Differential Diagnosis of Attentional Problems

The differential diagnosis is extensive because attention is easily perturbed. Vision and hearing deficits should always be considered in children with attentional problems. Seizures, both generalized, such as petit mal, and partial, can cause significant deficits in attention. Recently increasing data are pointing to sleep disorders, such as sleep apnea and narcolepsy, as significantly affecting attention. Recent studies provide evidence that snoring affects the quality of sleep, with resultant decrements in attention. Insufficient normal sleep should also be considered. Thyroid disease, such as hyperthyroidism or hypothyroidism, has an impact on attention. Toxins such as lead, alcohol, and prescribed medications and illicit drugs have all been associated with decreased attention.

One should also consider environmental causes of attentional problems, such as stress at home from illness, death, or marital issues, in addition to the possibility of physical and sexual abuse. Poverty with an inadequate diet or deficits in the availability of a place to sleep safely or to do homework obviously has an impact on attention. Finally, many genetic and medical problems have been associated with an increased prevalence in attentional problems, including but not limited to premature birth, surgery for congenital heart disease, neurofibromatosis, fetal alcohol syndrome, and prenatal and postnatal lead exposure. Temperamental differences must also be considered as part of the differential diagnosis (see Chapter 7). Clearly, many children who have reduced attentional focus and increased activity levels have age-appropriate function. In these cases, the characteristics may represent a variation of normal.

Clinicians also must consider other learning and emotional issues as causes of attentional weakness. Children with language disorders often present with attentional weakness. Their problems may be due to trouble understanding complex language in their classroom, home, and social environment or may be a coexisting issue with attentional weakness. Children with reading or math disabilities or problems with fine motor output may try to obscure their academic or production weaknesses by disrupting class and may appear to have very significant attentional problems. Also, children with cognitive impairment that is at the borderline or more severe levels may show attentional problems when they are presented with work beyond their ability. However, they may have attentional weakness as a coexisting issue with cognitive limitations. ADHD can coexist with learning disabilities, language impairments, and cognitive disorders. The presence of one of these diagnoses does not preclude the diagnosis of ADHD.

Children with behavior consistent with an autism spectrum disorder can appear to have severe attentional problems because they are often not motivated to please their family members, teachers, or even peers. Finally, children with depression often present with severe attentional problems. This list is not totally inclusive of all causes of attentional problems, but it highlights the many pitfalls in the commonly exhibited headlong rush to make the diagnosis of ADHD and suggests that clinicians consider ADHD a diagnosis used after many other causes have been considered and always with caution. Any suggestion of other causes of attentional problems in the history and physical examination needs to be followed up by specific testing before the diagnosis of ADHD is made.

Epidemiology of ADHD

There is considerable variation in the prevalence of diagnosis with ADHD between countries and even between different regions within the United States. This variance is thought to stem from the differences in the ratio of physicians to people in the region and the differences in applying diagnostic criteria. In the United States, ADHD is estimated to affect 3% to 7% of school-age children (Rappley, 2005; Satcher, 1999). Boys are more often described as meeting criteria for ADHD, but the reported male-to-female ratio varies widely (Rappley, 2005).

ADHD symptoms have their onset in preschool or early childhood. Many symptoms persist through adulthood. In individuals identified with ADHD as children, the rate of persistence to adulthood has been reported to be as high as 50%. On occasion, a person who has underachieved throughout life reaches adulthood and is then diagnosed with ADHD (Okie, 2006). A recent national survey in the United States found an estimated prevalence of ADHD of 4.4% of U.S. adults. The investigators emphasized that adult ADHD symptoms often coexisted with a range of other mental health disorders. The majority of adults were untreated for ADHD, although many were under treatment for the other comorbid mental health or substance-related disorders (Kessler, 2006).

GENETICS, ENVIRONMENT, AND ATTENTION

Both genetic and environmental influences are generally accepted to have an impact on one's attention abilities. Determination of the relative contributions of each and the interplay between genes and environment continues to be a significant research challenge.

Genetics and Attention

ADHD has been shown to run in families, and therefore genetic factors are thought to play an important role in the severity of attentional problems. This observation is based on analyses of the rates of the ADHD within families relative to degrees of relatedness and the incidence of ADHD in adopted children (Table 54-3). Multiple candidate genes have been suggested to contribute to symptoms of ADHD. It remains unclear if the genetics of ADHD may involve one or more genes acting individually, particular alleles of several genes interacting, or a variety of genetic mechanisms contributing to the spectrum of ADHD symptoms.

Our understanding of specific genes that may be involved in the presentation of attentional problems continues to evolve. Animal studies have suggested a role for genes controlling the dopaminergic and noradrenergic

Table 54-3. Summary of Family Studies and Diagnosis of Attention-Deficit/Hyperactivity Disorder

Parents of children meeting criteria for ADHD have an increased risk (2- to 8-fold increase) of meeting criteria for ADHD themselves.

Siblings of children with ADHD, after controlling for effects of social status, gender, and degree of genetic relatedness, also demonstrate an increased risk of ADHD symptoms (2.1 to 3.5 times the risk).

On the basis of *twin studies* of ADHD symptoms, heritability data pooled from 20 separate analyses suggest that approximately 80% of the heritability risk for ADHD diagnosis and symptoms (hyperactivity, inattentiveness) is attributable to genetic factors.

Adoption studies demonstrate that adoptive relatives of hyperactive children are less likely to meet criteria for ADHD, whereas biologically related individuals are more likely to have ADHD symptoms (suggesting a genetic rather than purely environmental etiology of ADHD symptoms).

Sources: Nigg et al, 1999; Durston, 2003; Castellanos et al, 2002; Faraone et al, 2006.

systems. Many specific genes have been implicated in contributing to meeting criteria for ADHD in humans For example, seven separate genes (in which the same variant has been studied in three or more case-control or family-based studies) show statistically significant evidence of association with ADHD on the basis of pooled odds ratios across studies: the dopamine D_4 receptor gene (*DRD4*), the dopamine D_5 receptor gene (*DRD5*), the dopamine transporter gene (*SLC6A3*, *DAT*), the dopamine beta-hydroxylase gene (*DBH*), the serotonin transporter gene (*SLC6A4*, *5-HTT*), the serotonin receptor 1B gene (*HTR1B*), and the synaptosomal-associated protein 25 gene (*SNAP25*) (Faraone et al, 2006).

Environmental Factors and Attention

Environment factors have also been implicated in the expression of attentional problems for any individual. It is unclear if environmental factors, including biologic and social factors, may be causative of ADHD or if they lead to gene expression in genetically predisposed individuals. Discrete prenatal and postnatal environmental risk factors associated with children's diagnosis with ADHD include parental tobacco and substance use. Whereas the prenatal or postnatal exposure to toxins, including lead and alcohol, may lead to presentation with attentional problems, the majority of children meeting criteria for ADHD do not have a history of lead or prenatal alcohol exposure. Similarly, specific prenatal or perinatal complications (toxemia, eclampsia, poor maternal health, and extremely low birth weight) have been implicated in contributing to later ADHD, but the majority of children with ADHD do not have known prenatal or perinatal complications.

Contemporary environmental influences for a child, including parenting strategies, environmental stressors, and parent-child temperament mismatches, may also contribute to a child's presentation with ADHD symptoms. It is unclear whether suboptimal parenting is causative of ADHD, but clearly it may exacerbate expression of attentional problems and functional impairment. Environmental stressors, including trauma and exposure to domestic violence, may also contribute to a child's presentation with vulnerable attention regulation, which may improve in a different environment.

ASSESSMENT FOR POSSIBLE ATTENTION DISORDERS IN CLINICAL SETTINGS

Consensus documents from the National Institutes of Health, the Centers for Disease Control and Prevention, and the American Academy of Pediatrics (Perrin, 2001) as well as the DSM-IV-TR (2000) describe diagnostic criteria and treatment strategies for clinicians. Evidence of symptoms consistent with a diagnosis of ADHD must be obtained from the affected individual (child, adolescent, adult) as well as from other observers including parents, teachers, and clinicians. A variety of questionnaires and checklists are available for children, parents, and teachers. Recent American Academy of Pediatrics guidelines (Perrin, 2001) describe one approach to a clinical assessment for symptoms of ADHD in a primary care setting:

1. use of explicit diagnostic behavioral criteria (as outlined in DSM-IV-TR);
2. elicitation of symptoms of impairment in more than one setting (home, school, office); and
3. consideration of coexisting conditions (diagnostic and treatment implications).

To consider "coexisting conditions" or a differential diagnosis, many experts suggest that a psychoeducational or mental health evaluation may be required.

Clinician's Role

A major challenge for the clinician is that many medical, behavioral, and learning problems can present as weaknesses of attention regulation. A major task is quantifying the pervasiveness, persistence, and impact of inattention and overactivity. It is important to identify treatable diagnoses for the cause of attentional problems (Table 54-4). It is also important to determine whether medical or psychotherapeutic treatment is necessary, whether there is or is not an identifiable cause. Key components of a clinical assessment for ADHD include a comprehensive history, a thorough physical examination, and a review of collateral information, such as school performance and testing results from other observers. Gathering of a comprehensive history includes a review of prenatal, perinatal, early childhood, extended family, and psychosocial factors. This history may also uncover possible comorbid conditions (Table 54-5). A thorough physical examination (see Chapter 76) should include a detailed neurologic examination and confirmation of a child's normal vision and hearing. No specific physical or laboratory findings are pathognomonic of a diagnosis of ADHD; hence, recent clinical guidelines do not suggest any particular routine medical assessment to confirm or to rule out a diagnosis of ADHD.

Parent and Teacher Questionnaires

Current ADHD diagnostic criteria require that an individual present with functional impairments in at least two of the three settings including home, school, and

Table 54-4. Differential Diagnosis of Attention-Deficit/Hyperactivity Disorder and Possible Symptom Overlap

ADHD Symptom Potentially Caused by or Overlapping with Another Concern	Alternative "Diagnosis" to Consider	Red Flags Not Characteristic of ADHD and Suggestive of a non-ADHD Diagnosis	Other Clinical Considerations
Inattention	Hearing impairment Visual impairment Seizure disorder Sleep disorders: sleep apnea and narcolepsy Anxiety disorders*	Excessive worries Fearfulness	Cognitive level (child not understanding? or child is bored?)
Talks excessively	Anxiety disorders* Bipolar disorder	Excessive worries Fearfulness Grandiosity	
School failure or underachievement	Learning disorders Adjustment disorder Psychosocial stressors	ADHD symptoms only in setting requiring academics (school; homework)	Consider behaviors during summer versus school year
Fidgety	Anxiety disorders* Tic disorder Stereotypical movement	Repetitive vocal or motor movements	High level of activity but not affecting performance

*Anxiety disorders including generalized anxiety disorder, obsessive-compulsive disorder, and post-traumatic stress disorder.

Table 54-5. Comprehensive History Components for Children with Possible Attention-Deficit/Hyperactivity Disorder

Prenatal and Birth History
- Prenatal exposure to substances associated with symptoms of ADHD (tobacco, cocaine, alcohol)
- Gestational age

Developmental and Behavioral History
- Motor skill development
- Language development
- History of onset of behavioral concerns
- Temperament
- Sleep habits
- Fears, worries, routines
- Social history (friends? bullying?)

Family History (3 Generations) Suggestive of Heritability
- Diagnosis of ADHD, anxiety, mood (depression, bipolar disorder), language, or learning disorders?
- Difficulty with completion of school, inconsistent job performance, substance abuse (suggestive of possible undiagnosed difficulties)

Psychosocial History to Evaluate Possible Stressors That May Affect a Child's Learning and Behaviors
- Frequent moves
- Changes in living or custody situation
- Exposure to domestic violence
- History of abuse, neglect
- Life stressors (moves of home, school)

work. Use of standardized rating scales (completed by parents and teachers) as part of a diagnostic work-up for ADHD provides documentation of symptoms of ADHD while also considering symptoms of alternative and comorbid diagnoses. A number of standardized questionnaires are available for parent, teacher, and child or adolescent report of symptoms of hyperactivity, impulsivity, and inattention. One example is a series of checklists for parents and teachers created by the National Initiative for Children's Healthcare Quality. The set may be obtained from the American Academy of Pediatrics. These checklists allow providers to review parents' and teachers' subjective reports of a child's behaviors (on a 4-point scale, rated never to very often) for consistency with a DSM-IV–based diagnosis of ADHD and to understand a child's current social and academic functioning. Follow-up questionnaires can be used to ascertain whether a child has improved with respect to behavioral ratings and academic or social functioning. Another more extensive set of questionnaires by Levine (ANSER System; see Chapter 55) looks more closely at specific areas of attention plus many functional academic areas that could contribute to attentional problems.

No specific tests can be used to confirm the diagnosis of ADHD. In the past, continuous performance tests were touted as objective methods to corroborate clinical evaluations. Continuous performance tests are generally long, boring tasks during which numbers, letters, or symbols are rapidly presented to a subject, usually by computer screen. The child is asked to press a response button when a specified target appears, such as when the letter A is followed by the letter X. In experimental situations, failure to press for the target, or omission error, was thought to reflect "inattention"; hitting for the wrong stimulus, or commission error, to reflect "impulsivity"; and the total number correct, to reflect "sustained attention." Unfortunately, from a clinical perspective, continuous performance tests are not sufficiently sensitive or specific to distinguish children with and without inattention, and they cannot determine whether poor performance is due to inattention or other causes (such as learning disabilities or emotional concerns).

SUPPORTING AND MANAGING CHILDREN'S ATTENTION SKILLS

Supporting a child in regulation of attention skills focuses on minimizing symptoms having an impact on a child's functioning or safety in the classroom, at home, and with transition to independent adulthood. Regardless of the treatment modality, measurable outcomes should be monitored at baseline and periodically during treatment of each child to assess efficacy of therapeutic changes. Guidelines of the American Academy of Pediatrics, the American Academy of Child and Adolescent Psychiatry,

Table 54-6. **Possible Treatment Outcomes for Patients with Attention-Deficit/Hyperactivity Disorder**

ADHD-Related Symptoms	Data-Gathering Approach
School related	
Fewer disruptive classroom behaviors	Obtain by standardized report
	Communication book
Improved quality of work	Review of report cards
Improved work completion (in class; homework returned)	Review of standardized assessments
	Standardized reports
Home related	
Improved efficiency of homework	Parent report during clinical interview
Improved completion of chores	Quality of life questionnaires
Decreased impulsive safety concerns	Standardized reports
Self-reported	Self-report during clinical interview
Improved self-esteem	
Improved relationships with peers	
Self-perception of improved efficacy of homework and daily tasks	

the European Society for Child and Adolescent Psychiatry, and the Scottish Intercollegiate Guidelines Network describe a range of "desirable outcomes" for children being treated for ADHD (Table 54-6).

A wide range of therapies have been advocated to address attentional problems in children and adults, including demystification (see Chapter 86), behavioral interventions (see Chapter 87), and psychoactive medications (see Chapter 90). Recent studies suggest that dietary changes, including reduction in food additives and improvements in nutrition, might benefit children with ADHD. Mind-body therapies (including but not limited to meditation and biofeedback) have been shown in some studies to offer benefit to children with ADHD. Complementary and alternative medicines have not been shown to improve symptoms or outcomes.

The first step, demystification, teaches the child, adolescent, or adult and the family about attentional issues by use of a nonpathologic approach (see Chapters 86 and 89). Levine has developed a series of tools helpful in this process, but the general approach is to discuss the patient's areas of relative strength and weakness and to make attentional problems a characteristic to improve rather than a source of shame (see Chapter 44).

Behavioral Approaches

At present, behavioral approaches are a starting place for addressing global attentional issues, especially in preschool but also in school-age children. Behavioral approaches have been shown to be better than placebo in multiple trials. Examples of behavioral strategies suggested for working with children with ADHD and their families include contingency management (e.g., point/token reward systems; time-out; response costs) and psychoeducation in home and school settings. Although it is efficacious for some comorbid symptoms (e.g., anxiety symptoms), cognitive-behavioral therapy including self-monitoring and verbal self-instruction has not been found to be effective for treatment of core symptoms of ADHD.

Several large randomized controlled trials compared behavioral therapy alone and psychopharmacologic therapy alone and considered the combination of behavioral and psychopharmacologic interventions for treatment of ADHD symptoms. Despite the intensity of these behavioral interventions (the MTA study "behavioral interventions" included 35 individual and group sessions, which tapered off during 14 months (Carey, 2000); the Abikoff study had weekly sessions for 1 year and then monthly in year 2) geared to psychoeducation, behavior management techniques, classroom consultation and support, and direct skill development, behavioral support alone was not as effective as medication for the core symptoms (activity and inattentiveness) of ADHD (Abikoff et al, 2004; Jensen et al, 2001). The combination of behavioral support with medication management of ADHD symptoms was comparable to medication only in terms of reduction of core symptoms in the MTA study. The combination was superior to medication alone for subclasses of children, including those with anxiety and reading problems. The combination was also better in cases of poor parent-child relationships. The combination was associated with greater family and teacher satisfaction. Unfortunately, behavioral support in community settings for children with ADHD and their families is generally far less intense than the behavioral strategies used in these studies. A 36-month follow-up of the original sample, however, showed no improvement from baseline in core symptoms of ADHD but no intervention group differences (Jenson et al, 2007). It remains unclear what accounted for the differences in short-term versus long-term findings, even after post hoc analyses of various theories, suggesting another reason for close monitoring for children receiving stimulant medication over time.

Psychological strategies and therapy are indicated for children with significant comorbid diagnoses (and their families), such as significant oppositional behaviors or anxiety disorders. Behavioral strategies should also be strongly considered in cases in which (1) a child or family prefers not to use a medication, (2) a child partially responds or does not respond at all to medication, (3) the therapeutic benefits of a medication for the child have worn off at the end of the day, or (4) the child cannot tolerate medication management (see Chapter 7 for more on the management of aversive temperament).

Although providers outside of the educational system cannot specifically "prescribe" interventions in a child's school setting, they can support parents advocating for their children to receive supportive services and reasonable accommodations. According to U.S. federal law (Individuals with Disabilities Education Act, 2004; see Chapter 93), children with health problems significant enough to have an impact on a child's educational performance qualify to receive services through their school program under the category of "other health impaired" to support their ability to make effective progress in an educational setting. Children may also receive special education if they meet one of the other eligibility criteria, such as learning disability or intellectual disability. However, ADHD does not itself qualify for special education.

Many children who are not eligible for special education can receive accommodations through Section 504 of the Rehabilitation Act. Accommodations include modifications of the environment, output expectations, or teaching methods. The ADHD kit from the American Academy of Pediatrics has sample letters for requesting both the multidisciplinary evaluation required to determine eligibility for special education and a so-called 504 Plan.

Pharmacologic Interventions

Numerous studies have suggested that medications, particularly psychostimulants, have an important role as part of a treatment plan for children, adolescents, and adults who have been carefully diagnosed with ADHD. All medications should be initiated in trial mode while baseline data are collected from as many sources as possible, at least home and one teacher. Careful attention to the nature and severity of adverse side effects is crucial for ultimate decisions about the use of medication. A reasonable approach to decisions about medication is to choose measurable target outcomes before the medication trial and to evaluate progress toward those outcomes with treatment. Several doses and formulations of medications may be required. Positive change should be demonstrated for medication to be continued. However, a favorable response to a stimulant is nonspecific and does not prove the diagnosis (Carey, 2000). Long-acting medications seem preferable to short-acting preparations to maximize blood levels of medication, to minimize decreased attention as medication wears off, and to eliminate the embarrassment of going to the school nurse for midday medication. Children should be seen regularly twice to four times per year to monitor vital signs, growth side effects, and comorbid conditions. The visit is an opportunity to make sure that academic and social successes are tracking with attentional improvement. A trial off of medication to determine whether the child or adolescent is still benefiting is desirable to some families. If children are not making progress toward target outcomes or if their academic or social experiences remain unfavorable, other interventions must be put in place on a timely basis. Approaches to the use of medication and treatment options are comprehensively reviewed in Chapter 90.

Complementary and Alternative Therapies

For many decades, numerous interventions beyond medications and behavioral support have been advocated for children with ADHD, including dietary replacement, exclusion, or supplementation; various vitamin, mineral, or herbal regimens; and biofeedback. Although some research has suggested possible benefits of some therapies (including yoga, massage, fatty acid supplementation), most studies have shown no effect, and more rigorously designed intervention studies are needed to consider the possible role of these therapies (see Chapter 95).

PREVENTING FUNCTIONAL PROBLEMS AND COMORBIDITY

Children with attentional problems often face academic and social difficulties. In comparison to children without attentional problems, children with ADHD earn poorer grades, fail more classes and grades, have higher rates of detention and expulsion, drop out of high school, and fail to go to college. Compared with children without attentional problems, children with ADHD have more difficulty with family relationships and fewer good friendships. The management of attentional problems requires choosing target symptoms for the intervention. The approaches will vary if the issues are narrowly restricted to attention or if they are pervasive, affecting academic and social life.

Increasing evidence suggests that early intervention to address attentional problems may prevent an individual's level of inattention or impulsivity from contributing to secondary concerns for children and adults, such as school failure, substance abuse, and motor vehicle accidents (Okie, 2006). Children with ADHD may experience long-term adverse effects on their self-esteem, academic performance, vocational success, and social-emotional development. Adolescents with a diagnosis of ADHD are more likely to report a negative outlook for the future, to have lower self-esteem, and to have an increased risk for motor vehicle accidents. As adults with ADHD, job performance, frequent job changes, and relationship difficulties are reported to be more common (Faraone et al, 2006).

Individuals with ADHD who receive treatment have reduced risk of substance use disorders and cigarette use compared with individuals with ADHD who are not treated. Adolescents and adults with ADHD are described as having increased rates of traffic accidents compared with non-ADHD peers. However, while stimulant medications are being taken, driving performance (both during driving simulation tests and observed on a driving course) is significantly improved (Barkley et al, 2002; Cox et al, 2004; Wilens et al, 2006).

Because school is a child's first job and attentional problems often negatively affect a child's success in that first job, it is essential to find areas of success for a child who has significant attentional issues. Constant recognition of even partial success on the part of family members is the first step in shaping behaviors and supporting self-esteem. An essential second step is finding areas in which the child feels pride. Success in sports is often a lifesaver in children with attentional issues, but for many others, nonathletic pursuits must be substituted because of developmental coordination difficulties or lack of interest. The area of success is not nearly as important as the fact that the child or adolescent finds success in some arena that is important to him or her.

SUMMARY

Evidence from neuroscience, neuropsychology, and genetics is refining our clinical understanding of the neurologic bases of attention and disorders of attention. Both genetic and environmental factors have an impact on attention abilities. Clinicians assessing children with attentional problems should gather key historical information in more than one setting (including home and school settings) and use explicit diagnostic criteria to make an accurate diagnosis. In addition, they should carefully consider alternative reasons for a child's presenting with challenges with attention regulation as well as possible confounding factors and potential comorbid diagnoses that may be important in treatment planning. Individuals diagnosed with ADHD can be treated with behavioral interventions and medication. The treatments play an important role in improving core symptoms of activity and inattentiveness and in decreasing secondary comorbidities in childhood, adolescence, and adulthood.

REFERENCES

Abikoff H, Hechtman L, Klein RG: American Academy of Pediatrics: Clinical practice guideline: Diagnosis and evaluation of the child with attention deficit/hyperactivity disorder. Pediatrics 105:1158-1170, 2000.

Abikoff H, Hechtman L, Klein RG, et al: Social functioning in children with ADHD treated with long-term methylphenidate and multimodal psychosocial treatment. J Am Acad Child Adolesc Psychiatry 43:820-829, 2004.

American Academy of Child and Adolescent Psychiatry: Practice parameter for the assessment and treatment of children and adolescents with attention-deficit/hyperactivity disorder. J Am Acad Child Adolesc Psychiatry 46:894-921, 2007.

Barkley RA, Murphy KR, Dupaul GI, et al: Driving in young adults with attention deficit hyperactivity disorder: Knowledge, performance, adverse outcomes and the role of executive functioning. J Int Neuropsychol Soc 8:655-672, 2002.

Carey WB: What the multimodal treatment study of children with attention-deficit/hyperactivity disorder did and did not say about the use of methylphenidate for attention deficits. Pediatrics 105:863-864, 2000.

Carey WB: Is ADHD a valid disorder? *In* Jensen PJ, Cooper J (eds): Attention Deficit-Hyperactivity Disorder: State of the Science, Best Practices. Kingston, NJ, Civic Research Institute, 2002. Available at: www.dbpeds.org/articles/detail.cfm?textid=128.

Casey B, Durston S: From behavior to cognition to the brain and back: What have we learned from functional imaging studies of attention deficit hyperactivity disorder? Am J Psychiatry 163:957-960, 2006.

Casey BJ, Forman SD, Franzen P, et al: Sensitivity of prefrontal cortex to changes in target probability: A functional MRI study. Hum Brain Mapp 13:26-33, 2001.

Castellanos FX, Lee PP, Sharp W, et al: Developmental trajectories of brain volume abnormalities in children and adolescents with attention-deficit/hyperactivity disorder. JAMA 288:1740-1748, 2002.

Cox DF, Merkel RL, Penberthy JK, et al: Impact of methylphenidate delivery profiles on driving performance of adolescents with attention-deficit/hyperactivity disorder: A pilot study. J Am Acad Child Adolesc Psychiatry 43:269-275, 2004.

Diagnostic and Statistical Manual of Mental Disorders, 2nd ed. Washington, DC, American Psychiatric Association, 1968.

Diagnostic and Statistical Manual of Mental Disorders, 3rd ed, revised. Washington, DC, American Psychiatric Association, 1987.

Diagnostic and Statistical Manual of Mental Disorders, 4th ed. Washington, DC, American Psychiatric Association, 1994.

Diagnostic and Statistical Manual of Mental Disorders, 4th ed, text revision. Washington, DC, American Psychiatric Association, 2000.

Dougherty DD, Bonab AA, Spencer TJ, et al: Dopamine transporter density in patients with attention deficit hyperactivity disorder. Lancet 354:2132-2133, 1999.

Durston S: A review of the biological bases of ADHD: What have we learned from imaging studies? Ment Retard Dev Disabil Res Rev 9:184-195, 2003.

Faraone S, Middleton F, Biederman J: An integrated neurobiological model of attention deficit/hyperactivity disorder. *In* Biederman J (ed): ADHD Across the Lifespan: An Evidence-Based Understanding from Research to Clinical Practice. Hasbrouck Heights, NJ, Veritas Institute, 2006, pp 73-87.

Green M, Wong M, Atkins D, et al: Diagnosis of Attention Deficit/Hyperactivity Disorder. Technical Review 3. Rockville, MD, Agency for Health Care Policy and Research, August 1999. IAHCPR publication no. 99-049.

Greenhill L, Pliszka S, Dulcan M, et al: Practice parameter for the use of stimulant medications in the treatment of children, adolescents, and adults. J Am Acad Child Adolesc Psychiatry 41(Suppl 2):26S-49S, 2002.

Hille E, den Ouden A, Saigal S, et al: Behavioral problems in children who weigh 1000 g or less at birth in four countries. Lancet 357:1641-1643, 2001.

Kessler R, Adler L, Barkley R, et al: The prevalence and correlates of adult ADHD in the United States: Results from the National Comorbidity Survey Replication. Am J Psychiatry 163:716-723, 2006.

Jensen PS, Hinshaw SP, Swanson JM, et al: Findings from the NIMH Multimodal Treatment Study of ADHD (MTA): Implications and applications for primary care providers. J Dev Behav Pediatr 22:60-73, 2001.

Jensen PS, Arnold LE, Swanson JM, et al: 3-year follow-up of the NIMH MTA study. J Am Acad Child Adolesc Psychiatry 46:989-1002, 2007.

Levine MD: All Kinds of Minds. Cambridge, MA, Educators Publishing Service, 1994.

Levine MD: The Concentration Cockpit. Cambridge MA, Educators Publishing Service, 1995.

Levy F, Hay D, McStephen M, et al: Attention-deficit hyperactivity disorder: A category or a continuum? Genetic analysis of a large-scale twin study. J Am Acad Child Adolesc Psychiatry 36:737, 1997.

Linnet K, Dalsgaard S, Obel C, et al: Maternal lifestyle factors in pregnancy risk of attention deficit hyperactivity disorder and associated behaviors: Review of the current evidence. Am J Psychiatry 160:1028-1040, 2003.

Mirsky A: Disorders of attention. *In* Lyon GR, Krasnegor NA (eds): Attention, Memory and Executive Function. Baltimore, MD, PH Brookes, 1996, pp 71-95.

MTA Cooperative Group: National Institute of Mental Health Multimodal Treatment Study of ADHD follow-up: 24-month outcomes of treatment strategies for attention-deficit/hyperactivity disorder. Pediatrics 43:802-811, 2004.

Nelson C, de Haan M, Thomas K: Neuroscience and Cognitive Development: The Role of Experience and the Developing Brain. New York, Wiley, 2006.

Nigg J, Quamma J, Greenberg M, et al: A two-year longitudinal study of neuropsychological and cognitive performance in relation to behavioral problems and competencies in elementary school children. J Abnorm Child Psychol 27:51-63, 1999.

Okie S: ADHD in adults. N Engl J Med 354:2637-2641, 2006.

Owens J: The ADHD and sleep conundrum: A review. J Dev Behav Pediatr 26:312-322, 2005.

Perrin J, Stein M, Amler R, et al: Clinical practice guideline: Treatment of school-aged children with attention deficit/hyperactivity disorder. Pediatrics 108:1033-1044, 2001.

Pliska S, McCracken J, Mass J: Catecholamines in attention-deficit hyperactivity disorder: Current perspectives. J Am Acad Child Adolesc Psychiatry 35:264, 1996.

Posner M, Rothbart M: Influencing brain networks: Implications for education. Trends Cogn Sci 9:99-103, 2005.

Rappley M: Attention deficit-hyperactivity disorder. N Engl J Med 352:165-173, 2005.

Rojas N, Chan E: Old and new controversies in the alternative treatment of attention-deficit hyperactivity disorder. Ment Retard Dev Disabil Res Rev 11:116-130, 2005.

Satcher D: Mental Health: A Report of the Surgeon General. 1999. Available at: http://www.mentalhealth.samhsa.gov/features/surgeongeneralreport/home.asp.

Still GF: Some abnormal physical conditions in childhood. Lancet 1:1008, 1902.

Vaidya C: Altered neural substrates of cognitive control in childhood ADHD: Evidence from functional magnetic resonance imaging. Am J Psychiatry 162:1605-1613, 2005.

Wilens TE, Prince JB, Spencer TJ, et al: Stimulants and sudden death: What is a physician to do? Pediatrics 118:1215-1219, 2006.

Wolraich ML: Felice ME, Drotar D: The Classification of Child and Adolescent Mental Diagnosis in Primary Care: Diagnostic and Statistical Manual for Primary Care (DSM-PC), Child and Adolescent Version. Elk Grove Village, IL, American Academy of Pediatrics, 1996.

55 DIFFERENCES IN LEARNING AND NEURODEVELOPMENTAL FUNCTION IN SCHOOL-AGE CHILDREN

MELVIN D. LEVINE

A school child's "balance sheet" of neurodevelopmental strengths and weaknesses is a prophetic marker of her or his readiness to succeed in school as well as in other areas of life. That profile of strengths and weaknesses will influence profoundly a wide range of academic, behavioral, emotional, and career outcomes.

A neurodevelopmental profile is composed of a child's abilities across eight interrelated constructs: attention, memory, language, temporal-sequential ordering, spatial ordering, neuromotor function, higher cognition, and social cognition (Levine, 2002). Weaknesses in one or more of these areas may be associated with academic underachievement, behavioral difficulties, or problems with social adjustment. It has been estimated that at least 15% of school-age children harbor one or more low-severity impairments of neurodevelopmental function. The actual prevalence may be even higher when one takes into consideration discrete dysfunctions that lead to a transient self-limited problem within a particular subject area or those weaknesses that are not readily captured on a diagnostic test (such as problems with organization, communication, or output).

Neurodevelopmental variations are associated with a wide range of preferred learning patterns, individual strengths, and impediments (Table 55-1). A variation that represents a developmental weakness (such as slow or imprecise word retrieval) is considered a dysfunction. If that dysfunction interferes with the acquisition of a particular skill (such as writing), it becomes a disability. If the skill impaired by the disability is particularly germane to productivity and the attainment of reasonable success in school and in our society in general, the disability constitutes a handicap. Neurodevelopmental variations also include areas of unusual strength or talent. In describing a child's neurodevelopmental profile, therefore, it is important to take into consideration his or her assets (such as notable creativity, strong spatial perception, or excellent nonverbal conceptual abilities). In capturing the individuality of a child, it is also critical to take into account his or her content affinities and areas of consistent interest (such as a fascination with cars, aviation, animals, or fashion design). Such areas should be helped to develop into passions and domains of expertise!

Most children enduring academic difficulties harbor more than one neurodevelopmental dysfunction. The additive effect of multiple dysfunctions may be sufficient to constrain the innate resiliency of a child, thereby generating academic underachievement. It is likely that most children are able to circumvent a single neurodevelopmental dysfunction to attain at least passable academic achievement.

Neurodevelopmental dysfunctions commonly result in the delayed or laborious acquisition of academic skills and in a notably reduced level of productivity or output in school and at home. When neurodevelopmental dysfunctions are overtly disruptive of learning, these problems are often referred to as learning disabilities. However, there is little or no agreement on the definition of this term (Bradley et al, 2002). Other labels, such as attention deficit disorder, dyslexia, and nonverbal learning disability, have also been applied to children with "low-severity" dysfunctions. These diagnostic labels may be required for obtaining services in school or for reimbursement purposes outside of school. They also may enable students to receive accommodations, such as extended time on tests. However, the diagnostic criteria for such labels are highly controversial and constantly changing. Most recently, children's eligibility for service has been based on their response to intervention ("RTI"). In this model, services are provided when children have failed to respond to interventions in school that have been "scientifically proven" (Fletcher et al, 2005).

Countless students with disheartening academic problems fail to meet their school's criteria and therefore tend to "fall through the cracks," as their learning needs go unrecognized and unfulfilled. Not only that, there are serious dangers inherent in applying fixed labels to children. These hazards include self-fulfilling prophesies, pessimism, a tendency to ignore multifactorial causes and manifestations of a child's problems (i.e., reductionism), and a widespread practice of neglecting children who are struggling but who fail to meet a school's criteria for

Table 55-1. A Hierarchy of Neurodevelopmental Status

Variation	An unusual pattern of neurodevelopmental function (e.g., a higher divergent mind)
Dysfunction	A distinct weakness within a neurodevelopmental function (e.g., weak retrieval memory)
Disability	A performance deficiency caused (at least in part) by a neurodevelopmental dysfunction (e.g., trouble throwing a ball)
Handicap	A disability occurring in a much-needed or critical performance area (e.g., a significant reading problem)

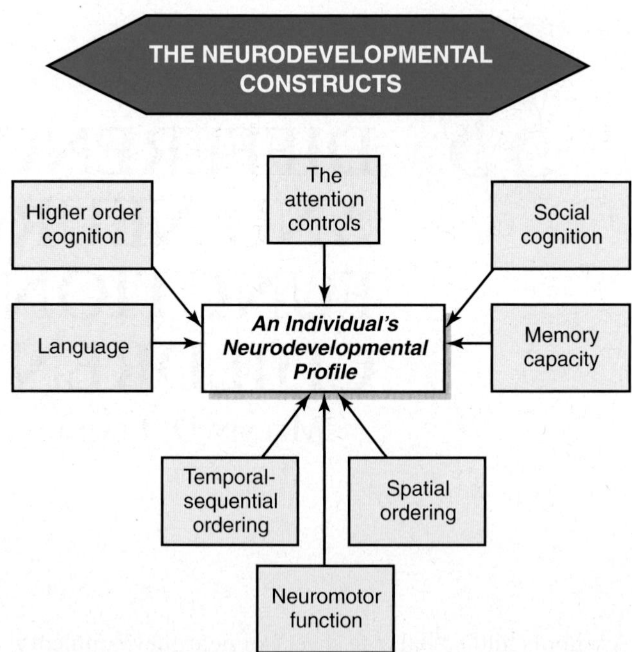

Figure 55-1. This diagram depicts the eight neurodevelopmental constructs, strengths and weaknesses of which contribute to a child's neurodevelopmental profile.

service eligibility. Under the Individuals with Disabilities Education Act legislation, some children may be able to receive services if a developmental delay can be demonstrated, that is, without the requirement of a label.

Labels fail to take into consideration the most important feature of any child, namely, his or her strengths! Consequently, this chapter shuns labeling and offers a phenomenologic approach to the neurodevelopmental dysfunctions that generate disabilities and significant handicaps.

CLINICAL MANIFESTATIONS OF DYSFUNCTION

Children with neurodevelopmental dysfunctions vary widely with regard to their clinical symptoms. Their specific patterns of academic performance and behavior represent final common pathways, the convergence of multiple genetic, health-related, environmental, and family-influenced factors. In addition, the manifestations of a particular dysfunction vary, depending on a child's strengths or weaknesses across other neurodevelopmental constructs. Thus, the manifestations of a memory dysfunction in a child with strong language skills will be different from those in a child whose memory problems are confounded by significant weaknesses of receptive language as well. Consequently, our broad interpretation of a child with neurodevelopmental dysfunctions must include consideration of strengths and weaknesses in the components of all the eight neurodevelopmental constructs summarized in Figure 55-1. In the following section, the basic manifestations of deficits and strengths in each of the key neurodevelopmental areas are described.

Attention

Dysfunctions of attention are, in all likelihood, the most common neurodevelopmental problems affecting children. Weaknesses of attention are especially incapacitating and are likely to have broad although often subtle and insidious impacts on day-to-day performance. Neurodevelopmental dysfunctions of attention are covered in Chapter 54.

Memory

As children proceed through school, there is a growing and potentially incapacitating strain on one or more of the numerous and varied components of memory (Levine, 2002). Students are expected to be increasingly selective, systematic, and strategic in contending with the imposed memory load. They must become deft when it comes to the organized storage of rules, facts, concepts, and procedures. By secondary school, rapid and accurate recall is an indispensable requisite for acceptable academic performance. Not surprisingly, some students experience tremendous frustration when their memory dysfunctions prevent them from meeting these ever-intensifying academic demands (Levine, 2003).

Table 55-2. Four Levels of Memory and Signs of Dysfunction

Level	Signs of Dysfunction
Short-term memory	Trouble following directions; need for repetition, difficulty studying for tests
Active working memory	Problems with mathematical computation; trouble remembering while reading; problems with writing
Consolidation in long-term memory	Overreliance on rote memory; inconsistent long-term recall; disorganization
Retrieval from long-term memory	Slow recall; problems in writing and mathematics

There are students who experience difficulty with the initial registration of information or skill in short-term memory (Table 55-2), as a result of which they fail to keep pace with the torrential information flow in a classroom. In some cases, children with attention deficits are insufficiently selective, alert, and reflective to register the most salient information in memory. They are likely to have generalized deficiencies of this initial registration process. Other students have more specific registration weaknesses (Vallar and Papagno, 1995). Some may have trouble registering only visual-spatial data in memory, whereas others may be ineffective at the entry of sequences of data or with their hold on verbal material. Some children ultimately can register data in short-term memory but cannot do so quickly enough, so they perpetually struggle to keep pace with instructions, explanations, or material they are expected to copy rapidly from a board. Still others have trouble capturing data arriving in "large chunks"; they simply are unable to register sizable portions of information compared with their classmates.

Many children experience problems with active working memory. They have difficulty suspending information in memory temporarily while they are in the process of making use of it. Ideally, active working memory should enable a student to keep in mind the various components of a task, such as a mathematics problem, while working to complete it. A student with an active working memory dysfunction, on the other hand, might carry a number and forget what it was that he or she intended to do after having carried the number. Active working memory enables children to remember the beginning of a paragraph while reading the end of it. Many students who are thought to have reading comprehension problems are actually enduring reading memory difficulties; they forget what they are reading while they are reading it! Thus, children with active working memory disorders can have trouble performing computations in mathematics and difficulty remembering or retelling what they have read.

Some children have agonizing problems consolidating information in long-term memory. They may have little or no trouble registering data initially in short-term storage, but their long-term retention cannot be relied on. Ordinarily, consolidation of data in long-term memory takes hours to days, often during non-REM sleep (Clemens et al, 2005). The filing of information and skill makes use principally of five main systems:

1. *Paired association*: linking two discrete bits of information (such as a cluster of letters with the sound it makes or a multiplication fact).
2. *Categories*: classifying facts in logically connected groupings (such as filing all insects together in memory).
3. *Patterns and rules*: linking new information to established rules or recurring patterns (so-called rule-based learning, such as spelling or punctuation rules).
4. *Procedures/skills*: the storage of ways of doing things—both motor (e.g., tying shoelaces and cursive writing) and nonmotor (e.g., reducing a fraction); arranging knowledge or skills, often represented by so-called linear chunks (such as the months of the year, the steps needed to tie your shoelaces or to form a letter).
5. *Narrative sequences*: the retention of stories, series of events, causal chains, and personal experiences.

An individual may exhibit serious gaps in any one or more of these five common forms of consolidation in long-term memory.

Although they may be able to register and to consolidate information in memory, some children have inordinate difficulty recalling data or skill, activating it on demand. Consequently, it may take them years to learn their multiplication facts (probably the clearest indicator of a long-term memory dysfunction in a child). Their recall may be painfully slow or inaccurate. Some of them encounter serious problems with simultaneous recall; they cannot retrieve several facts or procedures at once. This shortcoming can be especially disabling when it comes to writing, a task necessitating the concurrent remembering of spelling, capitalization, letter formation, punctuation, facts, ideas, vocabulary, and the directions or topic for the assignment. When they attempt to write, children with simultaneous-recall deficits suffer a disheartening memory overload, often manifesting illegibility (due to a crowding out of memory for letter formation), poor use of punctuation and capitalization, deficient spelling, and surprisingly primitive ideation. These children may stand accused of laziness, a lack of motivation, or a failure to strive because legibility or spelling is so poor in a paragraph and so far superior in isolation (such as on a list of spelling words). Such a student may sound brilliant in a class discussion, whereas what he or she transcribes on paper is woefully impoverished!

Students with memory *strengths*, on the other hand, can deploy these assets to overcome weaknesses or potential deficits in other components of their neurodevelopmental profiles. For example, a child who has difficulty understanding certain concepts in mathematics may compensate (at least in part) by having an excellent recall of mathematical facts and rules.

Language

Linguistically competent children have a distinct advantage in school because much of what gets taught is encoded in literate language. All of the basic academic skills are conveyed largely through verbal expression. Many important thinking skills are conveyed and applied through language (Nelson, 1996). Therefore, it is not surprising that children with language dysfunctions are susceptible to tumultuous academic careers (Paul, 2001).

There exist multiple forms and levels of language dysfunction. These are summarized in Table 55-3 (see also Chapter 72). Some children have problems with phonology, so that they are hampered in their appreciation and manipulation of discrete language sounds. They may have trouble discriminating between and forming associations with the sounds of their native language. Problems with phonologic awareness have been studied extensively in recent years and have been identified as one of the most common forms of learning disorder in childhood. Affected students have difficulty perceiving some or many of the 44 language sounds (phonemes) in the English language (Runge and Watkins, 2006). They may as well suffer from deficits in their phonemic awareness, their sense that words are made up of individual language sounds and can be taken apart into these and re-blended at will, another requisite for fluent decoding and accurate spelling. Children with weaknesses of phonologic and phonemic awareness may be forced to overrely on visual and context clues during reading. Many of them find it hard to hold language sounds in active working memory firmly enough to break a word down into its component sounds and re-blend

Table 55-3. Common Forms of Language Dysfunction

Specific Language Breakdown	Common Manifestations
Phonologic awareness	Difficulty processing, retaining, and manipulating language sounds, leading to trouble decoding words, spelling, learning a second language
Semantics	Trouble understanding word meanings, taking its toll on vocabulary growth and reading comprehension
Syntax	Problems understanding and formulating complex sentences, impairing ability to follow directions and verbal explanations, also undermining reading comprehension
Discourse	Poor processing and retention of language delivered in large amounts (extended passages, chapters, lectures)
Expressive language	Deficient encoding of thoughts into words and sentences, dysfluency, poor writing, lack of verbal participation in school
Receptive language	General weakness affecting ability to interpret accurately and with sufficient speed of the spoken or written language

them, a facility critical for decrypting new multisyllabic vocabulary.

It is common for children and adolescents with even mild phonologic difficulties to endure frustration and failure when they attempt to master a second language. Some bilingual children who have school problems do so because of phonologic dysfunctions in their underlying primary language.

Deficiencies at the semantic level of language represent another common language breakdown. By the end of second grade, most students know about 6000 root words; after that, they add approximately 1000 words per year. But some have mastered only 4000 or fewer words by the end of second grade; these students have been shown to be failing in most cases by the end of eighth grade, a finding that underlines the critical importance of vocabulary growth in elementary school (Biemiller, 2005). Students so impaired have rigid and restricted notions of word meanings. It is hard for them to incorporate new vocabulary, which becomes a major liability in high school and college, when there is a virtual explosion of key technical words that are essential to understanding complex subject matter.

Other language-based problems take in deficient understanding and use of syntax (sentence construction), reduced insight into how language works (weak metalinguistics), trouble with discourse (confusion when faced with language that goes beyond the boundaries of sentences—paragraphs, passages, chapters, lectures, and entire books), and lack of "higher language." The last includes such functions as the understanding and formulation of abstract language, the detection and resolution of ambiguity, the drawing of inferences (i.e., supplying missing information), the use of symbolic language (metaphors, analogies), the deployment of language to form abstract concepts, and the mastery of a second language. The attainment of these higher language levels becomes vital for success during secondary school. Students who proceed through high school lacking higher language sophistication often experience failure and commonly also develop signs of behavioral maladjustment or emotional instability.

A distinction can be made between receptive language dysfunctions (those affecting comprehension) and expressive language dysfunctions (those thwarting language production or communication). Children with primarily receptive language problems may have serious difficulty following instructions in the classroom, understanding verbal explanations, and interpreting what they read. Those with expressive weaknesses are likely to display weaknesses of word retrieval; despite an adequate vocabulary, their dysphasias make it hard for them to recall exact words on demand. This impairment can make it embarrassing and difficult for an affected student to participate in class discussions or to come up with precise answers on a quiz. Still others with expressive dysfunctions have trouble formulating sentences, using grammar effectively, and organizing spoken (and often written) narrative. Children with expressive language problems are likely to be hesitant when they speak. They may overindulge in circumlocutions. Their spoken narrative is often lacking in cohesive ties; it sounds as if they are reading a list of sentences when they talk. Words such as "then," "as soon as," "before," and "next" are used sparsely (if at all), resulting in a lack of narrative cohesion.

Some students with verbal dysfluency are noticeably passive, taciturn, and consistently nonelaborative in their communications. When asked what he or she did in school today, such a student is likely to respond "stuff"! Sometimes a child with expressive language dysfunctions speaks fluently with peers and family members, making use of limited vocabulary and simple or repetitive syntactic patterns. These same students may be poor at using more literate language.

Language dysfunctions range from blatant to subtle to barely discernible. They are frequently diagnostically elusive. Some students with mild language difficulties function reasonably well in school until they are required to master a second language. Other students with language dysfunctions may succeed until they reach late elementary or middle school, when language becomes increasingly decontextualized. That is, they can do well when language is used to describe familiar contents. When it becomes less predictable, such as when a teacher describes events that occurred long ago and far away, a language-impaired child may experience a steep decline in comprehension.

Students with notably strong language function may make use of their linguistic facility to overcome other learning problems. For example, it may be possible to verbalize one's way through the mathematics curriculum, thereby overcoming latent confusion over certain primarily nonverbal concepts (such as ratio, equation, and circumference).

Spatial Ordering

Most spatial data enter minds through visual pathways, but some are mediated through nonverbal conceptualization or propriokinesthetic pathways. Shape, position, relative size, foreground and background relations, and form constancy (the notion that a shape retains its integrity regardless of its position in space) are among the parameters of spatial ordering. Young children with visual-spatial dysfunctions may encounter problems with letter recognition. Spelling may be inaccurate, as some affected students fail to recall or to recognize the visual patterns formed by strings of letters that keep turning up in English words. In general, however, those who are confused about spatial attributes are unlikely to have long-standing or devastating academic problems unless their visual-spatial weaknesses are complicated by other neurodevelopmental dysfunctions. At one time, it was thought that visual-spatial dysfunctions were the leading cause of reading disabilities. Most recent research has refuted this view, although visual-spatial abilities clearly are by no means trivial or irrelevant, as they may play a major role in numerous careers. There are also indications that spatial thinking contributes substantially to effective mathematical reasoning (Van Garderen, 2006).

Children with spatial ordering dysfunctions may be late in discriminating between left and right. They may exhibit fine or gross motor clumsiness, or both, as they struggle to make use of visual-spatial data to program motor responses.

Students endowed with particularly keen spatial ordering may possess artistic and mechanical talents. Some may be able to use visualization to enhance their learning of even highly verbal concepts. This bypass route can be especially redemptive for students with strong visual-spatial ordering in the presence of a language disability.

Temporal-Sequential Ordering

The appreciation and application of time and sequence is an important neurodevelopmental function (Marshuetz, 2005). Students need to be able to preserve and to manage a vast range of practical and abstract sequences. They must tell time, process and produce multistep explanations and procedures, and register lengthy sequences in short-term memory. The curriculum demands the preservation of serial order in spelling, in narrative, and in mathematical algorithms. Therefore, an inability to work with sequences is likely to be associated with problematic writing, with mathematical deficiencies, and with generalized organizational problems.

Children who have difficulties with temporal-sequential ordering may be delayed in learning to tell time. They can also become confused over multistep inputs of various types. Thus, it is not unusual for a child with temporal-sequential disorganization to experience trouble following multistep instructions and processing complex sequential explanations. Sequencing weaknesses often result in the delayed mastery of multiplication facts as well as the performance of multistep computations. Over time, such a dysfunction can interfere with a student's ability to organize tasks in stages and to allocate time effectively. Thus, it is not unusual for children with temporal-sequential dysfunctions to be poor at time management, which in turn leads to frustrating delays and inefficiencies of work output.

Many children with sequencing problems exhibit overall difficulty with information that either enters, gets stored, or must be constructed in highly specific linear chunks. Spelling accuracy, the organization of writing, and the progression of steps in math procedures may all be negatively affected. When they spell, such students are likely to get the first two letters and the last two letters correct, with conspicuous inaccuracy in the middle. They may omit words from paragraphs and steps from a math computation. Interestingly, often these students are excellent with gestalts or configurations, sets of data configured in an overall pattern (such as a map or a chart or a work of art) rather than in a linear array.

Neuromotor Function

A child's motor skills can play a significant role in a wide range of academic and nonacademic pursuits (Denckla, 1985). Productivity in school becomes very dependent on efficient writing skills. The motor aspects of writing, known as graphomotor function, activate capacities that differ from fine motor function. In fact, it is not at all unusual for a student to display good fine motor function (such as in art and in repairing a bicycle) in the presence of poor graphomotor function. Because writing demands rapid and precise graphomotor coordination, it is not surprising that students with certain forms of dysfunction are prone to substantial academic underachievement. Such students have been described as having "developmental output failure." They seem to have far more trouble with productivity than with learning. The graphomotor dysfunctions that affect writing can be divided into eight subtypes, which are described as follows.

1. Some children have finger agnosia; they have trouble localizing their fingers in space while they write. There appears to be a breakdown of propriokinesthetic (re-afferent) feedback, resulting in poor appreciation of the precise location of the point of the writing utensil at any particular instant. Because of their impaired tracking, these children need to maintain their eyes very close to the page. Ultimately, their writing becomes agonizingly slow and laborious. Often these students develop a fistlike pencil grip that causes them to write with their wrists and their elbows rather than the distal joints of their digits. The wrists and elbows clearly have wider excursions during writing, so that propriokinesthetic feedback will be less subtle. Regrettably, the awkward pencil grip itself is a liability, making writing agonizingly slow, uncomfortable, and laborious. In particular, these students are likely to have trouble with lengthy writing, such as is needed to complete book reports in junior high school. In addition, children with finger agnosia tend to have other neurodevelopmental dysfunctions resulting in broad delays in academic performance.

2. Graphomotor production deficits affect many children, who have difficulty implementing the coordinated motor movements for writing. It is inordinately difficult for them to decide which muscles to facilitate (and which to inhibit) to form specific letters. It is hard for them to assign certain muscles to the stabilization of the writing utensil and others to its movement. They are motorically indecisive. During the early grades, they often exhibit an unstable pencil grip (occasionally dropping the pencil in the middle of a sentence). Eventually they compensate, often by developing a perpendicular, excessively tight and distal (or hooked) grasp as a means of overstabilizing the utensil, which can result in awkward, laborious movement. Many of these students also display an oromotor production deficit, resulting in speech articulation defects as well as writing problems.
3. Some students harbor a previsualization dyspraxia. They have difficulty visualizing and therefore planning the configurations of letters and words they are about to form. Because they do not have a clear and consistent visual plan or blueprint, their written output tends to be poorly or inconsistently legible. Often the same problem they experience when visualizing letters impedes the ability to visualize entire words. Consequently, they frequently exhibit spelling errors as well as legibility problems. Their spelling errors are likely to be phonetically correct but visually poor approximations (e.g., "brawt" for "brought"). Of interest is the fact that many children with previsualization weaknesses fluctuate in their picturing of letter configurations. As a result, their writing is inconsistent; while forming a letter, they often (but not always) forget the gestalt of that letter. Therefore, their writing is marked by hesitation, retracing, and erratic letter formation.
4. Some students have procedural memory dyspraxias. They are unable to recall and therefore to plan the precise sequences of motor movements required to form letters. These children also show letter formation inconsistencies, a poor writing rhythm, and erratic legibility. Their motor sequential recall may fluctuate from word to word or even letter to letter. They (as well as students with previsualization weaknesses) commonly prefer printing (manuscript) to cursive writing. Often students with procedural memory dyspraxias also endure difficulties in mathematics as a result of their weak recall of the multistep procedures in that content area.
5. Visual-motor dyspraxia occurs in children who have a great deal of difficulty using visual information to program a motor response. In this case, memory is not required. The child must copy from a board or a book with the information remaining in front of him or her. Some youngsters will have great difficulty making use of visual configurational data and the act of writing. They are likely to have trouble copying quickly and accurately in school.
6. Verbal-motor dyspraxia is found in students who appear to have tremendous difficulty listening and writing at the same time. They may experience extreme agony in trying to take notes in high school or in college. Some of these youngsters have underlying language problems. Others have difficulty with immediate verbal memory or active working memory. In many cases, they are students with good language and memory abilities who simply are unable to integrate verbal inputs with motor responses.
7. Pseudomotor dysfunction is encountered in children whose ideational fluency far exceeds the normal capacity of their fingers to transcribe thoughts on paper. Sometimes these students have excellent verbal abilities, fertile imaginations, and notable verbal fluency. Graphomotor output simply cannot keep pace with the accelerated rate of their thought processes. Sometimes these children exhibit stammering or stuttering during their preschool and early elementary school years. This, too, is a manifestation of a disparity between rapid ideational fluency and relatively slow motor (i.e., oromotor) speed. When they are able to decelerate their thought processes, both articulation and writing are likely to improve substantially.
8. Sometimes graphomotor abilities are compromised by functional undermining. In this case, one or more of the nonmotor components of writing are siphoning so much effort that motor precision is compromised. If a student has to struggle inordinately with the simultaneous memory demands of writing (as described previously in this chapter), letter formation may be secondarily compromised. That same student may be able to write a list of words legibly, that is, when he or she does not have to deal with multiple other simultaneous demands.

A student with a writing disability may suffer from one or more of the eight basic graphomotor dysfunctions. Many such students excel at fine motor activities that do not involve writing. Thus, a child with a procedural memory dyspraxia or with finger agnosia may be an excellent artist or mechanic despite difficulties with writing. Alternatively, a student may have eye-hand coordination problems but good motor memory and nonvisual finger localization. Such a child may be excellent at writing but clumsy or awkward when it comes to artistic endeavors, building a model, fixing things, or working with a computer.

Some children harbor underlying gross motor dysfunctions with or without fine motor or graphomotor incoordination. They may exhibit generalized gross motor delays or highly specific deficits (Sugden and Keogh, 1990). Some cannot program accurate motor responses based on the processing of certain kinds of input data. For example, some of them have difficulty using visual-spatial information to guide their gross motor actions. Consequently, they are inept at catching or throwing a ball. They simply do not make accurate judgments or estimates about trajectories in space. Others are poor at using "inner spatial" data, so they have trouble interpreting proprioceptive and kinesthetic information emanating from their muscles and joints. They are said to be lacking in body position sense, an impairment that compromises activities requiring balance and keen awareness of one's body movements. Still other children show evidence of a gross motor dyspraxia and have trouble implementing complex motor procedures demanding precise mobilization of specific muscle groups. They may be slow at acquiring skills for swimming, gymnastics, and dancing. Closely related to this phenomenon is one in which children cannot master gross motor sequences. They have trouble forming, automatizing, and sustaining complex rhythms.

Children with gross motor problems are at risk. Many of them suffer a significant loss of self-esteem, and their feelings of inadequacy erode self-concept (Shaw et al, 1982). They may incur considerable embarrassment in physical education classes. Their gross motor dysfunctions result in specific athletic disabilities, which in turn can become handicaps when they perpetuate social rejection or withdrawal.

Children who exhibit motor strengths have access to some valuable modes of gratification in life. Students who have academic disabilities and motor talents can use the latter to preserve their self-esteem while struggling with coursework. Motor competency can also enable a child to feel efficacious artistically as well as in the mechanical/spatial realm.

Higher Order Cognition

Higher order cognition is composed of a range of sophisticated thinking skills. Among the functions subsumed under this category of neurodevelopmental function are concept acquisition, systematic decision making, evaluative thinking, brainstorming (including creativity), and rule usage.

Children vary considerably in their capacities to understand the conceptual bases of skills and content areas in school. Concepts are groupings of ideas that somehow fit together. For example, the concept of furniture includes tables, chairs, beds, and bookcases. As students progress through their education, the concepts they encounter become increasingly abstract and complex. New concepts often contain preexisting concepts, and students are continually adding new elements to preexisting conceptual frameworks. Over time, they can identify perfect prototypes of a concept as well as imperfect prototypes of that concept, and they become increasingly able to distinguish between an idea that fits a concept and one that is beyond the realm of that concept. Such conceptual ability is critical for truly in-depth learning. Unfortunately, some students acquire only a tenuous grasp of concepts. Those who hold such chronically tenuous grasps are most likely ultimately to underachieve. Some of them may exhibit pervasively weak grasps, whereas others may have difficulty with conceptual grasps in circumscribed domains (such as mathematics, social studies, and science). There are students who much prefer to conceptualize verbally, whereas others are more comfortable forming concepts without the interposition of language. Many of the best students try to portray or to ponder concepts both verbally and nonverbally. Some students have serious trouble mastering abstract concepts. They tend to be overly concrete. Such a student may struggle to assimilate concepts such as liberalism, internal combustion, or equation.

Systematic decision making is an important part of mathematics as well as of virtually every other content area in school. Students with well-developed systematic decision skills are keen strategists. They are generally excellent at previewing or estimating answers, thinking about multiple alternative techniques to solve a problem, selecting the best technique, and monitoring what they are doing while they are doing it (Bloom and Broder, 1950). Poor decision makers, on the other hand, tend to be rigid, unsystematic, or impulsive. They often mismatch time allocation to the task at hand, either allowing too much or too insufficient time for problem solving. They fail to consider alternative strategic approaches, instead irreversibly committing themselves to an initial approach whether or not it is working. These students may encounter significant problems in coursework requiring the choice of appropriate strategies and flexible thinking.

Brainstorming gets activated whenever a student has to derive a topic for a report, think about the best way to fashion a project, or deal with myriad other open-ended academic and nonacademic challenges. Some children have difficulty generating original ideas. They much prefer to be told exactly what to do. They would always rather comply than innovate. They balk at having to choose a topic, speculate, develop an argument, or think freely and independently. They have trouble confronting a blank page and generating the ideas to fill it.

Making use of their *evaluative thinking,* successful students often demonstrate keen abilities to evaluate issues, products, and people (including, it is hoped, themselves), deploying objective criteria in doing so. They are able to tease out their own personal biases and the viewpoints of others. They are effective in comparing and contrasting their values and views with those of an author. They can think about and talk about the qualities of a person. They become adept at assembling criteria to judge the products they see in a store or on television. But some students are notably weak in their evaluative thinking. They have difficulty analyzing issues, developing arguments, and evaluating ideas. This can be especially handicapping in subjects (such as social studies) that often demand critical reading and analytical abilities.

Students adept at *rule usage* are sensitive to regularity and irregularity. They are able to develop their own rules based on consistent judgments or observations they have made. When two phenomena are seen as invariably associated, they may adhere as a rule in the mind of a student. Rules generally assume the configuration of "if . . . then." Students who are quick to discover rules are likely to have the learning process greatly facilitated for them. A student may come to notice that every time he or she encounters the name of a city in a book, it is capitalized. Such a student may discern this regularity before the formal rules of capitalization are explained by a teacher. In addition to being able to discern regularities or rules, students must understand and apply the rules they are taught. For some children, rules are appealingly logical. Some even crave rule-based learning. Others experience agonizing frustration in subjects that demand substantial rule application. Somehow grammatical rules, mathematical rules, and foreign language rules fail to clarify phenomena for them.

It should be clear that a student's strengths in any of these higher cognitive functions can go far to bypass weaknesses in other domains. Someone who is excellent at conceptualizing may not need to process or to memorize verbal material as thoroughly as a learner who is weak at conceptualizing. The strong conceptualizer does not need to rely as much on rote memory as does the student who has a poor or tenuous grasp of concepts. Similarly, systematic decision making ability, brainstorming effectiveness, metacognition, and rule usage can be facilitators of learning and academic productivity. They, too, can enable a student to bypass weaknesses in other neurodevelopmental areas. On the other hand, a student with higher cognitive weaknesses as part of a cluster of neurodevelopmental dysfunction is at a distinct disadvantage academically.

Social Cognition

A student's social abilities are stringently tested throughout the school day. There exists a discrete neurodevelopmental function of social cognition. Some children are extremely adept in their social cognitive abilities, whereas others exhibit debilitating social skill deficits. Social skill variations are discussed in detail in Chapter 38. An account of a child's social abilities is a critical component of any complete description of his or her neurodevelopmental profile.

ACADEMIC IMPACTS

The neurodevelopmental functions enumerated here are represented in varying clusters (of strengths and of weaknesses) within individual children. In fact, there are so many different combinations of dysfunctions operating in such diverse environmental and cultural contexts that an endless variety of performance and behavioral patterns is encountered. This heterogeneity constitutes further justification for avoiding the simplistic labeling or pigeonholing of struggling school-age children. Clusters of neurodevelopmental dysfunctions commonly result in academic delays, most conspicuously in the basic skills of reading, spelling, writing, and mathematics.

Reading

Reading can be significantly impaired in a child who struggles with language processing, especially at the phonologic and semantic levels. Problems with sentence comprehension and discourse likewise can thwart reading comprehension, especially as the demands for understanding complex text intensify through secondary school. Attention and various forms of memory also exert their influences, as students have to ferret out key details and recall the relevant contents of the top of the page while reading its last several lines so as to splice together the overall meaning (active working memory).

Spelling

Language also plays a pivotal role in the acquisition of accurate spelling abilities. Students with serious phonologic or semantic deficits are likely to be poor spellers. Weak spelling can also be found in those who have problems with pattern recognition, visualization, or rule application.

Writing

Written output demands the integration of multiple neurodevelopmental functions, including graphomotor skill, retrieval memory (for spelling, rules, facts, letter formation), expressive language, higher order cognition (to generate rich thoughts), and organizational abilities. A shortfall in any one of these areas can compromise writing and lead to "output failure," often accompanied by a recurring refusal to do homework.

Mathematics

Mathematics calls for its unique blend of neurodevelopmental functions. Some children fail in this area because they lack the long-term memory needed to recall math facts automatically and precisely; others have trouble with procedural memory (e.g., recalling the steps in long division). Math difficulties also ensue in the presence of weak pattern recognition or poor active working memory. Language also is a key player in math, and there are children who have trouble with the complicated semantics of the subject as well as difficulty at the sentence level (so important in word problems and in processing a teacher's verbal explanations). Some students encounter problems because they have trouble visualizing while solving word problems and grasping the spatial elements in mathematics (such as in measurement and in geometry). Finally, math demands a substantial level of attention to detail and prolonged focusing, which may cause children with attentional dysfunction to founder.

NONACADEMIC IMPACTS

In some instances, children with neurodevelopmental dysfunctions harbor excessive performance anxiety, overt clinical depression, or both. Sadness, self-deprecatory comments, diminished self-esteem, chronic fatigue, loss of interests, and sometimes even suicidal ideation may set in. Not uncommonly, children with neurodevelopmental dysfunctions lose motivation. As a result of their repeated failures, they harbor a diminished sense of self-efficacy (Schunk, 1991) and come to feel that it is futile to expend effort.

Many studies have documented a relationship between learning disorders of various types and juvenile delinquency. The so-called JD-LD link can occur on many levels. Highly impulsive children may be more likely to commit crimes. Those who experience excessive academic failure and embarrassment may feel a need to engage in "macho" acts aimed at impressing a peer group because they are unable to acquire respect through other means.

There is an intimate association between language dysfunctions and delinquent behavior. In some instances,

Vignette

At age 12, Joel, a sixth grader, became increasingly difficult for his parents and teachers to handle. He was starting to act out in school and failing to hand in assignments in English, social studies, and mathematics. His father and his English teacher insisted that Joel was a slacker, just plain lazy. A school social worker decided he had "oppositional defiant disorder."

Joel was interested only in his small gaggle of friends and his array of video games. He insisted that he could not stand school. This boy was a very good reader, although he seldom read independently. Joel would come alive during class discussions, as he has strong opinions that were eloquently stated; his verbal fluency is a prized asset. But he had problems in math since third grade; by sixth grade, he still did not know his math facts. Whenever he would seem to have mastered them, he would go on to forget them almost entirely. However, Joel's greatest academic difficulties were seen when he had to write; he despised writing in any form. Although he was able to copy from the board, Joel could not or would not tackle written reports or stories. He became overwhelmed when he tried to do so. Joel was able to spell words accurately on a spelling quiz but then would misspell the same words in a paragraph. He also had trouble recalling rules of punctuation and retrieving facts he needed in an essay. There was a gaping disparity between the wealth of Joel's ideas in a class discussion and the impoverished thoughts he could transcribe on paper. His writing was reminiscent of that of a second- or third-grade student.

Joel was evaluated by a team including a developmental-behavioral pediatrician, a psychologist, and an educational diagnostician. After history taking, testing, and careful examination of work samples, all concurred that this boy was having serious problems with recall from long-term memory, especially when he had to deploy this function rapidly with precision and also when he had to engage in simultaneous recall (as during writing). Joel revealed abundant strengths, especially in the language, spatial ordering, and social domains.

Joel was demystified so he could understand his difficulties as well as his strengths. He was taught various mnemonic strategies and encouraged to do his writing in stages, first brainstorming over a tape recorder and then using a step-by-step approach toward a finished product. After that, Joel showed steady improvement in writing, although mathematics remained a challenge for him. Joel was not labeled by the clinical team or his school. There was a marked change in Joel's moods, and he seemed motivated. He told his parents he was thinking of becoming a journalist.

a child or adolescent may commit antisocial acts simply because he or she cannot control circumstances verbally; more physical means then come forth. It is unlikely that learning disorders actually cause juvenile delinquency. On the other hand, they certainly represent risk factors that may be actuated, especially amid depriving or stressful environmental circumstances.

ASSESSMENT

Children with possible manifestations of neurodevelopmental dysfunction require meticulous multidisciplinary evaluations based on differential diagnoses appropriate for chronologic age and grade level. It is unlikely that any single professional can assess adequately the diverse sources and broad effects of academic underachievement. An optimal evaluation team should consist of a pediatrician or nurse, a psychologist or psychiatrist, and a psychoeducational specialist. The last should be either a special educator or an educational psychologist who can undertake a fine-grained analysis of academic skills and subskills. Other professionals can become involved as needed in individual cases. These additional clinicians might include a speech and language pathologist, an occupational therapist, a pediatric neurologist, and a social worker. The exact composition of teams and additional consultants depends largely on local needs and accessible resources in the school and in the community.

Many children undergo evaluations within a school setting. Such assessments are an entitlement in the United States under Public Law 94-142. Multidisciplinary evaluations conducted in schools are usually very helpful and are a requirement if a child is to qualify for special services. However, evaluations in school are susceptible to some biases or conflicts of interest. Available therapeutic resources, rigid regulations, and funding constraints may unduly influence the outcome of a school-based evaluation. Because of such limitations, there has been a growing demand for independent evaluations, for second opinions outside of the school. Pediatricians are often asked to become involved in such independent evaluations.

Commonly, children are determined to be eligible for services if they exhibit a significant discrepancy between IQ test results and achievement test scores. Such a discrepancy is interpreted as an indication of "learning disability." Unfortunately, with use of this paradigm, many students with dysfunctions "fall through the cracks" and are deemed ineligible for services in school. Certain clusters of neurodevelopmental dysfunctions may fail to create a sufficient disparity between an IQ result and an achievement test score. Clinicians need to be aware of those students who have significant neurodevelopmental dysfunctions and yet are turned down for help or accommodations in school.

The Pediatric Role

The pediatrician can play a prominent role in the evaluation and follow-up of a child with suspected neurodevelopmental dysfunctions. Any initial assessment ought to include a complete physical, neurologic, and sensory examination. Associated medical issues, such as allergies, sleep difficulties, neurologic disorders, delayed or precocious puberty, and depression, need to be ruled out.

Standardized questionnaires can be used by pediatricians to obtain historical data from the school, the parents, and even the child. Several pediatric neurodevelopmental examinations exist for those clinicians who wish to make direct observations of neurodevelopmental function. These examinations include the PEET, the PEER, the PEEX 2, and the PEERAMID 2. They allow pediatricians or other clinicians to observe or to sample directly key neurodevelopmental functions, such as attention, memory, language, and motor skills. Examinations of this type also permit direct behavioral observations as well as assessments of minor neurologic indicators (sometimes called soft signs) frequently associated with certain neurodevelopmental dysfunctions. These indicators include associated movements or synkinesias.

Additional Assessment Components

Intelligence testing can be helpful. Although an overall IQ may be misleading, the results of specific subtests often are helpful in providing evidence for one or more specific neurodevelopmental dysfunctions. Psychoeducational testing can yield highly relevant data, especially when such testing includes error analyses that pinpoint discrete breakdowns in reading, spelling, writing, and mathematics (see Chapter 82). A psychoeducational specialist, making use of input from multiple sources, can help formulate specific recommendations for regular and special educational teachers.

A mental health professional is valuable in identifying family-based issues complicating or aggravating neurodevelopmental dysfunctions. That professional also can diagnose any specific psychiatric condition contributing to the clinical picture in a child with academic problems.

Other "à la carte" assessments may be called for in individual cases. These would include a more detailed assessment from a speech and language pathologist, a social worker, a pediatric neurologist, or an occupational therapist.

MANAGEMENT

Just as assessment demands a multidisciplinary approach, the management of children with neurodevelopmental dysfunctions necessitates multimodal intervention. Most children with neurodevelopmental dysfunctions require at least several of the following 10 forms of intervention.

Demystification

Most children with neurodevelopmental dysfunctions have little or no understanding of the nature or sources of their difficulties. Once an appropriate descriptive assessment has been performed, it is especially important to explain a child's dysfunctions and strengths to that child. This explanation should be provided in nontechnical, optimistic, concrete, and nonaccusatory terms. Children can also be given an opportunity to read about neurodevelopmental dysfunction in its varied forms (Levine, 1990, 1994; Levine and Clutch, 2001). Parents and teachers also need to become knowledgeable (Levine, 2001).

Table 55-4. General Forms of Bypass Strategy Used in the Management of Children with Neurodevelopmental Dysfunctions

Form	Description or Examples
Rate adjustment	Allowing a child more time on a test or a longer interval to answer a question or presenting instructions and explanations more slowly
Volume adjustment	Reducing the length of a report or number of items on a test
Complexity adjustment; prioritizing	Simplifying directions or explanations; stressing or grading on fewer task components (such as ignoring spelling errors and emphasizing good ideas in a report)
Staging	Performing tasks in specific prescribed steps
Format shift	Presenting information in a child's strong learning mode (e.g., visually demonstrating a mathematical process to a child with a language dysfunction)
Affinity use	Teaching skills with materials that tap a child's interests or areas of expertise
Curriculum change	Selecting courses that do not overload a child's weak functions (e.g., avoiding too many memory-laden subjects at once)
Device use	Using a word processor, calculator, dictionary

Bypass Strategies (Accommodations)

Numerous techniques can enable a child to circumvent neurodevelopmental dysfunctions. Such bypass strategies should ordinarily be encouraged in the regular classroom; individualized intervention in other settings is aimed at strengthening deficient functions. The general forms of bypass are summarized in Table 55-4. Examples of specific bypass strategies include using a calculator while solving mathematics problems, writing essays with a word processor, presenting oral instead of written reports, assigning fewer mathematics problems, seating a child close to the teacher to minimize distraction, offering visually presented demonstration models of correctly solved math problems, and granting permission for a student to take scholastic aptitude tests (SATs) untimed or with extended time. These bypass strategies do not "cure" neurodevelopmental dysfunctions, but they minimize their academic and nonacademic impacts.

Remediation of Skills and Subskills

Tutorial programs are commonly used to bolster deficient academic skills. Reading specialists, math tutors, and other such professionals can make use of diagnostic data to select techniques that take advantage of a student's neurodevelopmental strengths and content affinities in an effort to improve decoding skills, writing ability, or mathematical computation. Remediation often takes place in a resource room or learning center at school. Remediation need not focus exclusively on specific academic areas. Many students need assistance to acquire study skills, cognitive strategies, and organizational habits.

Developmental Therapies

Considerable controversy exists regarding the efficacy of treatments to enhance weak neurodevelopmental functions. It has not been demonstrated convincingly that it is possible to improve substantially a child's graphomotor skills, active working memory, problem solving proficiency, or temporal-sequential ordering abilities. Nevertheless, some modes of developmental therapy are widely accepted. Speech and language pathologists commonly offer intervention for children with language dysfunctions. Occupational therapists strive to improve the motor skills of certain students with writing problems or gross motor clumsiness. Recently, there has been considerable interest in social skills training that usually takes the form of small group sessions in which school-age children are helped to become more aware of the dynamics of social interaction. Coaching has become another promising option for intervention. Students receive ongoing advice on their approaches to tasks as well as their plans for the future; they learn to think strategically while getting to know their own best ways of learning.

Curriculum Modification

Many students with neurodevelopmental dysfunction require alterations in the school curriculum. For example, high-school students with memory weaknesses may need to have their courses selected so that they do not have to contend with a cumulative memory overload in any one semester. The timing of a foreign language, the selection of a mathematics curriculum, and the choice of science courses are critical issues for many underachieving students.

Asset Management

In all cases, students with neurodevelopmental dysfunctions need to have their affinities and potential or actual talents identified and enhanced. It is more important to strengthen strengths than it is to remediate deficiencies. Athletic skills, artistic inclinations, leadership abilities, creative talents, or mechanical aptitudes are among the potential assets of certain students who are underachieving academically. Parents and school personnel need to create opportunities for such students to build on these proclivities and to savor respect and praise for their efforts. The strengthening of strengths is essential for preserving self-esteem and motivation.

Individual and Family Counseling

When learning difficulties are complicated by family problems or identifiable psychiatric disorders, psychotherapy may be indicated. Clinical psychologists or child psychiatrists are able to offer long-term or short-term therapies. Such interventions can involve the child alone, an entire family, or a small group of children with similar problems. It is essential that a therapist have a firm understanding of a child's neurodevelopmental dysfunctions. The parents and a child can become seriously confused if a psychotherapist attributes the child's learning difficulties exclusively to environmental factors, thereby ignoring the potent influence of underlying dysfunctions of attention, language, or memory. Most families do not require a heavily psychoanalytical or psychodynamic approach but instead can benefit from a counseling program that offers practical advice on behavioral management.

Advocacy

Children with developmental dysfunctions require informed advocacy. They must have their rights upheld in the school, in the family, and in the community. A physician can be especially helpful in advocating for a child in school. Some children, for example, are devastated by retention in a grade. The likelihood of benefit is minimal. A physician may need to represent the rights of a child in opposing such grade retention as well as other acts of public humiliation. A physician may also need to advocate strongly for a child to receive services in school or to benefit from modifications in the curriculum. Physicians can also advocate by becoming vocal citizens of their communities. Serving on a school board, for example, a physician can exert a major influence on local policy and on the allocation of resources to school-age children with special educational needs.

Medication

Certain psychopharmacologic agents can be especially helpful in lessening the toll of neurodevelopmental dysfunctions. Most commonly, stimulant medications are used as part of the management of attention deficits. They are never a panacea because most children with attention deficits have other associated dysfunctions (such as language disorders, memory problems, motor weaknesses, or social skill deficits). Nevertheless, the use of medications such as methylphenidate (Concerta), amphetamines (Adderall), atomoxetine (Strattera), and dexmethylphenidate (Focalin) can be an important adjunct to treatment because they seem to help certain youngsters focus more selectively and control their impulsivity. When depression or excessive anxiety is a significant component of the clinical picture, antidepressants can be prescribed. Pharmacotherapy is discussed in greater detail in Chapter 90. Children receiving medication need regular follow-up visits that include a review of current behavioral checklists, a physical examination, and appropriate modifications of medication dose. Treated children should be given periodic "medication holidays," drug-free intervals so that they can strive to be in control of themselves.

Longitudinal Case Management

All children with neurodevelopmental dysfunctions can benefit from the support and guidance of a service coordinator, a professional who can offer advice in a continuing manner and be available to monitor function over the years. The pediatrician may be an ideal professional to assume this responsibility. With time, new questions inevitably emerge, as a child's neurodevelopmental dysfunctions evolve while academic expectations undergo progressive change. Because children with neurodevelopmental dysfunctions represent such a heterogeneous group, no two call for identical management plans. Nor is it possible to predict with certainty at age 7 what the needs of a youngster will be when he or she is 14. Consequently, affected children and their families require vigilant follow-up plus individualized, objective advice and informed advocacy throughout their years in school. They can also benefit from discussion of a child's eventual career directions (Levine, 2005).

SUMMARY

Many children and adolescents face chronic frustration in school because they harbor subtle differences in learning. When properly evaluated, they are found to have one or more neurodevelopmental dysfunctions. These specific weaknesses, in such areas as attention, memory, language, or spatial ordering, may interfere with the acquisition of traditional academic skills and may compromise seriously a child's overall academic productivity. In addition, when unrecognized and improperly managed, the dysfunctions can result in behavior problems, low self-esteem, affective disorders, and delinquent tendencies. Pediatricians can play a role as an integral part of a team, helping to elucidate and manage these dysfunctions while uncovering contributing medical problems and complications. The pediatrician also can help "demystify" affected children and their parents, so that they can understand their issues. As well, a pediatrician can be vital in providing long-term follow-up care for these differences in learning.

REFERENCES

Biemiller A: Size and sequence in vocabulary development: Implications for choosing words for primary grade vocabulary instruction. *In* Hiebert A, Kamil M (eds): Teaching and Learning Vocabulary: Bringing Research to Practice. Mahwah, NJ, Erlbaum, 2005.

Bloom BS, Broder L: Problem Solving Processes of College Students. Chicago, University of Chicago Press, 1950.

Bradley R, Danielson L, Hallahan DP (eds.): Identification of Learning Disabilities: From Research to Practice. Mahwah, NJ, Erlbaum, 2002.

Clemens Z, Fabo D, Halasz P: Overnight verbal memory retention correlated with the number of sleep spindles. Neuroscience 132:529, 2005.

Denckla M: Motor coordination in dyslexic children: Theoretical and clinical implications. *In* Duffy FH, Geschwind N (eds): Dyslexia: A Neuroscientific Approach to Clinical Evaluation. Boston, Little, Brown, 1985, p 187.

Fletcher JM, Francis DJ, Morris RD, Lyon GR: Evidence-based assessment of learning disabilities in children and adolescents. J Clin Child Adolesc Psychol 34:506, 2005.

Levine MD: Attention and memory: Progression and variation during the elementary school years. Pediatr Ann 18:366, 1981.

†Levine MD: Keeping a Head in School: A Student's Book About Learning Abilities and Learning Disorders. Cambridge, MA, Educators Publishing Service, 1990.

†Levine MD: All Kinds of Minds. Cambridge, MA, Educators Publishing Service, 1994.

*Levine MD: Educational Care, 2nd ed. Cambridge, MA, Educators Publishing Service, 2001.

*Levine MD: A Mind at a Time. New York, Simon & Schuster, 2002.

*Levine MD: The Myth of Laziness. New York, Simon & Schuster, 2003.

*Levine MD: Ready or Not, Here Life Comes. New York, Simon & Schuster, 2005.

†Levine MD, Clutch J: Jarvis Clutch—Social Spy. Cambridge, MA, Educators Publishing Service, 2001.

Levine MD, Reed M: Developmental Variation and Learning Disorders, 2nd ed. Cambridge, MA, Educators Publishing Service, 1998.

Levine MD, Karnisky W, Palfrey J, et al: Risk factor complexes in early adolescent delinquents. Am J Dis Child 139:50, 1985.

Marshuetz C: Order information in working memory: An integrated review of evidence from brain and behavior. Psychol Bull 131:323, 2005.

Meltzer L: Strategic learning in children with learning disabilities. Adv Learn Behav Disabil 108:181, 1996.

Nelson K: Language in Cognitive Development. Cambridge, England, Cambridge University Press, 1996.

*Paul R: Language Disorders from Infancy Through Adolescence: Assessment and Intervention, 2nd ed. St. Louis, Mosby–Year Book, 2001.

Runge TJ, Watkins MW: The structure of phonological awareness among kindergarten students. School Psychol Rev 35:370, 2006.

Schunk DH: Self efficacy and academic motivation. Educational Psychologist 26:207, 1991.

Shaw L, Levine MD, Belfer M: Developmental double jeopardy: A study of clumsiness and self-esteem in learning disabled children. J Dev Behav Pediatr 4:191, 1982.

Sugden DA, Keogh JF: Problems in Motor Skill Development. Columbia, SC, University of South Carolina Press, 1990.

Swanson HL, Cooney JB: Learning disabilities and memory. *In* Reid DK, Hresko WP, Swanson HL (eds): Cognitive Approaches to Learning Disabilities, 3rd ed. Austin, TX, PRO-ED, 1996.

Torgeson JK: Memory processes in reading disabled children. J Learn Disabil 18:350, 1985.

Vallar G, Papagno C: Neuropsychological impairments of short-term memory. *In* Baddeley AD, Wilson BA, Watts FN (eds): Handbook of Memory Disorders. New York, John Wiley, 1995.

Van Garderen D: Spatial visualization, visual imagery, and mathematical problem solving of students with varying abilities. J Learn Disabil 29:496, 2006.

Weinert FE, Perlmutter M: Memory Development: Universal Changes and Individual Differences. Hillsdale, NJ, Erlbaum, 1988.

*These books can be recommended for reading by parents.
†These books are intended for children.

Part VII OUTCOMES—PHYSICAL FUNCTIONING

56 RECURRENT AND CHRONIC PAIN

Tonya M. Palermo and Lonnie K. Zeltzer

Vignette

Ashley is a 16-year-old girl with chronic daily headaches that have been nonresponsive to prophylactic migraine medications. Ashley misses several days of school each week and is no longer participating in competitive sports. She is also spending less time with peers. Ashley has developed a significant sleep disturbance in which it is taking her several hours to fall asleep at bedtime. She feels ineffective in her ability to manage headaches and holds a belief that she cannot participate in school and other important daily activities when she has head pain. Her parents feel overwhelmed by worry about her health and well-being.

An estimated 15% to 25% of children and adolescents suffer with recurrent and chronic pain conditions (Perquin et al, 2000; Roth-Isigkeit et al, 2005). These conditions may be part of an underlying chronic medical condition, or the pain itself may be the primary problem. A variety of recurrent and chronic pain conditions are commonly seen in pediatric offices and clinics. Evaluation and management of these conditions can present challenges for the pediatrician because of the unclear etiology, the fact that sensible treatments often fail, and the high level of child and family distress. In this chapter, we review the significance of recurrent and chronic pain for children, adolescents, and their families; the etiology and natural history of recurrent and chronic pain problems; and evaluation and management approaches.

TERMS AND DEFINITIONS

Chronic pain may or may not be symptomatic of underlying, ongoing tissue damage or chronic disease. It can persist long after an initial injury has healed or other event has occurred (typically longer than 3 months) and no longer serves a useful warning function. Children may experience pain related to conditions such as arthritis, cancer, nerve damage, and Crohn disease. Cancer-related pain and pain associated with life-limiting medical conditions, as in end-stage diseases, are other forms of serious chronic pain. Chronic and recurrent pain may be the problem itself, as in Ashley's case, without underlying, clearly identifiable metabolic, structural, inflammatory, or degenerative etiology, as in pain associated with functional dysregulation syndromes, including irritable bowel syndrome, chronic daily headaches, musculoskeletal pain, and complex regional pain syndrome.

SIGNIFICANCE OF RECURRENT AND CHRONIC PAIN

Chronic and recurrent pain is commonly experienced by children and adolescents. One population-based study reported a pain prevalence of 54% in youth aged 0 to 18 years, with a quarter of the respondents reporting chronic pain lasting more than 3 months (Perquin et al, 2000). The most commonly reported locations of pain are the head, abdomen, and limbs (Perquin et al, 2000). Girls tend to have more complaints of recurrent and chronic pain than do boys, and pain complaints peak between 12 and 15 years of age.

Impact on Children and Families

Recurrent and chronic pain can have a major impact on the daily lives of children, adolescents, and their families. Whereas some children experiencing pain symptoms develop minimal day-to-day impairment, other children with pain symptoms develop psychosocial difficulties, academic problems, peer and family disruptions, and anxiety and depression. The children who seek treatment for their chronic pain symptoms probably represent the group that is experiencing the most impairment. Unexplained chronic pain in adolescents has been associated with poor quality of life for the adolescent and his or her family (Hunfeld et al, 2001).

Disability that results from chronic pain is a separate concept from pain itself and equally important to consider in assessment and management of pediatric pain patients (Palermo, 2000). Disability refers to those areas in an individual's life that are limited by pain (i.e., the things that a person cannot do because of pain) (Walker and Greene, 1991). The domains of functioning that seem to be particularly affected by chronic pain are school and academics, participation in physical and social activities, sleep, and family functioning (Palermo, 2000). Missed schooling can have direct effects on academic performance and school success as well as important effects on socialization and maintenance of peer relationships. The majority of children with unexplained chronic pain also suffer impairment in sports activities and social functioning.

Persistent pain can also have a substantial impact on the emotional status of children and adolescents. In general, children with recurrent pain experience more stress and feel less cheerful and more depressed compared with children without pain (Langeveld et al, 1996). Chronic pain does appear to be associated with psychiatric comorbidity, particularly anxiety and mood disorders, at least in some selected populations. For example, in a sample of children seen in primary care for recurrent abdominal pain, 79% of children met criteria for an anxiety disorder and 43% for a depressive disorder (Campo et al, 2004). Pain can also interfere with the quality and quantity of children's sleep, and in turn, sleep deprivation can reduce children's ability to cope with pain and enhance pain sensitivity. More than half of children and adolescents with chronic pain report sleep difficulties (Roth-Isigkeit et al, 2005). These problems typically include difficulty initiating sleep, difficulty maintaining sleep, and early morning awakening.

Chronic pain can have a negative impact on family life, including increased restrictions on parental socialization, high parental stress levels, anger, and hostility. Parents also experience the financial burden of evaluation and management of recurrent and chronic pain, including direct costs of pain treatment such as hospitalization, visits to physicians, and costs of medications. Indirect costs include parental time off work, transportation costs, childcare, and incidental costs (Sleed et al, 2005).

ETIOLOGY OF CHRONIC PAIN

A number of models that fall under biobehavioral or biopsychosocial frameworks have been developed to understand children's recurrent and chronic pain. Central to these models are interrelationships among physical, cognitive, affective, and social factors that influence children's pain and disability. Sex and age differences have emerged in children's symptom reporting and development of endogenous pains. For example, in nonreferred samples, girls generally report higher pain intensity, longer lasting pain, and more frequent pain than do boys (Perquin et al, 2000). There is an increased prevalence of several pain problems in girls compared with boys, especially after puberty. For example, adolescents treated for complex regional pain syndrome, fibromyalgia, and migraine headaches are much more likely to be girls.

There are central nervous system pain mechanisms that may play a role in the persistence of pain. For example, in understanding functional bowel disorders, current theories suggest that the pain or symptoms are caused by abnormal brain-intestinal neural signaling that creates intestinal or visceral hypersensitivity. Abdominal pain is thought to be brought on by visceral hyperalgesia, which may be caused by alterations in the sensory receptors of the gastrointestinal tract, abnormal modulation of sensory transmissions in the peripheral or central nervous system, or changes in the cortical perception of afferent signals (Drossman, 2005). Modern imaging techniques have also identified a central neural circuitry contributing to maintenance of pain and the degeneration of certain pain inhibitory systems with persistent pain states, as found in adult fibromyalgia (Borsook and Becerra, 2006).

In considering etiologic factors in children's pain-related disability, a variety of factors have been conceptualized to play a role, including children's coping, anxiety and depressive symptoms, and family reinforcement of pain behavior (Palermo, 2000). Identification of factors that predict disability related to pain is an active area of pediatric pain research, particularly because many of these factors represent areas that can be directly targeted in behavioral interventions. Familial factors have been identified as potentially important in the etiology of pain-related disability, including parental responses to the child's pain (Palermo and Chambers, 2005; Walker et al, 1993). Positive behaviors demonstrated by a parent can be related to better child coping behaviors, whereas solicitous or overly reinforcing responses to the child's pain can be related to increased child functional impairment.

NATURAL HISTORY AND COURSE OF PAIN

Despite the tendency of physicians to reassure parents that their child will "outgrow" recurrent pain complaints, the symptoms of many children with pain complaints persist. Although the overall base of knowledge of the natural history and course of pain is limited, the data that are available suggest that early exposure to pain may alter later pain response, that initial pain complaints often persist over time or may occur in another part of the body, or that other somatic symptoms may develop in the child.

Early and prolonged exposure to pain might alter later stress response, pain systems, and behavior and learning in childhood. There is some evidence that children who undergo pain or tissue damage as neonates may have increased pain sensitivity later in childhood (Peters et al, 2005). This finding has important implications for the long-term care of these patients because they may be more likely to develop problems with chronic pain in later life.

In short-term follow-up studies of children with chronic pain, a significant number of children are found to have continuing complaints of pain during 1- to 2-year follow-up periods (Perquin et al, 2003). Children whose pain persists over time are reported to have more emotional problems; and depressive symptoms have predicted generalization of pain from one localized site (i.e., neck pain) to widespread pain at follow-up (Mikkelsson et al, 1999).

Long-term outcome studies suggest that children who present with chronic abdominal or headache pain continue into adulthood with chronic pain and physical and psychiatric complaints (Fearon and Hotopf, 2001). Children whose chronic pain limits their functioning may develop lifelong problems with pain and disability. It is unknown whether medical and psychological treatments alter these long-term outcomes.

EVALUATION

The evaluation of the child with recurrent or chronic pain complaints often falls on the office-based pediatric practitioner. All children with chronic pain that is interfering with functioning in day-to-day life can benefit from attention to the psychosocial as well as the biomedical aspects of their pain. Evaluation and management of these problems can be complex and time-consuming. Physicians often fear that they are missing an organic explanation, despite lengthy, expensive, and sometimes invasive workups. It can be difficult to identify the red flags in the history, physical, and laboratory investigations that may suggest additional investigation is needed. Table 56-1 presents an overview of diagnosis and management strategies, with use of abdominal pain as an example. There are no standard laboratory tests that are recommended for evaluation of chronic pain conditions. Rather, a comprehensive evaluation focused on identification of any comorbidity, such as anxiety disorder, depression, or pervasive developmental disorder, somatic, and psychosocial contributors is needed.

The initial evaluation and explanation to the child and family are important and set the stage for effectively addressing the pain problem. A biopsychosocial framework is helpful in explaining to the family that all pain has physical and psychological contributors. Therefore, any comprehensive evaluation and treatment plan should address both. It is also important to communicate to the patient and family that success should be measured not just by pain relief but by improvement in function. Extra attention should be given to communicating sensitively with parents who will need to "buy into" the evaluation and treatment plan because they play a critical role in decreasing pain and improving function for their child. It is often helpful to describe pain as a neurobiologic system that can continue with circuitry in the brain even after the reason for the initiation of the pain has long been gone (hence reasons for lack of findings despite multiple tests). It can be explained that the best way to alter these neural pain matrices (pain patterns in the brain) is through physical action (e.g., going to school) and changes in emotion and thinking.

Clinical Evaluation of Pain

Clinical evaluation of pain includes assessment of the following: pain and pain history; other physical symptoms; physical, social, academic, family, emotional, and cognitive functioning; coping style and problem solving

Table 56-1. Evaluation and Treatment Strategies At-a-Glance

Evaluation

History: listen to patient and to parent; need time alone with adolescent
- Hear narrative about the pain and its related problems
- Identify psychological-developmental comorbidities
- Identify psychosocial contributors, such as child coping, family and school contributors

Physical examination: look at patient's appearance, posture; examine for areas of hypersensitivity, tender points in muscles and tendon insertion areas

Laboratory and radiographic testing: only tests needed, if not recently done, are complete blood cell count with differential, sedimentation rate, and urinalysis; only if history and examination combined suggest a specific potential diagnosis, such as hypothyroidism in a child presenting with chronic fatigue, should further testing be done

Treatment

Education of patient and family about the reasons for the pain, with use of language describing temporarily dysfunctional nerve signaling

Enhancement of coping skills and development of a plan for improvement of function
- Enhance sleep (good sleep hygiene; psychological and pharmacologic methods for sleep induction and maintenance)
- Cognitive-behavioral therapy, hypnotherapy, relaxation strategies, biofeedback
- Consider Iyengar yoga, physical therapy
- School re-entry plan and plan for increasing academic, social, and physical activities (use of behavioral incentives, desensitization, approximating increasing function in graded steps)
- Develop a plan for eating if a food/eating aversion or panic has developed

Somatic treatments: consider massage therapy, abdominal heat

Other treatments: acupuncture, art therapy, aromatherapy, music therapy, and other creative ways to enhance coping and to reduce stress

Medication

See Table 56-4

capacity; perceived stressors; major life events; and pain consequences. For example, using the case example of Ashley, evaluation of a child who presents with headaches includes assessment of all of these factors and should not be aimed just at "ruling out organic pathology." Parents presenting with a child suffering from headaches do not just want a diagnosis but want the clinician's help in reducing pain and suffering for their child.

Assessment of Pain

Accurate assessment of children's pain should include evaluation of quality, duration, frequency, intensity, and location of the pain as well as environmental variables that may affect pain and the impact of pain on children's functional status. When possible, asking children directly is the best way to learn about their pain. For older children and adolescents, numerical pain scales, such as 0 to 10 rating scales, will be appropriate; for younger children, faces rating scales, which depict pictures of faces with different gradations of pain, are useful to elicit children's self-reported pain intensity. It is also important to learn what factors make pain worse and what helps, temporal qualities, description of the pain experience, and what treatment strategies (including medication and nonpharmacologic treatment) have been tried and failed and what has helped. Pain diaries may be useful for obtaining estimates of the frequency and duration of pain as well as possible patterns (e.g., differences between school days and non–school days) and triggers (e.g., exams, performance stress). If a diary is to be used, it should be for a short time only to understand more about the pain so that the child does not focus on the pain for the purpose of recording it.

History and Physical Examination

The most productive way to initiate the history is to elicit the patient's narrative about the pain, rather than beginning with targeted questions. Further prompts about the pain can then be provided, according to the characteristics described before. The next part of the history should bring forth the ways in which the pain has interfered with functioning, including sleep (onset and maintenance), eating, school attendance and performance, and activities (physical, social, and family). Current and past treatments, both pharmacologic and nonpharmacologic, will also help direct understanding and planning for treatment of the pain. Inquiries into nontraditional treatments, such as acupuncture and herbs, are also important. Typically, a review of systems will reveal other areas of the body that are experienced as problematic by the child. For example, it is not uncommon for a child with headaches to also have abdominal pain or leg pains or somatic symptoms of anxiety, such as dizziness, shakiness, tightness in the throat, sweaty palms, feelings of being too hot or too cold, and other sympathetically mediated symptoms. Social and academic function can be assessed next. For example, inquiry about school can be initiated by an open-ended "so tell me about school" with further inquiry about grades, favorite and most difficult subjects, bullies at school, perceived teacher problems, and the like. Such questioning can point to both potential academic (e.g., isolated learning disability) and social difficulties that make school an ongoing stressor for the child. Social function is also important, with questioning about friendships, having a best friend, ability to spend the night away from home, and sexual relationships (for adolescents). Other than for very young children, there should be some time to obtain history from the child without the parent present. Physical activity and family relationships can be elicited next.

There are questionnaires that can be sent to families in advance of an appointment for a pain problem to obtain past medical history, birth and developmental history, and family history. The physical examination should be thorough and also check for tender points in the muscles; traditional ones are found in the posterior cervical, suprascapular, and paraspinous areas. For children with abdominal pain, it is useful to palpate the rectus abdominis muscles because myofascial abdominal wall pain often can be a contributor to the belly pain. Children with complex regional pain syndrome may have hypersensitivity to light touch in the affected body part, which may have color and temperature changes and possible swelling.

With Ashley as an example, workup of her chronic headaches would not involve invasive medical tests as the first approach unless the history and physical examination findings suggest intracranial disease that can be visible on magnetic resonance imaging or computed tomographic scan, such as a hemorrhage, tumor, or other lesion. The initial thinking by the clinician during the evaluation should be to rule out something structural in the brain (e.g., tumor, traumatic brain injury), chemical (e.g., monosodium glutamate reactions), or other identifiable "causes" that can be readily treated if diagnosed (e.g., sinus infection, poor vision). Clearly, observation and a history of unusual or sudden symptoms or signs, such as fever, morning vomiting, visual disturbances, seizures, paralysis, weakness, loss of sensation, shaking, or any sudden changes in alertness, speech, or thinking, especially after head trauma, would suggest the need for urgent evaluation with further diagnostic tools.

However, most children presenting with chronic pain do not have easily identifiable single causes of the pain (e.g., sinus infection), and the longer pain has persisted, the more "baggage" the pain picks up along the way, such as secondary stressors of school absenteeism, muscle tension from restricting the painful body part, and pain-related anxiety, to name a few. At this point, most parents can be reassured that the cause of the pain is not an acute problem (e.g., appendicitis) and that further diagnostic tests are not needed for now. Monitoring for changes in symptoms will, however, continue on a routine basis.

Table 56-2 lists interview questions for obtaining a pain history from the child and parent.

Psychosocial Assessment

Some clinicians have recommended that psychosocial assessment begin as soon as noncoping occurs, meaning that a child begins to miss school or to curtail participation in regular activities because of pain. Whereas the primary care physician should gather psychosocial information as part of the clinical evaluation of the pain problem, a referral to a psychologist or psychiatrist for a psychosocial assessment can greatly extend this inquiry. We believe the process of how the physician makes the referral for a psychosocial assessment is critical to the subsequent acceptance of psychological conceptualizations for symptoms and to management approaches and thus should be done with appropriate care. Patients and their families are more likely to accept a psychological referral and not feel abandoned by their physician if it is presented early and as a routine procedure in all cases of persistent pain causing disruption of normal activities. It is critical that professionals avoid dichotomization between organic and psychogenic causes of pain and present the psychosocial assessment along with the physical investigation and follow-up. This procedure avoids the trap of waiting for psychosocial assessment as a last resort after all other physical attempts to understand the problem have failed.

Psychosocial assessment may consist of clinical interviews, record keeping, and observation of the interaction among family members. A detailed clinical interview

Table 56-2. Interview Questions for Obtaining a Pain History

How long has your child [have you] been bothered by the pain?
Does the pain occur at any particular time of day (e.g., when your child first awakens [when you first awaken]), week (e.g., school days only), or month (with menses, for girls)?
How often do the pain episodes occur and how long do they last?
Do they come on suddenly or gradually?
Is the pain preceded or followed by any other symptoms or unusual feelings?
Where is the pain located? What does it feel like (e.g., pounding, stabbing)?
What makes it worse, and what helps it feel better?
Did anything new or different, such as attending a new school, precede the pain? What do you think started the pain and what keeps it going?
What medications (name, dose, how often, and for how long) has your child taken for the pain and what is still being taken (and does it help)? What didn't help? [for the child: What do you think helped most?]
What herbs or nondrug therapies has your child tried for the pain (e.g., warm baths, ice packs, listening to music, physical therapy, massage, yoga, relaxation training, hypnotherapy, acupuncture, psychotherapy)? Did they help? Tell me more (Why do you think helped?) [Ask same of child.]
What does the pain stop your child [you] from doing (e.g., concentrating, doing homework, attending school, playing sports, attending social activities with friends, activities with family)?
Does the pain interfere with falling asleep or staying asleep? Does your child [you] wake up feeling tired or not rested?
Does the pain affect your child's [your] appetite? Has your child [have you] lost or gained weight because of the pain?
What do you think is causing the pain?

Modified from Zeltzer L, Schlank C: Conquering Your Child's Chronic Pain: A Pediatrician's Guide for Reclaiming a Normal Childhood. New York, HarperCollins, 2005.

should assess developmental, behavioral, or psychiatric concerns in the patient's and family's history and should identify potential stressors and areas of maladaptive coping around academic success, relationships, school absenteeism, and social activities. Observation and direct questioning concerning the roles of various family members toward pain and its management can uncover maladaptive patterns in how family members respond to the child's pain. Information concerning the parent's own emotional functioning, anxiety, and marital stress may also contribute to a more complete understanding of sources of stress within the child and family.

Standardized psychological measures may be administered to screen for mental health diagnoses, in particular, anxiety and depressive symptoms, to assess coping behaviors, functional disability, and family functioning. At this time, there is not a specific battery of psychological measures that has been identified as particularly useful for assessment of all patients with chronic pain. The choice of whether to administer such measures will depend largely on the presenting concerns within the child and family. For patients with long-standing difficulties related to academic performance, referral for formal academic testing may be a useful adjunct to assess whether children are functioning at grade level; undiagnosed learning disorders may hinder academic performance and contribute additional stress.

Because comorbid sleep disturbances are so prevalent in children with chronic pain, it is useful to obtain a detailed history of sleep patterns by clinical interview or a sleep diary. In particular, it is important to obtain description of any difficulties in falling asleep or staying asleep. Children with chronic pain may develop extended problems with sleep because of arousal at bedtime, in which negative thoughts and hypervigilance at bedtime are incompatible with settling to sleep. Many children will meet diagnostic criteria for a clinically significant sleep disturbance, especially insomnia, that may require separate intervention (see Chapter 64 on sleep disorders).

Allowing the child (and parent) to describe a typical day can be an informative and nonthreatening way of getting specific detail about how pain interferes with the child's normal daily routine and accommodations that child and family have made because of the pain problem. It is also useful in this context to understand how much time the child spends in activity versus bedrest as this may have important implications for the child's rehabilitation needs.

MANAGEMENT APPROACHES

Counseling by the Physician

Management usually starts with counseling by the physician and may include referral for other services if these are needed and available. It is wise to limit unnecessary referrals because it can help reduce cure-seeking and can discourage multiple medical investigations with unclear benefit. Brief counseling from a physician can be of great help to children with recurrent pain and to their parents. Some suggested content of this counseling follows. Compliment the parents on their tremendous efforts to help the child and let them know it is no longer necessary to treat the pain as an acute problem and that the good news is that further diagnostic tests are not needed for now. Reassure the parent and child, however, that you will continue to monitor for changes in symptoms on a routine basis. It can be helpful to set up routine follow-up visits with the child (every 2 weeks or so) to continue to monitor and to provide counseling.

Meeting separately with the child and parents allows both parties to speak freely about issues, events, and emotions when the other party is not present. Counseling can be directed toward sources of stress and other triggers of pain. Time should be spent with the parents to help establish a reduction of attention paid to pain symptoms, in favor of increased attention paid to functional improvement. Table 56-3 lists suggested pain management guidelines for parents.

Perhaps the most important element of treatment that can be provided in counseling is around a return to normal activity. Clear, graded plans for increasing activity should be constructed with the child and parents. It can be explained to children and parents that functional improvement often precedes rather than follows pain relief. It is important to prescribe setting of concrete goals and expectations around activities like school because many parents struggle and feel ineffective in trying to push their child to do more. Having the child hear this

Table 56-3. Pain Management Guidelines for Parents and Caregivers

The following are some general guidelines for how parents and caregivers can encourage optimal coping in children and teens with chronic pain.

When your child complains of pain, do not give excessive attention, such as special privileges, treats, or extra sympathy. Parents should focus on encouraging positive coping behaviors.

Encourage and expect normal activity during pain episodes, including attendance in school, completion of daily chores and responsibilities, and participation in regular extracurricular activities. Do not remove responsibilities because of pain.

Provide consequences for your child's participation in normal activities. This means that if school or other important responsibilities are missed because of pain, the child should not be permitted to do special things like watch TV or play games (even if pain resolves later in the day). A day with pain and accompanying difficulty participating in usual activities should be low-key, quiet, and not filled with reinforcing responses. Remember, the goal is for your child to want to engage in positive "well behaviors" that bring him or her out of the house.

Encourage independent management of pain. This means that if your child reports pain, then encourage your child to use a pain management strategy like distraction or relaxation and breathing skills. A good response to a complaint of pain is, "What do you think you can do right now to help your pain?"

Lessen the focus on pain. Try not to ask your child questions about whether he or she has pain or how much it hurts. Trust that your child will come to you for assistance if needed.

Reduce dependence on medicines. Do not immediately offer medication for breakthrough pain when your child complains. Ask your child what strategies he or she can use to manage pain. Then, if your child asks for medication, deliver it only as prescribed.

message about return to normal activity from the physician can be extremely helpful. Parents can be encouraged to provide incentives for the child's efforts toward functional improvement, such as earning special privileges for reaching a school attendance goal.

Some physicians have training in relaxation, biofeedback, hypnotherapy, and related approaches, which are effective and empirically validated tools for pain management. If they can be offered in the physician's office, this can be of great value to the child. If these approaches cannot be offered in the office, you may consider referral for psychological treatment.

Medications

The goals for pharmacologic treatments may include prevention by treating acute pain well, reduction of somatic contributors (e.g., inflammation), facilitation of nighttime sleep, treatment of comorbid psychological disorders including anxiety and depression, and reduction of neural transmission. The use of most medications for childhood chronic pain is based on anecdotal evidence rather than on controlled clinical studies. For example, medications aimed at re-regulating the neural signaling mechanism, such as low-dose amitriptyline, although used often in clinical practice, have never undergone empiric investigation in children with nonheadache chronic pain. Several case studies report success in treating children with complex regional pain syndrome (previously referred to as reflex sympathetic dystrophy) and other neuropathic pain with gabapentin, a novel agent developed for the treatment of seizures.

Whereas opioids are very helpful in relieving acute pain, they are less helpful in the management of recurrent and chronic pain. Opioids might be used in situations in which children with chronic pain have been taking opioids prescribed by another physician for more than 2 or 3 weeks and a plan for weaning the child off the opioids is needed. In this case, pure opioids, rather than mixed analgesic opioids (e.g., Lortab, Vicodin, Tylenol with codeine), should be used with a round-the-clock administration plan with a goal of reducing the total daily opioid dose by 10% to 20% per day until all opioids are discontinued. Children who have been receiving acetaminophen or nonsteroidal anti-inflammatory drugs for a long time can experience headaches or continued pain in other sites just related to the continued analgesic use and have rebound pain when they stop, so that the pain without the medication drives the continued use of the analgesics. Education and support for withdrawal of opioids and other analgesics can be very helpful. Addressing anxiety and depression both psychotherapeutically and, if needed, pharmacotherapeutically can also be of great benefit. Often the anxiety relief with opioids is what drives continued opioid use, and management of anxiety with more targeted pharmacotherapy can assist in reducing pain and perceived need for opioids.

Nonopioid analgesics, when they are taken early in the pain episode, may help in treatment of headaches. Tricyclic antidepressants (e.g., amitriptyline) and other prophylactic medications, such as anticonvulsants (e.g., topiramate, gabapentin), are indicated for many patients with migraines and chronic daily headache. Analgesics are not typically helpful for children with abdominal pain; rather, use of low-dose amitriptyline or other tricyclics at night as well as peppermint geltabs with meals, ginger for nausea, and tegaserod (Zelnorm) for the child with constipation-predominant irritable bowel syndrome can be helpful. Topical anesthetics, such as Lidoderm patches, can be useful over tender muscle areas and areas of hypersensitivity found in complex regional pain syndrome. See Table 56-4 for an overview of pharmacologic treatment approaches.

Children with anxiety or depressive disorders may require a psychiatry evaluation to optimize pharmacologic treatment of these comorbidities. There is some evidence that treatment of comorbid anxiety and depression in children with recurrent abdominal pain may result in reductions in pain (Campo et al, 2004). Campo and colleagues found improvements in self-reported pain levels, anxiety, depression, and functional improvements in children with recurrent abdominal pain after 12-week use of citalopram, a selective serotonin reuptake inhibitor used for anxiety and depression.

Referral

The majority of children with chronic or recurrent pain can be successfully managed in the pediatric office. Chronic and recurrent pain is most often managed with a combination of behavioral and psychological treatments, complementary therapies, and physical rehabilitation approaches, with fewer children requiring medications.

Table 56-4. **Pharmacologic Treatment Options**

Category of Medication	Medication	Indication	Special Notes
Nonsteroidal anti-inflammatory drugs	Ibuprofen	Inflammation, analgesia	
Tricyclic antidepressants	Amitriptyline (Elavil)	Irritable bowel syndrome, neuropathic pain, chronic daily headache	Use low dose at night
Selective serotonin reuptake inhibitors/serotonin and norepinephrine reuptake inhibitors	Citalopram (Celexa)	Comorbid anxiety disorders: generalized anxiety disorder, obsessive-compulsive disorder, social phobia, panic, separation anxiety, post-traumatic stress disorder	Lower gastrointestinal tract upset
	Escitalopram (Lexapro)		Newer drug, less sedating than citalopram; lower gastrointestinal tract upset; needs close monitoring
	Venlafaxine (Effexor XR)	Irritable bowel syndrome (if underlying anxiety disorder or depression)	Studied in adults with fibromyalgia
	Duloxetine (Cymbalta)		Purported to have lower side effect profile than venlafaxine; studied only in adults; needs close monitoring
	Mirtazapine (Remeron)	Weight loss, depression, poor sleep	Needs close monitoring
Neuroleptics	Quetiapine (Seroquel)		Psychiatry consult needed
	Chlorpromazine (Thorazine)		Psychiatry consult needed
	Risperidone (Risperdal)	Tics, pervasive developmental disorder, pain perseveration	Psychiatry consult needed
Antiseizure medications	Gabapentin (Neurontin)	Neuropathic pain, mood disturbance, anxiety	Sedating, low side effect profile
	Pregabalin (Lyrica)	Neuropathic pain	Studied in adult populations
	Topiramate (Topamax)	Migraine headaches, neuropathic pain	Can impair memory, concentration
Beta blockers	Propranolol	Migraine headaches	Helpful when child has high body focus
Muscle relaxants	Cyclobenzaprine (Flexeril)		Infrequently used in pediatric populations
	Baclofen		
	Tizanidine (Zanaflex)		
Topical agents	Lidoderm patches	Focal neuropathic pain	Up to 3 patches, on 12 hours and off 12 hours
α-Adrenergics	Clonidine patches	Weaning from opioids	Useful with opioid withdrawal
Benzodiazepines		Breakthrough panic episodes, pain or anxiety in patients taking selective serotonin reuptake inhibitors	Not good for sleep, blocks stage IV sleep; rarely used
Sleep medications	Diphenhydramine (Benadryl)	Sleep onset problems	Recommended for short-term use only
	Melatonin	Circadian rhythm disturbance Insomnia	Over-the-counter supplement, low side effect profile
	Desyrel (Trazodone)	Sleep onset problems	Sedating
	Zolpidem (Ambien)	Insomnia	No data available on long-term use

However, children with complex pain complaints, excessive disability, or comorbid psychiatric disturbance may require referral for specialized pain care. In general, these options will typically include referral to a pediatric pain clinic, mental health provider, physical therapy, or complementary and alternative therapies.

Referral to a Pediatric Pain Clinic

Children who receive care in a multidisciplinary pediatric pain clinic are typically offered a multicomponent treatment involving psychological therapies, physical therapy, and medication management under the philosophy of a rehabilitation approach to treatment. In this approach, pain is accepted as a symptom that might not be eradicated, and efforts are directed toward improvement of functioning. As functioning and coping skills are improved, pain often remits as well. The specific structure of each program differs; some provide inpatient rehabilitation, whereas other programs exclusively treat children on an outpatient basis. For example, the effectiveness of an inpatient residential pediatric pain program involving physiotherapy and psychological therapy was recently evaluated in a group of adolescents with chronic pain and pervasive disability, and good support was found for this multicomponent treatment (Eccleston et al, 2003). We refer the reader to Zeltzer and Schlank (2005) for a listing of pediatric pain and gastrointestinal pain programs in the United States, Canada, and internationally.

Referral to a Mental Health Provider

Referral for psychological treatment is often very helpful but may be difficult to arrange in many communities. It can be useful to talk with physician colleagues about their relationships with mental health care providers to identify recommended clinical psychologists, psychiatrists, social workers, or counselors. Many mental health professionals do not have adequate training in pain management or in a biopsychosocial model of care. For identification of appropriate mental health providers, it is useful to inquire about their experience with children and adolescents, with treatment of children with medical problems, and in use of cognitive-behavioral therapy. The best referral options will have affirmative responses to each of these areas of inquiry.

There have been numerous studies that focus on treatment of recurrent and chronic pain, especially abdominal pain and headaches, with psychological interventions. About a dozen controlled trials of psychological therapy for children and adolescents with chronic pain were recently reviewed (Eccleston et al, 2002). These authors concluded that there is strong evidence that psychological therapies, principally relaxation and cognitive-behavioral therapy, are effective in reducing the severity and frequency of chronic pain in children and adolescents. The cognitive-behavioral therapy interventions primarily involved brief, standardized treatments in which children were taught specific coping skills (e.g., positive self-statements, relaxation).

For example, in a recent study, cognitive-behavioral family intervention was compared with standard pediatric care for recurrent abdominal pain (Robins et al, 2005). Children in the cognitive-behavioral family intervention group received five 40-minute sessions and were trained in relaxation skills and positive self-talk, and parents were taught to limit secondary gains from sick behavior. The standard medical care group received customary medical treatment consisting of follow-up office visits, education, support, and medications as deemed appropriate by the treating physician. Children who received the cognitive-behavioral intervention reported significantly less pain after treatment and at 1-year follow-up compared with children receiving standard care, providing support for the use of cognitive-behavioral family interventions in children with abdominal pain (Robins et al, 2005).

Referral to Physical Therapy

Referral to physical therapy can be an important element of treatment for many children with chronic pain. If a child is extremely deconditioned, physical therapy can serve as one method in working toward a return to normal activities. Physical therapy and rehabilitation approaches typically focus on body conditioning, desensitization, enhancement of flexibility, and strength. Body conditioning may also be accomplished through gym, pool, Pilates, or yoga, although these approaches have not yet undergone empiric evaluation.

There have been several descriptions of intensive physical therapy and rehabilitation programs for the treatment of complex regional pain syndrome in children. In one study, 103 children diagnosed with complex regional pain syndrome were entered into an intensive physical therapy–based exercise program in which they participated in treatment for 5 to 6 hours per day for a period of 6 to 8 weeks (either as inpatients or as outpatients). Findings demonstrated that 92% of the children had their symptoms resolve and were able to regain full function after the intensive exercise treatment (Sherry et al, 1999). Similarly, the benefits of physical therapy and cognitive-behavioral treatment were demonstrated in a randomized controlled trial that included 28 children with complex regional pain syndrome (Lee et al, 2002). Each child was randomly assigned either to receive physical therapy once a week for 6 weeks or to receive physical therapy three times a week for 6 weeks. Both groups received weekly cognitive-behavioral treatment. In general, all children showed reduced pain and improved function from physical therapy and cognitive-behavioral therapy. The frequency of the physical therapy did not alter outcome.

Referral for Complementary Treatment (Biofeedback, Acupuncture, Yoga)

Many parents of children with chronic pain seek out complementary and alternative medicine (CAM) therapies. Most of these therapies require further study for their use to be recommended. Certain CAM therapies (e.g., herbals) may have the undesired effect of encouraging a physical understanding of the pain problem and may detract attention from important psychosocial contributors.

The one CAM therapy that has been found to be an effective and well-established treatment for pediatric pain is biofeedback. Thermal biofeedback involves teaching patients how to increase their peripheral temperature by use of electronic instruments (a temperature probe on the finger) to measure temperature and a computer monitor to display reinforcing information back to the patient. Relaxation training has also received evidence-based support and is often used in combination with thermal biofeedback. Biofeedback has undergone only empiric evaluation in children with migraine and tension headache. There is strong evidence, however, to recommend biofeedback and relaxation to any child who suffers from headaches. Other studies of CAM modalities for chronic pain in adult populations are increasing, such as Iyengar yoga for low back pain (Williams et al, 2005). See Tsao (2006) for a review of CAM studies for pain treatment in children.

SUMMARY

Recurrent and chronic pain in childhood is a frequent presenting problem and may be due to chronic disease or to functional causes. Most children will have no serious or easily treatable physical cause of the pain. Instead, a biopsychosocial understanding of the pain is needed for evaluation and management of the problem. Primary care physicians can help prevent and relieve children's pain. An approach that establishes trust, rapport, and acceptance by the child and family will facilitate functional recovery. Detailed clinical interviews with child and parent are important to identify possible psychosocial and family factors that may contribute to problems in coping with pain. Counseling by the physician should focus on guiding the child in a return to normal activity and aiding parents in encouraging adaptive coping in their child. Among the pharmacologic, psychological, rehabilitation, and complementary approaches that are used in clinical practice, those interventions that promote learning of relaxation skills and strengthening and flexibility are the best established.

REFERENCES

Borsook D, Becerra LR: Breaking down the barriers: fMRI applications in pain, analgesia and analgesics. Mol Pain 2:30, 2006.

Campo JV, Perel J, Lucas A, et al: Citalopram treatment of pediatric recurrent abdominal pain and comorbid internalizing disorders: An exploratory study. J Am Acad Child Adolesc Psychiatry 43:1234-1242, 2004.

Drossman DA: What does the future hold for irritable bowel syndrome and the functional gastrointestinal disorders? J Clin Gastroenterol 39(Suppl):S251-S256, 2005.

Eccleston C, Malleson PN, Clinch J, et al: Chronic pain in adolescents: Evaluation of a programme of interdisciplinary cognitive behaviour therapy. Arch Dis Child 88:881-885, 2003.

Eccleston C, Morley S, Williams A, et al: Systematic review of randomised controlled trials of psychological therapy for chronic pain in children and adolescents, with a subset meta-analysis of pain relief. Pain 99:157-165, 2002.

Fearon P, Hotopf M: Relation between headache in childhood and physical and psychiatric symptoms in adulthood: National birth cohort study. BMJ 322:1145, 2001.

Hunfeld JA, Perquin CW, Duivenvoorden HJ, et al: Chronic pain and its impact on quality of life in adolescents and their families. J Pediatr Psychol 26:145-153, 2001.

Langeveld JH, Koot HM, Loonen MC, et al: A quality of life instrument for adolescents with chronic headache. Cephalalgia 16: 183-196; discussion 137, 1996.

Lee BH, Scharff L, Setbna NF, et al: Physical therapy and cognitive-behavioral treatment for complex regional pain syndromes. J Pediatr 141:135-140, 2002.

Mikkelsson M, Sourander A, Salminen, JJ, et al: Widespread pain and neck pain in schoolchildren. A prospective one-year follow-up study. Acta Paediatr 88:1119-1124, 1999.

Palermo TM: Impact of recurrent and chronic pain on child and family daily functioning: A critical review of the literature. J Dev Behav Pediatr 21:58-69, 2000.

Palermo TM, Chambers CT: Parent and family factors in pediatric chronic pain and disability: An integrative approach. Pain 119: 1-4, 2005.

Perquin CW, Hazebroek-Kampschreur AA, Hunfeld JA, et al: Pain in children and adolescents: A common experience. Pain 87:51-58, 2000.

Perquin CW, Hunfeld JA, Hazebroek-Kampschreur AA, et al: The natural course of chronic benign pain in childhood and adolescence: A two-year population-based follow-up study. Eur J Pain 7:551-559, 2003.

Peters JW, Schouw R, Anand KJ, et al: Does neonatal surgery lead to increased pain sensitivity in later childhood? Pain 114:444-454, 2005.

Robins PM, Smith SM, Glutting JJ, Bishop CT: A randomized controlled trial of a cognitive-behavioral family intervention for pediatric recurrent abdominal pain. J Pediatr Psychol 30:397-408, 2005.

Roth-Isigkeit A, Thyen U, Stoven H, et al: Pain among children and adolescents: Restrictions in daily living and triggering factors. Pediatrics 115:e152-162, 2005.

Sherry DD, Wallace CA, Kelley C, et al: Short- and long-term outcomes of children with complex regional pain syndrome type I treated with exercise therapy. Clin J Pain 15:218-223, 1999.

Sleed M, Eccleston C, Beecham J, et al: The economic impact of chronic pain in adolescence: Methodological considerations and a preliminary costs-of-illness study. Pain 119:183-190, 2005.

Tsao JC: CAM for pediatric pain: What is state-of-the-research? Evid Based Complement Alternat Med 3:143-144, 2006.

Walker LS, Garber J, Greene JW: Psychosocial correlates of recurrent childhood pain: A comparison of pediatric patients with recurrent abdominal pain, organic illness, and psychiatric disorders. J Abnorm Psychol 102:248-258, 1993.

Walker LS, Greene JW: The functional disability inventory: Measuring a neglected dimension of child health status. J Pediatr Psychol 16:39-58, 1991.

Williams KA, Petronis J, Smith D, et al: Effect of Iyengar yoga therapy for chronic low back pain. Pain 115:107-117, 2005.

Zeltzer L, Schlank C: Conquering Your Child's Chronic Pain: A Pediatrician's Guide for Reclaiming a Normal Childhood. New York, HarperCollins, 2005.

57 "COLIC": PROLONGED OR EXCESSIVE CRYING IN YOUNG INFANTS

WILLIAM B. CAREY

Vignette

A frantic, disheveled mother has brought her 4-week-old infant to the pediatrician for a visit. "Doctor, we can't stand all this crying any more. He has been yelling ever since we brought him home. He will not let me put him down. I have to carry him around all the time. I am exhausted. My husband and I are fighting about what to do. Please help us now. We cannot wait until he is three months old."

"Colic" is a poorly defined and incompletely understood state of prolonged or excessive crying seen in young infants who are otherwise well (Fig. 57-1). Although widely regarded by pediatricians and parents as confusing and frustrating, it can usually be successfully improved in a few days.

DEFINITION

There is no standard definition of colic. Pediatrics texts and advice books for parents usually (but not always) present a brief section on a phenomenon variously designated by terms such as paroxysmal fussing in infancy, infantile colic, evening colic, or 3-month colic.

Usual descriptions of colic indicate that the condition begins soon after the infant comes home from the newborn nursery and is likely to persist until he or she is 3 or 4 months of age. The crying is characterized as intense, lasting for up to several hours at a time, and usually occurring in the late afternoon and evening. The affected infant is typically pictured as drawing up the knees against the abdomen and expelling much flatus. He or she can appear hungry but is not quieted for long by further feeding or other attempts at soothing. The infant eats well and grows normally, however. The usual explanation offered is that the crying is caused by abdominal pain of intestinal origin.

The standard textbook description in the preceding paragraph is inadequate on several counts:

1. Without a more precise definition of the duration of the crying, it can be extended to apply to almost all young infants at one time or another.
2. Such imprecision makes most studies of the phenomenon of questionable value. Writers on the subject often express strong convictions about favorite theories of cause and management that can be neither refuted nor verified because the infants studied are so poorly identified.
3. Figures relating to the incidence of colic are of little value.
4. Telling parents that their child has colic is at best a confusing message and may be misinterpreted as a diagnosis of an unproven physical problem.

The best definition available is still the one used by Wessel and colleagues (1954), that such a young infant is "one who, otherwise healthy and well fed, had paroxysms of irritability, fussing, or crying lasting for a total of more than three hours a day and occurring on more than three days in any one week." Some authors add another criterion of a duration of more than 3 weeks. The prolonged crying is thus identified in terms of total duration but neither as to the frequency of the bouts of crying nor as to its quality. Even this definition, however, is applied with difficulty at times. The term *colic* should ideally be eliminated from clinical use and perhaps restricted to research projects, in which it is important to describe accurately the population of subjects.

Any attempt at improving this definition should convey the idea that the child is otherwise well but is crying substantially more than the mean amount for infants of his or her age. The condition might then be better referred to as prolonged or excessive crying. The evidence to date does not justify any conclusion that the quality or pitch of the prolonged crying is any different from that of other infants. Most parents do find a high-pitched cry more unpleasant, but it seems to be the quantity that makes them more likely to complain to their child's physician. The flatus might be a consequence rather than the cause of the crying. It is not even

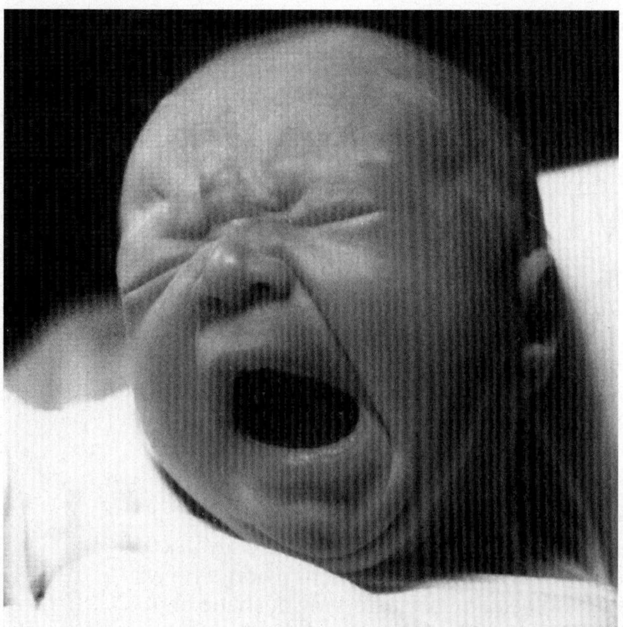

Figure 57-1. "I'm sensitive and irritable. Please stop jiggling." *(Photograph by H. Belluci.)*

certain that such infants are experiencing abdominal pain, as has been commonly assumed. Infants flex their legs in response to a variety of noxious stimuli, such as a pinprick. It will be difficult to answer with certainty the question of whether such infants are experiencing any kind of pain. Because the crying can generally be markedly diminished within a few days by management techniques that do not reduce pain, it is hard to maintain the view that pain is primarily responsible. The affected infant does not seem to have any disease or malfunction of the bowel or any other organ but differs from the norm only in regard to the amount of crying.

Most studies of prolonged crying have used referred populations, thereby introducing a selection bias. A clearer perspective comes from studies performed in primary care pediatric practices (Carey, 1968, 1972; Taubman, 1988) and from cross-sectional population studies. Such a study of 530 infants in London found that according to diaries kept by the mothers, 23% of the infants met the Wessel criteria for colic at 6 weeks but that "the overwhelming majority of the crying and associated behavior is unsettled, fussing, and irritable behavior, rather than paroxysmal, abnormally intense or inconsolable crying" (St. James-Roberts et al, 1995). All infants had periods of inconsolable crying. Those regarded as colicky had more of it but still spent only a small portion of their time in that intense, unsoothable state.

The best conclusion to be derived from these and other data is probably that what is being called colic today is the upper end of the normal range of crying rather than a discrete, categorical disorder. Barr (1990) has noted that as the total amount of crying increases or decreases, it is the duration of the bouts that changes rather than the number of separate bouts. Our current understanding of these phenomena is advancing but still far from complete (see review of research in Lester and Barr, 1997).

DIFFERENTIAL DIAGNOSIS

Because the phenomenon under discussion is prolonged or excessive crying in otherwise well young infants, this condition must be distinguished from two others: normal crying and secondary excessive crying resulting from faulty feeding techniques or physical problems in the infant.

Normal Crying

Brazelton (1962) assessed in detail the crying patterns in a middle class sample of 80 infants. Crying lasted a total of about 2 hours a day at 2 weeks, increased to a peak of almost 3 hours by 6 weeks, and then gradually decreased to about 1 hour by 3 months. The upper quartile of infants were crying 3½ hours per day at 6 weeks. Throughout these 3 months, the principal time for crying for all infants was in the evening. These findings have been supported by similar figures in Canada and England. Pertinence for other populations in other areas has yet to be determined.

Several observers have noted that for prematurely born infants, the crying peak occurs at a point 6 weeks after 40 weeks postconceptional age, but this conclusion requires further substantiation. No evidence has been published for gender or birth order differences based on objective data collection.

The amount of parental complaining about crying is not necessarily proportional to the extent of the crying. Some parents are upset about typical periods of fussing, whereas others might not seem disturbed by greater quantities. The first step in the differential diagnosis is to decide whether the crying is merely an ordinary amount that the parents cannot tolerate or is truly longer than average. There seems to be little doubt that parents with greater psychosocial stress are more likely to complain about their infants' crying.

Faulty Feeding Techniques

Underfeeding and overfeeding and inadequate burping or sucking are faulty feeding techniques that should be considered. These possibilities usually can be excluded by a routine history and physical examination. Some have suggested that the type of bottle used or breast versus formula feeding may affect the amount of crying, but these possibilities are not well supported by current evidence.

Physical Problems in the Infant

If colic or prolonged crying in infants is by definition found only in those who are otherwise well, various physical problems in the infant must be excluded before the diagnosis can be applied. Three kinds of problems are usually cited: (1) acute disorders, such as otitis media, intestinal cramping with diarrhea, corneal abrasion, hair tourniquet on a digit, and incarcerated hernia—all of which are relatively easily ruled out by the history and by the examination of the infant—and more chronic conditions, such as gastroesophageal reflux; (2) nutritional intolerances, such as cow's milk allergy, lactose intolerance, or transmission of irritating substances such as caffeine through breast milk, all of which appear to be relatively insignificant causes of prolonged crying in otherwise well infants; and (3) inadequately defined clinical entities, such as "immaturity" of the central nervous system or of the intestine, which have not been sufficiently studied. Premature infants may be more irritable than full-term ones but are not necessarily colicky.

Despite the widespread opinion that milk allergy can cause excessive crying in otherwise well infants, no study of acceptable design has confirmed this possibility (Carey, 1989). If such a connection should at some point become established in 5% to 10% of prolonged criers, as some believe, the diagnosis of such infants could not be colic if that term applies only to infants who are otherwise well. In those infants thought to have lactose intolerance, an elimination of lactose in the diet decreases breath hydrogen but has no effect on the crying.

CONTRIBUTORY FACTORS IN INTERACTION

If the infant is healthy but is irritable, fussing, and crying substantially more than most, there is usually no single clear-cut explanation for this behavior. The answer appears to lie in the interaction between factors in the infant and the environment. The two principal contributory elements to consider are a physiologic predisposition in the infant and inappropriate handling by the parents, both of which usually appear to be variations of normal rather than abnormalities. A third factor to bear in mind is that the first 3 months are a period of immaturity of the central nervous system, during which the infant may be transiently more vulnerable to the interactions of the first two factors (see Barr et al, 2000).

Infants vary considerably in their temperaments or emotional reactivity characteristics (see Chapter 7). The most likely contribution of the infant in colic is a normal predisposition to be more sensitive, more irritable, more intense, less adaptable, or less soothable than average for age. More perceptive infants with low sensory thresholds are prone to increased crying, apparently because they are more vulnerable to disorganization by excessive or inappropriate sensory input from the environment (Blum et al, 2002; Carey, 1972, 1984). This relationship between prolonged crying and temperament should become clearer when temperament is studied and clinically assessed before, during, and after the period of excessive crying in the same individuals.

Parents may not know at first which methods are most effective for quieting infants in general and theirs in particular. If they cannot understand or tolerate their infant's needs and react to them appropriately, they may engage in unsuitable manipulations that increase rather than decrease the duration of the bouts of crying. Inexperience and anxiety are factors that can make parents even less skillful at responding sensitively. Excessive and inappropriate handling of the infant, such as picking up a fussy, overtired baby, is frequently observed both as a causal factor and as a response to prolonged crying (Van IJzendoorn and Hubbard, 2001). Prolonged crying probably occurs most typically in the absence of any abnormality in the infant or parent but rather when the parents have not yet learned to interact harmoniously with their infant. This general interpretation has been reaffirmed by the large study by Papoušek and colleagues (2008).

The possible role of psychosocial factors in generating prolonged crying in young infants has been much debated in the literature. An important consideration has been the type of sample used. Infants who are referred to specialty clinics because of the severity of the crying are a selected subgroup of the total population and are probably more likely to demonstrate significant "destabilized maternal functioning" owing to the problems in their lives (Papoušek and von Hofacker, 1995). Primary pediatric care samples and cross-sectional studies, on the other hand, tend to find maternal anxiety and guilt, but it is uncertain how much this differs from what is seen in the general population.

MANAGEMENT

Most advice dealing with the management of prolonged or excessive crying is unreasonably pessimistic about the effectiveness of professional intervention. This defeatism is unjustified; appropriate measures are usually successful in reducing crying to acceptable amounts in 2 to 3 days.

History

Management begins, as elsewhere in pediatrics, with an adequate history. The first step is to define the symptom: the intensity, duration, and frequency of the crying. Parents often say that the baby is too "gassy" or too hungry, and the clinician must sift the evidence to discover that the crying is the real problem. A good way to make the parents' description of the infant more precise is to ask for a detailed narration of the infant's typical day or for a diary of the crying. Information about the infant's temperamental characteristics can usually be adequately based on brief descriptions of the infant's sensitivity, irritability, intensity, and soothability, but the clinician or researcher may choose to use a more detailed questionnaire (see Chapter 78). Having the parents demonstrate their soothing techniques during the examination can be helpful in revealing practices that require modification.

The rest of the medical history should be obtained in the usual manner but with an enrichment to include parental concern about the pregnancy and the child and anxieties related to their own experience as children or with rearing previous children or to inadequate family support and other stresses. Family psychosocial stressors should be sought and dealt with appropriately, but they will not necessarily be found, and if uncovered, they are not necessarily causative of or resulting from the prolonged crying.

Physical Examination

The physical examination seldom reveals anything useful in regard to the diagnosis or management of the crying but is an absolutely necessary part of the procedure. Most parents are doubtful about reassurance that is not preceded by a careful assessment of the infant. For example, a hasty prescription of sedative drops over the telephone is generally not successful.

Laboratory tests, however, are usually not necessary and should not be performed unless specifically indicated by the history and physical examination. A battery of tests would suggest the physician's concern that there is a serious possibility of an underlying physical problem.

Counseling

Counseling has proved to be the most effective method available for helping parents cope successfully with prolonged crying (Carey, 1994). Standard lectures on infant care and simple empathy with the distress of the parents have not been shown to be successful. Counseling should be individualized to the particular situation and should include these main topics:

1. The infant is not sick. The physician should reassure the parents that the physical examination has not revealed any problem in the infant's health. The crying may mean distress but is seldom due to pain. Antecedent fears about the infant and anxieties resulting from the crying can be allayed. Counseling about prolonged or excessive crying and its management should avoid "the medical model" that there is probably something, as yet unconfirmed, wrong with the infant's gastrointestinal tract, nervous system, allergic responses, or general viability. Similarly, the parents must be unburdened of unjustified worry or guilt about their caregiving abilities. Reassurance about their competence is helpful. Pertinent psychosocial stressors that possibly have contributed to the crying should be discussed.
2. Education about infant crying. A comparison of the particular infant's crying with the average for the age should be followed by an educational discussion that includes information such as the following: All young infants are irritable and fussy and cry to some degree, the average in this period being 2 to 3 hours a day. Normal infants vary in how much they cry, how intense the crying is, how sensitive they are to stimuli, and how easily soothed they are. Many parents do not know that fatigue is a common reason why infants cry. Infant crying affects parents' feelings and behavior, such as marital satisfaction and self-esteem. Parents react differently to infant crying, with varying amounts of guilt, anger, and fear and with stimulation, attempts at soothing, and often overfeeding of the infant. Thus, excessive crying is probably the result of a "poor fit" between the infant's needs and predispositions and the present parental response.
3. The excessive amount of crying can be reduced. As stated, parental handling of the infant may require alteration. Parents with fussy infants usually are doing too much or doing the right things at the wrong times and they need to shift their tactics. They usually will be successful if they soothe more—as with a pacifier, repetitive sound, swaddling, swinging, and a heating pad or hot-water bottle—and stimulate less—as with decreasing picking up and feeding the infant in response to every cry. Parents need to learn to be more selective as to when they pick up their crying infant and to refrain from responding to every whimper. This does not mean a lessening of expressions of affection. A quiet, dimly lit environment with a minimum of unnecessary handling and correction of any faulty feeding techniques without changing the composition of the feedings seem to be helpful. All of these instructions can be given without making the parents feel inadequate.

The essence of this individualized approach is in helping parents to become more skillful at meeting the needs of their infant by observing their infant carefully and interpreting more accurately the behavior their infant displays ("sensitive differential responding"). Perhaps the best way to accomplish this is to watch parent and infant interact during the office visit. Because this is at best a brief episode, however, a more practical method is to ask the parent to relate a typical day, with descriptions of what the infant does, how the parents respond, how the infant in turn reacts, and so on throughout the day. Such observations and descriptions usually reveal ways in which the transactions can be modified to be more soothing for the infant. Such specifically designed behavioral management of the infant has been shown to be more effective in reducing prolonged crying than simply expressing empathy with the parent about the stress of the crying or any other method (Barbero et al, 1957; Carey, 1968; McKenzie, 1991; Taubman, 1988; Wolke et al, 1994). No study has shown this method to be ineffective when it is properly applied. No other form of management has shown similar promise. These revisions of handling should not be thought of as changing the infants' temperamental predispositions but rather as altering the interaction of the caretakers with them and the resulting output of fussing and crying. The reduction in crying is usually achieved by decreasing the length of the bouts rather than the number of them.

The expression of optimism about the immediate outcome of the foregoing measures is justified and improves chances of success. Although acknowledging with the parents that prolonged crying in young infants is an incompletely understood phenomenon, the clinician is on firm ground in telling parents that if the recommended steps are followed, there is an excellent chance that the crying will diminish considerably in the next 2 or 3 days. This sanguine prophecy is based on experience and is usually correct. On the other hand, telling parents that the excessive crying will go away by 3 months of age, which may be a condemnation to 2 or more months of further screaming, is not comforting and is likely to be distressing.

Close, supportive follow-up of the excessively fussy infant is important. A convenient way to do this is by a telephone contact every 2 or 3 days until there is substantial improvement. On rare occasions, it is necessary to re-evaluate the child and the situation in a week or so. Referral of the infant or parents for further evaluation and management of physical or psychosocial issues should be pursued if indicated, but it usually is not.

Other Measures

The use of medication for temporary relief of excessive crying is controversial. Drugs are usually unnecessary. In extreme cases, however, such as with serious sleep deprivation in the parents, medication may have a place in management. The most often recommended drugs are phenobarbital elixir, 10 mg three times daily, or diphenhydramine (Benadryl elixir), 6 mg two or three times a day. Treatment for 1 week is usually sufficient. If excessive crying returns after that, the medication can be given for a second week. There might be some placebo effect in the administration of such substances, but it is likely that there is also a pharmacologic one. The use of a drug alone without the other more important measures, which were mentioned earlier, is only modestly effective. Simethicone has been shown to be of no value (Metcalf et al, 1994). Herbal tea preparations have been thought by some to be helpful in reducing the crying, but their varying constituents make these preparations unacceptable as a general recommendation. Medication, when considered, should be made optional, because some parents want to try first to lessen the crying without it.

Under very extraordinary circumstances and as a last resort, separation of the infant from the parents by a brief period of hospitalization or a stay with a competent relative or friend has been shown to be dramatically effective in reducing the infant's crying. If, however, parental feelings and handling of the infant are not dealt with effectively before the parents are reunited with their infant, the old pattern of interaction and crying is likely to resume (Barbero et al, 1957).

Several unsuitable forms of treatment should be mentioned, if only to discourage their use. A change in the composition of feedings, that is, from one formula to another, is seldom an appropriate solution. Almost any formula change—in fact, almost any altered procedure done with conviction—is likely to be followed by a temporary reduction in crying because of the placebo effect. But these transient improvements typically wear off in a few days. The lack of support for these techniques has been described elsewhere (Carey, 1989).

Although the use of rectal manipulations and enemas is widely supported by tradition, there is no published evidence to establish their value. Simply carrying the infant for more time each day, regardless of his or her state and needs, has not been demonstrated to be helpful.

PROGNOSIS

Standard pediatric texts and conventional wisdom repeat the notion that colic usually goes away by itself by 3 or 4 months of age and that little can be done to alter that fate. However, clinical experience and reported studies (Barbero et al, 1957; Carey, 1968; McKenzie, 1991; Taubman, 1988; Wolke et al, 1994) indicate that excessive crying in young infants can be sharply reduced within a few days in most instances if appropriate steps are taken. Some infants and some situations take longer, but virtually all respond to suitable management. Conversely, with inappropriate care, the prolonged crying is likely to continue until 3 or 4 months of age.

Some short-term consequences are commonly seen. A temperamental predisposition to be irritable or sensitive will probably continue to be evident for at least the next few months and probably longer. Parental overattentiveness to the infant or more serious destabilizations of maternal functioning may still be present unless the family and their professional advisors have been able to improve those situations. Both of these factors may have an impact on the infant's subsequent behavior in matters such as night waking in the second 6 months of life and later. If professional advice has not been sufficiently skillful, the parents may still believe that there is some subtle defect in the child, and a vulnerable child syndrome may have been fostered (see Chapter 34). If the parents' response to the prolonged crying has been too much feeding, the infant may by this time have gained excessive weight.

The long-term prognosis for individuals who as young infants cried more than average has not been sufficiently investigated. Any statement that these infants become more impatient or aggressive as children or adults is pure speculation. Anecdotal reports from parents indicate that they carry vivid memories of the colic with them into the future, but the effects on them as parents or adults need more documentation. Because retrospective data relating to amounts of crying tend to be highly inaccurate, only prospective studies will resolve this issue.

PREVENTION

No investigation has yet proved that any particular early measures will reduce the subsequent occurrence of colic or excessive crying. Some theoretical possibilities deserve mention.

We do not know how to alter the apparently predisposing temperamental or physiologic factors. We are not even fully certain which are the most important. It may become possible, however, by the use of a measure such as the Brazelton Neonatal Behavioral Assessment Scale or some derivative of it to identify infants in whom excessive crying is particularly likely to develop. So far, no such evidence has become available. Furthermore, traits determined in the newborn period have so far been shown to have very low stability.

It is possible to educate all parents, even starting prenatally, about infant crying and soothing. Some have no idea that even completely normal young infants cry about 2 hours or more a day. Parents often are unaware of the importance of infant fatigue and that a tired infant usually does better if not picked up.

The alert clinician also deals with parental anxieties whenever they are expressed. Concerns revealed prenatally or in the newborn nursery can lead to inappropriate handling of the infant if they are not resolved satisfactorily.

SUMMARY

Much of the general public and many primary care physicians regard colic as an incomprehensible and unmanageable condition that brings great distress to families. Unlike most discussions of this subject, this chapter reports that prolonged crying in young infants is sufficiently understandable in most cases to allow a rational approach that is usually effective. The strategy is to lessen the poorness of fit between the irritable or sensitive behavioral predisposition of the infant and the particular handling techniques of the family.

REFERENCES

Barbero GJ, Rigler D, Rose JA: Infantile gastro-intestinal disturbances: A pilot study and design for research. Am J Dis Child 94:532, 1957.

Barr RG: The "colic" enigma: Prolonged episodes of a normal predisposition to cry. Infant Mental Health J 11:340, 1990.

Barr RG, Hopkins B, Green JA (eds): Crying as a Sign, a Symptom & a Signal Cambridge, Cambridge University Press, 2000.

Blum NJ, Taubman B, Tretina L, et al: Maternal ratings of infant intensity and distractibility. Arch Pediatr Adolesc Med 156:286-290, 2002.

Brazelton TB: Crying in infancy. Pediatrics 29:579, 1962.

Carey WB: The effectiveness of parent counseling in the management of colic. Pediatrics 94:333, 1994.

Carey WB: Cow's milk formula and infantile colic [letter to the editor]. Pediatrics 84:1124, 1989.

Carey WB: "Colic": Primary excessive crying as an infant-environment interaction. Pediatr Clin North Am 31:993, 1984.

Carey WB: Clinical applications of infant temperament measurements. J Pediatr 81:823, 1972.

Carey WB: Maternal anxiety and infantile colic: Is there a relationship? Clin Pediatr 7:590, 1968.

Lester BM, Barr RG (eds): Colic and Excessive Crying. Report of the 105th Ross Conference on Pediatric Research. Columbus, OH, Ross Products Division, Abbott Laboratories, 1997.

McKenzie S: Troublesome crying in infants: Effect of advice to reduce stimulation. Arch Dis Child 66:1416, 1991.

Metcalf TJ, Irons TG, Sher LD, Young PC: Simethicone in the treatment of colic: A randomized, placebo-controlled, multicenter trial. Pediatrics 94:29, 1994.

Papoušek M, von Hofacker N: Persistent crying and parenting: Search for a butterfly in a dynamic system. Early Dev Parenting 4:209, 1995.

Papoušek M, Schieche M, Wurmser H (eds): Disorders of Behavioral and Emotional Regulation in the First Years of Life. Washington, DC, Zero to Three, 2008.

St. James-Roberts I, Conroy S, Wilsher K: Clinical, developmental, and social aspects of infant crying and colic. Early Dev Parenting 4:107, 1995.

Taubman B: Parental counseling compared with elimination of cow's milk or soy milk protein for treatment of infant colic syndrome: A randomized trial. Pediatrics 81:756, 1988.

Van IJzendoorn MH, Hubbard FOA: Infant crying and maternal responsiveness during the first year. The Signal 9:1, 2, 2001.

Wessel MA, Cobb JC, Jackson EB, et al: Paroxysmal fussing in infancy, sometimes called "colic." Pediatrics 14:421, 1954.

Wolke D, Gray P, Meyer R: Excessive infant crying: A controlled study of mothers helping mothers. Pediatrics 94:322, 1994.

58 COMMON ISSUES IN FEEDING

MARTIN T. STEIN

The feeding of infants and children by caregivers is a primary focus of their mutual interactions that is affected by many factors including the cultural setting, parental experience, the child's developmental level, and temperament. Parents experience a variety of satisfactions and worries and frequently turn to their medical caregivers for help. Concerns about the content and amount of the food consumed are frequent and include issues such as rate of weight gain, spitting up, fussiness, food dislikes, and pica. Opportunities for anticipatory guidance and prevention of behavior problems are numerous.

FEEDING: A MAJOR EVENT

Feeding infants and young children is a behavioral event. Beyond the need for adequate nutrients to ensure physical growth, the process of feeding is important in shaping the emotional and social development of children. The time spent feeding consumes an enormous part of an infant's life. Beyond the consumption of nutrients for growth, feeding time represents the earliest opportunity for an infant to experience novel social interactions.

The interplay between the child, parent, and environment begins during fetal life and accelerates immediately after birth. A prolonged gestation in humans provides time for the development of an intense attachment to the fetus that prepares a mother for the nurturing behaviors needed after birth. When the nursing infant sucks and swallows, the infant visually locks into the mother's face, hears her voice, and feels her skin. Nursing infants exhibit behaviors associated with specific tastes from foods consumed by the mother (Mannella and Beauchamp, 1991). An infant who is equipped with a mature neurologic system and ready to interact with the immediate environment experiences these sensory stimuli. The range of emotional responses experienced by the infant and the mother is broad. The feeding dyad is built on these reciprocal and contingent behaviors of an infant and mother.

An individual child's temperament, state regulation, physiologic variables, and behavioral organization contribute to the interactional process. The mother's or caretaker's unique characteristics also make an important contribution. The mother's psychological health, temperament, perspective on parenting, social support, and recovery period after delivery are important variables. To encourage a pleasurable experience associated with feeding, the child-parent dyad must find a common ground to maintain a nurturing encounter.

Individual variation in both child and parent temperaments guides the feeding interaction. Early in a child's life, effective parents learn to respond to subtle feeding cues that reflect hunger, satiety, and the desire to feed slower or faster. Infants and children often develop predictable patterns of feeding behavior, and parents participate by developing good observation skills and reading the infant's cues accurately. Whereas many parents naturally learn the value of monitoring and responding to behavioral cues, others benefit from a supportive family member or health care professional who can guide the process (Satter, 1990).

Multiple events in early childhood ensure the development of a sense of "basic trust." The achievement of this psychological task requires predictable, pleasurable, and secure feelings. At around 3 months of age, the child learns to anticipate feeding routines and is more interested in the feeding activities of others. The enormous pleasure derived from sucking when fed by a responsive caregiver and the self-satisfaction that comes later with independent feeding fuel the development of basic trust.

The introduction of solid foods between 4 and 6 months of age is a nutritional and social landmark. Solid foods provide the infant with an opportunity to explore new textures, smells, colors, and tastes of foods. Other than the requirement at 6 months for additional iron found in some solids, nutrients in breast milk alone are adequate for the first 12 months for full-term infants. Solids, however, promote development by encouraging the use of new motor skills, visual milestones, and social behaviors. At around 6 months of age, tongue thrusting behavior decreases as the ability to chew emerges, head and trunk control allow the infant to sit upright, and the ability to reach for and grasp objects develops in association with hand-eye coordination skills. Steady sitting is associated with readiness for the use of a cup. A pincer grasp and effective hand-eye coordination are requirements for eating finger foods. The infant has more control over choice of food type and amount with exploration and experimentation during feeding.

Similar to play in late infancy and among toddlers, feeding explorations are often accompanied by messy

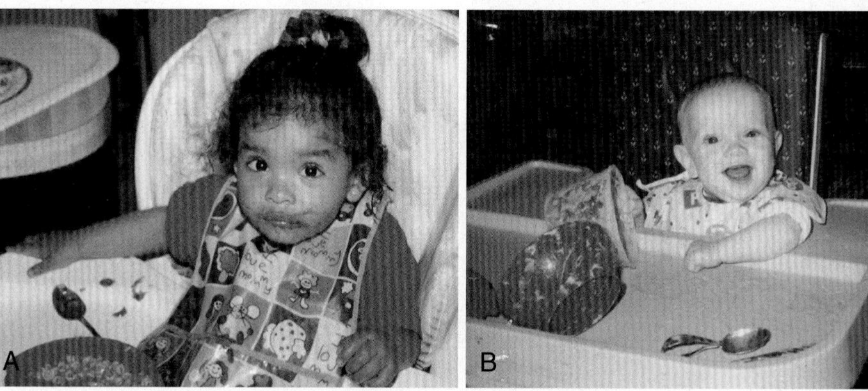

Figure 58-1. Typical toddler messiness.

tables and messy kids. Self-discovery and mastery of individual tasks inevitably require a messy environment (Fig. 58-1). Parental response to the events modulates the child's experience with exploration in general and with feeding specifically. Parents should be encouraged to respect the child's quest for autonomy and mastery over feeding. Parents can be advised that although new foods tend to be rejected initially, preference for novel foods increases with repeated exposure (Sullivan and Birch, 1994). Clinicians should be sensitive to temperament differences that may guide a child's interest, tempo, and responses to new foods.

Feeding is central to the development of autonomy in the second and third years of life. Motor skills (to independently discover, prepare, and pick up food), language skills (to express desires for food now!), and psychological development (to convey needs through strong feelings, to be a ggressive and egocentric) come together in the toddler to make feeding, at times, a dramatic family event. Independent feeding at this age can be viewed as one component of a child's journey toward self-regulation, self-determination, and psychological separation. Sleeping, playing, verbal expression, and toilet training are other components of this same journey. As with all these emerging skills, learning about feeding occurs at different rates, and setbacks (or regression) may follow intercurrent events in the family (Hammer, 1992).

Parents are most responsive to guidance around nutritional concerns when they can be framed in the context of developmental skills (Dixon and Stein, 2006). This approach to anticipatory guidance (and feeding problems) encourages parents to respond to a child's cues and needs at a particular developmental age. As illustrated in Table 58-1, the most significant changes and challenges to feeding occur in the first 3 years when the ground rules for feeding change frequently with emerging neurodevelopmental milestones.

FEEDING IN THE CONTEXT OF CULTURE

Culture dominates feeding practices and styles (see Chapter 19). There are many examples in both developed and developing countries. Breastfeeding was universal until the dairy industry and biochemical technologies produced infant formulas. That single innovation dramatically changed infant feeding. Among ancient hunter-gatherer societies, infants were fed frequent, small feedings while being carried throughout the day. Infants were in continuous skin contact with their mothers and fed at the slightest cue of hunger for most of human history. Children slept in proximity with parents and siblings (co-sleeping), which allowed frequent nighttime feeds. As many as 50% of African American young children co-sleep with their mothers. This same practice is found in Southeast Asian families and in other cultures.

Weaning is another feeding practice that varies significantly among cultures. In developing countries, weaning is delayed because breastfeeding remains the cheapest, most nutritious form of sustenance, serves as a form of birth control, and encourages survival of the child. Co-sleeping, traditionally discouraged in Western countries as a disincentive to mastering independence and self-regulation of sleep, promotes prolonged breastfeeding (Stein et al, 2001). In Western countries, early weaning from breast milk or formula to a cup has been viewed by many clinicians in the context of a toddler's quest for autonomy. If the breast or artificial nipple is an infantile symbol, the cup represents independence and encourages self-regulation. Yet there are no data that support a developmental advantage in children weaned at 12 months compared with those weaned at 24 months.

Clinicians should practice tolerance for the wide variety of early childhood feeding practices. Unless a particular practice is shown to affect adversely either the nutritional intake or the developmental progress of a child, culturally dependent feeding patterns should be encouraged, monitored for effects, and viewed by clinicians as a source of clinical insight.

The trend for mothers of infants and toddlers to work outside the home has had an impact on feeding patterns in developed countries. The increased use of daycare has been associated with earlier weaning from breast to formula as well as a social change in the feeding environment. Young children in daycare are fed by individuals other than parents or other family members, and by the age of 1 year, they experience feeding in groups. Neither developmental disadvantage nor clear advantages have been shown to come from these changes in feeding patterns.

Table 58-1. **Behavioral and Developmental Abilities Related to Feeding**

Age	Behavioral-Developmental Abilities
Newborn–2 months	Primitive reflexes (rooting, sucking, swallowing) facilitate feeding and quickly become organized into a whole pattern of behavior; hunger cry initiates feeding interaction; minimal vocal, visual, or motor activity during feeding
2-4 months	More alert and interactive during feeding; explosive cough to protect self from aspiration; beginning ability to wait for food; associates mother's smell, voice, and cradling with feeding; hand-to-mouth behavior quiets infant, increases interest in mouthing activities
4-6 months	Readiness for solids; excellent head and trunk control; reaching for objects; raking grasp; increased hand-to-mouth facility; loss of extrusion reflex of the tongue; may purposefully spit out food as part of food exploration; adaptation to introduction to solids may be affected by infant's temperament
6-8 months	Sits alone with a steady head during sitting feedings; chewing mechanism developed; holds bottle; vocal eagerness during meal preparation; much more motor activity during feeding
8-10 months	Finger food readiness; thumb-forefinger grasp (i.e., inferior pincer); grasps spoon but cannot use it effectively; feeds self crackers and so on; enjoys new textures, tastes; emerging independence
10-12 months	Increasing determination to feed self; rim pincer grasp; drops food off highchair onto floor to see where it goes; holds cup but frequently spills it; more verbal and motor behavior during feeding
12-15 months	Demands to feed self without help; decreased appetite and nutritional requirements; improved cup use (both hands); uses spoon, fills poorly, turns at mouth; can use spoon as extension of hand; messy play
15-18 months	Eats rapidly, short feeding sessions; wants to be motorically active (too busy to eat); fairly good use of spoon and cup; enhanced ability to wait for food; plays with food to elicit response from parent
18-24 months	Feeds self, using combination of utensils and fingers; verbalizes "eat, all gone"; asks for food; negativism emerges, says no when really wanting offered food; wants control of feeding situation
2-3 years	Uses fork; ritualistic, repetitive at mealtimes; food jags, all one food at a time; dawdles; likes to help set and clear table; may begin to help self to refrigerator contents
3-4 years	Spills little; uses utensils well; washes hands with minimal help; likes food preparation; reasonable table manners when eating out
4-5 years	Serves self; choosy about food; resists some textures; begins to request foods seen on television ads (especially junk food); makes menu suggestions; likes to assist in washing dishes; helps in food preparation
5-6 years	Uses knife; assists in preparing and packing own box lunch; can be responsible for setting and clearing table; aids younger siblings' request for food or drink
6-8 years	Does dishes independently and willingly; increases pressure to buy junk food; interested in, often critical of, and attempts to negotiate about daily menu; manages money for school meal ticket
8-10 years	Enjoys planning and preparing simple family meals; wants supplemental spending money to buy snacks when away from home; more reticent to try new foods; resists kitchen chores

Modified from Dixon SD, Stein MT: Encounters with Children: Pediatric Behavior and Development, 4th Ed. Philadelphia, Elsevier Mosby, 2006.

OPPORTUNITIES FOR PREVENTING FEEDING PROBLEMS

Primary prevention through anticipatory guidance can limit or eliminate many common feeding problems. Education about early infant feeding begins at the prenatal visit and newborn examination. Plans for feeding should be explored, and breastfeeding should be encouraged by emphasizing nutritional, immunologic, and psychological benefits. Realistic expectation for nursing and instructions to ensure proper latching on and effective sucking by the infant should be reviewed before mother and infant are discharged home. A follow-up office visit within 1 week should be encouraged for first-time nursing mothers. Lactation counseling by the infant's clinician or another person assists many mothers and prevents early discontinuation of breastfeeding (Powers and Slusser, 1997).

Clinicians can assist parents to prepare for each stage in feeding by reviewing anticipated milestones that change a feeding pattern (see Table 58-1). Temperament variations and cultural differences should be evaluated and incorporated into recommendations.

When talking directly to school-age children and adolescents, nutritional counselors should take into consideration cognitive stages of development in terms of the child's ability to understand cause and effect (concrete operations) and to hypothesize an outcome (formal operations) (see Chapters 5 and 6).

PARENTAL CONCERNS ABOUT FEEDING

My child is not gaining enough weight.

Standard growth measurements and monitoring practices during health supervision visits allow tracking of growth on height and weight charts. When a concern about growth is expressed by the parent of a child who is growing at an expected rate, the visual image of growth illustrated by a chart is often therapeutic. It is also useful to ask the parent to describe a meal in terms of the child's behavior and the immediate environment. Curious and active children may show so much interest in the surrounding environment during feeding that they may only appear to be undereating. Parental expectations may be a clue to developmentally inappropriate goals. Concerns about too-frequent meals, picky eating patterns, spitting up, and food preferences or aversions may provide an opening to discuss behaviors that have an impact on broader aspects of the child's development.

Failure-to-thrive, defined as weight loss that crosses at least two major percentile lines on a standard growth chart or weight lower than the 5th percentile, is discussed elsewhere (see Chapter 60). Milder forms of weight loss secondary to *underfeeding* are frequent in the first 3 years of life. A pediatric approach to a mild form of failure-to-thrive requires a comprehensive medical and psychosocial evaluation. Caution should be taken in assuming that a behavioral or interactional problem is the cause for underfeeding. A common form of mild failure-to-thrive can be seen in infants and toddlers who exhibit a transient but dramatic weight loss after a series of common intercurrent infections. These frequent febrile illnesses may be associated with irritability, painful oral lesions, sore bottoms, and anorexia. Even though the infant or toddler may recover quickly from the illness, feeding patterns may not rebound as efficiently, especially when a parent perceives the child as vulnerable or fragile. A parent at risk for depression, substance abuse, or other significant psychosocial stress may not adapt effectively to the child's changing feeding behaviors. Attentive observations of parent-child interactions in the office, a 2-day nutritional diary, and a clear explanation of the effect of illness on appetite and temporary weight loss begin the evaluation and treatment process.

My baby is spitting up all the time.

Spitting up (or regurgitation) is common during infancy. In the absence of projectile vomiting and poor weight gain, it usually is a result of gastroesophageal reflux. The main mechanism of gastroesophageal reflux is transient lower esophageal relaxation. Regurgitation is a common maturational process in healthy infants. It occurs at least once daily in 50% of infants younger than 3 months, peaks at 4 months (67%), and decreases to 20% at 6 months. At 12 months, less than 5% of infants are symptomatic (Gershman, 2005).

When infants regurgitate with every feeding, especially in association with irritability, a parent is usually concerned about a serious disease. In a thriving infant with normal findings on physical examination, gastroesophageal reflux is the likely cause. A diagram that illustrates the course of a meal from the mouth to the stomach allows the clinician to illustrate the anatomy and function of the lower esophagus and gastroesophageal sphincter and its predictable maturation during infancy. Smaller, more frequent feeds and holding the infant's head steady above the abdomen during feeding diminish spitting up in most infants. Thickening a formula with rice cereal decreases the frequency of regurgitation but not other symptoms. Medications that suppress gastric acid (H_2-receptor antagonists and proton pump inhibitors) are prescribed in the most severe case. Formula change is not indicated unless there is a strong family history of allergy or intolerance to dairy products. Gastroesophageal reflux is an example of a common developmental problem with a physiologic cause that may be associated with significant parental concerns and anxiety. This is especially true when more severe symptomatic reflux causes peptic esophagitis, "heartburn," and dramatic arching of the trunk and neck (Sandifer syndrome).

A related problem is the excessive air swallowed (*aerophagia*) by some infants during feeding. Fussiness, abdominal distention, and regurgitation may result from an overly distended stomach. Attention to the infant's latching on to the nipple during nursing, proper holding, feeding in a calm environment, and adequate burping are beneficial. When regurgitation or aerophagia does not respond to these techniques or when the feeding interaction is chaotic and stressful, an examination of maternal-child interactions and stresses in the family is usually helpful.

Regurgitation may also be a sign of *overfeeding*. At other times, the only clinical clue may be excessive weight gain. Caution in infancy is recommended because many breastfed infants are chubby in the first year. Bottle-fed infants who gain more than 1 ounce each day or who consume more than 35 ounces of formula each day may be overfeeding. In early childhood, overfeeding is usually responsive to education of parents about appropriate weight gain and alternative ways to comfort and soothe. A similar approach is appropriate for older children after an evaluation of the family's mealtime behaviors, the food quantities and types available to the child, and the child's functional psychosocial status (see Chapter 61).

My baby is so fussy. The formula isn't satisfying him.

Some parents may interpret prolonged periods of fussiness in a healthy infant as an expression of hunger. Even though this may be true in some infants, episodic fussiness in early infancy is more commonly a reflection of a child's inborn temperament (see Chapter 57). Frequent feeding that may lead to excessive weight gain is not in the best interest of the child.

I know she's growing, you've shown me her growth chart. But she only eats a few preferred foods and refuses most of the foods we serve. It's very frustrating.

The time and emotional energy spent feeding an infant during the first year of life changes dramatically when toddlers and preschool children make choices about content, amount, and timing of meals. For some parents, it is a difficult transition. In other families, mealtime is so central to family life that performance expectations are set high. Most parents find reassurance in a few important facts. First, when offered nutritional foods, without sweets, and an appropriate level of fat content, children select a balanced diet during a period of a few weeks (Pilner and Pelchat, 1986; Story and Brown, 1987). Second, growth rates for height and weight are expected to decrease after 1 year of age. Many children normally develop a leaner body at this time as activity level and energy output increase. Third, no parent has ever won "a battle" over food intake or preferences. By encouraging choice in the diet, parents promote autonomy, mastery, and self-esteem. Keeping healthy foods in the home for meals and snack time, limiting junk food for special occasions, and reviewing food choices among adults in the home promote adequate nutrition habits.

Less common than food fussiness are *food phobias* in which a child experiences anxiety or a tantrum related to a particular food. Avoidance of the food that elicits the phobic response is usually sufficient unless the phobia is associated with other psychological problems. For most children without a suggestion of disease after a complete medical history and physical examination, a parent's concern about a picky eating pattern or limited food preferences is a behavioral problem that should focus on developmental expectations and parent-child interactions. It should be seen as an opportunity for a behavioral intervention through education.

Parents can be advised not to use food as a reward for behavior and not to reward a child for finishing a meal. Most children respond when they see other children eating foods they have avoided (Davis, 1938). Meals that include a variety of foods served in a family setting, without television or video watching and without forcing, promote healthy eating habits.

My child will always choose junk foods over good foods.

Food preference is a learned behavior. The preferences of children (and adults) reflect their exposure to foods at mealtime and snack time and their exposure to food advertising. To prevent preferences for foods with excessive sugar and fat content, early counseling of parents about nutrition is appropriate in the first year of life and periodically after that during health supervision visits (Hagan et al, 2008). Office wall posters and literature for parents may be informative. When parents watch television with their children or see an advertisement for junk food in a magazine or on a billboard, they can be advised to comment and engage their child in a conversation about appropriate nutrition and health. Role modeling of parental snacking habits at home—especially eating high-fat, sweet, or salty foods while watching television—should be reviewed. Family meals without a television promote good nutrition habits.

When junk food intake is frequent and excessive, it may be helpful to review the parents' goals for nutrition and patterns of mealtime behaviors and snacking at home and away from home. Elimination of junk foods in the home is a good start. Encouraging fruit and vegetable sticks for snacks is helpful. For older children, a reward program of self-directed healthy eating can be initiated. Realistic counseling goals inform parents that they can control the availability of food in the home and give their child appropriate nutrition information. Eating behaviors outside the home may be influenced, but not entirely controlled, by parental guidance.

Pica is seen in children who frequently ingest nonfood substances. It is found in all children in the first 2 years as a reflection of normal hand-to-mouth exploratory behavior. When pica occurs persistently, beyond the age of 2 years, or involves dangerous substances, it is a medical and behavioral problem. Children with intellectual disability, significant psychological disorders, autism, and sensory impairment may exhibit pica extensively. Children with insufficient emotional or intellectual stimulation ingest nonfood substances as well. This practice may be harmful when it involves lead in peeling paint, dirt, or other toxic substances (see Chapter 31).

ALTERNATIVE DIETS—NUTRITIONAL AND BEHAVIORAL CONSIDERATIONS

For a variety of reasons, some parents and older children choose to consume foods in a pattern outside the cultural mainstream. These alternative diets are embraced by a subset of the population, either temporarily or long term. A religious, ethical, or cultural context often guides the choice for these diets. Other parents and older children may sublimate a desire to gain control over their lives through a commitment to an alternative nutrition system. Concern for environmental pollution in the food chain or water supply initiates the decision for others. Even though most of the diets are not harmful, pediatric clinicians should be aware that specific nutrient deficiencies could occur with some alternative diets. A lacto-ovo-vegetarian diet (which includes dairy and egg consumption) may be iron deficient. Vegans (no animal products at all) benefit from iron and vitamin B_{12} supplements. Megavitamin diets may cause vitamin D toxicity, decrease vitamin B_{12} absorption (ascorbic acid excess), and decrease breast milk production (pyridoxine excess). A macrobiotic diet may be deficient in calories, protein, and some minerals and vitamins (American Heart Association, 2006).

Food fads are common beginning at the age of puberty. The decision to break away from family tradition and begin some form of a vegetarian diet is linked closely with an age-appropriate quest for independence. Pediatricians can support the adolescent at the time of this decision, as well as reassure parents, by reviewing both the benefits and the potential nutritional deficiencies in the diet. The most frequent choice, a lacto-ovo-vegetarian diet, is healthy and without risk except for the need for a supplemental iron source. A pure vegetarian diet (vegan) requires more nutritional knowledge to ensure adequate protein and calorie intake for the growing body. A diet diary for a few days may be useful when there is concern about excessive restriction of essential nutrients. Self-imposed limits on calorie intake may be an early sign of anorexia nervosa (see Chapter 59).

SUMMARY

Healthy feeding patterns and feeding associated with physical and behavioral symptoms during childhood can be understood in the context of a child's development and parent-child interactions. This chapter reviews the components of the parent-child dyad that affect the feeding process with an emphasis on attachment, temperament, the environment, and the parent's psychological health. Cultural factors (e.g., co-sleeping) and social trends that have an impact on feeding are discussed. Common feeding concerns that parents bring to pediatricians are reviewed from the perspective of an interaction between a child's development, physiology, and parental responses.

REFERENCES

American Heart Association, Dietary Recommendations for Children and Adolescents: A Guide for Practitioners. Pediatrics 117:544-559, 2006.

Davis CM: Self-selection of diet experiment: Its significance for feeding in the home. Ohio State Med J 34:862, 1938.

Dixon SD, Stein MT: Encounters with Children: Pediatric Behavior and Development, 4th ed. Philadelphia, Elsevier Mosby, 2006.

Gershman G: Gastroesophageal reflux. *In* Osborn LM, DeWitt TG, First LR, et al (eds): Pediatrics, Philadelphia Elsevier, Mosby, 2005 p 658-665.

Hagan JF, Shaw JS, Duncan PM: Bright Futures: Guidelines for the Health Supervision of Infants, Children, and Adolescents, 3rd ed. Elk Grove Village, IL, American Academy of Pediatrics, 2008.

Hammer LD: The development of eating behavior in childhood. Pediatr Clin North Am 39:379-394, 1992.

Mannella JA, Beauchamp GK: Maternal diet alters the sensory qualities of human milk and nursling's behavior. Pediatrics 88:737-744, 1991.

Pilner P, Pelchat ML: Similarities in food preferences between children and their siblings and parents. Appetite 7:333, 1986.

Powers NG, Slusser W: Breastfeeding—update 2: Clinical lactation management. Pediatr Rev 18:147-161, 1997.

Satter EM: The feeding relationship: Problems and interventions. J Pediatr 117:5181-5189, 1990.

Stein MT, Colaruso C, McKenna JJ, et al: Cosleeping (bedsharing) among infants and toddlers. J Developmental Behav Padiatr 18: 408-412, 1997.

Story M, Brown JE: Do young children instinctively know what to eat? The studies of Clare Davis revisited. N Engl J Med 316:103, 1987.

Sullivan SA, Birch LL: Infant dietary experience and acceptance of solid foods. Pediatrics 93:271-277, 1994.

59 DISORDERED EATING BEHAVIORS: ANOREXIA NERVOSA AND BULIMIA NERVOSA

Eric Sigel

OVERVIEW

The eating disorders represent one of the most complex biopsychosocial illnesses that children and adolescents experience. They are challenging to understand and not easy to treat. Youths who are struggling with an eating disorder are often secretive about their illness, so parents and health care providers often do not recognize it until there are serious medical effects. This chapter outlines the context in which eating disorders develop, explains the differences between the eating disorders, and increases the clinician's ability to recognize and to treat eating disorders.

ETIOLOGY

In general, it is thought that patients have a genetic susceptibility to development of eating disorders. Factors from the environment—stressors such as changes at home or social pressure to be thin—influence the biologic milieu, setting into motion a process that ultimately leads to the development of eating disorders.

Genetic Contribution

Evidence supports a genetic predisposition for development of eating disorders (Bulik and Tozzi, 2005). There is a 7% incidence of anorexia nervosa in first-degree relatives of anorexic patients compared with a 1% to 2% incidence in the general population. Twin studies have shown a 55% concordance rate in monozygotic twins compared with 7% in dizygotic twins. Twin studies estimate the heritability of anorexia nervosa (AN) to be between 33% and 84% and that of bulimia nervosa (BN) to be between 28% and 83%. A study of males with AN showed a relative risk of 20% for first-degree female relatives. Genomic regions on chromosome 1 for AN and chromosome 10 for BN are likely to harbor susceptibility genes.

Neurohormonal Contribution

Leptin, a hormone secreted by adipocytes that regulates energy homeostasis and satiety signaling, is abnormal in patients with AN (Chan and Mantzoros, 2005), mediating energy changes that affect the hypothalamic-pituitary axis while playing a role in the perpetuation of AN. Leptin levels decrease as individuals lose weight and increase to excessive levels as weight is restored. The idiosyncratic higher levels of leptin may contribute to the difficulty patients have in trying to regain weight, as higher leptin signals the body to decrease energy intake. Leptin also plays a role in some of the sequelae of AN, with low levels signaling the hypothalamus to inhibit reproductive hormone production.

There is evidence of persistently altered serotonergic and dopaminergic function in AN and BN (Bosanac et al, 2005) as well as alterations in gut peptides. Patients with BN or binge-eating disorder appear to have a blunted serotonin response to eating and satiety. With a decreased satiety response, patients continue to eat, leading to a binge. Treatment with selective serotonin reuptake inhibitors (SSRIs) tends to equilibrate satiety regulation. An alteration in dopamine has also been recognized (Bailer and Kaye, 2003), although its significance has not been elucidated. Ghrelin, a gut peptide, is elevated in patients with AN. Ghrelin does not decrease in the normal fashion after a meal in patients with AN. Adiponectin appears elevated in AN, although it is unclear as to whether it is due to the malnourished state or elevated independently of malnourishment. Cholecystokinin is decreased in BN, perhaps contributing to the lack of post-ingestion satiety that perpetuates a binge. Although significant research has been done on the neurobiology of eating disorders, it remains unclear whether alterations contribute to the development of eating disorders or are present as a consequence of the physiologic changes that occur.

Psychological Factors

Traditional psychological theory has suggested several factors that might contribute to the development of eating disorders. Enmeshment of mother and daughter to the point that the teenager cannot develop her own identity (a key developmental marker of adolescence) may be a predisposing factor. The teenager may cope by asserting control over food, as she senses her lack of control in the developmental realm. A second theory involves father-daughter distancing. As puberty progresses and a girl's sexuality blossoms, a father may experience difficulty in dealing with his daughter as a sexual being and may respond by withdrawing both emotionally and physically. The teenage girl may intuitively recognize this and subconsciously decrease her food intake to become prepubertal again. A third theory is related to puberty itself. Some teenagers may fear or dislike their changing bodies. By restricting food intake, they lose weight, stop menstruating, and effectively halt pubertal development.

Societal Influence

Society has provided the message that being thin or muscular is necessary for attractiveness and success. Youths are bombarded by images throughout all types of media that highlight body types that are unrealistic to attain but serve as models of beauty and masculinity. Messages about fat being bad and ugly are pervasive, and modern society has created readily available tools that contribute to the evolution of eating disorders, including fat-free foods, diet aids, and pro-anorexia Web sites that teach youths how to have an eating disorder. Genetic predisposition, psychological factors, and environmental pressures combine to create a milieu that allows eating disorders to develop in today's youth.

INCIDENCE

Among teenage girls in the United States, AN is the third most common chronic illness. The incidence in the United States has been increasing steadily since the 1930s. Most studies show that 1% to 2% of teenagers develop AN and 2% to 4% develop BN (Yager and Anderson, 2005). Adolescents outnumber adults 5 to 1, although the number of adults with eating disorders is rising. The incidence is also increasing among younger children. Prepubertal youths often have significant associated comorbid psychiatric diagnoses. Men represent approximately 10% of the total eating disorder population, although recent studies show increasing prevalence in men (Woodside et al, 2001). The increasing number of men diagnosed with eating disorders correlates with the increased media emphasis on muscular, chiseled appearance as the male ideal. Binge-eating disorder has a 1.1% incidence in teenagers.

Many youths engage in eating disorder behaviors. In the recent Youth Risk Behavior Survey (Centers for Disease Control, 2006) of U.S. teenagers, 62% of girls and 30% of boys were attempting to lose weight during the preceding 30 days of the survey. Twelve percent of youths fasted for more than 24 hours to lose weight; 6.1% of youths had used diet pills, powders, or liquids to lose weight (8.1% of girls and 4.6% of boys). Self-induced vomiting or laxative use (or both) is common; 6.2% of girls and 2.8% of boys used one or the other. Forty-six percent of girls and 30% of boys reported at least one bingeing episode during their lifetime. Although the number of youths with full-blown eating disorders is low compared with these practices, it is alarming that so many youths experiment with unhealthy weight control habits. These signs certainly may be precursors to the development of eating disorders, and clinicians need to explore these practices with all of their adolescent patients.

ANOREXIA NERVOSA

Demographics

Anorexia is found in all racial and ethnic groups (Shaw et al, 2004), although diagnosis is more common in middle–upper middle class, white girls. Youths diagnosed with AN are typically high achieving academically. Those involved in gymnastics, figure skating, and ballet—activities that emphasize (and in which coaches often require) thin bodies—are at higher risk for AN than are children in sports that do not emphasize body image. Sudden changes in dietary habits, such as becoming vegetarian, may be a first sign of AN, especially if the change is abrupt and without good reason.

Diagnosis

Table 59-1 lists the diagnostic criteria for AN according to the *Diagnostic and Statistical Manual of Mental Disorders*, 4th edition (DSM-IV). There are two forms of AN. In the restricting type, patients do not regularly engage in binge eating or purging. In the purging type, classic AN is combined with binge eating or purging behavior (or both). Differentiation of the two is important because of differing implications for prognosis and treatment. In addition, there is debate about criteria for AN; some experts have argued to eliminate amenorrhea as a specific criterion. Although patients may not demonstrate all features of AN, they may still exhibit the deleterious symptoms associated with AN.

Clinical Presentation

Recognition of the clinical features of AN (Miller et al, 2005; Rome et al, 2003) is crucial, especially in assessing those with developmental disabilities who may not be able to clearly state intentional weight loss. In addition, those with AN are often secretive about their

Table 59-1. Diagnostic Criteria for Anorexia Nervosa

A. Refusal to maintain body weight at or above a minimally normal weight for age and height (e.g., weight loss leading to maintenance of body weight less than 85% of that expected; or failure to make expected weight gain during period of growth, leading to body weight less than 85% of that expected).
B. Intense fear of gaining weight or becoming fat, even though underweight.
C. Disturbance in the way in which one's body weight or shape is experienced, undue influence of body weight or shape on self-evaluation, or denial of the seriousness of the current low body weight.
D. In postmenarcheal females, amenorrhea, i.e., the absence of at least three menstrual cycles. (A woman is considered to have amenorrhea if her periods occur only following hormone, e.g., estrogen, administration.)

illness, and a clinician will need to recognize the symptoms and signs of AN first to arrive at a diagnosis. In the teenager who is not ready to share his or her concerns about body image, the clinician may find clues by carefully considering presenting symptoms. Any significant weight loss should lead the clinician to consider AN, and weight loss from a baseline of normal body weight is an obvious red flag. Keeping up-to-date growth charts is essential to help interpret any changes that may have occurred (Fig. 59-1). In addition, AN should be considered in any girl presenting with secondary amenorrhea. Physical symptoms are usually secondary to weight loss and proportional to the degree of malnutrition and the rate of weight loss. The body effectively goes into hibernation, becoming functionally hypothyroid (euthyroid sick) to save as much energy as possible. Body temperature decreases, patients report being cold, and they may present with cold and blue hands and feet. Patients become bradycardic, especially in the supine position. Dizziness, lightheadedness, and occasional syncope may ensue, as orthostasis and hypotension secondary to impaired cardiac function occur. Left ventricular mass is decreased (as all striated muscle throughout the body loses mass), stroke volume is compromised, and peripheral resistance is increased, contributing to left ventricular systolic dysfunction. Patients can develop prolonged QT syndrome and increased QT dispersion, putting them at risk for cardiac arrhythmias (Panagiotopoulos et al, 2000). Hair thins, nails become brittle, and the skin is dry. Lanugo develops as a primitive response to starvation. The gastrointestinal tract may be affected (Benini et al, 2004). Inability to take in normal quantities of food, early satiety, and gastroesophageal reflux can develop as the body adapts to reduced intake. The normal gastrocolic reflex may be temporarily lost because of lack of stimuli, leading to delayed gastric emptying and constipation. Neurologically, patients may experience decreased cognition, inability to concentrate, increased irritability, and depression, which may be related to structural brain changes and decreased cerebral blood flow.

A combination of malnutrition and stress causes hypothalamic hypogonadism. The hypothalamic-pituitary-gonadal axis shuts down as the body struggles to survive, directing finite energy resources to support more vital functions. Both boys and girls experience decreased libido and interruption of pubertal development, depending on the timing of the illness. Skeletal growth may be interrupted. Amenorrhea is due to the hypothalamic hypogonadism as well as the loss of adipose tissue. Adipose tissue is needed to convert estrogen to its activated form. When weight loss is significant, adipose tissue is lost and there is not enough substrate to activate estrogen.

Making the Diagnosis

There are two common ways that clinicians start to diagnose AN. One is recognizing the clinical signs, and the other is responding to a parent's report of weight loss and change of eating habits. Regardless, once a clinician suspects AN, determination of whether a patient meets DSM-IV criteria will lead to a diagnosis. As with all diagnoses, a careful history and physical examination are essential (Table 59-2).

The first diagnostic criterion for AN is being less than 85% ideal body weight (see Fig. 59-2 for an example of extreme malnutrition). Calculation of body mass index (BMI)—weight in kilograms divided by height in meters squared—is the way to assess the degree of malnutrition. A BMI less than the 25th percentile (using BMI growth curves) indicates risk for malnutrition, and less than the 5th percentile indicates significant malnutrition. Ideal body weight (IBW) is calculated by using the 50th percentile of BMI for age and determining the corresponding weight. Current weight divided by IBW then provides

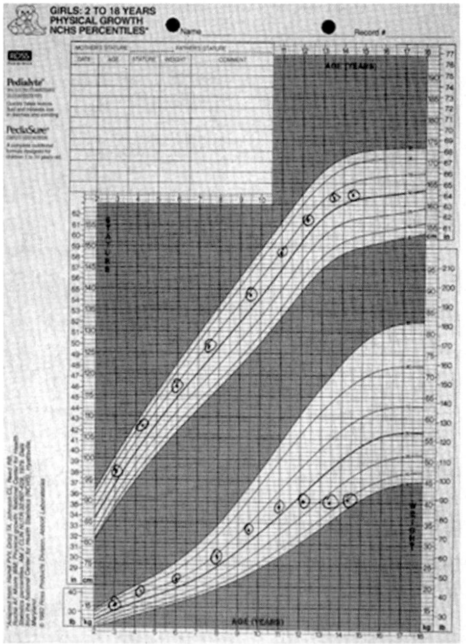

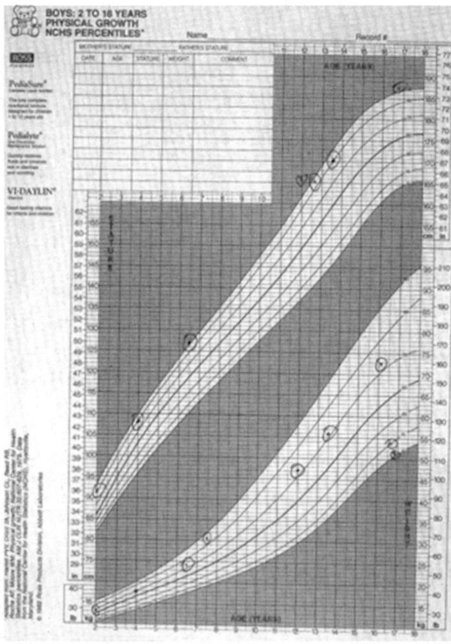

Figure 59-1. Examples of growth charts in patients with anorexia nervosa.

the percent IBW. Weighing youths with suspected AN can be tricky. A gown-only weight after urination is the most accurate way to assess weight. Patients tend to wear bulky clothes and may hide weights in their pockets or drink excessive amounts of fluid (water loading) to trick the practitioner.

The second diagnostic criterion is fear of fat—either in their food or on their bodies. Nutritional assessment is vital. Often patients eliminate fat from their diets, eating less than 5 grams of fat and as little as 100 to 200 kcal per day.

The third criterion, body image distortion, is the hallmark feature of AN. It is believed that those with AN truly have a biologically based distorted body image, not just a feeling of being overweight. They see themselves bigger and fatter than they truly are, and they see fat in places that is nonexistent to any outside observer. Asking youths how they see themselves in a mirror—either about the right size, smaller than average, or larger than average—can determine their body image. Asking parents as well about what youths say about themselves can provide insight, as they frequently comment at home about being fat and needing to lose weight. The clinician should recognize that adolescents do not necessarily need to see themselves as fat to have a distorted body image; if they happen to be 75% of IBW and they see their weight as normal, those individuals have a distorted body image as well.

Table 59-2. Screening Questions to Help Diagnose Anorexia and Bulimia Nervosa

How do you feel about your body?
Are there parts of your body you might change?
When you look at yourself in the mirror, do you see yourself as overweight, underweight, or satisfactory?
If overweight, how much do you want to weigh?
If your weight is satisfactory, has there been a time that you were worried about being overweight?
If overweight/underweight, what would you change?
Have you ever been on a diet?
What have you done to help yourself lose weight?
Do you count calories or fat grams?
Do you keep your intake to a certain number of calories?
Have you ever used nutritional supplements, diet pills, or laxatives to help you lose weight?
Have you ever made yourself vomit to get rid of food or to lose weight?

The last diagnostic criterion for AN is amenorrhea for 3 months. This criterion is being debated among the experts in the field and in the future may not be necessary to diagnose AN. In addition to figuring out whether a child meets the four specific criteria for AN, the clinician needs to determine if there are behaviors that are associated with the other eating disorders; this helps with diagnosis as well as guides the physician toward anticipating other medical sequelae.

For the initial assessment as well as routine medical follow-up, there are several essential components to the medical visit (Rome et al, 2003). It is necessary to obtain a gowned weight and vital signs including orthostatic heart rate, blood pressure, and body temperature. In addition, assessment of nutritional intake (general calorie level), amount of exercise, binge eating, and any other purging behaviors helps determine current medical status and guides the clinician to the appropriate next step in management.

Laboratory Findings

Most organ systems can potentially suffer some degree of damage in the anorexic patient (Table 59-3), related to both severity and duration of illness (Miller et al, 2005). Initial screening should include complete blood cell count with differential; serum levels of electrolytes, blood urea nitrogen/creatinine, phosphorus, calcium,

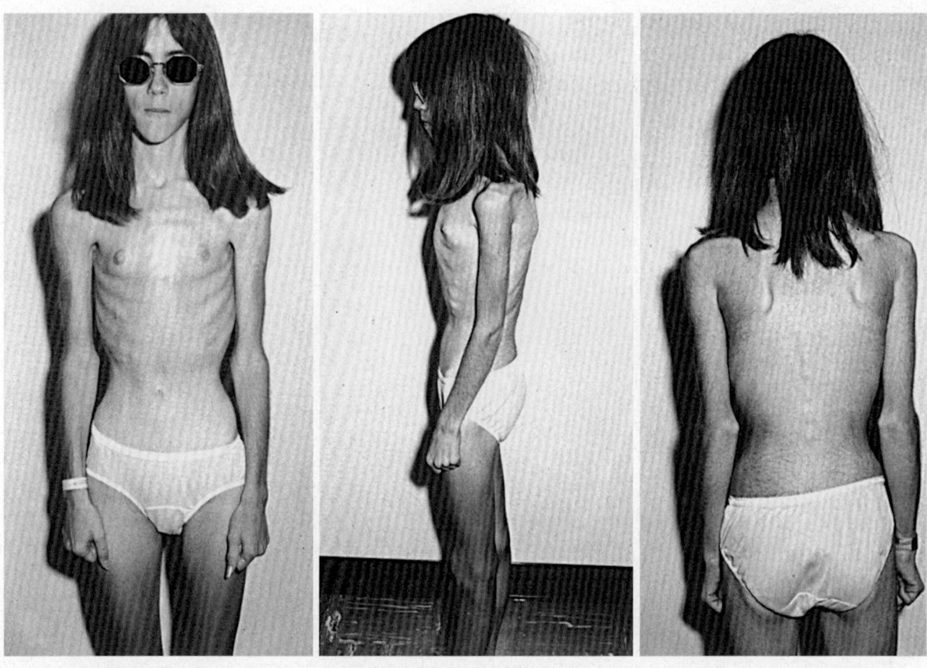

Figure 59-2. Severe emaciation with characteristic physical findings of anorexia nervosa.

Table 59-3. Laboratory Findings: Anorexia Nervosa

↑Blood urea nitrogen/creatinine secondary to renal insufficiency
↓White blood cells, platelets, and less commonly red blood cells/hematocrit secondary to bone marrow suppression
↑AST and ALT secondary to malnutrition
↑Cholesterol, thought to be related to fatty acid metabolism
↓Alkaline phosphatase secondary to zinc deficiency
Low to low-normal thyroid-stimulating hormone and thyroxine
↓Follicle-stimulating hormone, luteinizing hormone, estradiol, and testosterone secondary to shutdown of hypothalamic-pituitary-gonadal axis
↓Na, K, Cl related to hydrational and nutritional status
↓Phosphorus
↓Insulin-like growth factor
↑Cortisol
↓Urine specific gravity in cases of intentional water intoxication

ALT, alanine aminotransferase; AST, aspartate aminotransferase;

magnesium, and thyroid-stimulating hormone; and liver function tests and urinalysis. Electrocardiography should be performed because significant electrocardiographic abnormalities may be present, most importantly prolonged QT syndrome. Bone densitometry should be done if amenorrhea has persisted for 6 months because patients begin to accumulate risk for osteoporosis.

Differential Diagnosis

If the diagnosis is unclear (i.e., the patient has lost a significant amount of weight but does not have typical body image distortion or fat phobia), the clinician must consider the differential diagnosis for weight loss in adolescents. This includes inflammatory bowel disease, diabetes, hyperthyroidism, malignant disease, and depression. Less common diagnoses include adrenal insufficiency and malabsorption syndromes such as celiac disease. The history and physical examination findings should direct laboratory and radiologic evaluation.

Management and Treatment

Practitioners need to address the detailed medical complications of AN (Table 59-4) as well as help families work toward recovery. There are a variety of treatment approaches to AN, and intervention depends on the severity of illness. Intervention early in the course of illness geared to weight restoration leads to a better prognosis. A multidisciplinary team approach, with psychologists, psychiatrists, and nutrition therapists with expertise in eating disorders, provides the most comprehensive treatment.

Many treatment modalities are available. Factors that determine treatment interventions are severity of illness, length of illness, specific manifestations of disease, prior treatment, outcomes, program availability, financial resources, and insurance coverage. Treatment options include outpatient management, day treatment hospitalization, and inpatient hospitalization of either a medical or psychiatric nature. Residential treatment is most often used when outpatient management or short-term hospitalization fails and the eating disorder becomes chronic. Residential treatment usually lasts 2 to 6 months. Day treatment programs are a good intervention for patients who do not yet need inpatient care but who are not

Table 59-4. Complications of Anorexia and Bulimia Nervosa

Cardiovascular

Bradycardia
Postural hypotension
Arrhythmia, sudden death
Congestive heart failure (during refeeding)
Pericardial effusion
Mitral valve prolapse
Electrocardiographic abnormalities (prolonged QT, low voltage, T-wave abnormalities, conduction defects)

Endocrine

↓LH, FSH
↓T_3, ↑rT_3, ↓T_4, TSH
Irregular menses
Amenorrhea
Hypercortisolism
Growth retardation
Delayed puberty

Gastrointestinal

Dental erosion
Parotid swelling
Esophagitis, esophageal tears
Delayed gastric emptying
Gastric dilatation (rarely rupture)
Pancreatitis
Constipation
Diarrhea (laxative abuse)
Superior mesenteric artery syndrome
Hypercholesterolemia
↑Liver function test results (fatty infiltration of the liver)

Skeletal

Osteopenia
Fractures

Hematologic

Leukopenia
Anemia
Thrombocytopenia
↓Erythrocyte sedimentation rate
Impaired cell-mediated immunity

Metabolic

Dehydration
Acidosis
Hypokalemia
Hyponatremia
Hypochloremia
Hypochloremic alkalosis
Hypocalcemia
Hypophosphatemia
Hypomagnesemia
Hypercarotenemia

Neurologic

Cortical atrophy
Peripheral neuropathy
Seizures
Thermoregulatory abnormalities
↓REM and slow-wave sleep

Renal

Hematuria
Proteinuria
↓Renal concentrating ability

FSH, follicle-stimulating hormone; LH, luteinizing hormone; T3, triiodothyronine; rT3, reverse T3; T4, thyroxine; TSH, thyroid-stimulating hormone.

improving with outpatient management. Treatment is costly. Many patients do not have insurance benefits that adequately cover the cost, leaving parents and practitioners with profound dilemmas as to how to best provide treatment in the face of financial constraints.

The key to determining level of intervention depends on the degree of malnutrition, the rapidity of weight loss, the degree of medical compromise, and the presence of life-threatening electrolyte abnormalities (Rome et al, 2003). No absolute criteria determine level of intervention. The practitioner must assess the degree of medical compromise, consider immediate risks, and assess the potential for an individual to reverse the situation on his or her own. An initial decision point is determination of whether medical compromise is severe enough to necessitate an inpatient hospital admission. Table 59-5 lists the criteria for hospital admission generally used in the medical community. It is usually quite difficult for a patient who is losing weight rapidly (>1 kg/week) to reverse the weight loss because the body is in a catabolic state. Details of inpatient management are not addressed here, but the important medical issues that a practitioner needs to manage at an outpatient level are discussed.

Outpatient Treatment

Once the need for inpatient medical care is ruled out, practitioners and families together can pursue treatment in the outpatient setting. It is generally recommended to use a multidisciplinary team approach if it is available. Overriding goals of treatment are to have patients achieve at least 90% to 95% of their healthy body weight, resume menstruation, eat in a normal manner, and be free of the persistent eating disorder thoughts that dominate their thinking. Weekly goals should be discussed with youths and their parents as well as with other team members. The initial goal is to reverse the catabolic state and weight loss. Patients in general should increase calorie intake 250 kcal every 2 to 3 days, depending on their present calorie intake and degree of medical side effects, until they start gaining weight consistently. Weight restoration goals can be 0.2 to 0.5 kg per week, which often requires 2500 to 3000 kcal per day. The practitioner usually needs to recommend cessation of physical activity as well. Activity can then be slowly introduced back into the daily routine once a patient demonstrates steady weight gain. Careful monitoring for medical instability and weight loss is important in determining whether an increased level of care is needed at any time during outpatient management. Expectations should be spelled out, and lack of achieving goals certainly may necessitate a more intense level of care to help the patient with AN get better.

Table 59-5. **Criteria for Inpatient Treatment of Anorexia Nervosa**

Criteria
Body weight < 75% of ideal body weight
Supine heart rate < 45/min
Symptomatic hypotension or syncope
Hypokalemia: potassium concentration < 2.5 mEq/L
Rapid weight loss that cannot be interrupted on outpatient basis
Failure of outpatient management
Acute food refusal

Common Issues in Outpatient Management of Anorexia Nervosa

Refeeding Syndrome

During the initial introduction of food, the clinician needs to monitor the patient for refeeding syndrome, a phenomenon that occurs if calorie intake is increased too rapidly. Signs of refeeding syndrome are decreased serum phosphate (as the body finally starts making adenosine triphosphate), decreased serum potassium (as increased insulin causes shifting of potassium from extracellular fluid into potassium-depleted cells), and edema related to fluid shifts as well as from congestive

Vignette

The parents of Jake, a 15-year-old boy, have been concerned about his energy level. He has recently started to get tired easily, and although he continues tennis practice (#2 singles varsity squad), he falls asleep before all his homework is done. He had a severe cold 3 months ago and has not seemed to recover his energy level. He lost about 10 pounds, but he and his parents are pleased about that; he had been 75th percentile BMI, a bit overweight, and 2 years ago he decided he needed to eat healthier and exercise. Talking with Jake alone, you discover that his moods are a bit flat, but he is not depressed. He likes the fact that he has gotten skinnier but still is unhappy with the flabbiness of his stomach and thighs; he wants a "six-pack," which he has not been able to achieve despite doing 500 sit-ups per day. He eats healthy foods, five times a day; he does not eat fast food or desserts anymore. On examination, his vitals are normal: heart rate, 60 supine, 70 standing; blood pressure, 102/68; temperature, 96.5°F. His height is 159 cm, 10th percentile; weight is 45.2 kg, 10th percentile; BMI is 17.9, 20th percentile. Two years ago, he was 153.5 cm tall, 40th percentile; weight, 53.7 kg, 75th percentile; BMI, 22.8. He is SMR 1 for pubic hair on genital examination.

Take Home Points

Commonly, parents are in search of a medical cause; certainly, with crossing height percentiles, one needs to consider hypothyroidism or inflammatory bowel disease. His lack of puberty development/delayed puberty could be the cause of his decreasing height percentiles. However, you, the clinician, recognize that the timing of his becoming more fit corresponds to changes in growth parameters. He is overly focused on his body and has some signs of body image distortion because he certainly does not have any apparent flabbiness on his abdomen. He has a major fat avoidance, and although he is eating about 1800 kcal per day, his needs, playing 2 hours of tennis, would be at least 2750 kcal/day. He is 90% of healthy body weight, so he does not meet full criteria for AN but has eating disorder not otherwise specified. His moods are flat because of his poor nutritional status. Although it was not wrong for his parents to encourage him to lose a little weight, he enjoyed the positive feedback and became chronically deficient in overall calories and fat intake. His relative malnutrition then has caused both decreased height velocity and delayed onset of puberty. Because he has not had significant weight loss, he has not experienced the typical symptoms associated with rapid weight loss. Intervention with nutrition therapy, psychotherapy, and medical monitoring should help reverse the physical impact of this eating disorder. The clinician needs to decrease his physical activity until his eating improves. Outcomes: His moods improve after 2 to 3 weeks of nutritional rehabilitation; 6 months later, after he reaches a healthy body weight, signs of puberty begin.

heart failure. Laboratory parameters (potassium and phosphate concentrations) should generally be monitored until youths are tolerating at least 1500 kcal per day and gaining weight.

Early Satiety

Patients may have significant difficulty digesting modest quantities as their bodies adapt to increased calorie intake. Patients may benefit from a gastric-emptying agent such as metoclopramide. This complication usually resolves after a patient has become used to larger meals.

Constipation

Patients may have prolonged constipation, often not having a bowel movement for a week or longer. Two mechanisms contribute to this symptom: loss of gastrocolic reflex and loss of colonic muscle tone. Stool softeners typically do not help because the colon has decreased peristaltic amplitude. Agents that induce peristalsis, such as bisacodyl and polyethylene glycol–electrolyte solution (MiraLax), are helpful. Constipation can persist for up to 6 to 8 weeks after refeeding. On occasion, patients need enemas.

Rare Complication

Superior Mesenteric Artery Syndrome

As patients become malnourished, the fat pad between the superior mesenteric artery and the duodenum may shrink, compressing the transverse duodenum and causing vomiting and intolerance of oral intake, especially solids. Diagnosis is made by an upper gastrointestinal tract series, which shows to and fro movement of barium in the descending and transverse duodenum proximal to the obstruction. Treatment involves a liquid diet or nasoduodenal feedings until restoration of the fat pad has occurred, coincident with weight gain.

Long-term Issues

Amenorrhea

Amenorrhea is a general indicator of a woman's overall health status, and return of menses is an important marker of physical recovery from AN (if menarche has occurred). Resumption of normal menses depends on increase of both body weight and body fat. Approximately 73% of postmenarcheal girls will resume menstruation if they reach 90% of their IBW. An adolescent girl needs, on average, 17% body fat to restart menses and 22% body fat if she has primary amenorrhea. In general, target weights for return of menses are approximately 1 kg greater than the weight at which menses was lost. This may be mediated by the effect of low levels of leptin on the hypothalamic-pituitary axis. Treatment styles differ, but a minimum weight goal for patients generally should be 90% of the healthy body weight. If they remain at 90% for 2 to 3 months without restarting menses, the target weight should be increased to 95% IBW. Signs of estrogen activation include a reappearance of physiologic leukorrhea. There are no specific laboratory evaluations needed for the presence of amenorrhea in a patient with AN; however, if a youth has had sexual intercourse, pregnancy should be ruled out. Also, some clinicians obtain bone densitometry if amenorrhea has persisted for 6 months or more. Risperidone and other atypical antipsychotics can cause an elevation in prolactin levels. If a girl is weight recovered and continues to be amenorrheic, an amenorrhea evaluation, including prolactin levels, should be pursued.

Osteopenia and Osteoporosis

Approximately 90% of girls with AN have reduced bone mass at one or more sites. The development of osteopenia and osteoporosis is multifactorial (Golden, 2003). Estrogen and testosterone are essential to potentiate bone development. Higher ghrelin level is an independent predicator of bone density in healthy adolescents; however, it does not appear to contribute to bone loss in patients with AN. Teenagers are particularly at risk because they accrue 40% of their bone mineral during adolescence. Low body weight is most predictive of bone loss. Duration of amenorrhea is also highly correlated with osteoporosis. Bone minerals begin to resorb without estrogen. Elevated cortisol levels and decreased insulin-like growth factor 1 also contribute to bone resorption. Studies show that as little as 6 months of amenorrhea can lead to osteopenia or osteoporosis. In one study, 44% of adolescents with AN had osteopenia of the lumbar spine. Boys also can develop osteoporosis (Castro et al, 2002) because of decreased testosterone and elevated cortisol. A recent finding has shown that the presence of depression in adolescent girls with AN contributes to higher risk of osteoporosis compared with AN alone (Konstantynowicz et al, 2005).

The only proven treatment of osteoporosis for girls with AN is regaining of sufficient weight and body fat to restart the menstrual cycle. Controversy exists about the use of hormone replacement therapy. Most studies (Golden, 2003; Karlsson et al, 2000) do not support use of hormone replacement therapy to improve bone recovery; however, some evidence indicates that hormone replacement therapy may stop further bone loss and may be of particular benefit for patients with extremely low body weight (<70% IBW). Some practitioners use hormone replacement therapy if amenorrhea is prolonged (>1 year) and the patient is not able to achieve normal body weight. The bisphosphonates used to treat postmenopausal osteoporosis are currently being studied in adolescents. Two small randomized controlled trials have shown small but positive effect on bone density with two of the bisphosphonates, alendronate (Golden et al, 2005) and risedronate, although clinical effectiveness has not yet been determined. Newer treatments in research trials have shown some promise, including recombinant insulin-like growth factor 1 injection and dehydroepiandrosterone, but both are still experimental.

General Growth Issues

For those who have not achieved final adult height, skeletal growth can be affected, depending on the timing, extent, and duration of the malnutrition. The longer an individual stays malnourished, the more impact there will be on height growth. Puberty can be delayed related to the degree of malnourishment and should be assessed initially. Careful documentation of height periodically, at least every 3 months, can provide insight into the changes on height velocity. Depending on how rapid a recovery, final adult height may be less than predicted. This information should be conveyed to the patients and their families to alert them to the impact the eating disorder may have on achieving final height.

Brain Changes

As malnutrition becomes more pronounced, brain tissue—both white and gray matter—is lost, and a concomitant increase in cerebrospinal fluid occurs in the sulci and ventricles (Kerem and Katzman, 2003). Follow-up studies of weight-recovered anorexic patients show a persistent loss of gray matter, although white matter returns to normal. Functionally, there does not seem to be a specific relationship between cognition and brain tissue loss, although studies have shown a decrease in cognitive ability as well as decreased cerebral blood flow in the more severely malnourished states. Communicating to the patient and the family that brain tissue can be lost can have a significant effect on the perception of the seriousness of this disorder.

Psychological Intervention

Teaming up with a therapist is critical to help youths and families recover from their eating disorder. Ideally, the therapist specializes in working with youths as well as with patients with an eating disorder. There are a variety of psychological approaches to youths with eating disorders (Rome et al, 2003).

Family therapy is especially helpful with younger teenagers, whereas older teenagers tend to benefit more from individual therapy, although both should be encouraged. Family therapy is an important means by which to help families understand the development of the disease and address the issues that may be barriers to recovery. Both therapies are used in most treatment programs, and recovery without psychotherapy is unusual. The average length of therapy is roughly 6 to 9 months, although some individuals continue therapy for extended periods. Adjunctive modalities include art and horticulture therapy, therapeutic recreation, and massage therapy.

A newer family therapy approach, manualized family therapy, developed in Britain by Maudsley and adapted by Lock and Le Grange (Le Grange et al, 2005), has shifted the therapeutic approach to youths with AN. Traditional therapy allowed the adolescents to control their eating and the parents to back off the food portion of recovery. This manualized approach gives power and control back to parents. Treatment is prescribed for 20 weekly sessions. The first 10 are devoted to empowering parents, putting them in control of their child's nutrition and exercise. Parents are educated about the dangers of malnutrition and supervise each meal. The next phase, sessions 11 to 16, returns control over eating to the adolescent once the adolescent accepts the demands of the parents. The last phase of treatment, sessions 17 to 20, occurs when the patient is maintaining a healthy weight, shifting the focus away from the eating disorder and examining the impact that the eating disorder has had on establishing a healthy adolescent identity. This approach has led to 90% of adolescents achieving good or intermediate-level recovery.

Nutrition Counseling

Appropriate nutrition counseling is vital in guiding a patient and family through the initial stages of recovery. Careful instruction is important to help the teenager and family dispel misconceptions about nutrition, identify realistic nutritional goals, and normalize eating. Initially, nutrition education may be the most important intervention as the teenager slowly works through his or her fears of fat-containing foods and weight gain. The teenager begins to trust the nutrition therapist and begins to restore body weight by eventually eating in a well-balanced, healthy manner. To help address the malnourished state, a multivitamin with iron and zinc supplementation may be beneficial. Zinc has been found to be depleted in those with AN. Supplementation helps restore appetite as well as improve depressive moods.

Use of Medication

Use of psychotropic medications has been commonplace in attempting to treat AN, despite lack of solid evidence. The most promising class of medication has been the atypical antipsychotics. Several open label trials (Mondraty et al, 2005; Newman-Toker, 2000) support the use of atypical antipsychotics (risperidone, olanzapine), which target specifically the body image distortion that these patients experience. A recent pilot study, the first randomized controlled trial of olanzapine in patients with AN, showed a decrease in rumination in those who received olanzapine. Further studies need to be done before there is enough scientific evidence to support the use of atypical antipsychotics.

Although vigorously studied, SSRIs repeatedly have been shown not to be helpful in treating AN initially. However, once the patient has achieved approximately 85% IBW, then SSRIs (fluoxetine, citalopram, or sertraline) help prevent relapse.

Outcomes

Outcomes in eating disorders, especially AN, have been studied extensively (Fischer, 2003; Strober et al, 1997). Most studies, however, have focused on specific inpatient treatment programs, and few have evaluated the less ill patients who do not need hospitalization. About 40% to 50% of patients receiving treatment recover; 20% to 30% have intermittent relapses; and 20% have chronic, unremitting illness. As time from initial onset lengthens, the recovery rate decreases and mortality associated with AN increases.

The course of AN often includes significant weight fluctuations over time, and it may be years until recovery is certain. Up to 50% of anorexic patients may develop bulimia as well as major psychological sequelae, including depression, anxiety, and substance abuse disorders.

It is unclear whether age at onset affects disease course. Shorter length of time between symptom onset and therapy tends to improve outcome. Various treatment modalities can be equally effective. Favorable outcomes have been found with brief medical hospitalization and long psychiatric or residential hospitalization. Higher discharge weight from the hospital seems to improve the initial outcome. It is difficult to compare treatment regimens because the numbers are small and the type of patient and illness vary between studies.

Patients with eating disorders are at a higher risk for dying than the general population. Meta-analysis has shown the risk for dying to be 5.9% in patients with eating disorders; estimates vary between 0% and 18%, depending on the patient population studied and the length of the study (Herzog et al, 2000). Death in anorexic patients is due to suicide, abnormal electrolyte levels, and resultant cardiac arrhythmias.

BULIMIA NERVOSA

The typical bulimic is more impulsive, tending to engage in risk-taking behavior such as alcohol use, drug use, and sexual experimentation, compared with the individual with AN. Bulimic patients (Fairburn et al, 2000) are often an appropriate weight for height or slightly overweight, and they get average grades. Some studies have found that 50% of bulimic patients have been sexually abused. Patients with diabetes also have an increased risk for BN. In boys, wrestling and homosexual orientation predispose to BN.

Evaluation and Diagnosis

Diagnosis of BN (Schneider, 2003) can be difficult unless the teenager is forthcoming or parents or caregivers can supply direct observations. Often, bulimic patients are average or slightly above average in body weight, without any physical signs of illness. Screening of all teenagers for body image concerns is essential. If the teenager expresses concern about being overweight, the clinician needs to screen the patient about dieting methods. Asking whether patients have binge eaten, feel out of control while eating, or cannot stop eating can clarify the diagnosis. Parents may report that significant amounts of food are missing or disappearing more quickly than normal. If the physician is suspicious, direct questioning about all the ways to purge should follow. By indicating first that the behavior in question is not unusual can make the questioning less threatening and more likely to elicit a truthful response. For example, the clinician might say, "Some teenagers who try to lose weight make themselves vomit after eating. Have you ever considered or done that yourself?" (See Table 59-2 for additional questions.)

Table 59-6 lists the diagnostic criteria for BN (American Psychiatric Association, 2000). Binge eating is either eating excessive amounts of food during a normal mealtime or having a meal (or other eating episode) last longer than usual, consuming food throughout. Bulimic individuals feel out of control while eating, unable or unwilling to recognize satiety signals. Any type of food may be included in a binge, although typically it is either carbohydrates or junk food. Extreme guilt is often associated with the episode. At some point, either before or during a binge, bulimic individuals often decide to purge. The amount of food consumed feels overwhelming, and they do not want to gain weight. The most common ways to purge are self-induced vomiting, exercise, and laxative use. Some individuals will vomit multiple times during a purge episode, after using large amounts of water to cleanse their system. This can induce significant abnormalities of electrolytes, such as sodium and potassium, which may put the patient at acute risk for arrhythmia or seizure. Other methods of purging include diuretics, diet pills, cathartics, and nutritional supplements.

Table 59-6. Diagnostic Criteria for Bulimia Nervosa

A. Recurrent episodes of binge eating. An episode of binge eating is characterized by both of the following:
   (1) eating, in a discrete period of time (e.g., within any 2-hour period), an amount of food that is definitely larger than most people would eat during a similar period of time and under similar circumstances
   (2) a sense of lack of control over eating during the episodes (e.g., a feeling that one cannot stop eating or control what or how much one is eating)

B. Recurrent inappropriate compensatory behavior in order to prevent weight gain, such as self-induced vomiting; misuse of laxatives, diuretics, enemas, or other medications; fasting or excessive exercise.

C. The binge eating and inappropriate compensatory behaviors both occur, on average, at least twice a week for 3 months.

D. Self-evaluation is unduly influenced by body shape and weight.

E. The disturbance does not occur exclusively during episodes of anorexia nervosa.

Clinical Presentation

Symptoms (Mehler, 2003; Schneider, 2003) seen clinically are related to the mechanism of purging. Gastrointestinal problems are most prominent, with abdominal pain being a frequent complaint. This can be due to gastroesophageal reflux, as the lower esophageal sphincter is compromised by repetitive vomiting. Frequent vomiting may result in esophagitis or gastritis, as the mucosa is irritated from increased exposure to acid. Early satiety, involuntary vomiting, and complaints of food "coming up" on its own are frequent. Less common but more serious is hematemesis or esophageal rupture. Patients may report bowel problems (diarrhea or constipation) if laxatives have been used. Sialadenosis (parotid pain and enlargement) may occur secondary to frequent vomiting. Erosion of dental enamel may result from increased exposure to acidity during vomiting. Because comorbid depression is common in BN, patients may report trouble sleeping and decreased energy. Lightheadedness or syncope may develop secondary to dehydration.

Most purging methods are ineffective. When patients binge, they may consume thousands of calories. Digestion begins rapidly. Although the patient may be able to vomit some of the food, much is actually digested and absorbed. Laxatives work on the large intestine, leading to fluid and electrolyte loss; calories eaten are still absorbed from the small intestine. Use of diuretics may result in decreased fluid weight and electrolyte imbalance but not a loss of calories.

On physical examination, bulimic patients may be dehydrated and have orthostatic hypotension. Sialadenosis, tooth enamel loss, dental caries, and abdominal tenderness are the most common findings. Abrasion of the proximal interphalangeal joints may occur secondary to scraping of the fingers against the teeth while inducing vomiting. An irreversible cardiomyopathy can develop secondary to ipecac use. Tachycardia and hypertension may occur secondary to caffeine and diet pill use.

Laboratory Findings

Electrolyte disturbances are characteristic of bulimic patients. The method of purging results in specific laboratory abnormalities. Vomiting causes metabolic alkalosis, hypokalemia, and hypochloremia. If laxatives are used, a metabolic acidosis can develop with hypokalemia and hypochloremia. Amylase may be increased secondary to chronic parotid stimulation.

Management and Treatment

Vignette

A 17-year-old female patient was diagnosed with BN 4 months ago. You have admitted her to the hospital twice for hypokalemia, with potassium levels being 1.9 to 2.1 mEq/L. She insists that she vomits only once per day. You have taken care of other bulimic patients and have never seen that degree of hypokalemia, despite reports of self-induced vomiting occurring three or four times per day. You are puzzled. You decide to review her history again. She insists that she does not use laxatives, diet pills, or other dietary supplements. Her self-induced vomiting occurs after a nightly binge episode. As you dig deeper, you find that "once" means one episode of purging. She typically will vomit, drink water, vomit again, drink water, and so on until her emesis is absolutely clear. This adds up to vomiting 8 to 10 times per "episode."

Take Home Points

Use of fluids such as water to clean out the stomach increases the rate of potassium and chloride loss, as electrolytes equilibrate with free fluid in the stomach. The number of episodes of vomiting adds to the electrolyte loss. Careful questioning about exact method of purging, dosage taken (diet pills and laxatives), and frequency can help the clinician assess the true medical risk. In this case, knowledge about the consequences of her purging method may have an impact because she does not like to be hospitalized. An interim step would be to suggest she not use water to clean out her stomach and to decrease the number of times she vomits per episode.

Treatment of BN depends on the frequency of bingeing and purging, the severity of biochemical and psychiatric derangement, and the chronicity of illness. Similar levels of care described in the AN section are available to patients with BN (Rome et al, 2003). Outpatient management is usually the first intervention, with a multidisciplinary team. Medical hospitalization is indicated for significant electrolyte disturbance, most commonly related to hypokalemia; a potassium level of less than 3.0 mEq/L indicates a need for inpatient treatment. The binge-purge cycle is addictive and can be difficult for patients to interrupt on their own. If outpatient management fails, hospitalization can offer a forced break from the cycle, allowing patients to normalize their eating, to interrupt the addictive behavior, and to regain ability to recognize satiety signals. Medical monitoring consists of checking electrolyte values periodically for patients who are purging and monitoring weight trends. Observation for weight loss and the symptoms associated with it is important, as is monitoring for other psychiatric comorbidities. The common symptoms that medical practitioners encounter are as follows.

Hypokalemia

Aside from being able to treat hypokalemia with supplementation, admission of patients to an inpatient setting allows close monitoring of self-induced vomiting. Cessation of vomiting alone goes a long way to correcting hypokalemia and alkalosis (Rome et al, 2003). If potassium concentration is less than 3.0 mEq/L, inpatient medical admission is warranted. General treatment guidelines for hypokalemia are as follows: if potassium concentration is less than 2.5 mEq/L, intravenous therapy is recommended; if potassium concentration is 2.5 to 2.9 mEq/L, oral supplementation is suggested. Typically, extracellular potassium is spared at the expense of intracellular potassium, so that a patient may become hypokalemic several days after the serum potassium concentration appears to be corrected. Supplementation can be stopped once potassium levels are greater than 3.5 mEq/L. Once serum potassium concentration is corrected and remains normal 2 days after supplements are stopped, the clinician can be confident that total body potassium concentration has returned to normal. A potassium concentration between 3.0 and 3.5 mEq/L can be treated on an outpatient basis; a short course of potassium supplementation is reasonable to pursue. Many eating disorder specialists will not treat adolescents with chronic potassium supplementation because it allows teenagers to treat the medical problem while continuing to purge.

Fluid Accumulation

Many patients who abuse laxatives or vomit frequently may become chronically dehydrated. The renin-angiotensin-aldosterone axis as well as the antidiuretic hormone level may be elevated to compensate. These systems do not shut down automatically when laxatives are stopped, and fluid retention of up to 10 kg/week may result. This puts patients at risk for congestive heart failure and can scare them as their weight increases dramatically. A diuresis often occurs after approximately 7 to 10 days. Parents and patients should be advised of this possible complication of initial therapy to help maintain their confidence in the care plan.

Constipation

Constipation may be seen in chronic laxative abusers, as the natural regulation of their gastrointestinal system has been lost. Practitioners need to determine whether a patient truly has constipation or is attempting to convince the practitioner in order to continue to purge. The physical examination findings and radiographs can be helpful in determining need for treatment. Practitioners need to be judicious when treating laxative abusers and should inform parents as to what they are prescribing.

Sialadenosis and Dental Caries

The pain and swelling of enlarged parotid glands can be helped by sucking on tart candy and by the application of heat. On occasion, parotid glands enlarge after self-induced vomiting has stopped. Development of caries and tooth enamel loss is related to the frequency and duration of self-induced vomiting. The most common teeth to show signs of enamel loss are the upper molars. Referral to a dentist is important to evaluate extent of damage.

Table 59-7. Diagnostic Criteria for Eating Disorder Not Otherwise Specified (Atypical Eating Disorders)

The eating disorder not otherwise specified category is for disorders of eating that do not meet the criteria for any specific eating disorder. Examples include

1. For females, all of the criteria for anorexia nervosa are met except that the individual has regular menses.
2. All of the criteria for anorexia nervosa are met except that, despite significant weight loss, the individual's current weight is in the normal range.
3. All of the criteria for bulimia nervosa are met except that the binge eating and inappropriate compensatory mechanisms occur at a frequency of less than twice a week or for duration of less than 3 months.
4. The regular use of inappropriate compensatory behavior by an individual of normal body weight after eating small amounts of food (e.g., self-induced vomiting after the consumption of two cookies).
5. Repeatedly chewing and spitting out, but not swallowing, large amounts of food.

Reprinted with permission from the American Psychiatric Association: Diagnostic and Statistical Manual of Mental Disorders, 4th ed, text revision. Washington, DC, American Psychiatric Association, 2000. Copyright 2000.

Psychotherapy

Cognitive-behavioral therapy is the most common psychotherapeutic approach used to help bulimic patients understand their disease and to offer suggestions for decreasing bingeing and purging. Dialectic behavior therapy, which teaches specific skills to patients confronted by certain stressors, also may be used. Family therapy is important as well to help empower the family in limit setting and to help address any family dynamic that may have contributed to the development of the eating disorder.

Nutrition Therapy

Nutrition therapy guides patients in ways to regulate eating patterns so that they can avoid the impulse to binge. Frequently, those with BN feel guilty about the previous day's binge, so they restrict eating the following day, until the impulse to binge eat appears again. Regular eating with three meals and two snacks per day, including breakfast, is important to help break the binge-purge pattern. Encouraging some satiety (fat) in the meal plan will also help regulate appetite.

Medications

SSRIs (Mehler, 2003; Schneider, 2003) are generally quite helpful in treating the binge-purge cycle. Fluoxetine has been studied most extensively; a dose of 60 mg/day is most effective in teenagers. Other SSRIs are thought to work similarly and are worth trying if the patient experiences side effects while taking fluoxetine. The course of medication should continue until the patient is symptom free for at least 3 or 4 months.

Outcomes

With appropriate intervention, patients with BN tend to recover more rapidly than do those with AN (Herzog et al, 1999). However, relapse is common, and patients should be monitored for extended periods. The mortality rate in bulimic patients is similar to that in anorexic patients. Death usually results from suicide or electrolyte derangements. Bulimic patients also develop similar psychological illness but rarely develop anorexia.

EATING DISORDER NOT OTHERWISE SPECIFIED

An additional diagnostic category is eating disorder not otherwise specified (EDNOS) (Table 59-7). Patients do not meet all the criteria for either AN or BN but have features of either or both (Chamay-Weber et al, 2005). EDNOS has been described as an atypical eating disorder or partial syndrome eating disorder. The incidence of EDNOS appears significant; studies show a range of 0.5% to 14% in the general adolescent population. Although patients may not have full syndrome AN or BN, their medical symptoms may be just as severe.

Symptoms and side effects are related to the specific eating disorder behavior. Monitoring and treatment discussed in the AN and BN sections apply and are guided by the specific manifestations of behavior. Careful attention by clinicians to patient concerns about body weight and dieting behavior can provide clues to the diagnosis. Some patients with EDNOS will go on to develop full-blown AN or BN, and early recognition and treatment may decrease further complications.

BINGE-EATING DISORDER

The diagnostic category of binge-eating disorder was created in DSM-IV (Table 59-8). Officially, it is still considered a research diagnosis. Studies show that most adults who have binge-eating disorder (a prevalence of 2% to 4%) develop symptoms during adolescence.

Clinical Presentation

Binge-eating disorder most often is recognized in patients who are overweight or obese. Eighteen percent of such patients report bingeing at least once in the past year.

Table 59-8. Diagnostic Criteria for Binge-Eating Disorder

A. Recurrent episodes of binge eating. An episode of binge eating is characterized by both of the following:
   (1) eating, in a discrete period of time (e.g., within any 2-hour period), an amount of food that is definitely larger than most people would eat in a similar period of time under similar circumstances
   (2) a sense of lack of control over eating during the episode (e.g., a feeling that one cannot stop eating or control what or how much one is eating)
B. The binge-eating episodes are associated with three (or more) of the following:
   (1) eating much more rapidly than normal
   (2) eating until feeling uncomfortably full
   (3) eating large amounts of food when not feeling physically hungry
   (4) eating alone because of being embarrassed by how much one is eating
   (5) feeling disgusted with oneself, depressed, or very guilty after overeating
C. Marked distress regarding binge eating at present.
D. The binge eating occurs, on average, at least 2 days a week for 6 months.
E. The binge eating is not associated with regular use of inappropriate compensatory behaviors (e.g., purging, fasting, excessive exercise) and does not occur exclusively during the course of anorexia nervosa or bulimia nervosa.

Patients with binge-eating disorder have an increased incidence of depression and substance abuse. By use of the DSM-IV diagnostic criteria as a guide for evaluation, the suspicion of binge-eating disorder should be raised for any significantly overweight patient. Asking patients about binge eating, which can be secretive, determines the diagnosis.

Treatment

A combination of cognitive-behavioral therapy and antidepressant medication has been helpful in treatment of binge-eating disorder in adults (McElroy et al, 2003). Use of SSRIs for binge-eating disorder in adolescents has not been studied; but in adults, fluoxetine and citalopram help decrease binge episodes and improve depression and the decreased appetite that contributes to weight loss. This evidence suggests that SSRIs in adolescents with binge-eating disorder may be helpful as well. Binge-eating disorder has been recognized only recently, and outcomes have not been studied. Intervention with an SSRI appears to help the binge eating, but little is known about long-term prognosis.

SUMMARY

Clinicians need to be aware of the spectrum of eating disorders as they commonly occur in adolescents as well as in younger children. It is essential to screen all teenagers about body image and dieting behavior. Obtaining history from parents is essential, as adolescents may be reticent to discuss their illness. Being aware of the short-term and long-term consequences of the eating disorders is important to help treat youths and their families. Clinicians should be aware of resources in their community; many larger cities have eating disorder treatment programs. Teaming up with specialists in the eating disorder field—therapists, psychiatrists, and dietitians—will help the clinician provide the best services possible. Becoming familiar with outpatient management will help the primary care provider feel confident being the primary medical person overseeing treatment of adolescent patients with eating disorders, serving as a valuable resource to families and patients alike.

REFERENCES

American Psychiatric Association: Diagnostic and Statistical Manual of Mental Disorders, 4th ed, text revision. Washington, DC, American Psychiatric Association, 2000.

Bailer UF, Kaye WH: A review of neuropeptide and neuroendocrine dysregulation in anorexia and bulimia nervosa. Curr Drug Targets CNS Neurol Disord 2:53-59, 2003.

Benini L, Todesco T, Dalle Grave R, et al: Gastric emptying in patients with restricting and binge/purging subtypes of anorexia nervosa. Am J Gastroenterol 99:1448-1454, 2004.

Bosanac P, Norman T, Burrows G, Beumont P: Serotonergic and dopaminergic systems in anorexia nervosa: A role for atypical antipsychotics? Aust N Z J Psychiatry 39:146-153, 2005.

Bulik CM, Tozzi F: Genetics in eating disorders: State of the science. CNS Spectr 9:511-515, 2005.

Castro J, Toro J, Lazaro L, et al: Bone mineral density in male adolescents with anorexia nervosa. J Am Acad Child Adolesc Psychiatry 41:613-618, 2002.

Centers for Disease Control: Youth Risk Behavior Surveillance—United States 2005. MMWR Surveill Summ 55(SS05):1–108, June 9, 2006. Available at: http://www.cdc.gov/mmwr/preview/mmwrhtml/ss5505a1.htm.

Chamay-Weber C, Narring F, Michaud PA: Partial eating disorders among adolescents: A review. J Adolesc Health 37:417-427, 2005.

Chan JL, Mantzoros CS: Role of leptin in energy-deprivation states: Normal human physiology and clinical implications for hypothalamic amenorrhoea and anorexia nervosa. Lancet 366:74-85, 2005.

Fairburn CG, Cooper Z, Doll HA, et al: The natural course of bulimia nervosa and binge eating disorder in young women. Arch Gen Psychiatry 57:659-665, 2000.

Fisher M: The course and outcome of eating disorders in adults and in adolescents: A review. Adolesc Med 14:149-158, 2003.

Golden NH: Osteopenia and osteoporosis in anorexia nervosa. Adolesc Med 14:97-108, 2003.

Golden NH, Iglesias EA, Jacobson MS, et al: Alendronate for the treatment of osteopenia in anorexia nervosa: A randomized, double-blind, placebo-controlled trial. J Clin Endocrinol Metab 90:3179-3185, 2005.

Herzog DB, Dorer DJ, Keel PK, et al: Recovery and relapse in anorexia and bulimia nervosa: A 7.5 year follow-up study. J Am Acad Child Adolesc Psychiatry 38:829-837, 1999.

Herzog DB, Greenwood DN, Dorer DJ, et al: Mortality in eating disorders: A descriptive study. Int J Eat Disord 28:20-26, 2000.

Karlsson MK, Weigall SJ, Duan Y, Seeman E: Bone size and volumetric density in women with anorexia nervosa receiving estrogen replacement therapy and in women recovered from anorexia nervosa. J Clin Endocrinol Metab 85:3177-3182, 2000.

Kaye WH, Nagata T, Weltzin TE, et al: Double blind placebo-controlled administration of fluoxetine in restricting- and restricting-purging-type anorexia nervosa. Biol Psychiatry 49:644-652, 2001.

Kerem NC, Katzman DK: Brain structure and function in adolescents with anorexia nervosa. Adolesc Med 14:109-118, 2003.

Konstantynowicz J, Kadziela-Olech H, Kaczmarski M, et al: Depression in anorexia nervosa: A risk factor for osteoporosis. J Clin Endocrinol Metab 90:5382-5385, 2005.

Le Grange D, Binford R, Loeb KL: Manualized family-based treatment for anorexia nervosa: A case series. J Am Acad Child Adolesc Psychiatry 44:41-46, 2005.

McElroy SL, Hudson JI, Malhotra S, Welge JA: Citalopram in the treatment of binge-eating disorder: A placebo-controlled trial. J Clin Psychiatry 64:807-813, 2003.

Mehler P: Bulimia nervosa. N Engl J Med 349:875-881, 2003.

Miller KK, Grinspoon SK, Ciampa J, et al: Medical findings in outpatients with anorexia nervosa. Arch Intern Med 165:561-566, 2005.

Mondraty N, Birmingham CL, Touyz S, et al: Randomized controlled trial of olanzapine in the treatment of cognitions in anorexia nervosa. Australas Psychiatry 13:72-75, 2005.

Newman-Toker J: Risperidone in anorexia nervosa. J Am Acad Child Adolesc Psychiatry 39:941-942, 2000.

Panagiotopoulos C, McCrindle BW, Hick K, Katzman DK: Electrocardiographic findings in adolescents with eating disorders. Pediatrics 105:1100-1105, 2000.

Rome ES, Ammerman S, Rosen DS, et al: Children and adolescents with eating disorders: The state of the art. Pediatrics 111:e98-108, 2003.

Schneider M: Bulimia nervosa and binge eating disorder in adolescents. Adolesc Med 14:119-131, 2003.

Shaw H, Ramirez L, Trost A, et al: Body image and eating disturbances across ethnic groups: More similarities than differences. Psychol Addict Behav 18:8-12, 2004.

Strober M, Freeman R, Morrell W: The long-term course of severe anorexia nervosa in adolescents: Survival analysis of recovery, relapse, and outcome predictors of 10-15 years in a prospective study. Int J Eat Disord 22:339-360, 1997.

Swenne I: Weight requirements for return of menstruations in teenage girls with eating disorders, weight loss, and secondary amenorrhoea. Acta Paediatr 93:1449-1455, 2004.

Yager J, Anderson AA: Anorexia nervosa. N Engl J Med 353:1481-1488, 2005.

Woodside DB, Garfinkel PE, Lin E, et al: Comparisons of men with full or partial eating disorders, men without eating disorders, and women with eating disorders in the community. Am J Psychiatry 158:570-574, 2001.

60 FAILURE-TO-THRIVE

PATRICK H. CASEY

Failure-to-thrive (FTT) is a traditional term used in clinical settings to describe infants and toddlers who do not grow at the expected rate for children of similar age and gender (Fig. 60-1). This clinical problem, which usually comes to the attention of primary care pediatricians and family physicians, is a diagnostic and therapeutic challenge because of the broad array of medical and environmental causes. The current incidence of this condition is difficult to ascertain. Although population-based data are not available, a community-based study found prevalence of 3% to 4% in the first year of life (Skuse et al, 1994). FTT occurs frequently, with an estimated 10% prevalence in outpatient settings (Altemeir et al, 1985). Certain clinical populations, such as low-birth-weight preterm infants and children with developmental disabilities like cerebral palsy (Sullivan et al, 2005), have a higher incidence, as much as 21% in preterm infants (Kelleher et al, 1993). Whereas older publications suggest that FTT accounted for 3% to 5% of admissions to academic hospitals, 34.9% of hospitalized children younger than 2 years demonstrated some degree of malnutrition (Hendricks et al, 1995). Although not well documented, the prevalence of FTT may be increasing because of the increasing number of preterm (12.5% of all births in 2004) and low-birth-weight (8.1% in 2004) infants with increased survival and perhaps higher rates of neurodevelopmental disability (Horbar et al, 2002; Wilson-Costello et al, 2005).

DEFINITION

The term *failure-to-thrive* is generally used to describe an infant or toddler whose weight is abnormally two standard deviations less than the mean (i.e., less than the 5th percentile) for gestation-corrected age and sex or whose weight crosses two major percentiles downward on a standardized growth grid. In addition, the ratio of weight to length is low, less than the 10th percentile. Height, head circumference, and developmental skills can also be affected, depending on severity, duration, age at onset, and cause of the clinical condition.

All children who fit these criteria, whether because of organic or nonorganic causes, are considered to have FTT. The term *abnormal* in the definition has two implications. Children who are genetically short because they have small parents are often *normal,* although they are less than two standard deviations from the average for gender and age. Also, infants who are growth retarded at birth may never rebound to normal for population. The definition suggests the importance of correcting for the degree of prematurity in plotting on a growth grid. Finally, this definition of FTT suggests that the *rate* or velocity of growth of the child is not adequate. Reference to percentile lines on the growth grid (90%, 75%, 50%, 25%, 10%, and 5%) is suggested to monitor rate of growth for at least 2 months because there are no objective data on how long a growth concern should exist before a child meets criteria for FTT. Short-term weight loss related to acute or subacute illness should not be considered FTT. A heavy infant might cross percentile lines as a normal growth pattern during a process of trimming weight. Also, some children are born larger than their long-term growth potential and may cross weight and length percentile lines in the first 2 years of life as a normal pattern for them (Mei et al, 2004).

In summary, FTT implies abnormal weight growth status and velocity disproportionate to height growth, taking into account genetic growth potential, appropriateness of size at birth for gestational age, and degree of prematurity at birth. Figure 60-2 displays a typical pattern of growth in an infant with FTT compared with the growth pattern of a premature infant and an infant with an endocrinopathy.

ETIOLOGY

Inadequate nutrition is recognized as the central cause of FTT (Wright et al, 1994). Children with FTT may suffer the biologic insult of calorie deprivation, whether inadequate calories are delivered or more than normal calories are required. Whether or not a biologic disease is present, most children with FTT demonstrate catch-up growth when adequate calories are provided (Bithoney et al, 1989; Wright et al, 1998).

CLINICAL CATEGORIES

Pediatricians historically dichotomized the etiology of FTT into organic and nonorganic causes. Organic FTT includes any biomedical condition that is severe enough to result independently in the growth problem. Disease in any organ system can cause FTT. Pediatricians

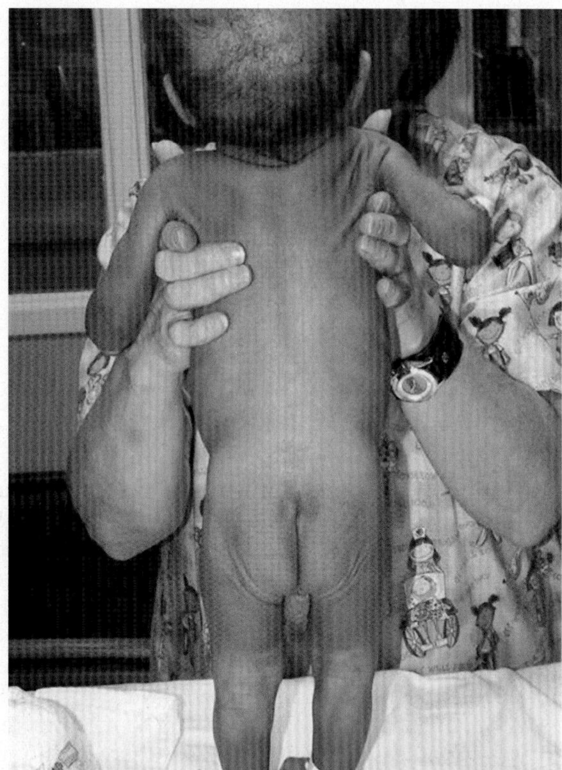

Figure 60-1. Infant with significant failure-to-thrive.

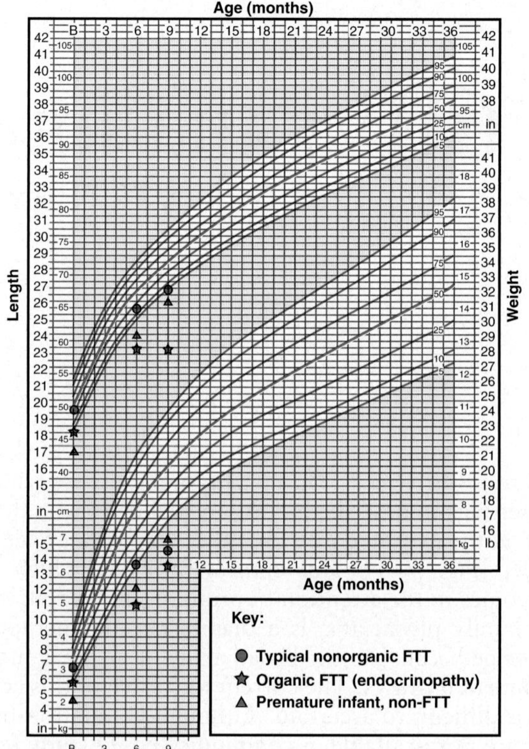

Figure 60-2. Failure-to-thrive (FTT) versus premature infant growth curves. *(Modified from Hamill PVV, Drizd TA, Johnson CL, et al: Physical growth: National Center for Health Statistics percentiles. © Am J Clin Nutr 30:607, 1979, American Society for Clinical Nutrition. Data from the Fels Research Institute, Wright State University School of Medicine, Yellow Springs, Ohio.)*

typically attribute the child's FTT to nonorganic causes when problems in the child's environment are judged to be the primary cause of FTT, in the presence or absence of medical disease. A third category of mixed-cause FTT has been described for children whose FTT results from a combination of organic and environmental causes (Homer and Ludwig, 1981). Most children with FTT suffer from nonorganic FTT, and no more than 30% of children with FTT suffer from organic causes alone. Of 131 children seen in a referral clinic, 17% had organic disease only, 45% had nonorganic FTT, and 35% had a mixed cause; for 3%, the cause was unknown (Casey et al, 1984). These percentages are likely to vary according to how a sample is identified. Children diagnosed and treated in a clinical or hospital sample are more likely to have physical or psychoemotional disease compared with those identified in a community setting.

The exclusionary diagnostic approach presents several problems. The symptoms of the child with FTT at presentation, such as persistent vomiting or diarrhea, are often not clearly caused by either organic or nonorganic problems, and uncertainty persists about the cause of the FTT. In addition, few features of the family other than overt parental poverty or emotional instability are used to make a positive diagnosis of nonorganic FTT. Although significant weight gain during a hospital stay is often the most positive clinical feature used to diagnose nonorganic FTT, this approach is subject to error. Some children with nonorganic FTT require weeks to gain weight. Likewise, some children with growth problems resulting from physical disease can demonstrate rapid growth when they are hospitalized. Even the "mixed cause" terminology is problematic as it suggests only a "blending" of biomedical and environmental psychosocial causes.

There is increasing recognition that some infants may inherently have poor appetite and inability to feed normally, which may play an important role in the development of FTT (Kasese-Hara et al, 2002; Wright et al, 1998). Psychiatrists have developed specific diagnoses in their *Diagnostic and Statistical Manual of Mental Disorders* (fourth edition, revised) that may be used in children with FTT. Criteria for the diagnosis of feeding disorder of infancy or early childhood include the following: (1) feeding disturbance manifested by persistent failure to eat adequately with significant failure to gain weight or significant weight loss during at least 1 month; (2) not due to associated gastrointestinal or other medical conditions; (3) not better accounted for by another mental disorder or lack of foods; (4) onset before 6 years of age. This diagnosis would include many children who pediatricians consider to have nonorganic FTT, but the feeding disorder diagnosis is rarely used by pediatricians.

Interactional Model

Whereas the term *maternal deprivation* was used almost interchangeably with FTT decades ago, research and experience have subsequently demonstrated that overt neglect of the infant is infrequently associated with FTT, and the use of that term is not appropriate. Clinicians

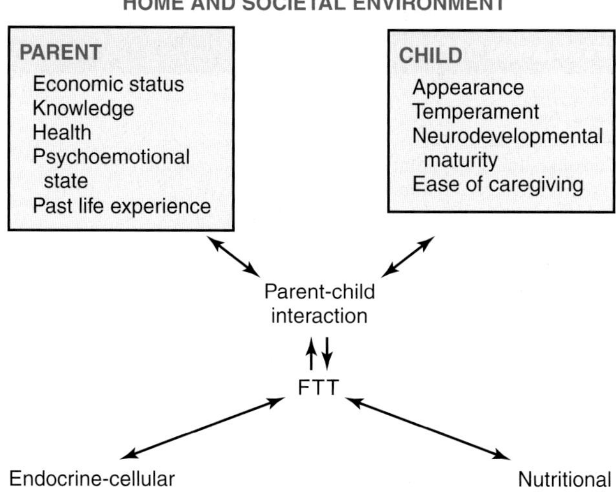

Figure 60-3. Interactional model of failure to thrive. *(From Casey PH: The family system and failure to thrive. In Ramsey CN [ed]: Family Systems in Medicine. New York, Guilford, 1989, p 348.)*

and theoreticians are increasingly using an interactional-transactional model of the causation of FTT, except in those infants with overt organic or nonorganic causes (Casey, 1989; Frank and Zeisel, 1988). The model in Figure 60-3 conceptualizes interaction at several levels. The central cause of FTT is viewed as a breakdown in the parent-infant interaction. The parent does not "read" or respond to the infant appropriately, and the infant has difficulty in eliciting attention and appropriate care from the parent. This bidirectional problem ultimately results in nutritional and nurturing deficiencies that then result in FTT. Certain extreme physical, emotional, or social problems in the parent cause unidirectional effects that would result in FTT in any child. This parent-to-child effect has dominated the literature on nonorganic FTT. More commonly, minor or subtle abnormalities in physical, temperamental, or emotional aspects of the parent, or all of these factors, combine with real or perceived similar abnormalities in the infant to result in interactional FTT. For example, infants who are difficult to care for, such as in feeding or soothing, place stress on the parent-infant interaction. Infants who are unpredictable and have difficulty signaling their needs can also impede a mutually rewarding relationship. Such problems occur more commonly in premature infants, infants born small for gestational age, drug-exposed infants, children with difficult or placid and easy temperaments, and children with neurologic dysfunction. Undernutrition in infants may have an independent detrimental effect on parent-infant interaction as early as the first 6 months of life. Finally, the interaction between the parent-child pair is viewed in the context of their microenvironment and macroenvironment. Physical aspects of the home provide the milieu in which the parent-infant interaction occurs. The number of people present in the home, the physical adequacy of the house (such as heating, cooling, and crowdedness), the home's organization, and the availability of support all affect parent-infant interaction and the parent's ability to meet the infant's needs. Strengths (supports) and weaknesses (stressors) in the home, the marital relationship, extended family, neighborhood, and workplace enhance or impede the quality of parent-child interaction and can have a direct impact on the development of FTT. This interactional model of FTT implies a multifactorial causation mediated by the maladapted parent-infant interaction. The maladapted interaction may result in nutritional and perhaps endocrine-cellular abnormalities, which in turn lead to FTT. This clinical model supersedes the organic versus nonorganic diagnostic dichotomy.

Special Clinical Populations

Several clinical populations are at particular risk for the development of FTT, including low-birth-weight infants and children with neurologic dysfunction. Up to 40% of infants with birth weight of less than 1500 g have been described as having "growth failure" at age 22 months (Dusick et al, 2003), and 21% of infants with birth weight of less than 2500 g developed FTT at 36 months of age (Kelleher et al, 1993). Also, children born small for gestational age are at risk for development of postnatal growth problems that may be diagnosed as FTT. Children with a chronic neurodevelopmental disability, such as cerebral palsy, are at increased risk for FTT. These clinical groups are at greater risk for medical problems such as chronic lung disease, gastroesophageal reflux, and swallowing dissonance. These may present challenges to their caregivers based on difficulty of feeding adequately or temperamental dissonance. In addition, the families of these children are at greater risk for psychological problems ranging from distress to depression, which may make it difficult for them to adequately care for their children.

Household food insecurity is another concern that may be associated with the development of FTT. Household food insecurity is defined by national experts as limited or uncertain availability of nutritionally adequate and safe foods and limited or uncertain ability to acquire acceptable foods in socially acceptable ways (Keenan et al, 2001). Food insecurity is considered a marker for the adequacy and stability of the household food supply during the preceding months for active and healthy living of all household members. National data in 2004 indicated that 11.9% of all U.S. households (13.5 million) were food insecure and 17.6% of households with children were food insecure. The prevalence is higher in African American (23.7%) and Hispanic (21.7%) households; 35.8% of households below the federal poverty line were food insecure. Food insecurity has been associated with negative child health, development, and behavior (Casey et al, 2005; Jyoti et al, 2005). Whereas no association has yet been found with food insecurity and FTT, it is likely that the adequacy of household food supply is linked to the evolution of FTT in certain children and families.

DIAGNOSTIC EVALUATION

The diagnostic approach to a child who presents with FTT requires a thoughtful medical, developmental-behavioral, nutritional, and social evaluation to recognize etiology, to develop a treatment plan, and to understand prognosis. Data collection in all of these areas should occur simultaneously, if possible, to develop a comprehensive interactional-transactional perspective based on positive findings, rather than a medical exclusionary diagnostic approach. Almost all of the initial data can be collected in the pediatrician's office.

As noted earlier, most children with FTT do not have a specific treatable medical cause. It is, of course, incumbent on the pediatrician to recognize and to manage any condition or circumstance that results in FTT. Whereas it is typical in chapters that describe FTT to provide long lists of potential medical diseases associated with FTT, the diagnostic approach to follow is process focused rather than disease oriented.

Medical Evaluation

Growth Status

The presence of FTT is documented by applying the definition described earlier, including current weight status for gestation-adjusted age, weight compared with length, and growth velocity over time. Accurate measurements of height, weight, and head circumference with use of standard collection techniques are critical. Growth charts developed by the National Center for Health Statistics are recommended for reference; they include the most recent reference growth data from a representative national sample of children. Growth grids for use with low-birth-weight preterm children based on a longitudinal sample are available to provide reference data for such children younger than 3 years (Sherry et al, 2003). The infant's height, weight, and head circumference are plotted to determine the percentile for age (corrected for gestational age if necessary) and the percentile for weight for height. Weight for age less than the 5th percentile suggests undernutrition. Weight-to-height ratio less than the 5th percentile, even in a short child, suggests acute recent malnutrition. Is the child gaining weight at an average rate, paralleling the growth curve, whether above or below typical weight and length for age, or is there a gradual decrease in the velocity of weight gain over time? Crossing percentile lines on the growth grid suggests a growth velocity problem. Velocity growth curves are available for use in assessing weight and length gain over time at various ages for infants younger than 2 years.

The weight percentile usually decreases before a change in the length or head circumference percentile in a child with FTT. The length and ultimately head circumference percentiles also drop if the problem is severe and chronic enough. Some term infants with weight, length, or head circumference less than normal at birth (small for gestational age) demonstrate a stable rate of growth, with normal weight for length, but remain at less than the 5th percentile for age. Often these children have had a problem in utero that precludes typical growth; these children do not have FTT. On occasion, a child demonstrates a normal weight-to-height ratio but a progressive deterioration of length percentile. This situation suggests an endocrinopathy or constitutional short stature. Some children whose weight and height percentiles at birth are greater than their ultimate growth potential cross growth curve percentiles downward between the ages of 6 and 24 months as a normal growth pattern (Mei et al, 2004). It is thus critical to take into account the heights of both parents in assessing normal growth expectations before determining the presence of FTT.

Table 60-1. Template of Medical History for Evaluation of Failure-to-Thrive

Prenatal

Maternal health
Chronic illness, e.g., diabetes mellitus, human immunodeficiency virus infection, cytomegalovirus infection
Habits, e.g., nutrition, alcohol, cigarettes, drugs
Environmental exposure
Obstetric complications, e.g., toxemia, hemorrhage, multiple pregnancies

Perinatal

Labor and delivery complications, Apgar score
Birth weight, gestational age (small for gestational age?)

Neonatal

Length of stay
Specific problem, e.g., intraventricular hemorrhage, seizures, hypoxia, extreme hyperbilirubinemia, infections

Postnatal Health

Growth trajectory and nutrition
Serious (e.g., meningitis) or recurrent infection (e.g., otitis media)
Recurrent symptoms, e.g., vomiting, diarrhea, wheezing, snoring
Chronic conditions, e.g., cerebral palsy, gastroesophageal reflux, chronic lung disease, upper airway obstruction

Developmental Trajectory and Temperamental Style

Family history
Size and growth
Developmental disabilities
Disease that may affect growth and development, e.g., hemoglobin sickle cell disease, cystic fibrosis
Social history (see text)

History

The medical history and physical examination should identify any condition or cluster of symptoms that negatively affects the infant's growth potential (such as in utero growth retardation), increases the child's basic calorie requirement (such as chronic infection), decreases the availability or use of calories (such as malabsorption), negatively affects the child's ability or willingness to feed (such as gastroesophageal reflux), or negatively influences the parents' ability to meet nutritional needs. An outline for some important aspects of the history is presented in Table 60-1. The medical history begins with the description of the development of the growth problem. How do the parents perceive the problem and its cause, and if both parents are present, how do they relate in describing this problem? How old was the infant at the beginning of the problem, and what medical conditions and symptoms were present? Were problematic feeding or behavioral styles present? A complete review of systems elicits information about recurring symptoms that might have been omitted from the general history. Organic problems that most likely result in FTT are gastrointestinal diseases that result in recurring diarrhea and vomiting, neurologic disease (particularly early cerebral palsy), and chronic upper airway disease (otitis media) and obstruction (Bithoney and Newburger, 1987). A thorough past medical history is established. Some past conditions, like gastroesophageal reflux, may result in ongoing food aversion, even if the condition is not active. Children with no medical cause of their FTT tend to have been smaller at birth and to have had more illness than children who grow normally (Altemeir et al, 1985). Birth weight, gestational age, and complications in the prenatal, perinatal, and postnatal periods are noted. In utero toxin exposure (e.g., alcohol, cigarettes, cocaine) and infection (e.g., acquired immunodeficiency syndrome, cytomegalovirus infection) are causes of FTT. Such conditions also increase the burden of caring for the infant, which stresses the parents' ability to provide. For example, some premature infants or infants who have been exposed to toxins can be hyperirritable and demonstrate deficient responses to visual, auditory, or tactile stimuli. Their unpredictable behavior, difficulty in signaling needs, and problems in coordinating suck and swallowing interfere with parent-child interaction and the feeding event.

The child's developmental milestones and progress are substantiated. Children with FTT commonly demonstrate developmental delays and subtle deviations from normal behavior (Raynor and Rudolf, 1996). A description of the child's behavioral style and eating ability and the presence of problems like "colic" is solicited. Normal children might have behavioral traits that stress parents beyond their ability to cope (Bithoney and Newberger, 1987). They might feed with difficulty, be poorly able to modulate their moods and whine or show other evidence of irritability, and be excessively clinging. In contrast, some children described as "good" babies might actually be withdrawn, depressed, or unable to place normal demands on their environment.

Finally, a family history is obtained to detect inherited problems such as cystic fibrosis, sickle cell disease, diabetes mellitus, or other endocrine, metabolic, neurologic, or gastrointestinal diseases that can affect ultimate growth. The physical size of the parents, siblings, uncles, aunts, and grandparents assists in predicting growth prognosis.

Physical Examination

Careful evaluation for minor dysmorphic features can suggest syndromes associated with short stature, such as fetal alcohol syndrome or Russell-Silver syndrome. Head size, configuration of the eyes and ears and mouth, proportion of trunk to extremities, and abnormalities of digits and extremities require particular attention. Specific organ diseases are sought, particularly those that can be asymptomatic, such as chronic serous otitis media, congenital heart disease, or abdominal masses. A neurologic examination evaluates the child for cranial nerve or motor tract dysfunction, particularly abnormalities of muscle tone and peripheral reflexes. Cranial nerve dysfunction associated with difficulty in swallowing can result in FTT. Hypertonicity and hyperreflexia, sometimes prematurely diagnosed as cerebral palsy, can actually result from progressive undernutrition in infancy. Finally, the child is evaluated for evidence of physical abuse, such as unexplained burns or skin lesions, fractures, or retinal hemorrhages.

Developmental and Behavioral Assessment

Because developmental problems are common in children with FTT, documentation of the child's developmental status with use of a screening instrument is important (American Academy of Pediatrics, 2006) (see also Chapter 79). Referral to a pediatric psychologist to document developmental status with a standardized technique, such as the Bayley Scale of Infant Development, may be useful. Assessment of oral-motor function, including lip and tongue coordination and swallowing, can yield relevant data, particularly in infancy (Reilly et al, 1999). An array of atypical behaviors seen in infants with nonorganic FTT has been described, including general inactivity, flexed hips and knees, expressionless face, gaze aversion, and lack of motor activity in response to stimulus, among others. These behaviors may differentiate children with FTT from children without FTT (Powell et al, 1987). Finally, behavior at mealtime and general behavioral style are of particular importance to the assessment of the child with the onset of FTT in the second year of life. Observation of behavior at mealtimes to assess problems such as food refusal, spitting, throwing, and oral retention may be useful in this diagnosis.

Laboratory Analysis

The results of the history and physical examination guide the laboratory evaluation. A thorough history and physical evaluation detect most organic causes of FTT, and laboratory tests almost never contribute to the diagnosis independently (Homer and Ludwig, 1981; Sills, 1978). When no significant symptoms or physical findings are present, a stepwise laboratory approach is recommended. Some conditions, like lead poisoning, tuberculosis, and giardiasis, can be endemic in certain geographic areas and require routine laboratory assessments. Laboratory evaluation can also be useful to document nutritional status. The albumin level is used to assess protein status in severe FTT. Deficiency in minerals, particularly iron and zinc, can have an independent detrimental effect on the development of FTT. Interpretation of growth patterns on growth grids can assist in decisions about laboratory evaluation. A child with a decreasing height growth velocity with a symmetric weight-to-height ratio might require bone age and thyroid studies and perhaps growth hormone evaluation. Conversely, these endocrine studies are not warranted in a typical FTT growth pattern.

An appropriate initial assessment in a child with FTT with no obvious problems identified in the medical history and physical examination, seeking to identify conditions that may be nonsymptomatic, includes the following: complete blood cell count; urinalysis; brief chemical panel including electrolytes, calcium, glucose, and renal function; and serum zinc level in toddlers. If concerns persist after a period of management, further laboratory evaluation to be considered might include sweat test, serologic screening for celiac disease, radiologic evaluation for gastroesophageal reflux, studies for gastrointestinal malabsorption, and even brain scan in the rare case of diencephalic syndrome.

Nutritional and Feeding Evaluation

A nutritional and feeding history assesses the calorie, protein, and micronutrient intake; the quality and appropriateness of food for age; the ability of the child to swallow and to chew normally; and the social nature of the feeding event. A first-level evaluation can be performed by a pediatrician or nurse. Children with FTT may have a lower intake of calories, protein, and certain vitamins and minerals than do normal children. The average daily requirement for infants younger than 6 months is 100 to 120 kcal/kg per day; for children 6 through 12 months, this amount decreases to about 105 kcal/kg per day, and it is somewhat less for children older than 1 year. It is helpful to use a 24-hour diet recall for infants. For infants younger than 6 months who receive formula or breast milk, the frequency and amount of feedings are recorded, along with how the formula was prepared (i.e., too diluted or concentrated) and delivered (propped or not), the infant's skill in sucking and swallowing, and whether the feedings are retained. Observation of a bottle feeding is useful to assess the parent's style. How long did it take and how much did the infant consume? Was there a good suck without vomiting? Was the social interaction (i.e., eye and body contact) good? Was the parent excessively stimulating, withdrawn, or disruptive?

A 3-day diet recall or food diary is used to ascertain intake for older children who are eating solid foods. Some children are described as good eaters who eat "all the time." Children who demonstrate this "grazing" pattern might nibble on non-nutritious foods throughout the day but fail to meet daily requirements. Drinking an excessive amount of fruit juices or other sweet liquids may be particularly problematic. One should inquire about the feeding event for the toddler taking solid foods. Are three meals provided per day? Are they eaten in a highchair or in a chair at the table and are they supervised by an adult? Children with FTT often suffer in these contextual aspects of the feeding event.

The parents' understanding of and attitude toward normal nutrition and feeding are ascertained. Some families adhere to atypical feeding practices because of lack of knowledge or experience; but in some cases, it is because of excessively zealous application of breastfeeding, vegetarian diets, diets to prevent obesity or cardiovascular disease, or medical regimens to treat diarrhea or suspected food allergies.

Social History

There are few specific socioenvironmental causes of FTT (e.g., extreme poverty, parent with intellectual disability or psychosis), and there is no single set of factors that routinely results in FTT. Most controlled research has found no difference between families with children with FTT and controls in maternal age, marital status, knowledge, stress, mental health, number of family members, birth order of index child, or number of rooms in the household (Wright and Birks, 2000). However, mothers who have children with FTT report more negative perceptions of their own childhood and their relationship with the child's father (i.e., arguments and separations) (Altemeier, 1985) and demonstrated more disorganized homes (Casey, 1989), more neglectful and less nurturing styles, and more social isolation and less support from families and neighbors (Bithoney and Newberger, 1987).

The social work interview solicits information about the parents, the family, and their environment, which may potentiate (vulnerability factors) or compensate (protector factors) the development of FTT. Historical features of specific importance are maternal and paternal education; household income and income/capita; availability of adequate food in the house; marital status; number of people and rooms in the child's home; presence of parental psychoemotional dysfunction, such as depression or habit disorder (e.g., alcohol or drug use); history of neglect or abuse with the parents' other children; history of parental abuse as a child; history of major stress to the parents, such as spousal abuse, loss of job, or recent death; atypical family feeding and cultural practices and problems in family routines and organization; and presence of emotional, financial, and physical support available to the primary provider. Children with FTT are often cared for by daycare providers, relatives, or neighbors, and the primary problem might lie outside the immediate household. The clinician interprets the interaction of the relative strengths and weaknesses in these various areas in determining their contribution to the development of FTT.

Parent-Child Interaction Assessment

There is no generally accepted clinical approach to assess the quality of parent-child interaction, despite its theoretical and practical value. Such an assessment can occur at home or in a clinical setting, by a pediatrician, nurse, social worker, or psychiatrist, in a feeding event or nonstructured situation, with a standardized instrument or global clinical judgment. In general, one attempts to assess the appropriateness, warmth, sensitivity, and responsiveness of the interaction between parent and child. There is no substitute for a home visit to observe the child and parent in the context of their own environment. An instrument for assessing a child's physical and social environment for use by pediatricians in clinical settings has been shown to predict child development status (Casey et al, 1993). Attention to the parent-child interaction during a feeding event is of particular relevance in FTT.

MANAGEMENT

Need to Hospitalize

The first decision after the initial outpatient evaluation is whether to hospitalize the child to initiate management. Successful outpatient management of most children with FTT has been demonstrated in settings with multidisciplinary groups (Bithoney et al, 1989; Casey et al, 1984; Wright et al, 1998). Physicians can attempt to manage in outpatient settings children who are mildly to moderately underweight (more than 60% average weight for age) and mildly wasted (more than 80% average weight for height), who constitute the majority of all FTT children (Wright et al, 1994). This outpatient intervention has the advantages of being less costly, of working with the family in the reality of their own environment, and of keeping the parent and child together as the focus of the intervention. The need for hospitalization is not common, but hospitalization is required for the following: (1) to protect the child from abuse when evidence of nonaccidental trauma is found at the time of initial evaluation; (2) to protect a severely malnourished child from the sequelae of further starvation; (3) in extremely problematic parent-child interaction, particularly toddlers with feeding behavior problems; (4) when practicality of distance and transportation preclude outpatient management; and (5) after failure of an adequate attempt at outpatient management. Inpatient care allows completion of the medical evaluation, observation of the child's spontaneous feeding ability and style, more detailed observation of parent-child interaction and parenting style, and development of a realistic nutritional plan based on these observations. These goals require the presence of the parent during the hospitalization. Involving the parents in the development of the treatment plan and educating them about the details of this plan are more likely to ensure cooperation and follow-through on discharge.

Nutritional Rehabilitation

Nutritional rehabilitation is at the core of the management of FTT (Table 60-2), whether it is inpatient or outpatient management (Frank and Zeisel, 1988). To allow weight growth to compensate toward normal, one attempts to provide more than expected calorie intake for average gain for age. Depending on the age of the child, the following are the general goals of nutrition management: stabilize a feeding schedule to encourage the development of the rhythm of appetite/satiation; diminish or eliminate between-meal junk foods and sweet liquids; increase beneficial calorie intake with a goal of 130 to 150 calories per kilogram per day; encourage parents to use positive reinforcement of positive eating behaviors and to avoid aggressive feeding styles. Enriched formulas (24 to 30 calories per ounce) with carbohydrate, triglyceride, or dried milk added to normal formula are used for young infants. Recipes for the preparation of higher calorie formula and a variety of high-calorie nutrition supplements are shown in Tables 60-3 and 60-4. A specific plan of quantity and frequency to achieve the nutritional goal is suggested as a minimum. Formula beyond this goal and solid food, if needed, are encouraged. Vitamin and mineral deficiencies, such as iron or zinc, can negatively affect behavior, appetite, and growth, and supplementation might be required. A randomized controlled study of zinc supplementation in children with FTT demonstrated a significant increase in weight gain in the zinc-supplemented children (Walravens et al, 1989).

Attention to the environmental context of feeding is required. Some infants and toddlers require a quiet setting with little distraction, and some toddlers need to be restrained in a highchair. Anorexic infants and toddlers with feeding and behavioral problems present particular challenges in nutritional rehabilitation. Elimination of non-nutritious intake (colas, Kool-Aid, juice drinks) and structuring of the timing and environment are first steps. Behavioral protocols to modify mealtime behavior and the use of nasogastric feeding tubes to expand intake are occasionally required.

Monitoring of daily weight gain during hospitalization or during a 1- to 3-week follow-up visit in the outpatient setting allows determination of the success of this nutritional protocol. Typical daily weight gain by age is shown on Table 60-5. Although catch-up growth can occur rapidly, up to 2 weeks can pass before growth occurs in the child with more involved FTT. The ultimate goals for catch-up growth are to achieve symmetry of weight to height and for height to attain genetic growth potential. For some children with significant feeding or behavioral problems, average weight gain

Table 60-2. Management of Failure-to-Thrive

Nutritional rehabilitation—establishing appropriate intake, restoration, and maintenance
Improved parent-child interaction
Developmental stimulation of infant in some cases
Management of organic disease
Amelioration of social-family problems
Mental health support for parents when indicated
Regular follow-up

Table 60-3. Increased Calorie Formula Preparation

24 calories/ounce: one can (13 oz) formula concentrate + 9 ounces water
27 calorie/ounce: 24 calories/ounce as above + ¼ cup Polycose powder
30 calorie/ounce: 27 calorie/ounce as above + 20 mL microlipids

Table 60-4. High-Calorie Nutrition Supplements

High-calorie beverages with vitamins and minerals
- PediaSure (with fiber): 30 kcal/ounce
- Kindercal (with fiber): 32 kcal/ounce
- Instant Breakfast: 32 kcal/ounce

High-calorie puddings
- Sustacal (Boost) pudding
- Ensure pudding

Powder additives for beverages and moist foods
- Polycose (carbohydrate)
- Scandical (carbohydrate and fat)

High-calorie beverages with no added nutrients
- ScandiShake (high-calorie powder added to 8 oz milk = 600 kcal/glass)
- Resource fruit beverage (22.5 kcal/oz in fruit flavors)

Table 60-5. Expected Average Weight Gain

Age (months)	Grams/day
0-3	25-30
3-6	15-20
6-12	10-15
>12	5-10

without catch-up may be an acceptable short-term goal, which suggests that they are able to accept average calories and to translate that into average growth. There has been recent concern that excessive weight gain in the first year of life, particularly in low-birth-weight infants, increases the probability of obesity and cardiovascular disease in adult years (Barker et al, 2005). Caution should be used in the nutritional rehabilitation of FTT infants so as not to overshoot the compensatory weight gain, resulting in overweight status in a young child.

Other Management Needs

Other aspects of the management plan are based on the problems identified in the initial evaluation. The goals of treatment are to improve parent understanding of child care, nutrition, and health and development of their child and to minimize stressors and to stabilize the home environment, all with the focus of improving parent-child interaction. For example, helping the parent understand the child with difficult or very easy temperament and offering management techniques for these temperaments may be helpful (see Chapter 7). Aggressive management of organic diseases associated with FTT is warranted. For example, placement of ventilation tubes in a child with recurrent otitis media might result in a striking return of appetite. Adenoidectomy in young children with upper airway obstruction and associated feeding problems should be considered. The use of gastrostomy tube to facilitate nutritional needs and to avoid aspiration in children with severe neurodevelopmental disability like cerebral palsy, with associated feeding problems, should be considered (Samson-Fang et al, 2003). Children with FTT in the toddler years may have significant behavioral problems that are manifested at mealtimes. Referral to a pediatric psychologist for assistance with behavioral management may be critical in this situation. A social worker or nurse, or both, often in conjunction with community social workers or public health nurses, works with the family for ongoing education and support and to stabilize the home environment. Use of an array of appropriate community resources (e.g., community financial supports; the Women, Infants, and Children [WIC] program; housing authority; homemaker assistance) may be helpful. Referral for mental health support might be necessary for some parents. Particularly in families with stress and psychological dysfunction, the child with FTT might benefit from out-of-home care at a developmental stimulation program. Controlled research with home-based intervention and center-based educational stimulation has resulted in improved growth (Wright et al, 1998) and developmental status in children with FTT (Casey et al, 1994; Hutcheson et al, 1997).

FOLLOW-UP

All of these steps, along with ongoing monitoring in the clinical setting, serve to provide the family an anchor to the world to minimize social isolation. The relationship of the physician and other health care workers to the family during this monitoring process is a supportive one, which increases the likelihood of compliance with the management plan and clinical follow-up. The frequency of follow-up is based on the course of the child's and the family's response to the plan. All aspects of the management plan are modified on the basis of the course.

PROGNOSIS

The outcome of children with FTT is predictably quite variable, given the broad range of severity, age at onset, and etiology. Even in the absence of diagnosable disease, children with FTT vary considerably in degree of malnutrition, subtle neurodevelopmental abnormality, and quality of nurturance and stimulation of their home environments, all of which independently contribute to ultimate outcomes in growth, development, and behavior.

Most controlled follow-up studies of children with FTT in this country and undernourished children in developing countries generally document negative long-term effects on growth and cognitive development. Most studies of children with FTT into school years have found them to be shorter and lighter than controls with a higher prevalence of stunting and wasting (Boddy et al, 2000; Drewett et al, 1999). Also, many of these long-term reports found that children with FTT functioned in the lower range of normal in cognitive measures, although lower than the control groups (Boddy et al, 2000; Rudolf and Logan, 2005). Negative effects of early FTT have recently been demonstrated on growth status, cognitive status, and academic achievement at 8 years of age in a longitudinal cohort of low-birth-weight preterm children (Casey et al, 2006). Long-term outcomes, of course, may be affected positively by treatment. Several randomized controlled interventions have been performed with benefits on growth and development with malnourished children in developing countries, using nutrition and psychosocial stimulation (Black and Dubowitz, 1991).

Concern has risen in recent years that children who have poor weight gain in the early years of life, particularly if they have later rapid and excessive weight gain, are at greater risk for an array of diseases in adult years, including cardiovascular disease, obesity, hypertension, and diabetes (Barker, 2003). Further longitudinal research will be required to confirm these associations; this concern warrants caution by pediatricians in their nutrition management approach.

SUMMARY

Most children with FTT can be expected to achieve normal growth and developmental status. In contrast, many children remain small and continue to be at risk for long-term negative developmental and behavioral sequelae. Because of the variation in clinical subtypes and etiologic contributors on the transactional spectrum, no generalization of prognosis is adequate for an individual child. Nutritional, family support, and childhood stimulation intervention will likely improve outcomes of children with FTT.

REFERENCES

Altemeir WA, O'Connor SM, Sherrod KB, et al: Prospective study of antecedents for nonorganic failure to thrive. J Pediatr 106:360-365, 1985.

American Academy of Pediatrics: Policy Statement. Identifying infants and young children with developmental disorders in the medical home: An algorithm for developmental surveillance and screening. Pediatrics 118:405-420, 2006.

Barker JDP: Low birth weight, early growth and chronic disease in later life. J Pediatr Nutr Dev 104:12-20, 2003.

Barker DJP, Osmond C, Forsen TJ, et al: Trajectories of growth among children who have coronary events as adults. N Engl J Med 353:1802-1809, 2005.

Bithoney WG, Newberger EH: Child and family attributes of failure to thrive. J Dev Behav Pediatr 8:32, 1987.

Bithoney WG, McJunkin J, Michalek J, et al: Prospective evaluation of weight gain in both nonorganic and organic failure to thrive children: An outpatient trial of a multidisciplinary team intervention strategy. J Dev Behav Pediatr 19:27-31, 1989.

Black M, Dubowitz H: Failure to thrive: Lessons from animal models and developing countries. J Dev Behav Pediatr 12:259-267, 1991.

Boddy J, Skuse D, Andrews B: The developmental sequelae of nonorganic failure to thrive. J Child Psychol Psychiatry 41:1003-1014, 2000.

Casey PH: The family system and failure to thrive. *In* Ramsey CN (ed): Family Systems in Medicine. New York, Guilford, 1989, pp 348-358.

Casey PH, Wortham B, Nelson JY: Management of children with failure to thrive in a rural ambulatory setting. Clin Pediatr 23:325-330, 1984.

Casey PH, Barrett KW, Bradley RH, et al: Pediatric clinical assessment of mother-infant interaction: Concurrent and predictive validity. J Dev Behav Pediatr 14:313, 1993.

Casey PH, Kelleher KJ, Bradley RH, et al: A multifaceted intervention for infants with failure to thrive: A prospective study. Arch Pediatr Adolesc Med 148:1071-1077, 1994.

Casey PH, Szeto K, Robbins JM, et al: Child health-related quality of life and household food security. Arch Pediatr Adolesc Med 159:51-56, 2005.

Casey PH, Whiteside-Mansell L, Barrett K, et al: Impact of prenatal and/or postnatal growth problems in low birth weight preterm infants on school-age outcomes: An 8-year longitudinal evaluation. Pediatrics 118:e1406-1413, 2006.

Drewett RF, Corbett SS, Wright CM: Cognitive and educational attainment at school age of children who failed to thrive in infancy: A population based study. J Child Psychol Psychiatry 40:551-561, 1999.

Dusick AM, Poindexter BB, Ehrenkranz RA, Lemons JA: Growth failure in the preterm infant: Can we catch up? Semin Perinatol 27:302-310, 2003.

Frank DA, Zeisel SH: Failure to thrive. Pediatric Clin North Am 35:1187-1206, 1988.

Hendricks KM, Duggan C, Gallagher L, et al: Malnutrition in hospitalized pediatric patients. Arch Pediatr Adolesc Med 149:1118-1122, 1995.

Homer C, Ludwig S: Categorization of etiology of failure to thrive. Am J Dis Child 135:848, 1981.

Horbar JD, Badger GJ, Carpenter JH, et al: Trends in mortality and morbidity for very low birth weight infants. Pediatrics 110:143-151, 2002.

Hutcheson JJ, Black MM, Talley M, et al: Risk status and home intervention among children with failure to thrive: Follow-up at age 4. J Pediatr Psychol 22:651-668, 1997.

Jyoti DF, Frongillo EA, Jones SJ: Food insecurity affects school children's academic performance, weight gain and social skills. J Nutr 135:2831-2839, 2005.

Kasese-Hara M, Wright C, Drewett R: Energy compensation in young children who fail to thrive. J Child Psychol Psychiatry 43:449-456, 2002.

Keenan DP, Olson C, Hersey JC, et al: Measures of food insecurity/security. J Nutr Educ 33(Suppl):S49-S58, 2001.

Kelleher K, Casey PH, Bradley RH, et al: Risk factors and outcomes for failure to thrive in low birthweight preterm infants. Pediatrics 91:941-948, 1993.

Mei Z, Grummer-Strawn LM, Thompson D, et al: Shifts in percentiles of growth during early childhood: Analysis of longitudinal data from the California Child Health and Development Study. Pediatrics 113:e617-e627, 2004.

Powell GF, Low JF, Speers MA: Behavior as a diagnostic aid in failure to thrive. J Dev Behav Pediatr 8:18-24, 1987.

Raynor P, Rudolf MCJ: What do we know about children who fail to thrive? Child Care Health Dev 22:241-250, 1996.

Reilly SM, Skuse DH, Wolke D, et al: Oral-motor dysfunction in children who fail to thrive: Organic or non-organic? Dev Med Child Neurol 41:115-122, 1999.

Rudolf MCJ, Logan S: What is the long term outcome for children who fail to thrive? A systemic review. Arch Dis Child 90:925-931, 2005.

Samson-Fang L, Butler C, O'Donnell M: Effects of gastrostomy feeding in children with cerebral palsy: An AACPDM evidence report. Dev Med Child Neurol 45:415-426, 2003.

Sherry B, Mei Z, Grummer-Strawn L, et al: Evaluation of and recommendations for growth references for very low birth weight (< or = 1500 grams) infants in the United States. Pediatrics 111:750-758, 2003.

Sills RH: Failure to thrive: The role of clinical and laboratory evaluation. Am J Dis Child 132:967-969, 1978.

Skuse D, Pickles A, Wolke D, et al: Postnatal growth and maternal deprivation: Evidence for a "sensitive period." J Child Psychol Psychiatry 35:521-527, 1994.

Sullivan PB, Juszczak E, Bachlet AME, et al: Gastrostomy tube feeding in children with cerebral palsy: A prospective longitudinal study. Dev Med Child Neurol 47:77-85, 2005.

Walravens PA, Hambidge KM, Koepfer DM: Zinc supplementation in infants with a nutritional pattern of failure to thrive: A double-blind, controlled study. Pediatrics 83:532-536, 1989.

Wilson-Costello D, Friedman H, Minich N, et al: Improved survival rates with increased neurodevelopmental disability for extremely low birth weight infants in the 1990s. Pediatrics 115:997-1003, 2005.

Wright C, Callum J, Birks E, Jarvis S: Effect of community based management of failure to thrive: A randomised controlled trial. BMJ 317:571-574, 1998.

Wright C, Birks E: Risk factors for failure to thrive: A population based survey. Child Care Health Dev 26:5-16, 2000.

Wright JA, Ashenburg CA, Whitaker RC: Comparison of methods to categorize undernutrition in children. J Pediatr 145:944-946, 1994.

61 CHILD AND ADOLESCENT OBESITY

Lawrence D. Hammer and Thomas N. Robinson

Vignette

T. R. presented to the pediatric weight clinic at 16 years of age with a weight of 169 kg and a body mass index (BMI) of 60 kg/m^2. Her mother had an unremarkable pregnancy, labor, and delivery, with the exception of gestational diabetes. T. R. had a birth weight of 3.7 kg and was euglycemic during her first few days of life in the hospital. By 3 years of age, her pediatrician noted that her weight and height were both accelerating above the 95th percentile, and at 6 years of age, her BMI was 30 kg/m^2, well above the 95th percentile for age. At 12 years of age, she began attending a local Weight Watchers program with her mother. Despite her efforts at dietary control and exercise, her BMI continued to increase at a rate of about 3 kg/m^2 per year. Her family history was remarkable for diabetes, hypertension, and hyperlipidemia in both of her parents and all of her grandparents. Her mother had a Roux-en-Y gastric bypass when T. R. was 14 years of age. Her review of systems was positive for snoring, daytime somnolence, limited exercise tolerance, and oligomenorrhea.
She was an excellent student but shied away from after-school activities and was uncertain about attending college after high-school graduation. On physical examination, she had hypertension, acanthosis nigricans, and extensive striae. Laboratory studies revealed insulin resistance, normal 2-hour glucose tolerance test result, elevated total and low-density lipoprotein cholesterol levels, and elevated alanine and aspartate aminotransferases. Her electrocardiographic and echocardiographic recordings were normal; however, polysomnography revealed a markedly elevated apnea-hypopnea index with multiple apnea events associated with oxygen desaturation. She and her mother requested that she be evaluated for bariatric surgery. After a 6-month period of weight maintenance, supported by dietary modification and limited exercise, she underwent a Roux-en-Y gastric bypass. Postoperatively, she was prescribed a restricted diet, supplemented with protein, minerals, and vitamins. Subsequently, she was able to reintroduce a wide variety of foods. Six months after surgery, her weight was 110 kg, her BMI was 43, and all laboratory studies had normalized, including polysomnography. As a valedictorian at her high-school graduation, 18 months after surgery, her weight was down to 87 kg and her BMI was 35.4. With improvement in her self-esteem, she looked forward to entering an out-of-state college soon thereafter.

PREVALENCE

The United States is experiencing a dramatic increase in pediatric obesity. Since 1971, the prevalence of overweight has increased from below 5% to almost 20% for non-Hispanic white children aged 6 to 11 years and from just above 5% to 17% among 12- to 17-year-olds (Ogden et al, 2002). Similar increases occurred for non-Hispanic black and Mexican American youth. Although the risk of overweight varies with gender, socioeconomic status (SES), and ethnicity, these associations have weakened over time and, in some cases, reversed. Non-Hispanic white boys 2 to 9 years of age of lower SES are at greater risk of overweight, whereas non-Hispanic white girls in this age group with higher SES are at greater risk than those of lower SES. This trend among girls reverses with age, such that lower SES non-Hispanic white girls 10 to 18 years of age are at greater risk than non-Hispanic white girls of higher SES. For non-Hispanic black girls 10 to 18 years of age, the reverse is true, with greatest risk seen in the higher SES group. In the period 1999-2002, the highest rates of overweight were seen among the groups of non-Hispanic black girls 10 to 18 years of age of higher SES (38%) and the middle SES Mexican American boys 10 to 18 years of age (35.2%).

MEDICAL AND PSYCHOLOGICAL SEQUELAE

Obesity is associated with a variety of medical and psychological sequelae, all of which may begin in childhood (Must and Strauss, 1999). It is no longer unusual to encounter overweight children with type 2 diabetes, obstructive sleep apnea, nonalcoholic steatohepatitis, pseudotumor cerebri, hypertension, hyperlipidemia, polycystic ovary syndrome (girls), and the metabolic syndrome.

Obesity in childhood and adolescence may have long-term consequences on adult health. Not only is the likelihood of adult obesity greatly increased for adolescents who are overweight, but so too is the presence of cardiovascular risk factors during the adolescent years, all of which, including hypertension, elevated low-density lipoprotein levels, elevated triglyceride levels, and reduced high-density lipoprotein levels, remain significant risk factors for adult cardiovascular disease. The severity of atherosclerotic lesions in coronary arteries and the aorta is associated with body mass index in autopsy studies of children and young adults.

The social and psychological sequelae of obesity in childhood and adolescence also deserve attention. Increased body fatness is associated with earlier physical and sexual maturation, which in turn may have social consequences, including poor self-esteem and disturbed body image. Preoccupation with weight is often accompanied by abnormal eating behaviors, leading to binge eating, unhealthy dieting, and, in some cases, anorexia. The stigma of obesity may lead to difficulty in establishing peer relationships and social isolation. Rejection on the basis of body size and shape begins during the preschool years and can continue throughout life, even leading to discrimination in college acceptance and employment. These social and psychological consequences also extend into adult life, including lower household income, fewer years of education, higher rates of poverty, and lower marriage rates, for adults who were overweight at age 16 years (Gortmaker et al, 1993). Overweight concerns, body dissatisfaction, and depressive symptoms are prevalent among school-age boys and girls of varying ethnicity and socioeconomic status (Erickson et al, 2000; Robinson et al, 2001a). In a sample of severely overweight adolescents evaluated for bariatric surgery, 30% met criteria for clinically significant depression with use of a self-report measure and 45% met criteria based on parent report (Zeller et al, 2006). Quality of life measures also suggest that health-related quality of life is affected by obesity and that the effect may be as great as that seen for children and adolescents diagnosed with cancer (Schwimmer et al, 2003).

DIAGNOSIS OF OBESITY

Body mass index (BMI) is the currently recommended metric for the assessment of overweight in the pediatric age group. Although methods exist for the estimation of body fatness, including skin fold thickness, underwater weighing, air plethysmography, and bioelectric impedance, these are not widely employed in clinical care. In this chapter, the term *obesity* is used in reference to a condition of excessive body fatness; the term *overweight* is used in reference to individuals or groups of individuals whose BMI is in excess of the 85th percentile for their age and gender.

BMI, calculated by the formula [BMI = weight (kilograms) divided by the square of height (meters)], should be plotted on a standardized gender-specific percentile curve by age, such as those currently available from the Centers for Disease Control and Prevention (Figs. 61-1 and 61-2). BMI at or above the 95th percentile for age and gender is defined as obese, whereas BMI at or above the 85th percentile and below the 95th percentile is defined as overweight.

DEVELOPMENT OF ADIPOSITY

Dietz (1994) has suggested that there may be three "critical periods" in the development of obesity, corresponding to periods of adipose tissue proliferation: gestation and early infancy, ages 5 to 7 years, and adolescence. The role of the prenatal period in the later development of obesity is still unclear, although metabolic influences on the developing fetus, such as those that occur in the presence of gestational diabetes, may have long-term consequences (Whitaker et al, 1998). During the first year of life, children tend to accumulate "baby fat," followed by a relative reduction in body fatness during the next several years, followed again by an increase in their BMI beginning at 5 to 6 years of age and continuing through puberty. Longitudinal studies of risk factors for adult obesity have generally shown that with increasing age, the overweight child or adolescent has an increasing likelihood of obesity in adult life, thereby providing justification for counseling of any child whose BMI exceeds the 85th percentile about risk of later overweight.

ETIOLOGIC FACTORS

The multifactorial nature of child obesity suggests an important interaction of genetic predisposition, family environment, and individual behavior. Whether the etiology of obesity is more genetic or behavioral, the clinical approach to the evaluation and treatment of this problem requires that all factors be acknowledged. Dietz and Robinson (1993) suggested that as in other diseases reflecting an interaction of host and environment, the most appropriate perspective is that genetics influences susceptibility to obesity but that the genetic predisposition to obesity can be modified by attention to environmental factors affecting calorie intake or energy expenditure.

Factors influencing the development of body fatness during childhood and adolescence include calorie intake and energy expenditure. Although differences in calorie intake or energy expenditure might account for differences in body fatness between individuals, it has been difficult to consistently demonstrate such differences, even in well-performed naturalistic studies. Small differences in daily food intake or physical activity, when extended for long periods, may account for the excessive weight gain of some children.

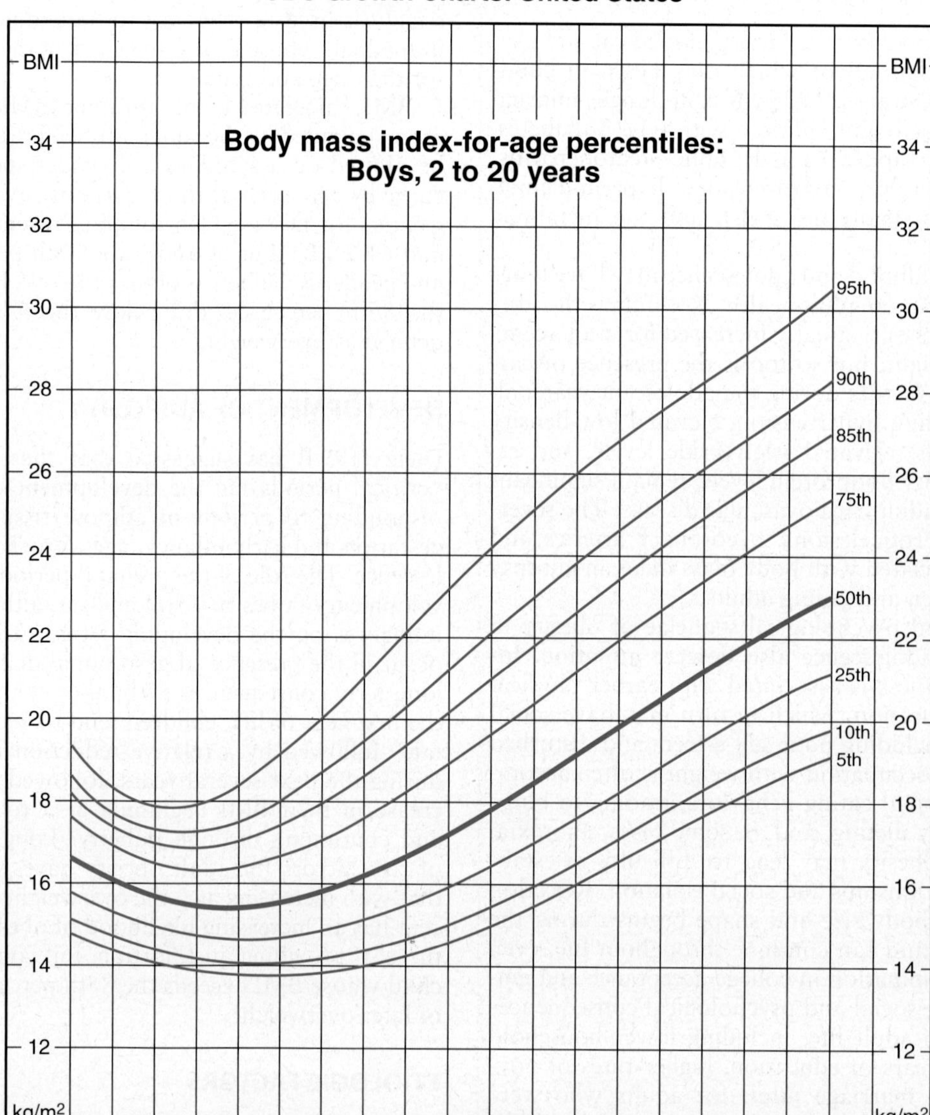

Figure 61-1. Percentiles of BMI for boys 2 to 20 years of age. (*From http://www.cdc.gov/growthcharts.*)

Excessive parental control rather than self-regulation of dietary intake may also be an important risk factor for overweight. Johnson and Birch (1994) studied the relationship of adiposity to children's ability to self-regulate dietary intake and found that overweight girls were less likely to compensate for their intake at a previous meal than were thinner girls. Parents may influence their children's eating behavior without clearly influencing their risk of overweight (Drucker et al, 1999). The effect of parental control on food intake remains somewhat uncertain, as it was not seen in an ethnically diverse sample with greater variability in socioeconomic status (Robinson et al, 2001b).

Child temperament may also play a role in feeding and weight gain. During infancy, difficult children (those with higher negativity and intensity and lower rhythmicity, approaching, and adaptability) may be more irritable, with parents then using feeding as a soothing technique (Carey, 1985). This hypothesized relationship was supported by a longitudinal study of children from birth to 9.5 years of age; children whose parents reported tantrums over food and whose temperament scores were higher on anger and frustration and lower on soothability had an increased risk of later overweight (Agras et al, 2004).

Inactivity may also contribute to increased weight gain. Excessive television viewing has received attention as a potential cause of obesity. In the Framingham Children's Study, time spent watching television was associated with changes in body fatness over time (Proctor et al, 2003). Interventions to decrease sedentary behaviors, including television viewing, or to increase physical activity are associated with changes in percent overweight and aerobic fitness (Epstein et al, 2000). Likewise, efforts to reduce television viewing can directly influence

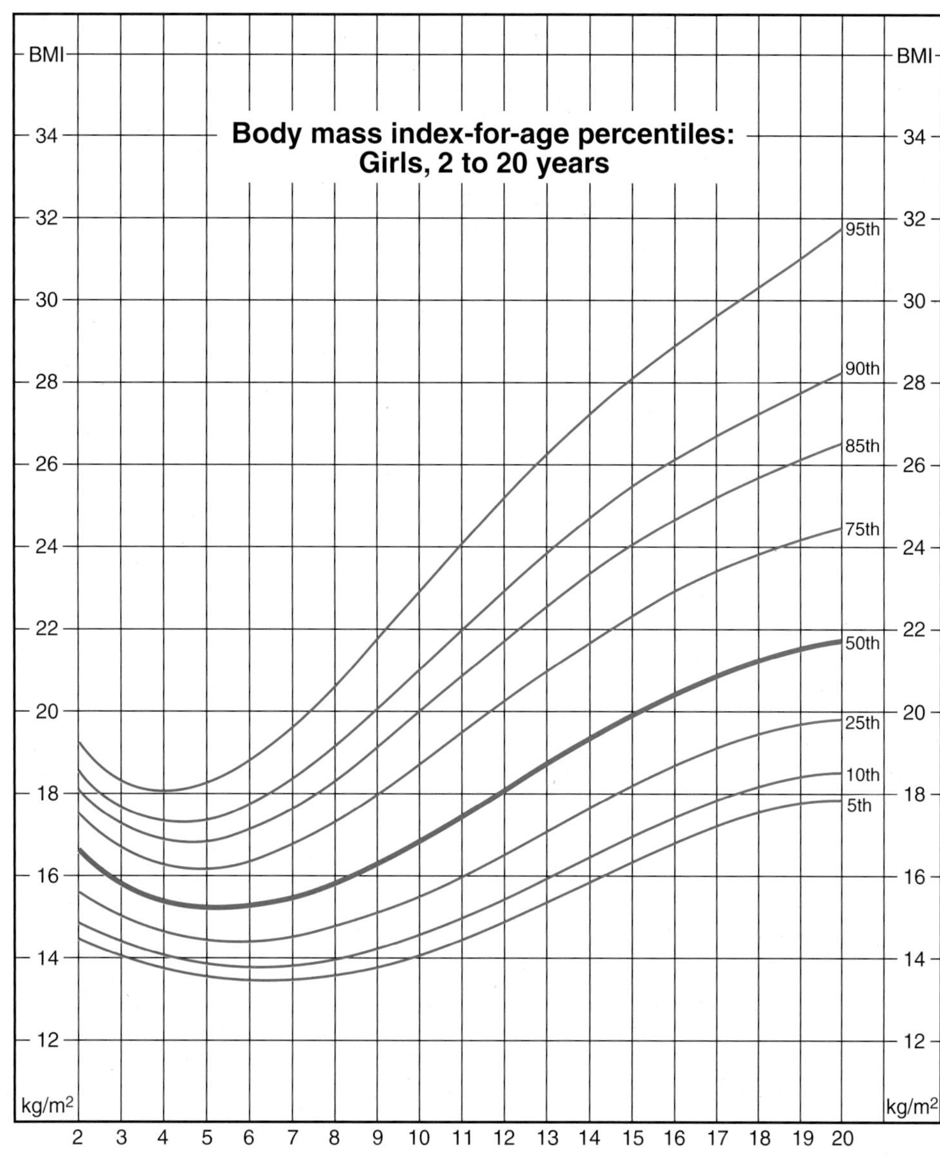

Figure 61-2. Percentiles of BMI for girls 2 to 20 years of age. (*From http://www.cdc.gov/growthcharts.*)

change in BMI and prevalence of obesity over time in nonclinical populations (Robinson, 1999).

ROLE OF THE PRIMARY CARE PHYSICIAN IN THE MANAGEMENT OF CHILD AND ADOLESCENT OBESITY

The primary care physician has a number of important roles in the care of overweight children, beginning with calculation of the BMI at each visit and the identification of overweight children. Although physicians may be reluctant to raise the issue of overweight in an effort to avoid labeling of the affected child, without such identification, it is unlikely that the child's weight status will be addressed in the office setting. A comprehensive history and physical examination are generally sufficient to rule out underlying endocrine and obesity disorders, and the primary care physician can focus on the medical and psychological comorbidities of obesity during the evaluation process. Depending on the availability of other resources in the community and the needs of the child or family, the physician might consider the additional consultation of a dietitian, psychologist, family therapist, and group treatment program. Even if the child engages in a weight management program independent of the physician's office, it remains important to monitor the nutritional adequacy of any dietary changes and safety of exercise and other physical activity accompanying the program and to monitor the child's BMI over time.

Pediatricians often express frustration in their efforts to engage patients and their parents in meaningful weight management efforts. This frustration may also be linked to a lack of confidence in their own or others' ability to successfully provide weight management counseling. Patients and their parents often appear to lack sufficient motivation to make significant change in eating behaviors, dietary composition, and physical activity. There is a growing interest in the application of motivational interviewing techniques to pediatric obesity treatment (Resnicow et al, 2006). Motivational interviewing uses a nonjudgmental and supportive mode of communication between physician and patient, designed to enhance motivation for behavior change, rather than the more traditional emphasis on the transfer of information about healthy diet or exercise. The physician must engage in active reflective listening to respond effectively to the patient's or parent's questions and statements. Once the patient or parent acknowledges both concern about the problem of overweight and a belief that behavior change will be effective in overcoming the problem, it then becomes much more likely that goals for behavior change can be articulated, agreed on, and ultimately achieved.

The pediatrician may wish to engage the consultation of other clinicians in the treatment of his or her overweight patients. In particular, the use of pediatric specialists for assistance with the management of comorbidities, such as diabetes, hypertension, sleep apnea, pseudotumor cerebri, and polycystic ovary syndrome, should be considered. In caring for patients with very severe overweight, consultation with a pediatric obesity specialist should also be considered, especially if the need for pharmacotherapy or bariatric surgery is under discussion.

DIAGNOSTIC EVALUATION

History

Less than 2% of overweight children have an underlying endocrinopathy, such as hypothyroidism or Cushing disease, or one of the recognized obesity syndromes, such as the Prader-Willi or Bardet-Biedl syndrome (Table 61-1). In general, nondysmorphic overweight children with normal or above-average height, normal intelligence, and normal gonadal development do not require further laboratory investigation for underlying genetic or endocrine disorders.

The child's past medical history should be reviewed with attention to early hypotonia, feeding difficulties, or developmental delay. Current and past medication use, suspected food allergies, hospitalizations, and surgeries should also be noted. The review of systems should include particular attention to symptoms associated with comorbidities of obesity, such as persistent headaches, as seen in pseudotumor cerebri; excessive daytime sleepiness, snoring, and enuresis, all of which may suggest the possibility of obstructive sleep apnea; persistent hip or knee pain, as seen with slipped capital femoral epiphyses or tibia vara; and, for pubertal girls, oligomenorrhea or amenorrhea, hirsutism, and excessive acne, which may suggest the presence of polycystic ovary syndrome.

The child's pattern of eating should be reviewed with attention to rapid eating, large portion sizes, multiple frequent meals throughout the day, excessive snacking, binging, and nighttime eating. A common pattern seen among older children and adolescents involves skipping breakfast and lunch, followed by a large dinner and after-dinner snacking. Diet records, kept for a period of weekend and weekdays, can be used to analyze the nutritional composition of the child's diet and to identify opportunities for dietary modification, as with poor food selection or excessive portion sizes.

The child's physical activity should also be reviewed, supplemented by a physical activity record, to describe the amount and intensity of physical activity. It is important to document periods of inactivity, including use of video games, computers, and television, as these are discrete sedentary behaviors that can be targeted for change.

Evaluation of the overweight child should include a psychological assessment, which should focus on ways in which the child's weight, or that of other family members, might influence the family's functioning as well as any factors that may influence eating habits or affect the ability to participate in a treatment program. This is an opportunity to discuss how the child's eating habits or obesity has an impact on the other family members and ways in which the child's obesity may affect peer relationships. The presence of significant psychopathology, including prior eating disordered behaviors, in the child or parents necessitates further psychiatric evaluation.

Table 61-1. Examples of Obesity Syndromes

Prader-Willi Syndrome
Early hypotonia
Early feeding difficulty
Early failure-to-thrive
Developmental delay
Later profound hyperphagia
Bardet-Biedl Syndrome
Intellectual disability
Hypogonadism
Polydactyly
Retinitis pigmentosa
Optic atrophy
Cataracts
Microphthalmia
Colobomas

Physical Examination

A careful general physical examination should be geared to the identification of underlying endocrine or other syndromes and to the identification of problems that may contribute to or be a consequence of the child's obesity (Table 61-2). Patients with normal stature, normal cognitive development, and normal gonadal development are unlikely to have a primary endocrine or genetic diagnosis underlying their obesity.

Laboratory Evaluation and Diagnostic Studies

In patients suspected of having the Prader-Willi syndrome, fluorescent in situ hybridization analysis has become the recommended approach to the laboratory diagnosis. Hypothyroidism can be assessed by serum levels of thyroxine, triiodothyronine (by radioimmunoassay), and thyroid-stimulating hormone. In patients with possible Cushing syndrome, cortisol levels and a dexamethasone suppression test should be obtained.

Given the increasing prevalence of many of the comorbidities of obesity in the pediatric age range, laboratory and diagnostic studies are indicated for all children whose BMI exceeds the 95th percentile for age as well as for children with BMI above the 85th percentile and clinical signs of any comorbidities (Table 61-3).

Psychological Assessment

A psychological assessment of the child and family can be very helpful and may provide important information about the family's concerns and ability to participate in further evaluation and in treatment. It is useful to observe the interaction of family members and to observe their expressions of concern for and criticism or support of the child in dealing with this problem. If the opportunity presents itself, it is also useful to note parents' responses to the child's requests for food during the visit. If there is any suspicion of child or family psychopathology, an experienced psychologist or family therapist should be consulted during this process.

TREATMENT APPROACHES

Recent publications provide a series of recommendations for the management of overweight children and adolescents. The Expert Panel on Child Obesity of the Maternal and Child Health Bureau met in March 1997 and agreed on the use of BMI to assess overweight status and on an algorithm based on BMI percentile, age, and associated comorbidities. The Panel emphasized that intervention should begin early, rather than waiting for the development of worsening overweight or associated comorbidities. The Panel also recommended that clinicians evaluate the family's readiness to participate in a program dependent on behavior change and that all family members should be involved in the weight management process, including dietary change and physical activity (Barlow and Dietz, 1998). The Panel's recommendations have been updated and expanded recently (Barlow and the Expert Committee, 2007).

Goals

Treatment should aim for modest, gradual change over time, with an emphasis on implementing small, permanent changes in diet and activity. Families should learn to use self-monitoring as a key component of the behavior change process and should set reasonable targets for weight maintenance or weight loss, depending on the age of the child and the severity of his or her overweight. Recommendations based on age and BMI are included in the new Expert Committee Report. Children 6 years of age and older should be encouraged toward weight loss if their BMI is at or above the 95th percentile, as should those 12 years of age and older with a BMI between the 85th and 94th percentiles in the presence of a comorbidity. Children between 2 and 5 years of age should be encouraged to lose weight only in the presence of a BMI at or above 21 kg/m^2.

It is not always easy to set a specific target weight for the child. One approach is to use the child's BMI curve to identify the current thresholds for 85th percentile and 95th percentile BMI for age. The current height is then used to calculate the weight loss that would put the child at each of these thresholds. Such a goal may be achievable with periods of weight loss alternating with periods of weight maintenance.

Behavioral treatment should support change in diet and exercise without placing the child at risk for calorie insufficiency. Depending on the age of the child and the severity of obesity, change in behavior may be used to maintain a young child's weight, allowing linear growth to proceed (producing a change toward lower degree of overweight or fatness), or to foster moderate weight loss in the older child (½ to 1 pound per week) or adolescent (1 to 2 pounds per week). By closely monitoring

Table 61-2. Important Physical Findings Related to Obesity

- Short stature (underlying endocrine or genetic diagnosis)
- Blood pressure (hypertension)
- Papilledema (pseudotumor cerebri) and retinitis pigmentosa (Bardet-Biedl syndrome)
- Thyromegaly
- Loud pulmonic second sound (increase in pulmonary vascular resistance)
- Hepatomegaly (enlarged fatty liver)
- Hypogonadism (Prader-Willi syndrome and other genetic disorders)
- Buffalo hump, truncal obesity, and striae (Cushing syndrome)
- Acanthosis nigricans (type 2 diabetes mellitus or insulin resistance)
- Hirsutism and excessive acne (polycystic ovary syndrome)
- Small hands (Prader-Willi syndrome)
- Bowing of the legs (Blount disease)

Table 61-3. Recommended Laboratory Studies for Comorbidities

Suspected Comorbidity	Laboratory or Diagnostic Study
Type 2 diabetes mellitus	Fasting blood glucose concentration; if elevated, add 2-hour glucose tolerance test*
Insulin resistance	Insulin level*
Hyperlipidemia	Fasting lipids (total cholesterol, low-density lipoprotein, high-density lipoprotein, triglycerides)*
Nonalcoholic fatty liver disease	Liver function tests (aspartate and alanine aminotransferases)*
Polycystic ovary syndrome	Abnormal levels of testosterone, free testosterone, dehydroepiandrosterone sulfate, and sex hormone–binding globulin, with normal levels of prolactin, insulin-like growth factor 1, thyroid hormones, and 17-hydroxyprogesterone
Obstructive sleep apnea	Polysomnography, electrocardiography
Blount disease	Knee radiographs
Slipped capital femoral epiphyses	Hip radiographs
Heart failure	Chest radiography, echocardiography
Pseudotumor cerebri	Computed tomography of the head

*Indicates studies recommended for all patients with BMI greater than 95th percentile; all others if suspected by history or physical examination findings.

the child's diet, rate of weight loss, and continuing growth in height, nutritional adequacy of the diet can be confirmed.

In addition to weight loss, it is important to emphasize associated goals of improved fitness, self-esteem, social interaction, and family harmony. These outcomes can all be achieved without an emphasis on weight loss and may be enhanced by a focus on the development of healthier eating habits and increased physical activity for the whole family.

A general word of caution should also be emphasized with regard to the overzealous application of any weight management strategy for the child or adolescent. Reports of significant retardation of growth, associated with the dietary treatment of hypercholesterolemia and with fear of the development of obesity, should be viewed as the adverse outcomes of inadequately supervised or misguided attempts at dietary manipulation. In addition, 20% of 137 patients who were followed up after participation in family-based group treatment reported being treated for psychiatric disorders during the 10-year follow-up (Epstein et al, 1994).

Family Involvement

Child and adolescent obesity is situated within a family context. There are typically other family members who have struggled with weight and whose experience can be extremely valuable in helping develop a realistic set of goals for the child and family. The tendency for families to feel defeated by obesity comes from their unrealistic expectation of dramatic and continued change.

The family's involvement is critical to the evaluation and management of child obesity. Parents are often confused by what they have read and thought about the origins of their child's obesity. Because obesity has both strong genetic and behavioral contributions, parents often feel guilty about their child's obesity and may have already experienced failure in trying to intervene. Because obesity is so resistant to intervention, the family may feel hopeless and at a loss. Efforts to explain the causes of the child's obesity are rarely successful and often lead to confusing or inadequate explanations for the family. For example, rather than using the dietary history as a means of proving the presence of excessive dietary intake, one should use the dietary history as a means of identifying opportunities for dietary change. Likewise, in discussing the child's regular physical activity, it should be possible to identify opportunities for increasing physical activity. One can approach intervention as a process of gradually modifying the child's eating behavior and physical activity over time, in the context of the whole family. It is critical that the family engage in this process in an active way and agree to initiate and to maintain change in the whole family's food and exercise habits.

Behavioral Intervention

For families who appear to be reasonably functional and motivated, the initial strategies are focused on gradual alterations in the child's eating and physical activity (Table 61-4). These behavioral strategies include goal setting, self-monitoring, record review, contracting, praise, environmental control, cognitive restructuring, anticipation, periodic reassessment, and maintenance.

Intervention does not require "calorie counting" or specific calorie intake reduction. An alternative approach is to categorize foods as more or less desirable and to use behavioral techniques that lead to the reduction of less desirable foods and encouragement of more desirable foods. One such system of categorization, the "stoplight diet," categorizes foods as "red light," "yellow light," and "green light" (Epstein et al, 1994). By identifying foods in this way, parents can support the child's efforts to reduce intake of red-light foods and increase intake of foods from the other two categories. Gradual reduction in intake of red-light foods can be rewarded and sustained in association with goals of weight loss or maintenance.

A discussion of dietary approaches to weight management in children would not be complete without some

Table 61-4. Behavioral Treatment Components

Goal setting	Set weekly challenging but achievable goals for change in diet, physical activity, and sedentary behavior.
Self-monitoring	Self-monitoring increases behavioral awareness of behavior change and facilitates reinforcement. Without self-monitoring or monitoring by parents, it is impossible to assess progress in behavior change over time.
Daily record review	Daily review with a parent helps provide feedback and reinforcement for behavior change.
Contracting	After setting of realistic and explicit goals each week, the parent and child contract for agreed on behavior change. Rewards should be simple, easy to administer, and inexpensive. Rewards should be deliverable immediately (i.e., weekly or daily).
Praise	Parents can learn to use praise as a powerful tool to reinforce and to maintain desired behavior change. Praise should be specific to the behavior. Criticism and punishment are less effective and may be detrimental.
Environmental control	Parents can help by identifying factors within the environment that promote overeating or inactivity. Examples of environmental control include removal of high-fat, high-calorie foods from the household, increasing the availability of cut-up vegetables rather than chips or sweets for snack time, avoidance of television viewing during mealtimes, reducing the amount of time indoors during daylight hours, and increasing the expectation for daily physical activity.
Cognitive restructuring	Parents and children learn alternative ways to think about their beliefs and behaviors to reduce the tendency to feel bad about their struggle with weight.
Anticipation	It is important to anticipate obesity-promoting situations and to plan specific strategies for parties, travel, and holidays.
Reassessment	Periodic reassessment enables the child and family to identify lapses in desired behavior change and to reinstitute previously successful strategies, before feelings of frustration and failure develop.
Maintenance	Ongoing reassessment of goals, strategies, and progress

mention of low-carbohydrate or low–glycemic index diets. Although the "low-carb" diet achieved enormous popularity in the United States during the 1990s, its use among children and adolescents has been more limited. A low–glycemic index diet is one that emphasizes foods that produce only a small increase in blood glucose concentration after consumption of a standard amount of carbohydrate. Examples of high-glycemic carbohydrate-containing foods are highly refined grains and potatoes; nonstarchy vegetables, legumes, and fruits produce smaller increases in blood glucose concentration and are considered to be low-glycemic foods. The "stoplight approach" has been applied in a study evaluating the feasibility of using a low–glycemic index diet for children 5 to 12 years of age (Young et al, 2004).

Unfortunately, there have been relatively few controlled studies of behavioral treatment for child and adolescent obesity. A recent meta-analysis identified treatment studies published between 1966 and 2005, of which only nine studies met all of the criteria specified by the authors, including use of a described dietary intervention, inclusion of a comparison group (either untreated or treated with an alternative approach), and use of weight change or BMI change as an outcome (Gibson et al, 2006). These studies varied in duration from 8 to 40 weeks and in duration of initial follow-up from none to 24 months and provided support for energy restriction as being useful in short-term weight loss, but no conclusions could be drawn with regard to longer term weight loss or maintenance of weight loss.

Epstein and coworkers (1994) have reported follow-up results of their family-based group treatment program. Combining subjects from a number of their treatment studies, at the 5-year follow-up they found that reinforcement of both child and parent behavior or reciprocal targeting of children and parents yielded better results than did a nonspecific control condition in which children were reinforced only for attendance at treatment meetings. Predictors of child success included self-monitoring of weight, changing eating behavior (eating fewer red-light foods and more selection of low-calorie snacks), parent-reported use of praise, and change in parent percent overweight. At the 10-year follow-up, about one third had maintained a decrease in percent overweight of 20% or more, and nearly 30% were no longer overweight.

Very Low Calorie Diets

Very low calorie diets, generally providing fewer than 800 kcal per day, became widely available for outpatient use in the treatment of adult obesity in the 1980s. These diets, sometimes called protein-sparing modified fasts, were associated with significant medical risks (electrolyte abnormalities, arrhythmias, and sudden death) but became widely marketed as part of many commercial weight loss programs. Despite their general success in supporting rapid weight loss, most patients experienced subsequent weight regain once the very low calorie diet was discontinued. These extremely hypocaloric diets have been used on a limited basis in the pediatric population, generally in an inpatient setting, with close medical supervision.

Surgery

Bariatric surgery includes any surgical procedure performed with the intention of inducing or supporting weight loss among overweight individuals, including procedures that foster a reduction in calorie intake by restricting the size of the stomach or that induce a malabsorptive state by excluding varying portions of the bowel. Although developed and modified over the years to be used primarily with adult patients, these procedures have become increasingly applied to the treatment of severely overweight adolescents. The bariatric surgery most commonly performed today is the Roux-en-Y gastric bypass, which combines elements of both gastroplasty (15- to 30-mL pouch) and intestinal bypass (75 to 150 cm). Recent improvements in laparoscopic techniques and equipment have made it possible for the Roux-en-Y to be performed with the laparoscope.

An alternative procedure, which does not permanently alter the anatomy of the stomach and intestine, involves placement of a band around the upper stomach with the option of using saline injected into a subcutaneous reservoir to adjust the tightness of the band. Although adjustable gastric banding can be reversed by removal of the band, its use in adolescent populations has been limited by lack of Food and Drug Administration approval of the device for patients younger than 18 years.

In 2004, an expert panel of surgeons and pediatricians developed a practice guideline for bariatric surgery in adolescent patients (Inge et al, 2004). On the basis of evidence available at that time, the group recommended the Roux-en-Y as having the best efficacy and safety of the procedures available and stressed the importance of gathering additional data concerning other procedures, such as the adjustable band. The importance of evaluating and treating adolescents in a pediatric setting rather than in an adult setting was also emphasized. The criteria for performance of bariatric surgery in adolescent patients emphasize physical and psychological maturity (Table 61-5).

Data concerning outcomes of bariatric surgery for adolescents have begun to emerge in terms of outcome and safety. A group of 10 patients, 15 to 17 years of age, had a Roux-en-Y bypass at one center and had a mean weight loss of 54 kg, with only one of the 10 failing to achieve weight loss in excess of 10 kg; however, four patients suffered late postoperative complications, including an incisional hernia, cholelithiasis, protein-calorie malnutrition, and small bowel obstruction (Strauss et al, 2001). Another series published in 2006 described 1-year outcomes for 39 patients operated on at three centers between 2001 and 2003, ranging in age from 13 to 21 years and all meeting the criteria described before (Lawson et al, 2006). Postoperative weight loss produced a change in mean BMI for the group from 56.5 kg/m^2 to 35.8 kg/m^2 with significant improvements in insulin sensitivity and lipid profiles. Postoperative complications included one death due to *Clostridium difficile* infection in a patient also under treatment for osteodystrophy.

Drug Treatment

Only two drugs currently have approval of the Food and Drug Administration for obesity treatment in the pediatric age group, sibutramine (age 16 years) and orlistat

Table 61-5. Criteria for Bariatric Surgery in Adolescents

The adolescent patient should:
Have a BMI > 40 kg/m^2 with one of the specified serious obesity-related comorbidities (obstructive sleep apnea, pseudotumor cerebri, or type 2 diabetes mellitus) or have a BMI > 50 kg/m^2 with less severe comorbidities (e.g., hypertension, nonalcoholic steatohepatitis, gastroesophageal reflux disease, dyslipidemia, venous stasis disease, weight-related arthropathy, or impairment of activities of daily living)
Have attained or nearly attained physiologic maturity
Have had a minimum of 6 months in supervised weight management as determined with the assistance of the patient's primary care physician
Demonstrate commitment to comprehensive medical and psychological evaluation before and after surgery
Agree to avoid pregnancy for at least 1 year postoperatively
Be able and willing to adhere to nutritional guidelines postoperatively
Demonstrate decisional capacity and provide informed consent
Have a supportive family environment

(age 12 years). In a randomized, double-blind, placebo-controlled trial involving 82 adolescents in a behavioral treatment program, the group that received sibutramine (Meridia), a norepinephrine-serotonin reuptake inhibitor, experienced greater weight loss during the initial 6 months of treatment, but no difference was detectable after a 6-month open label treatment period (Berkowitz et al, 2003). Side effects led to discontinuation of the drug or reduction in dosage in 40% of participants. Although orlistat (Xenical), a gastrointestinal lipase inhibitor, has been available by prescription, it has recently been approved for over-the-counter sale, despite the known risk of unpleasant gastrointestinal side effects, including fatty/oily stools and fecal incontinence. Another drug available in the pediatric age group, metformin (Glucophage), is currently approved for pediatric use in type 2 diabetes mellitus, but its potential value in weight management is currently under investigation.

Follow-up

The primary care provider should provide regular follow-up for the child who is involved in either an office-based or a group treatment program. This follow-up can include periodic monitoring of the child's weight and height as well as review of the child's self-monitoring records for diet and physical activity. For the child who is involved in a community-based, school-based, or hospital-based group treatment program, the primary care provider can provide added support, reinforcement, and encouragement to the child and family and help the family monitor their goals and progress along the way. Regular follow-up is suggested for at least 1 year and longer if possible.

PREVENTION

In 2003, the American Academy of Pediatrics issued a policy statement emphasizing the importance of accurately identifying children who are overweight and beginning efforts to increase physical activity and to reduce excessive calorie intake (American Academy of Pediatrics, 2003). Four specific behaviors that affect energy balance can be addressed during routine well-child care, including television viewing, outdoor play, breastfeeding, and limiting the consumption of sugar-sweetened drinks (Whitaker, 2003). In a 2005 report, the Institute of Medicine's Committee on Prevention of Obesity in Children and Youth similarly recommended that health care professionals routinely track BMI, offer relevant evidence-based counseling and guidance, serve as role models with their own behaviors, and provide leadership in their communities (Institute of Medicine, Committee on Prevention of Obesity in Children and Youth, 2005). The Committee also recommended that medical professional organizations disseminate evidence-based clinical guidance, establish programs on obesity prevention, and coordinate with each other to present a consistent message and that educational and accreditation entities include obesity prevention knowledge and skills across the spectrum of professional education and in their certification examinations.

A number of community- and school-based initiatives have been developed and tested during the past 10 years and found to have some impact on physical activity, television viewing, or dietary intake. In a school-based program designed to influence television viewing, students who were part of the intervention school not only decreased their television viewing but also showed less increase in BMI during the study period than did children in a control school, thereby demonstrating the potential for programs targeting specific behaviors rather than weight management (Robinson, 1999). Efforts to reduce access to soft drinks and other nutrient-poor products in the school environment are actively under way. Likewise, the influence of the physical environment on children's physical activity is a focus of efforts toward increasing access to safe, accessible playgrounds, playing fields, and parks.

SUMMARY

Although it is not a new problem, obesity among children and adolescents has reached a level of prevalence and severity never before seen in the United States and throughout the world. As a result of this "epidemic," it is estimated that the current generation of U.S. children, born after the year 2000, will have a shorter lifespan than that of their parents and that one third of these children are likely to develop type 2 diabetes during their lifetimes! Other comorbidities of obesity, including hypertension, hyperlipidemia, nonalcoholic steatohepatitis, and obstructive sleep apnea, are being seen in a large number of overweight youth. A general lack of physical activity, coupled with increasing use of electronic media, and the increase in family meals eaten out of the home, especially at fast-food restaurants, have likely contributed to the problem. Treatment efforts have been generally disappointing, except for intensive family-based behavioral group programs, whereas efforts at prevention, particularly on a school or community basis, have shown short-term promise.

REFERENCES

Agras WS, Hammer LD, McNicholas F, et al: Risk factors for childhood overweight: A prospective study from birth to 9.5 years. J Pediatr 145:20-25, 2004.

American Academy of Pediatrics, Committee on Nutrition: Prevention of pediatric overweight and obesity. Pediatrics 112:424-430, 2003.

Barlow SE, Dietz WH: Obesity evaluation and treatment: Expert committee recommendations. Pediatrics 102:e29, 1998. Available at: http://www.pediatrics.org/cgi/content/full/102/3/e29.

Barlow SE, and the Expert Committee: Expert Committee recommendations regarding the prevention, assessment, and treatment of child and adolescent overweight and obesity: Summary report. Pediatrics 120:5164-5192, 2007.

Berkowitz RI, Wadden TA, Tershokovec AM, et al: Behavior therapy and sibutramine for the treatment of adolescent obesity. A randomized clinical trial. JAMA 289:1805-1812, 2003.

Carey WB: Temperament and increased weight gain in infants. J Dev Behav Pediatr 6:128-131, 1985.

Centers for Disease Control and Prevention, National Center for Health Statistics: CDC growth charts: United States. May 30, 2000. Available at: http://www.cdc.gov/growthcharts/.

Dietz WH: Critical periods in childhood for the development of obesity. Am J Clin Nutr 59:955-959, 1994.

Dietz WH, Robinson TN: Assessment and treatment of childhood obesity. Pediatr Rev 14:337-344, 1993.

Drucker RR, Hammer LD, et al: Can mothers influence their child's eating behavior? J Dev Behav Pediatr 20:88-92, 1999.

Epstein LH, Valoski A, Wing RR, et al: Ten-year outcomes of behavioral family-based treatment for childhood obesity. Health Psychol 13:373-383, 1994.

Epstein LH, Paluch RA, Gordy CC, et al: Decreasing sedentary behaviors in treating pediatric obesity. Arch Pediatr Adolesc Med 154:220-226, 2000.

Erickson SJ, Robinson TN, Haydel F, et al: Are overweight children unhappy? Body mass index, depressive symptoms, and overweight concerns in elementary school children. Arch Pediatr Adolesc Med 154:931-935, 2000.

Gibson LJ, Peto J, Warren JM, et al: Lack of evidence on diets for obesity for children: A systematic review. Int J Epidemiol advance access. September 19, 2006. doi:10.1093/ije/dyl208.

Gortmaker SL, Must A, Perrin JM, et al: Social and economic consequences of overweight in adolescence and young adulthood. N Engl J Med 329:1008-1012, 1993.

Inge TH, Krebs NF, Garcia VF, et al: Bariatric surgery for severely overweight adolescents: Concerns and recommendations. Pediatrics 114:217-223, 2004.

Institute of Medicine, Committee on Prevention of Obesity in Children and Youth: Preventing Childhood Obesity: Health in the Balance. Washington, DC, The National Academies Press, 2005.

Johnson SL, Birch LL: Parents' and children's adiposity and eating style. Pediatrics 94:654-661, 1994.

Lawson ML, Kirk S, Mitchell T, et al: One-year outcomes of Roux-en-Y gastric bypass for morbidly obese adolescents: A multicenter study from the Pediatric Bariatric Surgery Study Group. J Pediatr Surg 41:137-143, 2006.

Must A, Strauss RS: Risks and consequences of childhood and adolescent obesity. Int J Obes Relat Metab Disord 23(Suppl 2):S2-S11, 1999.

Ogden CL, Flegel KM, Carroll MD, et al: Prevalence and trends in overweight among U.S. children and adolescents, 1999-2000. JAMA 288:1728-1732, 2002.

Proctor MH, Moore LL, Gao D, et al: Television viewing and change in body fat from preschool to early adolescence: The Framingham Children's Study. Int J Obes Relat Metab Disord 27:827-833, 2003.

Resnicow K, Davis R, Rollnick S: Motivational interviewing for pediatric obesity: Conceptual issues and evidence review. J Am Diet Assoc 106:2024-2033, 2006.

Robinson TN: Reducing children's television viewing to prevent obesity: A randomized controlled trial. JAMA 282:1561-1567, 1999.

Robinson TN, Chang JY, Haydel F, et al: Overweight concerns and body dissatisfaction among third-grade children: The impact of ethnicity and socioeconomic status. J Pediatr 138:181-187, 2001a.

Robinson TN, Kiernan M, Matheson DM, et al: Is parental control over children's eating associated with childhood obesity? Results from a population-based sample of third graders. Obes Res 9:306-312, 2001b.

Schwimmer JB, Burwinkle TM, Varni JW: Health-related quality of life and severely obese children and adolescents. JAMA 289:1813-1819, 2003.

Strauss RS, Bradley LJ, Brolin RE: Gastric bypass surgery in adolescents with morbid obesity. J Pediatr 138:499-504, 2001.

Whitaker RC: Obesity prevention in pediatric primary care. Four behaviors to target. Arch Pediatr Adolesc Med 157:725-727, 2003.

Whitaker RC, Dietz WH: Role of the prenatal environment in the development of obesity. J Pediatr 132:768-776, 1998.

Young PC, West SA, Ortiz K, et al: A pilot study to determine the feasibility of the low glycemic index diet as a treatment for overweight children in primary care practice. Ambul Pediatr 4:28-33, 2004.

Zeller MH, Roehrig HR, Modi AV, et al: Health-related quality of life and depressive symptoms in adolescents with extreme obesity presenting for bariatric surgery. Pediatrics 117:1155-1161, 2006.

62 URINARY FUNCTION AND ENURESIS

Ramzi Nasir and Alison Schonwald

Vignette

Jamal is 8 years old and his sister Shayna is 6 years old. Their mother is concerned about Jamal's frequent bed-wetting and Shayna's frequent daytime urinary accidents as well as nightly bed-wetting. A detailed history and physical examination and a simple laboratory test enable the pediatrician to exclude serious pathologic causes and confidently devise a therapeutic plan for each child.

DEVELOPMENT OF URINARY CONTINENCE

Like all areas of neurologic development, urinary continence progresses through a complex dynamic of biologic maturity and environmental opportunities. The bladder holds urine by detrusor relaxation (mediated by sympathetic fibers from spinal cord segments T10-L2) and external urinary sphincter contraction (mediated by the pudendal nerves from S2-4). Infant voiding is controlled by spinal cord reflex, with central nervous system mediation. The sensation of bladder fullness is relayed to the brain by afferent nerves in the bladder wall. By 2 years of age, 30% of children sense bladder fullness, and by 4 years, all typical children detect the urge to void (Jansson et al, 2005). Emptying of the bladder involves detrusor contraction (mediated by parasympathetic cholinergic nerves from S2-4) and relaxation of the external urinary sphincter. This centrally mediated process can be suppressed voluntarily (Chapple and MacDiarmid, 2000).

Daytime dryness is usually complete by 3½ years, with nighttime dryness following within a year (Jalkut et al, 2001). By 5 years, about 85% of children are dry at night. Typical children older than 5 years void five to eight times per day.

DISORDERS OF DAYTIME CONTINENCE

The most common definition of daytime incontinence is repeated voiding of urine into clothes that occurs at least twice a week for at least 3 consecutive months or that causes clinically significant distress or impairment of function in children 5 years of age chronologically or developmentally. The International Children's Continence Society adopts 5 years as the age when daytime incontinence merits evaluation without defining a frequency of events for diagnostic purposes.

Epidemiology

Prevalence of childhood daytime incontinence is estimated at 8% overall, with 13% of 4-year-olds affected, decreasing to 4% in 13-year-olds and 2% in those older than 18 years. Girls are about twice more likely to have symptoms than boys are.

Pathophysiology and Common Presentations

Daytime urine incontinence can reflect several pathologic processes disrupting the systems involved in continence.

Loss of cortical control can be due to brain lesions and intermittent alteration of consciousness (i.e., in epilepsy) that interrupt the cortical regulation of continence.

Spinal cord lesions, such as tethered cord or other dysraphisms, can interfere with bladder control, mainly as growth and movement stretch the cord and its blood supply.

Abnormalities of the peripheral nerves from traumatic lesions of the pudendal nerve or peripheral neuropathies (e.g., long-standing diabetes mellitus) impair involuntary sphincter contraction necessary for urine holding.

Acquired or congenital anatomic abnormalities of the lower urinary tract include ectopic ureter, posterior urethral valves, urethral stenosis or diverticula, labial adhesions, and traumatic lesions of the urethral sphincter, which may act as mechanical disruptions.

- Labial adhesions can limit urination to a small opening, with urine accumulation into the pocket behind the adhesed labia and then slow leakage after voiding. Stagnant urine predisposes children to urinary tract infections. Topical estrogen creams lyse the adhesions.
- Vaginal reflux occurs commonly in obese or younger girls who fail to fully spread the labia

while voiding. Urine refluxes from redundant folds into the vagina and later leaks. Children should spread the labia widely while urinating (by dropping the underwear to the ankles or sitting backwards on the toilet).

- Ectopic ureter (the ureter inserts just distal to the external urethral sphincter) is suggested by continuous dribbling of urine. It is more common in girls than in boys.
- Posterior urethral valves can present with continuous dribbling due to bladder outlet obstruction. Treatment is surgical for both valves and ectopic ureter.
- Stress incontinence results from insufficiency of the intrinsic urinary sphincter in girls and presents as leakage of urine during Valsalva maneuvers. As stress incontinence may reflect abnormalities of the spinal cord or pelvic floor, further urologic or neurologic referral is recommended.

Excessive urine production can overwhelm an otherwise functional lower urinary tract, as seen with diabetes mellitus, diabetes insipidus, sickle cell disease with reduced urine concentration, volume overload, and diuretic agents.

Bladder wall irritability may result from irritants (e.g., bacteria, viruses, calciuria).

Constipation commonly causes enuresis, apparently because the stool mass irritates the bladder and decreases its storage volume.

Emotional stress, such as post-traumatic stress disorder, sexual abuse, or other major life changes, can lead to regressive behaviors such as incontinence.

Functional voiding disorders are a heterogeneous group of disorders that account for daytime incontinence in most children. Typically, the findings on physical and neurologic examinations are normal. Robson (1997) suggested that the independent preschooler is more interested in his or her environment, ignoring the body's signal to void. Children with attention-deficit/hyperactivity disorder (ADHD) may have a higher incidence of dysfunctional voiding symptoms, perhaps related to inattention to body signals.

Follow-up data suggest remission/improvement rates of 60% to 91% of functional voiding symptoms within a few years of medical attention (Hellerstein and Zguta, 2003; Saedi and Schulman, 2003; Wiener et al, 2000). Retrospective studies link childhood urinary symptoms to adult urinary symptoms, indicating potential long-term morbidity.

The following categories are often used to classify functional voiding disorders, although, practically, there is frequent overlap in clinical presentations.

- Overactive bladder or urge incontinence reflects excessive bladder irritability. To suppress the urge to urinate, children hold the perineum, cross their legs, or squat on their heels. If the child is picked up while squatting, an immediate accident ensues (Robson, 1997).
- Giggle incontinence is characterized by complete emptying of the bladder while laughing and usually comes with other daytime symptoms (urgency, hesitancy, and urge incontinence). When these conditions are treated, giggle incontinence may improve.
- Underactive bladder is characterized by infrequent voiding and the need to increase intra-abdominal pressure to urinate; urodynamic studies typically show detrusor underactivity. Affected patients are typically girls whose incontinence is triggered by physical activity. Children may delay the first morning void and avoid using the school toilet. Urine infections, constipation, and encopresis are commonly associated (Casale, 2000).
- Hinman syndrome, a rare but serious disorder, is characterized by infrequent urination, urge incontinence, recurrent urinary tract infections, constipation, and encopresis. Bladder imaging shows a thickened bladder wall with reflux and hydronephrosis. Urodynamic studies confirm incoordination between the bladder and the external urinary sphincter, resulting in detrusor contraction in the face of a narrowed sphincter.
- Voiding postponement, a behavioral problem, is similar to functional voiding disorders. Affected children are often preschoolers who delay urination and assume holding postures until "the last minute." They may restrict fluid to avoid urinating.

Extraordinary daytime urinary frequency presents with small-volume voids more than once per hour. Those affected may have comorbid incontinence, particularly if they are unable to reach the bathroom on time. The disorder is self-limited, spontaneously resolving after weeks to months. Typically, no abnormalities are found on evaluation. Suggested causes are cystourethritis and emotional stress; some recommend anticholinergic treatment.

Evaluation

Children who fail to develop daytime urine continence by 5 years or who develop incontinence after an interval of complete dryness should be evaluated (Fig. 62-1).

History

A history should include review of the following signs and symptoms.

A voiding diary with timing, presence of urgency, hesitancy, dysuria, quality of stream, hematuria, straining, and squatting may suggest etiology. Urgency, frequency, and dysuria are common with urinary tract infections. Hesitancy, straining, and a weak urinary stream suggest urethral obstruction. Children with labial adhesions or vaginal reflux dribble urine shortly after leaving the toilet. Children with ectopic ureter or posterior urethral valves may be constantly wet. Boys often have a drop of urine in their underwear after using the bathroom; however, the stain dries quickly and causes no distress and thus is easily distinguished from enuresis.

Back pain and gait abnormalities with incontinence suggest spinal cord disease and direct urgent neurologic or neurosurgical evaluation.

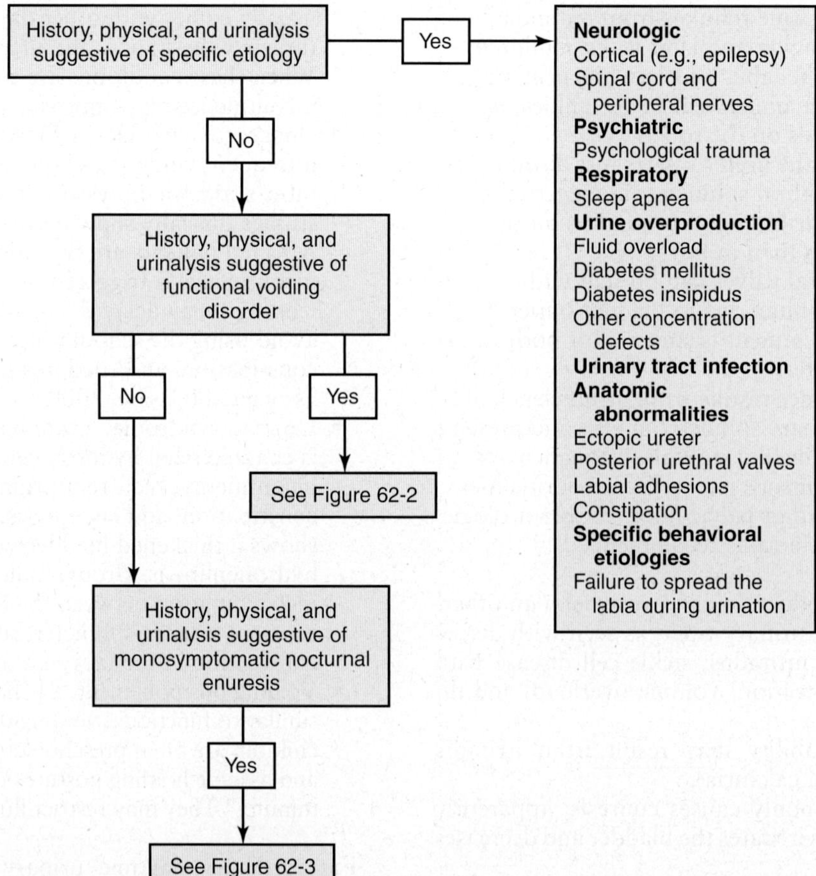

Figure 62-1. Initial approach to a child with voiding difficulties (see text for details).

Triggering psychological events, family response to a child's incontinence, and the emotional impact of incontinence on the child must be assessed. Ask both the caregiver and the child about sexual or physical abuse.

Physical Examination

A detailed physical examination is essential. Elevated blood pressure might reflect renal dysfunction; signs of fluid overload may indicate renal failure or congestive heart failure. Palpation of the abdomen allows identification of constipated stool masses, and bladder percussion may find distention from outlet obstruction or neurogenic disease. Examination of the back can detect vertebral anomalies or cutaneous markers of spinal dysraphisms, such as hemangiomas or hair tufts. Neurologic examination of the perineum involves assessment of the sacral reflexes, including anal wink and cremasteric reflexes in boys. Rectal examination may be performed in the cooperative child to confirm sphincter tone and the extent of constipation. Neurologic examination of the lower extremities can detect abnormalities related to spinal cord disease (altered strength or gait, diminished muscle stretch reflexes, and up-going toes).

Initial Diagnostic Studies

All children presenting with daytime incontinence require urinalysis. A random specific gravity of less than 1.002 (or less than 1.025 after 12 hours of fluid restriction) suggests inability to concentrate urine and is confirmed with serum electrolyte determinations and osmolality. Glucosuria likely indicates diabetes mellitus; nitrites or white blood cells suggest a urinary tract infection.

Management

In most cases, history, unremarkable physical examination, and normal urinalysis suggest that the voiding disorder is functional or behavioral (Fig. 62-2). Treatment of constipation often resolves urinary symptoms. For children with concomitant daytime and nighttime symptoms, address daytime symptoms first and then the night symptoms, which may remit after daytime symptoms are treated.

Behavioral Approaches

All behavioral approaches require active participation of the child. The child is expected to attempt to void at regularly scheduled times every 2 to 3 hours, regardless of the sensation of the need to go. Positive reinforcement encourages motivation. A wrist alarm watch that sounds at set intervals minimizes child-parent conflict, optimizes a child's sense of achievement, and may serve as an additional reward for compliance with the plan. In school, the assistance of the teacher to encourage the child to go to the bathroom at routine intervals is essential. Regular voids can be scheduled around natural breaks in the day, such as meals, recess, and snack. Arranging to use a private (nurse's or staff) bathroom can improve program adherence.

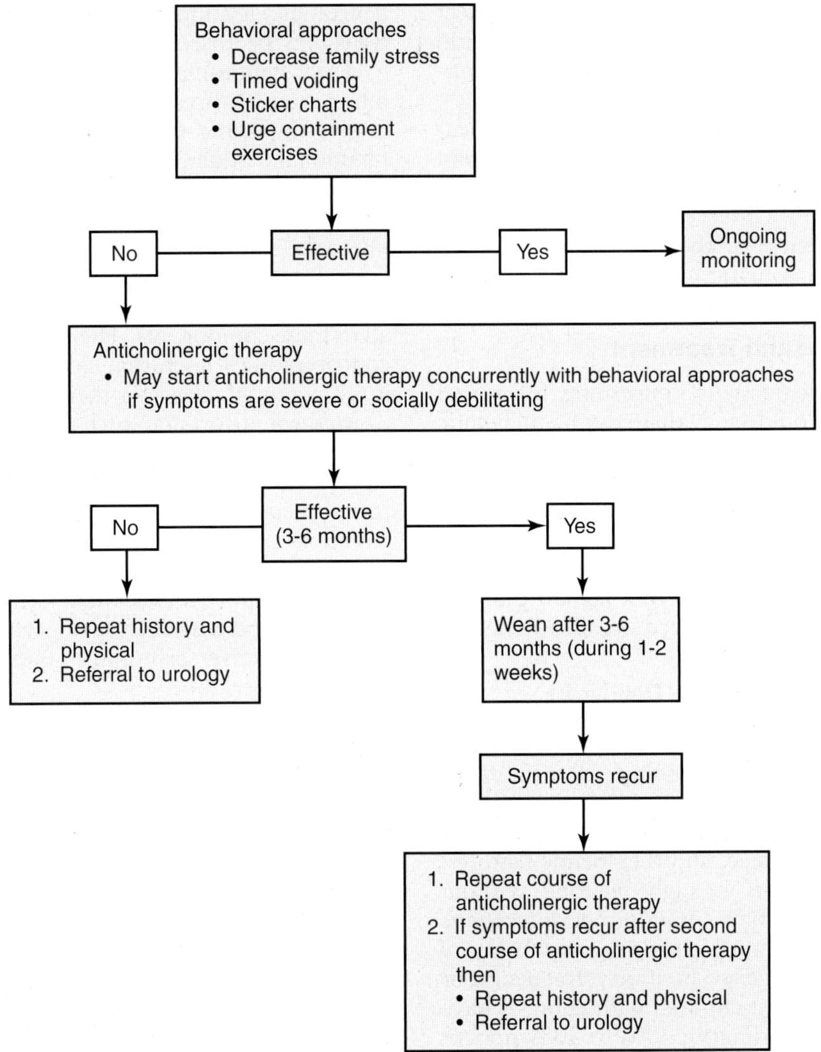

Figure 62-2. Initial assessment suggestive of functional voiding disorder (see text for details).

Stressful family dynamics must be addressed; resolution may take weeks to months. Parents may be frustrated with the child's incontinence, and their negative affect may become an obstacle that prevents the child from overcoming this problem. Instruct families not to punish the child; the disorder is neither the fault of the child nor under his or her voluntary control. Eliminate arguing and disparaging remarks when the child has an accident. Accidents should be handled in a matter-of-fact manner, with the child taking responsibility to change his or her clothes after wetting. Motivating strategies, such as a sticker chart for bathroom visits, can help motivate and empower the reluctant child. With significant family stress, we recommend a period of days to weeks of "cooling off" before interventions begin, when no discussion of accidents is allowed. Referral to family therapy is indicated at times.

Children with functional incontinence may benefit from urge containment exercises to increase the functional capacity of the bladder and to avoid detrusor contractions at low urine volume. During urination, the child stops and starts the urinary stream by contracting the muscles of the pelvic floor. Measurement of the volume of urine voided at the beginning of therapy and at intervals of the treatment course may document improvement. An estimate of bladder capacity up to 12 years is [30 + (age in years × 30)] in milliliters. After 12 years, capacity is stable at about 390 mL. The estimated volume is not an absolute therapy target; it may be unachievable by many symptomatic children.

Medication

Oxybutynin (Ditropan and Ditropan XL) is an antispasmodic, anticholinergic medication approved by the Food and Drug Administration (FDA) for treatment of overactive bladder. The short-acting preparation is approved for children older than 5 years; initial dosing is 2.5 mg twice daily, titratable to 5 mg three times a day. The long-acting preparation is dosed at 5 mg once a day, titrated to 20 mg once a day. Tolterodine (Detrol and Detrol LA) is not FDA approved for children but is often used in children intolerant to oxybutynin.

Anticholinergic agents can be used at the beginning of therapy with behavioral approaches in children whose symptoms are severe or socially debilitating and can be added in those with urge symptoms failing to respond to several weeks of behavioral interventions. The effect of medication should be evident within a few days, and dosage can be titrated while observing closely for anticholinergic side effects.

In our practice, we continue anticholinergic medications and behavioral therapy for up to 6 months and then slowly taper medication during a few weeks while maintaining behavioral interventions. If symptoms recur, we repeat a course of therapy, after which we refer persistently symptomatic children for a urologic evaluation.

Intensive Evaluation and Treatment

Children with neurologic signs concerning for spinal cord abnormalities should be evaluated with magnetic resonance imaging of the lumbosacral spine to assess for tethering or other abnormalities. Lack of improvement after a few months of behavioral or medical therapy should prompt further investigation of underlying emotional needs and difficulties with compliance. In our clinic, we also refer these children to a pediatric urologist for investigation of unrecognized organic disease.

ENURESIS (NOCTURNAL INCONTINENCE)

Enuresis is defined as urinary incontinence during sleep in children older than 5 years of chronologic or mental age. In the absence of clear medical or psychological causes, children with enuresis are grouped into two categories with distinct clinical, etiologic, and therapeutic features. *Monosymptomatic enuresis* is night wetting without other urinary tract symptoms. *Non-monosymptomatic enuresis* includes night wetting coexisting with urinary tract symptoms, such as urgency, hesitancy, frequency, or daytime incontinence. Most children with enuresis have never been dry at night (primary); 20% to 30% present with symptoms after a period of at least 6 months of dry nights (secondary).

Epidemiology and Natural History

Enuresis occurs at similar rates across cultures, causing similar parental concern (Hjalmas et al, 2004). It occurs in about 15% to 20% of 5-year-olds, with a 15% annual spontaneous remission rate; 0.5% to 3% remain enuretic as adolescents and adults. Boys are more commonly affected than are girls.

Genetics

Enuresis is heritable, usually autosomal dominant (although approximately 30% of cases are sporadic). If one parent is affected, the risk that a child is affected approximates 44%; if both parents are affected, that risk nears 77%. Four chromosomes are linked to the trait, but no candidate genes have been identified (von Gontard et al, 2001).

Pathophysiology

Nighttime continence typically develops as several systems mature. With age, urine production during sleep decreases, mediated by antidiuretic hormone. In addition, growing children have increased bladder capacity as well as greater *functional* bladder capacity due to neurologic development. Such adaptations and maturations may be absent in children with enuresis.

Monosymptomatic enuresis results from the complex interaction of three physiologic processes: nocturia (excessive nighttime urine production); reduced nocturnal functional bladder capacity, provoking detrusor contraction at lower than expected volumes; and difficulties with arousal, preventing the child from appropriately responding to the stimulus to urinate. The extent of the contribution of any of these factors may be difficult to elucidate in an individual child. Treatment strategies affect some or all of these components. There is increasing interest in the contribution of nocturnal calciuria to enuresis, and thus it is a potential target for therapy (Aceto et al, 2003).

Medical disorders, such as nocturnal epilepsy and obstructive sleep apnea, can present with bed-wetting. Many neurologic disorders cause both diurnal and nocturnal incontinence as described before. Similarly, constipation can cause bed-wetting because of decreased bladder capacity and increased irritability. There are anecdotal reports of secondary enuresis associated with pinworms and with the use of psychoactive medications, such as selective serotonin reuptake inhibitors, valproate, and risperidone.

Enuresis can be due to psychological trauma, such as child abuse, witness to violence, or other extraordinary stress (Fritz et al, 2004). Conversely, children with enuresis express distress about their symptoms, and treatment of enuresis can improve behavioral symptoms. ADHD symptoms, such as inattention and hyperactivity, are more common in children with enuresis (Baeyens et al, 2004), and enuresis may be more difficult to treat in children with ADHD. In the majority of affected children, enuresis resolves with age, suggesting developmental and maturational factors in its pathogenesis.

Evaluation and Management

Both nocturnal enuresis and daytime incontinence require a detailed history and physical examination. When symptoms are limited to nighttime, additional questions about snoring, abnormal breathing patterns while asleep, and abnormal nighttime events (seizures or parasomnias) may clarify concerns. Psychological triggers should be reviewed. All children with bed-wetting need a urinalysis to assess for concentrating defects, pyuria, or glucosuria. More intensive evaluation is dictated by findings on history and physical examination (see Fig. 62-1).

Treatment Guidelines

Medical disorders such as sleep apnea and epilepsy require appropriate referral. Constipation management often ameliorates symptoms. Children with a history of trauma should be referred for mental health evaluation and treatment. In general, treat daytime bladder symptoms before addressing nighttime symptoms.

Treatment of Monosymptomatic Nocturnal Enuresis

Children who are 7 years old developmentally and interested in ending bed-wetting are candidates for intervention (Fig. 62-3). Initial treatment involves demystification—careful explanation of the problem

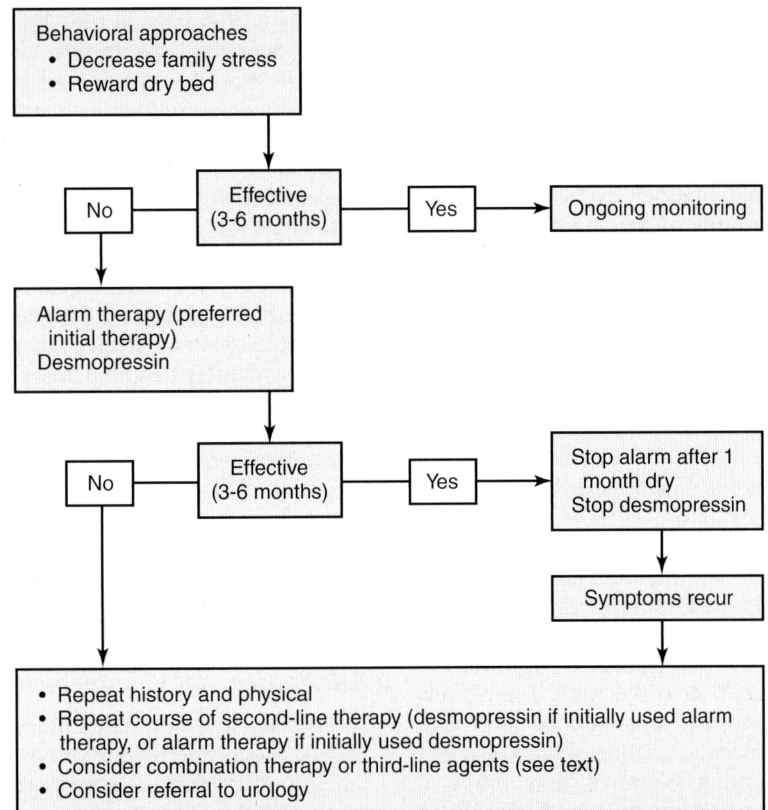

Figure 62-3. Initial assessment suggestive of monosymptomatic nocturnal enuresis (see text for details).

and its excellent prognosis. Clarify that enuresis is not volitional, the child does not have full control over the symptoms; punishment or reprimands have no role in the management of the disorder.

Simple behavioral strategies are safe and effective in some children with enuresis (Glazener and Evans, 2004). In our practice, we encourage children to use visual imagery at bedtime, to picture a full bladder and how they will wake up and go to the bathroom in response. They imagine waking up to a dry bed. Common initial interventions with anecdotal support include limiting excessive fluids (particularly those with caffeine, calcium, and sodium) in the evening hours and waking the child to urinate as the parents go to bed. However, if fluid restriction is difficult or stressful, it should be abandoned as there is little supportive evidence of efficacy.

The child should be responsible for helping with wet linens as a way to be "in charge of your body" rather than as punishment. Plastic mattress liners under the sheets can ease morning clean up for everyone. The child can place wet bedclothes in the washing machine. Sticker charts can be motivating; the child is offered a sticker or a star for completing the imagery, for helping with wet linens, and later for each dry night. Helping the child and family manage the incontinence so that the child's self-worth and family relationships are maintained is vital. Emphasis is on success and competence.

Some families, particularly those with younger children, are reassured by demystification and the optimistic prognosis, thus desiring no further interventions. Follow-up visits for ongoing support are helpful. For older children or those whose symptoms cause family or social distress, further therapy is indicated.

If no decrease in wet nights follows a few weeks of simple strategies, consider additional interventions that promote arousal in the setting of a full bladder, increased functional bladder capacity, or reduced volume of urine produced at night.

Enuresis Alarms

Numerous studies, including randomized controlled trials, support the use of alarm therapy in nocturnal enuresis and indicate overall efficacy approximating 68% (Glazener et al, 2005b). A typical alarm has a moisture sensor (activated when it is exposed to a small amount of urine) attached to the child's pajamas or underwear. A speaker, connected to the moisture sensor, attaches to the pajama top in the shoulder area. As the child urinates during sleep, the alarm sounds or vibrates. Many children initially sleep through the alarm, requiring parents to wake the child and walk the child to the bathroom to complete voiding. In the first week, the size of the puddle shrinks, and then during the following weeks, the child begins to wake at the sound of the alarm as the urine accident shrinks to a small spot. Within a few months of consistent alarm use, the child begins waking spontaneously to urinate when the bladder is full or may sleep through the night without urinating. We suggest a sticker reward the first week for waking to the alarm with help, the second week for waking without help, and the third week for dry nights. The alarm should be used until the child completes one full month of uninterrupted dryness.

Bed-wetting alarms require significant commitment of time and effort by families and may take several months to be effective. Frequent office visits are recommended at the start of therapy to provide ongoing encouragement.

Alarm therapy seems to increase arousal in the setting of a full bladder, although some studies demonstrate increased functional bladder capacity, allowing the storage of a larger volume of urine before detrusor contraction (Hvistendahl et al, 2004). Alarm therapy continues for 3 to 6 months. If no improvement occurs within 2 months, pharmacotherapy or combination therapy should be considered. Relapse occurs in about 50% of children when alarms are stopped but often responds to a repeated treatment course.

Desmopressin

This analogue of antidiuretic hormone is approved by the FDA for children older than 6 years with nocturnal enuresis. Administration of desmopressin before bedtime reduces urine production at night, counteracting the nocturia in some enuretic children. Desmopressin can be used daily or as needed for camp or sleepovers. Desmopressin is available as a nasal spray (dose range, 10 to 40 μg) or an oral tablet (dose range, 0.2 to 0.6 mg). A relatively safe medication, desmopressin's most serious (although rare) side effect is hyponatremic seizures. Hyponatremia can be avoided by preventing excessive fluid intake at night and by parental supervision of administration to prevent overdose. A practical approach includes allowing 8 ounces of fluid at dinner and another 8 ounces afterward, without fluid intake 2 hours before administration of the medicine at bedtime and for 8 hours thereafter.

A subset of children experience a prolonged half-life of intranasal desmopressin and may develop water intoxication from daytime fluid intake. These children may have delayed first-morning voids and symptoms of hyponatremia (headaches, nausea, altered mental status, or seizures), which should be discussed with families.

Long-term effects of desmopressin are unclear. Consistent desmopressin use for 2 years without reported adverse sequelae is documented (Kano and Arisaka, 2006). One study of 32 patients found increased urinary calcium excretion during desmopressin treatment without change in blood calcium levels. Further studies are needed to determine if desmopressin has a meaningful impact on calcium homeostasis.

Failure of Alarms or Desmopressin

Lack of response after 2 to 3 months calls for reevaluation, particularly for symptoms of constipation, mechanical dysfunction, or daytime voiding dysfunction. Combination therapy, with use of both an alarm and desmopressin simultaneously for up to 3 months, is often considered after failure of monotherapy, but supporting evidence for this practice is limited.

Anticholinergics

Anticholinergics can be helpful in cases of reduced functional bladder capacity at night or for a child with comorbid daytime voiding symptoms (i.e., urgency). A nighttime dose of the short-acting preparation may be given with the option of changing to the long-acting preparation if enuresis occurs later in the night. Long-term administration is relatively safe, but monitoring for postvoid urine residuals should be considered. Furthermore, constipation induced by anticholinergic agents can worsen enuresis.

Imipramine

Imipramine in this scenario is dosed considerably lower than when it is used for depression. The mechanism of action appears related to anticholinergic and central nervous system effects. It is used for children older than 6 years at an initial dose of 10 to 25 mg at bedtime. If the response is inadequate after 1 week of therapy, the dose is increased by 25 mg per day to a final dose that should not exceed 2.5 mg/kg per day or 50 mg at bedtime for 6- to 12-year-olds, 75 mg for children older than 12 years. In recalcitrant cases, imipramine has been used in conjunction with desmopressin. Given the potential for cardiac toxicity, screening and follow-up electrocardiography and plasma drug level determinations are recommended. In our practice, we generally do not use imipramine; anticholinergics, desmopressin, and behavioral interventions are largely successful with safer side effect profiles.

Alternative and Complementary Therapy

Alternative and complementary therapy is described in a 2005 Cochrane review of complementary and miscellaneous interventions for nocturnal enuresis (Glazener et al, 2005a). This meta-analysis finds weak evidence in support of the use of hypnosis, psychotherapy, acupuncture, and chiropractics. Trials were characterized by small size and weak methodology.

Approach to Nonresponders

Children who do not respond to enuresis therapies may benefit from taking a treatment break for a few months, with reassurance of the 15% yearly rate of spontaneous resolution. If difficulties persist, urologic referral is indicated to assess the anatomy and function of the lower urinary tract.

SUMMARY

Daytime incontinence and nocturnal enuresis are common pediatric disorders. The majority of cases can be managed successfully by pediatricians after a thorough history, physical examination, and urinalysis exclude significant disease. First-line interventions involve behavioral therapies, starting with the formation of a caring therapeutic alliance with the child and family. Several pharmacologic agents can be used as adjuncts to behavioral strategies (including enuresis alarms), and specialist referrals are reserved for patients with concerning presentations and failure to respond to studied interventions.

REFERENCES

Aceto G, Penza R, Coccioli MS, et al: Enuresis subtypes based on nocturnal hypercalciuria: A multicenter study. J Urol 170: 1670-1673, 2003.

Baeyens D, Roeyers H, Hoebeke P, et al: Attention deficit/hyperactivity disorder in children with nocturnal enuresis. J Urol 171: 2576-2579, 2004.

Casale A: Daytime wetting: Getting to the bottom of the issue. Contemp Pediatr 17:107, 2000.

Chapple CR, MacDiarmid SA: Urodynamics Made Easy, 2nd ed, London, Harcourt, 2000.

Fritz G, Rockney R, Bernet W, et al: Practice parameter for the assessment and treatment of children and adolescents with enuresis. J Am Acad Child Adolesc Psychiatry 43:1540-1550, 2004.

Glazener CM, Evans JH: Simple behavioural and physical interventions for nocturnal enuresis in children. Cochrane Database Syst Rev 2:CD003637, 2004.

Glazener CM, Evans JH, Cheuk DK: Complementary and miscellaneous interventions for nocturnal enuresis in children. Cochrane Database Syst Rev 2:CD005230, 2005a.

Glazener CM, Evans JH, Peto RE: Alarm interventions for nocturnal enuresis in children. Cochrane Database Syst Rev 2:CD002911, 2005b.

Hellerstein S, Zguta AA: Outcome of overactive bladder in children. Clin Pediatr (Phila) 42:553-556, 2003.

Hjalmas K, Arnold T, Bower W, et al: Nocturnal enuresis: An international evidence based management strategy. J Urol 171: 2545-2561, 2004.

Hvistendahl GM, Kamperis K, Rawashdeh YF, et al: The effect of alarm treatment on the functional bladder capacity in children with monosymptomatic nocturnal enuresis. J Urol 171:2611-2614, 2004.

Jalkut MW, Lerman SE, Churchill BM: Enuresis. Pediatr Clin North Am 48:1461-1488, 2001.

Jansson UB, Hanson M, Sillen U, et al: Voiding pattern and acquisition of bladder control from birth to age 6 years—a longitudinal study. J Urol 174:289-293, 2005.

Kano K, Arisaka O: Efficacy and safety of nasal desmopressin in the long-term treatment of primary nocturnal enuresis. Pediatr Nephrol 21:1211; author reply 1212, 2006.

Robson WL: Diurnal enuresis. Pediatr Rev 18:407-412; quiz 412, 1997.

Saedi NA, Schulman SL: Natural history of voiding dysfunction. Pediatr Nephrol 18:894-897, 2003.

Van Leerdam FJ, Blankespoor MN, Van Der Heijden AJ, et al: Alarm treatment is successful in children with day- and night-time wetting. Scand J Urol Nephrol 38:211-215, 2004.

von Gontard A, Schaumburg H, Hollmann E, et al: The genetics of enuresis: A review. J Urol 166:2438-2443, 2001.

Wiener JS, Scales MT, Hampton J, et al: Long-term efficacy of simple behavioral therapy for daytime wetting in children. J Urol 164:786-790, 2000.

63 BOWEL FUNCTION, TOILETING, AND ENCOPRESIS

LAURA WEISSMAN AND CAROLYN BRIDGEMOHAN

Encopresis and toileting failure are common problems in children. The incidence varies with age, affecting approximately 2.8% of 4-year-olds, 1.5% of 7- to 8-year-olds, and 1.6% of 10- to 11-year-olds (Loening-Baucke, 2001). Preschoolers typically present with constipation and toileting refusal; school-age children may also have encopresis. Although these problems often cause a great deal of stress to children and families, most cases are not the result of an organic illness (with the exception of constipation) and are curable with appropriate and diligent treatment. However, many children with encopresis are also vulnerable to developmental, behavioral, and emotional problems (Joinson et al, 2006), and their functioning should be monitored over time.

BOWEL PATHOPHYSIOLOGY AND EMERGENCE OF ENCOPRESIS

To better understand abnormal bowel function, let us first review normal bowel function (Fig. 63-1). Stool moves from the small to large intestines. The role of the large intestines is to remove water from the stool and to hold stool until the time of evacuation. As the stool enters the rectum, most of the water is removed, resulting in a semisolid bolus. The stool is held in the rectum by the internal anal sphincter, which is innervated by ganglion cells and is under involuntary control, and the external anal sphincter, which is under voluntary control by the pudendal nerve (S2-4). When the rectosigmoid colon becomes distended, it stimulates the rectorectal reflex. The portion of bowel above the bolus of stool contracts and the portion below the bolus relaxes. This is followed by a reflex relaxation of the internal anal sphincter that results in the urge to defecate. The child then voluntarily releases the external anal sphincter, and with increased abdominal pressure created by the Valsalva maneuver, the child defecates. A child can withhold stool by voluntarily contracting the external anal sphincter and puborectalis (part of the levator ani and innervated by a branch of the fourth sacral nerve). This voluntary contraction then decreases the rectorectal reflex (returning the rectorectal inhibitory reflex), and the internal anal sphincter contracts and the subsequent urge to defecate passes (Yamada et al, 2003). A child who is toilet trained or in the process of toilet training has the ability to keep the external sphincter closed until he or she has the opportunity to release. However, if a child develops constipation because of either diet changes or stool withholding, stool remains in the rectum. As stool remains in the colon, more water is absorbed, and it becomes harder and subsequently more difficult to pass. This results in pain with defecation, and more withholding ensues. The rectum dilates as more stool collects. The muscles and nerve fibers stretch and do not function appropriately. This means that it is difficult both to control the external anal sphincter and to sense the urge to defecate as the reflex arc becomes less sensitive. When the child squeezes the external anal sphincter to retain stool, some stool may be ejected into the underwear, resulting in staining. Children may also have leakage of wet stool that makes its way past the harder bolus of stool, or they may have complete stool accidents resulting from inability to appropriately control defecation (Fig. 63-2).

TOILET TRAINING

In the United States, toilet training typically occurs from 2.5 to 3 years of age, although in other countries it is earlier. In the early 20th century, a strictly scheduled, parent-centered approach was used for toilet training. Typically, training was initiated before 18 months. In the 1940s, some pediatricians began advocating a less rigid approach that emphasized developmental readiness (Brazelton, 1962). Although many different approaches to toilet training exist, the current model endorsed by most experts as well as by the American Academy of Pediatrics is a child-centered process emphasizing developmental readiness as a precursor to toilet training. As part of this approach, three factors must be in place: the developmental and physiologic skills needed for toileting, the ability to understand instruction, and the motivation to perform the task. Children typically reach the developmental milestones needed for toilet training between 18 and 30 months of age (Brazelton et al, 1999). The development of nighttime bowel continence is usually followed by daytime bowel continence, then daytime urine continence, and last, nighttime urine continence. The readiness skills that a child needs to toilet train include motor, language, and social skills. A child must have the motor skills needed for ambulating, sitting, and assisting with removal of clothing. These skills are usually attained by the age of 18 months. To maintain continence, a child must have voluntary control of the bowels and bladder (usually emerging at 9 months, although it

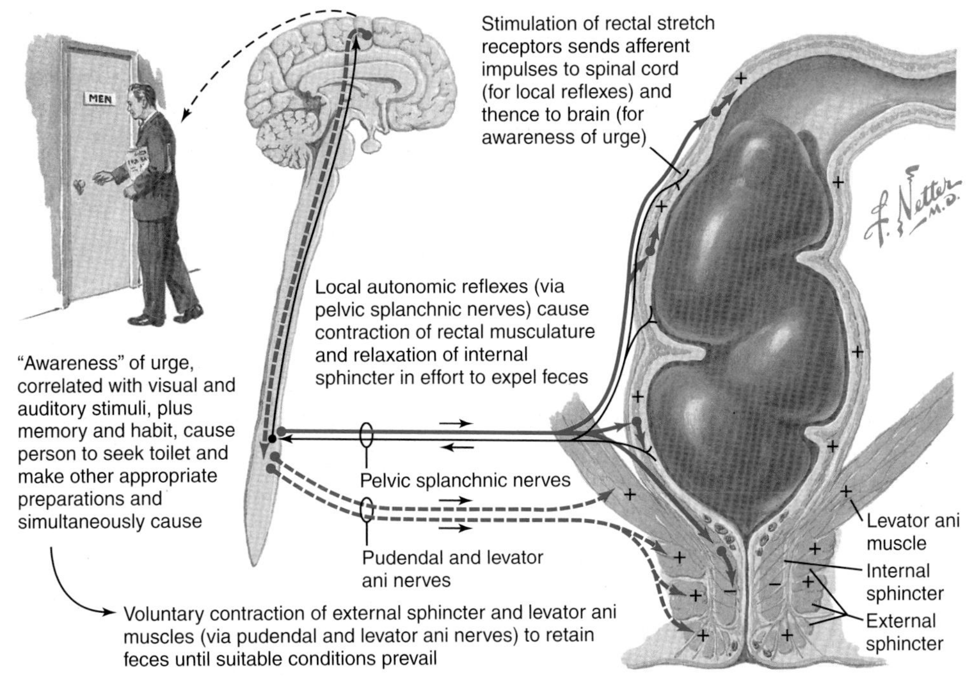

Figure 63-1. Normal bowel function. *(Netter diagram from http://www.netterimages.com/image/6739.htm.)*

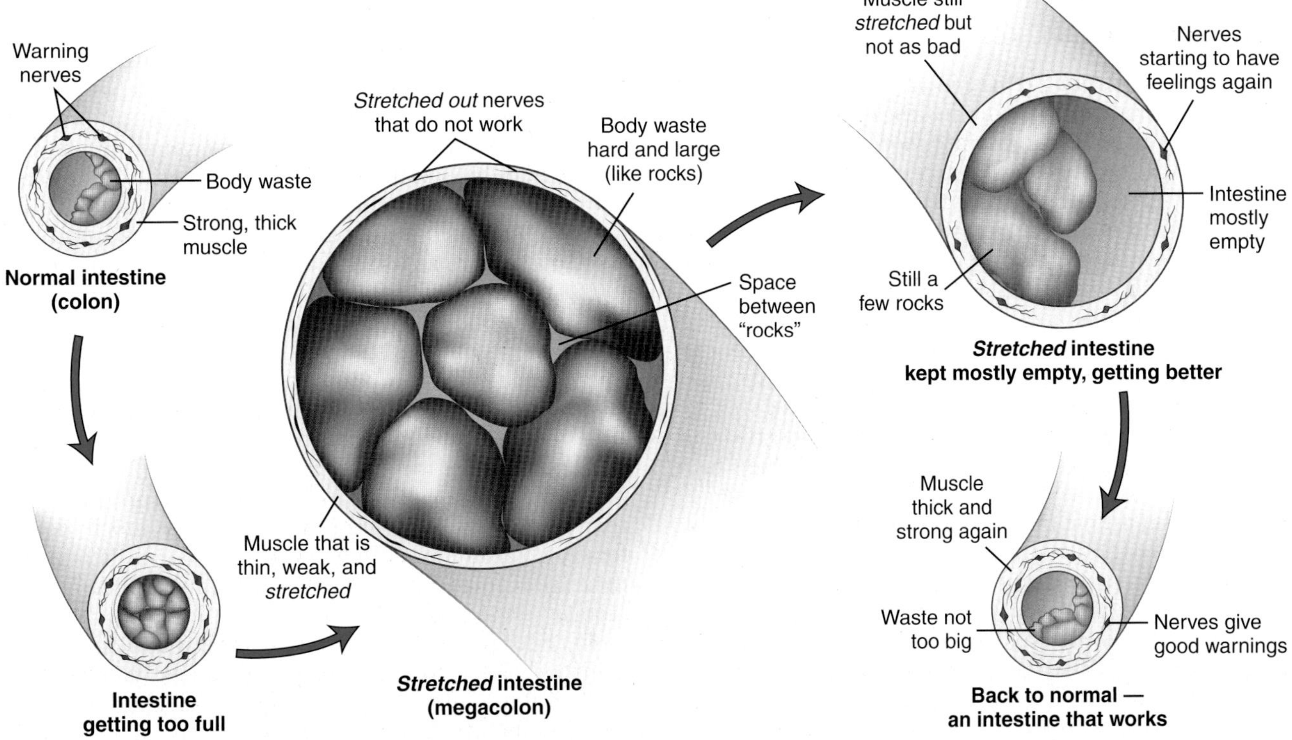

Figure 63-2. Encopresis: patient training diagram.

must be combined with other described skills for full continence to be achieved) and then be aware when he or she needs to defecate (usually attained at 18 months). The child must have a way of indicating to caregivers that she or he needs to use the toilet. Cognitively, the child must understand that certain things go in certain places. Socially, the child needs to recognize the behavior of others and possess the motivation to attain continence.

Once a child has achieved the readiness skills, a step-by-step approach can be used to introduce, model, and facilitate appropriate toileting behavior. A regular discussion in a story format can introduce and normalize toileting behavior for the child. At the same time, the toilet or potty seat can be introduced. This should be a comfortable place to sit, and the child should have a place to rest his or her feet. In the case of a potty chair, this would be the floor; and with a toilet seat, this should be a stool or other support. The child should have time to sit on the potty or toilet either with or without a diaper or pull-up on and with no specific expectation for voiding. As the child becomes comfortable, regular sitting times can be created. During this time, there can be books or quiet activities to facilitate and to reinforce sitting. The optimal time for these sittings is approximately 20 to 30 minutes after meals as the gastrocolic reflex increases the urge to defecate. When the child has success on the toilet or potty, she or he should be rewarded with verbal praise or a small token. Over time, a child will learn to request toilet time outside of scheduled sittings. This behavior should also be rewarded. When the child is starting to use the toilet on a regular basis, the diaper or pull-up can be removed and the child can move to underwear.

Children learn how to toilet train at different rates. Some children learn quickly in a few days, and others may take a few months. If at any point in time a child is resistant to toileting or demonstrates negative behaviors around toileting, active training should be discontinued temporarily. Research shows that constipation (Blum et al, 2004; Schonwald et al, 2004) and difficult temperament traits are associated with challenges in toilet training (Schonwald et al, 2004).

TOILETING REFUSAL

In some ways, toileting refusal is a unique form of encopresis, so it presents its own challenges to treatment. In young children who are resistant to toileting, toilet training should be discontinued for a period of months and the child returned to diapers. Younger children who have toileting refusal should also be assessed for constipation and treated appropriately (Blum et al, 2004) before continuing with training. For children with toileting refusal who are developing typically and are older than 3 years, management is similar to that for children with encopresis but requires some modification. These children often have acquired the basic skills needed for toilet training, but for some other reason, whether it is related to constipation, withholding, temperament, or other conflict, they have been unsuccessful. As with young children, they should be assessed for constipation and treated appropriately (see the section on encopresis for treatment). Also evaluate medically for any contributing organic causes (refer to the encopresis portion of this chapter for details). The next step to management involves a behaviorally based program to desensitize a child's toileting aversion by decreasing anxiety around toileting. Start with whatever portion of toileting a child is willing to perform. For example, some children will be stooling in a pull-on diaper or underpants at this time. The first goal might be to have them stool in the diaper or underpants in the bathroom or on a specific mat or while sitting on the toilet. The care provider can use a reward system to encourage completion of the goal. Once the goal is obtained, a new goal is developed by use of a stepwise approach. For example, a child may next sit on the toilet wearing a diaper in which a small hole has been cut. The size of the hole can be enlarged over time until the child is no longer wearing a diaper. The specifics of the plan and the approach depend on where the child starts as well as the temperament of the child. Group toileting programs for children who are late to toilet can be extremely helpful. The peer interaction around the topic can help decrease anxiety for both parents and children.

TOILET TRAINING IN SPECIAL POPULATIONS

Some children have developmental conditions that make toilet training more challenging. For example, children with chronic illness, children in daycare, children with developmental disabilities, and those with neurologic impairment may take longer or need special guidance to master toileting. First, it is important to start out with the same general principles described before. If a child has acquired some but not all of the readiness skills described, the strategy to toilet training may be more flexible. For example, a child with developmental delay may have difficulty making the connection between the urge to defecate and the social need to hold. In this case, frequent sitting at 1- to 2-hour intervals may be appropriate. Verbal praise for success should continue. Some children will toilet train this way; others may not be able to use the toilet of their own initiation consistently but will stay dry and soil free between sits, thus enabling them to wear underwear. Some children may have difficulty understanding the concepts of being wet and dry, and these may also need to be taught.

Toilet training can be particularly challenging in children with autism spectrum disorders because of decreased social and communication skills as well as behavioral rigidity. Children with autism spectrum disorders may be overly sensitive to the sensation of defecating, and they may not know to communicate the urge to void. Children with autism spectrum disorders are also more prone to anxiety around toileting. It is useful in this case to work with the school or an autism consultant or behavioral specialist to design a structured plan for toilet training. These children require a behavioral approach in which training is broken into incremental steps. If the child uses a picture exchange communication system or other communication system, this should be appropriately incorporated into training. This might include the development of a story or picture sequence that demonstrates toileting instruction. If the child suffers from firm stools that might increase resistance to defecation, medications can be used for softening the stools.

In children who have a physical disability, such as a spina bifida or cerebral palsy, neurologic factors may make it more difficult or impossible for a child to maintain continence. Although social motivation is likely to be less of a problem, neurologic difficulties present unique challenges, and these children are often at risk for constipation. Stool softening agents should be used when needed to make stools soft enough to pass with minimal effort (see Table 63-3 for specific medications). It is also important to consult the child's specialty providers to determine whether being accident free is an achievable goal. If a child is unable to maintain voluntary continence, timed sittings can help to keep a child dry in between sittings and possibly allow the child to wear underwear, which may be important socially for the child. Catheterization may also be an appropriate option and, in some cases, medically necessary. Try to find out the importance of remaining accident free for the child as this will affect success. If a child does not care about accidents, the child is less likely to be compliant with timed sittings. There are also other medical therapies that may be helpful, such as medications to reduce bladder spasms or to induce longer periods of dryness and surgeries to allow independence with toileting.

ENCOPRESIS, CONSTIPATION, AND TOILET TRAINING FAILURE

Overview

Constipation is defined by the North American Society for Pediatric Gastroenterology and Nutrition as delayed or difficult defecation for more than 2 weeks. Functional constipation is that which is not due to an organic or physical condition or medication.

The *Diagnostic and Statistical Manual of Mental Disorders* defines encopresis as "the repeated passage of feces into inappropriate places (e.g., clothing or floor). Most often this is involuntary but occasionally may be intentional. The event must occur at least once a month for at least 3 months, and the chronological age of the child must be at least 4 years (or for children with developmental delays, a mental age of at least 4 years). The fecal incontinence must not be due exclusively to the direct physiological effects of a substance (e.g., laxatives) or a general medical condition except through a mechanism involving constipation." Most commonly, encopresis is associated with functional constipation; and in rare cases, encopresis is seen without constipation.

Etiology

Encopresis is a complex disorder likely resulting from physical vulnerability in the context of potentiating environmental and behavioral factors. The primary cause is a physical predisposition to constipation, reduced bowel regularity, and ineffective evacuation. In some cases, there may be a history of painful bowel movement with subsequent withholding. Children with attentional deficits, obsessions and compulsions, and oppositional behavior are more prone to encopresis (Joinson et al, 2006). Children with attention deficits may be less attuned to body signals around toileting and may have trouble establishing a regular toilet routine. In addition, individuals with challenging or difficult temperament traits may be more prone to encopresis and toileting delays (Schonwald et al, 2004). Certainly, environmental factors such as lack of access to the toilet, disorganized home setting, and exposure to trauma or violence can contribute to the development of encopresis. However, a majority of children with encopresis do not have a history of emotional disturbance.

Diagnosis

Diagnosis of encopresis and constipation starts with a thorough history and physical examination. In most cases, this is sufficient to identify any organic disease.

History

Some patients do not present with encopresis until school age, but many have had a history of stool withholding or initial toileting refusal. Some children may have had a history of mild soiling, such as smearing, and are not identified as having encopresis until the condition progresses to more frequent or larger accidents or their soiling affects their functioning with peers or in other settings.

In some children with constipation or encopresis, parents can target a specific illness or other situation that may have immediately preceded withholding behavior. Ask about frequency of symptoms, whether there are entire bowel movement accidents or just staining, consistency of bowel movements (hard, soft), size, and ease of passage. A child with constipation and encopresis may stool daily but pass only small, hard stools. Ask about times that stool accidents occur. Most children soil between 3 and 7 PM or specifically after or on the way home from school. Soiling at school is usually a marker of a more severe problem. Very rarely do children soil during sleep. Children with significant withholding may soil just as they fall asleep when they finally relax. However, nocturnal soiling can also be a sign of seizures.

Questions about urine accidents are also important. Children with constipation may have urine accidents caused by bladder spasms resulting from pressure to the bladder. Girls with encopresis are also at risk for urinary tract infections from contamination or poor hygiene. In taking the history, ask about any previous interventions tried. Take a diet history and include intolerances or allergies to any foods. Past medical history should review any concerns about growth. Short stature may be a clue to thyroid disease as a cause of constipation. A history of weight loss soon after introduction of solids may be a clue for celiac disease. The neurologic history should include questions about clumsiness or newly acquired lower extremity problems, which might be present in the case of a tethered cord. The gastrointestinal history should also include any history of explosive stools after retention or thin-caliber stools, which may indicate Hirschsprung disease. The family history should include questions about constipation, encopresis, colitis, irritable bowel syndrome, thyroid disease, or similar concerns. Social history should include screening for history of trauma or ongoing trauma. Sexual or physical abuse is too important to miss. It is often difficult to ask about these sensitive questions, but they need to be part of the history. The abuse may be from someone other than the parents, so ask about concerns for the child with any other caregivers.

Physical Examination

Providers should complete a full physical examination with focus on assessment of the abdomen and genitourinary and neurologic systems. The first part of the examination should include a look at the overall appearance, including physical habitus and growth parameters, possible dysmorphism, and behavior and social interaction. Abdominal examination may reveal fullness, distention, or a nontender sausage-shaped mass in the lower left quadrant. The absence of this finding does not rule out constipation and may be difficult to appreciate in a child who is overweight or cannot tolerate an abdominal examination. The neurologic examination needs to be thorough and should include assessment of gait as well as lower extremity reflexes and strength. Increased reflexes or decreased tone could signal a spinal cord abnormality.

Inspect the position of the anus and also look for evidence of soiling. Be alert for any signs of trauma, such as scarring, tears, or reduced rectal tone. Also see Chapter 10 for further guidance on the evaluation of suspected trauma or abuse. In girls, the distance between the posterior fourchette and the anus should be at least one-third the distance between the posterior fourchette and coccyx; in boys, the distance between the scrotum and anus should be half the scrotococcygeal distance (Reisner et al, 1984). A rectal examination should be performed (Baker et al, 1999). This is sometimes difficult during the first visit, but a rectal examination needs to be performed during the course of treatment. Increased rectal tone with a history of small-caliber stools and delayed passage of meconium may be a sign of Hirschsprung disease. Decreased rectal tone might be a sign of neurologic concern, such as spinal cord tethering or anomaly, although decreased tone can also be seen with prolonged constipation. Digital rectal examination should also include assessment of the rectal content. A large amount of stool in the rectum has a high positive predictive value for the presence of fecal retention, although absence of stool in the rectum does not rule out fecal retention (Rockney et al, 1995). Intact neurologic sensation of the anus can be tested by eliciting the anal wink reflex, which involves lightly touching the anus with a cotton swab; this should result in closing of the sphincter. A cremasteric reflex in boys is another way to test lower sacral function; gently stroke the inner thigh and observe for testicular retraction. See Table 63-1 for a listing of organic causes of stool withholding and leakage as well as red flags.

Laboratory Evaluation and Imaging

In most cases, children presenting with constipation and encopresis do not require routine laboratory evaluation or imaging. However, if there is clinical suspicion of an organic cause, further investigation is warranted. Laboratory testing might include thyroid function studies and determination of calcium, magnesium, and electrolyte values, depending on history and examination findings. If the history is unclear and physical examination does not confirm constipation, abdominal radiography may be helpful to determine the amount of retained stool (Fig. 63-3). A baseline radiograph can also be useful to have as a reference after a clean out is performed. For children who present with urinary incontinence as well as constipation, urinalysis and urine culture may be useful. Constipation can result in pressure on the bladder and may also lead to urinary tract infection. If a child has any lower extremity symptoms, lumbosacral spinal films and lumbosacral magnetic resonance imaging may be useful to rule out a tethered cord or spinal dysraphism. If there is increased rectal tone and a history of

Table 63-1. Other Causes of Fecal Incontinence

Disorder or Condition	Historical and Physical Findings
Malformations	
Anal stenosis Partial imperforate anus	Abnormality on inspection and examination of the anus
Neurogenic	
Occult spinal dysraphism Tethered cord	Increased lower extremity tone
Tumor	Recent onset of symptoms with neurologic signs, back pain, trouble walking up stairs, new-onset incontinence
Endocrine-metabolic	
Multiple endocrine neoplasia III	Variable presentation including constipation
Thyroid disorder	Constipation, weight gain, decreased energy, cold intolerance
Electrolyte imbalance	Variable presentation, depending on electrolyte affected
Neuromuscular	
Muscular dystrophy	Presents in boys aged 3-5 years; lower extremity proximal muscle weakness
Hirschsprung disease	History of constipation from birth followed by explosive stools; delayed passage of meconium, thin-caliber stools
Medications	Variable presentation, depending on medication
Sexual abuse	Physical signs of trauma or history of abuse; see Chapter 10
Diarrheal disease	In the case of celiac disease, may present as constipation or diarrhea with growth concerns

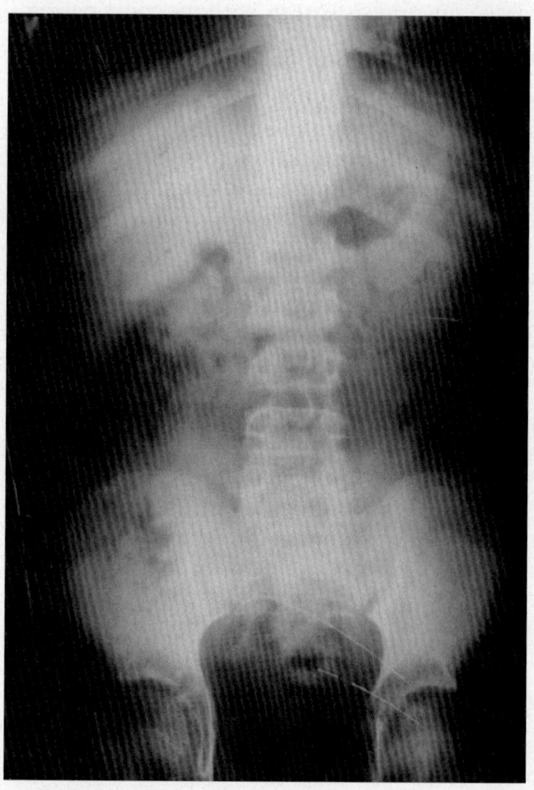

Figure 63-3. Plain abdominal radiograph.

inconsistent explosive stools, anal manometry may be useful to rule out Hirschsprung disease.

Treatment

Once the diagnosis of encopresis is confirmed by thorough history and physical examination, a multimodal treatment program ensues (Fig. 63-4). This requires both medical management of the underlying constipation, if present, and behavioral intervention to encourage the child to use the toilet regularly. In fact, resolution of encopresis is most dependent on diligent adherence to a regular sitting regimen (Brooks et al, 2000).

Education

Encopresis can be emotionally overwhelming for a child and family. Many families do not understand the underlying pathophysiologic mechanism of this disorder. As a result, by the time most families seek medical attention, the child may have been punished or continually reprimanded for accidents. The first step in treatment therefore is education to explain the cause and process of encopresis. Explain the cycle of stool retention illustrated in Figure 63-2 and discuss how physical factors, predisposition to constipation, and in some cases emotional or temperamental traits contribute to encopresis. Let them know that there are many other children with the same problem and that there are many things you and they can do to make things better. Emphasize to the family that this is not the child's fault and explain the relapsing and remitting course of this disorder both before and after treatment. Although this portion of treatment may seem intuitive, it is integral to helping a family remain with the treatment program. The family and child may be quite frustrated by this time and have tried other therapies. The use of pictures and handouts can be helpful to moving a family toward understanding.

Clean Out

In children with constipation, intervention includes the clean out of retained stool and a regimen to maintain regular passage of stool so as not to exacerbate the underlying problem. In most cases, this clean out can be performed at home. There are many different ways to perform a bowel clean out. The plan you choose depends on the severity of the constipation as well as on the comfort level of the child and family. Discuss the options with the child and family and consider factors specific to the child, such as maturity, motivation, and emotional functioning. For severe constipation, a more aggressive clean out with enemas alone or in conjunction with oral cathartics may be useful (see Table 63-2 for regimen). We do not recommend use of enemas in children younger than 5 years or in children with a history of abuse or trauma, however.

Another option is to use a stronger medication more commonly employed in the inpatient settings, such as magnesium citrate or polyethylene glycol with electrolytes taken by mouth or nasogastric tube. For less severe constipation, a child may benefit from a daily medication to soften the stool, such as an osmotic laxative or lubricant in conjunction with a mild to moderate bowel stimulant to encourage stool passage until there is clean out. This less intensive approach is milder and will take longer than the aggressive clean out. Possibilities include mineral oil, polyethylene glycol without electrolytes, and lactulose in conjunction with senna or bisacodyl tablet. See Table 63-3 for examples of medications as well as the potential uses.

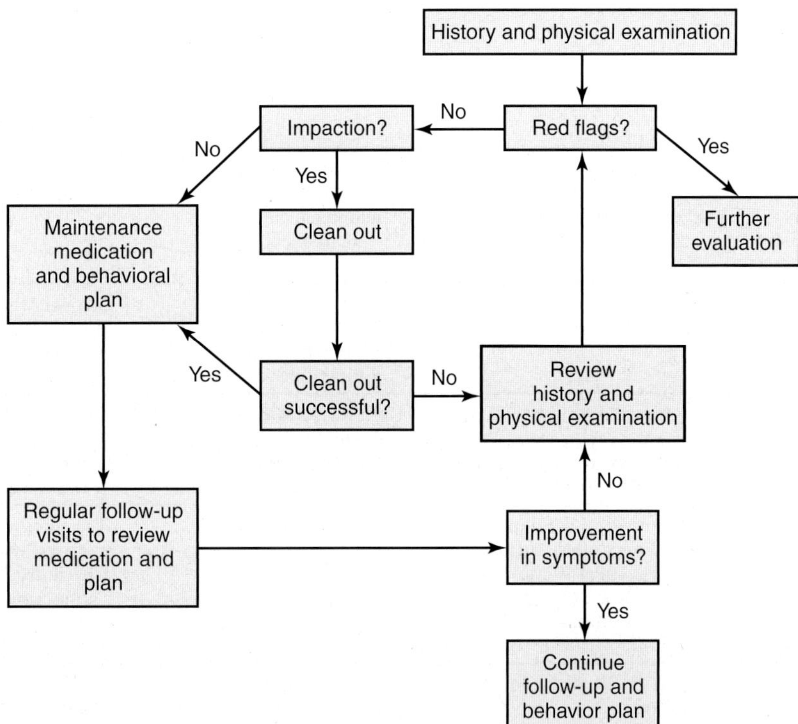

Figure 63-4. Algorithm for treatment of encopresis.

Table 63-2. Sample Clean Out with Oral Medication and Enemas

Day 1: bisacodyl pill Day 2: bisacodyl suppository Day 3: 1 adult Fleet* enema (repeat days 1-3 three times for a total of 12 days and then return to office)

*Monobasic sodium phosphate.
Based on a table from Schonwald A, Rappaport L: Consultation with the specialist. Encopresis: Assessment and management. Pediatr Rev 25:278-282, 2004.

Clean out can be brief in some children and longer in others. For severe constipation, a child may require reexamination or repeated abdominal radiography to confirm the clearance of stool. Initially, accidents may appear to increase with the introduction of a clean out regimen. For children who attend school, one option is to use an agent to soften the stool during the week and add a stimulant on the weekends in hopes of decreasing the likelihood of an accident during the school day (Table 63-4).

Table 63-3. Medications Used for the Treatment of Constipation and Encopresis

Medication	Type of Laxative	Dose	Use	Comments
Fiber supplement	Bulk-forming agent	Depends on form and brand	Use for maintenance or as daily supplement for children with low-fiber diets	Many different forms are available, including wafers, powders, tablets, and liquids
Mineral oil	Softener	5-11 yr: 1-3 teaspoons daily >12 yr: 1-3 tablespoons per day	High dose for clean out Lower dose for maintenance use Titrate to effect	May cause leakage of stool and oil Medication best disguised in cold yogurt or pudding Do not use if child is at risk for aspiration Decrease dose if leaking occurs
Docusate sodium	Softener	Given once daily or divided up to 4 times a day <3 yr: 10-40 mg/day 3-6 yr: 20-60 mg/day 6-12 yr: 40-150 mg/day	Use for maintenance therapy	
Lactulose	Osmotic	0.5-1.0 mL/kg/dose, qd or bid Maximum: 60 mL/day	Use for maintenance therapy	
Magnesium hydroxide (milk of magnesia)	Osmotic	1-2 mL/kg/dose 1-2 times daily	Use for maintenance therapy	Side effects can include cramping, diarrhea, nausea, and vomiting and also fluid and salt losses with prolonged use
Monobasic sodium phosphate enema	Osmotic, enema	1 adult enema (120 mL)	Use for clean out	A pediatric enema (65 mL) is often insufficient for treatment of encopretic children Avoid prolonged use Avoid enemas in younger children and children with a history of sexual abuse
Polyethylene glycol (PEG) without electrolytes	Osmotic	0.8 g/kg/day Typically 8.5-17 g/dose Every 17 g needs to be mixed in 8 oz of water or juice	High dose for clean out Lower dose for maintenance Titrate to effect	Taste and texture usually well tolerated
Bisacodyl	Stimulant	<12 yr: 5-10 mg PO/PR qd >12 yr: 5-15 mg PO	Use for clean out as described above Use for extra clean out during times of relapse	Stronger than senna product Avoid long-term continuous use as this may lead to dependence
Senna product	Stimulant	15-mg tablets or chocolate squares ½-2 chocolate squares per day ½-2 tablets per day	Used for extra clean out in child who does not tolerate enemas	Comes in liquid, tablet, or chocolate square Avoid prolonged continuous use as this may lead to dependence
Magnesium citrate	Osmotic	2-5 yr: 2-4 mL/kg/d qd or BID max 60-90 mL/kg 6-12 yr: 100-150 mL PO × 1 or div BID >12 yr: 150-300 mL PO × 1 or div BID	Used for clean out	Taste improved when cold and mixed with lemon-lime soda Check drug interactions before prescribing
PEG with electrolytes	Osmotic	>6 yr: 25-40 mL/kg/hr PO until clear Maximum: 4 liters for children > 12 yr	Used for clean out	NPO 3-4 hr before ingestion of solution

Table 63-4. Sample Treatment Plan for Patient Presenting with Encopresis

Family education
Clean out
- Treatment plan A (see Table 63-2)
- *or*
- Osmotic laxative with stimulant
- *or*
- Magnesium citrate
- *or*
- PEG with electrolytes

Maintenance
- Osmotic laxative (i.e., PEG without electrolytes); titrate to maintain soft daily stool and to minimize leakage (see Table 63-3 for other maintenance medications)

PEG, polyethylene glycol.

Table 63-5. Maintenance Plan for Encopresis

- Medication for maintenance therapy titrated to effect
- Behavioral plan including daily sitting with developmentally appropriate reward
- Discussion of diet changes, including increasing fiber and water content
- Encourage increasing activity
- Regular visits with provider to reinforce the plan and continually educate the family

In a majority of cases, hospitalization or inpatient treatment is never necessary. Aggressive outpatient treatment with a clear treatment plan is typically appropriate. Hospitalization itself can be traumatic and further add to the problem and therefore should be avoided if at all possible. Only severe cases, such as extreme abdominal distress, risk of obstruction, vomiting of feculent material, or extreme parental noncompliance, necessitate hospitalization.

Maintenance

Once clean out is achieved, or if a child does not require a full clean out, the next step is maintenance therapy (Table 63-5). Many of the medications used for maintenance are the same as those used for clean out, such as mineral oil or polyethylene glycol without electrolytes, but at a lower dose. Other osmotic laxatives, such as lactulose, or stimulants such as senna-based products can also be useful. The goal of maintenance therapy is to encourage regular evacuation of soft bowel movements and to prevent recurrence of constipation. Often, medications need to be titrated to effect, and the dose may change over time and with change in diet. The choice of medication is often made on the basis of what a child will take on a regular basis. Some children experience gastrointestinal distress with stimulants or strong cathartics. Individuals have varied preferences for pills, liquid preparations, or drinks. Polyethylene glycol without electrolytes is a good choice as it has minimal taste. It can also be safely used up to 12 months (Loening-Baucke, 2002b). Mineral oil is another option, but the taste is often more difficult to disguise and is best used when cold and disguised in yogurt or pudding or flavored with chocolate or maple syrups. Prior concerns about the impact of mineral oil on absorption of fat-soluble vitamins are unfounded and supplementation is not necessary (Sharif et al, 2001).

As the constipation resolves, children can be slowly weaned off of medications as tolerated. The length of use depends on need as well as on the safety of the medication used. The prolonged use of stimulants and enemas should be avoided because of the side effects and potential for dependence. However, what constitutes prolonged used is difficult to ascertain. To avoid concerns about dependence, stimulants can be used intermittently as described before.

Diet

Include a discussion of diet as part of education and maintenance therapy. If possible, parents should encourage high-fiber foods including fruits, vegetables, and whole grains as well as fluids. For very mild cases of constipation, diet changes or a fiber supplement alone may be all that is required.

Behavioral Plan

The behavior component of treatment is essential, but it is not necessarily complex. A child requires a regimen of regular sitting on the toilet for two reasons: first, to encourage the evacuation of stool; and second, to help the child become comfortable with using the toilet. Initially, a child may be resistant to sitting on the toilet for many reasons. For one, the child may have developed a fear or aversion to use of the toilet. In addition, the child may have become overwhelmed by the long-standing nature of the problem and is less willing to perform a sitting task. The chronicity and nature of the disorder may have also led to disrupted family dynamics and struggles between parent and child around use of the toilet. However, no matter what the source of the behavior, the plan remains essentially the same.

The behavior plan includes motivating and rewarding a child for sitting on the toilet. The best time to sit is 20 to 30 minutes after meals as the gastrocolic reflex encourages defecation; however, it is not necessary to do it at this time only. It may be more convenient for sitting to occur in the morning or directly after school. Depending on the age of the child, she or he should be encouraged to sit on the toilet one to three times a day for 5 to 10 minutes at a time. The child may have a specific toy, book, or desired object during that time. The child is not required to stool but should try if able. There are many different ways to reward and to reinforce sitting behaviors. For preschoolers, a sticker chart can be used as a reward, and special toys or books can be used as reinforcers. For school-age children, stickers and small sweets may also still be useful, but they can earn special time or desired items by sitting. It is important to try to minimize conflict during sitting times. The reward system should be determined collaboratively with the parent and child, and the child needs to voice his or her agreement and understanding. The child then receives a reward for performing the sitting task. If the child does not perform the task, she or he should not be punished or reprimanded. The child should be gently reminded that if she or he does not complete the task, she or he will not receive the reward.

Regular scheduled visits with a provider are key to maintain motivation, to clarify the plan, and to provide encouragement. Often, it is easier for a child to perform the task for the provider rather than for a parent. If there is a great deal of conflict or resistance, consider eliciting the aid of a psychologist or behavioral specialist. See Chapter 87 for more in-depth behavioral strategies.

Other Therapies

As is common for all children with chronic medical conditions, parents often seek complementary and alternative therapies for their children. The literature is not extensive in regard to complementary and alternative treatment of encopresis. One review of nine randomized controlled studies found that biofeedback did not provide an additional advantage compared with a standard medical-behavioral approach. The authors also found no advantage to prokinetics or acupuncture (Brooks et al, 2000).

Outcome

Encopresis tends to be a relapsing and remitting disorder. Increased soiling and accidents are common during times of stress, for example. Most children will improve and many will have resolution of symptoms with treatment. The cure rate is variable but has been reported as 30% to 50% by 1 year and 48% to 75% by 5 years in clinic samples of children with chronic constipation (Loening-Baucke, 2002a). Outcomes vary, depending on the medical complexity of the case as well as other emotional and psychosocial factors involved. The longer the condition is present, the greater the impact on child and family functioning and overall treatment. It is important therefore to recognize and to treat this disorder as soon as possible. This also includes helping parents anticipate challenges to toilet training.

SUMMARY

The principles for successful toilet training include recognition of readiness skills and following a stepwise process that recognizes individual developmental, behavioral, and temperamental variation. Management of toilet refusal includes ensuring soft stools and using a stepwise approach with positive behavioral strategies. Encopresis is common in the pediatric population and may or may not be associated with constipation, withholding, or toilet refusal. Encopresis is rarely caused by organic illness, and careful history and physical examination are usually sufficient to rule out organic disease. Management of encopresis includes treatment and alleviation of constipation and the use of a structured sitting program with positive behavioral strategies.

REFERENCES

Baker SS, Liptak GS, Colletti RB, et al: A medical position statement of the North American Society for Pediatric Gastroenterology and Nutrition. Constipation in infants and children: Evaluation and treatment. J Pediatr Gastroenterol Nutr 29:612-626, 1999.

Blum NJ, Taubman B, Nemeth N: Relationship between age at initiation of toilet training and duration of training: A prospective study. Pediatrics 111:810-814, 2003.

Blum NJ, Taubman B, Nemeth N: During toilet training, constipation occurs before stool toileting refusal. Pediatrics 113:e520-e522, 2004.

Brazelton TB: A child-oriented approach to toilet training. Pediatrics 29:121-128, 1962.

Brazelton TB, Christophersen ER, Frauman AC, et al: Instruction, timeliness and medical influences affecting toilet training. Pediatrics 103:1353-1358, 1999.

Brazzelli M, Griffiths P: Behavioural and cognitive interventions with or without other treatments for defaecation disorders in children. Cochrane Database Syst Rev 4. CD002240, 2001.

Brooks RC, Copen RM, Cox DJ, et al: Review of the treatment literature for encopresis, functional constipation, and stool-toileting refusal. Ann Behav Med 22:260-267, 2000.

Joinson C, Heron J, Butler U, et al: Avon Longitudinal Study of Parents and Children Study Team: Psychological differences between children with and without soiling problems. Pediatrics 117:1575-1584, 2006.

Levine MD, Bakow H: Children with encopresis: A study of treatment outcome. Pediatrics 58:845-852, 1976.

Loening-Baucke V: Constipation and encopresis. *In* Lifschitz CH, (ed): Pediatric Gastroenterology and Nutrition in Clinical Practice. New York, Marcel Dekker, 2001, 551.

Loening-Baucke V: Encopresis. Curr Opin Pediatr 14:570-575, 2002a.

Loening-Baucke V: Polyethylene glycol without electrolytes for children with constipation and encopresis. J Pediatr Gastroenterol Nutr 34:372-377, 2002b.

Reisner SH, Sivan Y, Nitzan M, Merlob P: Determination of anterior displacement of the anus in newborn infants and children. Pediatrics 73:216, 1984.

Rockney RM, McQuade WH, Days AL: The plain abdominal radiograph in the management of encopresis. Arch Pediatr Adolesc Med 149:623, 1995.

Schonwald A, Rappaport L: Consultation with the specialist. Encopresis: Assessment and management. Pediatr Rev 25:278-282, 2004.

Schonwald A, Sherritt L, Stadtler A, Bridgemohan C: Factors associated with difficult toilet training. Pediatrics 113:1753-1757, 2004.

Sharif F, Crushell E, O'Driscoll K, et al: Current topic. Liquid paraffin: A reappraisal of its role in the treatment of constipation. Arch Dis Child 85:121-124, 2001.

Yamada T, Alpers DH, Kaplowitz N, et al: Textbook of Gastroenterology. Philadelphia, Lippincott Williams & Wilkins, 2003.

64 SLEEP AND SLEEP DISORDERS IN CHILDREN

Judith A. Owens

Vignettes

Gregory

Gregory is 7 years old and is repeating first grade. He cannot sit still and has problems paying attention. His parents say that he has always been like this, as long as they can remember. He was recently diagnosed with ADHD, and his parents and teachers have seen some positive changes since they started treatment. However, his parents are still having major problems at night, which the medication is making worse. Gregory often refuses to get into bed, and even after they turn out the lights, it can be hours before he is finally asleep. Both of his parents are exhausted and dread what they call the "beastly hours" of the day.

Augustin

Augustin is 7 years old and was diagnosed with autism when he was 3 years old. He falls asleep with little problem at 8:30 at night but invariably is awake by 3:00 in the morning. Most nights he does not fall back to sleep until 5:00 AM, although there are some nights when he is up at 3:00 AM "for the day." He frequently falls asleep on the long bus ride home after school.

NORMAL SLEEP IN INFANTS, CHILDREN, AND ADOLESCENTS

To fully appreciate both the trajectory of normal sleep development and the causes and effects of sleep disturbances and inadequate sleep in children and adolescents, some basic understanding of the structure of sleep and familiarity with the mechanisms that regulate sleep are extremely helpful. Sleep and wakefulness are regulated by two basic, highly coupled processes operating simultaneously: the homeostatic process or "sleep drive," which is dependent on length of time awake and primarily regulates the length and depth of sleep; and endogenous circadian rhythms (biologic time clocks), which influence the internal organization of sleep and timing and duration of daily sleep-wake cycles. Intrinsic circadian rhythms (which govern many other physiologic systems in addition to sleep-wake cycles) are also synchronized to the 24-hour day cycle by environmental cues (*zeitgebers*), such as timing of meals and other activities; the most powerful circadian cue is the light-dark cycle, which exerts a powerful influence on melatonin secretion by the pineal gland ("light—on, darkness—off").

Whereas sleep in neonates and infants is quite different from that in adults, the structure of children's sleep and sleep-wake patterns begin to resemble those of adults as they mature (Mindell et al, 1999). In terms of sleep architecture, there is a dramatic decrease in the proportion of both slow-wave and rapid eye movement (REM) sleep from birth through childhood to adulthood. Because ultradian sleep cycles lengthen, there is often a concomitant decrease in the number of end-of-cycle arousals. Several general trends in the maturation of sleep patterns over time may also be identified. First, there is a decrease in the 24-hour average total sleep duration from infancy through adolescence, with a less marked and more gradual continued decrease in nocturnal sleep amounts into late adolescence, as well as a significant decline in daytime sleep (scheduled napping) between 18 months and 5 years (Iglowstein et al, 2003). There is also a gradual but marked circadian-mediated shift to a later bedtime and sleep onset time that begins in middle childhood and accelerates in early to mid adolescence. Finally, sleep-wake patterns on school nights and non–school nights become increasingly irregular from middle childhood through adolescence.

The following section provides a more detailed description of normal sleep behaviors and patterns in different age groups.

Sleep in Newborns

Newborns sleep approximately 16 to 20 hours per day, generally in 1- to 4-hour sleep periods followed by 1- to 2-hour periods awake, and sleep amounts during the day approximately equal the amount of nighttime sleep. Sleep-wake cycles are largely dependent on hunger and satiety; for example, bottle-fed infants generally sleep in longer bouts (3 to 5 hours) than breastfed infants do (2 to 3 hours). Newborns have two sleep states that are essentially analogous to adult REM and non-REM sleep, active (REM-like; characterized by smiling, grimacing, sucking, and body movements; 50% of sleep) and quiet (non–REM-like), as well as a third "indeterminate" state. Unlike adults and older children, newborns and infants up to the age of approximately 6 months enter sleep through the active or REM state.

Sleep in Infants (1 to 12 months)

Infants generally sleep about 14 to 15 hours per 24 hours at 4 months and 13 to 14 hours total at 6 months; however, there appears to be a very wide intraindividual variation in parent-reported 24-hour sleep duration. Sleep periods last about 3 to 4 hours during the first 3 months and extend to 6 to 8 hours by the age of 4 to 6 months. Most infants between 6 and 12 months of age nap between 2 and 4 hours divided into two naps per day.

Two important developmental "milestones" are normally achieved during the first 6 months of life; these are known as *sleep consolidation* and *sleep regulation*. Sleep consolidation is generally described as an infant's ability to sleep for a continuous period that is concentrated during the nocturnal hours, augmented by shorter periods of daytime sleep (naps). Infants develop the ability to consolidate sleep between 6 weeks and 3 months, and approximately 70% to 80% of infants achieve sleep consolidation (i.e., "sleeping through the night") by 9 months. Sleep regulation refers to the infant's ability to be able to control internal states of arousal both to fall asleep at bedtime without parental intervention or assistance and to fall back asleep after normal brief arousals during the night. The capacity to "self-soothe" begins to develop in the first 12 weeks of life and is a reflection of both neurodevelopmental maturation and learning. However, the developmental goal of independent self-soothing in infants at bedtime and after night wakings may not be shared by all cultures and families, and voluntary or "lifestyle" bed and room sharing of infants and parents is a common and accepted practice in many cultures and ethnic groups. Sleep behavior in infancy, in particular, must also be understood in the context of the relationship and interaction between child and caregiver, which has a great impact on the quality and quantity of sleep, as well as of other important factors affecting sleep, such as child temperament, breastfeeding practices, and environmental factors (Fig. 64-1).

Sleep in Toddlers (12 to 36 months)

Toddlers sleep about 12 hours per 24 hours. Napping patterns generally consist of ½ to 3½ hours per day, and most toddlers give up a second nap by 18 months. During this stage, both developmental and environmental issues begin to have more of an impact on sleep; examples include an increase in separation anxiety, which may lead to bedtime resistance and problematic night wakings; the development of imagination, which may result in increased nighttime fears; the increased understanding in toddlers of the symbolic meaning of objects, which can lead to increased interest in and reliance on transitional objects to allay normal developmental and separation fears; and an increased drive for autonomy and independence, which may result in increased bedtime resistance. Sleep problems in toddlers are very common, occurring in 25% to 30% of this age group; bedtime resistance is found in 10% to 15% of toddlers, and night wakings in 15% to 20%.

Sleep in Preschoolers (3 to 5 years)

Preschool-age children typically sleep about 11 to 12 hours per 24 hours; most children give up napping by 5 years, although approximately 25% of children continue to nap at the age of 5 years, and there is some evidence that napping patterns and the preservation of daytime sleep periods into later childhood may be influenced by cultural and ethnic differences (Jenni and O'Connor, 2005). Difficulties falling asleep and night wakings (15% to 30%), in many cases coexisting in the same child, are still common in this age group. Developmental issues

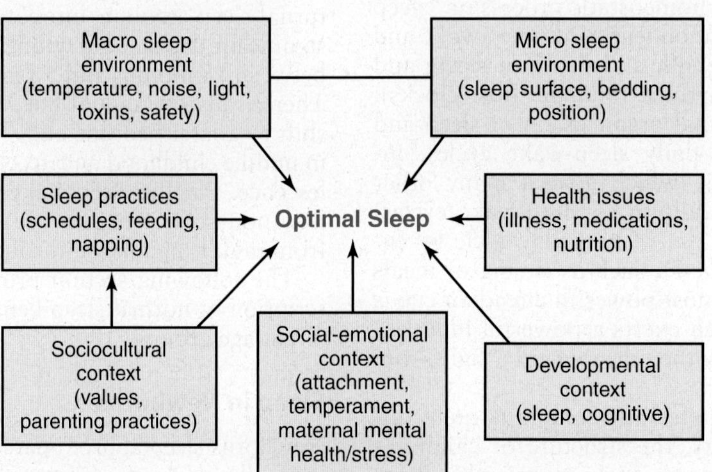

Figure 64-1. Factors influencing sleep quality in children and adolescents.

affecting sleep include expanded language and cognitive skills, which may lead to increased bedtime resistance, as children become more articulate about their needs and may engage in more limit testing behavior; developing capacity to delay gratification and to anticipate consequences, which enables preschoolers to respond to positive reinforcement for appropriate bedtime behavior; and increasing interest in developing literacy skills, which reinforces the importance of reading aloud at bedtime as an integral part of the bedtime routine. Bedtime routines and rituals, use of transitional objects, and sleep-wake schedules are all-important sleep-related issues at this developmental stage.

Sleep in Middle Childhood (6 to 12 years)

Most children this age sleep between 10 and 11 hours a night. Because a high level of physiologic alertness during the day is characteristic of school-age children, the presence of daytime sleepiness in an elementary school–age child is likely to be indicative of significant sleep disruption and fragmentation or insufficient sleep. Middle childhood is also a critical time for the development of healthy sleep habits. Increasing independence from parental supervision and a shift in responsibility for health habits as children approach adolescence may result in less enforcement of appropriate bedtimes and inadequate sleep duration; parents may also be less aware of sleep problems if they do exist. Although it was previously believed that sleep problems are rare in middle childhood, recent studies have reported an overall prevalence of significant parent-reported sleep problems of 25% to 40%, ranging from bedtime resistance to significant sleep onset delay and anxiety at bedtime.

Sleep in Adolescents (12 to 18 years)

Although a number of significant sleep changes occur in adolescence, adolescent sleep needs do not appear to differ dramatically from sleep needs of preadolescents, and optimal sleep amounts remain at about 9 to 9¼ hours per night. However, a number of studies across different environments and in different cultures have suggested that the average adolescent typically sleeps about 7 hours or less per night and that this accumulating sleep debt may have a significant impact on functioning, performance, and quality of life. Biologically based pubertal changes also significantly affect sleep. In particular, around the time of onset of puberty, adolescents develop as much as a 2-hour sleep-wake "phase delay" (later sleep onset and wake times) relative to sleep-wake cycles in middle childhood. Environmental factors and lifestyle and social demands, such as homework, activities, and after-school jobs, clearly also significantly affect sleep amounts in adolescents, and early start times of many high schools may contribute to insufficient sleep. There is also significant weekday and weekend variability in sleep-wake patterns in adolescents, often accompanied by weekend "oversleep" in an attempt to address the chronic sleep debt accumulated during the week; this further contributes to circadian disruption and associated decreased daytime alertness levels. All of these factors often combine to produce significant sleepiness in many adolescents.

NEUROBEHAVIORAL AND NEUROCOGNITIVE IMPACT OF INADEQUATE AND DISRUPTED SLEEP IN CHILDREN

There is clear evidence from both experimental laboratory-based studies and clinical observations that insufficient sleep and poor-quality sleep result in daytime sleepiness and behavioral dysregulation and affect neurocognitive functions in children, especially those functions involving learning and memory consolidation and those associated with the prefrontal cortex (e.g., attention, working memory, and other executive functions) (Fallone et al, 2002). Sleep loss and sleep fragmentation are known to directly affect mood and mood regulation (increased irritability, decreased positive mood, poor affect modulation). Behavioral manifestations of sleepiness in children are varied and range from those that are classically "sleepy," such as yawning, rubbing eyes, and resting the head on a desk, to externalizing behaviors, such as increased impulsivity, hyperactivity, and aggressiveness to increased distractibility and off-task behavior. Sleepiness may also result in observable neurocognitive performance deficits, including decreased cognitive flexibility and verbal creativity, poor abstract reasoning, impaired motor skills, decreased attention and vigilance, and memory impairments. Finally, other postulated health outcomes of inadequate sleep in children include potential deleterious effects on the cardiovascular, immune, and various metabolic systems, including glucose metabolism and endocrine function, and an increase in accidental injuries; recently, for example, several studies have suggested a link between shortened sleep duration and overweight and obesity in children. In addition, studies have documented secondary effects of children's sleep problems on parents (e.g., maternal depression), particularly on caregivers of special needs children as well as on family functioning.

ETIOLOGY, EPIDEMIOLOGY, PRESENTATION, EVALUATION, AND TREATMENT OF COMMON SLEEP DISORDERS IN CHILDREN

First, it is helpful to understand that four basic etiologic mechanisms essentially account for most sleep disturbances in the pediatric population, as follows: sleep is either *insufficient for individual physiologic sleep needs* (e.g., "lifestyle" sleep restriction, sleep onset delay related to behavioral insomnia) or adequate in amount but *fragmented or disrupted* by conditions that result in frequent or prolonged arousals (e.g., obstructive sleep apnea and periodic limb movement disorder, which cause frequent or prolonged arousals). Third, *primary disorders of excessive daytime sleepiness* (e.g., narcolepsy) are less common but important and underrecognized causes of sleep disturbance in children and adolescents. Finally, *circadian rhythm disorders,* in which sleep is usually normal in structure and duration but occurs at an undesired time (e.g., delayed sleep phase syndrome) may result in daytime sleepiness. For practical purposes, sleep disorders may also be defined as primarily "behaviorally based" versus organic or "medically based," although, in reality, these two types of sleep disorders are often influenced by similar psychosocial and physical-environmental factors and frequently coexist.

Obstructive Sleep Apnea and Sleep Disordered Breathing

Sleep disordered breathing (SDB) in childhood includes a spectrum of disorders that vary in severity, ranging from obstructive sleep apnea (OSA) to primary snoring (defined as snoring without ventilatory abnormalities) (Schechter, 2002). The prevalence is also variable, from 10% in habitual snoring to 1% to 3% in OSA. The basic pathophysiologic process of OSA involves cessation of airflow through the nose and mouth during sleep (pathologic duration of apnea is determined by age-appropriate norms) despite respiratory effort and chest wall movement; this disrupts normal ventilation during sleep, resulting in hypoxemia or hypoventilation and a sleep pattern characterized by frequent arousals. Common manifestations of SDB in childhood include loud, nightly snoring; choking or gasping arousals; and increased work of breathing characterized by nocturnal diaphoresis, paradoxical chest and abdominal wall movements, and restless sleep. However, SDB may be manifested primarily with neurobehavioral symptoms, including inattention, hyperactivity, and poor academic functioning.

Common risk factors for SDB are those contributing to a reduced upper airway patency and include obstructive features (e.g., adenotonsillar hypertrophy, allergies, reactive airway disease), reduced upper airway size (e.g., obesity, craniofacial syndromes, midfacial hypoplasia, or retrognathia or micrognathia), and reduced upper airway tone (e.g., neuromuscular disorders characterized by hypotonia, Down syndrome). Racial (e.g., African American) and genetic factors (family history of SDB) as well as environmental factors (e.g., secondary smoke exposure) may also play a role.

Specific physical examination findings (growth abnormalities such as obesity or failure-to-thrive, nasal obstruction with hyponasal speech and "adenoidal facies" or mouth breathing, enlarged tonsils) may suggest OSA. However, the presence of large tonsils and adenoids does not necessarily mean the patient has OSA, and in fact, there is no constellation of presenting symptoms and physical findings that have reliably been found to differentiate between OSA and primary snoring in the ambulatory setting. Overnight polysomnography remains the gold standard for evaluation and diagnosis of pediatric SDB. Overnight polysomnography documents physiologic variables during sleep, including sleep stages and arousals (electroencephalographic montage, eye movements, chin muscle tone), cardiorespiratory parameters (airflow, respiratory effort, oxygen saturation, transcutaneous or end-tidal carbon dioxide concentration, and heart rate), and limb movements, and allows both confirmation of the diagnosis and assessment of severity of OSA.

Successful treatment of OSA has been shown in a number of studies to fully or partially reduce associated neurobehavioral and neurocognitive deficits. Adenotonsillectomy is generally the first line of treatment for pediatric SDB, although adenoidectomy alone may not be curative when other risk factors, such as obesity, are present. Nutrition and exercise counseling should be a routine part of treatment in pediatric SDB in obese children. Positive airway pressure, as either continuous or bi-level positive airway pressure (the most common treatment of OSA in adults), can be an effective and reasonably well tolerated treatment option for those children and adolescents for whom surgery is not an option or in children who continue to have OSA despite surgery.

Parasomnias

Parasomnias are defined as episodic, often undesirable nocturnal behaviors that typically involve autonomic and skeletal muscle disturbances as well as cognitive disorientation and mental confusion. The most common parasomnias in childhood may be further categorized as occurring primarily during stage 4 slow-wave or deep (delta) sleep (partial arousal parasomnias), during REM sleep, or at the sleep-wake transition. The *partial arousal parasomnias,* which include *sleepwalking and sleep terrors,* typically occur in the first third of the night at the transition out of slow-wave sleep and thus share clinical features of both the awake (ambulation, vocalizations) and the sleeping states (high arousal threshold, unresponsiveness to the environment, amnesia for the event). Sleep terrors are typically characterized by a very high level of autonomic arousal; sleepwalking, by definition, usually involves displacement from bed. Both are more common in preschoolers and school-age children and generally disappear in adolescence, at least in part because of the relatively higher percentage of slow-wave sleep in younger children and probably also as a corollary of neurodevelopmental maturation. Sleep terrors are considerably less common (1% to 3% incidence) than is sleepwalking (40% of the population has had at least one episode). Furthermore, any factors that are associated with an increase in the relative percentage of slow-wave sleep (certain medications, previous sleep deprivation, sleep fragmentation caused by an underlying sleep disorder such as OSA syndrome) may increase the frequency of either of these events in a predisposed child (Sheldon, 2005). Finally there appears to be a genetic predisposition for both sleepwalking and night terrors, and it is not uncommon for individuals to have both types of episodes.

In contrast, *nightmares,* the most common REM-associated parasomnia in childhood, are very common, occur primarily during the last third of the night when REM sleep is most prominent, generally include vivid recall of dream content, and are more likely to be triggered by anxiety or a stressful event. In general, nightmares are fairly easily managed with a combination of behavioral, cognitive, and relaxation strategies. However, frequent and persistent nightmares in a child warrant further investigation of possible trauma, such as sexual abuse, or evaluation for a more global anxiety disorder.

Atypical presentations of partial arousal parasomnias are sometimes difficult to distinguish from nocturnal seizures; the index of suspicion for a seizure disorder should be higher in the presence of a previous history of or risk factors for seizures, any unusual or stereotypic movements accompanying the episodes, or postictal phenomena. Subsequent daytime sleepiness is also much more likely with nocturnal seizures. Home videotaping of the episodes may be helpful in making the diagnosis, but overnight polysomnography (with a full electroencephalographic seizure montage) may be necessary.

Management of partial arousal parasomnias should first include reassurance and education of the child and family about the benign and self-limited nature of the disorder. Parents may be told that most children stop having sleepwalking episodes or sleep terrors by adolescence. Interim management should include institution of appropriate safety measures, including gates (doorways, top of staircases), locking of outside doors and windows, lighting of hallways, and ensuring safety of the sleeping environment (e.g., clutter on floors), and parent notification measures, such as alarm systems or a bell attached to the bedroom door. Avoidance of possible trigger or exacerbating factors (e.g., sleep deprivation, change in sleeping environment) as well as avoidance of awakening a child during an event should be discussed with parents. In the case of frequent (e.g., nightly) events, a technique called scheduled awakenings, which involve having the parent wake the child approximately 15 to 30 minutes before the time of night that the first parasomnia episode typically occurs, can be quite effective. Pharmacotherapy (with a slow-wave sleep–suppressing drug such as a benzodiazepine or tricyclic antidepressant) may be indicated in severe or chronic cases.

Rhythmic movement disorders, including *body rocking, head rolling, and head banging,* are parasomnias that occur largely during sleep-wake transition and are characterized by repetitive, stereotypic movements involving large muscle groups. They are much more common in the first year of life and generally disappear by the age of 4 years, although they may persist into adulthood in rare cases. Although occasionally associated with developmental delay, most occur in normal children and do not result in physical injury to the child. Treatment is generally parental reassurance and, if appropriate, judicious padding of the sleeping surface.

Bruxism, or repetitive nocturnal teeth grinding, occurs in as high as 50% of normal infants during eruption of primary dentition, and the incidence of at least occasional episodes approaches 20% in older children. There is some speculation that the underlying pathophysiologic mechanism may be linked to alterations in central nervous system serotonergic and dopaminergic neurotransmission. Symptomatic treatment (e.g., for temporomandibular joint pain, wearing of teeth surfaces) generally involves the use of occlusal splints, and behavioral treatment (e.g., biofeedback) may also be useful.

Restless Legs Syndrome and Periodic Limb Movement Disorder

Restless legs syndrome and periodic limb movement disorder (RLS/PLMD) are related sleep movement disorders that are frequently overlooked in both adult and pediatric clinical practice. RLS/PLMD is estimated to affect about 10% of adults; although the prevalence of these disorders in the pediatric population is unknown, retrospective reports given by affected adults suggest that symptoms (such as restless sleep and discomfort in the lower extremities at rest) frequently first appear in childhood and can result in significant sleep disturbance. As in adults, RLS symptoms in children and adolescents are typically worse in the evening and are exacerbated by inactivity, leading to significant difficulty in falling asleep. Individuals with RLS describe uncomfortable "creepy-crawly" tingling sensations in the lower extremities rather than pain per se; however, these symptoms are often poorly articulated by the children themselves and may be expressed as "growing pains" (Picchietti and Walters, 1996). Periodic limb movements, which often co-occur with RLS (as many as 80% of adults with RLS also have periodic limb movements), are characterized by brief, repetitive, rhythmic jerks primarily of the lower extremities during stages 1 and 2 of sleep; these may result in sleep fragmentation related to nocturnal arousals and awakenings. Additional diagnostic clues may include iron deficiency anemia (specifically, a low ferritin level), exacerbation of symptoms by caffeine intake, and positive family history of RLS/PLMD. Periodic limb movements in particular have been associated with attention-deficit/hyperactivity disorder (ADHD) symptoms in children and are more frequently found in children with ADHD. Whereas RLS is a clinical diagnosis, documentation of periodic limb movements associated with arousals requires an overnight sleep study. Pharmacologic management with a variety of agents, such as dopamine agonists, opioids, and anticonvulsants as well as iron supplementation if appropriate, and avoidance of exacerbating factors are often quite helpful.

Narcolepsy

Narcolepsy is a rare primary disorder of excessive daytime sleepiness that affects an estimated 125,000 to 200,000 Americans (Dahl et al, 1994).

Narcolepsy is rarely diagnosed in prepubertal children, but retrospective surveys nonetheless suggest that it frequently first is manifested in late childhood and early adolescence. However, both pediatric and adult patients with narcolepsy often delay in seeking medical attention and are frequently labeled as having mood disorders, learning problems, and academic failure before the underlying etiology is identified, as long as several decades later. In about 25% of cases, there is a family history of narcolepsy; secondary narcolepsy after brain injury or in association with other medical illnesses may also occur.

The cardinal and usual initial presenting feature of narcolepsy is repetitive episodes of profound sleepiness that may occur both at rest and during periods of activity (talking, eating). These "sleep attacks" may be very brief (3 seconds or "microsleeps"), resulting primarily in lapses in attention. Other features of the so-called narcoleptic tetrad essentially represent "uncoupling" of REM phenomena or the intrusion of REM sleep features (muscle atonia, dream mentation) into wakefulness. In addition to daytime sleepiness, the tetrad includes cataplexy (sudden loss of total body or partial muscle tone, usually in response to an emotional stimulus); hypnagogic (at sleep onset) or hypnopompic (on waking) visual, auditory, or tactile hallucinations; and sleep paralysis (temporary loss of voluntary muscle control) at sleep onset or offset. These symptoms of narcolepsy are also frequently misdiagnosed as part of a psychiatric or neurologic disorder, such as psychosis or a conversion reaction. The pathophysiologic mechanism of narcolepsy is thought to involve alterations in the hypocretin-orexin sleep neuroregulatory system. The gold standard of diagnosis is overnight polysomnography followed by a multiple sleep latency test. The multiple sleep latency test involves a series of opportunities to nap, during which patients with narcolepsy will demonstrate a pathologically shortened sleep onset latency (<5 minutes) as well as periods of REM sleep occurring immediately after sleep onset. The treatment of narcolepsy generally involves a combination of medications to combat daytime sleepiness (stimulants) and REM sleep suppressants (such as selective serotonin reuptake inhibitors) to prevent cataleptic attacks.

Delayed Sleep Phase Syndrome

Delayed sleep phase syndrome is a circadian rhythm disorder that involves a significant and persistent phase shift in sleep-wake schedule (later bedtime and wake time) that conflicts with the individual's school, work, or lifestyle demands (Herman, 2005). Thus, it is the *timing* rather than the quality of sleep that is problematic; sleep *quantity* may be compromised if the individual is obligated to wake up in the morning before adequate sleep is obtained. Individuals with delayed sleep phase syndrome may complain primarily of sleep initiation insomnia; however, when they are allowed to sleep according to their preferred later bedtime and wake time (e.g., on school vacations), the sleep onset delays resolve. The typical sleep-wake pattern in delayed sleep phase syndrome is a consistently preferred bedtime/sleep onset time after midnight and wake time after 10 AM on both weekdays and weekends. Adolescents with delayed sleep phase syndrome often complain of sleep onset insomnia, extreme difficulty waking in the morning, and profound daytime sleepiness. Delayed sleep phase may be treated with a combination of the imposition of a strict sleep-wake schedule, exogenous melatonin in the evening, and bright light therapy in the morning to help "reset" the clock. Teenagers with a severely delayed sleep phase (more than 3 or 4 hours) may benefit from a technique called chronotherapy, in which bedtime ("lights out") and wake time are successively delayed (by 2 to 3 hours per day) during a period of days until the sleep onset time coincides with the desired bedtime. If the adolescent has school avoidance or a mood disorder as part of the clinical picture, which is commonly the case, noncompliance with treatment is typical, and more intensive behavioral and pharmacologic management strategies as well as referral to a sleep specialist may be warranted.

Behavioral Insomnia of Childhood (Sleep Onset Association and Limit Setting Subtypes)

As in adults, "insomnia" in children and adolescents should be viewed as a constellation of sleep-related symptoms that result from a wide range of possible causes, and not as a diagnosis per se. The causes of childhood insomnia are varied and include both medical (i.e., drug related, pain induced, associated with primary sleep disorders such as obstructive sleep apnea) and behavioral (i.e., associated with poor sleep hygiene or negative sleep onset associations) issues and are often the result of a combination of these factors. Practically speaking, the most frequent clinical manifestations of childhood insomnia, particularly in younger children, are bedtime refusal or resistance, delayed sleep onset, and prolonged night wakings requiring parental intervention.

It is estimated that overall, 20% to 30% of children in cross-sectional studies are described to have some significant bedtime problems or night wakings (Mindell and Owens, 2003). However, because these two sleep complaints frequently coexist and similar treatment strategies may be used for both, many studies do not approach them as separate concerns, and thus individual prevalence rates are difficult to estimate. Difficulties falling asleep and night wakings (15% to 30%) are common in toddlers and preschoolers as well as in middle school–age children. Furthermore, studies suggest that that lifetime prevalence of insomnia in 13- to 16-year-old adolescents is greater than 10%.

In general, behavioral insomnia of childhood is a disorder of young children (0 to 5 years) but may persist into middle childhood and beyond. The presenting problem in the sleep onset association subtype of behavioral insomnia is generally one of prolonged night waking resulting in insufficient sleep. In this disorder, the infant learns to fall asleep only under certain conditions or in the presence of specific sleep associations, such as being rocked or fed, which are usually readily available at bedtime. During the night, when the child experiences the type of brief arousal that normally occurs at the end of each ultradian sleep cycle or awakens for other reasons, the child is not able to get back to sleep (self-soothe) unless those same conditions are available to him or her. The infant then "signals" the caregiver by crying (or coming into the parents' bedroom if the child is no longer in a crib) until the necessary associations are provided.

The limit setting behavioral insomnia subtype is a disorder most common in children of preschool age and older and is characterized by active resistance, verbal protests, and repeated demands at bedtime ("curtain calls") rather than night wakings. If it is sufficiently prolonged, the sleep onset delay may result in inadequate sleep. This disorder most commonly develops from a caregiver's inability or unwillingness to set consistent bedtime rules and enforce a regular bedtime, often exacerbated by the child's oppositional behavior. In some cases, however, the child's resistance at bedtime is due to an underlying problem in falling asleep caused by other factors (e.g., medical conditions such as asthma or medication use, a sleep disorder such as restless legs, or anxiety) or a mismatch between the child's intrinsic circadian preferences ("night owl") and parental expectations.

Successful treatment of behavioral insomnia of childhood generally involves a combination of these behavioral strategies aimed at eliminating inappropriate sleep onset associations or reducing undesirable nighttime behaviors. A recent review of 52 treatment studies indicates that behavioral therapies produce reliable and durable changes for both bedtime resistance and night wakings in young children (Mindell et al, 2006). Most of the interventions described in these studies could be placed into the following categories: extinction and its variants (i.e., unmodified extinction, extinction with parental presence, graduated extinction), positive bedtime routines, scheduled awakenings, bedtime fading with response-cost, positive reinforcement, and parent education/prevention. The introduction of more appropriate sleep associations that will be readily available to the child during the night (transitional objects such as a blanket or toy) in addition to positive reinforcement (e.g., stickers for remaining in bed) is often beneficial. Problems with limit setting generally respond to some combination of decreased parental attention for bedtime-delaying behavior, establishment of a consistent bedtime routine that does not include stimulating activities such as television viewing, bedtime fading (temporarily setting bedtime to the current sleep onset time and then gradually advancing bedtime), and positive reinforcement (e.g., sticker charts) for appropriate behavior at bedtime (Morgenthaler et al, 2006).

Most sleep disturbances in children are successfully managed with behavior therapy alone, although a combination of behavioral and pharmacologic intervention may be appropriate in selected clinical situations and in specific populations (e.g., children with attention-deficit/hyperactivity disorder [ADHD], autism spectrum disorders). Furthermore, education of parents and children about normal sleep development and good sleep hygiene is key to successful treatment. The institution of appropriate sleep hygiene measures that revolve around the basic environmental, scheduling, sleep practice, and physiologic factors promoting optimal sleep are a necessary component of every treatment package (Table 64-1).

SLEEP ISSUES IN SPECIAL POPULATIONS, INCLUDING CHILDREN WITH MEDICAL, PSYCHIATRIC, AND DEVELOPMENTAL DISORDERS

Chronic health conditions such as asthma, diabetes, sickle cell disease, and juvenile rheumatoid arthritis in children (Lewin and Dahl, 1999) may predispose children to sleep problems, which in turn are likely to have a further impact on morbidity and quality of life. A number of patient and environmental factors, such as the impact of repeated hospitalization, family dynamics, underlying disease processes, comorbid mood and anxiety disorders, and concurrent medications, are clearly important to consider in assessing the bidirectional relationship of insomnia and chronic illness in children. Specific medical conditions that may also have an increased risk of sleep problems include allergies and atopic dermatitis, migraine headaches, seizure disorders, other rheumatologic conditions such as chronic fatigue syndrome and fibromyalgia, and chronic gastrointestinal disorders such as inflammatory bowel disease. In addition, many over-the-counter and prescription drugs have potentially significant effects on sleep and alertness in children, including direct pharmacologic effects, disruption of sleep patterns (e.g., night wakings), exacerbation of a primary sleep disorder (e.g., obstructive sleep apnea or restless legs syndrome), withdrawal effects, and daytime sedation. Drugs commonly used in children that may have effects on sleep include psychotropic drugs such as stimulants and antidepressants, antihistamines, corticosteroids, opioids, and anticonvulsants.

Sleep disturbances often have a significant impact on the clinical presentation and symptom severity as well as on the management of psychiatric disorders in children and adolescents. Virtually all psychiatric disorders in children may be associated with sleep disruption (Dahl et al, 1996; Owens, 2005). Studies of children with major depressive disorder, for example, have reported a prevalence of insomnia of up to 75% of depressed adolescents. Sleep complaints, especially bedtime resistance, refusal to sleep alone, increased nighttime fears, and nightmares, are also common in anxious children and children who have experienced severely traumatic events. Parents of children with ADHD consistently report an increased prevalence of sleep problems, including delayed sleep onset, poor sleep quality, restless sleep, frequent night wakings, and shortened sleep duration, although more objective methods of examining sleep and sleep architecture (e.g., polysomnography, actigraphy) have overall disclosed minimal or inconsistent differences between children with ADHD and controls. Conversely, growing evidence suggests that "primary" insomnia (i.e., insomnia with no concurrent psychiatric disorder) is a risk factor for later developing psychiatric conditions, particularly depressive and anxiety disorders.

The high prevalence rates for sleep problems found in children with neurodevelopmental disorders such as intellectual disability and autism spectrum disorders, ranging from 13% to 85%, may be related to any number of factors, including intrinsic abnormalities in sleep regulation and circadian rhythms, sensory deficits, and medications used to treat associated symptoms (Johnson, 1996). The types of sleep disorders that occur in these children are generally not unique to these populations but rather are more frequent and more severe than in the general population and typically reflect the child's developmental level rather than chronologic age. Significant problems with initiation and maintenance of sleep, shortened sleep duration, irregular sleeping patterns, and early morning waking, for example, have been reported in a variety of different neurodevelopmental disorders, including Asperger syndrome, Angelman syndrome, Rett syndrome, Smith-Magenis syndrome, and Williams

Table 64-1. Sleep Hygiene

Sleep Hygiene for Children	
Sleep schedule	Bedtime and wake-up time should be about the same time everyday. There should not be more than an hour difference in bedtime and wake-up time between school nights and non–school nights.
Bedtime routine	A 20- to 30-minute bedtime routine that is the same every night is important in setting the stage for sleep. The routine should include calm activities, such as reading a book or talking about the day, with the last part occurring in the room where the child sleeps.
Bedroom	A child's bedroom should be comfortable, quiet, and dark; a dim nightlight is fine. Children also sleep better in a room that is cool (below 75°). Avoid using a child's bedroom for time-out or as a punishment. You want your child to think of his or her bedroom as a good place, not a bad one.
Snack	A light snack (such as milk and cookies) before bed is a good idea. Heavy meals within an hour or two of bedtime, however, may interfere with sleep.
Caffeine	Children should avoid caffeinated beverages in general and particularly for at least 3 to 4 hours before bed. Caffeine can be found in many types of soda, coffee, iced tea, energy and "performance" drinks, and chocolate.
Evening activities	The hour before bed should be a quiet time. Avoid high-energy activities, such as rough play or playing outside, or stimulating activities, such as playing computer games.
Television	Keep the television set out of a child's bedroom. Children can easily develop the bad habit of "needing" the TV to fall asleep. It is also much more difficult to control TV viewing if the set is in the bedroom.
Naps	Naps should be geared to a child's age and developmental needs. However, very long naps or too many naps should be avoided, as too much daytime sleep can result in a child's sleeping less at night.
Exercise	Children should spend time outside every day and get daily exercise.
Sleep Hygiene for Adolescents	
Sleep schedule	Wake up and go to bed at about the same time on school nights and non–school nights. Bedtime and wake time should not differ from one day to the next by more than an hour or so.
Weekends	Do not sleep in on weekends to "catch up" on sleep. This makes it more likely that you will have problems falling asleep at bedtime.
Naps	If you are very sleepy during the day, nap for 30 to 45 minutes in the early afternoon. Do not nap too long or too late in the afternoon or you will have difficulty falling asleep at bedtime.
Sunlight	Spend time outside every day, especially in the morning, as exposure to sunlight, or bright light, helps keep your body's internal clock on track.
Exercise	Exercise regularly. Exercise may help you fall asleep and sleep more deeply.
Bedroom	Make sure your bedroom is comfortable, quiet, and dark. Make sure that it is also not too warm at night, as sleeping in a room that is more than 75° will make it difficult to sleep.
Bed	Use your bed only for sleeping. Do not study, read, or listen to music on your bed. Keep the "electronics" (TV, computer, DVD player) to a minimum or, better yet, out of the bedroom altogether.
Bedtime	Make the 30 to 60 minutes before bedtime a quiet or wind-down time. Relaxing, calm, enjoyable activities like reading a book and listening to calm music help your body and mind slow down enough to let you get to sleep. Avoid watching TV, studying, exercising, or getting involved in "energizing" activities during the 30 minutes before bedtime.
Snack	Eat regular meals and do not go to bed hungry. A light snack before bed is a good idea; eating a full meal in the hour before bed is not.
Caffeine	Avoid eating or drinking products containing caffeine in the late afternoon and evening. These include caffeinated sodas, coffee, tea, and chocolate.
Alcohol	Avoid alcohol. Alcohol disrupts sleep and may cause you to awaken throughout the night.
Smoking	Smoking disturbs sleep. Do not smoke at least 1 hour before bed (and preferably, not at all!).
Sleeping pills	Do not use sleeping pills or other over-the-counter sleep aids to help you sleep. These may be dangerous, and the sleep problems often return when you stop the medicine.
Do not drive drowsy	Teenagers are at the highest risk for falling asleep at the wheel, so do not drive when you have not gotten enough sleep.

syndrome. Sleep problems, especially in children with special needs, are often chronic in nature and unlikely to resolve without aggressive treatment. In addition, sleep disturbances in these children often have a profound effect on the quality of life of the entire family. Higher degrees of cognitive impairment tend to be associated with more frequent and severe sleep problems. Comorbid psychiatric disorders in children and adolescents with special needs and psychotropic medications used to treat these disorders may further contribute to sleep problems.

IMPLICATIONS FOR CLINICAL CARE AND RESEARCH

Every child who presents with mood, learning, or behavioral issues should be screened for sleep problems. Parents and the children themselves may not recognize the connection between behavioral and learning disorders and sleep problems and thus may fail to spontaneously volunteer such information. Furthermore, because parents of older children and adolescents, in particular, may not be aware of any existing sleep difficulties, it is also important to directly question the patient as well about sleep issues. A number of parent-report sleep surveys for use in primary care settings as well as several clinical screening tools exist. The latter category includes an instrument called BEARS. Key areas of inquiry are **B**edtime resistance/delayed sleep onset; **E**xcessive daytime sleepiness (difficulty in morning awakening, drowsiness); **A**wakenings during the night; **R**egularity, pattern, and duration of sleep; and **S**noring and other symptoms of sleep disordered breathing (Owens and Dalzell, 2005).

If a sleep problem is identified, a comprehensive evaluation includes assessment of current sleep patterns, usual sleep duration, and sleep-wake schedule, often best assessed with a sleep diary in which parents record daily sleep behaviors for an extended period (2 to 4 weeks). A review of sleep habits (such as bedtime routines), daily caffeine intake, and the sleeping environment (temperature, noise level) may reveal environmental factors that contribute to the sleep problems. Additional diagnostic tools, such as polysomnographic evaluation, are seldom warranted for routine evaluation but may be appropriate if organic sleep disorders such as obstructive sleep apnea and periodic limb movements are suspected. Finally, referral to a sleep specialist for diagnosis or treatment should be considered in children or adolescents with persistent or severe bedtime issues that are not responsive to simple behavioral measures or that are extremely disruptive.

SUMMARY

Sleep problems in children are highly prevalent and may have a major impact on development, mood, and behavior. Differential diagnosis and systematic evaluation of presenting sleep complaints are key; polysomnography should be considered to evaluate for sleep disordered breathing and movement disorders. All children presenting with learning, attention, and behavior problems should be screened for primary and comorbid sleep disorders.

REFERENCES

Dahl RE, Holttum J, Trubnick L: A clinical picture of child and adolescent narcolepsy. J Am Acad Child Adolesc Psychiatry 33:834-841, 1994.

Dahl RE, Ryan ND, Matty MK, et al: Sleep onset abnormalities in depressed adolescents. Biol Psychiatry 39:400-410, 1996.

Fallone G, Owens JA, Deane J: Sleepiness in children and adolescents: Clinical implications. Sleep Med Rev 6:287-306, 2002.

Herman J: Circadian rhythm disorders. *In* Sheldon S, Ferber R, Kryger M (eds): Principles and Practice of Pediatric Sleep Medicine. Philadelphia, Elsevier Saunders, 2005, pp 101-112.

Iglowstein I, Jenni OG, Molinari L, Largo RH: Sleep duration from infancy to adolescence: Reference values and generational trends. Pediatrics 111:302-307, 2003.

Jenni OG, O'Connor BB: Children's sleep: An interplay between culture and biology. Pediatrics 115(Suppl):204-216, 2005.

Johnson C: Sleep problems in children with mental retardation and autism. Child Adolesc Psychiatr Clin North Am 5:673-681, 1996.

Lewin DS, Dahl RE: Importance of sleep in the management of pediatric pain. J Dev Behav Pediatr 20:244-252, 1999.

Mindell J, Owens J: A Clinical Guide to Pediatric Sleep: Diagnosis and Management of Sleep Problems in Children and Adolescents. Philadelphia, Lippincott Williams & Wilkins, 2003.

Mindell J, Owens J, Carskadon M: Developmental features of sleep. Child Adolesc Psychiatr Clin North Am 8:695-725, 1999.

Mindell JA, Kuhn B, Lewin DS, et al: Behavioral treatment of bedtime problems and night wakings in infants and young children. Sleep 29:1263-1276, 2006.

Morgenthaler TI, Owens J, Alessi C, et al: Practice parameters for behavioral treatment of bedtime problems and night wakings in infants and young children. Sleep 29:1277-1281, 2006.

Owens JA: The ADHD and sleep conundrum: A review. J Dev Behav Pediatr 26:312-322, 2005.

Owens JA, Dalzell V: Use of the "BEARS" sleep screening tool in a pediatric residents' continuity clinic: A pilot study. Sleep Med 6:63-69, 2005.

Picchietti D, Walters A: Restless legs syndrome and period limb movement disorders in children and adolescents. Child Adolesc Psychiatr Clin North Am 5:729-740, 1996.

Schechter M: Section on Pediatric Pulmonology, Subcommittee on Obstructive Sleep Apnea Syndrome, American Academy of Pediatrics: Diagnosis and management of childhood obstructive sleep apnea. Pediatrics 9:704-712, 2002.

Sheldon S: The parasomnias. *In* Sheldon S, Ferber R, Kryger M (eds): Principles and Practice of Pediatric Sleep Medicine. Philadelphia, Elsevier Saunders, 2005, pp 305-316.

REFERENCES FOR PARENTS

Ferber R: Solve Your Child's Sleep Problems. New York, Simon & Schuster, 2006.

Mindell J: Sleeping Through the Night: How Infants, Toddlers, and Their Parents Can Get a Good Night's Sleep. New York, HarperCollins, 2006.

Owens J, Mindell J: Take Charge of Your Child's Sleep: The All-in-One Resource for Solving Sleep Problems in Kids and Teens. New York, Marlowe & Company, 2005.

65 REPETITIVE BEHAVIORS AND TICS

NATHAN J. BLUM

Vignettes

A 4½-year-old sucks her thumb at bedtime and while watching TV or riding in the car.

An 18-month-old bangs his head on his mattress each night as he is falling asleep. He has caused erythema on his forehead but no bruising or swelling.

A 3-year-old has pulled out the hair on the left lateral side of her scalp and her eyebrows. She tends to pull her hair while sucking her thumb.

A 6-month-old regurgitates his food, rechews it, and then swallows it or spits it out.

All of the children described in these vignettes are engaged in repeated and rhythmic behavior that at least on initial appearance seems purposeless. These types of behaviors are often referred to as repetitive or stereotypic behavior. Assessment of children with repetitive behaviors is complex because although this type of behavior is a universal component of typical child development, repetitive behaviors can also occur across a wide spectrum of developmental, emotional, and physical disorders. In addition, the behavior itself may be a concern because it causes tissue damage, is socially undesirable, or causes the individual distress. The four cases described represent a range of behaviors with at least one that is very likely to be benign and self-limited, one that is very concerning, and two others that require further assessment. In this chapter, I briefly review the etiology of repetitive behaviors and then discuss the assessment and management of these behaviors, including the ones described in the vignettes.

ETIOLOGY

Both biologic and environmental factors are important in causing or maintaining repetitive behaviors. Studies of infants have found that repetitive behaviors are nearly universal phenomena that occur with a distinctive developmental progression. For example, hand sucking occurs in most typically developing infants within 2 hours of birth; foot kicking begins between 2 and 3 months of age; object banging and body rocking begin at approximately 6 months of age; and hand clapping begins at 7 to 8 months of age (Kravitz and Boehm, 1971; Thelen, 1996). The nearly universal occurrence of these behaviors in the first year of life and their distinctive developmental progression have led to the theory that rhythmic behaviors represent movement patterns encoded in the brain that serve as a transition between uncoordinated movements and more mature goal-directed behaviors (Thelen, 1996). Further facilitating the development of more complex behaviors is the brain's ability to create sequences of behavior that link sensory cues with motor behavior without requiring thought. This ability is critical for learning such complex adaptive behaviors as walking or riding a bike but may also facilitate the development of habits (Leckman and Riddle, 2000). In addition, although habits are often viewed as purposeless, they may serve some adaptive functions as individuals often report that these behaviors reduce feelings of anxiety or fear and increase feelings of security and control.

Pharmacologic, functional neuroimaging, neuroanatomic, and animal studies are beginning to elucidate brain structures and pathways involved in habits, tics, compulsions, and other repetitive behaviors. Much of this research is focused on the cortical-striatal-thalamic-cortical pathways and the dopamine neurotransmitter systems. The striatum is believed to be responsible for habit learning (as opposed to explicit memory based in the hippocampus), and dopamine-containing neurons from the substantia nigra modulate the activity of striatal neurons. Activation of striatal dopamine receptors has been demonstrated to produce stereotypic behaviors in laboratory animals, and some functional neuroimaging studies of individuals with Tourette syndrome suggest that there is increased striatal dopaminergic innervation in this disorder (Albin and Mink, 2006). Furthermore, administration of stimulant medications that increase dopamine levels produces tics or repetitive picking behaviors in some individuals. Inputs to the striatum from the frontal cortex are thought to inhibit the development of repetitive behaviors, and neurologic disorders associated with degeneration of the frontal lobes in humans have also been reported to cause repetitive behaviors.

Although the cortical-striatal-thalamic-cortical pathways may provide the biologic substrate that predisposes the brain to manifest repetitive behaviors, environmental factors also influence these behaviors. Both high and low levels of arousal may increase the frequency of repetitive behaviors. Severe sensory deprivation has been shown to produce these behaviors in both laboratory animals and humans. In the first year of life, most repetitive behaviors are associated with either a change in stimuli (e.g., appearance of a caretaker, presentation of a toy) or a nonalert (usually fussy) state (Thelen, 1996). In older individuals, repetitive behaviors are reported to occur most frequently either during periods of low arousal such as when tired, bored, or distracted by other stimuli (e.g., reading, television) or during periods of high arousal such as when concentrating, angry, or frustrated (Sallustro and Atwell, 1978).

The environmental response to repetitive behaviors may also be important in maintaining these behaviors. For example, repetitive behaviors such as those associated with self-injurious behavior in individuals with disabilities are often reinforced by caretakers who respond to the behaviors by providing attention or other reinforcers (discussed later and in Thompson and Caruso [2002]). In toddlers, similar factors may reinforce head banging associated with temper tantrums. Thus, in both typically developing children and those with disabilities, environmental variables play an important role in determining the rate at which repetitive behaviors occur.

CLASSIFICATION

Classification of repetitive behaviors is a complex and controversial topic. A system that adequately accounts for all of the following facts has not been developed: (1) some repetitive behaviors occur almost universally during typical child development; (2) some individuals experience repetitive behaviors as adaptive, whereas others experience the behaviors as intrusive; (3) repetitive behaviors usually appear not to have a function but in some cases serve an important communicative function or serve to relieve stress; (4) repetitive behaviors occur in many different forms; and (5) the form of the behaviors occurring across a wide range of developmental, medical, and psychiatric disorders may be very similar in appearance.

The classification system for repetitive behaviors used in the fourth edition of the *Diagnostic and Statistical Manual of Mental Disorders* (DSM-IV-TR; American Psychiatric Association, 2000) and *The Classification of Child and Adolescent Mental Diagnoses in Primary Care: Diagnostic and Statistical Manual for Primary Care (DSM-PC), Child and Adolescent Version* (Wolraich et al, 1996) is shown in Table 65-1. This system emphasizes some forms as separate disorders (e.g., trichotillomania) but lumps many other topographies together under the category of stereotypic movement disorder or ignores them entirely. For a repetitive behavior to be classified as stereotypic movement disorder, it must be viewed as purposeless and cause impairment. Repetitive behaviors are also subclassified as normal variations, as problems, or as disorders primarily on the basis of the degree of dysfunction or stigmatization that is associated with the behaviors. However, this classification system does not provide recommendations on how to systematically determine whether a behavior is purposeless or to assess the degree of dysfunction associated with the behavior. In addition, repetitive behaviors that occur as part of a general medical or neurologic condition, in response to medications, or as part of a developmental disorder, sensory impairment, or psychiatric disorder are not given a separate diagnosis if the repetitive behaviors that cause dysfunction are thought to be part of the underlying condition. This may occur in the pervasive developmental disorders, obsessive-compulsive disorder, body dysmorphic disorder, or some other conditions.

Given some of the problems associated with classification based on form and degree of dysfunction, some have recommended classification based on the function of the behavior (Rapp and Vollmer, 2005). This classification system would use functional analysis procedures (discussed in the section on self-injury) to identify repetitive behaviors that serve a social communication function, and these behaviors would not be considered stereotypic behaviors. Stereotypic behaviors could be further classified on the basis of whether they provided pleasure to the individual (positive reinforcement) or escape from some adversive experience such as stress or pain (negative reinforcement). Although this classification system would provide a systematic method for determining if repetitive behaviors serve a communicative function, methods for assessing the internal experience leading to the behavior are only beginning to be studied.

REPETITIVE BEHAVIORS

Sucking

Sucking of the hand, fingers, or thumb has been observed in utero as early as 29 weeks of gestation and is a nearly universal phenomenon in healthy neonates within hours after birth (Kravitz and Boehm, 1971). Sucking is viewed as a biologically driven behavior that develops into a habit in some children. Both genetic and environmental factors contribute to thumb sucking as one twin study found that 58% of monozygotic twins were concordant for frequent thumb sucking compared with only 33% of dizygotic twins (Ooki, 2005).

Thumb or digit sucking may be adaptive for many infants and toddlers in that it may provide stimulation to delay the onset of boredom during periods of low stimulation, and it may help soothe the child when he or she is tired, sick, or upset. In some children, thumb sucking may occur in response to emotional stress or anxiety, but thumb sucking has not been found to be consistently associated with specific behavioral or emotional disorders. The habit is usually harmless in infants and young children, but it has been associated with a number of sequelae when it persists, especially at high frequency or intensity, beyond the age of 4 to 6 years. Some of the most frequent sequelae of thumb sucking involve dental problems, such as an anterior open bite, decreased

Table 65-1. Classification of Repetitive Behaviors

Repetitive Behaviors—Variation (V65.49)
Sporadic repetitive movements are of limited duration, cause no physical harm, and do not impair normal development or activities.
Repetitive Behaviors—Problem (V40.3)
Repetitive behaviors cause some social disruption and/or dysfunction that results from the behavior itself and from the response of others to that behavior but is not sufficiently intense to qualify for a diagnosis of a repetitive behavior disorder.
Repetitive Behaviors—Disorders
Stereotypic movement disorder (307.3)
Motor behavior that is repetitive, often seemingly driven, and nonfunctional. The behaviors are clearly associated with social dysfunction and stigmatization.
Trichotillomania (312.39)
Recurrent pulling out of one's hair, resulting in noticeable hair loss. Associated with tension before hair pulling and gratification or relief after pulling.
Transient tic disorder (307.21)
Single or multiple motor and/or vocal tics that occur many times a day, nearly every day, for at least 4 weeks, but for no longer than 12 consecutive months.
Chronic motor or vocal tic disorder (307.22)
Single or multiple motor or vocal tics, but not both, have been present at some time during the illness. The tics occur many times a day nearly every day or intermittently throughout a period of more than 1 year.
Tourette syndrome (307.23)
Similar to chronic motor or vocal tic disorder except that both multiple motor and one or more vocal tics have to be present at some time during the illness.
Repetitive Behaviors Associated with General Medical Conditions
Examples: multiple sclerosis, postviral encephalitis, head injury, Sydenham chorea, Huntington chorea, Lesch-Nyhan syndrome
Repetitive Behaviors Associated with Sensory Impairments
Examples: repetitive behaviors occur with increased frequency in children with hearing impairment and children with visual impairment
Repetitive Behaviors Associated with Substances
Examples: stimulants, seizure medications, hypnotics, anxiolytics
Repetitive Behaviors Associated with Developmental Disorders
Examples: intellectual disability, pervasive developmental disorder
Repetitive Behaviors Associated with Psychiatric Disorders
Examples: obsessive-compulsive disorder, schizophrenia

Data from Wolraich ML, Felice ME, Drotar D (eds): The Classification of Child and Adolescent Mental Diagnoses in Primary Care: Diagnostic and Statistical Manual for Primary Care (DSM-PC), Child and Adolescent Version. Elk Grove Village, IL, American Academy of Pediatrics, 1996; and American Psychiatric Association: Diagnostic and Statistical Manual of Mental Disorders, 4th ed, text revision. Washington, DC, American Psychiatric Association, 2000.

alveolar bone growth, mucosal trauma, and even altered growth of the facial bones. Thumb or digit sucking is a common cause of paronychia in children, and it may be associated with an increased incidence of accidental ingestion. Deformities of the fingers and thumb may occur. Finally, thumb or digit sucking persisting into the elementary school years may have psychological sequelae. Peers may view these children as less desirable playmates, and frequent reprimands or nagging from parents may lead to unhappiness or insecurity.

Treatment of thumb sucking is rarely indicated in children younger than 4 years. In older children, if thumb sucking occurs infrequently (e.g., only at night) or only as a temporary response to a significant stressor, treatment is not usually indicated. Treatment is indicated if thumb sucking causes dental problems, digital malformations, or distress to the child. Children older than 4 years who suck their thumb in multiple settings or both during the day and at night are at increased risk for medical and psychological sequelae, and treatment should be considered.

A variety of successful treatments for thumb sucking have been described (Table 65-2). If thumb sucking has resulted in significant negative reactions from the parents, a moratorium on parental comments on the thumb sucking should precede any other treatment. This reduces tension between the parent and child and may decrease the sucking if it had been reinforced by parental attention. If other sources of stress or anxiety are thought to be related to the thumb sucking, a plan to manage these stressors should be developed, before the sucking is treated. All of the treatments are most effective when the child is a willing partner in the treatment.

Banging

Rhythmic banging behaviors, such as the banging of one's hand or an object against a surface, occur commonly during the development of typical infants and are not discussed further.

Head banging is the most dramatic banging behavior and the one that is most likely to elicit concern from parents. Head banging involves the rhythmic hitting of the head against a solid surface, often the crib mattress but sometimes harder surfaces. It occurs in 5% to 19% of children during the infancy and toddler years. Most often, it occurs when the child is tired or alone, such as at bedtime, but it may also occur as part of a tantrum (Sallustro and Atwell, 1978). Many

Table 65-2. **Treatments for Thumb or Digit Sucking**

Treatment	Description	Efficacy and Comments
Reminder therapy and rewards	Combine praise and rewards when not sucking with "devices" that remind child not to suck: Band-Aids on digit Loose-fitting socks over the hand at bedtime Thumb splint	Efficacies of different reminder devices have not been compared. The device the child is willing to accept will likely be the most effective.
Elastic bandage approach	Increase praise when not sucking At bedtime, an elastic bandage is wrapped from mid-arm to mid-forearm (child must request the wrap) Rewards given if child asks to have wrap and if child reports not sucking during night Professionals check on progress weekly	Most effective when habit is primarily nocturnal Do not wrap too tightly. When the arm is wrapped, the child can get the thumb in the mouth, but it requires increased effort. Success rate of 35%-60%
Aversive taste treatments	Coat thumb nail with aversive taste substance in morning, in evening, and if sucking is observed Small rewards offered to child for not sucking during specified intervals	Success rate 12/22 at 3 months and 20/22 at 1 year Aversive taste products such as Thum are commercially available.
Intraoral appliances	A variety of appliances that must be placed by a dentist; some types of appliances have resulted in injury to the child Appliance interferes with child's placement of the thumb or finger in the mouth	Efficacy is high when children want to stop sucking, but appliances can be avoided, bent, or broken by children who do not want to cooperate with treatment.

children who bang their heads have had other rhythmic behaviors, often body rocking or head rolling, earlier in infancy. Each episode of head banging usually lasts for less than 15 minutes, but episodes lasting a few hours may occur. Although the frequency of head banging declines rapidly after 18 months of age, 1% to 3% of children continue the behavior after the age of 3 years, and uncommonly it persists into the elementary school years.

Although most children who bang their heads do not have physical illness, in some cases, the onset of head banging has been associated with episodes of otitis media and with teething. In these cases, head banging has been postulated to serve as a pain-relieving function.

Head banging when a child is relaxed is not a sign of a developmental or emotional disorder. In addition, this type of head banging does not cause injuries to the brain, although occasionally it can result in callus formation or abrasions at the site of the banging. Typically developing children who head bang during tantrums do not usually injure themselves, although occasionally they may make a mistake and bang on a surface that is harder or sharper than they expect, causing a bruise or laceration. They do not usually bang on this surface a second time. Thus, with the exception of children with severe developmental disabilities (most commonly autism) or bleeding disorders, head banging does not usually result in significant injury.

Treatment primarily involves reassurance of the parents that head banging alone is not a sign of another disorder and that injury is unlikely. If the child is banging against a hard surface, padding the surface decreases the chance of abrasions or contusions. In most cases, parents should be counseled to ignore the behavior while it is occurring. This is especially true for head banging during tantrums, which may be inadvertently reinforced by the parent. This may occur if the head banging results in parental attention in the form of concern or punishment or causes a parent to give into a child's demands in an attempt to stop the head banging. In children with developmental disabilities, severe and persistent head banging may place the child at risk for significant intracranial or retinal injury and may necessitate the use of helmets and pharmacologic treatment in some cases (see the section on repetitive behaviors in children with developmental disorders in this chapter and also Chapter 74).

Body Rocking

Body rocking occurs in most infants during the first year of life. It usually begins around 6 months of age and has been reported to occur most frequently when infants are listening to music or are alone in their cribs. It usually involves a rhythmic forward and backward swaying of the trunk at the hips that occurs most frequently in a sitting position but also in the quadruped position. It can be gentle or violent enough to shake or even move a crib. The peak prevalence has been variably reported to be between 6 and 18 months of age, with a rapid decline in the prevalence of the behavior after 18 months of age. Most episodes of uninterrupted body rocking last for less than 15 minutes, but Sallustro and Atwell (1978) found that 12% of parents reported that their children had episodes lasting 15 to 30 minutes.

Body rocking persists beyond the age of 2 years in approximately 3% of typically developing children, and its prevalence may increase again at school age. On self-report measures, more than 20% of adults and college students state that they engage in body rocking. A variety of functions of rocking behaviors have been proposed, including self-stimulation and tension reduction. In children with developmental disorders and children with visual impairments, body rocking has been associated with a lack of environmental stimulation.

In most cases, body rocking does not cause significant functional impairment or stigmatization. However, cases in which rocking occurs throughout most of the day, interfering with functional activities and causing significant impairment or stigmatization, have been described in children and adults. These cases meet criteria for stereotypic movement disorder.

Breath-Holding Spells

Breath-holding spells (BHS) are not typically thought of as a repetitive behavior, but they do have some similarities to repetitive behaviors in their management. BHS are reflexive events in which the child becomes apneic at end-expiration. Typically, there is a provoking event that causes anger, fear, frustration, or minor injury and results in the child's beginning to cry. The crying may be brief or prolonged and gradually intensifying. In either case, the crying stops at end-expiration when the child becomes apneic and cyanotic or pale. In some cases, the spell resolves at this point as the child takes a deep breath (simple BHS); whereas in other cases, the event continues and the child may lose consciousness and fall to the ground. On occasion, the child may have a brief seizure. After the event, there may be a period of drowsiness.

BHS are generally reported to occur in 4% to 5% of the pediatric population. Rarely, they may begin in the first month of life but most frequently begin between 6 and 18 months of age. Approximately half of children will have resolution of their BHS by 4 years of age, and it would be very unusual for the spells to persist beyond 8 years of age (Dimario, 1999).

BHS may be divided into three subtypes: cyanotic spells, pallid spells, and mixed spells. Autonomic dysregulation is thought to play a role in all three subtypes. Cyanotic spells are the most common, and the autonomic dysregulation is thought to lead to inhibition of respiratory effort. In addition, abnormalities in pulmonary reflexes may lead to ventilation-perfusion mismatches that cause cyanosis. Pallid spells are related to an overactive vagal response leading to bradycardia or brief asystole. Children with pallid BHS may be at increased risk for having episodes of vasovagal syncope as adolescents or adults. Children with mixed spells may have both inhibition of respiratory effort and bradycardia. There is a genetic predisposition to BHS, with a positive family history found in 20% to 35% of those with BHS (Dimario, 1999).

The differential diagnosis of BHS includes seizures, cardiac arrhythmias, and a brainstem tumor or malformation (e.g., Arnold-Chiari malformation). Anemia may increase the frequency of BHS, and treatment with ferrous sulfate (5 mg/kg per day) has been reported to decrease the frequency of the spells (Daoud et al, 1997). BHS have also been reported to occur with increased frequency in children with familial dysautonomia and Rett syndrome, but they would not be the sole manifestation of these disorders. Usually, the history of a provoking event and the presence of color change before the loss of consciousness allow one to distinguish BHS from seizures on clinical grounds, but electroencephalography is occasionally helpful. If a child has pallid spells, one should consider obtaining an electrocardiogram to evaluate the child for conditions associated with cardiac arrhythmias, such as long QT syndrome.

BHS are frightening to parents. Treatment primarily involves reassurance that the spells will not harm the child and demystification of the events leading to the loss of consciousness. Parents should understand that if the child does lose consciousness, he or she will begin breathing at that time. If parents remain fearful of the events, they may try to prevent the child from experiencing pain, fear, minor injury, anger, or frustration. In trying to prevent these events, the parents may unnecessarily restrict some activities, may have difficulty setting consistent limits when the child has tantrums, or may provide attention in response to tantrums. In these cases, the parents' behavior may reinforce the tantrums, and the child may learn to trigger the BHS during tantrums to get the desired response from his or her parents.

For children with BHS who are anemic, treatment with iron is indicated, but the role of iron for children with BHS who are not anemic is less clear. Daoud and colleagues (1997) found that iron was effective in decreasing BHS even in some children who were not iron deficient. The mechanism by which iron decreases BHS is not fully understood, but it may improve some aspects of the autonomic dysregulation (Kolkiran et al, 2005). In cases of very frequent and severe (i.e., associated with seizures) pallid BHS, treatment with atropine or scopolamine may decrease the frequency of the seizures (Dimario, 1999). In very rare cases, cardiac pacemaker implantation has been used. In children with cyanotic spells, there are preliminary reports that tetrabenazine or piracetam may be beneficial.

Nail Biting

Nail biting is uncommon in preschool children but is common in school-age children, occurring in 30% to 60% of children at the age of 10 years. The incidence then decreases to about 20% during adolescence and about 10% during adulthood (Leung and Robson, 1990). During childhood, the incidence of nail biting is similar in boys and girls; but during adolescence and adulthood, more boys than girls bite their nails. Nail biting is often thought to be an indication of tension or anxiety. In some cases, the habit itself may be the source of tension within the family. It has been reported that monozygotic twins show concordance for the habit about twice as frequently as dizygotic twins do, suggesting a possible genetic contribution (Ooki, 2005).

Nail biting is usually confined to the fingernails, and most individuals bite all 10 nails equally. On occasion, specific fingernails are bitten (or avoided) selectively, and some individuals bite toenails. The bitten nails are short and irregular. Sometimes the skin margins of the nail bed or the cuticle are bitten. This may result in paronychia or, in cases of oral herpes, development of herpetic whitlow on the bitten finger. In severe cases, nail biting may cause scarring of the nail bed, bleeding, and damage to the dentition.

When specific stressors related to nail biting can be identified, treatment should be directed at helping the child to cope with these stressors. Efforts should be made to be supportive of the child because punishments, nagging, and ridicule related to the nail biting are likely to worsen the behavior or to create other difficulties in the parent-child relationship. Good nail hygiene is recommended because the rough nail edges may be irritating and worsen the behavior. In adolescents and adults, the habit reversal procedure (described later) can be effective.

Rumination

Rumination is characterized by the regurgitation of food into the mouth followed by rechewing and reswallowing or expulsion. Rumination has been described most frequently in infants and in individuals with intellectual disability, although recent reports have emphasized that it can also occur in typically developing youth (Chial et al, 2003; Khan et al, 2000).

Infant rumination syndrome is characterized by stereotypical and repetitive contraction of abdominal and related muscles leading to the regurgitation of food as described before. Typically, the onset is between 3 and 8 months of age, and the regurgitation is not associated with signs of distress. Infant rumination syndrome is associated with severe sensory and emotional deprivation causing failure-to-thrive and, if untreated, potentially lethal dehydration and malnutrition. The diagnosis can usually be made by observation of the feeding and the rumination episodes and by the fact that it does not occur during sleep or when the infant is actively involved in engaging activities. Exclusion of medical causes of regurgitation, such as pyloric stenosis, esophageal obstruction, or gastroesophageal reflux, can usually be done by history. Infant rumination syndrome should be considered in the differential diagnosis of children diagnosed with gastroesophageal reflux as many infants with rumination are initially misdiagnosed as having reflux.

Infant rumination syndrome has been described in both severely deprived home situations and neonatal intensive care units. In the latter setting, efforts to promote parent-infant bonding and to make intensive care units more responsive to the needs of infants have made infant rumination syndrome rare. Treatment involves increasing the nurturing of the infant. This may involve use of a temporary mother-substitute to hold, comfort, and feed the infant while the mother is taught to recognize and to respond to the infant's physical and emotional needs.

Rumination has been reported to occur in up to 10% of individuals with severe intellectual disability living in institutions (Fredericks et al, 1998). These individuals need a thorough evaluation for medical conditions possibly associated with rumination, such as gastroesophageal reflux, esophagitis, and anatomic defects. The possible role of medications that may alter esophageal function, such as antipsychotics and benzodiazepines, needs to be considered. Complications associated with rumination in these cases include weight loss, malnutrition, electrolyte disturbances, halitosis, and dental erosions.

As in infants, rumination is thought to begin as a self-stimulatory behavior when it occurs in individuals with intellectual disability. If rumination results in social attention or leads people to avoid asking the individual to engage in tasks, these responses may reinforce the behavior. Increasing overall levels of environmental stimulation and providing reinforcement for alternative behaviors may be effective interventions. A novel behavioral intervention is food satiation, in which large or unlimited quantities of food are provided at the meal. It is not clear exactly how increased food consumption affects rumination. Some studies suggest that a rapid increase in food consumption is necessary and that foods of a thick consistency are most effective, but further research is needed (Fredericks et al, 1998).

Rumination also occurs in typically developing youth, although it is rare. It is usually described as effortless regurgitation that occurs 5 to 30 minutes after a meal and persists for about an hour (Chial et al, 2003). Abdominal pain has been reported to occur in 40% to 80% of patients and weight loss in 40% to 60%; up to 33% will have other gastrointestinal disorders including constipation, nausea, or diarrhea. Estimates of the prevalence of coexisting psychiatric disorders have varied from less than 20% to more than 50% (Chial et al, 2003; Khan et al, 2000). A variety of relaxation therapies in combination with cognitive-behavioral therapy have been reported to be effective treatments.

Bruxism

Bruxism refers to the grinding and clenching of teeth. It is common in both children and adults. In children, the incidence of bruxism has been reported to vary between 7% and 88%, with most studies reporting an incidence between 15% and 30% (Cash, 1988). During childhood, bruxism increases in frequency, reaching a peak between the ages of 7 and 10 years and then decreasing after that. The peak at 7 to 10 years has been postulated to be related to the mixture of deciduous and permanent teeth that are present at this age.

Diurnal (daytime) bruxism should be distinguished from *nocturnal bruxism*. Nocturnal bruxism is associated with both grinding and clenching of the teeth and generates tremendous forces that produce audible grinding sounds. In general, each episode of nocturnal bruxism is brief, and during a night of sleep, an average of 42 seconds of bruxing occurs (Attanasio, 1991). In contrast, diurnal bruxism usually does not produce grinding sounds (except in individuals with central nervous system dysfunction) because it is associated primarily with clenching of the teeth, and the forces generated are less than those produced during nocturnal bruxism. Diurnal bruxism is thought to be related to other oral habits such as nail biting or lip biting and chewing on objects as these behaviors tend to occur in similar settings.

Symptoms from bruxism are less common in children than in adults. In children, the most common symptom is pain on palpation over the muscles of mastication (Cash, 1988). Other symptoms, such as dysfunction of the temporomandibular joint, recurrent headaches, and thermal hypersensitivity of the teeth, may be related to bruxism in some cases. The most common sign of bruxism is abnormal wearing of the teeth. Hypermobility of the teeth, injury to the periodontium, fractured teeth, and pulpitis may also occur.

Investigations of bruxism have not identified clear etiologic factors, and it is likely that its cause is multifactorial in most cases. Studies have centered on dental occlusion problems and psychological factors. The role of dental occlusal discrepancies in bruxism remains controversial. Whereas some studies have suggested that the creation of occlusal discrepancies in laboratory animals and in humans may lead to bruxism, many studies have failed to identify a direct relationship between nocturnal bruxism and an individual's dental occlusion. Nonetheless, evaluation of dental occlusion in individuals with bruxism is important because the occlusion affects the distribution of the forces generated by the bruxism.

Many psychological factors have been thought to be related to the occurrence of bruxism. Most frequently, bruxism is associated with emotional stress, such as frustration, anger, anxiety, or fear. Children who have experienced more unpleasant life events have been found to be more likely to have bruxism. However, many studies are limited in that they have failed to distinguish between nocturnal and diurnal bruxism. When studies are limited to individuals with nocturnal bruxism, the finding of a relationship between nocturnal bruxism and emotional stressors is less consistent (Cash, 1988). A small study suggests that there may be an association between certain psychopharmacologic treatments, including stimulants, and bruxism (Malki et al, 2004).

Treatment of bruxism in children needs to be considered carefully because bruxism is often transient and children are less likely to have symptoms than adults are. Thus, reassurance is often the only treatment that is needed. If the child is having significant symptoms, a thorough medical and dental evaluation should occur before treatment. If treatment is indicated, the options include occlusal adjustment of the dentition, interocclusal dental appliances, psychological therapies, physical therapy, and pharmacologic treatment.

Occlusal adjustment involves altering the teeth and is permanent. It should be considered only when there is an obvious interference with occlusion. A variety of interocclusal devices worn over the surface of the teeth have been developed. They have been reported to decrease bruxism in about 50% of individuals but to reduce symptoms of bruxism in an even greater number of individuals. In these latter cases, it may be the redistribution of masticatory forces that is responsible for the benefit (Attanasio, 1991).

Psychological treatments aimed at decreasing stress or teaching the individual to manage stress are helpful in some cases. Nocturnal alarms that arouse the individual during bruxing events have been shown to decrease the frequency and duration of bruxing during treatment, but the gains may not be maintained after treatment. Relaxation training and biofeedback have also been reported to have at least short-term benefit in adults, but they have not been studied in children. Exercises, heat applications, ultrasound, and transcutaneous electric stimulation are treatments that may be used by physical therapists to help manage pain associated with bruxism. Nonsteroidal anti-inflammatory agents may also be helpful for pain management.

Picking

Picking behavior may involve picking at the skin or nose. There has been little systematic study of nose picking, although survey studies suggest that more than 90% of adolescents and adults report nose picking and 4% to 8% report eating what they picked (Andrade and Srihari, 2001). Young children are often observed to pick their noses in public, whereas older children are more likely to do so when they are alone or when they feel protected from public view. Nose picking may begin in association with rhinorrhea and nasal irritation or itchiness. The most common complication of nose picking is epistaxis, and recurrent epistaxis in children is often attributed to nose picking. Other complications, such as infections or perforation of the nasal septum, are much less common but can occur. When nose picking is associated with allergic symptoms or rhinorrhea resulting from a cold, treatment with antihistamines or decongestants may be helpful.

Individuals may also pick at their skin or at scabs, resulting in excoriations, which at times may become infected. Problematic skin picking has been reported to occur in 2% to 4% of adolescents and adults (Bohne et al, 2005). The skin picking has been described either as a habit occurring during periods of stress and anxiety or as a symptom occurring in the context of obsessive-compulsive disorder or body dysmorphic disorder. In body dysmorphic disorder, skin picking occurs in response to an imagined or slight defect in the appearance of the body or skin. In some cases, skin picking may occur in response to or be exacerbated by treatment with stimulant medications. Skin picking occurs relatively commonly in adolescents and adults with Prader-Willi syndrome.

Little systematic information on the treatment of skin or nose picking is available. Emphasizing good hygiene and, with skin picking, blocking access to the picked site until it heals will be sufficient for some children. In more difficult cases, behavioral treatment using the habit reversal procedure (see the section on habit reversal) could be attempted. There are reports of treatment with serotonin reuptake inhibitors improving skin picking (Bohne et al, 2005).

Trichotillomania

Trichotillomania is a disorder characterized by recurrent pulling of one's own hair, resulting in alopecia (Fig. 65-1). Typically, hair is pulled from the scalp, eyebrows, or eyelashes, but hair pulling can involve any site in which hair grows, including axillary and pubic hair. On occasion, hair may be pulled from dolls, pets, or other materials. Many will tickle their lips or nostrils with the hair, and 5% to 18% engage in trichophagia (Tay et al, 2004). The DSM-IV classifies trichotillomania as an impulse control disorder and requires that individuals experience an increasing sense of tension before pulling out their hair and a sense of gratification or relief when pulling out their hair. However, both of these aspects of DSM-IV are controversial as trichotillomania has also been described as part of the obsessive-compulsive disorder spectrum of behaviors, and a significant portion of individuals with clinically significant hair pulling do not report this sense of tension and gratification (Bohne, 2005). Thus, the prevalence of trichotillomania depends on the criteria used to make the diagnosis. Using DSM-IV criteria, Christenson and colleagues (1991) found a lifetime prevalence of trichotillomania of 0.6% in college freshman. However, hair pulling resulting in alopecia is

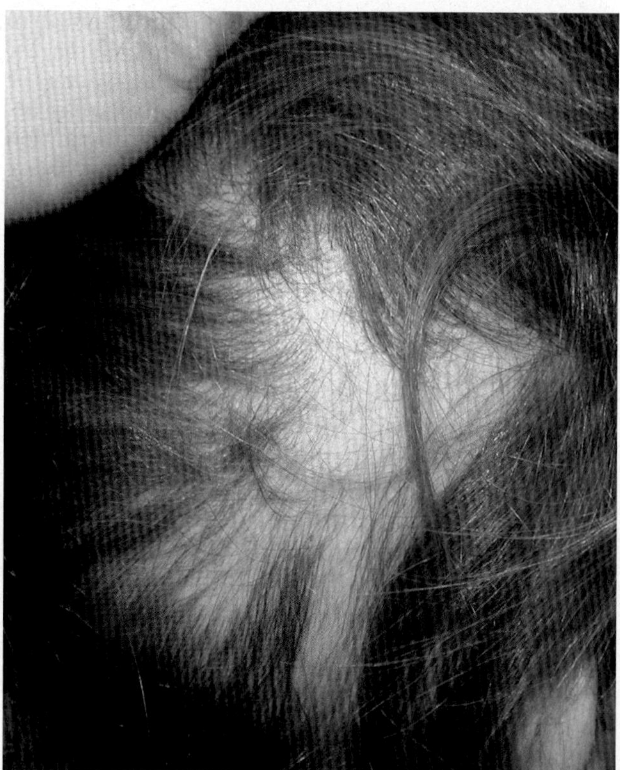

Figure 65-1. Hair loss due to trichotillomania. Note the nonanatomic distribution of the hair loss and the hairs of multiple different lengths. *(Photograph courtesy of Dr. Albert Yan.)*

more common, occurring in 1% to 2% of individuals, and hair pulling that does not result in alopecia may occur at some point during childhood or adolescence in 10% or more of the population.

The diagnosis of trichotillomania can be difficult. It is not unusual for individuals with trichotillomania to deny hair pulling and to engage in the behavior surreptitiously. Trichotillomania must be distinguished from other causes of alopecia in children, most commonly tinea capitis or alopecia areata. In both trichotillomania and tinea capitis, the hair loss is usually patchy, but tinea capitis is usually associated with scaling of the scalp and broken hairs at the scalp. In alopecia areata, the hair loss is usually complete in the affected area; whereas in trichotillomania, the hair loss is usually incomplete, and hairs of various length are present in the area of alopecia. General thinning of the hair may occur in response to severe stressors, hypothyroidism, hyperthyroidism, and certain medications.

Clinical reports suggest that at least two subtypes of trichotillomania may exist. One form that tends to begin in younger children (usually younger than 6 years) is viewed as a benign habit that is self-limited or easily treated with behavior modification or counseling. In these cases, the behavior often occurs in association with thumb sucking and may be most frequent during periods of low stimulation, such as at naptime or bedtime. When trichotillomania begins in older children and adolescents, it appears more likely to become a chronic condition and more likely to be associated with an anxiety disorder or depression. Most adults with trichotillomania describe its onset during childhood or adolescence. In all cases, the clinician should inquire about trichophagia because treatment is more urgent in children who are eating their hair to prevent formation of a trichobezoar.

A variety of treatments for trichotillomania have been described. Behavioral treatments have the best demonstrated efficacy. In young children who suck their thumb while pulling their hair, treatment of the thumb sucking (see Table 65-2) often stops the hair pulling. For others, behavioral treatments using variations of the habit reversal procedure (see the section on habit reversal) or habit reversal in combination with cognitive-behavioral therapy (Woods et al, 2006) are often effective. Treatment with hypnosis has also been described. Randomized placebo-controlled studies of selective serotonin reuptake inhibitors in adults with trichotillomania have produced equivocal results, and comparisons with the behavioral treatments have found the behavioral treatments to be more effective (Woods et al, 2006). No randomized trials of selective serotonin reuptake inhibitors in children with trichotillomania have been completed at this time.

Habit Cough

Habit cough or "psychogenic" cough has been described in children, adolescents, and rarely adults. The cough usually begins after an upper respiratory infection, but the cough persists long after the other respiratory symptoms resolve. Typically, the cough is harsh, barking, and nonproductive. Characteristically, it disappears during sleep or distraction and is not exacerbated by physical exercise. However, the ability of these symptoms to distinguish habit cough from pathologic causes of cough in children has not been systematically evaluated (Irwin et al, 2006). Thus, the diagnosis of habit cough requires a thorough evaluation to rule out other causes of chronic cough, but it also requires the clinician to consider this diagnosis when these symptoms are observed. Many children with a habit cough are misdiagnosed and treated as if they have asthma. Further complicating the diagnostic evaluation is the possibility that the child may have both a medical disorder, such as asthma or sinusitis, and habit cough.

Habit cough may be associated with psychosocial stressors. The most common are school problems as the frequent loud coughing can be very disruptive in a classroom and may lead to school absenteeism, which can reinforce the cough. Treatment of habit cough associated with school absenteeism has been found to be more difficult than when the child is still attending school. Some children with habit cough also have anxiety disorders or conversion disorder, but many children with a habit cough do not have other behavioral or emotional disorders.

If habit cough is associated with school avoidance, school problems, or other emotional or behavioral problems, a comprehensive plan to treat these problems should be developed. When habit cough is not associated with these complicating factors, an explanation and reassurance will often result in a decrease in symptoms over time. Lokshin and colleagues (1991) described one approach in which the cough is described as related to a cycle in which coughing leads to bronchial irritation, which leads to further coughing. They provided the patient a distractor to "help decrease the irritation" (e.g., breathing nebulized medicine, sipping warm water). The patient is praised for resisting the urge to cough and told that each second of delay makes further inhibition easier. When some ability to suppress the cough is noted, which usually takes about 10 minutes, they are asked, "You are beginning to feel that you can resist the urge to cough, aren't you?" When the patient goes for 5 minutes without a cough, he or she is asked, "Do you feel you can resist the urge to cough on your own?" When the patient answers this question affirmatively, the session ends and the patient is advised to repeat the procedure for any recurrence of the cough. All nine children and adolescents had a significant decrease in symptoms 1 week after treatment and at follow-up a median of 3.4 years later.

Lavigne and coworkers (1991) described an alternative behavioral treatment. Parents were instructed to monitor the frequency of the symptom during a 30-minute period of the evening. Goals were then set for a 10% reduction in the frequency of the coughing with further 10% reductions occurring when the child met the goal for 3 days. In some cases, parental praise for reaching the goal was the only reinforcer needed; in other cases, tangible rewards were offered for reaching the goal. The decrease in coughing generalized to other times of the day in all four patients in the study. Self-hypnosis has also been found to be effective for some children.

TICS AND TOURETTE SYNDROME

Tics are involuntary, brief, rapid, repetitive, nonrhythmic movements or vocalizations. Individual tics are usually classified as motor or vocal (if they involve the movement of air through the mouth or nose) and as simple or complex. Simple motor tics are those that involve an individual muscle group and include blinking, shoulder shrugging, squinting, and lip licking. On occasion, they may be a slower movement resulting in a briefly sustained abnormal posture (dystonic tics). Complex motor tics involve either a cluster of simple tics or a more coordinated pattern of movements such as touching, jumping, manipulating clothing, or facial grimacing. Simple vocal tics involve making sounds such as grunting, sniffing, and throat clearing. Complex vocal tics involve saying words, parts of words, or phrases; palilalia (repeating one's own words); or echolalia (repeating other's words). Tics are often mild and may hardly be noticed by the child or others, but on occasion they may be so severe that they interfere with classroom activities, speech, walking, and driving or cause physical injury. During the course of the day, tics tend to occur in bouts with tic-free periods in between.

Tics may be preceded by an unpleasant feeling that may be described as a pressure, urge, burning, or itch that becomes progressively more bothersome until the tic is performed. Often, individuals can temporarily suppress tics, and typically there is a reduction in the frequency and severity of tics when individuals are concentrating on mental or physical tasks and during sleep. Tics may be exacerbated by anxiety, stress, excitement, or fatigue. Tics are suggestible, and talking about the tics often increases their frequency.

Individuals with tics may be classified as having one of three tic disorders (see Table 65-1) on the basis of both the duration and the type of tics that are present. *Transient tic disorder* requires that single or multiple motor or vocal tics be present for less than 1 year. Because there is no accurate way to predict whether tics will resolve or become chronic, the diagnosis of transient tic disorder can be made only in retrospect. Nonetheless, transient tic disorder is the most common tic disorder, occurring in 12% to 24% of school-age children (Scahill et al, 2005). *Chronic tic disorder* is diagnosed when single or multiple tics, which are only motor or less commonly only vocal, occur for more than 1 year. Chronic tic disorder occurs in 1% to 2% of the school-age population. *Tourette syndrome* is diagnosed when both motor and vocal tics occur and tics have been present for more than 1 year. Tourette syndrome occurs in 0.1% to 1% of children (Scahill et al, 2005). A substantial amount of evidence from genetic studies suggests that chronic tic disorder and Tourette syndrome are part of the same spectrum of tic disorders, whereas questions remain as to whether transient tic disorders represent the mildest end of the Tourette syndrome spectrum or an unrelated tic disorder.

The modal age at onset is 7 years for motor tics and 9 years for vocal tics, but tics may occur as early as 2 years of age, and in rare cases, the new onset of tics has been described as late as the early 20s. Tourette syndrome usually has a gradual onset with one or more episodes of transient tics followed by more persistent motor and vocal tics. The tics have a waxing and waning course, tending to get worse through the late childhood and tending to improve during adolescence. By adulthood, half of patients with Tourette syndrome are free of tics (Jankovic, 2001). Over time, new tics may replace old tics or be added to the preexisting repertoire of tics. Even within the group of children with Tourette syndrome, there is a lot of variability in the severity of the tics. On occasion, complex tics involve obscene gestures (copropraxia) or obscene words (coprolalia). Even though coprolalia was included in the initial description of Tourette syndrome, it is not part of the diagnostic criteria and occurs in less than 10% of individuals with Tourette syndrome in primary care settings.

Tourette syndrome is often associated with other behavioral or learning problems. Obsessive-compulsive behaviors have been described in more than half of affected individuals, and approximately 33% meet criteria for obsessive-compulsive disorder. Attention-deficit/hyperactivity disorder (ADHD) is diagnosed in more than 50% of children with Tourette syndrome, and the ADHD symptoms often predate the onset of the tics. Anxiety disorders, depression, and learning disabilities occur in about 20% to 30% of individuals with Tourette syndrome (Freeman et al, 2000).

The familial nature of Tourette syndrome is well established. Ten percent to 15% of first-degree relatives of probands with Tourette syndrome will be diagnosed

Table 65-3. Medications Commonly Used in the Treatment of Tics

Medications	Usual Dose Range*	Potential Adverse Effects
Atypical Antipsychotics		
Risperidone	0.5-3.0 mg/day in 1-2 doses Initial dose: 0.25-0.5 mg/day	Weight gain, acute dystonia, akathisia, neuroleptic malignant syndrome, withdrawal dyskinesia, tardive dyskinesia, hyperglycemia, sedation, hypotension, amenorrhea, erectile dysfunction, decreased libido, galactorrhea
Olanzapine	2.5-20 mg/day in 1-2 doses Initial dose: 1.25-2.5 mg/day	Similar to risperidone, but fewer sexual side effects More weight gain, dyslipidemia, sedation, and anticholinergic effects
Ziprasidone	2.5-40 mg/day in 1-2 doses Initial dose: 2.5 mg/day	Similar to risperidone, but less weight gain and fewer sexual side effects More likely than risperidone to prolong the QTc interval
Typical Antipsychotics		
Haloperidol	0.5-3.0 mg/day in 2-3 doses Initial dose: 0.25 mg/day	Similar to risperidone but more extrapyramidal symptoms, dyskinesia, akathisia, fatigue, and cognitive blunting
Pimozide	1.0-6.0 mg/day in 1-2 doses Initial dose: 0.5 mg/day	Same as haloperidol and prolongation of the QTc interval
α_2-Adrenergic Agonists		
Clonidine	0.05-0.3 mg/day *or* 0.003-0.01 mg/kg/day in 3-4 doses per day	Sedation, dry mouth, constipation, irritability, sleep disturbance, nightmares, hypotension, anxiety, depression, hallucinations (rare), rebound hypertension if stopped suddenly
Guanfacine	0.5-3.0 mg/day *or* 0.015-0.05 mg/kg/day in 2-3 doses per day	Similar to clonidine, but with less sedation

*Doses above these ranges are often accompanied by significant side effects.

with Tourette syndrome, and up to 20% will have a tic disorder (Pauls, 2003). Although early studies suggested a pattern consistent with autosomal dominant inheritance, more recent studies suggest a more complex inheritance pattern involving a number of different genes. Genetic studies have also pointed to a relationship with obsessive-compulsive disorder as first-degree relatives of individuals with Tourette syndrome have a much higher incidence of obsessive-compulsive disorder than is found in the general population. A subgroup of individuals who may develop obsessive-compulsive disorder or tics after group A beta-hemolytic streptococcal infection have also been described and identified by the acronym PANDAS (pediatric autoimmune neuropsychiatric disorders associated with streptococcal infections). It is hypothesized that antibodies against streptococcal antigens cross-react with antigens in the basal ganglia, producing symptoms (Snider and Swedo, 2004), although the existence and pathophysiologic mechanism of PANDAS remain somewhat controversial (Hoekstra et al, 2004). Given that both tics and streptococcal infections are common, the diagnosis of PANDAS is complicated (see Snider and Swedo [2004] for diagnostic criteria).

Treatment of children with Tourette syndrome must focus on determining the impact of the tics as well as the impact of comorbid conditions on the child's functioning. Often, the comorbid conditions have a greater impact on the child's functioning than the tics do, and treatment should focus on the management of the identified comorbid conditions (management of the various comorbid conditions is discussed elsewhere in this book, especially Chapters 47 and 48).

The presence of tics alone is not a reason for treatment. However, when the tics cause significant disruption in motor or speech functions or are interfering with the child's social or emotional development or interpersonal relationships, then treatment is indicated. Thus, even in a referred population of children with Tourette syndrome, a significant portion are not treated with medications.

Pharmacologic treatments for tics (Table 65-3) have the best documented efficacy. Both traditional antipsychotics and the newer atypical antipsychotics that block the dopamine D_2 receptor have been demonstrated to decrease the frequency of tics in double-blind placebo-controlled trials (Scahill et al, 2006). Of the atypical antipsychotics, risperidone has been the most extensively evaluated in Tourette syndrome, and these studies suggest on average it decreases tic frequency by 35% to 50% (Scahill et al, 2006). Small placebo-controlled trials of ziprasidone and olanzapine and open label studies of some of the other atypical antipsychotics have suggested that they may also decrease tic frequency. The traditional antipsychotics haloperidol and pimozide are the only medications approved by the Food and Drug Administration for Tourette syndrome.

Potential adverse effects limit the use of antipsychotic medications. Compared with the typical antipsychotics, the atypical antipsychotics have a lower incidence of neurologic side effects, such as cognitive blunting, extrapyramidal effects, and akathisia, and probably a lower risk of tardive dyskinesia, but these adverse effects can occur. Weight gain, social phobia, and prolonged cardiac conduction times (particularly the QTc interval) can be a problem with these medications (see Table 65-3). When antipsychotics are used, they should be started at a low dose, which can be increased on a weekly basis to find the lowest effective dose. Although

Table 65-4. Components of Habit Reversal Procedure

Increase Individual's Awareness of Habit
Response description—have individual describe behavior to therapist in detail while re-enacting the behavior and looking in a mirror.
Response detection—inform individual of each occurrence of the behavior until each occurrence is detected without assistance.
Early warning—have individual practice identifying earliest signs of the target behavior.
Situation awareness—have individual describe all situations in which the target behavior is likely to occur.
Teach Competing Response to Habit
The competing response must result in isometric contraction of muscles involved in the habit, be capable of being maintained for 3 minutes, and be socially inconspicuous and compatible with normal ongoing activities but incompatible with the habit (e.g., clenching one's fist, grasping and clenching an object). For vocal tics and stuttering, deep relaxed breathing with a slight exhale before speech has been used as the competing response.
Sustain Compliance
Habit inconvenience review—have individual review in detail all problems associated with target behavior.
Social support procedure—family members and friends provide high levels of praise when a habit-free period is noted.
Public display—individual demonstrates to others that he or she can control the target behavior in situations in which the behavior occurred in the past.
Facilitate Generalization—Symbolic Rehearsal Procedure
For each situation identified in situation awareness procedure, individual imagines himself or herself beginning the target behavior but stopping and engaging in the competing response.

doses higher than those listed in Table 65-3 are sometimes used, it is unusual to have a dramatic decrease in tics at higher doses. In some cases, it can be difficult to distinguish between a response to medication and the natural waxing and waning that occurs with tics.

A small placebo-controlled trial of the dopamine D_2 receptor blocker metoclopramide demonstrated that this medication also decreased the frequency of tics (Nicolson et al, 2005). Although this medication may be less likely to cause the cognitive blunting and dysphoria that can be seen with antipsychotic medications, it can cause the extrapyramidal effects seen with antipsychotics.

The α_2-adrenergic agonists clonidine and guanfacine are less effective than antipsychotics in suppressing tics but still may be used as the first-line medication because they have fewer side effects. In addition, these medications may help decrease hyperactivity and are often used in children with ADHD and a tic disorder. Maximum efficacy of these medications may not be seen for 3 to 4 weeks; but even at this point, 50% to 75% of individuals report little or no improvement in tic symptoms. The most common side effect of these medications is sedation, which, although it tends to decrease during the first 3 to 4 weeks of treatment, still limits the use of these medications in some children. Rapid discontinuation of these medications can produce rebound hypertension as well as worsening of the tics, and thus the medications should be tapered before they are discontinued.

Injection of botulinum toxin into the muscle group involved in the motor tic or into the laryngeal folds in the case of a vocal tic has been shown to decrease tic frequency. Benefit is limited to the anatomic site of the injections, and thus this treatment is most useful for individuals with one or two problematic tics. Injections need to be repeated every 3 to 9 months. Adverse effects include weakness of the injected muscle or loss of voice volume when the laryngeal folds are injected (Scahill et al, 2005).

Nonpharmacologic treatments for tics, including habit reversal (see the section on habit reversal), relaxation training, biofeedback, and hypnosis, have been reported to decrease the frequency of tics in some individuals.

HABIT REVERSAL

Habit reversal is a multicomponent behavioral treatment (Table 65-4) that has been demonstrated to be effective for a wide variety of repetitive behaviors including thumb sucking, nail biting, hair pulling, and tics (Miltenberger et al, 1998). The components of the treatment are designed to accomplish four goals: (1) to increase the individual's awareness of the habit, (2) to teach individuals a competing response to engage in when they feel as if they are about to engage in the habit, (3) to help sustain compliance, and (4) to facilitate generalization.

Since the original description of the habit reversal, modifications of the procedure have also been demonstrated to be effective. Studies that have evaluated components of the original procedure suggest that the training to increase awareness of the habit and the use of the competing response are the most important components of the treatment. The social support procedures may have particular importance in children. Other studies have added components to the habit reversal procedure, including progressive muscle relaxation, relaxed breathing, and visual imagery.

Studies of habit reversal in young children (younger than 6 to 7 years) and those with developmental disabilities suggest that habit reversal may not be as effective in these groups as in adolescents and adults. If a child is not motivated to change the behavior or if the repetitive behavior is resulting in significant conflict between the parent and child, these issues need to be managed before attempting to implement this treatment. Teaching patients the habit reversal procedures takes some time and experience. Most often, patients are taught the habit reversal procedure by a behavioral psychologist, but other clinicians interested in treating habits can learn to use the procedure effectively.

REPETITIVE BEHAVIORS IN CHILDREN WITH DEVELOPMENTAL DISORDERS

Individuals with developmental disorders such as autism, intellectual disability, and severe visual impairments have higher rates of repetitive behaviors than are found in the general population. These behaviors may be of concern because they are stigmatizing, because they occur to the exclusion of more adaptive behaviors, or because they result in self-injury. Self-injury is the most severe form of repetitive behavior and is the focus of this section.

Self-injurious behaviors include a wide range of behaviors, such as repeated wetting and rubbing of the hands in the mouth, causing maceration of the skin; biting or picking skin, resulting in open lesions that may become infected; and violent banging of the head or other body parts against hard surfaces, which may result in fractures, retinal detachments, intracranial hemorrhages, and even death. Self-injury is a major reason for intensive special education programming and hospitalization, thus greatly increasing the costs of an individual's care.

Environmental and biologic factors are associated with repetitive behaviors in general and self-injurious behaviors in particular. Increases in repetitive behaviors have been shown to be a response to the level of environmental stimulation. Prolonged institutionalization, especially when it is associated with low levels of stimulation or confinement of the individual, has been shown to increase repetitive behaviors, which may be fulfilling a self-stimulatory function. For example, visually impaired individuals may compress the optic globe (which may result in injury to the eye) because such an action stimulates the retina. In this type of situation, increasing environmental stimulation may decrease the repetitive behaviors. On the other hand, high levels of stimulation that produce anxiety, stress, or frustration may also increase repetitive behaviors. Individuals with severe disabilities may have limited abilities to describe their experiences, requiring clinicians and caretakers to observe carefully and describe the individual and situations that elicit the repetitive behaviors.

Studies of self-injurious behavior have demonstrated that the predictable reactions of caretakers to the behavior often reinforce the behaviors. For example, this may occur when self-injury results in care providers' giving attention to the individual or responding to the behavior by allowing the individual access to materials or activities that may be otherwise restricted (e.g., food, going on a walk). Self-injurious behavior may also be reinforced when it causes care providers to remove task demands. In these cases, the self-injurious behaviors are best viewed as learned behaviors that serve as a form of nonverbal communication (Thompson and Caruso, 2002).

Biologic factors are also important in the occurrence of self-injurious behavior. Alterations in neurotransmitter systems are thought to contribute to some self-injurious behaviors. Dopamine deficiency early in development is thought to cause the nearly universal occurrence of self-biting in individuals with Lesch-Nyhan syndrome (Breese et al, 1995). It has been hypothesized that in some cases, the ability of self-injurious behavior to release endogenous opiates may maintain the behavior, and effective treatment with the opiate antagonist naltrexone has been described (Thompson and Caruso, 2002). Other biologic variables may affect the likelihood that an individual will engage in self-injurious behavior. Increased rates of self-injurious behavior have been suggested to occur in association with menstruation, physical conditions such as otitis media, fatigue, and allergies. Although it is unlikely that these factors directly cause self-injury, they could certainly decrease one's tolerance for task demands or frustration and thus alter the likelihood of a specific event's triggering self-injurious behavior.

For a review of the assessment and treatment of self-injurious behavior, see Schroeder, Oster-Granite, and Thompson (2002). Briefly, the treatment plan must first protect the individual from significant injury. In some cases, this may involve the use of helmets or even restraints, but these devices limit adaptive functioning and thus are best used as temporary measures to protect the individual until an assessment is completed and an effective treatment plan is implemented.

An assessment must include an evaluation of the potential communicative role for the behaviors. Although in some cases the communicative role of the behaviors may be clear to care providers, in many cases it is not. When it is not clear, a functional analysis may be necessary. The procedure uses interviews in combination with observation of the behavior across the day and in some cases observation of the behavior under controlled conditions to identify its communicative function. When a communicative function is identified, treatment should focus on training the individual to use more adaptive means for communicating his or her needs.

On occasion, a communicative function for the self-injurious behaviors is not identified or the self-injury is so severe that pharmacologic intervention is required. Atypical antipsychotics are the most frequently used medication in this situation. However, these medications must be used with caution because of their potential for severe side effects (see Table 65-3). Research into the use of other medications, such as mood-stabilizing anticonvulsants, opiate antagonists, serotonin reuptake inhibitors, and beta-blockers, may allow more targeted pharmacologic treatment for self-injury in the future.

SUMMARY

A wide variety of repetitive behaviors are common during childhood. They are often normal variations, such as thumb sucking and rocking, requiring only reassurance and counseling of adults not to reinforce the behaviors. However, at times, repetitive behaviors may be a sign that a child is experiencing significant distress, or the behaviors may occur in conjunction with a significant developmental, behavioral, or emotional disorder. In addition, the repetitive behaviors may become problematic because they cause stigmatization, subjective distress, or tissue damage. Evaluation of all of these possibilities is necessary for clinicians to help families develop a plan for effective intervention.

REFERENCES

Adair SM: The Ace Bandage approach to digit-sucking habits. Pediatr Dent 21:451-453, 1999.

Albin RL, Mink JW: Recent advances in Tourette syndrome research. Trends Neurosci 29:175-182, 2006.

American Psychiatric Association: Diagnostic and Statistical Manual of Mental Disorders. 4th ed, text revision. Washington, DC, American Psychiatric Association, 2000.

Andrade C, Srihari BS: A preliminary survey of rhinotillexomania in an adolescent sample. J Clin Psychiatry 62:426-431, 2001.

Attanasio R: Nocturnal bruxism and its clinical management. Dent Clin North Am 35:245-252, 1991.

Bohne A, Keuthen N, Wilhelm S: Pathologic hairpulling, skin picking, and nail biting. Ann Clin Psychiatry 17:227-232, 2005.

Breese GR, Criswell HE, Duncan GE, et al: Model for reduced dopamine in Lesch-Nyhan syndrome and the mentally retarded: Neurobiology of neonatal–6-hydroxydopamine lesioned rat. Ment Retard Dev Disabil Res Rev 1:111-119, 1995.

Cash RG: Bruxism in children: Review of the literature. J Pedodont 12:107-127, 1988.

Chial HJ, Camilleri M, Williams DE, et al: Rumination syndrome in children and adolescents: Diagnosis, treatment, and prognosis. Pediatrics 111:158-162, 2003.

Christenson GA, Pyle RL, Mitchell JE: Estimated lifetime prevalence of trichotillomania in college students. J Clin Psychiatry 52:415-417, 1991.

Daoud AS, Batieha A, Al-Sheyyab M, et al: Effectiveness of iron therapy on breath-holding spells. J Pediatr 130:547-550, 1997.

Dimario FJ: Breath-holding spells in childhood. Curr Probl Pediatr 29:281-299, 1999.

Fredericks DW, Carr JE, Williams WL: Overview of the treatment of rumination disorder for adults in a residential setting. J Behav Ther Exp Psychiatry 29:31-40, 1998.

Freeman RD, Fast DK, Burd L, et al: An international perspective on Tourette syndrome: Selected findings from 3500 individuals in 22 countries. Dev Med Child Neurol 42:436-447, 2000.

Friman PC, Leibowitz J: An effective and acceptable treatment alternative for chronic thumb and finger sucking. J Pediatr Psychol 15:57-62, 1990.

Hoekstra PJ, Anderson GM, Limburg PC, et al: Neurobiology and neuroimmunology of Tourette's syndrome: An update. Cell Mol Life Sci 61:886-898, 2004.

Irwin RS, Glomb WB, Chang AB: Habit cough, tic cough and psychogenic cough in adult and pediatric populations: ACCP evidence-based clinical practice guidelines. Chest 129:174s-179s, 2006.

Jankovic J: Tourette's syndrome. N Engl J Med 345:1184-1192, 2001.

Khan S, Hyman PE, Cocjin J, Di Lorenzo C: Rumination syndrome in adolescents. J Pediatr 136:528-531, 2000.

Kolkiran A, Tutar E, Atalay S, et al: Autonomic nervous system functions in children with breath-holding spells and effects of iron deficiency. Acta Paediatr 94:1227-1231, 2005.

Kravitz H, Boehm JJ: Rhythmic habit patterns in infancy: Their sequence, age of onset, and frequency. Child Dev 42:399-413, 1971.

Lavigne JV, Davis AT, Fauber R: Behavioral management of psychogenic cough: Alternative to the "bedsheet" and other aversive techniques. Pediatrics 87:532-537, 1991.

Leckman JF, Riddle MA: Tourette's syndrome: When habit-forming systems form habits of their own? Neuron 28:349-354, 2000.

Leung AKC, Robson LM: Nailbiting. Clin Pediatr 29:690-692, 1990.

Lokshin B, Lindgren S, Weinberger M, et al: Outcome of habit cough in children treated with a brief session of suggestion therapy. Ann Allergy 67:579-582, 1991.

Malki GA, Zawawi ZH, Melis M, Hughes CV: Prevalence of bruxism in children receiving treatment for attention deficit hyperactivity disorder. J Clin Pediatr Dent 29:63-68, 2004.

Miltenberger RG, Fuqua RW, Woods DW: Applying behavior analysis to clinical problems: Review and analysis of habit reversal. J Appl Behav Anal 31:447-469, 1998.

Nicolson R, Craven-Thuss B, McKinay DB: A randomized, double-blind, placebo-controlled trial of metoclopramide for the treatment of Tourette's disorder. J Am Acad Child Adolesc Psychiatry 44:640-646, 2005.

Ooki S: Genetic and environmental influences on finger-sucking and nail-biting in Japanese twin children. Twin Res Hum Genet 8:320-327, 2005.

Pauls DL: An update on the genetics of Gilles de la Tourette syndrome. J Psychosom Res 55:7-12, 2003.

Rapp JT, Vollmer TR: Stereotypy I: A review of behavioral assessment and treatment. Res Dev Disabil 26:527-547, 2005.

Sallustro MA, Atwell CW: Body rocking, head banging, and head rolling in normal children. J Pediatr 93:704-708, 1978.

Scahill L, Sukhodolsky DG, Williams SK, et al.: Public health significance of tic disorders in children and adolescents. Adv Neurol 96:240-248, 2005.

Scahill L, Erenberg G, Berlin CM, et al: Contemporary assessment and pharmacotherapy of Tourette syndrome. J Am Soc Exp Neurother 3:192-206, 2006.

Schroeder SR, Oster-Granite ML, Thompson T (eds): Self-Injurious Behavior. Washington, DC, American Psychological Association, 2002, pp 3-22.

Snider LA, Swedo SE: PANDAS: Current status and directions for research. Mol Psychiatry 9:900-907, 2004.

Tay YK, Levy ML, Metry DW: Trichotillomania in childhood: Case series and review. Pediatrics 113:e494-498, 2004.

Thelen E: Normal infant stereotypes: A dynamic systems approach. *In* Sprague RL, Newell KM, (eds): Stereotyped Movements: Brain and Behavior Relationships. Washington, DC, American Psychological Association, 1996, pp 139-164.

Thompson T, Caruso M: Self-injury: Knowing what we are looking for. *In* Schroeder SR, Oster-Granite ML, Thompson T, (eds): Self-Injurious Behavior. Washington, DC, American Psychological Association, 2002, pp 3-22.

Wolraich ML, Felice ME, Drotar D (eds): The Classification of Child and Adolescent Mental Diagnoses in Primary Care: Diagnostic and Statistical Manual for Primary Care (DSM-PC), Child and Adolescent Version. Elk Grove Village, IL, American Academy of Pediatrics, 1996.

Woods DW, Flessner C, Franklin ME, et al: Understanding and treating trichotillomania: What we know and what we don't know. Psychiatr Clin North Am 29:487-501, 2006.

Part VIII OUTCOMES—DEVELOPMENTAL

66 MOTOR DEVELOPMENT AND DYSFUNCTION

Paul H. Lipkin

Vignette

Daniel has been referred by his pediatrician for a neurodevelopmental consultation because of concerns noted at his 9-month preventive care visit. At his 6-month visit, he was able to roll in both directions and sit with two-arm support. He could grab a toy with each hand and transfer it from one hand to the other. Dr. Gordon noted then that Daniel's tone was slightly increased at his hips, but he was meeting gross and fine motor milestones close to the usual time. At the 9-month visit, the office staff administered developmental screening, and Dr. Gordon noted concerns in the area of gross motor development. Daniel was unable to sit without support and could not crawl on his hands and knees. He passed his screening in all other areas of development, including fine motor. During the physician's examination, Daniel's tone remained increased at the hips, and his deep tendon reflexes in the legs were brisk. Dr. Gordon referred Daniel for further medical consultation and to a local physical therapist and the county early intervention program.

At the neurodevelopmental consultation, Dr. Barthel confirmed Daniel's delay in gross motor development and found that Daniel had strong and persistent asymmetric tonic neck and tonic labyrinthine reflexes and bilaterally increased hip adductor and ankle tone. She explained to Daniel's parents that his gross motor delay was due to cerebral palsy, primarily affecting his legs. A magnetic resonance imaging scan was performed later, verifying that Daniel had periventricular leukomalacia. Daniel began an active treatment program of physical therapy. He pulled himself to stand at 10 months, but did not sit without support until 15 months. By 24 months, Daniel was walking on his toes with two-hand support. After medical treatment for the increased tone, Daniel began walking independently at 2½ years of age.

Development of the core competencies of movement and posture, commonly referred to as *motor development*, emerges from the development of the central and peripheral nervous systems and the musculoskeletal system. The term *coordination* is often used synonymously. Movement begins early in the intrauterine period and continues throughout childhood, with completion of development achieved in the early adult years.

Motor development is typically subdivided into gross motor and fine motor skills. Gross motor development involves large full body movements, primarily involving the trunk and legs, and culminates during the aptly named "toddler" years with independent walking, climbing, and running. Fine motor development is centered on shoulder, arm, and hand use, with refinement of movement into small hand and arm movements such as the pincer grasp of late infancy or throwing during the toddler and preschool years. Delays in the acquisition of these skills result from slow or disrupted maturation of the nervous or musculoskeletal system, causing a spectrum of motor disorders. These motor dysfunctions range from mild motor coordination disorders to the more severe disorders of central nervous system–based cerebral palsy or peripheral motor system–based neuromuscular disease.

INTRAUTERINE AND NEONATAL MOTOR DEVELOPMENT

The development of movement in the fetus occurs in response to the neurologic maturation of the subcorticospinal system and ascending myelination from the spinal cord between 24 and 34 weeks of gestation (Allen, 2005; Amiel-Tison and Gosselin, 2001). The subcorticospinal, or extrapyramidal, system originates in the brainstem and connects to the thalamus and cerebellum. It serves to maintain posture against gravity and upper extremity flexor tone. With the upward progression of myelination, tone progresses in a caudocephalic direction.

In the past, with the inability to examine tone, movement, and posture in the fetus directly, insight into the early foundations of the development of children's motor skills depended on the recognition by the pregnant woman of fetal movement. This recognition typically occurs with the onset of quickening at approximately 16 to 18 weeks' gestation, when the mother perceives large amplitude and prolonged fetal movements. Greater understanding of intrauterine motor development in the embryonic and fetal periods emerged with advances in intrauterine monitoring and imaging (DiPietro, 2005). Spontaneous movement is now observable with real-time ultrasound, as are elicited movements occurring in response to stimuli such as light, sound, or vibration. Frequency and amplitude of fetal movements can be measured with Doppler actigraphy.

Specific movement patterns of increasing complexity across time have been recognized in the fetus. Movements are first discernible on ultrasound at 7 weeks' gestation. Over the course of the next 8 to 10 weeks, a large variety of specific movements of the head, trunk, and limbs emerge (Table 66-1) (de Vries et al, 1984). Quick, jerky startles or twitches begin at the same time that rapid and smoother large amplitude general movements of the limbs, trunk, and head are seen. Across time, these general movements become more graceful and flowing, and more variable in speed and amplitude, forming the basis for Prechtl's assessment of general movement (Einspieler and Prechtl, 2005). Isolated jerking arm or leg movements have their onset between 9 and 12 weeks, varying from small to large amplitude, and may involve extension, flexion, rotation, abduction, or adduction. These progress to smoother movements and extend to the hand with development of a clasp or grasp by approximately 18 to 19 weeks of gestation. Isolated head flexion and rotation are seen at 9 to 14 weeks, with complete fetal rotation seen during this same period. The fetal hand makes contact with the face at 10 to 16 weeks.

Subsequent intrauterine motor development evolves into the more complex movements visible in preterm infants and typical during infancy. The emergence of thumb sucking, grasping, and generalized rotation and writhing movements is seen, and motor activity related to other functions, such as eye movement, breathing, and swallowing (DiPietro, 2005; Einspieler and Prechtl, 2005). Prechtl postulated a functional significance to fetal movement (Prechtl, 1984). Some movements may serve an intrauterine function, such as the prevention of adhesions and the stasis of skin circulation. Fetal turning in the second half of pregnancy may assist in intrauterine positioning, including the more common vertex presentation and the less common breech presentation. Other movements may serve later postnatal functioning, such as intrauterine breathing and ocular movements, or may promote structural development, such as shaping of the skeletal system.

Primitive reflexes also emerge during the intrauterine period and play an important role in later motor development. These are stereotyped, complex, automatic movement patterns that are suppressed during infancy by higher cortical functions, allowing the emergence of voluntary movement (Capute et al, 1982, 1984). Mouth opening in response to perioral stimulation, equivalent to the postnatal rooting response, emerges at 9.5 weeks, and head turning emerges at 11.5 weeks. The palmar grasp emerges at 10.5 weeks, with finger flexion in response to palm stroking, and the plantar grasp is seen at 11.5 weeks, with toe flexing in association with sole stimulation (Allen, 2005; Peiper et al, 1963). By 25 to 30 weeks of gestation, the Moro reflex, asymmetric tonic neck reflex (ATNR), and Galant (lateral trunk incurvature) reflex have been observed in preterm infants (Allen and Capute, 1986). The lower extremity placing, positive support, and stepping reflexes are in place before term.

As a result of previously described neurologic development, tone and deep tendon reflex development in preterm infants occurs in a specific order and pattern in a caudocephalad direction, from the lower to the upper extremities, and a centripetal pattern, from distal to proximal (Allen and Capute, 1990). Allen and Capute (1990) noted lower extremity flexor tone at 29 weeks' gestation–age equivalent, with strong tone noted by 36 to 38 weeks' gestation–age. In the upper extremities, flexor tone was first noted at 31 weeks' gestation–age, and strong tone was seen at 37 to 39 weeks' gestation–age, slightly behind the lower extremities. Trunk tone developed later than extremity tone, at nearly term-age (36 to 40 weeks). A similar pattern was observed for all reflexes, including deep tendon reflexes, primitive reflexes, and pathologic reflexes, with lower extremity development occurring before upper and with distal reflexes emerging before proximal.

Table 66-1. Onset of Fetal Movements

Fetal Movement	Week of Onset (Approximate)
First movements	7
Startle or twitch	8-16
General movements	8-16
Isolated arm or leg movements	9-12
Finger movements	12-14
Hand-face contact	10-16
Stretch	10-16
Rotation	10-13

Adapted from de Vries JIP, Visser GHA, Prechtl HFR: Fetal Motility in the First Half of Pregnancy: Continuity of Neural Functions from Prenatal to Postnatal Life. London, Spastics International Medical Publications, 1984, pp 46-64.

The evolution of movement, tone, and reflexes in preterm and newborn infants serves as the foundation for the neonatal developmental measures, including measures for full-term infants and measures for infants at high risk for developmental disabilities, particularly preterm. The most widely used measures have drawn on the observations of pioneers such as Gesell, André-Thomas, Saint-Anne Dargassies, and Brazelton (Lipkin, 2005). The Dubowitz examination has become incorporated into practice in newborn nurseries and neonatal intensive care units around the world (Dubowitz et al, 1999, 2005). Originally published in the 1970s, this examination is now in its second edition. Conceived of as a neurologic examination of the newborn, the examination looks at motor development through measurement of spontaneous movement, trunk, neck, and extremity tone and posture; deep tendon and primitive reflexes; and protective responses.

Similarly, the examination of Amiel-Tison (Amiel-Tison and Gosselin 2001; Gosselin et al, 2005) looks at posture and tone of the trunk and limbs, active movement (referred to as active tone), and primitive reflex development. The Prechtl examination is centered on spontaneous general movement (Einspieler and Prechtl, 2005). Other examinations now available that specifically look at early motor development include the Einstein Neonatal Neurobehavioral Assessment Scale, the Neurobehavioral Assessment of the Preterm Infant, the Test of Infant Motor Performance, and the Alberta Infant Motor Scale (Darrah et al, 1998; Majnemer and Snider, 2005; Piper et al, 1992).

INFANT AND EARLY TODDLER MOTOR DEVELOPMENT

Motor development of the fetus occurs in response to maturation of the subcortical pathways and ascending myelination from the spinal cord, whereas motor development from birth reflects myelination of the corticospinal, or pyramidal, and corticobulbar tracts (Allen, 2005; Amiel-Tison and Gosselin, 2001; Sarnat, 1989). The pyramidal tract originates in the motor and premotor cortex, then connects to the basal ganglia, crosses at the medulla, and descends laterally in the spinal cord (Allen, 2005; Sarnat, 1984, 1989). Myelination occurs upward to the cortex and in a descending fashion from the pons to the spinal cord, beginning at approximately 32 weeks of gestation with rapid progression through 2 years of age, but continuing at a slower rate until at least 12 years of age (Allen, 2005; Amiel-Tison and Gosselin, 2001; Sarnat, 1989). This process results in inhibition of the subcortical system, including the primitive reflexes, and promotes development of the postural responses and upright posture, walking, and fine motor control.

At birth, a newborn term infant has the same repertoire of movement as that seen in a fetus and a preterm infant, consisting of the generalized and reflexive movements described previously. The change in environment from the uterus to the extrauterine world does not effect a change in these movements, suggesting a neurologic predeterminism (Prechtl, 1984). The environmental changes are vast, however, from submersion in amniotic fluid in a dark, restricted cavity to the experience of exposure to gravity; changing light, sound, and temperature; and absence of spatial restriction. The adaptive roles of these movements adjust with the environmental change. Although the movements assist in fetal positioning during the intrauterine period, they play new roles after birth (Einspieler and Prechtl, 2004). Alternating fetal leg movements become the stepping reflex. Finger and toe flexion become the newborn's palmar and plantar grasps. Lateral head movements turn toward stimulated perioral areas as the rooting reflex used in the newborn's feeding. Intrauterine sucking and swallowing of amniotic fluid similarly serve in feeding. New responses to the changed environment are identifiable in neonates. New respiratory function requires the protective reflexes of coughing and sneezing. Vestibular responses, including the tonic labyrinthine reflex and the Moro response, assist in spatial orientation and protection.

In the first 2 months after birth, the predominant observable spontaneous movements are the general movements described in Prechtl's method (Einspieler and Prechtl, 2004, 2005). From term birth to 6 to 9 weeks of age, these movements are writhing in nature, small to moderate in amplitude and speed. The writhing movements evolve into fidgety movements, small movements of the neck, trunk, and limbs in an awake infant, of moderate speed and variable acceleration. From 3 to 6 months, fidgety movements occur together with saccadic arm movements, wiggling-oscillating, swipes, finger manipulation, reaching and touching, leg lifting, hand-knee contact, trunk rotation, and axial rolling. The fidgety movements persist until approximately 20 weeks, when intentional antigravity movements dominate.

The brainstem-mediated primitive reflexes that emerged during the intrauterine period peak or increase in intensity during early infancy (Capute, 1986, Capute et al, 1984). The Moro response that results in arm abduction followed by adduction and flexion with sudden head extension is strongest at term. The ATNR, the "fencer" posture of ipsilateral limb extension and contralateral flexion produced with lateral head rotation, peaks at 8 to 10 weeks. The tonic labyrinthine reflex is produced with head extension or flexion with the infant and results in leg extension and shoulder retraction with head extension or leg flexion and shoulder protraction with head flexion. It peaks at approximately 5 weeks in an infant lying supine and 20 weeks in an infant lying prone. Other notable reflexes that can be elicited in early infancy include the Galant, positive support response, symmetric tonic neck reflex, lower and upper extremity placing responses, stepping, crossed extension, and downward thrust response (Capute, 1986).

At approximately 8 to 10 weeks after birth, the infant's pattern of movement alters. The changes now result in new movement and activity centered on adaptation to the extrauterine environment. Antigravity responses emerge owing to advancing central neural development and increased muscle power (Prechtl, 1984). The primitive reflexes are progressively suppressed and later inhibited by higher cortical pathways by approximately 6 months post-term, allowing for the progressive emergence of volitional movement (Capute et al, 1982, 1984).

Rolling from prone to supine is associated with a marked decline in the Moro response and lesser decreases in the ATNR and tonic labyrinthine reflex. Rolling from supine to prone occurs in association with a decrease in the tonic labyrinthine and Moro reflexes. Marked diminutions of the ATNR and its eventual absence and a decrease in the tonic labyrinthine reflex are necessary for independent sitting.

Postural and protective responses emerge with the developmental of voluntary motor activity, allowing the infant to maintain equilibrium and righting (Capute, 1986). They promote the acquisition of the gross motor skills represented as developmental milestones in infancy. The Landau reaction appears between the second and third month of life. This midline righting response consists of neck, trunk, and leg extension in response to voluntary neck extension, best observed in prone suspension. The derotative righting response is a segmental rolling reaction in the axial plane that follows development of the Landau response and is a precursor to voluntary rolling. With head rotation, segmental derotation occurs in the opposing direction from the shoulders, followed by the trunk, hips, and lower extremities. With leg rotation, similar segmental derotation occurs in a caudocephalad direction. Upper extremity protective extension is seen anteriorly by 6 months and serves to maintain the seated infant upright. It occurs posteriorly at approximately 10 months, allowing for pivoting while sitting and protection for the standing child when cruising and walking.

Gross Motor Milestones

The development of voluntary movement occurs in a predictable, sequential fashion tied to the decline of the primitive reflexes and the emergence of the postural responses. The sequence and pattern reflect the ongoing maturation of the nervous system discussed previously. In a tradition harking back to the early 20th century works of pediatric child development pioneers such as Gesell (Gesell, 1925; Gesell and Amatruda, 1941; Gesell et al, 1940), specific skills or "milestones" are used to mark the progress of a child's development. Although motor development is clearly a slow and progressive series of small changes and advancements, identification of readily observable milestones assists in the monitoring of a child's development by clinicians evaluating the health and well-being of the child. The age at which these milestones occur also can assist the diagnostic evaluation of a child who is delayed for age in motor skills (Table 66-2).

Although milestones are presented as occurring at distinct ages, these typically represent a mean age of accomplishment of these skills. As a mean, these ages are ideally established through large population sampling with calculation of a statistically defined normal range of accomplishment, including the general population mean and standard deviation. Such norms were first established on North American infants by the observations of Gesell in the early 20th century (Gesell et al, 1940), with more recent updating by Capute and colleagues (Capute et al, 1985). Broader geographic norms now also have been obtained by the World Health Organization, with data derived from Ghana, India, Norway, Oman, and the United States (WHO Multicentre Growth Reference Study Group, 2006). In the discussion that follows, milestone ages are based on the mean ages reported in these data. Although these samples represent the strongest scientifically derived clinical information on normal motor development, these norms are based on modest population sizes, from distinct geographic, social, and demographic communities.

Table 66-2. Gross Motor Developmental Milestones*

Gross Motor Skill	Mean Age
Rolling prone to supine	3.6
Rolling supine to prone	4.8
Sitting supported	5.3
Sitting unsupported	6.3
Commando crawling	6.7
Coming to sit from lying	7.5
Crawling	7.8
Pulling to stand from sitting	8.1
Cruising	8.8
Walking independently (unsupported)	11.7
Walking backward	14.3
Running	14.8

*Mean age in months based on 381 children.
Adapted from Capute AJ, Shapiro BK, Palmer FB, et al: Normal gross motor development: The influences of race, sex and socio-economic status. Dev Med Child Neurol 27:635-643, 1985.

Motor development of an infant typically occurs in the cephalocaudad and proximodistal directions, with the first voluntary movements beginning in the head, shoulder, trunk, and hips. As discussed earlier, this pattern is linked to the process of myelination of the nervous system's central and peripheral pathways. The first 2 months of an infant's life are dominated by the general writhing and fidgety movements described by Prechtl (1984). Discerning specific milestones in a young infant is readily accomplished through observation of the infant in the prone position. In a series of changes, the infant progresses from minimal volitional head movement to head and chest elevation by 4 months.

The newborn begins simply turning the head to the side and clearing his or her nose. By 1 month of age, the infant lifts the head upward off a flat surface, and at 2 months, the infant lifts the head and chest off the surface. At 3 months, tone and strength extend to the shoulders and upper arms, as the infant lifts the head and upper trunk high and props on the elbows. Prone strength extends to the lower trunk as the 4-month-old infant props himself on extended arms. With this newly acquired strength in arm extension and flexion, the infant now can accomplish at 3 to 4 months the easily observable skill of rolling from prone to supine. Within the next month, at approximately 5 months of age, antigravity strength is extended to the hips, and derotative righting emerges, allowing the child to roll voluntarily from supine to prone.

Further advancement in the postural righting of the trunk and the lateral protective responses (upper extremity protective extension), along with inhibition of primitive reflexes, promotes the development of sitting (Capute et al, 1982). The infant can sit propped at 5 months, with the development of independent unsupported sitting at 6 months. Both of these sitting milestones require the infant to be placed in the sitting upright position. By 7 to 8 months, the infant can move from the lying to the sitting position.

From birth to 6 months old, the infant is primarily stationary, with minimal ambulation beyond the short distance achieved with rolling. Beginning at 7 months of age, the infant strives to explore the environment, first by pulling his or her body through arm flexion and extension in prone, or commando, crawling (also referred to as creeping and combat crawling). As tone and strength progress caudally, the infant develops the ability to stand on hands and knees (quadruped stance). Alternating reciprocal movements emerge at a mean age of 8 months, and crawling begins, allowing the infant to move greater distances with greater efficiency and with independence around a room. This same strengthening that occurs in the lower trunk, hips, and upper legs, coupled with the greater strength of the arms and shoulder girdle, also enables the infant to pull himself or herself from the sitting or quadruped position to standing. Self-achievement of this standing position at 8 months represents a crucial, often unnoted milestone in the infant's development, as he or she achieves the upright erect posture unique to humans and some primates. With its development, the infant is prepared for greater motor independence.

The infant's movement is initially restricted by limits in lower leg, ankle, and foot strength and in reciprocal leg movements. By 9 months, the infant takes his or her first steps, however, relying on upper trunk and arm support, commonly referred to as cruising, and usually seen occurring along furniture. These cruising movements rely primarily on sets of leg abduction and adduction movement emanating from the hip. With strengthening of hip and knee flexion and extension and ankle dorsal and plantar flexion, the infant propels himself or herself forward toward independent walking. The infant begins walking dependent on others for upper extremity and trunk support, similar to that needed in cruising. As greater strength emerges in the lower extremities, the child progressively loosens his or her grip from the supporting person. The child's dependence changes progressively from two supportive hands with the child's arms held high to a single supportive hand held low. At an average age of 12 months, the infant releases hand support and becomes a toddler, walking by taking his or her first independent steps.

Demographic differences in ages of motor skill development have been noted. Studies of these factors have shown race differences consistently favoring black over white, whereas gender and socioeconomic status do not seem to affect age of motor milestone achievement (Capute et al, 1985; Kelly et al, 2006). Ethnic differences also have been reported, but these often disappear when socioeconomic status is factored in (Kelly et al, 2006).

Independent walking begins with the toddler maintaining balance with his or her hands in a "high-guard" posture, with the arms elevated near the shoulder line, and a wide base, with the legs maintained apart. With advancing motor skill, the toddler's arms progressively lower from mid guard to eventual low guard, with the hands placed alongside the lower trunk. The legs also shift toward the midline across time, narrowing the walking base. At approximately 14 months, the newly independent toddler can walk backward. Early gross motor development culminates when the toddler begins to run at 15 months of age, propelling himself or herself forward with both feet briefly off the ground.

Table 66-3. **Fine Motor Developmental Milestones***

Fine Motor Skill	Mean Age
Unfisting	2.7
Manipulates fingers in midline	3
Transfer across the midline	4.1
Whole-hand object grasp	4.7
Overhand raking grasp	5.7
Three-finger pincer grasp	7.8
Isolated finger use	9.4
Mature two-finger pincer grasp	9.9
Voluntary object release	11
Makes mark with crayon	11.5
Places 10 cubes in a cup	16
Spontaneously scribbles	17.5
Builds 3-cube tower	21.3
Builds horizontal train with blocks	22.3
Makes horizontal and vertical strokes	25.1
Builds block train with chimney	29.6
Builds 3-cube bridge	31.1
Draws circle	32.6
Draws person with head plus one other body part	35.7

*Mean age in months based on 1239 children.
Adapted from Accardo PJ, Capute AJ: The Capute Scales: Cognitive Adaptive Test/Clinical Linguistic and Auditory Milestone Scale (CAT/CLAMS). Baltimore, Paul H. Brooks, 2005.

Fine Motor Milestones

Fine motor development progresses in the upper extremity most notably in the proximodistal direction, beginning at the shoulder girdle and progressing to the crucial milestone of the mature pincer grasp. When first observed in the newborn, the primitive reflexes limit the purposeful arm movements to general writhing movements, as previously described, with all other movements being obligatory and reflexive. The palmar grasp reflex allows a newborn to clench an object when pressure and touch are applied to the palm; however, this is not volitional in nature.

The first readily recognizable fine motor skill that is crucial to normal development is unfisting. With the loss of palmar grasp reflex, the infant can extend the fingers and maintain the hand in an open position at 4 months of age, paving the way for further progressive fine motor development (Accardo and Capute, 2005). The child's generalized writhing and fidgety movements, emanating primarily from the shoulder and upper arm, advance with the diminishing of the ATNR, tonic labyrinthine, and Moro reflexes into more refined and purposeful movements in the distal direction. These advances are first shown at 3 to 4 months when the infant can bring his or her hands to midline and manipulate and play with his or her fingers (Accardo and Capute, 2005) (Table 66-3). Infants typically put their hands in their mouth at this time. While placing the hands in midline position, the infant's fine motor skills remain unilateral at this time with an inability to cross this midline. Improved control of movements from the shoulder girdle and upper arm allows the infant to swipe crudely and imprecisely at dangled objects.

At 5 months, the infant can take an object offered close to the chest and held at midline and grasp it in a single hand through simple unfisting on the other side. The skills advance across the midline at 6 months with the development of the corpus callosum. At this time, the infant is no longer bound to ipsilateral grasping. Dangled objects such as rings and held objects such as 1-inch blocks are easily grabbed. The infant can be observed grabbing an object with one hand, passing it to the midline, and transferring it to the contralateral side. As grasping skills and arm control advance, transfer of smaller objects is seen.

The infant's grasp progresses from the proximal palm toward the distal fingertips over the next several months and from the ulnar (medial) to the radial (lateral) side. The first grasping at 5 months involves an overhand raking movement. A large object is approached with the palm from above, the fingers flexing together and grasping the object. With the skills advancing more distally and in a radial or lateral direction, the infant relies less on palm support and gains control of movement of individual fingers originating on the ulnar side with the fifth digit. Beginning first with five-finger grasping, the child develops increasing finger strength, allowing him or her to grasp progressively smaller objects with fewer fingers, shifting from five to three or four and then two fingers.

The infant's grasp reaches the crucial milestone of the mature pincer grasp at 10 months, when the child can grasp a small object, such as a bead or small food snack, through apposition of the thumb and first finger only. This mature finger control also is observable at this age with isolated first finger pointing ("the pointer") and placing of the finger in small holes (testable in a pegboard). Infant fine motor development culminates with the crucial and often unnoted voluntary release response at 12 months, shown with purposeful dropping of an object, handing it to another person, or placing it.

LATE TODDLER AND PRESCHOOL MOTOR DEVELOPMENT AND BEYOND: HIGHER ORDER MOTOR DEVELOPMENT

After children accomplish the crucial gross motor milestone of independent walking and fine motor skills of the mature pincer grasp, pointing, and voluntary release, further development centers on adaptation to the ambulation and prehension demands of daily life. New skills acquired are centered on functional independence in the home and community. Recognized milestones beyond infancy and the early toddler years are commonly centered on such activities of daily living. Given that children who acquire these skills are not affected by major disability, such as cerebral palsy, norms for these milestone are not well established. The ages typically stated, including the ages stated here, are accepted estimates of the mean age of acquisition of these skills.

Gross Motor

In gross motor development, advancement occurs in strength and balance. A child advances from walking to running at 15 months. A child can creep upstairs and descend them backward at this age. At 18 months, the child can walk up the stairs with hand assistance and may descend through bouncing on the buttocks. The toddler becomes a facile climber onto higher surfaces and in and out of chairs. A squatting position can be assumed and used during exploratory play. By 24 months of age, the child can sit on a riding toy and propel himself or herself forward with his or her feet. The child gains ease and speed in running and climbing, and these are actively used in outdoor play. At 2½ years, the toddler confidently climbs and descends stairs using two feet per step while holding the railing. The toddler can jump with two feet down a step. A large ball can be kicked.

A 3-year-old ascends and descends stairs using alternating feet. The child can run faster and turn with ease, pedal a tricycle ("3 wheels at 3 years") with appropriate steering, and kick a ball with greater force. Brief one-legged standing can be elicited, and cross-legged sitting is observed. At 4 years, the child ascends and descends stairs similar to an adult. Climbing slides, ladders, and trees can be achieved. The 4-year-old typically advances in riding skills to a "four-wheeled" bicycle with training wheels ("4 wheels at 4 years"). One-legged standing, hopping, and jumping can be accomplished for several seconds. By the time a typical child is 5 years old and is entering elementary school, he or she is capable of refined gross motor skills, allowing various indoor and outdoor skills to develop for athletic activities, such as ball play and gymnastics, or musical activities, such as dance (Sheridan et al, 1997).

Fine Motor

After achieving development of the mature pincer grasp, further skill development is observable through object manipulation, easily incorporated into tasks observed at home or tested by a developmental examiner. At this point, fine motor development evolves into more advanced visual motor development, relying on these motor skills and visual perception and intellectual problem solving. Developmental professionals use the monitoring of fine motor development during the toddler years and beyond in the evaluation of intelligence and prehension and graphomotor skill. Adults observe the child using these skills in play, daily living tasks, and learning.

Gesell's early observations (Gesell et al, 1940) established patterns for childhood graphomotor development. Current norms from the Capute Scales (Accardo and Capute, 2005) establish that the average toddler can pick up a large crayon and make a mark at 12 months. At 15 months, the toddler scribbles in imitation. The toddler develops spontaneous scribbling by 18 months. At 24 months, the toddler holds a pencil and imitates a stroke, and then draws specific horizontal and vertical strokes at 30 months. By age 3 years, the child draws a circle and begins to draw a human figure. Continued graphomotor development results in the child drawing increasingly complex geometric figures, commonly referred to as the Gesell figures, including a square at 4 years old, triangle at 5 years, vertical diamond at 7 years, cylinder at 9 years, and three-dimensional cube at 12 years (Taylor, 1959), as well as advanced human figures (Goodenough, 1975).

The child begins to use blocks in play and advances in constructions of increasing complexity (Accardo and Capute, 2005; Gesell et al, 1940). When the child is 15 months old, he or she can stack two cubes, advancing to three cubes at 21 months (Capute and Accardo, 1996a). At 18 months, the child can place 10 cubes into a cup. At 24 months, the child can build a horizontal four-cube train, adding a chimney at 30 months. At 3 years, the child can build a bridge with three cubes, and at four can build a complex gate figure with five cubes. By age 5, the child can build stairs with six cubes.

Other key fine motor milestones include development of clear handedness for play and writing at 24 months. The toddler also first throws a ball at 18 months. The child attempts to fold paper at 24 months, and achieves folding with a crease at 2½ years.

In activities of daily living or adaptive skills, advances in eating and dressing skills are observable by parents. With the mature pincer grasp in place, the infant first eats with his or her fingers at 9 months. By 15 months, the child can drink from a cup without assistance and can scoop with a spoon. The child achieves spearing with a fork at approximately 24 months and spreads with a knife by age 4. In dressing, the toddler removes clothing at 24 months and dresses himself or herself at 3 years. The child can achieve zipping and buttoning of clothing at an average of 4 years of age, and learns to tie shoes at approximately 5 years.

MEASURING MOTOR DEVELOPMENT: IDENTIFYING CHILDREN WITH MOTOR DISABILITIES

Understanding normal or typical motor development offers the pediatric health care provider and other early childhood professionals an opportunity to provide families anticipatory guidance related to typical development and related home safety. The motor milestones also serve to identify children with neurodevelopmental disabilities in developmental surveillance, screening, and evaluation. A child with a motor disability, ranging from high prevalence minor neuromotor abnormalities and coordination disorders to more severe and lower prevalence disorders such as cerebral palsy, the myopathies, and the muscular dystrophies, deviates from the typical pattern.

These disabilities, whether mild or severe, also may serve as a marker for other neurodevelopmental disabilities, including the spectrum of intellectual and communication disabilities. Delays in motor development and associated hypotonia are typical in children with genetic disorders and intellectual disabilities, such as Down syndrome, fragile X syndrome, and Prader-Willi syndrome, often bringing these diagnoses to light. Similarly, motor ataxia associated with delays is seen in children with Angelman syndrome. Although Down syndrome is typically identified through physical stigmata, hypotonia and motor delay are important factors in the developmental pattern of affected children.

Developmental Surveillance

Pediatricians and other child health care professionals perform developmental surveillance at every well-child preventive care visit (American Academy of Pediatrics Council on Children with Disabilities et al, 2006). Surveillance is defined as a flexible, longitudinal, continuous, and cumulative process whereby knowledgeable health care professionals identify children who may have developmental problems. Surveillance consists of five components: (1) eliciting and attending to the parents' concerns about their child's development, (2) documenting and maintaining a developmental history, (3) making accurate observations of the child, (4) identifying risk and protective factors, and (5) maintaining an accurate record of documenting the process and findings. Through obtaining the developmental history based on the norms of early motor development, and through the observation of a child's motor skills, the primary care provider can begin the process of early identification in the medical home of children with motor disabilities.

The history and observation can help determine whether a child has developmental delay, deviancy, dissociation, or regression in motor development (American Academy of Pediatrics Council on Children with Disabilities et al, 2006; Capute and Accardo, 1996b). A child most commonly is found to be delayed in milestone attainment across several visits, or developmentally delayed, acquiring skills later than do age peers. Other children may be noted to achieve milestones out of the typical order, defining developmental deviancy or deviation. In the spastic diplegia form of cerebral palsy, a child may be noted to have deviancy in gross motor development, as when a child rolls and crawls, but does not sit. Deviancy also can be seen in fine motor development, as when a child with the spastic hemiplegic form of cerebral palsy can grasp with the left hand, but remains fisted on the right.

Developmental dissociation is commonly observable, as when a child with delayed or deviant motor development has a different pattern of development in other areas. A child with cerebral palsy may have delays or deviancy in motor skills, while having better skills in language and intellect. A child with intellectual disability or a child with an autism spectrum communication disorder may have typical or mildly delayed motor development, while experiencing delays or deviancy in attaining language skills. Finally, a child who plateaus in motor development or frankly loses motor skills has developmental regression, suggestive of a serious metabolic or neurodegenerative disorder, such as a leukodystrophy. Surveillance can be a powerful tool for the pediatric health care provider for the early identification of neurodevelopmental disabilities.

Developmental Screening

Developmental screening involves the administration of a brief standardized tool to identify children at risk for a developmental disorder. Screening is performed when surveillance suggests that the child may be at risk for a motor disability and at the routine scheduled well-child visits at 9, 18, and 24 or 30 months (American Academy of Pediatrics Council on Children with Disabilities et al, 2006). Children with severe neurodevelopmental motor disorders typically present during the first year of life and would be identifiable through screening at the 9-month visit, whereas children with milder motor problems may be identified at the later screening visits.

Developmental screening tests vary from general tests that screen multiple areas of development to tests that are domain-specific or disorder-specific (American Academy of Pediatrics Council on Children with Disabilities et al, 2006). They also vary in style, with some based solely on parental report, while others require direct testing of the child. In the screening of motor development, all of the general instruments include screening of gross motor and fine motor development, although specific sensitivity, specificity, and validity for the screening of motor disorders vary from limited to unknown.

Although there are no disorder-specific tools that screen for cerebral palsy or other motor disorders, two screening tests specific to motor development have been published. The Motor Quotient (Capute and Shapiro, 1985) uses normed gross motor milestones to calculate developmental ages and quotients. Based on its single study of 144 children, it has been noted to have moderate sensitivity and specificity (American Academy of Pediatrics Council on Children with Disabilities et al, 2006). The Early Motor Pattern Profile (Morgan and Aldag, 1996) is a physician-administered standard examination of movement, tone, and reflex development with a simple 3-point scoring system. In its single published study of 1247 high-risk infants, moderate to high sensitivity was reported (American Academy of Pediatrics Council on Children with Disabilities et al, 2006).

Medical and Developmental Evaluation of Motor Development

When a child is identified as at increased risk for a developmental disorder through surveillance or screening, he or she should be referred for further medical and developmental evaluation (American Academy of Pediatrics Council on Children with Disabilities et al, 2006). These evaluations seek to identify the specific developmental disorder at the root of the child's problem in motor development. A detailed medical evaluation includes in-depth investigation of a child's medical and developmental history and detailed physical and neurologic examinations, including assessments of tone, reflex, posture, and movement (Amiel-Tison and Gosselin 2001; Capute et al, 1984; Hadders-Algra, 2005; Touwen, 1979). Age-specific standardized neuromotor examinations have been developed and show promise for prognosticating a child's motor outcome (Hadders-Algra, 2005). In its aims to establish the cause of a child's motor problems and to diagnose specific medical conditions, this examination may call for further laboratory investigation, including neuroimaging, cytogenetic testing, blood chemistries, and metabolic testing (Shevell et al, 2003; Ashwal et al, 2004).

The developmental evaluation of motor skill may provide prognostic information to a family through the standardized measurement of function and severity. It also can be useful for the initiation of appropriate early childhood therapeutic interventions. Several standardized instruments are available for the detailed developmental evaluation of a child's motor development (Tieman et al, 2005). The Bayley Scales of Infant Development (Bayley, 1993), Peabody Developmental Motor Scales (PDMS-2) (Folio and Fewell, 2000), and the Toddler Infant Motor Evaluation (TIME) (Miller and Roid, 1994) are widely used norm-referenced tests typically administered by psychologists, physical therapists, or occupational therapists. Each instrument requires up to 1 hour for completion. Test results are given as standard scores, percentile ranking, or age-equivalent performance.

Other instruments, such as the Pediatric Evaluation of Disability Inventory (PEDI) (Haley, 1992) and the Gross Motor Function Measure (GMFM) (Russell et al, 2002), have been developed for measurement of motor function, intervention planning, developmental progress, and motor outcome in children with cerebral palsy and related motor disabilities. These norm-referenced and criterion-referenced instruments are used primarily by physical therapists. Scoring of the PEDI includes standard, scaled, and fit scores and reflects functional skills attained. The GMFM is designed for measurement of motor change using a percentage score and an interval-level score.

The wide spectrum of motor disabilities can be identified through the combination of detailed diagnostic medical and developmental evaluation of a child with delay, deviancy, or regression in motor development. This methodology is capable of identifying severe motor disabilities, such as cerebral palsy and the neuromuscular disorders. It also can identify children with milder delays, as seen in children with hypotonia and in children with other associated developmental disorders. Finally, medical and developmental motor evaluation also may recognize children with coordination and graphomotor disorders, which primarily affect school function, adaptive skills, and athletic abilities. This group of children also is at high risk for associated developmental disorders in learning, language, and behavior.

Monitoring a child's motor development through surveillance; use of standardized screening of motor development at periodic intervals; and performance of medical and developmental evaluations of children recognized with delay, deviancy, dissociation, or regression in motor skills can identify children with neurodevelopmental motor disabilities. Through identification of these disabilities, early medical treatments and developmental interventions can be promptly initiated in the affected child, offering the child and the family the best hope for optimal long-term outcome.

SUMMARY

A child's motor development is a continuous process from fetal life to maturity, evolving from development of the central and peripheral nervous systems. Fetal movement serves as the foundation for newborn motor skills, through the emergence of tone, primitive reflexes, and general fetal movements. From the newborn period through early infancy, inhibition of the fetal reflexes and increasing strength and tone lead to progressive advancement in voluntary gross motor and fine motor skills. Gross motor skills develop during infancy toward independent walking, followed by expanded ambulation skills, including running, climbing, and engagement in community-based activities such as athletics and dance. Surveillance, screening, and evaluation of gross motor and fine motor skills from fetal life into later childhood are used in the identification, treatment, and intervention of children with neurodevelopmental motor disabilities.

REFERENCES

Accardo PJ, Capute AJ: The Capute Scales: Cognitive Adaptive Test/ Clinical Linguistic and Auditory Milestone Scale (CAT/CLAMS). Baltimore, Paul H. Brookes, 2005.

Allen MC: Assessment of gestational age and neuromaturation. Ment Retard Dev Disabil Res Rev 11:21-33, 2005.

Allen MC, Capute AJ: The evolution of primitive reflexes in extremely premature infants. Pediatr Res 20:1284-1289, 1986.

Allen MC, Capute AJ: Tone and reflex development before term. Pediatrics 85(3 Pt 2):393-399, 1990.

American Academy of Pediatrics Council on Children with Disabilities, Section on Developmental and Behavioral Pediatrics, Bright Futures Steering Committee, and Medical Home Initiatives for Children with Special Needs Project Advisory Committee: Identifying infants and young children with developmental disorders in the medical home: An algorithm for developmental surveillance and screening. Pediatrics 118:405-420, 2006.

Amiel-Tison C, Gosselin J: Neurological Development from Birth to Six Years: Guide for Examination and Evaluation. Baltimore, Johns Hopkins University Press, 2001.

Ashwal S, Russman BS, Blasco PA, et al: Practice parameter: Diagnostic assessment of the child with cerebral palsy: Report of the Quality Standards Subcommittee of the American Academy of Neurology and the Practice Committee of the Child Neurology Society. Neurology 62:851-863, 2004.

Bayley N: Bayley Scales of Infant Development. New York, Psychological Corporation, 1993.

Capute AJ: Early neuromotor reflexes in infancy. Pediatr Ann 15:217-218, 221-223, 226, 1986.

Capute AJ, Accardo PJ: The infant neurodevelopmental assessment: A clinical interpretive manual for CAT-CLAMS in the first two years of life, part 1. Curr Probl Pediatr 26:238-257, 1996a.

Capute AJ, Accardo PJ: A neurodevelopmental perspective on the continuum of developmental disabilities. *In* Capute AJ, Accardo PJ (eds): Developmental Disabilities in Infancy and Childhood. Baltimore, Paul H. Brookes, 1996b, pp 1-22.

Capute AJ, Palmer FB, Shapiro BK, et al: Primitive reflex profile: A quantitation of primitive reflexes in infancy. Dev Med Child Neurol 26:375-383, 1984.

Capute AJ, Shapiro BK: The motor quotient: A method for the early detection of motor delay. Am J Dis Child 139:940-942, 1985.

Capute AJ, Shapiro BK, et al: Motor functions: Associated primitive reflex profiles. Dev Med Child Neurol 24:662-669, 1982.

Capute AJ, Shapiro BK, Palmer FB, et al: Normal gross motor development: The influences of race, sex and socio-economic status. Dev Med Child Neurol 27:635-643, 1985.

Darrah J, Piper M, Watt MJ: Assessment of gross motor skills of at-risk infants: Predictive validity of the Alberta Infant Motor Scale. Dev Med Child Neurol 40:485-491, 1998.

de Vries JIP, Visser GHA, Prechtl HF: Fetal motility in the first half of pregnancy. *In* Prechtl HFR (ed): Continuity of Neural Functions from Prenatal to Postnatal Life. London, Spastics International Medical Publications, 1984, pp 46-64.

DiPietro JA: Neurobehavioral assessment before birth. Ment Retard Dev Disabil Res Rev 11:4-13, 2005.

Dubowitz LMS, Dubowitz V, Mercuri E: The Neurological Assessment of the Preterm and Full-term Newborn Infant. London, Mac Keith Press, 1999.

Dubowitz L, Ricci D, Mercuri E: The Dubowitz neurological examination of the full-term newborn. Ment Retard Dev Disabil Res Rev 11: 52-60, 2005.

Einspieler C, Prechtl HFR: Prechtl's Method on the Qualitative Assessment of General Movements in Preterm, Term, and Young Infants. London, Mac Keith Press, 2004.

Einspieler C, Prechtl HF: Prechtl's assessment of general movements: A diagnostic tool for the functional assessment of the young nervous system. Ment Retard Dev Disabil Res Rev 11:61-67, 2005.

Folio MR, Fewell RR: Peabody Developmental Motor Scales-2 (PDMS-2). Texas, Pro-Ed, Inc, 2000.

Gesell A: The Mental Growth of the Pre-school Child: A Psychological Outline of Normal Development from Birth to the Sixth Year, including a System of Developmental Diagnosis. New York, Macmillan, 1925.

Gesell A, Amatruda CS: Developmental Diagnosis: Normal and Abnormal Child Development, Clinical Methods and Practical Applications. New York, PB Hoeber, 1941.

Gesell A: The First Five Years of Life: A Guide to the Study of the Preschool Child, from the Yale Clinic of Child Development. New York, Harper & Row, 1940.

Goodenough FL: Measurement of Intelligence by Drawings. New York, Arno Press, 1975.

Gosselin J, Gahagan S, Amiel-Tison C: The Amiel-Tison Neurological Assessment at Term: Conceptual and methodological continuity in the course of follow-up. Ment Retard Dev Disabil Res Rev 11:34-51, 2005.

Hadders-Algra M: The neuromotor examination of the preschool child and its prognostic significance. Ment Retard Dev Disabil Res Rev 11:180-188, 2005.

Haley SM: Pediatric Evaluation of Disability Inventory (PEDI): Development, Standardization and Administration Manual. Boston, New England Medical Center Hospital, Department of Rehabilitation Medicine. PEDI Research Group, 1992.

Kelly Y, Sacker A, Schoon I, et al: Ethnic differences in achievement of developmental milestones by 9 months of age: The Millennium Cohort Study. Dev Med Child Neurol 48:825-830, 2006.

Lipkin PH: Towards creation of a unified view of the neurodevelopment of the infant. Ment Retard Dev Disabil Res Rev 11:103-106, 2005.

Majnemer A, Snider L: A comparison of developmental assessments of the newborn and young infant. Ment Retard Dev Disabil Res Rev 11:68-73, 2005.

Miller LJ, Roid GH: The T.I.M.E. Toddler and Infant Motor Evaluation, a Standardized Assessment. Tucson, Therapy Skill Builders, 1994.

Morgan AM, Aldag JC: Early identification of cerebral palsy using a profile of abnormal motor patterns. Pediatrics 98(4 Pt 1):692-697, 1996.

Peiper A, Nagler B, Nagler H: Cerebral Function in Infancy and Childhood. New York, Consultants Bureau, 1963.

Piper MC, Pinnell LE, et al: Construction and validation of the Alberta Infant Motor Scale (AIMS). Can J Public Health 83(Suppl. 2): S46-S50, 1992.

Prechtl HFR: Continuity of Neural Functions from Prenatal to Postnatal Life. London, Spastics International Medical, 1984.

Russell DJ, Rosenbaum PL, et al: Gross Motor Function Measure (GMFM-66 and GMFM-88) User's Manual. London, Mac Keith Press, 2002.

Sarnat HB: Topics in Neonatal Neurology. Orlando, Grune & Stratton, 1984.

Sarnat HB: Do the corticospinal and corticobulbar tracts mediate functions in the human newborn? Can J Neurol Sci 16:157-160, 1989.

Sheridan MD, Frost M, Sharma A: From Birth to Five Years: Children's Developmental Progress. London, Routledge, 1997.

Shevell M, Ashwal S, Donley D, et al: Practice parameter: Evaluation of the child with global developmental delay: Report of the Quality Standards Subcommittee of the American Academy of Neurology and The Practice Committee of the Child Neurology Society. Neurology 60:367-380, 2003.

Taylor EM: Psychological Appraisal of Children with Cerebral Defects. Cambridge, MA, Published for the Commonwealth Fund [by] Harvard University Press, 1959.

Tieman BL, Palisano RJ, et al: Assessment of motor development and function in preschool children. Ment Retard Dev Disabil Res Rev 11:189-196, 2005.

Touwen BCL: Examination of the Child with Minor Neurological Dysfunction. London, Heinemann Medical [for] Spastics International Medical Publications, 1979.

WHO Multicentre Growth Reference Study Group: WHO Motor Development Study: Windows of achievement for six gross motor development milestones. Acta Paediatr Suppl 450:86-95, 2006.

67 CEREBRAL PALSY

LAURIE GLADER AND ANN TILTON

Vignette

David is a 7-year-old boy with spastic diplegic cerebral palsy. He was born at 29 weeks' gestation and had early difficulties with airway management and feeding. An ultrasound revealed periventricular cystic formation, but no evidence of bleeding. David ultimately did well and was discharged home from the neonatal intensive care unit at the gestational age of 38 weeks. He was able to breastfeed and had no need for oxygen.

David developed a quick social smile and clearly indicated interest in his environment early on. He developed good facility with his hands, playing with toys and feeding himself. He was delayed, however, in his ability to sit, crawl, and pull to stand. A brain magnetic resonance imaging study at age 2 years indicated periventricular leukomalacia, and he was diagnosed with cerebral palsy.

Now in first grade, David is a happy student who participates in the regular academic curriculum. He continues to have motor symptoms, primarily in his lower extremities. David walks with a walker and wears ankle foot orthoses to optimize his gait. He has received botulinum toxin A (Botox) injections on several occasions to reduce the tone in his calves. Drooling has been an indolent problem, and his parents have spoken with the pediatrician about the possibility of starting treatment with an anticholinergic medication. David also wears glasses for esotropia. He attends multiple medical and therapeutic appointments for issues related to his cerebral palsy. Overall, however, David is thriving and has frequent play dates with classmates after school.

DEFINING TERMS

Cerebral palsy (CP) is the most common motor disorder in children; current prevalence estimates range from 1.5 to 2.5 of every 1000 live births (Surveillance of Cerebral Palsy in Europe, 2000). The definition of CP has evolved over time, but has been updated more recently. "CP describes a group of disorders of the development of movement and posture, causing activity limitations that are attributed to non-progressive disturbances that occurred in the developing fetal or infant brain. The motor disorders of CP are often accompanied by disturbances of sensation, cognition, communication, perception, and/or behaviour, and/or by a seizure disorder" (Bax et al, 2005).

CP represents a group of movement disorders diverse in their etiologies, but with the commonality that they are caused by static change to the young developing brain. A period of observation is required to make the definitive diagnosis. If there is clinical indication of progressive symptoms, another diagnosis must be considered. Although the more recent definition preserves the motor disorder as a prominent feature, it emphasizes the likelihood of other impairments, which may be even more significant functionally or developmentally.

This expanded definition includes a classification scheme with reference to motor abnormalities, associated impairments, anatomic and radiologic findings, and causation and timing. In this scheme, the movement disorder is classified as spastic, dystonic, athetotic, ataxic, or mixed (Table 67-1). An emphasis was placed on the need to address formally the functional impact of all of the impairments with objective scales.

ETIOLOGY

CP encompasses a heterogeneous group of etiologies and a wide variation in clinical presentation. Despite advances in medical care, CP seems to have been increasing in prevalence since the mid-1970s because of advances in neonatal care for premature infants. The risk of CP is 90 per 1000 live births if the birth weight is less than 1500 g, and 50% of CP cases occur in infants with a birth weight of less than 1000 g (Miller, 1998).

Neuroimaging supports the current thought that antepartum causes of CP, such as brain malformations, intrauterine vascular malformations, and infection, are far more common than birth asphyxia (Truwit et al, 1992). Although intrapartum asphyxia originally was thought to be a major contributor to CP, it accounts for only 10% to 20% of cases (Nelson and Ellenberg, 1986). The most frequent perinatal/neonatal etiologies in low-birth-weight infants are periventricular leukomalacia, periventricular hemorrhage, and cerebral infarction, whereas in infants of normal birth weight, hypoxic-ischemic encephalopathy is most often the cause. Postnatal causes, such as meningitis, typically result in

Table 67-1. **Classification of Movement Disorders in Cerebral Palsy**

Spastic	83%
Diplegia: legs more involved than arms	44%
Quadriplegia: all four extremities equally involved	6%
Hemiplegia: one-sided involvement, usually arm more than leg	33%
(Double hemiplegia: arms involved more than legs, usually asymmetric)	
Dyskinetic	17%
Hyperkinetic or choreoathetoid	
Dystonic	
Ataxic	
Mixed	

Table 67-2. **Possible Presentations of Cerebral Palsy**

Abnormalities in muscle tone (high and low) or involuntary movements
Delay in motor milestone acquisition or qualitative differences in motor development
Persistent primitive reflexes
Delay in development of protective reflexes
Hallmarks of spasticity (upper motor neuron signs)
- Increased deep tendon reflexes
- Clonus
- Extensor plantar response

No signs of developmental regression

Table 67-3. **Evaluation of a Child with Cerebral Palsy**

Brain MRI if prior neuroimaging is not conclusive or etiology is unclear
Audiologic assessment
Visual assessment
Developmental assessment
In children with hemiplegia: evaluation for coagulopathy

MRI, magnetic resonance imaging.

spastic CP and represent only about 10% to 18% of cases (Pharoah et al, 1989). Overall, this disorder affects more than 100,000 Americans younger than age 18 years. The 30-year survival rate is approximately 87%. The economic impact of CP on society is significant.

IDENTIFICATION AND MANAGEMENT

It is important for the general practitioner to recognize a child with evolving signs and symptoms of CP (Table 67-2). Generally, the diagnosis is made when a child presents with delays in motor milestone acquisition and abnormalities of tone, coupled with specific findings on examination that indicate a cerebral origin. Even if skills are not delayed chronologically, they may be qualitatively affected (e.g., a hemiplegic infant crawls in an asymmetric manner). It is important to establish that there has been no loss of previously acquired function or sign of progressive neurologic dysfunction, eliminating neurodegenerative disorders that may masquerade as CP.

The history provides an important context for making the diagnosis of CP. Details about birth, such as prematurity, complications of labor and delivery, or multiple gestation, are red flags. Feeding difficulties are another red flag. Poor latching onto the breast or bottle, choking while eating, or difficulty keeping food in the mouth all may reflect oromotor dysfunction. Concerns about a child's reduced or exaggerated response to sound or visual input are important to pursue given the prevalence of sensory deficits in children with CP, as is any report of stigmata of seizure activity.

On examination, the key to identifying an infant with CP generally lies in the neurologic presentation. General appearance may reveal dysmorphic features, which can be helpful in identifying a genetic etiology. Most often, however, a child with early signs of CP presents with abnormal tone. Even in a child who ultimately develops spasticity, tone may be diminished. Increased deep tendon reflexes, clonus, and persistent primitive reflexes are classic hallmarks of upper motor neuron dysfunction. Pathologic reflexes always should raise concern, such as a crossed adductor response, in which tapping the reflex on one leg elicits a response in the opposite leg. This response indicates a lack of appropriate inhibition of the reflex and pathologic overflow. An important concept in the neurologic development of children with CP is the combination of delay or qualitative difference in motor milestone acquisition accompanied by persistent primitive reflexes (i.e., tongue thrust, asymmetric tonic neck reflex), along with the delay in the development of protective reflexes (i.e., righting response, parachute response) (Dorman and Pellegrino, 1998).

When CP is suspected, the workup always must seek an explanation for the underlying etiology because it may have implications for prognosis, risk of recurrence, family counseling, and medical management. Toward this end, a neuroimaging study almost always should be obtained (Table 67-3). Magnetic resonance imaging (MRI) is the preferred modality. Studies indicate that in 89% of cases of children with CP there are abnormal findings on MRI (Russman and Ashwal, 2004). MRI is superior to CT in identifying the timing of the insult.

Because of the association of hearing and visual impairments with CP, hearing and ophthalmologic assessments should be obtained. Similarly, developmental testing to look at cognitive skills and language disorders is indicated because of their high prevalence in CP. Laboratory studies are not needed to confirm the diagnosis. The exception is children with hemiplegia, who warrant evaluation for coagulopathy (Mercuri et al, 2001). Other studies, such as electroencephalogram, chromosomal analysis, metabolic workup, and TORCH (toxoplasmosis, other [congenital syphilis and viruses], rubella, cytomegalovirus, and herpes simplex virus) titers, should be pursued on a case-by-case basis, depending on clinical suspicion. Referral to a neurologist is often warranted for assistance in clarifying the diagnosis. Even if the diagnosis of CP is not confirmed, therapeutic interventions to work on general developmental stimulation and motor milestone acquisition are indicated. Toward this end, the primary care provider can assist the family in obtaining prompt referral to early intervention services.

ROLE OF THE PRIMARY CARE PROVIDER

The role of the primary care provider includes careful monitoring of the child along with synthesizing information from the plethora of subspecialists, therapists, and teachers who become involved in a child's overall management. Knowing the potential secondary complications allows for optimal medical management. Because the caregiver plays the central role in the day-to-day management of the child, he or she should be a central figure in setting treatment goals. At each stage of goal setting, treatment planning, and plan modification, it is vital to obtain complete information from the caregiver regarding the effects of previous treatments and the details of the child's current situation.

The comprehensive treatment of a child with CP requires a team approach with multiple professionals, including an educational or developmental specialist, the child's primary care physician, a pediatric neurologist, a pediatric orthopedic surgeon or physiatrist, a physical therapist, an occupational therapist, a social worker, and other professionals cognizant of the child's home, leisure, medical, and school environment. A primary focus on reducing muscle overactivity is common, but in the best situation should be only one aspect of the overall treatment plan. Multiple factors influence the determination of the goals and the approach to the individualized treatment plan. These factors include the age of the child, the presence of complicating issues (e.g., seizures, cognitive or sensory impairment, respiratory compromise, and gastrointestinal difficulties), the family's financial capabilities, and the ability to comply with home treatments or return for regular follow-up. The priority is always whether the proposed treatments would benefit quality of life and function.

SPASTICITY AND INVOLUNTARY MOVEMENTS: NEUROMUSCULAR COMPLICATIONS AND MANAGEMENT

A child with CP by definition has abnormal posture and movement, and virtually all children with the disorder have neuromuscular and orthopedic sequelae. Typical orthopedic complications include extremity contractures, hip subluxation or dislocation, and scoliosis, depending on the type and severity of the CP. Frequently, as the mechanical relationships of the body change over time, a child also can develop chronic pain. This pain may be secondary to positioning, muscle spasms, or fractures, as osteopenia secondary to disuse is a common problem in nonambulatory children with CP. Twenty-five percent of adults with CP report chronic pain (Odding et al, 2006). Understanding the manifestations and complications of these symptoms is invaluable in developing an effective treatment plan. Most children with CP should be followed by an orthopedic surgeon for routine surveillance. The goals of treatment include optimizing skeletal alignment, mobility, and postural control.

Spasticity and Dystonia

Spasticity is defined as an increase in velocity-dependent tonic stretch reflexes with exaggerated tendon jerks. The term *spasticity* is often meant to include other forms of muscle overactivity within the upper motor neuron syndrome (i.e., clonus, flexor spasms, dystonia, and cocontraction of agonists and antagonists). Cocontraction leads to rigidity, characterized by low-velocity resistance, lack of synergistic movement around the joint, and absence of return of the limb to a fixed posture or angle (Sanger et al, 2003). Dystonia is defined as a movement disorder in which involuntary, sustained, or intermittent muscle contractions cause twisting and repetitive movements, abnormal postures, or both. The distinctions between these various forms of muscle overactivity may be clinically relevant because certain medications or other treatment modalities may produce better results with some forms than others.

The Modified Ashworth scale, a 6-point measure of limb resistance to passive movement, is a simple and clinically useful tool for quantifying spasticity (Table 67-4). Resistance that is due to spasticity, which is medically amenable to treatment, must be distinguished from resistance that is due to muscle fibrosis, which does not respond to pharmacologic interventions and may require orthopedic surgery to address.

In upper motor neuron disorders such as CP, symptoms reflect increased muscle activity ("positive" symptoms) and loss of function ("negative" symptoms). Positive symptoms include increased reflexes, spasticity, and dystonia, and negative symptoms include weakness and loss of fine motor dexterity. Positive symptoms are generally amenable to treatment, whereas negative symptoms are not. The negative symptoms typically have the largest effect on function.

Table 67-4. **Modified Ashworth Scale**

For Evaluating Resistance to Passive Stretch in an Isolated Muscle Group	
0	No increase in muscle tone
1	Slight increase in muscle tone, manifested by a catch and release or by minimal resistance at the end range of motion when the part is moved in flexion or extension/abduction or adduction
1+	Slight increase in muscle tone, manifested by a catch, followed by minimal resistance throughout the remainder (less than half) of the ROM
2	More marked increase in muscle tone through most of the ROM, but the affected part is easily moved
3	Considerable increase in muscle tone, passive movement is difficult
4	Affected part is rigid in flexion or extension (abduction or adduction)

ROM, range of motion.

From Bohannon RW, Smith MB: Interrater reliability of a modified Ashworth scale of muscle spasticity. Phys Ther 67:206-207, 1986.

Evaluation and Treatment of Neuromuscular Complications

Motor impairment is frequently the most visible sign of CP, and reducing tone is often the first priority. Reducing tone is not always synonymous with improvement, however. The goal of treating muscle overactivity in CP is to improve function, comfort, and care. The hope is that appropriate intervention would prevent future musculoskeletal complications, such as fixed contractures and subluxation. In the broad view, a physical therapy program and regular physical activity form the basis of every treatment program.

Many treatment modalities are available to address the problem of muscle overactivity. Oral medications act systemically and may have a role in global tone reduction. The well-described cognitive and other systemic side effects are likely to limit their use, however. Injections of botulinum toxin (BTX), alcohol, or phenol may be delivered to specific muscle groups and provide focal tone reduction. Intrathecal baclofen offers a modality to reduce tone in patients with significant and widespread muscle overactivity, especially in the lower extremities. Selective dorsal rhizotomy may be considered for a subset of young patients with good underlying strength and no contribution to their impairment from dystonia. Treatment with any of these therapies at an early stage may postpone or reduce the need for orthopedic surgery later on.

Physical Therapy and Equipment Use

Physical therapy programs focus on maintaining and improving strength, range of motion, balance, and coordination. The hope is that the patient can accomplish these goals while being engaged in activities he or she naturally enjoys. Although active play may promote these goals, compensatory strategies and postures may prevent the full range of motion of some affected muscle groups, which sets the stage for development of contractures. An aggressive home program of stretching under the direction of a physical therapist is standard and necessary, although often difficult. An often underrecognized difficulty in patients with CP is accompanying weakness. Strengthening offers direct benefits and improvement in the overall feeling of well-being. Additional approaches provided by physical therapists include use of orthotics, hydrotherapy, and horseback riding, and modalities such as biofeedback, heat, cold, electrical stimulation, and massage.

There is renewed interest in constraint-induced therapy for children with hemiplegia, based on new understanding of brain plasticity and clinical results in stroke patients. Constraint-induced therapy forces the patient to perform functional tasks with the less capable limb by constraining the use of the more functional one. Despite its promise, the use of constraint-induced therapy in patients with CP is challenging because 6 hours per day of inhibited movement is required. It remains to be seen whether a less rigorous treatment program may be able to offer similar benefits (Taub et al, 2004).

Children with CP are often weak, which may be especially significant in the trunk muscles, affecting posture, head control, and upper extremity movements. The stiffness produced by muscle overactivity may be used by the patient to compensate for this weakness, and tone reduction, especially with systemic medication, may unmask underlying, previously unrecognized weakness. Strength training may improve ambulation and other functional activities and may provide psychological benefits as well, especially in adolescents, increasing the ability and willingness to participate in school or community activities (McBurney et al, 2003).

An ankle-foot orthosis is often used to treat dynamic equinus, in which toe strike replaces heel strike at the beginning of the stance phase in ambulation. Ankle-foot orthoses can significantly improve ankle dorsiflexion at foot strike, although it has been more difficult to show gait improvements (Carlson et al, 1997). For a child with spastic diplegia, for whom posterior or lateral balance is impaired, a walker may improve mobility and standing ability. Crutches may be required if forward balance also is impaired.

Prevention of fixed contracture is a significant concern in a child with CP. Dynamic contracture resulting from muscle overactivity may not respond fully to stretching or tone reduction medications. In such cases, serial casting to restore the full range of motion may be considered. Typically, a joint (e.g., the ankle) is placed in a cast in maximal extension for 1 week. The range of motion at the joint is then reassessed, and often the cycle is repeated until maximal stretching has occurred. In recent years, serial casting has often been replaced with or become an adjunct to BTX type A injections (see later). Several randomized controlled trials have compared the efficacy of casting alone, BTX type A alone, or both treatments together. The results have been mixed.

Oral Medications

Oral medications are often tried for relief of muscle overactivity, although their usefulness is often limited by their tendency to produce sedation and drowsiness, along with exacerbation of gastroesophageal reflux, constipation, and hypoventilation or upper airway obstruction. The principal medications are benzodiazepines, baclofen, tizanidine, and dantrolene sodium. The choice of medication is empiric, and rigorous studies supporting their efficacy are sparse, with many trials dating from the 1970s and 1980s (Gracies et al, 1997).

Benzodiazepines

The benzodiazepines increase γ-aminobutyric acid (GABA)–induced inhibition through their facilitative action at GABA-A receptors, a major kind of inhibitory synapse in the central nervous system (Simonds, 2005). Diazepam is the most commonly used benzodiazepine in clinical use. Its effectiveness in spasticity reduction in children, especially children with athetosis, was shown in trials from the 1960s. Clonazepam also has been shown to be effective in children with CP.

Baclofen

The GABA-B agonist baclofen is widely used in children with CP, although only a single placebo-controlled trial of oral baclofen in CP has shown its ability to reduce spasticity and improve passive and active limb movements.

Tizanidine

Studies in adults have shown the clinical efficacy of tizanidine, an α_2-adrenergic agonist, which acts on spinal interneurons to inhibit release of excitatory amino acids. Support for the use of tizanidine in CP is primarily based on these adult studies and case reports in children.

Dantrolene Sodium

In contrast to other antispasticity medications, dantrolene exerts its effects at the level of the muscle, reducing calcium efflux and decoupling excitation and contraction. Although there is physiologic evidence supporting reduced force and spasticity, clinical and functional improvement has not been as convincingly shown.

Botulinum Toxin and Phenol Injections

Chemodenervation—the focal reduction of neuromuscular excitation through injection into nerve or muscle—has been used for 5 decades or more in spastic conditions, including CP. The introduction of BTX in the late 1980s and early 1990s revolutionized the practice of chemodenervation, however, by providing much more finely graded reduction in muscle activity, with fewer adverse effects, than was possible with early chemodenervation agents, phenol and ethyl alcohol.

Botulinum Toxin

Pharmacology

The bacterium *Clostridium botulinum* produces seven serotypes of BTX, A through G, each of which is a proteolytic enzyme. Each serotype targets one or more of the vesicle fusion proteins that allow acetylcholine vesicles to fuse with the membrane at the neuromuscular junction. BTX prevents release of acetylcholine, weakening the muscle.

Two serotypes, A and B, are approved by the U.S. Food and Drug Administration and by European regulatory agencies for use in humans. In the United States, neither is approved for use in CP. Each serotype differs in its exact target, duration of action, antigenicity, and adverse effects profile. The clinical effects of injection are usually seen within several days, with the peak effect at approximately 4 weeks. There is a gradual loss of benefit over time, as the nerve terminals recover, and the muscle strengthens again. Reinjection is typically required at 3 to 6 months. Experience has shown the importance of reinjecting no more frequently than every 3 months, and keeping the dose to the minimum, to reduce the risk of development of neutralizing antibodies. Switching to the alternative serotype is possible if antibody-based resistance occurs, but may not provide long-lasting benefit (Brin and Aoki, 2002).

Clinical Practice

In the CP population, the most appropriate candidate for BTX injection is one for whom the weakening of a few muscles has the potential to provide meaningful benefit in care, comfort, or function. Because it is a focal treatment, BTX does not affect cognition, and side effects (excess weakness, occasional mild flulike symptoms) are usually minimal and well tolerated. BTX may be combined with other treatments, including oral medications or intrathecal baclofen, providing targeted tone reduction against a backdrop of generalized reduction in muscle overactivity.

Phenol and Ethyl Alcohol

Phenol and ethyl alcohol are injected onto nerves, causing nerve degeneration and consequent muscle weakness (Gracies et al, 2005). Although their use has never been widespread, and has declined with the introduction of BTX, they still offer an alternative, especially for the treatment of powerful muscles that would require too high a dose of BTX, or when cost is an issue, or when BTX no longer can be used because of antibody-based resistance. Injection requires greater skill and training, and the risk of adverse effects is greater, than with BTX. Pain and dysesthesia, especially after injection onto a mixed nerve, are significant risks. The duration of benefit ranges unpredictably from several weeks to many months.

Intrathecal Baclofen

The amount of baclofen needed to reduce tone can be dramatically reduced, and adverse effects minimized, by directly delivering it to the intrathecal space. Intrathecal baclofen is delivered with the SynchroMed infusion system (Medtronic, Minneapolis, Minnesota). In this system, a pump and drug reservoir are implanted subcutaneously in the abdomen, and a catheter is inserted into the intrathecal space at the mid to upper thoracic level. The pump can be remotely programmed with a handheld device, and the reservoir can be refilled percutaneously, usually every 12 to 24 weeks.

Intrathecal baclofen is most useful in patients with significant muscle overactivity, with involvement of multiple upper and lower muscle groups and lower extremity spasticity of 3 or greater on the Ashworth scale. Screening is performed with a bolus infusion, with a threshold of reduction of 1 unit on the Ashworth scale being the usual standard for proceeding with pump implantation.

Intrathecal baclofen has been shown in clinical trials to reduce muscle overactivity, particularly in the lower extremities, and to improve long-term function. The most significant gains are in reduced spasticity, easier care and transfers, and reduced pain, whereas the effects on ambulation may be unpredictable and variable. Complications include infection, pump malfunction, catheter kinking or breakage, and drug withdrawal. The family must be educated about the signs of and response to withdrawal, which may be life-threatening (Murphy et al, 2002).

Selective Dorsal Rhizotomy

In selective dorsal rhizotomy, the overactive dorsal nerve rootlets are severed to reduce afferent activity from muscle spindles, reducing spasticity. In most centers, the individual nerve rootlets from L4 or L5 to S1 are electrophysiologically stimulated during surgery to identify overactive rootlets (typically 25% to 60% of all nerve rootlets), which are then severed.

Improvements shown in controlled trials include reduced lower limb spasticity, increased range of motion (Steinbok, 2001), improved gross motor function, better self-care, and improved gait. Children 3 to 7 years old, with spastic diplegia, good trunk control, good leg strength, and isolated leg movements (i.e., leg movements without involuntary involvement of other limbs) are considered the best candidates for surgery. Rigorous physical therapy after the operation mobilizes the patient to maximize the potential for regain of preoperative motor function. Increased risk of scoliosis has been raised as a concern after selective dorsal rhizotomy, owing to increased weakness. Further long-term studies are needed to address this issue. Some studies indicate that selective dorsal rhizotomy may delay or avoid the need for later orthopedic surgery.

Orthopedic Surgery

With the advent of better treatments and the recognition of the importance of early intervention, the need for orthopedic surgery to correct fixed contracture in CP has declined sharply, from 40% for children born in 1990-1991 to 15% for children born in 1994-1995 (Hagglund et al, 2005). Nonetheless, even with early tone intervention and optimal care, many children with CP eventually require orthopedic surgery. Equinus or equinovarus are the most common deformities, necessitating lengthening of the heel cords.

COMMONLY ASSOCIATED CONDITIONS

Virtually all children with CP have orthopedic concerns as a result of the abnormal tone or movement associated with the disorder. For some children, these orthopedic concerns may be the extent of the effect of CP. Many are at risk, however, for associated medical concerns as well. Virtually any system can be affected, and most children with CP have at least one additional disability. For many children, the additional disability may be more significant from a functional or quality-of-life perspective than the neuromotor impairments that define the condition. It is important for the primary health care provider to be aware of potential associated disabilities and medical complications so that the child can be monitored in a proactive manner.

Primary Effects: Neurologic Sequelae

From a neurologic perspective, numerous primary issues may arise as a result of the underlying injury causing the CP. Major manifestations include seizures, intellectual and learning disabilities, neurobehavioral concerns, sensory impairment, and effects of bulbar palsy (Table 67-5).

Table 67-5. Primary Neurologic Complications of Cerebral Palsy

Muscle tone abnormalities	100%
Seizure disorders	43%
Intellectual disability	65%
Neurobehavioral problems	
Learning disabilities	
Hydrocephalus	
Sensory impairment	
Vision	28%
Hearing	12%
Bulbar palsy	38%
Speech impairment	
Swallowing difficulties	
Drooling	

Seizure Disorders

Forty-three percent of children with CP have seizure disorders, most commonly children with spastic quadriplegia and hemiplegia where there is more cortical injury (Russman and Ashwal, 2004). Control of seizures is crucial. Seizures can have a considerable effect on a child's level of alertness and overall developmental presentation. Treatments vary in their effectiveness. They range from anticonvulsant medications to more aggressive measures for children who have refractory seizure disorders. Such measures include the ketogenic diet, vagus nerve stimulator implantation, and ablative surgery.

Intellectual Disability and Learning Disabilities

About 65% of children with CP meet criteria for intellectual disability (Miller, 1998). There is some, but no absolute, correlation between intellectual disability and the subtype of CP. Children with spastic quadriplegia have the highest likelihood of having an intellectual disability. There also is some indication that the presence of epilepsy correlates more strongly with intellectual disability.

Language-based learning disabilities occur in children with CP, and seem to correlate with general cognitive function. Controversy exists over whether children with a right-sided hemiplegia have increased prevalence of language disorders based on a left-sided injury (Trauner et al, 1996). Low-birth-weight infants with CP have increased risk for educational impairments (Fennell and Dikel, 2001).

Neurobehavioral Concerns

Numerous neurobehavioral concerns arise in children with CP. Typical manifestations include inattention, internalizing behavioral problems, immature adaptive skills, and self-injurious behaviors. Inattention may be primarily neurologic, consistent with a diagnosis of attention-deficit/hyperactivity disorder. It also may indicate subclinical seizures, depression, discomfort, anxiety, or fatigue. The interplay between a myriad of medical realities can result in some of these maladaptive behaviors such that they are of a secondary rather than primary etiology. This situation demands a different approach to treatment and knowledge of the potential associated medical concerns. It can be challenging to elucidate the etiology of neurobehavioral symptoms in a child with CP, particularly if communication impairment exists. The diagnosis of neurobehavioral origin is generally one of exclusion, after other explanations, such as discomfort or fatigue, have been ruled out.

Hearing Impairment

Some degree of hearing loss occurs in 12% of children with CP. Most commonly, hearing loss relates to a history of kernicterus, very low birth weight, meningitis, or

Table 67-6. Secondary Complications of Cerebral Palsy

Orthopedic complications
Respiratory issues
  Aspiration pneumonia
  Reactive airway disease
  Restrictive lung disease
Gastrointestinal issues
  Poor growth and nutrition
  Gastroesophageal reflux and dysmotility
  Constipation
Upper airway obstruction
Sleep disorders
Osteopenia
Tooth decay/gum disease
Bladder control issues
Decubitus ulcers
Discomfort
Fatigue

severe hypoxic-ischemic injury. Because of its prevalence, it is crucial to obtain a hearing evaluation in any child suspected to have CP.

Visual Impairment

At least 28% of children with CP have some sort of visual impairment, and some studies place the prevalence at closer to 40%. Patients with a history of periventricular leukomalacia seem to be particularly vulnerable to visual impairment. The range of ophthalmologic problems encountered includes retinopathy of prematurity, nystagmus, amblyopia, refractive errors, optic nerve atrophy, and cortical blindness (Rudank et al, 2003). All children diagnosed with CP must be screened by an ophthalmologist. A functional vision assessment looks for the presence of visual field cuts and behaviors, such as the use of peripheral vision and gaze preference. All of these can affect a child socially and academically.

Pseudobulbar Palsy

Pseudobulbar palsy, or deranged lower brainstem function caused by bilateral corticobulbar disruption, affects the oromotor musculature in children with CP and is present 38% of the time. From a functional standpoint, it affects speech production and intelligibility, chewing, swallowing, and drooling.

Secondary Effects: Medical Complications

In addition to primary neurologic complications in a child with CP, numerous potential secondary complications occur that are more medical in nature (Table 67-6). Presentation can include virtually any organ system. Although the underlying lesion that causes CP is static, a child's manifestations of the complications often evolve over time.

Respiratory and Upper Airway Complications

Children with CP are at risk for intrinsic and extrinsic lung disease. Intrinsic disease results from chronic aspiration in a child with oromotor dysfunction and poor airway protection (Shaw, 1996). It can be compounded by recurrent pneumonias and bronchospasm. Treatment involves reducing the risk of aspiration and controlling the associated bronchospasm.

When considering a child's risk for chronic aspiration, the primary care provider needs to be aware of the effectiveness of a child's chewing and swallowing abilities, the possible presence of gastroesophageal reflux disease, and possible poor secretion management. A videofluoroscopic swallowing test or modified barium swallow (often under the direction of a speech or occupational therapist in conjunction with a radiologist) can delineate the extent of a child's dysphagia. Dietary modifications, such as thickening feeds or avoiding certain food textures altogether, may be indicated. For more profound cases, direct enteral feeds through a gastrostomy tube may be necessary to protect the lungs. Gastroesophageal reflux disease should be treated to reduce damage to lung parenchyma by means of aspiration from below. A wide range of antacid treatments are available, including proton-pump inhibitors and H_2 blockers.

Thirty-five percent of children with CP have excessive sialorrhea, which can lead to chronic aspiration. An anticholinergic drying agent can be effective in reducing symptoms, but is frequently associated with unacceptable side effects. Aggressive pulmonary toileting includes not only chest physiotherapy, but also postural drainage and suctioning. Some children with regular need for pulmonary toileting respond well to mechanical chest physical therapy vests.

Restrictive lung disease also is a problem in some children with CP. Progressive neuromuscular scoliosis can gradually change the thoracic cavity, having a significant effect on ventilation. Underlying weakness of intercostal and accessory muscles of respiration also contribute to restrictive disease.

Sixty-three percent of parents who have a child with CP report that their child snores loudly at night (Zucconi and Bruni, 2001). Parents may also report pauses in their child's breathing pattern while asleep. Clinicians may observe stridor in an office visit. Any of these presentations merits evaluation for the possibility of upper airway obstruction. The presence of obstruction may be mechanical, such as enlarged adenoids or tonsils. Sometimes craniofacial differences play a role. Decreased tongue control may result in the tongue falling into the posterior oropharynx, obstructing the airway during sleep. Tracheomalacia may be present.

Diagnostically, concern about the possibility of upper airway obstruction should be pursued through sleep study evaluation. Up to 19% of children with CP have some degree of obstructive sleep apnea. Interventions can be determined based on results. At times, a simple surgical intervention may be curative, such as adenoidectomy. Mandibular advancement or glossopexy may be effective. At other times, positive airway pressure, such as continuous positive airway pressure or biphasic positive airway pressure, must be considered.

On occasion, the child with severe upper airway obstruction or difficulties with poor secretion control may benefit from a tracheotomy to assist with management. Treatment of severe restrictive or obstructive disease may require endotracheal ventilatory assistance through a tracheotomy.

Decisions about proceeding with tracheotomy are complex and highly personal. Various physiologic and psychological considerations, such as quality of life, have an impact on the child's function and independence and overall state of health and prognosis (Simonds, 2005). The goal of long-term mechanical ventilation is to correct chronic respiratory failure and to allow a child to reach his or her developmental potential within the context of optimal quality of life. It is crucial to discuss all options before moving forward with long-term mechanical ventilation or tracheotomy.

Gastrointestinal Issues

Numerous gastrointestinal issues are present in a child with CP. Poor growth and nutrition are common (Sullivan et al, 2000). The sequelae of malnutrition are important to recognize. Endurance and ability of a child to perform to the best of his or her developmental potential can be affected. Postoperative wound healing can be compromised, and susceptibility to infection may be increased.

Decreased oral intake may reflect underlying gastrointestinal disorders, particularly conditions relating to dysmotility. A child with poorly controlled gastroesophageal reflux or constipation may be quite uncomfortable. Treatment of these underlying disorders can have a marked effect on appetite. An appetite stimulant can be effective sometimes as adjunctive therapy. Caloric enhancement and work with a nutritionist to optimize caloric goals can be central to helping a child to overcome a malnourished state.

A common reason for decreased oral intake is oromotor dysfunction, which can be exaggerated by challenges with overall tone and poor positioning. Treatments to enhance oromotor control and safety include modification of food textures, feeding techniques, and seating. A therapist with expertise in feeding can play an invaluable role for a child struggling with oral feeding. In more extreme cases, feeding orally cannot be managed safely, and evaluation for direct enteral feeds (e.g., placement of a gastrostomy tube) must occur.

Many children with CP struggle with difficulty gaining weight; however, on occasion, obesity is a problem. When it occurs, the child faces increased challenges to overall motor activity and coordination. Again, involving a nutritionist to identify ideal caloric goals can be quite useful.

Sleep Disorders

Sleep disorders are prevalent in children with CP. Etiologies include, among others, primary obstructive sleep apnea; discomfort, which requires thorough evaluation for a wide range of medical risks; and a primary neurologic manifestation of sleep-wake cycle abnormality or even seizures. Soporifics may be effective, but airway obstruction, pain, and seizures must be ruled out before initiating treatment.

DEVELOPMENTAL CONCERNS

Impact on the Child

A child with CP is at risk for various developmental concerns, limitations in autonomy, and, subsequently, compromised self-esteem (Table 67-7). Because of the fundamental manifestations of CP, motoric delays or disabilities are ubiquitous. Coupled with the prevalence of intellectual disability, many children show significant restriction in activity and social participation (Beckung and Hagberg, 2002). Functionally, children can be limited in their abilities to eat, dress, perform school tasks, and participate in some forms of play. Oromotor dysfunction can have a tremendous impact on speech production, affecting a child's ability to communicate effectively. Additionally, a child may be dependent on assistance to eat. Children may be aware of their differences from peers. Matters that are usually private, such as personal hygiene, may require assistance. Social relations, self-esteem, and mood are affected. As adolescents approach adulthood, consideration must be given to how safely they may be able to live independently, and the realities of potential vocational opportunities.

One of the most important developmental concerns for a child with CP is the ability to communicate. A child's ability to communicate is crucial to how he or she is perceived in the world and links directly to his or her sense of autonomy. Communication impairment can be underappreciated. This is particularly true in a child with choreoathetotic CP, who may have tremendous mechanical challenges with speech production, but whose cognition and receptive language skills may be strong.

Medical influences on communication in children with CP abound. Receptively, a child's ability to understand and react to his or her environment may be clouded by intellectual disability, visual or auditory impairment, seizures, inattention, discomfort, or fatigue. Expressively, speech is affected by issues relating to pseudobulbar palsy. Breath control provides the power for speech and relies on a complex integration of many structures in the head, neck, and trunk, which might be altered in a child with CP. Breath volume may be decreased, the rate may be too rapid, and exhalation may be poorly controlled. Craniofacial differences, such as cleft lip or palate, also may interfere with speech production or breath control.

A multitude of augmentative technologies exist to enhance a child's ability to communicate. These

Table 67-7. **Developmental Concerns for a Child with Cerebral Palsy**

Developmental Area Affected by Cerebral Palsy	Ramifications
Physical ability	Eating, dressing, mobility, school activities, play, personal hygiene
Communication	Social interaction
Cognition	Social interaction, academics
Self-esteem	Social interaction, mood disorders
Adult development	Transition planning

technologies may be quite simple, ranging from sign language to picture exchange systems. Many technologically complex computer-based systems also are available. These may use switches that take advantage of a child's volitional movement (e.g., head control, leg movement, eye gaze) to control a computer mouse. Synthetic voice production may be used. Specialists in augmentative technology encourage early referral, even at younger than 1 year, to assist children in developing invaluable communication skills.

Impact on Families

Having CP can affect virtually every aspect of daily life for a child and his or her family. The stresses families grapple with are wide ranging and include medical concerns for their child; interfacing with multiple medical, therapeutic, and educational providers; managing multiple agencies (e.g., medical suppliers, nursing); coordination nightmares; financial hardship; multiple insurers; exhaustion and lack of community supports or services. The National Survey of Children with Special Health Care Needs reflects concerning financial realities (Haflon and Olson, 2004). According to the study, 39.5% of families of children with special health care needs indicate their child's or youth's condition impacts the family's financial situation; 13.5% say they spend 11 or more hours per week coordinating care for their child or youth; 24.9% indicate they cut back on work because of their child's or youth's condition; and 28.5% indicate they stop working because of their child's or youth's condition. Understanding these stresses helps the primary care provider guide families toward appropriate support services. This can include agency support for funding and case management and psychosocial support.

EDUCATION AND SERVICES

Virtually all children with CP are followed by some constellation of therapists on an ongoing basis. At a minimum, physical therapy is usually involved. Other services may include occupational, speech, oromotor, augmentative technology, and vision therapies. Access to services should begin as soon as developmental delays or concerns arise. For children younger than age 3, federally funded early intervention programs provide a range of supportive services. Between the ages of 3 and 22, services are obtained through the public educational system.

Classroom placement can be complex. For many children with cerebral palsy, participating fully in an integrated setting is appropriate. For others, a small substantially separate placement may be more beneficial, with therapists and nursing services more readily available throughout the school day. This decision usually is made collaboratively between a school and a family. Primary care providers may be included in this process, particularly as the need for input regarding a child's medical needs arises.

Many families are pursuing a growing number of alternative therapies for their children with CP (Liptak, 2005). Hippotherapy, or therapeutic horseback riding, has been studied and has documentable benefits for improving balance and truncal strength. Music therapy, massage, Reiki, and craniosacral therapy have been studied to a lesser extent. Hyperbaric oxygen treatment has been heavily sought by families of children with CP, but further data is needed at this point to support its utility.

SUMMARY

CP is prevalent. Primary care providers need to be aware of its early manifestations and proactive in its identification and management. Initial workup should include brain MRI as well as vision, hearing, and developmental assessments. A child with hemiplegia also should undergo evaluation for coagulopathy. Knowledge of commonly associated neurologic and medical complications allows for vigilant monitoring and early referral for appropriate intervention. The developmental effects of medical problems commonly associated with CP cannot be overstated, and early intervention is indicated to support a child in exploring his or her full potential. Although there currently is no cure for CP, prevention and slowing of the associated medical and developmental complications can dramatically enhance the quality of life for a child. Ultimately, the focus of care is to promote health, function, and independence for all children with CP.

REFERENCES

Bax M, Goldstein M, Rosenbaum P, et al: Proposed definition and classification of cerebral palsy, April 2005. Dev Med Child Neurol 47:571-576, 2005.

Beckung E, Hagberg G: Neuroimpairments, activity limitations, and participation restrictions in children with cerebral palsy. Dev Med Child Neurol 44:309-316, 2002.

Brin MF, Aoki KR: Botulinum toxin type A: Pharmacology. *In* Mayer NH and Simpson DM (eds): Spasticity: Etiology, Evaluation, Management, and the Role of Botulinum Toxin. New York, WE MOVE, 2005, pp 110-124.

Carlson WE, Vaughan CL, Damiano DL, et al: Orthotic management of gait in spastic diplegia. Am J Phys Med Rehabil 76:219-225, 1997.

Dorman J, Pellegrino L: Making the diagnosis of cerebral palsy. *In*: Caring for Children with Cerebral Palsy. Baltimore, Brookes Publishing, 1998, pp 31-54.

Fennell EB, Dikel TN: Cognitive and neuropsychological functioning in children with cerebral palsy. J Child Neurol 16:58-63, 2001.

Gracies JM, Elovic E, McGuire J, et al: Traditional pharmacologic treatments for spasticity, part I: Local treatments. *In* Mayer NH and Simpson DM (eds): Spasticity: Etiology, Evaluation, Management, and the Role of Botulinum Toxin. New York, WE MOVE, 2005, pp 44-64.

Gracies JM, Nance P, Elovic E, et al: Traditional pharmacological treatments for spasticity, part II: General and regional treatments. Muscle Nerve Suppl 6:S92-S120, 1997.

Haflon N, Olson LM: Introduction: Results from a new national survey of children's health. Pediatrics 113:1895-1898, 2004.

Hagglund G, Andersson S, Duppe H, et al: Prevention of severe contractures might replace multilevel surgery in cerebral palsy: Results of a population-based health care programme and new techniques to reduce spasticity. J Pediatr Orthop B 14:269-273, 2005.

Liptak GS: Complementary and alternative therapies for cerebral palsy. Ment Retard Dev Disabil Res Rev 11:156-163, 2005.

McBurney H, Taylor NF, Dodd KJ, et al: A qualitative analysis of the benefits of strength training for young people with cerebral palsy. Dev Med Child Neurol 45:658-663, 2003.

Mercuri E, Cowan G, Gupte G, et al: Prothrombotic disorders and abnormal neurodevelopmental outcomes in infants with neonatal cerebral infarction. Pediatrics 107:1400-1404, 2001.

Miller G: Cerebral palsies: An overview. *In* Miller G, Clark GD (eds): The Cerebral Palsies: Causes, Consequences, and Management, Boston, Butterworth-Heinemann, 1998, pp 1-35.

Murphy NA, Irwin MC, Hoff C: Intrathecal baclofen therapy in children with cerebral palsy: Efficacy and complications. Arch Phys Med Rehabil 83:1721-1725, 2002.

Nelson KB, Ellenberg JH: Antecedents of cerebral palsy—multivariant analysis. N Engl J Med 315:81-86, 1986.

Odding E, Roebroeck ME, Stam HJ: The epidemiology of cerebral palsy: Incidence, impairments and risk factors. Disabil Rehabil 28:183-191, 2006.

Pharoah P, Cooke T, Rosenbloom L: Acquired cerebral palsy. Arch Dis Child 64:1013-1016, 1989.

Rudank SL, Fellman V, Laatikainen L: Visual impairment in children born prematurely from 1972-1989. Ophthalmology 110:1639-1645, 2003.

Russman BS, Ashwal S: Evaluation of the child with cerebral palsy. Semin Pediatr Neurol 11:47-57, 2004.

Sanger TD, Delgado MR, Gaebler-Spira D, et al: Classification and definition of disorders causing hypertonia in childhood. Pediatrics 111:e89-e97, 2003.

Shaw BN: The respiratory consequences of neurological deficit. *In* Sullivan PB, Rosenbloom L (eds): Feeding the Disabled Child. Clinics in Developmental Medicine No. 140. New York, Cambridge University Press, 1996, pp 40-46.

Simonds AK: Ethical aspects of home long-term ventilation in children with neuromuscular disease. Paediatr Respir Rev 6:209-214, 2005.

Steinbok P: Outcomes after selective dorsal rhizotomy for spastic cerebral palsy. Childs Nerv Syst 17:1-18, 2001.

Sullivan P, Lambert B, Rose M, et al: Prevalence and severity of feeding and nutritional problems in children with neurological impairment: Oxford Feeding Study. Dev Med Child Neurol 42:674-680, 2000.

Surveillance of Cerebral Palsy in Europe: A collaboration of cerebral palsy surveys and registers. Surveillance of Cerebral Palsy in Europe (SCPE). Dev Med Child Neurol 42:816-824, 2000.

Taub E, Ramey SL, DeLuca S, et al: Efficacy of constraint-induced movement therapy for children with cerebral palsy with asymmetric motor impairment. Pediatrics 113:305-312, 2004.

Trauner DA, Ballantyne A, Friedland S, et al: Disorders of affective and linguistic prosody in children after early unilateral brain damage. Ann Neurol 39:361-367, 1996.

Truwit CL, Barkovich AJ, Kock TK, et al: Cerebral palsy: MR findings in 40 patients. AJNR Am J Neuroradiol 13:67-78, 1992.

Zucconi M, Bruni O: Sleep disorders in children with neurologic disease. Semin Pediatr Neurol 8:258-275, 2001.

68 INTELLECTUAL DISABILITY

Ellen Roy Elias and Allen C. Crocker

Intellectual disability is a new term for what was formerly called mental retardation. The old term, mental retardation, was often employed in a fashion that was prejudicial and personally limiting, whereas the new term strives to define a group of disorders categorized particularly by exceptionality in cognitive function. Intellectual disability is defined as significant limitations in intellectual functioning and adaptive behavior, which originate before age 18 (Luckasson et al, 2002).

There are many underlying causes of intellectual disability, including genetic causes, environmental factors, and prenatal and postnatal insults to the central nervous system (CNS). For many individuals with intellectual disability, the cause is unknown. Services and supports have expanded significantly for individuals with intellectual disability and their families.

DEFINITION OF MENTAL RETARDATION

A functionally oriented and dynamic definition of mental retardation was proposed by the American Association on Mental Retardation (AAMR), historically the leading professional organization in this field, in 1992 (American Association on Mental Retardation, 1992), and last revised in 2002 (Luckasson et al, 2002). The AAMR has been renamed the American Association on Intellectual and Developmental Disabilities, but the concepts in the underlying definition are still pertinent.

Mental retardation refers to substantial limitations in present functioning. It is characterized by significantly subaverage intellectual functioning, existing concurrently with related limitations in two or more of the following applicable adaptive skills areas: communication, self-care, home living, social skills, community use, self-direction, health and safety, functional academics, leisure, and work. Mental retardation manifests before age 18 (American Association on Mental Retardation, 1992). The change of the term *mental retardation* to *intellectual disability* is discussed in detail by Schalock and colleagues (2007). This change in nomenclature occurred after extensive study and survey. A comparable shift has occurred in other organizations as well (e.g., the President's Committee on Intellectual Disability) and in the language used by families, individuals, and workers. This is now a cultural revision with earnest humanistic origins.

When assessing an individual for an intellectual disability, per the American Association on Intellectual and Developmental Disabilities definition, it is essential to measure the intellectual and adaptive limitations within the context of the individual's age, peers, and culture, to and address the following four points:

1. Valid assessment considers cultural and linguistic diversity and differences in communication and behavioral factors.
2. The existence of limitations in adaptive skills occurs within the context of community environments typical of the individual's age-peers and is indexed to the person's individualized needs for supports.
3. Specific adaptive limitations often coexist with strengths in other adaptive skills or other personal capabilities.
4. With appropriate supports over a sustained period, the life function of an individual with intellectual disability generally improves (American Association on Mental Retardation, 1992; Luckasson et al, 2002).

The characteristics and measurement of intelligence are considered in Chapters 77 and 81; the utility and the limitations presented there are related to the concept of the *intelligence quotient (IQ)*. Although these constraints are admitted, the basic degree of cognitive or intellectual disability is commonly discussed in terms of IQ ranges. An accepted convention is to view intelligence in a distribution, with the level of concern beginning at 2 standard deviations below the median IQ score of 100, and with subsequent categories charged at 3, 4, and beyond. In applying results from the Wechsler Intelligence Scale for Children, these groups would be as follows:

- Mild disability (or retardation): IQ 50-70
- Moderate disability: IQ 35-49
- Severe disability: IQ 20-34
- Profound disability: IQ <20

It has long been usual practice to refer to IQ measurements of 70 or less as compatible with intellectual disability (or mental retardation). It is important to acknowledge the imprecision of IQ determination, however, and to use "approximately 70 to 75 or less" as a psychometric boundary. If taken literally, this determination would move many individuals from the borderline normal range into intellectual disability, but the point is well taken that preoccupation with small number differences does not do justice to the basic principles of this field. At any age, 1% to 2% of the population tests in the range of intellectual disability, with most (85% to 90%) falling in the area of "mild" disability.

Many children with mild and moderate intellectual disability are included in regular ("inclusive") classrooms, rather than being segregated to a special education setting. The use of segregated classes is greatly reduced across all ranges of intellectual disability, and expectations for important progress are now much more open and supportive (see Chapter 80).

The "adaptive skills" concerns in the definition of intellectual disability acknowledge that "retardation" has cultural and personal aspects as well. Some of these components are easier to measure than others. Relevant instruments exist for the general assessment of adaptive behavior, such as the Vineland Social Maturity Scale and the AAMR Adaptive Behavior Scale. In typical situations, adaptive and social skills parallel closely the intellectual capacity of the young individual. In exceptional situations (with unusually creative or unusually desultory support, or in some idiosyncratic settings), there may be notable deviation. It is crucial that one reflect on the setting of learning and living for an individual with intellectual disability, that evaluation be carried out in an equitable fashion, and that the needs for services and supports be evaluated.

In a young child, *adaptation* implies achievement of useful coordinated psychomotor skills, then communication capacity, and finally gains in "activities of daily living" (self-help and independence in eating, dressing, and toileting). These skills and capacities are related to basic neurologic issues as well. In older children, one looks to broad social skills, accommodation to the educational environment, achievement of prevocational and vocational competence, and ability to manage independent living requirements. In the latter sequence, experiential and mental health factors are important.

Individuals with intellectual disability, their families, and persons who are involved in professional or voluntary efforts have come to realize that there is a subculture associated with "subaverage intellectual functioning" among people. It has its own special warmth and special desperation. Human rights efforts in the past 3 decades have brought a particular grace to the field of intellectual disability. One hopes that the new atmosphere of individual consideration, active support, and freedom from prejudicial generalizations will prevail in our culture.

ORIGINS OF INTELLECTUAL DISABILITY

When intellectual disability is identified in a child, there is a sense of urgency to determine the causative factor or factors. This sense of urgency derives primarily from a need to guide and counsel the family accurately, but also pertains to the eventual ability to plan appropriate interventions and training. In the broader view, the settings for intellectual disability must be understood as a basis for public health and preventive activities (Crocker, 1989).

Tremendous advances in many fields, including molecular biology, cytogenetic testing, and radiology, all have led to a better understanding of the underlying etiologies of intellectual disability. Significant progress also has been made in the clinical arena toward understanding rare genetic metabolic disorders, which allow for definitive diagnostic testing unavailable a decade ago. This section delves into the genetic causes of cognitive disabilities in greater detail, and concludes with recommendations for genetic evaluation in a child diagnosed with intellectual disability.

Chromosomal Abnormalities

Patients with chromosomal abnormalities, including trisomy, duplications, deletions, and unbalanced translocations, generally present with the following constellation of findings: unusual facial appearance (dysmorphic facies), unusual limbs, growth failure, anomalies involving internal organs (e.g., CNS dysgenesis, congenital heart disease, renal dysplasia), and developmental/cognitive disabilities. Any child presenting to the developmental pediatrician with this constellation of findings warrants a formal genetic assessment and genetic testing. Unusual features may be quite subtle, such as mild webbing of the second and third toes or a bifid uvula, and sometimes may be missed by providers not experienced in dysmorphology examinations. This is why a formal genetic consultation is often helpful. The developmental pediatrician often has a good sense, however, that the child does have unusual findings, and it is appropriate to secure basic genetic testing if there is a suspicion of a problem.

Advances in technology have led to a gradual change in the recommendations as to which specific genetic tests should be considered and are most likely to result in a clear diagnosis. The following tests are recommended in the evaluation of a child with cognitive/developmental disabilities who also has other unusual features, growth issues, or birth defects.

Chromosomes with High-Resolution Banding

Obtaining a karyotype with high-resolution banding detects most chromosomal rearrangements, such as unbalanced translocations and larger deletions or duplications. Cytogenetic karyotyping is still considered the gold standard for chromosomal abnormalities, although it may be replaced some day by comparative genomic hybridization microarray, a newer and more sensitive tool (see subsequently).

Fluorescent In Situ Hybridization

Fluorescent in situ hybridization (FISH), available since the 1990s, is a helpful, simple, and quick technology that can detect tiny chromosomal changes, particularly microdeletions, which may not be visible using traditional chromosomal analysis. If the child's phenotype suggests a specific common genetic disorder, such as velocardiofacial syndrome or Williams syndrome, FISH testing can provide rapid confirmation of a diagnosis. It also is useful to provide rapid confirmation of a suspected trisomy diagnosis in a critically ill newborn.

FISH testing of the tips of the chromosomes, called *subtelomeric FISH,* has been widely used since the late 1990s to identify subtle microdeletions in a region of the genome that may not be well seen with standard karyotype testing. This testing is being supplanted, however, by the new comparative genomic hybridization microarray (see next). Multicolor FISH testing is a useful technology that can help define further complex chromosomal rearrangements.

Comparative Genomic Hybridization Microarray

Comparative genomic hybridization microarray is a powerful new technology that has become more readily available and cost-effective in recent years. This technology uses a computer CytoChip array of Bacterial Artificial Chromosomes to screen thousands of genes from the patient's DNA and compare with normal reference DNA. This technology can detect subtle chromosomal changes too tiny to be discerned on traditional chromosomal analysis, and detect microdeletions traditionally detected by FISH. Many geneticists believe that comparative genomic hybridization microarray may someday supplant the genetic testing formally used.

Molecular Testing

Molecular testing is the direct DNA testing of a specific gene to detect changes or mutations. Common examples include testing for the specific changes that cause fragile X syndrome (expansion of the CGG trinucleotide repeat and methylation of the gene) and mutational testing to detect changes in the *MECP2* gene, which causes Rett syndrome.

Molecular testing also can be helpful for certain conditions that are known to be associated with imprinted genes, such as Angelman syndrome. Many patients with Angelman syndrome have a deletion on chromosome 15 in the Prader-Willi/Angelman syndrome region, detectable by FISH or microarray. A subset of patients have Angelman syndrome because the DNA has been mismarked, however, or the patient has inherited two copies of DNA from the father (uniparental disomy), which appears normal on FISH testing, but is detectable with methylation testing of the gene.

Metabolic Testing

Most metabolic disorders are rare, and it would not be cost-effective or sensible to screen all children with cognitive disabilities for all metabolic disorders. Certain symptoms and physical features should trigger concern, however, for the possibility of a metabolic disorder and prompt additional workup (see Chapter 30). Clinical findings that should increase suspicion for a metabolic disorder include the following:

- Unusual features and organomegaly, which raise concern for a possible storage disorder
- A loss of milestones, or a neurodegenerative course
- Severe hypotonia
- Unusual movements, such as choreoathetosis
- Autonomic instability, visual abnormalities, and stroke in infancy, which all raise concern for a possible mitochondrial disorder
- Neurologic examination and developmental history that are inconsistent with the patient's medical history (i.e., no history of birth trauma or head trauma or severe infection)

Certain metabolic disorders, such as Smith-Lemli-Opitz syndrome, have a spectrum of severity, and the mild end of the spectrum may manifest with only cognitive disabilities and subtle features, such as second and third toe syndactyly. The input from a clinical geneticist and sometimes a metabolic geneticist is often helpful with these patients because a simple blood test can detect this disorder, which has a 25% recurrence risk in future pregnancies (Elias et al, 1997).

Head Imaging

The technology of head imaging has seen major advances in the past 10 years. There have been significant advances in computed tomography and magnetic resonance imaging, the two major imaging techniques that are readily available in most medical centers. These advances allow very detailed visualization of subtle CNS abnormalities, vascular malformations, and even metabolic derangements.

Because it is expensive, and often requires sedation in young infants or older, less cooperative patients, head imaging is not indicated in every child diagnosed with cognitive disabilities. Imaging may be quite helpful, however, in certain circumstances as detailed subsequently, and may provide the clues toward making a correct, definitive diagnosis. A computed tomography scan is helpful for eliminating acute pathology, such as an intracranial hemorrhage or stroke or hydrocephalus, but magnetic resonance imaging is the preferred study in most cases because it allows for more detailed imaging and a much better view of the posterior fossa. The following findings in a child with cognitive disabilities should prompt the developmental pediatrician to consider obtaining head imaging:

- Dysmorphic facial features, including hypotelorism (eyes too closely spaced), midline cleft lip/palate, and microcephaly, suggesting the possibility of holoprosencephaly
- Significant microcephaly of unclear etiology, suggesting CNS dysgenesis, such as lissencephaly
- Hypotonia and movement disorder, suggesting abnormal brainstem formation
- A neurodegenerative process, to look for signs of leukodystrophy or other white matter changes
- An asymmetric neurologic examination or asymmetric seizures, to rule out asymmetric CNS dysgenesis or vascular malformation or stroke

Other Issues

Obtaining accurate and detailed information regarding maternal obstetric history, pregnancy, delivery, and family history is essential. A maternal history of multiple miscarriage or infertility increases the possibility of a chromosomal or other genetic problem being present. Use of advanced reproductive techniques, such as in vitro fertilization (IVF) or gamete intrafallopian transfer (GIFT), is now believed to be associated with an increased risk of disorders related to epigenetic errors such as imprinting errors. If the medical history or family history reveals this information, consultation with a geneticist may be indicated (Table 68-1).

Table 68-1. Genetic Evaluation of a Child with Intellectual Disability

Obtain comprehensive history
- Birth and delivery history
- Past medical history
- Family history

Perform detailed physical examination
- Growth factors
- Abnormal skin findings
- Unusual features of the face or limbs

Obtain laboratory testing
- DNA studies for fragile X syndrome
- Comparative genomic hybridization microarray*

Formal genetic assessment and specialized testing may be indicated in certain situations
- Fluorescent in situ hybridization testing may be helpful to confirm a suspected diagnosis of common genetic disorders such as VCFS or Williams syndrome if suspected
- DNA testing for Rett syndrome in girls with degenerative course, progressive microcephaly
- Methylation testing for patients with seizures and features suggestive of Angelman syndrome
- Metabolic testing for children with findings such as coarse features, organomegaly, or neurodegenerative course
- Head imaging such as MRI is helpful if the skull shape is unusual, or OFC is unusually large or too small

*If comparative genomic hybridization microarray is unavailable, obtain chromosomes with high-resolution banding.

MRI, magnetic resonance imaging; OFC, occipitofrontal circumference; VCFS, velocardiofacial syndrome.

Although genetic factors are extremely important, other elements, including culture and environment, affect developmental outcome. Impressions about the mechanisms of intellectual disability are influenced by the circumstances in which children are seen. Professionals who work in the child study sections of school systems see large numbers of children with mild, more dynamic disabilities of apparent cultural and environmental origin. Workers in community health clinics or mental health clinics are impressed by the frequency of troubled support systems for families and of polygenic inheritance. Pediatricians and hospital clinicians see a disproportionate number of children with organic difficulties and complications of illness. Finally, child development centers and centers for evaluation of intellectual disability tend to draw the complex child, with mixed biologic and social liability, who has bewildered the educational and health care systems. In the last-mentioned setting, some of the most analytical studies are undertaken, and the lessons from this work are emphasized here. The findings in Table 68-2 reflect the diagnostic experience of a university-affiliated program for intellectual disability, as it carefully evaluated children referred for developmental review from community, school, and residential programs.

Other causes of intellectual disability include fetal malnutrition, which refers to diminished support for fetal growth as pregnancy proceeds, especially regarding factors in placental integrity or vascular configuration. Reduced size of the infant or the early onset of labor may result, sometimes with untoward developmental consequences directly or as listed in the following section.

Perinatal stresses, considered in detail in Chapter 27, affect particularly the vulnerable infant. Perinatal stress refers to premature birth or obstetric complications in a full-term infant. There is a potentially compromising complex of troubling events—anoxia, trauma, CNS hemorrhage, acidosis, hypoglycemia, and sometimes infection—that can operate negatively on the extrauterine adjustment of the immature infant brain. These important issues can produce immediately recognizable complications for development or place the child in an uncertain "at risk" status.

Specific conditions acquired in childhood cause intellectual disability in relatively few instances. Most significant are complications of CNS infections (encephalitis, meningitis) and cranial trauma (household and motor vehicle accidents) (see Chapter 23). The role of toxins is often less discrete, but unquestionably important (see Chapter 31).

Deprivation in children constitutes a vast area of varying characteristics, which include psychosocial disadvantage and disordered parenting. Specific issues of inadequate stimulation, deficient interpersonal nurturance, physical abuse, and malnutrition may affect developmental progress. Family chaos, cultural maladjustment, poverty, and inept support systems are common. (See Chapters 10 and 29 for specific analyses of these potential developmental deterrents.) Such situations also may complicate the course in children who already have specific disabilities.

Any schema that outlines the backgrounds or the occurrence of intellectual disability inevitably becomes a checklist for disordered human development in general. As such, it chronicles all the steps in the developmental sequence at which pernicious influences can intrude. The clinical outcome may be predominantly intellectual disability, but it may just as well be cerebral palsy, epilepsy, blindness, deafness, physical disability, emotional disturbance, or learning disability (with any combinations thereof). Refer to other chapters in this book for further discussion about related situations and syndromes (see Chapters 22, 24 through 26, 49, 67, 69 through 71, and 74).

Psychiatric Disorders

Various psychiatric disorders in the child, parents, or both also can lead to a modified developmental course and ultimate intellectual disability. Maternal schizophrenia can be such a setting, as can a serious intrinsic psychic atypicality in the child. The autism spectrum disorders are a group of disorders with multiple underlying etiologies, which in most instances manifest behavioral/psychiatric and cognitive disabilities. Children with velocardiofacial syndrome also may manifest cognitive disabilities and psychiatric disorders, such as schizophrenia or bipolar disorder.

Many patients with intellectual disability have significant behavioral issues, such as hyperactivity, self-stimulatory or self-injurious behaviors, and sleep disorders which are quite challenging for their families and themselves. The input of a child psychiatrist in the management of patients with "dual diagnosis" (i.e., intellectual disability and psychiatric problems) can be particularly

Table 68-2. **Settings in Which Mental Retardation (Intellectual Disability) Occurs***

	Percentage of Total Group
Hereditary Disorders	5
(preconceptional basis; variable expression, multiple somatic effects, sometimes a progressive course)	
Inborn errors of metabolism (e.g., Tay-Sachs disease, Hurler syndrome, phenylketonuria)	
Other single gene abnormalities (e.g., neurofibromatosis, tuberous sclerosis, diverse syndromes)	
Chromosomal aberrations, including translocation, fragile X syndrome	
Polygenic familial syndromes, including some causes of autism	
Mitochondrial disorders	
Early Alterations of Embryonic Development	32
(sporadic events affecting embryogenesis; phenotypic changes, usually a stable developmental disability)	
Chromosomal changes, including trisomy (e.g., Down syndrome, microdeletion disorders)	
Prenatal influence syndrome (e.g., intrauterine infections, drugs, unknown forces)	
Multifactorial disorders (e.g., spina bifida)	
Other Pregnancy Problems and Perinatal Morbidity	11
(impingement on progress of fetus during the second half of pregnancy or in the newborn period; neurologic abnormalities frequent, disability stable or occasionally with increasing problems)	
Fetal malnutrition—placental insufficiency	
Perinatal difficulties (e.g., prematurity, hypoxia, trauma)	
Acquired Childhood Diseases	4
(acute modification of developmental status; variable potential for functional recovery)	
Infection (e.g., encephalitis, meningitis, encephalopathy of various causes including HIV)	
Cranial trauma	
Other (e.g., asphyxia, near-drowning, intoxications)	
Environmental Problems and Behavioral Syndromes	18
(dynamic influences, operational throughout development; commonly combined with other disabilities)	
Psychosocial deprivation	
Parental neurosis, psychosis	
Emotional and behavioral disorders	
Autism, childhood psychosis	
Unknown Causes	30
(no definite hereditary, gestational, perinatal, acquired, or environmental issues; or else multiple elements present)	

*Experience of the Developmental Evaluation Center, Children's Hospital, Boston (3000 children with intellectual disability).
Adapted from Crocker AC: The causes of mental retardation. Pediatr Ann 18:623, 1989.

helpful. Newer medications that have greater efficacy with fewer ill effects have been developed to assist in the management of these behavioral problems.

MEANING OF INTELLECTUAL DISABILITY FOR THE CHILD AND FAMILY

Psychology of Exceptionality

Children and adults with intellectual disability share an attribute with all other minority groups: they are different. The difference may be real or perceived, but the effect is substantial. Difference begins with the altered expectations of parents when they learn about the prospect of cognitive disabilities. A newborn with Down syndrome may lack none of the capabilities of other newborns, but that infant is perceived as different. Deeply entrenched cultural attitudes may serve to assign a negative connotation to this difference and reinforce the parents' sense of alarm. Counselors assisting parents during the period of diagnostic crisis, whether this be in early infancy or in later years, must reckon with the personal significance of difference.

When one examines the characteristics of difference for an individual with intellectual disability, one notes several components, all of which are to some extent dynamic. First is the matter of *achievement* and *performance,* in the measured or standard sense. This matter is linked to the functional limitation present, of cortical origin. As mentioned previously, however, the final effects of constraints in intelligence are modulated by concurrent attainments in adaptation. If expectations remain low, elements of self-fulfilling prophecy intrude on performance.

The second dissimilarity is that of *requirements for services* provided to the individual and family to allow maximal realization of potential. This is real and not always easy, but fits justifiably within the spectrum of contributions expected among people and their agencies. All of us draw on inside and outside services in this social world; for individuals with significant exceptionality, the urgency is greater.

A third difference can be that of *participation* in life events and sequences, or involvement in the usual experiences of growth and daily living. For a child with intellectual disability, this has a considerable cultural prescription. Descriptors such as normalization, communitization, least restrictive environment, and inclusive society speak to the current resolve to provide an enhanced setting for participation in usual form. In the external sense, the victories of the past several decades in the human rights area provide assurance that joining in school, community, and residential settings will be guaranteed. The right to establish contracts (e.g., marriage and ownership), with guidance as appropriate, also assists in the reversal of historical limitations.

The fourth or final difference could be that of *connectedness*. Here there can be no fundamental or primary defense, although societal weakness or clouded vision has often deprived us all of full fellowship.

It is conceded that difference is present in the best of times. Thinking about the difference in the context of its components (mentioned previously) may diminish the first impressions of oppressiveness and give some guidance about best plans for helpful actions. When one shares time and experiences with families who have children with intellectual disability, one is taught some precious lessons about the ultimate meaning of the residual differences. It becomes clear that the importance of less-than-superior skills is a matter of personal interpretation and is not absolute. If the job is well done within the context of native talents, and if the pursuit of referenced happiness and best quality of life is honored, the measured features of performance seem less prominent. Diversity among humans is a richness. When appropriate support systems are in place, and a cordial environment exists, parents come to assign uncommon value to their exceptional family member. The differences are often accommodated with grace. Professionals frequently damp the natural strengths of families to love and succeed.

Infants and Young Children at Risk for Intellectual Disability

For the past 25 years, a great deal of attention has been focused on infancy and toddlerhood, acknowledging this period as dynamic for the establishment of developmental patterns. Serious concerns are raised by the presence of congenital anomalies and chromosomal aberrations; bewilderment exists about possible sequelae from stressful perinatal experience; and there is discomfiture about dysfunctional circumstances of infant nurturance and stimulation. The impression persists that devoted investment in infant support and training can draw on a measure of plasticity still present in the young nervous system and avoid or reduce the occurrence of developmental disability.

Early speculation in this area devised a concept of particular infants being specifically "at risk" for developmental disorder. Three categories of circumstances have been widely employed in research and planning. The first refers to infants at *established risk,* by virtue of the presence of biomedical conditions known to affect personal progress. The second, that of *biologic risk,* refers to children who have had a history of events with a significant potential for brain impairment or whose early functioning gives concern about development. The third, *environmental risk,* notes young children being reared with incomplete supports or compromised settings.

It is difficult to produce certain figures for the prevalence of these situations. The smallest number would be those with established risk. Down syndrome, with an incidence of 1 in 1000 births, accounts for 0.1% of newborns. Other congenital anomaly syndromes are individually less frequent, but in the aggregate represent an additional 0.2% to 0.3%. Serious inborn errors of metabolism and prenatal syndromes producing hypotonia or cerebral palsy–like pictures may add another 0.1% to 0.2%. In sum, the incidence of established risk is less than 1% of infants.

Infants born prematurely are the major component for those regarded to be at biologic risk. From the large number with nominal low birth weight (6% to 7%), only a fraction are developmentally threatened (possibly 15%), in particular, infants who are most seriously preterm (see Chapter 27). About 1% of all infants qualify for inclusion in biologic risk. Another 0.5% may have developmental delay of diverse origins and be at biologic risk as well.

Reckoning is difficult in the area of environmental risk. Teenaged motherhood (13%), single parenthood (20%), child rearing in poverty, illicit drug use, and developmental disability in the parents, singly or in combinations, can add to 10% or more of young children with serious concern in current times. The meaning, or irreversibility, of those risks is unknown, but experience suggests that currently intellectual disability is disproportionately represented among the outcomes.

Public and private programs of early intervention (training, health promotion, family support) have been widespread in the United States for more than 20 years. In these programs, infants typically receive home visits by educators or therapists in the early months and training in small groups in centers as the next several years proceed. Currently, various states have enrolled 2% to 6% of all infants in early intervention programs. This percentage usually accounts for one half or more of infants at established or biologic risk, but irregular or smaller numbers from the environmental risk category. Commitments from Public Law 105-17 embody involvement of a larger percentage of infants and toddlers, especially from the environmental risk category; this is a courageous and commendable resolve. See Chapter 92 for further discussion of early education.

The current concern with services for infants in educationally oriented programs has served other purposes as well. For families, this interest has provided endorsement of their own hopes for the children's best progress. Direct family assistance in practical matters, personal counseling, and parenting instruction has relieved isolation and troubled circumstances. Physicians have been involved in "child find" screening and infant tracking activity, which have given particular attention to medical interventions as well (Nelson, 1989). The American Academy of Pediatrics has strongly endorsed developmental screening during infancy and early childhood, even altering the traditional well-child screening schedule to include an additional recommended screening at 30 months (Committee on Children with Disabilities, 2006). Preventive health care has been reinforced and monitored, including consideration of hearing, vision, seizures, orthopedic issues, nutrition, growth, intervention for physical anomalies, and behavioral issues.

Effects of Intellectual Disability and Its Causes on the Child

The central figures in this life story are the young individuals themselves. While we analyze the consequences of exceptionality, they are living it. It seems reasonable to state that the results are better than we as "others" might have predicted. Some of the poignant aspects of being different have been mentioned; they are not all unfavorable. The key issues are understanding, support, and respect. The social revolution of the 1960s and 1970s infused our culture with a critically valuable and long overdue level of compassion for rights and opportunities. For children with intellectual disability, the new world has been more nurturing; the quality of life has gained greatly.

Much of the action in the child's life plays out in the school. What was formerly a curtailed number of years has now come to extend from infancy to early adulthood. School districts have gradually moved their pupils with special needs from segregated to mainstreamed to integrated class designs, with increasing capacity for a common learning environment and social experience. The most creative conception, the truly inclusive class, has a challenging assignment and a growing adherence (see Chapter 93). These later models have a potential for familiarity and friendships among students with and without special needs (and out of school as well), with each learning from the other. The degree of attainment of the hoped-for outcomes varies, as could be expected. The old isolation has been permanently relieved.

Currently, about 10% to 20% of schoolchildren have special "education plans," formulated jointly by the school district and the families. Most of these are for students with learning disabilities or speech or language impairments; about 18% are for children with intellectual disability. These plans contain concrete information on educational techniques and goals, with a capacity for assessment and modification as required. In a 1990 study of five large school districts, Palfrey and colleagues (1990) found that most students with intellectual disability were being provided concurrent habilitative therapies—18% received occupational or physical therapy, 34% received counseling services, and 57% received speech and language therapy. Such studies have shown that for children with particular developmental needs, the schools continue to be the major providers of therapeutic services.

As personal progress in education has moved forward, the process of inclusion can be seen in the community also. Children with developmental disabilities are increasingly a part of neighborhood life and engage in a variety of sports and other extracurricular activities with their typically developing peers. Special activities such as hippotherapy (teaching children with disabilities to ride horses) have proven to be particularly enjoyable and valuable. As children with intellectual disability reach young adulthood, they often look forward to more independent living. Many young adults with intellectual disability have become spokespersons, locally or with a larger audience (books, television, national groups). Special cause for celebration is the strength seen now from the 20 years of growth of the self-advocacy movement. The various People First organizations and others, such as Self Advocates Becoming Empowered, are assisting all of us toward better understanding (Dybwad and Bersani, 1996).

Needs of Families and Their Responses

In establishing arrangements for the necessary support systems for their children with special needs, parents suddenly become expert "caregivers" and even "case managers." It is an enormous tribute to parental love and resiliency that this adaptation is achieved so strongly (Taylor et al, 1990). Among the many assignments that parents characteristically perform are those that relate to

- Physical maintenance of the child (diets, adaptive equipment, home modifications, and access to specialized health care)
- Emotional and psychological support (assistance in emerging self-concept, personality definition, developing autonomy, and interactive skills)
- Ensuring access to appropriate education (advocacy, conferencing, and monitoring)
- Social and recreational opportunities (finding possibilities for groups, camps, and sports)
- Ensuring the transition to adulthood (living, vocational, and personal components)

Coordination of medical care also may be a major responsibility. The professions have traditionally underestimated the magnitude of parental contributions to the success of a child's course (Crocker, 1997).

When one interviews families about the pressures felt and the supports desired, the most prominent strategic requirements are the following:

- Parent education of rights and entitlements
- Financial counseling
- Information on community resources
- Recreational opportunities
- Parent support groups
- Parent training for child's health needs
- Transportation
- Respite care
- Legal services

These reflect the diverse areas of activity and outreach enjoined by a family with a child who has a developmental disability. The search for special knowledge is discussed in two books by and for parents: *A Difference in the Family: Life with a Disabled Child* by Featherstone, and *Since Owen: A Parent-to-Parent Guide for Care of the Disabled Child* by Callanan.

Particular regard is due for brothers and sisters, as they grow up and help in households with children who have intellectual disability (Powell and Gallagher, 1992). These young individuals ultimately have the longest term relationships with the child with intellectual disability, and their understanding and support traditionally have not received appropriate attention. Brothers and sisters often must deal with alterations in the normalcy of family rhythm, competition for parental resources and attention, possible misconceptions about the origins or outcome of the syndrome of the involved child, and an obligation to meet enhanced parental expectations. They also may receive mixed messages about double standards on compliance and behavior and on the competency of the affected child. Brothers and sisters gain significantly by being provided meaningful information in suitable form, being involved in decision making, and having counseling or group activity with similar peers when appropriate. Most studies show a favorable long-range adaptive outcome for these brothers and sisters, which is a tribute to their strength and to the complex, often positive, effects of living with difference (Orsmond and Seltzer, 2000).

During the past 25 years, there has been a slowly growing number of families who have adopted children with intellectual disability. Although to some degree this outreach has been promoted by the reduced availability of normal infants and children, another, more specific motivation is generally at work. Children with special needs are discretely chosen in an earnest expression of caring, and many times more than one child is eventually adopted by one family (Lightburn and Pine, 1996). The families are predominantly from moderate-income to low-income groups. Physician assistance is needed in preadoption reformation transfer and in postplacement supportive services, but pediatricians have been slow to realize the extent of this movement. In many metropolitan areas there are waiting lists for infants and young children with Down syndrome, a fact that should be acknowledged during genetic counseling. The adoption of children with intellectual disability validates their dignity and provides credibility to their value in the community.

Transitions

In the first full definition of developmental disabilities, included in 1978 in Public Law 95-602, it was understood that the need for special services is "lifelong." School and agency programs tend to build discrete units of activity oriented to particular age periods—infancy, preschool, school years, young adult, adult, and elderly—with limited provision for coordination of the carryover periods. The two periods of transition for young individuals with intellectual disability that prove to be the most pressing are (1) movement from early intervention services to public preschool at 3 years of age, and (2) graduation of youth from education services (and entitlements) at 21 years into the potential for further vocational training and employment as an adult.

For youth and young adults in the latter circumstance, there are many chances for discontinuity. This is an interval of notable personal challenge for intrinsic reasons. Adolescents with mild and moderate disabilities are confronted with difficulty in relating to their impetuous normal peers. Their thinking is often different than that of typical teenagers, and behavior may be altered by comorbid affective disorders, such as depression and anxiety (Dekker and Koot, 2003). The emergence of sexual feelings is bewildering because these are seldom realistically acknowledged by parents or service providers (Murphy and Elias, 2006). Pubertal individuals with intellectual disability are often treated by society with silence, overprotection, and covert alarm; meaningful exchange and education, plus the guided opportunity for positive experience, would be preferable.

In the search for suitable autonomy, youth with intellectual disability have need of numerous assisted preparations. It can be claimed that we are often guilty of holding young people hostage to dependency, and in this sense society has a developmental disability. The American Academy of Pediatrics strongly recommends a transition plan for children with developmental disabilities and chronic medical conditions. Transition planning, including emphasis on independence; continuation of coordinated medical and supportive services; and attention to changes in insurance coverage, educational supports, and employment opportunities, requires intensive coordination on the part of the patient, family, and pediatrician (Committee on Children with Disabilities, 2000).

Since the 1970s, important changes have occurred in the fields of rehabilitation and vocational counseling, including stronger identification with young individuals who have intellectual disability. There also have been improvements in the commitment to prevocational and vocational training in the public schools. It was optimistically believed that with the development of assisted employment and supported employment, virtually all individuals with mild intellectual disability could be established in gainful jobs (Kiernan, 1992). This goal has been achieved only for a few, however. Further facilitation is needed in the early and continuing school vocational experiences, with thoughtful personal choices and broadly based counseling ensured. State agencies also must begin promptly with their incorporation of young adults in community support services, to avoid possible waiting lists. Transition planning should begin by age 14 years. A greater variety of options for community living has made transitional planning more comprehensive than in the past.

Consumer Activism and Organizations

Finally, vigorous accolades must be paid to the army of parents, relatives, friends, and sympathizers who have done so much to change the milieu in which children with intellectual disability now live. Singly or in small groups, these individuals have worked as program volunteers, advocates, peer supporters, and authors. They have served endlessly on advisory groups, human rights committees, and developmental disabilities councils. In many communities, parents have performed the necessary work to begin group homes, including arrangement for property acquisition, long-term financing, and staffing. Their public voice has served to hearten other, less articulate, families; to educate government officials and agency personnel; and to prod the conscience of professionals. They have planned programs, written legislation, and launched class action suits. These private individuals have raised money for research, joined in projects, and been responsible for the creation of prevention endeavors. Their activities have gone far beyond any prospects of particular assistance to their own family members. The list could be vast, but special acknowledgment must be made at least to The Arc (national, state, local), United Cerebral Palsy Association, Epilepsy Foundation, National Down Syndrome Congress, Parent to Parent, Federation for Children with Special Needs, TASH, Association for the Care of Children's Health, Alliance of Genetic Support Groups, National Tay-Sachs and Allied Diseases Association, and the National MPS Society.

SEVERE AND PROFOUND INTELLECTUAL DISABILITY

In the total spectrum of intellectual disability, a minority exists within the minority whose disability is of unusually serious nature: children (and adults) who have severe or profound retardation. This group—at most 5% of all individuals with cognitive disabilities—raises special issues because of the magnitude of their quantitative and qualitative atypicality. Their need for us to teach them is extraordinary, and their ability to teach us is equally remarkable. The general public, and many professionals as well, are bewildered by individuals with IQs less than 35 (or, particularly, <20) and lack frames of reference for interaction with them. Notable features of individuals with profound intellectual ability are the following:

1. Lack of self-care and even survival skills. These are individuals with a truly pervasive disability who often are unable to dress, feed, or toilet themselves, even in adult life, and who have a compelling dependency on others throughout their lives.
2. Communication blockade. Inadequate language is invariable, and often there is no successful verbal communication whatsoever. This can lead to social difficulties, complicated by the incomplete ability of others to interpret the individual's feelings.
3. Deviant behavior. With blunted exchange and reward on other levels, there is often a resort to bizarre repetitive or stereotypic behavior, sometimes self-stimulating. This behavior can include rocking, twirling, and posturing, with alarm induced when actions become self-injurious.
4. Serious organic pathology. Although severe or profound retardation is found in all segments of the causation schema (see Table 68-2), it is more frequent in individuals with hereditary or malformation problems. Usually there are combined disabilities (including seizures and sensory problems) and often serious health issues. Motor function difficulties or complications often reduce the individual's potential for ambulation.
5. Greater commitment for intervention. Incidental learning (e.g., learning that from ambient experiences and social exchange) is reduced, so that efforts for progress require more discrete programming.
6. Teacher confusion regarding potential. Standard test instruments are less relevant at this far end of the spectrum, and personal progress and its documentation are slow and irregular. Disagreements have often erupted in determination of public policy regarding the educational investment.

Individuals with these serious degrees of developmental disability raise special personal challenges. It is axiomatic in human development (and in education) that continued learning and progress are a fundamental response to adequate stimulation for all except those who are in coma, but in these situations the gains can be painfully slow, and the feedback not of the conventional sort. Individual interactions have their own language and their own special rewards. Most clinical psychologists restrict the use of the term *profound mental retardation* to individuals in whom the adaptive components are extremely restricted, rather than using the IQ definition primarily. *Profound disability* is a more reasonable term because in these individuals complexity of problems is the rule. Since the 1970s, the promulgation of "no reject" programs for education, family support, and general activities has allowed many quiet miracles of personal triumph to occur; this refers to fulfillment for the individuals with severe special needs as well as for the individuals who relate to them or work with them.

On a historical note, individuals with developmental disabilities, particularly on the more severe end of the spectrum, were formerly placed in state residential institutions where they received basic shelter and care, but very little in the way of individualized services or comprehensive medical care. This was referred to as "congregate care." By the last quarter of the 20th century, however, the pendulum of public opinion had shifted away from institutionalization and toward a community-based environment, where people with disabilities could receive educational interventions, therapeutic services, and good medical care while living at home with their parents or in small community-based supportive homes. The improvements in medical care have led to a significantly increased life expectancy, and improved quality of life overall for individuals with intellectual disability (Braddock et al, 2004).

PREVENTION OF INTELLECTUAL DISABILITY

On first consideration, the achievement of prevention regarding intellectual disability would seem to consist of identifying a causation of relevance, devising an interventionist strategy, and applying the strategy in the appropriate setting. In practice, this approach only occasionally works. Problems come in the wide variety of etiologies, some of them multifactorial; frequent conundrums about affecting the process; and competition for resources or priority for application. Actually, we have done quite well in a number of low-volume/high-intensity disorders with intellectual disability (e.g., molecular, viral), but in the subtler, high-volume disorders, we are not doing so well.

The assignment, basically, is to provide protection and sustenance to the developing CNS. In the larger arena, this means support to pregnant women and younger children (Crocker, 1992; Wallace and Nelson, 1994). It is generally believed that the basic maternal and child health services construct must be maintained, and that the particular activities of greatest ultimate value are (1) family life education in public school (in parenting skills); (2) early, high-quality, and affordable prenatal care; (3) regional newborn intensive care units;

(4) generously supplied early intervention programs; (5) a "medical home" for each child, with continuity of care; and (6) effective services for children and families where there is disability. With moderately diligent use of these principles, many of the most important risk indicators are not changing appreciably (teenage fertility, racial disparity in infant mortality, preterm birth, child abuse) (Crocker, 1994). More recently, much energy has been directed to the prevention of secondary conditions (complications or contingencies of primary disabilities), and this can be expected to have valuable conserving effects.

Following is the current status of prevention work:

NEARLY TOTAL ELIMINATION

- Congenital rubella—by early immunization and antibody screening
- Phenylketonuria, galactosemia, and congenital hypothyroidism—by newborn screening followed by dietary management or replacement therapy
- Kernicterus—by reduction of sensitization through the use of globulin therapy, and more effective neonatal treatment with phototherapy and exchange transfusion

MAJOR REDUCTION

- Tay-Sachs disease—by carrier screening and prenatal diagnosis in individuals with increased risk
- Morbidity from prematurity—through newborn intensive care nurseries
- Measles encephalitis and *Haemophilus influenzae* meningitis—by early vaccination

SIGNIFICANT CURRENT EFFORTS UNDER WAY

- Neural tube defects—by folic acid supplementation and by maternal serum α-fetoprotein screening and prenatal diagnosis
- Down syndrome—through counseling of older pregnant women and prenatal diagnosis guided by marker screening
- Lead intoxication—through environmental improvement, screening of lead levels, and chelation when necessary
- Prenatal alcohol effects and syndrome—through public education
- Morbidity from head injury—through the use of child restraints in automobiles and bike helmets
- Child neglect and abuse—through family life education in public schools that assists youth in preparation for parenthood

SPECIAL ASSISTANCE AND RELIEF

- Prompt identification and early intervention for infants with disability or at risk
- Support to families with children who have disabilities to provide guidance and resources
- Genetic counseling when special risk is involved
- Improved management for difficult pregnancies

There are many children whose disability cannot be prevented by usual means. These include most children with congenital anomalies from unknown prenatal influences; most children with nonfamilial chromosomal disorders (including children with Down syndrome born of younger mothers [≥80% of the total]); most children with serious childhood neuroses and psychoses, which interfere with development; and all children in whom the basis of intellectual disability cannot be identified at all, even on careful study.

The outlook is good for continuing improvement in the prevention of intellectual disability syndromes. Childcare professionals can assist in this movement by promoting immunization, performing newborn screening, providing guidance during pregnancy, and promoting the use of child safety measures. Gains also would be made through the wider employment of early developmental screening, comprehensive assessment of children with known disabilities, and thoughtful genetic counseling. Public support should be marshaled for programs for infants and young children. Basic and applied research regarding the nature of cortical impairment must not lapse.

REFERENCES

American Association on Mental Retardation: Mental Retardation: Definition, Classification, and Systems of Supports. Washington, DC, American Association on Mental Retardation, 1992.

Braddock D, Hemp R, Rizzolo MC: State of the states in developmental disabilities. Ment Retard 42:356-370, 2004.

Callanan CR: Since Owen: A Parent-to-Parent Guide for Care of the Disabled Child. Baltimore, Johns Hopkins University Press, 1990.

Committee on Children with Disabilities: The role of the pediatrician in transitioning children and adolescents with developmental disabilities and chronic illnesses from school to work or college. Pediatrics 106:854-858, 2000.

Committee on Children with Disabilities: Identifying infants and young children with developmental disorders in the medical home: An algorithm for developmental surveillance and screening. Pediatrics 118:305-420, 2006.

Crocker AC: The causes of mental retardation. Pediatr Ann 18:623, 1989.

Crocker AC: Data collection for the evaluation of mental retardation prevention activities: The fateful forty-three. Ment Retard 30:303, 1992.

Crocker AC: Prevention of disability. *In* Wallace HM, Nelson RP, Sweeney PJ (eds): Maternal and Child Health Practices, 4th ed. Oakland, CA, Third Party Publishing Co, 1994, pp 705-710.

Crocker AC: The impact of disabling conditions. *In* Wallace HM, Biehl RF, MacQueen JC, Blackman JA (eds): Mosby's Resource Guide to Children with Disabilities and Chronic Illness. St. Louis, Mosby–Year Book, 1997, pp 22-29.

Dekker MC, Koot HM: DSM-IV disorders in children with borderline to moderate intellectual disability, I: Prevalence and impact. J Am Acad Child Adolesc Psychiatry 42:915-922, 2003.

Dybwad G, Bersani H (eds): New Voices: Self-Advocacy by People with Disabilities. Cambridge, MA, Brookline Books, 1996.

Elias ER, Irons MB, Hurley AD, et al: Clinical effects of cholesterol supplementation in six patients with the Smith-Lemli-Opitz syndrome (SLOS). Am J Med Genet 68:305-310, 1997.

Featherstone H: A Difference in the Family: Life with a Disabled Child. New York, Basic Books, 1980.

Kiernan WE: Vocational rehabilitation. *In* Levine MD, Carey WB, Croaker AC (eds): Developmental-Behavioral Pediatrics, 2nd ed. Philadelphia, WB Saunders, 1992, pp 734-736.

Lightburn A, Pine BA: Supporting and enhancing the adoption of children with developmental disabilities. Children Youth Serv Rev 18:139, 1996.

Luckasson RA, Schaleck RL, Snell ME, et al; American Association on Intellectual and Developmental Disabilities: Mental Retardation: Definition, Classification, and Systems of Supports Manual. 2002.

Murphy NA, Elias ER: Sexuality of children and adolescents with developmental disabilities. Pediatrics 118:398-403, 2006.

Nelson RP: Community services for children with mental retardation. Pediatr Ann 18:615, 1989.

Orsmond GI, Seltzer MM: Brothers and sisters of adults with mental retardation: Gendered nature of the sibling relationship. Am J Ment Retard 105:486-508, 2000.

Palfrey JS, Singer JD, Ralphael ES, Walker DK: Providing therapeutic services to children in special educational placements: An analysis of the related services provisions of P.L. 94-142 in five urban school districts. Pediatrics 85:518, 1990.

Powell TH, Gallagher PA: Brothers and Sisters: A Special Part of Exceptional Families, 2nd ed. Baltimore, Paul H. Brookes, 1992.

Schalock RL, Luckasson RA, Shogren KA, et al: Understanding the change to the term intellectual disability. Intellect Dev Disabil 45:116-124, 2007.

Taylor AB, Epstein SG, Crocker AC: Health care for children with special needs. *In* Schlesinger M, Eisenberg L (eds): Children in a Changing Health Care System: Prospects and Proposals. Baltimore, Johns Hopkins University Press, 1990, pp 27-48.

Wallace HM, Nelson RP: Emerging priorities in maternal and child health services. *In* Wallace HM, Nelson RP, Sweeney PJ (eds): Maternal and Child Health Practices, 4th ed. Oakland, CA, Third Party Publishing Co, 1994, pp 120-130.

HISTORICAL REFERENCES OF NOTE

Crocker AC: Sisters and brothers. *In* Mulick JA, Pueschel SM (eds): Parent-Professional Partnerships in Developmental Disabilities. Cambridge, MA, Ware Press, 1983, pp 139-148.

Crocker AC: Societal commitment toward prevention of developmental disabilities. *In* Pueschel SM, Mulick JA (eds): Prevention of Developmental Disabilities. Baltimore, Paul H. Brookes, 1990, pp 337-343.

Guralnick MJ: The Effectiveness of Early Intervention. Baltimore, Paul H. Brookes, 1997.

Lewis RG: Adoption and mental retardation. Pediatr Ann 18:637, 1989.

Nelson RP, Crocker AC: The medical care of mentally retarded persons in public residential facilities. N Engl J Med 299:1039, 1978.

Szymanski LS: Emotional problems in a child with serious developmental handicap. *In* Levine MD, Carey WB, Crocker AC, Gross RT (eds): Developmental-Behavioral Pediatrics. Philadelphia, WB Saunders, 1983, pp 839-846.

Turnbull AP, Turnbull HP: Developing independence. J Adolesc Health Care 6:108, 1985.

69 AUTISM AND RELATED DISORDERS

Fred Volkmar and Lisa Wiesner

EVOLUTION OF DIAGNOSTIC CONCEPTS

Autism and the related disorders are conditions characterized by deviance and delay in the development of social and communication skills associated with unusual, restricted patterns of behavior and interests. Autism is the best-known disorder in this group. In addition, several other conditions are currently recognized, including Rett syndrome, childhood disintegrative disorder (CDD), Asperger syndrome, and "subthreshold" autism (pervasive developmental disorder–not otherwise specified [PDD-NOS]). This chapter reviews these conditions with a focus primarily on autism, and discusses aspects of screening and treatment.

DEVELOPMENT OF DIAGNOSTIC CONCEPTS

Autism was first recognized by Kanner (1943), who reported 11 children with "autistic disturbances of affective contact"; the term *autistic* was intended to convey the profound social isolation that Kanner believed was a hallmark of the condition. Although children with autism had likely been observed before, Kanner's ability to describe the condition so precisely sets his work apart. He suggested that the condition was congenital, and noted that in addition to marked social problems, the children had unusual difficulties with change and "insistence on sameness." His report also noted that many children did not communicate verbally, and children who did had unusual language with atypical intonation, a tendency to echo, and confusion of personal pronouns.

Kanner's description remains classic, although some aspects of it proved misleading. Parents in the original cohort were well educated and successful; this led to the notion that there might be some social class bias in autism and to the idea that perhaps autism stemmed from deviant parenting (neither notion is correct). Kanner also noted that *some* intellectual skills were preserved and presumed that this meant intelligence was likely normal, and he noted that the children did not have an unusual appearance or obvious associated medical conditions. It is now clear that many children with autism do exhibit significant intellectual impairments, and that they are prone to specific medical problems and conditions.

Before and after Kanner, other clinicians described syndromes with some similarities to autism. In 1908, Heller described the condition now referred to as CDD (previously referred to as *disintegrative psychosis*). In this rare condition, children develop a severe autistic-like condition after some years of normal development (Volkmar et al, 2005). The year after Kanner's paper on autism, a Viennese medical student, Asperger, described a small group of boys with marked social problems, unusual interests, and motor clumsiness, but with good language and vocabulary skills (Asperger, 1944). Unaware of Kanner's work, Asperger termed the condition *autistic psychopathy*. His description had points of similarity (social difficulties) and difference (preserved language skills) to Kanner's, but was little recognized until publication of a review by Wing (1981). Essentially, this term referred to children with severe social disability but good language abilities.

Rett (1966) reported an unusual syndrome in girls with a history of early normal development followed by head growth deceleration and developmental deterioration. Rett speculated initially that this might be a form of autism, but as more extensive information became available, it became clear that the more "autistic-like" phase of the syndrome was brief. An abnormal gene has now been observed in many cases (Amir et al, 1990).

The term PDD-NOS (also referred to as atypical PDD or atypical development) is used for children with some, but not all, features of autism. This condition is undoubtedly more common than classic autism, but it is much less frequently studied. PDD-NOS is now of greater interest because of potential genetic links with autism and the "broader autism phenotype" (Rutter, 2005a). Characteristics of these conditions are summarized in Table 69-1.

Confusion about the continuity of autism and childhood schizophrenia complicated early work on autism. As children with autism were followed over time, it became clear they differed from children with schizophrenia in their course and in clinical features and family history. The high rates of epilepsy noted in longitudinal samples suggested the importance of brain mechanisms, and high concordance rates for identical twins suggested a strong genetic component. The term *pervasive developmental disorder* was itself coined as a class term for the entire group of disorders in 1980, when autism was first officially recognized. As a practical matter this term is synonymous with autism and related conditions or autism spectrum disorders.

Table 69-1. **Diagnostic Features of Autism and Nonautistic Pervasive Developmental Disorders**

Feature	Autistic Disorder	Asperger Disorder	Rett Disorder	Childhood Disintegrative Disorders	Pervasive Developmental Disorder–NOS
Age at recognition (mo)	0-36	Usually >36	5-30	>24	Variable
Sex ratio	M > F	M > F	F >> M	M > F	M > F
Loss of skills	Variable	Usually not	Marked	Marked	Usually not
Social skills	Very poor	Poor	Varies with age	Very poor	Variable
Communication skills	Usually poor	Fair	Very poor	Very poor	Poor to good
Circumscribed interests	Variable (mechanical)	Marked (facts)	NA	NA	Variable
Family history of similar problems	Sometimes	Frequent	Not usually	No	Unknown
Seizure disorder	Common	Uncommon	Frequent	Common	Uncommon
Head growth slows	No	No	Yes	No	No
IQ range	Severe ID to normal	Mild ID to normal	Severe ID	Severe ID	Severe ID to normal
Outcome	Poor to good	Fair to good	Very poor	Very poor	Fair to good

ID, intellectual disability; NA, not applicable; NOS, not otherwise specified.
Adapted from Volkmar FR, Cohen D: Nonautistic pervasive developmental disorders. *In* Michaels R, Cooper AM, Guze SB, et al (eds): Psychiatry. Philadelphia, Lippincott-Raven, p 4.

DEFINITIONS

The definition of autism has evolved over time. Presently, the American (DSM-IV) (American Psychiatric Association, 2000) and international (ICD) approaches to diagnosis of autism are the same. Social factors are weighted more heavily than communicative or behavioral features because they are more strongly predictive of diagnosis. The current diagnostic approach works reasonably with two important exceptions (Volkmar and Klin, 2005). Since the time this approach was originally proposed (Volkmar et al, 1994), there has been a major effort to diagnose autism in the first year or two of life, although it is clear that some children do not exhibit all features of autism until around age 3. Also, the issue of possible overlap of autism and Asperger syndrome remains a topic of debate—whether Asperger syndrome is best viewed as high functioning autism (Klin et al, 2005).

EPIDEMIOLOGY AND DEMOGRAPHIC AND CULTURAL ISSUES

More than 30 studies of the epidemiology of autism are now available. Estimates of prevalence range widely from 0.7/10,000 to 72.6/10,000, and vary depending on differences in definitions and methods (Fombonne, 2005a) with a median prevalence estimate of 13/10,000. More recent studies of autism report higher rates, leading some to worry that autism may be increasing in frequency, but this issue is unresolved given the major changes in definition and improved case detection (Fombonne, 2005b). Except for PDD-NOS (which may apply to 1 in 150 children), other disorders in the autism spectrum group are less common than autism.

Autism is three to five times more common in boys than girls, but girls with autism are more likely to be more severely intellectually impaired (Fombonne, 2005a). Females may have a higher threshold for expressing the disorder, and a greater "dose" of whatever causes autism is required. Male predominance also is the rule for the other disorders in this group except for Rett syndrome, where male cases are only rarely seen.

Current approaches to the diagnosis of autism work well around the world (Volkmar and Klin, 2005), but treatment practices in relation to cultural and ethnic differences have not received much attention (Ozonoff et al, 2003). Within the United States, children living in poverty may be less likely to be diagnosed with autism (Mandell et al, 2006).

CLINICAL AND DEVELOPMENTAL FEATURES

Clinical features of these conditions are summarized in Table 69-1. Autism is first and foremost a disorder of "affective contact," and social dysfunction (autism) is the central defining feature of the condition. This disability appears, in most cases, to exist from birth (Table 69-2). In contrast to typically developing infants, infants with autism have limited social interest in the human face and voice—skills important for many other aspects of development (Chawarska and Volkmar, 2005). Although prospective studies are needed, available data reveal many early social-communicative warning signs of autism that should prompt additional assessment (Table 69-3).

In autism, delays in development of spoken language are a common cause for initial evaluation. Communication difficulties also are central in autism, and many (now probably less than half) individuals with autism do not use speech as a primary mode of communicating; this number seems to be decreasing with early intervention (Paul and Sutherland, 2005). Children who do speak have language that is unusual in many ways (e.g., idiosyncratic language, echolalia, unusual monotonic voice, overly literal language) and severe difficulties with social language use. A child may have a good vocabulary, but have severe difficulties in carrying on a conversation (Paul and Sutherland, 2005).

In contrast to their lack of social responsivity, children with autism are often acutely responsive to small changes in the nonsocial environment. They exhibit unusual mannerisms, such as body rocking or hand flapping, and are often intolerant of change and insistent on routine. These behavioral features are required for a diagnosis of autism, although they sometimes are observed in other disorders by themselves. A child with autism may seem to have little interest in family members, but be highly attached to an unusual inanimate object (a type of magazine, bundle of twigs, hard metal toy). Similarly, the child may not consistently respond to his or her name and may not imitate speech sounds, but he or she may be very upset with the sound of the vacuum cleaner. The unusual stereotyped movements seen in older children (>3 years) with autism are likely preceded by unusual perceptual interests (Chawarska and Volkmar, 2005). Unusual affective responses (e.g., throwing a tantrum in response to a small change) may be a source of great distress to parents. Play skills tend to remain underdeveloped, with objects used more for simple sensorimotor or functional play, rather than more symbolic activities (Chawarska and Volkmar, 2005), and are important areas for early intervention (National Research Council, 2001).

Cognitive development in autism is unusual. Generally, children with autism do best with tasks that involve perceptual-motor or motor abilities, and do poorly with tasks that involve social judgment, abstract thinking, and use of symbolic information or verbal abilities (Prior and Ozonoff, 1998). When the highly discrepant results of various subtests are averaged, IQ scores are often within the range of intellectual disability/intellectual deficiency (Klin et al, 2005). With earlier intervention, there seems to have been a trend toward decreased rates of associated intellectual disability, likely reflecting changes in diagnostic practice and the results of earlier intervention (National Research Council, 2001). As children with autism reach school age, scores become more stable. Unusual islets of ability are sometimes observed (e.g., children with autism may have amazing abilities to do calendar calculation or drawing abilities) (Hermelin, 2001). Such individuals (usually referred to as *autistic savants*) can be quite impaired in other areas.

Although children with Asperger syndrome also are severely socially disabled, they usually are highly verbal, and their difficulties are not a source of concern until the child is exposed to peers (i.e., typically in the preschool years). In contrast to autism, motor clumsiness

Table 69-2. **Key Clinical Features of Autism***

Significantly Impaired Social Interaction (Two of the Following)
Markedly impaired nonverbal behaviors (e.g., eye gaze)
Lack of expected peer relations
No spontaneous sharing of pleasure/joint attention
Social-emotional reciprocity impaired
Impaired Communication (at Least One)
Delayed/absent spoken language
Inability to have a conversation (for those who can talk)
Repetitive, stereotyped, idiosyncratic language
Relative to developmental level lack of imaginative play
Restricted Behavior/Interests (at Least One)
Preoccupation with stereotyped and restricted interest
Inflexible adherence to nonfunctional rules
Stereotyped motor mannerisms
Preoccupation with parts of object

*For a DSM diagnosis of autism, a total of at least six features required with onset before age 3.
Adapted from American Psychiatric Association: Diagnostic and Statistical Manual of Mental Disorders, 4th ed, rev ed. Washington, DC, American Psychiatric Association, 2000.

Table 69-3. **Symptoms Differentiating Infants and Toddlers with Autism from Typical and Developmentally Delayed Peers**

	Social Interaction	**Communication**	**Stereotypical and Repetitive Behaviors**
First Year	Limited ability to anticipate being picked up Low frequency of looking at people Little interest in interactive games Content to be alone	Poor response to name Infrequent looking at objects held by others	Excessive mouthing Aversion to social touch
Years Two to Three	Abnormal eye contact Limited social referencing Limited interest in other children Limited social smile Low frequency of looking at people Limited range of facial expressions Limited sharing of affect/enjoyment Little interest in interactive games Limited functional play No pretend play Limited motor imitation	Low frequency of verbal or nonverbal communication Failure to share interest (e.g., by pointing, giving, showing) Poor response to name Failure to respond to communicative gestures (showing, pointing, giving) Use of other's body as tool (e.g., takes hand to get object without making eye contact—as if hand is the agent) Unusual vocalizations (may not produce entire range of language sounds)	Hand/finger mannerisms Inappropriate object use Repetitive interests/play Unusual sensory behaviors (hypersensitivity/hyposensitivity to sounds, texture, taste, or visual preoccupations) Unusual attachment to objects (hard not soft, the specific object is less important than category of object)

Adapted from Chawarska K, Volkmar FR: Autism in infancy and early childhood. *In* Volkmar F, Klin A, Paul R, Cohen D (eds): Handbook of Autism and Pervasive Developmental Disorders, 3rd ed. Hoboken, NJ, John Wiley, 2005, p 230.

is frequent, as are all-encompassing interests; the latter interfere with functioning and often intrude on family life. The pattern on cognitive testing also is different: In contrast to autism, verbal skills are often an area of significant strength for the child; this pattern sometimes is referred to as nonverbal learning disability (see vignette) (Rourke, 1988). Individuals with Asperger syndrome are much less likely to function in the intellectual disability range.

Vignette

Autobiographical Statement of a 10-Year-Old Boy with Asperger Disorder*

My name is Robert Edwards. I am an intelligent, unsociable but adaptable person. I would like to dispel any untrue rumors about me. I cannot fly. I cannot use telekinesis. My brain is not large enough to destroy the entire world when unfolded. I did not teach my long-haired guinea pig, Chronos, to eat everything in sight (that is the nature of the long-haired guinea pig).

*Name changed.
From Volkmar FR, Klin A, Schultz RT, et al: Asperger's disorder: Clinical case conference. Am J Psychiatry 157:262-267, 2000.

In Rett syndrome, early development is normal, then head growth decelerates, and the child loses purposeful hand movements; over time, severe psychomotor retardation and numerous other difficulties are evident, including breathing problems and characteristic hand washing/hand wringing mannerisms (VanAcker et al, 2005). The original impression that Rett syndrome is exclusively found in girls has been re-evaluated in light of the discovery of a gene involved in most cases (Amir et al, 1990); it is now clear that boys also may exhibit the mutation, but with different clinical manifestations (Volkmar et al, 2005). CDD is a rare condition in which a syndrome identical to autism develops after a prolonged period (at least 2, but usually 3 to 4 years) of normal development. The child then deteriorates behaviorally, typically losing social and language abilities (Volkmar et al, 2005). In Rett syndrome and CDD, significant intellectual impairment and severe communication problems are typical.

In PDD-NOS, the clinical picture is much more variable. Various subtypes are likely to be identified eventually within this broad category. By definition, the child's difficulties are not severe enough to justify a diagnosis of autism or Asperger syndrome. There have been some suggestions that at least in some cases there is a significant overlap with attentional disorders (Towbin, 2005).

ONSET OF AUTISM AND RELATED CONDITIONS AND REGRESSION

Kanner (1943) originally believed that autism was a congenital disorder, but subsequent work suggests that in perhaps 25% of cases the child develops normally for a time before exhibiting either a loss of skills or a pattern of developmental stagnation (Rogers, 2004). A major limitation of the available research has been a lack of prospective data. More than half of parents report being worried by the time the child is 1 year old, and almost 90% report being worried by age 2 (Chawarska and Volkmar, 2005). Common initial concerns include lack of social engagement, delayed speech, or worries about deafness. Sometimes parents report a regression in development, but careful history reveals preexisting delays. Regression is a universal phenomenon in Rett syndrome and CDD. In Asperger syndrome, parents typically become worried only when the child is exposed to same-age peers (e.g., in preschool) (Klin et al, 2005).

Developmental Change

In autism, the most "classic" presentation is typically assumed to be between ages 3 and 5, although variability also is seen (Fig. 69-1) (Charman et al, 2005). Although infants are now being diagnosed with autism, sometimes only some of the required diagnostic features are present (e.g., motor mannerisms may not emerge until age 3) (Lord, 1995). Often by school age, increased social interest has developed along with more sophisticated cognitive and communication skills (Loveland and Tunali-Kotoski, 2005). In adolescence, some children make gains, whereas others sometimes exhibit losses (Shea and Mesibov, 2005). In Asperger syndrome and PDD-NOS, outcome is probably better than in more classic autism (Howlin, 2005). Poor outcome is characteristic of CDD and Rett syndrome.

Neurobiology

Genetics

Autism is a strongly genetic disorder. The risk for parents who have had one child with autism for having a second is 2% to 10%. Monozygotic twins have substantially increased concordance for autism (around 90%),

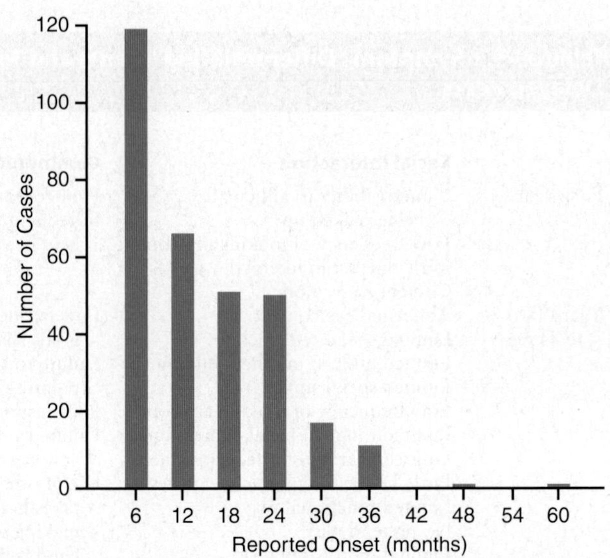

Figure 69-1. Age of onset (cases with clinical diagnosis of autism in DSM-IV field trial). *(From Volkmar F, Klin A: Issues in the classification of autism and related conditions. In Volkmar F, Klin A, Paul R, Cohen D [eds]: Handbook of Autism and Pervasive Developmental Disorders, 3rd ed. Hoboken, NJ, John Wiley, 2005, p 20.)*

and siblings are at risk for a broader range of social and developmental difficulties (Rutter, 2005b). Presently, it seems likely that multiple genes are involved, and that a broader phenotype of related difficulties may be inherited (Rutter, 2005a). Regions of interest have been identified on various chromosomes, and as specific genes are identified, animal models can be developed, and fundamental mechanisms can be examined. In most cases of Rett syndrome, mutations in the gene *MeCP2* (methyl-CpG-binding protein 2) are present (Amir et al, 1990).

Neuroimaging and Brain Function

Several lines of evidence strongly implicate brain mechanisms in the pathogenesis of autism. Longitudinal studies revealed that children with autism were at high risk for developing epilepsy (Fig. 69-2) (Volkmar and Nelson, 1990) and other neurologic signs and symptoms (Minshew et al, 2005). With the advent of magnetic resonance imaging (MRI), it has become possible to study brain morphology with improved resolution, and the advent of functional MRI has made it possible to study discrete brain systems in vivo.

Given the diverse expression of autism and its impact on diverse aspects of development, various neural systems likely are involved. It also is clear from the study of children who have good cognitive abilities that some systems must be relatively spared. Various models have been proposed, based on sensory and complex information processing or emphasizing the difficulties with social-affective engagement. Animal models of the disorder also have been attempted (Bachevalier and Loveland, 2003), although the representativeness of such approaches has been questioned (Amaral et al, 2003).

In his original article, Kanner (1943) noted that children with autism had enlarged heads. This finding was replicated, but only as MRI and neuropathologic studies become available did interest in it increase. Among toddlers with autism, the brain may be enlarged by 10% (Courchesne et al, 2001), but by adolescence and adulthood, the effect is substantially reduced. Head size is not increased at birth, suggesting the operation of factors in the first months of postnatal life (e.g., possibly reflecting a failure of normal neural pruning). It also is unclear whether the brain size increase is a generalized versus localized phenomenon (Horwitz et al, 1988). Macrocephaly is observed in some other conditions associated with autism (e.g., fragile X syndrome).

Abnormalities in areas included with the limbic system have included reduced density, cell size, and dendritic arborization (Bauman and Kemper, 2005) with alterations in cortical architecture (minicolumns) as well (Casanova et al, 2002). Studies using functional MRI have revealed many interesting findings; for instance, the fusiform gyrus (an area of the brain typically highly engaged by human faces) is hypoactive in autism (Schultz et al, 2000). Other areas of the brain are being investigated, including the superior temporal sulci and the dorsomedial prefrontal cortex. Research on the social brain also has shown differences in the ways individuals with autism view social scenes (Klin, 2004) (Fig. 69-3)—an observation with potential importance for screening.

About one third of children with autism exhibit peripheral hyperserotonemia (Anderson and Hoshino, 2005). Although the significance of this finding is unclear, studies of potential basic genetic mechanisms that might underlie it have now begun to appear (Veenstra-VanderWeele et al, 2002). A role for the dopaminergic system is suggested because of its importance in movement problems and the potential behavioral benefits of the atypical neuroleptics in treatment (Anderson and Hoshino, 2005). Speculation also has focused on endogenous opioid systems and the use of opioid antagonists in treatment (e.g., of self-abuse); controlled studies have not been positive (Buitelaar et al, 1998).

Obstetric and Environmental Risk

Beginning in the 1980s, a series of studies suggested increased rates of prenatal, perinatal, and neonatal complications in the histories of children with autism. Glasson and colleagues (2004) reported increased risk for experiencing complications during the prenatal and perinatal periods in large series of cases of individuals with

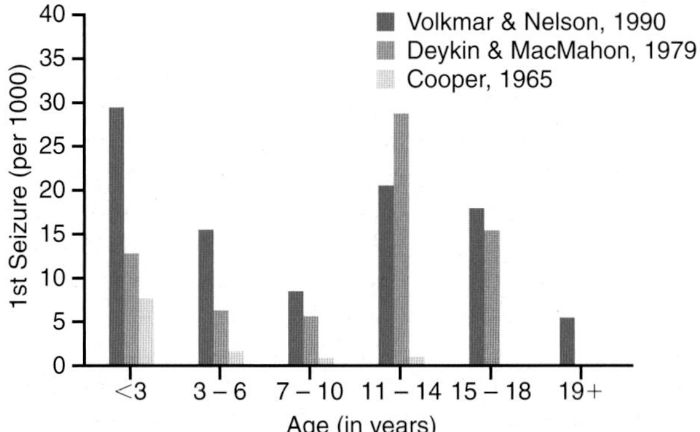

Figure 69-2. Rates of epilepsy (recurrent seizures) in two samples of individuals with autism/pervasive developmental disorder (Volkmar and Nelson, 1990, and Deykin and MacMahon, 1979) and a normative British sample (Cooper, 1965). *(Data from Volkmar FR, Nelson DS: Seizure disorders in autism. J Am Acad Child Adolesc Psychiatry 29:127-129, 1990.)*

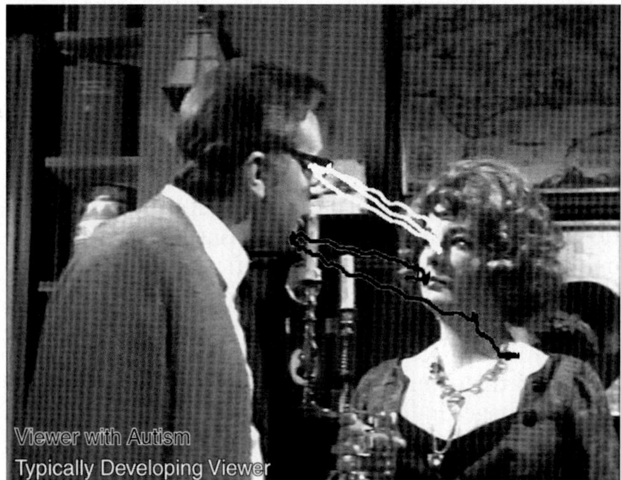

Figure 69-3. Visual focus of an autistic man *(black line)* and a normal comparison subject *(white line)* shown in a film clip of a conversation. *(From Klin A, Jones W, Schultz R, et al: Defining and quantifying the social phenotype in autism. Am J Psychiatry 159:895-908, 2002.)*

autism spectrum disorders and a similarly large sample of unaffected siblings compared with a large, randomly selected, population-based control group. The increased risk in the affected and unaffected siblings also is compatible with a strong genetic contribution (Hultman and Sparen, 2004).

Interest in possible environmental factors and autism has been stimulated by occasional lay press reports of cluster cases and by the controversy regarding measles-mumps-rubella (MMR) vaccination and thimerosal. Wakefield and colleagues (1998) suggested that regression autism might result from MMR immunization. Concern also arose about the possibility that thimerosal (an ethyl mercury compound long used as a preservative) might be involved. These concerns received considerable attention in the lay press, and as a result rates of measles vaccination have decreased in the United States and United Kingdom, with an associated increase in rate of measles infection. A series of studies has failed to confirm the hypothesis that vaccines cause autism and there is clearly no evidence that vaccinations have any role in the etiology of autism. Rates of autism do not seem to change with differences in vaccine (with or without thimerosal), and changes in rates of "late-onset" or "regressive" autism have not been observed. Thimerosal has now been removed from all single-dose vaccines, and substantive subsequent data have not supported either hypothesis (Fombonne et al, 2006; Rutter, 2005b).

Although various other environmental factors have been suggested to be associated with autism, evidence for environmental etiologies is weak (Wing and Potter, 2002). Many parents remain concerned, however, because of continued media attention.

TREATMENT AND OUTCOME

Behavioral and Educational Interventions

Autism is a disorder that affects development and interferes with learning. Essentially, the major goal of treatment is to minimize this interference and to maximize positive developmental change and learning. Treatment should be individualized taking into account the particular strengths and weaknesses of the child. In most cases, a structured and intensive intervention program is needed. Usually the efforts of multiple care providers (speech pathologists, special educators, occupational therapists, and physical therapists) are needed. The National Research Council report (2001) on early interventions in autism summarized aspects of effective practice in various treatment models (Table 69-4). The increasing focus on early screening and case detection is likely to have a substantial impact on an already stressed educational system in the coming years.

For younger individuals with autism, there is often a focus on teaching "learning to learn skills"; behavioral approaches can be particularly effective in this regard (National Research Council, 2001). For children with autism who are unable to communicate verbally, augmentative communication strategies (picture exchange, computer-generated speech, visual aides, and schedules) can be extremely helpful (Paul and Sutherland, 2005); it is important for parents (and others) to realize that the use of such strategies only makes it more likely the child will eventually speak.

Table 69-4. Characteristics of Effective Intervention Programs for Young Children with Autism*

Intensive
Structured
Family involvement
Individualized
Explicit teaching of
Social skills
Communication
Play
"Learning to learn" skills

*Programs differ in some respects, and not all features of effective programs are listed.
From National Research Council: Educating Young Children with Autism. Washington, DC, National Academy Press, 2001.

Effective programs share many commonalities and some areas of difference; behavioral programs tend to focus more on goals set by the adult for the child's learning, whereas more developmentally oriented programs explicitly encompass the child's interests and motivations when possible (National Research Council, 2001). As children become older, there should be a greater focus on practical skills (to foster as much adult independence as possible) and careful consideration of adult vocational and educational opportunities (Shea and Mesibov, 2005).

Often children are placed in available programs with minimal consideration of the importance of the individual child's need. Although behavioral programs (e.g., programs using applied behavior analysis) have been shown to be effective, other programs that are more eclectic or developmentally based also can be effective. For children at all ages, it is important that the family be involved because a major area of difficulties is the child's ability to generalize skills across settings often resulting in severely delayed abilities to adapt to "real world" settings (National Research Council, 2001). The question of "how much" is enough is difficult to address—this depends on the individual child's needs and the nature of the program (some of which include a large home component). In the National Research Council report, the typical effective program was about 25 hours a week (National Research Council, 2001).

For the other disorders on the autism spectrum, goals for intervention vary depending on the specific clinical context and age of the child. For children with Rett syndrome, the support of other medical specialists, such as orthopedists and respiratory therapists, is often needed. In Asperger syndrome, the better verbal ability of the child can potentially be a major asset for intervention, through explicit, verbally based teaching of social and other skills (Fig. 69-4) (Klin et al, 2005).

Partly as a result of earlier intervention and service provision, more children with autism and related conditions are now able to attend college, although often additional supports are needed. Psychotherapy (of a highly structured type) sometimes can be helpful

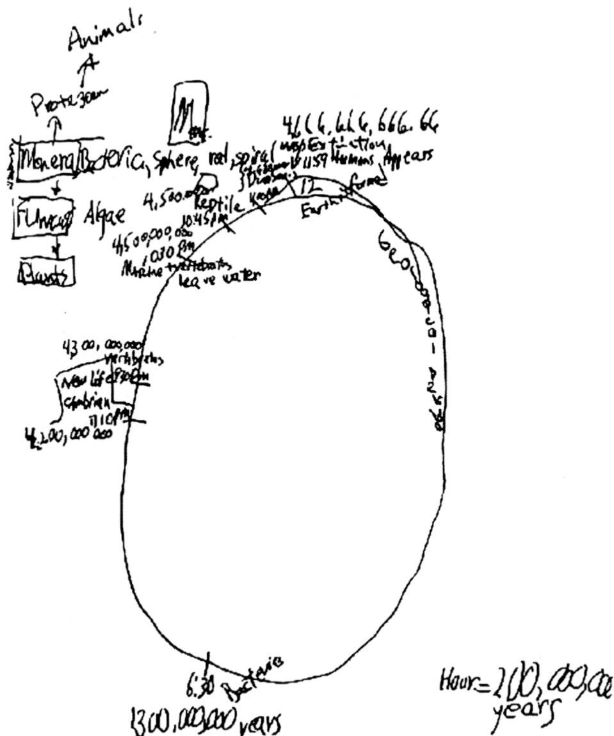

Figure 69-4. Drawing made by a boy with Asperger syndrome, illustrating his interest in time. The drawing illustrates the history of the universe from the moment of its creation (12:00 midnight) through geologic time (e.g., the appearance of bacteria) (6:30 A.M.). It illustrates the patient's interest (and knowledge) regarding this topic, which tended to be all-encompassing, and his less-developed fine motor abilities. *(From Volkmar F, Klin A, Schultz R, et al: Asperger's disorder: Clinical case conference. Am J Psychiatry 157:262-267, 2000.)*

for older children and adults. Various approaches to social skills teaching have appeared in recent years, although most of the currently available research has focused on the youngest age groups, who clearly can learn social skills from typical peers, if the child and the typical peer are appropriately supported (Paul, 2003). Coordination of services is often a problem for families, and the pediatrician has an important role to play in securing, maintaining, and coordinating services.

Drug Treatments

Pharmacologic interventions that address the core social-communication problems have not yet been developed. There are effective treatments, however, for the problem behaviors (agitation, stereotyped movements) that often interfere with learning (Scahill and Martin, 2005). In the last several years, a series of well-designed, placebo-controlled studies have appeared (McCracken et al, 2002). As with any drug treatment, the risk-benefit ratio should be considered as part of the process of obtaining informed consent. Depending on the agent chosen, baseline laboratory studies (tests of liver and renal function, electrocardiogram, urinalysis, blood count, weight, blood pressure) may be indicated, and periodic examination for abnormal movements may be performed (this is particularly important for the use of neuroleptics). Table 69-5 summarizes selected drug treatments.

Table 69-5. Drug Treatments in Autism and Related Conditions

Category of Agent (Example)	Uses	Adverse Effects/ Comments
Atypical neuroleptics (Risperidone*)	Agitation, aggression, stereotyped movements	Sedation, weight gain
Traditional neuroleptics (Haloperidol*)	Stereotyped mannerisms	Sedation, extrapyramidal symptoms, tardive dyskinesia
Stimulants (Methylphenidate*)	Hyperactivity/ inattention (in about 50% of cases)	Many children unable to tolerate owing to agitation and increased stereotyped movements
SSRIs (Fluoxetine*)	Repetitive behaviors/ mood and anxiety problems	Agitation, behavioral deterioration

*Randomized, controlled data available
SSRIs, selective serotonin reuptake inhibitors.

Presently, the atypical neuroleptics (e.g., risperidone) have been the most intensively studied agents (McCracken et al, 2002); these newer agents have largely supplanted the first-generation neuroleptics in terms of reduced side effects. Their main mechanism of action (and side effects) is dopamine receptor blockade. A series of carefully designed, placebo-controlled studies has shown that these agents promptly reduce agitation and stereotyped mannerisms. Side effects include sedation, movement problems, and weight gain. The U.S. Food and Drug Administration has approved the use of risperidone in the treatment of autism.

Next to the atypical neuroleptics, the selective serotonin reuptake inhibitors are probably the most commonly used agents in the treatment of autism spectrum disorders; their use was prompted by the similarities with the behavioral rigidity of obsessive-compulsive disorder (Scahill and Martin, 2005). Data are not as extensive for children as for adults, and usually some weeks are required for an adequate dose to be achieved and the child's response to be determined (Scahill and Martin, 2005). Behavioral activation may be a side effect, and prepubertal children may respond less well (Gordon et al, 1993).

Problems with affective lability or with depression and anxiety may prompt the use of other agents, such as mood stabilizers or antidepressants, but data are even more limited. Various agents have been used (e.g., anxiolytics, β-blockers, clonidine, and naltrexone), but their use is reported largely in case reports, and efficacy is not clearly established. Stimulant medications are sometimes used, particularly in children with less classic autism, but in more classic cases of autism, activation and increased difficulties are common (Scahill and Martin, 2005).

Alternative/Complementary Treatments

Nonestablished treatments are used by many parents—particularly of younger children. Given the important role of the primary health care provider, it is essential that parents be able to discuss such treatments in a frank, open, nonhostile manner. The quality of the evidence used to justify such treatments and potential risks and benefits can be discussed. Parents should be encouraged to pursue traditional treatments with demonstrated benefits—pursuit of nontraditional treatments should not come at the price of loss of treatments with established potential benefits (Hyman and Levy, 2005; Volkmar and Wiesner, 2004). Although limited in number, a few objective resources are available to physicians (Jacobson et al, 2005).

Media attention is easily directed to dramatic claims and may understandably arouse high levels of parental interest. In a few instances (e.g., the more recent double-blind studies of the gut hormone secretin), it was clear that there was no significant improvement overall compared with placebo (Unis et al, 2002). The robust placebo response rate in such studies underscores the importance of controlled research. Occasionally, treatments are proposed that pose danger to the child (e.g., nutritional deficiencies have been observed with restrictive diets) (Arnold et al, 2003). More commonly, the danger is of removing children from programs with proven effectiveness.

OUTCOME AND PROGNOSIS

Earlier diagnosis and more effective interventions have significantly improved the long-term prognosis for many individuals with autism (Howlin, 2005). Significantly more adults are now able to achieve independence and self-sufficiency, and more individuals with autism spectrum problems are now going to college. Despite these important gains, not every child is able to achieve such gains—even when provided with good intervention programs (National Research Council, 2001). Most individuals exhibit improved social-communicative and self-help skills over time. Maximizing the potential for independence is the main long-term goal whenever possible; for individuals unable to achieve total independence, the goal is help the individual have as much self-sufficiency as possible. In more classic autism, factors that predict long-term outcome include some communicative speech by age 5 and nonverbal abilities within the normal range (Howlin, 2005).

Although early intervention is important, gains in social-communication skills continue to be made by children and adolescents if structured, individualized, and intensive interventions are in place. Kanner noted (1971) that some children make gains during adolescence, whereas others exhibit a decline in functioning.

Individuals with Asperger syndrome and PDD-NOS generally seem to have more positive outcomes, although symptoms of depression and anxiety are often apparent in more able adolescents (including individuals with autism) as they sometimes become very aware of their differences from others. The outcome in Rett syndrome and CDD is poor with most individuals requiring lifelong support.

SPECIAL CONSIDERATIONS FOR HEALTH CARE PROVIDERS

Screening

Various approaches to screening have been developed for children with autism and, to a lesser extent, related disorders. These approaches vary in several ways (e.g., specific autism screen or more general developmental screen, age of the child at assessment, organization and format of the screener) (Coonrod and Stone, 2005). Such instruments augment, but do not replace, clinical judgment. Table 69-6 briefly describes selected instruments. Instruments vary in the nature of the intended informants, age group screened, and format. New approaches to screening are actively being developed. It is hoped that these new approaches will rely less on paper and pencil assessment, and be more physiologically based (Klin et al, 2003). The Centers for Disease Control and Prevention (http://www.cdc.gov/ncbddd/dd/ddautism.htm) also provides a body of useful information including materials (in English and Spanish) for distribution to parents.

Medical Issues and Evaluations

Kanner's initial impression that autism was not associated with other medical conditions proved incorrect. As children with autism were followed over time, it became clear that they were at significantly increased risk for developing all types of seizure disorders with peaks of onset in early childhood and adolescence (see Fig. 69-2). The question of whether medical conditions might be causative of autism has been more controversial. Some authors have argued for associations with a host of other medical conditions; the strongest associations of autism with other medical conditions include fragile X syndrome and tuberous sclerosis (Fombonne, 2005a). Medical assessments typically should include physical examination, hearing and vision screening, and screening for fragile X syndrome, if these have not been obtained previously (Volkmar et al, 2006). Lead testing is indicated because of frequent pica in this group of children. For various reasons, there has been increased interest in possible gastrointestinal factors associated with autism, but little rigorous scientific research on this issue exists (Erickson et al, 2005).

Genetic or neurologic consultation may be suggested by examination or history; a strong family history of developmental difficulties, unusual dysmorphic features in the child, or symptoms suggestive of seizure should prompt intensive evaluation. For children with histories of regression, the evaluation should include electroencephalogram and metabolic screens with referral for genetic or neurologic consultation if indicated, such as screening for the *MECP-2* gene in Rett syndrome and for potentially contributory medical conditions in CDD or Landau-Kleffner syndrome (acquired aphasia with epilepsy) in children with sudden loss of language. It is hoped that the next years will see the advent of more specific tests for genes involved in autism. Guidelines for genetic evaluation of children with intellectual disability may be appropriate, particularly for children with some

Table 69-6. **Selected Screening and Diagnostic Instruments**

Instrument/Developer	Format	Setting, Training, and Intended Ages	Comment
Communication and Symbolic Behavior Scales Developmental Profile (CSBS DP); Wetherby and Prizant, 2002	24 items, parent report	Pediatric office setting, 6-24 mo	Information on sensitivity and specificity needed
Checklist for Autism in Toddlers (CHAT); Baird et al, 2000	Parent report and interactional items, few items	Used by health care visitor at 18 mo	Considerable research, high specificity, low sensitivity
Modified Checklist for Autism in Toddlers (MCHAT); Robins et al, 2001	Parent report version of CHAT with additional items	24 mo screening	Initially good sensitivity and specificity, good ease of use
Screening Tool for Autism in Two-year-olds (STAT); Stone et al., 2000; Stone and Ousley, 1997	12 items (about 20 min to administer), play-based	Requires training in administration and score, 24-36 mo	Good sensitivity and specificity and reliability, but more data needed
Autism Behavior Checklist (ABC); Krug et al, 1980	57 items, yes/no, teacher report	Applicable over wide age range (not just preschool)	Readily used, reliability issues, may have high false-negative rate
Childhood Autism Rating Scale (CARS); Schopler et al, 1988	15 items, rating scale, observation and parent report	Requires some training, can be used with preschool children	Good reliability, probably overdiagnoses autism among very young and children with greater ID
Gilliam Autism Rating Scale: Second Edition (GARS-2); Gilliam, 2006	42 items, behavior checklist, parents/teachers	3-22 yr, teachers, parents, clinicians	Questionable as a screener before age 3

ID, intellectual disability.

"autistic-like" features who also exhibit cognitive delay (Moeschler et al, 2006).

Challenges for Providing and Obtaining Quality Health Care

Challenges for provision of high-quality care in this population arise as a result of problems in social interaction and communication and limited tolerance for change. Other problems are posed by the more general problems individuals with disabilities have in obtaining quality health care. As noted elsewhere, the nonverbal child's illness may manifest as behavior change (Volkmar et al, 2006). Table 69-7 lists obstacles to providing health care. It is important to emphasize the central importance of regular pediatric care, including well-child visits (to help the child accommodate to the office setting), preventive care (including dental care), and concern by the pediatrician with advocacy and provision of appropriate information. Accidents are the leading cause of death in this population, and safety considerations should be paramount for parents of younger children; as children become older, help with behavior problems and then emerging sexuality becomes more important (Volkmar and Wiesner, 2004). Information for parents and health care providers is increasingly available (Batshaw, 2002; Exkorn, 2005; Powers, 2000).

Table 69-7. **Challenges to Providing Quality Health Care**

Area of Difficulty	Possible Solutions
Marked social difficulties	Familiarity with providers (well-child checks) Have familiar staff/family available Slow down pace, exaggerate social cues
Problems with communication	Use visual supports (picture books, visual schedule) Keep instructions simple Break procedures into small steps Give ample wait time, talk before touching
Difficulties with novelty	Familiarize child with office/setting (if possible) Picture books, visual supports, stories As appropriate allow child to manipulate instruments and materials
Difficulties with organization/attention	Minimize extraneous distractions Use separate waiting area Use picture schedule/visual aids

Adapted from Volkmar FR, Wiesner LA, Westphal A: Healthcare issues for children on the autism spectrum. Curr Opin Psychiatry 19:361-366, 2006.

SUMMARY AND DIRECTIONS FOR THE FUTURE

Considerable progress has been made over the last decade in understanding autism and related disorders. Advances in neurobiology and genetics have increased understanding of the fundamental basis of the disability. Earlier diagnosis and intervention have reduced the negative impact that autism can have on development. The core features of these conditions pose important obstacles for provision of high-quality health care. Physicians can improve long-term outcome with early diagnosis and can facilitate provision of high-quality health care services to children with these conditions.

REFERENCES

Amaral DG, Bauman MD, et al: The amygdala and autism: Implications from non-human primate studies. Genes Brain Behav 2:295-302, 2003.

American Psychiatric Association: Diagnostic and Statistical Manual of Mental Disorders, 4th ed, rev ed. Washington, DC, American Psychiatric Association, 2000.

Amir RE, Van den Veyver IB, Wan M, et al: Rett syndrome is caused by mutations in X-linked MeCP2, encoding methyl-CpG-binding protein 2. Nat Genet 23:185-188, 1990.

Anderson GM, Hoshino Y: Neurochemical studies of autism. *In* Volkmar F, Klin A, Paul R, Cohen D (eds): Handbook of Autism and Pervasive Developmental Disorders, 3rd ed. Hoboken, NJ, John Wiley, 2005, pp 453-472.

Arnold GL, Hyman SL, et al: Plasma amino acids profiles in children with autism: Potential risk of nutritional deficiencies. J Autism Dev Disord 33:449-454, 2003.

Asperger H: Die "autistichen Psychopathen" im Kindersalter. Arch Psychiatr Nerve 117:76-136, 1944.

Bachevalier J, Loveland KA: Early orbitofrontal-limbic dysfunction and autism. *In* Cicchetti D, Walker E (eds): Neurodevelopmental Mechanisms in Psychopathology. New York, Cambridge University Press, 2003, pp 215-236.

Batshaw ML: Children with Disabilities. Baltimore, Brookes Publishing, 2002.

Bauman ML, Kemper TL: Neuroanatomic observations of the brain in autism: A review and future directions. Int J Dev Neurosci 23(2-3):183-187, 2005.

Buitelaar JK, Willemsen-Swinkels S, et al: Naltrexone in children with autism [letter; comment]. J Am Acad Child Adolesc Psychiatry 37:800-802, 1998.

Casanova MF, Buxhoeveden DP, et al: Clinical and macroscopic correlates of minicolumnar pathology in autism. J Child Neurol 17:692-695, 2002.

Charman T, Taylor E, et al: Outcome at 7 years of children diagnosed with autism at age 2: Predictive validity of assessments conducted at 2 and 3 years of age and pattern of symptom change over time. J Child Psychol Psychiatry 46:500-513, 2005.

Chawarska K, Volkmar F: Autism in infancy and early childhood. *In* Volkmar F, Klin A, Paul R, Cohen D (eds): Handbook of Autism and Pervasive Developmental Disorders, 3rd ed. Hoboken, NJ, John Wiley, 2005, pp 223-246.

Coonrod EE, Stone WL: Screening for autism in young children. *In* Volkmar F, Klin A, Paul R, Cohen D (eds): Handbook of Autism and Pervasive Developmental Disorders, 3rd ed. Hoboken, NJ, John Wiley, 2005, pp 707-729.

Courchesne E, Karns C, et al: Unusual brain growth patterns in early life in patients with autistic disorder: An MRI study. Neurology 57:245-254, 2001.

Erickson CA, Stigler KA, et al: Gastrointestinal factors in autistic disorder: A critical review. J Autism Dev Disord 35:713-727, 2005.

Exkorn KS: The Autism Sourcebook. New York, Harper Collins, 2005.

Fombonne E: Epidemiological studies of pervasive developmental disorders. *In* Volkmar F, Klin A, Paul R, Cohen D (eds): Handbook of Autism and Pervasive Developmental Disorders, 3rd ed. Hoboken, NJ, John Wiley, 2005a, pp 42-69.

Fombonne E: Epidemiology of autistic disorder and other pervasive developmental disorders. J Clin Psychiatry 66(Suppl 10):3-8, 2005b.

Fombonne E, Zakarian R, et al: Pervasive developmental disorders in Montreal, Quebec, Canada: Prevalence and links with immunizations. Pediatrics 118:e139–e150, 2006.

Glasson EJ, Bower C, et al: Perinatal factors and the development of autism: A population study. Arch Gen Psychiatry 61:618-627, 2004.

Gordon CT, State RC, et al: A double-blind comparison of clomipramine, desipramine, and placebo in the treatment of autistic disorder. Arch Gen Psychiatry 50:441-447, 1993.

Hermelin B: Bright Splinters of the Mind: A Personal Story of Research with Autistic Savants. London, Jessica Kingsley, 2001.

Horwitz B, Rumsey JM, et al: The cerebral metabolic landscape in autism: Intercorrelations of regional glucose utilization. Arch Neurol 45:749-755, 1988.

Howlin P: Outcomes in autism spectrum disorders. *In* Volkmar F, Klin A, Paul R, Cohen D (eds): Handbook of Autism and Pervasive Developmental Disorders, 3rd ed. Hoboken, NJ, John Wiley, 2005, pp 201-222,

Hultman CM, Sparen P: Autism—prenatal insults or an epiphenomenon of a strongly genetic disorder? Lancet 364:485-487, 2004.

Hyman SL, Levy SE: Introduction: Novel therapies in developmental disabilities—hope, reason, and evidence. Ment Retard Dev Disabil Res Rev 11:107-109, 2005.

Jacobson JW, Foxx RM, et al (eds): Controversial Therapies for Developmental Disabilities: Fad, Fashion and Science in Professional Practice. Mahwah, NJ, Lawrence Erlbaum Associates, 2005.

Kanner L: Autistic disturbances of affective contact. Nervous Child 2:217-250, 1943.

Kanner L: Follow-up study of eleven autistic children originally reported in 1943. J Autism Child Schizophr 1:119-145, 1971.

Klin A: Defining and quantifying the social phenotype in autism: Reply. Am J Psychiatry 161:933-934, 2004.

Klin A, Jones W, et al: The enactive mind, or from actions to cognition: Lessons from autism. Philos Trans Roy Soc Lond Series B Biol Sci 358:345-360, 2003.

Klin A, McPartland J, et al: Asperger syndrome. *In* Volkmar F, Klin A, Paul R, Cohen D (eds): Handbook of Autism and Pervasive Developmental Disorders, 3rd ed. Hoboken, NJ, John Wiley, 2005, pp 88-125.

Klin A, Saulnier C, et al: Clinical evaluation in autism spectrum disorders: Psychological Assessment within a transdisciplinary framework. *In* Volkmar F, Klin A, Paul R, Cohen D (eds): Handbook of Autism and Pervasive Developmental Disorders, 3rd ed. Hoboken, NJ, John Wiley, 2005, pp 772-798.

Lord C: Follow-up of two-year-olds referred for possible autism. J Child Psychol Psychiatry 36:1365-1382, 1995.

Loveland KA, Tunali-Kotoski B: The school-age child with an autistic spectrum disorder. *In* Volkmar F, Klin A, Paul R, Cohen D (eds): Handbook of Autism and Pervasive Developmental Disorders, 3rd ed. Hoboken, NJ, John Wiley, 2005, pp 247-287.

Mandell DS, Ittenbach RR, et al: Disparities in diagnoses received prior to a diagnosis of autism spectrum disorder. J Autism Dev Disord 37:1795-1802, 2007.

McCracken JT, McGough J, et al: Risperidone in children with autism and serious behavioral problems.[see comment]. N Engl J Med 347:314-321, 2002.

Minshew NJ, Sweeney JA, et al: Neurologic aspects of autism. *In* Volkmar F, Klin A, Paul R, Cohen D (eds): Handbook of Autism and Pervasive Developmental Disorders, 3rd ed. Hoboken, NJ, John Wiley, 2005, pp 453-472.

Moeschler JB, Shevell M, et al: Clinical genetic evaluation of the child with mental retardation or developmental delays. Pediatrics 117:2304-2316, 2006.

National Research Council: Educating Young Children with Autism. Washington, DC, National Academy Press, 2001.

Ozonoff S, Rogers SJ, et al (eds): Autism Spectrum Disorders: A Research Review for Practitioners. Washington, DC, American Psychiatric Publishing, 2003.

Paul R: Promoting social communication in high functioning individuals with autistic spectrum disorders. Child Adolesc Psychiatr Clin North Am 12:87-106, vi-vii, 2003.

Paul R, Sutherland D: Enhancing early language in children with autism spectrum disorders. *In* Volkmar F, Klin A, Paul R, Cohen D (eds): Handbook of Autism and Pervasive Developmental Disorders, 3rd ed. Hoboken, NJ, John Wiley, 2005, pp 946-976.

Powers MD (ed): Children with Autism: A Parents' Guide, 2nd ed. Bethesda, MD, Woodbine House, 2000.

Prior M, Ozonoff S: Psychological factors in autism. *In* Volkmar FR (ed): Autism and Pervasive Developmental Disorders. Cambridge, Cambridge University Press, 1998, pp 64-108.

Rett A: Uber ein eigenartiges hirntophisces Syndrome bei hyperammonie im Kindersalter. Wein Med Wochenschr 118:723-726, 1966.

Rogers SJ: Developmental regression in autism spectrum disorders. Ment Retard Dev Disabil Res Rev 10:139-143, 2004.

Rourke BP: The syndrome of nonverbal learning disabilities: Developmental manifestations in neurological disease, disorder, and dysfunction. Clin Neuropsychol 2:293-330, 1988.

Rutter M: Genetic influences and autism. *In* Volkmar F, Klin A, Paul R, Cohen D (eds): Handbook of Autism and Pervasive Developmental Disorders, 3rd ed. Hoboken, NJ, John Wiley, 2005a, pp 425-452.

Rutter M: Incidence of autism spectrum disorders: Changes over time and their meaning. Acta Paediatr 94:2-15, 2005b.

Scahill L, Martin A: Psychopharmacology. *In* Volkmar F, Klin A, Paul R, Cohen D (eds): Handbook of Autism and Pervasive Developmental Disorders, 3rd ed. Hoboken, NJ, John Wiley, 2005, pp 1102-1122.

Schultz RT, Gauthier I, et al: Abnormal ventral temporal cortical activity during face discrimination among individuals with autism and Asperger syndrome. Arch Gen Psychiatry 57:331-340, 2000.

Shea V, Mesibov GB: Adolescents and adults with autism. *In* Volkmar F, Klin A, Paul R, Cohen D (eds): Handbook of Autism and Pervasive Developmental Disorders, 3rd ed. Hoboken, NJ, John Wiley, 2005, pp 288-311.

Towbin KE: Pervasive developmental disorder not otherwise specified. *In* Volkmar F, Klin A, Paul R, Cohen D (eds): Handbook of Autism and Pervasive Developmental Disorders, 3rd ed. Hoboken, NJ, John Wiley, 2005, pp 165-200.

Unis AS, Munson JA, et al: A randomized, double-blind, placebo-controlled trial of porcine versus synthetic secretin for reducing symptoms of autism. J Am Acad Child Adolesc Psychiatry 41:1315-1321, 2002.

VanAcker R, Loncola JA, et al: Rett syndrome: A pervasive developmental disorder. *In* Volkmar F, Klin A, Paul R, Cohen D (eds): Handbook of Autism and Pervasive Developmental Disorders, 3rd ed. Hoboken, NJ, John Wiley, 2005, pp 126-164.

Veenstra-VanderWeele J, Kim SJ, et al: Transmission disequilibrium studies of the serotonin 5-HT2A receptor gene (HTR2A) in autism. Am J Med Genet 114:277-283, 2002.

Volkmar FR, Klin A: Issues in the classification of autism and related conditions. *In* Volkmar F, Klin A, Paul R, Cohen D (eds): Handbook of Autism and Pervasive Developmental Disorders, 3rd ed. Hoboken, NJ, John Wiley, 2005, pp 5-41.

Volkmar FR, Klin A, et al: Field trial for autistic disorder in DSM-IV. Am J Psychiatry 151:1361-1367, 1994.

Volkmar FR, Koenig K, et al: Childhood disintegrative disorder. *In* Volkmar F, Klin A, Paul R, Cohen D (eds): Handbook of Autism and Pervasive Developmental Disorders, 3rd ed. Hoboken, NJ, John Wiley, 2005, pp 70-78.

Volkmar FR, Nelson DS: Seizure disorders in autism. J Am Acad Child Adolesc Psychiatry 29:127-129, 1990.

Volkmar F, Wiesner E: Health Care for Children on the Autism Spectrum. Bethesda, MD, Woodbine Publishing, 2004.

Volkmar FR, Wiesner LA, Westphal A: Healthcare issues for children on the autism spectrum. Curr Opin Psychiatry 19:361-366, 2006.

Wakefield AJ, Murch SH, et al: Ileal-lymphoid-nodular hyperplasia, non-specific colitis, and pervasive developmental disorder in children [retraction in Murch SH, Anthony A, Casson DH, et al: Lancet 363:750, 2004]. Lancet 351:637-641, 1998.

Wing L: Asperger's syndrome: A clinical account. Psychol Med 11:115-129, 1981.

Wing L, Potter D: The epidemiology of autistic spectrum disorders: Is the prevalence rising? Ment Retard Dev Disabil Res Rev 8:151-161, 2002.

70 HEARING IMPAIRMENT

Desmond P. Kelly

Hearing impairment in childhood can have a significantly negative impact on language, social, and emotional development, and subsequent academic achievement. Early identification of hearing loss and prompt intervention to augment hearing abilities and promote language development can minimize these risks, however. There is considerable heterogeneity among children with hearing loss, in etiology and in functional profiles, and the success of many of these children, even children with profound hearing loss, illustrates the potential for neuronal plasticity and their individual resilience.

TERMINOLOGY

Although the term *hearing impairment* covers the range from mild to profound hearing loss, the designation *deaf* is generally reserved for children whose hearing loss is in the severe to profound range, and who can at best hear only a few prosodic and phonetic elements of speech. Children who are *hard of hearing*, with hearing loss below the severe range, can at least partially understand spoken language. Sounds consist of complex combinations of pure tones that vary in frequency or pitch (measured in Hertz) and intensity or loudness (measured in decibels). Hearing is commonly measured by pure tone audiometers, and the results of hearing tests are graphically represented by means of pure tone audiograms. Typical conversational speech occurs in the range of 30 to 50 dB. The loudness and pitch of common sounds and the functional impact of varying degrees of hearing loss are illustrated in Figure 70-1.

Classification systems are usually based on the average hearing threshold in decibels for pure tones presented at 500 Hz, 1000 Hz, and 2000 Hz. The range for normal hearing is 0 to 15 dB. Although the threshold for classification as hearing impaired has generally been defined as 25 dB, most experts agree that any hearing loss greater than 15 dB in an infant or young child could impede speech perception and language development. Degrees of hearing loss can be categorized as follows (American Speech Language and Hearing Association, 2006):

- Mild hearing loss: 20-40 dB
- Moderate hearing loss: 41-60 dB
- Severe hearing loss: 61-90 dB
- Profound hearing loss: >90 dB

Hearing loss is traditionally subtyped as either *conductive* or *sensorineural*, but frequently there is a combination of these components, or *mixed* hearing loss. *Conductive* hearing loss results from an interruption in the mechanical components responsible for conducting sound waves in the air to the inner ear, where they become hydraulic waves that stimulate the hair cells within the cochlea. These include the pinna, external ear canal, eardrum, ossicles, and middle ear cavity. The degree of conductive loss is usually limited, with some conduction via the temporal bone to the cochlea occurring if sounds are louder than 50 dB. Children with conduction defects can discriminate speech if it is loud enough and may be soft-spoken because they hear their own voice more loudly. *Sensorineural* hearing loss occurs if there is dysfunction of the inner ear (cochlear apparatus) or interruption of the neural pathways to the auditory cortex. The higher frequency ranges are usually affected most. Comparison of air and bone conduction hearing levels is used to differentiate the type of loss. In the treatment of children with sensorineural hearing loss, the clinician should monitor for *mixed* loss with associated conductive hearing loss that might be amenable to medical or surgical intervention.

Auditory neuropathy (also referred to as *auditory dys-synchrony*) is now a better recognized entity and reflects dysfunction of the nerve conduction to the cortex (Berlin, 1996). *Cortical* deafness is rare, but occurs in the context of diffuse brain damage with difficulty related to auditory perception or discrimination at the central level.

EPIDEMIOLOGY

Although profound hearing loss is rare, milder degrees of hearing impairment, particularly conductive hearing loss secondary to otitis media with effusion, are common. Estimates of the prevalence of hearing impairment are beset by inconsistencies in classification and reporting, and vary in different regions of the world. In the United States and England, the estimated incidence of deafness at birth (sensorineural hearing loss >35 to 40 dB) is 1.3 to 1.8 per 1000 children. The prevalence of permanent sensorineural hearing loss increases to 2.7 per 1000 by 5 years of age and 3.5 per 1000 in adolescence (Morton and Nance, 2006). Five to 10 times as many children experience lesser degrees of impairment (Brookhouser, 1996). In underdeveloped countries, sensorineural hearing loss is almost twice as common, with greater risk of suppurative complications of otitis. Although preventive techniques, such as immunizations against rubella and *Haemophilus influenzae* type B, and improved antibiotic and surgical interventions

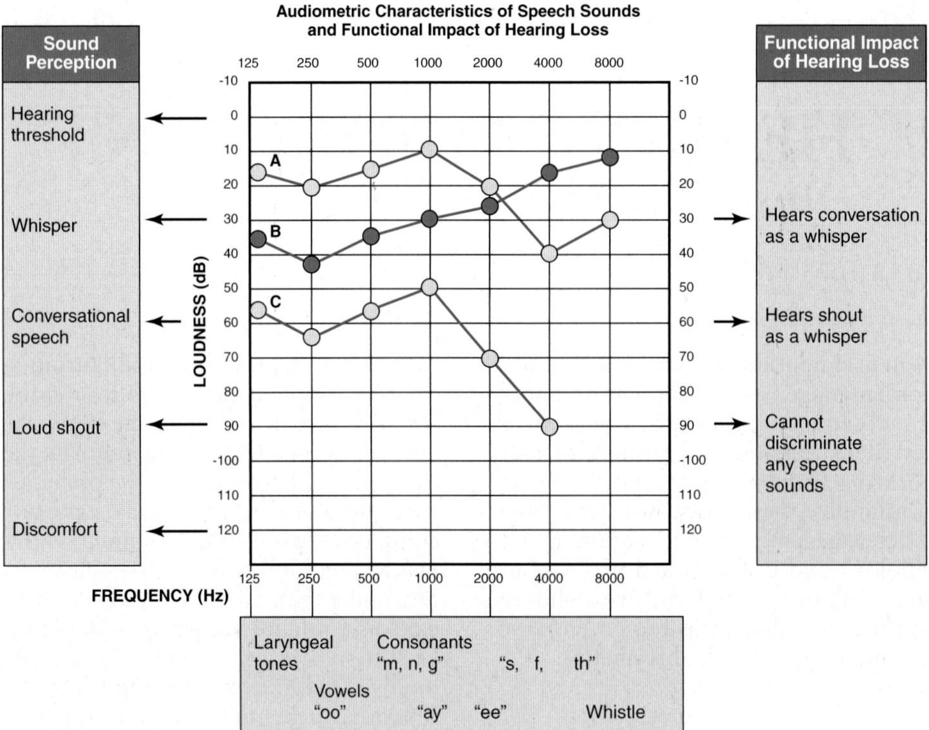

Figure 70-1. Audiometric characteristics of speech sounds and functional impact of hearing loss. Audiograms *A* and *C* reflect mild and moderate-to-severe hearing loss. Note the greater deficits in the higher frequency ranges that particularly affect appreciation of consonants. Audiogram *B*, mild conductive loss, is notable for greater involvement at lower frequencies. *(Adapted from data in Ballantyne J, Martin JAM: Deafness, 4th ed. New York, Churchill Livingstone, 1984.)*

have reduced the incidence of some forms of hearing impairment, the increasing number of children surviving extreme prematurity or complex medical conditions suggests that the overall prevalence is unlikely to decline significantly. The prevalence of acquired immunodeficiency disease in developing countries also has contributed to higher incidence of sensorineural and conductive hearing loss in those settings.

ETIOLOGY

Genetic

Deafness can be inherited as an autosomally dominant or recessive, or X-linked, condition, and can be an isolated trait or constitute one component of a recognizable syndrome. More than 300 forms of hearing loss related to syndromes with distinctive clinical features have been described. Pendred syndrome is the most common. Table 70-1 describes the more prevalent forms and their clinical features. Most cases of genetic hearing loss are nonsyndromic, however.

Molecular genetic testing has enabled identification of more than 100 chromosomal loci and 65 genes associated with nonsyndromic hearing impairment (Morton and Nance, 2006). Autosomal recessive patterns of inheritance account for 70% to 80% of cases. Mutations in the gap junction proteins beta 2 and beta 6 (GJB2 and GJB6) are known to cause hearing impairment, with a mutation of GJB2, which encodes the Connexin protein 26 (one of the primary proteins involved in potassium homeostasis in the cochlea), reported as responsible for 50% of recessively inherited hearing loss (Frei et al, 2005). More than 90 mutations have been described, of which the 35delG is the most common. The hearing loss is usually moderate to severe and bilateral, but it can be mild, asymmetric, and progressive. Mutations in two genes of the SLC26 anion transport gene family also have been implicated in hearing loss. One of these, *SLC26A4,* is associated with Pendred syndrome and nonsyndromic sensorineural hearing loss. Mitochondrial DNA mutations also have been found in individuals with hearing loss. These mutations can cause deafness directly or increase vulnerability to the ototoxic effects of aminoglycoside antibiotics (Gardner et al, 2006).

Further identification of all the genes involved in hereditary hearing loss would help in the understanding of the basic mechanisms of normal hearing and would aid in early diagnosis and targeted therapy (Petersen and Willems, 2006). Table 70-2 provides an overview of the frequency of the currently recognized causes of hearing loss.

Acquired

Prenatal causes of hearing impairment include maternal infections, such as toxoplasmosis, rubella, cytomegalovirus, and herpes simplex, and exposure to toxins, such as alcohol, trimethadione, and mercury (Roizen, 1999). Of these causes, cytomegalovirus is the most frequently identified. The most common perinatal cause of hearing loss is extreme prematurity with its associated risks, including hypoxia, acidosis, hypoglycemia, high levels of ambient

Table 70-1. Common Syndromic Forms of Hearing Impairment

Syndrome	Inheritance	Relative Frequency*	Clinical Features
Alport syndrome	XL or AR	1%	Hematuria; progressive renal failure; late-onset high-frequency sensorineural hearing loss
Brachio-oto-renal syndrome	AD	2%	Preauricular pits; malformed pinnae; branchial fistulae; renal anomalies (structural malformations to agenesis)
Fabry disease	XL	1/40,000	Vascular skin lesions; nephropathy (renal failure); corneal dystrophy; cardiomyopathy; high-frequency sensorineural hearing loss
Jervell and Lange-Nielsen syndrome	AR	0.5%	Prolonged QT interval; syncope; sudden death; profound sensorineural hearing loss
Pendred syndrome	AR	4-10%	Goiter; cochlear malformations; enlarged vestibular aqueduct in carriers; sensorineural hearing loss
Treacher Collins syndrome	AD	1%	Malformed ossicles; microtia; cleft palate; micrognathia; downward slanting eyes; coloboma; conductive hearing loss
Usher syndrome	AR	4-6%	Retinitis pigmentosa; sensorineural hearing loss and vestibular symptoms (type 1, onset in first decade; type 2, stable moderate-to-severe hearing loss; type 3, progressive hearing loss; variable onset of retinitis pigmentosa). Most common cause of deafness with blindness
Waardenburg syndrome (type 1)	AD	1-4%	Neural crestopathy; unilateral or bilateral hearing loss; hypopigmentation of eyes, skin, or hair; occasional—Hirschsprung disease and spina bifida

*Relative frequency among individuals with hearing loss.
AD, autosomal dominant; AR, autosomal recessive; XL, X-linked.
Adapted from Morton CC, Nance WE: Newborn hearing screening—a silent revolution. N Engl J Med 354:2156, 2006.

Table 70-2. Estimated Causes of Deafness at Birth

	%
Genetic	68
Pendred syndrome	3
Other syndromic	14
GJB2 mutation	21
Other nonsyndromic	30
Acquired	32
Cytomegalovirus	21
Clinically apparent infection	10
Clinically inapparent	11
Other environmental causes	11

GJB2, gap junction protein beta 2.
Adapted from Morton CC, Nance WE: Newborn hearing screening—a silent revolution. N Engl J Med 354:2156, 2006.

noise, and ototoxic drugs such as aminoglycosides. These influences likely are additive (Roizen, 1999). Hyperbilirubinemia remains a risk for hearing impairment even though kernicterus is now much less common. It is uncertain which levels of bilirubin are harmful in premature infants with associated stresses such as infection and acidosis. Neonatal infections, including meningitis, carry a high risk of hearing loss.

Postnatally, bacterial meningitis is associated with sensorineural hearing loss in 9% of cases. The introduction of immunizations has decreased the incidence of some forms of meningitis, but 7% of children who have survived non–*H. influenzae* type B meningitis develop sensorineural hearing loss (Koomen et al, 2003). Children who contract meningitis require close audiologic follow-up because the hearing loss can be progressive. Viral infections, such as mumps, can cause hearing impairment, although this is a rare complication. Acquired immunodeficiency syndrome has become a more frequent cause of acquired hearing loss. Prolonged exposure to loud noise, such as personal audio players, often with earphones worn within the external ear canal, poses an increasing, but highly preventable, risk for hearing loss. Acquired causes of conductive hearing loss include otitis media, ossicular discontinuity (owing to infection, trauma, or cholesteatoma), tympanosclerosis, tumors (e.g., histiocytosis), otosclerosis, fibrous dysplasia, and osteopetrosis (Kenna, 2004).

DEVELOPMENTAL AND BEHAVIORAL OUTCOMES

So many variables influence the impact of hearing loss on development that generalizations regarding outcomes for children with deafness are largely unrealistic. Each child deserves individual consideration. Factors that have been clearly implicated can be categorized as follows (Meadow, 1980):

1. Degree of hearing loss. A child with a mild hearing loss corrected by amplification at an early age is at very little risk developmentally, in contrast to a profoundly deaf child in whom hearing loss is not diagnosed early.
2. Etiology. Children with inherited deafness whose parents are deaf have usually fared better academically and behaviorally than children with acquired deafness. It has been assumed that this difference reflects the benefits of early diagnosis and appropriate communication and family support. This difference is likely to be less pronounced since the advent of universal newborn hearing screening with earlier diagnosis and intervention. In contrast to inherited deafness, which might affect only a discrete neurologic component of the hearing pathway, acquired deafness, such as that secondary to a congenital

infection, carries with it a higher risk for additional neurologic dysfunction. Maternal rubella has been a prototypical example of the acquired etiology with potential for multisystem involvement, including visual problems, heart disorders, intellectual disability, and emotional and behavioral problems.

3. Age at onset of deafness. Lack of exposure to language during the critical early developmental years places children who are *prelingually* deaf (generally defined as <2 years old) at significant disadvantage compared with children who have been able to assimilate a language structure before losing their hearing.
4. Family climate. Children born into families with other members who are deaf generally benefit earlier from adaptations and efforts to facilitate communication and other aspects of development. In families without prior experience of deafness, early efforts by parents and other members to learn sign language and foster communication provide similar benefits. In contrast, children raised in a home environment where they are unable to engage in any substantive communication, and who cope with the multiple disability of sensory and psychosocial deprivation, are at grave risk for poor outcome.
5. Timing and appropriateness of educational interventions. Early diagnosis and intervention are central to achieving optimal outcome in the language and social areas. Controversy persists regarding which educational settings facilitate optimal development, and individual factors need to be considered.

Language

In children who are profoundly deaf, the primary impact is not merely that they are unable to hear sounds, but that their ability to develop spoken language is impeded (Kennedy et al, 2006). Children who are prelingually deaf are deprived of auditory memories, images, and associations. Not only are they unable to communicate their thoughts and needs or readily acquire information verbally, but also inner language development, including the ability to translate experience into verbally mediated thoughts and memories, is impeded. The role of standard language in thought processes and "intelligence" has not been clearly established. Studies of deaf children show that they place greater reliance than hearing children on visuospatial short-term memory than on temporal-sequential coding (Marschark, 1993).

It is known that infants can recognize their mothers' voice from birth, and much of early parent-child interaction involves soothing talk and vocal interactions. It is a marvel to realize that by 4 years of age the average child has a complete grasp and knowledge of his or her native language that has been assimilated without the aid of any formal teaching. A child with profound deafness is at a great disadvantage without appropriate efforts to foster communication. Children whose hearing loss is identified early (especially infants <6 months old) have been shown to have significantly higher language developmental quotients than children identified at a later age (Yoshinaga-Itano, 2003).

Cognitive Development

Determination of the intellectual abilities of children who are deaf can prove elusive. Most of the cognitive assessment instruments in common use are based on the ability to read a standard language, and comparison of verbal intelligence scores is not practical. On the nonverbal, or performance, sections of tests, children who are deaf generally fall within the normal range of intelligence, but score consistently below hearing age-mates (Marschark, 1993). Expression of many abstract concepts depends on a system of symbolic language that a child with deafness might not have had the opportunity to develop.

Although expert opinions have varied over the years, it is now agreed that deafness per se does not impart limitations to intelligence (Vernon, 2005). Children who are deaf show qualitative differences, however, in the interrelations among their abilities. In particular, they are likely to be less competent in language abilities and cognitive flexibility. Lack of auditory input also has been associated with lower (but not pathologic) scores in visuospatial praxis tasks and sustained attention (Schlumberger et al, 2004). Measured levels of academic achievement are generally lower for deaf school-age children. Early schooling for children with deafness concentrates heavily on development of communication skills, leaving less time for instruction in other areas. Leaders in deaf education also have voiced concern that goals and expectations for students with deafness are unnecessarily low. In reading comprehension, the mean grade equivalent for 18-year-old students with deafness in special educational settings has been reported to be at the fourth-grade level, with math at the seventh-grade level. There also is the risk that some children with deafness have difficulty with balance, equilibrium, and other motor skills reflecting associated vestibular dysfunction (Rapin, 1993).

In contrast, research has suggested the development of compensatory skills in children deprived of hearing. Some studies indicate more efficient visual processing abilities. By use of brain electric activity mapping techniques, investigators have shown differences in cortical organization between deaf and hearing children, with the former generally showing compensatory changes in the right hemisphere and visual processing areas (Wolff and Thatcher, 1990).

Social and Emotional Development

Although generalizations should be avoided, studies have suggested that individuals with deafness are less "socially mature" (a culturally derived term). This global description would seem to reflect the fact that opportunities for usual social interaction are limited, and parents generally tend to be more protective of children who are deaf. Language and communication is a central component of all social exchanges. Other descriptors include egocentricity, rigidity, and suggestibility.

In extensive studies of children with deafness secondary to rubella, Chess and Fernandez (1980) noted deficits in internal controls, or impulsivity with aggressive behavior. A more recent population-based study based

Table 70-3. Associated Disabling Conditions in Children with Hearing Impairment

Condition	Prevalence (%)*
Visual impairment	4.6
Developmental delay	1.8
Autism	1
Orthopedic impairment	3.7
Learning disability	9.2
Attention-deficit/hyperactivity disorder	6.3
Intellectual disability	8.2
Emotional disturbance	1.9
Other health impairment	1
"Other conditions"	6.9

*Prevalence among 37,500 students in a national survey. From Gallaudet Research Institute: Regional and National Summary Report of Data from the 2004-2005 Annual Survey of Deaf and Hard of Hearing Children and Youth. Washington, DC, GRI, Gallaudet University, 2005.

on parental reports for children who had been fitted with hearing aids indicated that more than half were viewed as manifesting significant behavioral problems. Emotional problems were most prevalent (56%), followed by conduct problems (25%) (Wake et al, 2004). It has been postulated that deficits in verbal mediation of self-control contribute to increased levels of impulsivity, and that aggressive behavior might reflect frustrated attempts to express emotions verbally (Cohen, 1980). Even in nonconfrontational interactions, children who are deaf are likely to initiate more physical contact, such as touching others to gain their attention.

Associated Challenges

The percentage of hearing-impaired school-age children with educationally significant associated disabilities is considerably higher than that for the general population. The *Annual Survey of Deaf and Hard of Hearing Children and Youth* continues to report such difficulties in 43% of deaf children, with many of these problems being related to the same factor that caused the deafness (Table 70-3) (Gallaudet Research Institute, 2005). The term *multiply-handicapped hearing-impaired children* has evolved to describe this group. Additional conditions include visual problems, epilepsy, cerebral palsy, intellectual disability, and specific learning disabilities.

It is important to evaluate each child fully and to be aware of conditions that might have an impact on development and performance. A child with deafness and associated visual-perceptual deficits might have great difficulty processing sign language and speech reading. Such a child might be incorrectly classified as cognitively impaired. Although there has been a paucity of research regarding attention deficits in children who are deaf, a child who is reliant on visual input for learning and communication would be at double jeopardy for learning problems if he or she had attention weaknesses. Studies at a residential school for children who are deaf, using parent and teacher questionnaire ratings, have suggested that although the overall prevalence of attention deficits in children who are deaf is not higher than for the general population, children with acquired deafness, such as secondary to bacterial meningitis, are at significantly increased risk (Kelly et al, 1993).

Many questions remain regarding the impact of fluctuating degrees of conductive hearing loss on subsequent language and learning abilities. Conductive hearing loss of 20 to 30 dB, and even up to 50 dB, can be associated with middle ear effusions. There are conflicting reports, but otitis media with effusion does seem to be one of multiple risk factors that influence the early development of language and reading skills, with home environment being the most significant contributor to outcomes (Roberts et al, 2002).

EVALUATION

Screening

The health professional must maintain an index of suspicion regarding hearing loss in infants and young children. Careful consideration of risk factors coupled with astute observation and attention to parental concerns is the key to successful early diagnosis. With the advent of universal newborn hearing screening, the average age at which hearing loss is diagnosed has decreased from 30 months to 2 to 3 months (Morton and Nance, 2006). In its "Year 2000 Position Statement," the Joint Committee on Infant Hearing (2000) endorsed early detection of, and intervention for, infants with hearing loss through integrated interdisciplinary state and national systems of universal newborn hearing screening. More than 40 states have adopted legislation mandating universal screening of newborns for hearing loss, and 5 states have achieved universal screening without legislation.

It also is recommended that all infants who have risk indicators for delayed onset or progressive hearing loss should have regular assessment of hearing every 6 months until age 3 years. The Centers for Disease Control and Prevention Early Hearing Detection and Intervention (EHDI) program has set "1-3-6" goals—hearing screening before *1* month of age, diagnostic audiologic evaluation for children with hearing loss before *3* months of age, and early intervention for these children before *6* months of age (Dorros et al, 2007).

The use of a "high-risk register" was previously promoted to identify children at most significant risk for hearing loss who should have evaluation of hearing and close follow-up. The factors originally recommended by the Joint Committee on Infant Hearing in 1990 and revised in 1994 and 2000 position statements are listed in Table 70-4, and include factors related to family history, prematurity, low birth weight, infections, trauma, or the diagnosis of a neurodegenerative disorder. Because only 50% of infants or young children with profound hearing loss manifest one of these risk factors, the clinician should still have a low threshold for ordering a full audiologic examination in any child with language delays, regardless of the results of newborn screening or the presence of risk factors. In all situations, the health professional must initiate further testing if there is any degree of parental concern, or any suspicion of hearing loss.

Table 70-4. Risk Factors for Late-Onset or Progressive Hearing Loss

Parental or caregiver concern regarding child's hearing, speech, language, or development
Family history of permanent childhood hearing loss
Craniofacial anomalies or stigmata of syndromes associated with hearing loss
TORCH infections (toxoplasmosis, other agents, rubella, cytomegalovirus, herpes simplex virus)
Ototoxic medications (including aminoglycosides, diuretics)
Bacterial meningitis
Persistent pulmonary hypertension, prolonged ventilator use, or extracorporeal membrane oxygenation
Syndromes associated with progressive hearing loss (e.g., neurofibromatosis, osteopetrosis)
Hyperbilirubinemia (requiring exchange transfusion)
Neurodegenerative disorders (Hunter syndrome, Friedreich ataxia, Charcot-Marie-Tooth disease)
Head trauma
Recurrent or persistent otitis media with effusion (lasting ≥3 months)

From Joint Committee on Infant Hearing: Year 2000 Position Statement: Principles and guidelines for early hearing detection and intervention programs. Pediatrics 106:798, 2000.

Delayed acquisition of language skills may be the first sign of hearing impairment. Parent-completed developmental screening questionnaires uncover concerns regarding delays in communication and language development. Informal assessments of hearing in the office setting, such as reactions to a bell or jingling keys, can be misleading because of the high intensity and limited frequency range of many of these noises. Office screening of hearing using portable screening devices with cooperative preschoolers is a valuable adjunct to the well-child evaluation, but if there is any question about hearing abilities, evaluation by an experienced audiologist is essential.

Evaluation of Hearing

With appropriate equipment and professional expertise, reliable assessments of hearing can be performed on children of any age. Antenatal diagnosis of hearing loss in high-risk pregnancies is becoming an accepted procedure.

In infants younger than 6 months of age, objective measurement of hearing abilities by means of auditory brainstem response testing is preferred. This procedure makes use of surface recording electrodes and microcomputer averaging and enhancement of signals to extract the responses of the brainstem to sound. Potentials evoked by up to 2000 separate auditory stimuli are stored and averaged to produce one waveform, which is analyzed for its overall morphology. This waveform contains seven peaks, of which three are analyzed closely for latency and amplitude characteristics. One of the most significant benefits of this test is that it does not rely on the cooperation of the patient. There are pitfalls, however, including subjectivity involved in interpretation of the waveforms, and the fact that other conditions affecting the brainstem might result in abnormal waveforms. Conversely, because responses are being measured below the level of the auditory cortex, this test does not indicate that the subject is correctly interpreting sounds.

Evoked otoacoustic emissions testing is a physiologic test that is used frequently, especially in newborn screening for hearing loss. Evoked otoacoustic emissions are a form of acoustic energy produced by active movements of the outer hair cells of the cochlea in response to sound. Testing involves measurement of emissions from the inner ear after presentation of a click from a probe placed in the ear canal. The technique does not require advanced training and is sensitive to hearing loss greater than 30 dB. Refinements in the procedure and technologic advances are increasing its accuracy with fewer false-positive results. A combination of evoked otoacoustic emissions and auditory brainstem response testing can establish the diagnosis of auditory neuropathy/auditory dyssynchrony. In this condition, evoked otoacoustic emissions testing is normal, reflecting normal function of the outer hair cells, but auditory brainstem response testing is abnormal, reflecting the dysfunction in neural conduction pathways.

Audiometry measures the response of a child to sound presented either through headphones or through speakers. In children younger than 2 years old, behavioral conditioning by use of visual reinforcers can be used to train children to localize by turning their heads to the direction of the sound. Depending on the skill and persistence of the audiologist, very reliable estimates of hearing can be obtained in young children. From 2 years of age, children can be engaged in play audiometry, in which they are conditioned to provide a specific response to sounds. In older children, speech recognition threshold is tested by having them repeat words or carry out performance tasks such as pointing to body parts or pictures.

Tympanometry assesses middle ear status by determining whether a normally mobile tympanic membrane is absorbing acoustic energy, or whether this energy is being reflected back by an immobile membrane. Measures include the flow of acoustic energy into the middle ear system (static admittance), an estimate of middle ear pressure (the location of the peak pressure when admittance is highest), ear canal volume, and the presence and threshold of the acoustic reflex. Physical conditions, such as middle ear fluid, negative pressure, and ossicular discontinuity, can be measured. Although the acoustic reflex correlates with hearing capacity, it should not be used as an indicator of normal hearing.

Medical Evaluation

If hearing loss has been confirmed, the medical evaluation should be directed toward establishing a cause and ruling out any associated health problems that could impede communication further or have long-term health implications. Evidence of a potentially correctable condition such as middle ear dysfunction warrants consultation with an experienced otolaryngologist to elucidate potential benefits of surgical intervention. Determination of etiology has important implications with regard to genetic counseling and prognostication regarding potential outcomes or associated physical problems.

Routine evaluation should include close attention to vision status, given the vital importance of this sensory modality to individuals who are hearing impaired. Early diagnosis of a condition such as Usher syndrome, with progressive loss of vision in addition to deafness, would have important treatment implications. It is widely recommended that children with hearing impairment have an assessment of vision annually to monitor visual acuity and to check for retinal changes. Other aspects of the medical examination warranting close attention include possible craniofacial anomalies, presence of goiter (Pendred syndrome), pigmentary changes (Waardenburg syndrome), and assessment of renal function (Alport syndrome). A history of syncopal episodes or other unexplained changes in level of consciousness should raise suspicion of cardiac arrhythmias secondary to prolongation of the QT interval, seen in Jervell and Lange-Nielsen syndrome. A detailed neurologic examination also is necessary, particularly in individuals with acquired deafness who might be at risk for other neurologic or vestibular dysfunction.

Special Investigations

Computed tomography of the temporal bone or magnetic resonance imaging can reveal Mondini dysplasia (an incomplete number of turns in the cochlea), which is seen in Pendred syndrome, or other structural anomalies of the inner ear, such as fistulae, which would have management implications. Genetic testing has become a crucial component of the medical workup, with two thirds of cases of deafness likely related to genetic causes, and new gene mutations associated with hearing loss being discovered at a rapid rate. Diagnostic microarray panels are now available that can test for 200 mutations in multiple genes associated with hearing loss (Gardner et al, 2006).

Developmental Assessment

Formal assessment of cognitive, language, and social abilities should be carried out by professionals who have experience in testing children with hearing impairment. Tests of cognition include the Hiskey-Nebraska Test of Learning Aptitude (specifically developed for children with hearing impairment), the performance scales of the Wechsler Intelligence Scales–Fourth Edition (WISC-IV), the Leiter International Performance Scale, and the Kaufman Assessment Battery for Children. Visuomotor tasks, including the Bender-Gestalt and Developmental Test of Visual Motor Integration, also are used frequently. Projective techniques can be helpful (if not entirely reliable) in assessing emotional status, in addition to use of instruments such as the Meadow/Kendall Social-Emotional Assessment Inventory for Deaf Children (Meadow, 1980).

Vignette

Mary was born at term without apparent medical complications before the advent of universal newborn hearing screening. She had frequent episodes of otitis media during the first year of life. Her parents are medical professionals. At 15 months of age, she was not using any single words, and her parents had concerns about her response to environmental sounds. Behavioral audiometry indicated hearing loss, and auditory brainstem response testing at the time of myringotomy and insertion of ventilation tubes indicated severe hearing loss in one ear and profound loss in the other.

Mary was fitted with hearing aids and an FM system, and was enrolled in an intensive program of speech and language therapy, including the use of sign language. Her parents decided at an early stage to promote oral communication as much as possible. After initial gains in language skills (using a limited 1-word vocabulary consistently), there was regression in communication abilities. Repeated testing indicated progression of the hearing loss to a profound degree bilaterally. Mary's parents had her evaluated at numerous medical centers, and she was deemed eligible for cochlear implantation. At surgery, there was evidence of new bone formation in the cochlea, suggesting an infectious etiology for the deafness, probably bacterial meningitis (although there had been no recognized symptoms of such an illness).

Immediately after the implant, Mary showed improved perception of environmental sounds. Language skills progressed slowly initially. Evaluation at another center indicated a need for remapping of the processor. Mary has since made steady gains. She receives individual and group speech and language therapy and separate weekly sessions of auditory-verbal training. She has attended regular preschool classes and is currently functioning well in a prekindergarten educational program at a private school. Two years after receiving the implant, her expressive language has advanced to 2- to 4-word combinations. Receptively, she is able to identify two-key verbal elements, such as "red book," without any visual cues. Her cognitive abilities have been measured to be in the average range, and she increasingly enjoys academic activities. There are mild behavioral challenges with limit-testing and occasional noncompliance. She enjoys social interaction.

Mary's history highlights many key issues, including the challenge of early diagnosis, the risks of progressive hearing loss, multiple modalities of treatment, and the large commitment of energy and resources by parents seeking an optimal outcome for their child.

MANAGEMENT

Optimal outcome for a child with hearing impairment is facilitated by attention to all areas of functioning (Fig. 70-2).

Prevention

Preventive efforts are crucial, including rubella immunization and other measures to decrease the risk of prenatal infections and minimize the other risk factors previously listed. Immunization against *H. influenzae* type B infection has significantly decreased the incidence of this form of bacterial meningitis and the deafness associated with it. The physician also should counsel regarding risks of exposure to loud noises such as firecrackers and loud music. Advances in knowledge regarding genetic mutations associated with hearing

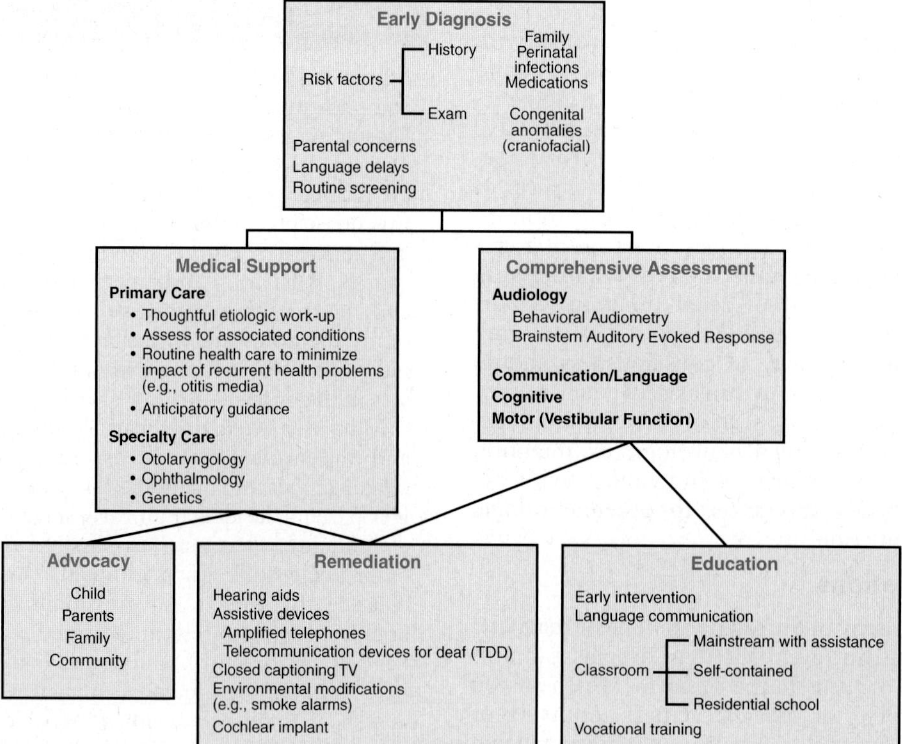

Figure 70-2. Steps to optimal outcome for a hearing-impaired child. An integrated multimodal approach to management aids adaptation and achievement of full potential.

loss enable more accurate genetic counseling for parents who already have a child with hearing impairment or who have members of their extended families with deafness.

Medical Management

Routine health screening and prompt treatment interventions should be coupled with focused anticipatory guidance. The primary care physician is in a unique position to interpret findings of other specialists during the diagnostic process and to function as care coordinator (Dorros et al, 2007). Steps should include prompt referral to the local early intervention entity; referral for otolaryngology and ophthalmology examinations; medical clearance for hearing aids or cochlear implants if chosen by the family; and other medical referrals as indicated, including genetics, neurology, and developmental-behavioral pediatrics. Other medical management interventions include surgery by an otolaryngologist or continued ophthalmologic follow-up. The physician should ensure that there are no delays in having a child who is deaf fitted with hearing aids; the physician can consult with an audiologist in this regard.

Cochlear Implants

Cochlear implants can provide useful hearing to many children with profound hearing loss. This treatment modality has received much attention and evoked considerable debate in recent years and is being performed with increasing frequency. The device consists of an internal component that is surgically implanted and an external component that is worn by the child. Sounds are received through an external microphone, and processed and encoded into radiofrequency signals that are transmitted across the skin to a magnetic receiver situated near the mastoid. From there, an electric signal is sent to a multichannel electrode that is implanted in the cochlea through the round window. The electrode directly stimulates the spiral ganglion cells of the cochlear nerve, with higher frequency sounds stimulating the basal turn and lower frequencies activating the apical turn.

Candidates for cochlear implantation should be carefully selected from among children who have bilateral profound sensorineural hearing loss and have shown little or no benefit from hearing aids. Associated cognitive or behavioral problems must be considered, and there must be family commitment to the intensive training and habilitation program that is an essential component of the process. Follow-up studies have indicated very promising results related to better appreciation of environmental sounds and significant long-term gains in speech perception and intelligibility and in expressive language abilities (Svirsky et al, 2004; Haensel et al, 2005).

In addition to specialized interventions, children with hearing impairment require the same routine health supervision and management of acute illnesses that any other children do. Special consideration is required to ensure that the child who is deaf is not excluded from conversations with parents during these encounters. The pediatrician or family physician also should provide anticipatory guidance regarding behavioral and developmental challenges. Inadequate communication between parents and child can heighten the stresses associated with mastering skills such as toilet training. The physician also might be called on to advise regarding treatment of more significant neurobehavioral problems, such as attention deficits. Although controlled studies are lacking, it seems that medications such as stimulants have a similar spectrum of activity and efficacy in children with hearing impairment.

Developmental Interventions

Three factors have been described that have central implications for optimal development of children who are deaf and should be incorporated into management plans (Marschark, 1993). Early language experiences, particularly linguistic interaction with parents from an early age, are critical. These interactions result in gain of facts, cognitive strategies, and social skills, and knowledge of self and a sense of being part of the world. The second factor is diversity of experience that shapes basic perceptual, learning, and memory processes. Active exploration of the environment and experience with people promotes problem-solving skills and flexibility. Social interaction is the third essential element. In addition to the cognitive functions of social interactions, these relationships help to develop bases for exploration and provide emotional support. Self-esteem, motivation, and moral development are promoted.

Early intervention should focus on development of communication skills for the child and the parents. Options include American Sign Language (ASL), auditory-oral, auditory-verbal, cued speech, and total communication. Opinions have differed among the deaf community and educators regarding the most appropriate instructional methods. The first efforts at deaf education by French monks in the late 1700s expanded on the native forms of sign language already being used by individuals with deafness. The concept of *oralism* subsequently came to the fore in the United States. This approach uses lip reading and vocal expression rather than manual signs and was advocated as offering the best opportunity for integration of children who are deaf into society. Acquisition of understandable speech proves an almost insurmountable task, however, for children with profound prelingual deafness without treatment such as a cochlear implant.

In contrast, proponents of manual communication point out that children who are deaf may develop a broader appreciation for "language" much earlier through the use of signs and can more easily communicate with other individuals with deafness with whom they might share a common identity (Ziring, 1983) or with hearing individuals who have signing skills. *Total communication,* which combines speech reading, manual communication, and oral expression, has emerged as a compromise and is the predominant approach currently used in deaf education. There also is considerable disagreement regarding sign language, however. There is no universal sign language, with each country having its own adaptations and forms of sign. In the United States, ASL is a unique form of communication and a complete language system of its own that is used by many members of the deaf community as an alternative to "Signed English" or other manual communication such as finger spelling. In this regard, a growing number of individuals with hearing impairment identify themselves as members of a deaf community with a distinct set of cultural values and ways of behaving. For them, ASL is a mark of distinction and a source of pride (Moores, 1987).

Education

The passage of Public Law 94-142, the Education for All Handicapped Children Act, since reauthorized as the Individuals with Disabilities Education Act (IDEA), has had a significant impact on deaf education. Free public education for all students who are deaf has broadened the available services and opportunities. Part H of this legislation mandates services from infancy, or the time of diagnosis. Families are entitled to assistance from a multidisciplinary team of professionals who can determine eligibility for services and work with the family to develop an individualized family service plan. Ideally, this team should consist of a physician with expertise in otologic disorders, an audiologist, a speech-language pathologist, and an educator. Primary care physicians should consult and collaborate with this team in the development of treatment and education plans.

As children approach school age, parents encounter differences of opinion among professionals regarding whether special school programs or mainstreaming in regular school programs provides the better educational environment. Residential schools for children who are deaf have been the traditional means of providing education for children who have profound hearing impairment and usually number teachers who are deaf among their faculty. With interpreters and other increased services for students who are deaf provided by public schools, and the mandate for education in the least restrictive environment, has come an increasing emphasis on mainstreaming of students who are deaf. Most children with hearing impairment receive their education in regular school settings. This mainstreaming does carry the risk, however, of social isolation inherent in being one of a small number of students, or the only student, who are deaf in a school or classroom.

The final decision regarding which educational setting is most appropriate for the individual child is influenced by many factors, including the resources and qualifications of professional staff in the different potential settings, the philosophy of educational approaches, goals of parents and educators, and the capability of the family to invest fully in the supportive components. Regardless of the setting, it is crucial that young children with hearing impairments receive appropriate intensive training in language development.

Increasing numbers of students who are deaf are pursuing higher education. There is a wide variety of post–secondary education programs for students who are deaf, and more than 1000 colleges and universities in the United States report supportive programs, including note-taking and interpreter services and availability of telecommunication devices. Gallaudet University in Washington, DC, and the National Technical Institute for the Deaf in Rochester, New York, serve more than half of the students who are deaf now in college.

Habilitation

Many resources are available for maximizing hearing potential. Hearing aids consist of a microphone for converting acoustic energy into electric energy, an amplifier powered by a battery, and a receiver or earphone for converting the amplified electrical energy back into acoustic energy and channeling this into the child's ear canal. If there is absence of the ear canal, a bone conduction oscillator is used. The four different types of hearing aids include body-worn (with a flexible cord leading from the microphone and amplifier to the button-sized receiver, used mostly by younger children), behind-the-ear (with all components contained in a small curved case), in-the-ear (with all components contained within a plastic shell fitted into the outer ear), and eyeglass aids (with the components built into the frame). The amount of sound amplification (gain) and the frequency response of the aid can be varied depending on the characteristics of the individual's hearing loss. Generally, higher frequencies are amplified more. Free-field FM systems can be used in the classroom setting as an effective means of amplification. These operate similar to a miniature radio transmitter with a unit worn by the teacher transmitting the speech to a receiver worn by the student that amplifies and transfers it to small earphones or the student's own hearing aid.

Other assistive listening devices and systems include telephone hand set amplifiers or hearing aid–compatible telephones. Closed-caption television supervised by the National Captioning Institute (established by Congress in 1979) has significantly increased access to news and entertainment. Alerting and warning assistive devices include those that convert the ring of a telephone into a low-pitched warble, strobe light, or flashing household lamp. Similar devices are available for doorbells, wake-up alarms (including vibrotactile devices), smoke detectors, and adverse weather warning systems.

New technologic developments in our digital world have reshaped the landscape for individuals with hearing impairment and have replaced earlier adaptive techniques such as telecommunication devices for individuals who are deaf. Electronic mail communication has become more prevalent and has more recently been superseded by text messaging by mobile telephones, which currently seems to be the preferred method of communication among teenagers and young adults. Participation in social networking sites on the Internet also is not limited by hearing abilities. Caution is warranted with supervision to ensure the safety of children who are already more vulnerable because of the challenges of their disability. As technology continues to advance, hearing impaired individuals should have increasing access to social communication with prototypes on the horizon including devices such as glasses with a receiver and processor that translates spoken input into printed representations of words, displayed on a screen across the bottom of the lenses.

Support and Advocacy

Comprehensive management of the services needed by a child with hearing impairment mandates a commitment to advocacy and support. In addition to medical management, the health professional can fill an important role as educator, not only of the family, but also of the community, regarding the special needs of these children. Families of children with hearing impairment need support, guidance, and training during many difficult periods of adjustment. This coordination of services and information is best achieved in the primary care medical home (Dorros et al. 2007) and by consultants such as developmental-behavioral pediatricians. More than 90% of children who are deaf are born to hearing parents, and the resultant changes in the family milieu are far-reaching. The diagnostic process is often delayed and traumatic for parents, who might have previously received false reassurances for their concerns. With numerous different specialists, including audiologist, otolaryngologist, and pediatrician or family practitioner, involved, it is not unusual for parents to receive the diagnosis in a fragmentary way with continuing hope that yet another specialist would be able to offer a cure.

There is much new information to be learned regarding all aspects of hearing impairment. Enrollment in an early intervention program carries additional burdens with many prescriptions and suggestions that might seem overwhelming or conflicting to parents. Questions regarding the appropriateness of cochlear implantation and the timing and associated rehabilitation challenges are daunting. As children progress through school, questions arise regarding the most appropriate educational approaches and services, and the controversies within the deaf education community in this regard only add to the uncertainty faced by parents. The advent of adolescence raises more questions regarding how much independence to allow a child who is deaf, and highlights the conflicts and concerns faced by all parents at this developmental stage. If the parents are fluent in their child's primary language, the issues may be comparable to those in a hearing family. In all these areas, empathy and advice from the primary physician who has ongoing contact with the family can be of great assistance.

Ziring (1983) noted the special difficulties faced by children with deafness in hospital wards or emergency departments, where communication problems add stress and where preparation of the nursing staff or provision of an interpreter is so important. Consultation with educators and other professionals regarding medical issues affecting children who are deaf is another important support component.

Ultimately, the unique characteristics and strengths of each child must be fostered as he or she grows into adulthood and plans for an independent life and career. Role models, such as deaf lawyers arguing cases before the Supreme Court, artists receiving national awards, and successful professionals or artisans in all walks of life, underline the growing opportunities available. The challenges are real, but the outlook is promising.

SUMMARY

Profound hearing loss is rare, but milder degrees of hearing impairment are more common. All clinicians who treat children encounter patients with hearing loss. Greater than 50% of childhood hearing impairment is due to genetic factors, and more than 20% is due to prenatal, perinatal, or postnatal environmental influences.

The outlook for children with hearing impairment has improved dramatically over recent decades. Increased knowledge related to the genetic basis of hearing loss has facilitated more accurate diagnosis and genetic counseling. Efforts at primary prevention, such as immunizations against the infectious agents responsible for meningitis, and counseling regarding the negative effects of exposure to loud sounds can decrease further the incidence of acquired deafness. Hearing impairment poses significant challenges for language development, social-emotional adjustment, and academic achievement. There are very positive outcomes, however, related to early identification and intervention for children with hearing loss.

Cochlear implants have revolutionized the treatment of hearing impairment in childhood. New technology has broadened the opportunities for communication for individuals with hearing impairment. Physicians have a critical responsibility to be alert to early signs of hearing problems, and to ensure that children with these problems have access to all the advances in management that would enable them to be successful.

REFERENCES

American Speech Language and Hearing Association: Available at: www.asha.org. Accessed December 2006.

Berlin CI: Role of infant hearing screening in health care. Semin Hearing 17:115-123, 1996.

Brookhouser PE: Sensorineural hearing loss in children. Pediatr Clin North Am 43:1195, 1996.

Chess R, Fernandez P: Impulsivity in rubella deaf children: A longitudinal study. Am Ann Deaf 125:505, 1980.

Cohen BK: Emotionally disturbed hearing impaired children: A review of the literature. Am Ann Deaf 125:1040, 1980.

Dorros C, Kurtzer-White E, Ahlgren M, et al: Medical home for children with hearing loss: Physician perspectives and practices. Pediatrics 120:2-288, 2007.

Frei K, Ramsebner R, Lucas T, et al: GJB2 mutations in hearing impairment: Identification of a broad clinical spectrum for improved genetic counseling. Laryngoscope 115:461-465, 2005.

Gallaudet Research Institute: Regional and National Summary Report of Data from the 2004-2005 Annual Survey of Deaf and Hard of Hearing Children and Youth. Washington, DC, GRI, Gallaudet University, 2005.

Gardner P, Oitmaa E, Messner A, et al: Simultaneous multigene mutation detection in patients with sensorineural hearing loss through a novel diagnostic microarray: A new approach for newborn screening follow-up. Pediatrics 118:985, 2006.

Haensel J, Engelke JC, Ottenjam W, et al: Long-term results of cochlear implantation in children. Otolaryngol Head Neck Surg 132:456-458, 2005.

Joint Committee on Infant Hearing: Year 2000 Position Statement: Principles and guidelines for early hearing detection and intervention programs. Pediatrics 106:798, 2000.

Kelly DP, Kelly BJ, Jones ML, et al: Attention deficits in children and adolescents with hearing loss: A survey. Am J Dis Child 147:737, 1993.

Kenna MA: Medical management of childhood hearing loss. Pediatr Ann 33:822-831, 2004.

Kennedy CR, McCann DC, Campbell MJ, et al: Language ability after early detection of permanent childhood hearing impairment. N Engl J Med 354:2131-2142, 2006.

Koomen I, Grobbee DE, Roord JJ, et al: Hearing loss at school age in survivors of bacterial meningitis: Assessment, incidence and prediction. Pediatrics 112:1049-1053, 2003.

Marschark M: Psychological Development of Deaf Children. New York, Oxford University Press, 1993.

Meadow KP: Deafness and Child Development. Berkeley, CA, University of California Press, 1980.

Moores DF: Educating the Deaf, 3rd ed. Boston, Houghton Mifflin, 1987.

Morton CC, Nance WE: Newborn hearing screening—a silent revolution. N Engl J Med 354:2151-2164, 2006.

Petersen MB, Willems PJ: Non-syndromic, autosomal recessive deafness. Clin Genet 69:371-392, 2006.

Rapin I: Hearing disorders. Pediatr Rev 14:43, 1993.

Roberts JE, Burchinal MR, Zeisel SA: Otitis media in early childhood in relation to children's school-age language and academic skills. Pediatrics 110:696, 2002.

Roizen NR: Etiology of hearing loss in children: Nongenetic causes. Pediatr Clin North Am 46:49-61, 1999.

Schlumberger E, Narbona J, Manrique M: Non-verbal development of children with deafness, with and without cochlear implants. Dev Med Child Neurol 46:599-606, 2004.

Svirsky MA, Teoh S, Neuberger H: Development of language and speech perception in congenitally profoundly deaf children as a function of age of cochlear implantation. Audiol Neurotol 9:224-233, 2004.

Vernon M: Fifty years of research on the intelligence of deaf and hard-of-hearing children: A review of the literature and discussion of implications. J Deaf Studies Deaf Educ 10:225-231, 2005.

Wake M, Hughes EK, Poulakis Z, et al: Outcomes of children with mild-profound hearing loss at 7 to 8 years: A population study. Ear Hearing 25:1-8, 2004.

Wolff AB, Thatcher RW: Cortical reorganization in deaf children. J Clin Exp Neuropsychiatry 12:2, 1990.

Yoshinaga-Itano C: From screening to early identification and intervention: Discovering predictors to successful outcomes for children with significant hearing loss. J Deaf Studies Deaf Educ 8:11-30, 2003.

Ziring PR: The child with hearing impairment. *In* Levine MD, Carey WB, Crocker AC, Gross RT (eds): Developmental-Behavioral Pediatrics, 1st ed. Philadelphia, WB Saunders 1983, p 770.

HELPFUL WEB SITES

Alexander Graham Bell Association for the Deaf: Available at: http://www.agbell.org.

American Academy of Audiology: Available at: http://www.audiology.org.

American Society for Deaf Children: Available at: http://www.deafchildren.org.

American Speech-Language-Hearing Association: Available at: http://www.asha.org.

Beginnings for Parents of Children Who Are Deaf or Hard-of-Hearing: Available at: http://www.beginningsvcs.com.

Boys Town National Research Hospital: Available at: http://www.boystownhospital.org.

Centers for Disease Control and Prevention Early Hearing Detection and Intervention: Available at: http://www.cdc.gov/ncbddd/ehdi.

Family Voices: Available at: http://www.familyvoices.org.

Marion Downs National Center for Infant Hearing: Available at: http://www.colorado.edu/slhs/mdnc.

My Baby's Hearing: Available at: http://www.babyhearing.org.

National Association of the Deaf: Available at: http://www.nad.org.

National Center for Hearing Assessment and Management: Available at: http://www.infanthearing.org.

Laurent Clerc National Deaf Education Center: Available at: http://www.clerccenter.gallaudet.edu/InfotoGo.

National Institutes of Health, National Institute on Deafness and Other Communication Disorders: Available at: http://www.nidcd.nih.gov.

71 BLINDNESS AND VISUAL IMPAIRMENT

Stuart W. Teplin, Judith Greeley, and Tanni L. Anthony

Although considered a "low-incidence" neurologic disability in children and adolescents, blindness and visual impairment comprise a range of ophthalmologic and central nervous system (CNS) conditions that can result in significant morbidity for and remarkable adaptations by affected children and their families. Excluding the much more ubiquitous conditions of strabismus and amblyopia, the prevalence of significant visual impairment in developed countries is approximately 1 to 3 per 10,000 children (birth to 15 years old). The prevalence of visual impairment in American children younger than 5 years old is 0.42 to 0.86 per 1000 (Kirchner, 1989). In Asia (excluding Japan) and Africa, the prevalence is approximately 6 to 15 per 10,000 children.

It is estimated that each year, about 500,000 children worldwide, most of whom live in underdeveloped regions, become blind or severely visually impaired. Of the latter, it is estimated that approximately 40% have conditions that are considered preventable. These preventable conditions include nutritional problems (e.g., vitamin A deficiency), bacterial infections (e.g., trachoma), parasitic infestations (e.g., *Toxoplasma*), and endemic infections (e.g., onchocerciasis or "river blindness"). Other contributing factors are poverty and limited access to health care (e.g., amblyopia secondary to long-standing refractive errors or strabismus), and some recessive genetic conditions that are more prevalent owing to higher rates of consanguinity in some cultures.

For children and adolescents in developed countries, the epidemiology of blindness is quite different and primarily related to underlying CNS disorders affecting vision, complications of prematurity after prolonged neonatal intensive care unit courses, and congenital/genetic disorders of the eye. In the United States, approximately half of children with visual impairment have genetic/heritable conditions. Among preschool children in the United States, the most prevalent conditions are (1) cortical visual impairment, (2) retinopathy of prematurity, and (3) optic nerve hypoplasia.

Congenital causes include many types of cataracts, metabolic disorders (e.g., albinism, Hurler syndrome, Tay-Sachs disease), retinal dystrophies (e.g., Leber congenital amaurosis, retinitis pigmentosa), and sequelae of congenital infections. Other congenital abnormalities include malformations of the eye and related brain structures (e.g., coloboma, micro-ophthalmia or anophthalmia, and optic nerve hypoplasia). These abnormalities may be an isolated condition or part of a complex of other congenital abnormalities, as occurs in certain syndromes (e.g., CHARGE association) and chromosomal disorders (e.g., trisomies 13, 18, and 21). Perinatally timed causes of visual impairment include hypoxic-ischemic CNS injury and retinopathy of prematurity (ROP).

As the technology and quality of intensive care for premature infants in developed countries has improved over the past 50 years, the risk of a premature infant acquiring ROP has become limited primarily to infants with birth weights less than 1000 g, particularly those with other severe complications of prematurity and its treatments. Yet, as noted, ROP continues to be one of the top three causes of visual impairment in children. Medical understanding of the pathogenesis of ROP is still unfolding; more recent research has documented a complex interaction between genetic predisposition, immature retinal vascular endothelium, oxygen exposure, and regulation of neovascularization by local levels of vascular endothelial growth factor (VEGF) at the junction of vascular-avascular retina. Surgical treatments (retinal cryotherapy and laser) aimed at the neovascular pathology have been shown to decrease the risk of unfavorable outcomes (i.e., detachment of the visually important posterior retina) by nearly half, when applied at the optimal timing of the pathogenetic process. Surgical attempts to reattach already detached retinas (e.g., through vitrectomies) have not been associated with significant improvements in visual outcomes. Even after the acute period is over, children with a history of ROP remain at some risk for late complications, including myopia, decreased visual field, strabismus, cataracts, and later retinal detachments.

Major postnatal causes of significant visual impairment include CNS infections, eye or brain damage secondary to accidental or inflicted trauma (e.g., shaken baby syndrome), and tumors (e.g., retinoblastoma). Amblyopia, a common cause of unilateral, mild-to-moderate visual impairment in children, is characterized by reduced visual acuity and depth perception secondary to abnormal visual development caused by lack of patterned visual stimulation during the critical early developmental period of the brain's visual pathways (i.e., birth to 7 to 8 years old). Amblyopia is usually the result of persistent uncorrected strabismus, unilateral obstruction of vision (e.g., dense cataract), or significant discrepancies in refraction between the two eyes. Treatment in young children is aimed at removal of any significant opacities in the pathway of light and forcing the use of the amblyopic eye, usually by occlusion of the better eye.

For 50% to 75% of children who are blind or significantly visually impaired, their diagnostic evaluations, medical care, and developmental-behavioral management are complicated further by comorbid chronic illnesses or neurologic disabilities or both, including intellectual disabilities (mental retardation), autism spectrum disorders, cerebral palsy, seizure disorders, hearing loss, chronic lung disease, cardiac conditions, and metabolic disorders. For children with multiple disabilities including visual impairment, clinicians often may fail to recognize or underestimate the impact of the visual problems because of other, more obvious or medically acute conditions (see Vignette).

Vignette

Billy is a 3½-year-old boy who has been followed by his primary care pediatrician for spastic quadriparetic cerebral palsy and significant cognitive impairments associated with severe perinatal hypoxia. He was referred to a developmental-behavioral pediatrician because of increased frequency and intensity of behavioral outbursts over the past 6 months. In response to the consultant's careful survey of the past history and review of systems, Billy's mother acknowledged frustration and confusion about his vision. Billy always seemed to be alert to sounds, but as an infant and toddler, he often failed to notice nearby objects. During the past year, his visual recognition of nearby toys and people had begun to improve, but Billy still sometimes seemed to "ignore" stationary objects that were on the tray of his wheelchair. He apparently has no difficulty tracking the movements of people or objects, especially if they are brightly colored and highly contrasted against their visual background. Neurologic assessment of the visual system showed normal pupillary responses to light and normal extraocular muscle function. On attempted visual acuity assessment (using a picture symbol system), Billy's responses were inconsistent and difficult to interpret. Based on his history of initially poor acuity that improved spontaneously, associated with an apparently intact anterior visual system (normal pupillary responses), the likelihood of cortical/cerebral visual impairment was discussed with Billy's parents, and two referrals were made: (1) a pediatric ophthalmologist for further assessment of the visual system and (2) a preschool teacher with specialized training and experience in working with children with visual impairments.

Table 71-1 provides an overview of the range of medical conditions in children for which there is co-occurrence of severe visual impairment and other developmental disabilities. Table 71-2 summarizes major conditions causing blindness or significant visual impairment in children, including the pathogenesis; genetics; associated eye, brain, and somatic complications; and developmental-behavioral implications.

PEDIATRIC SCREENING RESPONSIBILITIES

Visual screening begins the process of identification of early-onset vision problems or impairment. Early referral of children whose eye or vision screens are abnormal by the pediatrician to a pediatric ophthalmologist for an eye examination is crucial. Family history of vision problems or impairment, caregiver concerns, and observations of poor visual performance are often discussed with or detected by a pediatrician. All young children, including children who are nonverbal or who have additional disabilities, can be screened for their visual health. Tools such as Teller Cards, Lea, and Lighthouse acuity cards can provide key information about the child's visual performance. It is recommended practice that all children receive an eye examination by age 3 years, or earlier if there are noted concerns.

For the nonophthalmologist physician, a routine eye screen includes the following:

- Naturalistic observations of the child's use of vision for reaching, mobility, eye contact with parents, obvious ocular abnormalities (e.g., ptosis, nystagmus, pupillary defects)
- Assessment of visual fixation and following, keeping in mind that poorly executed following could be a sensory problem (i.e., poor visual acuity), a motor problem (e.g., oculomotor apraxia), or both.
- Observation of pupillary responses to bright light to learn about the intactness of the anterior visual pathway (ocular structures and optic nerves, anterior to the optic chiasm).

CHARACTERISTICS AND DEFINITIONS OF BLINDNESS AND VISUAL IMPAIRMENT

Visual impairment may manifest in poor visual acuity, reduced visual field, photophobia, poor depth perception, or poor eye teaming and motility. The extent of these difficulties is highly individualized and tied to the actual diagnosis. A child may have a permanent visual impairment, yet still may benefit from prescriptive lenses to correct a concomitant refractive error.

For the pediatric age group, and especially for nonverbal and preverbal children, there is no universally acceptable definition of the term *blindness*. *Legal blindness* refers to best corrected distance visual acuity in the better eye of 20/200 or less or a visual field restriction in the better eye of less than 20 degrees, or both. These criteria, originally established as governmental guidelines in determining eligibility for disability services in adults, are used for children, but often do not "translate" effectively when applied to the unique medical and developmental circumstances of infants and children with visual difficulties. Students with *low vision* have corrected acuities in the 20/70 to 20/200 range and, although not considered legally blind, meet eligibility requirements for special education services within a public

Text continues on p. 710

Table 71-1. **Common Eye Conditions and Their Syndromic, Visual, Neurologic, and Behavioral Associations**

Condition	Genetics	Pathophysiology	Common Ocular/ Visual Problems	Possible Associated Neurologic and Somatic Problems	Common Developmental, Cognitive, and Behavioral Features	Comments
Conditions Involving Multiple Regions of Eye or Brain or Both						
Oculocutaneous albinism	AR; multiple subtypes, including abnormal tyrosinase gene on chromosome 11q or other abnormal genes on 15q, 9p, and 5p	Deficient prenatal production of melanin pigment in retina, hair, and skin. Results in maldevelopment of retina, hypoplastic macula	Variable reduction in corrected visual acuity (20/40 to 20/400)	Skin and hair are very fair, with heightened susceptibility of skin to ultraviolet injury	No direct effect on mental development. In early infancy, infant may not make eye contact with others. Some may show mild, transient developmental and fine motor delays owing to difficulties with tracking and depth perception. May have head tilt	Advocacy and Parent Support available from National Organization for Albinism and Hypopigmentation (NOAH), PO Box 959, East Hampstead, NH 03826-0959. Phone: 800 473-2310 (U.S. and Canada), 603 887-2310. Fax: 800-648-2310. URL: http://www.albinism.org
		Anomalous routing of optic nerve fibers to contralateral side	Difficulty reading typically sized fonts and viewing low-contrast materials	Oculocutaneous albinism can be isolated disorder, or part of multisystem syndrome, e.g., Chediak-Higashi syndrome (immune defects, ataxia, intellectual disability), Hermansky-Pudlak syndrome (platelet dysfunction, prolonged bleeding time)	Regardless of visual function, with appropriate functional vision assessment, low-vision aids, and minor curricular and classroom adaptations, most children with albinism can be successful students	
			Problems with depth perception		May struggle with stigma of appearing "different," especially children of darker skinned racial groups. May become targets of social ostracism or bullying or both	
			Difficulties tracking objects that are small and rapidly moving Variable difficulty recognizing people at a distance Photophobia Pendular nystagmus from birth, most prominent in infancy Significant refractive error Astigmatism Strabismus		Benefit from consistent support from parents, teachers, and accepting peers	

Ocular albinism	XR; female carriers may have depigmented patches of skin and mottled retinal pigmentation	Deficient prenatal melanin production causes macular hypoplasia. Deficient melanin in skin and hair is apparent only microscopically	Same as listed for oculocutaneous albinism, above	Skin and hair pigment may be normal, but likely to be fairer than that of other family members	Same as listed for oculocutaneous albinism. If still undiagnosed, there may be more confusion on the part of teachers and others as to why the child might be having vision problems because many people are unaware of albinism that does not affect the skin and hair.	
				Heightened susceptibility of skin to ultraviolet injury		
Microphthalmia	Variable	Axial length of eyeball is shorter than normal for age	Vision can range from normal to severely impaired, often depending on absence or presence of associated ocular and CNS abnormalities	Variable, depending on associated CNS abnormalities	Highly variable	
		Can be unilateral or bilateral		Eyelids may appear sunken owing to absence or small size of eye		
		Can be isolated defect or part of multiple congenital anomalies. Coloboma and cataracts are most commonly associated ocular abnormalities				
Coloboma	Unknown or sporadic (e.g., part of CHARGE* association)	Failure of fusion of the embryonic choroidal fissure (5-6 wk gestation), resulting in a cleft of variable length and severity	In mildest form, defect limited to "keyhole" notch in iris (teardrop-shaped pupil). Most severe visual impairment when the cleft interrupts retinal tissue, particularly near fovea	Depends on associated CNS abnormalities	Behaviors associated with photophobia (e.g., keeping eyelids partially closed, excessive blinking)	Contact lenses may be used for cosmetic purposes and to reduce photophobia
	Associated with genetic or chromosomal syndromes (e.g., trisomy 13, Meckel-Gruber syndrome)		Can be isolated defect or associated with other ocular or systemic anomalies (e.g., CHARGE association)		Other, depending on associated anomalies	

*CHARGE, *C*oloboma, *H*eart disease, *A*tresia choanae, *R*etarded growth/developmental anomalies, *G*enital anomalies and/or hypogonadism, and *E*ar anomalies and/or deafness.

Continued

Table 71-1. **Common Eye Conditions and Their Syndromic, Visual, Neurologic, and Behavioral Associations—cont'd**

Condition	Genetics	Pathophysiology	Common Ocular/ Visual Problems	Possible Associated Neurologic and Somatic Problems	Common Developmental, Cognitive, and Behavioral Features	Comments
			Ophthalmoscopic features of macular colobomas; abnormal red reflex, large optic nerve head, and white retinal defect (bare sclera)			
Anterior Segment Abnormalities						
Glaucoma	Either sporadic or multifactorial with reduced penetrance (90%)	Persistently elevated intraocular pressure secondary to inadequate drainage of aqueous humor from anterior chamber	Variable visual impairment, secondary to associated corneal clouding, optic neuropathy, or associated amblyopia	None specific to glaucoma	Behaviors associated with photophobia (e.g., keeping eyelids partially closed, excessive blinking)	When suspected by primary care physician, prompt referral to pediatric ophthalmologist is indicated. For a pediatric patient, glaucoma can be identified by an eye examination under anesthesia
	Other 10% familial; usually AR, usually associated with gene defect in chromosome 2p21 region	Uncontrolled pressure leading to corneal clouding; irreversible damage to the optic nerve	Peripheral vision is affected first; tunnel vision at end stages		Frequent rubbing of eyes	Treatment for children usually requires surgery and sometimes medical therapy to control intraocular pressure. If treated early in course, visual loss usually can be prevented. Follow-up includes monitoring for and aggressive management of myopia and any amblyopia
		May also be part of a complex of multiple congenital eye abnormalities (e.g., associated with aniridia, retinopathy of prematurity, congenital rubella, Rubenstein-Taybi syndrome), metabolic disorders (e.g., Lowe syndrome, mucopolysaccharidosis) or acquired in association with other conditions (e.g., trauma, aphakia after cataract surgery, dislocated lens in Marfan syndrome)	May not see objects to side and below face			

			Significant visual impairment can be prevented if underlying glaucoma treated promptly Common initial symptoms in infants: enlarged cornea, excessive tearing, corneal clouding, conjunctival injection, photosensitivity, and blepharospasm (excessive blinking) Eye pain is not typically prominent initially			
Aniridia	AD in 66%. Sporadic in 33%	Congenital absence of all or part of iris	Variable visual function, including severe visual impairment owing to foveal hypoplasia	Increased risk of Wilms tumor		Physician needs increased index of suspicion for associated Wilms tumor; requires serial renal ultrasounds or cytogenetic tests or both for early detection
	Deletion or mutation of a transcription factor gene, *PAX6* (on chromosome 11p), is often present May be associated with deletion of Wilms tumor gene, also on chromosome 11p		Photophobia common Congenital nystagmus Possible cataracts Possible glaucoma Optic nerve hypoplasia Corneal opacification			
Peters anomaly	AD; multiple genes involved	Congenital whitish corneal scar resulting from incomplete separation of developing cornea from overlying surface ectoderm	High risk for glaucoma	Possible skeletal dysplasia with short stature		
			Possible underlying iridocorneal adhesions Possible anterior displacement of lens Possible cataract Possible aniridia or microphthalmia or both	Sometimes associated with facial, dental, or skin anomalies		

Continued

Table 71-1. **Common Eye Conditions and Their Syndromic, Visual, Neurologic, and Behavioral Associations—cont'd**

Condition	Genetics	Pathophysiology	Common Ocular/ Visual Problems	Possible Associated Neurologic and Somatic Problems	Common Developmental, Cognitive, and Behavioral Features	Comments
Cataract	Cataracts that are hereditary are usually AD	Cloudiness of crystalline lens	Small opacifications in the anterior or posterior poles of lens ("polar cataracts") generally do not cause visual impairment	Variable, depending on degree of visual impairment and presence of associated CNS abnormalities	Variable, depending on degree of visual impairment and presence of associated CNS abnormalities	Lack of a normal red reflex by an infant's primary care physician is an indication for prompt referral to pediatric ophthalmologist If the cataract is dense and present at birth, it is crucial to remove it surgically before 2 months of age (preferably in first few weeks of life) to prevent irreversible, severe amblyopia and to allow near-normal visual development
	AR and X-linked patterns also possible	Can be unilateral or bilateral	Congenital, dense cataracts, if not treated very early, can produce severe visual impairment and nystagmus			Untreated, later acquired cataracts still can cause lesser degrees of amblyopia up to age 7-8 yr
	Nonhereditary forms	Isolated lens defect versus part of many ocular malformations (e.g., microphthalmia, Peters anomaly, aniridia)	Significant unilateral visual impairment secondary to cataract can result in permanent visual loss owing to severe deprivation amblyopia			The postsurgical aphakic eye requires eyeglasses or contact lens to allow usable vision After removal of a unilateral cataract, patching of the normal eye is often necessary to counteract the child's natural tendency to rely exclusively on that eye, and prevent amblyopia
		Can be part of systemic condition, including Chromosomal anomalies (e.g., Turner syndrome; cri du chat syndrome; trisomies 13, 18, and 21) Metabolic disorders (e.g., Lowe syndrome, galactosemia, homocystinuria)				

		Multisystem syndromes (e.g., Apert syndrome, incontinentia pigmenti, osteogenesis imperfecta, Smith-Lemli-Opitz) Intrauterine infections (e.g., rubella, cytomegalovirus) Vitamin deficiency (A, D) Eye trauma Exposure to toxins Acquired cataracts can be associated with radiation and steroids				
Persistent hyperplastic primary vitreous	Apparently sporadic	Failure of normal involution of the primitive hyaloid vascular system during 7th gestational month Leads to formation of opaque fibrovascular membrane on posterior capsule of lens If untreated, pulling of ciliary body can later cause glaucoma and loss of the eye	Leukocoria (white pupil) Usually unilateral; involved eye is usually microphthalmic Also can be associated with cataracts, glaucoma, retinal detachment, and amblyopia Visual function varies from adequate (after cataract surgery and rehabilitation) to impaired (if retina/optic nerve involved)	Usually not associated with other CNS abnormalities	No behaviors specific to persistent hyperplastic primary vitreous	
Retinal Disorders						
Retinopathy of prematurity	Although primarily nongenetic, genetic factors may increase vulnerability among affected premature infants	Retinal neovascular proliferative disorder limited almost exclusively to premature infants	May be associated with cerebral visual impairment	Often associated with additional developmental disabilities	Sometimes associated with fine and gross motor and spatial awareness difficulties that are more pronounced than in comparably visually impaired children owing to other causes	Long-term (15 yr) outcomes after cryotherapy in neonatal intensive care unit versus matched group who did not receive cryotherapy: Unfavorable visual acuity outcomes found in 44.7% of treated and 64.3% of control eyes ($P < .001$) New retinal detachments, even in eyes with good structural findings at age 10 yr, suggest value in long-term, regular follow-up of eyes that experience threshold retinopathy of prematurity

Continued

Table 71-1. **Common Eye Conditions and Their Syndromic, Visual, Neurologic, and Behavioral Associations—cont'd**

Condition	Genetics	Pathophysiology	Common Ocular/ Visual Problems	Possible Associated Neurologic and Somatic Problems	Common Developmental, Cognitive, and Behavioral Features	Comments
		Risk and severity associated primarily with: premature gestational age and retinal tissue hyperoxia via VEGF; hyperoxia → VEGF is down-regulated → retinal vessel growth stops → retinal tissue hypoxia → VEGF up-regulated → if large area of avascular retina, then VEGF is overstimulated → neovascularization → scarring, retinal detachment	Potential visual complications (during childhood and adolescence)	Deafness	Self-stimulatory eye pressing is common	For all retinal disorders, research and support through Foundation Fighting Blindness, 11435 Cronhill Drive, Owings Mills, MD 21117. Phone: (800) 683-5555. URL: www.blindness.org
		Overall incidence: approximately ⅔ of infants with birth weight <1251 g and 90% of infants with birth weight <750 g	Severe myopia	Cerebral palsy	In middle childhood (age 10 yr), neonatal threshold retinopathy of prematurity (stage III or greater) is associated with functional limitations in health attributes and reduced health-related quality of life Among children who developed threshold retinopathy of prematurity, there is greater overall developmental impairment among children with a poor visual outcome compared with children with better sight	
		Significant visual impairment is generally limited to stages IV-V (i.e., partial or complete retinal detachment)	Astigmatism	Autism		
			Anisometropia Amblyopia Strabismus	Intellectual disability Learning disabilities Attention-deficit/hyperactivity disorder		
			Late retinal detachments			

Leber congenital amaurosis	AR; associated with at least 4 genes, located on different chromosomes (including 1, 17 and 19)	Group of conditions characterized by abnormal development of photoreceptor cells in retina, with secondary degenerative changes in several cell layers in the retina. Diagnosis may change over time as other ophthalmologic or systemic symptoms become apparent; these include retinitis pigmentosa, Joubert syndrome, and Alström syndrome	Typically results in roving nystagmus by early infancy and visual impairment, ranging from mild to severe. Children with residual functional vision are extremely farsighted. Degree of vision loss remains stable through young adulthood, but may progressively worsen in older adulthood	Approximately 20% have associated CNS disorders (e.g., seizure disorders, intellectual disability, autism, and motor disorders)	Some children are extremely photophobic	
			Examination of fundus during infancy is normal, but electroretinography shows minimal to no retinal activity Often associated with deep-set eyes, keratoconus (cone-shaped cornea), and cataracts		Often associated with frequent eye pressing	
Retinitis pigmentosa	AD (20%), AR (20%), XR (10%), and sporadic (50%)	A group of inherited disorders affecting the retinal pigment epithelium, causing dysfunction of outer portions of the rods and cones, eventually causing blindness	In isolated form, onset of visual symptoms is typically during adolescence	Wide heterogeneity of associated neurologic and somatic symptoms, particularly when retinitis pigmentosa is part of a syndrome	Variable, depending on degree of visual impairment and presence of associated CNS abnormalities	Some syndromes (partial list) that can be associated with retinitis pigmentosa
	Main defect for many forms is defect in gene for rhodopsin, a protein important for function of rods		Visual symptoms usually emerge earlier when retinitis pigmentosa is part of a syndrome (see list in last column)			Joubert syndrome
			Initially destruction of rods; may eventually affect cone function as well			Batten disease
			Poor night vision and defective dark adaptation			Zellweger syndrome
			Tunnel vision (loss of peripheral visual fields)			Bardet-Biedl syndrome
			Acuity and color vision present early on, but lost as disease progresses			Usher syndrome

Continued

Table 71-1. Common Eye Conditions and Their Syndromic, Visual, Neurologic, and Behavioral Associations—cont'd

Condition	Genetics	Pathophysiology	Common Ocular/ Visual Problems	Possible Associated Neurologic and Somatic Problems	Common Developmental, Cognitive, and Behavioral Features	Comments
			Initial ophthalmoscopic examination of retina may appear normal. Eventually see dark "bone-spicule"–shaped densities of pigment and attenuated blood vessels			Refsum disease Hurler syndrome (mucopolysaccharidosis II) Friedreich ataxia Kearns-Sayre syndrome
Congenital Abnormalities of Optic Nerve						
Optic nerve hypoplasia	N/A	Prenatal underdevelopment of optic nerve. Sometimes is unilateral, but more commonly affects both eyes. Causes are unknown. Some association with young maternal age, maternal diabetes mellitus, maternal alcohol abuse, maternal use of antiepileptic drugs	Wide range of visual function, from normal acuity to total blindness Nystagmus is usually present in association with any visual acuity deficits Visual field cuts may range from significant limitations in central or peripheral fields to subtle peripheral field loss Photophobia occasionally noted Stability of visual function (no deterioration over time). Nystagmus and visual acuity sometimes spontaneously improve over time	Can be associated with CNS and endocrine abnormalities (e.g., septo-optic dysplasia, with variable hypoplasia or absence of septum pellucidum) plus low levels of some or all of hormones controlled by pituitary gland (e.g., growth hormone deficiency, diabetes insipidus, hypothyroidism, insufficient adrenal response to stress)	Often have history of feeding/eating problems, particularly limited repertoire of acceptable foods. Requires patience and sometimes nutritional consultation to maintain adequate nutritional quality, particularly if there is endocrine risk of hypoglycemia	Early symptoms of septo-optic dysplasia may include neonatal hypoglycemia, temperature instability, hyperbilirubinemia, or failure to thrive during infancy. All children diagnosed with optic nerve hypoplasia should have cranial imaging to check for integrity of midline structures and a referral to a pediatric endocrinologist to monitor for emerging hormonal deficits Family Support site: http://www.focusfamilies.org/focus/

Cortical/Cerebral Causes of Visual Impairment						
Cortical/cerebral visual impairment	Variable, depending on associated conditions	Injury or abnormal prenatal development of optic radiations or visual cortex or both	Visual function is highly variable; even in same child, visual function often varies from hour-to-hour or day-to-day Classic features Diminished visual function despite normal function of anterior visual system (anterior to optic chiasm) Normal pupillary reactions to light Normal retinal function Absence of nystagmus Frequent associated visual dysfunctions or behaviors Difficulties with facial recognition Difficulty interpreting others' facial expressions Problems with visual attention Visual function much better for moving target than for stationary Visual function often better for targets in peripheral field than centrally Visual function may improve during first 1-2 yr of life Often associated with comorbid ocular disorders Strabismus Nystagmus Cataracts Glaucoma High myopia/hyperopia Optic nerve disorders Retinal disorders (e.g., retinopathy of prematurity)	Can be associated with Intellectual disability Cerebral palsy Autism Deafness Learning disabilities	Variable, depending on degree of visual impairment and types of associated CNS abnormalities	Some aspects of visual function may improve over the first few years of life

*CHARGE, *C*oloboma, *H*eart disease, *A*tresia choanae, *R*etarded growth/developmental anomalies, *G*enital anomalies and/or hypogonadism, and *E*ar anomalies and/or deafness.
AD, autosomal dominant; AR, autosomal recessive; CNS, central nervous system; VEGF, vascular endothelial growth factor; XR, X-linked recessive.
Data from Bizzarro et al, 2006; Good and Hoyt, 1989; Good et al, 2001; Holbrook, 1996; Kipp, 2003; Levin, 2003; Palmer et al, 2005; Quinn et al, 2004; Stout and Stout, 2003; Thompson and Kaufman, 2003; Warren, 1994; Wright, 2008.

Table 71-2. **Central Nervous System Conditions Often Associated with Severe Visual Impairment and Other Developmental or Chronic Disabilities**

Central Nervous System Disorders (Classified by Cause)	Associated Eye Conditions	Associated Neurodevelopmental and Other Chronic Disorders
Primary abnormal prenatal development of brain (e.g., congenital hydrocephalus, absence of corpus callosum, congenital microcephaly	Cortical visual impairment, optic atrophy, nystagmus, anophthalmia, microphthalmia, optic nerve hypoplasia	Intellectual disability, cerebral palsy, behavioral problems, epilepsy, endocrinologic disorders (e.g., hypothyroid, diabetes insipidus)
Prenatal exposure to maternal viral infections (e.g., rubella, cytomegalovirus, herpes)	Cataracts, retinopathy, microphthalmia, glaucoma, chorioretinitis	Hearing impairment, intellectual disability, behavioral problems, epilepsy
Genetic inborn errors of metabolism and single-gene disorders (e.g., Hurler syndrome, Tay-Sachs disease, Marfan syndrome, Lowe syndrome, Zellweger syndrome, CHARGE association, Usher syndrome)	Glaucoma, ectopic lens, corneal clouding, optic atrophy, retinitis pigmentosa, coloboma	Hearing impairment, intellectual disability, behavioral problems, epilepsy, renal problems, poor growth
Chromosomal abnormalities (e.g., Down syndrome, trisomy 13, cri du chat syndrome, cat-eye syndrome	Coloboma, microphthalmia, cataracts, corneal clouding, strabismus	Intellectual disability, behavioral problems, epilepsy, cardiac problems, cleft palate, poor growth
Other congenital ophthalmologic syndromes of uncertain etiology (e.g., Leber congential amaurosis, optic nerve hypoplasia)	Retinal dysfunction, optic nerve hypoplasia, coloboma, corneal abnormalities	Intellectual disability, poor growth, endocrinologic abnormalities
Prematurity and perinatal hypoxia	Retinopathy of prematurity, secondary glaucoma, strabismus, cortical blindness	Intellectual disability, cerebral palsy, chronic lung disease, poor growth, hydrocephalus
Bacterial meningitis (e.g., *Haemophilus influenzae*, group B streptococcus)	Cortical visual impairment, strabismus, optic atrophy	Intellectual disability, cerebral palsy, hydrocephalus, epilepsy, behavioral problems, hearing impairment
Head trauma (e.g., accidental and nonaccidental, shaken baby syndrome, near-drowning	Cortical visual impairment, strabismus, optic atrophy, retinal hemorrhage (usually transient)	Intellectual disability, cerebral palsy, behavioral problems, epilepsy

Adapted from Kelly DP, Teplin SW: Disorders of sensation: Hearing and visual impairment. *In* Wolraich M (ed): Disorders of Development and Learning, 3rd ed. Hamilton, Ontario, Canada, BC Decker Inc., 2003, pp 329-343.

school setting. Ascertainment of visual acuity is often difficult in young children, and criteria for itmpairment based solely on acuity neglect the importance of other determinants of visual function.

Approximately 75% of *legally blind* children have some remaining vision that is functional and can provide the foundation for individually tailored learning plans, including environmental and curricular adaptations at home and school. Ultimately, the most important criteria for provision of services specific to blindness or visual impairment at home and school should be based on how the child is actually functioning, not solely on visual acuity measurements. To qualify for such services within a public school setting, a child must have a diagnosis that results in uncorrectable diminished visual acuity or visual field or the confirmation of a degenerative visual condition *and* show an educational need for the special education services.

INTERVENTIONS AND MANAGEMENT

National legislation has asserted the direction for services for family and children with visual impairments since implementation of the Individuals with Disabilities Education Act (IDEA), originally started as Public Law 94-142 in 1975; it guaranteed free and appropriate public education for children with disabilities in the least restrictive environment. All students receiving special education have an Individualized Education Program (IEP), which details assessment findings and service needs. The IEP is based on parent input and professional assessment findings.

Through reauthorizations and amendments, gradually realization of additional or different needs for children with visual impairments are being regarded by law, usually as a result of advocacy by such groups as the National Association of Parents of Children with Visual Impairments (NAPVI), and position statements from teaching associations and other advocacy groups. By 2000, Public Law 105-17 made mandatory services for children birth through 5 years of age who have a visual disability. The current law mandates Braille instruction for students deemed by a team to need it, and highlights orientation and mobility as a related service. Part B of IDEA describes services for children 3 to 21 years old; Part C relates to infant and toddlers, reflecting the importance of family as central to programming.

Part C is a major influence in service provision to families with children birth through age 3 years who have developmental delay or a disability such as blindness and visual impairment. Part C requires interagency coordination with parent representation at all times, service referral and smooth transitions (such as hospital-to-home), legal rights protection through due process, and institution of an Individual Family Service Plan (IFSP). Coordination and collaboration at the state and administration levels includes a single point of entry, usually a district's Child Find. This is where a medical referral should be directed to start the process. Assessment and service delivery is usually through a transdisciplinary team approach. It is important that a certified teacher of students with visual impairments (TVI) be part of the team from the start. A team serving a young child who is blind or visually impaired with possible other impairments may include parents; TVI; orientation and mobility instructor; special education teacher or early interventionist; ophthalmologist; optometrist; developmental pediatrician or primary care physician; physical, occupational, and speech therapists; psychologist; nurse; social worker, parent or child advocate; and others as appropriate.

In determining the best programming for their child, families have an array of options that include service delivery in the home, center-based programs specifically for serving children with visual disabilities, and more generic center-based programs serving children with various special needs with input from a TVI or a certified orientation and mobility specialist (COMS). Integration with nondisabled peers can occur in various center-based and community programs with TVI support. It is important for any system to embrace parent support and involvement. Parents of children with visual disabilities are grateful for opportunities to meet and exchange ideas and mutual support with other parents through parent groups and conferences such as those sponsored by national and state parent organizations (e.g., NAPVI and Parents of Blind Children). Newsletters and Internet links have made it easier for parents to connect, especially when they are in rural, isolated areas.

DEVELOPMENTAL AND EDUCATIONAL IMPLICATIONS OF VISUAL IMPAIRMENT

The impact of visual impairment on a child's development is highly individual, and is related to the age of onset, severity of vision loss, and any other concurring conditions. No other sense can trigger curiosity, integrate information, and invite exploration to the extent that vision does. Vision is usually the main venue for communication and learning in the first years of life and remains crucial into adulthood. Vision makes a significant contribution to rate and sequence of normal development (Sonksen, 1982).

Severely visually impaired children lose thousands of hours of incidental learning and learning from visual imitation. They require more "hands-on," meaningful experiences and guidance from adults knowledgeable in training the effective use of vision, hearing, touch, smell, and taste. Efficient sensory compensations for visual impairment do not develop automatically. Deliberate care must be taken to provide accessible and meaningful learning situations for the child (Figs. 71-1 and 71-2).

Data from a longitudinal study of the first 5 years of 248 children with visual impairments, Project PRISM, showed that developmental scores and growth are significantly lower than for children with typical vision. Visual function at the 20/800 level also seemed to be associated with developmental patterns or sequences that differed from those of children with normal vision. Communication was less affected by level of vision, whereas performance in the adaptive and motor domains seemed to be most sensitive to level of vision.

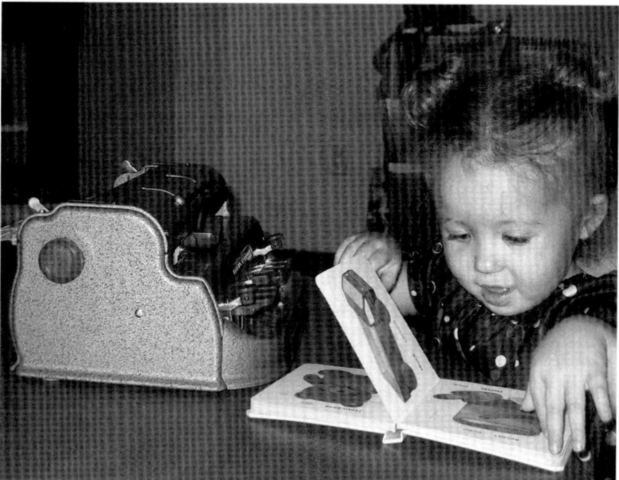

Figure 71-1. This toddler enjoys reading and writing, both visually and tactilely (Braille). Her Twin Vision book has the book's original print and pictures plus transparent Braille pages. This allows a sighted caregiver to read aloud while the child with visual impairment reads along. (For more information on Twin Vision books, American Action Fund for Blind Children and Adults, Baltimore, MD, see www.actionfund.org.)

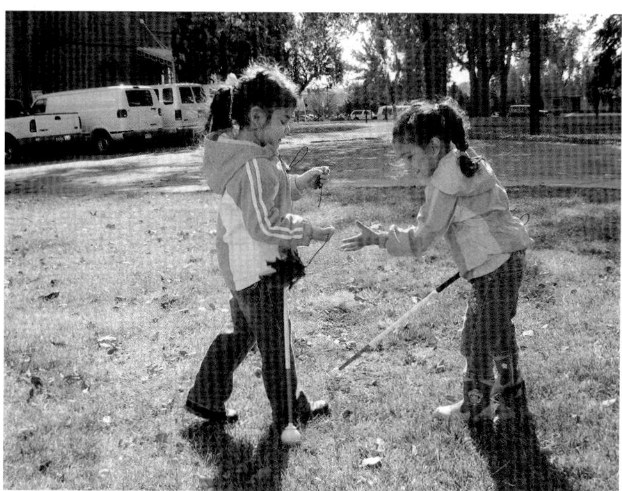

Figure 71-2. Two visually impaired girls enjoying their use of mobility, language, and social interactions through mutual play.

The age at which the blindness or visual impairment occurs is crucial; even a brief period of usable vision can help an infant develop, especially with regard to spatial concepts and motor functions. Most causes of visual impairment in children are congenital or of very early onset. In the presence of nystagmus or with an infant's inability to fix and follow visually, eye-to-eye contact may not occur or becomes more fleeting and less reliable as a social cue. Similarly, smiling in infants who are severely visually impaired is often muted or fleeting and could lose some of its typical power as a social cue in the parent-infant attachment process. Parent-infant bonding and attachment occur, but may proceed a bit more precariously and deliberately as the parent learns to attend to unique, more subtle, or alternative social-communicative signals the infant is sending and responding to. This is one of many developmental domains in which early intervention with a teacher experienced in working with infants and preschoolers with severe visual impairments can provide specialized guidance and support for parents. The interventionist can help parents recognize and capitalize on their own infant's bonding and communicative behaviors. Leaning an ear toward a parent's voice, certain hand postures, and skin-to-skin touching are examples.

Beginning with cries and cooing, sounds grow into language, a powerful tool for a child who is blind or visually impaired for communication and for building the conceptual linkages that develop into cognitive understanding. Articulation may develop normally with recitations of familiar phrases and songs, but the ability to put words into sentences may require a prolonged period of echolalia and of confusion about reversals of pronouns. This often results in verbatim repetitions of what the child has heard (e.g., a child who wants a cookie is likely to request it by saying, "Do you want a cookie?" repeated in same questioning intonation used by the mother). Concepts need to be developed through multiple, meaningful adult-initiated "lessons" that are verbalizations paired with hands-on experiences. A noun such as "button" can refer to a shirt button, push-button on TV, or a bellybutton; likewise, a verb such as "push" can mean to walk a stroller forward, press down the top of a pop-up toy, or squeeze feet into socks.

It is important that interventionists and parents provide extra time and varieties of experiences so that language concepts can be generalized. As the child gets older, this role needs to include verbal descriptions of play areas and what classmates are doing so that social skills can be developed and practiced. The auditory channel plays a strong role in communication and cognition for a child who is blind or visually impaired. Unable to synthesize sensory information through vision, a child may be observed to grow quiet to concentrate on listening, rather than vocalize or move. It is important for parents and teachers not to misinterpret this quietness as "withdrawal" or "sadness." Later, the child may use auditory memory to show an ability to participate in story time with classmates, for example, by showing the motion to match the vocabulary the child knows about his or her body parts in the song "Head, Shoulders, Knees, and Toes."

Motor milestone attainment is usually impacted most by early-onset blindness or visual impairment. It is common for physical and occupational therapists to use sensory integration and neurodevelopmental techniques to ensure that the child from earliest infancy experiences full developmental sequences. The sequence of motor milestone attainment may vary, however, from that typically seen in infants and toddlers with normal vision. Without being able to rely on seeing a desired object or person as an automatic motivator to move through space, the infant often is sedentary with flexed postures and a reduced incentive to move. Visual deprivation can be responsible for low arousal and "sleepy" state. If left in the crib without sufficient sensory stimulation to activate the brain's regulatory systems, the infant with visual impairment may present with low muscle tone, offbeat sleep patterns, or the reputation for being a "good" or "quiet" infant. The following are components that, without specific intervention, can be missing in the child's movement repertoire: sensory integration; optical righting antigravity flexion and extension in head, shoulder, trunk, and pelvis; proximal stability of head, neck, scapula, trunk, and pelvis; grading of movement (i.e., movements tend to be "all or nothing"); lateral and diagonal weight shift; and rotational, protective and balance reactions.

Spatial concepts are derived for a child with visual impairment through movement, hearing, and touch, starting with orientation activities in special play areas rich in sensory opportunities, such as Lilli Nielsen's popular "little room" (Nielsen, 1992). Spatial concepts lead to cognitive development and to efficient orientation and mobility. For spatial experiences, high color contrasts, special illumination, sound cues, and low-vision devices such as monocular telescopes make movement within the child's environment purposeful. The acquisition of certain cognitive concepts, such as object permanence, recognition of "I" as separate from the greater world, and ways to explore and control, may be delayed for a child with visual impairment until sufficient sensory experiences are gained. For a child with visual impairment, who is relying primarily on auditory and tactile cues, the motor milestones of reaching for a sound cue or purposeful movement to get an object may seem delayed. In contrast to vision, auditory and tactile cues are noncontinuous and lack the power to synthesize other sensory experiences. A child must first have many opportunities to handle and listen to a bell before the child realizes that its tactile properties are matched to the sound it makes (i.e., understanding of object permanence must be present before auditory localization of the ringing bell would be a motivator for mobility).

Purposeful movement leads to orientation and mobility in the larger world. COMS have special training in working to develop the child's functional use of residual vision (if any is present) and to train safe and independent movement. "Push toys" such as a hula hoop pushed in front by the child becomes a traditional white cane as the child masters traveling in environments outside familiar rooms. Good orientation and mobility techniques are necessary for safe and independent travel at home, school, and workplace. This is true also for an adult with blindness who must be trained how to use a guide dog efficiently.

Stereotypic behaviors, such as rocking, eye pressing, head weaving, and perseveration of certain movements (e.g., finger-flicking), are theorized to be attempts to gain additional sensory input that a child who is blind or visually impaired does not gain through typical experiences. Another view is that sensory modulation may be difficult for the child, and these self-stimulatory behaviors may help maintain arousal/calming and attention. These "blindisms" have become less frequent in children with visual impairments now than in the past as early intervention and better understanding of motor development of children with severe visual impairments have been implemented over the 2 to 3 decades. Eye pressing and "poking" remain the exception when retinal diagnoses are present, especially in children with ROP and Leber amaurosis. In persistent cases, the child's face can be damaged by the behavior, the retina can detach, motor development is affected, and the activity can become a socially liability when the child is among sighted peers.

SCHOOL-AGE CHILDREN AND ADOLESCENTS

School services to meet the unique needs of students with visual impairments, which often begin during the preschool years, include direct service and consultation service models. These are provided, as needed, by two professionals who are specifically trained to understand the educational and mobility needs of students who are blind/visually impaired: a TVI and a COMS. A TVI provides information and training about possible developmental and academic challenges, provides specialized instruction such as teaching Braille codes or training the use of prescribed low-vision devices, and procures needed specialized equipment. A COMS determines the need for equipment, such as adapted mobility devices or a long cane; this specialist also teaches about concepts of space and directionality and specific strategies for safe and efficient travel within familiar and unfamiliar environments.

Students with visual impairments have instructional needs beyond the scope of the general curriculum content; the concepts that are incidentally learned by sighted students must be systematically and sequentially taught to a student who is blind or visually impaired. The *Expanded Core Curriculum* (American Foundation for the Blind, 2007) addresses nine additional learning needs for children and adolescents with visual impairments: (1) compensatory or functional academic skills, including communication modes (e.g., skills in organization, listening, Braille, low-vision devices, augmentative or alternative communication systems); (2) orientation and mobility; (3) social interaction skills; (4) independent living skills; (5) recreation and leisure skills; (6) career education; (7) use of assistive technology; (8) visual efficiency skills; and (9) self-determination.

Access to appropriate educational services must include an assurance that instructional materials are available to students in the appropriate media and at the same time as their sighted peers (Huebner et al, 2004). Daily instructionally related print materials may be produced in Braille by the TVI or by a district Braillist. Many states have instructional resource centers, which work directly with school district TVIs to process orders for Braille books (see Fig. 71-1). One helpful solution on the horizon to increase availability of new textbooks in large print or Braille is the National Materials Accessibility Standard, mandated by the 2004 revisions of the IDEA. This law requires textbook publishers to provide an electronic copy of their textbooks to instructional resource centers for the purpose of translation into large print, Braille, audio, and digital formats.

Students who are blind or visually impaired also may receive services from specialized programs unique to children with visual impairments and educational programs open to all children in communities and public schools. There is a wide range of placement options depending on the collected input of teams of professionals who meet with parents to formulate the IFSP (for children birth to 3 years old) and IEP (for students 3 to 21 years old).

Several states have specialized early intervention programs for only infants, toddlers, and preschoolers with visual impairments. Preschool-age children also may be served in a community preschool or a public preschool setting. Most primary school–age children with visual impairments are educated in their home schools. Another option for placement is a day or residential school for the blind. About 8% of students with legal blindness are educated in special schools, such as state schools for the blind (American Printing House for the Blind, 1997).

ASSESSMENT AND EVALUATION OF CHILDREN WITH VISUAL IMPAIRMENTS

School-age children and adolescents who are blind or visually impaired have the same educational assessment needs as their sighted peers. Classroom, district, and state assessments must be adapted, as needed, for the student's participation. An assessment may be adapted into Braille or large print. The student may need to use a low-vision device or screen reading program and extended time to access the assessment materials. In addition to the traditional assessments used within a school setting, the student who is blind or visually impaired usually needs educational assessments unique to this population.

A TVI has the expertise and responsibility to conduct a Functional Vision Assessment (FVA) with children who are visually impaired. The purpose of a FVA is to assess the daily visual skills of a child and to identify what assists the child's visual performance (Anthony, 2000). FVAs can substantiate qualifications for services for visually impaired students. The FVA findings should be used in developmental and academic testing and should serve as a basis for programming of visual efficiency training and compensatory skill development. An FVA provides information on the following functional-visual performance abilities: (1) appearance of eyes; (2) visual reflexes; (3) visual responsiveness to light, color, and form; (4) muscle balance; (5) eye preference; (6) eye movement behaviors; (7) field of vision; (8) color vision; (9) depth perception and figure-ground perception; (10) light sensitivity; (11) functional visual acuity; (12) visuomotor coordination; and (13) visual-cognitive skills (e.g., visual imitation, visual pattern sequencing).

A companion assessment to the FVA is the Learning Media Assessment, which allows for systematic selection of learning and literacy media for students who are blind or visually impaired (Koenig and Holbrook, 1995). Learning media include real objects, models, rulers, worksheets, and tools used for promoting literacy in print and Braille. The decision as to which literacy media to use (e.g., Braille versus large print versus optical modifications of regular print, or combinations of these modes) must be based on much more than the child's visual acuity.

Because of the low incidence of blind and visually impaired children in the population and small sample sizes, standardization of scores on assessments, especially at the youngest ages, has not been possible. Adaptations are often not developmentally appropriate, especially if any additional disabilities are present. Additionally, infant assessments, such as the Bayley Scales of Development, often used in neonatal units and in clinical settings are not good predictors of later function for a child with visual impairment. Criterion-referenced, developmentally sequenced assessments, such as the Hawaii Early Learning Profile, which offer small steps of progression, seem to fit into programming best. Later, testing (e.g., IQ) is complicated by verbal versus performance issues; often only the verbal component is administered, giving a skewed picture of what the child may be able to do. Standardized testing scores are currently important criteria for educational accountability at a national level; developing tests with adaptations and timing appropriate for different levels of mastery for children with various visual impairments has become a priority issue. Results still must be reviewed with caution. It is imperative that personnel trained to work with young children who have visual impairment be included in any formal assessment procedure conducted by Child Find Teams at early ages and by educational institutions; without access to this special expertise, assessment teams are likely to make educational planning decisions that fail to meet the child's needs.

A team needs to provide a thorough medical, developmental, and academic evaluation of the student to determine needs. An optimally comprehensive evaluation of the child with visual impairment involves assessments by specialists from multiple disciplines, including the pediatric ophthalmologist, pediatrician, TVI, and other school personnel. Depending on the child's presenting difficulties, other disciplines that may be crucial are occupational or physical therapist, COMS, social worker, and speech-language pathologist. Synthesis of the evaluation findings requires effective communication between all involved professionals. With this information, the TVI is equipped to make recommendations for adaptations that allow optimal learning and skill development within the child's natural environments and routines at home, school, and community. Contrary to what primary care physicians often assume, the ophthalmologist's expertise does not usually include knowledge about the cognitive, educational, emotional, and social implications of visual impairment in children.

Although the primary care physician does not need to attain expertise in these areas, as the provider of the child's "medical home," he or she is well prepared for the role of providing ongoing family support and learning about developmental and special educational resources for children with visual impairment in the community. Consultation with a developmental-behavioral or neurodevelopmental pediatrician, particularly when this subspecialist works in an interdisciplinary environment, is another way that the family can obtain additional information about their child's unique developmental strengths and needs; how the child's visual function affects his or her behavior and learning; whether there are any genetic considerations; and whether the nature of the child's eye or CNS conditions suggest that further medical, metabolic, or genetic workup is indicated.

SECONDARY TRANSITION AND EMPLOYMENT

Data collected in 1994-1995 indicated that 46% of individuals in the United States between the ages of 18 and 54 years with visual impairment were unemployed (Kirchner et al, 1999). Providing appropriate literacy and career-linking experiences during the formative years improves employment outcomes (Wolffe, 1999). IDEA 2004 mandates that school personnel work with high school students and others such as rehabilitation counselors to develop and implement a transition plan for career exploration and preparing for postschool activities such as attending a university or securing employment.

SUMMARY OF PHYSICIAN AND EDUCATOR ROLES

The child's primary care physician, as the medical home for the child, plays a key role in helping the child to function as ably as possible. In addition to the obvious routine and continuous medical care and preventive health services that any child requires, the primary care physician (sometimes in collaboration with a consulting developmental-behavioral pediatrician) can be the source of many features of tailored care for the child with visual impairment. These features include the following:

- Provide emotional support and help parents become active advocates for their child. Family support services are crucial, particularly during the weeks and months following the often-shocking news about a child's impaired vision. Local, regional, and national parent groups and agencies are available to help link "new" with "veteran" parents for the purposes of support and education (see References).
- Help direct family to relevant parent support groups and local/national organizations (see References).
- Encourage discussion of the child's developmental status (strengths and weaknesses); when appropriate or requested by parents, referral to other developmental or behavioral specialists is helpful (e.g., developmental-behavioral or neurodevelopmental pediatrician, psychologist, occupational therapist, ophthalmologist, low-vision optometrist, ocularist [fashions and maintains prosthetic eyes]).
- Explore emotional impact of the child's disability on siblings.
- Become knowledgeable regarding school-based, community, and national resources (see References), including early intervention programs, statewide services, and eligibility for specialized materials and accommodations at school.
- Maintain communication with the child's ophthalmologist, teachers (including TVI), community-based service agencies.
- Help prepare family members for major developmental transition times (e.g., from early

intervention/preschool program to elementary school, from middle school to high school, from high school to postsecondary learning or living as independently as possible as a young adult).

The role of the TVI is to work closely with medical personnel to assist with the identification of the student's visual condition; to complete needed assessments to determine the child's developmental and, later, academic needs; and to provide specialized instruction and equipment. An educational program for the student who is blind or visually impaired should reflect the general education and expanded core curriculum.

SUMMARY

With proper identification, appropriate medical and family supports, early referral to and the provision of educational services, children who are blind and visually impaired can experience learning and living to their full potential.

REFERENCES

American Foundation for the Blind. 2007. Available at: http://afb.org/Section.asp?SectionID=44&TopicID=189&SubTopicID=4.

American Printing House for the Blind. 1997. Available at: www.aph.org/

Anthony TL: Performing a functional low vision assessment. *In* D'Andrea FM, Farrenkopf C (eds): Looking to Learning: Promoting Literacy for Students with Low Vision. New York, American Foundation for the Blind Press, 2000, p 32-83.

Bizzarro MJ, Hussain N, Jonsson B, et al: Genetic susceptibility to retinopathy of prematurity. Pediatrics 2006; 118;1858-1863, 2006.

Good WV, Hoyt CR: Behavioral correlates of poor vision in children. Int Ophthalmol Clin 29:57-60, 1989.

Good WV, Jan JE, Burden SK, et al: Recent advances in cortical visual impairment. Dev Med Child Neurol 43:56-60, 2001.

Holbrook MC (ed): Children with Visual Impairments—A Parents' Guide, 2nd ed. Bethesda, MD, Woodbine House, 2006.

Huebner KM, Merk-Adams B, Stryker D, Wolffe K: The National Agenda for the Education of Children and Youths with Visual Impairments, Including Those with Multiple Disabilities, rev ed. New York, AFB Press, 2004.

Kipp MA: Childhood glaucoma. Pediatr Clin North Am 50:89-104, 2003.

Kirchner C: National estimates of prevalence and demographics of children with visual impairments. *In* Wang MC, Reynolds MC, Walberg HJ (eds): Handbook of Special Education Research and Practice, Vol 3. Low Incidence Conditions. Oxford, Pergamon, 1989, pp 135-153.

Kirchner C, Schmeidler E, Todorov A: Looking at Employment through a Lifespan Telescope: Age, Health and Employment Status of People with Serious Visual Impairment. Mississippi State, MS, Rehabilitation Research and Training Center on Blindness and Low Vision, 1999.

Koenig AJ, Holbrook MC: Learning Media Assessment of Students with Visual Impairments: A Resource Guide. Austin, TX, Texas School for the Blind and Visually Impaired, 1995.

Levin AV: Congenital eye anomalies. Pediatr Clin North Am 50: 55-76, 2003.

Nielsen L: Space and self: Active learning by means of the little room. Copenhagen, Sikon, 1992.

Palmer EA, Hardy RJ, Dobson V, et al: 15-year outcomes following threshold retinopathy of prematurity: Final results from the multicenter trial of cryotherapy for retinopathy of prematurity. Arch Ophthalmol 123:311-318, 2005.

Quinn GE, Dobson V, Saigal S, et al: Health-related quality of life at age 10 years in very low-birth-weight children with and without threshold retinopathy of prematurity. Arch Ophthalmol 122:1659-1666, 2004.

Sonksen PM: The assessment of 'vision for development' in severely visually handicapped babies. Acta Ophthalmol Suppl 157:82-90, 1982.

Stout AU, Stout T: Retinopathy of prematurity. Pediatr Clin North Am 50:77-87, 2003.

Thompson L, Kaufman LM: The visually impaired child. Pediatr Clin North Am 50:225-239, 2003.

Warren DH: Blindness and Children—an Individual Differences Approach. Cambridge, Cambridge University Press, 1994.

Wolffe KE: The importance of career education. *In* Wolffe KE (ed): Skills for Success: A Career Education Handbook for Children and Adolescent with Visual Impairments. New York, American Foundation for the Blind Press, 1999, pp 12-26.

Wright KW: Pediatric Ophthalmology for Primary Care, 3rd ed., Elk Grove Village, IL, American Academy of Pediatrics, 2008.

SUGGESTED READINGS

Holbrook MC: Children with Visual Impairments: A Parent's Guide. Bethesda, MD, Woodbine House, 2006. This book is authored by an expert team of parents and professionals. It offers jargon-free advice to parents of young children with visual impairments from birth to age 7.

Lueck AH, Chen D, Kekelis L: Developmental Guidelines for Infants with Visual Impairment: A Manual for Early Intervention. Louisville, KY, American Printing House for the Blind, 1997. This manual was written for professionals working with children with visual impairments from birth through 2 years of age. The manual includes narrative chapters and developmental charts in the domains of social-emotional, communication, cognitive, and motor development.

Pogrund RL, Fazzi DL: Early Focus: Working with Young Children Who Are Blind or Visually Impaired and Their Families, 2nd ed. New York, American Foundation for the Blind Press, 2002. This book addresses young children with visual impairments, including children with additional disabilities. It addresses challenges and intervention recommendations in all developmental domains, including early literacy, daily living skills, and orientation and mobility.

AGENCIES AND WEBSITES

American Association for Pediatric Ophthalmology and Strabismus. Available at: http://www.aapos.org. This website provides information about latest research efforts, and concise overviews of common conditions causing visual impairment in children, and treatment approaches.

American Foundation for the Blind. Available at: www.afb.org. The American Foundation for the Blind provides a variety of services including policy development, publications, and services for people of all ages with visual impairments; provides resources, materials, educational devices and toys, and useful suggestions for parents and teachers.

American Printing House for the Blind. Available at: www.aph.org. This website is a source of publications and adapted educational equipment for children and adolescents who are visually impaired.

Assist the Development of Visually Impaired Students through Online Resources. Available at: www.e-advisor.us. Sponsored jointly by the Department of Ophthalmology at Boston Children's Hospital and Perkins School for the Blind, the ADVISOR project's website has separate tabs for parents, teachers of visually impaired young children, and physicians, with the goal of facilitating effective communication among these three groups. Resources for physicians aim to further understanding of vision and eye disorders. It is not intended to provide medical advice.

Blind Babies Foundation. Available at: http://blindbabies.typepad.com/resources/. This website provides excellent fact sheets summarizing major conditions of visual impairment in children.

National Association of Parents of Children with Visual Impairments (NAPVI). Available at: http://www.spedex.com/napvi/index.html. NAPVI is a nonprofit organization of, by, and for parents committed to providing support to the parents of children who have visual impairments. It has publications specific to children with visual impairment.

National Federation of the Blind. Available at: www.nfb.org/. The National Federation of the Blind is a membership organization of blind people in the United States. It has numerous publications for parents and professionals on blindness and visual impairment and includes a national parent organization.

Texas School for the Blind and Visually Impaired. Available at: http://www.tsbvi.edu. This is a comprehensive website with many instructive articles on topics related to visual impairment in children, medical and educational approaches, and glossaries of terms.

72 LANGUAGE AND SPEECH DISORDERS

Heidi M. Feldman and Cheryl Messick

Vignette

Travis was a handsome, social 26-month-old child. His speech and language skills lagged far behind those of his older sister when she was that age. His mother had discussed her concerns about Travis's language development on several occasions with his pediatrician. The pediatrician insisted that boys develop more slowly than girls, and besides his chatty sister spoke for him. Then, Travis began to tantrum in frustration if he was not understood. His mother learned from a neighbor that she could make her own referral to the publicly financed early intervention service program for evaluation.

The speech-language pathologist confirmed that Travis' expressive language skills were comparable to a child 14 months of age, although receptive skills and cognition were near age appropriate. His hearing was rechecked despite a normal screen at birth and was found to be adequate for speech perception. He was enrolled in a toddler communication group, 2 hours per session, two sessions per week, with a speech-language pathologist. Slowly, Travis began to increase his vocabulary and build grammatical skills. At 36 months of age, his vocabulary was greater than 250 words, and he was speaking in short phrases. At 48 months old, he had residual immaturities in speech sounds, but had caught up with peers in all other domains of communication. At age 7 years, his second grade teacher called his parents in for a conference because he still made some articulation errors and his reading skills were below age expectations.

DEFINITIONS

Language is the symbolic and systematic communication system through which humans share ideas, thoughts, emotions, and beliefs. Language is symbolic because meaning is conveyed through arbitrary sounds and words, which have no direct connection to their meanings. Language is systematic in that each language has its own distinctive rules, which govern the placement of sounds in words and words in sentences. Order cannot be altered without changing the meaning or violating a rule. Using arbitrary signs and combinatory rules, humans have the capacity to create and understand an infinite number of messages.

Speech refers specifically to oral or verbal output of language. Speech results from a complex interaction of the respiratory system, larynx, pharynx, mouth structures, and nose. Alternative outputs of the language system are sign language and written language.

Language is subdivided into components to facilitate description for clinical and research purposes. Receptive language refers to the ability to understand or comprehend words, sentences, discourse, and conversation. Expressive language refers to the ability to produce words, sentences, discourse, and conversation. Receptive and expressive language typically progress in relative synchrony, with receptive skills more advanced than their expressive counterparts in the early phases.

Language is subdivided further into components based on the size and function of the unit. Table 72-1 lists the terms used to describe components of language, their definitions, and examples. Comprehensive evaluations of language development require assessment of most of these components. Speech also can be conceptualized as having multiple features. Table 72-2 lists these features and their definitions. Evaluations of speech typically include assessments of many or all of these features.

NORMAL DEVELOPMENT

Newborns show the social and auditory building blocks for language development. At birth, they prefer to look at the human face over other visual stimuli and to listen to the human voice over other auditory stimuli. Infants show the ability to discriminate similar speech sounds (*/ba/*versus*/pa/*). They also can use the statistical properties of sound co-occurrences in continuous streams of

Table 72-1. Terms to Describe Components of Language

Term	Definition	Examples
Phoneme	Smallest unit of the sound system that can change meaning	/*p, b, i, a, t,* and *n*/ differentiate the meaning of *pit, bit, pat,* and *pan*
Phonology	Inventory of phonemes within a specific language and the rules for combining them	In English: /*st*/ and /*fr*/ can occur sequentially, /*sht*/ or /*bt*/ cannot
Morpheme	Smallest unit of meaning in a language, including words and word parts	Prefixes (*un-, dis-*), suffixes (*-ly, -ness*), grammatical markers (plural *-s,* past tense *-ed*), articles (*a, the*)
Lexicon (vocabulary)	Inventory of words	Early words: *mama, bye, more* Late words: adverbs
Syntax (grammar), also known as morphosyntax	Rules for combining words and morphemes	"*The cat is eating*" is a sentence (but "*cat the eating is*" is not)
Semantics	The meaning of words and sentences	Early meanings: *attribution* ("*big ball*"), *possession* ("*my ball*"), and *agent* + *action* + *object* ("*daddy throw ball*")
Pragmatics	Social aspects of language use that affect the effectiveness of communication	Intonation, politeness, appropriateness, turn-taking, and communicative functions

Table 72-2. Elements of Normal and Disordered Speech

Element	Definition
Speech sound inventory	Set of phonemes used by the speaker in total and as a function of placement within a syllable (initial versus final)
Articulation errors	Speech sound errors based on incorrect motor patterns (e.g., /*sh*/*for*/*s*/ in syllable initial and final positions)
Phonologic errors	Speech sound errors based on inappropriate use of language rules, such as reducing consonant clusters (*tick* for *stick* and *bum* for *broom*) and deleting the final consonants (*da* for *dog*)
Intelligibility	Understandability of speech, which can be measured as the percent of words understood by the listener
Stimulability	Ability to imitate a sound correctly in a hierarchy of increasing linguistic complexity (e.g., sound level /*s*/; syllable level /*sa*/, /*su*/; single syllable word *sit, see*; multisyllabic word *sucker, silly*; phrase *sit down, see it*)
Fluency	Flow of language. Dysfluency can be erratic pacing or stuttering
Voice and resonance	Vocal quality of speech sounds, including characteristics of hoarseness, breathiness, and hyponasality or hypernasality

speech to group syllables into wordlike units (Saffran et al, 1999). These nonspecific perceptual mechanisms assist children in parsing the continuous sound stream into recognizable chunks, an initial step in learning language.

The language in the verbal environment refines innate speech perception mechanisms. By the time they are about 9 months old, infants show greater precision in differentiating the phonemes of their native language than phonemes from other languages. American and Japanese infants younger than 6 months old are equally accurate at discriminating between /*r*/ and /*l*/. At 9 months of age, in contrast to American infants, Japanese infants no longer make the distinction because /*r*/ and /*l*/ are used interchangeably in Japanese (Kuhl, 2004). At approximately 9 months of age, infants learn to produce actions in response to verbal commands ("*wave bye-bye*").

Table 72-3. Stages in the Development of Speech Sounds in the First Year of Life

Stage (Age)	Type of Vocalization	Description
Stage 1 (birth to 1 mo)	Vegetative and reflexive vocalizations	Crying, fussing, coughing, and burping Normal phonation, limited resonance Vocalizations with closed or nearly closed small mouth
Stage 2 (2-3 mo)	Cooing	Sounds produced in the back of the mouth Primitive consonant-vowel syllables without timing of articulatory gestures for adult consonants
Stage 3 (4-6 mo)	Vocal play	Experimentation with sounds, including repetition of vowel-like elements Squeals, yells, raspberries, and clicks Adult-like vowels and consonant-vowel syllables without regular-syllable timing
Stage 4A (6-8 mo)	Canonical or reduplicated babbling	Strings of repeated true consonant-resonant vowel sequences (/*bababa*/, /*dididi*/)
Stage 4B (8-12 mo)	Variegated babbling	Large variety of consonants and vowels within a single utterance Sentence-like intonation (jargon)

They also begin to show emerging linguistic comprehension of common words such as *no, mama,* and *daddy.*

During the first year of life, infants learn to produce the sounds of their native language (Table 72-3) (Oller, 1980; Stark, 1980). During the first 6 months, infants learn how to control the mouth to produce vowels and some consonants, loudness, pitch, and intonation. During the second 6 months of life, infants learn how to produce chains of syllables and the intonation patterns of sentences. At the end of their first year, infants

Table 72-4. **Receptive Language Development: Average Age of Acquisition and Age Indicating Significant Delay or Red Flag**

Receptive Language Milestones	**Average Age of Acquisition**	**Significant Delays and Red Flags**
Alerts or quiets to sound	Birth to 1 mo	2 mo
Turns to the source of sound	Birth to 1 mo, then again 3-5 mo	6 mo
Responds to own name	6-8 mo	10 mo
Follows verbal routines/games ("*Wave bye-bye*")	8-10 mo	12 mo
Understands simple questions ("*Where's mommy?*")	9-11 mo	15 mo
Stops when told "*No*"	9-10 mo	15 mo
Understands at least 3 different words	10-13 mo	15 mo
Points to 3 different body parts	12-16 mo	18 mo
Follow simple commands ("*Show me the ball*" or "*Get your shoes*")	12 mo	18 mo
Follows 2-part commands ("*Get your shoes and give them to Dad*")	24 mo	30 mo
Answers simple questions ("*Who is that?*" or "*What are you doing?*")	24-30 mo	36 mo

Table 72-5. **Expressive Language Development: Average Age of Acquisition and Age Indicating Significant Delay or Red Flag**

Expressive Language Milestones	**Average Age Range**	**Significant Delays and Red Flags**
Cooing	2-3 mo	6 mo
Babbling	6-8 mo	10 mo
Nonverbal purposeful messages (requests with a reach; shows objects)	9-10 mo	12 mo
Pointing	10-11 mo	14 mo
Says 3 different spontaneous words	12-15 mo	16 mo
Vocabulary at least 35-50 words	18-22 mo	24 mo
Production of 2-word phrases ("*Mommy sock*"; "*No water*")	18-22 mo	24 mo
Simple sentences ("*I want juice*"; "*Where's my ball?*")	24-30 mo	36 mo
Intelligibility to unfamiliar adult at >50%	30-36 mo	42 mo
Able to tell about a past event with parent asking questions (personal narrative)	24-30 mo	36 mo
Able to tell or retell a familiar story	36-48 mo	54 mo
Fully intelligible to an unfamiliar adult (despite some immature sounds, such as consonant clusters or /r/ and /l/)	48-54 mo	60 mo
Fully mature speech sounds	Up to 72 mo	>72 mo

typically convey meaning with nonverbal methods, such as pointing, shrugging, nodding, and iconic gestures.

The process of language learning proceeds predictably in an orderly fashion in most children. At age 1 year, typically developing children are just beginning to understand and produce words of their language. During the first half of the second year, children learn a handful of words every month. In the second half of the year, they learn a handful of words every day. The rapid increase in vocabulary typically occurs the same time they begin stringing words together in two-word phrases (Fenson et al, 1994). By age 3 years, children produce simple complete sentences. By age 4 to 5 years, they have mastered the rules of language. They participate actively in conversations and construct narrative discourses. Although they may continue to have a few immaturities in speech sound production, their speech is nearly 100% intelligible to unfamiliar people.

Table 72-4 describes key developments in receptive language, the range of normal acquisition, and red flag signs that development is not typical or delayed, which should prompt an evaluation. Table 72-5 describes key developments for expressive language. The most important red flags are failure to acquire vocabulary beyond *ma-ma* and *da-da* by 15 months of age, failure to follow any commands by 18 months of age, failure to achieve a vocabulary of at least 35 to 50 words plus emergence of word combinations by 24 months of age, and failure to progress to four-word and five-word sentences by 36 months of age. Children exhibiting delays of this magnitude warrant a comprehensive speech-language assessment.

DEVELOPMENTAL VARIATIONS

The rate of language and speech development varies, even among children who ultimately exhibit normal skills. Many children build a vocabulary of object names (*ball, dog, shoe*) and progress from a clear one-word phase to a clear two-word phase ("*Mommy shoe*"). Other children first learn fixed social expressions ("*thank you,*" "*gimmedat,*" or "*whazat*"), using language to express needs or to interact with others. They may not go through a clear one-word and two-word phase. These early stylistic differences do not seem to predict major differences in later development (Bates et al, 1994).

Studies consistently document that girls are ahead of boys during the early stages of language development.

Differences in vocabulary size and grammatical complexity are minor, however, equivalent to about 1 to 2 months of developmental progress (Fenson et al, 1994). Because boys are more likely than girls to develop language disorders, a substantial delay in the early stages of language development for boys or girls warrants prompt evaluation, rather than watchful waiting.

Studies have found minor, stylistic differences in the language development of first-born and later born children. These differences are likely related to differences in the environments of children of different birth orders (Hoff-Ginsburg, 1998). Children usually find great utility in speaking for themselves, however, rather than letting an older sibling guess what they want.

Children in bilingual households often show language mixing in the early phases of language development. As they acquire more language skills, they begin to segregate the two languages into separate systems. Their developmental rate is not substantially delayed, however, if the accomplishments of the two languages are added together (Pearson et al, 1993). Substantial delay in bilingual children requires a comprehensive evaluation.

The rates of vocabulary and syntactic development are associated with the amount of child-directed language in the environment of the child. On average, parents in the lower socioeconomic strata provide less child-directed language than middle-class parents (Hart and Risley, 1995). As a group, children from the lower socioeconomic classes show slower language development, reduced vocabulary, and less developed syntax than children from middle-class families (Dollaghan et al, 1999). Improvements in the quality and quantity of environmental input can improve at least the short-term prognosis (Huttenlocher et al, 1998, 2002).

DEVELOPMENTAL DELAY

A child's communication may be considered delayed when it is noticeably behind age-matched peers. There is no consensus on the degree of delay that is clinically significant. For some purposes, the criterion for language delay is performance 1.5 to 2 standard deviations or greater below the population mean on standardized tests of speech or language. In some states, a developmental delay of at least 25% in one or more domains of functioning, calculated from the ratio of developmental age to chronologic age, renders the child eligible for early intervention services. Using this latter definition, a 24-month-old who is functioning at the level of a 17-month-old in at least one aspect of language development has a significant delay.

It is exceedingly difficult to predict which children who show initial delays are destined to develop language disorders. Approximately half of children delayed at 2 years of age catch up to peers by 3 years of age. Resolution of the delays has been weakly associated with good receptive language and mature symbolic play skills. For this reason, assessment of language in toddlers includes an evaluation of comprehension and play. Language is used for a variety of purposes, including expressing wants and needs, greeting others, describing objects or actions, and answering questions. If the range of communicative functions and social skills is restricted, the child is likely to have a language disorder. Finally, the more components of language affected and the greater the severity of deficit, the higher is the likelihood that the child will have long-term communication deficits.

EVALUATION PROCEDURES

Assessment procedures vary as a function of the age, cognitive level, and social characteristics of the children. In addition, the purpose of evaluation must be considered in the selection of assessment procedures.

Screening

Screening establishes whether asymptomatic children are at high risk for language or speech impairment. Screening procedures rely heavily on parent reports or interviews because direct assessment of children at young ages is time-consuming and not likely to produce representative samples of the child's capacities. The *Early Language Milestone (ELM)* test, a test that is used as a screening instrument in some pediatric practices, combines parent interview with direct observation. The *Pediatric Evaluation of Developmental Status* and the *Ages and Stages* questionnaires include speech and language items, and assess other domains using parent reports.

Diagnostic Testing

Diagnostic testing establishes the clinical status of the child in terms of multiple aspects of communication abilities and performance. In infants, toddlers, and young preschoolers, the purposes of assessment are identifying children with delays and disorders who could benefit from early intervention services, determining eligibility for early intervention services, designing intervention strategies and targets, monitoring the effectiveness of treatment, and educating parents about strategies for facilitating communication development. In older preschoolers and school-age children, the purpose of assessment is often to explain academic, social, or communication difficulties, and to identify children in need of therapeutic and support services. Children with reading and spelling problems may have underlying speech and language disorders. Children with behavior difficulties may have comprehension and pragmatic deficits, or slow and effortful expressive language contributing to the behavior disorders. Evaluations at these ages are used to establish the nature of intervention and specific target outcomes. As children get older, assessments are more likely to provide insights into the prognosis for future functioning. At all ages, language and speech assessments are prerequisites for monitoring progress.

Accurate assessment of infants and toddlers is challenging because of the low frequency of verbal output and the difficulty that young children have in cooperating with clinicians. Informal observations, parent interview tools, and natural assessments play an important role in the evaluation of young children. Formal assessments become more central to evaluation as the child reaches preschool age and beyond. The specific assessment protocol should be individualized and usually integrates more than one approach.

Observational and Interview Assessment Strategies

Table 72-6 summarizes observational and interview methods. Conversation sampling assesses functional communication in a naturalistic setting. Speech-language pathologists transcribe and analyze the conversation in real time or create audio or video tapes for detailed linguistic analysis. Advantages of this approach are that multiple components of language can be assessed concurrently, and that pragmatics and speech in connected discourse can be assessed. Parental language can be examined at the same time as child language, providing the clinician with insight into the quality of the language environment. Syntax and vocabulary diversity can be measured and compared with normative data. Observation is a good way to assess pragmatic behaviors (e.g., communicative functions, topic initiation, topic maintenance). Conversation sampling must be supplemented by other methods to have comprehensive and standardized measures across receptive and expressive language skills.

Parent report inventories and interviews circumvent some of the challenges of conversational analysis and have proven to be valuable tools, particularly for evaluating children in the birth through 36-month age range. They tap into a parent's extensive knowledge and frequent observations of his or her child's abilities. To improve reliability and validity, these tools ask about current abilities, rather than past skills or age of acquisition. Parent report inventories have been shown to have good to excellent reliability and concurrent validity in relation to direct assessments and analysis of conversational samples, although accuracy may vary by age and social class (Feldman et al, 2000). Predictive validity is only fair to good, usually because some delayed children catch up with peers during the preschool period.

Table 72-6. **Observational and Interview Assessment Strategies**

Strategy	Procedures and Specific Instruments
Language (conversation) samples	50-100 child utterances gathered during parent/clinician and child interaction
Parent-report inventories of lexicon	MacArthur-Bates Communicative Development Inventories (CDI): *Words and Gestures* (8-16 mo); *Words and Sentences* (16-30 mo); III (30-42 mo) (available at: http://www.brookespublishing.com/store/books/fenson-cdi/index.htm)
	Language Development Survey (LDS) (18-35 mo) (available at: http://www.aseba.org/research/language.html)
Parent interviews	Receptive-Expressive Emergent Language (REEL)
	Autism Diagnostic Interview (ADI)
Child observations	Communicative and Symbolic Behavior Scale
	Autism Diagnostic Observation Scale (ADOS)
	Symbolic Play Scale (Westby)

Direct child observation is another strategy of evaluation for young children. The *Communication and Symbolic Behavior Scales (CSBS)* and the *Autism Diagnostic Observation Schedule* combine parent interview with professional observations of the child's social and communicative behaviors under semistructured situations. They are valuable in the evaluation of children who may be along the autism spectrum.

Norm-Referenced Formal Measures

Norm-referenced measures require standardized procedures for administration and scoring, and generate age-adjusted standard scores. They allow comparison of an individual child with children of the same age. Norm-referenced tests are often used to qualify a child as eligible for early intervention services or other supports, such as Supplemental Security Income, and to compare the relative level of language skills in relation to other abilities, such as cognition or motor skills. Norm-referenced formal measures play an increasingly prominent role in the evaluation of children as they grow older and their skills become increasingly differentiated. Table 72-7 includes examples of norm-referenced measures. Receptive and expressive skills are usually evaluated in separate subtests, and the tests may generate subscale scores and a composite score. The pattern of subtest scores and the composite score is used to diagnose the nature of the child's communication problems and to determine eligibility for service and treatment plans.

In some situations, speech-language pathologists supplement comprehensive norm-referenced tests with measures of specific domains. This procedure can be used to test specific hypotheses about a child's functioning. The evaluator may decide to confirm the domains of language in which delays or disorders were identified by using a second specific measure. Such assessments include formal measures of preliteracy or literacy skills. Table 72-8 lists components of language and the measures that selectively assess them.

Criterion-Referenced Measures

Criterion-referenced tests measure what skills the child has mastered from either the set of skills in development sequence or from a curriculum used to treat children

Table 72-7. **Norm-Referenced Comprehensive Measures of Language and Speech**

Age Range	Specific Instruments
Birth to 3 yr	Assessing Prelinguistic and Early Linguistic Behaviors (ALB)
	Rosetti Infant Toddler Language Scale
	Reynell Developmental Language Scales III
Birth to 6 yr	Preschool Language Scale–4
Preschool	Test of Emergent Language Development (TELD-3)
	Clinical Evaluation of Language Fundamentals–Preschool (CELF-P)
School-age	Clinical Evaluation of Language Fundamentals (CELF-IV)
	Test of Language Development–Primary (TOLD-P)
	Test of Language Development–Intermediate (TOLD-I)

who are delayed in development. Criterion-referenced measures allow adjustment in the administration of items for children with sensory or motor impairments. Criterion-referenced measurement emphasizes the specific behaviors that have been mastered, rather than the relative standing of the child in reference to the group. They can be used to compare children with themselves, allowing longitudinal tracking of changes in development. That makes these measures useful for planning interventions and monitoring progress after treatment. Many federally funded early intervention programs use measures to determine if children qualify for services, to generate the objectives on the Individualized Family Service Plans (IFSP), and to monitor progress. Often criterion-referenced tests generate age equivalents or developmental quotients, rather than or in addition to scaled scores. Examples of criterion-referenced assessments are the *Hawaii Early Learning Profile* and the *Battelle Developmental Inventory, Second Edition.*

Table 72-8. **Norm-Referenced Assessment of Selective Language Components**

Domain	Specific Instruments
Receptive language	Peabody Picture Vocabulary Test (PPVT-3) Bracken Basic Concept Scale (Receptive and Expressive) Assessing Semantic Skills through Everyday Themes, Receptive subtest (ASSET) Test of Word Knowledge (Receptive subtests)
Expressive vocabulary	Expressive Vocabulary Test (EVT) Assessing Semantic Skills through Everyday Themes, Expressive subtest (ASSET) Test of Word Knowledge (Expressive Subtests)
Morphosyntax	Structured Photographic Expressive Language Test (SPELT) Test for Examining Expressive Morphology (TEEM)
Pragmatics	Test of Pragmatic Skills (Revised) Test of Pragmatic Language (TOPL)
Language comprehension	Test of Auditory Comprehension of Language (TACL-3) Token Test for Children Miller Yoder Language Comprehension Test
Word finding skills	Test of Word Finding Test of Word Finding in Discourse
Phonologic analysis/awareness	Children's Language Process Inventory (CLPI) Lindamood Auditory Conceptualization Test–Revised (LAC)

Assessment of Speech

Tests are available to assess speech sound development. These tests typically assess speech sound production in single words, but not in connected discourse, and overestimate the child's overall speech abilities and level of intelligibility for speech. Examples of such tests are the *Goldman-Fristoe Test of Articulation–2* and the *Photo Articulation Test.* Conversational analysis is a useful adjunct to identify children with a few selected articulation problems or to characterize the speech problems that emerge as words and sentences increase in length.

LANGUAGE DISORDERS

Causes

Table 72-9 summarizes the requirements for normal language development. First, children need to interact with responsive adults, ideally in an unstressed environment. Second, they must hear an ample corpus of language. Third, they must use cognitive and neural processes to derive meaning from sound and to learn the combinatorial rules for sounds, words, and sentences. Finally, they must be able to organize their pharynx, tongue, mouth, and breathing apparatus to produce speech quickly and accurately. Table 72-9 also provides examples of problems within the social environment, verbal environment, hearing apparatus, cognitive/neurologic system, and speech production mechanisms that lead to language delays and disorders. These conditions constitute the differential diagnosis of language and speech disorders. The main causes of language and speech delay are unresponsive social interaction and impoverished verbal input, hearing loss, cognitive impairment (which may occur in isolation or in the context of a neurologic or genetic condition), autism, and specific language impairment (SLI).

Table 72-9. **Causes of Delays and Disorders in Language and Speech as a Function of Fundamental Requirements**

Requirements	Social Interactions	Verbal Input	Hearing	Neural Processing	Speech Apparatus
Normal	Responsive	Adequate	Threshold <20 dB across frequencies	Intact neural pathways	Intact oral and respiratory mechanisms
Causes of delays and disorders	Unresponsive social interactions Psychosocial deprivation Child abuse and neglect Stressful environment	Impoverished verbal input	Hearing loss Auditory neuropathy Auditory processing disorder	Cognitive impairment Chromosomal or genetic disorder Neural injury Seizure disorders Autism Specific language impairment Dysarthria Childhood apraxia of speech	Cleft lip and cleft palate Velopharyngeal insufficiency Anatomic disorders of any structure within the speech system Oral motor dysfunction

Unresponsive Social Environment and Impoverished Language Environment

Children raised in orphanages with multiple caregivers and limited adult contact are likely to experience language and speech disorders, in addition to other developmental disorders and poor health. Language skills also are often delayed in children who have experienced child abuse and child neglect. In cases of less severe environmental deprivation, such as low socioeconomic status and poor verbal input, language skills are often delayed, particularly in the semantic and syntactic domains (Hart and Risley, 1995).

Hearing Loss

Normal conversation averages 40 to 60 dB in intensity and clusters in the range of 500 to 2000 Hz in frequency. Some speech sounds, such as vowels and the consonants /*m, n,* and *b*/, are relatively low frequencies and high intensity, rendering them easy to hear. Other sounds, such as the consonants /*s, f,* and *th*/, are high frequency and low intensity, rendering them more difficult to hear.

The degree of hearing loss and the range of frequencies affected determines the amount of speech readily perceived (see Chapter 70). In mild hearing loss, the quietest sound that a person can hear is 25 to 40 dB. At this degree of loss, some high-frequency speech sounds may be difficult to detect, especially in background noise, and other sounds may be distorted. In moderate hearing loss, the quietest sound that a person can hear is 40 to 60 or 70 dB, depending on the specific standards used. With this degree of hearing loss, many to all speech sounds in normal conversations would be difficult to detect. In severe hearing loss, the quietest sound that a person can hear is 70 to 90 dB, and in profound hearing loss, the quietest sound is greater than 90 dB. At these levels, almost all conversational language cannot be perceived without amplification.

Children with bilateral severe-to-profound sensorineural hearing loss generally have difficulty in comprehending and producing oral language. Their success at learning language depends on multiple factors, including the extent of the hearing loss, the age of receiving amplification for treatment, and the consistency of use of amplification. Currently, many children with sensorineural hearing loss have their loss detected in the newborn period as the result of Universal Newborn Hearing Screening. Data suggest that this public policy results in better outcomes in some domains for children with hearing loss than in the past, when losses were often not detected until language delays were identified, often when children were 2 to 3 years old (Kennedy et al, 2006). Children with bilateral severe-to-profound sensorineural hearing loss may be candidates for cochlear implantation, a prosthetic device that allows perception of the auditory signal. Cochlear implantation dramatically improves the prognosis for speech and language skills in children with profound hearing loss (Spencer et al, 2003).

Children with mild-to-moderate hearing loss have variable outcomes in terms of language. Some may show normal vocabulary, sentence comprehension, and achievement of literacy. Some may have difficulty with aspects of language and speech. Their success at phonologic discrimination and their phonologic memory are associated with their language skills. Children with mild-to-moderate sensorineural hearing loss may have a speech disorder, but not a language disorder (Briscoe et al, 2001). The sounds that are most vulnerable are sounds at high frequencies and low intensities.

Randomized clinical trials of tympanostomy tubes for persistent middle ear effusion have found that prompt tube insertion does not improve the outcomes for language or speech over watchful waiting, even though the tubes successfully reduced the number of days of effusion and presumably the associated intermittent conductive losses. These results suggest that otitis media with effusion does not cause language disorders. The associations of otitis media and unfavorable outcomes may be related to common underlying factors, such as low socioeconomic status, rather than to a causal relationship (Paradise et al, 2005).

Speech-language therapy is indicated for children with hearing loss associated with language or speech impairment. For children with severe-to-profound hearing loss, a debate rages about whether children should be receive Total Communication or Oral Education. Total Communication incorporates all types of modalities of communication to teach children with hearing impairments speech and language skills: sign language, oral speech, and tactile cues (using a hand symbol on the body to represent characteristics of a sound). The underlying concept is that multiple modalities result in overall improvement of communication skills. Oral Education focuses on oral speech and language skills with the emphasis on verbal input only, excluding the use of sign language, gestures, or any augmentative forms of communication. From an intervention point of view, it is important that families learn about the options available to their children with hearing impairments, and learn about all of the available community resources and make their decision based on the family's goals and desires.

Cognitive Impairment

Developmental delays in language learning are often the presenting complaint for children with mild-to-moderate overall cognitive impairment because language skills represent one of the early milestones in cognitive development. If cognitive impairment is severe and persistent, and if adaptive behaviors are affected, the diagnosis of intellectual disability may be appropriate.

Children with mild cognitive impairment typically show normal progression of speech and language skills at a slow developmental rate. Vocabulary and grammar are typically affected, although pragmatic skills may be preserved. Abstract language concepts may present severe challenges. Parents of children who function in the range of mild intellectual disability are more likely to have cognitive impairments than parents of children of normal intelligence, and may not provide stimulating verbal input, adding environmental factors to any genetic contributions to the language disorder. Early intervention services may improve the quality and quantity of language input to children with mild cognitive impairment or mild intellectual disability, either by directing services to the parents or to the children. In either case, the services tend to improve the children's skills.

Moderate, severe, and profound intellectual disability is often associated with a single biologic cause, such as genetic disorders, metabolic diseases, or neural malformation. The prognosis for language skills depends on the cause and is less favorable than for mild retardation. Social interactions with typically developing peers and speech-language therapy may improve functional communication, however. Treatment typically focuses on promoting communication skills in different environments (e.g., at home; at school) and on improving effectiveness of nonverbal communication for children with poor speech. Low-technology alternative or augmentative means may be incorporated to help improve communication. A child might be trained to hit a switch as a means of activating a tape recorder to offer a social greeting. This approach provides a method for teaching cause-effect relationships and for motivating communication.

Chromosomal and Genetic Causes of Cognitive Impairment

Some chromosomal and genetic conditions with associated cognitive impairment have distinctive behavioral phenotypes in terms of language. Children with Down syndrome typically show more significant impairments in speech and language development than would be predicted on the basis of the level of their cognitive abilities or receptive language skills. Grammatical skills are particularly weak. Children with Down syndrome also often have poor speech skills and dysfluency, rendering their speech unintelligible or difficult to understand. Early intervention for children with Down syndrome often incorporates Total Communication techniques. The goal of the treatment is to build communication skills, while preventing the frustrations and behavioral problems that sometimes result from the protracted period of poor verbal communication. As the children begin to acquire verbal language, their use of signs typically decreases.

Boys with fragile X syndrome learn to speak late. Their vocabulary and grammatical skills eventually seem to be consistent with their level of nonverbal intelligence. The rate and rhythm of their language is characterized by frequent rapid bursts and phonologic disorders, however, making them unintelligible to unfamiliar listeners. Boys with fragile X syndrome also exhibit echolalia, or repetition of words. The perseveration of the words or sounds at the end of sentences, can become so dramatic that they cannot complete sentences. These boys have poor pragmatic skills, associated with poor eye-to-eye gaze and heightened anxiety. Some boys talk incessantly or fail to maintain the topic of conversation.

Children with Williams syndrome show better expressive language skills than would be expected from their cognitive abilities. Children with Williams syndrome may be quite delayed initially in language abilities at a young age, indistinguishable from children with Down syndrome. As they develop, language and social skills develop at a faster rate than visuospatial skills. Fluent conversational abilities often mask difficulties in other domains of language, including grammatical knowledge and language comprehension.

Genetic causes of language disorders are assumed because of the high rates of disorders within some families, but the specific deficit is unknown. A large multigeneration family, called the KE family, has been identified in whom impairments in the ability to sequence verbal movements is inherited as an autosomal trait. In this case, genetic analysis determined that the affected members of this family have a point mutation on chromosome 7 in the *FOXP2* gene, a transcriptional factor, suggesting that the difficulties with speech and language in this family may result from other genetic or neurologic factors, rather than this mutation per se (Lai et al, 2001).

Autism

Autism is characterized by qualitative impairments of communication. Autism should be considered in the differential diagnosis for children with primary language delays or regression of skills in the language and social domains (see Chapter 69).

In the most severe cases of autism, children totally lack a means of communication, including verbal language, sign language, or gestures. They often use nonsymbolic communication, such as dragging a parent to a desired object and whining until the parent figures out what they want. Many children with autism eventually may learn some rudimentary language, but they do not engage in social interactions with others beyond making requests or demands. They lack the ability to establish a joint focus of attention. In moderately severe cases, children with autism may show limited vocabulary and grammar skills; poor pragmatic skills; and stereotyped, repetitive, or idiosyncratic uses of language. At the mild end of the spectrum, children may show an inability to initiate or sustain a conversation with others. Their ability to engage in conversational exchanges with peers and unfamiliar adults is constrained because they cannot maintain the topic of conversation. Poor communication further compromises their social interactions, limiting their ability to develop friendships with peers.

The prognosis for language and communication for children with autism is evolving as the definition of the disorder changes and intensive early intervention services become routine. In adults with autism who have become successful communicators, pragmatic skills typically remain underdeveloped. They have difficulty understanding humor or metaphor. They continue to have problems reading the social cues of their listener, modifying the topics of communication, and engaging in social interactions. Intonation remains flat or unchanging.

Neurologic Conditions

Distinctive patterns of language use have been associated with specific neurologic conditions. Hydrocephaly, the abnormal accumulation of the cerebrospinal fluid in isolation or in association with other disorders, such as myelomeningocele, is associated with what has been described as "cocktail party chatter." These children develop diverse vocabularies and appropriate syntax, but exhibit difficulties with semantics and pragmatics. Conversations are verbose and superficial, often consisting of repeated verbal routines. They struggle to understand the meaning of discourse, including figurative language, such as idioms, and may be weak at drawing inferences from facts. Some children with hydrocephalus have language-related academic difficulties, including difficulty with reading comprehension, despite average nonverbal intelligence.

Landau-Kleffner syndrome is a rare acquired seizure disorder that manifests with an abrupt disruption of receptive language functioning in a child who had previously displayed normal language development. The disorder has been called an acquired verbal agnosia, emphasizing the poor comprehension abilities of affected children. Imaging studies typically show no clear abnormality, and the abnormalities on electroencephalography vary. Although the prognosis for seizures is generally favorable, the long-term outcomes of cognition and language are highly variable.

Electric status epilepticus in slow wave sleep or continuous spike and wave in slow wave sleep is another rare acquired seizure disorder that affects cognitive and language functioning. Age of onset is typically 5 to 7 years. Atrophy and neural injuries on imaging studies of the brain are more likely than in Landau-Kleffner syndrome. Language abnormalities may be accompanied by memory disturbances and behavioral disorders of varying severity.

Children with severe traumatic brain injury are very likely to show persistent disorders in speech and language. The language and speech characteristics of children with traumatic brain injury vary substantially, based on multiple factors, including the severity, type, and location of injuries. The features of communication also evolve in the period after injury, associated with additional factors, such as the age of injury and the socioeconomic factors of the family. Among children with severe injury, residual deficits in speech are common (Campbell and Dollaghan, 1995).

Children with focal left hemisphere injuries may show less severe disturbances in language functioning than adults with comparable injuries. Their language and speech skills are only mildly delayed in development and only subtly different at older ages (Feldman et al, 1992). Functional imaging studies of children with congenital left hemisphere injury typically show that language processing occurs in the right hemisphere (Booth et al, 1999). These findings show the plasticity of the nervous system for language and speech when neurologic injury occurs in early childhood.

Specific Language Impairment

Specific language impairment (SLI), also known as developmental language disorder, refers to children with impairments in language skills despite normal intelligence, hearing, neurologic functioning, and oral mechanisms. Although a heterogeneous disorder, most children with SLI have greater difficulty with expressive skills than receptive skills. Morphology and syntax are the most vulnerable parts of the language system, although the precise grammatical structures that are most vulnerable vary across languages. Some affected children also have difficulty with the phonologic rules of language, resulting in decreased intelligibility of speech. Some children with SLI also have significant comprehension deficits resulting in pragmatic irregularities, in addition to grammatical deficits.

The prevalence of SLI among children in kindergarten was found to be 7.4% (Tomblin et al, 1997). Children with SLI also are at high risk for reading disorders, emphasizing that reading disorders are more related to language than to visual skills. Some children whose early delays in language and speech apparently resolve during the preschool years have reading disorders at school age, indicating that the initial delay was indicative of a fundamental, although subtle long-standing disorder.

The underlying processing mechanisms that give rise to SLI are incompletely understood. One major theory is that the language deficits are secondary to more fundamental auditory perceptual processes that affect nonlinguistic and linguistic stimuli. A related theory is that these children have difficulty in processing rapid or brief stimuli, whether in the auditory or other sensory systems (Tallal, 2004). The results of this processing issue would be most dramatic in speech because discriminations require perception of multiple and rapidly changing stimuli.

Electrophysiologic and functional neuroimaging studies of auditory perception in humans have suggested that two pathways arise from primary auditory cortex: a ventral stream, which is involved in mapping sound onto meaning, and a dorsal stream, which is involved in mapping sound onto articulatory-based representations. The ventral stream projects toward inferior posterior temporal cortex and ultimately links to widely distributed conceptual representations. The dorsal stream connects posteriorly via the inferior parietal lobe or Wernicke area and ultimately to the frontal lobes, including Broca area. Each pathway is sensitive to different characteristics of the signal and different modes of processing. Differences in the relative balance of information processing between them may explain some of the phenomena of SLI. Most children with SLI show gradual improvement over time, although language processing, reading, and writing remain areas of relative weakness as they age.

Management of Language Disorders

The treatment of language disorders are predicated primarily on the child's language profile and level of communication skill, regardless of etiology. In many cases, the first focus of management is to create an optimal language learning environment, capitalizing on the importance of environmental stimulation to the process of language learning. One component of therapy is to teach family members how to stimulate language development. Parents are coached to expand a child's utterances; if the child uses single-word utterances (*"ball"*), the parent can respond with a longer phrase (*"yes, a big ball"*). Parents might be taught to create opportunities for the child to communicate and to reinforce their child's communication attempts. They also may be taught to slow down their own rate of speech, use exaggerated stress and intonation patterns, and articulate their own language clearly.

Other foci of intervention address specific areas of deficit. The goal of treatment may be increasing the child's vocabulary, varying the sentence structure, or lengthening conversations. The techniques involve direct engagement with the child to facilitate learning. Focused stimulation is a technique in which the speech-language pathologist provides an intensive level of modeling a target behavior, on the assumption that a child with language delay needs a higher level of exposure to terms and grammatical structures to learn them. A child may be asked to show comprehension or to produce a target structure in appropriate contexts. Modeling and imitation are other useful strategies. Rules of grammar may be explained, then practiced using drill work to teach structures. Subsequently, the speech-language pathologist provides structured opportunities to use the structures frequently in conversational exchanges in the clinic and then in other environments (i.e., classroom, playground, and home). This strategy increases the likelihood that the child will generalize new abilities to everyday situations.

The outcome of therapy varies. Children with mild-to-moderate disorders are more likely to resolve their difficulties than children with severe disorders. Currently, there is little evidence of which treatment strategies are the most effective for which types of language disorders. Children who participate in speech-language treatment show better improvement than children who have no treatment. Additionally, children enrolled in early intervention services show stronger language skills and academic performance than children who did not receive early intervention.

SPEECH SOUND DISORDERS

A speech sound disorder represents impairment in the ability to produce the sounds of the words of the language. A primary symptom of speech impairment is often unintelligible speech. Speech disorders are described in terms of the characteristics of the speech sound errors or the cause of the problem. Speech disorders include problems with articulating sounds, using speech rules (phonologic rules), or planning and executing speech sounds (childhood apraxia of speech). Speech sound disorders also may include disorders in voice and resonance, or dysfluent speech.

Speech sound disorders may be the result of hearing loss; anatomic abnormalities, such as cleft palate or velopharyngeal insufficiency; or neuromotor disorders. In many cases, an underlying cause for the speech sound disorder cannot be identified. The term *functional articulation disorder* is reserved for children whose speech fails to mature at the rate of their age-matched peers for no apparent reason.

Articulation Disorders

The inability to produce sounds correctly in speech is referred to as an articulation disorder. Children with articulation disorders typically exhibit errors on a small subset of sounds (e.g., */r, l, s/*). In most cases, there is no known cause of an articulation disorder, and they are presumed to be the result of mis-learning. An articulation error may occur in all contexts (e.g., at the beginning, middle, or end of a word) or in a single position (e.g., at the end of a word). Children with articulation disorders typically have mild-to-moderate deficits in speech, and most of their speech may be intelligible to unfamiliar listeners despite the errors.

One known cause of articulation disorders is permanent bilateral mild-to-moderate hearing loss. Children with mild hearing loss may benefit considerably from amplification with hearing aids. They also may benefit from speech therapy to correct inaccurate speech sound productions. Children with severe-to-profound hearing losses have severe speech sound errors and language deficits, and show resonance difficulties characterized by hypernasal speech patterns.

Phonologic Disorders

When a child shows speech errors based on patterns or implicit rules, despite the ability to produce the same sounds correctly in other contexts, the problem is labeled a phonologic disorder. A child with this disorder says *"pi"* for *"pig,"* although he or she can say *"go,"* or *"tuh"* for *"tub,"* although he or she can pronounce *"bee."* These are examples of *final consonant deletion.* The child seems to be applying an incorrect rule (e.g., "it is permissible to drop the last sound of a word), rather than showing an inability to produce the sound correctly. When asked to imitate nonsense syllables (e.g., *"mib," "bup"*), the child does not use the rule and produces the syllable correctly. When asked to imitate real words (e.g., *"mob," "beep"*), the child applies the rule, and in this case drops the final consonant.

Most commonly, children continue to follow a rule that was age appropriate at an earlier time. In some situations, they produce errors atypical of normal development (e.g., *deletion of initial consonants*). Children with phonologic errors typically have moderate-to-severe deficits in speech skills, which have a significant impact on their overall intelligibility and communication effectiveness. Research has suggested that children with phonologic disorders need on average 21 to 42 sessions to advance from being understood by unfamiliar listeners less than 50% of the time to being understood 75% of the time (Campbell, 1999).

Anatomic Disorders

Children with cleft palate are at extremely high risk for phonologic disorders and language deficits. Even after early and appropriate repair of an isolated cleft palate, the children may exhibit unusual or idiosyncratic patterns of articulation. The main problem for these children is that the velopharyngeal structures function abnormally, resulting in an inability to generate adequate intraoral air pressure for the production of consonants. They may produce only consonants made in the back of the mouth (e.g., */k, g, u/*), or may use consonants that do not appear in the English language (e.g., pharyngeal fricatives and nasal snorts).

Some children have isolated velopharyngeal insufficiency for unknown reasons. These children are at risk for speech sound disorders similar to those of children with cleft palate. The velum is supported in early childhood by the adenoids. As the adenoids shrink with age, the speech disorder may become more severe. This speech problem is not amenable to the usual articulation therapy and may require surgical correction. Adenoidectomy might exacerbate speech problems in children with velopharyngeal insufficiency. For that reason, otolaryngologists should attempt to evaluate the velum before adenoidectomy.

Neurologic Disorders

Dysarthria is a speech disorder associated with neuromotor disorders or dysfunction. Children with cerebral palsy may present with dysarthria. High muscle tone, poor coordination of motor movements, and poor coordination of respiration and sound production result in slow muscular movements and limited range of motion. Dysarthric speech has a slurred and strained quality, affecting not only the accuracy of speech sound production, but also rate, pitch, and intonation. Speech therapy for such children can help them to slow the pace of speaking, improve respiratory control for phrase production, and improve the intelligibility of their output. For children whose speech intelligibility is severely compromised despite intact language skills, an assistive or augmentative communication device, such as a picture exchange system or a computer device, may improve their functional communication.

Childhood apraxia of speech, known alternatively as developmental verbal apraxia or dyspraxia, is a condition in which children have difficulty with the controlled production of speech sounds. The presumed etiology is neurologic in origin, although imaging studies do not find consistent anatomic lesions. Criteria for diagnosis vary among clinicians. The first symptoms of apraxia may be a lack of expressive vocabulary despite normal hearing, language comprehension skills, and social interaction skills. As expressive language emerges, speech may consist of primarily vowel sequences, with very few consonants produced, even in babbling. Affected children make errors in producing vowels and consonants, and show enormous variability in terms of phonemes, loudness, and related features. The inconsistency in their production makes interpretation of their speech very challenging. When they are able to produce a sound correctly in a single word (e.g., /m/ in *mom*), they may not be able to produce the same sound in other words, particularly longer words (e.g., *mama, moon, broom*).

In some children, apraxia of speech seems to be an isolated speech deficit. In other children, it is associated with cognitive, learning, motor, or social-emotional abnormalities.

Intensive levels of treatment are needed to help children with childhood apraxia of speech learn to produce sounds in syllables of increasing complexity. Research has suggested that children with apraxia needed on average 144 to 168 sessions to move from 50% of their speech being understood by unfamiliar listeners to 75% of their speech being understood, fivefold more sessions than needed for a phonologic disorder (Campbell, 1999). In the initial phases of treatment, each phoneme, in increasing levels of complexity, must be taught because the child may have no ability to generalize production of the sound in one syllable to varied syllables. Treatment integrates motor learning, strategies with multimodality input, and language enrichment. Many affected children have residual speech sound errors and exhibit difficulties in comprehension and narrative skills in school-age years.

Stuttering

Dysfluency is a disruption in the ongoing flow of speech. Children between 3 and 4 years old frequently show developmental dysfluency, often repeating whole words, phrases, or sentences. This dysfluency occurs as they try to put more complex meanings into longer sentences, while their proficiency in production remains limited. Fluency in a normal child improves at age 4, although many adults display continued bursts of dysfluency when trying to explain difficult material or speaking under stress.

Stuttering is the most common cause of significant dysfluency, manifested by repetition of sounds and syllables and prolongation of vowels or consonants made with a continuous airflow (e.g., /s, f/). Stuttering is often accompanied by inappropriate pauses, repetitive facial expressions, or other behavioral routines (i.e., arm jerks or knee slapping). Approximately 1% of people stutter. The degree of stuttering varies across individuals, ranging from a mild annoyance to a severe disruption of speech. The degree of stuttering also varies within individuals, subsiding in relaxed conversation and flaring on the telephone or during public speaking. Stuttering disorders may co-occur with speech sound disorders or language disorders or both. They also are common in children and adults with developmental disabilities owing to cognitive impairments.

The cause of stuttering is unknown. Some cases are associated with known neural injury, fueling the speculation that the disorder represents a neural timing disorder. Stuttering also is associated with anxiety, however, and it remains unclear which is the primary cause and which the effect. In most studies, individuals who stutter do not differ from control populations in terms of anatomy, physiology, or personality.

Speech therapy started at very young ages has been shown to improve stuttering. If stuttering is accompanied by behavior routines, treatment is indicated as soon as possible. In young children, treatment typically focuses on teaching family members to provide an environment to facilitate fluent speech behaviors. Total elimination of stuttering is not a realistic goal. Intervention focuses on teaching compensatory strategies, and becoming comfortable interacting and communicating in different environments despite the disability.

Voice and Resonance

Voice disorders are abnormalities in the production of vocal tone. They include abnormalities in the volume of the voice (inordinate loudness or softness) and abnormalities of the vibratory quality of the vocal cords (hoarseness, harshness or aphonia, the lack of sound). Voice depends on the vibratory characteristics of the vocal folds, setting the air above the level of the larynx into vibrations as well. The intonation and stress patterns of conversation and connected discourse require rapid changes in the delicate laryngeal musculature.

A common voice problem seen in children is due to stress on the laryngeal tissues from excessive screaming and shouting. Loudness can be generated without damage, as in the case of actors or opera singers. In young untrained children, the effect may be edema and inflammation of the vocal chords. Over the long-term, such vocal abuse can cause polyps, requiring surgical intervention. Referral of a child with a voice disorder to an otolaryngologist can determine the etiology of the disorder and the appropriate course of treatment. Voice therapy can re-educate children to vary their voice patterns to prevent these complications.

Management of Speech Sound Disorders

Speech therapy plays a key role in the management of speech sound disorders. Regardless of the nature of the disorder, speech therapy is particularly useful in helping affected children to identify and practice the mature patterns of speech.

Articulation therapy typically progresses from practice of target sounds or words in limited contexts to practice of larger units (phrases and sentences) in increasingly wider arrays of context. Treatment techniques include instructions on how to produce target consonants, modeling, imitation, and using sequential steps toward approximating accurate sound production. Phonologic disorders, in contrast, are treated by teaching the child that use of the target rule results in a difference in meaning. Activities pair words where the phonologic process such as *final consonant deletion* results in different meanings (*bee* versus *bead* and *cake* versus *cape*).

The goal is always improvements in functional communication. In some cases, if extensive speech treatment and focused practice does not improve the speech sound disorder, individuals may learn strategies to bypass their problem areas. Children and adults with speech disorders often experience embarrassment and poor self-esteem. Therapy is designed to reduce the negative psychological consequences of the disorder and direct remediation.

SUMMARY

Language and speech are important developmental skills. Most children acquire mastery of language by age 5 years and speech by age 7 years without specific instruction. Delays at age 2 years represent a significant risk factor for speech and/or language disorders, but prediction of which children will progress normally is difficult. Language and speech sound disorders are prevalent in children, and can adversely affect other domains of functioning, including learning, communication, and social relationships, and response to therapy.

A child such as Travis in the vignette at the beginning of this chapter, who shows early delays, warrants a prompt assessment. The fact that he is a second-born male child is not adequate explanation for the degree of delays. Proper diagnosis of the language and speech disorder entails formal and informal assessments of multiple domains of communication, and evaluation of play and receptive language. Speech and language disorders are generally caused by unresponsive social interactions or inadequate verbal input, hearing loss, cognitive and neurologic disorders including autism, specific language impairment, and anatomic disruptions. Table 72-10 provides an approach to the assessment of a child with language and speech delays based on this differential diagnosis. The assessment evaluates cognition, social skills, family history, physical examination, and neurologic examination. A team approach is ideal.

Table 72-10. Evaluation of a Preschool Child with Delayed Language or Speech

Evaluation	Proposed Evaluator(s)	Areas and Techniques of Assessment	Follow-up of Abnormal Findings
Hearing	Audiologist for children <4 yr Physician, SLP, or school nurse conducts hearing screening for children >4 yr	Do not rely on newborn screen OAE and ABR for infants Visual reinforcement, conditioned play, or conventional audiometry for children >1 yr	Audiologist for amplification Genetic evaluation for cause ENT evaluation for structural abnormalities or evaluation for cochlear implants
Developmental status	Primary care clinician Early intervention Psychologist Developmental-behavioral pediatrician	Social skills Cognition/problem-solving/play skills Adaptive skills	Early intervention, special education, and occupational therapy, as indicated
Medical and neurologic issues	Primary care clinician Developmental-behavioral pediatrician Child neurologist Geneticist	Family history General health Growth parameters Dysmorphic features Skin Neurologic examination	Subspecialty follow-up, as indicated Laboratory and neuroimaging evaluations, as indicated
Psychosocial conditions—quality of social interaction; amount of verbal input	All evaluators Social workers	Quality and quantity of verbal input Quality of social interactions, including warmth, responsivity, reciprocity, and safety	Education about importance of verbal input Parent-to-parent support Social service, as indicated Child Protective Services, as indicated

ABR, auditory brainstem response; ENT, ear, nose, and throat; OAE, otoacoustic emission; SLP, speech-language pathologist.

Therapy and other management strategies are predicated primarily on the level of functioning across domains and occasionally based on the specific diagnosis. Intensive early treatment provides children with the best opportunities for normalization of language and speech. A child such as Travis in the vignette should be enrolled in a treatment program. Close monitoring of functional improvement is necessary to refine management strategies, combat poor self-esteem, and provide alternative communication strategies if verbal language would be impossible. Ongoing monitoring can detect complications early on and early problems, such as academic difficulties, that also must be evaluated and managed. Neuroscience and genetics are contributing to the understanding of normal speech and language development and disorders. The future may bring new assessment procedures or treatment approaches.

REFERENCES

Bates E, Marchman V, Thal D, et al: Developmental and stylistic variation in the composition of early vocabulary. J Child Lang 21:85-123, 1994.

Booth JR, Macwhinney B, Thulborn KR, et al: Functional organization of activation patterns in children: Whole brain fMRI imaging during three different cognitive tasks. Prog Neuropsychopharmacol Biol Psychiatry 23:669-682, 1999.

Briscoe J, Bishop DV, Norbury CF: Phonological processing, language, and literacy: A comparison of children with mild-to-moderate sensorineural hearing loss and those with specific language impairment. J Child Psychol Psychiatry Allied Discipl 42:329-340, 2001.

Campbell TF: Functional treatment outcomes in young children with motor speech disorders. *In* Caruso AJ, Strand EA (eds): Clinical Management of Motor Speech Disorders in Children. New York, Thieme, pp 385-396.

Campbell TF, Dollaghan CA: Speaking rate, articulatory speed, and linguistic processing in children and adolescents with severe traumatic brain injury. J Speech Hear Res 38:864-875, 1995.

Dollaghan CA, Campbell TF, Paradise JL, et al: Maternal education and measures of early speech and language. J Speech Lang Hear Res 42:1432-1443, 1999.

Feldman HM, Dollaghan CA, Campbell TF, et al: Measurement properties of the Macarthur communicative development inventories at ages one and two years. Child Dev 71:310-322, 2000.

Feldman HM, Holland AL, Kemp SS, Janosky JE: Language development after unilateral brain injury. Brain Lang 42:89-102, 1992.

Fenson L, Dale PS, Reznick JS, et al: Variability in early communicative development. Monogr Soc Res Child Dev 59:1-173; discussion 174-185, 1994.

Hart B, Risley TR: Meaningful Differences in the Everyday. Baltimore, Paul H. Brookes, 1995.

Hoff-Ginsburg E: The relation of birth order and socioeconomic status to children's language experience and language development. Appl Psycholing 19:603-629, 1998.

Huttenlocher J, Levine S, Vevea J: Environmental input and cognitive growth: A study using time-period comparisons. Child Dev 69:1012-1029, 1998.

Huttenlocher J, Vasilyeva M, Cymerman E, Levine S: Language input and child syntax. Cogn Psychol 45:337-374, 2002.

Kennedy CR, McCann DC, Campbell MJ, et al: Language ability after early detection of permanent childhood hearing impairment. N Engl J Med 354:2131-2141, 2006.

Kuhl PK: Early language acquisition: Cracking the speech code. Nat Rev Neurosci 5:831-843, 2004.

Lai CS, Fisher SE, Hurst JA, et al: A forkhead-domain gene is mutated in a severe speech and language disorder. Nature 413:519-523, 2001.

Oller DK: The emergence of the sounds of speech in infancy. *In* Yeni-Komshian G, Kavanaugh J, Ferguson C (eds): Child Phonology: Volume 1. Production. New York, Academic Press, 1980, pp 93-112.

Paradise JL, Campbell TF, Dollaghan CA, et al: Developmental outcomes after early or delayed insertion of tympanostomy tubes. N Engl J Med 353:576-586, 2005.

Pearson BZ, Fernandez SC, Oller DK: Lexical development in bilingual infants and toddlers: Comparison to monolingual norms. Lang Learn 43:93-120, 1993.

Saffran JR, Johnson EK, Aslin RN, Newport EL: Statistical learning of tone sequences by human infants and adults. Cognition 70: 27-52, 1999.

Spencer LJ, Barker BA, Tomblin JB: Exploring the language and literacy outcomes of pediatric cochlear implant users. Ear Hear 24:236-247, 2003.

Stark RE: Stages of speech development in the first year of life. *In* Yeni-Komshian G, Kavanaugh J, Ferguson C (eds): Child Phonology: Volume 1. Production. New York, Academic Press, 1980, pp 73-90.

Tallal P: Improving language and literacy is a matter of time. Nat Rev Neurosci 5:721-728, 2004.

Tomblin JB, Records NL, Buckwalter P, et al: Prevalence of specific language impairment in kindergarten children. J Speech Lang Hear Res 40:1245-1260, 1997.

73 OTHER SENSORY PROBLEMS

Jane Case-Smith and Karen Ratliff-Schaub

Sensory processing disorders (SPDs), sometimes termed *sensory integration disorders,* can be present in children with autism, learning disabilities, developmental coordination disorder, or other diagnoses. This chapter describes children whose primary diagnosis is SPD, referring predominantly to children with problems in somatosensory and vestibular system processing and integration. Children with SPD also may have secondary problems in visual perception, auditory processing, or olfactory/gustatory system processing without impairment of hearing or visual acuity. Because SPDs cannot be directly observed, they are identified through atypical behavioral patterns (e.g., irritability or aggressiveness) or deficit performance (e.g., clumsiness).

Examples of behaviors that characterize SPD include extreme aversion to touch, smells, tastes, or sounds that are acceptable to others, or expressed fear of movement, touch, or sounds that typify everyday life. Performance problems that may indicate this diagnosis are poor motor planning, poor coordination, or immature balance reactions without evidence of frank central nervous system impairment. This chapter focuses on children whose difficulty with sensory processing causes behavioral or performance problems that limit or disrupt participation in everyday life activities or school performance.

TYPES OF SENSORY PROCESSING DISORDERS

Sensory processing problems can be categorized into two groups: (1) sensory-based motor disorders and (2) sensory modulation disorders (SMDs) (Schaaf and Miller, 2005). The categories can describe SPD in children with a specific diagnosis (e.g., children with autism often have sensory modulation problems, and children with learning disabilities may have sensory-based motor problems); however, each category can describe a child whose primary problem is sensory processing. One estimate of the prevalence of SPDs suggests that they are present in 5% of all children (Ahn et al, 2004) with a high proportion of boys (i.e., 70%) (Mulligan, 2000). Because SPD is conceptualized as a continuum from severe (i.e., causing serious behavioral or performance dysfunction) to mild (i.e., causing behavioral quirks or minor difficulty in everyday life), published estimates should be viewed with caution. In addition, many of these children are not diagnosed, further clouding an understanding of prevalence. Sensory-based motor disorders and SMDs are described with examples in the following sections.

SENSORY-BASED MOTOR DISORDERS

Sensory-based motor disorders can be categorized as (1) vestibular-based postural disorders (children with balance and postural deficits) and (2) dyspraxia (children with motor planning problems). Both groups of children may exhibit discrimination deficits in perception of vestibular, proprioceptive, and tactile input such that feedback from movement and touch is less accurately interpreted. With limited perception of somatosensory feedback, manipulating objects or moving through the environment becomes slower and less precise. Sensory memories of movements are less reliable when the same or similar task is presented to the child, slowing development of skill. In vestibular-based postural disorders, children show balance problems and postural instability. They often exhibit bilateral coordination delays and ocular motor deficits. In dyspraxia, children exhibit motor planning problems with delays in skillful movement and learning of multistep complex movements.

Vestibular-Based Postural Disorder

A child with vestibular-based postural disorder tends to have poor awareness of where his or her body is in space. The child exhibits delayed or deficit balance when asked to perform a dynamic balancing task (e.g., walking heel to toe or walking on a line). The following vignette provides an example of this problem. When testing balance by standing on one foot or by walking on an unstable surface, performance is markedly poorer with eyes closed compared with eyes open. With immature balance mechanisms, the child's movements appear awkward or rigid. The child may stiffen or lock legs and spine to balance rather than move smoothly in and out of positions using trunk rotation. Reciprocal and coordinated movements of arms and legs may be delayed or impaired (e.g., a 6-year-old child cannot perform jumping jacks or a hop-skip-jump sequence). The child may be fearful on unstable surfaces or high surfaces (e.g., the child clings to the rail and proceeds slowly when descending the stairs). The child is slow to register when his or her balance is challenged and often overuses the visual system to compensate for lack of specific information from the vestibular-proprioceptive systems.

Vignette

Thom, 8 years old, reportedly does well academically and is a "sweet kid." Although a good student, Thom's mother explains that he is clumsy and sometimes trips or falls for no reason. He did not learn to ride a bike until this year. He cannot sequence a hop, skip, and jump, and is poor at catching a ball. Thom compensates for his poor body awareness by moving slowly and cautiously on stairs and unstable surfaces. Movements that others make automatically seem to require greater conscious effort and planning. Although Thom does well in school, his parents worry about his self-esteem and wish he could participate more in sports and the active play of his peers. On examination, Thom has poor posture, low trunk extension tone, and poor postural stability, as evidenced by his slightly kyphotic posture. He has no evidence of central nervous system impairment.

Dyspraxia

Children with dyspraxia or motor planning problems generally have concurrent deficits in somatosensory discrimination. Poor tactile discrimination has been associated with delays in development of fine motor skill (Case-Smith, 2001) and with dyspraxia (Ayres, 1977). A child with dyspraxia has difficulty recognizing shapes or textures by touch and manipulation alone and seems to receive less accurate feedback from fine movements. The child generally has normal intelligence and achieves motor milestones at typical ages; however, skilled manipulation and complex multistep movements are limited, and achievement of activities of daily living, such as dressing, buttoning, and shoe tying, is delayed. Teachers note that the child's drawing, and writing are immature.

Children with dyspraxia take more time and require more practice to learn new motor skills; they may require compensatory methods (e.g., use their eyes or "self talk" to guide their movements). These children are often reticent to try new tasks or look perplexed when presented with a multistep motor task. They are vulnerable to poor self-esteem because they struggle in learning new skills, and show poor ability in sports, motor-based games, drawing, and writing. Because they do not receive precise feedback from movement and touch, they often have less confidence and diminished body awareness. As school tasks become increasingly demanding, these children may be unable to keep up with the amount of work required, resulting in poor academic performance and possible loss of motivation and less self-esteem (Levine, 1984, 1987). Children with dyspraxia have been shown to be more introverted and to have few social interactions in environments where motor skill is the focus of interaction (e.g., on the playground) (Smyth and Anderson, 2000). Table 73-1 lists secondary issues associated with sensory-based motor disorders.

SENSORY MODULATION DISORDER

Sensory modulation refers to the ability to regulate the degree, intensity, and nature of responses to sensory input. This basic physiologic ability allows individuals to respond appropriately and adaptively to the sensory experiences of everyday life. Ability to modulate falls on a continuum of overresponsiveness (hypersensitivity) to underresponsiveness (hyposensitivity), with most individuals functioning in a midrange. In children with SMD, their sensitivity is beyond the normal range such that they have difficulty adapting to the sensations of everyday activities. Most children with SMD are overreactive or underreactive (or both) to more than one sensory modality (e.g., tactile, smells, sounds, and touch). Universally, these children have difficulty modulating, organizing, or making meaning of sensory input. As a result, sensory input, which typically produces pleasure in children, is aversive, uncomfortable, and even painful to these children. The following vignette presents an example of a child with SMD.

Table 73-1. Characteristics Associated with Sensory-Based Motor Disorders

Primary Problem	Performance Consequence	Secondary Issues
Vestibular-postural disorder	Poor balance Low or low normal muscle tone Mild-to-moderate postural instability Primitive equilibrium responses May exhibit delayed oculomotor control (related to vestibular system influence on ocular movements)	May be frightened on unstable surfaces or seek a low level (grounded) posture when on an unstable surface May exhibit delays in bilateral coordination (related to lack of body rotation and use of hands in contralateral body space) May show delays in visuomotor skills
Dyspraxia	Poor motor planning when presented with a novel task Decreased bilateral coordination and sequenced actions Delays in activities of daily living Poor handwriting Difficulty conceiving complex motor actions Difficulty planning and performing projected action sequence	Resistance to attempting novel tasks Poor skills in ball play, jumping rope, other sports or games Poor self-esteem Difficulty in writing assignments and tests—grades suffer because of poor handwriting Parents are frustrated, and may not understand child's poor performance Lack of acceptance by peers

Vignette

Mornings tend to be stressful for the Towson family because 4-year-old Bethany's sensory modulation problems insert chaos into their everyday routine. Although she is often the first to awaken, getting dressed tends to be a battle because Bethany prefers to stay in her soft nightgown and refuses to don her preschool clothes, which feel "scratchy." Despite her mother using softeners to make new clothes more acceptable to her, Bethany has a dresser full of clothes that she refuses to wear. She does not wear socks with seams; clothes that are stiff, textured, or rough; or shirts with tags. She refuses to wear clothes washed in "smelly" (fragrant) detergent. Breakfast also is a struggle because Bethany rejects the foods that the other family members enjoy. She prefers totally bland and soft foods, stating that other foods "do not feel right" or "smell yucky." Although Bethany's parents do their best to accommodate her pickiness, she often arrives late at school, hungry and wearing her outfit from the previous day.

Overresponsiveness is generally heightened when the child is tired, when the input is unexpected, or when stimulation is repeated. Children with SMD who are overreactive may show difficulty with common everyday experiences, such as riding in a car, shopping in a crowd, eating food with a variety of textures, standing in a line where they are lightly touched by others, or brushing their teeth. Dunn (2001) characterized these children as overaroused. The overaroused child tends to become quickly disorganized and anxious, and has difficulty calming and reorganizing when overaroused. Common behaviors include flight responses (e.g., running without a specific destination), aggressive responses (e.g., biting or hitting a peer or parent), emotional responses (e.g., a temper tantrum or crying), or complete shutdown (e.g., a child may cope with overstimulation by falling asleep). Because the hypersensitive child is motivated to avoid sensory input, he or she may resist activity transitions, have a temper tantrum in the grocery store, refuse to dress or brush his or her teeth, or refuse to eat certain foods. Opportunities for the child to remove himself or herself from the overstimulating environment or tasks may help the child calm and reorganize.

Children who are underaroused need more intense sensory stimulation to show an adaptive response. They may appear either (1) lethargic and unresponsive or (2) hyperactive and sensory seeking. The lethargic and unresponsive child is passive and sedentary. This child lacks alertness and attentiveness, is difficult to engage, and needs intensive support to participate in activities (Parham and Mailloux, 2005). Sensory-seeking children are very active and crave intensive sensory experiences to maintain arousal. These children may run into others, stomp instead of walk, chew on inedible objects, or risk fast movement. Behaviors that indicate a child who is sensory seeking include purposely falling or bumping into others, intense wrestling and tumbling play, or constant rocking movements. The behaviors of sensory-seeking children can be disruptive or inappropriate in social situations. In extreme cases, safety is a concern. One objective of intervention is to identify strategies that meet the child's need for sensory input through socially acceptable and safe activities.

Children with SMD have been shown to have a different pattern of physiologic response to sensory input. McIntosh and colleagues (1999) found that children with SMD exhibited heightened and sustained galvanic skin response to a sensory stimulation challenge. Specifically, their electrodermic reactivity showed higher magnitude of response to tactile and visual inputs. This physiologic response was shown to correspond to children's behavioral overreactivity to sensation. Secondary issues arise for these children because of their atypical behavioral response to sensory input. When touch and movement are aversive for the child, typical peer interactions and play may be difficult to establish. Their temper tantrums or aggressive behaviors may inhibit further positive relationships with peers. Parents also may misinterpret the child's hyperactivity, irritability, or resistance to specific activities or environments. With limited positive social interactions, the child's social-emotional development is at risk (Table 73-2).

ASSESSMENT

Evidence that SPD is a causative factor in a child's performance or behavior problems can be extracted from a detailed history and parent interview. Referral to an occupational therapist for standardized testing can confirm the diagnosis.

History

The parent's history of the child's birth and developmental milestones may reveal an unremarkable birth and typical achievement of motor milestones in the first years of life. The parents of children with SMD often describe them as difficult, irritable, and anxious infants. They describe an infant with persistent sleeping and eating problems. As toddlers and preschoolers, the parents frequently describe a defiant, irritable, stubborn or rigid child who does not tolerate certain activities or environments and resists transitions. Sleeping and eating problems may continue into the preschool years. By asking about antecedent factors to specific instances of sleeping or eating problems, patterns emerge suggesting that the child's behaviors are associated with specific sensory experiences. Parents of children with SMD often describe a passive child who seems reluctant to try new activities and who struggles to learn new skills.

The interview also may reveal an association between sensory experiences and reluctance to participate, avoidance, or noncompliance. Infants who originally were resistive to touch or refused certain food textures often become less sensitive as they mature; however, they may maintain the negative and defiant behaviors when these are reinforced by adult attention or parents' emotional responses. The interview may reveal that sensory processing problems in infants become behavioral problems in preschoolers that are self-sustaining because they create multiple layers of reactions from others.

Table 73-2. Primary and Secondary Issues in Sensory Modulation Disorder

Primary Problem	Behavioral Consequence	Secondary Issues
Tactile hypersensitivity	Avoidance of or unusual preference for certain textures of clothing Appears uncomfortable with sudden touch Appears aversive to daily living tasks such as bathing, dressing, tooth brushing Responds with inappropriate aggression to light touch or being close to people	May prefer solitary play Delayed in establishing peer relationships or support is needed to establish peer relationships Experiences stress, anxiety in daily routines Mealtime is stressful; child has limited diet and may have poor weight gain
Vestibular hypersensitivity	Aversive response to movement, being on an unstable surface Expressed fear of everyday experiences that involve movement, particularly head movement Small movements are perceived as greater than they are Movement within a vehicle (e.g., riding in a car) may cause strong feelings of discomfort, nausea, and dizziness	May not trust the environment, may be extraordinarily anxious in a new environment or one where the walking surface is unstable Reluctant to explore environment Is passive and sedentary Seems to have a poor sense of where his or her body is in space and so may bump into objects Is clumsy
Taste or smell hypersensitivity (generally seen when other hypersensitivities are present)	Avoids certain tastes or smells Overly responsive to common tastes or smells by refusing to eat, throwing a temper tantrum, vomiting	Pickiness creates frustration at mealtime Food refusal can become a battle ground between parent and child When extreme, may be associated with failure to thrive

Table 73-3. Interview Questions to Screen for Sensory Processing Problems

System	Questions
Auditory	1. Does your child have trouble understanding what other people mean when they say something? 2. Is your child bothered by any household or ordinary sounds, such as the vacuum, hair dryer, or toilet flushing? 3. Does your child respond negatively to loud noises, as in running away, crying, or holding hands over ears? 4. Is your child distracted by sounds not usually noticed by other people? 5. Does your child seem overly sensitive to sounds?
Gustatory/olfactory	6. Does your child gag, vomit, or complain of nausea when smelling odors such as soap, perfume, or cleaning products? 7. Does your child like to taste nonfood items such as glue or paint? 8. Does your child gag when presented with certain foods?
Proprioception	9. Does your child sometimes grasp objects so tightly that they break? 10. Does your child grind his or her teeth? 11. Does your child seem driven to seek activities such as pushing, pulling, dragging, lifting, and jumping? 12. Does your child seem to exert too much pressure for a task, such as slamming doors or pressing too hard when using pencils or crayons? 13. Does your child have difficulty positioning himself or herself in a chair? 14. Does your child bump or push other children?
Tactile	15. Does your child pull away from being touched lightly? 16. Does your child seem to lack the normal awareness of being touched? 17. Does your child react negatively to the feel of new clothes? 18. Does your child show an unusual dislike for having his or her hair combed, brushed, or styled? 19. Does it bother your child to have his or her face touched or washed? 20. Does your child avoid foods of certain textures?
Vestibular	21. Is your child excessively fearful of movement, such as going up and down stairs, or riding swings, slides, or other playground equipment? 22. Does your child exhibit distress when he or she is riding on moving equipment? 23. Does your child have poor balance? 24. Does your child spin and whirl his or her body more than other children? 25. Does you child rock himself or herself when stressed?

Adapted from Parham LD, Ecker C: Clinical observations of neuromotor performance, evaluation of sensory processing and touch inventory for elementary school children. *In* Bundy A, Lane S, Murray E (eds): Sensory Integration Therapy and Practice. Philadelphia, FA Davis, 2002, Appendix 7-IE.

A detailed history can identify problems in sensory processing. Table 73-3 lists potential interview questions.

Examination

An in-depth examination and extensive observations are required to analyze sensory processing problems. Referral to an occupational therapist, particularly one trained in administering the *Sensory Integration and Praxis Tests* (Ayres, 1989), is optimal for comprehensive evaluation and intervention. Table 73-4 lists standardized assessments administered by therapists that are helpful in confirming this diagnosis and developing an intervention plan. The examination can include assessment of neurologic soft signs to screen for possible SPD. Table 73-4 also lists clinical observations and neurologic soft signs associated with each SPD.

Table 73-4. **Evaluations to Identify and Analyze Sensory Processing Problems**

Type of Instrument	Diagnostic Tests/Scales	Type of Sensory Processing Disorder Evaluated
Observation	*Sensory Integration and Practice Tests (SIPT)* (Ayres, 1989) *Bruininks Oseretsky Test of Motor Proficiency (2nd ed) (BOT-2)* (Bruininks and Bruininks, 2006) *Motor Assessment Battery for Children (MABC)* (Henderson and Sudgen, 1992)	Sensory-based motor disorder Dyspraxia Vestibular-based postural disorder
Parent or caregiver report	*Sensory Profile* (Dunn, 1999) *Evaluation of Sensory Processing* (Parham et al, 2006)	Sensory modulation disorder
Teacher report	*Sensory Processing Measure Main Classroom Form* (Miller-Kuhaneck et al, 2006)	Sensory modulation disorder
Screening methods: soft neurologic signs	Walking and running gait Skipping, hopping Standing on 1 foot Stressed walking (on toes, heels, inner and outer aspects of feet—observing upper extremity posturing) Right-left determination (ability to discriminate right from left on self and examiner) Hand, foot, eye dominance Synkinesia (abnormal mirror movements/ overflow of finger movements) Diadochokinesia (ability to perform rapid alternating movements, such as rapid pronation/supination)	Sensory-based motor disorders Dyspraxia Vestibular-based postural disorder

INTERVENTION

Occupational therapists are the primary professionals to provide services to children with SPD; referral to speech pathology or physical therapy services may be appropriate. Services are directed to the child, the family, and other adults who teach or care for the child. A priority goal of intervention is to promote the child's integration of sensation and ability to show adaptive and organized responses to sensory input (Ayres, 2005). Equally important goals are to help the child learn to compensate for SPD, to help parents understand and reframe the problem, and to modify the child's environments and routines to improve goodness-of-fit. The intervention plan should consider the child's multiple environments (e.g., home and school), and should emphasize caregivers' understanding of the problem such that they learn to accommodate the child's sensory needs. Optimal timing for sensory integration intervention is 2 through 7 years of age (generally SPD is not identified before age 2 years). Children may receive services beyond 7 years if more involved, identified at an older age, or according to the family's preference.

Children with significant SPD may receive occupational therapy services at school and in a clinic. Generally, these services complement each other; the school-based occupational therapist helps the teachers and aides accommodate to the child's sensory needs and recommends modifications to the classroom environment and routines. The clinic-based occupational therapist has opportunities to work directly with the child and family to improve performance and behaviors through one-on-one sensory integration treatment. Services should emphasize the family's education about the disorder and should teach parents strategies that help the child improve arousal, alertness, attentiveness, and performance (Bundy and Koomar, 2001).

One typical recommendation to family members is to provide a "sensory diet" to the child. This diet helps the child's arousal and organization throughout the day and generally includes activities that provide deep pressure, heavy work, linear vestibular input, and sometimes rhythmic movement such as bouncing. The goals of these activities are to increase arousal, calm, help organize, increase attentiveness, improve alertness, and decrease activity level (Koomar and Bundy, 2002). Sources of sensory stimulation believed to help children better modulate sensory input include filtered (modulated) music through head phones, weighted vests, therapy balls, deep pressure, and massage. Sensory diets should be closely monitored and modified over time; they should fit easily into the family's daily routine.

Table 73-5 lists the principles of sensory integration intervention. Sensory integration intervention includes activities that directly promote skill building (e.g., practice of balance, visuomotor skills, handwriting, or activities of daily living). Parents have defined the outcomes that they value for sensory integration intervention. Cohn (2001a) found that parents valued most (1) reframing of their children's behavioral and performance problems as SPD; (2) learning to accommodate to their children's sensory needs; (3) learning strategies, tools, and language for advocating for their children; and (4) observing improvements in their children's self-esteem, confidence and social skills. Resources for parents are provided at the end of this chapter.

Table 73-5. Principles of a Sensory Integrative Approach

Principle	Description
Intervention takes place in a sensory-rich environment	In this sensory-rich environment, play choices at or slightly above the child's developmental levels are available
Just right challenge	Therapist creates playful activities with achievable challenges
Child achieves an adaptive response	In response to a challenging activity, the child adapts his or her behavior and shows mastery of the activity
Active engagement	The child is presented with activities that are motivating, developmentally appropriate, and playful; the child is cued and supported to become actively engaged in the activity
Child directed	Activities are selected because they match the child's preferred interests; therapist allows the child to take the lead in directing the activity and in creating play scenarios; therapist follows the child's selection of play activities

Adapted from Schaaf R, Miller LA: Occupational therapy using a sensory integrative approach for children with developmental disabilities. Ment Retard Dev Disabil Res Rev 11:143-148, 2005.

OUTCOMES OF SENSORY INTEGRATION INTERVENTION

Two meta-analyses (Ottenbacher, 1982; Vargas and Camilli, 1999) and one systematic review (Polatajko et al, 1992) of sensory integration intervention have been published. These reviews have shown that the effects of sensory integration are positive but modest. Gains were primarily in motor skills; however, behavioral organization and self-esteem measures have rarely been used in clinical trials. Vargas and Camilli (1999) found that average effect sizes for motor performance and cognition measures (0.39 to 0.40) were higher than average effect sizes for language and perceptual skills (0.13 to 0.14). Because a primary outcome of sensory integration intervention is goodness-of-fit among parent, child, and environment, interactional variables should be assessed, but rarely have been.

Although behavior and performance improvements are modest, parents have indicated that they are important and relate to significant changes in their children's self-esteem, peer relations, and confidence. In two qualitative studies that involved interviewing parents whose children received sensory integration intervention (Cohn, 2001a, 2001b), parents expressed that their children's participation in a range of activities had increased, and their perception of self-worth seemed to improve. Equally important outcomes for parents were (1) increased understanding of their children, (2) ability to establish expectations for their children, (3) validation of their parenting experiences, and (4) learning strategies for supporting and advocating for their children.

SUMMARY

Children with SPDs present with a range of behavioral and performance consequences. Identification requires history and examination, and when suspected, SPD should be confirmed by standardized sensory-motor-perceptual scales administered by an occupational therapist. Essential elements of intervention include educating the family members about SPD and how it affects the child's behaviors; recommending modifications to the child's environment and routines; helping all caregivers accommodate to the child's sensory processing needs; and giving the child methods to maintain optimal levels of arousal, attentiveness, organized behavior, and skillful performance.

REFERENCES

Ahn RR, Miller LJ, Milberger S, McIntosh DN: Prevalence of parents' perceptions of sensory processing disorders among kindergarten children. Am J Occup Ther 58:287-293, 2004.

Ayres J: Cluster analysis of measures of sensory integration. Am J Occup Ther 31:362-366, 1977.

Ayres J: Sensory Integration and Praxis Tests. Los Angeles, Western Psychological Services, 1989.

Ayres J: Sensory Integration and the Child. Los Angeles, Western Psychological Services, 2005.

Bruininks R, Bruininks B: 2006. Bruninks Oseretsky Test of Motor Proficiency, 2nd ed. Circle Pines, MN, AGS Publishing, 2006.

Bundy A, Koomar JA: Orchestrating intervention: The art of practice. *In* Bundy AC, Lane SJ, Murray EA (eds): Sensory Integration: Theory and Practice, 2nd ed. Philadelphia, FA Davis, 2001, pp 242-259.

Case-Smith J: The effects of tactile defensiveness and tactile discrimination on in-hand manipulation. Am J Occup Ther 45:811-818, 2001.

Cohn ES: From waiting to relating: Parents' experiences in the waiting room of an occupational therapy clinic. Am J Occup Ther 55:167-174, 2001a.

Cohn ES: Parent perspectives of occupational therapy using a sensory integration approach. Am J Occup Ther 55:285-294, 2001b.

Dunn W: The Sensory Profile: Examiner's Manual. San Antonio, TX, The Psychological Corporation, 1999.

Dunn W: The sensations of everyday life: Empirical, theoretical, and pragmatic consideration. Am J Occup Ther 44:608-620, 2001.

Henderson SE, Sugden DA: Movement Assessment Battery for Children Manual. New York, Psychological Corporation, 1992.

Koomar JA, Bundy AC: Creating direct intervention from theory. *In* Bundy AC, Lane SJ, Murray EA (eds): Sensory Integration: Theory and Practice, 2nd ed. Philadelphia, FA Davis, 2002, pp 261-308.

Levine M: Cumulative neurodevelopmental deficits: Their impact on productivity in late middle childhood. *In* Levine MD, Satz P (eds): Middle Childhood: Development and Dysfunction. Baltimore, University Park, 1984, pp 227-243.

Levine M: Motor implementation. *In* Levine MD (ed): Developmental Variation and Learning Disorders. Cambridge, Educators Publishing Service, 1987, pp 208-239.

McIntosh D, Miller LJ, Shyu V, Hagerman R: Sensory modulation disruption, electrodermal responses, and functional behaviors. Dev Med Child Neurol 41:608-615, 1999.

Miller-Kuhaneck H, Henry DA, Glennon TJ: Sensory Processing Measure Main Classroom Form. Los Angeles, Western Psychological Services, 2006.

Mulligan S: Cluster analysis of scores of children on the Sensory Integration and Praxis Tests. Occup Ther J Res 20:256-270, 2000.

Ottenbacher K: Sensory integration therapy: Affect or effect? Am J Occup Ther 36:571-579, 1982.

Parham LD, Ecker C: Clinical observations of neuromotor performance, evaluation of sensory processing and touch inventory for elementary school children. *In* Bundy A, Lane S, Murray E (eds): Sensory Integration Therapy and Practice, 2nd ed. Philadelphia, FA Davis, 2002 Appendix 7-IE.

Parham LD, Ecker C, Miller-Kuhaneck H, et al: Sensory Processing Measure Manual. Los Angeles, Western Psychological Services, 2006.

Parham LD, Mailloux Z: Sensory integration. *In* Case-Smith J (ed): Occupational Therapy for Children. St. Louis, Mosby, 2005.

Polatajko HJ, Kaplan BJ, Wilson BN, et al: Sensory integration treatment for children with learning disabilities: Its status 20 years later. Occup Ther J Res 12:323-341, 1992.

Schaaf R, Miller LA: Occupational therapy using a sensory integrative approach for children with developmental disabilities. Ment Retard Dev Disabil Res Rev 11:143-148, 2005.

Smyth MM, Anderson HI: Coping with clumsiness in the school playground: Social and physical play in children with coordination impairments. Br J Dev Psychol 18:389-413, 2000.

Vargas S, Camilli G: A meta-analysis of research on sensory integration treatment. Am J Occup Ther 53:189-198, 1999.

RESOURCES FOR PARENTS

Ayres J: Sensory Integration and the Child. Los Angeles, Western Psychological Services, 2005.

Biel L, Peske N: Raising a Sensory Smart Child: The Definitive Handbook for Helping Your Child with Sensory Integration Issues. New York, Penguin Books, 2004.

Kranowitz CS: The Goodenoughs Get in Sync. Las Vegas, NV, Sensory Resources, 2004.

Kranowitz CS: The Out-of-Sync Child: Recognizing and Coping with Sensory Integration Dysfunction. New York, Penguin Group, 2005.

Kranowitz CS: The Out-of-Sync Child Has Fun: Activities for Kids with Sensory Integration Dysfunction. New York, Penguin Group, 2006.

Miller LJ: Sensational Kids: Hope and Help for Children with Sensory Processing Disorder. New York, Penguin Group, 2006.

SPD Network: Available at: www.SPDnetwork.org.

SPD Parent Connections: Available at: www.KIDfoundation.org/parentconnection.

74 CHILDREN WITH MULTIPLE DISABILITIES AND SPECIAL HEALTH CARE NEEDS

Ellen Roy Elias

The medical management of a child with multiple disabilities can present a very complex and challenging set of issues to the pediatrician. Children with multiple disabilities fall under the classification of *children with special health care needs (CSHCN)*. The formal definition of CSHCN adopted by the American Academy of Pediatrics in October 1998 is as follows: "Children with special health care needs are those who have or are at increased risk of having a chronic physical, developmental, behavioral or emotional condition and who also require health and related services of a type or amount beyond that required by children generally"(McPherson et al, 1998).

The prevalence of CSHCN is astounding. More recent figures indicate that almost 13% of children in the United States have special health care needs (SHCN), which corresponds to greater than 9 million children nationwide. Approximately 20% of U.S. households have a child with SHCN. With a problem of this magnitude, caring for CSHCN is something that all pediatricians need to grapple with on some level. It is crucial particularly for the developmental pediatrician to establish a set of strategies and a model for how to address the needs of a child with SHCN to create a functional medical home for the child and family.

COMPLEXITY OF DIAGNOSES AND MANAGEMENT

A major challenge of caring for a child with SHCN is that the child rarely has just one problem, but more often has at least several comorbid diagnoses. More than half of children with cerebral palsy also have cognitive disabilities (intellectual disability). Children with cerebral palsy also may have sensory deficits, including poor vision or hearing impairment. A child might have more than one sensory impairment; A child with CHARGE (coloboma, heart disease, atresia choanae, retarded growth and retarded development, genital hypoplasia, and ear anomalies) syndrome might have visual impairment secondary to retinal colobomas and sensorineural hearing loss. Table 74-1 presents common associations of comorbid conditions. The importance of understanding these associations cannot be overemphasized because the comprehensive evaluation of the child and referral for appropriate services are contingent on recognizing that more than one condition may coexist.

Even more challenging than the combination of physical plus cognitive disabilities, with or without sensory impairment, is the "dual diagnosis" combination of cognitive disabilities plus behavioral disorders. Children with cognitive disabilities may display various mental health issues, including significant depression, attention-deficit/hyperactivity disorder, and obsessive-compulsive disorder, which may be more functionally disabling than the underlying cognitive problems. Children with intellectual disability at the more severe end of the spectrum may present with extremely challenging self-stimulatory and self-injurious behaviors and significant sleep problems, which may be amenable to medication. Finding mental health providers who are knowledgeable and skilled in the behavioral management of and psychopharmacology for children with intellectual disability is often quite difficult.

Caring for a child with SHCN and multiple disabilities can provide great satisfaction to the pediatrician. These are children and families who really need their health care providers. Numerous particular issues regarding the care of CSHCN require special mention, however. A child who is medically fragile requires a higher level of input from the provider. Visits often last longer, and the number of issues that need to be dealt with at each visit are more numerous and more complex. Children with SHCN often require more frequent visits to the health care provider than typical healthy children. They also require hospitalizations at a much higher rate, with admission to regular pediatric services and to the intensive care unit. During hospitalizations, it is often crucial for the pediatrician who knows the child and family best to be available for difficult discussions about end-of-life issues, or for care conferences to help plan future medical interventions. Care coordination is an important part of the process.

Not only are multiple lengthy visits, hospitalizations, and care conferences time-consuming, and often difficult to schedule, but they also are poorly reimbursed. Because many CSHCN have Medicaid insurance rather than private payers, the reimbursement to care providers for these services is often minimal. For this reason, many physicians make a conscious decision *not* to care for patients with SHCN, often leaving families searching for providers who are knowledgeable and willing. Although CSHCN constitute an ever-increasing proportion of hospitalized children, very few pediatric training programs in the United States offer a consistent

Table 74-1. **Comorbid Diagnoses**

Condition	Common Associated Diagnosis	Etiology
Cerebral palsy	Intellectual disability	CNS dysgenesis Anoxic injury CNS infection Chromosomal/syndromic disorder Metabolic disorder
	Hearing loss	Kernicterus CNS dysgenesis Anoxic injury
	Visual loss	CNS dysgenesis (septo-optic dysplasia) Anoxic injury Metabolic
	Seizures	Stroke Anoxic injury Metabolic disorder
Intellectual disability	Multiple congenital anomalies	Chromosomal abnormalities Syndromic disorders Metabolic disorders
	Cerebral palsy	See above
	Seizures	Syndromic disorders (tuberous sclerosis or Angelman syndrome) See above for cerebral palsy
	Visual loss	CNS dysgenesis (septo-optic dysplasia or occipital abnormalities) Metabolic (peroxisomal) disorders Syndromic disorders (CHARGE or Prader-Willi syndrome) Chromosomal abnormalities (trisomy 13 or trisomy 21) Anoxic injury
	Hearing loss	Syndromic disorders (CHARGE or Stickler syndrome) Chromosomal abnormalities (trisomy 13 or trisomy 21) Anoxic injury Metabolic
	Behavioral disorder	Chromosomal abnormalities (22q deletion) Syndromic disorders (Angelman syndrome) Metabolic disorders (Sanfilippo syndrome or Smith-Lemli-Opitz syndrome) Anoxic injury CNS dysgenesis

CNS, central nervous system.

approach to training pediatric residents in the care and management of CSHCN. Family medicine and internal medicine residents receive even less training in the management of patients with SHCN than pediatricians. Many CSHCN who are dependent on assistive medical devices, such as ventilators and feeding tubes, are entering the public school system, and pediatricians are being asked to assist the schools in their management. The role of the developmental pediatric consultant in the management of CSHCN has become even more crucial for these patients.

ETIOLOGY

As noted earlier, children with SHCN often present with complex and multiple concurrent problems. There may be a clear underlying etiology to the child's issues, such as documented anoxia at birth, closed head trauma, or a confirmed genetic disorder. Often there is not a clear underlying etiology for the child's medical and developmental problems, however. Intellectual disability and cerebral palsy have multiple causes and are clinical descriptors, but are not etiologic diagnoses. It is crucial for the physician caring for a patient with intellectual disability and cerebral palsy always to ask whether there is a known etiology for the child's medical issues. Obstetricians have been falsely blamed for birth injuries, when there may be clear indication of a prenatal problem or genetic disorder that is the true etiology. Having an index of suspicion is important, especially if there is no history of difficulty at the time of delivery, and no neonatal respiratory or feeding issues.

Making the correct diagnosis is important for many reasons. Certain genetic diagnoses carry with them known associated medical problems that may develop in the future, and having a diagnosis allows the clinician to prognosticate accurately and intervene at an earlier stage when those problems do develop. The correct diagnosis allows for more effective and appropriate medical interventions.

Of great importance to the families is that having a correct underlying diagnosis allows for appropriate genetic counseling and determination of recurrence risks. It is a tragedy for a family to have a second affected child with special needs, who has an underlying diagnosis that could have been prenatally detected, because no one thought to test the older child or make a correct diagnosis in a timely way. This situation has occurred frequently for rare autosomal recessive disorders. Even for diagnoses as common as Down syndrome or spina bifida, many families are unaware of their recurrence risks, of available means of prenatal detection in future pregnancies, or of the possibilities of certain interventions to reduce the recurrence risk, such as folic acid in neural tube defects.

When caring for a child with SHCN, if there is no clear underlying etiology for those needs, or the suggested etiology is inconsistent with the history, the pediatrician should be suspicious. A genetic consultation should be requested for any child with dysmorphic features or known birth defects. Metabolic testing should be considered for a child with a history of a change in neurologic status or loss of milestones, or a change in developmental status associated with intercurrent illness. The pediatrician should obtain a good family history: Are there other individuals in the family with similar symptoms, or a history of consanguinity, infertility, fetal loss, or death during early infancy? Has the microcephalic child with no history of brain injury ever had a good head imaging study such as magnetic resonance imaging (MRI) to look for central nervous system dysgenesis? The more severe the disabilities and medical problems, the more likely that an etiology will be found. See Chapter 30 for a detailed discussion of the workup of inborn errors of metabolism.

APPROACH TO A CHILD WITH SPECIAL HEALTH CARE NEEDS

Children with developmental disabilities frequently have symptoms that lead to complicated medical problems. Feeding problems (see later) can be difficult to manage and lead to failure to thrive. Respiratory issues leading to chronic lung disease also are quite common. Comorbid neurologic conditions, particularly seizures, are common and often require medication management.

The following is an approach by system to address the medical management of CSHCN. Many of these topics are covered in greater detail in separate chapters, but an overall approach to the medical evaluation of CSHCN is presented here.

Feeding Problems

Nutritional concerns are common in CSHCN. Feeding disorders, in which the child is unable to consume safely and efficiently a sufficient number of calories to grow and adequate fluid volume to maintain good hydration status, may be due to various underlying causes, including oromotor dyscoordination, low muscle tone, and anatomic abnormalities of the palate or airway or both.

Closely following the child's growth velocity and plotting weight, height, and weight for height are important. Children who are unable to maintain a normal growth velocity or who fall off the curve for weight and weight for height may require caloric supplementation. Many formulas now are available for children who require caloric supplementation, and caloric additives can be easily added to the child's regular feedings. The caloric needs of a child are associated with the child's underlying developmental status and motor function. A child who is overactive, or has spasticity, may have greater caloric needs than a severely hypotonic child who moves very little. Plotting the growth parameters on a standard growth curve allows the clinician to determine if the child's particular needs are being met in an appropriate way. Also available are specialized growth curves for children with specific genetic diagnoses, such as Down syndrome and achondroplasia.

Sometimes poor oromotor function affects the ability to consume adequate calories in a reasonable time. A child who takes an hour to consume just a few ounces may be burning off so many calories by the efforts expended with feedings that it becomes impossible to take in adequate nutrition. Of particular concern are children who have respiratory symptoms associated with feedings, including choking, coughing, gagging, and wheezing. These symptoms may represent insufficient protection of the airway with swallowing, leading to aspiration. Obtaining a modified barium swallow is indicated for these symptoms. If aspiration is documented, an alternative route to oral feedings is generally recommended.

Feeding Tubes

A variety of options are available for a child who is unable to consume adequate calories safely by mouth.

Nasogastric Tube Feedings

Nasogastric feeds can be safely accomplished for many weeks to months. Generally considered a short-term option, the primary caregiver needs to be taught how to place the tube safely into the stomach. The child may inadvertently pull out the tube or dislodge it from an appropriate position, requiring it to be replaced frequently, a major disadvantage to this option. Children fed via nasogastric tube may develop significant issues with gastroesophageal reflux disease (GERD) (see later), which complicate this feeding route. The feeds may be given via a bolus, or may be run in more slowly using a feeding pump. Children with lethal diagnoses (e.g., trisomy 18 or type II osteogenesis imperfecta) and children who are medically fragile and not surgical candidates can be fed via nasogastric tube for months to years.

Nasojejunal Tube Feedings

Nasojejunal feeds are a good option for children who manifest significant GERD with nasogastric feeds. The end of the tube is advanced past the pylorus, and the feeding cannot be easily refluxed or vomited. A nasojejunal tube requires placement by a radiologist to ensure correct positioning. The major disadvantage to this feeding approach is that if the tube is inadvertently pulled out, or pulled back into the stomach, it cannot easily be replaced. Nasojejunal feeds are given continuously using a pump and cannot be given as a bolus because they are given directly into the intestine. This can be an issue for a child who cannot receive feedings at certain times (i.e., when at school or out at the playground).

Gastrostomy Tubes

Gastrostomy tubes require surgical placement, but when this is accomplished, they have the advantage of staying in position and are not routinely pulled out by the child. Feedings can be administered either via bolus feedings or more slowly using a pump. Feedings also can be given as a slow drip overnight, to catch up on calories and fluids that a child might be unable to take in during the day. Primary caregivers require teaching to learn how to administer the feeds, and how to care for the skin around the tube. GERD is a common problem in children who are tube fed (see later) and may require treatment with medications such as acid blockers and metoclopramide (Reglan). If medical management is unsuccessful, a surgical fundoplication may need to be considered. Gastritis also is a frequent complication and may progress to a gastrointestinal bleed.

Gastrojejunal Tube

Gastrojejunal tubes are options for children who require tube feedings, have significant GERD, and are not surgical candidates for a fundoplication. The child requires a surgical procedure to place a gastrostomy tube, and then an interventional radiologist can pass the jejunal part of the tube into the correct position. Similar to nasojejunal feeds, gastrojejunal feeds are drip feeds requiring a pump, and boluses cannot be used. A limitation of this kind of tube is that the child must be old enough and large enough because no gastrojejunal tubes are manufactured that are small enough to be used in infants and very young children. Another limitation of gastrojejunal feeds is that, similar to nasojejunal feeds, the distal portion of the jejunal tube can become dislodged, and replacement requires fluoroscopic assistance and the services of a radiologist.

Gastrointestinal Complications

Gastrointestinal issues are common and may significantly complicate feedings. The gastrointestinal issues most frequently encountered are discussed.

Gastroesophageal Reflux Disease

GERD is extremely common in children with abnormal muscle tone (spasticity and hypotonia). Symptoms include gagging, retching, and often frank vomiting. If chronic GERD has occurred, esophagitis may develop and cause irritability, arching with feeds, and food refusal. The mainstay of treatment for GERD is suppression of gastric acid production. Ranitidine (Zantac) is often helpful, but stronger agents such as proton pump inhibitors (omeprazole [Prilosec] or lansoprazole [Prevacid]) are often needed.

GERD may be exacerbated by poor gastrointestinal tract motility. Several agents enhance gastrointestinal tract motility, including metoclopramide, bethanechol, and erythromycin. The latter two are often difficult to titrate and may cause gastrointestinal tract upset. There may be significant side effects with metoclopramide, including a lowering of seizure threshold, which may become problematic. If the GERD is severe enough to affect weight gain and quality of life of the child, and medical management is ineffective, a surgical fundoplication may be indicated. Previously considered a major surgical intervention, the advent of newer laparoscopic surgical techniques has allowed this procedure to be done less invasively. Fundoplication may worsen problems with oral secretion management, particularly in children with severe sialidosis (drooling). There also may be increased retching and gagging if the wrap is too tight.

Constipation

Constipation is common in children with motor disabilities, especially children with low muscle tone. It also is associated with spina bifida and other myelodysplasias, and certain syndromic disorders such as FG syndrome. If severe enough, constipation can lead to food refusal and feeding intolerance. Milder cases often can be managed with dietary modifications and increased fluid intake. More severe cases often require treatment with medications such as polyethylene glycol (MiraLAX) or Senokot.

Gastritis

Irritation of the gastric mucosa is often seen in children with gastrostomy tubes. This irritation can evolve into a frank ulcer with gastrointestinal bleeding. The parents may notice coffee-ground gastrostomy tube drainage, or melenotic stools. Acute treatment with sucralfate is often helpful, but long-term sucralfate interferes with the action of acid-blocking medications and the absorption of other medications (including digoxin and phenytoin). Careful timing of the dose and only short-term use of sucralfate are recommended.

Respiratory Issues

Respiratory issues also are quite common among CSHCN. The etiologies are multiple and include abnormalities of the airway and diseases of the lung. These are addressed separately, but it is important to realize that a child might have more than one respiratory problem.

Abnormalities of the Airway

The most serious of the anatomic airway abnormalities manifest at birth and may require immediate intervention, including intubation and sometimes tracheostomy. Certain airway issues are commonly associated with malformations because of an underlying genetic disorder. Probably the most common of these is Pierre-Robin anomalad, which is the association of cleft palate, microagnathia and glossoptosis, leading to airway obstruction. Infants with severe Pierre-Robin anomalad often require tracheostomy in the newborn period. The prognosis for eventual decannulation, given growth of the lower jaw over time, is excellent. Pierre-Robin anomalad may be associated with an underlying genetic disorder, such as Stickler syndrome. Genetic evaluation is important to ensure that comorbid conditions, such as cataract and hearing loss, are sought.

Choanal atresia is another anomaly of the airway that requires intervention at birth, and is associated with underlying genetic conditions, including CHARGE association and certain craniosynostosis disorders. A genetic consultation is helpful to determine the correct underlying etiology.

More subtle airway issues may develop over time. Children with conditions associated with midface hypoplasia (Down syndrome is the most common example) are prone to the development of upper airway obstruction from adenoidal and tonsillar hypertrophy. The symptoms include noisy breathing or snoring at night, often with restless sleep. The child might be quite lethargic during the day because of sleep deprivation. Evaluation with a sleep study is indicated, and removal of the enlarged tonsils and adenoids is often indicated.

Laryngomalacia and tracheomalacia are common airway abnormalities in children with abnormal muscle tone, particularly hypotonia. These conditions may be seen more commonly in infants born preterm, who required long-term intubation in the neonatal intensive care unit. Children present with inspiratory noisy breathing that is often positional, worse in supine and better in prone. Anatomic abnormalities (e.g., laryngeal clefts) of the lower airway may mimic the symptoms of laryngomalacia or tracheomalacia and require evaluation by an ear, nose, and throat surgeon.

Lung Diseases

Diseases of the lung also can cause significant respiratory issues. A commonly seen problem is recurrent aspiration pneumonia in a child with feeding/swallowing dysfunction. The child often shows increased respiratory symptoms, such as noisy breathing or coughing in association with feedings. The right upper lobe is particularly affected in cases of aspiration pneumonia because of the anatomic ease of aspiration at that site. Evaluation with a modified barium swallow, often performed by a feeding therapist along with a radiologist, is indicated for a child who has experienced recurrent aspiration pneumonias.

Children born prematurely also are at risk for chronic lung disease, following issues with surfactant deficiency at birth. Difficulty tolerating upper respiratory infections is more common in former preterm newborns, and many of these patients require consultation by a pulmonologist and long-term therapy with bronchodilators and inhaled steroids. Supplemental oxygen often is required in children with airway issues or chronic lung disease and recurrent respiratory infections. Some premature infants are discharged home from the nursery on oxygen via nasal cannula and require this for some time after birth; this is particularly true for patients who live at high altitude. Other patients who are successfully weaned from oxygen therapy may require intermittent oxygen use in association with intercurrent illness. Children with congenital heart disease also may have respiratory symptoms and issues and require diuretic treatment in addition to pulmonary medications and oxygen.

Tracheostomy and Ventilatory Support

Children with airway and respiratory issues severe enough to require placement of a tracheostomy are often quite challenging (and sometimes a little frightening) for the pediatrician to manage. Children with anatomic anomalies of the airway are often identified at birth and require tracheostomy on a fairly emergent basis. In many CSHCN, airway issues develop more gradually, however, and the decision for tracheostomy may be more elective. This situation may arise in a child with severe brain injury who cannot protect his or her airway and manifests significant upper airway obstruction. This patient should be evaluated by specialists including ear, nose, and throat surgeons and pulmonologists, to assess whether the airway obstruction is severe enough to merit intervention. A sleep study is often required to rule out airway obstruction.

Tonsillectomy and adenoidectomy are often first-stage interventions, but when this intervention does not solve the problem, tracheostomy may be considered. Sometimes a child develops a severe respiratory illness (i.e., respiratory syncytial virus infection) requiring endotracheal intubation and ventilation, and then cannot be weaned off the ventilator and extubated despite numerous attempts. Children with muscular dystrophies, congenital myopathies, or other neuromuscular disorders (e.g., mitochondrial myopathies) may develop severe muscular weakness of the respiratory musculature over time, requiring tracheostomy and long-term ventilatory support.

The decision to perform a tracheostomy is a major one, which should be made after careful consideration of the child's medical status and prognosis. Having a tracheostomy significantly complicates the level of home medical care that the child requires and may lead to the need for home nursing support. Because of the shortage of qualified home care personnel, much of the complex medical management for CSHCN with a tracheostomy falls to the parents to provide. Parents need to learn how to care for a child with a tracheostomy, including how to suction the tracheostomy, change the tracheostomy if necessary, and care for the skin around it. No parent is able to provide complex medical care to his or her child around the clock, however, every day.

Caregivers and medical providers for a child with a tracheostomy also need to be aware of changes in respiratory status that require evaluation and treatment. These changes include symptoms such as increased respiratory rate and work of breathing; increase in tracheostomy secretions, particularly if associated with a change in color of secretions (green or yellow secretions often indicate bacterial infection); cough; increased oxygen requirement; and fever. These symptoms should prompt evaluation, including culture of tracheostomy secretions, possible chest x-ray, and consideration of antibiotic usage.

Other specialized equipment that may be used for respiratory support in CSHCN are biphasic positive airway pressure (BiPAP) and continuous positive airway pressure (CPAP). Children with upper airway obstruction that is not ameliorated by tonsillectomy and adenoidectomy often benefit from these interventions, which are usually worn at night during sleep. Using positive pressure to keep the airways open can be extremely beneficial to certain children, especially children with craniofacial anomalies causing hypoplasia of the midface and children with neurologic issues and weakness of the respiratory muscles who cannot keep their air passages open on their own. Use of either BiPAP or CPAP can improve symptoms to the point that tracheostomy sometimes can be averted. The use of these interventions is limited in children who are very small, for whom appropriately sized masks are unavailable, and in children with significant behavioral issues, who would not leave the mask in place.

A more recent intervention that also can be extremely helpful is the use of a vest, which is a mechanical device that vibrates around the thorax and helps clear secretions. This technology is now replacing, and seems more effective than, the older practice of chest physiotherapy. This technology has been used for many years in children with chronic respiratory diseases such as cystic fibrosis, and more recently has become available for CSHCN. The development of smaller, child-sized vests has enabled this technology to be used in much younger patients. Vests are particularly helpful for children with severe hypotonia or neuromuscular diseases, who have difficulty clearing secretions on their own. The major disadvantage of the vest is its expense.

OTHER SPECIALIZED EQUIPMENT AND SPECIAL HEALTH CARE NEEDS

In addition to feeding tubes and respiratory supports, such as oxygen, tracheostomy, and ventilators, CSHCN often have other pieces of medical equipment or have undergone specialized surgical procedures that affect their home care and medical needs. The next section addresses a few of the more common of these, including ventriculoperitoneal shunts, urologic devices, and ambulatory equipment. The neural tube defect, myelomeningocele (or spina bifida), is used as a model in this section.

CHILD WITH MYELOMENINGOCELE (SPINA BIFIDA)

The patient with spina bifida is a classic example of a child with SHCN, who requires a multidisciplinary approach to management. A child with spina bifida has many complex concurrent issues that require surgical intervention, including the neurosurgical closure of the open back lesion, and placement and management of hydrocephalus. The child with spina bifida also has many orthopedic concerns, including management of foot deformities and scoliosis. Neurogenic bowel and bladder are usually present, which requires specialized management by a urologist.

The role of the developmental pediatrician in the management of a child with spina bifida is crucial. The pediatrician needs to have a basic understanding of the surgical interventions that the child has undergone, and when to contact the surgical specialist should a complication arise. The pediatrician is the member of the team who can truly assess the child's overall state of health, including nutritional status, particularly if the child has feeding problems related to Arnold-Chiari II malformation. The developmental pediatrician also is often required to play an important role in the assessment of therapeutic interventions and specialized classroom supports for the child with spina bifida, who often has associated learning disabilities. The pediatrician also should be aware of the genetic implications of this diagnosis, and understand the recurrence risk in future pregnancies (2% to 3%, or greater if other family members also have neural tube defects) and the importance of folate prophylaxis to reduce this risk (when taken by the mother for a minimum of 3 months before conception and during the first month of pregnancy, an appropriate dose of folic acid can reduce the recurrence risk by >50%). Neural tube defects may occur as a primary birth defect, as part of an underlying genetic syndrome, or as a teratogenic consequence of maternal alcohol abuse or valproic acid use during pregnancy. Referral to a geneticist may be indicated in certain cases. Comorbid diagnoses such as seizures are common. Lastly, the child with spina bifida has a risk of developing latex sensitivity, owing to repeated exposure to latex in the medical environment, a preventable complication.

Patients with neural tube defects are often diagnosed prenatally on ultrasound. With the advent of prenatal maternal serum screening, now done fairly universally, the presence of spina bifida can be prenatally suspected on the basis of an elevated maternal serum α-fetoprotein and confirmed with ultrasound and sometimes amniocentesis. Prenatal detection of a neural tube defect may lead to a change in mode of delivery because there is some evidence that delivery by cesarean section may lead to better motor outcome than vaginal delivery.

Children with spina bifida are often followed in a multidisciplinary spinal defects clinic, where the pediatrician and surgical subspecialists see the child during one clinic session, usually several times a year. This model has been used for many years and is often appreciated by the families. It may not be the most efficient approach to multidisciplinary management from the clinician's standpoint, however, and many medical insurance providers often do not cover all the services provided in such a model.

Vignette

Timmy was born at full term by vaginal delivery, and noted at birth to have an open L4-5 level myelomeningocele, an enlarged head circumference, and bilateral clubfeet. His family lived in a rural area, and the mother had not undergone prenatal screening. Timmy was transported to a tertiary medical center after birth, where he underwent neurosurgical closure of his spina bifida and placement of a ventriculoperitoneal shunt on day 1 of life. During his first year of life, he was healthy and fed well, although he had trouble transitioning to table foods of higher texture, related to Arnold-Chiari malformation. He required serial casting and eventual surgery for his clubfeet. At age 1 year, he presented with lethargy, vomiting, and mild stridor. A computed tomography scan showed ventricular enlargement and he underwent shunt revision with resolution of his symptoms.

His developmental milestones were met except for gross motor skills, which were delayed. He has been receiving developmental services through his local early intervention program, specifically physical therapy to help him ambulate with the assistance of ankle-foot orthoses and a walker, and occupational therapy to address his feeding issues.

Timmy has received routine pediatric care through his pediatrician, and attends a multidisciplinary spina bifida clinic every few months, where he is followed by a developmental pediatrician, neurosurgeon, orthopedist, and urologist. Timmy has a neurogenic bowel and bladder, has problems with chronic constipation, and has had one urinary tract infection. Timmy's physicians, his parents, and personnel at his school all use latex precautions. Timmy's mother takes 4 mg of folic acid per day, as do her siblings, to decrease the risk of neural tube defects in future pregnancies.

The child with spina bifida has often undergone multiple surgical procedures. The more common of these procedures and the associated medical equipment are discussed next.

Ventriculoperitoneal Shunts

Approximately 85% of children with spina bifida and some children with other disorders, such as multiple suture craniosynostosis syndromes, have associated hydrocephalus requiring shunt placement. Children with severe head injuries leading to increased intracranial pressure, premature infants with severe intraventricular hemorrhage, and children with genetic diagnoses associated with congenital hydrocephalus, such as aqueductal stenosis, also may require shunt placement. The most common form of shunt is the ventriculoperitoneal shunt. This shunt consists of tubing that is inserted into one of the lateral ventricles and is connected to a shunt reservoir and a one-way valve, allowing cerebrospinal fluid (CSF) to drain out of the ventricle, but not back into the brain. The fluid runs through subcutaneous tubing, which is passed over the ribs and inserted into the peritoneal cavity, where extra tubing is placed to allow for growth of the patient. A more recent development in shunt technology is the programmable shunt. This type of shunt allows the degree of shunt drainage to be regulated (increasing or decreasing as needed), without requiring an additional surgical procedure.

The major complications of shunts are malfunction and infection. The symptoms of shunt malfunction are related to increased intracranial pressure and include severe headache, vomiting, and lethargy. In an infant, the symptoms are often lethargy, irritability, vomiting, and a bulging fontanelle. Shunt malfunction may be acute or more chronic, as with a distal shunt problem, such as blockage of the tip of the ventriculoperitoneal shunt in the peritoneal cavity, leading to cyst formation known as a "CSF-oma." Evaluation of possible shunt malfunction generally includes a head computed tomography scan to evaluate the size of the ventricles and may include a shunt series (x-rays to look for discontinuity in the tubing) or an abdominal ultrasound study if a distal shunt problem is suspected. Intermittent shunt malfunction also may occur and be associated with a worsening in school performance or personality changes.

Shunt infection often manifests with similar symptoms to shunt malfunction, plus fever. It is often difficult to determine if a child with a known shunt and fever is presenting with a shunt infection or fever from some other source. If all other sites of infection have been ruled out, and the child is presenting with symptoms suggestive of shunt problems, a shunt tap is indicated, with analysis of the CSF for possible shunt infection. The CSF studies associated with shunt infection generally show a less pronounced leukocytosis and lower glucose than is associated with meningitis. The typical bacteria causing shunt infection are skin flora, such as staphyloccocal epidermitis. The most common time for a shunt infection to manifest is in the several-week period following a shunt revision. Treatment of shunt infection generally requires removing the old shunt hardware and tubing and replacing with a completely new system, after the CSF has been sterilized.

A special complication of shunt dysfunction in children with spina bifida must include discussion of the associated anomaly known as Arnold-Chiari type II malformation, which is seen in children with myelomeningocele. Arnold-Chiari type II malformation is seen on MRI as herniation of the cerebellum and brainstem through the foramen magnum into the upper part of the cervical spinal canal. With an acute shunt malfunction and increased intracranial pressure, this herniation may become more pronounced, and blood supply to this critical region may be compromised, leading to ischemic damage of critical structures such as the respiratory center in the brainstem and important cranial nerves. Ensuing vocal cord paralysis, inability to suck and swallow, and paralysis of the abducens nerve are common in children who have a "Chiari crisis." Immediate shunt revision is indicated in such a situation, which may lead to improvement or resolution of these symptoms. Some children may have permanent neurologic dysfunction following a Chiari crisis, however, necessitating tracheostomy, ventilation, and feeding tube placement.

Urologic Procedures in Children with Neurogenic Bowel and Bladder

Clean Intermittent Catheterization

Children who are unable to empty their bladders, and who especially have a history of vesicoureteral reflux or urinary tract infection (UTI), or both, may require clean intermittent catheterization. This is a simple procedure that can be easily taught to the primary caregivers. By early elementary school age, most children can learn to catheterize themselves independently. Children with neurogenic bladders always should be screened for UTI if they develop fever, gastrointestinal symptoms such as vomiting or diarrhea, or a change to the color or odor of the urine. Children who are insensate may experience some abdominal discomfort, but may not appreciate typical dysuria associated with UTI.

Bladder Augmentation and Artificial Sphincters

Many children with spina bifida undergo continence surgical procedures to enhance bladder capacity and prevent leakage of urine. They often must catheterize to drain urine from the bladder. Symptoms of possible UTI as noted previously should prompt a catheterized urine culture to rule out infection.

ACE Procedure

The ACE procedure, or bringing the appendix to the surface of the abdominal wall to create a stoma through which medication such as GoLYTELY can be administered, can be an enormously helpful procedure for children with neurogenic bowel who have severe, chronic constipation. The typical management of neurogenic bowel relies on the concept of controlled constipation and normal gastrocolic reflexes to train the child to evacuate stool on a regular schedule. Some children cannot be regulated with this minimalist approach, however, and develop severe obstipation, which can complicate appetite and growth, and lead to a worsening of bladder control as well. The ACE procedure has been helpful in this subset of patients.

Orthopedic Procedures in Children with Spina Bifida

Clubfeet Management

Children with spinal cord defects and congenital paralysis frequently develop foot deformities related to decreased fetal movement and malpositioning of the foot in utero. After birth, these deformities are often treated with serial casting to bring the foot position gradually into more normal alignment. Surgical intervention is frequently required, however, if casting is not fully successful.

Ambulation Management

Various approaches are used, depending on the motor level of the child's spinal defect. Children with lower lumbar and sacral level lesions often may ambulate quite well with the use of such minimal support as ankle-foot orthoses. Children with mid to upper level lumbar lesions often require more support. They may be able to ambulate for short distances with the use of more elaborate bracing support and crutches or walkers or both. Children with higher level lesions are typically wheelchair ambulators. Wheelchairs may be manually operated or power-operated. The latter provide more independence for the patient, but are very expensive. The need for careful measurements by trained therapists and equipment vendors to ensure the equipment fits the child, medical orders from the physician for these pieces of durable medical equipment, and the necessity for insurance prior approval, may delay and complicate the time frame between when the equipment is first recommended and when the child actually receives it.

Scoliosis Management

Scoliosis is a common complication in children with vertebral anomalies and is often progressive. In contrast to idiopathic scoliosis, which generally starts in the teenage years and is more common in girls, the scoliosis associated with spinal defects may be seen at a very young age and in boys and girls. Conservative management with physical therapy and the use of spinal orthoses such as "scoli jackets" are often part of the initial management. Surgical intervention is often required, however. The rapid progression of scoliosis in a child with spina bifida, especially if it is associated with back pain, change in bowel or bladder function, or neurologic changes in the lower extremities, may be the result of a tethered spinal cord. This condition may require evaluation with MRI, and treatment may require intervention from the neurosurgeon.

General Developmental and Medical Concerns and Needs of a Child with Spina Bifida

In addition to the medical and surgical issues noted earlier, children with spina bifida have many developmental issues and needs. Children with congenital paralysis related to spina cord defects require physical therapy starting during infancy and continuing through school age. Physical therapy is provided by early intervention programs during the first 3 years of life, and then by the school system thereafter. The physical therapist assesses interventions to enhance ambulation and treat scoliosis. An occupational therapist also is often required, particularly to address feeding issues in children with symptoms related to Arnold-Chiari malformation.

Most children with spina bifida are cognitively normal, although children with higher level lesions, other central nervous system malformations, or history of central nervous system infection may show cognitive delays. There is an association between spina bifida and learning disabilities. Children with spina bifida generally can be included in a normal classroom setting, but may require special learning services and an aide in the classroom to facilitate safe use of a wheelchair or braces or walker. Adaptive physical education is often necessary.

Precocious Puberty

Precocious puberty is increased in incidence in children with spina bifida, up to 20% (versus 1 in 1000 incidence in the general pediatric population). The cause of this is unknown, although it is thought possibly to be associated with hydrocephalus, a known risk factor for precocious puberty. Endocrine evaluation and treatment with the gonadotropin-releasing hormone antagonist leuprolide acetate (Lupron) may be indicated.

Growth Issues

There may be concerns about growth at both ends of the spectrum in children with spina bifida. Infants have a higher incidence of feeding problems, inability to transition to higher levels of textured foods, and slow growth, related to Arnold-Chiari type II malformation. Adolescents may develop problems with obesity, related to decreased activity level and nonambulatory status. Nutritional consultation is often helpful in both of these situations.

Sexuality

Children with spina bifida have unique issues related to sexuality. Because of neurogenic bowel and bladder issues, they are often in diapers until a much older age than is typical. Occasional incontinence of either urine or stool may be devastating for a teenager. In older patients, there are other concerns. A female patient who is insensate may require alternative measures to achieve sexual pleasure. A male patient may be unable to achieve erection or ejaculation. These issues often require the intervention of a urologic consultant. Latex sensitivity may complicate the use of condoms. An individual with spina bifida has a 5% chance of having a child with a neural tube defect, and female patients should be offered counseling and discussion regarding folic acid prophylaxis and prenatal testing. These are issues that are important for the pediatrician to discuss with adolescent patients.

SUMMARY

Caring for CSHCN and multiple disabilities requires great dedication, compassion, and some specialized areas of knowledge. A physician who cares for these patients must assess the basic needs of the child for adequate nutrition and growth and respiratory function. The physician must be cognizant of associated comorbid conditions and diagnoses. A thoughtful assessment of the underlying diagnosis should be made so that appropriate medical care and counseling to the family can be offered.

It is often necessary to care for CSHCN with the support of numerous pediatric and surgical subspecialists. The child also might use multiple pieces of medical equipment, such as feeding tubes, oxygen, tracheostomy, and ventilatory support, and require home care nursing and therapies. The child might be on multiple medications. All of these are necessary interventions, but may be remarkably stressful for the parents and primary caregivers to handle.

The patient with multiple disabilities and SHCN and his or her family require the support of a physician who is able to see the big picture, prioritize interventions, evaluate the recommendations of multiple consultants and help the family make informed and reasonable decisions, assist the family in coordination of medical interventions, and help the family through difficult times. Doing all of this is challenging, especially given insufficient time to address multiple problems during clinic sessions and inadequate reimbursement for activities such as care coordination.

Some physicians have been able to provide this kind of medical care in private practice, with the support and understanding of sympathetic colleagues who are willing to accept Medicaid reimbursement. More often, this challenge is met within a tertiary medical center with access to multiple medical and surgical specialists, and the ability to group and coordinate appointments for the family. This requires a commitment on the part of the institution to support medical providers willing to provide this type of care, with the understanding that such providers will never be able to meet their salaries in terms of their billing. Given the large and growing number of CSHCN, pediatric and family medicine training programs need to reassess the training of residents so that more physicians can learn the skills necessary to care for these patients in the future.

SUGGESTED READINGS

American Academy of Pediatrics Council on Children with Disabilities: Care coordination in the medical home: Integrating health and related systems of care for children with special health care needs. Pediatrics 116:1238, 2005.

Batshaw ML: Children with Disabilities. Baltimore, Brookes Publishing, 2002.

Bent N, Tennant A, Swift T, et al: Team approach versus ad hoc health services for young people with physical disabilities: A retrospective cohort study. Lancet 360:1280, 2002.

Berman S, Rannie M, Moore L, et al: Utilization and costs for children who have special health care needs and are enrolled in a hospital-based comprehensive primary care clinic. Pediatrics 115:e637, 2005.

Jones KL: Smith's Recognizable Patterns of Human Malformation. 6th ed. Philadelphia, Elsevier, 2006.

McPherson M, Arango P, Fox HB, et al: A new definition of children with special health care needs. Pediatrics 102:137, 1998.

Medical Home Initiatives for Children with Special Needs Project Advisory Committee, American Academy of Pediatrics: The medical home. Pediatrics 110(1 Pt 1):184, 2002.

Newacheck PW, Inkelas M, Kim SE: et al: Health services use and health care expenditures for children with disabilities. Pediatrics 114:79, 2004.

Newacheck PW, Kim SE: A national profile of health care utilization and expenditures for children with special health care needs. Arch Pediatr Adolesc Med 159:10, 2005.

Rosenberg RN, Prusiner SB, DiMauro S, et al: The Molecular and Genetic Basis of Neurologic and Psychiatric Disease, 3rd ed. Philadelphia, Butterworth Heinemann, 2003.

Rubin IL, Crocker AC: Medical Care for Children and Adults with Developmental Disabilities, 2nd ed. Baltimore, Brookes Publishing Co, 2006.

Van Dyck PC, Kogan MD, McPherson MG, et al: Prevalence and characteristics of children with special health care needs. Arch Pediatr Adolesc Med 158:884, 2004.

WEB RESOURCES

American Academy of Pediatrics: Available at: www.medicalhomeinfo.org.

National Information Center for Children and Youth with Disabilities: Available at: www.nichcy.org.

Part IX ASSESSMENT

75 INTERVIEWING: A CRITICAL SKILL

Esther H. Wender

The interview is a conversation between the clinician and the patient aimed at gathering and imparting information used to diagnose and treat the patient's problems. As the term *conversation* suggests, the interview is an interaction. Clinicians not only question, but also listen and comment on what is being said. Patients not only answer questions, but also inquire and explain.

In the practice of developmental-behavioral pediatrics, the information needed is often accompanied by strong emotion, such as guilt, embarrassment, or sadness. As in all areas of pediatrics, interviewing is complicated by the fact that the parent or other caregiver is usually the source of information and responsible for adherence to treatment recommendations. Under these circumstances, skillful interviewing is especially critical.

Teaching the skill of interviewing can be challenging. One reason is that talking to patients and asking questions seems to be simple. The most important skill of interviewing is listening and observing. Initially, trainees may be preoccupied with the task of obtaining answers to a list of questions and fail to listen for the cues the patient gives when answering those questions. Similarly, when imparting information about a diagnosis or treatment, the trainee may focus on the information to be given and miss the patient's reaction to what is being said.

Interviewing is an art. Learning this skill requires practice under supervision. Written suggestions such as those given in this chapter can only provide a starting point for developing proficiency.

IMPORTANCE OF THE EFFECTIVE INTERVIEW

Studies have repeatedly shown that skillful interviewing improves the quality of the information obtained and the degree to which patients adhere to treatment recommendations (Mumford et al, 1982; Roter et al, 1995; Stewart, 1995). Pediatric interviewing has been studied extensively by Korsch and her group. These studies looked at the effect of interviewing style on parents' satisfaction and compliance, and documented the importance of skillful interviews (Francis et al, 1969; Korsch et al, 1968). Although speaking directly with children is important, research has not been done on this aspect of interviewing. Investigators such as Ginott (2003) and Gordon (2000) have carefully evaluated children's responses to different styles of questioning, however, and have written extensively about the strategies that seem most effective.

In the sections that follow, vignettes are used to illustrate strategies that enhance effective interviewing (Table 75-1). Throughout, the term *patient* may refer either to the caregiver, usually a parent, or the child or adolescent.

STRATEGIES THAT PROMOTE EFFECTIVE INTERVIEWING

Setting

The characteristics of the room, the arrangement of furniture, the posture of the participants, and the presence of distracters can profoundly affect the quality of the interview. Following a few fundamental guidelines, such as the following, greatly enhances most interactions.

1. The interviewer should be sitting facing the patient at a comfortable distance with no furniture between the two parties. The usual office setting with the physician behind a desk is not optimal. In most offices, it is easy to move the clinician's chair out from behind a desk to face the patient directly.
2. The interviewer should be at the same height as the individual being interviewed. The clinician should not stand to talk to patients who are seated. At a hospital bedside, the clinician should draw up a chair to sit at the bedside with the bed lowered to place the patient at eye level.

Table 75-1. Strategies That Promote Effective Interviewing

Establishing an optimal physical setting
Initiating and supporting the clinician-patient relationship:
- Empathic support
- Repetition and review
- Clarifying language
- Content and process
- Active listening
- Keeping the interview interesting
- Remaining patient-centered

3. If there are multiple family members present, sufficient chairs should be obtained to accommodate all.
4. It is often helpful to have younger children present when parents are being interviewed. If old enough to participate, they should be in chairs alongside the parents. If too young to participate through conversation, toys and sufficient room should be provided for the child to play while the parent is interviewed. The toys should be chosen carefully to prevent excited play that would disrupt the conversation. Drawing materials are usually a good choice.
5. When the interview is emotionally charged, such as when giving bad news, privacy must be assured, and tissues should be available. In a hospital setting, this means moving to a separate room away from the bedside.
6. Finally, distractions, such as phones ringing or people knocking on the door, should be avoided whenever possible. Beepers should be put on vibration. Room-in-use signs should be used to prevent unnecessary intrusions from outside.

Who Should Be Interviewed?

In pediatrics, the strategy of obtaining and imparting information changes as the child patient grows and develops. Beginning in infancy until children are able to verbalize at simple levels, information is obtained primarily from the caregiver, although much can be learned by observing the child interacting with the caregiver in the interview setting. When children have enough language to express some wishes and feelings—usually around age 5 or 6 years—they should be included in the verbal interview. Because attention spans are inherently short at this age, toys or drawing materials allow children some physical activity while the parent is interviewed at length. Clinicians should attempt to control overactive children by removing from reach items that could be broken or by placing themselves or the parents as barriers from areas that are off limits.

In some situations, the young child should remain in the waiting room under someone else's care while the parent is being interviewed. One such circumstance is when the young child is sufficiently disruptive to prevent the clinician and caregiver from conversing. Another circumstance is when the caregiver is observed to be angry and hurtful in what they say about the child. Finally, sometimes the information to be obtained is emotionally charged, such as sexual behavior, and the caregiver does not feel free to discuss the history in the child's presence. Often in developmental-behavioral pediatrics, the sensitive history is already known to the child, however, and may be discussed in the child's presence.

When children are able to provide meaningful information about themselves—usually about age 9 years and older—they should be interviewed separately as well as in the presence of the caregiver.

Initiating and Supporting the Relationship

Much of the information sought during the interview may be difficult for the patient or the caregivers to reveal. The facts of the illness may be embarrassing. Important information may seem private and excessively revealing. The parent may have to reveal mistakes that were made. The information sought and the advice given may provoke strong emotions within the parent or child. And, when the clinician is in the role of giving an opinion or advice, patients should trust that such advice is in their best interest. For all of these reasons, an effective interview requires warmth and trust between the clinician and the patient. If the interviewer is cool, business-like, or judgmental, the patient is likely to distort or withhold information. Establishing, and then supporting, the clinician-patient relationship is vital in accomplishing all the goals of the interview. Following are some of the most important techniques that promote a helpful relationship between clinician and patient.

Empathic Support

Empathy is based on understanding, with sincerity, another's feelings or ideas. This understanding can be expressed verbally or nonverbally. Following is an example of verbal empathy: The mother of a sick child explains that her husband was out of town when her child became ill. The clinician notes that her eyes begin to tear and responds, "You must have felt awfully alone." One can sense that this mother will be able to reveal much more about the child's illness following this support. A nonverbal response might be a hand placed briefly on the parent's arm and a facial expression of concern.

Empathy must be sincere to enhance the interview. To understand someone's predicament but not feel it emotionally is more akin to pity than to empathy. Empathy is enhanced by, but does not require, sharing the patient's experience. One young physician related that she never felt comfortable managing child abuse cases until, being a parent herself, she came to understand how feelings that lead to abuse could develop even in a loving, caring parent. A genuine curiosity about people and a willingness to listen to their thoughts and feelings also promotes empathic understanding.

It is important for the clinician to understand the barriers to providing empathic support. These barriers include being too hurried or reluctant to abandon the formal and factual communication style learned in medical history taking. Also, clinicians may be uncomfortable with tears and other signs of emotion that are often elicited by empathic support. The skilled interviewer must learn to manage emotional situations rather than avoid them. Frequently, the best response to tears is to remain silent, while maintaining eye contact, until the patient regains control. This behavior conveys the unspoken message that such emotions are not out of place and will not impair the patient-clinician communication.

Repetition and Review

Communication is greatly enhanced if the interviewer truly listens to what the parent or patient is saying. One way to indicate directly that the patient has been heard is to repeat what has been said. This repetition can be a succinct summary of a history narrative. In this case, the patient also has the chance to correct any misunderstandings. This technique is particularly helpful in keeping the patient on track, while indicating that the interviewer is listening. Sometimes the most effective repetition is of just one word or phrase repeated with a questioning intonation. Such a repetition invites the patient to clarify what has just been said. The following are examples of these techniques:

Clinician: Tell me about Johnny's illness.
Mother: He started a fever last night. He was up most of the night crying. Actually I wondered if he was sick before that. On Friday he didn't seem hungry, and he vomited after his lunch. His sister, Liz, has been sick all week. Last night he didn't want anything to eat at all. He only drank a little juice. He kept pulling on his ear. Finally he got to sleep in the early morning, but today he has no energy.
Clinician: Let me repeat what I've heard. You first noticed something Friday when he seemed less hungry and vomited once. Then yesterday he developed a fever in the evening and was up most of the night crying. He was also pulling on his ear and wouldn't eat, though he drank a little. How was he during the day yesterday?

This mother rambles a little at the beginning. The clinician's summary clarifies the sequence, lets the mother know he is listening, and gives her the opportunity to correct the story.

In the next example, only one word is repeated:

Clinician: How does he do in school?
Mother: He loves school. He gets almost straight A's. The teacher says he's one of the hardest working boys in his class.
Clinician: Does he have any difficulty in handling gym?
Mother: He tries hard, but most things he just can't do. The teacher lets him do other things like keeping score whenever the games are too hard for him.
Clinician: Does he seem to you to be happy?
Mother: Oh, yes! We don't let his illness get him down.
Clinician: We?

This technique requires careful listening for statements that seem inappropriate or require explanation. It is a technique that can be used frequently and is often quite helpful.

Clarifying Language

A skillful interviewer learns to adapt his or her language to a style and complexity that is familiar to the patient. The way one talks to a college graduate who is a scientist would be different than how one speaks to a manual laborer with little education. It also is important for the interviewer to be aware of words that have many shades of meaning. Words that identify behaviors or emotions are likely to be misunderstood or may mean different things to different people. Words such as *lazy, sensitive, spoiled,* or *angry* should be clarified when they occur during an interview. The interviewer may ask, for example, "What do you mean by lazy?" or, "What makes you think Suzie is spoiled?"

In developmental-behavioral pediatrics diagnostic terms often mean something quite different to patients than to clinicians. It is helpful to ask patients about their understanding of terms such as *retarded, autistic,* or *hyperactive.*

Content and Process

The interviewer should learn to shift back and forth between what is being said (*content*) and how it is being presented (*process*). This skill requires careful listening. Listening to content is straightforward. Listening for process requires paying attention to body language and looking for patterns in a series of responses. The following conversation between the clinician and a mother illustrates this issue:

Mother: I think Bobbie is just too skinny.
Clinician: On my physical exam he looked just fine.
Mother: But his ribs stick out so much.
Clinician: It's okay for his ribs to show that much.
Mother: My friend Jane's boy is just his age and he weighs 5 pounds more.
Clinician: Her son's build may be different. On the growth chart, Bobbie's weight is just right for his build.
Mother: But he eats hardly anything. For breakfast I can't get him to finish even one piece of toast.
Clinician: You know, Mrs. Smith, each time I say that Bobbie seems fine, you bring up another concern. I get the feeling that nothing I say could make you stop worrying about him.

Until this last statement, the physician had been responding each time to what the mother said (content). A pattern of interaction is being established (process), however, and the last statement acknowledges and describes that pattern. Such a comment at this point in the interchange suddenly shifts the focus of communication and usually helps to reveal the real concerns.

Whenever the clinician senses mounting frustration in an interview situation, he or she should consider not only what is being said (content), but also the way it is conveyed (process). Focusing on the quality rather than the content of communication can be seen as critical or intrusive, however, and the patient may become defensive. Timing and the quality of the relationship are important factors to consider. In this next sequence, a straightforward initial history session seems to call for a comment on the style rather than the content of the mother's replies, yet a process statement in this situation would be premature.

Clinician: How long has he had asthma?
Mother: Three or four years. His other doctor said he shouldn't play any sports because he starts wheezing whenever he runs around.
Clinician: Is he on any medicines?
Mother: Yes. He takes an antihistamine, and we keep a nebulizer at home to use whenever he starts to wheeze. He's missed a lot of school. His other doctor said I should keep him home whenever the weather is bad.
Clinician: How many attacks did he have, say, in the last year?
Mother: Just one or two. He's supposed to stay in bed at the first sign of a cold because if he gets an infection you can be sure he'll have a bad attack.

The pattern of the mother's response indicates considerable anxiety, perhaps to the point of overprotection. At this early stage of a new patient-clinician relationship, it would be premature to comment, for example, that "every time I ask a question you are anxious to tell me how easily he gets sick." Instead, an empathic statement such as, "I can see that his asthma has been a real worry," would be more appropriate.

Generally, shifting the focus of attention from what is being said to how it is communicated helps to reveal hidden issues and feelings, which then can be handled more directly. This is one of the most useful techniques in managing a difficult interview, such as when the patient is angry or depressed. This subject is discussed later.

Active Listening

Active listening refers to a response—usually a statement on the part of the interviewer—that indicates the interviewer is hearing the patient and understanding the patient's feelings. This is an especially effective technique when interviewing children. Consider the following example:

Clinician: How are you feeling today?
Patient (a 10-year-old boy hospitalized with cystic fibrosis): I don't like that new intern.
Clinician: Oh? He seems pretty nice to me.
Patient: He poked me five times to get my IV started.
Clinician: I'm sure he tried his best.
Patient: They shouldn't let him start my IV's. He doesn't know how to do it.
Clinician: I bet it really feels good when your IV gets started right the very first time.
Patient: Yeah!

The clinician's comment to this child acknowledges the underlying wish that procedures would go smoothly. A simple, supportive statement, such as "I know it must hurt," would not be as effective as this more active response indicating what a good experience would be like.

Another example is as follows:

Patient (an 8-year-old girl with osteomyelitis, being given antibiotics intravenously): My brother's birthday party is tomorrow.
Clinician: How old will he be?
Patient: He's gonna be six. They're going to a movie. I sure wish I could go.
Clinician: Maybe both of you can go to a movie with your Mom when you get out of the hospital.
Patient: Yeah, but I won't get to see him open his presents.
Clinician: It's kind of lonely being here in the hospital, isn't it?
Patient (tears in eyes): I miss everybody at home. [Pause, followed by brightening.] Judy [the child life worker] is going to help me make a yarn picture for his present.

In this sequence, the active listening consists of hearing the loneliness behind the complaints and apparent refusal to be comforted. When the underlying emotion is acknowledged, one frequently sees the phenomenon illustrated here. The child leaves the complaints behind and involves herself with present activities.

Keeping the Interview Interesting

Often an interview session becomes factual and dry, and the sensitive interviewer becomes aware of feeling bored. By contrast, a lively interview is interesting, and the interviewer and patient are alert. Liveliness stems from patients' emotional involvement with what they are saying. This involvement is particularly important when the goal of history taking is exploration of the interaction between the psychological and physical aspects of the illness. Information related in a dry factual way is likely to be safe material that is easy for the patient to discuss, but not very useful. All of the techniques described earlier serve to make the interview lively. To change the atmosphere of a dry interview, the physician should be observant and prepared to respond to subtle cues indicating the feelings that underlie the patient's words. The skilled interviewer notices the patient's use of unusual words or phrases or subtle changes in facial expression. The following interview of parents of a 12-year-old girl with chronic abdominal pain illustrates this approach:

Clinician: Do you know of anything that might be bothering Mary?
Mother: That's what we can't figure out. She seems so well adjusted.
Father: She plays in the school band. She has lots of friends, and she gets good grades.
Mother: She's really helpful around the house. I can always count on Mary when I need a job done.
Father: She's always been the easy one to discipline. She never seems to complain when we ask things of her. Sometimes I come down kind of hard on the kids, but never with Mary. I don't have to.
Mother (one corner of her mouth turning up to a slight smile).
Clinician: Did you think of something amusing?

Mother: I was remembering the kids last week joking around, mimicking their father being heavy-handed. Mary was joking most of all. Maybe being strict bothers her more than we think.

During this segment of the interview, the parents are painting an idyllic picture of Mary. The clinician just listens and observes closely. The slight change in the mother's expression gives a clue about an intruding thought. Commenting on the changed expression is often all one needs to do to encourage more meaningful information.

Remaining Patient-Centered

Physicians see themselves as givers of expert advice, and medical training reinforces that self-image. The advice-giving role seems to be successful when the patient is accepting and compliant. Two problems develop, however, when the physician-patient interaction is based primarily on the giving and accepting of advice. First, patients may question or reject the advice, but remain reluctant to do so openly because the physician occupies a position of superiority. Instead, the advice is rejected covertly and is manifested in noncompliance. Second, patients may adopt a passive role in the management of health problems and fail to contribute to their own care. It is wise to encourage the resourcefulness and independence of parents and patients. It also is important to solicit patients' ideas about their problem and its treatment.

One technique that fosters the patients' independence is to ask for their thoughts about the nature of the illness—what caused it and how it should be managed. Two useful questions are: "What did you think might be the problem?" and "What did you hope to get from this visit?" The patient might respond that he or she expected the clinician to determine the nature of the problem. A response to this might be: "It is my job to find out what's wrong, but sometimes parents have a notion about what might be the problem, and it would be helpful to know about your thoughts."

In the following example questioning the parent about her thoughts reveals concerns often categorized as "the vulnerable child syndrome" (Green and Solnit, 1964).

Mother (of a 2-year-old with fever): He became ill so suddenly!
Clinician: He has a fever of 103°F, but I don't find any signs of bacterial infection, so it is probably a virus.
Mother: He seems to be breathing funny.
Clinician: I've checked his lungs and heart, and both are okay.
Mother: Why would he get sick so quickly?
Clinician: Viruses often affect a child that way.
Mother: Are you sure there isn't any infection?
Clinician: Yes. [Pause.] What do you think might be wrong?
Mother: He was premature and had trouble breathing in the nursery. He was so sick! They had him on a respirator for several days. I worry so that his lungs are weak because of that.

Because of the patient's earlier problem as an infant, this mother is now sensitive that any illness may be a sequel of that episode. The clinician's question helps to bring out the reason for her unrealistic worries. Because the mother's concerns have been revealed, the clinician knows that whenever this child becomes ill he or she should respond by specifically reassuring the mother about the consequences of the problem in infancy.

Another helpful technique is to encourage and support the patient's attempt to find solutions to the problem. This approach is illustrated in the following exchange:

Father: I've been concerned about Mark's wheezing whenever he runs hard. I'm afraid he's not going to learn to play and interact with the other boys.
Clinician: Does he stay away from the other kids when they're having fun?
Father: Well, yes; he hasn't gone out for soccer or football.
Clinician: Does he do anything else with other children?
Father: Yeah. He wrestles around, and he rides his bike. He asked us the other day if he could take karate or wrestling.
Clinician: What did you think about that?
Father: You know, I think he's figuring out how to pick sports that don't have a lot of running. Maybe we should let him try those and see if his asthma will be okay.

By remaining noncommittal and encouraging the father to continue his own internal conversation, the clinician has helped him come to his own conclusions. The father's solutions are more likely to be acted on than any ideas the clinician might generate.

Difficult Interview

In this section, the techniques already described are brought to bear on three of the most commonly encountered difficulties in the interview situation—the patient who talks too much, the patient who talks too little, and the angry patient. The patient who talks too much produces frustration because the clinician cannot control the interview, and precious time is used in unproductive ways. Patients who talk too little provoke the clinician into overly dominant participation, asking more and more questions and even suggesting responses. Most clinicians experience the greatest difficulty, however, in handling the angry, demanding patient. This patient provokes the clinician into a defensive stance and feelings of irritation and anger.

Overly Talkative Patient

When excessive talking is encountered, one should determine if this pattern is due to the patient's style, which means it is typical of that individual's verbal interaction in all situations. Alternatively, there may be emotional reasons for excessive talkativeness in the particular interviewing situation. The overly talkative individual is often tangential and verbally disorganized. An overly talkative individual also may obsessively overqualify everything he or she says.

In the case of the loosely organized and disjointed account, it is useful to interrupt, using the technique of repetition and review to do so tactfully. The following exchange illustrates this approach:

Clinician: How long has she been sick?
Mother: About 2 days, No, maybe a week or so. Last week she didn't look good on Tuesday. I thought she might be coming down with something then. Dr. Jones told me that I should watch if she ever got diarrhea. You know she had a really bad bout of that a couple of years ago.
Clinician (interrupting): You're uncertain, then, whether her illness began 2 days ago or started last week?
Mother: No. The fever began 2 days ago.
Clinician: After you noted the fever, what happened next?

The next vignette illustrates the obsessive verbal style. The best approach is to interrupt while repeating the question and giving permission to omit detail:

Clinician: When did you first notice his school problem?
Mother: He's always had trouble in school. Well, actually, it's only been since kindergarten, about the middle part of kindergarten. Let's see—was it before Christmas? No, he still had Mrs. Brown as a teacher then. No, Mrs. Brown didn't start until February some time.
Clinician (interrupting): I wondered when you first noticed his problem. I only need to know in a general way.
Mother: Oh. [Pause.] Somewhere in the middle of kindergarten.

Sometimes, excessive talking reflects the parents' need to ventilate. This is more likely to be the case in a first interview or when an emotional incident is part of the account. A statement that acknowledges the need to ventilate (a process statement) can sometimes shorten this period, while still satisfying the parents' emotional need. The following interview with parents of a 7-year-old-boy who is having problems in school illustrates these points:

Clinician: Tell me about Adam's problems.
Mother: We were really shocked. The teacher told us last week that they want to hold him back. Up until then we had no idea he was having difficulty.
Father: His kindergarten teacher said he was a little immature, but would probably grow out of it, but they didn't do anything else. We asked if he should be tested, but they said "no."
Mother: I think the kindergarten teacher just let him play with blocks while the others did their school work. We were really mad when we found that out.
Father: We think he might have been okay if they had helped him. Instead they just let him do what he wanted.
Mother: This year we wanted to be sure they didn't ignore him, so we asked the teacher to keep in touch with us. She kept saying not to worry. Then they dropped this bombshell on us. We're about to take this whole thing to the superintendent.
Clinician: I can see that you are very upset with the school. I would like to hear more about that, but first I wonder if you think Adam has any kind of problem. Did you come mainly because of the school's concerns?
Father: Oh, no. We've been concerned about how hard it seems for him to learn his letters.
Mother: And sometimes he seems so much younger than the others in his grade.

In this example, the parents indicate their willingness to shift the focus to their child. Sometimes the need to ventilate is so strong that the parent cannot shift attention elsewhere. In this case, the interviewer may need to be more direct: "I can see that you would like to talk about this. However, we have only 15 minutes. Should we use that time to discuss this subject?" This is an effective way of handling such a situation. The clinician establishes the limits and gives the patient the choice of how to use the time.

Reticent Patient

Talking very little also may stem from the patient's long established style or reflect psychological factors operating in the particular interview setting. The patient who is stylistically nontalkative has a long history of poor verbal skill. Such people may have a limited vocabulary and difficulties with grammar and syntax. These problems may be accentuated by low self-esteem in the presence of the more verbal clinician. If style is the basis of the reticence, the clinician should resist the natural tendency to ask more questions and instead learn to cultivate silences punctuated by facilitative phrases, such as, "Tell me more about that." Or "What's that like for you?" Empathic statements may be helpful, such as, "I know this must be hard to talk about," or "It's difficult to find the right words."

When reticence is due to psychological factors, the nontalkative response is usually based on lack of trust, especially when psychosocial information is being sought. Patients with a history of problems with authorities are particularly likely to be distrustful and nontalkative. Increasing trust is usually a long-term goal, but a more immediate technique is to comment on the style of the interview (process) as it begins to emerge out of the content. The following interview, with a 16-year-old boy living in a drug rehabilitation unit, referred because of stomach pain, illustrates this technique:

Clinician: Tell me about your stomach pain.
Patient: What do you want to know?
Clinician: When did it start? What was it like?
Patient: I dunno. Just a pain.
Clinician: Could you describe it for me?
Patient: Nothing special.
Clinician: Does anything make it better or worse?
Patient: Nope.
Clinician: I've asked several questions and you haven't said very much. I get the feeling this pain hasn't bothered you.
Patient: That's right. They made me come.

When it is clear to the physician that very little information is going to be offered, it is helpful, as illustrated here, to comment on the style of the interaction. This boy's response confirms the hunch that his reticence is due to psychological factors. It may not be true that he is unconcerned about his pain, but this is the stance he has chosen to take, and the history will continue to be unproductive unless his feelings change. Sometimes the confrontation of a process statement improves communication because the patient, after he has asserted his rebellion, may experience less need to maintain it.

Angry Patient

Patients who are angry seem to aim that anger at the clinician, but frequently these patients are frustrated by their inability to affect what is happening to them. They may be upset with the medical problem that has so disrupted their lives and the low income that fails to meet their needs. The anger often provokes a defensive response in the clinician. It is important to avoid this defensive reaction. The most useful technique is to recognize and then identify the demand that is implicit in the expression of anger. While the patient is talking, it helps to ask oneself, "What does this person want?" and "What does he or she want from me?" The following sequence illustrates this point:

Father: This hospital is run by a bunch of incompetents.
Clinician: What's the problem?
Father: We've been waiting an hour. My boy is in pain and no one seems to care. They haven't even given him any pain medicine, though I begged them to.
Clinician: I can see he is in pain. The staff has instructions not to give medicines before he is examined, and everyone has been tied up with a very bad accident.
Father: I've seen several people just standing around. Someone could have called another doctor. I asked them to.
Clinician: I came as quickly as I could.
Father: Why didn't they call someone else?
Clinician: I don't know. [Pause.] What would you like me to do?
Father: I know it's not your fault. I've been sitting around here fuming, and I had to get it off my chest.

Some individuals are continually frustrated by their inability to affect what happens to them and respond habitually by making demands of others. Such individuals are usually ineffectual and have difficulty in accepting responsibility for their own choices. Instead they find it easier to blame their frustrations on others. The following interview illustrates a typical situation with this type of parent, in this case, a mother of a 6-year old-boy with school problems. Attention-deficit/hyperactivity disorder has been diagnosed, and treatment with stimulant medication has begun.

Mother: What am I going to do when the teacher calls and wants me to take him home because she can't handle him?
Clinician: Hopefully the medication will help, and that won't happen anymore.
Mother: It happened last week. Sometimes the medicine doesn't help enough.
Clinician: We've talked to the school about different methods of handling him. They will put him with the resource teacher when he is difficult.
Mother: Yeah, but she's not any good at managing him.
Clinician: Is there anyone at the school who you think can handle him well?
Mother: No.
Clinician: Well, then, maybe he's better off coming home when that happens.
Mother: But I can't be around all the time just in case they can't manage.
Clinician: What would you like to see happen?
Mother: I don't know.
Clinician: Do you see any alternatives other than those we've discussed?
Mother: I guess I could let the school try their plan.

In the middle of this discussion, the clinician should sense that he is responding with suggestions that the mother repeatedly rejects. This style is best handled by encouraging the parent to take responsibility for developing approaches to the problem.

History Taking—Effective Questioning

All of the above-described strategies that promote the clinician-patient relationship also enhance the ability to obtain useful information. In addition to those techniques, this section addresses the issue of skillful questioning.

Open-ended questions are questions that allow the patient a wide latitude of response. This type of question is especially important at the beginning of a history-taking session. Examples include: "What brings you to the clinic today?" or "What can I do for you today?" Such general questions encourage patients to explain issues in their own words. When such a question begins an interview, it is tempting for the clinician, especially if rushed, to interrupt by asking specific questions, such as, "Is she having trouble learning?" or "Is he overly active?" When patients are allowed to complete their opening complaint, they often answer such questions. More importantly, they often provide additional information that might not otherwise be given.

When the patients have completed their opening statement, the clinician may ask progressively more specific questions to help clarify the story. This sequence is referred to as the "open-to-closed cone" (Cole and Bird, 2005).

In addition to questions, many phrases can be used to encourage patients to say more. Examples include: "And then ..."; or "Tell me more." Such phrases should be followed by a pause long enough to allow the patient to respond. These facilitative phrases are especially helpful when the patient is reticent or relatively nonverbal.

Toward the end of an interview, a very useful phrase is, "What else?" or "Is there anything more?" Patients often hold back on part of the story because they are embarrassed, or they think their ideas are not important. Such phrases may lead to important information.

In developmental-behavioral pediatrics, it also is important to ask, "What brings you here now?" because the problem has usually been present several months, or even years. It also may be helpful to ask, "What did you hope would happen as the result of today's appointment?" This is another way to learn about the family's expectations.

Leading questions should be avoided. Patients often respond to leading questions by giving the clinician the answer they believe the clinician wants. The following is an example:

Clinician: Did he begin the medication last month?
Mother: Yes. He's been taking it every day.
Clinician: Did it help him with his behavior?

The clinician, by asking this way, implies that he expects the medication to help, and it may be hard for the mother to give an honest answer. A better question would be, "Did the medicine seem to do anything to change his behavior?" If the mother responds in the affirmative, a good follow-up question would be, "What change did you notice?"

Discussing Diagnosis and Treatment

At the conclusion of the assessment process, the clinician is charged with providing a diagnosis or conclusion and a plan for treatment. Initially, trainees may approach this task from the vantage point of authority—knowing what is best for patients or their parents. The experienced clinician learns that soliciting feedback during these conversations leads to better acceptance of the diagnosis and better compliance with recommendations. This section reviews some techniques that enhance this aspect of communication.

Soliciting Patient's Ideas and Understanding

Before giving a diagnostic conclusion or a treatment suggestion, it is always best to hear the patient's thoughts (see the earlier section on remaining patient-centered). Almost always patients come to the diagnostic process with ideas or fears about what is wrong and opinions about how the condition should be treated. These ideas often come from relatives, friends, or the child's teacher. If such ideas support the clinician's conclusions, they can be used to enhance the treatment recommendations. Often the patient's ideas are misunderstandings of the condition or its treatment, however, and this misunderstanding needs to be addressed if treatment is to be successful.

Similarly, there may be several possible approaches to treatment and patients or their families may be willing to accept some and not others. Knowing their thoughts before entering a discussion of treatment helps clinicians to direct their plan first to what is acceptable to the family.

The clinician also should be aware of the need to address patients' fears. Frequently, parents are unwilling to voice their fears, which may seem to them to be silly or scary. Parents may fear, for example, that their child may be crazy or may end up just like Uncle Joe who is in jail. The clinician might ask, for example, "What do you think Jimmy's problem might be?" and, "What are your thoughts about what will happen to Jimmy in the future?"

Discussing Diagnostic Conclusions

Clinicians should begin the discussion with a clear and straightforward statement of their conclusions. Especially when the diagnosis means giving bad news, this statement should be accompanied by additional hope-giving information, such as, "There is much we can do for this condition," or "I will work with you to do as much as we can for Johnny." At this point, the clinician should pause and assess the parent's or patient's reaction. The response may range from stunned silence to tears or an immediate torrent of questions. These reactions would each require a different response. If silence is the response, it would be helpful to ask something such as, "What are you thinking?" Tears would require an empathic response, allowing parents time to get their emotions under control. This process of checking for reactions and responding accordingly should be followed throughout the discussion. Of course, questions should be answered, and it is a mistake not to allow sufficient time for questions.

Discussing Treatment Plans

Clinicians should outline their treatment plans clearly and briefly, perhaps modifying them based on the family's ideas and understanding of the condition. The clinician should pause to assess the patient's response. A general question might be, "How does this seem to you?" Then, as more detail is discussed, clinicians should check for reactions and respond accordingly. It is particularly important to determine if the family has tried any of these suggestions previously. If so, the clinician should learn what happened, and how the family perceived the attempt. It also is helpful to see if the parent or patient has ideas about other treatments not mentioned by the clinician. An open-ended question might be, "Do you have any other thoughts about treatment?"

Motivational Interviewing

Motivational interviewing is a special approach that employs most of the techniques discussed earlier, but also employs some special strategies. The goal of motivational interviewing is to improve adherence with behavioral change recommendations. To accomplish this goal, motivational interviewing helps patients explore and resolve their ambivalence about change. When the ambivalence has been identified, the clinician and patient explore the negative and positive aspects of behavioral change choices made by the patient and the relationship between proposed behavioral change and the patient's personal values ("change talk"). Motivational interviewing has been studied in adult populations, but has not yet been evaluated in children, where the parents must be the focus of the approach. The technique shows promise, however, in addressing behavioral change in adolescents. The interested reader should explore the appropriate references (Miller and Rollnick, 2002; Rollnick et al, 1999).

SUMMARY

The interview is described as a conversation between clinician and patient aimed at (1) establishing a relationship, (2) collecting information, and (3) imparting information about diagnosis and treatment. Techniques that enhance effective interviewing include providing a supportive setting, deciding whom to interview, and initiating and supporting the relationship. The relationship is enhanced by (1) empathic support, (2) repetition and review, (3) clarifying language, (4) attending to content and process, (5) use of active listening, (6) keeping the interview interesting, and (7) remaining patient-centered. Interviewing a difficult patient is reviewed using these relationship-enhancing techniques. Suggestions are given on how to question effectively and how best to impart information or advice. In addition, strategies are described to enhance the discussion of diagnostic conclusions and treatment plans. Finally, the more recently developed area of motivational interviewing is briefly described.

REFERENCES

Cole SA, Bird J: The Medical Interview, 2nd ed. St. Louis, Mosby, 2005.

Francis V, Korsch BM, Morris MJ: Gaps in doctor-patient communication: Patient's response to medical advice. N Engl J Med 280:535-540, 1969.

Ginott H: Between Parent and Child: The Bestselling Classic That Revolutionized Parent-Child Communication. New York, Three Rivers Press, 2003.

Gordon T: Parent Effectiveness Training: The Proven Program for Raising Responsible Children. New York, Three Rivers Press, 2000.

Green M, Solnit AJ: Reactions to the threatened loss of a child: The vulnerable child syndrome. Pediatrics 34:58-66, 1964.

Korsch BM, Gozzi EK, Francis V: Gaps in doctor-patient communication, 1: Doctor-patient interaction and patient satisfaction. Pediatrics 42:855-871, 1968.

Miller WR, Rollnick S: Motivational Interviewing: Preparing People for Change, 2nd ed. New York, Guilford Publications, 2002.

Mumford E, Schlesinger HJ, Glass GV: The effects of psychological intervention on recovery from surgery and heart attacks: An analysis of the literature. Am J Public Health 72:141-151, 1982.

Rollnick SR, Mason P, Butler C: Health Behavior Change. Edinburgh, Churchill Livingstone, 1999.

Roter DL, Hall JA, Kern DE, et al: Improving physicians' interviewing skills and reducing patients' emotional distress. Arch Intern Med 155:1877-1884, 1995.

Stewart MA: Effective physician-patient communication and health outcomes: A review. Can Med Assoc J 152:1423-1433, 1995.

GENERAL REVIEWS

Coleman WL: The interview. *In* Levine MD, Carey WB, Crocker AC (eds): Developmental-Behavioral Pediatrics, 3rd ed. Philadelphia, WB Saunders, 1999, pp 663-676.

Dixon SD, Stein MT: Encounters with Children, 4th ed. St. Louis, Mosby, 2005.

Korsch B: Talking with Parents. *In* Parker S, Zuckerman B, Augustyn M (eds). Developmental and Behavioral Pediatrics, 2nd ed. Philadelphia, Lippincott Williams & Wilkins, 2005.

76 THE LAYING ON OF HANDS: THE PHYSICAL EXAMINATION IN DEVELOPMENTAL AND BEHAVIORAL ASSESSMENT

RANDALL PHELPS AND HEIDI M. FELDMAN

Vignettes

Terri

Terri is a quiet 6-year-old girl, brought by her parents to the developmental-behavioral pediatrician because they want to know the cause of her developmental delays and unusual behaviors. She has a history of seizures, currently well controlled on anticonvulsants. Her parents describe her as slow to warm up, socially limited in interactions with other children, and unable to communicate fully her needs and wants.

When the pediatrician approaches her, Terri averts her gaze and stiffens. He offers his hands and patiently waits until the child places her hands on his. Using a calm and reassuring tone of voice, he prepares the child for each maneuver. She gradually calms and passively allows him to complete the examination, including an examination of her skin using a Wood's lamp. He notes several small, hypomelanotic macules with irregular borders on her trunk and lower extremities. He also notes a smooth, firm, flesh-colored plaque over her sacrum. The parents comment that their daughter had never before allowed a physician to complete a comprehensive physical examination.

Jason

Jason is a 10-year-old boy who has been diagnosed with attention-deficit/hyperactivity disorder, oppositional defiant disorder, and conduct disorder. He is on multiple medications. His mother brings him to the pediatrician, asking whether he might have bipolar disorder. When the pediatrician enters the room, Jason and his mother are sitting on opposite sides of the room. He shoots the pediatrician an angry stare and does not offer his hand when she offers hers for a handshake. He glowers when she asks him questions. His mother quickly answers for him. His mother enumerates his many behavioral difficulties and cannot identify any of Jason's assets when asked directly. After the history, the pediatrician asks Jason's mother to go to the waiting room so that she can complete a physical examination.

Alone with the boy, the pediatrician fails to break the ice with her usual questions. After explaining what she will do, she begins the physical examination by first asking to see his hands. He reluctantly complies. She then asks him to squeeze her fingers. He seems to relish squeezing them a little too hard. She laughs, compliments his strength, and playfully asks him to stop before he breaks her fingers. She tests strength of multiple muscle groups of the upper extremities. Jason begins to smile, and then to laugh, as he pushes and pulls against her resistance. His expression softens. She offers him the opportunity to listen to his heart, which he accepts and enjoys. By the time she has completed the physical examination, the glower is gone. She repeats questions that she had asked previously. Jason admits he is angry because his father got custody of his younger brother and his mother got custody of him. Now, he cries, he doesn't even have his brother as a buffer from his mother.

Developmental-behavioral diagnosis is primarily based on history. Some professionals in developmental-behavioral medicine, such as psychiatrists and psychologists, have largely dispensed with the physical examination. The information obtained during a physical examination may not be diagnostic or essential. Even if there are revealing physical findings, when children are followed closely in a competent medical home or seen by many different subspecialists, many of those findings may have been previously enumerated and interpreted.

Nevertheless, the physical examination serves as a valuable component of the diagnostic workup in developmental-behavioral pediatrics for three reasons.

First, the examination may reveal subtle or previously missed findings that provide the explanation for a developmental disorder. In the first vignette, the examination provided information leading to the diagnosis of tuberous sclerosis. Second, the physical examination offers the clinician an opportunity to model for caregivers approaches that promote calmness and cooperation. In the first vignette, the examination showed how an uncooperative child could be gently encouraged to cooperate. Third, the physical examination offers an opportunity to create an emotional connection with a child. Particularly after the physician has obtained a long history in which the child has been only rarely involved, the physical examination allows the clinician to link back with the child, using a combination of physical and nonphysical means. In the second vignette, the examination eventually relaxed the oppositional child and allowed him to reveal his true feelings. The response of the child to kind and supportive interactions in such cases provides a wealth of information, often as relevant to diagnosis as the physical findings.

When done skillfully, the physical examination contributes to the positive relationship between clinicians, parents, and children, increasing the chances that the child and family will participate in treatment planning and adhere to the management plans. The physical examination may be particularly useful for generalists and subspecialists in evaluating new patients and evaluating new problems in established patients.

CONDUCTING THE PHYSICAL EXAMINATION

The physical examination is usually best done after the history. Information collected during the interview guides the physical examination. By the completion of the interview, especially if the clinician makes efforts to engage the child in the discussion, a shy or fearful child may have had an adequate chance to warm up or relax.

To establish a positive relationship, the physical examination should begin with conversation with the child. Simple questions, such as the child's favorite foods or the name of the family's pet, serve to show the supportive nature of the interaction. Repositioning of seating may be helpful to demarcate the actual physical examination from the conversational part of the assessment. Whenever possible, the examiner should be seated comfortably at eye level with the child. The examination should proceed in a systematic and calm manner, allowing the examiner to introduce each part of the examination as it proceeds and to provide reassurance when necessary.

In examining preschoolers, school-age children, and adolescents, we advocate starting with a request to see the patient's hands. Many pediatricians begin the examination of older children similar to the way they examine an infant—by laying a stethoscope on the chest. The advantage of starting with the hands is that the maneuver is unintimidating, akin to familiar acts, such as shaking hands. For a shy or fearful child, the clinician can remain relatively remote, moving closer only as the child's behavior suggests he or she is ready. After the child places his or her hands in the clinician's, the clinician may ask a question about a ring or a bruise or some other distinctive features of the hands. This moment provides an opportunity to assess social and communication skills.

We proceed to test upper extremity tone and strength, joint range of motion, dexterity, rapid alternating movements, and right-left discrimination. These tasks are almost invariably amusing to preschoolers and school-age children, and yet are not as arousing as gross motor testing. If the child is uncooperative or highly impulsive, this part of the examination allows the clinician to try various maneuvers to encourage cooperation or organization. The clinician can impose physical limits on the child so that he or she cannot grab at tools, or the clinician can offer social rewards in the form of praise for cooperation. The child is typically visibly relaxed after this portion of the examination.

With a cooperative school-age child, we proceed from evaluation of the upper extremities to various maneuvers to assess informally neurologic soft signs, working memory, short-term memory, verbal abilities, organizational skills, and spontaneous recall from categories (Holden et al, 1983; Stinnett et al, 2002). Neurologic soft signs are not pathognomonic of disorders. Also, behavior in the office may not be representative of functional abilities in the world. These maneuvers allow the clinician to sample behaviors, however, and to observe how the child handles a set of challenges. These procedures often show the symptoms that brought the child to the evaluation, demonstrating to parents that the clinician understands their concerns.

We ask the child to show right-left discrimination on body parts, progressing from single body parts ("show me your left hand"), to crossed commands ("put your right hand on your left ear"), to right-left discrimination on others ("show me my left hand") and crossed commands ("shake my right hand with your right hand"). Some children can perform accurately at first, but then impulsively begin to anticipate the command before it is actually given. Other children cannot remember the crossed commands. We also ask the child to do a digit span forward, expecting that he or she will be able to recall about 2 less than his or her age to a maximum of 6 to 7. We follow this task with digit span backward, expecting the child to do 2 less than he or she did on digit span forward. Some children with apparently good attention are unable to remember more than a couple of digits. Some children with a good forward digit span cannot perform the reverse span, suggestive of problems of short-term memory and executive function (Stinnett et al, 2002).

It also is informative to see how the parents relate to the child during these maneuvers. Some parents reprimand the child when he or she becomes impulsive or giggle when the child makes a mistake. When parents are present, we ask whether the behaviors we are observing seem characteristic of their child and related to their concerns.

With the patient still seated, we proceed with the standard pediatric physical examination, from head to toe. We conclude the examination by assessing the patient's

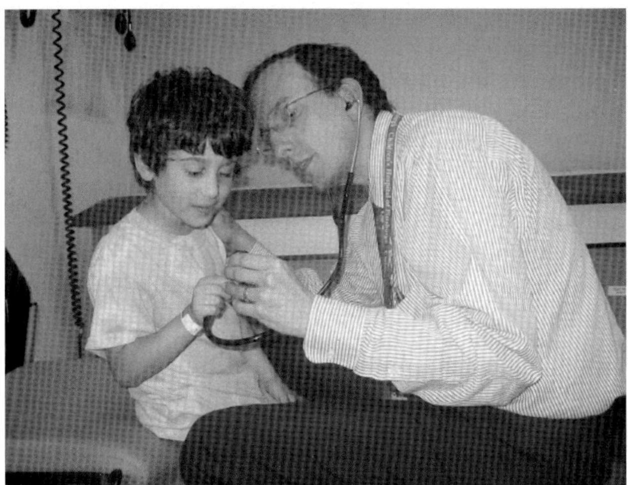

Figure 76-1. Physical examination of a child with a high activity level and poor attentional skills may be facilitated through physical containment by body positioning and engaging the child's interests.

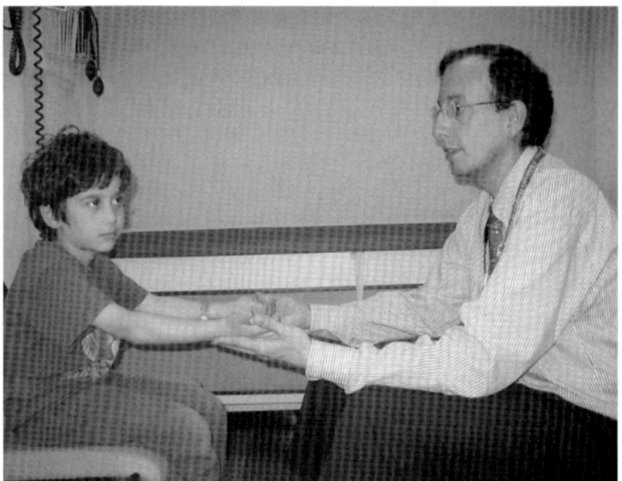

Figure 76-2. Physical examination of a child who is fearful, worried, shy, or socially unskilled may be facilitated by maintaining distance, avoiding the child's eye-to-eye gaze, and minimizing physical contact.

gross motor skills, concurrent with his or her ability to follow a set of commands and to hold postures for long periods despite noises and distractions. These maneuvers again provide insight into the child's ability to remember commands, coordinate movements, and control impulses (Holden et al, 1983; Stinnett et al, 2002). Throughout the examination, we continue to prepare the patient for each step. We voice appreciation for cooperation, and remark on positive features or good performances.

For children with behavioral problems, the physical examination allows the clinician to model effective, creative, and compassionate behavioral approaches for families. Containment by strategic positioning, engaging the child's interests, and gentle but firm redirection promote participation in a child with hyperactivity and impulsivity (Fig. 76-1). Playful transitions can lure an oppositional child into participation. A preschooler who refuses verbal entreaties to participate in testing and continues to loll around on the floor may respond positively to the offer to "fly in a helicopter" over to the table. Children who are shy and slow to warm up may respond to a gentle, calm approach. Children with autism may require some maneuvers to be done at a distance without any physical touch (Fig. 76-2). Children who have difficulties with transitions benefit from frequent reminders of what comes next.

BEHAVIORAL OBSERVATION

Informal and semistructured behavioral observations during the history and physical examination are essential to the diagnostic evaluation. We carefully observe children from the moment we first see them. We typically have toys available in the examination room. How the child plays, the activity level of the child, and the child's attention span may be interpreted, with some caution, from watching the child during the visit. Although a child may play differently in the clinic than at home, observations of unstructured play are a useful complement to parent and teacher reports. In addition to insights into play skills and interests, free play offers a prime opportunity to watch for stereotypic or other repetitive movements, hyperactivity, impulsivity, oppositionality, and tics.

We routinely ask children to work on drawings of themselves and their families during the history. Drawings provide insights regarding family dynamics and visuomotor development and attention span. Asking children about their drawings is a way to obtain a language sample from a child who is unwilling to engage in other conversations (Dixon and Stein, 2006). Some children do not like to draw. It is informative to see how they handle frustration or stress.

It is useful to organize behavioral observations into functional domains to complement data collected during the interview and questionnaires. The activities and participation domains of the International Classification of Functioning, Disability and Health (ICF) (Table 76-1), developed by the World Health Organization in 2002 (World Health Organization, 2003), provide a useful organizing framework for the data. The ICF is designed to assess function regardless of health condition or diagnostic labels. The ICF interprets functioning at three levels of analysis: body structures and functions, activities of daily living, and social participation. The findings within activities and social participation domains can serve as a "review of functioning," which complements the "review of systems" of the traditional medical model.

We pay particular attention to communication skills throughout the interview and during the physical examination because of the importance of communication in children's lives and the underidentification of communication disorders. We consider the size and diversity of the vocabulary; the length, complexity, and grammaticality of sentences; and the intelligibility and accuracy of articulation. In addition to the quality and quantity of speech, how the child uses speech and nonverbal communication to participate in conversation or regulate his or her own behavior is telling. Prosody (intonation) and semantics (meaning) of speech

Table 76-1. **Behavioral Observations of Functional Abilities, Organized According to the Domains of Activity and Participation from the International Classification of Functioning, Disability, and Health (ICF)**

ICF Domain	Preschool Children	School-Age Children
Learning and applying knowledge	Quality of drawings Ability to identify letters and numbers and to count Ability to remember the name of the reflex hammer	Skills in reading, writing, and arithmetic Quality of drawings Memory of the drawing assignment
General tasks and demands	Activity level Degree of impulsivity Ability to handle frustrations, such as waiting or stress, such as an otoscopic examination	Ability to entertain self with play or schoolwork Activity level Ability to focus and remember Organization of thought and verbal communication
Communication	Maturity and clarity of speech Use of nonverbal communication Ability to initiate conversation and maintain topic Diversity of communication functions	Conversational ability Pragmatic skills Ability to relate stories or describe events Sample of written communication
Self-care	Toileting, including use of diaper or request to use bathroom Dressing after examination Level of hygiene	Grooming Ability to tie shoes after examination
Mobility	Walking Running Hopping or skipping	Stressed gaits Fine motor control
Interpersonal interactions	Greetings Response to praise Ability to maintain joint focus of attention Nature of parent-child interactions	Humor Empathy Initiation of conversation Response to conversation Nature of parent-child interactions

also can be an important clue in diagnostic assessment (see Chapter 72).

The evaluation of self-care skills relies heavily on parent report. Informal observations during the interview and the physical examination can add valuable information, however. How independent is the preschooler in initiating a request to go to the bathroom or to have a snack? How much help does the child receive in eating? Does the child participate in clean-up afterwards? How does the child manage dressing after the physical examination? How is the school-age child dressed? Are the child's hands clean?

The physical examination offers opportunities for assessing mobility. In addition to moving about through space, we try to assess fine motor skills in the physical examination, particularly in school-age children, for whom writing and drawing are important tasks.

Direct observations of parent-child interactions and clinician-child interactions contribute significantly to the assessment of social skills. The child may act quite differently in the clinic than in his or her natural environment. Nervousness may induce unusual awkwardness or silliness. Fear may inspire compliance with requests. The clinician must acknowledge that a child's interactions with him or her may not accurately reflect that child's social skills with family at home or with peers. Nevertheless, observations of social interactions even in the clinic setting can be very informative. Does the child notice when the examiner enters the room? How does the child respond to a greeting? How does the child respond to humor? Does the child look to parents for reassurance? Does the child look to parents for comfort? Does the child initiate social interactions or seek to share success? Finally, how does the parent interact with the child?

RELEVANT PHYSICAL FINDINGS

Growth and Physical Maturity

Crucial data that should be collected in every developmental assessment are growth measurements and indicators of physical maturity. Physical development including height and weight, head size, and sexual development may provide clues important to diagnosis. Head size should be measured in all patients presenting for developmental assessment, regardless of age. The thyroid should be consistently evaluated, which includes not only palpation of the gland itself, but also assessment of hair and skin texture and evaluation of the relaxation phase of the deep tendon reflexes. Table 76-2 summarizes the implications of various features of growth and maturity.

Abnormal Findings

A set of major and minor malformations may allow for the diagnosis of a specific syndrome, such as Down syndrome, fragile X syndrome, fetal alcohol syndrome, or Williams syndrome. Identifying the specific syndrome in the case of children with multiple dysmorphic features has implications for the assessment of current functioning, prognosis, and recurrence risk in the family. Children with abnormal findings should be referred for a comprehensive genetic evaluation. Some major and minor dysmorphic features do not point to a specific diagnosis, but indicate possible abnormalities of brain morphogenesis, and have implications for developmental evaluation and prognosis (Table 76-3) (Jones, 2006). Interpretation of any specific finding must be made carefully because many of these features occur in a small percentage of individuals with typical development.

Table 76-2. **Possible Diagnostic Significance of Abnormal Findings in Growth and Sexual Maturation**

Abnormal Findings	Possible Significance
Short stature, height percentile > weight percentile	Calorie deficiency
Short stature, height percentile < weight percentile	Endocrine abnormality
Short stature, height percentile = weight percentile	Genetic or constitutional causes
Tall stature	Fragile X syndrome, Weaver syndrome, Sotos syndrome
Microcephaly	Abnormal brain development
Macrocephaly	Abnormal brain development, autism spectrum disorder
Enlarged fontanelle	Thyroid deficiency

Table 76-3. **Nonspecific Dysmorphic Features Associated with Anomalous Brain Development**

Body Part	Dysmorphic Features	Pathogenesis/Possible Significance
Cranium	Microcephaly	Reduced brain growth
	Asymmetry	Premature suture fusion, deforming external forces, or abnormal underlying brain growth
Hair	Absent or multiple (>2) parietal whorls	Abnormal brain development 10-16 weeks' gestation
	"Cowlick," or anterior upsweep of scalp hair	Posterior displacement of junction of parietal and frontal hair streams, resulting from reduced frontal brain development
Eyes	Short palpebral fissures	Deficient frontal brain growth
	Up-slanted palpebral fissures	Relatively deficient frontal brain growth compared with midface growth
Ears	Low set (below top of helix below outer canthi)	Delayed morphogenesis, fetal pattern of ear position
	Posterior rotation (axis tilted backward >15 degrees	Delayed morphogenesis, fetal pattern of posterior ear rotation
Mouth	High arched	Persistent lateral palatal ridges, indicative of oral hypotonia or other oral-motor dysfunction

Table 76-4. **Miscellaneous Physical Examination Findings of Developmental or Behavioral Significance**

Finding	Possible Significance
Tonsillar hypertrophy	Obstructive sleep apnea
Alopecia	Trichotillomania, stereotypies involving scalp
Ecchymoses over soft tissues	Nonaccidental trauma
Bitten nails, cuticles, calluses	Self-mutilation, stereotypies
Characteristic scars	Self-cutting
Discoloration of dorsum of hand, posterior molar acid damage, parotid hyperplasia	Bulimia nervosa

Findings on dermatologic examination may be indicative of various neurocutaneous syndromes. In the first vignette at the beginning of the chapter, the findings are consistent with the diagnosis of tuberous sclerosis. Many other findings on the general physical examination are pertinent to developmental assessment. Table 76-4 presents examples of such findings.

Neurologic Examination

The neurologic examination is a crucial component of the developmental assessment because it may provide evidence for neurologic immaturity or focal neurologic injury. A systematic assessment of the evolution of complex reflexes can indicate neurodevelopmental delay, such as is seen in global developmental delay, or neurodevelopmental deviance, such as is seen in cerebral palsy. A systematic approach, as in the Milani-Comparetti Motor Development Screening Test, evaluates the child's posture and tone in many different positions, the development of motor skills, the evolution of primitive reflexes, and protective responses to rapid movement (Trembath et al, 1977).

Careful examination of cranial nerve function may help in elucidating focal lesions. Table 76-5 provides

Table 76-5. Significance of Findings on Examination of Cranial Nerves

Finding	Possible Significance
Vertical nystagmus	Brainstem dysfunction
Horizontal or rotary nystagmus	Congenital abnormality, vestibular abnormality, medication side effect
Pupil asymmetry	Intracranial mass effect, midbrain dysfunction, optic nerve abnormality, medication side effect Associated with ptosis and anhydrosis: Horner syndrome (*Note*: 10% of children have subtle baseline pupil asymmetry)
Ptosis	Impaired sympathetic innervation, myasthenia gravis, cranial nerve III dysfunction
Increased width of palpebral fissure	Upper motor neuron dysfunction, cranial nerve VII dysfunction
In-turning of eye or impaired abduction	Cranial nerve VI dysfunction
Positive cover test	Esophoria or exophoria
Upper and lower facial weakness	Cranial nerve VII dysfunction
Isolated lower facial weakness	Stroke

Table 76-6. Key Findings on Neuromuscular Examination and Associated Diagnoses

Key Findings	Possible Significance
Asymmetry of muscle tone, bulk, or range of motion	Cerebral palsy, stroke, peripheral lesion
Weakness Most sensitive: deltoids, wrist extensors, hamstrings, ankle dorsiflexors Least sensitive: handgrip, biceps, quadriceps, gastrocnemius	Neuromuscular disorders
Asymmetry of rapid alternating movements	Dyscoordination, associated with many disorders, including ADHD, ASDs
Slowness of attempted rapid pincer movements or toe-tapping	Upper motor neuron dysfunction
Irregularity of attempted rapid pincer movements or toe-tapping	Cerebellar dysfunction
Abnormal finger-nose-finger testing	Tremor, dysmetria, dyscoordination
Decreased deep tendon reflexes	Muscular, peripheral nerve, acute upper motor neuron or cerebellar abnormality
Increased deep tendon reflexes, clonus	Brain or spinal cord lesion, such as cerebral palsy

ADHD, attention-deficit/hyperactivity disorder; ASDs, autism spectrum disorders.

examples of some findings on cranial nerve examination with the corresponding significance (Maria, 2005). Clues to developmental diagnoses may be provided by abnormalities of tone, strength, coordination, or deep tendon reflexes. Systematic examination of each of these features should be included in developmental assessments. Table 76-6 summarizes key findings with their corresponding significance.

SUMMARY

Many clinicians who complete developmental and behavioral assessments of children do not perform physical examination as part of their routine diagnostic workup. Physical examination is a valuable feature of the developmental-behavioral evaluation. The physical examination may uncover the cause of a developmental or behavioral problem, allowing families to know the reason for the disorder, the prognosis, and the recurrence risk in other family members. Parents can observe approaches to assist their children with developmental-behavioral problems, such as maintaining composure, complying with requests, and responding to positive reinforcement. In addition, the laying on of hands facilitates the creation of a relationship between the clinician and the child. When we touch our patients, we make a literal connection that can serve as a warm beginning of a therapeutic alliance.

REFERENCES

Dixon SD, Stein MT: Encounters with Children: Pediatric Behavior and Development. Philadelphia, Elsevier Science Health Science, 2006.

Holden EW, Tarnowski KJ, Prinz RJ: Reliability of neurological soft signs in children: Re-evaluation of the panels. J Abnorm Child Psychol 10:163-172, 1983.

Jones KL: Smith's Recognizable Patterns of Human Malformation. Philadelphia, WB Saunders, 2006.

Maria BL: Current Management in Child Neurology, 3rd ed. London, BC Decker, 2005.

Stinnett TA, Oehler-Stinnett J, Fuqua DR, Palmer LS: Examination of the underlying structure of the NEPSY: A developmental neuropsychological assessment. J Psychoed Assess 20:66-82, 2002.

Trembath JT, Kliewer D, Bruce W: The Milani-Comparetti Motor Development Screening Test. Omaha, NE, Media Resource Center, C Louis Meyer Children's Rehabilitation Institute, University of Nebraska Medical Center, 1977.

World Health Organization: (2003). International Classification of Functioning, Disability and Health. ICF CHECKLIST website. Available at: http://www3.who.int/icf/checklist/icf-checklist.pdf. Accessed November 15, 2006.

77 GENERAL PRINCIPLES OF PSYCHOLOGICAL TESTING

RAYMOND STURNER

RELEVANCE TO PRIMARY CARE AND DEVELOPMENTAL BEHAVIORAL PEDIATRICS PRACTICE

The application of psychological tests and principles is essential to connecting developmental care to traditional medicine. In primary care, the primary care physician or nurse practitioner, traditionally trained in the use of stethoscopes and otoscopes, needs to use or at least understand a new set of tools to probe in the "new morbidities" of child health, including developmental delays, learning disabilities, attentional problems, and cognitive impairment. Psychological testing is one such tool. Although the primary care physician may not personally administer the tests, it is imperative that the physician or nurse practitioner understand basic psychometric principles and the implications of test scores to evaluate and manage children with such disorders.

Concepts of validity and reliability govern psychological testing in much the same way they govern any medical laboratory test. The probability of error in an individual test result may be calculated in the same way that it is calculated for any medical test result. The principles of psychological testing are based on the same scientific and statistical basis of other parts of medicine. New pediatric practice guidelines call for use of previsit parent questionnaires to screen for developmental and behavioral concerns and for primary care practitioners to review the school reports and Individual Education Plans that parents are requested to bring to checkup visits. Compliance with these clinical guidelines to understand the child's functioning and monitor how needs are being addressed requires a solid understanding of the basic psychometric properties of psychological tests and a familiarity with the most commonly used tests.

Developmental-behavioral pediatricians often choose to administer psychological tests themselves. That level of competency requires not only an understanding of psychometrics, but also training in test administration by observing an experienced tester, practicing under the scrutiny of an experienced practitioner, and demonstrating reliability in test administration and scoring. Further training and experience usually is needed for a good tester to evolve into a skilled evaluator. A skilled evaluator not only administers tests reliably, scores accurately, and interprets soundly, but also remains sensitive to way the child's behavioral style or coping capacities are displayed in the nonscored aspects of the test, such as how the child manages moments of frustration or recognition of a previous error. In such evaluations, aspects of child-examiner interaction become markers of difficulties that show up in other parts of the child's life, and may help explain key difficulties underlying presenting concerns.

REASONS FOR FORMAL TESTING

The purpose of psychological testing is to obtain the data needed to make clinical decisions about children. Reasons for formal testing include the following:

1. To identify groups of children who are at risk for problems for which extensive and costly further evaluations are warranted
2. To diagnose a problem and determine how serious it is
3. To compare individual children with a normative group
4. To determine the appropriate intervention program and eligibility for the program
5. To determine the child's knowledge of specific skills and relative strengths and weaknesses for educational planning
6. To evaluate treatments that are aimed at preventing or improving developmental outcomes
7. To determine if the child is making adequate progress as a way to monitor the educational or medical intervention

PSYCHOMETRIC CONSIDERATIONS

Psychological tests result in statistically based conclusions about the child, and as such require an understanding of the underlying principles of measurement, which are briefly reviewed here. An important resource to be considered for an in-depth and current consensus regarding test issues is the *Standards for Educational and Psychological Testing* (1999), which reflects a consensus of expert opinion.

Standardization and Sampling

A child usually is considered for testing because the clinician wants to know if the child functions differently from other children of the same age or circumstance, or is experiencing a different or deviant developmental process than that experienced by children from the population at large. The measurement question may be likened to conducting a hypothetical scientific experiment with the goal of changing an individual's developmental functioning. In psychological test jargon, the randomly chosen "control group" for the "experiment" is called the *standardization* or *normative sample*.

Types of Scores

Some clinical questions require comparison of how well the child does in different areas of functioning as measured by different tests. This comparison would not make sense if the differences between the tests were due to idiosyncrasies of test construction and scoring, rather than to the child's performance in two different constructs of psychological functioning. Instead, scores are created that follow a common, "normal" (also known as gaussian) distribution of results as illustrated by a curve in the shape of a bell. In Figure 77-1, the well-known bell curve is depicted divided into equal intervals—called "standard scores"—that can be used for all tests. Choice of metric depends on how fine a gradation in performance variability needs to be communicated.

In medicine and research, test results generally are communicated using the standard deviations to describe the probability that there are statistically and clinically "significant" differences in any experimental testing. The interval of a standard deviation is sometimes referred to as a *Z score*. A *T score* is the Z score expressed in a different numerical form (10 × Z + 50). A "standard score" refers to a convention where a mean of 100 corresponds to a Z score of 0 and a standard deviation of 15 is a Z score of ± 1. For example, an intelligence quotient (IQ) is typically described with a mean of 100 and a standard deviation of 15. Because these tests have been carefully designed to generate scores on the bell-shaped curve, the implication is that 95% of children earn scores between 70 and 130. The approximately 2.5% of children scoring higher than 130 are considered gifted. The approximately 2.5% of children scoring lower than 70 are considered cognitively impaired or intellectually disabled (see Chapters 68 and 81).

In the educational field, sometimes the range of scores is divided into nine equal intervals known as *stanines* (for standard nines). Standard scores are often accompanied by a confidence interval expressed as a percent (e.g., 90% or 95% confidence level) indicating the degree of certainty that the individual's score reflects his or her true ability and not just random fluctuation. Standard scores also are accompanied by a standard score range within which the true score is likely to fall. This score is derived from comparison with a population of age-matched "controls" from the normative sample. If a child has the

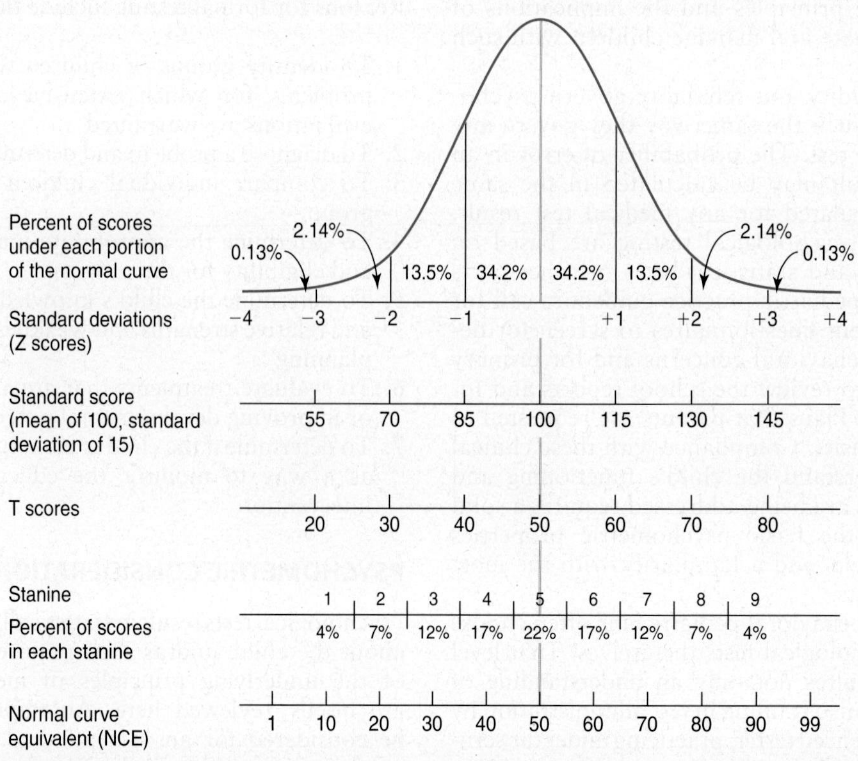

Figure 77-1. Depiction of the well-known bell curve. An individual's raw score can be converted to derived scores, which compare that individual's performance to the standardization sample. This figure shows the relationship of derived scores in a normal distribution.

same score when tested one year (e.g., 94) and again the next year (i.e., again 94), that indicates 1 year of normal progress, rather than lack of progress. The narrower the interval used in the measurement, the more likely it is to show year-to-year fluctuation. The narrowest interval generally used to show rank order in performance is the familiar percentile score. Although they provide a familiar perspective on rank order, percentiles are not equal-interval standard scores and cannot be arithmetically manipulated and cannot be used to compare results of different subtests. "Normal curve equivalents" are based on percentiles, but have been statistically converted to an equal-interval scale. Only normal curve equivalents of 1, 50, and 99 correspond directly to percentiles.

Reliability

Reliability of a test refers to the tendency for its results to be reproducible or consistent despite artifacts of testing conditions. Being tested a second time on a different day is called *test-retest reliability*. Comparison of results from different respondents or observers is called *intertester reliability*. The term *reliability* also may refer to the consistency of a set of items in its tendency always to "go together" when the test is performed on different individuals with similar problems. This characteristic is known as *internal consistency*. *Validity*, discussed in more depth later, refers to the accuracy with which a test measures the intended psychological process. A test can be perfectly reliable and consistent, but not be a useful or valid measure of what it is intended to assess. A test can never be valid, however, if its measurement cannot be counted on to give consistent results.

Often a simple correlation coefficient is used to describe the extent to which the scores on one instance of measurement predict the score on a second administration, with 0.0 showing a total lack of association and 1.0 showing perfect agreement. When reviewing these kinds of data, one not only should look for the highest positive number for a correlation coefficient, but also note the statistical significance of the correlation, which takes into account the number of subjects that were studied and the strength of the correlation.

When internal consistency refers to how each item relates to the total overall score, it is called an *item-total correlation*. This correlation is used by test developers to decide if items are redundant. To get a general sense of how consistent all the items intended to measure the same concept are within the test, "split-half reliability" may be calculated by randomly choosing half of the items and determining the average correlation between the two halves. Cronbach α may be thought of as an estimate of the average of all split-half estimates of reliability. It is derived from the average inter-item correlation.

Standard error is another indicator of reliability because it expresses the range within which the real score of a test falls. A test score of 100 with a standard error of 5 suggests that the real score lies in the range of 95 to 105.

Validity

The most important thing to know about a test is whether it actually does what it sets out to do. At the outset, experts may make judgments regarding "test content evidence," or whether the test contains items that represent the construct or trait that the test was intended to measure. What the test promises to accomplish is described by the proposed interpretation of its scores. Consider the situation of a program that requires an IQ test score cutoff for entry. A test that is constructed to be a screening test must establish the cutoff scores for eligibility. In this case, validity is how well the screening tool result predicts that criterion IQ test when it is administered concurrently. If the purpose of a test is to predict a later occurring outcome, such as a readiness test to determine later school functioning, the most relevant aspect of validity is predictive, rather than concurrent, validity.

Prediction of any single concurrent or later occurring measure is less relevant for a test designed to be a diagnostic tool (e.g., one that tests for specific types of neuropsychiatric functioning). For such a diagnostic test that includes multiple scales, a thorough examination of its internal structure would be an important piece of evidence for validity. Here validity hinges on examination of internal structure using the statistic Cronbach α when the test constructs are represented by discrete scales. If the constructs are ambiguous, or there are no scales, data regarding the internal structure can be obtained and analyzed by factor analysis to determine if items group together in potentially meaningful ways.

Sensitivity and Specificity, and Positive and Negative Predictive Validity

When comparing a continuous measure with the criterion of test accuracy, or *gold standard*, a correlation statistic is usually reported. For categorical outcome measures, however, such as diagnostic conclusions or continuous measure tests with a cutoff score for screening, the "utility measures" such as sensitivity and specificity are used to describe how accurately the test predicts the group of individuals with the target condition in a population. *Sensitivity* estimates the proportion of true-positive cases that would be correctly identified by the cutoff score. *Specificity* refers to the proportion of individuals without the disorder or condition that would be correctly identified. When thinking about the accuracy of the test for predicting that an individual patient will be correctly diagnosed by the criterion gold standard, the term *positive predictive value* is used as an estimate of the likelihood that the patient has the disorder or condition if the test is positive, and *negative predictive value* is the probability that a negative test result corresponds to a noncase.

TYPES OF TESTS

The choice of the type of test or other approach to evaluation depends on the type of clinical questions being addressed. For detailed reviews of individual tests, readers are referred to comprehensive reviews, such as the *Mental Measurements Yearbook* (Spies and Plake, 2005), the *Handbook of Psychiatric Measures* (Rush et al, 2000), and *Children's Psychological Testing* (Wodrich, 1997). Two major categories of tests to consider are norm referenced and criterion referenced.

Norm-Referenced and Criterion-Referenced Tests

Sometimes the purpose of testing is to determine where an individual child performs compared with a national sample or to establish if a clinically or educationally important criterion has been met. To understand that individual within the group or the range of abilities within a group of students, a norm-referenced test would be needed. Norm-referenced tests also would be required if one wanted to determine if a child's poor math skills are discrepant enough from his or her other abilities to meet criteria for a math learning disability. Norm-referenced tests typically provide a standard or a T-score in an absolute way, rather than determining rank order in ability.

A criterion-referenced test is appropriate for determining mastery of specific skills within an expected sequence or curriculum, such as basic skills needed for activities of everyday living (e.g., buttoning and shoe tying). It is the kind of testing that is often needed to make decisions about how to group students for instruction. An advantage of criterion-referenced, or curriculum-based, assessment is that the method of administration can vary to bypass sensory or motor disabilities. It also is very useful for monitoring progress. Criterion-referenced tests often provide an age-equivalent or percentile score.

Measures of Intellectual Ability

Currently, the IQ score is based on the standard statistical distribution of scores around a mean of 100 as described earlier in the section on types of scores. One implication of clinical importance is that at the statistical scoring extremes of a population, a few points of change can greatly affect school placement decisions, whereas a few points of change around the population average can be dismissed as random error. A new treatment that shifts the mean of the affected population from 94 to 100 substantially reduces the proportion of affected children with cognitive impairment.

One advance in the development of intelligence scales has been a greater attempt to organize test items into groupings that can remain consistent throughout the age span. This improvement, developed by Wechsler, may be responsible for the continued dominance of his series of tests including the *Wechsler Adult Intelligence Scale (WAIS)*, which preceded the development of the comparable scales for children, now the *Wechsler Intelligence Scale for Children–IV (WISC-IV)* and the *Wechsler Preschool and Primary Scale of Intelligence–Revised (WPPSI-R)*. Another important trend in intelligence test construction is the notion of subtypes of intelligence. In contrast to the original Stanford Binet, which yielded one global IQ score, measures that divide performance into at least two domains of verbal and nonverbal or performance abilities are now favored. These subtests of intelligence tests provide insight into the strengths and weaknesses of a child.

Sometimes intelligence tests are supplemented by additional measures of special ability, such as *Visual Motor Integration, Wide Range Assessment of Memory and Learning,* measures of information processing such as the *Detroit Tests of Learning Aptitude–3,* or language tests, to describe a child's skills or deficits further. A detailed review of various cognitive tests and approaches to administration and interpretation may be found in Sattler's authoritative text (Sattler, 2001) (see also Chapter 81).

Some limitations of attempts to divide intelligence into multiple domains may be related to measurement limitations, rather than the actual nature of individual abilities. When subscales contain few items, they are less likely to be reliable. They also are more likely to be in error. Some purported subtests do not prove to be statistically distinct. Using data from a variety of sources, however, Gardner (1983) has shown evidence for distinct "multiple intelligences." The different abilities include logical-mathematical, spatial, bodily kinesthetic, musical, interpersonal, intrapersonal, and naturalist. Intelligence tests provide only a limited view of the abilities of individuals.

IQ test scores may be invalid if the child has a sensory or motor impairment that limits his or her ability to understand instructions and other such factors can adversely affect IQ test results. The diagnosis of intellectual disability or cognitive impairment requires not only low IQ test scores, but also comparable scores on a test of adaptive behavior (see Chapter 68). Some tests of adaptive behavior, such as the Vineland, generate standard scores, facilitating comparisons with IQ test scores.

Adaptive Behavior

According to the American Association for Individuals with Developmental Disabilities 2002 definition, limitations in adaptive behavior should be determined using measures standardized in the general population and disabled individuals. Limitations in adaptive behavior are "operationally defined as performance that is at least 2 standard deviations below the mean of either (a) one of the following three types of adaptive behavior: conceptual, social, or practical, or (b) an overall score on a standardized measure of conceptual, social, and practical skills" (American Association for Individuals with Developmental Disabilities). Conceptual skills include receptive and expressive language, reading and writing, money concepts, and self-directions. Social skills include interpersonal, responsibility, self-esteem, gullibility, naiveté, follows rules, obeys laws, and avoids victimization. Practical skills include activities of daily living, occupational skills, and maintaining a safe environment. The *Vineland Adaptive Behavior Scales–Revised* may be the most popular adaptive behavior measure. It is based on a large national normative sample, uses an interview format, and has a teacher evaluation version.

Problems of available adaptive measures include limited usefulness in planning interventions for children (Reschly and Gresham, 1988); reliance on third-party report, rather than direct observation over various settings and samples of time; and scoring based on typical performance, rather than peak performance, which might be a better reflection of the child's potential (Reschly and Gresham, 1988). These issues should still be considered especially when there is a question regarding the reliability of the observer and are required for diagnosis of intellectual disability.

Measures of Infant Development

Situational variables, such as fatigue, emotional status, or unfamiliarity of the environment or tester, can always compromise optimal performance in a given testing session, especially in testing infants and young children. Testing is often done to determine the child's optimal level of functioning, not just a random sample of skills. In addition, for the youngest children, optimal functioning requires the immediate support and comfort of an adult attachment figure—typically a parent. Also, it is within the interaction with the parent that many emerging capacities are displayed, and where much of the child's future "curriculum" and education occur. For these reasons, participation of the parent is a necessary part of a complete evaluation of an infant or young child. Forming an alliance with the parent is an essential part of the evaluation and any subsequent intervention. A full assessment should include multiple sources of information to ensure further that the test results are representative of the child's typical behavior and capabilities in various areas of development and to elucidate parent concerns. (Also see Meisels and Fenichel, 1996, for a general discussion of infant test issues.)

Newborns may be assessed for current functioning using the well-researched *Brazelton Neonatal Behavioral Assessment Scale*. This structured examination has proven to be especially valuable as a clinical intervention by providing a demonstration of the unique capacities of the infant, promoting better interaction between at-risk mothers and their infants. Scores do not have predictive validity (see also Chapter 79).

Beyond the newborn period, the *Bayley Scales of Infant Development–II* has become the dominant instrument because of its comprehensiveness and updated norms. In contrast to the *Brazelton Neonatal Behavioral Assessment Scale,* it uses standardized administration. It generates standard scores.

Intellectual Testing in Special Populations

New assessment tools are becoming available that provide several distinct advantages for assessing children with disabilities. First, in contrast to most standardized tests, normal children and children with impairments are included in the "normative" sample. Second, items are organized so that one can document what the child can do with and without assistance, which can include electronic assistive devices. This feature is akin to criterion-referenced testing. Third, items may be broken down into the discrete steps required to achieve the function being assessed. These fine gradations in performance, or "component analyses," provide guidance for a specific "curriculum" of instruction to attain these end points of functioning. Scales of items of this type may be referred to as growth-scaled or ability-scaled scores because they reflect growth or progress attained by individual children, but do not compare the child with a "norm group."

Another important strategy for assessing children with impairments is to include assessment within their natural environment of family and childcare or school. This assessment is especially necessary to get a closer look at the how the child accomplishes activities of everyday living and potential strategies for integrating intervention goals into daily routines. This assessment can be done with an assessor who "shadows" the child through part of a typical day aided by a standardized approach for documenting progress. (see Murphy, 1987, for a review of this approach.) The *Pediatric Evaluation of Disability Inventory (PEDI),* a functional measure, is an example of such a test covering ages 6 months through 7 years and including a Level of Caregiver Assistance and Modifications subtests. The *Toddler and Infant Motor Evaluation (TIME)* for children 4 months to 3 1/2 years old contains scales that document not only the motor activities the child can accomplish, but also how the child does it. This differentiates normal from atypical motor patterns and motor responses the child may accomplish with examiner-prompted, parent-facilitated or aide-facilitated movements.

The *Leiter International Performance Scale* is an important measure that has long been available to assess cognitive abilities in children (ages 2 through 21 years) with motor impairments, nonverbal hearing-impaired children, and children who are non–English speaking. This test allows children to illustrate their understanding of concepts through a series of matching tasks that can be responded to in various ways, including directing eye gaze. This test was first devised in the 1930s, but was revised and renormed in 1995.

Neuropsychologic Testing

Child neuropsychologic tests have clinical utility in situations where it is important to understand the child's level of functioning in a wide range of domains, such as memory, reasoning, attention, and language. Sophisticated neuroimaging techniques do not yet reveal the impact on functioning determined through neuropsychologic testing. Questions that might be addressed include: Does the child show signs of brain injury after a known trauma? How might a child be affected by brain surgery? How can we monitor the progress of a child who has sustained a known brain injury? Does the child have evidence for a nonverbal learning disorder (a sometimes subtle condition with implications for learning and social functioning)?

A few neuropsychologic tests are commonly used and warrant mention. The *Halstead-Reitan* (covering ages 9 to 14 years) and the *Reitan-Indiana* (ages 5 to 6 years) *Neuropsychological Test Batteries for Children and Older Children* were refined from studies on adult patients known to have sustained brain injuries. Some additional unique subtests were developed to assess children. These tests include subtests that assess abstract reasoning, conceptual ability, and language resembling traditional IQ tests, but have a greater emphasis on subtests that emphasize motor speed and strength, sensory awareness of bilateral and pattern recognition, attention, laterality, and perceptual skills. The specific items have been designed to capture distinct syndromes of brain dysfunction. Patterns of performance have implications for localization of brain lesions and some pathognomonic signs, rare signs, and symptoms that indicate pathology regardless of the results of the rest of the test battery. The reliability of some of the items has been called into question, and validity data and norms are limited, especially in younger children. The batteries also are time-consuming and require special equipment.

The *Luria-Nebraska Neuropsychological Battery* is suitable for children 8 to 12 years old and is very similar to the adult version. In contrast to the empirically based Reitan authored tests, this test is based on the work of the famous Russian theorist Luria, who tested his theories in individuals with brain injury. This test also has been criticized for limited norms and evidence for reliability, but it does seem to discriminate children with brain injury and can assist in monitoring their progress over time. It has an advantage over the Reitan batteries in taking less time (but still 2 to 3 hours) and less equipment.

The *NEPSY: A Developmental Neuropsychological Assessment* represents a compilation of various tests that had been developed for young children combined into a battery and normed from ages 3 to 12 years. The NEPSY also takes some of its inspiration from Luria's theories, but with redesign of pass-fail items into a psychometrically normed approach, retaining Luria's format of including subtests that are used only to verify hypotheses generated by the initial battery. The various subtests cover the domains of Attention/Executive functioning, Language, Sensorimotor, Visual-motor, and Memory/Learning. The conclusions generally are given in terms of strengths and weaknesses of functions and processes. The test is better suited to answer specific questions about what may have been damaged, or what processes are getting in the way, rather than to provide an overall assessment of global functioning or even assess more integrative functions, such as attention or memory (see Chapter 83).

Measures of Academic Achievement

In recent years, there has been increasing emphasis on use of group achievement testing, such as the *Iowa* or *Stanford Achievement Tests,* as a measure of school accountability and student progress. Some children (e.g., with attention-deficit/hyperactivity disorder [ADHD]) may underperform because of time limitations and a distracting classroom environment, rather than lack of mastery of the academic content. Although group testing screens for children having academic difficulties, individually administered tests are preferable for determining eligibility for services because they can be used to pinpoint the educational diagnosis or provide remediation suggestions. The *Woodcock-Johnson Psycho-Educational Battery–Revised* (including a cognitive measure in addition to 17 achievement subtests) and the *Kaufman Test of Educational Achievement (K-TEA)* are commonly used diagnostic achievement tests.

The limitation of academic achievement testing is that students' capacities are assessed with a single snapshot of performance under artificial circumstances. Such test results may not be representative of the child's abilities. An alternative to achievement testing is performance monitoring with ongoing curriculum adjustment or "authentic performance assessment," such as the *Work Sampling System,* used in some preschool and elementary schools (Meisels et al, 2001) (see also Chapter 82).

Measures of Attention

Although the DSM-IV-TR (*Diagnostic and Statistical Manual of Mental Disorders, 4th edition, Text Revision*) criteria for ADHD make no mention of psychological test performance, many well-standardized parent and teacher questionnaire measures are available to aid in this diagnosis. The most useful child-administered tests for diagnosis are cognitive and achievement screening or diagnostic tests to determine the presence of learning problems as a cause or result of inattentiveness.

Clinicians continue to attempt to diagnose ADHD by direct testing of children. One approach has been to look for patterns within intelligence test performance. In particular, it was suggested that children with ADHD had more difficulty on three particular subtests (Arithmetic, Digit Span, and Coding), so these subtests were averaged to create a "Freedom from Distractibility" index. Numerous studies (Kaufman, 1994) show, however, that this was not an accurate way to diagnose ADHD as is the case with other psychological test measures of executive functioning (Barkley and Grodzinsky, 1994).

Another approach that has been attempted to diagnose ADHD is the use of tests of vigilance and impulse control, putative psychological processes underlying the disorder. Continuous performance tests require that the child focus attention in a laboratory-type setting for a period of time on an auditory or visual stimulus with occasional interruptions and background stimuli. The child has specific instructions about when to push the button, and the distractors may result in errors of commission or omission, which can be compared with established norms. Examples of continuous performance tests include the *Gordon Diagnostic System, Test of Variables of Attention (TOVA),* and the *Conners' Continuous Performance Test.* These tests do not adequately differentiate the performance of children with ADHD from that of controls. They may not add significantly to the diagnostic process because ADHD is a clinical phenomenon, with multiple and diverse underlying psychological processes, many of which depend on specific environmental conditions and contextual expectations (see Chapter 54).

Projective Tests

In contrast to the previously described tests, projective measures are not primarily based on norm-referenced empiric research, but rather on a hypothesis that an individual will "project" his or her feelings, thoughts, needs, attitudes, and conflicts onto an ambiguous stimulus. Some popular projective measures include Rorschach inkblot technique, in which individuals tell what they see in a standard inkblot; thematic apperception tests, in which children make up stories about standard pictures illustrating people interacting; incomplete sentences, in which children complete brief standard sentence fragments covering latent themes; and drawing techniques, in which children are asked to draw a person, family members, or a house, tree, and person together. These techniques all have the advantage of being less threatening than direct questioning and more likely to engage otherwise reticent children. These techniques include specific guidelines for administration and directives for coding data and comparing with responses from normative and clinical populations. They rely on the experience and interpretative skill of the clinician and do not meet the psychometric standards of other instruments. For these reasons, these approaches should not be used to make clinical decisions without other collaborating evidence from interviews and more objective measures.

DIAGNOSING MENTAL OR PERSONALITY DISORDERS VIA STRUCTURED INTERVIEWS OR DIMENSIONAL RATINGS

When clinicians disagree after diagnostic interviewing, the problems often can be traced to differences in questions asked and in judgments about when symptoms meet diagnostic criteria. The goal of using interview protocols is to enhance reliability of data collection with the ultimate goal of improving diagnostic agreement and accuracy. They have a potential adverse effect on rapport, but advocates note that with sufficient practice the structured nature can become invisible.

Numerous standardized structured interviews, validated in children, are available to diagnose psychopathology according to DSM criteria. (see Rogers, 2001, for a detailed review.) Two popular ones are the *Schedule of Affective Disorders and Schizophrenia for School-Age Children (Kiddie-SADS)* and the *Diagnostic Interview Schedule for Children (DISC)*. These measures are specifically linked to DSM-IV, and changes in diagnostic approaches or criteria would occasion the need for a new measure. Numerous structured interviews also are available to assist in making a schedule II or personality diagnosis, such as the *Diagnostic Interview for Borderlines (DIB)*. None of the personality interviews have been validated to any extent in pediatric populations.

Symptom checklists (e.g., *Child Behavior Checklist*) and self-reporting personality measures (e.g., *Minnesota Multiphasic Personality Inventory [MMPI-2]*) represent time-honored alternative approaches to assessing psychopathology. Use of temperament rating scales is a similar approach, following a more normal range and less pathology-oriented framework (see Chapter 78). Advocates for these approaches argue that the criteria for making categorical disorder diagnoses are often arbitrary, and mental disorders are best understood as a continuum of symptom severity, better suited for more sophisticated analyses.

Computerized previsit symptom ratings or computerized interviews followed by open-ended confirmatory interviews or structured follow-up interviews are now available (e.g., *Child Health and Development Interactive System [CHADIS]*) and may be a way in which the benefits of both of the aforementioned approaches to mental health diagnoses can be adapted into primary care pediatrics within the typical time constraints.

SUMMARY

Administering, obtaining, and interpreting psychological testing are important components of general and developmental-behavioral subspecialty clinical practice. Psychological testing represents an important approach for the field of developmental-behavioral pediatrics to ensure that a standardized, reproducible, and scientific basis is built into clinical practice. Appropriate use of a test requires attention to its psychometric properties, including reliability, validity, sensitivity, and specificity. Psychological tests are now available to address almost all developmental-behavioral clinical issues, including intelligence, learning, communication, motor skills, self-help skills, behavioral adjustment, temperament, and other adaptive functions.

REFERENCES

American Association on Intellectual and Developmental Disabilities: Available at: http://www.aaidd.org/. Accessed October 26, 2008.

American Educational Research Association, American Psychological Association, National Council on Measurement in Education: Standards for Educational and Psychological Testing. Washington, DC, American Educational Research Association, 1999.

American Psychiatric Association: Diagnostic and Statistical Manual of Mental Disorders, Fourth Edition, Text Revision (DSM-IV-TR). Arlington, VA, American Psychiatric Association, 2000.

Barkley RA, Grodzinsky GM: Are tests of frontal lobe functions useful in the diagnosis of attention deficit disorders? Clin Neuropsychologist 8:121-139, 1994.

Gardner H: Frames of Mind: The Theory of Multiple Intelligences. New York, Basic Books, 1983.

Kaufman AS: Intelligent Testing with the WISC-III. New York, John Wiley & Sons, 1994.

Meisels SJ, Fenichel E: New Visions for the Developmental Assessment of Infants and Young Children. Washington, DC, Zero to Three Press, 1996.

Meisels SJ, Jablon JR, Marsden DB, et al: The Work Sampling System. New York, Pearson Early Learning, 2001.

Murphy G: Direct observation as an assessment tool in functional analysis and treatment. *In* Hogg J, Raynes N: Assessment in Mental Handicap. Cambridge, MA, Croom Helm Ltd, 1987, pp 190-238.

Reschly DJ, Gresham FM: Adaptive behavior and the mildly handicapped. *In* Kratochwill RR (ed): Advances in School Psychology, Vol 4. Hillsdale, NJ, Erlbaum, 1988, pp 249-282.

Rogers R: Handbook of Diagnostic and Structured Interviewing. New York, Guilford Press, 2001.

Rush AJ, Pincus HA, First MB, (eds): Handbook of Psychiatric Measures. Washington, DC, American Psychiatric Association, 2000.

Sattler JM: Assessment of Children's Intelligence and Special Abilities, 4th ed.San Diego, Jerome M. Sattler Publisher, 2001.

Spies RA, Plake BS: Mental Measurements Yearbook, 16th ed. Lincoln, University of Nebraska Press, 2005.

Wodrich DL: Children's Psychological Testing, 3rd ed. Baltimore, Paul Brooks Publishing, 1997.

78 ASSESSMENT OF BEHAVIORAL ADJUSTMENT AND BEHAVIORAL STYLE

William B. Carey

This chapter presents suggestions on how a pediatrician in private or clinic practice can evaluate children's behavior competently without the aid of allied disciplines. Techniques used by those specialists are discussed in later chapters.

Some terms should first be clarified. Elsewhere in this book, the point has been made that development and behavior are intertwined in the individual. Nevertheless, they can be assessed separately. *Development* refers to the evolution of capacities that is a reflection of the maturation of the central nervous system (see Chapter 79). The term *behavior* refers to the content and style of the actions of a child in his or her relationships, the way abilities are used. The first part of this chapter discusses assessment of behavioral adjustment, which is the content of these actions. The second part deals with temperament, which is the style with which they are performed.

BEHAVIORAL ADJUSTMENT

Challenge and Obstacles

The proficient evaluation by the pediatrician of behavior in children is a complex challenge. Much is expected of the pediatrician. Ideally, every comprehensive pediatric appraisal and especially every investigation of a specific problem with possible developmental-behavioral components, such as headaches or scholastic difficulties, should include a clear picture of the child's behavioral adjustment pattern; the physical, developmental, temperamental, and environmental factors interacting with them; and a plan for possible alteration of these factors for the benefit of the child. An astute clinician should have the child's development and behavior in mind in every encounter. Besides well-developed interviewing and counseling skills, this expectation presumes an understanding of whether specific behaviors are normal, and, if not normal, a judgment as to how severe they are, why they have developed, and what to do about them. These objectives represent a major shift for the practice of pediatrics, which emerged a century ago as the subdivision of medical science dealing with the nutritional and growth problems and physical diseases then prominent in childhood.

In rising to meet this challenge, the pediatrician is confronted with major obstacles, as follows:

1. *Unclear presentation of concern by parents.* Compared with most common physical illnesses, behavioral problems are likely to manifest clinically in confusing, unorganized forms. The concern may be evident, but its real focus may be obscure. The parent might ask the pediatrician for advice on discipline, when the true distress is marital discord and the accompanying disputes over childrearing. Another parent might request a different formula or complain about intestinal gas, when the actual problem is excessive crying in the infant. The concern must be clarified before the diagnosis can begin.
2. *Undefined parental expectations.* A parent's mention of certain behavioral issues does not mean that he or she is asking for or expects the involvement of the pediatrician. The parent may simply be ventilating dissatisfaction. The expectations of the parents may be inappropriate. A discussion must occur as to what the parents want and what the pediatrician can offer.
3. *Skill and time required.* As with any other area of clinical competence, evaluation of behavior requires training to achieve the necessary skill. Most pediatric residency programs expose trainees to an abundance of tertiary care of major illnesses, but to a minimum of experience fostering the knowledge and skills of behavioral pediatrics. Graduates of these programs report an understandable feeling of inadequacy. Even a pediatrician with the requisite skills is confronted with many competing responsibilities during the available time with the patient, and with a reimbursement system that at present overvalues mechanical procedures and underpays for time spent in diagnostic interviewing and counseling.
4. *Frequently confusing advice from mental health specialists.* Conflicting theories about the origins of behavior problems and their management often leave pediatricians confused. Examples of differing opinions are evident in advice about sleeping arrangements, handling of excessive crying, and the use of spanking. The techniques suggested by spokespersons of those disciplines may be unsuitable for pediatric settings.

Confronted with these obstacles, some pediatricians are tempted to avoid asking parents about behavioral issues or try to evade them when brought up. Some pediatricians give standard prescription advice for the problem without fitting it to the needs of the particular child. Other pediatricians refer immediately to a mental health specialist all parents concerned about their children. The extent of this common suboptimal performance is not easily determined, but it is probably not as great as has been estimated by more severe critics (Costello, 1986; Horowitz et al, 1992; Lavigne et al, 1993). Following is a discussion of the available diagnostic classification systems and some existing techniques for obtaining the data needed for classification.

Diagnostic Classification Systems

Diagnostic and Statistical Manual of Mental Disorders, 4th Edition

The most widely known of the diagnostic systems for behavioral and emotional problems is the DSM-IV (*Diagnostic and Statistical Manual of Mental Disorders, 4th edition*) by the American Psychiatric Association (1994). This volume was preceded by several versions, starting with the DSM-I in 1952, and has been most recently updated by a minor revision, the DSM-IV-TR in 2000. The current version subdivides overall diagnoses into five components or axes: (1) clinical disorders, (2) personality disorders and intellectual disability, (3) general medical conditions, (4) psychosocial and environmental problems, and (5) global assessment of functioning. In the last of these measures, the clinician indicates a general judgment from 1 (persistent danger to self or others) to 100 (superior functioning without any symptoms). Normality is not specifically defined, but is assumed to be the lack of any of the conditions listed.

Because the DSM system has been virtually the only one available to physicians in the United States for decades, many have assumed that it is the best one possible. Clinicians in pediatric care have increasingly become aware of its limitations, however, as follows:

1. The DSM system is primarily intended for adults and does not deal sufficiently with the variety of problems and concerns facing children, their parents, and the professionals trying to help them in primary care.
2. DSM diagnoses use the categorical "medical model"—the diagnosis is either present or absent—a view that does not fit well with the primary care pediatrician's experience with the wide variation of children's adjustment along several dimensions of function.
3. The DSM system does not recognize or describe normal variations of behavior. The most favorable rating under Axis V is "Superior functioning in a wide range of activities, life's problems never seem to get out of hand, is sought out by others because of his or her many positive qualities." Temperament is not even mentioned. Consequently, many normal variations of temperament are overdiagnosed, such as an inattentive child who is functioning normally, but who is supposed to be given the "subthreshold" diagnosis of "attention-deficit/hyperactivity disorder, not otherwise specified," rather than simply being considered normal.

The content of the new DSM-V is not fixed yet, but there are signs that some leaders of American psychiatry are dissatisfied with the current system of static, categorical disorders. Jensen and colleagues (2006) have proposed changing to a system that is dimensional and adaptational and takes into consideration the child's context and interaction with it.

Diagnostic and Statistical Manual for Primary Care: Child and Adolescent Version

The American Academy of Pediatrics Task Force on Mental Health Coding for Children (1996) developed and published the DSM-PC (*Diagnostic and Statistical Manual for Primary Care: Child and Adolescent Version*). The principal aim was to overcome all three limitations mentioned regarding the DSM-IV and its predecessors, and "to help primary care clinicians better identify psychosocial factors affecting their patients so that they can provide interventions when appropriate, be reimbursed for those interventions, and identify and refer patients who require more sophisticated mental health care." This was an interdisciplinary effort in which psychiatrists and psychologists collaborated with pediatricians on an approximately equal footing.

The DSM-PC includes two principal parts, a listing of environmental situations that may affect children's behavior (e.g., caregiving changes, educational challenges) and a longer child manifestations section of problems in 10 different areas (e.g., negative/antisocial behaviors, somatic and sleep behaviors). Within each of these 10 "behavioral clusters," the presentation of symptoms is subdivided into three levels: (1) developmental variations, by which is meant normal behavioral variations that nevertheless may attract the concern of the clinician or the parent; (2) problems, which are behaviors serious enough to disrupt the child's social or scholastic functioning, but are not severe enough to warrant a diagnosis of a mental disorder (e.g., a child who gets into fights intermittently in school or in the neighborhood); and (3) disorders, as defined by the DSM-IV. The framers of the DSM-PC were required by the American Psychiatric Association to incorporate the entire DSM-IV terminology unaltered as the standard inventory of behavioral diagnoses.

The DSM-PC was a big step forward toward designing a diagnostic system more appropriate for use by physicians for all sorts of behavioral concerns with children. Some of the major limitations of the DSM series have been eliminated. Many pediatricians have found it useful. There are still some significant limitations, however, that must be overcome before it can achieve its maximum value. These limitations are as follows:

1. Physical status. There should be a place to incorporate a consideration of the great variety of general physical and neurologic factors affecting behavior. The environment is not the only influence.
2. Temperament. The relegation of the formal presentation of temperament to two paragraphs in the

preamble of the environmental situations section and scattered brief mention later betrays an insufficient recognition of its importance. Temperament variations are one of the three principal sources of behavioral concern that parents bring to pediatricians (the others being actual behavior dysfunction and misperceptions of abnormality). Shyness and moodiness are mentioned in the DSM-PC, but most important traits, such as high intensity, unpredictability, high persistence, and sensitivity, are not included. The particularly important trait of adaptability appears nowhere in the DSM-PC. Through interactions with the environment, temperament participates in the formation of physical, developmental, and behavioral problems; it affects children's responses to physical illnesses and use of medical care; and it can alter the child's environment, with which he or she is interacting (see Chapter 7).

3. Development. The child's developmental status would be better listed as a component contributing to the behavioral outcome, rather than as simply another child manifestation.
4. Parent-child interactions. No suggestions are offered as to how to describe the parent-child interactions and the ways in which the environmental situations may be influencing the symptoms in the child manifestations. This should be a primary focus of intervention efforts, which necessitates its inclusion in the diagnostic process.
5. Service needs. The DSM-PC has a useful section on determining the severity of the behavioral problem, but no place to indicate the service needs of the child. The clinician who has evaluated the child should indicate what level of care is needed, including (a) anticipatory guidance or brief educational counseling; (b) reassurance or individualized counseling for bothersome normal variations; (c) intervention counseling for mild to moderately severe situations or behavior problems, which need more time; and (d) referral counseling for major behavioral or emotional disorders. The clinician generating the diagnosis is the individual best qualified to make this determination about service needs. If the clinician does not make the determination, that function would be left to others, such as health insurance companies.
6. Summary profile. The DSM-PC resembles the DSM-IV in presenting long lists of possible problems. In contrast to the DSM-IV system with its five axes, however, the DSM-PC does not suggest a way to put all the findings together into a diagnostic profile (see Chapter 85 for an example of how this could be done in a pediatric setting).
7. Omission of ratings of strengths. The DSM-PC system is still basically oriented toward the abnormal in that there is no opportunity for the clinician to make note of positive aspects of behavioral adjustment, such as social competence, task performance, self-assurance, and general contentment.
8. Omissions of influences and problems. The list of possible problems is long, but there are important gaps. The powerful and pervasive environmental influence of television is not mentioned. Colic, the most common behavior problem in the first few months of life, does not appear in either the index or the list of presenting complaints.

The developers of the DSM-PC acknowledged that this was a first attempt, and that revisions are inevitable. Usefulness of the DSM-PC in its present state has not been established. Plans for revision still are not evident more than a decade later.

International Statistical Classification of Diseases and Related Health Problems, 10th Revision

The ICD-10 (*International Statistical Classification of Diseases and Related Health Problems, 10th revision*) by the World Health Organization (1992) is, along with the DSM series, the other best-known diagnostic scheme. As the name implies, it also deals only with disorders. The disorders listed as having their onset in childhood and adolescence include hyperkinetic disorders, conduct disorders, mixed disorders of conduct and emotions, emotional disorders, disorders of social functioning, and tic disorders. Much effort was expended by the developers of this system and of the DSM-IV to make the two classification systems as convergent as possible. Nevertheless, some significant differences can be found in criteria for diagnoses, such as with the unequal definitions of hyperkinesis and attention-deficit/hyperactivity disorder.

The International Classification of Functioning, Disability and Health (ICF) offers a comprehensive summary of physical and mental functions, activity limitations, and environmental factors (World Health Organization, 2001). However, it has few applications in general pediatrics practice.

Diagnostic Classification: 0-3. Diagnostic Classification of Mental Health and Developmental Disorders of Infancy and Early Childhood

Another of the diagnostic procedures available to child health care practitioners is the DC: 0-3 (*Diagnostic Classification: 0-3. Diagnostic Classification of Mental Health and Developmental Disorders of Infancy and Early Childhood*) by the National Center for Clinical Infant Programs (1994). The DC: 0-3 was offered as "a systematic, developmentally based approach to the classification of mental health and developmental difficulties in the first four years of life." Following the example of the DSM series, it offers the advantage of organizing the diagnosis into five axes: (1) the primary diagnosis; (2) the relationship classification; (3) physical, neurologic, and developmental disorders and conditions; (4) psychosocial stressors; and (5) functional emotional developmental level. The breadth of this approach is promising, but it has some drawbacks. The DC: 0-3 also fails to include temperament in any appropriate way. There is brief mention of it in the introduction, but it is not incorporated into the model except as traits such as sensory threshold and adaptability become entwined as part of the abnormality in the "regulatory disorders" diagnoses.

A revision, the DC: 0-3-R, was published in 2005. It makes some important changes in terminology, but not in the general format. There is still room for improvement, such as the addition of child and parent strengths (Sturner et al, 2007).

Comprehensive Child Assessment

Reasonable expectations for the performance of pediatricians and the actual conditions of pediatric practice call for a kind of diagnostic classification plan different from those described previously. In an effort to overcome all the defects in the systems mentioned, a comprehensive child assessment is offered here.

A good starting point in defining the relevant areas of adjustment is to decide on what constitutes normality. In Chapter 7, the point was made about how hard it is to find a satisfactory definition of normality in children's behavior. Chess and Thomas (1986) have proposed that social competence and task mastery be taken as criteria for current normality and as goals of future achievement. Chess also has revised an earlier textbook definition of normality (see Chapter 7).

Building on these guidelines, one can tentatively construct six general criteria for the assessment and rating of behavioral adjustment. There is no one definitive way to do this; the scheme proposed in Chapter 7 represents a suggestion to be considered until something better evolves. The following criteria are suitable for pediatric use in that they include positive and negative aspects of the major areas of adjustment and are easily applied (Table 78-1):

1. Behavior: relationships with parents, siblings, teachers, other adults, peers, and others—social competence versus undersocialization (aggressiveness or withdrawal).
2. Achievements: task performance, including work and play—achievement versus underachievement or excessive preoccupation with work or play.
3. Self-relations—self-assurance versus poor self-relations or overconcern for self. Included here are self-care, self-esteem, and self-regulation.
4. Internal status—reasonable contentment versus symptoms of distress in feelings or thoughts.
5. Coping patterns: strategies typically used to deal with the problems confronted in daily life—direct and appropriate engagement versus ineffective, maladaptive problem solving with overuse of defense mechanisms, such as denial, avoidance, or repression. This poorly studied aspect of a child's personality is probably derived from temperament, cognitive capacities, and experience, especially parental rearing practices.
6. Symptoms of physical functions: eating, sleeping, elimination, gender/sex, unexplained physical complaints, and repetitive behaviors—comfort versus discomfort (Carey & McDevitt, 2004).

The internal consistency of these areas has been established, and their assessment has been standardized with a 48-item questionnaire developed on a sample of 412 children 4 to 14 years old seen in general pediatrics practices. This scale is described further in the following section.

Table 78-1 provides a possible plan for organizing information and judgments about a child's behavioral adjustment. The profile is separated into these six areas of adjustment, and each of them is subdivided into five levels of function, from excellent to good to satisfactory to unsatisfactory to poor. Precise behavioral descriptions for placement along these continua cannot be supplied for all children, although it would be helpful if that were possible. Criteria for these judgments depend on various circumstances, such as age, sex, family, and cultural settings. Strengths and liabilities are included. Problems are considered as disruptions of various areas of function, not with regard to the presence or absence of "psychiatric" disorders. When these conclusions are incorporated into a comprehensive diagnostic formulation (see Chapter 85), they are accompanied by separate judgments regarding the child's physical health, neurologic status, developmental level, temperament, and interaction with the environment; a summary; and a statement of service needs.

Child health profiles of this sort are rare in the medical and mental health literatures (see Chapter 7). (Chapter 87 also describes behavioral assessment.)

Diagnostic Techniques

The usual techniques for obtaining data about children's behavioral adjustment to be incorporated into whatever classification system is used are observations, questionnaires, and interviews. Observations of the child's behavior and of the parent-child interaction in the office setting can be highly illuminating to the diagnostic process. These data are usually based on relatively brief contacts, however, and might be atypical of the overall picture. Long-term observations reported by teachers and other caregivers can be more helpful. The physician's own observations can confirm or raise doubts about the history, but are seldom sufficient to replace the history as the basis of the diagnosis.

Questionnaires concerning the child's behavior can make a useful contribution to the diagnosis if they are descriptive and are used as part of the data-gathering process, rather than by themselves as an oversimplified diagnostic mechanism.

Interviewing is the pediatrician's most powerful tool for the assessment of behavior in children. No other technique has the flexibility and subtlety of skillfully allowing the parent or patient to describe and express feelings about what is going on.

The two principal techniques for gathering diagnostic information about behavior in common usage today are (1) brief questionnaires for screening for psychopathology for the purpose of referral or longer ones for greater detail, and (2) a comprehensive pediatric assessment primarily by interview that allows and promotes pediatric management for most parental concerns about behavior.

Psychopathology Categorization Method

A common view of the role of pediatricians in behavioral matters is that they should screen for behavioral disturbances, as they do for developmental delay and various physical problems, so that they can refer troubled children to mental health specialists who are more

Table 78-1. Comprehensive Profile of Behavioral and Emotional Adjustment

Areas of Adjustment/Definitions	Ratings and Comments
Behavior, Social Competence—Relationships with People: How Well Does Child Get Along with People? High social skills versus deficit Caring versus hostile, aggressive, destructive Cooperation versus opposition, defiance, manipulation Involvement versus withdrawal Autonomy versus dependence, overconformity	a) Highly competent, pleasant, likable b) More pleasing, likable than average c) Gets along moderately well; average d) Some significant relationship problems, not major e) Generally unpopular, often rejected *Comments*:
Achievements—Task Performance—School, Home, Other: How Well Does Child Do Tasks and Play? Extent of achievement Skill development, use Motivation, effort, interest, responsibility Satisfaction, pride in accomplishment	a) Excellent achievement b) Good achievement c) Average, satisfactory achievement d) Underachievement, not failing; excessive striving e) Poor achievement, failing; truancy *Comments*:
Self-Relations—Self-Assurance and Management: How Does Child Feel About and Manage Self? Self-esteem—mental and physical abilities, appearance, social worth Self-care versus neglect, abuse, risks, overconcern Self-regulation—appropriate versus overregulation or underregulation	a) Excellent self-esteem, self-care, and self-regulation b) Good status in these areas c) Variable, average status d) Below average in some of these matters e) Poor; problems in some or all these areas *Comments*:
Internal Status—General Contentment versus Disturbance in Feelings or Thinking: How Does Child Feel and Think? Feelings—degree of comfort or discomfort Thinking—clarity and reality versus distortion	a) High but reasonable contentment b) Comfortable feelings and thinking c) Average mixture of concerns d) Unsatisfactory; disturbing but not crippling feelings of fear, anxiety, depression, anger, guilt; or reality distortions, phobias, obsessions, compulsions, delusions; post-traumatic stress disorder e) Poor; major disturbance of feelings or thinking *Comments*:
Coping—Problem Solving: How Well Does Child Identify and Solve Problems? Identify problems versus denial Plan solution versus avoidance Work on solution versus passivity Persist at solution versus give up Make needed revisions versus perseveration Seek appropriate help versus not	a) Highly effective coping b) Generally effective coping c) Satisfactory; average; variable d) Unsatisfactory coping e) Poor problem solving; excessive use of defensive strategies, such as denial, giving up *Comments*:
Symptoms of Body Function—General Comfort of Body Functions versus Discomfort or Dysfunction Eating Sleeping Elimination Gender/sex Pains Repetitive behavior	a) Comfortable in all areas b) Generally good function; only minimal concern c) Some concern; within normal range d) Significant concern; not severe e) Major concern *Comments*:
General Assessment	
Main Service Needs	

proficient with these issues (Costello, 1986; Jellinek et al, 1986). A dozen or more of these screening checklists are available—brief checklists (<10 minutes), longer ones, and ones designed for special areas of function. Detailed analyses of their characteristics can be found periodically in various reviews in the *Journal of the American Academy of Child and Adolescent Psychiatry* and in *Pediatrics in Review* (Glascoe, 2000; Perrin and Stancin, 2002).

Among the best known of the brief checklists are the *Pediatric Symptom Checklist* (Jellinek et al, 1986), *Eyberg Child Behavior Inventory* (Eyberg and Ross, 1978), *Conners Parent Rating Scale* (Goyette et al, 1978), and *Parents' Evaluations of Developmental Status (PEDS)*

(1997). Some screening scales requiring more time include the *Child Behavior Checklist* (Achenbach and Edelbrock, 1983), *Behavior Assessment System for Children (BASC)* (Reynolds and Kamphaus, 1992), *Brief Infant-Toddler Social and Emotional Scale (BITSEA)* (Briggs-Gowen et al, 2004), *Ages and Stages Questionnaire: Social Emotional (ASQ:SE)* (Squires et al, 2002), *Devereux Early Childhood Assessment Program (DECA)* (LeBuffe and Naglieri, 1999), and *Vineland Socio-Emotional Early Childhood Scale* (Sparrow et al, 1998).

Some additional scales are designed to evaluate specific areas of function, such as coping, self-esteem, or social skills or of malfunction, such as depression, inattention, or autism. The reader is directed to specific chapters addressing these matters for more extensive information. The question of the accuracy and ethics of screening all teenagers with a brief questionnaire to discover early signs of depression is discussed elsewhere.

The proposed advantages of these behavioral rating scales are as follows:

1. They gather information from the informants with the greatest experience with the child.
2. They include some behavior not likely to be observed by the clinician, such as sleep.
3. They are inexpensive and efficient.
4. Some available normative data allow determinations of deviations.
5. They provide quantitative assessments concerning qualitative aspects of behavior.

Perhaps the most important use of such a screening scale by a pediatrician may be to facilitate communication between the physician and the parent or teacher, in that it indicates the physician's concern for behavioral issues and promotes discussion of them. Despite their value in psychiatric research and practice, however, these questionnaires all have significant problems that interfere with their use in pediatric primary care, as follows:

1. The data produced are of little assistance in the identification and management of the common behavioral concerns parents bring to pediatricians, such as sibling quarrels and resistance to toilet training. Screening and referral for major behavioral problems is only a small part of the appropriate mental health role of the pediatrician.
2. Although various claims are made of their psychometric qualifications, no proof has been offered that these questionnaires detect important abnormalities any better than do a few appropriately phrased and directed interview questions, or that they result in an improvement in physician performance (Stancin and Palermo, 1997). The true efficiency of these scales in pediatric practice remains to be shown.
3. With rare exceptions, the available scales rate only abnormalities and do not evaluate positive evidence of behavioral adjustment, such as social competence or self-esteem. The few questionnaires that evaluate positive aspects include the *Strengths and Difficulties Questionnaire* (Goodman, 2001) and *Behavior and Emotional Rating Scale (BERS)* (Epstein and Sharma, 1998).
4. They are highly impressionistic. An item such as "talks too much" measures the caregiver's judgment of what constitutes an excess of talking as much as it does the actual quantity of the behavior in the child. The parents are exercising the diagnostic judgment that should be made by the clinician.
5. They usually give equal weight to ratings of problems of unequal significance, such as nose picking and fire setting.
6. They typically ask about the overall frequency of the behavior without regard for its varying significance in different settings, such as whether trouble paying attention is a problem with listening to safety rules or learning irregular verbs as well as with video games.
7. The context and the parent-child interaction are typically neglected. Two exceptions are the *Child and Adolescent Psychiatric Assessment (CAPA)* (Wamboldt et al, 2001) and *Keys to Interactive Parenting Scale* (Comfort et al, 2006). Because pediatric counseling is likely to deal with the parent-child interaction, any diagnostic system failing to uncover that would be of limited value.

Critics in the mental health professions have complained that pediatricians are not doing a good job in this screening process and are failing to detect substantial numbers of problems present. These conclusions may be correct to some extent, but they say little about the types and significance of problems being missed or the consequences of delay in detection. A more appropriate analysis of this situation (Horowitz et al, 1992) showed "when using a classification system developed specifically for primary care settings, clinicians do identify a large number of children (with) psychosocial and developmental problems." Appropriately directed interviewing has been shown to produce a higher yield of the existing problems (Wissow et al, 1994).

Comprehensive, Dimensional View of Behavior

The *BASICS Behavioral Adjustment Scale (BBAS)* (Carey & McDevitt, 2004) was developed in an effort to overcome as many as possible of these problems for children 4 to 14 years old. This scale was based on the view of adjustment involving the six BASICS areas (*B*ehavior in social relationships, *A*chievements, *S*elf-relations, *I*nternal status, *C*oping, and *S*ymptoms of body functioning) (see Chapter 7). This new scale is comprehensive (covering all these areas), dimensional (positive and negative), descriptive, and useful for clinical practice. It was standardized on a sample of more than 400 children seen in general pediatric practices. It can be completed by the parent in about 15 minutes and scored by a secretarial helper in 2 to 4 minutes. Psychometric qualities are good internal consistency and retest reliability and discriminant validity. It can be used as a further assessment of adjustment after the clinician has determined some degree of parental concern about the child and desires an efficient way to obtain a broader inventory. Clinicians can use these ratings as a starting point to focus for further interviewing and observations.

The Psychodynamic Diagnostic Manual (PDM) of the PDM Task Force (2006) is a welcome psychoanalytical addition to comprehensive systems in that it considers both healthy and disordered personality functioning. Its applications in pediatrics have not yet been evaluated.

Diagnostic Procedure

This chapter urges the view that pediatricians should make use of a comprehensive child health profile, such as the one outlined in this chapter, and that the best way to obtain the necessary data is by parent interview as supplemented with interview data from others, observations, and appropriate information from questionnaires. Before undertaking the actual assessment of the behavioral adjustment, the clinician is well advised to take two preliminary steps: defining the concern and clarifying the goals (Fig. 78-1).

Define the Concern

The first step in the clinical assessment of behavioral adjustment is to clarify what areas of behavior arouse concern either from the caregivers or from the clinician. General parental concern is easily derived from a few introductory questions, such as "How are things going?" or "What sorts of things bother you at this point?" or "What kinds of problems are particularly troublesome now?" Queries more focused on behavior include "What is your child like these days?" or "How is your child's behavior now?" or "How is your child getting on with life these days?" or "How has your child been treating you lately?" This part of the diagnostic process is neither difficult nor time-consuming. The pediatrician can talk with the parent or child about the general nature of outstanding problems in a few minutes.

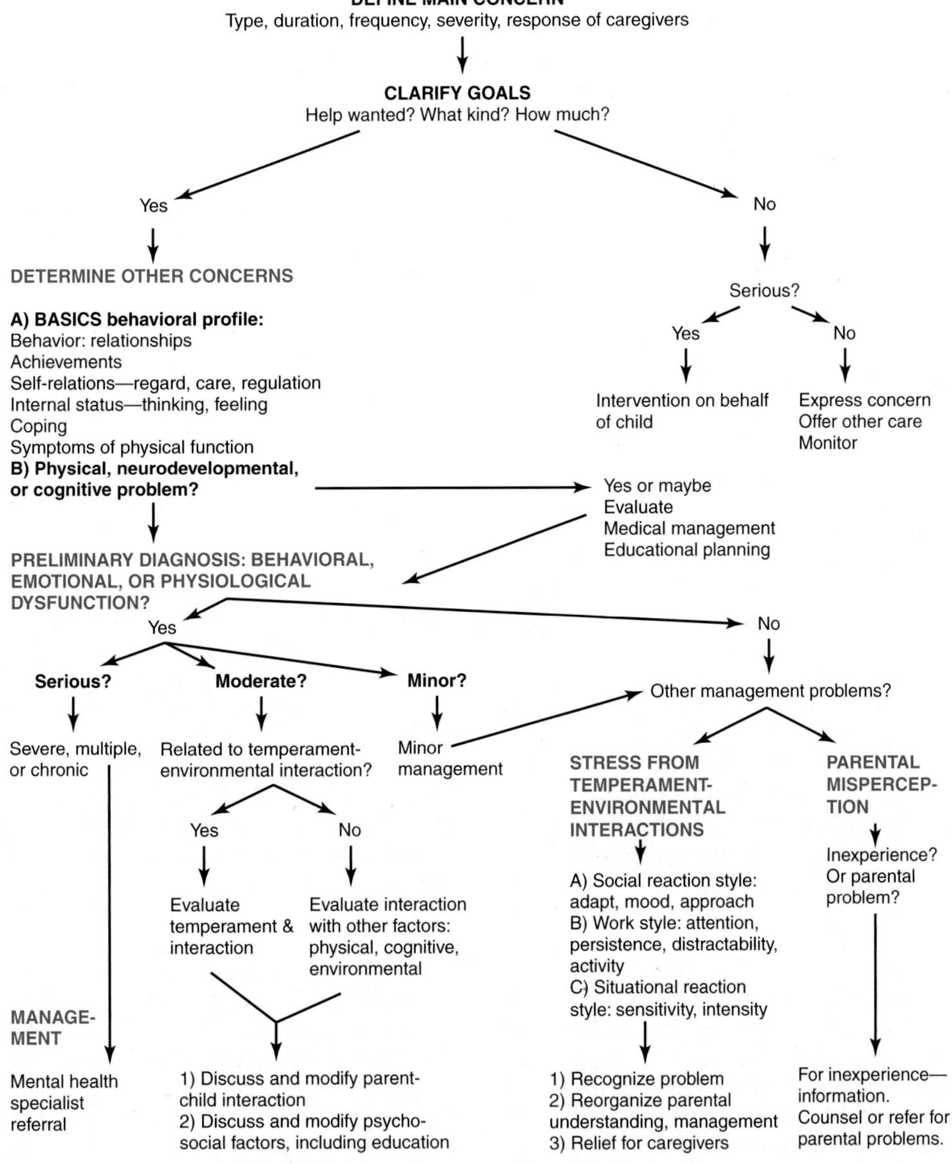

Figure 78-1. Algorithm for management of parental concerns about a child's behavior.

If concern about behavior either is expressed as the reason for the visit or comes up in the course of this initial inquiry, the interviewer should find out who has the concerns, what the concerns involve, where the concerns come from, and why the concerns emerge at this time. If at the outset of a general examination, the caregiver (or patient) reports complete satisfaction with the child's status and progress in all areas, the questioning can be greatly abbreviated from what is described here.

Clarify the Goals and Make an Agreement

When the concern has been discovered, the next step is to determine whether and to what extent family members wish to have the clinician help them with it. The behavioral issue may have been mentioned without any desire for or expectation of intervention by the clinician. The clinician must clarify the objectives of family members and set goals for management. For behavioral issues, the pediatrician does not simply take charge of the diagnostic and therapeutic procedure as when presented with physical illnesses such as otitis media or pneumonia. For behavioral issues, the process of evaluation and management is shared with family members, and an agreement must be established as to what family members expect and what the physician will provide. If family members do not want help, the physician can only express appropriate concern and monitor the problem, unless it is so severe that intervention on behalf of the child is mandatory. When this agreement is reached, the process of diagnosis can continue: determining the child's general physical-developmental-behavioral profile, and establishing the preliminary diagnostic impression and disposition.

Determine the General Physical-Developmental-Behavioral Status: What Else Is Going On?

By means of the history, physical examination, and sometimes laboratory data, the clinician needs to find out what else is going on in the child's life. In particular, more should be learned about function in the other six BASICS areas previously mentioned and presented in Table 78-1.

There is no established set of questions to open and explore these areas. An inquiry regarding social competence might be: "How skillful is your child at getting along with people?" or "How is your child getting on with adults these days?" or "How socially mature does your child seem for a child of his or her age?" or "How does your child get along with other children?" or "What sorts of things happen between your child and other people that do not seem right?"

The pediatrician can inquire as to task performance with questions such as these: "How are things going at school?" or "What does your child do best or least well at school?" or "What does your child like most or least about school?" or "To what extent is your child's performance up to his or her abilities?"

Self-assurance can be assessed by asking: "How does your child seem to feel about himself or herself?" or "What is your child most or least proud of?" or "How well does your child take care of himself or herself?" or "How much trouble does your child have controlling impulses?"

Regarding internal status one might ask: "How happy a child is your child?" or "What sort of worries does your child have?" or "How mature is your child's thinking?"

Coping strategies can be sampled by asking questions such as: "How does your child go about solving a tough problem?" or "What does your child generally do when things are not going well for him or her?"

Symptoms of physical functioning can be assessed with various approaches such as: "What sort of physical complaints does your child have that puzzle you?"

With an older child, the interview also should involve the patient directly. With adolescents, the topics covered may be more specifically directed by the HEADSS approach (*H*ome, *E*ducation/employment, *A*ctivities, *D*rugs, *S*exuality, *S*uicide) or one of the variations on this plan (see Chapter 7), but the results still can be contained in the suggested diagnostic profile.

Assessment of the child's interaction with the caregivers and larger psychosocial situation generally suggests directions for counseling.

Establish Preliminary Diagnostic Impression and Disposition

It should be possible at this point to categorize the parental concern as a parental misperception of a problem (annoying but normal temperament, related to their inexperience, or distortions owing to their own problems) or into one of three levels: a minor problem, which can be dealt with adequately at the time; a more complex issue requiring further attention from the primary care physician at that time or later (mild to moderately severe dysfunction in the child, such as colic or night waking); or a major disturbance needing the more advanced skills or greater time allotments provided by a mental health specialist (significant dysfunction in the child, such as persistent antisocial behavior, declining school performance, or depression).

The objective of this diagnostic process is not only to screen for psychopathologic conditions, as some critics have suggested, but also to develop a more complete picture of the child's status: successes and failures of all types and degrees. The specific tactics and amount of time required for an individual child vary from several questions in a few minutes to extensive interviewing for more than an hour. A second or third visit might be necessary to complete the evaluation, but a preliminary diagnostic impression generally can be gained in several minutes by a skillful interviewer who knows the family.

Judgments as to whether the behavior described is a variation of normal, a temporary or isolated disruption, or a deviation requiring pediatric or psychiatric intervention depends on a knowledge of the range of normal behavior in the child's particular context, as is described in Chapters 2 through 6, and on the application of the criteria of satisfactory adjustment listed previously. The more numerous, severe, and chronic the behavioral symptoms, the greater the need the pediatrician has for seeking help from a mental health specialist. One cannot suggest a simple formula, such as a score on a behavior checklist, for defining indications for referral for concerns about behavior; much depends on the nature and extent of the symptoms, the skills of the pediatrician, and the quantity and quality of referral resources available. These matters are discussed further in Chapter 75 and Chapter 86.

BEHAVIORAL STYLE OR TEMPERAMENT

Because temperament is defined and described in Chapter 7, this section is limited to a discussion of the indications and techniques for temperament assessment.

Indications for Assessment

Routine Professional Care

Pediatricians can and should include a few screening questions about temperament in their periodic evaluations to know what kind of child they are dealing with, and to look for evidence of stressful traits and concerns requiring further investigation. Although routine formal determinations of temperament of all children at certain regular times by pediatricians or schools might become an accepted practice some day, they are not now. No convincing case has been made for such detailed assessments if caregivers are generally satisfied with a child's current behavioral status and there are no discernible areas of malfunction in the child. Possible problems of compliance, uncertain value of the data, and misuse by inexperienced individuals outweigh the potential advantages at present (Carey and McDevitt, 1995).

Nevertheless, the general education of parents and other caregivers about temperament is an important anticipatory guidance role for pediatricians. Because these discussions are not specific, they can be accomplished without a formal assessment. Several books are available for more extensive parent education (Carey and Jablow, 2005; Chess and Thomas, 1987; Keogh, 2003; Kristal, 2004; Kurcinka, 1998; Turecki and Tonner, 1989).

When Child Arouses Concerns

There are two principal indications for formal clinical temperament determinations in children. In cases of behavioral adjustment problems, it is helpful to determine the contribution of the child's temperament to the situation. Such information can provide help in explaining the magnitude and direction of the child's symptoms, and it assists the setting of realistic goals for any therapeutic intervention. With appropriate alteration of the management by caregivers, the reactive symptoms in the child should diminish or disappear. Meanwhile, the parents and other caregivers must learn to live in a more tolerant manner and be more flexible with the child's temperament, which is evidently less changeable (Carey and McDevitt, 1995). It is hard to determine how often this practice is followed.

The other principal situation for temperament determinations is when there is caregiver concern about the child's behavior or the parent-child interaction, but no definite behavioral adjustment problem is evident yet. If the child has a "difficult" temperament or one of the other "temperament risk factors," and these traits are causing a stressful "poor fit" (incompatible relationship) with the values and expectations of the parents or other caregivers, even without a secondary or reactive behavior disorder, it is important for the pediatrician to be fully aware of the child's participation in the problem. If the friction is coming from such a disharmonious interaction, the appropriate management consists of (1) recognition of the true nature of the dissonance, (2) revision of the understanding and management by the caregivers, and (3) some suggestions to the parents and others on how to find relief from their own feelings of stress. Punitive discipline for the child or psychotherapy for the parent or child would be inappropriate. Figure 78-1 shows the timing of these two uses of temperament data. Greater detail about these techniques is available in several books (Carey and McDevitt, 1995; Chess and Thomas, 1986; Turecki and Tonner, 1989).

Techniques for Temperament Determinations

As mentioned earlier, there are three principal methods for obtaining data relating to behavior: interviews, observations, and questionnaires. This is true for temperament and behavioral adjustment.

Interviews

The best-known interview technique for obtaining temperament data is the one devised more than 50 years ago by the New York Longitudinal Study by Thomas and colleagues (see Chapter 7). Although this interview was sufficient for the needs of the New York Longitudinal Study, neither it nor any adaptation of it has found wide usage in research or clinical practice (Chess and Thomas, 1996). Its flexibility makes it more sensitive to varying situations, but it also is less capable of standardization. Its length of 1 to 2 hours (plus ≥1 hours for dictation and rating) allows great richness of detail to be developed in behavioral descriptions, but renders it impractical in any clinical and most research settings.

Nevertheless, clinicians can and often do use these concepts in a much abbreviated form in practical situations. A much shortened interview of the clinician's own construction can yield usable data as long as the clinician resists the temptation to generalize too readily from insufficiently comprehensive descriptions, such as just one instance of a trait. A parental impression of a trait should be supported by illustrations in several settings. Table 78-2 presents suggested areas of function to investigate. The interview approach, adapted to the particular needs of the occasion, is the most convenient way to screen routinely for a "poor fit" or to obtain abbreviated temperament data when there is no need for a more detailed analysis (Carey and McDevitt, 1995).

Observations

Daycare workers and teachers generally have extensive contact with children, placing them in a good position to form sound judgments of individual children. Pediatricians should make use of their contributions. Primary care clinicians usually witness only brief, sometimes atypical samples of behavior. There is still no standardized comprehensive observation technique for assessing

Table 78-2. **Clinician's Impressions of Child's Temperament**

Based on interview and office observation.

Name of child:
Age:
Date:
Professional rater:
Parental informant:

Instructions—This checklist is designed to aid child health professionals in obtaining a rapid survey of any temperament traits causing concern. It reminds the clinician of the main areas where the trait may be described or observed. All items for each trait may not apply to all children, especially younger ones. Items appropriate for infants and toddlers come first. It produces a broad description, not a score or diagnosis.

Activity—Amount of Physical Motion	**High**	**Medium**	**Low**	**?**	**B**
During sleep					
During meals					
During play					
During car ride					
During dressing					
Rate of eating					
While waiting					
Going up, down stairs					
Walking with family					
Listening to music					
Watching TV					
Entering, leaving house					
Talking with parents					

Approach/Withdrawal—Initial Reaction to Novelty	**Approach**	**Medium**	**Withdrawal**	**?**	**B**
New foods					
New sitter					
New place					
New clothes					
Visitors in home					
Strangers elsewhere					
Unfamiliar children					
New toy, game					
New group activity					
Arrival social event					
New situation					

Rhythmicity, Predictability—Physical and Behavioral-Regularity	**Regularity**	**Medium**	**Irregularity**	**?**	**B**
Sleeping times					
Hunger times					
Amount eaten					
Food choices					
Response to parent					
Bowel habits					
Play schedule					
Doing chores					
Doing homework					
Care of possessions					
Order in own room					
Keep appointments					

Adaptability—Flexibility, Ease of Adjustment to Change	**High**	**Medium**	**Low**	**?**	**B**
Change meal time					
Change activities					
Change routines					
Calming if upset					
New places					
Change family plans					
Settling arguments					
Accepting new rules					
Response to coaxing					
Response to mild punishment					
Response to firm punishment					
Major setbacks					

Intensity—Energy of Responses to	**Intense**	**Medium**	**Mild**	**?**	**B**
Hunger					
Pain					
Happiness					
Anger					
Surprise					
Scolding					
Disappointment					
Praise					
Likes and dislikes					
Teasing					
Disapproval					
Discovery					

Distractibility—How Easily External Stimuli Affect Activities	**Distractible**	**Medium**	**Nondistractible**	**?**	**B**
Soothability during pain or fear					
While playing alone					
Playing with friends					
Household noises					
Somebody walks by					
By TV when reading					
By conversation when reading					

Table 78-2. Clinician's Impressions of Child's Temperament—cont'd

Mood—Observed Reactions Positive and Friendly or Negative	Positive	Medium	Negative	?	B
On awakening					
At bedtime					
When tired					
When hungry					
During, after meals					
Frustrated					
Sick or injured					
When corrected					
During play					
Asked to do chores					
During chores					
Denied permission					
New visitors in home					

Sensory Threshold—Sensitivity to Stimuli, Notices	High	Medium	Low	?	B
Changes in taste					
Changes in lighting					
Changes in sound					
Water temperature					
Room temperature					
Texture of clothes					
Odors					
Soiled diapers					
Soiled clothes					
Minor injuries					
Mild parental disapproval					

Persistence/ Attention Span—How Long Activities Pursued	Persistent	Medium	Nonpersistent	?	B
Practice physical activity					
Interest in new toy					
Look at, read book					
Watch TV					
Learning special skill					
Listening to parent					
Household chores					
Work on own project					
Doing homework					
Care of pet, garden					
Difficult project					
Resume task after interruption					
Resume play after interruption					

Comments-

Concerns of caregiver-

Impressions of clinician-

Service needs and other plans-

? = Does not apply or do not know.
B = Bother—refers to whether this specific item is a problem for the caregiver. If so, make a check mark.
For standardized questionnaires assessing temperament or behavioral adjustment, go to www.b-di.com.

temperament for clinical purposes. Various studies have devised methods for use with particular investigations, but these are not easily applicable elsewhere. Matheny (1980) developed an elaboration of the behavioral items on the Bayley development scale for ratings of temperament in the study of twins. This method requires trained observers and has not been applied clinically.

Brazelton's *Neonatal Behavioral Assessment Scale* (1973) is regarded by some clinicians as an appropriate way to determine "constitutional temperament." Despite its considerable value for studying and dealing with neonatal problems and for helping parents understand their newborns, however, newborn behavior is primarily affected by nongenetic prenatal and perinatal factors, is not very stable even from one day to the next, and does not provide an adequate view of the primarily genetically determined temperamental characteristics that emerge in the next few weeks. Comparison between newborn behavior, as measured by the Brazelton scale, and later temperamental traits has been hindered by these factors, and by the fact that some of the newborn measures, such as muscle tone, are not temperament variables, and that

Table 78-3. **Questionnaires for Measuring Temperament**

Principal Questionnaires in English Using New York Longitudinal Study Categories*

Age Span	Name of Test	Authors	No. Items	Retest Reliability	Alpha	References
1-4 mo	*Early Infancy Temperament Questionnaire (EITQ)*	Medoff-Cooper et al	76	0.69m	0.62m	J Dev Behav Peditr 14:230, 1993
4-11 mo	*Revised Infant Temperament Questionnaire (RITQ)*	Carey and McDevitt	95	0.86t	0.83t	Pediatrics 61:735, 1978
1-3 yr	*Toddler Temperament Scale (TTS)*	Fullard et al	97	0.88t	0.85t	J Pediatr Psychol 9:205, 1984
3-7 yr	*Parent Temperament Questionnaire for Children*	Thomas et al	72	NA	NA	Thomas and Chess: Temperament and Development. New York, Brenman/Mazel, 1977
	Teacher Temperament Questionnaire	Thomas et al	64	NA	NA	Thomas and Chess: Temperament and Development. New York, Brenman/Mazel, 1977
	Teacher Temperament Questionnaire short form	Keogh et al	23	0.69-0.88	NA	J Ed Meas 29:323, 1982
	Behavioral Style Questionnaire (BSQ)	McDevitt and Carey	100	0.89t	0.84t	J Child Psychol Psychiatry 19:245, 1978
	Temperament Assessment Battery for Children	Martin	48	0.53-0.81	0.6-0.9	Dept. of Psychology, Univ. of Georgia, Athens, 1988
8-12 yr	*Middle Childhood Temperament Questionnaire (MCTQ)*	Hegvik et al	99	0.87m	0.82m	J Dev Behav Pediatr 3:097. 1982
13-17 yr	*Adolescent Temperament Questionnaire*	McDevitt and Shacknai	NA	NA	NA	In press
18-60 yr	*Adult Temperament Questionnaire*	Chess and Thomas	54	0.76m	0.82m	Behavioral-Developmental Initiatives, 1998

Other Principal Questionnaires Generally not Using New York Longitudinal Study Dimensions†

Colorado Childhood Temperament Inventory (CCTI)
Infant Characteristics Questionnaire (ICQ)
Infant Behavior Questionnaire (IBQ)
Reactivity Rating Scale (RRS)
Emotionality, Activity, and Sociability Scale (EAS)
Dimensions of Temperament Survey (DOTS)
Toddler Behavior Assessment Questionnaire (TBAQ)
Children's Behavior Questionnaire (CBQ)
School Age Temperament Inventory (SATI)
Infant, Toddler, and Preschooler Questionnaires
Temperament and Atypical Behavior Scale

*Retest reliability and internal consistency (alpha) are given as median category *(m)* or total *(t)* values.
†Primarily for research rather than for clinical use.
NA, data not available.
The EITQ, RITQ, TTS, BSQ, MCTQ, Adolescent and Adult Questionnaires, and scoring software may be obtained through Behavioral-Developmental Initiatives (B-DI), 14636 North 55th Street, Scottsdale, AZ, 85254. Telephone 800-405-2313. Web address: www.b-di.com. Online assessment of patients can be approved by registering at www.ipasscode.com/register.

none of the scale items or clusters is the same in content and dimensions as the nine temperament characteristics of the New York Longitudinal Study.

Questionnaires

With the increased recognition of the theoretical and clinical importance of temperament, and the lack of practical ways of measuring it accurately by interview or observations, a series of parent and teacher questionnaires has been developed. Table 78-3 lists a selection of the currently available scales. Most are intended for completion by parents, but some are designed for ratings by teachers, including the *Temperament Assessment Battery for Children* by Martin (1988). Table 78-3 does not include (1) scales based only on observations, such as those by Matheny or Brazelton; (2) techniques possibly assessing temperament, but ostensibly measuring something else, such as the *Conners Parent and Teacher Rating Scales*; (3) scales in foreign languages; (4) unpublished scales; and (5) earlier scales intended primarily for adults such as those by Eysenck in 1956, Guilford and Zimmerman in 1956, Thorndike in 1963, and Strelau in 1972.

Sample items from a scale based on the New York Longitudinal Study view, the MCTQ, are (1) "Runs to where he/she wants to go" and (2) "Avoids (stays away from, doesn't talk to) a new sitter on first meeting." These two items are assessing activity and initial response or approach/withdrawal. They are rated as to frequency from almost never, to rarely, to variable, usually does not, to variable, usually does, to frequently, to almost always.

The questionnaires using the New York Longitudinal Study formulation have several advantages, as follows:

1. They are briefer and more efficient than comparable interview and observation techniques in that they require only 20 to 30 minutes for the caregiver to complete and about 10 to 15 minutes for the clinician or an assistant to score. They are low in cost and high in acceptability. Yet they are not excessively simple; all but one have more than 48 items, and most have 90 to 100 items.
2. They are based on clinically relevant variables. All nine characteristics, such as adaptability and mood, have been shown to be clinically observable and sometimes related to clinical problems. Most of the other research scales available use computer-derived composite constructs, such as "surgency" and "effortful control," which are of uncertain clinical clarity or pertinence (see Chapter 7).
3. They consist of specific behavioral descriptions (e.g., "The infant moves about much [kicks, grabs, squirms] during diapering and dressing"), rather than parental perceptions or general impressions of the child's behavior (e.g., "Child is very energetic").
4. They are standardized as to norms for characteristics at various ages from 1 month through 12 years and beyond.
5. They have adequate psychometric characteristics regarding retest reliability and internal consistency and validity as far as it can be evaluated.

Persisting uncertainties about this set of questionnaires include the following:

1. The question remains unresolved as to whether parents with less than a high school education can respond accurately to these scales. Parents with below average verbal skills may not be able to handle adequately the formation of balanced generalizations and the various shades of meaning, leading to distortions.
2. Parents in cultures or subcultures different from those of the standardization samples might understand the items in dissimilar ways, especially when translated. Not only translation, but also restandardization of the entire scale is indicated in these situations (Carey and McDevitt, 1995).
3. The issue of validity is not easily resolved. Behavioral scientists currently have tended to speak of any parental judgments of temperament as "perceptions," and of their own data, no matter how brief and unrepresentative, as scientific "observations." It would be more appropriate to say that perceptions are general or hasty impressions, and that ratings are a series of more carefully considered judgments of certain behavioral patterns in specific settings. Parents and professionals can have perceptions and make ratings. The ideal test of the validity of the parental ratings on a temperament questionnaire would be a comparison with a comprehensive standardized observational rating scheme. As already mentioned, there is no appropriately matched one in existence now. Every adequately designed test so far has shown at least moderate validity of parental reports, however. Data from parents must be contemporaneous and relate to specific behavioral patterns, rather than general impressions. Comparisons of parental and professional ratings must involve the same content and dimensions of behavior, a requirement overlooked in the few published reports claiming to discredit the validity of parental ratings (Carey, 1983). Clinical users of temperament questionnaires can be reassured of at least a moderate degree of validity. Although distortions can occur, they can be minimized by the interviewing and observations that should always accompany the use of a questionnaire.
4. Several critical reviews of these and other psychometric properties of the existing questionnaires have been published by academic psychologists (Carey and McDevitt, 1995). Although one can agree with them that all the scales have their shortcomings, these reviews suffer from a superficiality of analysis and the absence of a clinical perspective.

In situations of clinical concern about behavior, the best way to measure the contribution of the child's temperament to the interaction is by using one of the more sophisticated questionnaires supplemented by observations and further history as needed. The briefer or more impressionistic questionnaires used by some clinicians in research, and the questionnaires presented in most popular books and articles for parents are not likely to be sufficiently objective and detailed for clinical use.

SUMMARY

Many pediatricians are unsure about how best to evaluate the behavior of their patients. For assessment of behavioral adjustment, this chapter does not encourage the use of screening checklists designed simply to select children for referrals, and it does not support the exclusive use of the categorical pathology diagnostic model. Instead, it recommends a primary reliance on interviewing of the parent directed toward constructing a comprehensive descriptive behavioral profile with a limited use of labels. For determinations of temperament in routine care, a few interview questions generally are sufficient, but in case of parental concern, a standardized questionnaire provides a fuller picture of the child's contribution to the interaction. This enhanced evaluation puts pediatricians in a better position to fulfill their expected role in dealing appropriately with parental concerns, most of which do not need referral.

ACKNOWLEDGMENTS

My thanks to my colleague, Sean C. McDevitt, Ph.D., of Scottsdale, Arizona, for his helpful critical review if this chapter.

REFERENCES

Achenbach TM, Edelbrock CS: Manual for the Child Behavior Checklist and Revised Child Behavioral Profile. Burlington, VT, University of Vermont, Department of Psychiatry, 1983.

American Academy of Pediatrics Task Force on Mental Health Coding for Children: Diagnostic and Statistical Manual for Primary Care: Child and Adolescent Version (DSM-PC). Elk Grove Village, IL, American Academy of Pediatrics, 1996.

American Psychiatric Association: Diagnostic and Statistical Manual of Mental Disorders, 4th ed (DSM-IV). Washington, DC, American Psychiatric Association, 1994.

Brazelton TB: Neonatal Behavioral Assessment Scale. Philadelphia, JB Lippincott, 1973 [Revised version published as Lester B, Tronick E: The Neonatal Intensive Care Unit Network Neurobehavioral Scale (NNNS). Pediatrics 113 (No. 3 Suppl), 2004].

Briggs-Gowen MJ, Carter AQS, Irwin JR, et al: The Brief Infant-Toddler Social and Emotional Assessment: Screening for Social-Emotional Problems and Delays in Competence. J Pediatr Psychol 29:143, 2004.

Carey WB: Some pitfalls in infant temperament research. Infant Behav Dev 6:247, 1983.

Carey WB, Jablow M: Understanding Your Child's Temperament. Philadelphia, XLibris, 2005.

Carey WB, McDevitt SC: Coping with Children's Temperament. New York, Basic Books, 1995.

Carey WB, McDevitt SC: The BASICS Behavioral Adjustment Scale. Test Manual. Scottsdale, AZ, Behavioral-Developmental Initiatives, 2004. Available at: http://www.b-di.com.

Chess S, Thomas A: Temperament in Clinical Practice. New York, Guilford, 1986.

Chess S, Thomas A: Know Your Child. New York, Basic Books, 1987 [republished New Brunswick, NJ, Jason Aronson, 1996].

Chess S, Thomas A: Temperament: Theory and Practice. New York, Brunner-Mazel, 1996.

Comfort M, Gordon PR, Unger DG: The Keys to Interactive Parenting Scale. Zero to Three May: 37-44, 2006.

Costello EJ: Primary care pediatrics and child psychopathology: A review of diagnostic, treatment, and referral practices. Pediatrics 78:1044, 1986.

Epstein MH, Sharma JM: Behavior and Emotional Rating Scale: A Strength-Based Approach to Assessment. Austin, TX, Pro-Ed, 1998.

Eyberg SM, Ross AW: Assessment of child behavior problems: The validation of a new inventory. J Clin Child Psychol 7:113, 1978.

Glascoe FP: Early detection of developmental and behavioral problems. Pediatr Rev 21:272, 2000.

Goodman R: Psychometric properties of the Strengths and Difficulties Questionnaire. J Am Acad Child Adolesc Psychiatry 40:1337, 2001.

Goyette CH, Conners CK, Ulrich RF: Normative data on revised Conners parent and teacher rating scales. J Abnorm Child Psychol 6:221, 1978.

Horowitz SM, Leaf PJ, Leventhal JM, et al: Identification and management of psychosocial and developmental problems in community-based, primary care pediatric practices. Pediatrics 89:480, 1992.

Jellinek MS, Murphy JM, Burns BJ: Brief psychosocial screening in outpatient pediatrics. J Pediatr 109:371, 1986.

Jensen PS, Knapp P, Mrazek DA: Toward a New Diagnostic System for Child Psychopathology: Moving beyond the DSM. New York, Guilford, 2006.

Keogh BK: Temperament in the Classroom. Baltimore, Brookes, 2003.

Kristal J: The Temperament Perspective. Baltimore, Brookes, 2004.

Kurcinka MS: Raising Your Spirited Child. New York, HarperCollins, 1991 [reissued 1998].

Lavigne JV, Binns HJ, Christoffel KK, et al: Behavior and emotional problems among preschool children in pediatric primary care: Prevalence and pediatricians' recognition. Pediatrics 91:649, 1993.

LeBuffe PR, Naglieri JA: The Devereux Early Childhood Assessment (DECA). Devereux Institute of Clinical Training and Research. Lewisville, NC, Kaplan Press, 1999. Available at: www.devereuxearlychildhood.

Martin RP: The Temperament Assessment Battery for Children. Athens, GA, University of Georgia, Department of Psychology, 1988.

Matheny AP Jr: Bayley's Infant Behavior Record: Behavioral components and twin analyses. Child Dev 51:1157, 1980.

National Center for Clinical Infant Programs: Diagnostic Classification: 0–3. Diagnostic Classification of Mental Health and Developmental Disorders of Infancy and Early Childhood (DC: 0-3). Arlington, VA, National Center for Clinical Infant Programs, 1994.

Parents' Evaluations of Developmental Status (PEDS). Nashville, Ellsworth & Vandermeer Press, 1997.

Perrin EC, Stancin T: A continuing dilemma: Whether and how to screen for concerns about children's behavior. Pediatr Rev 23:264, 2002.

Psychodynamic Diagnostic Manual Task Force: The Psychodynamic Diagnostic Manual. Silver Spring, MD, Alliance of Psychoanalytic Organizations, 2006.

Reynolds CR, Kamphaus RW: Behavior Assessment Scale for Children. Circle Pines, MN, American Guidance Service, 1992.

Sparrow S, Balla D, Chichetti D: The Vineland Social-Emotional Early Childhood Scale. Circle Pines, MN, American Guidance Service, 1998.

Squires J, Bricker D, Twombly E: Ages and Stages Questionnaires: Social-Emotional. Baltimore, Brookes, 2002.

Stancin T, Palermo T: A review of behavioral screening practices in pediatric settings: Do they pass the test? J Dev Behav Pediatr 18:183, 1997.

Sturner R, Albus K, Thomas J, Howard B: A proposed adaptation of DC: 0-3R for primary care, developmental research, and prevention of mental disorders. Infant Mental Health J 28:1, 2007.

Turecki S, Tonner L: The Difficult Child (revised). New York, Bantam Books, 1989.

Wamboldt MZ, Wamboldt FS, Gavin L, et al: A parent-child relationship scale derived from the Child and Adolescent Psychiatric Assessment (CAPA). J Am Acad Child Adolesc Psychiatry 40:945, 2001.

Wissow LS, Roter DL, Wilson MEH: Pediatrician interview style and mothers' disclosure of psychosocial issues. Pediatrics 93:289, 1994.

World Health Organization: International Statistical Classification of Diseases and Related Health Problems, 10th revision (ICD-10). Geneva, WHO, 1992.

World Health Organization: International Classification of Functioning Disability and Health (ICF). Geneva, WHO, 2001.

BOOKS RECOMMENDED FOR PARENTS

Carey WB, Jablow M: Understanding Your Child's Temperament. Philadelphia, XLibris, 2005.

Keogh BK: Temperament in the Classroom. Baltimore, Brookes, 2003.

Kristal J: The Temperament Perspective. Baltimore, Brookes, 2004.

Kurcinka MS: Raising Your Spirited Child. New York, HarperCollins, 1991. Reissued 1998.

Turecki S, Tonner L: The Difficult Child (revised). New York, Bantam Books, 1989.

79 DEVELOPMENTAL SCREENING AND ASSESSMENT: INFANTS, TODDLERS, AND PRESCHOOLERS

MARTIN T. STEIN AND MEGHAN KOREY LUKASIK

The fundamental principles of pediatrics can be conceptualized as promotion of optimal physical and psychological health, monitoring developmental maturation, and effective use of the therapeutic relationship that evolves over time. These three core concepts converge in pediatric practice many times each day during the process of developmental screening.

Developmental screening refers to the process of monitoring the maturation of the central nervous system as the environment influences brain maturation. Motor, language, social, and cognitive skills are documented at a particular age and compared with the range of expected maturation. Early recognition of the importance of developmental screening has its roots in the work of Gesell, who developed a neuromaturational model for clinical ascertainment of emerging skills. Although Gesell viewed maturation as primarily biologic, more recent research supports the continuous interaction between a child's social, physical, and emotional environment and brain maturation (see Chapter 8). Synaptogenesis and pruning is the process of forming new neuron connections and the loss of other neuronal connections that constructs the brain's architecture, especially in early childhood. It is a product of interactions between a child's experiences and genetic endowment.

DEVELOPMENTAL SURVEILLANCE, DEVELOPMENTAL SCREENING, AND DEVELOPMENTAL ASSESSMENT

Surveillance, screening, and assessment are different methods used by clinicians to understand the development of children. *Developmental surveillance* is a flexible, longitudinal, continuous, and cumulative process whereby a clinician identifies a child who may be at risk for developmental delays or may have developmental problems (American Academy of Pediatrics, 2006; Dworkin, 1989). To achieve effective surveillance, a pediatrician thinks about a child's development at each clinical encounter. The focus of surveillance is on supporting healthy development, providing parent education, determining the need for referral for further evaluation or treatment, and monitoring early intervention and therapy. Developmental surveillance includes the following five components:

1. Eliciting and attending to parents' concerns
2. Maintaining a developmental history
3. Making accurate and informed observations of the child
4. Identifying risk and protective factors
5. Documenting the process and findings

Mechanisms used for developmental surveillance include a clinical interview in which specific milestones are assessed, a brief neurodevelopmental screen using a predetermined list of milestones, or a standardized screening instrument. The former two methods have strong historical precedent in pediatrics. More recently, these methods have been criticized for lack of standardization and accuracy. Many pediatric practices now use a standardized developmental screening instrument at specific times in the first 3 years of life.

Developmental screening is the use of standardized instruments to identify and refine a developmental risk or potential problem that emerges from surveillance. A psychometric evaluation to establish an acceptable sensitivity, specificity, validity, reliability, and predictive values is a requirement for a "standardized" screening test. These evaluations are typically brief and simple to administer and completed by either a parent or the clinician. Most developmental screening tests are composed of questions directed to a parent or other caregiver about specific areas of development; others require demonstration of specific developmental milestones. A screening test does not yield a diagnosis; rather, it is a process by which a child's development in one or more domains may be identified as atypical compared with children of the same age. Developmental screening may be performed at specific ages or may be used to target an area of concern identified during developmental surveillance.

Developmental evaluation is a diagnostic *assessment* of one or more developmental delays or problems discovered during developmental surveillance or screening. A comprehensive developmental assessment is an evaluation of a child's skills in multiple areas of function, including cognition, communication, motor skills, daily living skills, and social and behavioral skills. Specific tests are available for each of these domains of development. To be considered an evaluation or assessment instrument, these tests must achieve a high level of psychometric quality that ensures validity, reliability, and reproducibility. A developmental assessment is typically performed by a professional with special training in the administration of developmental assessment.

PROCESS OF DEVELOPMENTAL SURVEILLANCE

Every pediatric encounter is an opportunity to consider the development of a child at a moment in time. The most effective and efficient pediatricians monitor current developmental achievements at each office visit. When child development is viewed at the core of primary care pediatrics, asking and making careful observations about developmental progress becomes an integral part of each clinical encounter. Developmental surveillance does not wait for a formal screening examination, but is built into the medical history and clinical observations. Although development refers to brain maturation in motor, language, social, and cognitive domains, experienced pediatricians include behavioral observations that monitor social reciprocity, mood, and the social context of language.

It is often useful to include a general question about concerns directed to parents early in a clinical encounter: "Do you have any concerns about your child's development or behavior?" Research suggests that the language used by clinicians is crucial to accurate responses from parents. The word *concerns* in English and its equivalent in other language elicits the most reliable responses (Glascoe, 1999). Combining *behavior and development* is useful because some parents do not easily differentiate between behavior and development, and developmental delays may manifest through an atypical behavior pattern. A 2-year-old with a language delay resulting from a hearing deficiency may present with either withdrawn or disruptive behaviors.

Developmental surveillance in primary care pediatrics depends on the interviewing skills of the clinician. Clinical encounters with parents and children generally are enhanced by continuity of care when a trusting relationship between a clinician and family is developed over time. Inquiring about a parent's concerns calls for sufficient time to allow the parent to tell his or her story. In most cases, a parent's description of a concern provides the elements of an initial impression that leads to further questions or a screening test at the same visit. To acquire the most accurate information about a young child's development, careful attention to the interpersonal process of the interview should simultaneously encourage empathy, enhancement of trust, limitation of anxieties that restrict information exchange, and active participation of the parent. Effective interviewing during an encounter that monitors early child development includes the following components:

1. Establishing the agenda: "What concerns to you have about your child?"
2. Open-ended questions: "What changes have you seen in your child's development since the last visit?"
3. Close-ended questions: "Tell me about how your child is talking—what words does your child use?"
4. Pauses and silent periods allow the parent to collect thought and express feelings.
5. Repetition of important phrases encourages further exploration and clarification: "Tell me more about that."
6. Active listening involves undivided attention to what the parent is saying through the clinician's words and body (nonverbal) language.
7. Communication of trust and respect includes sensitive awareness of parent's needs, expectations, and concerns, and their resources and limitations.
8. "Time with the patient will remain the currency of medical care." (Eisenberg L: Personal communication, 2002)

Developmental surveillance may occur during a well-child visit, an illness visit, when monitoring a chronic physical condition, in the hospital or emergency department, and even when talking to a parent on the telephone. There are numerous opportunities in the work of a primary care clinician that should encourage effective surveillance for developmental monitoring or the determination of a potential problem (Table 79-1).

An alternative method of developmental surveillance is the use of a "developmental theme" for each well-child visit (Dixon and Stein, 2006). Rapid changes in neurodevelopmental capacities and behavior during childhood allow clinicians an opportunity to conceptualize a unique developmental or behavioral theme at each well-child visit. Recognizing that a child evolves along several dimensions at any one time, specific strands of development emerge as prominent at particular, predictable times. The clinical relevance of a topic at a moment in time allows the clinician to review the full range of a developmental theme at a particular age. In this way, each visit opens up new information and perspective at a time when a particular theme is important to a family and easy to see in a child. When the focus is on a specific developmental theme, the clinician is ready to take on concerns, problems, deviations from typical development, and the issues of children in unusual circumstances.

Using this method of surveillance, questions to parents and children, clinical observations, physical and neurodevelopmental examinations, and anticipatory guidance may be guided by the developmental-behavioral theme. In this way, surveillance for age-expected milestones can be monitored in a broader context. Through focused observations, questions, and a few interactions, a child can teach us what we need to know. These clinical probes allow easy access to understanding what a child and family is about. It is the children that allow pediatric clinicians to practice this form of developmental surveillance.

Table 79-1. **Examples of Opportunities for Developmental Surveillance in Primary Care Pediatrics**

Presentation	Implications for Screening
At a 4-month well-child visit, the pediatrician observes a remarkably quiet infant with limited spontaneous movements when held by the mother and when placed on the examination table	A quiet, slow-to-warm-up temperament; generalized hypotonia or hypertonia and weakness; central depression from nonaccidental brain injury
The parent of a thriving 6-month-old infant is asked, "Does he reach out for things?" Following a positive response, the pediatrician asks, "Does he prefer one hand over the other?" The mother responds, "Yes, he seems to use his left hand more"	Occult nonaccidental trauma; hemiparesis from a fetal stroke or congenital brain anomaly of development
The parent of an 18-month old toddler, who was observed to walk well and climb onto her mother's lap, is asked, "Tell me about her use of words." The father responds that she says only 2 words ("dada" and "ba" for milk)	Significant expressive language delay
A 20-month-old child was seen in the emergency department for a high fever, rhinorrhea, and irritability. The clinician made a diagnosis of acute otitis media. The clinician then asked the parent if there were any other concerns. When the response was negative, the clinician followed with a few developmental screening questions: "When did he walk?" "How many words is he saying?" "Does he use a cup and spoon to feed himself?" The parent responded that the child does not walk, and that she has been worried about limited use of his legs for a long time. A screening neuromuscular examination revealed mild symmetric, increased tone and hyperreflexia of all extremities	Spastic cerebral palsy

Children always practice the leading edge of their developmental competency, working at an emerging or newly acquired skill and delighting in a toy or activity that is just a little new and challenging. Through knowledge of developmental sequences, a wise clinician sets up toys or asks questions aimed at that developmental edge. The office visit should be orchestrated so that the assessment occurs automatically, seemingly incidentally through the processes of checking in, weighing, measuring, playing in the waiting room, and being in the examination room. The clinician should set the agenda, set the stage, and then let the drama begin. Through this proactive, automatic, and easy approach, rich information is gathered with no extra time or ongoing effort. This process depends, however, on the clinician knowing what to look for, what to ask, and what simple maneuvers can be done quickly with a child and family (Dixon and Stein, 2006).

Providing a developmentally focused name for each well-child visit expands a clinician's ability as he or she approaches each child with a framework that discovers the connections between individual milestones and events in a child's life. The following examples of developmentally focused surveillance themes among infants, toddlers, and preschool children illustrate this method:

Prenatal visit: making an alliance with a family
6 Months: reaching out
8 to 9 Months: exploring and clinging
15 to 18 Months: declaring independence and pushing the limits
2 Years: language leaps
3 Years: the emergence of magic
4 Years: A clearer sense of self

DEVELOPMENTAL SCREENING

Experienced pediatricians may perform a comprehensive interview and a standard neurologic examination, including developmental milestones, as a method of developmental screening. More recently, developmental screening refers to questionnaires in the form of a checklist completed by parents. *Checklists are effective as an adjunct to the clinical interview.* They may be completed before a visit (at home or while waiting in the office; with paper and pencil or through a computer database). In some pediatric offices, an individual with nursing or child development training is responsible for systematic screening for developmental (and behavioral) problems during well-child visits.

When administered before interviewing and examining a child, standardized developmental screening tools may focus the clinical interview in areas of importance to the parents. It also may encourage the clinician to focus clinical observations and interactions with the child and parent on specific areas of development. Screening tests may trigger questions, raise issues, and prevent omissions in data collection. Validated screening tests should have good reliability and predictive value. A screening test is not diagnostic, however. A positive developmental screening test suggests a problem that must be evaluated further through either a comprehensive, focused interview and neurodevelopmental examination by the primary care clinician or a referral for a developmental assessment by a developmental-behavioral pediatrician or a child psychologist. To ensure the value of screening, pediatricians must be aware of available specialty resources in their community to refer a child for a more comprehensive developmental assessment.

Developmental screening instruments have some distinct advantages and limitations. They provide a standardized database that may serve some clinicians as an organizing strategy for health supervision visits. Screening tests prevent omissions that may occur during an interview alone. They provide potential educational value as a parent or older child answers questions that raise a concern that may not have been considered previously. During the process of completing the screening, a parent may become a better observer of the child's developmental changes and behaviors. In this way, the process of screening is an opportunity to communicate with parents about a child's developmental strengths. Maintaining copies of the screening checklist in the medical record has been used to monitor quality assurance.

A potential disadvantage of relying only on a screening tool is that a parent's agenda for the visit may be missed by not permitting an individualized focus for each visit. A checklist without a therapeutic interview encourages an emphasis on content at the expense of process and a false sense of completeness (Perrin and Stancin 2002). In addition, a standardized screening test may not be sensitive to cultural differences that have an impact on developmental trajectories.

Pediatricians generally rely on developmental surveillance. Less than 25% of primary care pediatricians routinely use a standardized test for developmental screening during well-child visits (Sand et al, 2005). The American Academy of Pediatrics recommends that, in addition to developmental surveillance at each well-child visit, a standardized developmental screening tool should be administered at 3 visits during the first 3 years of life: 9 months, 18 months, and 30 months (American Academy of Pediatrics, 2006). These stages in a child's early development represent a time when particular domains of developmental achievement may be accurately assessed: gross/fine motor skill and early social skills at 9 months; early language and emerging social skills at 18 months, when signs of autistic spectrum disorder may be detected; and expressive/receptive language at 30 months, especially among the 15% to 20% of "late-talking" toddlers at 24 months, many of whom are normal at 30 months (Table 79-2).

Developmental screening instruments are categorized in four areas: general developmental, language/cognitive development, motor development, and autism screening. Most of the tests rely on questions directed to parents. Some tests include eliciting developmental achievements from the child (see Table 79-2). A unique form of general developmental screening is the *Parents' Evaluation of Developmental Status (PEDS)*; the parent is asked specifically about "concerns" in eight developmental, behavioral, and learning domains. All of the developmental screening tools, with the exception of those that focus on autism, derive their organizing framework from Gesell's neuromaturational model of developmental milestones. They are different with regard to age range, administration time, psychometric properties, and number of milestones ascertained. It is useful for primary care pediatricians to develop expertise in one test in each of the categories. To ensure the regular use of screening tests, the staff and organization of an office or clinic must be responsive to the routine use of these tests, including scoring and follow-up.

DEVELOPMENTAL ASSESSMENT

Developmental assessment describes a comprehensive evaluation of a child's skills, including cognition, communication, motor skills, daily living skills, and social and behavioral skills. A developmental assessment typically includes one or more standardized tests. Although

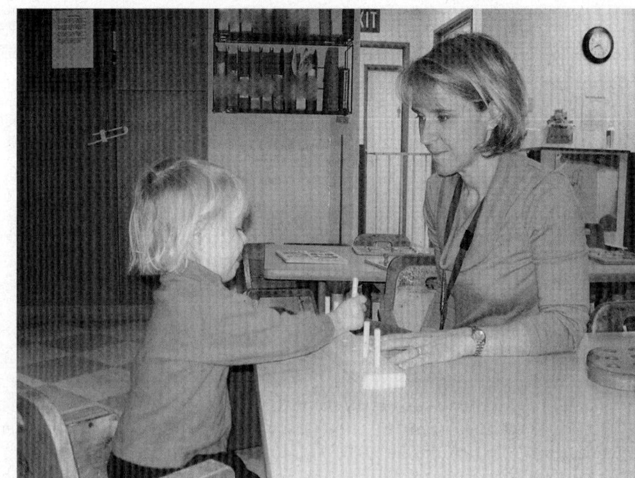

Figure 79-1. Administration of a standardized developmental assessment.

professionals with specific training perform developmental assessments, understanding the essential elements of a developmental assessment allows pediatric clinicians to provide parents with accurate information and to make effective referrals (Fig. 79-1).

The selection and administration of appropriate standardized tests are crucial components of a developmental assessment allowing comparison of one child's responses with a clearly defined normative sample of same-aged peers. A standardized test measures a sample of behavior at a particular moment in time. Each test is limited by what it was designed to measure, and no one test captures all aspects of a child's functioning. Poor cooperation and low motivation can affect performance. Interviews with the child, parent, and other individuals consistently involved with the child also are important components of developmental assessment. Behavioral observation during testing and in more familiar settings (home, daycare, school) provides information about the child in various environments and conditions. An informal assessment of play skills and the use of language supplements standardized procedures. At the end of the testing period, an opportunity is provided for the parents and professionals to review the results.

In most cases, a written report is generated using language that is tailored to the intended audience (i.e., parents, teacher, pediatrician). A clear and concise written report serves as a valuable communication tool; provides information about the child's current functioning; and, most importantly, can be used to direct appropriate treatment recommendations and measure progress following early intervention (Sattler, 1988).

Quality Control

In an effort to promote professional and ethical standards with regard to the administration of developmental and other psychological tests, the American Psychological Association (2006) developed specific guidelines. Most publishers of standardized tests have adopted a standard language that consists of three levels of user qualifications (levels A, B, and C). The definition of the levels of user qualification can be found on the companies' websites, catalogues, or in the testing manual. Most developmental and cognitive tests require a graduate level education and specific training.

Psychometric Assessment and the Flynn Effect

When interpreting results of psychological tests, it is important to consider the date of publication of the normative sample. Typically, tests are renormed every 15 to 20 years (Kanaya et al, 2003). Flynn showed that intelligence scores for a population increase over time 5 to 25 points (the "Flynn effect"). The cause of this increase is uncertain. Flynn compared IQ scores on a popular test used in the United States where the test was not renormed for 25 years. At the beginning of the normative cycle, the number of individuals classified as intellectually disabled was 8.8 million compared with 2.6 million after restandardization (Plucker, 2003).

Similarities and Differences between Developmental Tests and Measures of Cognition and Intelligence

Pediatricians should be knowledgeable about what a test was designed to measure. Developmental tests measure motor, social, language, and nonverbal skills in infants and toddlers. The Gesell (not reviewed in this chapter owing to outdated norms) and the Bayley Scales are two of the most well-known measures of development. The Gesell was the first test to measure predictable neuro-maturational milestones of development (Gesell and Amatruda, 1941). The current Bayley Scales measures cognition and language, play, and motor abilities. In contrast, the *Wechsler Preschool and Primary Scale of Intelligence, Third Edition (WPPSI-III)* is a *cognitive* or *intelligence* test with scores provided using an intelligence quotient (IQ). The WPPSI-III emphasizes problem-solving and communication skills, rather than motor play and behavioral issues. The WPPSI-III and other cognitive measures also include assessment of developmental progress in young children.

Test scores of young children provide information about the current level of developmental functioning. They should not be used to make predictions about future performance (Sattler, 1988). With the exception of young children with severe developmental delays, test results in infants and toddlers typically do not correlate well with later performance. It is not until age 5 that scores on standardized tests begin to show some stability (Handen, 1997). Despite lack of predictive validity, testing young children is helpful in identifying early indications of concern, which can direct intervention at a time in children's lives when the brain is rapidly growing, synaptogenesis is robust, and therapeutic interventions are most effective.

Frequently Used Standardized Tests for Developmental Assessment

Bayley Scales of Infant and Toddler Development, Third Edition

The Bayley Scales has become a gold standard for assessment of early child development (Table 79-3). The popularity of this measure is attributed to sound psychometric properties, child-friendly materials, and usefulness in providing benchmark information at various stages of intervention. The third edition of the *Bayley Scales of Infant and Toddler Development* is an individually administered test of developmental functioning for infants and young children 1 to 42 months of age. The original *Bayley Scales of Infant Development* was published in 1969. The test was developed to reflect the significant changes that occur in development during the first few years of life.

The Bayley Scales is administered individually to identify children with developmental delays, to initiate early intervention services, and to chart progress after intervention. The third edition has an increased focus on the toddler years. A primary goal of the third edition was to update the normative sample. New distinct composite areas include measures of cognition, expressive and receptive language, fine and gross motor skills, social-emotional aspects, and adaptive behavior. Race, ethnicity, parent education, and geographic region closely correspond with the 2000 U.S. Census. Children with risk factors that could potentially affect performance were excluded. A separate normative database for children at risk for developmental delay is included. Expected test performance differences are found between the clinical group and the normative group indicating that this is an excellent assessment tool for determining developmental functioning in children with special needs and for determining their eligibility for services (Bayley, 2006a, 2006b).

Leiter International Performance Scale–Revised

The *Leiter International Performance Scale–Revised* is a nonverbal test of cognitive abilities. This test does not require any spoken language by the examiner or the individual taking the test. It has been normed on individuals 2 to 20 years, 11 months old, which is a younger start point than other nonverbal tests. The theoretical basis of the Leiter-R has its foundations in hierarchical models of cognitive abilities similar to the *Kaufman Assessment Battery for Children-II (KABC-II), Stanford Binet 5,* and WPPSI-III. General intelligence ("g") in children 2 to 5 years old is measured by assessing fluid reasoning, fundamental visualization, and attention.

Twenty subtests are grouped evenly in two overall areas: visualization and reasoning and attention and memory. The batteries can be administered separately or together depending on the referral question. For the visualization and reasoning battery, overall results are reported using a full-scale IQ score. There also are four behavioral rating scales (examiner, parent, self, and teacher) and a brief IQ screener for the visual and reasoning battery and a brief memory process screener. The Leiter-R was standardized using population samples from the 1993 U.S. Census. The Leiter-R has been normed on children with several chronic conditions, including severe speech and language impairment, severe hearing impairment, severe motor delay or deviation, traumatic brain injury, mild-to-moderate or severe intellectual disability, attention-deficit/hyperactivity disorder, gifted, nonverbal learning disabilities, verbal learning

Table 79-2. **Developmental Screening**

General Developmental Screening Tool	Description	Age Range	No. Items	Administration Time
Ages and Stages Questionnaires (ASQ)	Parent-completed questionnaire; series of 19 age-specific questionnaires screening communication, gross motor, fine motor, problem-solving, and personal adaptive skills; results in pass/fail score for domains	4-60 mo	30	10-15 min
Battelle Developmental Inventory Screening Tool, 2nd edition (BDI-ST)	Directly administered tool; designed to screen personal-social adaptive, motor, communication, and cognitive development; results in pass/fail score and age equivalent; can be modified for children with special needs	Birth to 95 mo	100	10-15 min (<3 yr) or 20-30 min (≥3 yr)
Bayley Infant Neurodevelopmental Screen (BINS)	Directly administered tool; series of 6 item sets screening basic neurologic functions (visual, auditory, and tactile input); expressive functions (oral, fine and gross motor skills); and cognitive processes; results in risk category (low, moderate, high risk)	3-24 mo	11-13	10 min
Brigance Screens–II	Directly administered tool; series of 9 forms screening articulation, expressive and receptive language, gross motor, fine motor, general knowledge, personal social skills, and preacademic skills (when appropriate); for 0-23 mo, can also use parent report	0-90 mo	8-10	10-15
Child Development Inventory (CDI)	Parent-completed questionnaire; measures social, self-help, motor, language, and general development skills; results in developmental quotients and age equivalents for different developmental domains; suitable for more in-depth evaluation	18 mo to 6 y	300	30-50 min

Psychometric Properties	Scoring Method	Cultural Considerations	Purchase/ Obtainment Information	Key References
Normed on 2008 children from diverse ethnic and socioeconomic backgrounds, including Spanish speaking; sensitivity 0.70-0.90 (moderate to high); specificity 0.76-0.91 (moderate to high)	Risk categorization; provides a cutoff score in 5 domains of development that indicates possible need for further evaluation	English, Spanish, French, and Korean versions available	Paul H. Brookes Publishing Co: 800-638-3775; www.brookespublishing.com	Squires J, Potter L, Bricker D: The ASQ User's Guide, 2nd ed. Baltimore, Paul H. Brookes Publishing Co, 1999
Normed on 2500 children, demographic information matched 2000 U.S. Census data; additional bias reviews performed to adjust for gender and ethnicity concerns	Quantitative; scaled scores in all 5 domains are compared with cutoffs to determine need for referral	English and Spanish versions available	Riverside Publishing Co: 800-323-9540; www.riverpub.com	Newborg J: Battelle Developmental Inventory, 2nd ed. Itasca, IL, Riverside Publishing, 2004
Normed on ~1700 children, stratified on age, to match 2000 U.S. census; sensitivity 0.75-0.86 (moderate); specificity 0.75-0.86 (moderate)	Risk categorization; children are graded as low, moderate, or high risk in each of 4 conceptual domains by use of 2 cutoff scores	English and Spanish versions available	Psychological Corp: 800-211-8378; www.harcourtassessment.com	Aylward GP: Bayley Infant Neurodevelopmental Screener. San Antonio, TX. Psychological Corp. 1995; Aylward G, Verhulst SJ, Bell S: Predictive utility of the BSID-II Infant Neurodevelopmental Screener (BINS): Risk status classifications, clinical interpretation, and application. Dev Med Child Neurol 42:25-31, 2000
Normed on 1156 children from 29 clinical sites in 21 states; sensitivity 0.70-0.80 (moderate); specificity 0.70-0.80 (moderate)	All results are criterion based; no normative data are presented	English and Spanish versions available	Curriculum Associates Inc: 800-225-0248; www.curriculumassociates.com	Glascoe FP: Technical Report for the Brigance Screens. North Billerica, MA: Curriculum Associates Inc, 2005; Glascoe FP: The Brigance Infant-Toddler Screen (BITS): Standardization and validation. J Dev Behav Pediatr 23:145-150, 2002
Normative sample included 568 children from south St. Paul, MN, a primarily white, working-class community; Doig et al included 43 children from a high-risk follow-up program, which included 69% with high school education or less and 81% Medicaid; sensitivity 0.80-1.0. (moderate to high); specificity 0.94-0.96 (high)	Quantitative; provides age equivalents in each domain and SDs	English and Spanish versions available	Behavior Science Systems Inc: 612-850-8700; www.childdevrev.com	Ireton H: Child Development Inventory Manual. Minneapolis, MN, Behavior Science Systems Inc, 1992; Doig KB, Macias MM, Saylor CF, et al: The Child Development Inventory: A developmental outcome measure for follow-up of high risk infant. J Pediatr 133:358-362, 1999

(Continued)

Table 79-2. Developmental Screening—cont'd

	Description	Age Range	No. Items	Administration Time
Child Development Review–Parent Questionnaire (CDR-PQ)	Parent-completed questionnaire; professional-completed child development chart measures social, self-help, motor, and language skills	18 mo to 5 yr	6 open-ended questions and a 26-item possible problems checklist to be completed by the parent, followed by 99 items crossing the 5 domains, which may be used by the professional as an observation guide or parent-interview guide	10-20 min
Denver-II Developmental Screening Test	Directly administered tool; designed to screen expressive and receptive language, gross motor, fine motor, and personal social skills; results in risk category (normal, questionable, abnormal)	0-6 yr	125	10-20 min
Infant Development Inventory	Parent-completed questionnaire; measures social, self-help, motor, and language skills	0-18 mo	4 open-ended questions followed by 87 items crossing the 5 domains	5-10 min
Parents' Evaluation of Developmental Status (PEDS)	Parent-interview form; designed to screen for developmental and behavioral problems needing further evaluation; single response form used for all ages; may be useful as a surveillance tool	0-8 yr	10	2-10 min
Language and Cognitive Tools				
Capute Scales (also known as *Cognitive Adaptive Test/Clinical Linguistic Auditory Milestone Scale [CAT/CLAMS]*)	Directly administered tool; measures visuomotor/problem solving (CAT), and expressive and receptive language (CLAMS); results in developmental quotient and age equivalent	3-36 mo	100	15-20 min
Motor Screening Tools				
Early Motor Pattern Profile (EMPP)	Physician-administered standard examination of movement, tone, and reflex development; simple 3-point scoring system	6-12 mo	15	5-10 min
Motor Quotient (MQ)	Uses simple ratio quotient with gross motor milestones for detecting delayed motor development	8-18 mo	11 total milestones; 1 per visit	1-3 min

From American Academy of Pediatrics: Identifying infants and young children with developmental disorders in the medical home: An algorithm for developmental surveillance and screening. Pediatrics 118:405-420, 2006.

Psychometric Properties	Scoring Method	Cultural Considerations	Purchase/ Obtainment Information	Key References
Standardized with 220 children 3-4 y from primarily white, working-class families in south St. Paul MN; sensitivity 0.68 (low); specificity 0.88 (moderate)	Risk categorization; parents' responses to the 6 questions and problems checklist are classified as indicating (1) no problem, (2) a possible problem, or (3) a possible major problem	English and Spanish versions available	Behavior Science Systems Inc	Ireton H: Child Development Review Manual. Minneapolis, MN, Behavior Science Systems, 2004
Normed on 2096 term children in Colorado; diversified in terms of age, place of residence, ethnicity/cultural background, and maternal education; sensitivity 0.56-0.83 (low to moderate); specificity 0.43-0.80 (low to moderate)	Risk categorization; pass or fail for each question, and these responses are compared with age-based norms to classify children in the normal range, suspect or delayed	English and Spanish versions available	Denver Developmental Materials: 800/419-4729; www.denverii.com	Frankenburg WK, Camp BW, Van Natta PA: Validity of the Denver Development Screening Test. Child Dev 42:475-485, 1971; Glascoe FP, Byrne KE, Ashford LG, et al: Accuracy of the Denver-II in developmental screening. Pediatrics 89:1221-1225, 1992
Studied in 86 high-risk 8-mo-olds seen in a perinatal follow-up program and compared with the Bayley scales; sensitivity 0.85 (moderate); specificity 0.77 (moderate)	Risk categorization; delayed or not delayed	English and Spanish versions available	Behavior Science Systems Inc	Creighton DE, Sauve RS: The Minnesota Infant Development Inventory in the developmental screening of high-risk infants at 8 mo. Can J Behav Sci 20(special issue):424-433, 1988
Standardized with 771 children from diverse ethnic and socioeconomic backgrounds, including Spanish speaking; sensitivity 0.74-0.79 (moderate); specificity 0.70-0.80 (moderate)	Risk categorization; provides algorithm to guide need for referral, additional screening or continued surveillance	English, Spanish, Vietnamese, Arabic, Swahili, Indonesian, Chinese, Taiwanese, French, Somali, Portuguese, Malaysian, Thai, and Laotian versions available	Ellsworth and Vandemeer Press LLC: 888-729-1697; www.pedtest.com	
Standardized on 1022 North American children 2-36 mo; correlations high with Bayley Scales of Infant Development; sensitivity 0.21-0.67 in low-risk populations (low); specificity 0.95-1.00 in low-risk population (high) and 0.82-0.98 in high-risk populations (moderate to high)	Quantitative (developmental age levels and quotient)	English, Spanish, and Russian versions available	Paul H. Brookes Publishing Co	Voight RG, Brown FR III, Fraley JK, et al: Concurrent and predictive validity of the cognitive adaptive test/clinical linguistic and auditory milestone scale (CAT/CLAMS) and the Mental Developmental Index of the Bayley Scales of Infant Development. Clin Pediatr (Phila) 42:427-432, 2003
Single published report of 1247 high-risk infants; sensitivity 0.87-0.92 (moderate to high); specificity 0.98 (high)	Risk categorization (normal/suspect/ abnormal	English version available	See key references	Morgan AM, Aldag JC: Early identification of cerebral palsy using a profile of abnormal motor patterns. Pediatrics 98:692-697, 1996
Single published report of 144 referred children; sensitivity 0.87 (moderate); specificity 0.89 (moderate)	Quantitative (developmental age levels and quotient)	English version available	See key references	Capute AJ, Shapiro BK: The motor quotient: A method for early detection of motor delay. Am J Dis Child 139:940-942, 1985

disabilities, and English as a second language. Individuals with a pervasive developmental disorder such as autistic disorder were not included. A limitation of the Leiter-R is the extensive time necessary to administer the visualization and reasoning and attention and memory batteries (Roid and Miller, 1997).

Mullen Scales of Early Learning

The *Mullen Scales of Early Learning* is a measure of cognitive functioning for infants and preschool-age children from birth through age 68 months (see Table 79-3). Although the Mullen Scales is not defined as a developmental or intelligence test, components of each are found in the test. Information about cognitive functioning is generated in four distinct areas (visual reception, fine motor, receptive language, and expressive language scales). There also is a measure of gross motor skills. In contrast to other developmental tests, the Mullen Scales provides a composite score that is referred to as an estimate of overall intelligence.

The theoretical foundation of the Mullen Scales is based on the concepts of neurodevelopment and intrasensory and intersensory learning. The decision to emphasize separate and distinct scales of learning over a single measure of intelligence was based on research in the area of infant and toddler intelligence that suggests a single score can be misleading and mask uneven abilities by lumping them all into one score. The Mullen Scales results are reported using T scores to interpret results and target intervention with an emphasis on a child's strengths as building blocks for weaker areas. The standardization sample for the Mullen Scales included 1849 children 2 days to 69 months of age (Mullen, 1995). As a test of cognitive function, the Mullen Scales has numerous strengths, including separate standard scores for expressive and receptive language and fine and gross

Table 79-3. Frequently Used Standardized Tests of Development and Cognition in Young Children

Test	Age Range	Description/Comments	Administration Time	Publisher, Date	Relationship to Similar Measures
Bayley Scales of Infant and Toddler Development, Third Edition	1-42 mo	Measures multiple developmental domains: cognitive, receptive, and expressive language; fine and gross motor; social-emotional and adaptive behavior	30-90 min	Harcourt Assessments, 2005	High correlations with the WPPSI-III; high correlations between the language composite and a similar measure of receptive and expressive language; moderate correlations for the motor composite and similar test of motor skills
Mullen Scales of Early Learning	Birth to 68 mo for cognitive scales; birth to 33 mo for gross motor scales	Measures four cognitive domains: fine motor, visual reception, receptive and expressive language, and gross motor skills; concerns raised that normative sample is becoming outdated	15-60 min	Pearson Assessments, 1995: originally published by American Guidance System, Inc, publishing	Good reliability with the original Bayley and other tests measuring specific areas of functioning
Peabody Picture Vocabulary Test–IV	2 yr 6 mo to >90 yr	Measures understanding of single word vocabulary	Averages 10-15 min	Pearson Assessments, 2006	
Stanford-Binet Intelligence Scale, Fifth Edition	2 yr to >85 yr	Measure of general cognitive ability	Approximately 5 min per subtest	Riverside Publishing, 2003	High correlations with previous WPPSI-R and with other similar measures for older children and adults; more research needed comparing preschool-age children
Wechsler Preschool and Primary Scale of Intelligence, Third Edition	2 yr 6 mo to 7 yr 3 mo (divided into 2 age bands)	Measure of general cognitive ability using 4 composite scores (full-scale IQ, verbal IQ, performance IQ, processing speed quotient)	30-60 min (depending on child's age)	The Psychological Corporation, a Harcourt Assessment Company, 2002	High correlations with *Bayley Scales of Infant Development, 2nd Edition, and Differential Ability Scale*
Woodcock-Johnson III	2 yr to >90 yr	Measure of intellectual functioning, oral language, and achievement	35-45 min for cognitive, 55-66 min for achievement	The Riverside Publishing Company, 2001	High correlations with other similar measures, but no available comparisons for children <4 yr

motor skills and a large age band for following children over time with the same measure. Many studies of children with autistic spectrum disorders use the Mullen as its primary measure of cognition. A weakness of this test is that studies of children with specific conditions (e.g., children with language delay, cerebral palsy) were not completed at the time of the standardization process. It is unclear how useful such measures are for these subgroups.

Peabody Picture Vocabulary Test, Fourth Edition

The *Peabody Picture Vocabulary Test, Fourth Edition (PPVT-IV),* measures listening and understanding of single-word vocabulary (see Table 79-3). It was developed for individuals 2 years 6 months old through greater than 90 years old. A similar test is appropriate for Spanish-speaking individuals, the *Test de Vocabulario en Imagenes Peabody (TVIP)*. The administration and scoring procedures of this version are similar to the third edition, with added color, a larger easel size, and a new metric for measuring growth, called the growth scale value. A strength of the PPVT-IV is the speed of administration. It does not require the child to speak, read, or write. Although most examinees respond by touching or pointing to pictures, the test can be administered to individuals with significant motor impairment. In those circumstances, the examiner provides the vocabulary word and the examinee signals "yes" or "no" as the examiner points to each picture option (Pearson Assessment, 2006).

Stanford Binet Intelligence Scale, Fifth Edition

Now in its fifth edition, the Stanford Binet Intelligence Scales (SB5) have made a significant contribution to intelligence testing (see Table 79-3). The earliest edition (1916) was the first formal intelligence test published in the United States and was a revision of the Binet-Simon scale developed in France in 1905 (Piotrowski, 2003). It was the first test to describe the term *intelligence quotient* by calculating the ratio of a person's mental age (based on test performance) divided by chronological age and multiplied by 100 (Roid, 2003a). The test has undergone many revisions. Calculation of composite scores is now performed by comparing scores of same-aged peers from a normative population sample. The current edition of the SB5 (2003) is a test of intelligence and cognition. It has been standardized on individuals 2 to greater than 85 years old.

The current edition includes five factors: fluid reasoning, knowledge, quantitative reasoning, visuospatial processing, and working memory. Each of the factors includes separate subtests that are grouped into one of two domains. These two domains were developed to provide a balance between tasks that involve language skills and tasks that ae less verbally dependent. A single composite or full-scale IQ score, a verbal IQ, and a nonverbal IQ are provided. The five factors are based on the Cattell-Horn-Carroll hierarchical model of general intellectual ability, similar to the KABC-II and Leiter. Some factors provide a predictive measure of achievement in school, whereas others measure higher order reasoning, acquired knowledge (*crystallized intelligence*) or thinking and reasoning abilities for novel tasks that are independent of acquired knowledge (*fluid intelligence*). The visuospatial processing factor provides a measure of spatial abilities with limited requirements for vocal responses The SB5 was standardized with 4800 individuals representative of variables including age, sex, race/ethnicity, geographic region, and socioeconomic level reflected in the 2001 U.S. Census. The SB5 has a strong correlation with other intelligence tests. Special populations were included during the standardization process, including intellectually gifted, intellectually disabled, learning disabled, and individuals with autistic disorder (Roid, 2003b).

Wechsler Preschool and Primary Scale of Intelligence, Third Edition

Wechsler is a name associated with the most widely used intelligence tests for individuals from preschool age through adulthood (see Table 79-3) (Piotrowski, 2003). Wechsler defined intelligence as "the capacity to act purposefully, to think rationally, and to deal effectively with his [or her] environment" (Lichtenberger and Kaufman, 2004). The original Wechsler test used multiple scales to group skills that were divided into three areas: verbal IQ, performance IQ (nonverbal) and an overall IQ (full-scale IQ). The shift from a single composite score to use of multiple global scales laid a foundation for subsequent tests and theoretical models of intelligence (Lichtenberger and Kaufman, 2004). The WPPSI-III is one of the most widely used tests of cognitive functioning with young children (2 years, 6 months through 7 years, 3 months). The age range is divided into two bands with core subtests designated for children ages 2 years 6 months to 3 years 11 months and 4 years to 7 years, 3 months, based on empiric studies of differences in reasoning and language skills between the two age groups (Wechsler, 2002a).

The WPPSI-III subtests are organized into composite scores (verbal IQ, performance IQ, and full-scale IQ). A general language composite score also is calculated for younger children, and a processing speed quotient is calculated for children 4 years and older. Compared with the Bayley Scales, which provides a measure of multiple areas of development including, but not limited to, cognition, the WPPSI-III focuses primarily on cognitive functioning. Although both instruments assess cognitive functioning, the Bayley Scales is often selected for children with a possible developmental delay, and the WPPSI-III is recommended for children with higher abilities. The WPPSI-III includes specific scales that assess *fluid reasoning* ("manipulating abstractions, rules, generalizations, and logical relationships") and *processing speed.* Research suggests that processing speed in infants may have some predictive value for future intelligence and is sensitive to certain neurologic profiles, such as attention-deficit/hyperactivity disorder. The WPPSI-III was standardized on 1700 young children who reflect the 2000 U.S. Census (Wechsler, 2002b). Consistent with some other cognitive tests, although the WPPSI-III is useful in diagnosing mild-to-moderate levels of intellectual disability, standard scores do not extend down far enough to substantiate diagnoses in the severe-to-profound range.

Woodcock-Johnson III

The *Woodcock-Johnson III* (WJ-III) includes two sections: tests of cognitive abilities and tests of achievement (see Table 79-3). These tests provide information about intellectual functioning, oral language, and achievement. The WJ-III was developed for use with individuals 2 years to greater than 90 years old (McGrew and Woodcock, 2001). Although the WJ-III is often selected for school-age children, it is used less often among preschool-age children. The *Bateria III Woodcock-Munoz* is the Spanish version of the cognitive and achievement batteries that parallels the WJ-III (Riverside Publishing, 2006).

PARENT RESOURCES

The role of a child's pediatrician is to help a family understand what to expect in a developmental assessment. Many helpful websites have been specifically designed to support and educate parents about development in young children. Zero To Three is a national organization with a website (www.zerotothree.org) that provides information specific to developmental assessment, including "New Visions: A Parent's Guide to Understanding Developmental Assessment." This resource was written by parents. It provides definitions of frequently used terms, understanding the referral process, tips for parents before and after an evaluation, and information about public funding and laws. It also includes information about warning signs of an inappropriate assessment (e.g., the expectation that a young child should be separated from the caregiver during an evaluation).

SUMMARY

Developmental surveillance, screening, and assessment provide a framework for clinicians to incorporate their knowledge about child development into pediatric practice. Surveillance of developmental progress, by obtaining a history of developmental milestones and focused observations, is the core of pediatric medicine. As a part of all pediatric clinical encounters, monitoring a child's development promotes the exchange of knowledge between pediatricians and parents, while recognizing children who may be at risk of developmental delay. Standardized questionnaires are the tools typically used for developmental screening. Many experienced pediatricians rely on a comprehensive interview and a neurologic examination of developmental milestones.

An assessment of development refers to a more comprehensive evaluation of motor, language, social, and cognitive skills usually performed by a specialist. This chapter reviews the principles of developmental surveillance, screening, and assessment. Suggestions for selecting methods and specific tests are made. Knowledge about developmental assessment tools promotes communication about child development between pediatricians and developmental-behavioral pediatricians, mental health professionals, and parents.

REFERENCES

American Academy of Pediatrics: Identifying infants and young children with developmental disorders in the medical home: An algorithm for developmental surveillance and screening Pediatrics 118:405-420, 2006.

American Psychological Association. Available at: www.apa.org. Accessed December 2006.

Bayley N: Bayley Scales of Infant and Toddler Development, Third Edition, Administration Manual. San Antonio, TX, The Psychological Corporation, 2006a.

Bayley N: Bayley Scales of Infant and Toddler Development, Third Edition, Technical Manual. San Antonio, TX, The Psychological Corporation, 2006b.

Dixon SD, Stein MT: Encounters with Children: Pediatric Behavior and Development, 4th ed. Philadelphia, Mosby Elsevier, 2006.

Dworkin PH: British and American recommendations for developmental monitoring: The role of surveillance. Pediatrics 84:1000-1010, 1989.

Gesell A, Amatruda CS: Developmental Diagnosis: Normal and Abnormal Child Development. New York, Hoeber, 1941.

Glascoe FP: The value of parents' concerns to detect and address developmental and behavioral problems. J Pediatr Child Health 35:1-8, 1999.

Handen B: Mental retardation. *In* Mash EJ, Terdal LG (eds): Assessment of Childhood Disorders, 3rd ed. New York, Guilford Press, 1997, pp 397-407.

Kanaya T, Scullin MH, Ceci SJ: The Flynn effect and U.S. policies: The impact of rising IQ scores on American society via mental retardation diagnose. Am Psychol 58:778-790, 2003.

Lichtenberger EO, Kaufman AS: Essentials of WPPSI-III Assessment. Hoboken, NJ, John Wiley & Sons, 2004.

McGrew K, Woodcock RW: Technical Manual. Woodcock-Johnson III Tests of Cognitive Abilities. Itasca, IL, Riverside Publishing, 2001.

Mullen EM: Mullen Scales of Early Learning Manual. Circle Pines, MN, American Guidance Service, Inc, 1995.

Pearson Assessment. Available at: www.pearsonassessment.com. Accessed December 2006.

Perrin EC, Stancin T: A continuing dilemma: Whether and how to screen for concerns about children's behavior. Pediatr Rev 23:264-275, 2002.

Piotrowski NA: Magill's Encyclopedia of Social Science Psychology, Vol 2. Pasadena, CA, Salem Press, 2003.

Plucker JA (ed): Human Intelligence: Historical Influences, Current Controversies, Teaching Resources. 2003. Available at: http://www.indiana.edu/~intell. Accessed December 2006.

Riverside Publishing. Available at: www.riverpub.com. Accessed December 2006.

Roid GH: Stanford-Binet Intelligence Scale Fifth Edition, Examiner's Manual. Itasca, IL, Riverside Publishing, 2003a.

Roid GH: Stanford-Binet Intelligence Scale Fifth Edition, Technical Manual. Itasca, IL, Riverside Publishing, 2003b.

Roid GH, Miller LJ: Leiter International Performance Scale–Revised. Wood Dale, IL, Stoelting Co, 1997.

Sand N, Silverstein M, Glascoe PP, et al: Pediatricians' reported practices regarding developmental screening: Do guidelines work? Do they help? Pediatrics 116:174-179, 2005.

Sattler JM: Assessment of Children, 3rd ed. San Diego, JM Sattler JM, 1988.

Wechsler D: WPPSI-III Technical Interpretive Manual. San Antonio, TX, The Psychological Corporation, 2002a.

Wechsler D: WPPSI-III Administration and Scoring Manual. San Antonio, TX, The Psychological Corporation, 2002b.

80 DEVELOPMENTAL ASSESSMENT OF THE SCHOOL-AGE CHILD

Kathleen Selvaggi Fadden

GETTING READY FOR DEVELOPMENTAL ASSESSMENT

Developmental assessment of a school-age child, by definition, requires the examination of school functioning because success at school is the main task of children age 5 through the teenage years. A third-grader who complains, "My stomach hurts" on school mornings could be in actuality telling the clinician, "The complex synthesis of material learned in third grade is beyond my coping strategies, and furthermore, I'm being bullied on the bus." A comprehensive evaluation requires historical information regarding school functioning, medical issues, behavioral issues, and family and genetic issues (Table 80-1), in addition to neurodevelopmental testing. The Maternal and Child Health Bureau initiative Bright Futures (Hagan et al, 2007) contains questions for gathering information from parents and children at each age range and checklists and rating scales, with a specific publication for mental health concerns (Jellinek et al, 2002). Collection of information, scoring of behavior questionnaires from parents and teachers, and assessment of psychosocial risk factors frequently can be done by a social worker. Alternatively, the history and physical examination can be done at one visit, neurodevelopmental testing can be done at another visit, and diagnosis and treatment options can be discussed with parents at a third visit.

School Functioning

When assessing school functioning, it is helpful to examine performance and behavior history grade by grade, starting with preschool. A child who is asked to leave a preschool because of behavior concerns requires close examination regarding the reasons, such as aggression or separation anxiety. Repeating the kindergarten year needs to be examined for whether academic, behavioral, or social concerns were in evidence. Review of report cards and standardized testing from all grades gives valuable information. A child who does not have sound/symbol recognition of letters or does not know simple addition in first grade is at risk for learning problems. Because a diagnosis of attention-deficit/hyperactivity disorder (ADHD) requires that symptoms must be present before age 7, obtaining history about kindergarten and first-grade behavior is important. Bullying peaks at second and third grade, and significant problems may occur at these ages. Learning disabilities frequently manifest in third grade when learning is less rote. Difficulties with organizational skills become significant in fifth grade when maintenance of a locker and changing classes occurs. Burgeoning adolescence in seventh and eighth grades presents children with the task of reconciling peer pressure to perhaps conflicting family values. In adolescence, children with Asperger syndrome have a higher chance of suicide because of rigidity and misperception of social cues.

Not only are peer relationships important, but also the teacher-student relationship is crucial. Some teachers intrinsically understand a child who may need a unique approach (e.g., authoritative versus nurturing, structured versus free-flowing). Many teachers expect a significant amount of compliance, however, and do not automatically teach to a child's unique style. A questionnaire such as the *Learning Styles Inventory* (Dunn et al, 1989) can provide helpful information from the child about learning preferences. Behavior questionnaires from teachers allow a clinician to assess for externalizing behavior concerns, such as hyperactivity, and internalizing concerns, such as anxiety. Involving the teacher at the assessment phase can be crucial to developing viable treatment recommendations. Understanding environmental factors in the classroom, such as seating assignment and background noise, can be important. Excessive absences or more than three school moves can have a negative impact on acquisition of knowledge.

Knowledge of any academic supports or special education instruction that the child may be receiving is part of the assessment of school functioning. Many school districts provide basic skills instruction for reading or math, in which the same curriculum may be presented in a smaller group in a slower manner. Some children with a disability merely need accommodations in the classroom, guaranteed for any school receiving public funds under Section 504 of the Rehabilitation Act of 1973 and the Americans with Disabilities Act of 1990 (see Chapter 98). These accommodations may include a bypass ramp to the steps for a child with cerebral palsy, preferential seating for a child with ADHD, or opportunities to rest for a child with cystic fibrosis.

Table 80-1. Information Needed for Developmental Assessment

Birth history (records if born prematurely or if any concerns)
Developmental milestones
Early intervention reports
Reports from physical, occupation, or speech-language therapists or tutors
Report cards, progress notes, or special education plans from preschool to present
Behavior questionnaires from teacher and guardian
Primary care records, growth charts, and immunization records
Diet history
Reports from previous assessments, especially cranial imaging or special laboratory tests
Hearing and vision tests
List of family moves and how tolerated
List of child's interests and activities
Peer/sibling interactions
Homework/classwork samples
Guardianship/visitation papers if divorce, adoption, or foster
Educational/work history of parents
Family history of medical, developmental, or psychiatric issues

A specific learning disability is assessed initially by evaluating any discrepancy between intelligence testing and achievement testing (see Chapter 82). The Individuals with Disabilities Education Act (see Chapter 98) ensures the right of all children to a free and appropriate education in the least restrictive environment, and more recent legislation about minimum competencies ensures that "no child is left behind." Some children may receive services by a special education teacher team teaching in a regular education classroom (commonly called inclusion), whereas others may require a separate classroom or specialized school.

Under the Individuals with Disabilities Education Act, diagnostic health services may be requested by the school district, typically for ADHD or autism. Rarely does a child hold an uncomplicated diagnosis, and in addition to attention deficits or autism, learning deficits and anxiety may be present. A comprehensive view of the child is important.

Medical Issues

First, any treatable medical issues affecting development must be assessed. Obtaining previous medical records is important (e.g., a child who was being treated for lead poisoning in one foster home should not be treated as having ADHD in another foster home because of lack of records). Sometimes simple issues, such as not having breakfast and lunch, can be the cause of poor performance in the classroom. A specific medical diagnosis may not cause developmental concerns itself; but the chronic state could cause issues (e.g., children with type 1 diabetes for 6 years have been shown to have deficits in long-term memory and in attention, processing speed, and executive skills with lower verbal and full-scale IQ scores noted if severely hypoglycemic (Northam et al, 2001). For a premature birth, it is helpful to review the *Nursery Neurobiologic Risk Score* (Brazy et al, 1993), which rates seven risk factors (ventilation, pH, seizures, intraventricular hemorrhage, periventricular leukomalacia, infection, and hypoglycemia) as being concerns for poor development.

An audiogram by an audiologist to ensure appropriate sensory input should be done because screening tests can be inaccurate in a child with a developmental concern. Similarly, an eye examination with dilation is helpful to ensure acuity and rule out chorioretinitis or Lisch nodules. If a vision therapist is being considered for difficulty reading, psychoeducational assessment should be recommended first, and although an eye examination also is indicated, vision therapy in the form of eye exercises is not recommended (see Chapter 71). Appropriate growth charts can be downloaded from the Centers for Disease Control and Prevention website to evaluate for body mass index, and specialty growth charts can be found, including for children with Down syndrome or for children internationally adopted from China. A girl with short stature and specific deficits in math may need to be checked for Turner syndrome. Head circumference can be done in older children to document the microcephaly of fetal alcohol syndrome or megalencephaly, which is associated with learning deficits (Sandler et al, 1996). Children with cyanotic heart disease are at higher risk for learning disabilities. Ultraviolet (Wood lamp) testing can elucidate the hypopigmented lesions in tuberous sclerosis or the hyperpigmented lesions in neurofibromatosis (the axillary freckling of neurofibromatosis should be checked for while auscultating the heart and lungs). A child's gait should be observed for asymmetries and dyscoordination or for sensory problems such as toe walking. Snoring during REM sleep can herald sleep apnea, which can affect daytime attention. Assess sleep onset and duration.

Behavioral and Developmental History

Ascertaining a child's developmental milestones can be important for diagnostic purposes (e.g., a diagnosis of Asperger syndrome requires that single words be used before age 2 and communicative phrases by age 3). Understanding a child's cognitive-emotional development is important as well (e.g., a child's understanding that death is permanent may come at 8 years old, which is when questions can surface from a child about adoptive status as well). Piaget explained in his concrete operations stage how children move from intuitive thought at 4 to 7 years old (imitation of behavior) to concrete operations at 6 to 12 years (mastery of physical world) to formal operations at 12 years onward (understanding of complex interrelationships).

Asking about a child's daily routine can help elucidate such issues as sleep deprivation (10 to 12 hours needed during kindergarten and 10 hours at age 11 or 12). Behavior issues such as aggression or hyperactivity cannot be fully appreciated in a physician's office, and are best assessed by behavioral questionnaires and classroom observation. Many diagnoses require specific behavioral symptoms to be present for at least 6 months. Ideally, behavioral questionnaires should be obtained to elicit internalizing conditions (e.g., anxiety and depression) and externalizing conditions (e.g. aggression and hyperactivity). Organizational skills should be assessed, such as the child's ability to write down homework assignments accurately, bring home the appropriate books, plan for a long-term assignment, assemble appropriate tools, and follow detailed instructions. Missing homework and displaced notices may be an indication that a better system of keeping track of materials is needed.

A description of a child's temperament is useful in interpreting behavior. Almost as important is a description of the "goodness of fit" of temperamental tendencies between the child and the parent or teacher (see Chapter 7).

An important part of developmental testing is to question the child about whether or not he or she likes school and to determine a favorite thing to do at school and the hardest thing to do. Sometimes children can be rated not on their ability, but on the perception of their ability at school, changing children's expectations of themselves. How children complete homework can elucidate areas of educational weakness and organizational abilities. Children with ADHD may need supervision for homework at an older age than other children, and families must plan accordingly.

Divorce in the family during the school-age years can be quite disruptive because of extreme family stress, a possible move, change of school, and possible change of peer group because of visitation. The most successful divorce situation is when parents can communicate for the good of their children.

It is imperative to examine children's ability to interact with peers. Typically, 6- to 8-year-old children like to interact with same-sex peers and have one best friend and one enemy. Asking a child, "Who is your best friend?" and "What do you and your best friend play?" can give information about the child's leisure time and socialization skills. Any bullying should be elucidated, with second and third grades being the peek for this behavior; every school should have a "zero tolerance" policy, empowering the student body to treat each other with respect. A child with a family history of addictive illness may be prone to early experimentation with drugs and alcohol, and peer group changes should be monitored. Homosexuality or a sexual identity concern should be ascertained in preteen and teenaged children, and their social experiences should be explored. Isolating hobbies such as video games need to be discussed. Sibling relations need to be evaluated—a child with autism may have severe sibling rivalry for years when a sibling is born.

Family History

Because many disorders have familial tendencies, it is important to take a two generational family history. Any history of medical, mental health, or learning difficulties should be ascertained, asking about each family member separately, especially asking about any medication taken for a disorder, or medications that were not tolerated. A child whose family members have a history of dyslexia or learning problems may need to be watched more closely for the same. A family history of early cardiac death or arrhythmia may have important treatment implications. A family history of a maternal aunt having a son with developmental delay and a maternal grandfather with an early onset of ataxia before age 50 can be an indication of fragile X syndrome, the most common inherited cause of intellectual disability (Hagerman, 2007).

NEURODEVELOPMENTAL TESTING

Neurodevelopmental testing goes beyond soft neurologic signs broadly indicative of dysfunction, such as mixed dominance, synkinesia, finger agnosia, or dysdiadochokinesia. It is helpful to consider left brain (language processing) and right brain (visual processing) functioning. Language processing includes input skills (auditory processing, reading) and output skills (speech, written language). Visual processing also includes input skills (visuospatial and perception) and output skills (visuomotor integration). Testing language and visual processing for input and output skills summarizes neurodevelopmental assessment.

Although a child may be categorized as an auditory or visual learner, many complex factors affect developmental assessment of a school-age child, such as attention span, emotional factors, sensory processing, and environmental factors. Temperamental factors regarding the "goodness of fit" between the child and parent or teacher can have an impact on the child's development. The goal of neurodevelopmental testing is frequently not only the test results themselves, but also a description of how a child approaches a task, and the child's length of attention for a task, ability to shift sets, frustration tolerance, organizational skills, and processing speed, and assessment of emotional state, especially anxiety. The analysis of specific developmental complaints by Levine (1994) greatly aids in understanding a child's strengths and weaknesses.

Table 80-2 summarizes common assessment tools for neurodevelopmental testing. Assessment tools can be comprehensive in nature, where all aspects of neurodevelopmental functioning is explored in one test, or assessment tools can be for a specific skill assessment. More comprehensive assessments include the *PEER*, *PEEX 2*, and *PEERAMID 2* and the Slosson test *Einstein Assessment of School Related Skills*. Parts of these tests can be used to assess specific complaints, or the more specific testing tools can be used (see Table 80-2). Many evaluators use a combination of tools to test specific functioning. Commonly, the *Peabody Picture Vocabulary Test* is used to ascertain a verbal/cognitive level. The *Wide Range Achievement Test* may elucidate reading, writing, and math deficits. The *Diagnostic and Statistical Manual of Mental Disorders* should be used to determine common behavioral disorders, such as ADHD, pervasive developmental disorders, depressive disorder, anxiety disorder, and oppositional defiant disorders with the help of behavioral questionnaires obtained from parents and teachers. Specific tests such as the *Gilliam Autism Rating Scale* also can support a diagnosis such as Asperger syndrome. Goodenough-Harris scoring of a human figure drawing can estimate cognitive level, tap emotional functioning, and screen graphomotor abilities. A *Short Sensory Profile* can help assess a kindergartener with sensory processing problems.

Table 80-2. Common Assessment Tools for Neurodevelopmental Testing

Ability	Test
Language processing	
Reading	*Wide Range Achievement Test–Revised (WRAT)* *Woodcock Reading Mastery Tests–Revised* *Gray Oral Reading Test, Fourth Edition* *Roswell Chall*
Auditory sequence/memory	Digit span: 4 by age 8, 5 by 10, 6 by 12, 7 by 14
Receptive vocabulary	*Peabody Picture Vocabulary Test, Fourth Edition*
Visual processing	*Bender Visual Motor Gestalt Test* House, tree, person drawing *Wold Sentence Copy Test* Gesell figures *Beery-Buktenica Developmental Test of VMI*
Academic achievement	*Wide Range Achievement Test–Revised (WRAT)*
Comprehensive	*Pediatric Examination of Educational Readiness* *Pediatric Early Elementary Examination–2* *Pediatric Examination of Educational Readiness at Middle Childhood–2* *Einstein Assessment of School Related Skills*
Cognitive	*Kaufman Brief Intelligence Test, Second Edition* *Goodenough-Harris Drawing Test* *Peabody Picture Vocabulary Test, Fourth Edition*
School readiness	*Battelle Developmental Inventory, Second Edition*
Autism	*Gilliam Autism Rating Scale* *Autism Behavior Checklist* *Childhood Autism Rating Scale*
Learning style	*Learning Styles Inventory*
Sensory	*Short Sensory Profile*

LEFT BRAIN DYSFUNCTION (LANGUAGE AND AUDITORY PROCESSING)

Vignette

Steven is an 8-year-old in the second grade who tells you that he wants to read, but that he cannot sound out words the way his classmates do. His mother reports that Steven is smart and listens avidly when material is read to him, even through the fourth-grade level. Steven is noted to have difficulty reading even level 1 books by himself. His mother is concerned that this bright child was placed in the lower reading group in his second-grade class. He cannot generate rhyming words for you, and you suspect dyslexia. You refer him to the school system for further testing and a multisensory phonolinguistic reading program.

The child in this vignette is clearly intelligent, but lacks the tools to decode new words. Reading disabilities constitute at least 80% of learning disabilities (Lyon, 1995). Dyslexia is thought by some investigators to be a visual processing problem with reversals, possibly cured by eye exercises. More recent research shows that reading disability has a neurobiologic signature on functional magnetic resonance imaging scans, and it is characterized by difficulties with accurate or fluent word recognition and by poor spelling and decoding abilities remediable by provision of an evidence-based, effective reading intervention (Shaywitz and Shaywitz, 2005). Some children may hide their inability to read and reach fourth grade without detection of the extent of their disability. A careful history must be taken regarding a child's reading level, comprehension ability, and fluency.

Facility in language correlates most to intelligence and academic success. Language processing generally has many components, including phonology (associating sounds with symbols), semantics (vocabulary development), morphology (word roots), syntax (word order), discourse (larger volume of language), metalinguistics (grammatical expression), and pragmatics (social language) (Levine, 1994). Language output deficits specifically can have a complex etiology. Word retrieval problems are common, especially in children with attention deficits. Deficits in syntax and pragmatics may be seen in children with residual autistic spectrum disorder symptoms. Problems with written expression are frequently multifactorial because the child not only must think of what to express, but also how to organize it, how to spell it, how to make the letters, and how to be legible. Written language expression is perhaps the most difficult task of a school-age child. Children with apraxia (poor motor planning of central origin) have difficulty executing many motor tasks unless they are overlearned. Motor apraxia can have a negative impact on writing skills, whereas verbal and oral apraxia can have a significant impact on speech development.

Children requiring repetition of instruction and dampening of background noise may have deficits in auditory processing. Formal central auditory processing testing can be done by an audiologist in a soundproof booth. Central auditory processing testing assesses how a child hears and gives norms starting at age 8 on such parameters as auditory sequencing, auditory discrimination, and auditory figure-ground (i.e., white noise such as the paper shuffling in a classroom is pumped into the soundproof booth, and the child needs to try to distinguish a teacher's frequency to follow directions).

RIGHT BRAIN DYSFUNCTION (VISUAL PROCESSING AND ORGANIZATIONAL SKILLS)

Vignette

Jason is having significant difficulty with sixth-grade math so that he may need to go to summer school because of failing grades. He is a verbally precocious boy who has always gotten A's and B's on his report card except for math, where he achieved C's and recently D's. Last year, he started to show deficiencies owing to poor organizational skills. He is noted to make a lot of detail errors. He is slow with his writing and sometimes does not make lower case "p" and "q" correctly in cursive. Over the years, there has been some concern that he has ADHD, especially because he would frequently not look at the teacher and appear not to pay attention. Jason sometimes misinterprets what is needed for a project. He has some trouble with coordination and balance, and just learned to ride a bike last year. Socially, he does not know how to take a joke and is experiencing a lot of teasing from his peers this year (his failing math grade was originally attributed to this).

Jason had an emergency psychiatric visit when he was noted to say "I wish I were dead," but he was not found to be acutely suicidal. After this episode, the Child Study Team of the school district tested him and referred for a neurodevelopmental assessment of possible ADHD. The school psychologist's testing showed a high average verbal comprehension score, but a perceptual reasoning score low average on the *Wechsler Intelligence Scale for Children IV*. The learning disabilities teacher consultant found high average functioning on all aspects of the *Woodcock-Johnson* except math, which was low average. Because of his slow written output, the occupational therapist did the *Bender Visual-Motor Gestalt Test, Second Edition,* and all four scales were below average. You evaluate Jason with the *PEERAMID 2*. You find motor functioning and visual processing to be weak, but language processing to be strong. Items sensitive to attention, planning/organization, and rate/rhythmicity were problematic. On the Vanderbuilt behavior questionnaire, parent and teacher findings were consistent with ADHD, predominantly inattentive type. You confirm this diagnosis, but your primary diagnosis is a nonverbal learning disability.

Children with a nonverbal learning disorder have impaired ability to organize the visuospatial field, adapt to new or novel situations, or accurately read nonverbal signals or cues (Thompson, 1996). They are unique in that their language processing is quite strong, and so they are usually quite capable in the classroom. In later years, however, weaknesses in visual processing and perceptual organizational skills lead to noticeable deficits in performance. Appropriate visual acuity without strabismus needs to be confirmed, but visual processing deficits are rarely due to eye pathology per se. Deficits in visual processing tend to be more subtle in presentation and may manifest in an aversion for word searches and difficulty in blackboard copying. Math skills requiring perceptual functioning are problematic. Children frequently focus on details, but miss the big picture, and miss classroom instructions, do not finish their work, and misinterpret what needs to be done. Poor perceptual skills lead to missed social cues owing to lack of attention to facial expressions. Boys, especially, who have coordination and motor planning deficits (dyspraxia) may not have sports as an avenue for peer acceptance. A girl with short stature and perceptual learning deficits may have Turner syndrome. Social isolation and a concrete view of the world can lead to frustration and misunderstanding so that these children are at higher risk for suicide. ADHD can be comorbid with a nonverbal learning disability. A child with a nonverbal learning disability profile may qualify for Asperger syndrome depending on the degree of disorder of social interaction or presence of stereotyped/repetitive behaviors.

ANCILLARY ASSESSMENTS

Children who are delayed in input and output skills and have global memory problems frequently have intellectual disabilities and should be referred to a psychologist for intelligence testing and adaptive testing. Intelligence testing gives an IQ score, whereas adaptive testing assesses practical abilities such as self-care and socialization (see Chapter 81). If there is concern about a specific learning disability, psychoeducational testing would be done, including intelligence testing by a psychologist and achievement testing by a learning disabilities teacher consultant. Testing by a speech-language therapist may include scores for receptive and expressive language and specific assessments for auditory processing and pragmatic or social language skills. An occupational therapist assesses more carefully visual processing and graphomotor skills and any issues with sensory processing of the environment. A psychologist could look more at emotional functioning by doing a structured interview or projective testing. A family with complex stressors may require a social worker to assist. Comprehensive testing of all of these issues also can be done by a neuropsychologist. Children with severe mood disturbances, psychotic tendencies, or suicidal ideation should be referred to a child psychiatrist. To understand a child fully, comprehensive developmental assessment with synthesis of the above-mentioned information can be the key to vital intervention for a school-age child.

SUMMARY

Developmental assessment of a school-age child is a complex process of synthesizing data to describe a child's strengths and weaknesses in neurodevelopmental areas important in learning. School functioning, medical issues, developmental-behavioral history, and family history need to be assessed before testing. In a situation unique to childhood, children change and grow so that one developmental task may be problematic at a certain age and another problematic as the child gets older. Neurodevelopmental testing can simplistically be divided into assessment of left brain functioning (language and auditory processing) and right brain functioning (visuospatial and novel stimuli processing). Evaluating how the child can input and output information can document a child's unique abilities. Helping parents, teachers, therapists, and coaches to understand a child's unique abilities can provide a nurturing environment in which the child may thrive.

REFERENCES

Brazy JE, Goldstein RF, Oehler JR, et al: Nursery neurobiologic risk score: Levels of risk and relationships with nonmedical factors. Dev Behav Pediatr 14:375-380, 1993.

Dunn R, Dunn K, Price GE: Learning Styles Inventory. Lawrence, KS, Price Systems, 1989.

Hagan JF, Shaw JS, Duncan PM (eds): Bright Futures Guidelines for Health Supervision of Infants, Children, and Adolescents, 3rd ed. Chicago, American Academy of Pediatrics, 2007.

Hagerman PJ, Hagerman RJ: Fragile X-associated tremor/ataxia syndrome (FXTAS). 2007. Available at: http://fragilex.org/FXTAS.pdf.

Jellinek M, Patel BP, Froehle MC (eds): Bright Futures in Practice: Mental Health Vol I. Practice Guide. Arlington. VA, National Center for Education in Maternal and Child Health, 2002.

Levine MD: Educational Care: A System for Understanding and Helping Children with Learning Problems at Home and in School. Cambridge, MA, Educators Publishing Service, 1994.

Lyon GR: Toward a definition of dyslexia. Ann Dyslexia 45:3-27, 1995.

Northam EA, Anderson PJ, Jacobs R, et al: Neuropsychological profiles of children with type I diabetes 6 years after disease onset. Diabetes Care 24:1541-1546, 2001.

Sandler AD, Knudsen MW, Brown TT, et al: Neurodevelopmental dysfunction among nonreferred children with idiopathic megalencephaly. J Pediatr 131:320-324, 1996.

Shaywitz SE, Shaywitz BA: Dyslexia (specific reading disability). Biol Psychiatry 57:1301-1309, 2005.

Thompson S: Nonverbal learning disorders. 1996. Available at: http://www.nldontheweb.org/thompson-1.htm.

81 ASSESSMENT OF INTELLIGENCE

HELEN TAGER-FLUSBERG AND
DANIELA PLESA-SKWERER

For more than 100 years, the concept of intelligence has been at the center of debate among psychologists and educators. Controversies continue to dominate discussions about how to define intelligence, whether there are numerous independent intelligences, the biologic bases of intelligence, how culture may play a role in defining different conceptions of intelligence and influence its development, and how intelligence can be measured. There is still no general consensus on these issues, and there continues to be a skeptical view on the ethics and practice of intelligence testing. Today, it is widely acknowledged that conceptualizations of intelligence are at least partly culturally defined and dependent on sociohistorical contexts, and that intelligence testing, largely a Western phenomenon, may not fully capture sociocultural variations in cognitive style. Despite these concerns, testing intelligence is still a central component of how children are assessed in developmental settings, and the results of such testing are used to inform recommendations for educational and service-based interventions and programming.

This chapter provides an overview of the history, theory, and methods for testing children's intelligence. The chapter ends with a discussion of factors influencing individual variation in intelligence, and how measures of IQ have changed over time.

HISTORICAL VIEWS OF INTELLIGENCE

Galton, a cousin of Charles Darwin, is generally credited with first developing a scientific and theoretical interest in intelligence. He viewed intelligence as a hereditary trait that was best conceptualized in terms of energy and sensitivity to stimuli (Galton, 1883). A quite different conception of intelligence motivated the work of Binet, who developed the first comprehensive intelligence test for children in response to his commission to identify a method for differentiating students who were suspected of having intellectual or learning disabilities. Binet's work grew out of practical and educational concern about intelligence. Based on intuitions about what constituted academic intelligence, Binet and his collaborator, Simon, designed a battery of tests that tapped higher mental processes (including following directions, reasoning, memory, counting), which was highly reliable and showed substantial validity in predicting academic performance (Binet & Simon, 1916).

The success of Binet's work on measuring intelligence is still evident today; the content of most current comprehensive intelligence tests (e.g., the Stanford-Binet and the Wechsler scales) can be traced back to his original ideas. At the same time, creators of intelligence tests generally acknowledge that scores on such tests reflect not only intellectual abilities, but also motivation and adaptive personality factors (Wechsler, 1950). There also is a clear role for the effect of cultural and social/familial factors on test taking skills and attitudes toward the significance of academic achievement, which may influence the assessment of intelligence in children.

DEFINING INTELLIGENCE

From the beginnings of intelligence research with Galton and Binet, no unified definition of intelligence has guided researchers or theorists in this area. Only at the most general level of conceptualizing intelligence has any agreement emerged, according to Sternberg and Detterman (1986), who summarized the views held by a wide range of contemporary theorists. The main themes emphasized by these experts included the capacity to learn from experience, the capacity to adapt to the environment, and metacognitive abilities—understanding and controlling one's own problem solving, reasoning, or decision making. At the same time, more than two dozen additional attributes were mentioned (e.g., learning, reasoning, speed of processing, elementary attentional and perceptual abilities), but no consensus about their significance was reached.

Why is there no general agreement about how to define intelligence? Differences among theorists can be traced to several complex questions that can be raised in the way intelligence is conceptualized intuitively and empirically. First, should a definition of intelligence be limited to a construct that defines individual differences, or should it also reflect universal and relatively invariant human capacities? Most theorists focus their definition on individual differences, not including highly abstract and universal cognitive abilities, such the capacity to speak and comprehend complex grammatical sentences, as markers of intelligence.

Second, should intelligence be conceptualized as a basic low-level capacity (e.g., sensorimotor processes), as Galton did, or are higher level capacities (e.g., reasoning, problem solving, or abstract thinking) fundamental to its definition, as Binet argued?

Third, to what extent should a definition of intelligence be limited to what is measured on intelligence tests? Limiting the definition in this way reduces intelligence to a construct that is isomorphic with academic performance. Broader conceptions of intelligence might incorporate developmental changes in knowledge and thinking, cultural variation, and current ideas from the cognitive and neurologic sciences. The surge of interest in "emotional intelligence" also may be viewed as a backlash to the narrowed perspective presented by traditional cognitive-based views of intelligence (Humphrey et al, 2007). As various models of intelligence are reviewed in the next section, examples of how different approaches to these questions influence theories and definitions of intelligence, and how they affect approaches to its assessment are given.

THEORETICAL MODELS OF INTELLIGENCE

Theories or models of intelligence can be classified into four main groupings: psychometric, computational, neuroscience, and complex systems approaches.

Psychometric Models

Psychometric models of intelligence are generally concerned with the structure and organization of mental abilities (Table 81-1). They focus on conceptions of intelligence that depend exclusively on the basis of intelligence tests as measures of individual differences, and the models are derived from statistical manipulations of scores obtained within and across IQ tests. Spearman (1927), who is credited with being the inventor of factor analysis, the major statistical method used by psychometric theories, initiated this approach.

Spearman's model of intelligence emphasized the singular nature of intelligence, which he termed *g* for general intelligence, a trait that is normally distributed across populations. Although individuals' scores across numerous subtests of an intelligence battery may differ, one still finds positive correlations across subtests. At a technical level, *g* represents the first principal component of a factor analysis of subtest scores, accounting for the common variance among the subtests. For Spearman, *g* was the essence of intelligence—a single attribute, which he thought of as a kind of "mental energy." Despite years of debate and controversy about what *g* might represent, it is a statistical reality that is obtained from different populations with high and low levels of intelligence (Chabris, 2007), and is reflected primarily in full-scale IQ scores. At the same time, *g* accounts for only a portion of the variance across subtests; the residual variance remaining on each subtest was termed *s* by Spearman, to represent additional specific factors of intelligence, such as spatial or verbal ability, but these were of only incidental interest to him.

Other researchers in the psychometric tradition criticized the reductionist approach to intelligence, represented by Spearman's emphasis on *g*. For Thurstone (1938), intelligence was best captured by a set of primary mental abilities—seven factors that included verbal comprehension, verbal fluency, inductive reasoning, spatial visualization, number, memory, and perceptual speed. This perspective is reflected in the specific subtests that are found on comprehensive IQ tests. Scores on these subtests, such as verbal reasoning or block design, are highlighted to provide a profile of a child's strengths and weaknesses across different types of measures.

Cattell (1971) took an alternative psychometric approach, emphasizing the hierarchical structure of intelligence. In his model and others based on it (Vernon, 1971), general intelligence consists of two fundamental types of ability: fluid and crystallized intelligence. Fluid intelligence is defined as the understanding of abstract and sometimes novel relations that does not depend on particular content. It is best measured on analogy problems or series completion tasks, such as *Raven's*

Table 81-1. Concepts of Intelligence in Psychometric Models

Theorist	Concept	Definition
Spearman	*g*	General intelligence—a single factor that explains performance on all tests
	s	Specific factors that are involved on single tests of mental ability (e.g., arithmetic computation)
Thurstone	Primary mental abilities	Seven factors that together define intelligence
	Verbal comprehension	Measured on vocabulary tests (e.g., defining the meaning of a word)
	Verbal fluency	Ability to provide verbal responses in a limited time (e.g., say as many words as possible beginning with B in 1 minute)
	Inductive reasoning	Ability to solve analogy or completion tests (e.g., doctor: patient; teacher: [school; student; class])
	Spatial visualization	Measured on tests requiring mental rotation of pictures or letters
	Number	Arithmetic computations and problem-solving ability
	Memory	Ability to recall strings of words or pictures
	Perceptual speed	Measured on tests such as finding the difference between two highly similar pictures
Guilford	Structure of intellect	Three-dimensional model of intelligence composed of at least 120 factors
	Operations	Simple mental processes (e.g., cognition, memory, or evaluation)
	Contents	Terms that appear in problems (e.g., words, numbers, sounds, pictures)
	Products	Kinds of responses required (e.g., single words or numbers, classes, relations)
Cattell	Fluid intelligence	Requires understanding of abstract relations as in tests of inductive reasoning or analogies, or series completion tests
	Crystallized intelligence	Established knowledge as measured on vocabulary or information tests

Progressive Matrices and Vocabulary Scales (Raven et al, 1998). Crystallized intelligence reflects accumulated knowledge and well-established problem-solving procedures, as measured on tests of vocabulary, or general information. In a hierarchical model, there may be further subdivisions within each of these main types of intelligence. This distinction between fluid and crystallized intelligence is now well established, although the idea that tests of fluid intelligence may be purer measures of intelligence because they do not reflect social variables such as schooling or home environment (Jensen, 1980) has been seriously challenged (Ceci et al, 1994). Most IQ tests that are currently in use include fluid and crystallized intelligence items, but they typically do not provide measures that map directly onto these constructs.

Although psychometric models dominate the field of intelligence, they have not gone uncriticized. These models limit their definition of intelligence to what is measured on an intelligence test, and the emphasis is on the end product or test scores, rather than on the mental processes that underlie performance on the tests. Ceci and colleagues (1994) pointed out that this approach cannot capture contextual influences on intelligence. In other words, the same skill operates with differential effectiveness as a function of the social or physical context, which cannot be captured in a static psychometric instrument. These issues need to be considered in evaluating the choice of tests for assessing intelligence in children from different backgrounds and interpreting individual children's performance.

Computational Models

What kinds of cognitive processes underlie intelligent behavior? This is the kind of question that motivates computational models, which focus on the information processing requirements of performance on tests of intelligence. These models draw on current research and theory in the cognitive sciences, extending beyond the intelligence test and focusing on elementary processes involved in performance on basic cognitive experimental tasks, which correlate with scores on psychometric measures of intelligence such as *Raven's Progressive Matrices*. Hunt (1978) was the first to introduce a computational approach to intelligence. For Hunt, intelligence could best be defined as speed of processing.

Sternberg (1982) analyzed the set of mental processes that were needed to perform on conventional intelligence tests into four basic components: encoding the problem, inferring relations among terms in the problem, mapping the relations, and applying the relations to new situations. Sternberg found that individuals who scored higher on intelligence tests took longer at the encoding or planning stage, but less time on later stages in the computational process. Although these kinds of models provide a useful approach to understanding the cognitive processes underlying intelligence, they do not say much about the structure and organization of intelligent abilities.

Neuroscience Models

In recent years with the explosion of research in the neurosciences, there has been a parallel increase in interest in exploring neurobiologic correlates of intelligence. These newer models have their roots in the ideas initially proposed by Galton and Spearman, but those investigators did not have the means to investigate differences in the brains of individuals varying in intelligence. Current research on neurobiologic models rests on the assumption that there is some single general measure of intelligence, which is operationalized either as full-scale IQ score or as *g* (Bartholomew, 2004).

Jensen (1991) speculated that *g* represents a common underlying biologic resource pool, specifically, the speed and oscillation of central nerve conductance. Some evidence for this idea comes from studies showing that full-scale IQ correlates significantly with speed of peripheral neural conduction (Vernon and Mori, 1992) and with cortical evoked potential measures (Matarazzo, 1994). Other studies have found that IQ correlates positively with whole brain volume (McDaniel, 2005) and negatively with the rate of cortical glucose metabolism, as measured by positron emission tomography (Haier et al, 1988). This latter finding suggests that individuals with higher IQ scores may be using their brains more efficiently as reflected in lower consumption of cortical glucose. More recent research has attempted to identify the specific neural mechanisms that underlie intelligence using magnetic resonance imaging, with studies focusing on white matter integrity (Schmithorst et al, 2005) and specific regions of interest such as the prefrontal cortex (Gray et al, 2003).

Although these findings are intriguing, the magnitude of the correlations obtained between IQ and these various neurobiologic measures is modest, generally accounting for less than one quarter of the variance. These findings also do not provide a theoretical model that might account for how and why brains of more intelligent individuals might be related to higher levels of *g*.

Complex Systems Models

The final set of models of intelligence to be considered here views intelligence as a complex system, rather than a single entity as captured by *g*. These kinds of models take a broader view of intelligence, not limiting it to what is captured on conventional intelligence tests. The models have greater intuitive appeal than the more objective psychometric models and are grounded in theories derived from cognitive science (Table 81-2).

The best-known systems theory is Gardner's (1983) theory of multiple intelligences. Gardner based his theory primarily on neuropsychologic evidence from adults with brain damage and individuals with exceptional talents, and evidence from developmental psychology and evolutionary biology. According to Gardner, there are seven relatively independent intelligences: linguistic, logical-mathematical, spatial, musical, bodily-kinesthetic, interpersonal, and intrapersonal intelligences. Each of these intelligences is a separate system of functioning, although they can interact to produce intelligent behavior. Gardner criticized conventional intelligence tests because they only capture the first three of these intelligence systems.

Sternberg (1985) proposed a triarchic theory of intelligence composed of analytic or componential intelligence, which is tapped by intelligence tests; creative

Table 81-2. **Concepts of Intelligence in System Models**

Theorist	Concept	Definition
Gardner	Linguistic intelligence	Related to all language-based performance (e.g., writing a poem, reading)
	Logical-mathematical	Related to mathematic, arithmetic, and intelligence logical problem-solving abilities (e.g., balancing a checkbook)
	Spatial intelligence	Related to visuospatial problem solving (e.g., map reading)
	Musical intelligence	Related to all musical performances (e.g., playing violin)
	Bodily kinesthetic	Related to all physical and athletic intelligence performance (e.g., playing basketball)
	Interpersonal intelligence	Related to interactions with other people and interpreting others' behavior, motives, or desires
	Intrapersonal intelligence	Related to understanding the self, personal insight
Sternberg	Analytic intelligence	Solving problems using strategies that manipulate elements of the problem (e.g., comparing, evaluating)
	Creative intelligence	Solving new kinds of problems that require novel solutions (e.g., designing, inventing)
	Practical intelligence	Solving problems in everyday contexts by applying and using existing knowledge

intelligence, which is concerned with combining experiences in novel ways; and practical intelligence, which is concerned with how to manipulate and adjust to the environment in everyday contexts. Sternberg emphasized how these systems work together in dealing with different problems in various contexts.

Although many investigators view the broader conceptions of intelligence that are manifest in these complex systems models as a real advance with important educational implications, others raise the concern that they may be too unconstrained, not allowing for rigorous empiric testing. Neisser and coworkers (1996) suggested that some of the intelligences in Gardner's theory are more appropriately designated as simply special talents.

Across all the perspectives on intelligence that have been reviewed here, intelligence is primarily defined in terms of individual differences. No serious consideration is given to developmental changes in either the structural organization or processes involved in intellectual performance. A richer, more complex, and less quantitatively oriented view of intelligence would result from incorporating knowledge about developmental changes in cognitive abilities into conceptions of intelligence (Ceci et al, 1994), moving the field away from a static perspective on intelligence.

METHODS FOR ASSESSING INTELLIGENCE IN CHILDREN

The administration of a comprehensive intelligence battery provides a valid and reliable assessment, yielding information that is useful to clinicians and other professionals working with a child. A variety of such batteries are currently available, including the Wechsler scales, *Wechsler Preschool and Primary Scale of Intelligence, Third Edition* and *Wechsler Intelligence Scale for Children, Fourth Edition* (Wechsler, 2002, 2003); *Stanford-Binet Intelligence Scale, Fifth Edition* (Roid, 2003); *Differential Ability Scales, Second Edition* (Elliot, 2006); and *Kaufman Assessment Battery for Children, Second Edition* (Kaufman and Kaufman, 2004). The advantage of using one of these batteries is that they have excellent psychometric properties, and they provide updated norms against which a specific child's performance can be evaluated. Most importantly, these batteries include valid measures of numerous relevant constructs that provide profiles of functioning across different subtests, including verbal, perceptual, spatial, and mathematical knowledge and reasoning; working memory; and processing speed. These tests typically cover the age range from 2 years to late adolescence. Although there are tests that tap very early developmental skills (Mullen, 1995), these scales generally are not referred to as intelligence tests because they assess different constructs, and scores on these measures do not predict strongly to later IQ scores.

Selection of which IQ test to use may depend on many different factors, including the age of the child and the specific goals of the assessment. The tests vary in the degree to which verbal demands are high, inclusion of social content in the subtests, reliance on timed tests, and the total amount of time needed to complete the assessment. For children with limited language abilities, clinicians often turn to nonverbal tests, such as the *Leiter International Performance Scale–Revised* (Roid and Miller, 1997) or *Test of Nonverbal Intelligence, Third Edition* (Brown et al, 1997), or they depend on just the nonverbal subtests of the more comprehensive batteries (DeThorne and Schaefer, 2004). It is beyond the scope of this chapter to provide a detailed evaluation and discussion on selecting and administering IQ tests; more information may be found in Kamphaus (2005) or Sattler (2001).

Factors Influencing Assessment of Intelligence

Assessing intelligence using a standardized instrument requires the clinician to follow the administration procedures that are described in the test manual rigorously so that the validity and reliability of the results of testing are not compromised. At the same time, so many factors may influence a child's performance that the most important factor to keep in mind is how to interpret a child's scores. Performance during the administration of a test may be affected by the physical or social environment, rapport between the child and evaluator, distractibility, off-task behaviors, difficulty with prolonged testing, interest in the materials, and motivational and other child-related factors (Kamphaus, 2005).

Other factors that need to be considered in interpreting a child's profile of performance in an assessment of intelligence include broader cultural and sociodemographic factors. IQ scores are valid only for the population on whom the test was developed and normed. Special caution should be taken in interpreting test scores of children from sociocultural backgrounds that differ substantially from the types of knowledge and reasoning formats typical of the largely middle-class cultural practices on which IQ tests rely (Richardson, 2000). Ultimately, it is important to consider the goals of the assessment for a particular child and the extent to which those goals can be achieved by using the standard instruments for assessing intelligence.

Factors Influencing Individual Differences in Intelligence

It is no longer useful to engage in a debate about whether genes or the environment exert the most significant influences on intelligence. There is now ample evidence supporting the important roles played by both, although there is still considerable discussion about how best to conceptualize the ways in which genes interact with specific aspects of the environment and variations in experience.

Genetic Factors

Research on genetic influences relies exclusively on performance on intelligence tests that are typically used in behavioral genetics studies to provide estimates of the heritability of *g*, or general intelligence. Heritability is a technical construct that refers to the percentage of variation of a particular trait, in this case *g*, in a population that is associated with purely genetic differences among those individuals. It is widely accepted that heritability estimates for general intelligence are between 0.45 and 0.75, suggesting that about 50% of the variance of IQ scores can be explained by genetic factors.

Studies of genetic influences on intelligence have now moved beyond showing their existence toward identifying some of the specific genes that may be responsible for its heritability, using the power of new molecular genetic technology (Plomin et al, 1994). This research is complex and challenging because genetic influences on intelligence seem likely to involve multiple genes of varying effect size, which have been called *quantitative trait loci*. Some progress in finding quantitative trait loci for intelligence is now being made by many different research groups, and several candidate genes have been identified (Plomin and Spinath, 2004; Posthuma and de Geus, 2006).

Environmental Factors

From the moment of conception, phenotypes are influenced by the interactions between the genotype and a wide range of environmental effects. These can be divided into two categories: biologic and social. It is well known that prenatal and postnatal exposures to poor nutrition, lead, and alcohol can have measurable effects on intelligence scores because they influence brain development. Perinatal factors, such as oxygen deprivation, also are associated with poorer cognitive outcome. Social-environmental influences on intelligence scores also have been widely documented. IQ scores are significantly correlated with family and home variables, which may include important cultural influences, social and parental occupational factors, schooling, and specific intervention programs, such as Head Start (Neisser et al, 1996).

Genetic and Environmental Interactions

The old nature-nurture debates are now over, but differences remain among researchers in how they conceptualize the interactions between genetic and environmental influences on intelligence. Some emphasize a more biologic perspective, arguing that the environment exerts its influence as a result of genetically determined factors; that is, the environment itself is genetically loaded (Scarr, 1992). Other, more balanced interactionists may view biology as a set of genetically constrained cognitive potentials that are influenced and shaped as they develop in the context of specific experiences.

Bronfenbrenner and Ceci (1993) have proposed a more complex and ambitious interactionist model that has a clear developmental focus, which they call a bioecologic view. They hold that intelligence is a multiple resource system that is only imperfectly gauged by intelligence tests. From the beginning, biology and experience are interwoven, but their relationship continually changes; with each change, new possibilities are set in motion, until even small changes may lead to cascading effects over the course of development. Environmental influences are specific to each type of cognitive resource or potential in timing of onset and rate of development. The genetic influences may be limited to cognitive traits, but also could include temperamental and motivational variables that exert an influence on measured intelligence (Ackerman and Heggestad, 1997).

Changes in Intelligence Scores Across Generations

A recurring theme in this chapter has been the relative weight given to conventional intelligence tests in conceptions, theoretical models, and empiric research on intelligence. Despite the controversies that remain regarding the overreliance on intelligence tests, the fact remains that these tests are reliable and valid measures. Yet it is still unclear what these tests actually measure. One of most intriguing findings in studies of IQ is the gradual increase in test scores that has occurred over the past several decades, not only in the United States, but also in many nations around the world (Flynn, 1987). This increase, amounting to about 3 IQ points per decade, has been found on verbally loaded tests, but is especially apparent on nonverbal tests that tap primarily fluid intelligence, such as the *Raven's Progressive Matrices and Vocabulary Scales* (Raven et al, 1998). The so-called Flynn effect remains poorly understood, although many hypotheses have been proposed to explain why IQ scores are on the increase (Neisser et al, 1996), including increases in the complexity of our culture or increases in nutritional status, which also has led to significant gains in height in many populations.

Perhaps the most significant lesson to be learned from the Flynn effect is that intelligence, as measured by standard tests, does change over time—that IQ scores are not immutable either within an individual or across populations. Standard tests of intelligence are important tools for predicting academic performance in children and identifying learning or intellectual disabilities. At the same time, there is a clear need to develop further instruments that would measure intelligence in a broader way that can capture the dynamic developmental processes that underlie cognitive performance across many domains of functioning. If IQ test scores predict individual differences in school achievement moderately well, and indirectly adult occupational status (to the extent that it is strongly related to academic success), the predictive correlations between IQ and actual job performance seem to be substantially reduced over time. Research by Dweck and colleagues (Dweck et al, 2004; Mangels et al, 2006) has shown that, besides actual ability, individuals' own beliefs about the nature of intelligence (e.g., whether it is believed to be a fixed quantity or to be acquirable) may influence their performance in a learning situation through top-down biasing of attention and strategic processing.

More importantly, intelligence is only one way to assess children. There are so many other dimensions that affect a child's daily life at home and in school that go beyond intelligence, and may not even be associated with it, such as quality of life and positive emotional experience (Watten et al, 1995).

SUMMARY

The origins of intelligence testing date back to Alfred Binet's early work on developing measures to assess children's potential for academic success. This chapter summarizes current theoretical views on how to define intelligence. Although controversy persists, there is general agreement that intelligence includes the capacity to learn from experience, the capacity to adapt to the environment, and the ability to use metacognitive or problem-solving skills. Current models of intelligence are presented and methods for assessing children's intelligence using comprehensive test batteries are surveyed. The chapter ends with a discussion of the factors that influence test performance, individual variation in intelligence, and historical changes in test scores.

REFERENCES

Ackerman PL, Heggestad ED: Intelligence, personality, and interests: Evidence for overlapping traits. Psychol Bull 121:219-245, 1997.

Bartholomew G: Measuring Intelligence: Facts and Fallacies. Cambridge, Cambridge University Press, 2004.

Binet A, Simon T: The Development of Intelligence in Children (ES Kite Trans.). Baltimore, Williams & Wilkins, 1916.

Bronfenbrenner U, Ceci SJ: Heredity, environment, and the question "how"? A first approximation. *In* Plomin R, McLearn G (eds): Nature, Nurture, and Psychology. Washington, DC, American Psychological Association, 1993, pp 313-324.

Brown L, Sherbenou RJ, Johnsen SK: Test of Nonverbal Intelligence, 3rd ed. Austin, TX, Pro-Ed, 1997.

Cattell RB: Abilities: Their Structure, Growth, and Action. Boston, Houghton Mifflin, 1971.

Ceci SJ, Baker-Sennett JG, Bronfenbrenner U: Psychometric and everyday intelligence: Synonyms, antonyms and anonyms. *In* Rutter M, Hay DF (eds): Development Through Life: A Handbook for Clinicians. Oxford, Blackwell, 1994, pp 260-283.

Chabris C: Cognitive and neurobiological mechanisms of the law of general intelligence. *In* Roberts MJ (ed); Integrating the Mind: Domain General versus Domain Specific Processes in Higher Cognition. Hove, UK, Psychology Press, 2007, pp 449-491.

DeThorne LS, Schaefer BA: A guide to child nonverbal IQ measures. Am J Speech-Language Pathol 13:275-290, 2004.

Dweck CS, Mangels JA, Good C: Motivational effects of attention, cognition and performance. *In* Dai DY, Sternberg RJ (eds): Motivation, Emotion and Cognition: Integrated Perspectives on Intellectual Functioning. Mahwah, NJ, Erlbaum, 2004, pp 41-55.

Elliot D: Differential Ability Scales, 2nd ed. New York, Psychological Corporation, 2006.

Flynn JR: Massive IQ gains in fourteen nations: What IQ tests really measure. Psychol Bull 101:171-191, 1987.

Galton F: Inquiry into Human Faculty and Its Development. London, Macmillan, 1883.

Gardner H: Frames of Mind: The Theory of Multiple Intelligences. New York, Basic Books, 1983.

Gray JR, Chabris CF, Braver TS: Neural mechanisms of general fluid intelligence. Nat Neurosci 6:313-322, 2003.

Haier RJ, Siegel B, Nuechterlein K, et al: Cortical glucose metabolic rate correlates with reasoning and attention studied with positron emission tomography. Intelligence 12:199-217, 1988.

Humphrey N, Curran A, Morris E, et al: Emotional intelligence and education: A critical review. Edu Psychol 27:235-254, 2007.

Hunt EB: Mechanics of verbal ability. Psychol Rev 85:109-130, 1978.

Jensen AR: Bias in Mental Testing. New York, Free Press, 1980.

Jensen AR: General mental ability: From psychometrics to biology. Diagnostique 16:134-144, 1991.

Kamphaus R: Clinical Assessment of Child and Adolescent Intelligence. New York, Springer, 2005.

Kaufman AS, Kaufman NL: Kaufman Assessment Battery for Children: Manual, 2nd ed. Circle Pines, MN, American Guidance Service, 2004.

Mangels JA, Butterfield B, Lamb J, et al: Why do beliefs about intelligence influence learning success? A social cognitive neuroscience model. Soc Cogn Affect Neurosci 1:75-86, 2006.

Matarazzo JD: Biological measures of intelligence. *In* Sternberg RJ, Ceci SJ, Horn J, (eds): Encyclopedia of Human Intelligence. New York, Macmillan, 1994, pp 186-199.

McDaniel MA: Big-brained people are smarter: A meta-analysis of the relationship between in vivo brain volume and intelligence. Intelligence 33:337-346, 2005.

Mullen EM: The Mullen Scales of Early Learning. Circle Pines, MN, American Guidance Service, 1995.

Neisser U, Boodoo G, Bonchard T, et al: Intelligence: Known and unknowns. Am Psychol 51:77-101, 1996.

Plomin R, McLearn GE, Smith DL, et al: DNA markers associated with high versus low IQ: The IQ quantitative trait loci (QTL) project. Behav Genet 24:107-118, 1994.

Plomin R, Spinath FM: Intelligence: Genetics, genes and genomics. J Person Soc Psychol 86:112-129, 2004.

Posthuma D, de Geus E: Progress in the molecular-genetic study of intelligence. Curr Dir Psychol Sci 15:151-155, 2006.

Raven J, Raven JC, Court JH: Manual for Raven's Progressive Matrices and Vocabulary Scales. Oxford, UK, Oxford Psychologists Press, 1998.

Richardson K: The Making of Intelligence. New York, Columbia University Press, 2000.

Roid GH: Stanford-Binet Intelligence Scale, 5th ed. Itasca, IL, Riverside, 2003.

Roid GH, Miller LJ: Leiter International Performance Scale–Revised. Wood Dale, IL, Stoelting, 1997.

Sattler JM: Assessment of children: Cognitive applications, 4th ed. San Diego, JM Sattler, 2001.

Scarr S: Developmental theories for the 1990s: Development and individual differences. Child Dev 63:1-19, 1992.

Schmithorst V, Wilke M, Dardzinski B, Holland S: Cognitive functions correlate with white matter architecture in a normal pediatric population: A diffusion tensor MRI study. Hum Brain Mapping 26:139-147, 2005.

Spearman C: The Abilities of Man. New York, Macmillan, 1927.

Sternberg RJ(ed): Handbook of Human Intelligence. New York, Cambridge University Press, 1982.

Sternberg RJ: Beyond IQ: A Triarchic Theory of Human Intelligence. New York, Cambridge University Press, 1985.

Sternberg RJ, Detterman DK (eds): What Is Intelligence? Contemporary Viewpoints on Its Nature and Definition. Norwood, NJ, Ablex, 1986.

Thurstone LL: Primary Mental Abilities. Chicago, University of Chicago Press, 1938.

Vernon PE: The Structure of Human Abilities. London, Methuen, 1971.

Vernon PE, Mori M: Intelligence, reaction times, and peripheral nerve conduction velocity. Intelligence 16:273-288, 1992.

Watten RG, Syversen JL, Myhrer T: Quality of life, intelligence and mood. Social Indicators Research 36:287-299, 1995.

Wechsler D: Cognitive, connative, and non-intellective intelligence. Am Psychol 5:78-83, 1950.

Wechsler D: Wechsler Preschool and Primary Scale of Intelligence, 3rd ed. San Antonio, TX, Psychological Corporation, 2002.

Wechsler D: Wechsler Intelligence Scale for Children: Technical and Interpretative Manual, 4th ed. San Antonio, TX, Psychological Corporation, 2003.

82 EDUCATIONAL ASSESSMENT

Martha S. Reed

RATIONALES FOR EDUCATIONAL ASSESSMENT

Academic performance is the benchmark by which student, school, curriculum, and teacher competence is measured, and almost every school-age child undergoes some type of formal academic testing in addition to regular class quizzes, tests, and examinations. There are seven basic rationales for educational assessment: (1) measurement of group academic achievement level as an indicator of program effectiveness and teacher/school accountability; (2) measurement of individual achievement status and academic progress; (3) screening of children perceived to be at risk for learning problems; (4) determination of eligibility for specific programs, such as gifted/talented, special education services, and therapies; (5) diagnosis of learning and performance difficulties and analysis of patterns of strength and weakness; (6) instructional planning, including class placement, academic programming and intervention, and academic accommodations; and (7) high-stakes decision making, including grade retention/promotion/graduation diploma, education track or course of study, college/school acceptance, and evaluation of school and teacher quality. Different testing procedures are employed for each purpose; however, for all, traditional practice typically involves some use of formal educational measures. Formal testing usually refers to use of norm-referenced instruments with standardized procedures for administration and scoring.

TRADITIONAL ASSESSMENT PRACTICES

School systems have engaged in standardized achievement testing for decades. Standardized tests fall into two broad categories: group general achievement tests and individually administered instruments (often described as diagnostic tests). Most group achievement tests are grade specific and are used for measuring the general achievement status and academic progress of specified groups of students and of individual students at a particular grade level. Diagnostic tests most often cover several grade and age levels and are administered individually for purposes of providing more detailed information regarding a student's acquisition of specific skills and learning patterns for purposes of instructional planning and intervention. Within each category (group achievement and diagnostic) are survey tests that assess academic achievement and skill development across several domains, and tests that examine a specific skill area, such as reading, listening, writing, spelling, and mathematics. In addition, there are standardized group achievement tests that measure mastery of a specific content area (history, biology, chemistry, foreign language, English literature), such as advanced placement tests, college boards, and, more recently, state end-of-course tests. Many states also include a test of computer competence as requisite for a high school graduation diploma. The federal government's National Assessment of Educational Proficiency Tests (NAEP), which are administered nationwide to a selected sample of students in grades 4, 8, and 12, include a combination of skill and content assessments. Tests that are normed on a national population sample may provide norms based on age or grade level or both, and most frequently are expressed in terms of standard scores, age and grade equivalents, and age and grade percentile ranks.

Until the 1990s, schools and states commonly relied on nationally standardized group achievement tests, such as the *California Achievement Test, Stanford Achievement Tests, Iowa Test of Basic Skills,* and *Educational Records Bureau* (most frequently used by private schools), for measuring group/grade and student performance levels and individual academic progress. In recent years, states have developed their own measures of academic achievement and proficiency in response to federal and state mandates regarding student proficiency, school accountability, and funding policies. State-generated tests are primarily grade based and group administered, are constructed to reflect a particular state's elected curriculum objectives and materials, and are normed on a particular state's population. State norms frequently are expressed in terms of state-determined levels of performance proficiency (often on a scale of 1 to 4, 4 being advanced). State-normed and nationally normed group achievement tests are regularly machine scored by outside agencies. State tests tend to change frequently to reflect alterations in state measurement policy and curriculum. Nationally normed assessment instruments and the federal NAEP tests remain more stable and are updated only at intervals of several years. Because of their stability, these tests are more useful than state-developed tests for indicating longitudinal trends and progress for groups of students and individual students. Table 82-1 lists many of the commercially published tests most frequently used, their age or grade ranges, and content coverage.

Eligibility for special education services and academic accommodations traditionally has required individually administered, standardized measures of cognitive ability and academic achievement, and diagnosis of learning

Table 82-1. **Commonly Used Educational Assessment Instruments**

Test	Age (yr) or Grade	Skill Areas
Group Achievement*		
California Achievement Test	Grade K-12	Word analysis, vocabulary, reading comprehension, spelling, language mechanics, language expression, mathematics computation, mathematics applications, science, social studies
Comprehensive Test of Basic Skills	Grade K-12	Alphabet knowledge, word analysis, vocabulary, reading comprehension, language mechanics, language expression, spelling, mathematics computation, mathematics concepts and problem solving, science, social studies
Educational Records Bureau	Grade K-12	Word analysis, vocabulary, reading comprehension, spelling, language mechanics, language expression, mathematics computation, mathematics problem solving
Iowa Test of Basic Skills	Grade K-9	Word analysis, vocabulary, reading comprehension, language mechanics, spelling, mathematics computation, mathematics applications and concepts, science, social studies, listening
Metropolitan Achievement Test	Grade K-12	Word recognition (analysis), vocabulary, reading comprehension, mathematics concepts and problem solving, mathematics computation, prewriting/composing/editing, spelling, listening, science, social studies, research and thinking
Stanford Achievement Tests (3 levels)	Grade K-12	Sounds and letters, word analysis, word reading, vocabulary, reading comprehension, listening, language grammar and spelling, language mechanics, language expression, mathematics concepts and applications, mathematics computation, science, social studies, study skills
Tests of Achievement and Proficiency (upper level of Iowa)	Grade 9-12	Vocabulary, reading comprehension, written expression, mathematics, information processing, science, social studies
Test of General Educational Development (high school equivalence)	Age ≥16	Reading comprehension, writing, mathematics, science, social studies
Individual Achievement		
Diagnostic Achievement Battery–2	Age 6-14	Story comprehension, characteristics, synonyms, grammatic completion, word identification, reading comprehension, writing mechanics, spelling, written composition, mathematics reasoning, mathematics computation
Diagnostic Achievement Test for Adolescents–2	Age 12-19	Receptive and expressive vocabulary, receptive and expressive grammar, word identification, reading comprehension, mathematics computation, mathematics problem solving, spelling, written composition, science, social studies, reference skills
Kaufman Test of Educational Achievement–2	Age 4.6-25	Reading—letter and word recognition, reading comprehension; reading-related subtests—phonological awareness, nonsense word decoding, word recognition fluency, decoding fluency, associational fluency, naming fluency; math—math concepts and applications, math computation; written language—written expression, spelling; oral language—listening comprehension, oral expression; comprehensive achievement composite
Peabody Individual Achievement Test–Revised	Age 5-18	Word identification, reading comprehension, spelling, mathematics, general information, written expression
Scholastic Achievement Test for Adults	Age ≥16	Verbal reasoning, nonverbal reasoning, quantitative reasoning, vocabulary, reading comprehension, mathematics computation, mathematics problem solving, spelling, writing mechanics, written composition
Wechsler Individual Achievement Test–II	Age 4-85 or grade PK-16	Reading composite—word reading, reading comprehension, pseudoword decoding; mathematics composite—numerical operations, math reasoning; written language composite—spelling, written expression; oral language composite—listening comprehension, oral expression
Wide Range Achievement Test–3	Age ≥5	Word identification, spelling, mathematics computation
Woodcock-Johnson Tests of Achievement III (Third Edition)	Age ≥5 or grade K-12	Reading—word identification, reading fluency, reading comprehension, reading vocabulary, word attack; oral language—story recall, understanding directions, picture vocabulary, oral comprehension, sound awareness; mathematics—calculation, math fluency, applied problems, quantitative concepts; written language—spelling, writing fluency, writing samples, editing, spelling of sounds, punctuation and capitalization; academic knowledge—science, social studies, humanities
Domain Specific		
Reading		
Formal Reading Inventory—silent and oral	Age 6-19	Oral reading accuracy, oral reading comprehension, silent reading comprehension
Gates-MacGinitie Reading Tests (group or individual)—silent	Grade K-12	Reading vocabulary, comprehension
Gates-McKillop-Horowilz Reading Diagnostic Tests—oral	Grade 1-6	Sight word recognition—timed; word identification—untimed; word attack—syllabication, sound blending, phonetics, letter identification, auditory discrimination, spelling, writing

Table 82-1. **Commonly Used Educational Assessment Instruments—cont'd**

Test	Age (yr) or Grade	Skill Areas
READING—CONT'D		
Gray Oral Reading Test–4	Age 6-19	Reading accuracy, reading comprehension
Gray Oral Reading Tests–Diagnostic	Grade 1-6	Paragraph reading, decoding (phonogram recognition and blending), word identification and vocabulary, word attack (morphemic analysis, contextual analysis, word ordering)
Nelson-Denny Reading Tests—silent	Grade 9-college	Reading vocabulary, reading comprehension, reading speed
Slosson Oral Reading Test	Age ≥5 or grade K-12	Word identification
Test of Reading Comprehension–3—silent	Age 7-18	General vocabulary, syntactic similarities, comprehension, sentence sequencing, mathematics vocabulary, social studies vocabulary, science vocabulary, reading directions
Test of Early Reading Ability–3	Age 3-9	Construction of meaning—awareness of print, knowledge of vocabulary relationships, discourse comprehension; knowledge of alphabet—letter naming, oral reading (letter-sound associations); conventions of written language—book handling, response to convention of print, proofreading
Watson-Glaser Critical Thinking Appraisal—silent	Grade 9-college	Inferential comprehension, deductive comprehension, evaluating arguments, drawing conclusions
Woodcock-Johnson Reading Mastery Tests–Revised—oral and silent	Age ≥5	Visual-auditory learning, letter and word identification, word comprehension, passage comprehension
WRITING, SPELLING, AND LANGUAGE		
CELF-R (Clinical Evaluation of Language Fundamentals–Revised) Screening Test	Age 5-16	Oral—sentence completion, following directions, sentence repetition, word classes, semantic relationships, sentence formulation, story retelling; written expression—story organization, story details, sentence structure and meaning, writing mechanics
Oral and Written Language Scales	Age 3-21	Listening comprehension, oral expression, written expression
Test of Early Written Language–2	Age 3-10	Transcription (copying); conventions of print—paragraphs, capitalization/punctuation, spelling, proofing; communication (writing notes, lists); creative expression; record keeping
Test of Written Language–3	Age 7-18	Vocabulary, spelling, style, logical sentences, sentence combining contextual conventions, contextual language, story construction
Test of Written Spelling–4	Age 6-18	Rule-governed words, irregular words
Test of Written Expression	Age 6.6-14.11	Writing conventions, grammar, composition
Writing Process Test	Age 8-18	Written composition—development (purpose, audience, vocabulary, style, support, organization), fluency (sentence structure, grammar/usage, capitalization/punctuation, spelling)
MATHEMATICS		
Key Math Diagnostic Arithmetic Test–Revised	Age 5-22 or grade K-12	Basic concepts—numeration, rational numbers, geometry; operations—addition, subtraction, multiplication, division, mental computation; applications—measurement, money, time, estimation, interpretation of data, problem solving
Sequential Assessment of Mathematics Inventories	Grade K-8	Mathematics language, measurement, ordination, geometric concepts, number and notation, mathematical applications, computation, word problems
Stanford Diagnostic Mathematics Test–3	Grade 2-12	Number identification, numeration, computation, applications
Test of Early Mathematics Ability–2	Age 3-9	Concepts of relative magnitude, counting, knowledge of conventions (reading and writing numbers), number facts, calculation (written and mental), Base-ten concepts (place value and money)
Test of Mathematical Abilities–2	Age 8-18 or grade 3-12	Attitude toward math, vocabulary, computation, general information, story problems

*Other examples of group achievement tests include the *PSAT (Pre Scholastic Aptitude Test)*, grades 9-10; *SAT (Scholastic Aptitude Test)*, grades 11-12 for college entrance; *ACT (American College Testing)*, grades 11-12 for college entrance; and *GRE (Graduate Record Examination)*, graduate school entrance. These tests typically cover vocabulary, verbal reasoning, reading comprehension, mathematics computation, and mathematics problem solving. The SAT examination also includes a written composition.

disabilities has been based on models indicating a significant discrepancy between learning aptitude (IQ) and academic performance. Although the validity of the IQ-achievement discrepancy model for diagnosing learning disabilities and determining eligibility for special education services is presently being questioned (see section on new era of educational assessment and alternative assessment techniques), it is still widely used. Within this model, criteria for eligibility for special education services and the diagnosis of learning disabilities are set by individual states and vary widely. Some states use discrepancies based on age norms and others on grade level performance, and degrees of IQ-achievement difference that indicate a *significant* discrepancy differ markedly among states, school systems, and public and independent (private) schools.

The *Wechsler Intelligence Scales* (preschool age, WPPSI-R; ages 6 to 16, WISC-IV; and adult, WAIS-III) are the most frequently used measures of cognitive ability and require administration by a certified psychologist or psychometrician. The *Stanford Binet-4* and *Woodcock-Johnson Tests of Cognitive Ability III* are other instruments used for assessing general intellectual ability and information processing. Commonly used educational tests for documenting discrepant academic performance include the *Woodcock-Johnson Tests of Achievement III, Kaufman Test of Educational Achievement–2 (K-TEA II), Wechsler Individual Achievement Test–2 (WIAT-2), Woodcock Reading Mastery Tests–Revised, Test of Written Language–3,* and *Key Math Diagnostic Arithmetic Test–Revised.* Often, partly for the sake of efficiency, educational diagnosticians rely on these same individually administered, standardized tests for diagnosing the nature of specific learning problems and formulating instructional plans. Careful analysis of individual performance patterns can yield helpful diagnostic information. Sole use of these tests for diagnosis and instructional planning has serious drawbacks, however (see section on weaknesses of traditional assessment practices).

Recognizing the limitations of standardized diagnostic tests, many educational diagnosticians supplement standardized testing with informal assessment inventories. Typically, informal assessment inventories assess skills and performance patterns within a specific domain, most commonly reading, spelling, and mathematics. Tasks on informal inventories may be organized by grade level of difficulty, such as reading passages, or by specific skill sequence, as in math. Commercially published inventories usually provide guidelines for evaluating a student's performance; reading inventories often suggest indicators for determining independent reading level, instructional level, and frustration level. Guidelines and checklists also are included for miscue analysis of error patterns. Informal inventories do not produce formal scores and so cannot be used for determination of eligibility for special education services or formal diagnoses. They are more useful for clarification and instructional planning. Educational diagnosticians, teachers, and school systems also may develop their own informal inventories, either skill based or curriculum based, to measure student progress in skill development and content acquisition (see section on alternative assessment techniques).

WEAKNESSES OF TRADITIONAL ASSESSMENT PRACTICES

Review of the literature reveals considerable dissatisfaction with traditional standardized methods of measuring intelligence, assessing academic progress, and diagnosing learning problems (Algozzine and Ysseldyke, 1986; Gardner, 1993; Goetz et al, 1990; Hambleton and Jurgensen, 1990; Isaacson, 1984; Jordan and Reed, 1988; Keith and Reynolds, 1990; Lyon, 1994; Lyon et al, 1993; Sternberg, 1988; Tallal, 1988; Testing: Is There a Right Answer?, 1988). Many standardized tests present serious inadequacies with respect to reliability and validity, and may lead to faulty or inappropriate diagnoses, labeling, and instructional planning. School and federal requirements for regular standardized group testing may have additional counterproductive effects. They are expensive and take away time and money that could be used for teaching and learning. Such testing practices produce anxiety and may contribute to or reinforce equating test scores with ability and place overemphasis on competition and student comparison. Students, parents, and teachers may interpret low scores as meaning poor ability. This misconception when coupled with perceived failure to keep pace in the academic race frequently results in misplaced attributions of lack of effort, declining self-esteem, and diminished student motivation for learning, ultimately placing a student at risk for school dropout and more serious social consequences, such as substance abuse and delinquency.

Policies dictating evaluation of student eligibility for special programs and education services perpetuate the emphasis on categorization and quantification. This concern with numbers tends to augment the dangers of the labeling process and dependence on scores as a measure of ability or need. Labels and low test scores can become self-fulfilling prophecies constraining the perceptions, expectations, and efforts of teachers, parents, and students. Labels are only gross generalities that imply a common disorder, but subsume a wide variation in abilities, behaviors, and dysfunctions that require widely different interventions (Levine and Jordan, 1987). Finally, the lack of consistency between states in the methods and criteria for evaluating academic proficiency, diagnosing learning disabilities, and determining eligibility for services presents a major problem. A student might be determined proficient or receive a diagnosis and be eligible for services in one state, but not in another, and lose services if the family should move. The confusion experienced by affected students and parents could have serious negative repercussions, causing stress, anger, misplaced blame, and erroneous attributions regarding student effort, ability, and teaching quality.

Tests used to assess student academic status and progress produce labels (disability or gifted), and even tests purporting to be diagnostic contain inherent inadequacies involving content, scoring, and sensitivity. Content problems include format and skill coverage. The same techniques and task formats are used for assessing students at all grade levels, failing to reflect the changes in classroom performance expectations that occur as children progress through the grades. Yet these changes can have a profound impact on learning and academic success. Test items tend to be highly structured and present little demand for independent generation, elaboration, organization, and integration of information. Items tend to be short and place minimal demands on sustained attention, information processing and storage capacity, and retrieval memory. Memory demands are reduced further by the frequent use of multiple choice formats and the availability of material for rereading and reference. In addition, many of the subtests on individually administered "diagnostic" tests are untimed and do not reflect speed of processing and production.

Skill coverage often inadequately reflects the curriculum to which the student has been exposed and can yield false-negative and false-positive results. A study conducted by Jenkins and Pany (1978) vividly showed how reading test scores can vary according to the test and reading series used. Freeman and colleagues (1982) found striking differences in the math content covered by commonly used standardized achievement tests and concluded that "because of the profound variety in content taught in schools and content tested, significant mismatches between the content of classroom instruction and the content of a standardized test are likely." Tests that do not reflect the curriculum provide little information about the student's learning ability; a student has not failed what he or she has not been taught. In addition to lack of curriculum responsiveness, skill coverage is frequently spotty and inadequate. Tests also tend to assess skills in isolation and not within the context of actual use. A student might perform adequately when attention is directed to a single element, but be unable to analyze, recall, and manipulate multiple elements simultaneously, such as required in class work and, most particularly, in written expression.

The scoring and reporting methods of standardized tests present another area of difficulty. First, most standardized group achievement tests and even some individually administered tests require students to record answers to test items on a separate answer sheet. The process of transferring answers often results in inaccuracies, particularly for students with attention or spatial problems. Bubble sheets are especially vulnerable to recording errors. Students may be unfairly penalized and assigned lower scores than they merit.

Second, the common practice of machine scoring, either by individual home computer programs or outside agencies, presents further difficulties. Scoring agencies are frequently subject to errors in calculating and reporting scores. In addition, the results that are sent back to teachers and schools are simply scores. Although they may provide information regarding a student's or class's general level of academic performance or a school's general level of educational proficiency, they yield very little information that is useful for purposes of instruction. Scores do not indicate where breakdowns are occurring, or how to improve learning and instruction; this would require examination and analysis of student responses, and test booklets typically are not returned to teachers or schools.

Third, hand scoring of many diagnostic tests is often extremely complex and subject to evaluator variability and error, as is entering scores into a home computer scoring program. The printout of scores and availability of computer-generated reports may deter educational diagnosticians from close examination of performance patterns and engender faulty judgments. In addition, most computer-generated reports amount to gross generalities and provide no information about how a student responded (what strategies were used). The *how* is as important as the *what* in analyzing a student's performance.

Fourth, test scores are based on performance accuracy and the number of items completed, and might not reflect a student's actual conceptual understanding or skill acquisition. Another problem arises from the increasing use of cluster or composite scores. A cluster or composite score lumps performance on subtests measuring specific skills into a broad domain score and may mask significant strengths and weaknesses in subskills. Knowledge of specific skill patterns and discrepancies is crucial information for planning appropriate intervention.

Fifth, the criteria for scoring in some cases are questionable. One widely disputed example is evaluating vocabulary maturity in written expression by the use of words of seven or more letters, thus excluding numerous sophisticated but shorter words (*chaos, realm, acute, demise*).

Some issues concerning test sensitivity already have been touched on, including lack of responsiveness to school curriculum, to instructional goals and techniques, and to changing processing and performance demands. Also mentioned are the limited item pool for valid and reliable diagnosis and the weakness of most tests in evaluating or even eliciting use of planning, organization, and performance strategies. Test formats can be insensitive to or penalize individual learning styles. A creative, divergent thinker has little opportunity to show these abilities on short answer or multiple choice questions. Most diagnostic tests are untimed and fail to reflect rate of processing and production. Finally, a one-shot performance on a group or individually administered test can differ significantly from daily production in the classroom.

NEW ERA IN EDUCATIONAL ASSESSMENT: STANDARDS OF COMPETENCE, ACCOUNTABILITY, AND ELIMINATION OF IQ-ACHIEVEMENT DISCREPANCY

In recent years, the nature of school education and testing has changed in response to federal and state shifts in educational priorities, performance mandates, and funding policies. The trend has been toward nationalization of educational standards from preschool through high school, and issues pertaining to school accountability, educational standards, and student competency have become major foci of federal and state legislation and educational testing.

The process toward nationalization of educational standards formally began in 1969 when the federal government introduced the NAEP (National Assessment of Educational Progress), otherwise known as "The Nation's Report Card," to measure the standards of academic performance of the nation's students. The federally administered test program is conducted at regular designated intervals. Assessments of reading, mathematics, science, writing, U.S. history, civics, geography, and the arts are given to a sample of the nation's students in grades 4, 8, and 12 drawn from public and nonpublic schools. The NAEP does not provide scores for individual students or schools. Instead, it renders information regarding the performance levels for the nation, geographic regions, states, and specific populations (female/male, ethnic/low-income groups) in the grades tested. School systems, teachers, and parents are not allowed access to the contents of the examinations to maintain objectivity of measurement and prevent "teaching to the test."

The trend toward creating national education standards received further impetus with the passing of The Goals 2000: Educate America Act in 1994 (North Central Regional Educational Laboratory, 2006b). The Goals 2000 Act codified national educational goals that were to be achieved by 2000. In particular, it stated that all students will start school "ready to learn," and will leave grades 4, 8, and 12 having shown competency over challenging subject matter, including English, mathematics, science, foreign language, civics and government, economics, the arts, history, and geography. In response to the mandates of the Goals 2000 Act, states adopted systems of outcome-based education and measurement. Outcome-based education describes what a student should know and at what level a student should be able to perform at designated points during the educational process (North Central Regional Educational Laboratory, 2006a). Individual states set standards for what students should know and be able to demonstrate to progress to the next grade stage (from grade 4 to 5, grade 8 to 9, and on leaving the system [exit criteria]). These exit tests are commonly known as high stakes testing.

The most recent federal legislation governing student competency and school accountability is the No Child Left Behind Act of 2001 (NCLB). The intents of the NCLB Act are to eliminate achievement gaps prevalent among minority and low-income populations; to raise the achievement level of all students; and to hold states, school districts, and schools accountable for demonstration of measurable progress toward improved student outcomes (Yell et al, 2006). The end goal of the legislation is that all students will show proficiency in reading and math by the 2013-2014. The NCLB Act includes the following mandates (Wikimedia Foundation, Inc, 2006):

States must test all students, including those with disabilities, annually in reading and math in grades 3 through 8 and once during high school.

By the 2007-2008 school year, states must assess students in science at least once during each of the three grade spans: 3 to 5, 6 to 9, and 10 to 12.

States must determine levels of performance proficiency and set standards for school demonstration of adequate yearly progress in raising the achievement levels of subgroups of students, including minority, low-income, and special education students, to levels of proficiency. All students must be included in school accountability systems, and all students must be proficient by 2013-2014.

States and districts must provide data on student achievement by subgroup, inform parents in a timely manner about the quality of their child's school, disseminate clear and understandable school and district report cards, and provide parents and the public with an accurate assessment of the quality of their teaching forces.

Schools receiving Title I funds that do not meet adequate yearly progress requirements for 2 consecutive years will be identified as "in need of improvement" and required to offer parents supplemental services, such as tutoring or the option of sending their children to another public school within the district or both. If a school continues in "in need of improvement" status, it will be required to take corrective action, such as removing relevant staff, restructuring the school's management and internal organization, and appointing outside experts to advise the school. These sanctions apply only to schools receiving Title I funds.

States must implement a rigorous system for ensuring that teachers are highly qualified, and that all students have access to highly qualified teachers.

Federal funding will support only educational procedures, materials, and strategies that are backed by scientifically based research.

In addition to the NCLB mandates, individual states have imposed their own sanctions on schools failing to meet adequate yearly progress goals, including reducing funding, eliminating teacher bonuses, and restructuring or possibly closing schools.

The emphasis on outcome-based education and standards-based learning and assessment has encouraged states and school districts to implement additional systems of end-of-course tests in designated courses in high school. Graduating with a high school diploma often depends on passing these tests. The specific courses subject for end-of-course tests and the standards for passing them are set by individual states. Some states depend on end-of-course test scores alone for determining passing or failing a course, promotion, and high school graduation; others use the test results as a heavily weighted factor in calculating a student's course grade, but also include daily performance and attendance.

In addition to state shifts in systems of accountability and testing to conform with federal and state mandates, there have been changes in philosophies regarding the validity of the use of intelligence testing and IQ-achievement discrepancy models for assessing learning disabilities and determining eligibility for special education services (Fuchs and Young, 2006; Lyon, 1994). Many professionals argue that traditional standardized IQ tests merely assess what an individual has learned or been exposed to (crystallized intelligence), and not reasoning and problem solving ability. Gardner (1993) and Sternberg (1988) present alternative definitions of intelligence that do not fit the commonly used standardized instruments for measuring IQ.

In addition, research increasingly has indicated that a discrepancy between cognitive functioning as determined by IQ tests and performance on standardized achievement tests is invalid for identifying a student as learning disabled. Studies have shown a lack of qualitatively distinct cognitive profiles that differentiate learning disabled from low-achieving students and have been inconsistent in revealing a differential response between learning disabled and low-achieving students to intervention (Fuchs and Young, 2006; Kovaleski, 2004; Pasternak, 2002).

One new trend is to use *response to intervention (RTI)* as a more valid determinant of learning disabilities. The reasoning is that many low-performing children have not have had the benefit of instruction that meets their individual needs, and if a child responds to specifically targeted and individually tailored remedial intervention, that child cannot be diagnosed as learning disabled. In other words, a child cannot be diagnosed as disabled if he or she has not had the benefit of individualized special intervention. The RTI process is described subsequently in the section on alternative assessment techniques. The use of RTI has gained additional support from the Individuals with Disabilities Education Improvement Act of 2004. The regulations of the Act strongly encourage the use of RTI and prohibit states from requiring evidence of a severe discrepancy between aptitude and achievement as the basis for the diagnosis of a specific learning disability and eligibility for special education services (Zirkel, 2006). As a result, states and school systems increasingly are eliminating or delaying formal assessment of cognitive functioning as part of the initial process for diagnosing learning disabilities and providing academic intervention for students exhibiting learning delays.

PROBLEMS RELATED TO CURRENT PRACTICES OF ACCOUNTABILITY AND PROFICIENCY ASSESSMENT

Although the Goals 2000 and the NCLB Acts set federal guidelines for establishing standards and timelines for student demonstration of proficiency in mastering curriculum, particularly in reading and mathematics, individual states have been left to define their own criteria for what students must learn, what constitutes proficiency and adequate yearly progress, and how to measure school effectiveness and student proficiency in mastery of core skills. Every state now has established its own core standards of student competence for reading and mathematics in grades 3 through 8 and high school graduation, has set benchmarks for school demonstration of adequate yearly progress toward the goal of 100% student proficiency by 2113-2114, and has developed a program of assessment using state-developed standardized tests.

The standards of proficiency, yearly progress benchmarks, and corresponding tests vary dramatically from state to state (Maloney, 2006; Peterson and Hess, 2005). Some states have adopted more difficult curricula, more advanced levels of proficiency, and more stringent methods for measuring performance than others. These differences have been documented by studies that compare state reported percentages of student competence at specified grade levels with that state's student performance on the NAEP tests (Fuller et al, 2006). Generally, reported levels of performance on state tests are much higher than state performance levels on the NAEP, with a wide degree of variation between states. Because of the variability in state curricula, standards of competence, and competency tests, a student moving from one state to another may discover that although he or she was evaluated as being proficient in reading or math in one state, his or her skills may be below acceptable levels in the other.

Issues pertaining to scoring described in the section on weaknesses of traditional assessment practices also apply to state and federal systems of measuring student proficiency and school accountability. Scoring is done by machines and outside agencies and subject to error. The results sent back to schools are confined to numbers and percentages. Scores may indicate that students are not reaching the defined standards of learning, and schools are not achieving satisfactory levels of academic competence and yearly progress, but there is no analysis of student responses to indicate where breakdowns are occurring in the learning or teaching process and to provide information useful for selecting and implementing relevant methods for improving student learning or correcting deficiencies in school curriculum and instruction.

NCLB was built on a status model that compares a single snapshot of aggregate student proficiency at a given grade level with a predetermined standard set by the state and against which school accountability and adequate yearly progress is measured. A single test score achieved on a single day of testing may not show a student's overall performance throughout the year, however, or progress in skill mastery. The practice of evaluating student (school) performance by a single test score violates the American Psychological Association's Standards for Educational and Psychological Testing (American Psychological Association, 1999). See subsequent discussion regarding high stakes testing. In addition, the frequency with which state proficiency tests undergo change makes the quality and consistency of their reliability and validity subject to question.

A further problem concerns longitudinal analysis of student improvement and school progress in showing adequate yearly progress in meeting state proficiency benchmarks. States are continually altering curriculum, performance standards, and tests. No valid trends of school accountability, student levels of proficiency, or individual student performance can be formulated. The student makeup of a grade changes yearly, and there are multiple changes in teachers and school administrators. Each year is an island unto itself.

Outcome-based or standards-based education and end-of-course tests represent a top-down approach to teaching and learning that encourages teachers to teach to the test and students to learn for the test. Such an approach may limit the breadth and creativity of teaching and learning and discourage growth of critical thinking, generalization of concepts, and problem-solving skills. Annual testing and time spent on student coaching use up valuable time that could be spent on learning. The emphasis on annual numerical measurement of student and school competence puts enormous pressure on students and on teachers, which may have many of the counterproductive consequences described in the section on weaknesses of traditional assessment practices because it reinforces equating test scores with ability (student learning and teacher instruction).

NCLB requires that all students be tested, including students with disabilities, and that the results be included in reporting data and evaluating whether states and school systems are meeting goals for adequate yearly progress. For students with "significant cognitive disabilities," states may create alternative achievement standards that are assessed by alternative assessment measures. NCLB does not define what constitutes a significant cognitive disability, however, or what alternative measures or test accommodations are acceptable. These interpretations and decisions are left up to individual states, and could (and do) vary significantly (Kohl et al, 2006). It is left to the individual school individualized education program or 504 teams to make decisions about which and how students with disabilities will participate in the statewide assessment (Yell et al, 2006). Policies regarding testing of students with disabilities and the students in question could vary significantly among schools, school districts, and states, and from year to year according to the members that constitute the individualized education program or 504 teams.

The underlying goals to ensure that no child be left behind in the educational process and to improve the education and performance levels of all students are noble and worthy. The NCLB Act contains serious underlying flaws, however, as outlined in the following discussion of high stakes testing. It is against established testing principles (American Educational Research Association, 1999) that student (and school) performance on which crucial decisions are made be evaluated by performance on a single test. In addition, the mandate that all students show performance proficiency in reading, math, and science at specified grade levels (i.e., to be performing at grade level), the arbitrary performance standards set by states and the federal government, and the use of standardized assessment systems all assume that "one size fits all" and run contrary to everything that is known about child development and developmental variations. Not all children learn the same things, at the same rate, in the same way (Healy, 1994; Levine and Reed, 1998).

High stakes testing is a term commonly applied to tests and test programs on which critical decisions are made in the educational arena (student promotion/retention, high school graduation, college acceptance, school accountability). It includes end-of-grade proficiency tests; end-of-course tests; exit examinations; and tests such as the GED, SAT, ACT, advanced placement, college boards, and aptitude tests for graduate school programs. The system of high stakes testing presumes that a student's performance on a single test on a single day under highly pressured conditions is a valid representation of that student's knowledge and ability. What about "bad hair days"? A low performance on any high stakes test may have a significantly damaging effect on a student's self-esteem, motivation, and, possibly, educational future. The American Psychological Association press release "How Should Student Learning and Achievement Be Measured?" (2006) presents several potential problems with current systems of testing, especially high stakes testing, and outlines principles to promote fairness in testing as contained in the *Standards for Educational and Psychological Testing* (1999), created by the American Psychological Association, American Educational Research Association, and National Council on Measurement in Education. Those most pertinent to high stakes testing include the following:

Any decision about a student's continued education, such as retention, tracking, or graduation, should not be based on the results of a single test, but should include other relevant and valid information. (This also should apply to evaluation of school accountability and demonstration of adequate yearly progress.)

When test results substantially contribute to decisions made about student promotion or graduation, there should be evidence that the test addresses only the specific or generalized content and skills that students have had an opportunity to learn.

For tests that determine a student's eligibility for promotion to the next grade or for high school graduation, students should be granted, if needed, multiple opportunities to show mastery of materials through equivalent testing procedures.

Other issues pertaining to high stakes and proficiency testing that have been brought before the federal courts in assessing the legality of specific testing practices (National Conference of State Legislatures, 2006) concern the following:

The educational basis and validity for established passing or cutoff scores. When testing programs use specific scores to determine "passing" or to define reporting categories such as "proficient," the validity of these specific scores must be established.

The significance of any fairness problems, such as possible cultural biases in the test or test items or discrimination that singles out students on the basis of any disability.

The use of an educational test for a purpose for which the test was not designed or validated. If a student lacks mastery of the language in which a test is given, that test becomes, in part, a test of language proficiency. Unless a primary purpose of a test is to evaluate language proficiency, it should not be used with students who cannot understand the language of the test itself as a measure of other skills. Nevertheless, English as a second language students are required to be tested after just 1 year in a U.S. school, even though it has regularly been shown that such students need at least 3 years of instruction in English to become competently literate. Another example is states' use of the SAT and ACT to measure reading and math proficiency of high school students. These tests were not validated for that purpose.

Finally, the entire system of annual testing as mandated by NCLB is under criticism on numerous counts, as follows (NoChildLeft.com, 2005):

1. Lack of convincing evidence that annual testing actually improves learning
2. Annual testing is expensive
3. Annual testing reduces the amount of time for learning
4. Annual testing creates pressure to teach to narrow tests
5. Annual testing increases anxiety
6. Annual testing leads to cheating in some places
7. Annual testing diverts resources from capacity building to testing
8. Annual testing is a coercive strategy by which test results are used as a form of supervision and management control

ALTERNATIVE EVALUATION TECHNIQUES

Criterion-referenced tests, curriculum-based assessment and measurement, and portfolio assessment are more recent methods of evaluating student performance that eliminate some, but not all, of the shortcomings of standardized achievement tests.

Criterion-referenced tests measure student performance in comparison to pre-established goals (standards), rather than to the achievement of other students (norm referenced). They may be commercially produced or locally developed by teachers and school systems, and are designed to assess mastery of skills in very specific, well-defined domains. The term *criterion* applies to the specific skill or behavior being tested (i.e., addition with regrouping). Student performance is usually reported as the percent of items answered correctly, and frequently a cutoff score is established to denote mastery. Criterion-referenced tests typically include multiple items sampling the same skill and provide more reliable and useful information for purposes of diagnosis and instructional planning. Locally developed tests also are more directly reflective of the curriculum being taught. Nevertheless, there are no rules governing how many test items are sufficient to measure a skill, requiring common cutoff scores across domains, or designating common standards for judging mastery. Interpretation is subject to wide variability.

Curriculum-based assessment evaluates student performance and educational needs using the materials being employed for instruction (Fuchs and Fuchs, 1990). Tests may be designed by individual teachers, school systems, or developers of commercial instructional programs such as reading series. Curriculum-based assessment, being directly tied to what is being taught, can assist instructional planning in the regular classroom by indicating deficiencies on materials already covered and readiness for subsequent instruction. Nevertheless, the focus is on short-term goals, and assessment may fail to represent long-term teaching objectives, more global integration of skills and conceptual understanding, or general student progress. Also, performance indicators cannot be generalized from one set of materials to another, which can cause problems if a student changes schools or if a system adopts a new curriculum series or textbook.

Curriculum-based measurement, a variant of curriculum-based assessment, focuses on long-term instructional goals. Tests are designed to reflect the end objective, and the same test (or equivalent form) is administered at regular intervals throughout the year. Student performance is graphed to determine the amount and adequacy of progress. At the same time, student responses are analyzed to determine instructional needs. Although curriculum-based measurement is sensitive to classroom instruction, can indicate student progress toward long-term goals, and is less susceptible to content and administration variability than curriculum-based assessment, it also has shortcomings. Similar to curriculum-based assessment, evaluation results are not readily generalized. There are no established guidelines regarding the subcomponents or subskills of long-term objectives that should be measured, the format for assessing them, or the rate of progress deemed satisfactory. Rate of student progress also may be highly unstable depending on the variation in the difficulty of steps toward the final goal and student variables at the different administration intervals.

Portfolio assessment is a more recent addition to the field of educational evaluation. Portfolio assessment involves evaluating student performance and development through collected work samples. Decisions about what to include in portfolios are usually made by students and teachers in collaboration. In addition to reflecting "real world" performance (what is required in the classroom) and assisting in integrating assessment and instruction, a goal of portfolio assessment is to encourage student critical thinking and self-evaluation. Portfolio assessment is still in a stage of development, however, and there are many unanswered questions regarding its utility. The content of portfolios differs from one subject area to another, and each tends to be evaluated independently, preventing identification of performance patterns across the curriculum. There are no set criteria for what should be included in a portfolio, how frequently materials should be collected, what domains (skills) should be included in evaluating student performance, scoring procedures, or what constitutes satisfactory progress. The creation and evaluation of portfolios remains highly subjective, reducing the reliability and validity of interpretation, limiting generalization, and seriously confounding decision making for purposes of placement, making comparisons between students, and judging achievement levels. Even when given considerable training in methods of appraisal, raters have tended to yield highly variable evaluations of portfolios (Salvia and Ysseldyke, 1995). Finally, portfolio assessment is extremely time-consuming, especially without established guidelines for performance evaluation; although not as much an issue for teachers of self-contained classes, it places an unrealistic burden on content area teachers, who may teach 100 to 150 students per day.

The newest approach to educational assessment has been the introduction of RTI (response to intervention) as a method of diagnosing learning disabilities that does not involve cognitive (IQ) testing or IQ-achievement discrepancy models (see section on traditional assessment practices). The RTI method (Kovaleski, 2004) is based on a dual-discrepancy model for identifying students with learning disabilities. First, a student must be significantly below same-grade peers on measures of academic performance. Most approaches use curriculum-based measurement (see earlier) to make this determination. The second criterion is that the student performs poorly in response to targeted interventions that are delivered in the regular classroom. If a student continues to display academic performance deficiencies after group-based interventions, the student is referred for more individually tailored interventions. In this phase, the student's RTI is specifically described and quantified. Students who show acceptable progress are deemed to have good "RTI" and typically are not referred for further assistance. Students who show poor "RTI" or the need for ongoing intensive intervention may meet state-established qualifications for special education and criteria for the diagnosis of learning disabled. How well this approach succeeds would depend on the skill and accuracy with which students' learning and processing problems are identified, the appropriateness of the interventions, the quality of instruction, and how well student performance is monitored during intervention and thereafter.

DEVELOPMENTAL, PROCESS-ORIENTED ASSESSMENT: AN INTEGRATED PERSPECTIVE

Learning is a complex, evolving, cumulative, and interactive process (Levine et al, 1993; Levine and Reed, 1998). Each child brings to school his or her own innate capabilities, temperament, and prior experiences, which continue to evolve as they act on and are acted on by curriculum materials, different teaching styles, changing educational demands, and experiences beyond the school walls. Figure 82-1 illustrates this interactive model of learning. In addition to direct testing, a comprehensive educational evaluation needs to include examination of the student's background, educational history, and daily work samples, and the school environment (Wallace and Larsen, 1978). Educational assessment that leads to effective instructional planning and management and makes the goal of successful inclusion in the regular education program a reality for students with varying patterns of learning is a multifaceted process requiring integration of information from several sources. The result should be a descriptive profile of learning strengths and weaknesses from which a detailed program of instruction and intervention can be generated.

Family and developmental history may provide useful information regarding several parameters that can have an impact on learning, and the child's pediatrician can be a valuable member of the evaluation team. A review of school history and observations obtained from past and present teachers can yield valuable diagnostic information, especially when direct observation of the child in the classroom is unfeasible: Does the child exhibit particular patterns of performance over time and across subject areas? Are the problems long-standing? When did they begin to emerge? Under what circumstances do they occur?

The student is another valuable source of information. Self-ratings and descriptions of abilities in subject areas, modes of processing and expressing information, teaching techniques, materials that facilitate or impede learning, methods of studying, athletic and social skills, and general areas of interest can yield clues to preferred learning styles, learning difficulties, organizational skills, study habits, and metacognitive awareness. Structured student interviews (Alley et al, 1981; Levine, 1988, 1994; Wiener, 1986) are a helpful addition to a diagnostic educational evaluation. Even simple comments made in response to questions about school or to particular test items can be diagnostically revealing.

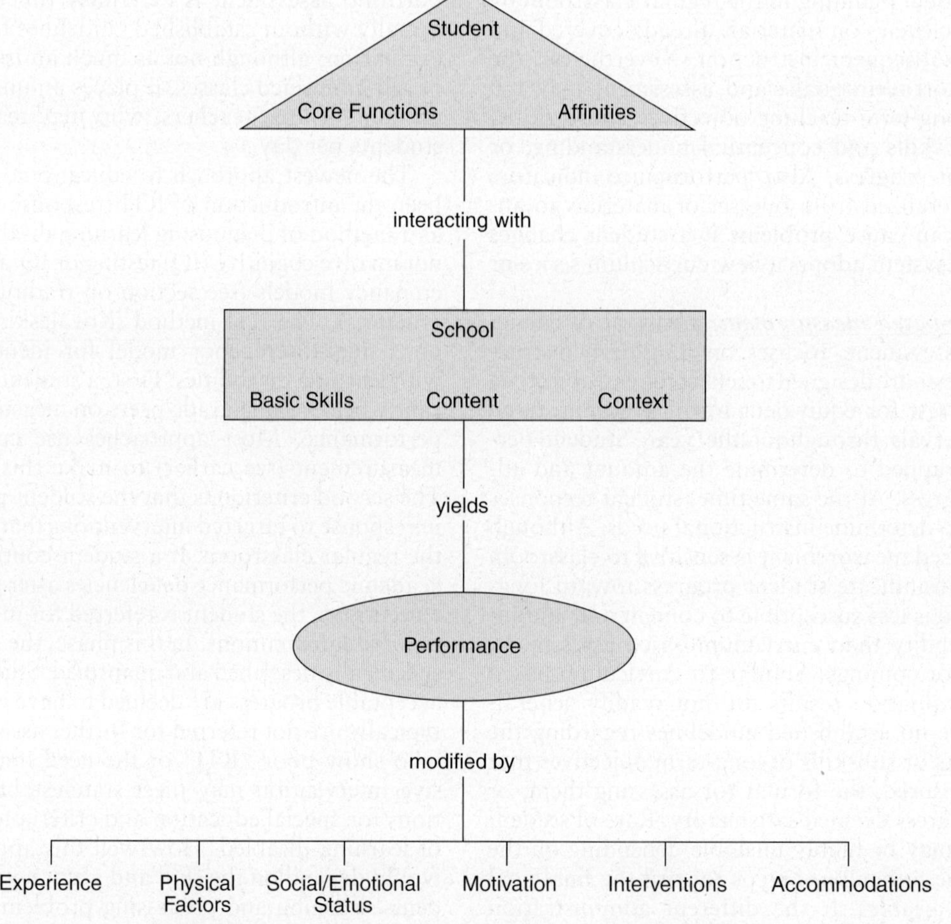

Figure 82-1. Inclusionary, interactive model of student performance.

A fine-tuned, direct examination of academic functioning is a four-dimensional process that (1) assesses specific skill acquisition and application; (2) reflects the developmental aspect of learning and changing demands on neurodevelopmental processing abilities imposed by the curriculum, teaching methods, task formats, and educational environment; (3) includes observation and analysis of behavior, error patterns, and performance strategies; and (4) incorporates student interests, affinities, and processing strengths and weaknesses. Tasks and materials used in the evaluation for the most part should be similar to those used in the classroom; however, novel tasks may provide insight into a student's problem-solving abilities, use of strategies, and generalization of learning (Silver, 1989; Swanson, 1991).

ASSESSMENT PARAMETERS AND INTERPRETATION OF PERFORMANCE

Table 82-2 defines the basic parameters of educational assessment. Evaluation of each parameter is discussed within an evolving educational timetable, an adaptation of the stages of reading described by Chall (1983).

Stage 1 (kindergarten to first half of second grade) is a period of skill acquisition. Emphasis is on learning the tools or codes of reading, writing, and mathematics. Learning is a bottom-up process in which content meaning is of relatively little importance. The focus of assessment is on the mechanics of reading, writing, and mathematics.

In reading, emphasis is given to evaluation of decoding skills, including phonologic awareness, symbol identification, knowledge and application of letter-sound associations, and sight word recognition. Confusions of letters that are similar in general form (*b/d, p/q, m/w/, n/h/u*) are common. In most cases, these confusions do not represent a visual-perceptual problem and usually reflect lack of visual attention, impulsiveness, weak spatial appreciation, or perhaps weakness in retrieval memory.

Most reading is oral, and the focus is on decoding accuracy. Typically at this stage, children rely heavily on sight recognition in reading, and errors tend to be substitutions based on whole word configuration or prominent visual elements. Comprehension commonly is measured by the ability to respond to specific questions. Problems may reflect weaknesses in receptive language, retrieval memory, or working memory.

Listening skills are crucial to successful performance in the classroom and are more regularly included in updated editions of standard educational assessment batteries. Having the child repeat sentences of varying length and syntactic complexity provides an indication of short-term retention capacity. Listening is a passive task and easily influenced by strength and length of attention. In the presence of poor listening skills, deficiencies in attention also warrant investigation.

Copying and handwriting skills are given highest priority. In view of the value placed on copying and neatness of writing, assessment of pencil grasp, pencil control, and motor patterns used to execute letter formations is very important.

Development of mathematics computation skills and understanding quantity occur at a concrete level. Evaluation should encompass basic concepts as outlined in Table 82-2, addition and subtraction without regrouping, and solving simple word problems.

Stage 2 (second half of second grade through fourth grade) is a period of continuing acquisition, practice, and consolidation of the basic tools of learning.

Assessment of reading decoding abilities should include words that must be learned by sight and words that adhere to regular phonetic and morphologic rules. Omissions of parts of words in the sounding process can indicate problems with sequencing.

Oral reading, in addition to being analyzed for patterns of decoding errors, should be evaluated for fluency and phrasing. Use of finger pointing or reduced accuracy in oral reading of connected discourse compared with identification of words in isolation can reflect erratic attention, poor visual scanning, or both.

Silent reading is introduced during this period. Silent reading speed can give additional evidence of decoding efficiency. Silent reading comprehension, similar to oral comprehension, should be assessed through unaided retelling and specific questions.

Writing requirements undergo greater change during this period. Cursive is introduced and imposes additional demands on fine motor control and fluency, motor planning, motor memory, and visual retrieval memory. A dysfunctional pencil grip becomes a great barrier to cursive writing speed and ease of production. Spelling requires knowledge and application of more advanced word analysis skills, more complex segmentation of multisyllable words, and greater revisualization capacity. Composition skills and writing mechanics receive more attention, placing greater demands on thought organization, grammatical understanding, attention, and working memory.

Mathematics also encompasses a growth in the complexity of demands. The introduction of multiplication and division toward the end of stage 2 presents multiple-step problems of increased complexity. Some children, although they can compute prewritten number problems, do not know how to set up equations by themselves, an indication of incomplete conceptual understanding or possibly poor spatial awareness or both.

Stage 3 (fifth grade through eighth grade) is a period when academic demands change dramatically, and students with an array of mild learning dysfunctions often become overwhelmed and falter for the first time. Learning increasingly becomes a top-down process in which the tools acquired during the early elementary years are applied for the purpose of acquiring new knowledge.

Reading becomes the avenue for most learning across the curriculum. The two most significant changes in reading occur in the volume and the nature of the content. With the increased amount of reading, it becomes paramount to evaluate rate of silent reading. Content switches from narrative to exposition, removing plot structure that may have aided comprehension and recall. Children with subtle language or attention problems, or both, can have difficulty determining saliency of information.

Table 82-2. **Parameters of Educational Assessment**

Reading

Word Recognition

Automatic sight recognition of high-frequency words as wholes; application of word analysis skills; vocabulary

Word Analysis

Knowledge of phonology (sound-symbol associations) and morphology (structural elements—suffixes, prefixes, syllables, root words); rule application; sound segmentation and resynthesis; vocabulary

Oral Reading

Rate, fluency, and expression; finger pointing and keeping place; accuracy and error patterns (omissions, substitutions, skipping lines); application of word analysis skills; semantic and syntactic awareness of errors; comprehension; recall of material

Silent Reading

Rate, finger pointing, subvocalization; summarization (accuracy, comprehensiveness, saliency, organization, expressive fluency); response to questions (grasp of main ideas, recall of detail, inferential reasoning, vocabulary); narrative versus expository content; length of passage; author tone, intent, bias; figurative language; poetry (meaning, meter, rhyme scheme)

Listening

Comprehension and recall of orally presented information; sentence repetition; following directions; summarization; response to questions (see under Reading); salience determination; narrative versus expository content; length; rate of processing; attention span

Writing

Spelling

Recognition (multiple choice) versus retrieval (dictation); rule application; application of word analysis skills (see under Reading); error patterns (phonetically correct or incorrect, visual configuration similarity, letter omissions, transpositions, impossible letter combinations)

Alphabet Writing

Knowledge of letter sequence and formations (manuscript and cursive); automaticity; reversals; method of forming letters

Copying

Visuomotor integration with reduced memory; rate; accuracy (omissions, additions, loss of place); spatial organization; legibility; handwriting; proofreading

Sentence Dictation

Memory of content; spelling; application of writing mechanics; handwriting

Proofreading

Recognition and correction of errors in spelling and writing mechanics (punctuation, capitalization, word usage, syntax, sentence structure); rule knowledge and application

Written Summary

Recall and organization of salient information; spelling; mechanics; proofreading; handwriting; rate of production; synchrony of subskills

Composition

Ideational fluency, elaboration, and organization; vocabulary; spelling; writing mechanics; syntactic maturity; usage; proofreading; rate of production; synchrony of subskills; narrative versus expository fluency

Handwriting

Pencil grasp; pressure and control; motor planning and patterns of forming letters; fluency; rate; legibility (accuracy of letter forms, consistency of size and spacing); automaticity

Word Processing

Knowledge of and fluency in use of a keyboard; composition skills (see under Composition); skill in use of commands; use of spelling and grammar checking; use of organizational software

Mathematics

Basic Concepts

Symbol recognition; counting; one-to-one correspondence; symbol-quantity associations; number sequencing; forming numbers (patterns, reversals); number vocabulary; clock time, money, units of measurement

Math Facts

Addition, subtraction, multiplication, and division; automatically and recall; use of concrete counting strategies

Basic Computation

Addition, subtraction, multiplication, and division with whole numbers, regrouping, decimals, and fractions; knowledge of correct algorithms; understanding of place value and regrouping; sequence of procedural steps; computation accuracy (fluency in recall of facts, use of counting strategies, alignment, attention to signs); legibility; self-monitoring

Advanced Computation

Understanding of fraction/decimal/percent equivalence; understanding of abstract symbols; solving equations for unknowns; computation with signed numbers; geometric functions and proofs; square roots; trigonometric functions; technical vocabulary; abstract, nonverbal reasoning; conceptual grasp of quantity and estimation skills

Word Problems

Reading skills; understanding of language; identification of salient information; selection of necessary operations and sequence of steps; equation construction; computation accuracy; self-monitoring; estimation skills; appreciation of quantitative relationships; logical reasoning; flexibility; use of alternative strategies

Table 82-2. Parameters of Educational Assessment—cont'd

Study Skills
READING
Previewing; note taking; underlining; paraphrasing and summarizing; salience determination; organization
LECTURE
See under Listening; note taking; organization; speed of writing; effective shorthand notation
PLANNING AND SETTING PRIORITIES
Scheduling, keeping track of assignments; time management
TEST PREPARATION AND TAKING
Knowing what to study; self-testing; memory strategies; time management; self-monitoring and metacognition
COMPUTER USE
Knowledge of websites for research

Written output emerges as the primary mode through which learning is evaluated, and any impediment to effective written expression can have devastating effects on academic success. Because a test setting is not conducive to creativity, a more valid indication of ideational and verbal fluency might be obtained from a preassigned writing task and examination of a collection of work samples.

Although use of computers often is introduced as early as kindergarten, it becomes more important during this stage and thereafter (high school, college, and adult career). Computer use can be grouped into two broad categories (Mathison and Lungren, 1989): general application, which includes word processing, database management, research, and graphics, and computer-assisted instruction, which focuses on content learning and specific skill acquisition and remediation.

Automaticity and integration become keys to success in mathematics as well. Complex multiplication, long division, and computation with decimals and fractions all require that basic facts be retrieved quickly and accurately, and a simple timed test of fact recall can provide helpful information. The student also must recall and apply several procedures in the correct sequence, placing a heavy demand on working and sequential memory.

Study skills take on major importance and warrant inclusion in the assessment process. Much valuable information can be obtained through interviewing the student regarding study habits and strategies for report writing and test preparation.

Stage 4 (ninth grade and beyond) is an ongoing period when previously learned skills must be used for various purposes. Emphasis is on interpretation, application, and manipulation of information. All subjects present increasing use of specialized vocabulary, and reading performance should be analyzed for word knowledge, use of context cues, and appreciation of word derivations and morphology for purposes of decoding and understanding. Reading no longer simply involves direct exposition of fact (Aaron and Baker, 1991; Chapman, 1993).

Listening skills take on added importance because a great deal of classroom instruction occurs via a lecture format. Sustained and selective attention, rapid processing, appreciation of language, interpretation of intent, and evaluation of saliency must be executed simultaneously and translated into some form of note taking.

Written expression becomes paramount for academic success. Writing must be used for a variety of purposes and includes different textual formats. Ideational fluency, elaboration, easy retrieval of vocabulary, and appreciation of language usage are essential (Warden and Hutchinson, 1992).

Success in mathematics depends heavily on abstract, logical reasoning; appreciation of quantitative and spatial relationships; understanding of concepts of equivalence and proportion; and cumulative, sequential memory.

Although students are often introduced to foreign language in kindergarten, it now becomes an integral part of the curriculum and a requirement for students planning to go on to college. Examination of the student's history in acquisition of speech, reading, spelling, and writing skills can provide valuable insights into the nature of difficulties in learning a second language.

Issues regarding attention may have their onset before school entry or may surface at any point during the school years or adulthood in response to the escalating demands of the curriculum, modes of instruction and production, or job requirements. It is crucial that any assessment of a student who is struggling in school or an adult who is experiencing difficulties in a job or daily activities include examination of attention capacities.

EDUCATIONAL MANAGEMENT OF LEARNING DIFFERENCES

Table 82-3 outlines the primary formal categories of educational diagnoses (American Psychological Association, 1994). A student may meet the criteria for more than one diagnostic category. Whether or not a formal educational diagnosis is formulated, educational management of learning differences (giftedness and dysfunctions) likewise requires a multifaceted approach. To be effective and to ensure successful participation of affected students in regular education programs, management must involve the collaborative efforts of the student, parents, teachers, therapists/tutors, and often the pediatrician, especially if medication

Table 82-3. Educational Diagnoses

Academically gifted in one or more areas
Academically gifted and learning disabled
Reading disorder
- Decoding
- Comprehension: passage, vocabulary
- Phonologic appreciation and phoneme/grapheme knowledge
- Reading fluency

Disorder of written language
- Spelling
- Writing conventions: grammar, capitalization, punctuation, syntax
- Written content
- Writing fluency

Mathematics disorder
- Computation
- Problem solving
- Quantitative reasoning
- Math fluency

Language disorder
- Receptive/listening
- Expressive/speaking
- Mixed receptive-expressive

Learning disorder not otherwise specified
- Academic fluency disorder: speed and accuracy in performing the basic skills of reading, written expression, and mathematics

Processing disorder that affects learning and interferes with academic achievement in multiple areas
- Memory
- Speed and accuracy of processing information: auditory, visual, verbal, nonverbal

Attention-based learning disorder: impaired learning and academic performance owing to attention deficits as opposed to specific skill deficiencies
Developmental coordination disorder: a disturbance in motor coordination (including handwriting and poor performance in sports) that significantly interferes with academic achievement or activities of daily living or both, and that is not due to a general medical condition

is involved. Because inconsistency, confusion, lack of communication, and disorganization often are primary problems that interfere with a child's ability to meet school expectations and potential for achievement, it is essential that these same problems not compromise the management efforts.

The descriptive performance profile developed from an integrated analysis of all the evaluation data should generate a detailed, multidimensional plan of management. A range of education services are available for students who qualify or are determined to be in need, including alternative educational programs, material and performance accommodations, consultation in the regular classroom, varying amounts of small group and individual instruction in a resource room, self-contained special class placement, specialized therapies, or a combination. Alternatives to public school services include private school programs, homeschooling, tutors, and therapists. Educational management typically involves some combination of individually tailored intervention and programming, direct remediation of specific skill deficits, instruction in study skills, employment of bypass strategies, and classroom accommodations. Medication also may be a part of the treatment plan; however, this is not the domain of the educator.

Selection of the modes, amount, and intensity of intervention depends on the student's needs, eligibility for special education services, severity and pervasiveness of the problem, prior remedial attempts and responsiveness, age of the student, and patterns of learning strength and weakness. For a younger child exhibiting learning differences, or a child who has received no prior intervention, class program adjustment may be the first course of action. In cases in which a learning deficit is very circumscribed and skill specific, direct remediation is usually implemented. Even in these cases, however, the child would benefit from some classroom modifications that allow successful participation without risk of humiliation.

In the upper grades, advanced placement classes and special school programs are available for more gifted students. For an older student with learning difficulties who has already received remedial work, or in cases in which the learning dysfunction is so severe or pervasive that it impedes acquisition and demonstration of knowledge in several subject areas, more emphasis is given to bypass strategies that provide continued access to new concepts and information and accommodations that enable productivity. Whether the focus is on advancement of special learning talents, direct remediation, accommodations, or a combination, the first step should be student demystification (explaining to the student his or her specific learning patterns). A student who understands his or her learning strengths and weaknesses is more receptive to intervention efforts, is able to help in the process, and is able to use the provided tools to better advantage. Other general principles and techniques of remediation and accommodation that facilitate effective management follow.

PRINCIPLES OF REMEDIAL INTERVENTION

1. Intervention should begin at the point of breakdown in the learning process—hence the need for careful analysis of error patterns, of student understanding of processes and underlying concepts, and of performance strategies being employed. A student who is good at math computation but is having trouble identifying the operations necessary to solve word problems might be asked to select from a group of word problems all those that require multiplication, or be asked to write word problems that involve a specified operation.
2. Methods and materials that use preferred learning styles, processing strengths, and interest affinities are more apt to be accepted, result in improvement, and promote maintenance and generalization of instruction. Visual learners and students with language or attention problems might grasp new concepts more effectively through graphic representation, models, demonstration, and manipulative materials. Topical magazines, comic books, TV and film scripts, technical manuals, and other high-motivation material often provide a more meaningful medium for instruction in basic skills.

3. To be effective, intervention efforts need to be directly relevant to classroom demands. Skills taught in isolation without application and practice within the context of regular use are less likely to be used, maintained, and generalized (Deshler et al, 1996).
4. Intervention efforts need to be coordinated between remedial-tutorial and regular classroom instruction so that skills and strategies are applied consistently and practiced across all subject areas. This requires close, regular contact and consultation among all teachers, tutors, and therapists. Parents also should be kept abreast of intervention goals and involved in their support at home.
5. Teaching techniques that involve active participation by the student promote greater understanding and retention of skills and concepts and, at the same time, provide a means of monitoring mastery. Cooperative small group learning activities, group problem-solving and critical thinking exercises, and opportunities for the student to explain or teach skills are examples. Including the student as a partner in developing the intervention plan promotes greater insight, investment, compliance, and feeling of self-worth.
6. Talking through thinking processes, modeling skills, providing guided practice, and giving immediate, constructive feedback have been shown to increase learning. The focus of instruction should begin with what the student is already doing correctly.
7. Preteaching activities to connect new learning with prior instruction, to clarify learning objectives, and to ensure that students have a sufficient knowledge base for comprehension, building new skills, and formulating new concepts have been shown to have a significant impact on facilitating successful learning.
8. Study skills need direct teaching. All students benefit from instruction in note taking, planning time and setting priorities, organizing workload, critical thinking, test-taking skills, use of mnemonic aids, metacognitive strategies, and self-monitoring of learning (Bragstad and Stumpf, 1987; Deshler et al, 1996).
9. Game formats can make skill drills more tolerable. Board games, flashcard games, games with dice and playing cards, word games such as Scrabble and Hangman, and computer software provide multiple possibilities (Mercer and Mercer, 1993).
10. Use of affinities and special interests can improve remediation efforts. A student is likely to become more engaged and exert greater effort and persistence when the subject matter of instruction and materials holds high personal interest.

TECHNIQUES OF ACCOMMODATION

First priority should be given to seeking out ways through which the child can experience success and avoid humiliation in front of peers. Specific talents should be exploited. Table 82-4 outlines basic categories of classroom accommodations and bypass strategies (Levine, 1994) that can improve a student's functional academic capability. Accommodations include assistive technology that encompasses nontechnologic items (pencil grips, slant boards, raised line paper, large print books) and high-technology devices (laptops, spell checkers, calculators, reading scanners, voice-activated computers). The Assistive Technology Quick Wheel available from the Council of Exceptional Children (www.cec.sped.org/law_res/doc/resources/tam;index.html) and the WATI Assistive Technology Checklist (http.//wati.org/loanlibrary/techchecklist.html) provide additional examples of accommodative devices.

Accommodations and bypass strategies should be used discretely so as to prevent public notice and discrimination. They may be arranged through a private agreement between the student and teacher. Often, however, these same accommodations can benefit all students at one time or another and might easily be made available to everyone on individual request. Tape-recorded notes and lectures can help a student who is slow in processing information or has difficulty with sustained attention or handwriting and aid students who have to miss class for some reason.

Provision of bypass strategies and accommodations should not be given freely as a matter of course, but carry a cost that ensures student accountability and shows respect for student integrity. If a student does fewer problems, the problems should carry heavier weight. Quality can substitute for quantity. A shorter written report might carry increased demands for graphic illustration and an accompanying model. More reading and references might be the payment for shortening the required length of a research paper. Flow charts might substitute for written explanations. Reduction in the amount of reading might carry a cost of extra time spent on drill practice in word identification.

SUMMARY

The processes of learning are highly complex and subject to individual variations in background, development, response to content, instructional methods, and educational environments. Learning differences and problems are multifaceted. They do not begin with entry into school, and they do not end when the first hurdle is surmounted. They can result from a wide variety of causes and do not always reflect a disability. In addition, the multiplicity and variability of testing practices and assessment instruments often render inconsistent or conflicting results regarding student mastery of skills, academic progress, diagnoses, and eligibility for programs and services. Nevertheless, whenever and as long as a student experiences difficulties or frustration in the learning process, it needs to be addressed seriously. Lack of motivation is rarely the original cause of a student's struggle in learning, but often may be the result if aid is not provided. Educational assessment and management should be viewed as ongoing, evolving processes through which a student's academic progress is closely monitored, learning patterns are analyzed, interventions are implemented and adjusted, and accommodations are provided to allow successful participation in regular education and enable the child to meet evolving academic expectations and his or her own learning potential.

Table 82-4. **Classroom Accommodations**

Accommodation Parameter	Example
Physical arrangement—alteration of seating and classroom furnishings to reduce distractions and facilitate student performance	Preferential seating: near to teacher; near to board; away from doors, windows, and noisy areas; among good role models Reduce amount of bulletin board and classroom display Study carrel, single desk versus table Take tests in separate room
Rate adjustment—additional time to process information, complete tasks, and demonstrate knowledge	Slowed rate of presentation with repetitions and summaries Extended time for tests Long response time to answer questions in class
Volume adjustment—smaller amounts of information to be processed or produced	Highlighted textbooks Selective sampling of task items (every odd number) Shorter reports
Complexity adjustment—reduced number of details, simplified language, more concrete examples and fewer abstract ideas	Simpler versions of textbooks Using shorter sentences and simple vocabulary to deliver information and give directions Illustrating concepts with examples from everyday experience
Staging—tasks broken down into a sequence of steps of smaller segments	Previewing material prior reading Answering questions while reading rather than at the end Writing reports in a series of steps so as to concentrate on one subcomponent at a time (ideas, planning, drafting, elaborating and revising, editing for mechanics, rewriting, proofing)
Prioritizing—emphasis only on selected components of a task	Not grading for spelling and mechanics when demonstration of knowledge is important Setting up the equation for solving a problem without having to perform the calculation
Format change	
Presentation of information in modes that facilitate understanding	Augmenting verbal delivery with visual materials (pictures, diagrams, demonstrations, video, and films) Tape recorded reading materials Large print texts Written copies of lectures or lecture notes
Production of information in modes that facilitate demonstration of competence	Replacing a written report with oral presentation, graphic depiction, demonstration model Giving open book and take home tests to offset memory problems Allowing students to write in test booklets to replace bubble sheets Yes/No or True/False responses to offset word retrieval or expressive language problems
Evaluation modification—different systems for assessing performance	Grading in stages, first for content then for mechanics Giving partial credit for self-correction Grading on display of progress toward goal, not absolute mastery Allowing retakes Options for earning back points for self-corrections
Curriculum alternatives—changes in course requirements or sequence	Substituting literature in tLranslation and history of a country for foreign language Deferring advanced mathematics courses, or substituting logic Altering the sequence of science or math courses
Material supports—devices that facilitate learning and demonstration of ability	Tape-recorded texts, reading scanners, calculators, word processors/laptop computers, taped lectures, note takers, scribes, printouts of class notes

REFERENCES

Aaron PG, Baker C: Reading Disabilities in College and High School: Diagnosis and Management. Parkton, MD, York Press, 1991.

Algozzine B, Ysseldyke J: The future of the l.d. field: Screening and diagnosis. J Learn Disabil 19:394, 1986.

Alley GR, Deshler DD, Warner MM: The Bayesian Screening Procedure for Identification of Learning Disabled Adolescents: Administration, Scoring and Interpretation. Monograph no. 10. Lawrence, University of Kansas, Institute for Research in Learning Disabilities, 1981.

American Educational Research Association; American Psychological Association; National Council on Measurement in Education: The Standards for Educational and Psychological Testing. Washington, DC, AERA Publications, 1999.

American Psychological Association: Diagnostic Criteria from DSM-IV. Washington, DC, 1994.

American Psychological Association: How Should Student Learning and Achievement Be Measured? 2006. Available at: www.apa.org/pubinfo/testing.html.

Bragstad BJ, Stumpf SM: A Guidebook for Teaching Study Skills and Motivation. Boston, Allyn & Bacon, 1987.

Chall JS: Stages of Reading Development. New York, McGraw-Hill, 1983.

Chapman A (ed): Making Sense: Teaching Critical Reading Across the Curriculum. New York, College Board Publications, 1993.

Deshler DD, Ellis ES, Lenz BK: Teaching Adolescents with Learning Disabilities, 2nd ed. Denver, Love Publishing, 1996.

Freeman DJ, Kuhs TM, Knappen LB, et al: A closer look at standardized tests. Arithmetic Teacher 29:50-54, 1982.

Fuchs D, Young C: On the irrelevance of intelligence in predicting responsiveness to reading instruction. Except Child 73:8-30, 2006.

Fuchs S, Fuchs D: Curriculum-based assessment. *In* Reynolds CR, Kamphaus RW (eds): Handbook of Psychological and Educational Assessment of Children: Intelligence and Achievement. New York, Guilford Press, 1990, pp 435-455.

Fuller B, Gesicki K, Kang E, et al: Is the No Child Left Behind Act Working? The Reliability of How States Track Achievement. Policy Analysis for California Education. Berkeley, University of California, 2006, pp 1-43.

Gardner H: Frames of Mind: The Theory of Multiple Intelligences. New York, Basic Books, 1993.

Goetz ET, Hall RJ, Fetsco TG: Implications of cognitive psychology for assessment of academic skill. In Reynolds CR, Kamphaus RW (eds): Handbook of Psychological and Educational Assessment of Children: Intelligence and Achievement. New York, Guilford Press, 1990, pp 477-503.

Hambleton RK, Jurgensen C: Criterion-referenced assessment of school achievement. *In* Reynolds CR, Kamphaus RW (eds): Handbook of Psychological and Educational Assessment of Children: Intelligence and Achievement. New York, Guilford Press, 1990, pp 456-474.

Healy J: Your Child's Growing Mind: A Practical Guide to Brain Development and Learning from Birth to Adolescence. New York, Doubleday, 1994.

Isaacson S: Evaluating written expression: Issues of reliability, validity, and instructional utility. Diagnostique 9:96, 1984.

Jenkins JR, Pany D: Standardized achievement tests: How useful for special education. Except Child 44:448, 1978.

Jordan NC, Reed MS: Reading disorders in early adolescence. *In* Levine MD, McAnarney ER, (eds): Early Adolescent Transitions. Lexington, MA, DC Heath, 1988, pp 227-244.

Keith T, Reynolds CR: Measurement and design in child assessment research. *In* Reynolds CR, Kamphaus RW (eds): Handbook of Psychological and Educational Assessment of Children: Intelligence and Achievement. New York, Guilford Press, 1990, 29-61.

Kohl FL, McLaughlin MJ, Nagle K: Alternate achievement standards and assessments: A descriptive investigation of 16 states. Except Child 73:107-124, 2006.

Kovaleski J: Response to instruction in the identification of learning disabilities: A guide for school teams. NASP Communiqué 32, 2004.

Levine MD: Survey of Teenage Readiness and Neurodevelopmental Status: STRANDS. Chapel Hill, NC, Clinical Center for the Study of Development and Learning, 1988.

Levine MD: Educational Care: A System for Understanding and Helping Children with Learning Problems at Home and in School. Cambridge, MA, Educators Publishing Service, 1994.

Levine MD, Hooper S, Montgomery J, et al: Learning disabilities: An interactive developmental paradigm. *In* Lyon R, et al (eds): Better Understanding Learning Disabilities: New Views from Research and Their Implications for Education and Public Policies. Baltimore, Brookes Publishing Co, 1993, pp 229-250.

Levine MD, Jordan NC: Learning disorders: Assessment and management strategies. Contemp Pediatr 5:31, 1987.

Levine MD, Reed MS: Developmental Variation and Learning Disabilities, 2nd ed. Cambridge, MA, Educators Publishing Service, 1998.

Lyon GR (ed): Frames of Reference for the Assessment of Learning Disabilities. Baltimore, Brookes Publishing Co, 1994.

Lyon GR, Gray DB, Kavanagh JF, et al: Better Understanding Learning Disabilities: New Perspectives from Research and Their Implications for Education and Public Policies. Baltimore, Brookes Publishing Co, 1993.

Maloney J: No child left behind. LDA Newsbriefs 41(3):16-17, 21, May/June 2006.

Mathison C, Lungren L: Using computers effectively in content area classes. *In* Lapp D, Flood J, Farnan N (eds): Content Areas Reading and Learning: Instructional Strategies. Englewood Cliffs, NJ, Prentice-Hall, 1989, pp 304-318.

Mercer CD, Mercer AR: Teaching Students with Learning Problems, 4th ed. New York, MacMillan Publishing, 1993.

National Conference of State Legislatures: State Assessments. 2008. Available at: www.ncsl.org/programs/educ/astateassessments.htm.

NoChildLeft.com: The Annual Testing Myth. NoChildLeft.com. 3, May 2005.

North Central Regional Educational Laboratory: "Outcome-Based" Education: An Overview. Madison, University of Wisconsin-Madison, Center on Education and Work, June 2006a.

North Central Regional Educational Laboratory: Summary of Goals 2000: Education America Act. Madison, University of Wisconsin-Madison, Center on Education and Work, June 2006b.

Pasternak R: The demise of IQ testing for children with learning disabilities. Distinguished Lecture, Chicago. NASP Communiqué 30, 2002, pp 41-42.

Peterson P, Hess F: Johnny can read ... in some states. Education Next 3, Summer 2005.

Salvia J, Ysseldyke JE: Assessment, 6th ed. Boston, Houghton Mifflin, 1995.

Silver L (ed): The Assessment of Learning Disabilities: Preschool through Adulthood. Boston, Allyn & Bacon, 1989.

Sternberg RJ: The Triarchic Mind: A New Theory of Human Intelligence. New York, Penguin Books, 1988.

Swanson HL: Handbook on the Assessment of Learning Disabilities: Theory, Research, and Practice. Austin, TX, PRO-ED, 1991.

Tallal P: Developmental language disorders. *In* Kavanagh J, Truss T (eds): Learning Disabilities: Proceedings of the National Conference. Parkton, MD, York Press, 1988, pp 181-272.

Testing: Is There a Right Answer? Harvard Education Letter 4:1, 1988.

Wallace G, Larsen S: Educational Assessment of Learning Problems: Testing for Teaching. Boston, Allyn & Bacon, 1978.

Warden MR, Hutchinson TA: Writing Process Test. Chicago, Riverside Publishing Company, 1992.

Wiener J: Alternatives in the assessment of the LD adolescent: A learning strategies approach. Learn Disabilities Focus 1:97, 1986.

Wikimedia Foundation, Inc: No Child Left Behind Act. Available at: http://en.wikipedia.org/wiku No_Child_Left_Behind. Accessed May 24, 2006.

Yell M, Katsiyannas A, Shiner J: The No Child Left Behind Act, adequate yearly progress, and students with disabilities. Teaching Exceptional Children 38:32-39, 2006.

Zirkel P: What does the law say? Teaching Exceptional Children 38:67-68, 2006.

83 NEUROPSYCHOLOGICAL ASSESSMENT OF THE DEVELOPING CHILD

JANE HOLMES BERNSTEIN

Assessing the behavior of a developing child—the psychologist's contribution to developmental-behavioral pediatrics—is a clinical activity that, similar to all other such activities, must be evidence-based (National Institute of Medicine, 2001). In neuropsychology, this means that the rapidly increasing knowledge base in neuroscience and the neural correlates of behavior need to be brought to bear on the behavioral assessment of the child. To be effective, this clinical endeavor requires an integration of the third-person perspective of scientific investigation and the first-person perspective that is the core of clinical work. Diagnostically, the critical investigative frame for clinical work is necessarily that of "individual difference." In the science frame, the experience of the individual is, however, all too likely to be relegated to the status of "error variance" in a group analysis. The clinician must resolve this tension in the collection and interpretation of data.

At the management stage, making meaning for the individual (and family members) is at the core of the client values expectation of evidence-based practice (National Institute of Medicine, 2001). A scientific explanation that cannot be meaningfully integrated into the ongoing narrative of a person's (and family's) life all too easily fails to provide clinical utility: Families ignore potentially valuable advice, fail to follow through, and do not understand their role in their own recovery or continued well-being (Bernheimer and Keogh, 1995). Evidence-based assessment in neuropsychology must incorporate the science of "brain" and the experience of the individual who has one.

DEFINITION OF NEUROPSYCHOLOGY

Neuropsychology is the study of brain-behavior relationships. The knowledge base for neuropsychology has been, and continues to be, derived from studies of behavior and behavior change—in humans and other animals; in infants, juveniles, adults, and elders across species; in sickness and in health; following lesions that occur naturally and lesions that are created under laboratory conditions; in "free-field" situations and in laboratory-based experimental paradigms, with or without concomitant use of neurodiagnostic techniques; in the context of atypical development in the course of disease; and in the case of failure of acquisition of expected skills under conditions of expectable experience (Banich, 1997; Kolb and Wishaw, 2003; Zillmer et al, 2007).

The clinical application of neuropsychological principles has changed the way in which children's behavior is evaluated. "Psychological evaluation" has given way to "neuropsychological evaluation" and "psychoeducational evaluation." In the clinical setting, neuropsychology is not simply a set of (more) tests. Third-party payers' reimbursement schedules notwithstanding, "neuropsychological testing" is itself arguably a misnomer. The instruments used to measure behavior are psychological tests. What makes a clinical evaluation neuropsychological is the ability of the clinician to make inferences about the central nervous system from observation of behavior.

In the clinical setting, application of neuropsychological principles has implications for the design of the assessment, most notably that it be appropriately inclusive of the range of functional skill that the brain supports. The basic neuropsychological assessment goes beyond the IQ and visuomotor tasks of traditional psychological measurement to include a comprehensive analysis of behavioral domains. In our approach (Bernstein, 2000; Bernstein et al, 2005), this analysis is achieved by a review of neurobehavioral systems (behavioral domains) that yields qualitative and quantitative data pertaining to emotional status, sensorimotor function, perceptual abilities, higher order information processing, cognitive level, and regulatory capacity. The target outcomes are not just academic success, but encompass the daily living skills, vocational and academic skills, and psychosocial competencies needed for optimal adaptation as an independent individual at the maximum level possible. A broad range of tools and techniques are employed in this endeavor, and create a problem of data management (Tversky and Kahneman, 1974) that the clinician must address (Bernstein, 2000). Table 83-1 presents an overview of behavioral domains, data sources, tools and techniques, and test variables.

Table 83-1. **Behavioral Domains, Data Sources, Data Types, Tools and Techniques, and Test Variables**

Behavioral Domains	Data Sources	Data Type	Tools/Techniques	Test Variables
Arousal	History	Qualitative	Analytic interviewing	Psychometric data
Attention	Family	Quantitative	Systematic observation	Levels of performance
Motivation	Demographic		Task analysis	Profiles of performance
Memory	Medical		Clinical limit testing	Behavioral data
Learning	Educational		Dynamic assessment	Elicited behaviors
Executive control	Psychological		Psychological tests	Problem-solving strategies
Exploratory capacities	Child		Educational tests	Task analysis data
Communication	Developmental		Behavioral rating scales	Task complexity
Language	Medical		Developmental questionnaires	Systemic variables
Speech	Educational			
Visuospatial processing	Psychological			
Sensory capacities	Observation			
Motor skills	Direct			
Social processing	In "free field"			
Social cognition	In test setting			
Emotional status	Indirect			
Temperament	Interview			
Personality characteristics	Telephone consultation			
	Tools/techniques			

REIMBURSEMENT OF NEUROPSYCHOLOGICAL SERVICES

Neuropsychological evaluation and assessment services are typically reimbursed at an hourly rate, which varies by geographic location, service location, negotiated contracts between insurance carriers and providers, and individual contracts with providers and education authorities or parents or both. Management/therapeutic services are billed and reimbursed in 15-minute units. The amount of time required to provide the service varies by (1) the nature of the information required to address the referral question, (2) the ability of the child to manage the demands of the evaluation (because of young age, lack of stamina, slow processing rate, dysregulated behavior), (3) the competence of the child in establishing baselines for psychological test scores, (4) the need for in-depth exploration of a particular behavioral domain, (5) the indication for detailed analysis of personality variables or emotional status or both, and (6) the availability of recently obtained psychological test data. Table 83-2 provides an approximate range of times per service for commonly requested neuropsychological evaluation services. The time-consuming nature of psychological test administration is documented in Table 83-3.

THE NEUROPSYCHOLOGIST

In contrast to medicine, psychology does not require board certification for the practice of a psychological specialty. A report entitled "report of neuropsychological testing (or evaluation or assessment)" can be produced by any psychologist. There are nonetheless three examining boards in clinical neuropsychology that evaluate competence for specialty practice in this area: the American Board of Clinical Neuropsychology, a member board of the American Board of Professional Psychology; the American Board of Pediatric Neuropsychology; and the American Board of Professional Neuropsychology.

Differences in background and training among individuals offering neuropsychological services have led to a range of applications of the neuropsychological knowledge base. Following a referral for neuropsychological services, the pediatrician can expect to receive a text labeled "report of neuropsychological testing/evaluation/assessment." The pediatrician can expect a description of the child's performance on a range of tasks tapping regulatory, cognitive, social, emotional, and sensorimotor capacities, and current achievement. There is, however, no guarantee that the physician will receive more

Table 83-2. **Billing/Reimbursement Units and Service Category**

Time Estimates (hr)	Nature of Service
1	Repeat test administration for medication/treatment monitoring with note
2-4	Initial consultation with report
3-8	Consultation with review of records, interview, feedback (interpretive) session, report, and collateral contacts as indicated for clinical management purposes*
4-10	Tailored evaluation protocol with interview, feedback (interpretive) session, report, and collateral contacts as indicated
8-16	Comprehensive evaluation protocol with interview, feedback (interpretive) session, report, and collateral contacts as indicated

*Forensic consultation can be expected to take longer.

Table 83-3. **Estimated Time for Administration of Partial Protocol**

Psychological Test	Time for Administration (Approximate)
IQ test	75 min
Selected language measures	20 min
Verbal learning	20 min + delay trials
Memory scale	35 min + delay trials
Complex figure copy	8 min
Continuous performance test	20 min
Finger dexterity	5 min

than a psychological analysis, that is, a more or less detailed analysis of the cognitive architecture (with no reference to the underlying brain—whether or not a brain condition is present).

Alternatively, the report may reflect a neuropsychological analysis in that the detailed description of the cognitive architecture is related specifically to brain systems, stating (where relevant) which behaviors are and are not consistent with a documented brain condition. Even here, however, the developmental-behavioral pediatrician may look in vain for the developmental context of the particular child's experience. This requires a different analysis, integrating knowledge of the child's developmental course to date, his or her profile of strengths and weaknesses, the contexts in which he or she operates, and the impact of the disorder (where relevant). This analysis is the basis on which the clinician characterizes the individual child's risks and protective factors and seeks to optimize the child's outcome by predicting future expectable challenges and creating a management plan to maximize the child's ongoing progress (Bernstein, 2000).

A good neuropsychological assessment provides a coherent description of the child; diagnostically relevant information; interpretation between physician and parents and educational system regarding the impact of the child's medical condition on his or her behavior; and a management plan to address the child's needs medically (where relevant), in the family setting, in school, and in the community. An inadequate neuropsychological evaluation often provides a lengthy list of test performances, no integrated diagnostic formulation, and no logical relationship between the diagnostic formulation and the recommendations.

Table 83-4. Neurodevelopmental Disorders

Category	Examples
Simple genetic syndromes	Down, Turner, Prader-Willi, fragile X, Williams
Complex genetic syndromes	Autism, specific language impairment, dyslexia, attention-deficit/ hyperactivity disorder
Structural brain abnormalities	Congenital hydrocephalus, agenesis or dysgenesis of the corpus callosum, Dandy-Walker, Arnold-Chiari, Sturge-Weber conditions
Acquired insults	Cerebrovascular accident, missile injury, motor vehicle accident, trauma, prematurity
Other disease insult	Secondary to compromised functioning of other organ systems: liver disease, kidney disease
Unavoidable treatment-related iatrogenic insult	Radiation, chemotherapy, steroids

Adapted from Tager-Flusberg H: Neurodevelopmental Disorders. New York, Guilford Press, 1999.

USE OF NEUROPSYCHOLOGICAL ASSESSMENTS

Children's abilities traditionally have been measured by psychological tests. In the educational setting, these tests were designed to allow for (and are good at) ranking a child relative to his or her age peers (an *inter-child analysis*) and predicting later academic achievement, the goal being to determine appropriate educational placement or to obtain services, or both. Psychological tests alone are inadequate, however, to the job of evaluating behavior within a brain-referenced framework, and they are insufficient for the clinical *intra-child analysis,* that yields a comprehensive portrait (Matarazzo, 1990) of the actively developing "whole child" (Holmes-Bernstein and Waber, 1990) as the basis for diagnostic classification and effective management.

Neuropsychological assessment applies neuropsychological principles to address the integrity and breakdown of behavior in light of what is currently known about the neural substrates for behavioral functioning and adjustment in normal development and disease. Developmental neuropsychological assessment further incorporates knowledge of change in behavior as a function of maturity in a developing child. A neuropsychological assessment is indicated whenever a child has a known or suspected medical or neurologic condition (or treatment) that can be expected to have an impact on the developing brain. Children with any of the well-known neuropathologies of childhood can benefit from a comprehensive neuropsychological assessment. Such neuropathologies are presented in Table 83-4.

The disorders for which neuropsychological analysis is appropriate are not only disorders that involve medical conditions. Neuropsychological assessment is now regularly sought for children whose presenting complaints involve academic skills and for children whose development has been threatened by early traumatic experiences (emotional, social, physical), the impact of which on developing biologic systems is being increasingly recognized (Nelson, 2000).

WHEN NEUROPSYCHOLOGICAL SERVICES ARE USED

Neuropsychological services typically are requested by physicians when they need an analysis of a child's behavioral status (portrait of child, baseline), when they seek to map behavior to the brain for diagnostic purposes, when they want an assessment of the impact of injury on behavior, when evaluation of the impact of treatment on behavior (prior, post) is required, when tracking of medication effects is indicated, and when management of behavioral outcomes is needed. The evaluation is the basis for determining an estimate of the general level of functioning, assessing the integrity of specific behavioral functions, evaluating functions believed to be sensitive to the impact of a given disorder, evaluating the child's psychological adjustment to a medical condition, assessing the family's capacity for support and advocacy on behalf of the child, and determining the services and supports needed from the school team or from other specialists. Parents and the educational team request neuropsychological evaluation when they seek to understand the impact of a disorder on a child's behavior and adjustment (now and in the future), when psychological test profiles provide no insight into the child's behavior and yet the child remains in distress, when behavioral outcomes need to be managed, and when they need help with appropriate parenting and behavior management strategies to support the child's adjustment and development.

When neuropsychological evaluations should be scheduled varies by the nature of the referral and the child's condition. Treatment monitoring that typically employs a brief protocol of targeted psychological instruments would be at shorter intervals as deemed appropriate given the expected action of a drug or treatment. Ongoing medical and behavioral management of disorders that can be expected to perturb developmental processes would need to incorporate repeat neuropsychological assessment throughout childhood, adolescence, and young adulthood (Rey-Casserly and Bernstein, 2007). In contrast to psychoeducational evaluation, which may be indicated on a regular yearly basis to document skill acquisition, we recommend repeat neuropsychological assessments at (more or less) 3-year intervals, typically before the major transition points that (grossly) reflect maturational stages and are defined by the educational system. We are available for consultation sooner if and when concerns arise.

PRACTICE OF NEUROPSYCHOLOGY

Diagnostic Environment

Neuropsychology is practiced within four different—frequently complementary—nosologic frameworks: medicine (referenced to the biologic substrate for disease), psychiatry (framed in terms of the behavioral clusters that are given status as disorders under the rubric of the *Diagnostic and Statistical Manual of Mental Disorders, Fourth Edition* [American-Psychiatric Association, 1994]), neuropsychology (referenced to brain-behavior relationships), and education (framed as failures of acquisition of expected academic and related skills under typical conditions of exposure). Under the influence of neuropsychology, the interaction of these nosologic frameworks has led to a shift from an earlier characterization of *learning disabilities,* whereby deficits in children's functioning were characterized primarily as they were manifest in the school context, to a more encompassing label, *learning disorders,* which reflects the role of the brain in learning—or not learning—the full range of behaviors that it supports. Learning disorders are framed in terms of biology (structural anomalies, genetic syndromes, acquired brain injury), psychological processes (disorders whose core symptoms suggest disruption of more or less specific behavioral systems that support attention, language, visuospatial functioning, social skills, and executive processes), behavioral clusters (attention-deficit disorder with and without hyperactivity, nonverbal learning disorders, Asperger syndrome), and manifest symptoms in particular settings (failure to acquire reading, math, organization, and social comportment skills as expected).

Theoretical Framework

The clinical neuropsychologist works within a theoretical framework that includes a theory of the organism itself, a theory of the potential disorders that affect children, and a theory of the assessment process. Knowledge of pedagogic theory also is important for the neuropsychologist in his or her role as a member of the child's treatment team.

A neuropsychological analysis starts with the premise that the organism in question, a human child, has a *brain.* Brains depend for their structure and their function in supporting behavior on interaction with a variety of expectable contexts. This necessary brain-context interaction is continually updated and shaped over the course of development. Analysis of behavior is scrutinized within this *brain-context-development* matrix (Bernstein, 2000).

A theory of the potential disorders (see Table 83-4) that can affect children's behavior and ongoing development is crucial to understanding perturbation or change in the way the child is developing. Different disorders involve different pathologic processes that can be relatively limited in their effects (at least initially) or can involve brain functioning system-wide. The occurrence of these disorders in the pediatric population entails, however, that they all occur in the context of dynamic change over the course of development. All of these disorders have potential for derailing behavioral development and changing behavioral outcomes. Genetic and structural disorders set up conditions for alternative developmental trajectories from the beginning of the child's interactions with the environment. Later acquired derailments have potential for resulting in so-called late effects. The pathology is or becomes part of the developmental course with important—not yet fully understood—implications for the understanding of brain-behavior relationships in the developing child.

The neuropsychologist not only must address the issue of potentially altered brain organization, but also must factor in the degree to which the insult is focal or systemic. The effects of more or less focal insults are likely to be reflected in disturbance of specific cognitive systems, but also can change the development of the system overall. Children with more or less focal insults typically stay "on developmental track"; their overall cognitive level stays with that of their peers. Specific cognitive issues are associated with specific deficits. Evidence of right hemisphere dysfunction accompanies deficits in conceptual organization, "big picture" thinking, math, social understanding, and aspects of attention. Evidence implicating left hemisphere dysfunction is associated with deficits in oral and written language, math, and sequential organization. Language deficits may lead to reading disability and to deficits in linguistic aspects of math.

Systemic insults, in contrast, typically undermine regulatory processes (attention and executive processes). Children may have difficulty maintaining state and managing the expectable sensory load of their environment; they may struggle to modulate emotion and fail to acquire age-expected control over motor and verbal activity. They are often "off developmental track" with cognitive level as indexed by psychometric tasks, typically declining relative to peers over time. Such children frequently are not "skill poor" under structured conditions, which can mask their need for educational services. Their major problem is one of overall behavior regulation secondary to pervasive problems with inhibitory control. Social behavior in particular is a significant problem; in contrast to written text that stays on the page and can be worked and reworked, the on-line nature of processing and responding to socially relevant information cannot easily be accommodated in any sort of structured format.

The impact of systemic insults interacting with developmental time itself shapes neural and behavioral pathology down the line. Developing skill-plus-insult can lead to a specific neuropsychological deficit later (Shaheen, 1984; Waber et al, 1992). Developing skill-plus-experience that is out-of-sync can lead to compromise of sequential skill development (see Dennis [1988, 1989] for an elegant analysis of the skills and deficits associated with the unhindered and perturbed acquisition of skills). Recognition of the potential threats to normal development is a crucial component of the pediatric neuropsychologist's training. Understanding the nature of the interactions of disorders and their treatments with normal developmental expectations is frequently the most important factor for outlining effective interventions (see Bernstein and Weiler [2000] for a discussion of the interaction with development of the multiple impacts of disorder and treatments in the case of myelodysplasia).

Knowledge Base

The rapidly developing knowledge base in the developmental neurosciences also is changing the way in which neuropsychology with children is practiced. Analysis of the components of specific behavioral domains using cutting-edge neurodiagnostic tools is becoming increasingly detailed and complements the findings of careful investigations of behavioral breakdown in the neuropathologies of childhood. The research program of Posner and colleagues has identified separable components of attention, validated them via functional imaging, documented differences in developmental trajectories for different components, and shown that different components respond differentially to interventions (Posner and Rothbart, 2007). Complementary to this work is the clinical research program of Dennis and colleagues (2005), who have examined the attentional capacities of children with spina bifida and shown different types of attentional breakdown in this population—with implications for medical and behavioral management. The identification of specific attentional difficulty is important for clinical practice. Equally close parsing of behavioral competencies in language, social information processing, and regulatory functioning can be expected to contribute to better understanding of disordered behavior and to the development of targeted intervention paradigms to promote children's progress.

CLINICAL EXAMPLES

The *brain-context* transaction that is the core of the clinical analysis provides the framework for the interpretation of behavioral data. It entails that the brain must be scrutinized as a dependent and an independent variable (Bakker, 1984). The apparent meaning of psychological test scores also needs to be scrutinized in light of this fundamental principle. Consider the observation of a verbal IQ > performance IQ profile after a left brain lesion that creates a frank aphasia, or the failure of a lesion that undermines language performance to compromise the verbal IQ score (Dlugos et al, 1999). Why is the verbal IQ score impervious to the impact of the damage? The damage has, after all, resulted in aphasia. The verbal IQ score is not a measure of language, however; it is correctly named as an index of *verbal knowledge*. Verbal knowledge depends for acquisition and maintenance on one's experience; it reflects the quality of that experience typically via education. Context (here, that of the individual's educational experience)—rather than biology—predicts the verbal IQ score.

In the pediatric context, consider the following scenario. An economically advantaged, home-based mother requests evaluation of her "gifted–learning disabled" 6-year-old daughter: "learning disabled," possibly; "gifted," unlikely. (A major challenge in working with a gifted–learning disordered child is that the giftedness frequently obscures the learning issues until the academic challenges become high—when it can be quite difficult to persuade a very bright teenager that he or she really does need to learn compensatory strategies for working at his or her conceptual level.) The "giftedness" in this scenario is likely to reflect the well-developed verbal knowledge of a usually female, often first, child whose development to date has been shaped by the context of multiple extended conversational interactions with an educated mother. At age 6, that is, at the beginning of formal education, this is what the verbal IQ would index—yielding an above-average score. By age 10, however, the verbal IQ score would reflect the child's success in acquiring verbal knowledge from the academic context—dependent on mastery of written language. To the extent that the child does have learning issues (after all, something has brought her to clinical attention), the likelihood is that she will acquire academic skills slowly. She will not have the "expectable" experience that is indexed by the IQ test; her rank relative to her peers will change, and she will lose points on the test. Her "loss of IQ" is not in this case a marker of change in the biologic substrate, but rather reflects test construction interacting with developmental expectations.

The *brain-context* transactional model not only requires reinterpretation of psychological test data, but also emphasizes the importance of the ecologic validity of the clinical analysis: "how the brain works" in the context of the real world, rather than just "what (this or that part of) the brain does." This stance requires the clinician to explain not only what the child cannot do, but also—and arguably more importantly—how the brain can do what it can do when other skills are apparently so limited. The former, deficit-based approach may be needed for diagnosis, but it is knowing the child's competencies, available strategies, and motivational capacities—a strength-based conceptualization—and the expectable challenges with which the child is likely to be faced that is the basis for effective rehabilitation, successful compensation, and maximization of outcome.

Failing to recognize the distinction between having the skill in a test condition (one context) and being independently able to use the skill on-line in real time and in the real world (involving quite different contextual demands) can result in costly clinical error. The evaluation of language is particularly prone to this. A child can have an average performance on psychological tests tapping specific linguistic skills administered one at a time in the quiet, structured, "artificial" setting of the psychologist's office and be functionally language-impaired in the rapid, on-line conditions of complex, reciprocal verbal exchanges in real-life situations, which typically occur against background noise and against competing stimuli. In contrast, a child's ability to use language in highly redundant social settings or to employ high-level vocabulary in very restricted content areas can mask a lack of understanding of the real world that may be profound. One child that I have followed over time was able to offer abstract dictionary-quality definitions on a vocabulary test, but asked her father while holding out her down jacket: "It's 89 degrees outside. Do I need this?" The clinician's repertoire must incorporate both analyses: Does the child have the skill? Can the child use the skill?.

Frequently psychological and psychoeducational test scores provide no insight into a child's struggle in school. Children sometimes acquire neurobehavioral problems subsequent to radiation therapy (which is thought to have a deleterious effect on myelination and undermine the efficiency of information transfer across brain systems (Moore, 2005; Mulhern and Butler, 2004). Review of a child's history indicates that he or she was treated with radiation therapy in the preschool period (Ah! That explains it!).

Why would no one have made such a connection before? Why was the impact of the radiation therapy not noted before? Answering both questions requires a developmental stance and careful education of the family. A *medical* condition that occurred, and was successfully treated, 8 years previously would not be the first thing the family would think of when *school* issues occur later. Also, it would not be appreciated that development brings change in expectations. In the *brain-context-development* analysis, however, the contextual demands of school grades are expected to change in response to the developmental gains in maturity and competence that come with increasing age (Holmes, 1987). Before, the teacher provided structured assignments whose parameters were well defined by the adult; the child's neuropsychological weakness was not challenged. Now, at the sixth-grade level, the child is expected to take on the responsibility for task organization, and the deficit is revealed.

The interaction of brain, context, and developmental variables in understanding a child's experience and providing adequately nuanced management also is highlighted in the following situation. Parents are concerned because their otherwise curious and thoughtful 7-year-old daughter is struggling to acquire reading skills. Family history is positive for written language difficulties, but is not otherwise remarkable. The developmental course has been normal. She seems to be of normal intellectual ability, taking part in conversation without difficulty. Social skills seem to be appropriate for age. Physical examination is noncontributory. Referral is made for psychological evaluation to try to understand the reason for the slow acquisition of reading.

The psychologist also sees a friendly, cooperative, and interested child whose social interaction is well developed. Testing supports the observation of the child as normally intelligent with scores in the average to above-average range for age. Reading skills are below grade expectancy with insecure mastery of sound-symbol relationships. The child relies heavily on sight word recognition to decode written text. Phonologic skills are poorly developed.

To address the presenting complaint, the psychoeducational evaluation supports the recommendation of a reading program that addresses phonologic relationships. From a neuropsychological perspective, however, it is unlikely that a "brain difference" sufficient to undermine reading would have no further impact on behavioral adjustment—and further information is available. The child's visuospatial skills are intact, as are executive skills. Gross and fine motor skills are normal. Subtle, but nonetheless clearly documentable language processing deficits are noted. Graphomotor control and output is very laborious with unevenly formed letters.

With this additional information, the neuropsychologist considers the child to be at increased risk for ongoing difficulties even as she makes effective progress in acquiring reading skills in the early grades. The pattern of intact and insecure skills makes up a diagnostic behavioral cluster (Holmes-Bernstein and Waber, 1990) that is consistent with less efficient input of left hemisphere brain systems to ongoing behavior. To the extent that other family members are reported to have had similar struggles with written language skills, this may be a familial condition. This diagnostic formulation sets the child up for difficulty as she faces the developmentally determined expectations of the upcoming school grades (Pardes, 1988). These expectations not only are framed in terms of academic skills, but also involve social, emotional, and regulatory capacities.

Table 83-5 presents an analysis of the demand characteristics of the content area itself and the requirements of the contexts in which the content is used. With language processing deficits/left hemisphere inefficiencies, the child is not only at risk for difficulty with written language skills (to the extent that these are based on oral language integrity), but also of math secondary to language demands and the linear output requirements

Table 83-5. **Context and Content Demands in Academic and Psychosocial Domains for a Developing Child with Insecure Language Processing**

Risks	Academic-Vocational	Social-Emotional
Context	Listening, learning in the classroom	Listening, participating in peer groups/ activities
Content	Reading decoding/fluency Reading comprehension Written expression Math	Self-regulation

of math algorithms. Language is a crucial element in the overall executive skill repertoire. Developmentally, it is crucial not only for communication and for academic achievement, but also as a necessary foundation for behavioral regulation and the development of social skills. Recognition of these risks forms the basis for the formulation of the management plan now and as the child faces expectable developmental demands in the future.

Identification of contextual demands—and change in contextual demands over time—is a critical part of the specification of risk. Risks also can "cascade" across a whole range of behaviors. One example of this on the child's developmental course is often seen in neurodevelopmental disorders, especially disorders in which there is involvement of the entire brain. The child is diagnosed as being a very slow processor of information. This can be characterized as a "taking-in" problem. To the individuals interacting with the child, he or she seems to talk adequately in ordinary conversation and can repeat instructions or directions when challenged. The child frequently fails to respond to the latter in the expected time frame, however. This situation can lead to frustration and anger on the part of teachers and parents, which itself has negative consequences, compounding the risk cascade. Lacking understanding of the child's problem, people do not wait for the child to respond. The result is that the child then fails to get the normal range of feedback needed to shape behavior effectively.

Repeated over time, this situation has an impact on attentional capacities, on behavioral modulation, and on memory and learning. The fact that people do not or cannot wait also means that the child fails to get coherent feedback that he or she is valuable as a person. This has an impact on emotional development, leading to misleading and deleterious attributions of self, and undermining self-efficacy and investment in the educational process (Palombo, 2001). Managing a child with slowed processing is a significant clinical challenge, primarily because the world simply cannot be slowed for one child. Understanding what is happening and educating parents and teachers can make an enormous difference, however, in how the child is viewed and limit unhelpful and damaging attributions of willfulness, lack of motivation, and oppositional behavior.

Table 83-6. Frequently Asked "Why" Questions

Why Does It Take So Long to Get an Appointment?

Because there are not enough neuropsychologists
Because the workload is extensive
Because reimbursement requires time-consuming preauthorization (from a clinician)

Why Does It Take So Long to Do the Evaluation?

Because the workload can be extensive (see Tables 83-1 and 83-2)
Because psychological tests take time to administer (see Table 83-3)
Because children can lack stamina, seize, process slowly, or resist

Why Does It Cost So Much?

Because it takes so long

Why Are the Reports So Long?

Because physicians, parents, and educators want comprehensive analyses
Because neuropsychologists must meet professional standards
Because what has been done must be documented
Because what needs to be done requires explanation and interpretation

SUMMARY

Assessment of a developing child in a neurodevelopmental framework can promote the child's progress and improve outcomes in significant ways. It requires, however, that the design and methodology of the assessment process be scrutinized and updated where indicated to do justice to the expanding knowledge base in the developmental neurosciences in the context of current requirements of evidence-based practice. Such assessment takes time: Consumers often query "why?" Table 83-6 offers answers to frequently asked "why?" questions.

REFERENCES

American Psychiatric Association: Diagnostic and Statistical Manual of Mental Disorders, 4th ed. Washington, DC, American Psychiatric Association, 1994.

Bakker DJ: The brain as dependent variable. J Clin Neuropsychol 6: 1-16, 1984.

Banich MT: Neuropsychology: The Neural Basis of Mental Function. Boston, Houghton Mifflin, 1997.

Bernheimer LP, Keogh BK: Weaving interventions into the fabric of everyday life: An approach to family assessment. Top Early Child Spec Ed 15:415-433, 1995.

Bernstein JH: Developmental neuropsychological assessment. *In* Yeates KO, Ris DM, Taylor HG (eds): Pediatric Neuropsychology: Research, Theory, and Practice. New York, Guilford Press, 2000, pp 405-438.

Bernstein JH, Kammerer B, Prather PA, Rey-Casserly C: Developmental neuropsychological assessment. *In* Koocher GP, Norcross JC, Hilt SS (eds): Psychologists' Desk Reference, Vol 2. New York, Oxford University Press, 2005, pp 28-32.

Bernstein JH, Weiler MD: "Pediatric neuropsychological assessment" examined. *In* Goldstein G, Hersen M (eds): Handbook of Psychological Assessment, 3rd ed. Amsterdam, Pergamon, 2000, pp 263-300.

Dennis M: Language and the young damaged brain. *In* Bolt T, Bryant BK (eds): Clinical Neuropsychology and Brain Function. Washington, DC, American Psychological Association, 1988, 85-123.

Dennis M: Assessing the neuropsychological abilities of children and adolescents for personal injury litigation. Clin Neuropsychol 3:203-229, 1989.

Dennis M, Edelstein K, Copeland K, et al: Covert orienting to exogenous and endogenous cues in children with spina bifida. Neuropsychologia 42:976-987, 2005.

Dlugos DJ, Moss EM, Duhaim, A-C, Brooks-Kayat AR: Language-related cognitive declines after left temporal lobectomy in children. Pediatr Neurol 21:444-449, 1999.

Holmes JM: Natural histories in learning disabilities: Neuropsychological difference/environmental demand. *In* Ceci SJ (ed): Handbook of Cognitive, Social and Neuropsychological Aspects of Learning Disabilities. Hillsdale, NJ, Erlbaum, 1987, pp 303-319.

Holmes-Bernstein JM, Waber DP: Developmental neuropsychological assessment: The systemic approach. *In* Boulton AA, Baker GB, Hiscock M (eds): Neuromethods, Vol 17: Neuropsychology. Clifton, NJ, Humana Press, 1990.

Kolb B, Wishaw IQ: Fundamentals of Human neuropsychology, 5th ed. New York, Worth Publishers, 2003.

Matarazzo JD: Psychological assessment versus psychological testing. Am Psychol 45:999-1017, 1990.

Moore BD: Neurocognitive outcomes in survivors of childhood cancer. J Pediatr Psychol 30:51-63, 2005.

Mulhern RK, Butler RW: Neurocognitive sequelae of childhood cancers and their treatment. Pediatr Rehabil 7:1-14, 2004.

National Institute of Medicine: Crossing the Quality Chasm: A New Health System for the 21st Century. Washington, DC, National Academy Press, 2001.

Nelson CA (ed): The Effects of Early Adversity on Neurobehavioral Development, Vol 31. Mahwah, NJ, Lawrence Erlbaum Associates, 2000.

Palombo J: Learning Disorders and Disorders of the Self in Children and Adolescents. New York, WW Norton, 2001.

Pardes JR: Beyond the diagnosis. *In* Rudel RG, Holmes JM, Pardes JR (ed): Assessment of Developmental Learning Disorders. New York, Basic Books, 1988, pp 205-234.

Posner MI, Rothbart MK: Educating the Human Brain. Washington, DC, American Psychological Association, 2007.

Rey-Casserly C, Bernstein JH: Making the transition to adulthood for individuals with learning disorders. *In* Wolf LE, Schreiber HE, Wasserstein J (ed): Adult Learning Disorders: Contemporary Issues. New York, Psychology Press, 2007, pp 363-388.

Shaheen SJ: Neuromaturation and behavioral development: The case of childhood lead poisoning. Dev Psychol 20:542-550, 1984.

Tversky A, Kahneman D: Judgment under uncertainty: heuristics and biases. Science 183:1124-1131, 1974.

Waber DP, Bernstein JH, Kammerer BL, et al: Neuropsychological diagnostic profiles of children who received CNS treatment for acute lymphoblastic leukemia: The systemic approach to assessment. Dev Neuropsychol 8:1-28, 1992.

Zillmer EA, Spiers MV, Culbertson W: Principles of Neuropsychology. Belmont, CA, Wadsworth, 2007.

84 DIAGNOSTIC METHODS FOR DISORDERS OF THE CENTRAL NERVOUS SYSTEM

David K. Urion

"What we observe is not nature in itself but nature exposed to our method of questioning."
—Werner Heisenberg

Neurology as a clinical discipline is just emerging from its semiotic phase of development: it is still centered to a great extent on the recognition and interpretation of signs. Despite this orientation, certain test procedures have evolved that aid the practitioner in the interpretation of the clinical picture the child presents. This chapter discusses these testing procedures and their appropriate uses. We discuss three main streams of evidence that can be of assistance to the clinician in elucidating pathologic processes in the nervous system: electrophysiologic measures; anatomic imaging; and direct measures of various attributes, such as cells, genes and their markers, and neurotransmitters.

Electrophysiologic measures include techniques such as electroencephalography, evoked potentials, electromyography, and nerve conduction studies and long latency responses.

Anatomic imaging includes techniques such as ultrasonography, computed tomography (CT), and magnetic resonance imaging (MRI).

Direct measures include assessment of various components of the cerebrospinal fluid, measurement of various metabolites in the blood, various genetic assessment techniques (including karyotyping, gene deletion analysis, fluorescent in situ hybridization, and detection of triplet repeats), measurement of various parts of extracerebral and cerebral blood flow, magnetic resonance spectroscopic evaluation of various regions of the brain, positron emission tomographic assessments for regional blood flow and metabolite uptake, and functional imaging techniques of the brain during various activity states.

GENERAL PRINCIPLES

When attempting to order a differential diagnostic process into likely and unlikely possibilities, history and physical examination are the crucial parameters. Although the diagnostic techniques discussed subsequently occasionally provide the answer to a poorly formed diagnostic question by a pathognomonic finding, "fishing expeditions" are to be avoided. It is more useful to generate a set of hypotheses and then investigate those conjectures with a series of diagnostic techniques. The goal is for one hypothesis to emerge as the most parsimonious explanation for the findings.

The examination techniques should be chosen so that some crucial aspect of a hypothesis may be tested. If one considers Tay-Sachs disease the leading possibility, immediate measurement of hexosaminidase A is indicated. If one suspects Duchenne muscular dystrophy, direct measurement for evidence of the genetic marker is indicated. Most situations are less clear.

The first general principle is to use a series of tests, often one from each of the three domains described to confirm or deny the leading hypothesis. The generation of leading hypotheses requires knowledge and discussion of which particular neurologic disorders produce a pattern of dysfunction compatible with the patient's history and presentation. Although that consideration is beyond the scope of this chapter and is discussed elsewhere (see Chapters 76 and 83), a paradigm can be offered to guide the generation of a reasonable differential diagnosis.

Kolodny (unpublished data, 1986) proposed a decision tree for approaching a patient with significant developmental delay and suspected neurologic disease. This paradigm has been modified (Weiner et al, 2003) and is presented in Figures 84-1 and 84-2. It uses points from the history and physical examination that are readily available to the clinician. It has advantages over other paradigms in that it does not require a decision regarding age at onset (Bresnan, 1986), which in our experience at the Children's Hospital in Boston has been a troublesome consideration.

The first decision point concerns the child's overall appearance. Although it is sometimes difficult in a young infant to decide whether certain physical features are dysmorphic or familial, in practice this decision

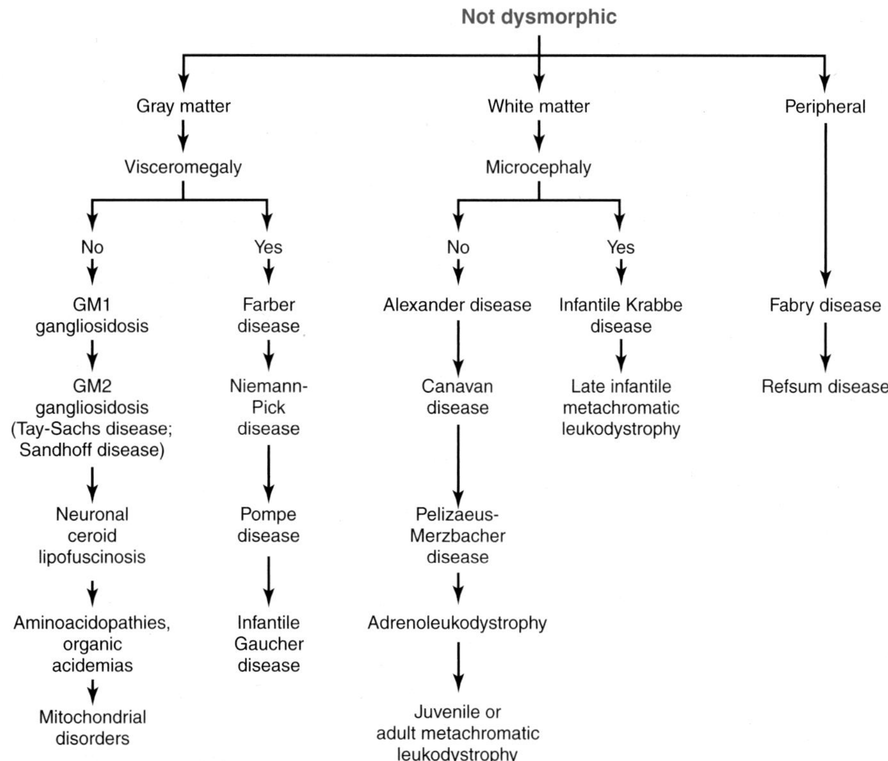

Figure 84-1. Algorithm for differential diagnoses of white matter and gray matter disease.

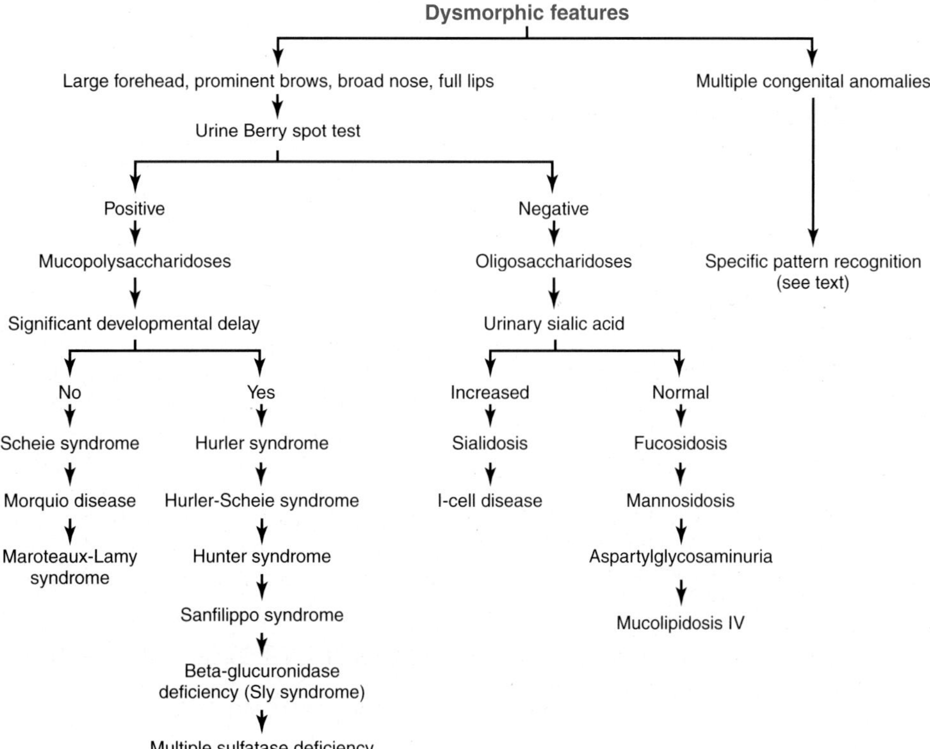

Figure 84-2. Algorithm for differential diagnoses in a child with dysmorphic features, such as Cornelia de Lange syndrome.

can usually be made. In a nondysmorphic child, the next important decision regards the localization of the bulk of clinical signs. In simple practice, the hallmark of gray matter disorders is the presence of seizures and loss of milestones early in the course of the process. In white matter disorders, spasticity is the cardinal early sign, with seizures and loss of milestones usually occurring late in these disorders. A child with peripheral nervous system disease usually presents with ataxia and areflexia. The decision regarding visceromegaly is made on the basis of general physical examination, whereas microcephaly is readily established with a tape measure and head circumference chart.

For a child with dysmorphic features, pattern recognition becomes an important tool. Certain features, collected together, represent recognizable syndromes. Examples of such pictures include Cornelia de Lange syndrome and fetal alcohol syndrome. Discussion of recognized patterns of human malformation is not feasible in this section (see Chapters 24 and 26).

In other instances, notable features include a large forehead, prominent brows, a broad nose, and full lips, previously referred to as a "coarse facies." For such a child, the Berry urine spot test is the first decision point. Children with a positive test result have one of the mucopolysaccharidoses; they can be subdivided further on the basis of their overall developmental history (the presence or absence of significant intellectual disability and developmental retardation). Dysmorphic children with negative Berry urine spot test results have one of the oligosaccharidoses, and can be subdivided further on the basis of urinary sialic acid excretion.

This paradigm may be considered the second general diagnostic principle. By using it and some simple findings from the physical examination and the laboratory tests, one can reduce the differential diagnosis into a manageable number of possibilities. The paradigm should not be viewed as anything other than an introductory schema by which one might approach thorny clinical problems with a certain pattern of priority.

Vignette

A 35-month-old boy is brought to the office for evaluation of irritability and developmental delay. The boy's mother, a 27-year-old primigravida, had had an uncomplicated pregnancy, labor, and delivery. His parents are nonconsanguineous; neither is Jewish, and both are of mixed Western European ancestry. The boy sat at age 6 months, walked at 17 months, never ran, and has recently begun stumbling. His first words emerged shortly after his first birthday, and he spoke in phrases by 2 years of age. Lately, however, his parents note that he has become difficult to understand and drools. Review of his history does not suggest seizures. Examination shows a nondysmorphic boy whose head circumference is at the 10th percentile. Old records suggest it was at the 50th percentile at birth and throughout the first year of life. When the child is suspended under the arms, his legs scissor. Deep tendon reflexes are absent in the legs, although the parents report that the last pediatrician had no difficulty obtaining them at the 2-year visit. Both great toes go up when the soles are stroked.

Using the paradigm from Figures 84-1 and 84-2, one can note in this case the absence of dysmorphic features, the presence of spasticity, and a loss of motor milestones without a history of seizures. These findings strongly suggest a white matter disease. This suggestion is buttressed by the developing dysarthria and apparent late-onset peripheral neuropathy (drooling and poor articulation and absent reflexes). One can note the presence of microcephaly. The differential diagnosis can be narrowed to two probabilities: infantile Krabbe disease and late infantile metachromatic leukodystrophy. Before embarking on enzymatic diagnostic tests, however, one would be well advised to check this differential diagnosis by the application of the first general diagnostic principle.

The suspicion of white matter disease given this picture is quite high, and the consideration of gray matter disease is not warranted. The head circumference data are, however, potentially "soft" because old records for well-child examinations are fraught with inconsistent recordings of head circumference. A series of referential and inferential tests would help confirm or deny the leading clinical possibilities.

White matter disorders usually are associated with an elevation of cerebrospinal fluid (CSF) protein without increased CSF cell count, and CSF examination would be the referential test of choice. The inferential physiologic test of choice would be electromyography and nerve conduction studies because most white matter diseases are accompanied by a peripheral neuropathy. This was suspected on the basis of clinical examination, and confirmation of this suspicion would validate the proposed differential diagnosis. The inferential anatomic test of choice would be MRI. Most white matter disorders show striking abnormalities on MRI because of this technique's great sensitivity to altered water content in tissue. In addition, four of the five nonmicrocephalic white matter disorders (Canavan disease, Alexander disease, Pelizaeus-Merzbacher disease, and adrenoleukodystrophy) have characteristic, if not pathognomonic, appearances on MRI. Use of the test would help to determine the validity of the original path through the diagnostic schema (i.e., toward a differential diagnosis between Krabbe disease and metachromatic leukodystrophy).

For the child in the vignette, use of this approach yielded the following results: increased CSF protein content, delayed nerve conduction velocities, and abnormal signal intensity in a nonspecific pattern on T2-weighted images of brain MRI. These results argue strongly for the process being either infantile Krabbe disease or late infantile metachromatic leukodystrophy. The final step in the diagnostic procedure would be tests for blood levels of galactosylceramidase (altered in Krabbe disease) and arylsulfatase A (altered in metachromatic leukodystrophy).

ELECTROPHYSIOLOGIC METHODS

Electroencephalography

Electroencephalography has a long history in pediatric neurology practice, which is elegantly reviewed by Holmes (1987). It is of great use in the diagnosis of seizure disorders and may be useful in the evaluation of encephalopathic states. The clinician should be aware of the reference laboratory's familiarity and comfort with pediatric patients; electroencephalographic technical production and interpretation are notably operator dependent.

Quantitative electroencephalography, called brain electric activity mapping in some places, is a technique whereby electric signals fast Fourier transform analysis, aided by computer; this creates a spectral density array map of the brain's electrical activity, similar to the weather map seen in the daily newspaper. This technique may be particularly useful in finding deep seizure foci, such as one sees in temporolimbic epilepsy, and subtle background changes associated with encephalopathy. Highly detailed evoked potentials can be done in this fashion; frequency-modulated auditory evoked responses have been useful in differentiating epileptiform aphasic disturbances, such as the Landau-Kleffner syndrome from other autism spectrum disorder syndromes (Stefanatos et al, 1997).

Evoked Potentials

The methods of somatosensory, visual, and auditory evoked potentials are generally applicable to children. Although normative data are still being developed in some age groups, the technique has applicability for auditory function evaluation, testing in certain settings of autism spectrum disorders as noted earlier, and in the assessment of various demyelinating conditions, such as multiple sclerosis.

Single-Photon Emission Computed Tomography and Positron Emission Tomography

Single-photon emission computed tomography (SPECT) and positron emission tomography (PET) are tomographically presented maps of cerebral function with radionuclide-labeled probes that allow measurement of blood flow, oxygen use, glucose metabolism, or specific ligand binding on a regional basis. Although these techniques are currently research tools in most institutions, examples from the adult literature suggest that when certain technical barriers are overcome, they would provide neurochemical data that could illuminate poorly understood disorders, the etiologies of which have been obscure to date (e.g., developmental language disorders, Gilles de la Tourette syndrome, dystonia musculorum deformans). SPECT and PET have been popularized by certain groups for the evaluation of subtypes of attention disorders (Amen, 2005), but many centers have had difficulty replicating this work (Biederman et al, 2006).

Magnetic Resonance Spectroscopy

Magnetic resonance spectroscopy is a technique to assess regional metabolism of the central nervous system, by examining tissue content for elements of energy transformation (adenosine triphosphate, adenosine diphosphate, adenosine monophosphate, and inorganic phosphate). It has proved particularly useful in evaluation of basal ganglia disorders and following the progression of brain tumors. It is increasingly being used for the evaluation of neurodegenerative disorders with known chemical profiles, such as *N*-acetyl aspartate accumulation in Canavan disease.

Functional Magnetic Resonance Imaging

Functional MRI is a technique of great research interest at present, but has yet to be developed sufficiently in pediatric practice to be put to routine clinical diagnostic use. This technique provides the same sort of information as SPECT or PET, that is, changes in regional blood flow that are associated with real-time changes in regional brain function. Functional MRI can provide insights into processes such as reading, naming, and memory. Although a research tool at present, its use in adult neurology suggests that when sufficient developmental normative data have been acquired, it would aid in the diagnosis of various neurocognitive disorders.

ANATOMIC METHODS

Ultrasonography

Cranial ultrasonography is the brain imaging screening technique of choice for fetuses and newborns (Hill and Volpe, 1989; Volpe, 1987). The window provided by the anterior fontanel provides the opportunity for excellent imaging without reconstruction in the sagittal, coronal, and horizontal planes. Periosteal and parameningeal regions are poorly imaged because of the angle with respect to the transducer and the echogenic properties of bone. Cranial ultrasonography images ventricular diameter, major malformations and dysgeneses, and intraparenchymal hemorrhages well, whereas subarachnoid and subdural fluid collections are poorly imaged.

Computed Tomography

CT is the imaging screening technique of choice for children younger than 10 months old (Barnes et al, 1990). It has the capacity to determine structural relationships in the horizontal plane directly and, with some difficulty, in the coronal plane. Sagittal views are produced through reformatting.

Limitations of CT scanning include poor imaging of the white matter compared with MRI and poor delineation of brainstem and cerebellar features. Bone can be simultaneously imaged, in contrast to MRI. Blood and blood-containing structures are well visualized on CT scans, and delineation is improved with intravenous administration of contrast media. The reader is referred to Barnes and colleagues (1990) for an exhaustive review of neuroimaging in pediatric practice.

Magnetic Resonance Imaging

MRI can provide better delineation of white matter, brainstem, and cerebellar structures, and primary imaging of the spinal cord. It can image the central nervous system in sagittal and horizontal presentations directly, providing valuable information regarding suspected midline pathology.

DIRECT MEASUREMENTS

Cerebrospinal Fluid Examination

CSF for examination is usually obtained with a lumbar puncture. Contraindications for lumbar puncture in children are few; posterior fossa mass, acute lead intoxication, Reye syndrome, and brain abscess are viewed as close to absolute contraindications because of the propensity of these situations to produce a "pressure cone" on lumbar puncture and lead to transtentorial or transmagnum herniation.

Measurement of CSF pressure is a useful, and usually neglected, maneuver. The CSF pressure is commonly elevated in meningeal disorders, including meningitis. Routine examination for cell count, protein, glucose, and microorganisms is well reviewed elsewhere (Barringer, 1970; Cole, 1969). Evaluation of CSF content of pyruvate and lactate has proved useful in the diagnosis of mitochondrial disorders (Jordan et al, 1983). Evaluation of the levels of certain neurotransmitters can be helpful in various metabolic disorders.

Biopsies

Tissue samples that provide direct morphologic data regarding the nervous system are an increasingly useful part of the clinician's armamentarium. Skin biopsy is of particular use in the diagnosis of diseases that produce intraneuronal inclusion material, such as neuraxonal dystrophy or neuronal ceroid lipofuscinosis (Carpenter et al, 1972). Skin biopsy specimens contain high concentrations of small nerve elements and sweat gland duct cells, which are useful because of the pathognomonic changes they show in certain conditions. Although light microscopy may provide some information, electron microscopy is more often the modality that provides the greatest insight into structural alterations. Methodologies for optimal technical conditions under which skin is obtained, preserved, and examined are reviewed elsewhere (Carpenter and Karpati, 1981).

Muscle biopsy is the test of choice for the evaluation of some suspected myopathies and mitochondropathies (Dubowitz and Brook, 1973). Structural evaluation with light and electron microscopy may yield pathognomonic features diagnostic of certain myopathic processes, including nemaline rod myopathy, central core disease, and the mitochondrial encephalomyopathies. In other instances, such as the muscular dystrophies, structural abnormalities may be consistent with, but not diagnostic of, the suspected disorder. Molecular diagnostic techniques evaluating cellular DNA are now generally considered more useful (Kunkel, 1986). The reader is referred to Jones and colleagues (2003) for a complete discussion of muscle biopsy. Finally, biochemical evaluation of muscle tissue for electron transport chain abnormalities is available in certain centers.

Nerve biopsy, separate from the examination of small nerve elements in skin biopsy, is useful in suspected peripheral neuropathies in childhood. The sural nerve, a pure sensory nerve accessed on the dorsal aspect of the foot, is usually the nerve of choice for biopsy. Structural analysis, including light and electron microscopy, is the usual diagnostic method. Teased fiber analysis, first used in the evaluation of adult peripheral neuropathies, is now coming into use in pediatric neurology (Gibbels et al, 1985).

Conjunctival biopsy is used for essentially the same indications as skin biopsy. For the clinician, the choice between skin and conjunctival biopsy is based on the expertise of the local reference laboratory. That is, one should obtain the sort of biopsy specimen one's pathologist likes to examine.

Quantitative Assays

Quantitative assays for the levels of specific enzymes, amino acids, organic acids, and urea cycle intermediary metabolites are of clear use in the diagnosis of specific metabolic disorders. Tissues sampled include plasma, serum, white blood cells harvested from blood, and urine. The most efficient use of these diagnostic modalities is to select a few assays for determination, rather than an "enzyme panel."

SUMMARY

This chapter reviews the methods available for investigating the central nervous system function in a child, with particular attention to disorders of development. The advantages and disadvantages of inferential and referential measures are considered and the methods reviewed.

REFERENCES

Amen, DG: Making a Great Brain Better. New York, Three Rivers Press, 2005.

Barnes PB, Urion DK, Share K: Clinical principles of pediatric neuroradiology and MR imaging. *In* Wolper R, Barnes PB, Strand RD (eds): MR in Pediatric Neuroradiology. St Louis, Mosby, 1990, pp 175-182.

Barringer R: A simplified procedure for spinal fluid cytology. Arch Neurol 22:305, 1970.

Biederman J, Monuteaux MC, Mick E, et al: Young adult outcome of attention deficit hyperactivity disorder: A controlled ten year follow-up. Psychol Med 36:167-169, 2006.

Bresnan MJ: Degenerative disorders. *In* Weiner H, Levitt L, Bresnan MJ (eds): Pediatric Neurology for the House Officer, 2nd ed. Baltimore, Williams & Wilkins, 1986.

Carpenter R, Karpati G: Sweat gland duct cells in Lafora body disease: Diagnosis by skin biopsy. Neurology 31:1564, 1981.

Carpenter R, Karpati G, Andermann F: Specific involvement of muscle, nerve, and skin in late infantile and juvenile amaurotic idiocy. Neurology 22:170, 1972.

Cole M: Examination of the CSF. *In* Toole J (ed): Special Techniques for Neurologic Diagnosis. Philadelphia, FA Davis, 1969.

Dubowitz V, Brook MH: Muscle Biopsy: A Modern Approach. Philadelphia, WB Saunders, 1973.

Gibbels E, Schaefer HE, Runne U, et al: Severe polyneuropathy in Tangier disease mimicking syringomyelia or leprosy: Clinical, biochemical, electrophysiological, and morphological evaluation. J Neurol 232:283, 1985.

Hill A, Volpe JJ: Fetal Neurology. New York, Raven Press, 1989.

Holmes OH: Diagnosis and Management of Seizures in Children. Philadelphia, WB Saunders, 1987.

Jones HR, DeVivo D, Darras BT: Neuromuscular Disorders of Infancy, Childhood, and Adolescence: A Clinician's Approach. Oxford, UK, Butterworth/Heinman, 2003.

Jordan GW, Statland B, Halsted C: CSF lactate in diseases of the CNS. Arch Intern Med 143:85, 1983.

Kunkel LM: Analysis of deletions in DNA in patients with Becker and Duchenne muscular dystrophy. Nature 322:73, 1986.

Stefanatos GA, Foley C, Grover W, Doherty B: Steady state auditory evoked responses to pulsed frequency modulations in children. Electronecephalopgr Clin Neurophysiol 104:31-42, 1997.

Volpe JJ: Neurology of the Newborn, 2nd ed. Philadelphia, WB Saunders, 1987.

Weiner H, Levitt L, Urion DK: Pediatric Neurology for the House Officer, 4th ed. Baltimore, Williams & Wilkins, 2003.

85 COMPREHENSIVE FORMULATION OF ASSESSMENT

William B. Carey

As the process of assessment nears completion, the clinician arranges and weighs evidence from various sources to compile a diagnostic formulation, one that evolves into a therapeutic plan. The preceding chapters have explored a wide range of biologic and psychosocial factors influencing the development and behavior of children. There has been extensive review of the many possible symptomatic manifestations of these factors, along with consideration of assessment techniques by which they may be evaluated. Only a comprehensive formulation that integrates pertinent information from these multiple sources can effectively coordinate the clinician's understanding and plan of management, while facilitating discussions about the child with family members and allowing for effective communication with colleagues and referral resources (Jellinek and McDermott, 2004). One approach to such a formulation is delineated here (see also Chapter 78).

DEFICIENCIES COMMONLY ENCOUNTERED IN PRESENT DIAGNOSTIC PRACTICE

Diagnostic reasoning commonly employed in clinical practice today may be susceptible to problems of oversimplification of various sorts and to a tendency to view the child too narrowly. Perhaps the most common weakness in current diagnostic practice is the use of the child's worst or most salient problem as the main or only diagnosis. To refer to a child as *CP, asthmatic, ADD*, or *drug abuser* may identify the most troublesome focus of parental and professional concern and even may be a useful form of mental shorthand for the clinician. Such labels fail to consider, however, the important array of relevant strengths and weaknesses of the child and his or her milieu. Because all children with a specific condition, such as asthma, are not the same, a false sense of homogeneity may be conveyed through inappropriate use of labels. Certain particularly meaningless and perhaps misleading labels are often used as summary statements about children. *Hyperactivity* is a prime example of this practice; the term is poorly defined and means different things to different people (Carey and McDevitt, 1995). *Emotionally disturbed* is another diagnosis that is too vague to convey a specific meaning and is potentially harmful to parents and children.

Another diagnostic distortion occurs when examiners put their own main interest or area of expertise first and give little or no attention to other aspects of the child. To the allergist, the child's hypersensitivities may be taken as his or her most pressing or only problem. To the family therapist, family dynamics are of paramount and sometimes exclusive significance. Although various aspects of the child and his or her situation may contribute to a comprehensive diagnostic formulation, no single facet should be mistaken as constituting an adequate account of the total child.

The problem-oriented approach has its supporters, who maintain that documenting specific clinical concerns ensures that they will be remembered and dealt with adequately. One cannot quarrel with that goal. The message of this chapter is that unless all pertinent strengths and weaknesses of the child and his or her situation are assembled into a single formulation, there is a real danger that some complication or critical, redeeming aspects of a child will be overlooked.

The inadequacies for pediatric practice of the currently available psychiatric diagnostic schemes are explored in Chapter 78. Even the pediatric modification of the DSM scheme, the *Diagnostic and Statistical Manual for Primary Care: Child and Adolescent Version (DSM-PC)* (American Academy of Pediatrics, 1996) presents only lists of "environmental situations" and "child manifestations," and does not offer any system for constructing a comprehensive formulation comparable to the one proposed in this chapter.

ELEMENTS OF A COMPREHENSIVE FORMULATION OF THE ASSESSMENT

Having strongly urged a comprehensive formulation, one must acknowledge that it is difficult, and perhaps impossible, to offer a single method on which all potential users can agree. One such diagnostic profile, favored by the author, is presented here (Table 85-1). Some might say that there is too much emphasis on temperament or not enough on various aspects of cognition. In any case, Table 85-1 shows that all the significant elements can be assembled on one page in a form that is comprehensive, dimensional, and interactional.

Table 85-1. Comprehensive Formulation of Assessment

Caregiver's main concern—type, duration, frequency, severity, antecedents, consequences, response of caregivers
Other caregiver concerns
Caregiver's goals and expectations

Significant Areas	Strengths, Assets	Satisfactory	Problems—Deficiencies, Deviations
Adjustment—Behavior, Emotional, Functional			
Behavioral competence in relationships—parents, sibs, peers, other adults	Skills, caring, cooperation, involvement, autonomy, amiable	Average	Aggression, opposition, withdrawal, unpopular
Achievements—task performance in school, home, community	High achievement, effort, motivation, satisfaction	Average	Poor achievement or failure
Self-relations—esteem, care, control of feelings and actions	Good self-esteem, care, control	Average or mixture	Poor esteem; self-neglect, abuse; overcontrol; under-impulsive
Internal status—feelings, thinking	Contentment; thought clarity	Average	Anxiety, depression, thought disturbance
Coping—identification and solution of problems	Effective coping	Average	Poor problem solving
Symptoms of body function—eating, sleeping, elimination, gender, sex, pain, tics	Comfortable function	Normal concerns	Moderate-severe symptoms—eating, sleep, elimination, gender, sex, pain, tics
Child Factors			
Physical—nutrition, growth, maturity, illness	Excellent health	Average	Significant health or nutrition problem
Neurologic—sensory, motor, reflex, coordination	Intact; good coordination, physical skills	Average	Central nervous system problems, especially sensory and motor
Development—motor, language, personal-social	Better than average	Average	Significant delay or deficiency
General cognitive skills (e.g., memory)	Good skills; above usual range	Normal	Deficit, disability
Specific cognitive skills—reading, spelling, writing, math	High level of skills	Average	Deficit, disability
Temperament			
Social style—approach, adaptability, mood	Flexible, pleasant	Average range	Rigid, irritable, "spirited"
Work style—persistence, distractibility, activity	High performance style; task oriented	Average range	Low performance style
Situational reaction style—intensity, threshold	Appropriate level of reactions	Average range	Explosive; overreactive or underreactive
Organizational style—regular, predictable, organized	Predictable, organized	Average range	Irregular, disorganized
Pervasive, extreme inattention or activity	Not present	Not present	"Hyperkinetic"
Environmental Factors			
Caregivers' contributions—structure-general capacity, commitment, availability, involvement	Good support	Adequate	Inadequate capacity, commitment, involvement; conflict
Sociocultural influences—relatives, neighbors, school, media, affluence/poverty	Supportive, not conflicting	Mixed	Major stressors (e.g., death, divorce, violence, conflict)
Physical—neighborhood, hazards, toxins	Good; healthy	Tolerable	Inadequate or hazardous
Interactions			
Goodness of fit—caregiver and child	Excellent; good	Adequate	Troublesome or poor
Contributions of caregiver to child—content			
Physical care (protection, food, housing, medical care)	Nourishing physical care	Adequate	Poor physical care
Stimulation—developmental, cognitive	Optimal quantity, quality	Adequate	Overstimulation or understimulation, neglect
Affection—acceptance, intimacy, warmth	Good timing, quality, amount	Adequate	Overaffection or underaffection, hostile, abuse
Guidance—approval, discipline	Attentive guidance	Acceptable	Overguidance, underguidance, or inappropriate guidance
Socialization—teaching social relations	Healthy familial and extrafamilial socialization	Average	Aberrant socialization
Effects of child on caregiver	Predominantly positive	Average, mixed	Predominantly stressful, challenging

Comments:

Summary and Diagnosis:

Plans—Service Needs:

For purposes of this diagnostic formulation, a four-part presentation is reasonable, as follows:
1. The child's developmental-behavioral adjustment
2. The various contributing child factors, including physical and neurologic health, developmental and cognitive skills, and temperament
3. The environmental factors, including family, sociocultural, and physical settings
4. The pattern of interactions among these factors that may participate in the child's adjustment.

Comments, summary, diagnosis, and plans complete the report.

Adjustment—Behavioral, Emotional, and Functional

The assessment of behavioral performance or adjustment, as described in several chapters (see especially Chapter 7), deals with the following BASICS elements:

1. Behavioral competence: the child's relations with others—the degree of social competence or undersocialization.
2. Achievements: performance of tasks, especially schoolwork, and play—the extent of task mastery or underachievement. Actual performance of tasks should be rated here and differentiated from the capacity to perform them, which is an aspect of development.
3. Self-relations: whether self-assured or troubled with problems in self-relations, such as self-neglect, poor self-esteem, and inadequate or excessive self-regulation.
4. Internal status: thoughts, feelings—a sense of well-being versus disturbed feelings (anxiety, depression) or disturbed thinking (phobias, obsessions).
5. Coping: an appraisal of the child's adaptive or coping style and abilities—effective or ineffective.
6. Symptoms of physiologic function or dysfunctions in sleep, elimination, eating, gender and sex, pains, and tics.

Motivation is an important dimension of personality, but because it is estimated only with great difficulty by the primary care clinician, it is not included as an element of this comprehensive profile. It may be possible to estimate it from other components of behavioral adjustment.

Child Factors

Physical Health

An appraisal of physical health describes the child's organic and functional condition and includes organic illness and malfunction or handicaps of various organ systems (e.g., the skin, respiratory system, and cardiovascular system), and nutritional status; growth and physical maturation; and problems such as malnourishment, obesity, disturbances of growth or bodily development, and evidence of substance abuse. Many of these conditions and their impacts are discussed in earlier chapters.

The neurologic status subsumes sensory and motor function, reflexes, and coordination. Problems in this area include sensory loss, including vision and hearing, "cerebral palsy," convulsive disorders, "soft signs" (minor neurologic indicators), or motor incoordination. These findings and the biologic influences affecting them are considered extensively in Part III of this book.

Developmental Function

The section of the diagnostic formulation on capacities includes the various elements of development and their current level and degree of appropriateness for age and the state of cognitive functions. Included are a child's gross motor function, fine motor skills, language proficiency, memory, spatial orientation, temporal-sequential organization, higher order conceptual abilities, and various aspects of social perception and skills. The child's level of academic performance skills and age-appropriate task performance capacities also are documented. The current status of the child's attention and organizational ability should be taken into account. These latter characteristics are hard to classify; they also are found in this comprehensive formulation under temperament. This section of the formulation is where one includes neurodevelopmental variations and specific skills and problems in learning, such as reading, spelling, writing, and math.

The diagnostician should undertake a careful search for developmental strengths, special talents, and content affinities. These highly individualized abilities that can serve as a crucial support system for self-esteem and motivation. In particular, the clinician needs to uncover strengths that are not being encouraged, a child's assets that are being neglected by parents and the school. Such abilities need ongoing nurturance. Assessment of these various capacities is discussed elsewhere, particularly in the other chapters of this section.

Instead of seeking to characterize a child's overall cognitive ability with a numeral (such as an intelligence quotient [IQ] score), it is far more beneficial to focus on a child's individual profile of strengths and weaknesses. There is growing recognition that many forms of intelligence exist (Gardner, 1983). An astute clinician should uncover and describe a child's unique areas of intellectual competence.

Temperament

The child's temperament or behavioral style should be considered and evaluated independently of his or her behavioral performance or adjustment. The various dimensions of temperament and the clinical clusters derived from them have been described fully in Chapter 7, and indications and techniques for their assessment are discussed in Chapter 78.

The previous discussion of temperament urges the avoidance of the use of the cluster labels of difficult, easy, and slow-to-warm up because they may encourage stereotypic thinking in the clinician and may be derogatory. Some other groups of traits may prove to be useful, however, if thought of as risk or protective factors, rather than categorical problems. The child's social style may consist of approach, adaptability, and mood. The work style would be affected by persistence/attention span, distractibility, and activity. Two others are situational reaction style with intensity and threshold, and organizational style, consisting of regularity or predictability and degree of organization.

As already noted, a quandary arises in regard to the placement of attention, considered to be an aspect of cognitive function and of temperament. There may be similarities or differences in the various components of attention required for specific learning tasks and those involved in a child's overall interaction with his or her social environment. For the present, the characteristic can tentatively appear under both headings, attention being more of an aspect of cognition, whereas persistence at tasks is more a part of temperament or behavioral style.

Environmental Factors

The concern is with the environmental factors that may be affecting the child. They are covered in Part II of this book.

Parents

Parental (or caregiver) care consists of parental attitudes, including expectations (how realistic and how supportive they are), parental feelings (the amount of attachment or detachment and of affection or anger and rejection), and the actual management of the child (the amount and quality of physical care, stimulation, affection, guidance, and socialization given to the child). Mrazek and colleagues (1995) suggested a parenting risk scale, which is an overall judgment of parenting divided into three levels of function: (1) adequate parenting, by which is meant either average or exceptional parenting; (2) concerns about parenting, which describes the situation with some degree of problems, such as intense marital conflict or parental emotional problems, but not serious enough for immediate intervention beyond close follow-up; and (3) parenting difficulties, which includes serious problems, such as punitive parenting and neglect.

The key dimensions of parenting used by Mrazek and colleagues (1995) in arriving at the general judgment of its adequacy are (1) emotional availability, or degree of warmth; (2) control, or degree of flexibility and permission; (3) parental psychosocial status, or the freedom from (or presence of) overt disorder in the parents; (4) knowledge base, or the parents' understanding of emotional and physical development and basic childcare principles; and (5) commitment, or an adequate prioritization of childcare responsibilities. These dimensions can be thought of in regard to their structure or presentation or their content or quality.

Sociocultural Milieu

The sociocultural situation describes the impact of brothers and sisters, other family members, peer group, neighborhood influences, television, school, and health care practices: Which are helpful and which are not? It is important to take into consideration the cultural background of a child and his or her family. A clinician should describe and respect behaviors, values, and attitudes that are a product of an individual's national or ethnic background. Bilingual children, including children born in other countries, should be thought about in terms of their adjustment to any divergent cultural demands and their success in forging an identity that bridges the two cultures.

Assessments of the general sociocultural situation should include a review of various extrafamilial factors, such as quality of the community, adequacy of educational services, parental employment status, housing, economic conditions, quality of health care, interactions with the legal system, and other issues. The available psychiatric diagnostic schemes (DSM-IV-TR, ICD-10, DC:O-3R) and the DSM-PC all have presented lists of environmental situations to consider in diagnosis, but all suggest ratings only of problems, without offering the clinician opportunities to make note of the acceptable or positive features in the child's environment.

Nonhuman Environment

An appraisal of the nonhuman environment rates the degree of value or hazard in housing, pets, environmental substances, disease exposure, climatic conditions, and natural disasters.

Interactions

We should estimate the goodness or poorness of the fit between the child with his or her temperament and other characteristics and the values and preferences of the caregivers. How well do the parents or teachers understand the child, tolerate what is not changeable such as temperament, and manage in ways that minimize the stressful interaction between them and promote harmony?

The essential components of parental contributions to the child are described in Chapter 10 and include physical care, stimulation, affection, guidance, and socialization. The impact of the child on his or her surroundings is a highly important part of the interaction that is frequently either ignored or not explicitly included in diagnostic formulations. One rates here the degree of pleasure or displeasure and satisfaction or dissatisfaction experienced by parents, teachers, and others who regularly encounter the child. A statement should be included about the aspects of the child that are most bothersome and that have led to clinical attention.

SUMMARY OF FINDINGS

At the end of the comprehensive diagnostic formulation, it is appropriate to summarize the various details in a single statement or two. An example follows:

This 8-month-old male infant is physically, neurologically, and developmentally normal and has a relatively easy temperament, but he has become very demanding of his mother's attention. He cries repeatedly and for prolonged periods, and his mother feels obliged to pick him up and comfort him whenever he cries. The mother has become angry about the infant's demands and thinks that there is something wrong with him. The reason seems to be that the authoritarian grandmother persuaded the mother that the infant should not be allowed to cry because of his umbilical hernia. The result was more crying and greater maternal distress.

Sometimes clinical syndromes emerge from certain combinations of findings. The so-called vulnerable child syndrome (see Chapter 34) characterizes the child who is physically and developmentally normal, but has a particular pattern of behavioral maladjustment related to the continuation of inappropriate parental concern and handling following full recovery from a worrisome early illness. The summary is the section in which such syndromes could be mentioned.

PLANS FOR SERVICE NEEDS

The clinician should select from the list of findings in the comprehensive diagnostic formulation the areas calling for action. Not all of the suspected or definite problems need be dealt with. If parents are coping well with a child with a difficult temperament, intervention is not indicated, as it would be if there were significant parental-child conflict because of the problem. Similarly, a pediatrician generally should not attempt to influence the course of a parental divorce, but should help the family understand and cope with its impact on the child. The service needs for the demanding infant in the previous example would include sufficient examination to reassure the clinician and the family that there is no physical problem with the child other than the umbilical hernia, suggestions to the mother about revision of her handling of the infant, and help for the mother in evaluating more critically the advice received from her own mother.

Having defined appropriate service needs, the clinician can proceed to implement them, which is the process of management described in Part X of this book. Plans for follow-up complete the formulation. Although the DSM-PC includes a section on estimation of the severity of the clinical problem, it does not suggest a way to formulate, prioritize, and execute the needs for clinical services (see Chapter 78).

ADVANTAGES OF A COMPREHENSIVE FORMULATION

The advantages in the use of the comprehensive diagnostic formulation can be found in practice, research, and education. In practice one gains the assurance in making a complex diagnosis that a broad range of pertinent factors is considered so that relevant issues are unlikely to be omitted. This inclusive view of the child enhances the clinician's diagnostic reasoning, his or her discussions with the patient and family members, and his or her communications with other professionals. One can reasonably argue that such a comprehensive evaluation is unnecessary in the immediate management of acute minor illnesses, such as otitis media or gastroenteritis. If professional contacts extend into well-child care or involvement with chronic physical problems, a broader evaluation becomes very helpful. With concerns in the area of development and behavior, this is a necessity, not a luxury. Plans for management of problems in the latter areas stand a far better chance of meeting the child's needs if they are based on a truly complete empiric assessment, rather than on incomplete data or stereotypic diagnostic labels.

In carrying out research, the use of this model of formulation encourages more precise definition of subjects, allowing studies to become more interpretable and more significant. As already mentioned, investigations referring to patients simply as *hyperactive* or *attention-deficit/hyperactivity disorder (ADHD)* without any further clarification of their overall function are of little value. In whose view is the child excessively active or inattentive, and how was that determined? What else is going on? Would not the study outcomes be affected by how a child stands in each of the components of the comprehensive formulation—physical and neurologic status, development and cognitive skills, temperament and behavioral adjustment, environmental factors, and interactions? There are serious dangers in attempting to study a child or a cohort identified by only a single symptom.

In medical education, the use of this approach to assessment would encourage teachers and students to think of children in terms of their true complexity and avoid overly facile diagnoses based on inadequate information or narrow observer bias.

PROBLEMS IN FORMULATION

Although primary care clinicians need to reason comprehensively, this admirable goal is not easily achieved. The various professional individuals dealing with the child's development and behavior may not agree that any one particular profile of the child's status is an acceptable one. Various settings and points of view may argue for modifications of contents and subdivisions. Advocates of neurology and psychiatry may plead for an expansion of their spheres of interest. One should not object to this as long as the other elements of the formulation are retained and considered in the final diagnosis and service plan.

Another problem is the lack of standardized criteria for diagnostic ratings in some areas, particularly behavioral adjustment. One can agree that this topic deals primarily with the child's relationship to others, to tasks, and to himself or herself, but the dividing line between normal and abnormal is broad and variable.

How is the clinician to arrive at a comprehensive diagnostic formulation if there is a major area of missing data, as with a pediatrician evaluating a problem of school adjustment without specific data about information processing skills? The pediatrician must refrain from proposing a final diagnosis until such assessments are available. The same information may be largely superfluous in other situations, as in the case of helping the child and surviving parent deal with the death of the other parent. All the areas of the formulation should be borne in mind, but clinical data in each are sought only to the extent appropriate for competent management of the child. Finally, a major problem in the use of this sort of diagnostic profile is its implementation—that is, in persuading oneself and others to give up old habits of abbreviated and distorted conceptualizations and to think comprehensively.

SUMMARY

Before proceeding from the diagnostic phase to management of problems or issues, the clinician has to bring together a wide range of information besides the overall adjustment status: environmental and biologic, developmental and behavioral, strengths and liabilities, major and minor, historical and observed. This chapter suggests a way to include all of these elements in an organized presentation that enhances understanding of the child and the situation by avoiding oversimplified labels, and that leads to optimal management.

ACKNOWLEDGMENTS

The author acknowledges the contributions of Melvin D. Levine, M.D., to the version of this chapter in the third edition of *Developmental-Behavioral Pediatrics*.

REFERENCES

American Academy of Pediatrics: The classification of child and adolescent mental diagnoses in primary care. *In*: Diagnostic and Statistical Manual for Primary Care (DSM-PC): Child and Adolescent Version. Elk Grove Village, IL, American Academy of Pediatrics, 1996.

Carey WB, McDevitt SC: Coping with Children's Temperament: A Guide for Professionals. New York, Basic Books, 1995.

Gardner G: Frames of Mind. New York, Basic Books, 1983.

Jellinek MS, McDermott JF: Formulation: Putting the diagnosis into a therapeutic context and treatment plan. J Am Acad Child Adolesc Psychiatry 43:7, 2004.

Mrazek DA, Mrazek F, Klinnert M: Clinical assessment of parenting. J Am Acad Child Adolesc Psychiatry 34:272, 1995.

Part X **MANAGEMENT AND TREATMENT**

86 PEDIATRIC COUNSELING

BARTON D. SCHMITT

Vignette

Samantha was born at 36 weeks gestation, weighing 4 pounds 4 ounces. The obstetrician attributed her small size to pregnancy-associated hypertension. After birth, Samantha took readily to breastfeeding. At her 4-month-old well-child visit, she was at the 25th percentile for weight and 50th percentile for length and head circumference. But her parents did not rejoice at this news. On probing, the pediatrician discovered that the parents had strong disagreements about whether Samantha should continue sleeping in their bedroom. There were other conflicts about child rearing as well. When the pediatrician seemed truly interested, the parents agreed they needed help with these issues.

Counseling is the clinician's most consistently effective management technique for developmental-behavioral issues. Pediatricians can help families to improve or resolve most of the behavioral problems they encounter by a combination of a basic knowledge of the field and skillful interviewing followed by individualized counseling. This chapter provides a comprehensive review of the essential components of this process and how to acquire them. As this competence increases, the practitioner is likely to deal more appropriately with parental concerns and to avoid excessive use of medication and referrals.

Behavior problems are common in childhood. Periodically, all children have behavioral symptoms. Ten percent to 15% of children develop behavioral problems that interfere with life adjustment. Physicians caring for children are called on to provide counseling about behavior and development many times each day.

Table 86-1 provides a definition of pediatric counseling. The fact that the pediatrician works with basically healthy families has a significant impact on the nature of counseling. In many cases, the pediatrician's role consists of delineating and clarifying problem behavior patterns and trying to change them through active advice. Frequently, this counseling requires only one or two visits, and usually such efforts are successful and highly efficient. The primary care physician has an advantage over many other counselors in knowing how the family operates and having their trust because of his or her previously established efficacy with physical illnesses. Families who do not respond to pediatric counseling can be referred for mental health services at a later time. A sensitive pediatrician often can detect more seriously disturbed families and refer them after the first visit.

This chapter reviews several types of pediatric counseling that fall within the primary care domain. The behavior problems selected as examples are common ones, and the counseling methods discussed can be integrated into the practicing pediatrician's office time frame. Levels of intervention are covered in approximate order of increasing complexity and time requirements. Generally, the pediatrician acts at the lowest level of intervention that is effective for the issue with which he or she is dealing. Pediatricians are in a unique position to be eclectic. Most problems require a combination of treatment approaches (e.g., education, reassurance, advice, and advocacy). Although every pediatrician provides some counseling, individual interest and training vary greatly. Each physician should participate in this aspect of health care only to the degree to which he or she feels comfortable.

When a meaningful alliance has been established, specific techniques of counseling can be employed. Most pediatricians tend not to adopt any stereotyped approach. The nature of the problems, the family's coping style, and the likelihood of a child's or parent's benefiting from various approaches are among the factors that need to be taken into consideration. General modalities of counseling are discussed in the following sections and are summarized in Table 86-2.

RELEASING PAINFUL FEELINGS

Some parents and patients are in acute emotional distress when they visit their physician. They are preoccupied with painful issues. Until these painful feelings find an outlet, the parent is likely to be unable to relate an accurate medical history or interpret medical advice. Also, any counseling that requires thinking (e.g., behavior modification) may be less successful until compelling emotional issues are dealt with.

The process of releasing painful feelings is usually called *ventilation,* a term that has numerous implications. An angry parent may need to ventilate about having to deal with their child's encopresis. A frightened patient may need to express fears (e.g., a hyperventilation attack). A mourning patient may need to grieve about a loss (e.g., sudden death of a parent). A patient who has been attacked (e.g., a rape victim) may need to pour out feelings about what has happened.

Table 86-1. Pediatric Counselor's Orientation (Relative to That of a Psychotherapist)

Works mainly with stable children and parents
Focuses more on the present
Focuses more on behavior than on thoughts or feelings
Focuses more on minor variations in behavior and development
Requires less extensive evaluations
Leads the interview more (provides less total listening time)
Uses more action-oriented, direct, specific approaches
Uses more empiric approaches (if an approach works, one does not need to know the theory behind it)
Uses more behavior modification
Relies more on education, reassurance, specific advice, and environmental intervention
Provides briefer follow-up visits (20-30 min)
Provides fewer visits (2-3 for most problems; 6 maximum)
Sets a shorter time frame for results or referral (usually 3 mo)

Table 86-2. Types of Pediatric Counseling

Releasing painful feelings	Dealing with all-consuming emotional issues first
Education	Supplying needed general information
Reassurance	Specific information that counteracts fears
Clarifying the problem and its cause	Providing parents with a clearer perspective about the child's problems
Approval of the parents' approach	Helping parents to use their own resources
Specific advice	Suggestions about altered parental handling of specific problems
Environmental intervention	Suggestions about other changes in the child's environment
Extended counseling	More visits for more complicated issues

For the process of ventilation to occur, the setting must be relaxed and private. The patient or parent is encouraged to talk. Usually ventilation begins spontaneously. If not, the process can be initiated by openers such as, "You look angry (worried or sad). Why don't you tell me what's troubling you?" The repetition of emotionally laden words that the parent has used helps to continue the process (e.g., "You felt put down"). The essential response to ventilation is noncritical listening. Any censure removes the invitation to talk freely. Even if the parent's feelings seem excessive, the physician must express agreement that the situation is "unfortunate." The parent or child does not want to hear that "It could be worse" or "Be grateful that (such and such) didn't happen." The success of ventilation depends on the patient's perception that he or she has expressed personal anguish to someone who really understands. As a distressed parent or child expresses deep feelings, there may be a recovery of composure and emotional equilibrium.

PROVIDING EDUCATION

Education involves the presentation of facts or medical opinions to a parent or child. Education is undertaken mainly to impart information, but it also plays a critical role in reducing anxiety, dispelling misconception, and fostering feelings of effectiveness on the part of a parent or child.

Requested Education

Education may be particularly effective when it has been asked for. In these instances, the timing of the education is optimal. Adolescents commonly have questions about acne, sexually transmitted diseases, the prevention of pregnancy, tattoos, and smoking. These topics deserve thoughtful answers. A family may ask a physician about the pros and cons of getting a dog. The physician can remind the parents that most children younger than 3 years of age cannot be taught to treat a dog appropriately and risk being bitten. If parents wish to have a dog during this developmental period, they can be advised not to leave their child alone with the dog at any time. The difficult situation of having to give parents bad news about the health of their child is discussed in various chapters about specific situations, such as the birth of a child with Down syndrome (see Chapter 25).

Anticipatory Guidance

Anticipatory guidance (or preventive counseling) is the advice pediatricians provide to avoid problems that could occur in the future. Topics such as nutrition, injury prevention, behavior management, developmental stimulation, sex education, and general health education all may be covered during every visit. Most expectant parents have many questions that can be discussed with their pediatrician several weeks before delivery. The most frequent concerns include arguments for and against breastfeeding and circumcision, hospital policies about rooming-in and the father's presence in the delivery room, ways of decreasing sibling rivalry, and essential infant equipment.

Printed or Audiovisual Approaches

Comprehensive education of the parents can be time-consuming for the physician. More efficient methods are available. Printed materials include information sheets written by the physician, health pamphlets, or books. Not only do information sheets save the physician's time, but they also give the father (or other family members who were not present during the office visit) the opportunity to read what the physician recommends. These handouts can provide more information than most physicians have the time to give, and they help to prevent recall problems for the mother. Some offices also have CDs or DVDs that are available in the waiting room to impart information. These aids may cover specific age groups (e.g., newborn care) or chronic diseases (e.g., asthma). These educational aids can supplement individualized discussion with the family.

PROVIDING REASSURANCE

Reassurance can be defined as a special kind of education that counteracts fears. Reassurance relieves or removes unnecessary anxiety, especially regarding one's physical or emotional health. Reassurance is the physician's most commonly used type of counseling. Reassurance is very therapeutic. Parents need some reassurance during almost every office visit or phone call. Reassurance is more likely to be effective if certain guidelines are followed (see also Chapter 32 in regard to the management of minor illnesses).

Precede by Data Collection

To be effective, reassurance must be properly timed. It should never be too hasty or offered too early. In patients with emotional concerns, a careful history should be elicited. Reassurance based on meager data is likely to be unconvincing to the parent. Only after the parent or child believes that the physician has explored the problem adequately and understands it will the reassurance be acceptable (see Chapter 75 on interviewing).

Be Specific

The most effective reassurance is specific and focused. The targeted concern or worry is identified by listening carefully. A parent may be afraid primarily of a brain tumor in a child with recurrent headaches, appendicitis in a child with recurrent abdominal pains, or a heart attack in a child with chest pains. When the precise overriding fear is identified, the physician can carefully investigate that specific concern and offer reassurance when the fear is unfounded. Blanket reassurance (e.g., "There's nothing to worry about," "Everything will be just fine," or other extravagant promises) leads the parent to suspect the physician of being insensitive or even dishonest, and dilutes the value of any specific advice.

Be Honest

What the physician tells the parents must be honest. If the physician is caught in one lie, the balance of his or her reassurance is thrown into question. The physician need not reveal everything he or she is thinking. Any nonessential data that would be anxiety producing can be withheld (e.g., the differential diagnosis).

Be Brief

Reassurance should be offered in as few words as possible. When reassurance is tenuous, the physician may be tempted to prolong the discussion of the aspects of the case that are reassuring. Most parents sense that the physician is hiding his or her real feelings and worries behind a long speech.

Universalize the Problem

Physicians can offer great comfort to parents and children by commenting on the universality of their problems (when appropriate). Statements such as, "Do you know any 3-year olds who don't have tantrums?" or "That argument goes on in every home where there's a 16-year-old" can alleviate much anxiety.

Provide Nonverbal Reassurance

Nonverbal messages often communicate more to the parent than the physician's words. The physician can show concern for the patient without expressing alarm. A physician can examine a patient's heart without wearing a worried facial expression. If a parent relates a history of symptoms that have frightened him or her to a physician who remains calm, he or she often concludes, "If this doesn't upset my doctor, I guess everything is going to be all right." Most parents and children believe body language more than words or logic.

Examples of Reassurance

Parents of infants need reassurance that their child's red face and grunting with bowel movements do not mean that the child is constipated. Head rolling and body rocking in infants do not represent an emotional problem, but are self-soothing methods for making a transition into sleep. Thumb sucking in young children is comforting, but does not mean that insecurity is present. This example also is a reminder that reassurance is age dependent, and that after age 5 or 6, thumb sucking should be discouraged because it can cause malocclusion of the permanent teeth. Although the parents of young infants should be reassured about postural abnormalities of the legs and feet (e.g., toeing-in or bowlegs), the physician must be careful not to raise false hopes about the rapidity of the self-correction. The parents can be reassured that the correction will be complete, but that it will not begin until the child starts to walk and then will take approximately 12 months or longer of walking before the child's legs and feet will begin to look straight.

School-age children who are reacting to a divorce need reassurance that visitation with both parents will continue, that their parents still love them, and that their school and friends will not change. Children with a history of retentive soiling need reassurance that their bowel movements will be pain-free if they take a stool softener, and that they do not need to hold back the bowel movements to protect themselves from pain. Adolescent patients are concerned often about rapid growth and body change. They need reassurance that their particular somatotype, genital size, breast size, and other body parts are normal.

CLARIFYING THE PROBLEM AND ITS CAUSE

Listening

To be effective at counseling, one needs a complete and accurate picture of a problem. A common error in giving advice is offering it too quickly. The parents and child should be listened to if one wishes to understand their worlds. Any conclusions about whether parents are reasonable or unreasonable should be delayed until they have been allowed to describe their unique situation. Listening in itself is therapeutic; it conveys respect and encourages independent decision making (see also Chapter 75).

Minimal Psychosocial Database

Children with one or two behavior symptoms (e.g., picky eater or nightmares) can be treated by offering direct advice if the physician observes a happy child and a positive parent-child interaction. An expeditious approach usually also can be taken with families whom the physician knows from long experience to be stable. In these cases, only three additional questions need to be asked: (1) "Does he (or she) have any other behavior problems?" (2) "Why do you think he (or she) is acting this way?" (3) "What have you already tried?" In this way, the physician avoids prescribing advice that has already failed. In children with multiple symptoms (e.g., multiple discipline problems) or complex problems (e.g., encopresis), a complete psychosocial database should be collected before advice is offered (see Chapters 75, 77, and 78).

Clarification of Problems

Clarification involves identification of the problem and an explanation of its possible causes and effects. The objective of clarification is to help parents understand their child's behavior. The physician must review carefully with the parents the behavior patterns they want changed. The parents have the final word about the selection of target behaviors. The physician can state, "If I understand you correctly, you are most concerned about ...." Pediatricians may not have enough time, however, to allow parents to work out their own understanding of the cause of their child's problems. When the physician understands the situation, he or she may explain it in general terms. In some cases, the parents are either too strict or too lenient Sometimes the central issue is a vicious cycle or power struggle (e.g., pressure brings resistance; constant criticism leads to giving up and depression). The parents should be given credit if their analysis of the problem seems correct. When the physician has presented an interpretation to the parents, he or she can ask whether it makes sense to them.

Reducing Parental Guilt Regarding the Cause

The parents of children with emotional problems usually take them personally and feel responsible for the problem. When the parent-child relationship has been examined, and parents have been advised to change what they are doing, this guilt is inevitable.

Guilt can be reduced in several ways. The physician would do best by keeping a no-fault attitude during counseling. The guilt can be universalized (e.g., "Everyone tries that."). The physician can absolve the parents (e.g., "I can easily understand why you tried that."). The blame can be shared with schools, relatives, siblings, and other etiologic factors (e.g., "Your actions were just one of the reasons behind this problem."). The parents can be reminded that the harm was not intentional. Also, the parents' errors can be relegated to the past (e.g., "That was long ago, and much has happened since then."). Most importantly, the physician can show empathy and emphasize, "All parents make some mistakes, and that is part of being an involved parent." Positive aspects of the parent-child relationship can be underscored. Sometimes problems stem from parental leniency and overindulgence, and the physician can state, "You love him too much" or "You tried too hard." One can end with the viewpoint that "The main need now is to look ahead rather than behind. Don't be too hard on yourselves."

APPROVING THE PARENTS' APPROACH TO TREATMENT

A definite trend in the delivery of health services is self-care. Parents are being encouraged to become active participants in their family's health service. Just as parents learn how to manage their child's coughs and colds by themselves, the common sense they possess about human behavior also should be supported. The physician is in a position to foster independent decision making. Not only is this approach sound economically, but it also enhances the parental sense of competency. Inexperienced new parents are often overanxious and insecure. They need to be temporarily dependent on their physicians. Bringing such parents to a level of independent problem solving and self-care is a gradual but achievable process.

Reinforce the Parents' Strategies

After clarification of a problem, parents may formulate their own treatment plan. Others can be encouraged to problem solve. The physician can ask, "Now that you understand the problem, what are your options?" The physician can endorse their plans (if they are reasonable) and encourage them to adhere to them. Often parents seek the physician's approval to do what they wanted to do anyway (e.g., using the pacifier). In this way, independent thought is encouraged, and the parents' self-confidence is strengthened. The physician constantly operates on the premise that a wide variation of workable approaches exists for most problems, and that the selection of a strategy must take into account the parents' lifestyle, culture, and value system. Because the parents will have to live with the consequences of the plan, they should be encouraged to arrive at final management decisions themselves. If the parent's plans are unlikely to be successful, however, the physician should discuss his or her reservations with them.

Approval of Parenting

Parents can be complimented regarding their parenting skills during every visit. Mentioning that a child is courteous, patient, brave, verbally interactive, or cooperative or shows other desirable personality traits in the office setting helps the parents believe they are doing a good job. Parents of children with emotional problems are usually on the defensive and need to hear that the physician knows they love their child.

Avoid Criticism

Criticism of parents has several adverse side effects. First, it engenders guilt. Many parents normally blame themselves for causing their child's symptoms (e.g., by losing their temper and yelling), and the physician should alleviate rather than accentuate such self-accusation. Second, parents who are criticized may become angry at the physician, and his or her medical advice then may be followed poorly. Even harmful approaches usually can be changed without confrontation by stating diplomatically, "Recently we have found that a different approach works better."

PROVIDING SPECIFIC ADVICE FOR MANAGEMENT

The physician should make specific recommendations for the relief of symptoms. Advice is indicated whenever a simple behavioral problem exists for which the parents are unable to devise an approach. The direct giving of advice is the mainstay of brief counseling. Suggestions about child rearing are among the most common types of advice offered. Standard advice can be given for symptoms with a clear etiology. More individualized advice must be prescribed for problems with a differential diagnosis of several etiologic subtypes. Practical, clear-cut instructions are more likely to be successful. Pediatricians should have treatment packages (consisting of 1 to 10 pieces of advice) for all common parental complaints. In emotionally healthy individuals, one does not need to worry about symptom substitution. The physician should restrict advice to his or her areas of expertise, and should avoid giving speculative advice in areas in which he or she is not trained or experienced, no matter what they may be. Examples of specific advice geared to the age of the child are presented in Chapters 2 to 6.

The following is a specific and very familiar advice-giving scenario: Negativism is a normal healthy phase seen in most children between 2 and 3 years old. First, the perspective that this phase is an important declaration of independence needs to be shared with parents. To the child, "No" means "Do I have to?" It should not be confused with disrespect. If the parent can keep a sense of humor about this phase, it will last only 6 to 12 months. Second, the child should not be punished for saying "No." Third, the parents should try to minimize their directives and rules; they should avoid unnecessary demands and keep safety as their main priority during this time. Fourth, the parents should give the child extra choices and alternatives to increase his or her sense of freedom. Examples are letting the child choose the book he or she wants to read, the toys that go into the bathtub, and the fruit he or she wants for a snack. The physician can ask which ear the child wants looked at first. The more quickly the child gains a feeling that he or she is a decision maker, the more quickly this phase passes. Fifth, the child should not be given choices when no choice exists. Buckling up a car seat and going to bed are not negotiable. Sixth, when a request must be made, the child can be given a 5-minute warning to help with the transition. The parent must avoid the two extremes of punishing the child or giving in to all of the child's "No's." See earlier parts of this book for discussions of helping children learn to cope with illnesses (see Part IV) and various social stressors (see Part II).

Gain the Parents' Acceptance of the Advice

The physician needs feedback from the parents about the advice that has been suggested. To avoid confusion, the physician can ask the parents to repeat the substance of what has been said. The physician can say, "Please review for me what our new plan is." If misunderstandings are present, they can be resolved before action is taken. To avoid noncompliance with advice, the physician also must ask whether this particular advice is acceptable to the parents. The physician can ask, "Does that seem reasonable to you?" or "How do you feel about that approach?" If the parents seem unconvinced, the physician must decide whether to persuade them to accept this particular advice or to suggest another option.

Write Down Advice for the Parents

The physician should write down the main suggestions that the parents have agreed on and give it to them as they leave, making a copy for his or her own records. Another option is to provide a parent handout on this subject. Exceptions to the generic advice can always be penciled in. In this way, the physician can be assured that the plan will not be undermined by forgetfulness. Parents usually appreciate this added demonstration of concern.

Follow-up Visits

If advice is given, the results of the advice should be learned. Advice should be followed by at least one visit or phone call. This approach is in contrast to prior approaches of reassurance and education in which follow-up visits are optional. If more than two follow-up visits are needed, probably the physician needs to acquire a more complete psychosocial database and a more precise concept of the etiology. The physician can ask the parent to keep a written record (diary or calendar) between visits; this provides material for discussion. The second visit should be scheduled approximately 1 week after the first. The problem identified should remain the focus of follow-up visits. One can assess progress on the basis of symptom elimination, symptom improvement, a lack of change, worsening of symptoms, or the occurrence of a new symptom. The physician can refine and recalibrate the treatment plan with the parents' contribution. The parents should be congratulated about any success they have had. If the treatment plan fails after several visits, and the problem is sufficiently severe, a family meeting may help, or the family can be referred to a mental health resource.

Parental Adherence to the Treatment Plan

Counseling does not become effective until the parent accepts the diagnosis and carries out the therapeutic recommendations (i.e., adherence or compliance). Treatment nonadherence takes many forms, including missed appointments, not implementing advice, not giving medications, and "doctor shopping." Adherence is improved by including the parents in goal selection and treatment planning, explaining the reason for each treatment, clarifying misconceptions, simplifying the treatment regimen, linking medication taking with daily routines, and providing written instructions. Excellent physician-parent communication and rapport also enhances compliance.

Pitfalls

A common pitfall in giving advice is rigidity on the part of the physician. The gap between the physician's request of the parents and the behavior that the parents are willing or able to provide should be kept to a minimum, If the physician's expectations are too high, he or she will lose the family to follow-up. Advice always should be presented as a consideration rather than a requirement or order.

An example of a situation in which physicians commonly give advice that is in conflict with parents' inclinations are the child's sleeping in the parents' room. Some mothers (especially those who are breastfeeding) prefer to have their infants sleep in a cradle in the parents' bedroom until they reach an age at which nighttime feedings are unnecessary (i.e., 3 or 4 months of age). No proven harm comes from this approach.

PROVIDING ENVIRONMENTAL INTERVENTION

Environmental intervention consists of recommendations for specific changes in the patient's physical or extrafamilial environments. These recommendations attempt to reduce factors that are contributing to the patient's problems or to mobilize individuals outside the family unit who can help. Environmental intervention is a part of many treatment plans. The physician becomes effective in this sphere after he or she acquires a thorough knowledge of the community's resources. Often a social worker can provide advice when the physician is uncertain about available help for a specific problem. Usually the school system and other agencies respond positively to the physician's suggestions.

In simple problems, environmental manipulation may be curative (e.g., a nightlight for a child who fears the dark). In children with multifactorial problems, it may offer temporary improvement while counseling paves the way to more permanent solutions (e.g., school attendance for school phobia). Environmental interventions on behalf of the patient at home, in the school, and in the community are best illustrated by the following specific examples.

Home Recommendations

Home recommendations can be used to change the home environment. For discipline problems, a time-out room can be designated and prepared. A quiet place can be provided for study. To prevent sleep deprivation, the television should be kept out of the bedroom, including teens' rooms. Chores or allowances can be increased or reduced, depending on circumstances. The television set might be disconnected temporarily to encourage studying or conversation.

School Recommendations

The following recommendations can be implemented to improve the child's school environment. Nursery school or Head Start may be indicated for a child who is overprotected or understimulated. Children with a learning disability may require remedial classes or tutoring after school (see Chapter 93). High school students may be enlisted as tutors for younger children. For the student who develops physical symptoms of anxiety while at school (e.g., abdominal pain), the physician may request that the school nurse permit the child to rest periodically in the nurse's office for 15 minutes, rather than sending the child home. For some anxious children, the physician may need to request a temporary shower excuse or gym excuse. Most children with problems can receive considerable support from their teachers if the pediatrician keeps them informed of the child's special needs (e.g., extra bathroom privileges).

Community Recommendations

The general advice for "full activity on doctor's orders" is especially beneficial for a depressed or overprotected child. Children with socialization or peer avoidance problems need more peer contact time. The possibility of joining clubs, teams, or other recreational outlets should be explored. A summer camp program serves a similar purpose, but the camp counselors must be prepared to deal with homesickness. Special camps exist for many children with chronic diseases or disabilities. Infants with developmental delays owing to environmental deprivation might be enrolled in stimulation programs.

Mobilizing a Support System

Physicians understand the value of support systems and can help mothers mobilize these. Taking care of a newborn during the first 3 months of life often requires at least two adults. The extended family may need to be enlisted if the mother has not done so. It is crucial that a relative or friend help care for siblings and assist the mother in obtaining naps, so that she does not become excessively fatigued. Sometimes a support system exists but needs to be consolidated. The father should be invited to come to a health supervision visit during the first year of life (as should a grandparent if one lives in the home), so that he knows his child's pediatrician values his input, and so that he is more accepting of the physician's telephone advice in future acute illnesses.

When no support group is available, the physician and public health nurse may temporarily provide a support system for the mother. Volunteers also may be helpful, especially mothers who have successfully managed a similar problem in their own child (e.g., colic, breastfeeding, breath-holding, or attention deficits). A physician may decide to keep a card file of the names and the phone numbers of successful mothers who are willing to provide such support and teaching. For the family in a serious crisis, temporary placement of the children with a relative, friend, or even foster home may need to be considered.

Implementation of Environmental Intervention

In order of increasing time commitment, environmental change can be initiated by having the parents do everything, making a telephone call oneself, writing a letter, or attending a conference. Having the parents explore the possibilities in their neighborhood and then coming up with a plan constitutes the easiest approach (e.g., finding an extracurricular activity for their child). If a parent-teacher conference is the recommendation, the parents can carry out this plan without the physician's further input. Telephone calls by the physician to other agencies or professionals can have an important impact (e.g., calling the psychiatrist when a child with bipolar disorder is expelled from school). More commonly, the physician makes phone calls to relatives (e.g., calling grandparents for support or calling the father if he is unreasonable about child custody or when the disciplinary approaches of the father and mother are polarized). A brief letter takes little more time than a telephone call. Often the physician writes the teacher, principal, school nurse, counselor, social worker, or several of these individuals regarding school recommendations. The physician may need to phone a camp director to gain special permission to allow a child with a handicap to attend camp. Scheduling a special conference in the physician's office may be the only way of dealing with an alcoholic father who is having a devastating impact on his son. Occasionally, the physician needs to attend a school staff meeting (e.g., when a patient has frequent seizures in school).

EXTENDED COUNSELING

In brief counseling, specific advice or options are offered for one or two behavioral symptoms. Good results are expected with one or two follow-up visits. Direct advice can be given after a minimal psychosocial database has been obtained. Every pediatrician should provide brief counseling and advice.

By contrast, extended counseling requires longer visits and more extensive contacts. Extended counseling is needed for children with multiple or complicated symptoms and should be preceded by the obtaining of a more complete psychosocial database. Extended pediatric counseling may require three to six visits (or more). Two examples of extended counseling that are common in the practice of pediatrics are psychosomatic counseling and discipline counseling.

Psychosomatic Counseling

Pediatricians must be fully trained to evaluate and treat children who have any symptom that might stem from psychological causes as well as organic ones (e.g., recurrent headaches, abdominal pains, and syncope). No other professional has the background to assess these complaints efficiently and completely. The main barrier to successful treatment is changing the family's focus from organic to nonorganic. Gaining the parents' confidence in a new diagnosis is usually the critical step for dealing with any psychosomatic symptom. Table 86-3 provides a helpful approach for these problems.

Discipline Counseling

Skills in discipline counseling or child management counseling are a prerequisite to the enjoyment of pediatric practice. Child rearing problems are mentioned during at least half of office visits. Table 86-4 lists the steps in discipline counseling. Parents need to be reminded that they must change their behavior and responses first. The child can only follow. A pediatrician can learn these skills by reading books for parents and taking appropriate courses.

Three additional areas in which counseling is most commonly requested center around divorce, school problems, and adolescence. Involvement in this additional counseling should be considered optional for a busy practicing pediatrician. It usually requires additional skills and training. A physician who elects to engage in these areas of expanded counseling must set attainable therapeutic goals regarding what will and will not be attempted. Although the physician may use some behavior modification and advice, most extended counseling entails active listening, family meetings, clarification, and support.

Table 86-3. Steps in Psychosomatic Evaluation and Counseling

1. Elicit a complete history
2. Perform a meticulous physical examination
3. Order sufficient laboratory tests to convince yourself of the child's physical health
4. Tell the parents the diagnosis after the evaluation is complete
5. Clarify that the child is in excellent physical health
6. Explain that emotions can cause physical symptoms
7. Tell the parents the reasons why the symptom is not the result of physical disease
8. Reassure the parents about any specific diagnosis they fear
9. Clarify for the parents that this condition occurs in normal children and in normal homes
10. Reassure the parents that you can treat this condition effectively
11. Encourage normal activities, especially full school attendance
12. Have the child spend more time with same-age peers

Table 86-4. Steps in Discipline Counseling

1. Teach the basic principles of behavior modification
2. List the types of problem behavior
3. Help the parent assign priorities to the problems
4. Devise a treatment plan or consequence for each target behavior
5. Demonstrate appropriate responses in the office
6. Correct the child in a kind way and with a quiet voice
7. Praise the child for adaptive behavior
8. Write down the treatment plan and use handouts for specific behaviors
9. Provide follow-up visits

One error in extended counseling is taking on a patient who needs long-term psychotherapy. A variation on this error is to remain involved with a case despite a lack of progress. Children with serious emotional problems should be referred to a mental health setting. Major education problems require educational specialists. Families with multiple problems should be referred to a social worker. If progress has not been accomplished by the fifth or sixth session of extended counseling, referral usually is indicated.

LOGISTICS AND ECONOMICS OF COUNSELING

Although some individuals may believe that it is unrealistic for a pediatrician to become involved with time-consuming behavioral problems, he or she is well suited for this role. Most primary physicians are efficient. If the physician is the child's regular physician, he or she has two advantages: he or she knows the family well, and the evaluation can be done in much less time. In addition, the parents already trust the physician's advice. The physician can attain the same results that it would take an unknown counselor much longer to achieve. This section reviews some aspects of office organization that may improve the physician's efficiency in counseling.

Counseling: Whom to Include

The counseling time spent with the child compared with the time spent with the parents increases with age. Children younger than 5 years of age theoretically can be treated by working exclusively with the parents (ideally both of them). The child can be left with a nonparental caregiver while the parents meet with the physician. Benefits of leaving the child with another person are that the child does not disrupt the adult conversation and is not exposed to negative comments about himself or herself. Disadvantages are that the physician does not get a true picture of the child's behavior and does not have an opportunity to demonstrate appropriate responses to it. The child definitely needs to come in if he or she needs to overcome a problem that requires special motivation (e.g., thumb sucking or encopresis).

Generally, it is advisable to have the child present at any age so that he or she can be made more accountable for change. By school age, the parent and children often are seen together and share the counseling time equally. If an adolescent has a personal problem, the parents may not be seen at all. If the difficulty is largely a family communication problem, the parents and adolescent come together during part of the visit, leaving some private time for the adolescent to meet with the physician. For parents who need individualized counseling, the presence of a part-time social worker in the physician's office is very helpful (e.g., for marital problems).

Data in Advance

The initial evaluation visit proceeds much more efficiently if the family or adolescent has completed a behavioral screening or descriptive questionnaire in advance (see Chapter 78). After scanning the results, the physician can focus the discussion on the main problem areas. More specific information also is helpful. Parents of a child with a bed-wetting problem may be asked for several bladder capacity measurements. Other important information to have the parents collect before being seen are a food intake diary for obesity, a school report for school problems, a pain diary for recurrent pains, and a sleep diary for sleep disorders. The results of previous laboratory or radiologic studies should be known. If time is short, this information may be gained by phone. The consulting physician should send a report to the referring professional or agency after his or her evaluation so that communication is optimal, and environmental intervention is maximized.

Scheduling Appointments

The initial evaluation commonly requires 45 to 60 minutes. A common error is to set aside inadequate time or to try to carry out an abbreviated evaluation during a visit for another purpose. If behavioral or psychosomatic problems are detected during a health supervision or acute illness visit, the patient should be rescheduled for a longer visit at a later time. Follow-up visits can usually be 20 to 30 minutes long, depending on the problem. Parents should be given an exact date and time for follow-up. Telling them simply to come back if advice does not work out is insufficient. If physicians agree that otitis media requires follow-up, they should readily see that a treatment plan for discipline problems or encopresis also needs to be monitored. Some physicians prefer to use the 5 P.M. to 6 P.M. time for initial evaluations because their office staff has left, and their overhead is reduced. Others find themselves more tired and less sensitive at that hour, however.

Fees for Counseling

Many physicians charge inadequately for the counseling they provide, and this may be one of the reasons they become disillusioned about dealing with psychosocial issues. Pediatricians must keep in mind that their productivity with counseling may be higher than that of any mental health professional. They should charge a reasonable amount for this time. The following is an oversimplified look at evaluation and management codes. An initial behavioral evaluation of 60 minutes would generate a 99205 CPT code. For a behavioral visit, at least half the time needs to be spent on counseling. A follow-up visit of at least 15 minutes generates a 99213 code and a 25-minute visit generates a 99214 code. The fees and the estimated total number of visits should be discussed with the family members before the initial evaluation is scheduled. The office manager usually can have this discussion with the family members. If the parents cannot afford to pay the physician for the amount of time he or she spends with them, they might be referred to a mental health clinic or another center with a sliding fee scale. If families are being seen in a prepaid health maintenance organization, such counseling fees can more readily be absorbed.

SUMMARY

Counseling is an intrinsic part of pediatric care. Parents often seek out physicians who feel comfortable dealing with physical and emotional issues. Optimal pediatric care requires competent counseling skills. Full enjoyment of a pediatric practice is enhanced through a knowledge of behavior modification principles (see also Chapter 87) and childrearing counseling techniques. Without such skills, physicians may turn excessively to psychotropic drugs and mental health referrals. Through clinical experience, seminars at medical meetings or local colleges, reading office handouts for various behavioral problems, reading parenting books (see list at end of chapter), and discussion groups, pediatricians can upgrade their counseling skills to match their competency in treating physical illness.

SUGGESTED READINGS

American Academy of Pediatrics: Diagnostic and Statistical Manual for Primary Care (DSM-PC): Child and Adolescent Version. Elk Grove Village, IL, American Academy of Pediatrics, 1996.

Bergman AS: Pediatricians as counselors: The relationship as treatment. Pediatrics 73:730, 1984.

Coleman WL: Family-Focused Behavioral Pediatrics. Philadelphia, Lippincott Williams & Wilkins, 2001.

Coleman WL, Howard BJ: Family-focused behavioral pediatrics: Clinical techniques for primary care. Pediatr Rev 16:448, 1995.

Dworkin PH: Detection of behavioral, developmental, and psychosocial problems in primary care practice. Curr Opin Pediatr 5:531, 1993.

Green M: No child is an island: Contextual pediatrics and the "new" health supervision. Pediatr Clin North Am 42:79, 1995.

Green M, Sullivan PD, Eichberg CG: What to do with the angry toddler. Contemp Pediatr 19:65, 2001.

Hickson G, Altemeir W, O'Connor S: Concerns of mothers seeking care in private pediatric offices: Opportunities for expanding services. Pediatrics 72:619, 1983.

Kalb LM, Loeber R: Child disobedience and noncompliance: A review. Pediatrics 111:641, 2003.

McCune Y, Richardson M, Powell J: Psychosocial health issues in pediatric practices: Parents' knowledge and concerns. Pediatrics 14:183, 1984.

Morgan ER, Winter RI: Teaching communication skills: An essential part of residency training. Arch Pediatr Adolesc Med 150:638, 1996.

Schmitt BD, Brayden RM, Kempe A: Parent handouts: Cornerstone of a health education program. Contemp Pediatr 14:120, 1996.

BOOKS FOR PARENTS ON CHILD REARING

American Academy of Pediatrics: Bright Futures Guidelines for Health Supervision, 3rd ed. Elk Grove Village, IL, AAP, 2008.

Brazelton TB: Touchpoints: Your Child's Emotional and Behavioral Development. Reading, MA, Addison-Wesley Publishers, 1994.

Chess S, Thomas A: Know Your Child. New York, Basic Books, 1987 [Republished, New Brunswick, NJ, Jason Aronson, 1996].

Christopherson ER: Little People: Guidelines for Common Sense Child Rearing. Kansas City, Westport Publishers, 1988.

Karp H: The Happiest Toddler on the Block. New York, Bantam, 2004.

Phelan TW: 1-2-3 Magic: Effective Discipline for Children 2-12, 3rd edition. Glen Ellyn, IL, Parentmagic, 2003.

Schmitt BD: Your Child's Health: A Pediatric Guide for Parents, 3rd ed. New York, Bantam Books, 2005.

87 BEHAVIOR MANAGEMENT

Jack H. Nassau, Gray M. Buchanan, and Pamela C. High

Because public health initiatives, immunizations, and therapeutics have been so effective in controlling infectious diseases in childhood, an increasing proportion of issues confronting today's clinicians are related to parenting, child development, and child behavior. Surveys of children's health show a high prevalence of emotional, developmental, and behavioral problems among children (Blanchard et al, 2006), and parents frequently consult pediatric providers about how to manage myriad childhood problems related to sleep, continence, thumb sucking, depressive symptoms, oppositional behavior, and risk-taking (Kelleher et al, 2000; Young et al, 1998). In addition, parents of children with chronic diseases seek guidance on how to implement treatment regimens that include symptom monitoring, medications, exercise, and diet, all of which have serious implications for their child's current and future health.

This chapter outlines behavioral principles and provides examples of how clinicians may implement behavioral interventions. It builds on Chapter 86, which describes generally how clinicians can use their interviewing skills and knowledge of child behavior and development to individualize counseling for families. We provide a general format for designing behavior management plans and discuss behavioral interventions in the context of three vignettes about children at different stages of child development, each highlighting specific behavioral considerations and interventions. Table 87-1 describes key types of learning on which many behavioral strategies are based, including clinical examples. Table 87-2 identifies key principles of operant conditioning because of the importance of this type of learning in behavior management. The examples and applications in these two tables underscore that behavioral therapies target specific behaviors, not their underlying causes. In addition, different types of interventions may be needed depending on the type of behavior being targeted, and several principles may be used in a coordinated way to change behavior. Table 87-3 lists commonly used behavioral strategies that derive from the principles outlined in Tables 87-1 and 87-2. Resources for clinicians and parents are provided at the end of the chapter.

The clinician is always faced with the task of developing an effective behavioral intervention or program that puts the principles and strategies outlined in Tables 87-1 through 87-3 into practice. This chapter outlines important components of developing any effective behavioral program. These include, but are not limited to, developing and maintaining positive parent-child interactions, defining the behavior to be changed, measuring and monitoring the target behavior, setting a behavior change goal, developing specific strategies to change the behavior, implementing and evaluating the behavior program, and maintaining behavior change (Table 87-4).

DEVELOPING AND MAINTAINING POSITIVE PARENT-CHILD INTERACTIONS

The importance of positive experiences in promoting cooperation in children is well established. Generally, the more parents provide opportunities for positive interactions with their children, the greater the likelihood that negative interactions will decrease. Enriched or enjoyable environments must be established before any time away or time-out can be an effective deterrent of negative behaviors. In many circumstances, success comes faster from rewarding what is desired, rather than from punishing what is undesired.

The clinician should be aware of factors that may be limiting positive interactions between parents and their children. Parents may be overwhelmed and frustrated with their struggles in managing their child and may face other stressors (e.g., single parenting, working multiple jobs) that make it more difficult to find the time and energy to have fun with their children. Importantly, parents may be inadvertently reinforcing their child's behavior problems by attending to the child when he or she is behaving poorly, even if that attention is in the form of telling the child to stop misbehaving, and ignoring the child or "leaving well enough alone" when he or she is behaving. In addition to teaching parents to attend to even small instances of positive child behavior, specific behavioral techniques such as "special time" (see Table 87-3) can be implemented to increase positive interactions between children and parents.

DEFINING THE BEHAVIOR TO BE CHANGED

Because behavioral treatments focus on changing specific behaviors, it is imperative to help parents define the behavior they wish to change. Although this sounds

Table 87-1. Types of Learning and Their Application

Types of Learning	Examples	Application
Classic conditioning (also called *respondent or pavlovian conditioning or stimulus-stimulus learning*) is a type of learning related to an automatic or reflexive response to a specific stimulus. A neutral stimulus is temporally paired with the specific stimulus (unconditioned stimulus [UCS]) so that it (the neutral stimulus) becomes also an elicitor (conditioned stimulus [CS]) of the reflexive response (conditioned response [CR]).	Basic: A loud sound (the UCS) causes a startle (the unconditioned response [UCR]). A neutral stimulus (e.g., the scent of an orange) is paired with the loud sound multiple times. The scent of the orange (CS) elicits a startle (now a CR). Clinical: A child comes to associate the pediatrician's office with painful immunizations. When the child goes to the office for any cause, the child becomes anxious, fearing getting a shot. Clinical: A child with leukemia becomes nauseated while dressing to go to a chemotherapy appointment.	This type of learning plays a role in the development of phobias, fears, food aversions, and school refusal. Interventions often include gradual exposure to the CS (feared stimulus—pediatrician's office) paired with a more desirable stimulus (children's book or sticker rather than immunization) to decrease the CR (fear). This is called *counter conditioning*. Classic conditioning also can teach desired behaviors: a bedwetting alarm wakes a child when the child begins to wet. The alarm is the US; waking is the UCR. Wetting becomes the CS leading to the CR of waking.
Operant conditioning (also called *instrumental conditioning or stimulant-response learning*) is a type of learning that occurs in response to environmental consequences. Operant behaviors are influenced either by *antecedent stimuli* (that precede the behavior) or by *consequences* (that result from the behavior). Consequences may either increase the behavior (reinforcement—positive and negative) or decrease the behaviors (punishment or deterrents).	Basic: A child who is rewarded for saying please increases the frequency of saying please. Desirable and undesirable behaviors may be learned and reinforced through operant conditioning. Clinical: A preschooler swears when he becomes frustrated. His older brother laughs when he hears it. The preschooler interprets his brother's laughter as approval and swears more because he enjoys his brother's positive attention. The older brother's laughter serves to reinforce positively the preschooler's operant behavior of swearing, even though this behavior is not necessarily desired by the older brother.	This type of learning often plays a role in the development of 3 types of behavioral concerns: (1) behavioral excess (e.g., aggression or tantrums); (2) behavioral deficiency (e.g., refusal to eat, toilet, or do homework or chores); (3) inappropriate behaviors (e.g., inappropriate dress, language, or touching). Interventions to increase or decrease the frequency of these behaviors focus on consequences following the behavior, whereas interventions aimed at changing the time or place of the behavior focus more on antecedent events.
Social or observational learning is a third type of learning that occurs through modeling or imitation. This learning may be either purposeful or incidental. It does not require reinforcement.	Basic: Parents model many behaviors and values, including tolerance, work ethic, manners, and interpersonal relationships. Clinical: Parents may inadvertently promote undesired behaviors such as smoking by modeling them, even while talking about the dangers of this habit. Actions often speak louder than words.	Children learn most commonly by watching those most important in their world (parents, siblings, friends) and then by emulating them. The influence of the model on the child's behavior increases with the child's perceived similarity to the model and the status and success of the model in the child's view.

like a straightforward process, it can be a difficult one. Behaviors can be discrete, such as saying "please" when asking for a toy, or more complex, such as being "polite." At the outset, it is often helpful to work collaboratively with parents to "break down" complex goals or behaviors into simpler component behaviors. Parents may want their child to "be good." Although this may be a desirable goal, it is not actually a discrete behavior, but a description of how one might interpret successful accomplishment of numerous other, smaller behaviors (e.g., listening the first time when asked to brush teeth). Even seemingly small behaviors (e.g., keep room clean) can be broken down into smaller ones (e.g., pick clothes up off floor, make bed), and it is often beneficial to begin an intervention with attempting to change small behaviors.

Success begets success. Success should be reinforced early and often. In addition, the initial target behaviors should be selected to allow a greater chance of success and less frustration for the child *and parent*. Finally, although the temptation may be to tackle the most bothersome behavior, it is helpful to choose a single, simpler, behavior to address initially even if the family has many issues of concern. Success with changing the initial behavior empowers parents to have more confidence and become more invested in addressing additional, more difficult, behaviors.

In addition to collaborating with parents, coordination with teachers and other school personnel is often necessary. In such cases, it is important for the clinician to determine what problematic behaviors occur in the classroom and to identify goals for target behaviors that complement goals established with the family. This is a complex process. Teachers often have many children in their classroom and can attend to the behaviors of an individual child only in a circumscribed manner; defining discrete, small behaviors that the teacher can attend to is necessary.

MEASURING AND MONITORING THE TARGET BEHAVIOR

A major benefit of defining a behavior as a target for intervention is that the behavior may be measured and monitored. If the behavior cannot be measured and monitored, one should not develop an intervention to

Table 87-2. **Behavior Management Techniques (or Principles of Operant Conditioning) and Applications**

Principles of Operant Conditioning	Examples	Application
Positive reinforcement refers to the provision of a favorable consequence or a reward in response to a behavior to increase that behavior. Positive reinforcers can be primary (candy, hugs, prizes, money) or secondary (stars, tokens, points). To be most effective, positive reinforcers must be given consistently soon after the behavior being reinforced (contingently) and should be withheld at all other times. Also, secondary reinforcers should be frequently and regularly converted to primary ones.	Whether a consequence is a positive reinforcer or a punishment depends on the child's perspective. Yelling at a child for misbehaving can serve to increase (positively reinforce) the misbehavior if a parent ignores the child when he or she is quiet and playing. To the child, negative attention may be preferable to no attention at all. Positive reinforcement can increase desired and undesired behaviors. Hugs may increase desired behaviors such as a child sharing toys with a playmate. Laughing while telling a child he or she is "bad" for jumping on the bed may be interpreted positively by the child and increase the child's interest in jumping on the bed.	Praise, time-in, sticker charts, rewards, point systems, and token economies all are forms of positive reinforcement that have varying degrees of success in increasing antecedent behavior depending on their design and application. The schedule of reinforcement is important. Typically, reinforcers are continuous (i.e., after each time the behavior happens) at the beginning and then are gradually given less frequently (e.g., the behavior needs to occur a number of times before the reinforcer is given). Satiation needs to be avoided.
Negative reinforcement refers to the removal or avoidance of an aversive consequence to a behavior, which increases that behavior. Negative reinforcement and punishment (see below) are two types of consequences with opposite effects. Negative reinforcement increases antecedent behaviors, whereas punishment aims to decrease antecedent behaviors with aversive consequences.	A toddler tantrums in public when his mom refuses to buy him a toy. His mother buys the toy to stop the tantrum, and the child calms down. The mom positively reinforced the tantrum, teaching that tantrums are rewarded with toys, which increases the chance the child will tantrum again. The child negatively reinforced the mom's toy buying, teaching the mom that buying toys stops tantrums.	We learn many lessons through negative reinforcement. We learn to wear coats in the snow to avoid getting cold. We learn to put on sunscreen to avoid getting sunburn. Undesirable behaviors may be negatively reinforced inadvertently. When a child with encopresis who does not like school is excused from class for soiling, the child learns how to avoid class.
Punishment is a consequence designed to be aversive and to decrease or extinguish a behavior. Although aversive, effective punishment should not be psychologically or physically hurtful or mean (see corporal punishment in Table 87-3).	Common examples of punishment are verbal reprimands, planned ignoring (extinction), removing a privilege or desired object (response cost), or time-out in response to an undesired behavior. One form of punishment is a logical consequence, a negative event logically tied to a misbehavior that is enacted in response to that misbehavior (e.g., removing a toy for 24 hours when siblings fight over it).	Often when parents are trying to decrease or extinguish a behavior, there is an initial intensification, or increase rather than decrease, of the target behavior. This is called an *extinction burst* and suggests the behavior plan is having an effect that the child is trying very hard to combat. Parents need to persevere through this time to see the targeted behavior begin to decrease. Punishment does not teach children appropriate behavior. It only teaches children what not to do.

change it because any objective change would be impossible to discern. Measuring and monitoring involves being able to count the frequency (and possibly the intensity and duration) of a behavior and the antecedents and consequences of the behavior. This process provides information regarding how often the behavior occurs, in what situation or context it occurs, and what learning and reinforcement mechanisms may be operating. When a family brings up a behavioral concern, such as sleep, as part of a busy health maintenance visit, the clinician can ask parents to monitor that behavior, preferably on a monitoring form. In this way, the clinician has efficiently and effectively recognized the parent's concern and started the process of behavioral intervention. At a follow-up visit, the monitoring can be reviewed, and a behavioral management plan can be developed.

Measuring and monitoring behavior is an ongoing process throughout a behavioral intervention. It is recommended that before initiating any other intervention, parents should measure and monitor the behavior for a few days to a week to learn about the baseline frequency. This useful first step allows a busy practitioner to attend to a parental concern quickly by enlisting the parent's assistance in collecting data important to development of treatment strategies. Also, knowing this baseline frequency helps in determining whether subsequent intervention is influencing the behavior in the desired way—either increasing it or decreasing it.

Asking parents "merely" to measure and monitor a behavior when they have typically come to the clinician wanting a quick cure for a problem that has been going on for a long time may frustrate some parents who wonder what and when something is going to be done to change the behavior. In such cases, parents can be reassured that measuring and monitoring the behavior is crucial to changing the behavior. Parents often learn about the behavior they are interested in changing during this step—realizing that it happens more or less often than they thought or has a certain pattern of antecedents or consequences associated with it. Parents may unintentionally exaggerate the intensity of difficulties.

Table 87-3. Commonly Used Behavior Management Techniques

Behavior Management Technique	Examples	Application
Time-in—refers to parents' interactions with their children when their children's behavior is acceptable, but not necessarily praiseworthy. Parents should be encouraged to have frequent, brief, positive physical, verbal, and visual contact with their child throughout the day, whenever the child is engaged in nonproblematic behaviors. In addition, when a child's behavior is praiseworthy, it deserves to be praised consistently. There are many variations of time-in that are commonly advocated to teach children desired behaviors. These include advice to "Catch them being good" and praise them, special time, or me time.	*Special time*—parents plan an opportunity to observe their child's positive behaviors, perhaps during a creative activity, and make sure that they praise the child for his or her effort and accomplishments. *Me time*—time in which the child generally gets what he or she wants within reason. The child is given choices from an array of desirable activities that usually include parental involvement. This should occur frequently, at least several times a week and optimally daily. Me time might be shorter on weekdays (reading a story or going for a walk together) and longer on a weekend (baking cookies or going to the park together). Naming the time "me time" often elevates it in stature in the child's view.	Time-in is an essential prerequisite for any behavioral management program. Special time should not be removed as a punishment. Time-in and special time are conducive to a child's learning appropriate behaviors and his or her motivation to cooperate.
Time-out—from positive reinforcers is one of the most common forms of punishment used in most behavior management programs. To be effective, time-out should happen immediately and consistently after the targeted misbehavior. The time is generally short (approximately 1 min per year of child age), but may need to be extended if the child continues to misbehave or protest when the time-out would be expected to conclude (using a timer is recommended). Time-out is most effective with concurrent use of time-in. Time-out is most effective when applied to infrequent dangerous or destructive behaviors.	Make a command/request of the child (short and clear statement—"if ..., then..."). Give a clear warning if the child does not respond to the request ("if you don't do ..., then you will have to sit in time-out"). If the child does not complete the command/request, administer time-out. Time-out is "time-out from positive reinforcement"; select a location with as few reinforcers as possible, and do not reason/verbally interact with the child. The child should be completely ignored during time-out.	Time-out is most effective in 2- to 6-year-olds, but can be effective in older children as well. Be prepared in case the child refuses to go to time-out. Effective alternatives are adding additional time, or if the child still refuses, giving the child a choice of either going to time-out or losing a privilege. Following time-out, the original command/request should be repeated. If the child does not comply, repeat the procedure.
Stimulus control—refers to controlling behavior by limiting access to antecedents that served to increase that behavior.	An overweight boy who drinks many sugar-filled sodas each day can be aided in decreasing this habit when his family decides that the whole family will be able to drink sodas only on Sundays. Sodas are available in the house only on that day.	As in any technique, collaboration is key. Making sure the child is aware of the rule/expectation before implementing the strategy is necessary to minimize protests from the child.
Differential reinforcement of incompatible behavior—refers to reinforcing a behavior that is incompatible with the behavior that is targeted for extinction.	A child with dermatitis exacerbates the condition by scratching in his or her sleep. Differential reinforcement of incompatible behavior might include praise and a desired outing after a specified number of successes in wearing cotton gloves at night to limit scratching.	There are several types of differential reinforcement; however, the overarching principles include reinforcing wanted behaviors and withholding reinforcement for unwanted behavior.
Shaping—gradually increasing a behavior by giving positive reinforcement to small increments (successive approximations) of the target behavior; most commonly used to develop a new behavior pattern.	A preschooler who is refusing to eat vegetables is rewarded with a sticker first for allowing the vegetable to sit on the plate, then for touching the vegetable, then for smelling it, then for licking it, then for tasting it, then for eating a bite. A row of stickers earns a trip to the ice cream store.	Steps (successive approximations) should be identified before attempting to shape a behavior. Carefully outlining small increments of the behavior facilitates success for the child and minimizes frustration in the process.
Systematic desensitization—gradually increasing a child's exposure to an anxiety-producing stimulus to enable the child to overcome the anxiety gradually. Also known as graduated exposure.	A child with school avoidance based on fear of bullying may be gradually exposed to school by attending one class on the first day, and two classes on the second day, while other supports such as counseling are in place.	Systematic desensitization is most commonly used in children who exhibit difficulties with anxiety. This technique usually includes careful instruction in relaxation training and the development of an anxiety hierarchy.
Fading—gradually decreasing a reinforcer as a desired behavior becomes integrated into routine. This is the natural response after a new behavior is learned. Fading also refers to changing something gradually.	When a toddler learns not to jump on the couch, he or she may not need to get hugs for each time period that he or she refrains from jumping. Gradually moving bedtime earlier by 15 minutes every 3 days is another use of fading.	Fading often can be used to reduce the level of protests displayed by a child. Gradually changing a behavior instead of abruptly changing it commonly results in less confrontation.

(Continued)

Table 87-3 Commonly Used Behavior Management Techniques—cont'd

Behavior Management Technique	Examples	Application
Planned ignoring (extinction)—withdrawal of all attention when a child is engaging in an unwanted behavior. Ignoring should be used only in situations that are nondangerous and nondestructive.	A toddler who often has a tantrum when wanting an unhealthy snack can be ignored by the parent, who continues to perform another act (e.g., reading book, cleaning up) until the child's escalation ceases. Most useful for behaviors such as whining, tantrums, pouting, and arguing.	Ignoring should include no physical contact, no verbal contact, and no nonverbal communication (i.e., no making faces, eye contact). Expect an "extinction burst" or an initial sharp increase in the child's unwanted behavior; however, with continued use, the unwanted behavior decreases.
Redirecting—refers to changing the child's attention from one interest to another.	A toddler sees a child eating an apple and whines for an apple herself. Her mother does not have an apple to give, and so she redirects her daughter's attention to the dogs across the street playing in the yard.	Redirection is generally most effective in younger children.
Corporal punishment (e.g., spanking)—application of physical pain with the goal of discouraging unwanted behavior. With recurring use, increasing intensity may be required to attain desired decrement in problem behavior. Can result in other discipline methods losing their effectiveness, and same effects can be attained through other methods.	Despite the ongoing use of this type of punishment, the American Academy of Pediatrics recommends that "parents be encouraged and assisted in the development of methods other than spanking for managing undesired behavior".	Research evidence suggests that corporal punishment can teach children that hitting is acceptable, can alter parent-child relationships, can result in aggression in children, and is no more effective than other discipline approaches.

Table 87-4. Developing an Effective Behavioral Program: Seven Steps to Behavior Management

1. Developing and maintaining positive parent-child interactions
2. Defining the behavior to be changed
3. Measuring and monitoring the target behavior
4. Setting a behavior change goal
5. Developing specific strategies to change the behavior
6. Implementing and evaluating the behavior program
7. Maintaining behavior change

Parents may have become so frustrated with a child's tantrums that they have developed a "negative bias" and have difficulty recalling positive experiences and report tantrum levels beyond what actually occurs. Conversely, parents may acclimate or become so accustomed to the tantrums that they underreport the intensity of the behavior. Objective assessment provides concrete evidence in regard to the necessity to change behavior or not. Likewise, teachers also may be influenced by their own biases, and it may be necessary to have an independent individual observe the child's behavior to obtain a more objective assessment.

Although monitoring a behavior may seem straightforward, the clinician should help parents and other caregivers develop an appropriate monitoring plan and anticipate challenges. At the most basic level, the clinician needs to help family members decide who will be responsible for monitoring the behavior and how the behavior will be monitored. Assessment of behavior often includes a simple frequency count, a tally of how often the behavior occurs. For some behaviors (e.g., tantrums), other parameters (e.g., the duration of the tantrum) need to be monitored too. In addition, parents, and teachers when appropriate, should be reminded of the "ABCs" (*antecedents, behaviors, consequences*) of behavior and encouraged to monitor the events that precede the behavior (antecedents) and the results of the behavior (consequences).

Whatever the behavior being monitored, parents must be instructed to record their data on a form, rather than relying on their memory and verbal report at the next visit. Forms such as behavior diaries and behavior charts, each of which allow parents to monitor behaviors over time, should be employed. Having the data on such forms allows parents to collect valuable information that they then help interpret. The act of objectively recording and monitoring behavior sometimes may result in a "reactive effect." That is, in the process of monitoring behavior, the behavior may change, either in a desired or undesired direction. Figure 87-1 is an example of a generic monitoring form that could be used as a cry/sleep diary.

SETTING A BEHAVIOR CHANGE GOAL

After a period of monitoring, the clinician should help the parent and teacher identify patterns in the occurrence of the observed behavior and help them develop a desired behavior change goal. Setting a goal helps families know what they are trying to achieve and when they have achieved it. It is important to set realistic goals so that the patient and family members can experience success early in the course of treatment. Success experiences reinforce the family, and patient, to continue the program. Over the course of an intervention, the patient and family members should be encouraged to set

During each 15 minute period of the day you are to indicate the main activity of your baby.

The baby behaviors you will record are: F = Fussing C = Crying S = Sleeping E = Eating A = Awake

______________ ______ ______ ______
Day of the Week Month Day Year

12MN 1AM 2AM 3AM 4AM 5AM 6AM 7AM

8AM 9AM 10AM 11AM 12noon 1PM 2PM 3PM

4PM 5PM 6PM 7PM 8PM 9PM 10PM 11PM

Where baby falls asleep (S = swing, A = arms, B = parents' bed, Ba = bassinette, C = crib, CS = car seat)
Place above the block designating onset of a sleep episode. If baby is bottle feeding, put volume that is taken above times he/she is eating.

Best 5 minutes of the day ______________________________

____

For Office Use Only:

Total Hours Fussing _____ Crying _____ Sleeping _____ Awake _____ Eating _____

Figure 87-1. Behavior diary.(*Courtesy of Brown Center for the Study of Children at Risk, Providence, RI.*)

intermediate goals on the way to achieving the goal that is ultimately desired. In the case of wanting a child to have a clean room at the end of the day, the family may set intermediate goals with respect to the different behaviors that compose this larger goal. These might include making the bed in the morning and picking up clothes at the end of the day before requiring the room be entirely clean. Intermediate goals with respect to the number of days each week the room needs to be clean could be 2 days per week, then 4 days per week, then 6 days per week thereafter. The goal may not increase to 7 days per week. The main problem with setting a goal of perfection is that when the child makes a mistake and cannot achieve perfection, motivation for continuing the behavior plummets.

Numerous factors should be considered at this stage of planning, including such issues as the severity of the behavior, the available treatment options (e.g., in-home services, school support), and the goals of all parties involved (e.g., preferences of parents versus teachers regarding initial target goals). Initial target goals may be different at home than at school; however, it also may be the case that goals will overlap, such as increasing compliance with adult requests, although the specific requests differ.

DEVELOPING SPECIFIC STRATEGIES TO CHANGE THE BEHAVIOR

When a goal has been established based on initial measuring and monitoring, specific strategies (see Tables 87-2 and 87-3) may be incorporated into a behavior plan aimed at changing the behavior to reach the established (and intermediate) goal. The selection of specific strategies should occur in consultation with parents and teachers with attention to what seems to maintain the unwanted behaviors. The effectiveness of specific strategies needs to be monitored so that interventions can be revised as necessary.

Altering the antecedents and consequences of the behavior (the ABCs) serves as the backbone of the plan, but may be emphasized differentially depending on the nature of the behavior and what has been learned from the initial monitoring period. One major strategy of altering antecedents to a behavior is stimulus control. Stimulus control refers generally to altering the environment in which the behavior occurs to change the behavior. If parents have the goal of reducing the number of bags of potato chips their child eats in a week, and potato chips are currently freely available at home, one stimulus control strategy would be to limit the child's access to potato chips, such as making them available only on Saturday and Wednesday. In this way, the parents have controlled the child's access to the potato chips, the stimulus. Numerous changes in the environment can be considered stimulus control strategies. Not allowing a teenager with bulimia who vomits in the bathroom immediately after eating to go into the bathroom until after a specified amount of time after meals is an example of controlling the environmental stimulus (access to the bathroom) to limit the vomiting behavior.

Major strategies for altering the consequences of behaviors include (1) providing attention or rewards, or both, for desired behaviors that parents want to increase (positive reinforcement) and (2) systematically withdrawing attention from or punishing (e.g., with time-out) undesired behaviors that parents want to decrease (extinction). Some parents and other caregivers are concerned that providing rewards for behavior that they perceive as "expectations" is tantamount to bribery. Clinicians should educate parents on the range of "rewards" that are available to encourage desired behavior. Reminding parents to use "social rewards," especially extra attention from or time with the parents, rather than relying solely on material rewards, such as candy and prizes, can help reduce the feeling that parents are "paying" for their child's good behavior. Parents also should be encouraged to use natural and logical reinforcements that are closely tied to the behavior they are trying to change, such as rewarding a child for going to sleep on time by letting the child have a friend sleep over on the weekend. It also can be helpful to educate parents and other caregivers about the value of rewarding and reinforcing behaviors that help the child acquire needed life skills.

In situations in which parents and other caregivers are attempting to decrease an undesired behavior, clinicians should provide education about the likelihood of an "extinction burst," a period when the frequency of the undesired behavior *increases* before decreasing. Consider a case in which a parent often gives a child what he or she wants after the child whines for it. The whining occurs after the parent has initially said "No" to the child's request. The child has received positive reinforcement (the desired object) for whining. Now the parent decides he or she wants to decrease the child's whining after the parent says "No." The parent chooses to ignore the child's whining as one strategy to achieve this goal. In such a case, the child's whining may initially increase (the extinction burst) because whining has previously been positively reinforced, and the child "believes" that if he or she just continues to whine long or loudly enough, he or she will be reinforced as usual. The good news is that if the parent consistently does not give into the child's whining, the extinction burst subsides, and the whining decreases.

Two more key points are as follows. First, most behavior plans include numerous behavioral strategies. In addition to controlling a child's access to potato chips, a parent could reward the child for meeting a goal of reducing the number of bags or potato chips eaten. In the case of a whining child, the child could be rewarded for reducing whining after being told "No." Second, parents may inquire about the use of corporal punishment to decrease negative behavior. Although this type of punishment is still employed by many parents, research suggests that corporal punishment can result in numerous deleterious outcomes (see Table 87-3). Most professionals and professional organizations, including the American Academy of Pediatrics, recommend that alternative methods of changing unwanted behavior be employed.

IMPLEMENTING AND EVALUATING THE BEHAVIOR PROGRAM

Following the development of specific behavioral strategies, parents are faced with the challenge of implementing the plan and evaluating their child's behavior change. The clinician must ensure that all involved caregivers agree with and are ready to implement the behavior program by verifying that they (1) have a clear understanding of the goals and techniques proposed and (2) are prepared to apply the techniques. Children are expert at finding the weakest link and taking advantage of any differences of adult opinion or readiness. Before implementation, it is necessary to review the plan with all caregivers in detail and allow for discussion of "what if" situations.

Clinicians should (1) educate parents and other caregivers about the techniques and possible initial effects, such as the likelihood of an "extinction burst"; (2) model appropriate use of the techniques; and (3) allow caregivers to practice using a technique, such as by giving a direction for the child to throw something in the trash can and then applying the appropriate consequence—positive reinforcement or punishment—depending on whether the child follows the direction in the office. Parents and older children also might work together to develop a specific behavioral contract that outlines the behavioral goals and the specific rewards and consequences that will be used; such contracts can be signed by parents and children to indicate their agreement with the plan.

For the implementation of any behavioral plan to be successful, three additional points need to be emphasized with parents and other caregivers: consistency, immediacy, and saliency. In the case of a 6-year-old who is described by parents as hitting his younger sibling every time they go to the grocery store, it is important for parents to know to interrupt the hitting every time it occurs (consistency) and to provide quickly (immediacy) a meaningful consequence (saliency) for the child's behavior. Allowing the child occasionally to "get away" with hitting would not lead to a reduction in hitting. It is likely that waiting until the child is out of the grocery store would make it more difficult to establish the connection between the behavior and consequence. Finally, providing a consequence that is not salient (e.g., something that the child does not find punishing) would not discourage the behavior from occurring again. A behavior plan should be implemented only when parents believe their actions can be consistent, immediate, and salient for the child. The clinician should carefully assess factors such as parental disagreement or exhaustion that might interfere with caregivers' abilities to be consistent and provide immediate and salient consequences.

When a program has been implemented for a specified period, usually a minimum of 1 to 2 weeks, behavioral change should be observable. The practitioner should have the family members and teacher carefully track targeted behaviors and should meet regularly with the family to assess the quality and effectiveness of the strategies being implemented. Comparisons with monitoring from before the plan was implemented help determine whether the behavioral goal is being met, and when additional behavioral goals may be set. If behavioral goals are not being met, the clinician must discuss this with the family, explore possible reasons, and modify the behavioral program, usually by modifying antecedents or consequences or both.

MAINTAINING BEHAVIOR CHANGE

The ultimate goal of a behavioral program is to maintain behavior change in the context of gradual withdrawal of systematic reinforcement—that is, to maintain behavior change in the "real world" where immediacy, consistency, and saliency are not always present. The hope of the family and clinician is that over time the child would be self-motivated to continue the behavior, rather than dependent on external reinforcement. When a behavior has been established at its goal level, the clinician can help the parents begin the process of *fading reinforcement* to decrease gradually reliance on immediate reinforcement to maintain behavior. Parents could offer reinforcement every two or three times a behavioral goal is met rather than every time; fading reinforcement would continue until the behavior is reinforced at a much lower rate. Other modifications with the goal of maintaining behavior change with less external reinforcement include reinforcing groups of behaviors rather than single behaviors (e.g., reinforcing the child once for performing three goal behaviors rather than separately for each one), and making the reinforcement less material and more social (e.g., reinforcing with desired privileges rather than material rewards).

Parents should be informed of three challenges to maintaining behavior change: (1) reinforcers losing their saliency, (2) parents not naturally maintaining new behavioral methods after adequate behavior change is established, and (3) children not maintaining behaviors as reinforcement is faded. Practitioners should talk with parents about these challenges in the context of follow-up appointments, the frequency of which would depend on how well the plan is working. The clinician can help the family develop new reinforcers, incorporate new parenting behaviors into daily routines, and assess the rate at which reinforcement is faded. Ideally, just as parents fade reinforcement of established behaviors over time, practitioners would adjust the schedule of follow-up appointments such that families are seen less frequently over time and ultimately receive only booster appointments as needed.

ENHANCING PARENTING USING BEHAVIORAL PRINCIPLES

Vignette

Daniel is a healthy 5-month-old infant who, by his mother Lynette's report, has a history of persistent fussing and crying for at least 6 hours a day. Daniel's father is fulfilling a month-long military reserve duty commitment in another state, from which he cannot be excused. Lynette is exclusively breastfeeding. Daniel has good weight gain and a normal physical examination. He is bright and alert and focused on his mother's face and voice. He is beginning to babble reciprocally and to reach for his toys. Daniel cries especially hard in the evenings and does not have a consistent bedtime. He has a hard time falling asleep at night and only catnaps in his mother's arms during the day. His mother sometimes resorts to running the vacuum close to him or taking him on a late-night car ride to get him to fall asleep. By his mother's description, Daniel is sleeping only 6 to 8 hours a day. Lynette reports that she is exhausted and near the end of her rope. She questions her adequacy as a mother.

Behavioral principles can be used to encourage the implementation of developmentally appropriate positive parenting strategies. Parents of infants and toddlers can be advised to begin developing dependable routines, such as regular bedtimes and soothing bedtime rituals. Family routines can be conceptualized as learning through classic conditioning, such as the child associating reading a book or two with the parent while being rocked in a rocking chair in his or her room at bedtime with falling asleep in his or her crib for the night. The pleasant interactions that occur during such routines or rituals also positively reinforce parents to maintain the routine. Routines provide consistency; set predictable limits; and, although they will change and will be challenged as the child grows, have the potential to become a time in the day that everyone in the family anticipates with great pleasure.

Developing and Maintaining Positive Interactions

The most important relationship for young children is with their parents (Shonkoff and Phillips, 2000). Pediatric providers are uniquely poised to identify strengths and to recognize and address emerging stresses in the parent-child relationship. They are often the only health professionals with long-term relationships with young families, and they can play an important role in educating parents about positive approaches to parenting through anticipatory guidance provided at each health maintenance visit. During this time, they have a special opportunity to compliment parents on their parenting successes. When clinicians support parents by pointing out their successes ("look how she can't take her eyes off of you" or "what a healthy and happy boy he is ... you can take a lot of credit for this"), they model how important praise can be for children, providing an opportunity for social learning. This kind of encouragement also positively reinforces the very parenting behaviors that promote the positive child behaviors appreciated by parents and providers.

In this first vignette, positive interactions between Lynette and Daniel may be limited owing to the stress of single parenting while Lynette's husband is completing military service, along with Daniel's sleep difficulties and Lynette's level of exhaustion as her own sleep is disrupted. A screening for postpartum depression may be important because depressive symptoms are common in new mothers and can potentially negatively affect parenting behaviors. The clinician should help Lynette identify times when she and Daniel are most calm, perhaps early in the day when she and Daniel are better rested, and encourage periods of simple positive interactions such as singing or cuddling together, "tummy-time," and other play activities.

Defining the Behavior to Be Changed

Lynette is clear that she wants Daniel to cry less and sleep more. During infancy, sleeping, crying, and feeding are closely associated with one another. Before attempting to change these behaviors, it would be most helpful to understand how much and when Daniel is crying and how much and where he is sleeping, and the association of these behaviors with his feeding schedule.

Measuring and Monitoring the Target Behavior

Because the behaviors that Lynette is trying to address are highly interrelated, a diary approach that allows for all the behaviors to be monitored simultaneously and in real time, such as one used to record feeding, crying, sleeping, and awake behaviors in 15-minute intervals (see Fig. 87-1), can be very useful. Diaries can be color-coded with highlighting markers for ease of interpretation and to facilitate comparisons across 2 to 4 days. Although monitoring behavior every 15 minutes for even 1 or 2 days is labor intensive, in clinical settings more than 80% of parents can collect these data dependably and find the results informative and helpful. Diaries also can be used to prompt parents to note the "best 5 minutes of the day." When parents are extremely stressed, appreciating that there is a good time in the day can be used to build in opportunities for positive interactions (as discussed in the section on developing and maintaining positive interactions).

Review of behavior diaries sometimes identifies behaviors that were not expected (the child woke up every 3 hours at night, not every hour), but often it confirms the report of parents, validating their concern. In this case, Daniel's baseline diaries showed that he was sleeping 10 to 11 hours out of 24, a little more than his mother's perception, but less than expected for his age. Daniel's sleep phase was shifted with a bedtime after midnight and late morning waking. Evenings were especially difficult with 3 to 4 hours of crying after 7 P.M.

Setting a Behavior Change Goal

Because of Lynette's current level of stress, it is especially important to set an initial behavior change goal that she thinks is attainable, even if it is only a small step toward her ultimate goal for Daniel. Based on review of the diaries, Lynette decides that she wants Daniel to fall asleep earlier in the evening, perhaps between 7 P.M. and 9 P.M. rather than after midnight, and to learn to fall asleep on his own. Intermediate goals, such as gradually shifting the evening bedtime from after midnight to the desired 7 P.M. to 9 P.M. time, an example of shaping a behavior to reach an ultimate goal, could be considered.

Developing Specific Strategies to Change the Behavior

With these behavior goals in mind, Lynette helps develop a plan that uses many behavioral management elements. The plan includes moving the crib from the parent's room into Daniel's room across the hall so that Lynette can respond to his clear signals, but sleep through his sighs and active sleep stages. This strategy is an environmental modification that allows Lynette to ignore systematically minor signals from her son in the night, addressing her own disrupted sleep and promoting independent sleeping for Daniel. She also agrees to shift Daniel's bedtime earlier gradually by about 30 minutes every few nights, while she also moves his wake time earlier in the morning, an example of gradually shaping a behavior. She plans to accomplish this by beginning a short bedtime routine comprising nursing, low lighting, and appealing sounds and interactions such as singing or reading together in Daniel's room that ends with him being put into his crib drowsy but awake. This is an example of learning through classic conditioning, pairing the soothing routine with falling asleep in his crib. She will check on Daniel regularly while he is falling asleep, but only enter his room when he is calm and not crying. This aspect of the plan uses operant conditioning by giving positive reinforcement for only his calm behavior. She also plans to keep any night awakenings "business only" by nursing Daniel and putting him back into his crib as quickly as possible, limiting positive reinforcement for waking in the night. After waking him in the morning, she will keep him active for several hours, which can be conceptualized as applying classic conditioning to set up consistent routines and operant conditioning to provide opportunity for positive interactions through play time. During the day, she will put him into his crib for naps after a shorter version of his bedtime routine at regular times, waking Daniel after any 2-hour nap. This step uses classic conditioning to set up consistent routines.

Implementing and Evaluating the Behavior Program

Lynette needs to continue to keep diaries of Daniel's behaviors and bring them to her next follow-up appointment. Based on progress, new intermediate goals can be developed and new strategies developed. In this case, at follow-up 2 weeks after implementing the plan, Daniel is falling asleep by 9:30 P.M. in his crib with only a little whimpering and waking three times at night to nurse. Naps are more problematic and sporadic. Daniel continues to fall asleep in his mother's arms or in his swing for afternoon naps, but is sometimes placed in his crib when asleep.

Maintaining Behavior Change

Lynette's ability to recognize improvement in Daniel's sleep, and its association with her own improved sleep and mood, will encourage her to set additional goals, such as providing a consistent routine for afternoon naps in Daniel's crib and increasing the frequency of daytime nursing. She decides to wait for stronger signals from Daniel at night before nursing him, stretching out times between feedings in the night, fading the reinforcement of prompt nursing in the night.

Vignette Summary

Daniel's bedtime routine and his mother's plan to encourage him to learn to fall asleep on his own in his crib uses classic and operant conditioning learning techniques as described in Table 87-1 and many of the common behavior management techniques described in Table 87-3. Daniel began to associate his sleepiness, his bath, his full tummy, the low lights, the music, the room, and his crib with sleep onset. When he wakes after any amount of sleeping and clearly signals, he is rewarded with nursing at night and playing in the day, and so this, as well as not being tired anymore, becomes positive reinforcement for sleeping in his crib. Lynette does not interpret putting Daniel down drowsy but awake and letting him settle and possibly fuss as a "time-out" or punishment, which would have been unacceptable to her. Instead she sees this strategy as teaching him an important skill—that he can put himself to sleep with supports and no longer need to be rocked for 30 to 60 minutes or listen to the vacuum to fall asleep. She may need to modify her responses in the night if Daniel gets a cold or if the family travels. Nonetheless, having successfully modified sleep behavior once, his parents have a good chance of revising their strategies to help their son get his sleep back on track when this kind of perturbation has resolved.

ADDRESSING COMMON BEHAVIOR PROBLEMS USING BEHAVIORAL PRINCIPLES

Vignette

Jeff is a single parent who is raising his 9-year-old son, Zachary. He complains that he cannot get Zachary to do anything, and that Zachary does not listen well. Jeff has to tell him over and over to do chores such as make his bed and do his homework, things that "kids his age should be able to do." Jeff constantly finds himself nagging Zachary, which results in Zachary frequently whining, arguing, and talking back. These behaviors also occur at Zachary's school according to reports from his teacher. In particular, Jeff often complains of Zachary fighting with him over bedtime and explains that most nights Zachary refuses to go to bed until 10 or 11 at night. Jeff describes similar difficulties with Zachary not wanting to get up in the morning and not completing his homework.

The practicing clinician is asked to help treat numerous behavioral problems such as those described by Zachary's father. Positive reinforcement strategies, such as social and material rewards, may be employed to increase or strengthen desired behaviors such as cleaning up and doing homework. Punishment strategies, such as systematic ignoring and time-out, may be used to decrease or weaken undesired behaviors such as whining and talking back. Many behavior management programs involve a combination of techniques. In this case, several of the commonly used strategies described in Table 87-3 can be used to improve behavioral compliance and enhance interactions between Zachary and his father.

Developing and Maintaining Positive Interactions

Following early childhood, parents continue to be faced with the burgeoning independence of their child, marked by events such as transitioning to school, participating in extracurricular activities, and developing closer peer relationships. Common challenges in behavior management often manifest as difficulties in children taking increased responsibility (e.g., for self-care, homework, household chores). Although it is developmentally appropriate for children to take increased responsibility and independence, it also is important to foster the development of these goals effectively by maintaining parental involvement.

In this case, in which Zachary presents with multiple noncompliant behaviors, it is particularly important to determine the extent to which Jeff provides opportunities for positive interactions. Any successful behavioral management plan should include regular, daily "special time" when the parent and child enjoy time together. The clinician also should consider factors influencing Jeff's desire for help. Often parents are overwhelmed and frustrated with their struggles in managing their child. In this case, in which Jeff is a single parent, these feelings may be intensified because of the increased responsibility of parenting alone; in dual parent homes, disagreement between parents regarding parenting strategies may be present. Because such factors can interfere with important aspects of implementing a behavior plan (e.g., consistency), they need to be addressed at the outset of developing the behavioral plan.

Defining the Behavior to Be Changed

Jeff may initially identify wanting Zachary to "do what he is told" or "listen" as the behaviors he wants to change. Although these are understandable parental desires, they are not clearly defined enough to be addressed in a behavior plan. The clinician needs to help Jeff define discrete, measurable behaviors that he would like to see Zachary improve or change. These behaviors might include getting up in the morning when called, making his bed each morning, doing homework when asked, going to bed when asked, less whining, and not talking back. Although Jeff can identify many behaviors that he would like Zachary to change, he should be encouraged to select initial behaviors to address. Jeff may decide to select Zachary getting up when called and making his bed in the morning as the initial target behaviors.

Measuring and Monitoring the Target Behavior

Because Jeff has chosen clearly observable behaviors (i.e., Zachary getting out of bed when called and making his bed), a useful monitoring tool could be a form on which Jeff simply records whether or not Zachary got out of bed when called and made his bed each morning. These data would provide a frequency count of the target behaviors. To gain a clearer picture of the context of Zachary's behavior, Jeff also could use an "ABC" chart such as the one in Figure 87-2.

From the "ABC" chart (see Fig. 87-2), the clinician can help Jeff identify several patterns, including that yelling does not seem to change Zachary's behavior, and that no consequences are given to Zachary for his noncompliance. When these patterns are identified, the task of setting a behavior change goal begins.

Setting a Behavior Change Goal

In Zachary's case, even though initial specific target goals may be different at home versus school, the larger goal (e.g., increasing Zachary's compliance with adult

Date/Time	Antecedent	Behavior	Consequence
3/1, 7:00 am	Asked Zachary to get up from bed	Refused to get out of bed for 30 min. and didn't make bed	Yelled at Zachary to make his bed
3/2, 6:45 am	Woke Zachary up and told him to get ready for school	Yelled at me and continued to sleep for another 40 min. and didn't make bed	Yelled and reminded him to get up and make his bed for 45 minutes

Figure 87-2. Antecedent, Behavior, Consequences, or "ABC" chart.

requests) may be similar. In Zachary's case, Jeff may identify several potential target goals in addition to getting out of bed when called and making his bed, including being more compliant throughout the day, reducing his whining, reducing his argumentativeness, going to bed at 9 P.M., and completing his homework on a daily basis. In the process of initially implementing and adding goals to a behavioral plan, the clinician needs to help Jeff break the goals down into smaller, intermediate steps that can be realistically achieved. Initially working on getting Zachary to make his bed every day would likely result in frustration and failure, but working toward getting Zachary to make his bed three times per week initially and then increasing his expectations to 4, 5, 6, and eventually 7 days per week would likely result in greater success and less frustration.

Developing Specific Strategies to Change the Behavior

From examining the behavioral record that Jeff made regarding Zachary's morning behaviors, several instances of parental behavior are apparently related to his noncompliance. Specifically, it seems that Jeff uses nagging (i.e., repeats instructions excessively), yelling, no consequences for noncompliance, and no positive reinforcement for compliance in his interaction. To change Zachary's behavior, the simplest approach would be to begin to address those issues. In addition, techniques such as "time-in," "special time," and "me time" would be a prerequisite to success in preparing Zachary for change via other intervention strategies. Jeff should be "coached" in how to implement these techniques before attempting to change unwanted behaviors.

Implementing and Evaluating the Behavior Program

When parents and teachers are fully informed regarding the behavioral approach chosen, the practitioner is charged with implementing the program. In Zachary's case and many others, noncompliance with requests is often a complaint. Commonly used strategies for increasing compliance employ operant conditioning principles. In Zachary's case, implementing a strategy that includes working with parents and teachers to begin to reinforce compliant behavior using praise and attention would be appropriate. The plan might include providing rewards (e.g., parent interaction, selection of favorite TV show, selection of dessert) for each compliant behavior Zachary displays. As Zachary displays noncompliance at home and school, it will be the task of the practitioner to help caregivers develop practical strategies to increase Zachary's compliance.

At school allowing Zachary to earn a small token (e.g., sticker) for compliance during class time might be difficult given that the teacher has numerous other children in the classroom who are behaving appropriately; however, simply praising Zachary for compliant behavior may be reasonable. In addition, a "daily report card" that records whether Zachary was compliant during different periods of the day and is sent home each day could be used to supplement the praise and enhance teacher-parent communication about how the plan is working. One key to success during this implementation stage will be continuing to keep in mind the principles of immediacy, consistency, and saliency across settings. It also will be necessary to tailor specific strategies to the individual family and setting. When a program has been implemented for a specified period, usually a minimum of 1 to 2 weeks, behavioral change should be observable. The practitioner should have the family and teacher carefully track targeted behaviors and should meet regularly with the family to assess the quality and effectiveness of the strategies being implemented. In many instances, this assessment may require the careful charting of behaviors (see resources at the end of the chapter for examples). If deficits in the program are apparent, the practitioner should be prepared and expect to make revisions to the plan as necessary.

Maintaining Behavior Change

Ultimately, the goal of the strategies implemented would be the gradual withdrawal of systematic reinforcement and the generalization of appropriate behaviors to "real-world" situations. This stage is often neglected in part because parents have already observed significant changes and may become more lackadaisical in their approach. Because the context in which behavior occurs is constantly evolving, it is necessary to plan for changes. The astute practitioner recognizes and expects new behavioral difficulties to appear. Careful planning is necessary. Typically, this planning should take the form of regular "check-in's" with the parent, along with scheduled booster sessions.

IMPROVING ADHERENCE TO MEDICAL REGIMENS USING BEHAVIORAL PRINCIPLES

Vignette

Angela is a 16-year-old girl with insulin-dependent diabetes. Although as a younger child she had periods of not wanting to test her blood glucose, by maintaining close supervision and structure, her family was able to manage her diabetes well. Similar to most teenagers, Angela now spends more and more time with her friends, and her parents no longer provide the supervision that they once did. Her parents also think they should not have to supervise Angela as they did when she was younger, that "Angela should understand that it's her responsibility to take care of her diabetes." Angela has not been testing her blood glucose or giving insulin as scheduled, and she has not been keeping to her diet, particularly when she is out with friends. As her diabetic control has deteriorated, arguments in the home have increased.

Adherence to medical regimens among children and adolescents with chronic medical conditions is another area in which clinicians have the opportunity to use behavioral principles in their interventions. Adherence to medical management is difficult for many children and families. First, consider what children and adolescents with medical conditions and their families are asked to do to care for the child's disease. In the case of asthma, the medical treatment plan is likely to include avoidance of various environmental triggers, administration of preventive medications on a daily basis, and administration of quick relief/rescue medications as needed. Although it may sound simple, this regimen is quite complex and difficult when one remembers that many preventive medications require multiple doses per day, and the "healing" effects of preventive medications are not immediately apparent to the child. The child does not receive positive reinforcement (i.e., does not notice an immediate improvement in breathing) when he or she takes preventive medication. Contrast this with the reinforcement, in the form of improved breathing, the child experiences when he or she administers rescue/quick relief medications. Other medical conditions, including diabetes and cystic fibrosis, provide additional examples of diseases that are treated with multiple interventions (e.g., nutrition, glucose testing and monitoring, and insulin injection in the case of diabetes; nutrition, enzymes and other medications, and chest percussion in the case of cystic fibrosis), the adherence to which may be influenced by behavioral treatment.

Developing and Maintaining Positive Interactions

Adolescence can be a time of increased parent-child conflict as adolescents are challenged with various developmental tasks that facilitate identity formation. Adolescents spend more time outside of their parents' care, asserting their independence by socializing with peers, participating in after-school activities or holding jobs, and challenging parental authority. For an adolescent with a chronic disease, adherence to treatment can become another context in which parent-child conflict arises. From the parental perspective, the difficulty of altering adolescent adherence behaviors may be increased because of less supervision and a desire for the adolescent to be more responsible; from the adolescent perspective, adherence behaviors may be difficult to maintain because of the increasingly social context in which adherence behaviors must occur, immature judgment and decision-making skills, lack of knowledge, and the desire to be like other kids and not have to perform such treatment.

As in other cases, developing and maintaining positive parent-child interactions is important to provide the base from which to enact a behavioral plan to improve adolescent treatment adherence. Taking advantage of the adolescent's natural drive for independence, the clinician can encourage parents to identify areas in which the adolescent can exercise independence without jeopardizing health. Such areas may include, but not be limited to, how the adolescent dresses or keeps his or her room. Parents also can be encouraged to provide positive reinforcement for particular ways that the adolescent has asserted independence or responsibility in an appropriate way, such as helping with a younger sibling or saving money over time to buy something.

Defining the Behavior to Be Changed

Ultimately, Angela's parents want her to take more independent responsibility for her diabetes management. Moving from a situation in which her parents have monitored and controlled all aspects of her care to one in which Angela assumes full responsibility is a big step, however. The clinician should help the family break down this ultimate goal into smaller parts by asking questions such as, "What does Angela need to do to take care of her diabetes?" or "What parts of her diabetes care is Angela doing better/worse with?" This step can have the effect of helping family members realize that adherence is difficult because of everything it entails, and aid in identifying areas of adherence that are more or less problematic. When the various aspects of adherence are outlined, and strengths and weaknesses are identified, the clinician can help Angela's family pick a specific aspect of adherence to be addressed initially (other areas would certainly be added as treatment progresses). In this case, the family decides to address the behavior of blood glucose testing and insulin administration when Angela is out with friends.

This case assumes that Angela has the knowledge and technical skills necessary to perform these behaviors. If this were not true, diabetic education to ensure skill development would be necessary before establishing the goal that Angela perform these skills in social situations.

Measuring and Monitoring the Target Behavior

A behavior chart that lists the adherence behaviors to be monitored and allows for record keeping each day as to whether the behavior was performed would be a useful way for Angela and her parents to monitor the chosen target behaviors. In addition, the family can use the blood glucose results from Angela's glucometer to verify when testing was done and what the result was.

Setting a Behavior Change Goal

Although the ultimate goal is for Angela to perform her diabetic care fully when with peers, the clinician can help family members agree on some intermediate goals. An initial goal could be for Angela to show increased independence in adherence behaviors at home. In addition, the family might agree to set a goal in which only a portion of adherence behaviors need to be done independently at the outset. Finally, the family could set goals for independent blood glucose testing or glucose monitoring in certain peer situations where success may be more likely (e.g., when Angela is with smaller groups of best friends who know about her diabetes), before setting the goal for this to occur in all peer situations.

Developing Specific Strategies to Change the Behavior

Angela has a strong desire to spend time with her friends, so the reward of increased freedom to be with friends is a strong motivator and could be used as potential positive reinforcement of success with the behavioral goals. Because data from the glucometer can confirm whether blood glucose testing was done when Angela is with her friends, time with friends also could be conceived as a logical consequence to adherence in that the consequence for lack of diabetic care when with friends could be less time with friends. Stimulus control techniques, such as setting up times with friends specifically to include circumscribed needs for adherence behaviors (e.g., meeting a friend for lunch for 1 hour, not spending an entire day with a friend) also might be employed.

Implementing and Evaluating the Behavior Program

With respect to implementation, Angela and her family could consider what role Angela's friends might play. Adolescents with diabetes receive support from their peers that may enhance adherence to blood glucose testing (Bearman and La Greca, 2002); Angela's peers may be in a position to encourage and support her in meeting her adherence goals. Other issues to consider are that Angela's parents may be setting increased limits about the amount of time she is allowed to spend with peers, and this could increase conflict between them and Angela. One strategy to reduce this conflict may be for Angela's parents to help her identify times she can be with friends when diabetic adherence behaviors are not routinely required (e.g., spending time with friends between eating times).

Because of the electronic recording of Angela's glucometer, there are ample concrete data to evaluate whether adherence behaviors are being conducted and in what contexts. With such information, Angela and her parents will know whether the goals are being met and when additional goals, either with respect to achieving the same behaviors more often or in new contexts, or becoming more independent in other adherence behaviors (e.g., accurate carbohydrate counting), can be introduced.

Maintaining Behavior Change

One specific issue to maintaining behavior change in this case is Angela's ability to generalize the skills of independent adherence behaviors to new contexts (e.g., summer or after-school job) as she develops. Similar strategies of having Angela gradually increase her involvement in such activities as she shows appropriate adherence could be considered. Another issue, which is similar to maintaining behavior change in other cases, is Angela's parents' ability to continue to monitor her success despite their desire for her to function with less involvement on their part. The clinician should provide praise and encouragement to the family, using the data of Angela's success as evidence of the importance of their efforts and to reinforce their continued involvement. Over time, the family can be guided to reduce their involvement and assess the effect of that change on Angela's adherence.

WHEN TO REFER

Given the constraints of the primary care clinician and the complexity of some cases, there are times when it is advisable to refer the family to a behavioral specialist. In particular, this course of action is recommended in cases where the behavioral concerns are complicated by significant family dysfunction or child psychopathology, or when the practitioner either is uncomfortable working within this framework or does not have adequate time to provide such treatment.

SUMMARY

The goals of this chapter were to highlight behavioral principles, provide an orientation to the steps involved in using behavioral strategies, and show how behavioral strategies can be implemented to address issues across the developmental spectrum. Using these principles, an effective and systematic approach to behavior management can be implemented in either primary care or subspecialty offices.

REFERENCES

Bearman KJ, La Greca AM: Assessing friend support for adolescents' diabetes care: The Diabetes Social Support Questionnaire–Friends Version. J Pediatr Psychol 27:417-428, 2002.

Blanchard LT, Gurka MJ, Blackman JA: Emotional, developmental, and behavioral health of American children and their families: A report from the 2003 National Survey of Children's Health. Pediatrics 117:e1202-e1212, 2006.

Kelleher KJ, McInerny TK, Gardner WP, et al: Increasing identification of psychosocial problems: 1979-1996. Pediatrics 105:1313-1321, 2000.

Shonkoff JP, Phillips DA (eds): From Neurons to Neighborhoods: The Science of Early Child Development. Washington, DC, National Academy Press, 2000.

Young KT, Davis K, Schoen C, Parker S: Listening to parents. Arch Pediatr Adolesc Med 152:255-262, 1998.

RESOURCES FOR PARENTS AND PROFESSIONALISM

Bloomquist ML: Skills Training for Children with Behavior Problems: A Parent and Therapist Guidebook (rev ed). New York: Guilford Press, 2005.

Christopherson ER, Mortweet SL: Treatments That Work with Children: Empirically Supported Strategies for Managing Childhood Problems. Washington, DC, American Psychological Association, 2001.

Clark L, Robb J: SOS Help for Parents: A Practical Guide for Handling Common Behavior Problems, 3rd ed. Bowling Green, KY, Parents Press, 2005.

Degangi GA, Kendall A: Effective Parenting for the Hard-to-Manage Child: A Skills-Based Book. New York, Routledge, 2008.

Drotar D(Ed): Promoting Adherence to Medical Treatment in Chronic Childhood Illness: Concepts, Methods, and Interventions, Mahwah, NJ, Lawrence Erlbaum, 2000.

Drotar D: Psychological Interventions in Childhood Chronic Illness. Washington, DC, American Psychological Association, 2006.

Silver LB: The Misunderstood Child: Understanding and Coping with Your Child's Learning Disabilities, 4th ed. New York, Three Rivers Press, 2006.

Webster-Stratton C: The Incredible Years: Parents, Teachers, and Children Training Series. Available at: http://www.incredibleyears.com.

88 CRISIS MANAGEMENT

Mirna Farah and Thomas Chun

In a crisis situation, parents often bring their children to the emergency department for prompt evaluation and timely care. Crisis can arise from many heterogeneous conditions; some are part of normal childhood development, and others are manifestations of an organic or psychiatric disorder. For all of these conditions, a carefully taken history, in a calming and supportive manner, is the essential part of the evaluation. Key information includes any precipitating factors, any history of similar symptoms in the child or family members, and any past medical history of a psychiatric or medical condition. This should be followed by a thorough physical examination to look for an organic cause of the behavior, particularly signs of neurologic deficit, intoxication, injury, or a source of pain and discomfort. Laboratory and imaging studies are not always necessary and should be guided by the history and physical examination findings. After documentation of these findings and institution of appropriate initial care, proper follow-up with the primary care physician or referral to a specialist for ongoing care is the basis of treatment for most of these conditions. Although this chapter is written from the emergency department point of view, it applies equally to the practitioner in his or her office.

THE AGITATED OR VIOLENT CHILD

Identification

Agitated or violent behavior covers a wide spectrum of behaviors. In its mildest form, a patient may appear only anxious, restless, or jittery. The patient might speak loudly, swear, or not speak at all. More severe forms include all manner of verbal or physical threats, self-injury, and physical assault on others. Alternatively, patients may be disoriented, combative, and unresponsive to direction. The paramount concern in evaluation and management of these patients is safety, not only of the patient but also of the treating staff and any other potential victims of violence. Because treatment options may range from simple removal of an instigating or exacerbating stimulus to five-point physical restraints with additional chemical restraint, differentiation between the possible causes of the behavior in a crisis situation is also crucial (Heyneman, 2003).

Differential Diagnosis

Agitated or violent behavior is not a diagnosis unto itself but rather the final common pathway for any number of medical, psychological, social, and environmental causes. In many cases, the cause of the behavior may be multifactorial. Medical causes of agitated or violent behavior include any condition that can alter a patient's cognitive or behavioral functioning. By far the most commonly encountered causes are intoxication and traumatic injuries, especially head injuries. Other possible causes include brain tumors, seizures, and any infections or medical condition causing delirium (toxic encephalopathy). The fact that the number of potential medical causes is so large underscores the importance of a careful and thorough history and physical examination.

Violence is an uncommon symptom of psychiatric illness, although agitation is frequently seen. Violence or agitation may be part of the underlying psychiatric condition or may be a manifestation of poor frustration tolerance. Psychiatric conditions that can present with violence or agitation include anxiety disorders, such as post-traumatic stress disorder; mood disorders, such as major depression and bipolar illness; psychotic disorders, such as schizophrenia; and disruptive disorders, such as attention-deficit/hyperactivity disorder, conduct disorder, and oppositional defiant disorder. Learning disorders and pervasive developmental disorders such as autism, Asperger syndrome, and Rett syndrome may also present in this manner.

Agitated or violent behavior may also be the result of social or environmental stressors. Children or adolescents who experience violence in their home setting (i.e., abuse inflicted on them or their family members) may respond with violence or agitation. Patients who feel unsafe in their home environments (e.g., fear of physical assault, drug- or gang-related behaviors) may also present with agitation or violence.

A patient must have his or her behavior under control before a medical and psychiatric examination can be performed. A calm, polite, respectful environment can be helpful in promoting safe behavior. The patient should be placed in a quiet, low-stimulus room, one that is free of any hazardous objects and in which the patient can be observed.

History taking should focus on risk factors for immediate and future violence. Past and recent histories of violent ideation and behaviors as well as access to weapons should be elicited. Current stressors and social situation, any history of impulsive or bizarre behavior, and impaired thought processes or judgment are all important for treatment planning.

A careful physical examination should be performed on all patients. Patients may have already injured themselves, which can be missed if they are not completely examined. In addition, they and their belongings should be searched for any weapons or objects that could be used as weapons. There is no standard laboratory evaluation of these patients. Laboratory evaluations should be obtained on the basis of clinical suspicion of possible underlying medical conditions.

Initial Management

As with other patients, the overall guiding principle for treatment of agitated or violent patients is to use the least restrictive methods possible. Nonrestrictive techniques may include providing a quiet space, offering choices, removing upsetting stimuli (which may include people in the patient's life), and clear, nonpunitive communication (e.g., expectations, rules, and limit setting). These measures facilitate the dignity and autonomy of patients and thus may help them control their behavior.

Table 88-1 lists medications commonly used for chemical restraint. Most experts consider these medications to be both safe and efficacious. Oral administration of medication is always the preferred route; however, in many situations, intramuscular administration may be necessary. The newer atypical antipsychotic medications appear to have better adverse effect profiles compared with older, "typical" antipsychotics. A common strategy favored by many experts is a combination of antipsychotic medication and benzodiazepine. This combination may be more effective than either drug alone and may result in less total medication needed to effectively restrain the patient (DeFruyt and Demyttenaere, 2004; Yildiz et al, 2003).

Studies of adverse outcomes due to the use of physical restraint have shown that these outcomes occur at greater rates in children than in adults. As a result, the Health Care Financing Administration and the Joint Commission on Accreditation of Healthcare Organizations now mandate that all hospital-based physical restraint adhere to strict standards and guidelines for the application and monitoring of such restraint.

A patient's ultimate disposition is contingent on whether the patient can be safely managed on an outpatient basis. If there is any question as to whether patients can be safe with themselves and in their home environment, mental health or social services consultation should be obtained. Chapter 40 offers further discussion on the subject of the agitated or violent child.

THE DEPRESSED OR SUICIDAL CHILD

Identification

The point prevalence of depression is approximately 2% of school-age children and 4% to 6% of adolescents. The lifetime prevalence of depression in adolescents is 20% to 25%. Suicide, unfortunately, is the third leading cause of death among children and adolescents.

The pathways to depression are complex and variable. Adoption, twin, and family studies all clearly demonstrate the significance of biologic factors. However, stressful environmental factors (e.g., parental divorce, school problems, relationship breakups, or maltreatment) often play critical roles in the onset of depressive episodes.

Depressive symptoms vary by age. Some, like hopelessness, hallucinations, and delusions, can be difficult to assess or absent in younger children. The younger the child, the more likely the child is to have somatic complaints. In older children, symptoms such as anhedonia, hopelessness, hypersomnia, weight gain, and social withdrawal may be more common. In adolescents, irritable mood may be as common as or more common than depressed mood.

Table 88-1. **Chemical Restraint Medications**

Medication	Dose	Route of Administration*	Comments and Adverse Effect
Diphenhydramine	<12 years: 1.25 mg/kg Teen: 50 mg	PO, IM, IV	
Hydroxyzine	<12 years: 1.25 mg/kg Teen: 50 mg	PO, IM, IV	
Lorazepam	<12 years: 0.05-0.1 mg/kg Teen: 2-4 mg	PO, IM, IV	May redose every 60 minutes
Midazolam	<12 years: 0.05-0.15 mg/kg Teen: 2-4 mg	PO, IM, IV	May redose every 60 minutes
Haloperidol	<12 years: 0.1 mg/kg Teen: 2-5 mg	PO, IM, IV	May redose every 60 minutes May prolong QTc
Risperidone	<12 years: 0.5 mg Teen: 1 mg	PO, IM, IV	
Olanzapine	<12 years: 2.5 mg Teen: 5-10 mg	PO, IM, IV	
Quetiapine	25 mg	PO	
Ziprasidone	<12 years: 5 mg Teen: 10 -20 mg	PO, IM, IV	May prolong QTc

*The preferred route of administration of the medications listed for an agitated patient is either oral (PO) or intramuscular (IM). Although it is probably safe to give them intravenously (IV), they are not approved by the Food and Drug Administration to be given by this route.

Differential Diagnosis

Comorbid psychiatric conditions are the rule rather than the exception. Substance abuse, anxiety, developmental, and post-traumatic stress disorders are also frequently present. The multitude of medical conditions that can present with depression merits a comprehensive and thorough history and physical examination.

Those who complete (as opposed to those who attempt but do not complete) suicide tend to be male and to have histories of persistent psychiatric problems (especially depression or bipolar disorder), substance abuse, antisocial behavior, use of more lethal methods to attempt suicide, and impulsive or obsessive traits. Lack of these risk factors does not automatically mean that a patient is "low risk" for suicide completion. All suicide attempts should be taken seriously and thoroughly evaluated. The large majority of these patients warrant an evaluation by a mental health professional.

Initial Management

As discussed, the primary objectives of an emergency evaluation center around ruling out acute medical conditions that may be causing the patient's symptoms and a careful safety evaluation of the patient and his or her home environment. To be discharged and safely treated on an outpatient basis, patients must be considered to be at low risk for future unsafe behavior as well as have home environments capable of adequately supervising them. All others should have an inpatient psychiatric evaluation and treatment once they are medically stable. "No suicide contracts" and "contracts for safety" have not been shown to prevent suicide. They are widely used, primarily as assessment tools, and should not be considered a substitute for a comprehensive and meticulous evaluation (Harrington, 2001). Chapter 47 offers further discussion on the subject of the depressed or suicidal child.

THE TRAUMATIZED CHILD

Identification

Psychological trauma can take many forms in childhood. Traumatic experiences can be a one-time event (e.g., a dog bite) or chronic and long-lasting (e.g., being raised by an abusive parent). The two most common types of trauma are being witnesses to violence (e.g., domestic or community violence) and being the victim of assault (e.g., physical or sexual abuse) or neglect. The cardinal features of post-traumatic stress disorder are exposure to an extreme traumatic stressor, intrusive re-experience of the trauma, persistent avoidance of stimuli associated with the trauma, and recurrent symptoms of physiologic arousal. Symptoms tend to vary by age. Avoidant symptoms may be absent or children may not report them. Physiologic symptoms may be headaches or stomachaches and not the classic symptoms of autonomic arousal. Fears and anxieties unrelated to the trauma may occur in younger children.

When child abuse is suspected, obtaining a detailed history of the events is the most important part of the medical evaluation and may be the only identifying factor of child abuse. For preverbal children, the history is obtained from the caregiver. Older children should be encouraged to vocalize what they witnessed. Asking age-appropriate, open-ended questions in a comforting, blame-free, and reassuring manner is essential. After the child is interviewed, careful documentation of the signs of injury, if any, by written descriptions with exact measurements or by taking pictures, is important and should be done in the presence of a trusted caretaker.

Differential Diagnosis

Comorbid psychiatric conditions, especially mood, anxiety, and impulse control disorders, are common. Psychotic disorders, borderline personality disorder, and dissociative disorders may also be comorbid although difficult to differentiate.

Initial Management

The emergent evaluation of a traumatized child should focus on detection of any underlying medical conditions and a safety assessment. Definitive psychiatric diagnoses can be deferred until a later time. Reassuring the patients that an abusive event was not their fault and encouraging them to talk about their feelings are helpful. Counseling parents to support their children by being available when needed, removing blame, and ensuring their safety decreases their sense of helplessness.

If there are no acute safety concerns, the patient can be discharged with a trusted caretaker with close counseling or psychiatric follow-up for further diagnostic evaluation and comprehensive treatment. Medications are usually not indicated, but on occasion, mild sedatives (see Table 88-1) such as an antihistamine or benzodiazepine may be considered (DeBellis and Van Dillen, 2005). Chapter 10 offers further discussion on the subject of the abused child.

THE NONCOMPLIANT CHILD

Identification

Compliance is broadly defined as the extent to which patients adhere to medical therapy as prescribed by their health care providers (Nevins, 2005; Osterberg and Blaschke, 2005). The term *compliance* has fallen out of favor as it is perceived to be authoritarian. The terms *adherence* and *concordance* are currently preferred synonyms that more clearly reflect the active involvement of the patient in medical decision making (Osterberg and Blaschke, 2005).

Nonadherence in medical therapy is a ubiquitous problem. In patients with chronic medical problems, rates of nonadherence have been reported to be as high as 30% to 50%. Nonadherence is less prevalent in patients with acute illnesses. Concurrent psychiatric diagnoses, especially depression, also affect adherence. Depressed patients are up to three times as likely to be nonadherent with medical therapy (DiMatteo et al, 2000). A clear sign of treatment nonadherence is worsening of symptoms despite supposedly adequate therapy, a discrepancy between the history and clinical picture.

Initial Management

Management of treatment nonadherence begins with an exploration of the reasons for noncompliance in the particular patient. Keeping in mind the prevalence of nonadherence, a nonjudgmental discussion should be held with the patient, identified issues addressed, and a tailored treatment plan created for each individual patient. It is imperative to avoid blame. Active participation and collaboration must be encouraged.

Adolescent patients are at especially high risk of nonadherence for a multitude of reasons, including peer pressure and the struggle for autonomy. It is therefore important to increase the teenage patient's involvement in his or her care. The teen should be evaluated alone at some point during the visit. Education should be provided at his or her level of understanding and concrete short-term goals agreed on. It is also useful to delineate a daily routine that involves the medication regimen and provides cues to remind the patient to take the medication. For example, a morning dose could be placed near the toothbrush as a cue. Pill boxes may also be useful as cues. As much as possible, the medication regimen should be simplified with the use of "forgiving drugs," that is, those drugs with long half-lives that therefore allow less frequent dosing, whenever feasible (Nevins, 2005; Yeo and Sawyer, 2005). Above all, an effective patient-provider relationship that lends itself to clear lines of communication and improved patient education and participation should be established. Chapter 39 offers further discussion on the subject of medical noncompliance.

THE INTOXICATED CHILD

Identification

The use of drugs of abuse in the pediatric and young adult population is a widespread problem. According to 2005 statistics from the National Institute on Drug Abuse, 50% of twelfth graders reported having used a drug of abuse in the past. Alcohol, tobacco, and marijuana were the top three most frequently reported illicit drugs used, but ecstasy, methamphetamines, and cocaine are also commonly used; 4.5% to 8% of all twelfth graders had used one of these (Johnston et al, 2006). Many of these substances can cause significant acute medical problems; cocaine, for instance, is associated with a risk of cardiac ischemia (Rimsza and Moses, 2005), and ecstasy is known to cause life-threatening hyperpyrexia and hyponatremia (Ricaurte and McCann, 2005). The topic of pediatric intoxications is also covered in Chapter 45. Here, the acute presentation and management are discussed.

Differential Diagnosis

Acute mental status changes in a previously healthy patient, especially after a social event, should prompt the clinician to evaluate for possible ingestions. In many cases, polydrug use occurs, and patients may not be able or willing to identify the specific drug (Ricaurte and McCann, 2005).

Table 88-2. Common Causes of Altered Mental Status

Stroke
Seizures
Intracranial bleed
Intracranial lesions or masses
Meningitis
Encephalitis
Traumatic head injury
Hypoglycemia
Electrolyte imbalances
Toxic ingestions

The differential diagnosis for a patient presenting with altered mental status is extensive, but history and physical examination and laboratory findings will aid in narrowing the list (Table 88-2). For example, infectious causes such as meningitis and encephalitis should be associated with other signs and symptoms of infection such as fever, and patients with stroke generally exhibit focal neurologic deficits.

Initial Management

Immediate stabilization of the patient is the highest priority. The airway is assessed for patency, breath sounds are auscultated, and the circulatory status of the patient is appraised through palpation of central pulses and evaluation of heart rate and blood pressure. Other vital signs should be assessed. Any disorder noted in this initial assessment is potentially life-threatening and must be addressed without delay. A thorough physical examination should follow. Mental status should be assessed, and the patient is evaluated for the presence of specific patterns of vital sign and examination findings characteristic of toxidromes.

Early consultation with the toxicology team or the local poison control center is warranted. If recent ingestion is obvious from the history and the patient is alert and cooperative, activated charcoal could be given after consultation with the toxicology team. If the patient is obtunded or poorly responsive, a dose of naloxone may be given to reverse a possible opioid overdose. Glucose and thiamine are administered to the adolescent or adult patient with suspected chronic alcohol abuse. In all patients with altered mental status, intravenous access should be obtained and oxygen administered. Initial laboratory investigation and testing include bedside serum glucose evaluation, electrocardiography, serum and urine toxicology, and serum electrolyte determinations. Once the patient is stabilized, a more thorough search for the etiologic agent is embarked on.

THE ANXIOUS AND HYPERVENTILATING CHILD

Identification

Anxious children may present to the emergency department for an unrelated medical condition or during an anxiety or panic attack. A variety of symptoms can be manifested, including dyspnea, tachypnea, breathlessness, chest tightness and pain, palpitations, anxiety, panic and a feeling of impending doom, paresthesias, coldness of the extremities, tetany, trembling, blurred vision, dry mouth, headache, lightheadedness, syncope, and seizure (Folgering, 1999). These symptoms can occur in "spells" lasting a few minutes to several hours each. They are due to the physiologic derangement produced by hyperventilation and the underlying psychiatric disturbance (Herman et al, 1981). Physical examination may reveal obvious hyperventilation, or more commonly, the patient may be observed to take periodic deep sighing respirations.

Differential Diagnosis

Intensive efforts should be made to diagnose functional symptoms at an early stage to prevent children from undergoing unnecessary and potentially harmful tests and therapies. Organic disorders that require serious consideration in the differential diagnosis include asthma, thyrotoxicosis, arrhythmia, metabolic acidosis, hyperammonemia, hypocalcemia, drug intoxication (including salicylism), hypercapnia, cirrhosis, organic central nervous system disorders, fever, and response to severe pain. A few paroxysmal disorders, such as hypotensive syncope, Stokes-Adams attacks, epilepsy, and migraine, should be ruled out.

Elements of history that suggest the diagnosis of hyperventilation syndrome include the lack of nocturnal symptoms, the sudden occurrence (even at rest without the typical trigger factors), the chronicity of the complaint, the unrelatedness of symptoms, the references to breathlessness, and the expressions of anxiety. Assessment of whether voluntary hyperventilation reproduces the patient's symptoms is also helpful. Termination of symptoms by rebreathing into a paper bag is another suggestive finding.

When the syndrome is recognized, extensive laboratory evaluation is rarely required in the pediatric population and may add to the child's overwhelming anxiety. The specific tests obtained should be determined by the patient's symptoms but will usually be selected from among chest radiography, electrocardiography, serum calcium and electrolyte determinations, and blood gas analysis.

Initial Management

The therapeutic approach to an anxiety attack has several stages or degrees of intervention: psychological counseling, physiotherapy, and pharmacotherapy.

Psychological Counseling

Reassurance by physicians, family, and professionals is the most prominent instrument to reduce or to diminish observed respiratory symptoms in the absence of significant organic abnormality. Children and adolescents need to be reassured in specific terms relevant to their fears. Counseling and psychiatric referral are necessary to discover the sources of the psychological disturbance experienced by the child.

Physiotherapy

The classic remedy for hyperventilation is relaxation and breathing into a paper bag. For adolescents in particular, emphasizing that the patient has control over the production of symptoms is important. This understanding is often accomplished by voluntary overbreathing, attribution of cause of symptoms to hyperventilation, and breathing training with emphasis on diaphragmatic breathing and slowing of expiration. Relaxation techniques such as self-hypnosis may positively influence the pathologic breathing pattern and slow the respiratory rate. Relaxation may also diminish the underlying anxiety. Parents and others should also be instructed to avoid reinforcing the patient's symptoms through attention.

Pharmacotherapy

A major goal is to avoid or to reduce the use of pharmacotherapy, limiting it to patients who fail to respond to education and counseling. Propranolol and anxiolytics have been used successfully in children to interrupt these spells. Chapter 47 offers further discussion on the subject of the anxious child.

THE CHILD WITH DISTURBED SLEEP

Identification and Management

Childhood sleep disturbances are common, occurring in 20% to 30% of children between the ages of 1 and 8 years. Some sleep disorders are based on disturbed sleep processes and may appear with dramatic, often paroxysmal clinical features that are frightening to the family and are likely to be seen in the emergency department (Howard and Wong, 2001).

Night terrors (pavor nocturnus) are dramatic events seen in as many as 20% of children between 5 and 7 years of age, but their frequency decreases as they get older. The child abruptly awakens 15 to 90 minutes after sleep onset with a piercing scream or cry, sits up in bed with wide-open eyes and extreme anxiety, and manifests many autonomic phenomena (sweating, flushing, racing heart beat, and rapid breathing). The child appears confused, is not able to recognize the parents, and is inconsolable for 10 to 15 minutes. Then the child relaxes and falls back to quiet sleep with no recollection of the event in the morning. Night terrors usually occur so rarely that treatment is not necessary (Wise, 1997). Attempts to waken the child and descriptions of the event to the child are not helpful.

Nightmares are unpleasant dreams from which the child is usually awake and responsive by the time the parents arrive and for which substantial recall can occur. Approximately 10% to 50% of children between the ages of 3 and 6 years experience a nightmare, but this frequency decreases over time. The child who just had a nightmare should be reassured with embraces and soothing words, and the parent should stay until the child is calm. Parents of children with occasional nightmares should be reassured about the benign nature of these episodes. Frequent nightmares may be a sign of distress that merits a psychological evaluation. Certain medications can trigger nightmares, such as levodopa, beta-blockers, and withdrawal from REM-suppressing drugs (Ward and Mason, 2002).

Obstructive sleep apnea syndrome affects 1% to 3% of all children and peaks between 2 and 6 years of age. It is caused by upper airway obstruction resulting in frequent apneic spells during sleep, hypoxia, hypercapnia, frequent arousals, and sleep fragmentation. Children may present with loud snoring, excess daytime somnolence, morning headaches, hypertension, cardiac arrhythmias, cor pulmonale, failure-to-thrive, enuresis, anoxic seizures, aggressiveness, decreased attention span, and poor school performance. Predisposing risk factors to obstructive sleep apnea include craniofacial abnormalities, hypotonia, and morbid obesity. Overnight polysomnography is the gold standard to confirm the presence and severity of obstructive sleep apnea. Management involves otolaryngologic consultation for thorough airway evaluation and appropriate measures to relieve obstruction, maintenance of continuous positive airway pressure, and initiation of weight loss in obese children. However, the most common treatment of obstructive sleep apnea is tonsillectomy and adenoidectomy, after which symptoms resolve in 70% of cases (Loughlin, 1992). Chapter 64 offers further discussion on the subject of sleep problems.

SUMMARY

We have discussed a wide selection of common behavioral emergencies that may be encountered in the emergency department or primary care setting. The general principles of evaluation and initial management of all such presentations are similar. In all cases, it is imperative to obtain a thorough history and to perform a physical examination to narrow the differential, which quite often involves myriad possible causes. Life- and limb-threatening problems should be identified and dealt with immediately. A thorough search should also be made for underlying organic causes of the behavioral abnormality. Finally, effective ongoing care beyond the acute setting is predicated on clear communication with the primary care physician and subspecialist team (if required) in addition to encouraging a strong patient-provider relationship between these providers and the patient.

REFERENCES

DeBellis MD, Van Dillen T: Childhood post-traumatic stress disorder: An overview. Child Adolesc Psychiatr Clin North Am 14:745-772, 2005.

DeFruyt J, Demyttenaere K: Rapid tranquilization: New approaches in the emergency treatment of behavioral disturbances. Eur Psychiatry 19:243-249, 2004.

DiMatteo MR, Lepper HS, Croghan TW: Depression is a risk factor for noncompliance with medical treatment: Meta-analysis of the effects of anxiety and depression on patient adherence. Arch Intern Med 160:2101-2107, 2000.

Folgering H: The pathophysiology of hyperventilation syndrome. Monaldi Arch Chest Dis 54:365-372, 1999.

Harrington R: Depression, suicide and deliberate self-harm in adolescence. Br Med Bull 57:47-60, 2001.

Herman SP, Stickler GB, Lucas AR: Hyperventilation syndrome in children and adolescents: Long-term follow-up. Pediatrics 67:183-187, 1981.

Heyneman EK: The aggressive child. Child Adolesc Psychiatr Clinics North Am 12:667-677, 2003.

Howard BJ, Wong J: Sleep disorders. Pediatr Rev 22:327-342, 2001.

Johnston LD, O'Malley PM, Bachman JG, Schulenberg JE: Teen drug use continues down in 2006, particularly among older teens; but use of prescription-type drugs remains high. University of Michigan News and Information Services, Ann Arbor, MI. Available at: www.monitoringthefuture.org. Accessed January 18, 2006.

Loughlin GM: Obstructive sleep apnea in children. Adv Pediatr 39:307-336, 1992.

Nevins TE: "Why do they do that?" The compliance conundrum. Pediatr Nephrol 20:845-848, 2005.

Osterberg L, Blaschke T: Adherence to medication. N Engl J Med 353:487-497, 2005.

Ricaurte GA, McCann UD: Recognition and management of complications of new recreational drug use. Lancet 365:2137-2145, 2005.

Rimsza ME, Moses KS: Substance abuse on the college campus. Pediatr Clin North Am 52:307-319, xii, 2005.

Ward T, Mason TB: Sleep disorders in children. Nurs Clin North Am 37:693-706, 2002.

Wise MS: Parasomnias in children. Pediatr Ann 26:427-433, 1997.

Yeo M, Sawyer S: Chronic illness and disability. BMJ 330:721-723, 2005.

Yildiz A, Sachs GS, Turgay A: Pharmacological management of agitation in emergency settings. Emerg Med J 20:339-346, 2003.

89 PSYCHOTHERAPY WITH CHILDREN AND ADOLESCENTS

Jane E. Caplan, Craigan T. Usher, and Michael S. Jellinek

> *"A sign of health in the mind is the ability of one individual to enter imaginatively and accurately into the thoughts and feelings and hopes and fears of another person; to allow the other person to do the same to us.... When we are face to face with a man, woman or child in our specialty, we are reduced to two human beings of equal status."*
>
> —D. W. Winnicott

Pediatricians are often asked to assess and to intervene in behavioral and emotional issues. Interventions include monitoring children, providing suggestions on negotiation of difficult transitions, prescribing psychotropic medication, and giving advice to parents and children on how to use "real-life" phenomena to bring about positive change. Advice about modifying rules or reframing a tension in the family is often therapeutic. Pediatricians often refer children and their families for formal "therapy" when the problems are severe, intractable, or dangerous. What constitutes therapy is often quite mysterious. It is this, the mystery of therapy, including the types, goals, and role of the pediatrician, that we hope to address in this chapter.

D. W. Winnicott, a British pediatrician and child psychotherapist who closely examined the inner lives of children, noted that the ability of a child or, for that matter, an adult to conceptualize "the thoughts and feelings and hopes and fears of another person" constitutes "health in the mind." The essence of what makes an intervention "psychotherapeutic" is that it repairs the ability "to enter imaginatively and accurately into the thoughts and feelings and hopes and fears of another person." Consider the teenager with an eating disorder who becomes so preoccupied with being thin, often to the point of starvation, that she is severely limited in seeing her own and others' needs. Similarly, parents who are in the process of divorce can sometimes become so focused on their own anger and sadness that they cannot feel empathy for their child. The child's fear and loneliness then overwhelm any ability to cope and are manifested in symptoms (Winnicott, 1965).

In this chapter, we define mental health; provide examples of when children's and teenagers' abilities to imaginatively and accurately perceive the thoughts and feelings of others go awry and demonstrate the therapeutic ways in which pediatricians routinely tackle these situations; offer practical advice on how to initiate the referral process; describe various forms of psychotherapy; provide guidelines for communication between therapists and pediatricians; and examine evidence regarding psychotherapy and what challenges lie ahead in better determining which types of psychotherapy work and for whom. Despite our recognition that practitioners from many different disciplines work in the care of children, we have employed the conventions of pediatrician (to describe any professional working on the pediatric medical team) and psychiatrist or therapist (to describe members of the mental health team).

MENTAL HEALTH

Winnicott offers that "a sign of health in the mind is the ability of one individual to enter imaginatively and accurately into the thoughts and feelings and hopes and fears of another person." By defining mental health in this way, neither Winnicott nor we are claiming that one need be 100% correct about what is on another person's mind, only "accurate enough."

With or without conscious awareness, pediatricians are Winnicottian. They develop a complex, psychologically rich view of children and parents. While taking histories and through observation, pediatricians often address whether the parent or child sees himself or herself in a reasonable manner, if there exist consistent unshakable distortions, and if the parent and child present a coherent narrative of the problem. Intuitively, pediatricians are mindful of "red flag" answers to these questions, acknowledging that sometimes there is more than meets the eye, inquire further, and intervene.

THE PEDIATRICIAN'S PSYCHOTHERAPEUTIC REPERTOIRE

Pediatricians use their own ability to imaginatively and accurately enter the thoughts and feelings of their patients and families to discern how relationships and interactions have gotten off track and offer psychosocial treatments that are "therapeutic," that is, interventions that help children or adolescents more accurately examine their own and others' thoughts, feelings, hopes, and fears. Healthier families possess the psychological capacity to listen and to modify their interactions with children in response to the child's behaviors and needs. Families who lack the capacity for empathy fall into rigid, maladaptive patterns of thinking, feeling, and acting. In these cases, more intensive treatment is warranted.

The following vignettes highlight the pediatrician's role in addressing mental and emotional problems, describe both the successes and limitations of those interventions, and provide guidance on when to refer for therapy. Later in the chapter, we examine how different forms of therapy would address these problems and refer back to these clinical studies.

Vignette

Aidan is a 7-year-old boy whose mother reported classic symptoms of attention-deficit/hyperactivity disorder both at home and in school. Aidan's pediatrician had encouraged his parents to use behavioral techniques to address his symptoms. Aidan's parents also worked hard to establish consistent routines and encouraged Aidan to learn organizational skills with his toys and school supplies. During the next month, marginal gains were seen in Aidan's behavior, and after discussion with his family, the pediatrician opted to prescribe a stimulant. Two months later, Aidan's mother described improvements in both Aidan's inattention and hyperactivity. For the first time, he received positive feedback from his teachers at school, and his parents and siblings found him more enjoyable to be around at home. Despite the positive attention he was receiving, Aidan was very self-critical. At times, Aidan deliberately drew negative attention to himself. As his mother described this, Aidan, who was playing with some toy cars in the office, crashed the cars so hard that one of the car doors fell off, and the other dented the wall. Aidan's mom yelled at him for breaking the toys, and Aidan sulked in the corner.

In Aidan's case, although the patient's primary symptoms of attention-deficit/hyperactivity disorder were treated effectively with a stimulant, he continued to have behavioral problems rooted in profound poor self-esteem (see Chapter 44). The pediatrician saw his behavior as serious and entrenched and referred him to a therapist.

Vignette

Jennifer is a 14-year-old girl whose parents are in the middle of a divorce. During her annual check-up, the pediatrician was surprised to discover Jennifer dressed seductively, a major change from her previous appearance. During her visit, Jennifer revealed that she had engaged in oral sex with a boy at school but had kept this a secret from her parents.

The pediatrician's first intervention was to provide sex education to Jennifer. He then attempted to understand the change in Jennifer's dress and behavior. When he asked Jennifer about the custody arrangement, Jennifer revealed how much she missed her father. Jennifer also shared that she had been afraid to tell her parents about her feelings for fear of hurting her mother. Understanding that part of Jennifer's dress and premature sexual activity was a reaction to the sporadic visitation with her father, Jennifer's pediatrician was able to work with her parents to find additional ways she could visit him. However, after a subsequent parental fight, Jennifer's mother refused to let her visit her father more often. In response, Jennifer escalated her behavior, and 2 weeks later, Jennifer's mother brought her back to the pediatrician's office because she was, in her mother's words, "demanding birth control pills!"

The pediatrician recognized that the parents were so desperately trying to meet their own needs that they were not able to empathize with Jennifer. The pediatrician suggested that Jennifer would benefit from formal psychotherapy so that she could learn an alternative solution to the loss in not seeing her father regularly and the sense that she played a less prominent role in his life, given his new romantic interest.

Vignette

Tina is a 16-year-old young woman with a 4-year history of chronic abdominal pain of unknown etiology as well as generalized anxiety. Her symptoms had been managed through the use of a serotonin reuptake inhibitor and relaxation techniques. However, after 2 years of stability, Tina's abdominal pain worsened and she began missing school. In the office, the pediatrician noticed that Tina's mother frequently spoke for her, including offering detailed reports on the degree of "Tina's" pain and also vehemently requesting additional workups and interventions. The pediatrician sensed that Tina and her mother were indirectly communicating a deeper truth that they "couldn't stomach."

The pediatrician speculated that Tina was defending against some hurt or loss by experiencing it as body pain. Tina's mother was similarly defending against something unspeakable, by talking extensively about Tina's problems. The pediatrician completed a few noninvasive tests. When no cause stood out, she referred Tina and her mother for family therapy.

Table 89-1. Attributes of Successful Psychotherapy Referrals

Have a vision in mind for how psychotherapy will be helpful and, as best as possible, describe this to the family.
Ask about the family's own worries for the child and the entire family.
Provide names and numbers of colleagues whom you recommend with confidence.
Maintain contact with the family by phone or follow-up appointment.
Offer the mental health colleague to whom you are referring specific information about your concerns.
Obtain the family's written consent for ongoing communication with the therapist. Ask to be notified if they do not keep their appointment.

Adapted from Jellinek M, Patel BP, Froehle MC (eds): Bright Futures in Practice: Mental Health, Vol. 1. Practice Guide. Arlington, VA, National Center for Education in Maternal and Child Health, 2002.

REFERRAL

Pediatricians frequently make referrals for children, parents, and families to see mental health practitioners. Several factors compose a successful referral, including an alliance with the family and establishment of a relationship with the colleague to whom one is referring a family or child (Table 89-1).

It is helpful for the pediatrician to be clear about the goals of the referral and to communicate those reasons to the parents. In practical terms, this means outlining the developmental goals the child is having trouble achieving. When families have an understanding of the goals of the referral and how the referral could result in better functioning for their child, seeing a therapist is less daunting. It might be helpful for the pediatrician to speak with the consultant first to discuss the case and to obtain suggestions on how to broach the subject with the family. For example, the pediatrician might say to Jennifer's family, "Jennifer's precocious sexual behavior might be related to the loss she feels from the divorce and may be an attempt to gain companionship or an identity away from all the tension. Talking it through may decrease or stop her potentially dangerous behavior." Sometimes the parents' most serious worry serves as the best therapeutic goal. Talking about psychotherapeutic treatment with a goal in mind offers parents a sense of hope about the referral.

Pediatricians are also successful in making psychotherapy referrals when they offer names and numbers of one or two mental health colleagues whom they can recommend with confidence. A pediatrician may provide a child or teenager instructions to "stick with" the person they find easiest to talk with. The referral process does not end with handing over names and numbers. A follow-up plan, in the form of a scheduled appointment or planned telephone call, should be established on the same day the referral is made. This helps prevent the family from feeling abandoned and increases adherence to the plan of seeking psychotherapeutic help.

Finally, psychotherapy referrals are successful when pediatricians provide mental health colleagues with information about their concerns for a child or family. The pediatricians can request to be contacted if the families or patients do not show up for their appointment.

RESISTANCE TO PSYCHOTHERAPY REFERRALS

Many parents and children are reluctant to see a "shrink" or therapist. In fact, a study conducted in 2002 of 206 primary care offices found that 650 of 4012 patients 4 to 15 years old were referred for mental health treatment, yet only 61% of the referred families actually saw a mental health provider in the 6-month period following the initial primary care referral (Rushton et al, 2002).

To reduce the stigma associated with seeing a mental health professional, the pediatrician can build into the entire practice a routine discussion of psychosocial issues, anticipatory guidance, and preventive measures. Pediatricians may also take advantage of screening tools, such as the Pediatric Symptom Checklist (*http://psc.partners.org*). When a family senses that emotional and relationship issues are a part of a normal office visit, they will often be more at ease if their pediatrician needs to question the child or parent more closely or offers referral to a mental health specialist.

Parents often feel a profound sense of helplessness and guilt about their child's physical or mental illness. Most pediatricians are quite comfortable reassuring parents that children's medical or mental illnesses are not the result of something they did or did not do. Even in dysfunctional family settings where some parental behavior patterns have clearly had an impact on a child, it should be noted that children respond differently to stress, and those who develop mental illness often have multiple vulnerabilities to illness. Acknowledging the parents' sense of caring, good intentions, and efforts made toward helping their children will go a long way in assuaging guilt and freeing the parent to go forward to obtain help.

Some children have already been through the mental health care system, and for various reasons, they or their parents failed to connect with the intended provider. On occasion, this is because a child needs a certain "subspecialist." For example, some psychotherapists work well with children with autism as opposed to helping children who have problematic personalities. Referral to a specialist often arouses a wish for a complete "cure." If it is not met, the child or family experiences overwhelming disappointment and ends the treatment prematurely. It is important that the receiving specialist understand a family's expectations and provide honest assessments of what will get better, how, and how soon, even if this means admitting uncertainty. Most important is a "goodness of fit" between the child, family, and psychotherapist.

Sometimes television programs and movies portray psychotherapists as caring and competent (*Good Will Hunting* and *Ordinary People*). Watching these movies may inspire some reluctant teenagers to attend their first appointment. In other films, psychiatrists are portrayed as incompetent or, worse, malevolent mind benders. It is helpful to ask what ideas come to mind when they think about seeing a psychiatrist or therapist. A family's cultural perspective, based on religion or ethnicity, can play a role in whether they accept a referral to see a psychotherapist. On occasion, a family may see psychotherapy as counter to how mental or behavioral problems are usually handled within their community. In such instances, be respectful of the family's values and beliefs; explore in a nonjudgmental fashion what they feel is wrong and how they would like to see their son or daughter improve. Families are very appreciative when physicians strive for cultural understanding. Pediatricians are often able to list the ways in which psychotherapy can be complementary, as opposed to antagonistic, to a family's cultural understanding of mental illness and treatment. Referral to a psychotherapist who can literally or culturally "speak the family's language" can be very helpful.

Parents with their own pervasively disruptive ways of thinking, feeling, and acting in the world, that is, those with personality disorders, are a difficult cohort. For these parents, the process of accepting referrals, finding therapists who are a "good fit," and sticking with a particular therapist is replete with roadblocks. Returning to their pediatrician's office, such parents often deride the therapist they were referred to and berate the pediatrician's sending them. To help avoid future therapist-child, therapist-parent blow-ups, a pediatrician can inquire about the nature of the problem with the previous practitioner, validate the problematic aspects of the relationship, and then suggest ways to deal with this obstacle in the future. It may be helpful to speak with previous providers to ascertain what went wrong from their perspectives. Given that people with personality disorders can be persistently aggravating and negative, many pediatricians tend to avoid rather than attempt to aggressively address problematic family dynamics. Common to these families is an initial idealization of the pediatrician and, later, a complete devaluation of the pediatrician by speaking negatively of the pediatrician in the community. A powerful therapeutic stance is to continue working with such families alongside a psychotherapist who is familiar with the dynamics of personality disorders by providing a "holding environment" in which both treaters withstand the emotional storms together.

Parents who grew up with a sibling, parent, or grandparent with a mental illness often fear that their child will develop that same illness. A seemingly innocuous referral to therapy by the pediatrician can provoke the parents' worst nightmare that their child is now destined to be just like their sibling, parent, or grandparent. Knowledge of the family history of mental illness allows the pediatrician to gently investigate the family's experience with an aunt, father, or brother who was treated in the past. The pediatrician can then help the parents put that experience into perspective and point out the differences between what happened to their loved one, what their child is experiencing in the here and now, and what modern psychotherapeutic treatment is like.

No matter how professionally, tactfully, or gently a pediatrician presents a recommendation for therapy, some families will be incredibly resistant. In desperate situations, one tried and true approach to resistant families is the "if ... then" approach. The pediatrician might start by expressing some concern about a particular behavior, using functional terms. "I've noticed that Tina's school attendance has slipped with the increase in abdominal pain. I am a little worried about it." This might be followed by a recommendation for psychiatric assessment and evaluation of need for treatment. The pediatrician may then pose the question to the family, "Although Tina has chronic abdominal pain, we should try to keep her development on track. Where do you think Tina should be in terms of school attendance and peer relationships in 1 month? 3 months? how about 6 months?" If the family points out that they would like to see Tina attending school more regularly and maintaining same-age peers, then the pediatrician may offer an "if ... then" proposal. "If, in 3 months, Tina has not made significant strides toward the goals she has for herself and you have for her, then would you consider referral to our psychiatric clinic?" Helping children and families generate their own goals and state what would constitute a problem for which they would need psychotherapeutic help can be very empowering and alliance building.

The severity of children's or teenagers' problems should dictate the timeline that the pediatrician suggests. If a child is at risk of failing school or causing irreparable damage to relationships, it is prudent to suggest a brief window of time. If the behavioral or psychological problem is less severe, then it may be more appropriate to suggest a timeline of 3 to 6 months. If the child is in immediate danger of hurting himself or herself or others or if the pediatrician is uncertain whether a child can wait days or weeks to see a psychiatrist, psychologist, or social worker, referral to an emergency department for immediate psychiatric consultation and possibly hospitalization is warranted.

THE VARIETIES OF THERAPEUTIC EXPERIENCE

D. W. Winnicott eloquently summarizes that the process of psychotherapy occurs over time, by a series of encounters between therapist and patient that can range from emotionally charged topics that directly address the referral question to subtle discussions about seemingly unrelated events. During these encounters, the therapist enters both imaginatively and accurately into the mind of the patient. The therapist must be free to fantasize without anxiety and must be able to imagine, either in conversation or in play with a child using dolls or cars, what the child may be feeling and thinking. The therapist must be relatively free of neurotic, psychotic, or characterologic distortions, which would undermine acceptance of the patient for who she or he is and what the patient is attempting to convey.

To accurately enter the mind of their patients, therapists must be able to challenge their own preconceived ideas and notions. As professionals, we may have biases about disorders and how therapy should proceed or toward a certain theoretical position. As members of society, we also come with a set of biases based on class, race, gender, and age. As therapists learn about the particulars of their patients, ideally these biases should

Table 89-2. Characteristics of "Good Enough" Psychotherapists

Readily build therapeutic alliances with patients and families
Tolerate closeness, even in light of significant pathology
Generally free of characterologic and perceptual distortions, such that the therapists' ways of perceiving the world do not impede therapeutic progress
Aware of their own potential biases
Empathic—free to explore and value patients' thoughts, feelings, hopes, and fears
Operate under a construct that allows them to formulate cases, offer diagnoses, establish criteria for completion of treatment, and measure progress along the way
Can effectively communicate with children or adolescents, their parents, pediatricians, and other care providers

fall aside and leave them face to face with individuals. As therapists learn about their patients, patients gain greater closeness with them. Soon the accoutrements that typically bestow status become irrelevant, and a therapist and patient sit together, "two human beings of equal status," left to face that which is most human.

After a series of encounters in which the therapist has entered imaginatively and accurately into the mind of the patient, change is possible. The therapist and patient have an opportunity to be together in a way that is different from most other relationships. With an intimate understanding of the child's conflicts, fears, and struggles, the work of therapy has begun and the situation has become ripe with the potential for change. The attributes of a "good enough" therapist are outlined in Table 89-2.

Because each child and family are unique and nearly every therapist blends psychotherapeutic treatment modalities, there are probably as many "types" of psychotherapy as there are therapists and patients. Nonetheless, individual psychotherapy can be subdivided into those treatments based on psychodynamic principles and those developed from the cognitive-behavioral tradition. Although most therapy takes place in the office setting (whether in an academic center, a community hospital, or a private practice), alternative settings such as schools and facilities with the capacity for structured sports or games are also employed.

Individual Psychodynamic Psychotherapy

The term *psychodynamic* refers to those mental phenomena that involve inner, often unconscious conflict. Born out of the Freudian tradition, the focus of psychodynamic psychotherapy (also referred to as psychoanalytic psychotherapy) is to help patients gain insight and mastery over those inner conflicts that trouble them. Through careful attention to a child's words and actions, the savvy psychodynamic therapist is able to make interpretations that transform a child's and family's understanding of the past, bring about awareness of psychological defenses the patient is using in the present, and offer the patient psychological skills to deal with difficult internal and interpersonal experiences in the future. In psychodynamic psychotherapy, there is a greater focus on the relationship between the therapist and child than on directly confronting problematic thoughts and feelings. Thus, this type of treatment may be best suited for children who are unable to tolerate direct dialogue about their problems but can address them indirectly through talk in displacement or by play.

Aidan, the 7-year-old with attention-deficit/hyperactivity disorder, was referred for psychotherapy because of ongoing behavioral issues thought to be secondary to low self-esteem. Aidan had been frequently reprimanded by parents and teachers for behaviors outside of his control. Receiving nearly constant redirection, which sometimes included soft-spoken reminders and at other times shouted reprimands, he grew frustrated, impatient, and angry that he could not control or anticipate what behavior would result in scolding. Unconsciously, when criticized, Aidan was faced with two options: "Are my parents or teachers bad?" or "Am I bad?" At 7 years of age, it made more developmental sense for Aidan to believe that the adults were right and that he himself was "bad." Accepting his "badness" led to low self-esteem and problematic behaviors that validated his underlying beliefs about himself.

In treatment, Aidan's psychotherapist attempted to help him discover accurate and imaginative ways of seeing himself. Slowly, in the displacement of play therapy, Aidan began having a different emotional experience from the one he had with other adults in life. During one session, Aidan smashed two cars together violently. At home and at school, violent play like this typically elicited comments like "Aidan! Stop, you're scaring the other children," causing Aidan to skulk away. In the office, the therapist enthusiastically exclaimed, "What a tremendous accident! What happens next?" Aidan was given permission to elaborate his play. During the next several sessions, Aidan would crash the cars, the police would come, and the "driver" would be arrested because he was "bad." Aidan's therapist expressed curiosity about the bad driver, who was frequently put in jail for car crashes he could not control. With empathy, the therapist would comment on how terrible it was for this poor driver who tried so hard but was not able to control his own car. The possibility of thinking about the driver in different ways was opened up, and soon Aidan (the driver) began to see himself in a more positive light. The driver began performing elaborate car stunts in the office. Mirroring this success, to his parents' surprise, Aidan also tried out different ways of playing and being at home and school.

After the therapist understood Aidan's plight, the therapist was able to share what was on his mind, including alternative ways of seeing the bad driver. Aidan was able to imaginatively work through his feelings of badness and come to a more accurate impression of his self.

Paradoxically, one of the major advantages of psychodynamic psychotherapy, its open-endedness and freedom for patient and therapist to "enter imaginatively" into others' minds, is also its chief drawback. Many complain that the therapeutic action of psychodynamic psychotherapy is too nebulous and nearly impossible to validate. Indeed, both the individualized narrative diagnostic formulations and the relatively high cost of frequent, longer term psychodynamic psychotherapy have rendered it exquisitely difficult to perform large-scale, standardized, reproducible studies on this form of child and adolescent therapy.

Cognitive-Behavioral Therapy

Cognitive-behavioral therapy (CBT) attempts to take into account a child's internal emotional and intellectual experience, examining how children perceive their external environment and alter distortions, which lead to anxiety, depression, or other symptoms. The role of the CBT psychotherapist is to address how children interpret the world around them and to help the child to think and then subsequently to feel and to act in ways that are less troubling.

Cognitive therapy is rooted in the theories of Aaron Beck, who postulated that anxiety and depression are the result of distorted thinking (see Chapters 47 and 48). Cognitive therapy takes a very direct approach toward understanding the thoughts and feelings, hopes and fears of the patient in the present. This direct approach involves the use of standardized, validated, manual directed treatments, providing children and adolescents with in-office and homework exercises that alter their understanding of the world. Meanwhile, the underlying principle of behavioral therapy is that if one responds to certain behaviors with rewards or punishments, the frequency and intensity of a child's behavior can be increased or reduced to desired effect. For example, in dealing with a boy who fervently believed that he would never get a cavity even if he did not brush his teeth, a pure behavioral therapist would not directly confront his cognitive distortions. The therapist would, instead, help the family create a reward system meant to inspire the child to brush his teeth, regardless of his thoughts on the matter.

In the case of Aidan, his symptoms were initially addressed by his pediatrician and parents by use of behavioral treatment. They began ignoring his troubling behaviors and rewarding his completion of tasks. Later, were he to have worked with a cognitive therapist on his poor self-image, the formulation and focus would have involved identifying and then challenging Aidan's negative cognitive distortions about himself in the present. Specifically, Aidan would be asked to accumulate evidence for and evidence against his "badness." With the help of the therapist, Aidan would start to self-correct his thoughts, realizing they were distortions of the truth. He would grow to believe that "although sometimes I do things that frustrate other people, in fact, there are a lot of things about me that my parents, teachers, kids in my class, and I really like."

Again, because CBT so directly confronts the thoughts, feelings, and behavior of patients, this type of psychotherapy can be completed quickly and is ideal for research studies. Whereas the goal-oriented approach of CBT appeals to many patients, others resent its approach as too eager to bring about change quickly, inadequately nuanced, and overly structured.

Dialectical Behavior Therapy

Dialectical behavior therapy (DBT) applies the principles and strategies of CBT to the treatment of borderline personality disorder, with a specific focus on reducing suicidal and self-harming behavior, such as cutting or burning. This focus makes it a particularly useful treatment for adolescents who engage in self-mutilating behaviors. The primary characteristic of DBT is its emphasis on "dialectics, the reconciliation of opposites in a continual process of synthesis" (Linehan, 1993). A fundamental dialectic of DBT is accepting and validating patients as they are while also encouraging them to change. Patients are given skills to manage their emotions, to increase their interpersonal effectiveness, and to tolerate distress more effectively.

In DBT, unlike in CBT, the therapeutic relationship is central, serving as therapy in itself, addressing the fundamental interpersonal deficits found in individuals with borderline personality disorder. These deficits can be so severe that they cause profound interpersonal problems, including difficulty distinguishing between one's own thoughts, feelings, hopes, and fears and another person's; vulnerability to feeling abandoned at every turn; and poor impulse control leading to relationships that are intense, volatile, and fleeting.

One note on the diagnoses of borderline personality disorder and other character disorders: they cannot be given to an adolescent with complete certainty. Adolescence for some is an identity "crisis," and the process of forming a stable, mature personality structure involves a period of trial and error often marked by various adaptive and maladaptive coping strategies. However, when an adolescent displays "a pattern of difficulties in interpersonal relationships, chronic low self-esteem, unusual response to losses, and a 'black and white' quality in thinking and judgment, the pediatrician has grounds to be concerned about his or her character development" (Jellinek and Ablon, 1998). DBT can be useful, as emerging character-disordered patients have difficulty tolerating open-ended discussions because of anxiety and feelings of being overwhelmed.

Jennifer, the 14-year-old girl in the vignette, had been referred for therapy after she started dressing provocatively and engaging in sexual activity in the aftermath of her parents' separation and divorce. When questioned by her therapist, Jennifer revealed that she felt overwhelmed by the events of the divorce and the absence of her father. Analyzing the chain of events, Jennifer learned that every time she began to have this feeling, she would engage in oral sex with boys because it would seem to calm her down. Jennifer occasionally drank alcohol and superficially cut her arm in an effort to alleviate profound inner tension. She was unable to stop herself.

A DBT therapist would help Jennifer get her destructive behaviors under control by learning new skills, such as emotion regulation, distress tolerance, interpersonal effectiveness, and mindfulness. These skills will provide her with a set of more adaptive coping skills to manage the emotions. Each time she engages in destructive behaviors, her therapist would have Jennifer do a chain analysis, a process that examines the events leading up to the behavior, to link underlying affects and thoughts with destructive behavior.

Family Therapy

In family therapy, an individual's symptoms are viewed as occurring within the system of the family. The family exerts a powerful influence over the individual, and it is theorized that some people cannot get better unless the family system also shifts toward health. An individual's symptoms may serve some larger purpose within the family structure. Despite the fact that the symptoms may be harmful to the individual, the family system (either knowingly or unknowingly) supports either the emergence or continuance of these symptoms. Common reasons for the development of symptoms in an individual are to divert marital conflict, to draw attention to another person in the family who needs help, to seek attention, and to avoid other conflicts or affects in the family that are too painful to address.

Family therapy attempts to change the pattern of relating and interacting within the family. The family therapist must attend to interpersonal dynamics between family members as well as the intrapsychic factors of each individual.

The family from the vignette presented for family therapy after the daughter's pain had worsened and no cause of the pain had been found. They were initially reluctant to go to family therapy, as they perceived her pain to be "real." The therapist did not challenge this notion because the pain was very real even if it was being generated or exacerbated by family-centered psychological factors. Tina's symptoms had been a way of avoiding talking about painful issues pertinent to her family life.

Eventually, Tina revealed that a friend was raped by a boy at their school. This had reminded Tina of her own trauma at age 11, when a neighbor touched her inappropriately. She had been holding onto this secret for years, burning with rage that her mother and father could not protect her. In therapy, Tina's mother admitted that she suspected this but had not been able to acknowledge the mere possibility of abuse. The therapist then pointed out that unknowingly, Tina's mother had overinvolved herself in Tina's medical care in an attempt to resolve her feelings of guilt—a process that Tina reinforced by having further abdominal pain. By the end of the treatment, Tina and her parents were better able to balance the intense feelings of love, rage, and hurt that had brought Tina to the physician's office for "stomachaches" many times.

Parent Guidance

Therapeutic work with parents is often helpful to the child who is also in his or her own treatment. The rationale of parent guidance is that parents can inadvertently re-enforce problems in their child. In turn, problematic children can make parenting quite difficult. In either case, the opportunity to talk over difficult parenting situations with a professional can be very helpful.

Once the parents come to a greater understanding of their childhood issues and conflicts, their own children will be free from the burden of helping the parent rework those issues by proxy (Armbruster et al, 2002).

Children with mental illnesses, especially those diagnosed at a young age, present many parenting challenges, even for the healthiest and most devoted of parents. The help of a therapist who is familiar with the child's diagnosis can provide psychoeducation and information on developmental norms. Although the parents might not know other children struggling with issues similar to those of their own child, a therapist will have seen multiple children with the similar diagnoses and can use those experiences in providing reference points for the parents.

Jennifer's divorced parents from the vignette were referred for parent guidance when the personal disputes between them interfered with their role as parents. With the help of parent guidance, Jennifer's parents were able to refocus on her need for them to continue to act in a parenting role, including keeping her needs primary. Jennifer's mother was able to see Jennifer's need to see her father as developmentally normal and agreed to regular visits When Jennifer's father discussed his own parents' divorce and his subsequent estrangement from his father, he discovered that he was in danger of unconsciously re-enacting the same situation with his daughter.

PSYCHOPHARMACOLOGIC INTERVENTIONS

Although psychopharmacologic interventions are beyond the scope of this chapter (see Chapter 90), it is important to acknowledge that medication can positively affect a child's ability to accurately and imaginatively enter into the minds of others and in this way are "psychotherapeutic." This is readily evidenced by the child, suffering an illness such as major depressive disorder or generalized anxiety, who after a trial with an antidepressant or anxiolytic no longer sees the world and others as menacing and can accurately assess what others are thinking and hence make new friends. Both the identification of mental illness in children and the prescription of symptom-relieving medications often fall on the shoulders of pediatricians. This has created a need for psychopharmacology training for pediatricians as well as the need for more accessible collaborative care between child psychiatrists and pediatricians.

PSYCHOTHERAPIST-PEDIATRICIAN COMMUNICATION

Greater communication of pediatricians with specialists often results in higher rates of referral completion (Rushton et al, 2002). The goal of the referral may not be complete for 1 or 2 years after the patient has been in treatment. Ongoing communication between a pediatrician and psychiatrist may be necessary to ensure that the family remains committed to treatment and that the goals of the treatment are completed.

Good communication between psychiatrist and pediatrician begins even before the time of the actual initial referral. Frequent points of communication include questions about how concerning the child's behavior appears, whether it would be an appropriate referral to that particular provider, how best to approach the family about the referral, and what the provider's availability is during the next few weeks. When contacted in person, many busy psychiatrists will find the time to meet with a patient about whom the pediatrician is concerned.

The psychiatrist can be helpful to the pediatrician in determining what type of treatment referral is needed. Psychiatrists can provide informal consultation without seeing the patient, one-time formal consultation by a meeting with the parents or child about a specific issue, psychopharmacologic management, or ongoing care of the child with both psychotropic medication and therapy. After the pediatrician and psychiatrist decide what role the psychiatrist should play, the pediatrician can relay this information to the parents, along with the message that communication has already occurred and the pediatrician has a sense of confidence that the psychiatrist will be helpful.

If the psychiatrist is going to observe the patient in an ongoing way, the pediatrician should be given a sense of how much of the therapeutic process is going to be shared. Psychiatrists have varying degrees of comfort with the disclosure of information learned during therapy sessions. Such information is an almost sacred aspect of the therapy that promotes the development of trust with and disclosure from the patient. Frequently, the psychiatrist will speak with the patient or family to discuss what information is to be shared with the pediatrician, thus preserving the sense of trust and alliance with the patient. Signed consent forms are an ingredient of good communication between therapist and pediatrician.

Communication between the pediatrician and psychiatrist can serve an important function for the psychiatrist as well. The pediatrician will be seeing the parents, child, and siblings in an ongoing way and may have developing information about family dynamics relevant to the care of the patient. The pediatrician can also support the work of the psychiatrist when the parents become frustrated by an overt lack of progress.

Unfortunately, communication between pediatricians and psychiatrists tends to be poor. In 2004, 100 pediatricians responded to a survey about their experiences in collaborating with psychiatrists. Only 14% of pediatricians reported receiving any type of information from the psychiatrist after the referral. More than 90% of pediatricians reported that they were more likely to receive communication from other medical subspecialists than from psychiatrists. Eighty-eight percent of pediatricians reported that the family is the primary source of information about the content of the psychiatric referral, but only 14% thought the family was a reliable source of information. Only 25% of pediatricians reported speaking with the psychiatrist before referral, although 66% thought that doing so might result in communication after the visit. Those who did report speaking with the psychiatrist before consultation were more likely to receive communication from psychiatrists after consultation (28%) than were those who did not communicate (9%) (Ross et al, 2004).

Factors that may hinder communication between pediatricians and psychiatrists include lack of time, concerns about confidentiality, limited access to the other provider, and financial pressures. In the era of managed care, families may be restricted by their insurance plan to certain mental health providers. In these cases, the pediatrician can ask the family for the list of eligible providers and help the family choose from those on the list. If the list is inadequate, advocacy may be necessary with the employer or insurer.

PSYCHOTHERAPY: THE EVIDENCE

Does Child and Adolescent Psychotherapy Work?

A major question posed to psychotherapists by pediatricians, parents, and kids is, Does psychotherapy make people better? At present, the research on child and adolescent psychotherapies clearly suggests that regardless of specific modality, psychotherapy treatment is better than no treatment (McCarty and Weisz, 2007). This claim is supported by four major meta-analyses (Casey and Berman, 1985; Kazdin et al, 1990; Weisz, et al, 1987, 1995) of child and adolescent psychotherapy research studies showing that mean unweighted effect sizes were all 0.71 or higher. When weighting is introduced to adjust for sample size, the effect sizes were more modest but still positive (Weisz et al, 2005). The most recent meta-analysis suggests that long-term therapy has an even stronger impact than previously reported (Leichsenring and Rabung, 2008). Further, it has been noted that not all disorders respond to psychotherapy, or at least the types of psychotherapy that have thus far been studied, with the same robustness (see Chapter 47 regarding the TADS study). CBT in combination with fluoxetine treatment was shown to be very effective, whereas patients treated with CBT did not show statistically significant improvement above the placebo group (Vitiello et al, 2006). Also discouraging, a recent meta-analysis of the effects of psychotherapy treatment for depression in children and adolescents showed an effect size of only 0.34, a much more modest effect (Weisz et al, 2006). However, an abundance of those treatment studies (33 of 44) involved CBT alone and not the blended (CBT with elements of psychodynamic psychotherapy and vice versa) versions of psychotherapy most representative of clinical reality. There are few definitive studies in this realm, and at present, nearly all treatment studies in youth psychotherapy end with a phrase calling for further, large-scale studies of this treatment in children and adolescents.

Challenges in Youth Psychotherapy Research

Several unique features of child and adolescent psychotherapy make it difficult to design and to draw meaningful, scientific conclusions from research studies. First, children and adolescents in psychotherapeutic treatment often do not meet clear diagnostic criteria. They have problems that on initial evaluation or even after multiple sessions defy categorization or elicit multiple diagnoses. Second, the process of getting into a research study may affect a child, whether the child is placed on a therapy waiting list, serves as a control, is placed in the treatment arm of a study, or is given a label or diagnosis to describe his or her symptoms. There is a difference between that child and someone who has never had contact with a mental health care provider. Another challenge in youth psychotherapy research is that unlike adults, children rarely refer themselves. The feelings and attitudes of the parents, teachers, pediatricians, and others surrounding a child (i.e., do they think psychotherapy works?) and the child (does the child think there is a problem and that psychotherapy can help?) are important in distinguishing what types of therapy work and for whom. A third issue is that children have very little control over what is happening in their lives. Given that factors such as abuse, neglect, divorce, substance abuse, bullying among peers, or other problems in the home have such a great impact, even the best psychotherapy may not be helpful in producing change in a child's life. Studies that hope to evaluate the benefits of child psychotherapy must also account for a child's home, academic, and after-school life—measuring these features in both the treated child and the child who is placed on a waiting list and receiving no psychotherapy. Children, adolescents, and their families are often not highly motivated to make it to psychotherapy appointments, which usually occur once a week, and hence retention, both in clinical practice and in research studies, is problematic.

It is hoped yet unlikely that large-scale research studies will be performed that are able to account for all major variables, including referral bias and preconceived notions of whether or not therapy will be helpful, comorbidity, concurrent pharmacotherapy, age, gender, socioeconomic class, family and home stability or fragility, culture, and therapist-related variables. Still, it is up to advocates for this doubly disenfranchised group (children who cannot vote and who suffer mental illness) to create studies that mimic clinical reality and to lobby for funds to carry out meaningful research studies.

SUMMARY

Pediatricians prescribe psychotherapeutic interventions to improve their patients' ability to accurately and imaginatively experience themselves and others. Pediatricians can help parents and children to understand therapy when they are referred. The central focus of all psychotherapies is to reconstitute a child's or adolescent's ability to examine the thoughts and feelings of others and to be free to let others do the same to them. Sometimes this must take place in psychodynamic psychotherapy; others benefit from cognitive-behavioral treatments. Troubles involving an entire family system may be best treated in family therapy or with individual therapy in conjunction with parent guidance. It is powerful when pediatricians and therapists practice the type of communication that they would like to foster in patients and families. Few large-scale studies validating the various forms of psychotherapy for most treatments have been undertaken. Some of those performed have shown only modest effect, whereas others demonstrate more promising results. Given our experience, a keenly interested therapist examining the thoughts, feelings, hopes, and fears can help guide children back onto a better developmental track. Pediatricians' understanding of mental health disorders and the role of therapies will help them deal with one of the most common concerns of primary care, psychosocial functioning, and will enrich the meaning of their daily practice.

REFERENCES

Armbruster M, Chock U, Tanner E, Holmes S: Parent work. *In* Lewis M, (ed): Child and Adolescent Psychiatry, 3rd ed. Philadelphia, Lippincott Williams & Wilkins, 2002, pp 1055-1068.

Casey RJ, Berman JS: The outcome of psychotherapy with children. Psychol Bull 98:388-400, 1985.

Jellinek M, Ablon S: Character disorders. *In* Friedman S (ed): Comprehensive Adolescent Health Care. St. Louis, Mosby, 1998, pp 911-920.

Kazdin AE, Bass D, Ayers WA, Rodgers A: Empirical and clinical focus of child and adolescent psychotherapy research. J Consult Clin Psychol 58:729-740, 1990.

Leichsenring F, Rabung S: Effectiveness of long-term paychodynamic. JAMA 300:151-1565, 2008.

Linehan M: Cognitive-Behavioral Treatment of Borderline Personality Disorder. New York, Guilford, 1993.

Massachusetts General Hospital: Pediatric Symptom Checklist (PSC). Available at: http://psc.partners.org. Accessed January 15, 2007.

McCarty C, Weisz J: Effects of psychotherapy for depression in children and adolescents: What we can (and can't) learn from meta-analysis and component profiling. J Am Acad Child Adolesc Psychiatry 46:879-886, 2007.

Ross W, Chan E, Harris S, Rappaport L: Pediatric experience with psychiatric collaboration. Dev Behav Pediatr 25:377-378, 2004.

Rushton J, Bruckman D, Kelleher K: Primary care referral of children with psychosocial problems. Arch Pediatr Adolesc Med 156:592-598, 2002.

Vitiello B, Rohde P, Silva S, et al: Functioning and quality of life in the Treatment for Adolescents with Depression Study (TADS). J Am Acad Child Adolesc Psychiatry 45:1419-1426, 2006.

Weisz JR, Doss AJ, Hawley KM: Youth psychotherapy outcome research: A review and critique of the evidence base. Annu Rev Psychol 56:337-363, 2005.

Weisz JR, McCarty CA, Valeri SM: Effects of psychotherapy for depression in children and adolescents: A meta-analysis. Psychol Bull 132:132-149, 2006.

Weisz JR, Weiss B, Alicke MD, Klotz ML: Effectiveness of psychotherapy with children and adolescents: A meta-analysis for clinicians. J Consult Clin Psychol 55:542-549, 1987.

Weisz JR, Weiss B, Han SS, et al: Effects of psychotherapy with children and adolescents revisited: A meta-analysis of treatment outcome studies. Psychol Bull 117:450-468, 1995.

Winnicott DW: The price of disregarding psychoanalytic research. *In* Winnicott DW: Home Is Where We Start From: Essay by a Psychoanalyst. New York, Norton, 1965, pp 172-182.

Winnicott DW: Cure; as quoted in Phillips A: Winnicott. Cambridge, Harvard University Press, 1970, pp 13-14.

90 CHILD AND ADOLESCENT PSYCHOPHARMACOLOGY

RICHARD E. D'ALLI

In 4 decades since the death of its cofounder, Henry Luce, the American edition of *Time* has devoted nearly 50 cover stories to topics unmistakably subsumed by developmental-behavioral pediatrics (*http://www.time.com*). The November 3, 2003, issue posed a bold question on its cover relevant to this chapter: Are we giving kids too many drugs? Community-based rates of prescribing psychotropic medications for mental illnesses in youth saw a sharp increase nationally in the 1990s with regional differences due to many factors, including access to treatment. Despite ostensibly balanced reporting, print and electronic media alike have succeeded in whipping this modern clinical practice phenomenon into a public controversy. As articulated in the press, the promise held out by psychotropic drugs of relatively quick and effortless relief from the pain of childhood mental illness is at odds with the popular belief that these same drugs are harmful to developing brains. The salient issue for clinicians, however, is whether this burgeoning prescribing practice is at odds with existing empiric evidence.

Empiricism in child and adolescent psychopharmacology arguably began in 1937 when Charles Bradley published his observation of "spectacular improvement in school performance" among behaviorally disordered children treated with Benzedrine, an amphetamine psychostimulant (Bradley, 1937). Bradley's paper describes a small, prospective, open label, nonrandomized trial in which drug response and adverse effects would be easily recognized today by any physician experienced in treating children with attention-deficit/hyperactivity disorder (ADHD). Inexplicably, this work would not be replicated by anyone other than Bradley himself for nearly a quarter century. Decades more would follow before formal programs of research on the efficacy and safety not only of psychostimulants but also of other psychotropic drugs in child and adolescent populations were given serious support by federal agencies.

Responding to escalating off-label use of psychotropic agents in children, the National Institute of Mental Health (NIMH) and U.S. Food and Drug Administration (FDA) jointly convened a 1995 consensus conference on overcoming obstacles to expanding the pediatric empiric data base (Vitiello and Jensen, 1997). One strategic recommendation, creating incentives for the pharmaceutical industry to support research, materialized in a series of congressional bills: the Food and Drug Administration Modernization Act of 1997 guaranteed a limited extension of patent life, also known as exclusivity, to any proprietary drug whose innovator voluntarily funded its study in youth; the Best Pharmaceuticals for Children Act of 2002 reauthorized the 1997 act and allocated new money for the FDA to contract for drug trials in youth that industry would not voluntarily conduct; and the Pediatric Research Equity Act of 2003 made FDA approval of a new drug contingent on completion of pediatric trials if the agent is likely to be used in children. The legislation had the intended effect of pumping private resources into scores of randomized, placebo-controlled trials of selected agents to treat child and adolescent depression, anxiety, and ADHD (Benjamin et al, 2006), but the payoff was not entirely satisfying. For example, industry-funded studies were designed to show statistical superiority of drug over placebo but not a meaningful measure of the magnitude of drug effect. Some industry-sponsored studies were never published, particularly negative trials, because the raw data were proprietary. The NIMH focused instead on funding multisite, multimodal, and occasionally novel intervention trials, hoping to capitalize on the power of these designs to quantify the relative effectiveness of various treatments (Table 90-1).

Taking a lesson from history, a collaborative academic, public, and private, if not integrated, action plan may be the most effective means going forward toward a robust national program of child and adolescent psychopharmacologic research (DeVeaugh-Geiss et al, 2006), the fruits of which could be more effective and better tolerated medicines to treat pediatric mental illnesses. On the other hand, accelerating the introduction of novel psychotropic technologies for youth is likely to strain the current FDA approval process to its limit.

BEFORE PRESCRIBING

Because sensitive and reliable blood, imaging, and genetic markers for psychiatric disorders are simply not yet available, a thorough and detailed patient history is the sine qua non of a thoughtful differential diagnosis. A child or adolescent psychiatric history demands collateral information from many sources, including parents, older siblings, extended relatives, other caregivers, babysitters, teachers, coaches, prior health care providers, or anyone else responsible for a young patient's nurturing,

Table 90-1. **Selected Samples of Completed, NIMH-Sponsored, Multisite, Randomized, Placebo-Controlled Clinical Trials in Child and Adolescent Psychopharmacology**

Study	N	Ages	Design
MTA* (Multimodal Treatment Study of Children with ADHD)	579	7-9	14-month randomized, parallel groups comparing efficacy of intensive medication management vs. intensive behavioral therapy vs. their combination vs. community practice
Methylphenidate in the treatment of hyperactivity and impulsiveness in children with pervasive developmental disorder	72	5-14	5-week randomized, placebo-controlled within subjects, plus open label maintenance, to test efficacy and tolerability of methylphenidate to treat comorbid ADHD in pervasive developmental disorder
Risperidone in conduct disorder in mild, moderate, and borderline intellectually disabled children	108	5-12	1-week run-in, followed by 6-week, placebo-controlled, parallel groups testing efficacy and tolerability of risperidone in conduct disordered, intellectually disabled children
Citalopram for children with autism spectrum disorders and high levels of repetitive behavior	149	5-17	12-week randomized, double-blind, placebo-controlled, parallel group to test efficacy of citalopram in reducing repetitive behaviors and improving functioning
TADS (Treatment for Adolescents with Depression Study)	439	12-17	12-week placebo-controlled, parallel groups, plus 24-week continuation comparing efficacy and safety of fluoxetine vs. cognitive-behavioral therapy vs. their combination vs. placebo in moderate to severe depression
TORDIA (Treatment of SSRI-Resistant Depression In Adolescents)	334	12-18	12-week randomized, factorial design comparing efficacy of alternative antidepressants alone and in combination with cognitive-behavioral therapy
Research Unit on Pediatric Psychopharmacology (RUPP) anxiety treatment study	128	6-17	8-week randomized, placebo-controlled, parallel group to test efficacy and tolerability of fluvoxamine in social phobia, generalized or separation anxiety
Fluoxetine after weight restoration in anorexia nervosa	80	16-45	12-month randomized, double-blind, placebo-controlled, parallel group after discharge from inpatient program at target weight to test efficacy of fluoxetine to reduce relapse rate
Galantamine in childhood autism	20	5-17	12-week randomized, double-blind, placebo-controlled, single group test of efficacy and safety of galantamine

*MTA study was not placebo controlled.
Adapted and modified from Vitiello B: An update on publicly funded multisite trials in pediatric psychopharmacology. Child Adolesc Psychiatr Clin North Am 15:2-4, 2006.

supervision, education, and well-being. During the first clinical encounter, it may be impossible to acquire and to organize such diverse reports into a formulation that lends itself to pharmacotherapy. Furthermore, functional impairment, a developmentally and contextually dependent variable, is critical to making a diagnosis, which means that treatment targets are sometimes moving ones. For these reasons and more, it is always best to resist the temptation to reach too quickly for the prescription pad.

Attempts to manage emotional or behavioral illness in youth with medication alone are likely to be inadequate. As discussed in Chapter 89, evidence-based psychosocial treatments merit strong if not first consideration in cases of mild to moderate mental illness. This chapter discusses pharmacotherapies supported by the gold standard of evidence, a double-blind, randomized, placebo-controlled trial (RCT). The preponderance of such studies presents evidence only for acute efficacy and safety of psychotropic medications in children and adolescents. Unfortunately, there are few data to guide physicians in either the proper sequencing or optimal duration of drug therapy, psychotherapy, or their combination.

When a decision has been made to treat with medication, a discussion of risks and benefits with the primary caretakers and with the patient, in words they can understand, is of paramount importance and part and parcel of informed consent. The potential benefits of treatment should be explained in terms of improved functioning that everyone can recognize. The more difficult discussion of risk may begin by considering the harm that doing nothing might cause but in short order must turn to the relative risk of harm posed by treatment itself. Open and honest medication education during a patient's visit and its documentation not only help ensure the patient's safety but also serve to remind the physician of that oldest of dictums, *primum non nocere*.

PHARMACOTHERAPY OF ATTENTION-DEFICIT/HYPERACTIVITY DISORDER

In a series of lectures delivered to the Royal College of Physicians of London more than a century ago, George F. Still argued "urgently for scientific investigation" of a pediatric condition he called a "defect of moral control" (Still, 1902). The children he described without "impairment of intellect" or "obvious physical disease" would today meet criteria of the *Diagnostic and Statistical Manual of Mental Disorders*, fourth edition, text revision (DSM-IV-TR), for attention deficit and disruptive behavior disorders. ADHD, discussed in Chapter 54, has long been recognized as a neurodevelopmental syndrome of inattention, impulsiveness, and hyperactivity. Complicating the diagnosis are other child and adolescent psychiatric disorders commonly comorbid with ADHD, especially disruptive and defiant behavior, anxiety, depression, learning disorders, and tic disorders.

The modern view of ADHD is that of dysregulated attention, orientation, and motor control and preparedness, mediated in part by neural circuits that loop from the prefrontal cortex through the striatum and thalamus back to motor, cognitive, and affective cortices with input from the cerebellum (Arnsten, 2006). The most important neurotransmitters driving these circuits are dopamine and norepinephrine. To date, every pharmacologic agent found to be effective in reducing the core symptoms of ADHD (many in off-label use) is a modulator of dopamine, norepinephrine, or both. Simultaneous treatment of ADHD and its common comorbidities does not lend itself to monotherapy, except in some cases of disruptive and defiant behaviors. Standard practice is concurrent treatment with agents for which there are convincing efficacy data in each impairing disorder, with careful attention paid to drug-drug interactions.

Psychostimulants

No pharmacotherapeutic agent or behavioral intervention has been shown to outperform the psychostimulants in treating the core symptoms of ADHD. Only two psychostimulant compounds are available today with FDA approval for the treatment of ADHD: methylphenidate and amphetamine, both of which have active levo- and dextro-isomers marketed in immediate release (IR) and long-acting formulations in a variety of delivery vehicles. A third psychostimulant, magnesium pemoline, was withdrawn from the market in 2005 after the FDA announced that its overall risk of liver toxicity outweighed any potential clinical benefit. A fourth psychostimulant, modafinil, although promising in pediatric clinical trials (Biederman et al, 2006), is stalled in the FDA approval process as of this writing because of associated serious skin reactions, including urticaria, erythema multiforme, and Stevens-Johnson syndrome.

Psychostimulants are generally believed to block the presynaptic dopamine and norepinephrine reuptake transporters and to stimulate the release of dopamine from presynaptic storage vesicles. They may also weakly stimulate the release of stored norepinephrine. There is a subtle difference between the dopamine storage sites at which methylphenidate and amphetamine act, but no difference in clinical effectiveness as a result has ever been appreciated. Amphetamine is approximately twice as potent as methylphenidate but has no advantage in either symptom selectivity or duration of action. Methylphenidate is metabolized by de-esterification to inactive ritalinic acid, which is almost entirely excreted in the urine; amphetamine is in large measure excreted unchanged in the urine with some deamination and hydroxylation into benzoic acid and hydroxyamphetamine. Psychostimulants have little plasma protein binding, are rapidly absorbed, exert their effect in the IR form within 30 minutes of ingestion, reach peak plasma concentrations in the 1- to 3-hour range, and have elimination half-lives in the 2- to 4-hour range.

The challenge to improve the clinical usefulness of these compounds has been twofold: parsing out the relative efficacy of their isomers and engineering delivery systems to sustain dosing automatically. Delivery vehicles currently used to extend the absorption time of psychostimulants are the wax matrix, double-pulse beaded, osmotic pump, transdermal, and lysine-bound systems. Double-pulse beaded long-acting systems package two doses of stimulant in a single, soluble capsule, the first dose in a set of immediate release spherules and the second dose in a set enterically coated to delay stimulant release for about 4 hours; thus, the duration of action of this delivery system is generally 6 to 8 hours. The osmotic pump system is an insoluble but permeable capsule that releases a stream of the medicine from a small outlet at one end as it migrates through the gut; the duration of action of this system, modulated in part by gut motility, is variable, from 6 to 12 hours. Highly concentrated psychostimulant in the adhesive layer of the transdermal system sets up a diffusion gradient driving medicine into the dermal capillaries, delaying its onset of action after application and protracting its action after removal. The lysine-bound system, an inactive prodrug, depends on differential absorption and cleavage of a bond between the amino acid and dextroamphetamine, thus releasing the stimulant in the gut over a 6- to 12-hour period. Essentially, all of these medications are restarted every day, permitting treatment to be interrupted on weekends or holidays with a predictable return to full daily effectiveness on resumption. Currently marketed psychostimulant preparations are summarized in Table 90-2.

Psychostimulant management involves optimizing both dose-response and time-action effectiveness while minimizing adverse effects. In medication naive school-age children and adolescents, it is equally reasonable to choose either an IR or a long-acting delivery system of either approved psychostimulant from the outset. It is prudent to initiate treatment of preschoolers, aged 3 to 5 years, with an IR preparation. Typical starting doses for children and adolescents are listed in Table 90-3. Preliminary results of the NIMH multisite Preschool ADHD Treatment Study suggest that 3- to 5-year-olds should be started at half those doses, with titration steps half those suggested for older children (Greenhill et al, 2006). The marketed doses of double-pulse beaded capsules are equivalent to half their value delivered twice in the IR form 4 hours apart. The contents may be sprinkled onto a spoonful of applesauce, yogurt, or similar creamy textured food for children who cannot swallow a capsule. The marketed doses of the osmotic pump are grossly equivalent to one-third their value taken three times in the IR form at 4-hour intervals. Every 10-mg step of the transdermal system, when it is worn for 9 hours, is roughly equipotent to an 18-mg step of the osmotic pump system. The 30-, 50-, and 70-mg capsules of lysine-bound *d*-amphetamine, which can be opened and their contents dissolved in water, are equivalent to the 10-, 20-, and 30-mg *d*-, *l*-amphetamine mixed salts double-pulse beaded capsules, respectively.

Titration, or incremental dose increases, is usually done weekly until one of three things occurs: a favorable response, the onset of intolerable adverse effects, or no response at the highest recommended dose. When an effective dose is reached, on average in the range of 1.0 mg/kg/day for school-age children or 0.75 mg/kg/day for preschoolers, no further titration is usually necessary

Table 90-2. Marketed Psychostimulant Preparations FDA Approved for ADHD

Brand Name	Active Isomers	Delivery System	Maximum Daily Dose: FDA	Available Strengths (mg)
Adderall	*d*-, *l*-Amphetamine mixed salts	IR tablet	40 mg	5, 7.5, 10, 12.5, 15, 20, 30
Adderall XR	*d*-, *l*-Amphetamine mixed salts	Double-pulse beaded capsule, sprinkles	30 mg	5, 10, 15, 20, 25, 30
Concerta	*d*-, *l*-Methylphenidate	Osmotic pump	72 mg	18, 27, 36, 54
Daytrana	*d*-, *l*-Methylphenidate	Transdermal patch	30 mg	10, 15, 20, 30 during 9 hours
Dexedrine	*d*-Amphetamine	IR tablet	40 mg	5
Dexedrine spansule	*d*-Amphetamine	Double-pulse beaded capsule, sprinkles	40 mg	5, 10, 15
DextroStat	*d*-Amphetamine	IR tablet	40 mg	5, 10
Focalin	*d*-Methylphenidate	IR tablet	20 mg	2.5, 5, 10
Focalin XR	*d*-Methylphenidate	Double-pulse beaded capsule, sprinkles	30 mg	5, 10, 15, 20
Metadate ER	*d*-, *l*-Methylphenidate	Wax matrix tablet	60 mg	10, 20
Metadate CD	*d*-, *l*-Methylphenidate	Double-pulse beaded capsule, sprinkles	60 mg	10, 20, 30, 40, 50, 60
Methylin	*d*-, *l*-Methylphenidate	IR tablet	60 mg	5, 10, 20
Methylin	*d*-, *l*-Methylphenidate	Liquid	60 mg	5 mg/5 mL, 10 mg/5 mL
Methylin ER	*d*-, *l*-Methylphenidate	Wax matrix tablet	60 mg	10, 20
Ritalin	*d*-, *l*-Methylphenidate	IR tablet	60 mg	5, 10, 20
Ritalin LA	*d*-, *l*-Methylphenidate	Double-pulse beaded capsule, sprinkles	60 mg	10, 20, 30, 40
Ritalin SR	*d*-, *l*-Methylphenidate	Wax matrix tablet	60 mg	20
Vyvanse	*l*-Lysine–bound *d*-Amphetamine	Microcrystalline soluble powder	70 mg	20, 30, 40, 50, 60, 70

IR, immediate release.

Table 90-3. Suggested Dosing of Agents Used in ADHD for Ages 6 and Above

Agent	Initial Dosing	Titration Steps
Psychostimulants	IR methylphenidate (MPH): 5 mg q 4 hr bid or tid	5 mg weekly
	IR dexmethylphenidate (*d*-MPH): 2.5 mg q 4 hr bid	2.5 mg weekly
	IR dextroamphetamine (DEX): 2.5 mg q 4 hr bid	2.5 mg weekly
	IR mixed amphetamine salts (MAS): 2.5 mg q daily	2.5 mg weekly
	Double-pulse beaded MPH: 10 mg q AM	10 mg weekly
	Double-pulse beaded DEX and MAS: 5 mg q AM	5 mg weekly
	Double-pulse beaded *d*-MPH: 5 mg q AM	5 mg weekly
	Osmotic pump MPH: 18 mg q AM	18 mg weekly
	Transdermal MPH: lowest marketed dose q AM	Next larger dose weekly
	l-Lysine-DEX: lowest marketed dose q AM	Next larger dose weekly
Atomoxetine	<70 kg child: 0.5 mg/kg/d divided q AM and afternoon × 4 d	Consolidate 1.0 mg/kg/d q d × 4 d; then 1.2 mg/kg/d q d
	>70 kg child: 18 mg capsule q AM and afternoon × 4 d	Consolidate 1.2-1.8 mg/kg/d; maximum = 100 mg/d
Tricyclic antidepressants*	Imipramine: 25 mg q d	25 mg weekly divided bid; maximum = 4 mg/kg/d (200 mg/d)
	Nortriptyline: 10 mg q d	10 mg weekly divided bid; maximum = 2 mg/kg/d (100 mg/d)
Bupropion*	50 mg q d	50 mg weekly; maximum = 300 mg/d
α_2-Adrenergic agonists*	Clonidine: 0.05 mg qhs × 3 d, then 0.05 mg tid	0.05 mg weekly; maximum = 0.4 mg/d
	Guanfacine: 0.5 mg qhs × 3 d, then 0.5 mg q 12 hr	0.5 mg weekly; maximum = 4 mg/d

*Not FDA approved for use in ADHD.
IR, immediate release.

in the short term. The choice of weekly titration steps is one of convenience and practicality. Not only is it easier for parents and teachers to remember to change doses on the same day each week, but also a true response, as well as its onset, duration, and fade out, that remains consistent for a week cannot have been due to sheer chance. Oral long-acting delivery systems are not always effective for the length of a school day (or, in the case of busy families, from before-school care through after-school care). The addition of an IR dose in the afternoon will serve to extend effectiveness, especially during homework time. Both psychostimulant compounds in all delivery systems carry the same risk of the adverse effects listed in Table 90-4, which resolve on discontinuation. The inability to tolerate one psychostimulant does not necessarily predict intolerance of the other.

The most common adverse effects of psychostimulants can be managed conservatively. To avoid weight loss due to appetite suppression, reducing the dose or supplementing the child's diet with high-calorie, enjoyable

Table 90-4. Adverse Effects of Pharmacotherapeutic Agents Used in ADHD

Agent	Adverse Effects
Psychostimulants	Agitation, appetite suppression, changes in pulse rate and blood pressure, chest pain, delay in sleep onset, emotional lability, formication, growth deceleration, hallucinations, headaches, irritability, lethargy, nail biting, nausea, paranoia, rash, skin picking, stomachaches, tics, transient depression
Atomoxetine	Abdominal distress, appetite suppression, cough, dizziness, growth deceleration, headache, hepatotoxicity (rare), hypertension, insomnia, irritability, moodiness, lethargy, nausea, suicidality (rare), tachycardia, vomiting, weight loss
Tricyclic antidepressants*	Arrhythmias, blurred vision, cardiac conduction slowing, cognitive dulling, constipation, death in overdose, dry mouth, hypertension, irritability, jaundice, postural hypotension, sedation, seizures, tachycardia, urinary retention, weight gain, withdrawal syndrome (flulike)
Bupropion*	Agitation, appetite suppression, constipation, dry mouth, hallucinations, headache, insomnia, irritability, nausea, rash, restlessness, seizures, tic exacerbation, tremor
α_2-Adrenergic agonists*	Appetite increase, behavioral activation, bradycardia (mild), constipation, depression, dizziness, dry mouth and eyes, fatigue, headache, hypotension (mild), irritability, rash, rebound hypertension, rebound tachycardia, sedation, stomachache

*Not FDA approved for use in ADHD.

foods may be helpful. Insomnia may resolve with earlier administration, by reducing the last of multiple daily doses, or by switching to an alternative psychostimulant or delivery system. Children who have a great deal of trouble settling for bed because of their ADHD may, in fact, be helped by a seemingly counterintuitive, small evening dose of IR psychostimulant. To avoid gastrointestinal distress, psychostimulants should never be taken on an empty stomach. Small tics induced by psychostimulants are best managed by dose reduction or by switching preparations. On the other hand, the comorbidity of a preexisting tic disorder, such as Tourette disorder, does not and should not preclude ADHD treatment with psychostimulants because they do not predictably exacerbate tics (The Tourette's Syndrome Study Group, 2002). Much has been written about a putative rebound phenomenon when a psychostimulant quickly loses its effectiveness. The observed behaviors, possibly due to the emergence of adverse effects but more likely due to the rapid recrudescence of ADHD symptoms, are best managed by either switching to another product or by adding an additional, small dose of IR psychostimulant.

The less common psychiatric adverse effects of these agents have generated much more provider and consumer concern. Emotional lability and irritability are occasionally induced by psychostimulants, often perceived by parents as a paradoxical exacerbation of ADHD and best addressed by either dose reduction or switching of preparations. On March 3, 2006, the FDA issued a memorandum summarizing its Adverse Events Reporting System data, which documented the emergence of manic and psychotic symptoms, especially visual hallucinations of insects and snakes, precipitated by usual doses of psychostimulants in the absence of any known risk factors. These symptoms always resolve when the offending agent is stopped.

The classification of psychostimulants by the U.S. Department of Justice as Schedule II controlled substances grew out of a concern for their potential diversion and abuse, which begged the question of whether early psychostimulant exposure increases the risk of later substance abuse. Meta-analysis of psychostimulant treatment studies in all age groups in which the emergence of substance use disorders was an outcome suggests that treatment of ADHD early and well actually reduces the risk of later alcohol and drug abuse (Wilens et al, 2003).

Changes in pulse rate and mean blood pressure due to these sympathomimetic agents are usually benign and rarely vary from baseline by more than about 5%, as measured by ambulatory blood pressure monitoring (Samuels et al, 2006). Once considered clinically insignificant during the 1990s, growth deceleration was found with chronic psychostimulant treatment in both the NIMH Multimodal Treatment Study of Children with Attention-Deficit/Hyperactivity Disorder (Swanson et al, 2007) and the Preschool ADHD Treatment Study (Swanson et al, 2006). There is no clear understanding of either the mechanism or longer term outcome of growth slowing after discontinuation of treatment.

Exceedingly rare cases of sudden death in children and adults who were taking psychostimulants have occurred, but at rates far below published background risk, which nevertheless has prompted the FDA to require a label warning. A review of the Adverse Events Reporting System data found that the majority of patients who died suddenly while taking mixed amphetamine salts had preexisting cardiac structural anomalies. A review of deaths associated with methylphenidate treatment similarly revealed cases in which cardiac structural anomalies were found. Motivated in part by these events and in part by practice in Japan and Europe, the American Heart Association Science Advisory and Coordinating Committee published a 2008 recommendation that all children, regardless of the absence of risk, have pretreatment ECG screening prior to starting stimulant medications (Vetter et al, 2008). The paper touched off a short-lived academic controversy that now appears settled with a careful approach, endorsed by the major stakeholding professional organizations, where positive patient and family-targeted cardiac histories or findings on examination would trigger further input from a pediatric cardiologist, but in the absence of risk, no pretreatment ECG is necessary (Perrin et al, 2008). The monitoring principles listed in Table 90-5, when performed at every clinic visit, will enhance the safety of psychostimulant treatment.

Atomoxetine

The only other medication with a current FDA indication for ADHD is atomoxetine, a nonstimulant first designed as a selective norepinephrine reuptake

Table 90-5. Basic Monitoring of Psychostimulant Treatment

Document height and weight on a growth chart at every visit. If a trend develops whereby the next lower, major percentile line is crossed, then a change in treatment is reasonable.
Document blood pressure and pulse at every visit, anticipating that a 5% change is possible. In rare cases of persistent tachycardia or hypertension, discontinue the offending stimulant.
Document any history of cardiac abnormalities and auscultate for worrisome murmurs before treatment. When in doubt, obtain a pediatric cardiology consultation. Routine electrocardiographic screening before treatment is neither necessary nor recommended for an otherwise healthy child with ADHD.
Always assess for persistent and pervasive changes in mood and do not hesitate to ask about suicidality when suspected.
Always talk to parents and caregivers about strengthening contingency behavioral management and encouraging structure in the child's life. This may permit treatment with the minimum possible stimulant dose to further reduce the risk of all adverse effects.

inhibitor antidepressant that failed to show efficacy in placebo-controlled trials in depressed patients. The efficacy of atomoxetine in ADHD is supported by RCTs, but with a smaller effect size than that of the psychostimulants (Michelson et al, 2001). Atomoxetine was studied as monotherapy for children with ADHD and comorbid anxiety, yielding a positive result (Kratochvil et al, 2005), but the trial was uncontrolled and will require replication. Older norepinephrine reuptake inhibitors have not been shown to be effective in child and adolescent anxiety (see the later section on pharmacotherapy of anxiety).

Atomoxetine binds extensively to plasma proteins and is metabolized by the hepatic cytochrome P-450 2D6 system to 4-hydroxyatomoxetine, an equally active norepinephrine reuptake inhibitor. The elimination half-life is a little more than 5 hours in patients with normal CYP 450 metabolic activity but climbs to 22 hours in those patients with slow metabolic activity. Any potent CYP 450 2D6 inhibitor, such as fluoxetine, will drive atomoxetine levels up. Atomoxetine must be administered daily, and maximum benefit may not be achieved until after several weeks of treatment. Dosing of atomoxetine, supplied in 10-, 18-, 25-, 40-, 60-, 80-, and 100-mg capsules, is related to body weight (see Table 90-3). There are no large RCTs at present to assess the practice or advisability of concomitant use of atomoxetine with psychostimulants.

With the exception of tics, the adverse effects of atomoxetine are remarkably similar to those of psychostimulants (see Table 90-4). The sympathomimetic effect of albuterol is potentiated by atomoxetine, so care should be taken in prescribing it to children with asthma. There has been no evidence for electrocardiographic changes due to treatment with atomoxetine. After receiving reports of hepatotoxicity in two patients taking atomoxetine, the FDA required a labeling change in 2004 warning of potentially severe liver injury. Physicians and caregivers alike were advised to monitor for itchy skin, jaundice, dark urine, upper right-sided abdominal tenderness, or unexplained "flulike" symptoms. In 2005, the FDA required a boxed warning about the increased risk, albeit very small, of suicidal thinking in children and adolescents taking atomoxetine, urging clinicians and parents to monitor closely for agitation, irritability, suicidality, or unusual behavioral changes for the first several months of treatment or after any dose change. The consent process for prescribing atomoxetine should therefore include discussion of this warning.

Antidepressants

Studies in the 1970s showed that imipramine, a tricyclic antidepressant (TCA), effectively treated hyperactive children (Waizer et al, 1974). Multiple trials have demonstrated the efficacy of TCAs in ADHD (Daly and Wilens, 1998), but the FDA has never approved them for this indication. The TCAs of choice, imipramine and nortriptyline, have been relegated to off-label, secondary use in ADHD practice guidelines when psychostimulants or atomoxetine have failed (see Table 90-3 for suggested dosing). The use of desipramine, one of the most effective tricyclics in ADHD, has largely been abandoned after reports were published of sudden death in children taking this medication (Biederman et al, 1995).

Imipramine and nortriptyline block both norepinephrine and serotonin reuptake transporters, but with different relative potencies. Both also act on presynaptic autoreceptors and antagonize histaminic and cholinergic receptors, which accounts for their less favorable adverse effects compared with psychostimulants and atomoxetine. TCAs are highly protein bound and are metabolized by demethylation of side chains and hydroxylation of ring structures by the CYP 450 2D6 system, posing a risk of significant drug-drug interactions. Elimination half-lives are 5 to 30 hours and 1 to 2 days for imipramine and nortriptyline, respectively.

The risk of cardiac conduction changes caused by TCAs demands electrocardiography before initiation, during titration, and periodically during treatment. If the PR interval widens beyond 210 msec and the QTc interval exceeds 450 msec, the TCA should be stopped. Heart rate and blood pressure should be measured routinely, with discontinuation recommended if blood pressure rises to 130/85 mm Hg during treatment. For additional safety, serum imipramine and nortriptyline trough levels should be measured at the effective dose and should not exceed 250 ng/mL or 100 ng/mL, respectively.

Bupropion, developed as a novel norepinephrine and dopamine reuptake inhibitor antidepressant in the 1980s, appears to be superior to placebo in the treatment of ADHD (Conners et al, 1996) but has not gained FDA approval for that indication. Marketing of bupropion was halted for 3 years because bulimic patients developed seizures taking the high doses recommended at the time. Bupropion should not be used in children or adolescents with a known seizure or eating disorder. Adverse effects are similar to those of the stimulants and atomoxetine, including the induction or exacerbation of tics, but excluding cardiovascular risk (see Table 90-4). It is available in immediate release, sustained release, and extended release delivery systems. Although bupropion has the FDA indication for smoking cessation programs in adults, there is no evidence to support its effectiveness in smoking prevention in youth with ADHD (Monuteaux et al, 2007).

None of the antidepressants in the selective serotonin reuptake inhibitor (SSRI) class is effective in treating the core symptoms of ADHD. Existing studies in which children with ADHD were given SSRIs are confounded by the comorbidity of depression, by lack of placebo controls, and by lack of power. Venlafaxine, a serotonin and norepinephrine reuptake inhibitor (SNRI), generated interest as a possible ADHD treatment because of its norepinephrine transporter antagonism, at first in very small trials with adults and later in youth (Olvera et al, 1996). However, no large-scale RCT is available to support the inclusion of venlafaxine in existing ADHD treatment protocols for children or adolescents. The same holds true for two other marketed SNRIs, duloxetine and desvenlafaxine. Finally, monoamine oxidase inhibitor antidepressants have promise as anti-ADHD medications but are neither approved nor suggested for use in children or adolescents because of dangerous adverse effects discussed later.

α_2-Adrenergic Agonists

Two agents in this class, clonidine and guanfacine, both with a primary indication for adult hypertension, have been used alone and in combination with stimulants to treat the hyperarousal, agitation, impulsivity, low frustration tolerance, and insomnia associated with ADHD. Clonidine is not FDA approved for ADHD, but guanfacine in a sustained release delivery vehicle is pending approval as of this writing. Clonidine and guanfacine are thought to work in specific brain regions in two ways: first, by presynaptic regulation of neuronal norepinephrine output from the locus ceruleus to reduce arousal; and second, by postsynaptic stimulation of prefrontal cortical neurons that regulate planning, impulse control, and to a lesser extent attention (Arnsten et al, 1996).

Many studies of clonidine have shown efficacy, with an effect size smaller than that of stimulants, in reducing the hyperactive-impulsive symptoms of ADHD, but not in improving attention (Connor et al, 1999). A recent multicenter RCT of guanfacine in an extended release delivery vehicle demonstrated its effectiveness in both improving attention and reducing hyperactivity (Biederman et al, 2008). Immediate release guanfacine is more rapidly absorbed than clonidine and has a significantly longer elimination half-life in children of 13 to 17 hours versus 6 to 12 hours for clonidine; thus, clonidine must be dosed more frequently than guanfacine to achieve a similarly consistent effect. Clonidine is approximately 10 times more potent than guanfacine and causes significantly more sedation, one of the reasons it is used as a hypnotic agent in hyperactive children. It may take several weeks at steady state for either agent to be effective. Clonidine is available in 0.1-, 0.2-, and 0.3-mg tablets and in a transdermal delivery system. Immediate release guanfacine has been available in 1-mg and 2-mg tablets, but the extended release formulation being prepared for market as of this writing will have additional available strengths.

Common adverse effects of both agents are listed in Table 90-4. The most concerning drug interaction is that with alcohol, in which dangerous central nervous system depression may occur. Although there is no clear or consistent evidence that either clonidine or guanfacine causes electrocardiographic changes, their associated mild hypotensive and bradycardic effects suggest a relative contraindication in patients with known sinus node or atrioventricular block or electrocardiography-demonstrated bradycardia. Pretreatment electrocardiography is not necessary, but taking a thorough cardiac history and routine monitoring of blood pressure and heart rate are essential. On discontinuation of α_2-adrenergic agonists after prolonged use, it is best to taper them to avoid rebound hypertension. In the mid-1990s, four cases of sudden death in children taking a combination of clonidine and methylphenidate were reported. In each case, preexisting cardiac disease precluded the FDA from finding that the cause of death was linked to the combination of these drugs (Popper, 1995).

Antipsychotics

The tranquilizing effects of the first-generation antipsychotics, now called the typical antipsychotics, including thioridazine, chlorpromazine, haloperidol, and others, made them attractive agents in the 1970s to target egregious hyperactivity, aggression, and agitation in ADHD that stimulants failed to ameliorate (Gittelman-Klein et al, 1976). These agents act primarily as antagonists at dopamine D_2 receptors (see pharmacotherapy of psychosis). Given this mechanism of action, it would seem counterintuitive to use these agents in the treatment of ADHD. Indeed, D_2 blockade in the mesocortical dopaminergic pathway may explain the cognitive blunting associated with typical antipsychotics.

The arrival of the second-generation or atypical antipsychotics, with the seductive promise of safety improvements, prompted interest in their use for refractory ADHD. The currently marketed atypical antipsychotics, including clozapine, risperidone, olanzapine, quetiapine, ziprasidone, aripiprazole, paliperidone, and iloperidone, have varying affinities for multiple types of dopamine, serotonin, α-adrenergic, cholinergic, and histaminic receptors. Among these atypicals, only risperidone has been well studied in children and adolescents with ADHD. Risperidone neither improves attention nor effectively controls impulsivity (Günther et al, 2006) but is effective in reducing the disruptive and aggressive behaviors associated with ADHD (see pharmacotherapy of disruptive behavior). Antipsychotics are not approved by the FDA for use in ADHD and do not appear in ADHD practice parameters.

Antiepileptic Drugs

The antiepileptic drug carbamazepine gained popularity as a potential treatment of ADHD in Europe, perhaps because its core molecular structure is that of a TCA. A dated meta-analysis of world literature suggested that carbamazepine is effective for ADHD (Silva et al, 1996), but a small, controlled study showed no value in disruptive behavior and aggression (Cueva et al, 1996). Because of its metabolic autoinduction and associated risks of agranulocytosis, aplastic anemia, exfoliative dermatitis, hyponatremia, and behavioral destabilization in children, carbamazepine is best avoided as a treatment of ADHD.

Non-Benzodiazepine Hypnotics

Insomnia is a common problem in children with ADHD, leading to the off-label use of the non-benzodiazepine hypnotics zolpidem and zaleplon in this population. A recent exclusivity RCT of zolpidem failed to demonstrate efficacy for insomnia associated with ADHD (U.S. FDA, 2006), and worrisome adverse effects emerged during treatment, including new-onset hallucinations, headache, and dizziness. The use of non-benzodiazepine hypnotics cannot be recommended in the pediatric population at present.

Complementary and Alternative Medicine

A review of existing, well-controlled complementary and alternative medicine studies of children with ADHD is beyond the scope of this chapter. Many complementary and alternative medicine studies begin with symptomatic patients in whom there is a preexisting vitamin or mineral deficiency or a metabolic derangement. Functional improvement after correction of these problems suggests that the ADHD-like symptoms in these patients had little to do with a neurodevelopmental etiology.

Psychosocial Treatments and Sequencing of Pharmacotherapy

In 1992, the NIMH launched the Multimodal Treatment Study of ADHD (MTA), the largest trial ever conducted to understand long-term, best practice approaches to its treatment. This uncontrolled study randomized 579 children aged 7 to 9 years into four treatment conditions: high-quality, intensive medication management alone (IR methylphenidate was the study drug); intensive, multicomponent behavioral therapy alone (such as social skills training and effective contingency management of disruptive behavior); their combination; and routine community care. The end point of treatment was at 14 months, when the two conditions containing high-quality stimulant management were clearly superior to either behavioral therapy alone or community care. Combination treatment resulted in better parent and teacher satisfaction as well as improvements in comorbidities like anxiety and disruptive behaviors (Jensen et al, 2001). After 14 months, families were free to choose their own follow-up treatment while continuing to be observed. At 24 months, the combination cohort and medication management alone cohort were still doing better than the other groups, but by 36 months, any differences had completely disappeared because of a natural regression of the groups initially treated with superior protocols toward a common outcome of improvement in all children compared to their status on entering the study (Jensen et al, 2007).

A helpful approach to sequencing medication trials is outlined in the ADHD practice parameter of the American Academy of Child and Adolescent Psychiatry Work Group on Quality Issues (Pliszka et al, 2007). In brief, after thorough assessment, a trial of psychostimulant is the first step, followed, if it is ineffective or not tolerated, in order by an alternative psychostimulant, atomoxetine, an effective antidepressant, an alternative antidepressant, and an α_2-agonist. This sequence mirrors not only expert consensus of best practice but also the order of decreasing effect size of these agents in efficacy studies.

PHARMACOTHERAPY OF DISRUPTIVE BEHAVIOR

The disruptive behavior disorders, discussed in Chapters 39 and 40, are first diagnosed in childhood and grouped together in the DSM-IV-TR with ADHD. They include oppositional defiant disorder, essentially recurrent, negativistic, hostile disobedience of authority figures; and conduct disorder, recurrent antisocial, sometimes aggressive behaviors that violate societal norms (American Psychiatric Association, 2000). Childhood oppositional defiant disorder is treated with evidence-based psychosocial interventions, for example, parent management training and school-based group therapies (Steiner et al, 2007). Pharmacotherapy in cases of oppositional defiant disorder is aimed at its common comorbidities, especially ADHD. The same is generally true for conduct disorder, but in this disorder, a growing body of evidence exists for pharmacotherapy of accompanying impulsive and predatory aggression.

Psychostimulants

Psychostimulants have long been considered a safe, effective, and rational first choice in treating the impulsive aggression associated with conduct disorder that is comorbid with ADHD (Campbell et al, 1992). Mild to moderate symptoms of disruptive behavior often remit when ADHD symptoms are fully treated.

Antimanic Agents

The antimanic agent lithium has been studied in hospitalized adolescents with aggression and conduct disorder since the 1980s. Relatively recent RCTs have demonstrated lithium's superiority to placebo in conduct disorder (e.g., Malone et al, 2000). The target dose of lithium for disruptive and aggressive behavior is the same as that for bipolar disorder, discussed in a later section (see pharmacotherapy of bipolar disorder).

Antipsychotics

The use of typical antipsychotics for severely disruptive behavior in childhood, substantiated by a few early trials of haloperidol, extends back 4 decades. The FDA has approved only chlorpromazine and thioridazine for this indication in children (see Table 90-11), but sufficient data from multiple, double-blind, controlled studies have shown that the atypical antipsychotic risperidone is well tolerated and acutely superior to placebo in reducing aggression and disruptive behavior in children and adolescents (Reyes et al, 2006), in children with subaverage intelligence (e.g., Aman et al, 2002), and in children with normal intelligence taking stimulants for ADHD (Armenteros et al, 2007). Risperidone, used off label for conduct disorder, may be dosed once or twice daily, generally not to exceed 4 mg daily. Even at low starting doses of 0.25 mg twice daily, the risks of extrapyramidal adverse effects and weight gain from risperidone are not insignificant. Only open trials of olanzapine and aripiprazole have been conducted for the acute treatment of adolescent conduct disorder. Despite the paucity of safety and efficacy data (with the exception of risperidone), the atypical neuroleptics are gaining popularity in practice, exposing children and adolescents, occasionally needlessly, to considerable risk.

PHARMACOTHERAPY OF DEPRESSION

After World War II, when psychoanalytic theory dominated American psychiatry, childhood depression, fully discussed in Chapter 47, was not thought possible because of psychological immaturity in the first decade of life. Ample research supports the validity of DSM-IV-TR diagnostic criteria for a major depressive episode in school-age children and adolescents but not in preschoolers or toddlers (Luby et al, 2002).

Findings in depressed adults of deficiencies in norepinephrine, dopamine, and serotonin neuroreceptor function and density, disturbances of the hypothalamic-pituitary-adrenal and hypothalamic-pituitary-thyroid axes, and structural differences in the medial prefrontal cortex, hippocampus, and amygdala have not yet been replicated in children and adolescents. Current pharmacotherapeutic strategies for the treatment of child and adolescent depression, therefore, were derived not from preclinical biologic models but instead from downward extensions of trials of effective drugs in adults.

In its practice parameters, the American Academy of Child and Adolescent Psychiatry divides the treatment of pediatric depression into three phases: an acute phase during the first 6 to 12 weeks; a continuation phase for 4 to 12 months; and a maintenance phase beyond 1 year (Birmaher et al, 1998). Nearly all existing drug trials of antidepressant efficacy in children and adolescents are limited to the acute phase.

Tricyclic Antidepressants

The impressive response rates of depressed adults to TCAs led to their early use in child and adolescent depression. A systematic review of all 13 published randomized, controlled trials of TCAs in pediatric depression revealed uniform failure of every trial, with response rates indistinguishable from placebo treatment (Hazell et al, 2002). Taken together with their problematic adverse effects (see Table 90-4) and potential lethality in overdose, this clear lack of evidence for efficacy argues strongly against the use of TCAs in depressed youth.

Selective Serotonin Reuptake Inhibitors

A surge in the use of SSRI antidepressants in adults beginning in the late 1980s, certainly because of their relative safety compared with TCAs, translated into enthusiasm for their use in the pediatric population. Although not as selective as the name implies, all SSRI antidepressants work primarily by blockade of the presynaptic serotonin transporter. The differences among SSRIs are in their relatively weak affinities for the norepinephrine and dopamine transporters and in their pharmacokinetics summarized in Table 90-6.

The first controlled study of fluoxetine in depressed 13- to 18-year-olds was disappointing (Simeon et al, 1990), in retrospect because of the small sample size. Subsequent, adequately powered RCTs of fluoxetine have demonstrated its uncontested efficacy in depressed children and adolescents in the acute phase of treatment (Emslie et al, 2002). These studies used a fixed dose of 20 mg given once daily. It has become clear in continuing work that for some unresponsive patients, well-tolerated dose titration up to 60 mg daily may be required to achieve benefit (Heiligenstein et al, 2006). Response rates in all pediatric studies of fluoxetine, in which response is defined as a 50% reduction in symptoms, have been consistently in excess of 60%, but interestingly, placebo response rates have also been large, on the order of 40%. This roughly 20% difference is a highly significant and replicated result, which led the FDA to approve fluoxetine as the first and, as of this writing, the only antidepressant for a major depressive episode in patients 7 to 17 years of age.

Fluoxetine is available in 10-, 20-, and 40-mg capsules, a 10-mg scored tablet, and a 20-mg/5 mL liquid. Initiation is usually at 10 mg daily; if tolerated, it is increased to 20 mg daily in 1 to 2 weeks. The adverse effects associated with fluoxetine and all SSRIs are listed in Table 90-7. In pediatric exclusivity studies, the FDA

Table 90-6. **Marketed Selective Serotonin Reuptake Inhibitor Antidepressants**

Agent	Parent Half-life	Metabolite with Antidepressant Effect?	Metabolic Inhibition*	Time to Steady State	Pediatric Indication
Fluoxetine	4-7 days	Yes; half-life, 4-16 days	CYP 2D6	4-6 weeks	MDD, OCD
Sertraline	27 hours	Yes; half-life, 66 hours	CYP 3A4	1 week	OCD
Paroxetine	21 hours	No	CYP 2D6	10 days	None
Fluvoxamine	15 hours	No	CYP 1A2	2 weeks	OCD
Citalopram	35 hours	Yes, negligible effect	CYP 2C19	1 week	None
Escitalopram	30 hours	Yes, negligible effect	CYP 2C19	1 week	None

*Most significant enzyme inhibition, among others.
MDD, major depressive disorder; OCD, obsessive-compulsive disorder.

found that weight loss, slight growth deceleration, behavioral activation, and higher plasma concentrations of drug occur in smaller children.

The emerging story of the remaining SSRIs in RCTs for pediatric depression is mixed. Two large, controlled studies of sertraline in depressed children and adolescents, aged 6 to 17 years, treated with a mean dose of 131 mg daily, were both negative when considered individually; but when the data were pooled in a repeated-measures, mixed model analysis, the drug appeared efficacious (Wagner et al, 2003). Three large, multisite, exclusivity studies of paroxetine in depressed children and adolescents, aged 7 to 17 years in aggregate, treated with 20 to 40 mg daily, failed to show a difference between drug and placebo response (U.S. FDA, 2002). Fluvoxamine has not been studied in a large RCT as monotherapy for pediatric depression. One positive exclusivity RCT of citalopram for pediatric depression yielded a response rate of 36% at 20 to 40 mg daily, compared with a placebo response rate of 24%, a statistically significant difference but not an impressive treatment effect (Wagner et al, 2004b). Escitalopram was recently found to be no more effective than placebo in a large RCT of depressed children and adolescents, aged 6 to 17 years, given 10 to 20 mg daily (Wagner et al, 2006).

Why should so many well-designed, well-controlled studies of these antidepressants yield negative results that run contrary to the experience of many clinicians in practice? Part of the reason may be buried in the rules of the studies. Study drugs were often titrated to the presumed target dose for effectiveness rather quickly, causing intolerability and study dropouts, especially among younger children. Differing methodologies, recruitment tactics, and exclusion criteria and the effect of conducting studies across multiple, sometimes international sites have all been suggested as confounding factors. The impressive placebo response rate in all studies makes it difficult to separate, borrowing a phrase from electrical engineering, the signal from the noise. These issues, as well as developmental immaturity of neural networks and pubertal effects on the brain, have been considered explanations for the many apparent failures of SSRI trials (Emslie et al, 2005). At present, SSRIs with some evidence for efficacy, specifically sertraline and citalopram, should be strongly considered in treatment of depressed children or adolescents who either cannot tolerate or do not respond to fluoxetine. A withdrawal syndrome is possible with abrupt discontinuation of all SSRIs except fluoxetine because of its long elimination half-life. In July 2006, the FDA issued an alert for the potential risk of serotonin syndrome when a 5-hydroxytryptamine receptor agonist used to treat migraine headaches is taken with any SSRI.

Table 90-7. Adverse Effects of SSRI Antidepressants

Dosing	Adverse Effects
Therapeutic	Abdominal discomfort, agitation, akathisia, anxiety, apathy syndrome, bruising, constipation, dizziness, drowsiness, dry mouth, epistaxis, fatigue, headache, hostility, insomnia, mania, movement disorders, nausea, sexual dysfunction, sweating, tics
Significant overdose*	Agitation, coma, diaphoresis, diarrhea, fever, hallucinations, hyperreflexia, incoordination, mental status change, myoclonus, shivering, tachycardia, tremor
Abrupt withdrawal†	Agitation, anxiety, crying spells, depression, disequilibrium, fatigue, insomnia, irritability, lethargy, migraine-like auras, myalgia, nausea, paresthesias, tremor, vivid dreams, vomiting

*Serotonin syndrome.
†Discontinuation syndrome.

Serotonin and Norepinephrine Reuptake Inhibitors

Venlafaxine, desvenlafaxine, and duloxetine are marketed representatives of antidepressants whose mechanism of action is serotonin and norepinephrine transporter antagonism (at higher doses, paroxetine, usually classified as an SSRI, acts as a serotonin and norepinephrine reuptake inhibitor). Venlafaxine, approved for use in adult depression, generalized anxiety disorder, and social phobia, is also a weak inhibitor of dopamine reuptake but has little affinity for other neuroreceptors. Venlafaxine is metabolized principally by the cytochrome P-450 2D6 system to O-desmethylvenlafaxine, also an active serotonin and norepinephrine reuptake inhibitor. The elimination half-lives of venlafaxine and its metabolite are 5 and 11 hours, respectively. Two large-scale, controlled, multicenter FDA pediatric exclusivity trials of venlafaxine for pediatric depression failed to show efficacy at doses ranging from 37.5 to 225 mg daily in 6- to 17-year-olds (U.S. FDA, 2003). Careful analysis revealed growth deceleration, hyperlipidemia, and hypertension in the treated group.

Monoamine Oxidase Inhibitors

The enzyme monoamine oxidase (MAO) occurs in humans in two forms, MAO-A and MAO-B. In neurons, MAO-A catabolizes norepinephrine and serotonin by deamination; both MAO-A and MAO-B destroy intraneuronal dopamine and tyramine. A class of drug called monoamine oxidase inhibitors developed in the 1950s created excitement after the serendipitous discovery of their antidepressant effect, hypothetically due to accumulation of neurotransmitters in the synaptic cleft by curtailing of their intracellular catabolism. Monoamine oxidase inhibitors have been synthesized with two important properties, reversibility and selectivity, to improve targeting of the central nervous system and to reduce their potentially dangerous drug-drug and drug-food interactions. Precisely because required dietary restrictions, avoidance of amphetamines, and severe central nervous system toxicity and cardiovascular instability in overdose present risky obstacles to the use of monoamine oxidase inhibitors in depressed, impulsive adolescents, there has been little interest in and no large scale RCTs in this age group.

Norepinephrine and Dopamine Reuptake Inhibitors

First synthesized in 1966, bupropion and its active hydroxylated metabolite inhibit the norepinephrine and dopamine reuptake transporters with little effect at other receptor sites. Largely protein bound, it is extensively metabolized by the hepatic CYP 450 2B6 pathway, resulting in significant drug-drug interactions. Its elimination half-life is about 12 hours. The launch of bupropion to market some 20 years after its synthesis was aborted because of reports of seizures in nondepressed, bulimic patients. Eventually introduced in 1989, the recommended maximum daily dose in adults was 450 mg, above which it becomes potentially epileptogenic. There is a paucity of studies, mostly open label, to support the use of bupropion in children and adolescents as monotherapy for a major depressive episode, and as of this writing, there have been no large-scale RCTs for this purpose registered with the FDA. Whether bupropion is any better than placebo in the treatment of pediatric depression is unknown.

Noradrenergic and Specific Serotonin Antagonists

Synthesized in the Netherlands in the late 1980s, mirtazapine was introduced to the United States in 1996 as a novel antidepressant that antagonizes α_2 and serotonin S_2 and S_3 receptors, increasing norepinephrine output presynaptically and selectively improving S_1 receptor neurotransmission. In multiple studies of depressed adults, mirtazapine proved to be as effective as SSRIs and serotonin and norepinephrine reuptake inhibitors, but it caused excessive somnolence in virtually one of every two treated patients as well as increased appetite and weight gain in one of four patients. Two pediatric exclusivity studies of mirtazapine were evaluated by the FDA, one for efficacy and safety and the other for pharmacokinetics. The efficacy study was a large RCT of depressed children and adolescents, aged 7 to 17 years, at 34 sites, who received 15 to 45 mg daily for 8 weeks. The result was a failure; patients randomized to mirtazapine responded indistinguishably from placebo-treated patients (U.S. FDA, 2004a). It is unwise to consider the use of mirtazapine as a hypnotic in adolescents as it will potentiate the effects of alcohol and other central nervous system depressants.

Serotonin S_2 Antagonist and Reuptake Inhibitors

Trazodone, synthesized in Italy in the 1960s, was the first of the serotonin S_2 antagonist and serotonin reuptake inhibitor antidepressants, followed years later by nefazodone. Trazodone differs from nefazodone in that trazodone also has antihistaminic action, whereas nefazodone has weak norepinephrine reuptake inhibition. Trazodone, avoided for treatment of depression in children and adolescents in part because of an associated risk of priapism, is sometimes used off-label at low doses, usually between 50 and 100 mg, as a hypnotic. Nefazodone was studied in two large exclusivity RCTs in 7- to 18-year-olds with depression at doses up to 600 mg daily, and both failed to show efficacy. Nefazodone carries a black box warning for the risk of liver failure, which combined with its lack of efficacy in exclusivity studies argues strongly against its use in children and adolescents.

Complementary and Alternative Medicine

Of all the oral "natural antidepressants" that have been promoted in mass media, at least two, St. John's wort and essential fatty acids, have generated considerable research interest. St. John's wort, or *Hypericum perforatum*, is a botanical that has been used for centuries for a multitude of ailments. It appears to have weak reuptake inhibition at serotonin, norepinephrine, and dopamine transporters and may also have effects at γ-aminobutyric acid (GABA) receptors. A relatively recent, extensive review of RCTs comparing *Hypericum* to placebo or to an active, evidence-based antidepressant revealed contradictory findings (Linde et al, 2005). No well-designed, controlled study of *Hypericum* has been conducted in depressed children or adolescents. Troublesome side effects of *Hypericum* relevant to adolescents include breakthrough bleeding on oral contraceptives and its induction of the CYP 450 system, specifically the 1A2, 3A4, and 2C9 enzymes, which reduces the effectiveness of many psychotropics, anticonvulsants, selected antibiotics, and other medications.

The source of long-chain fatty acids in Western diets has changed remarkably during the past century from fish and plants to bovine animals and vegetable oils. Speculation about the connection between higher fish consumption and lower rates of depression in non-U.S. populations led to studies whose findings were mixed at the level of inference. However, several researchers have found an association between depression and lower than normal plasma and erythrocyte membrane levels of omega-3 fatty acids. A recent review of small RCTs using fish oil versus vegetable oil augmentation of conventional psychotropic drug treatment for bipolar and depressed patients seems to suggest an additive antidepressant effect of omega-3 fatty acids (Parker et al, 2006). This intriguing result encouraged a group of Israeli investigators to pilot a small study of omega-3 fatty acids in depressed children that yielded a positive result (Nemets et al, 2006).

Psychosocial and Combination Treatment

In cases of mild to moderate depression, it is best to begin treatment with a psychosocial therapy. Multiple RCTs have demonstrated the efficacy of cognitive-behavioral psychotherapy (Compton et al, 2004) and interpersonal psychotherapy (Mufson et al, 2004) in treating adolescent depression. A groundbreaking, randomized, placebo-controlled study of moderately to severely depressed teenagers known as TADS (Treatment for Adolescents with Depression Study) examined the efficacy and cost-effectiveness of cognitive-behavioral therapy (CBT), the antidepressant fluoxetine, their combination, and placebo (March et al, 2004). At 12 weeks, the response rate in the fluoxetine monotherapy group was comparable to that of prior exclusivity studies of fluoxetine in depressed youth, whereas the response rate of the CBT monotherapy group was surprisingly closer to the placebo response rate. However, the synergy of simultaneous therapy with both CBT and fluoxetine (called combination treatment) resulted in a superior response on all outcome measures.

At 12 weeks, fluoxetine monotherapy was more cost-effective than combination treatment, but both proved to be at least as cost-effective as routine primary care for adolescent depression (Domino et al, 2008). Interestingly, by 36 weeks, the difference in response rates among the active TADS conditions essentially disappeared; however, response was accelerated in the conditions in which fluoxetine was used, whereas CBT appeared to confer enhanced safety with greater reduction in suicidal ideation in the conditions in which it was used (March et al, 2007). A British trial conducted with 208 moderately to severely depressed adolescents in which half were randomized to an SSRI (fluoxetine preferred) with routine care and half were randomized to an SSRI plus CBT and routine care showed neither a difference in outcome measures nor any protective effect of CBT at 12 weeks (Goodyer et al, 2007). The Treatment of SSRI-Resistant Depression in Adolescents (TORDIA) addressed the problem of depressed youth who do not respond to an initial adequate trial of fluoxetine (or other SSRI) monotherapy. The TORDIA study randomized 334 depressed adolescents to monotherapy with an alternative SSRI, monotherapy with venlafaxine, combination CBT plus the alternative SSRI, or combination CBT plus venlafaxine. Switching to any condition resulted in a significant response rate with fewer adverse effects due to the alternative SSRI compared with venlafaxine, but a clearly superior response, consistent with the TADS findings, resulted when either combination treatment was used (Brent et al, 2008).

Black Boxes and the Risk of Suicidality

When the FDA requested clarification of the term *emotional lability* describing a type of adverse event in exclusivity trials of paroxetine for pediatric depression, GlaxoSmithKline submitted a report on May 22, 2003, suggesting an increased risk of suicidality (suicidal thinking and behavior) in patients treated with drug compared with placebo. If ever there were a spark that ignited the current firestorm over the safety of antidepressants in children and adolescents, this was it. Six months later, the Medicines and Healthcare Products Regulatory Agency in the United Kingdom declared paroxetine, venlafaxine, sertraline, citalopram, and escitalopram (but not fluoxetine) to be contraindicated in pediatric depression. After a blue-ribbon advisory committee's meta-analysis of 24 U.S. exclusivity RCTs of antidepressants in pediatric depression, ADHD, and anxiety disorders, and after blistering congressional hearings, the FDA issued a public health advisory on October 15, 2004, directing manufacturers of all marketed antidepressants to include a black box package warning of an increased risk of suicidality in children and adolescents treated with these agents (U.S. FDA, 2004b). The average risk was small, 4% in patients exposed to antidepressants compared with 2% in patients treated with placebo (a risk difference of 2%), and none of the 4487 patients in the 24 studies completed suicide. The language in the black box has been modified twice, no longer implying causality and including young adults in the risk group.

A larger meta-analysis of 5310 children and adolescents in 27 RCTs of antidepressant treatment for depression, obsessive-compulsive disorder (OCD), and non-OCD anxiety disorders resulted in a pooled, overall risk difference of only 0.7% between drug- and placebo-treated depressed youth, lower than the FDA's original estimate of 2% (Bridge et al, 2007). This important review also demonstrated that SSRI antidepressants are more effective in anxiety disorders, especially non-OCD anxiety disorders, than in depression. In 2004, the FDA strongly recommended a rigid monitoring schedule for youth treated with SSRIs, namely, face-to-face visits each week for the first 4 weeks, followed by every-other-week office visits for the next month. In 2007, the FDA retracted these recommendations in favor of "appropriate monitoring" for clinical worsening during the initial months of treatment and at each dose change.

In the decade before the black box controversy, suicide rates in U.S. adolescents had been declining as antidepressant prescription rates were climbing (Olfson et al, 2003). Similarly, after adjustment for complicating factors, including access to health care, national suicide rates of children aged 5 to 14 years were shown to be lower in those counties with higher SSRI prescription rates (Gibbons et al, 2006). It now appears that after the first of the FDA warnings in 2003, a sharp drop occurred not only in prescription rates for antidepressants in youth but also in the diagnosis of depression itself (Libby et al, 2007). At the same time, the number of suicides in youth younger than 20 years rose dramatically in the United States (Hamilton et al, 2007), reversing the prior trend.

Many experts have concluded that despite a marginal increase in suicidality associated with antidepressant use, these drugs prevent completed suicides by treating depression, and any small increase in suicidality attributable to drug appears to be cancelled out by the positive effects of cognitive-behavioral psychotherapy in combination treatment (Emslie et al, 2006). A full discussion with the patient, if the patient is old enough to understand, and with the family of the risks and benefits of treatment with SSRIs should be the standard of care in modern practice. Monitoring by regular visits during the acute phase of treatment is a highly recommended part of the safety plan. Interested parents may go to *www.parentsmedguide.org* or to the FDA Web site at *www.fda.gov/cder/drug/antidepressants/default.htm* for further information.

PHARMACOTHERAPY OF ANXIETY

Anxiety, discussed more completely in Chapter 47, can range from a protective alerting signal to diffuse apprehension, tension, or fear in response to real or imagined threats. Anxiety can be impairing when the response, mediated through the autonomic nervous system, is excessive, involuntary, persistent, and pervasive, leading to avoidance and distress if not physiologic, emotional, cognitive, or behavioral dysfunction. The principal neurotransmitters involved, and the targets for modulation by effective anxiolytic agents, are serotonin, norepinephrine, and gamma-aminobutyric acid.

Tricyclic Antidepressants

Effective in adult anxiety disorders, TCAs were among the first agents considered in treatment of childhood anxiety. Imipramine was the most commonly studied

TCA in early trials for school refusal, formulated as separation anxiety (Gittelman-Klein and Klein, 1971). Carefully controlled follow-up studies of TCAs in this and other childhood anxiety disorders were unimpressive. Lack of evidence, unfavorable adverse effects, and potential lethality in overdose led to the dwindling use of TCAs in child and adolescent anxiety. The single exception is clomipramine, essentially imipramine with a unitary chlorine substitution on one of its aromatic rings, making it the most potent serotonin reuptake inhibitor of all the TCAs. Clomipramine, clearly effective in placebo-controlled trials for pediatric OCD (DeVeaugh-Geiss et al, 1992), gained FDA approval for this indication (but not for other childhood anxiety disorders). Clomipramine carries the same risks as all other TCAs.

Selective Serotonin Reuptake Inhibitor Antidepressants

OCD attracted the attention of many researchers interested in studying SSRIs in pediatric anxiety. Fluoxetine was the first SSRI antidepressant to be shown efficacious in child and adolescent OCD (Riddle et al, 1992), eventually gaining FDA approval for this indication. Similarly, sertraline (March et al, 1998) and fluvoxamine (Riddle et al, 2001) were found to be effective and approved for pediatric OCD (Table 90-8) in dose ranges remarkably similar to those for adults. Although not FDA approved for this indication, paroxetine also appears efficacious in a controlled study of pediatric OCD (Geller et al, 2004). To date, neither citalopram nor escitalopram has been well studied in pediatric OCD.

SSRIs have also been studied in the more common childhood anxiety disorders (Table 90-9). The first large-scale RCT targeting separation anxiety, social phobia, and generalized anxiety in children and adolescents was conducted by the Research Unit on Pediatric Psychopharmacology (RUPP), a consortium of investigators sponsored by the NIMH. The study drug, fluvoxamine at 50 to 300 mg daily, yielded a significant response rate of 76% with few side effects (RUPP, 2001). Fluoxetine at 20 mg daily is also effective for non-OCD pediatric anxiety disorders (Birmaher et al, 2003). Sertraline was shown to be effective at 50 mg daily in a small but exclusive study of generalized anxiety in children and adolescents (Rynn et al, 2001). A large-scale RCT of paroxetine for social phobia in 8- to 17-year-olds demonstrated its superiority to placebo at 10 to 50 mg daily (Wagner et al, 2004a).

In less common forms of child and adolescent anxiety, the data are few and weak. Studies of selective mutism,

Table 90-8. Anxiolytic Agents with FDA-Approved Pediatric Indications

Agent	Indication	Evidence in Anxiety Exclusivity Studies	Dose Range for Efficacy or Comments	Starting Dose (mg daily)*
Clomipramine	OCD	Positive RCT, ages 10-17 years	100-200 mg daily	12.5/25
Fluoxetine	OCD	Positive RCT, ages 7-17 years	20-60 mg daily	5-10/10-20
Sertraline	OCD	Positive RCT	50-200 mg daily	12.5/25
Fluvoxamine	OCD	Positive RCT, ages 8-17 years	50-200 mg daily divided bid	12.5/25
Doxepin	GAD	No studies, no evidence, >12 years	A tricyclic antidepressant	Not suggested
Meprobamate	GAD	No studies, no evidence, >6 years	Abuse potential, fatal in overdose	Not suggested
Hydroxyzine	GAD	No studies, no evidence	Bronchodilator, antihistamine	Not suggested

*Child/adolescent.
OCD, obsessive-compulsive disorder; GAD, generalized anxiety disorder; RCT, randomized, placebo-controlled trial.

Table 90-9. Other Selected Placebo-Controlled Pediatric Trials of Anxiolytic Agents

Agent	Off-Label Use	Evidence	Dose Range for Efficacy or Comments	Starting Dose (mg daily)*
Fluvoxamine	GAD, SAD, SoP	Positive RCT, ages 6-17 years	50-300 mg daily	12.5/25
Fluoxetine	GAD, SAD, SoP	Positive RCT, ages 7-17 years	20 mg daily	5-10/10-20
Sertraline	GAD	Positive RCTs, ages 5-17 years	50 mg daily	12.5/25
Buspirone	GAD	2 negative RCTs, ages 6-17 years	No better than placebo	Not suggested
Venlafaxine	GAD	Negative RCT, ages 6-17 years	Growth deceleration	Not suggested
Paroxetine	SoP	Positive RCT, ages 8-17 years	10-50 mg daily	5/10

*Child/adolescent.
GAD, generalized anxiety disorder; SAD, separation anxiety disorder; SoP, social phobia; RCT, randomized, placebo-controlled trial.

conceptualized as an extreme form of social phobia, have focused on the use of fluoxetine. One dated, small, controlled study of 6- to 12-year-olds treated with fluoxetine, 20 mg daily, was positive only by parent ratings, an effect that was lost at the end of the study (Black and Uhde, 1994). Panic disorder is relatively uncommon in children, which may explain the lack of pediatric exclusivity RCTs using any pharmacotherapeutic agent. Treatment of post-traumatic stress disorder in the pediatric population with SSRIs has not been carefully studied.

A suicidality signal was detected in the OCD and non-OCD anxiety studies included in the FDA meta-analysis that led to the black box warning on all antidepressants. The pooled risk difference between patients receiving active drug versus placebo was 0.7% in the OCD trials and 0.8% in the non-OCD trials (Bridge et al, 2007). Nevertheless, given their efficacy and tolerability, SSRIs should be considered first-line agents in treating child and adolescent non-OCD anxiety disorders (Seidel and Walkup, 2006).

Serotonin and Norepinephrine Reuptake Inhibitor Antidepressants

Although it is indicated for adult anxiety, two FDA exclusivity trials of venlafaxine in 6- to 17-year-olds with generalized anxiety yielded equivocal results, neither of which was published—one positive with a relatively low 46% response rate, and one negative with a lower response rate indistinguishable from placebo (U.S. FDA, 2003). In these trials, the same adverse effects and safety risks occurred as in the pediatric depression studies of venlafaxine.

Benzodiazepines

Benzodiazepines, first synthesized in the 1950s, have an affinity for a receptor complex that modulates GABA activity, inhibiting specific neurons that contribute to anxiety. In adults, benzodiazepines are also used to treat insomnia, agitation, seizures, and withdrawal syndromes and as preanesthesia and muscle-relaxing agents. Benzodiazepines are rapidly absorbed and have elimination half-lives, depending on the particular agent, ranging from 2.5 to 100 hours.

The literature on controlled trials of benzodiazepines in children and adolescents is, however, vanishingly small. This may be due to a concern for the development of tolerance or addiction as seen in some adults, a disinhibition phenomenon seen in children, or problematic adverse effects, including sedation, irritability, rage, hyperarousal, perceptual disturbances, and seizures on abrupt withdrawal. One dated RCT of alprazolam in children and adolescents with generalized anxiety disorder and social phobia failed to show any benefit of the drug over placebo (Simeon et al, 1992). Clonazepam seems to be of little use in separation anxiety disorder (Graae et al, 1994). At present, there are no data to support acute or long-term treatment of child and adolescent anxiety with benzodiazepines. Their utility in the pediatric population remains limited to special applications, such as rapid tranquilization, preanesthesia, and aborting seizures.

Buspirone

Buspirone is a serotonin receptor agonist and mixed dopamine agonist-antagonist. It has no activity at GABA receptors. Open trials during the 1990s suggested the efficacy of buspirone in pediatric anxiety, but two well-controlled FDA exclusivity studies failed to demonstrate any difference between drug and placebo treatment (U.S. FDA, 2007a). At present, there is little support for the use of buspirone in pediatric anxiety.

Antihistamines

Hydroxyzine, a histamine H_1 and muscarinic antagonist, has been shown to be effective in adults with generalized anxiety disorder (Llorca et al, 2002). This relatively recent finding cannot account for the decades' old practice of prescribing hydroxyzine or diphenhydramine to children for anxiety without any supporting data. Both antihistamines are used off-label as hypnotics in children and adolescents, and diphenhydramine is a well-known intervention for acute dystonias caused by typical antipsychotics. Adverse effects associated with antihistamines are legion, including, to list a few, sedation, gastrointestinal distress, anticholinergic effects, hallucinations, agitation, and even death in overdose.

Glutamate Antagonists

Treatment-resistant cases of pediatric OCD are not uncommon. Animal models of OCD have strongly implicated excessive production of the excitatory neurotransmitter glutamate in the pathogenesis of this anxiety disorder (McGrath et al, 2000). Preliminary studies of riluzole, a glutamate antagonist, have suggested its efficacy in adults with OCD. One open label trial of riluzole in a small pediatric sample of treatment-resistant children and adolescents provided further evidence of its potential efficacy and safety (Grant et al, 2007). As a result, a randomized, controlled trial of riluzole in children and adolescents with OCD, including those with autistic spectrum disorders, sponsored by the NIMH is in the recruiting phase as of this writing.

Psychosocial and Combination Treatment

In mild to moderate cases of anxiety, the first intervention should be evidence-based psychosocial therapy, usually CBT. In OCD, the combination of CBT with medication produces a better and more resilient outcome than either treatment alone (Pediatric OCD Treatment Study Team, 2004). Designed much like TADS, the Child/Adolescent Anxiety Multimodal Treatment Study is an RCT comparing the efficacy of CBT, sertraline, and their combination for separation anxiety disorder, social phobia, and generalized anxiety disorder in 7- to 17-year-olds (National Institute of Mental Health, 2007). Results of the CAMS study, published as this text was going to press, were remarkably similar to those of TADS, in that combination treatment of anxiety with CBT plus sertraline produced a robust response, monotherapy with either CBT or sertraline yielded an equivalent, good but less robust response, and all active treatments were superior to placebo treatment (Walkup et al, 2008). Importantly, there was no difference in harm-related adverse events, including suicidal ideation, between the sertraline and CBT groups.

PHARMACOTHERAPY OF PSYCHOSIS

Schizophrenia, discussed in Chapter 48, is exceedingly rare in childhood, generally being manifested in late adolescence and frequently comorbid with anxiety, depression, substance abuse, disruptive behavior, and learning disorders. A complex neuropsychiatric disorder, its treatment must be multimodal, including medication management, psychoeducation, psychotherapy, family support, and educational or vocational consultation.

Typical Antipsychotics

Chlorpromazine, the first typical antipsychotic discovered just after World War II, the impact of which on public health has been compared with that of penicillin, catalyzed the deinstitutionalization movement of chronically mentally ill patients in the United States. Chlorpromazine blocks dopamine D_2 receptors in mesolimbic dopamine pathways in the human brain, the mechanism believed to relieve the positive symptoms of schizophrenia. It also blocks neurotransmission in three other major dopamine pathways, namely, the mesocortical, nigrostriatal, and tuberoinfundibular tracts. The blockade of nigrostriatal dopamine receptors causes movement disorders, collectively known as extrapyramidal side effects. Chlorpromazine and all typical antipsychotics also antagonize muscarinic cholinergic, α-adrenergic, and histaminic neuroreceptors. The unpleasant adverse effects associated with all of these actions are summarized in Table 90-10. Among the most concerning adverse effects are involuntary, choreoathetoid movements of the head, limbs, and trunk known as tardive dyskinesia and a potentially fatal condition known as neuroleptic malignant syndrome, characterized by muscle rigidity, temperature to 107° F, altered consciousness, and autonomic instability. In addition, all typical antipsychotics have the potential to lower the seizure threshold.

Table 90-10. **Adverse Effects Associated with First-Generation Antipsychotic Receptor Antagonism**

Receptor	Adverse Effects Due to Receptor Antagonism
Mesocortical and mesolimbic dopamine	Anhedonia, ataraxia (indifference), cocaine-seeking, cognitive blunting, tranquilization
Tuberoinfundibular dopamine	Decreased follicle-stimulating hormone, decreased luteinizing hormone, hyperprolactinemia
Nigrostriatal dopamine	Acute dystonias, akathisia, bradykinesia, cogwheel rigidity, drooling, masked facies, muscle stiffness, oculogyric crisis, resting tremor, shuffling gait, stooped posture, tardive dyskinesia
Muscarinic cholinergic	Confusion, constipation, delirium, drowsiness, mydriasis (blurred vision), nausea, open-angle glaucoma exacerbation, QRS interval prolongation, sinus tachycardia, urinary retention, vomiting, xerostomia (dry mouth)
α_1-Adrenergic	Dizziness, dysrhythmias, incontinence, orthostatic hypotension, QTc prolongation, reflex tachycardia, sedation
α_2-Adrenergic	Anorgasmia, erectile dysfunction, priapism, retrograde ejaculation
Histamine H_1	Diabetes risk, sedation, weight gain

The typical antipsychotics for which there are trials in child and adolescent psychosis are listed in Table 90-11. Four of these agents have an FDA pediatric indication. The elimination half-lives are all in the 20- to 40-hour range, permitting once-daily dosing but requiring about 1 week to reach steady state. Virtually all typical antipsychotics are metabolized by the CYP 450 2D6 system, making them liable to significant drug-drug interactions. High-potency typical antipsychotics have a higher affinity for dopamine receptors (bind more tightly) than low-potency agents do. In general, higher potency typical antipsychotics, such as haloperidol, are less sedating, less cardiotoxic, and less anticholinergic than low-potency agents but more likely to cause extrapyramidal side effects.

Dosing of typical antipsychotics should be conservative, starting haloperidol at 0.25 mg daily in children or 1.0 mg daily in an adolescent. To reduce the risk of extrapyramidal side effects, titration of haloperidol should be gradual, increasing the dose in weekly increments. The target dose for psychosis is 3 to 6 mg daily in children and 10 mg daily in adolescents. Acute dystonias may occur early in treatment, especially after a dose change, but can be aborted by administration

Table 90-11. **First-Generation Antipsychotics with Trials in Children and Adolescents and Risks**

Agent	Metabolic Inhibition*	FDA Pediatric Indication?	Potency	EPS†	Sedation	Endocrine‡
Thioridazine	CYP 2D6	Yes, severe behavioral dyscontrol	Low	Low	High	High
Chlorpromazine	CYP 2D6	Yes, severe behavioral dyscontrol	Low	Low	High	High
Haloperidol	CYP 2D6	Yes, psychosis	High	High	Low	Low
Pimozide	CYP 3A4	Yes, Tourette disorder > age 12 years	Moderate	Moderate	Moderate	Moderate
Loxapine	CYP 2D6	No	Moderate	High	Moderate	Moderate
Fluphenazine	CYP 2D6	No	High	High	Low	Low

*Most significant enzyme inhibition, among others.
†EPS, extrapyramidal side effects; e.g., dystonias, akathisia, parkinsonism, tardive dyskinesia.
‡Endocrinologic effects; e.g., weight gain, galactorrhea.

Table 90-12. **The Atypical Antipsychotics**

Agent	Parent Half-life	Metabolic Inhibition*	Controlled Trials in Children and Adolescents
Clozapine	12 hours	1A2/3A4	Psychotic disorder
Risperidone	3 hours	2D6/3A4	Disruptive, autistic, Tourette, psychotic, bipolar disorders
Olanzapine	36 hours	1A2/2D6	Disruptive, autistic, psychotic, bipolar disorders
Quetiapine	6 hours	3A4	Bipolar disorder
Ziprasidone	4 hours	3A4 (slight)	Tourette disorder
Aripiprazole	68 hours	2D6/3A4	Unpublished RCT in adolescents
Paliperidone	23 hours	2D6/3A4	No published RCTs in children or adolescents at present
Iloperidone	14 hours	1A2/3A4	No published RCTs in children or adolescents at present

*Most significant enzyme inhibition, among others.
RCT, randomized, placebo-controlled trial.

of oral or intramuscular benztropine (1 to 2 mg) or diphenhydramine (25 to 50 mg). Rarely seen in children, akathisia is most often managed with low doses of propranolol.

Atypical Antipsychotics

Clozapine, synthesized in Switzerland in 1958, was the first of a second generation of antipsychotics, now called atypicals. Clozapine was removed from the European market in 1975 after the death of eight Finnish patients who developed agranulocytosis. Mandatory, intensive hematologic monitoring for agranulocytosis, shown to be reversible if it is discovered in time, was required by the U.S. FDA for approval of clozapine in 1990. Clozapine is still considered to be the most effective antipsychotic available for the treatment of refractory schizophrenia. Seven more atypical antipsychotics, shown in Table 90-12, have been brought to market in fairly rapid succession. Atypical antipsychotics are also known as dopamine-serotonin antagonists because of their affinity for dopamine D_2 and serotonin S_{2A} receptors. The difference among them is their variable effects, from negligible to significant, on α-adrenergic, muscarinic cholinergic, and histaminic receptors. The atypicals were initially touted as safer than the first-generation antipsychotics with respect to extrapyramidal side effects and risk of tardive dyskinesia. However, the atypical antipsychotic risperidone binds more tightly to dopamine receptors than dopamine itself and all of the other atypicals, making it at least as risky for extrapyramidal side effects as the drugs it was to replace (Seeman and Tallerico, 1998). Quetiapine is the least tightly bound atypical, suggesting that it has the lowest risk for extrapyramidal side effects, whereas olanzapine's affinity for dopamine receptors is about the same as that of many low-potency typical antipsychotics. In short, the risk for acute dystonias, akathisia, parkinsonism, and even tardive dyskinesia with the atypicals is not insignificant. Hyperprolactinemia and enuresis are also commonly seen in children treated acutely with risperidone.

All atypicals carry the risks of QTc prolongation, diabetes onset or exacerbation, weight gain, insulin resistance, and hyperlipidemia, the last three of which are collectively called a metabolic syndrome. Clozapine and olanzapine pose the greatest risk of weight gain and diabetes, risperidone and quetiapine a moderate risk, and ziprasidone and aripiprazole the lowest risk. The 2004 Consensus Development Conference on Antipsychotic Drugs and Obesity and Diabetes, jointly sponsored by the American Diabetes Association, the American Psychiatric Association, the American Association of Clinical Endocrinologists, and the North American Association for the Study of Obesity, published a set of monitoring guidelines applicable to patients of all ages treated with atypical antipsychotics. The guidelines recommend baseline measurement of body mass index, waist circumference, blood pressure, fasting plasma glucose concentration, and fasting lipid profile, to be repeated at 12 weeks and then annually, with the exception of fasting lipid profile at every 5 years (American Diabetes Association et al, 2004). Marked changes in any of these parameters warrant a switch to another agent.

Several early, small, retrospective and open label studies suggested the effectiveness of atypical antipsychotics in pediatric schizophrenia. In an NIMH short-duration study of treatment-resistant children, clozapine at an average dose of 176 mg daily was more effective in relieving symptoms than haloperidol at an average dose of 16 mg daily, but it caused more adverse effects, including neutropenia and tachycardia (Kumra et al, 1996). In a pilot study of 50 patients aged 8 to 19 years randomized to risperidone 4 mg daily, olanzapine 12.3 mg daily, or haloperidol 5 mg daily for 8 weeks, all groups improved regardless of the agent (Sikich et al, 2004), but those treated with olanzapine experienced a significant weight gain (average, 7.1 kg) and those receiving risperidone gained a moderate amount of weight (average, 4.9 kg); haloperidol caused the least weight gain (3.5 kg). On August 22, 2007, the FDA announced approval of risperidone for the treatment of schizophrenia in adolescents aged 13 to 17 years on the basis of two unpublished, industry-sponsored, double-blind, multicenter, international studies requested by the FDA under the Best Pharmaceuticals for Children Act (U.S. FDA, 2007b). In the first controlled study, 158 patients were randomized to placebo, risperidone 1 to 3 mg daily, or risperidone 4 to 6 mg daily. In the second study, 255 patients were randomized either to low-dose risperidone (maximum,

Table 90-13. **Agents with the FDA Indication for Bipolar Disorder**

Agent	Class	Indications	Pediatric Evidence	Pediatric Indication?
Lithium	Antimanic agent	Acute mania, maintenance	RCTs, open label, comparator study	Yes
Chlorpromazine	Typical antipsychotic	Acute mania	None	No
Risperidone	Atypical antipsychotic	Acute mania	RCTs, open label	Yes
Olanzapine	Atypical antipsychotic	Acute mania, maintenance	Open label	No
Olanzapine plus fluoxetine	Atypical antipsychotic and SSRI antidepressant	Bipolar depression	None	No
Quetiapine	Atypical antipsychotic	Acute mania	Comparison study	No
Ziprasidone	Atypical antipsychotic	Acute mania	Case report	No
Aripiprazole	Atypical antipsychotic	Acute mania, maintenance	RCT	Yes
Divalproex	Antiepileptic	Acute mania	Case reports, open label, comparator study	No
Carbamazepine	Antiepileptic	Maintenance	Case reports, comparison	No
Lamotrigine	Antiepileptic	Maintenance	Case reports, open label	No

RCT, randomized, placebo-controlled trial.

0.4 to 0.6 mg/day) or high-dose risperidone (maximum, 4 to 6 mg/day). In both studies, risperidone was titrated to the target dose within 2 weeks. A significant drop in the Positive and Negative Symptom Scale for schizophrenia (PANSS) score at 6 or 8 weeks was achieved at 3 mg/day, with no clear benefit in excess of that dose. The recommended starting dose of risperidone for psychosis, suggested by these studies, is 0.5 mg/day with titration steps of 0.5 mg/day. On October 29, 2007, the FDA announced approval of aripiprazole for the treatment of schizophrenia in adolescents on the basis of a single, unpublished, 6-week, multicenter, international, double-blind, parallel group trial in which 294 inpatients and outpatients were randomized to one of three conditions: placebo, high-dose (30 mg/day), or low-dose (10 mg/day) active drug. The end point reduction in PANSS score compared with baseline for patients receiving aripiprazole was significantly greater than that for patients treated with placebo, with only slightly better improvement in the high-dose group (U.S. FDA, 2007c).

Before any antipsychotic is administered, baseline examination of patients for involuntary movements, such as tics, stereotypies, or preexisting dyskinesias, is essential. During treatment, patients should be reassessed at each visit by a standardized involuntary movement rating scale, such as the Abnormal Involuntary Movement Scale (National Institute of Mental Health, 2000). Substantial work remains to be done with atypical antipsychotics to address questions of acute and long-term effectiveness, safety, potential for relapse prevention, and usefulness in the prodromal stage or whether they are any more efficacious than typical antipsychotics in childhood and adolescent-onset schizophrenia. New data suggest that they may not be. Results of the NIMH Treatment of Early Onset Schizophrenia Spectrum Disorders study (TEOSS), a double-blind, multisite, randomized comparison of olanzapine, risperidone, and molindone, an older, first-generation antipsychotic, in 119 youths aged 8 to 19 with schizophrenia or schizoaffective disorder, showed no significant differences in response as measured by reduction in the PANSS and clinical global impression scales (Sikich et al, 2008). Patients who received the atypical antipsychotics suffered remarkable signs of a metabolic syndrome, while those on molindone reported less problematic akathisia.

PHARMACOTHERAPY OF BIPOLAR DISORDER

The description of mania as an expansive or irritable mood state dates to writings of Hippocrates in the fourth century BC. In recent years, an increasing number of children and adolescents with explosive behaviors and "mood swings" have been diagnosed with the mixed manic state of bipolar disorder, more completely discussed in Chapter 47. Clearly, a subset of mood-dysregulated children and adolescents will meet DSM-IV-TR criteria for bipolar I disorder, but certainly other subsets will not. Whether pediatric mania is the same disease as adult mania is still debated (McClellan et al, 2007). Research efforts are focused on defining phenotypes of pediatric bipolar disorder, anticipating at least improved nomenclature (Liebenluft et al, 2003) and at most the identification of its neuropathologic substrates. Absent such a diathesis, there is a practical lower developmental limit at which current DSM-IV-TR bipolar criteria seem relevant. For the moment, the diagnoses of bipolar disorder made in preschoolers or toddlers should be viewed with skepticism.

Antimanic Agent

Lithium, the third simplest element in the universe and a monovalent alkali metal similar to sodium and potassium, was introduced into medicine in the 1800s, but credit for recognition of its calming effect in psychotic agitation (the manic state of bipolar disorder) is given to Australian psychiatrist John Cade, who published his findings in a landmark 1949 paper (Cade, 1949). Lithium's precise mechanism of action remains incompletely explained, but most investigators believe it directly or indirectly alters neuronal second-messenger systems and antagonizes serotonin S_{1A} and S_{1B} receptors, resulting in calming, antidepressant, and improved sleep cycle effects.

Extensively studied in adult bipolar disorder, there is only one published, prospective, 6-week, double-blind RCT of lithium in bipolar adolescents aged 12 to 18 years that demonstrated superiority to placebo at a serum level of 0.97 mEq/L (Geller et al, 1998). Other positive published trials were open label, randomized, controlled studies, brief discontinuation studies, and a head-to-head comparison of lithium to antiepileptic drugs (Table 90-13).

Lithium has an elimination half-life of about 20 hours, reaching steady state in 4 to 5 days. Lithium is not protein bound, distributes throughout body water, and is excreted almost entirely by the kidneys. The target therapeutic dose is generally considered to be 30 mg/kg/day, divided conveniently twice daily, or a serum trough level between 0.8 and 1.2 mEq/L. Adverse effects at low doses include acne, cognitive impairment, dry mouth, fine tremor, gastrointestinal distress, leukocytosis, polydipsia, polyuria, rash, and weight gain. Signs of lithium toxicity include alopecia, ataxia, coarse tremor, coma, confusion, dysarthria, electrocardiographic T-wave inversion, hyperreflexia, hypothyroidism, lethargy, nephritis, and seizures. A pretreatment work-up and periodic laboratory monitoring are mandatory, including electrocardiography, hematopoietic status, thyroid and renal function, and pregnancy testing in women. At present, the FDA has not recommended the use of lithium in patients younger than 12 years.

Antiepileptic Drugs

Divalproex was the first antiepileptic drug studied as a mood stabilizer in the 1960s. It is believed to block the catabolism of the inhibitory neurotransmitter GABA, to increase its release, and to increase $GABA_B$ receptor density. Its popularity in adult bipolar treatment translated into wide use in children and adolescents, yet there have been no published, adequately powered, prospective, double-blind, placebo-controlled studies of divalproex in pediatric bipolar disorder. Case reports, positive open trials, and retrospective chart reviews make up the bulk of the evidence on which this practice is built. In a randomized comparison of lithium, divalproex, and carbamazepine, all three agents were judged effective in a study of 8- to 14-year-olds with bipolar disorder (Kowatch et al, 2000). Nausea and sedation were the only adverse effects reported in the divalproex arm of the study, in which the target dose was 20 mg/kg/day. Carbamazepine, thought to inhibit neuronal voltage-dependent sodium channels, is less well studied in pediatric bipolar disorder. In the Kowatch trial, response rates were relatively lower for carbamazepine; the common adverse effects of nausea, dizziness, rash, and sedation occurred at the target serum level of 9 to 11 μg/L. Oxcarbazepine, an analogue of carbamazepine, failed to show efficacy in a large, double-blind RCT of 7- to 18-year-olds with bipolar disorder.

Lamotrigine is a novel antiepileptic drug that is believed to inhibit sodium flux in rapidly firing neurons, reducing a kindling effect that purportedly explains seizures and mood instability. It indirectly reduces the release of the excitatory neurotransmitter glutamate. In 2003, the FDA approved lamotrigine for maintenance treatment of bipolar I disorder in adults. Only case reports and open trials in adolescents with bipolar depression have been published. Topiramate, a GABAergic and glutamatergic antiepileptic drug, generated early interest in adult bipolar disorder but failed to show efficacy in controlled trials. A double-blind, placebo-controlled, large-scale RCT of topiramate in children with mania was cut short while in progress in light of the failed adult trials, so its potential efficacy in pediatric bipolar disorder is unknown (DelBello et al, 2005). Finally, because controlled trials of gabapentin have failed to show efficacy in adult mania, there has been virtually no interest in studying it in pediatric bipolar disorder.

Antipsychotics

The success of atypical antipsychotics across the board in gaining FDA indications for adult bipolar disorder stimulated interest in their use in children and adolescents. An open label monotherapy trial in 8- to 12-year-olds with mania and a randomized, open label comparison with olanzapine in preschoolers suggested the efficacy of risperidone in pediatric bipolar disorder. In the same August 22, 2007, announcement of its approval for use in pediatric schizophrenia, risperidone was given FDA approval for the acute treatment of manic or mixed episodes of bipolar I disorder in children and adolescents aged 10 to 17 years. The decision derived from a multisite RCT of 166 patients, aged 10 to 17 years in a manic or mixed state at the time of treatment, who were randomized to placebo, low-dose risperidone (0.5 to 2.5 mg daily), or high-dose risperidone (3 to 6 mg daily) and titrated to target doses within 7 to 10 days. The outcome measure was the change in the Young Mania Rating Scale at 3 weeks. Both active drug conditions were superior to placebo in efficacy, but there was no significant difference in improvement between high and low doses.

On February 29, 2008, the FDA similarly announced approval of aripiprazole for the acute treatment of manic or mixed episodes of bipolar I disorder in children and adolescents aged 10 to 17 years. In a multicenter, double-blind, unpublished U.S. study between 2005 and 2007, 296 patients in a manic or mixed manic state were randomized to low-dose aripiprazole (10 mg daily), high-dose aripiprazole (30 mg daily), and placebo (U.S. FDA, 2008). The outcome measure was mean change in the Young Mania Rating Scale score from baseline to 4 weeks. Both medication conditions were superior to placebo, but high-dose aripiprazole did not convey any additional benefit over the low-dose condition.

A double-blind, randomized, 28-day comparison of quetiapine to divalproex indicated that both agents were effective in reducing scores on a standard mania rating scale (DelBello et al, 2006). Neither this study nor any past study of divalproex monotherapy in pediatric mania has ever been placebo controlled. The data on ziprasidone in pediatric bipolar disorder are limited to case reports. On the basis of large, as yet unpublished RCTs, the FDA is reviewing at the time of this writing the manufacturer's request for olanzapine to be granted an indication for acute mania and schizophrenia in adolescents.

Augmentation Strategies

It has been estimated that up to half of all adults and adolescents with mania do not respond to monotherapy with an antimanic or antiepileptic drug (Kowatch et al, 2003). Thoughtful, treatment-specific algorithms, including augmentation strategies, are in continuing development for pediatric bipolar disorder. The reader is referred to the most recent treatment guidelines for children and adolescents with bipolar disorder (Kowatch et al, 2005).

PHARMACOTHERAPY OF TICS AND TOURETTE DISORDER

Tics are brief, sudden, repetitive movements or sounds that tend to be stereotyped, nonrhythmic, and despite being characterized as involuntary, suppressible. A fascinating subgroup of tic disorders known as pediatric autoimmune neuropsychiatric disorders associated with streptococcal infection (PANDAS), first described in the 1990s, is characterized by the abrupt and explosive onset of intense and frequent motor and vocal tics or OCD symptoms within 2 weeks of bacterial exposure (Pavone et al, 2006). Tics and Tourette disorder usually do not occur in isolation, and in fact, commonly comorbid psychiatric conditions, including ADHD, OCD, and other anxiety, mood, learning, sleep, and elimination disorders, tend to be the major sources of impairment and focus of clinical attention. The most effective treatment approaches to tic disorders are multidisciplinary, emphasizing support of the patient, psychoeducation about tics, and treatment of comorbidities. A full discussion of the epidemiology, clinical presentation, and evidence-based pharmacotherapy of tics and Tourette disorder may be found in Chapter 65.

α_2-Adrenergic Agonists

For the treatment of mild to moderate tics, clonidine and guanfacine are reasonable first choices among effective agents. Clonidine has long-standing evidence for efficacy in suppressing mild to moderate tics (Sandor, 2003). At least one RCT has shown guanfacine to be superior to placebo in treating both the symptoms of ADHD and comorbid tics (Scahill et al, 2006). Tics respond to clonidine and guanfacine at the same doses used for ADHD, but usually after several weeks of treatment.

Benzodiazepines

Several case reports suggest the utility of clonazepam in Tourette disorder, but no RCTs have confirmed this observation. As noted before, there is little to recommend the use of benzodiazepines for anxiety that accompanies tic disorders.

Antipsychotics

Converging findings from functional imaging studies have convinced some researchers that the abnormality in Tourette disorder lies in the dopamine pathways of the striatum (Frey and Albin, 2006). Others suggest instead that the apparent malfunction of the striatum is really the consequence of overloading by excessive input from the cerebellum, increasingly implicated in ADHD, OCD, autism, and other neuropsychiatric disorders (Lerner et al, 2007). Three typical antipsychotics, haloperidol, pimozide, and fluphenazine, have been shown to be highly effective agents in tic suppression, presumably by postsynaptic dopamine D_2 receptor blockade in the basal ganglia. At present, only pimozide has the FDA indication for Tourette disorder in children older than 12 years. The FDA issued a MedWatch warning on November 9, 1999, contraindicating pimozide with certain antibiotics. Pimozide also has calcium channel blocking effects, making electrocardiographic monitoring an important safety consideration with its use. An FDA MedWatch alert in April 2006 warned against the concomitant use of pimozide and fluoxetine because of the increased risks of QTc prolongation and erythema multiforme.

Among the atypical antipsychotics, risperidone has accumulated the most evidence for efficacy in several RCTs in Tourette disorder, including a crossover comparison to pimozide (Gilbert et al, 2004). Ziprasidone appeared superior to placebo in one controlled trial in 7- to 17-year-olds with Tourette disorder, in which the only significant adverse effect was somnolence (Salee et al, 2000). There are no available RCTs of olanzapine, quetiapine, aripiprazole, paliperidone, or iloperidone for children or adolescents with Tourette disorder. An open label, nonrandomized, industry-sponsored trial of aripiprazole in Tourette disorder with or without OCD and ADHD is in the recruitment phase at the time of this writing. The dosing and safety of both typical and atypical antipsychotics in Tourette disorder are more fully discussed in Chapter 65.

Other Dopamine Antagonists

Tetrabenazine, which reversibly depletes presynaptic dopamine stores (and to a lesser extent serotonin and norepinephrine stores) and weakly antagonizes postsynaptic dopamine receptors, is used primarily to treat movement disorders but may have promise in Tourette disorder. Two European neuroleptics, tiapride and sulpiride, both selective dopamine D_2 antagonists, unavailable in the United States, are reportedly effective in Tourette disorder.

Mixed Dopamine Agonist

Pergolide, a mixed dopamine agonist, had been used in high doses to treat Parkinson disease; but at lower doses, it appeared effective in two RCTs of children and adolescents with Tourette disorder (Gilbert et al, 2003). On March 29, 2007, pergolide was withdrawn from the American market because of a clear association with cardiac structural damage resulting in valve regurgitation.

Baclofen

In a large open trial, the muscle relaxant baclofen, which inhibits presynaptic release of excitatory amino acids, appeared to be efficacious in treating tics. However, a small RCT in children 8 to 14 years old failed to demonstrate any reduction in tic severity (Singer et al, 2001).

Nicotinergic Agents

Neither controlled studies of nicotine chewing gum augmentation of neuroleptic treatment nor controlled trials of mecamylamine, a nicotine antagonist, could demonstrate effectiveness of nicotinergic agents in the treatment of Tourette disorder.

Other Approaches

Somatic treatments promoted for Tourette disorder that have not withstood the test of a well-designed, randomized, placebo-controlled study include monotherapy with an androgen receptor antagonist, suggested by the extraordinary prevalence of Tourette disorder in boys; monotherapy with Δ^9-tetrahydrocannabinol, the active agent in marijuana, suggested by reports of tic relief during substance abuse; and repetitive transcranial magnetic stimulation of the motor cortex. For treatment-refractory cases of Tourette disorder, ablative surgery and deep brain stimulation, generally not studied in patients younger than 18 years, have produced notable results (Mink et al, 2006). Children with PANDAS and a positive throat culture should be treated with antibiotics and effective pharmacologic and behavioral therapies for OCD and tics. Severely affected children with PANDAS have responded to intravenous immune globulin and plasma exchange in a randomized, placebo-controlled trial (Swedo et al, 2004). An NIMH-sponsored RCT comparing efficacy and safety of the anticonvulsant levetiracetam to clonidine in children with Tourette disorder is in progress. An open label, nonrandomized, industry-sponsored efficacy study of topiramate in Tourette disorder is in the recruitment phase.

PHARMACOTHERAPY OF AUTISTIC SPECTRUM DISORDERS

Autistic spectrum disorders (ASD), fully discussed in Chapter 69, refer collectively to autistic disorder, Asperger disorder, and pervasive developmental disorder not otherwise specified. Findings of abnormalities in brain development in ASD are rapidly emerging, including cerebral overgrowth associated with a genetic variant of the serotonin transporter gene (Wassink et al, 2007) and uneven cellular growth in the amygdala, basal ganglia, and cerebellum (Bailey et al, 1998). The complicated neural connectivity problems whose final common pathway is ASD have so far eluded pharmacotherapeutic treatment. Dysfunction of cholinergic, glutamatergic, GABAergic, and serotonergic neurotransmitter systems has been implicated in ASD (Bethea and Sikich, 2007). Overall functioning can be improved by treating comorbidities common to ASD, such as aggression, inattention, hyperactivity, irritability, obsessional anxiety, insomnia, and others.

Antipsychotics

In parallel with the history of treatments for disruptive and aggressive behaviors, several of the first-generation antipsychotics were studied in ASD. The most systematic studies were of haloperidol, for which placebo-controlled trials in ASD during the 1970s and 1980s demonstrated efficacy in treatment of aggression, hyperactivity, and stereotypies (Campbell et al, 1996). Case reports of broader symptom improvement and fewer adverse effects appeared with the proliferating off-label use of atypical antipsychotics in ASD. In 1997, the NIMH created the Research Units on Pediatric Psychopharmacology Autism Network (RUPPAN), tasked with rigorous investigation of the safety and efficacy of the atypical antipsychotics in ASD. Risperidone was selected as the study drug in the first RUPPAN, multisite RCT in 101 children with ASD, aged 5 to 17 years. Significant reduction in aggression, irritability, and hyperactivity was obtained at 0.5 to 3.5 mg daily (McCracken et al, 2002). The most prominent adverse effect was an average weight gain of 2.7 kg after 8 weeks. In a nearly identical study published 2 years later, children and adolescents with ASD responded to risperidone at an average dose of 1.17 mg daily with dramatic global improvement and significantly reduced aggression, self-injurious behaviors, and tantrums (Shea et al, 2004). The most prominent adverse effect was somnolence, but the children also gained a significant amount of weight on average. Further analysis of the RUPPAN data made clear that risperidone had no effect on two core symptoms of ASD, namely, social relatedness and spoken language, but did reduce repetitive behaviors and stereotypies, consistent with the older studies of haloperidol (McDougle et al, 2005).

On October 6, 2006, the FDA approved the use of risperidone in children with ASD to treat irritability, aggression, self-injury, and temper tantrums. As of this writing, there are no other large-scale RCTs in the literature demonstrating safety and efficacy of other atypical antipsychotics in ASD. The FDA Office of Orphan Products Development is studying the efficacy and safety of olanzapine in ASD. An industry-sponsored, multisite, randomized, double-blind, placebo-controlled study of aripiprazole to reduce behavioral dyscontrol in children and adolescents with ASD is in progress.

Antidepressants

The Children's Health Act of 2000 mandated creation of an autism research network to facilitate a series of investigations called Studies to Advance Autism Research and Treatment (STAART). The reported dysfunction of serotonin in ASD as well as associated symptoms of anxiety, obsessional behavior, and irritability argued persuasively for trials of SSRIs in patients with ASD. The risk of such intervention is that the most common adverse effects of SSRIs, especially in vulnerable children, happen to be agitation, anxiety, and hostility. Nevertheless, STAART 1 was a randomized, controlled trial of citalopram in 149 pediatric patients with ASD targeting repetitive behaviors, presumably analogous to compulsions. The results had not been published at the time of this writing. Meanwhile, a controlled trial of liquid fluoxetine in 39 children with ASD published in 2005 demonstrated superiority to placebo in the treatment of repetitive behaviors at an average dose of 10 mg daily (Hollander et al, 2005). The effect size was high, and adverse effects reported in treated children were indistinguishable from those in the placebo group.

A significant finding in children with autism is that serotonin synthesis is abnormally low in the first year of life, climbing steadily through the first decade to adult production levels and then exceeding normal production by 20%. In normal infants, serotonin synthesis and frontal lobe synaptogenesis is extraordinarily high, which then decreases across the first decade to adult levels (Bethea and Sikich, 2007). These observations raise the intriguing possibility that early treatment with a serotonergic agent might alter the developmental trajectory of infant brains with ASD toward a more normal course. DeLong showed in an open label, uncontrolled, nonrandomized trial of fluoxetine in 2- to 7-year-olds with ASD that 59% of subjects had good to excellent improvement in language acquisition after a mean treatment duration of 21 months (DeLong et al, 1998). STAART 2, launched in July 2005, is an ambitious RCT of fluoxetine in young children 30 to 58 months of age with ASD. The objective is to assess the safety and impact of early SSRI treatment on neural plasticity with the hope of positively influencing development.

Antiepileptic Drugs

The comorbidity of seizures with ASD has been recognized since the days of Leo Kanner. Studies of the antiepileptic drug divalproex in ASD have generally been open label, and at least one has shown behavioral as well as electroencephalographic improvements (Plioplys, 1994). A controlled study sponsored by the National Institute of Neurological Disorders and Stroke to test the efficacy and safety of divalproex in children and adolescents with ASD, aged 5 to 17 years, is in progress. One small, double-blind, placebo-controlled study of lamotrigine titrated to 5 mg/kg/day in 28 children with ASD who did not have a seizure disorder failed to show improvement on any measure of the core symptoms of autism (Belsito et al, 2001).

Psychostimulants

Despite the high rate of inattention and hyperactivity in children with ASD, little systematic effort has been expended in studying the psychostimulants in this population. Early clinical studies and practical experience suggested that psychostimulants can be quite toxic, if not ineffective, in children with ASD. Consequently, the RUPPAN chose as their second study a randomized, placebo-controlled, crossover trial of IR methylphenidate in 72 children, aged 5 to 14 years, with pervasive developmental disorders and moderate to severe hyperactivity. Dosing was flexible but never exceeded about 75% of typical doses used in the MTA study of normal children with ADHD. Thirteen patients dropped out of the study because of adverse effects, and only 35 of the remainder, or 49%, were considered responders. This study may not generalize to all psychostimulants or delivery vehicles, but it seems clear that ASD conveys vulnerability to stimulant adverse effects, limiting conventional treatment for comorbid inattention and hyperactivity. There are two additional NIMH-sponsored RCTs of methylphenidate in autism and pervasive developmental disorder nearing completion as of this writing.

α_2-Adrenergic Agonists

When stimulants fail or cannot be tolerated by children with ASD and ADHD, the α_2-adrenergic agonists clonidine and guanfacine should be considered. The short half-life and sedative characteristic of clonidine may limit its usefulness in this population. An open label, 8-week, multisite trial of guanfacine was conducted as a companion to the RUPPAN methylphenidate study previously described for children who did not improve with methylphenidate or had failed methylphenidate treatment elsewhere (Scahill et al, 2006). Guanfacine was titrated in children over 25 kg exactly as described in the ADHD section of this chapter up to 5 mg/day; smaller children received half the starting dose, half the incremental increases, and a maximum of 3.5 mg/daily. Significant improvements in hyperactivity, impulsiveness, explosive behaviors, stereotypies, and social interaction were reported by parents and teachers. Guanfacine was generally well tolerated, with common adverse effects seen in normal children.

Other Approaches

Galantamine, an acetylcholinesterase inhibitor and nicotinic receptor modulator, increases acetylcholine release, theoretically involved in associative learning and perhaps attention. Open trials of galantamine suggesting positive effects in autism prompted a small RCT in autistic children aged 5 to 17 years sponsored by the National Alliance for Autism Research, the results of which were not available at the time of this writing. The potential therapeutic effect of hyperbaric oxygen in young children with autism is currently being explored.

Complementary and Alternative Medicine

News of alternative biologic, mechanical, and technologic treatments for ASD tends to proliferate easily and widely through the omnipresent Internet. The reader is referred to an excellent review by Levy and Hyman (2005) of the serendipity and science behind the generally unsupported promises of complementary and alternative medicine for ASD.

PHARMACOTHERAPY OF EATING DISORDERS

The two principal eating disorders affecting children and adolescents, anorexia nervosa and bulimia nervosa, are quintessential biopsychosocial syndromes. Anorexia nervosa, whose incidence has been increasing during the past 50 years, is a lethal illness with a suicide rate 32 times higher than that for the general population. Treatment, difficult at best, is multidimensional, emphasizing evidence-based psychotherapies. Pharmacotherapy, for which there is little evidence in anorexia nervosa, plays an adjunctive role in comprehensive treatment of bulimia nervosa.

Antipsychotics

Attempts to take advantage of the weight gain associated with typical antipsychotics motivated their use in anorexia nervosa as early as the 1960s. These agents, including chlorpromazine, pimozide, and sulpiride, failed to provide lasting results and caused many unpleasant adverse effects. Interest in atypical antipsychotics to induce weight gain, if not to mitigate core symptoms of anorexia nervosa, has been increasing, but as of this writing, there are no published, positive RCTs to support this practice (controlled trials of olanzapine and risperidone are nearing completion). Antipsychotics have no role in the treatment of the core symptoms of bulimia nervosa.

Serotonin Antagonists

Cyproheptadine, a histamine H_1 and serotonin S_{2A} antagonist generally used for allergies and known to cause weight gain, was considered for use in anorexia nervosa. In a dated, placebo-controlled, head-to-head trial with amitriptyline, cyproheptadine was weakly effective in decreasing the time to goal weight and at high doses seemed to have an antidepressant effect in anorectic patients (Halmi et al, 1986).

Antidepressants

A theoretical link between serotonin dysfunction and enhanced satiety as well as their convincing safety and efficacy record in the treatment of depression and anxiety made SSRI antidepressants logical choices for study in anorexia nervosa. A systematic review of the strongest existing RCTs in anorexia nervosa with fluoxetine was disappointing, in which neither core symptom reduction (Claudino et al, 2006) nor relapse prevention (Walsh et al, 2006) was shown. In contrast, the Fluoxetine Bulimia Nervosa Study Group demonstrated that fluoxetine at 60 mg daily was superior to placebo in reducing the frequency of bingeing and purging and was well tolerated (Fluoxetine Bulimia Nervosa Study Group, 1992). A subsequent meta-analytic review of 19 RCTs of antidepressants across nearly all classes (TCAs, SSRIs, monoamine oxidase inhibitors, serotonin S_2 antagonist and reuptake inhibitors, norepinephrine and dopamine reuptake inhibitors) found that treatment with these agents was superior to placebo in relieving the symptoms of bulimia nervosa (Bacaltchuk and Hay, 2003). Fluoxetine is the only medication with an FDA indication for bulimia nervosa.

Failed Approaches

Use of the prokinetic agent cisapride, a weak serotonin S_3 antagonist and smooth muscle stimulant, was conceived as a way to increase gut motility usually impaired in anorexia nervosa. A small RCT of cisapride in anorectic patients failed to improve gastric emptying or to cause weight gain (Szmukler et al, 1995), perhaps fortuitously, as cisapride was pulled from market shelves on June 14, 2000, because of its association with prolonged QT intervals, ventricular dysrhythmias, and deaths from torsades de pointes. A small RCT of lithium in anorexia nervosa was conducted, but the anticipated outcome of weight gain could not be shown (Gross et al, 1981). The appetite-stimulating effect of cannabis prompted a short-duration RCT comparing oral Δ^9-tetrahydrocannabinol to diazepam in anorexia nervosa, but no benefit was demonstrated (Gross et al, 1983). Finally, the association of appetite disruption and weight loss with zinc deficiency led to three RCTs of zinc supplementation in anorexia nervosa, none of which resulted in any difference in core symptoms (Lask et al, 1993).

SUMMARY

Psychopharmacologic agents available today offer symptom relief but not cures, sometimes accompanied by unknown risks that must be balanced against inaction. Neuroscientists think of psychotropic medications as potential mediators of neural circuits, biasing them toward normal information processing (March and Wells, 2003). Clinical practitioners see psychotropic medications as imperfect but powerful tools in a kit of interventions to facilitate a patient's return to health.

If evidence-based medicine has taught us nothing else, it has made clear that combination or multimodal treatments are generally superior to monotherapies and that targets of treatment are rarely singular. For example, the treatment of ADHD may seem as straightforward as titration of a medication to efficacy while minimizing adverse effects, but more often than not it requires management of comorbid conditions, liaison with schools for academic support, and assisting the family with organizational and structural challenges. In treating disruptive behavior and eating disorders, pharmacotherapy plays a limited role in the containment of severe aggression and in the reduction of bingeing, respectively, while all the rest is better addressed by a team of professionals with a variety of complementary skills.

In developmental terms, psychopharmacotherapy is somewhere in its early adolescence. What we know today is that some antidepressants and antipsychotics appear to be more effective than others in the pediatric age range, at least under the conditions of a controlled study, and that no antidepressant or antipsychotic can be deemed safer than any other. Untreated mood and psychotic disorders pose an inherent risk to patients, each with suicide rates approaching 15%, much greater by far than the risk posed by exposure to antidepressant and antipsychotic medications. Medicines developed for one syndrome are often found useful in other syndromes. A case in point is the SSRI class of antidepressants that now appear more effective for anxiety than for depression in children and adolescents. However, a one-psychotropic-fits-all mentality, suggested by the proliferating use of atypical antipsychotics, can be as dangerous as it is seductive. And then there are syndromes, such as anorexia nervosa, that seem invulnerable to attack by anything in pill form.

The common thread in these observations is that the biology of attentional, disruptive, mood, anxiety, psychotic, tic, autistic, and eating disorders is far from understood. Nevertheless, combining several psychotropic agents at once to treat child and adolescent mental illnesses has become rather commonplace (Safer et al, 2003). There is no evidence to validate the rationale, efficacy, and safety of this practice, but that will undoubtedly become a priority for researchers in the years ahead.

REFERENCES

Aman MG, De Smedt G, Derivan A, et al; Risperidone Disruptive Behavior Study Group: Double-blind, placebo-controlled study of risperidone for the treatment of disruptive behaviors in children with subaverage intelligence. Am J Psychiatry 159:1337-1346, 2002.

American Diabetes Association; American Psychiatric Association; American Association of Clinical Endocrinologists; North American Association for the Study of Obesity: Consensus development conference on antipsychotic drugs and obesity and diabetes. Diabetes Care 27:596-601, 2004.

American Psychiatric Association: Diagnostic and Statistical Manual of Mental Disorders, 4th ed, text revision. Washington, DC, American Psychiatric Association, 2000.

Armenteros JL, Lewis JE, Davalos M: Risperidone augmentation for treatment-resistant aggression in attention-deficit/hyperactivity disorder: A placebo-controlled pilot study. J Am Acad Child Adolesc Psychiatry 46:558-565, 2007.

Arnsten AF: Fundamentals of attention-deficit/hyperactivity disorder: Circuits and pathways. J Clin Psychiatry 67(Suppl 8):7-12, 2006.

Arnsten AF, Steer JC, Hunt RD: The contribution of $alpha_2$-noradrenergic mechanisms of prefrontal cortical cognitive function. Potential significance for attention-deficit hyperactivity disorder. Arch Gen Psychiatry 53:448-455, 1996.

Bacaltchuk J, Hay P: Antidepressants versus placebo for people with bulimia nervosa. Cochrane Database Syst Rev 4:CD003391, 2003.

Bailey A, Luthert P, Dean A, et al: A clinicopathological study of autism. Brain 121:889-905, 1998.

Belsito KM, Law PA, Kirk KS, et al: Lamotrigine therapy for autistic disorder: A randomized, double-blind, placebo-controlled trial. J Autism Dev Disord 31:175-181, 2001.

Benjamin DK, Smith PB, Murphy MD, et al: Peer-reviewed publication of clinical trials completed for pediatric exclusivity. JAMA 296:1266-1273, 2006.

Bethea TC, Sikich L: Early pharmacological treatment of autism: A rationale for developmental treatment. Biol Psychiatry 61:521-537, 2007.

Biederman J, Thisted RA, Greenhill LL, Ryan ND: Estimation of the association between desipramine and the risk for sudden death in 5 to 14 year old children. J Clin Psychiatry 56:87-93, 1995.

Biederman J, Swanson JM, Wigal SB, et al: A comparison of once-daily and divided doses of modafinil in children with attention-deficit/hyperactivity disorder: A randomized, double-blind, and placebo-controlled study. J Clin Psychiatry 67:727-735, 2006.

Biederman J, Melmed RD, Patel A, et al: A randomized, double-blind, placebo-controlled study of guanfacine extended release in children and adolescents with attention-deficit/hyperactivity disorder. Pediatrics 121:e73-84, 2008.

Birmaher B, Axelson DA, Monk K, et al: Fluoxetine for the treatment of childhood anxiety disorders. J Am Acad Child Adolesc Psychiatry 42:415-423, 2003.

Birmaher B, Brent DA, Benson RS: Summary of the practice parameters for the assessment and treatment of children and adolescents with depressive disorders. American Academy of Child and Adolescent Psychiatry. J Am Acad Child Adolesc Psychiatry 37:1234-1238, 1998.

Black B, Uhde TW: Treatment of elective mutism with fluoxetine: A double-blind, placebo-controlled study. J Am Acad Child Adolesc Psychiatry 33:1000-1006, 1994.

Bradley C: The behavior of children receiving Benzedrine. Am J Psychiatry 94:577-585, 1937.

Brent D, Emslie G, Clarke G, et al: Switching to another SSRI or to venlafaxine with or without cognitive behavioral therapy for adolescents with SSRI-resistant depression: The TORDIA randomized controlled trial. JAMA 299:901-913, 2008.

Bridge JA, Iyengar S, Salary CB, et al: Clinical response and risk for reported suicidal ideation and suicide attempts in pediatric antidepressant treatment: A meta-analysis of randomized controlled trials. JAMA 297:1683-1696, 2007.

Cade JFJ: Lithium salts in the treatment of psychotic excitement. Med J Aust 2:349-352, 1949.

Campbell M, Gonzalez NM, Silva RR: The pharmacologic treatment of conduct disorders and rage outbursts. Psychiatr Clin North Am 15:69-85, 1992.

Campbell M, Schopler E, Cueva JE, et al: Treatment of autistic disorder. J Am Acad Child Adolesc Psychiatry 35:134-143, 1996.

Claudino AM, Hay P, Lima MS, et al: Antidepressants for anorexia nervosa. Cochrane Database Syst Rev 1:CD004365, 2006.

Compton SN, March JS, Brent D, et al: Cognitive-behavioral psychotherapy for anxiety and depressive disorders in children and adolescents: An evidence-based medicine review. J Am Acad Child Adolesc Psychiatry 43:930-959, 2004.

Conners CK, Casat CD, Gualtiere CT, et al: Bupropion hydrochloride in attention deficit disorder with hyperactivity. J Am Acad Child Adolesc Psychiatry 35:1314-1321, 1996.

Connor DF, Fletcher KE, Swanson JM: A meta-analysis of clonidine for symptoms of attention-deficit hyperactivity disorder. J Am Acad Child Adolesc Psychiatry 38:1551-1559, 1999.

Cueva JD, Overall JE, Small AM, et al: Carbamazepine in aggressive children with conduct disorder: A double-blind and placebo-controlled study. J Am Acad Child Adolesc Psychiatry 35:480-490, 1996.

Daly JM, Wilens T: The use of tricyclic antidepressants in children and adolescents. Pediatr Clin North Am 45:1123-1135, 1998.

DelBello MP, Findling RL, Kushner S, et al: A pilot controlled trial of topiramate for mania in children and adolescents with bipolar disorder. J Am Acad Child Adolesc Psychiatry 44:539-547, 2005.

DelBello MP, Kowatch RA, Adler CM, et al: A double-blind randomized pilot study comparing quetiapine and divalproex for adolescent mania. J Am Acad Child Adolesc Psychiatry 45:305-313, 2006.

DeLong GR, Teague LA, McSwain-Kamran M: Effects of fluoxetine treatment in young children with idiopathic autism. Dev Med Child Neurol 40:551-562, 1998.

DeVeaugh-Geiss J, Moroz G, Biederman J, et al: Clomipramine hydrochloride in childhood and adolescent obsessive-compulsive disorder—a multicenter trial. J Am Acad Child Adolesc Psychiatry 31:45-49, 1992.

DeVeaugh-Geiss J, March JS, Shapiro M, et al: Child and adolescent psychopharmacology in the new millennium: A workshop for academia, industry, and government. J Am Acad Child Adolesc Psychiatry 45:261-270, 2006.

Domino ME, Burns BJ, Silva SG, et al: Cost-effectiveness of treatments for adolescent depression: Results from TADS. Am J Psychiatry 165:588-596, 2008.

Emslie GJ, Heiligenstein JH, Wagner KD, et al: Fluoxetine for acute treatment of depression in children and adolescents: A placebo-controlled, randomized clinical trial. J Am Acad Child Adolesc Psychiatry 41:1205-1215, 2002.

Emslie GJ, Ryan ND, Wagner KD: Major depressive disorder in children and adolescents: Clinical trial design and antidepressant efficacy. J Clin Psychiatry 66(Suppl 7):14-20, 2005.

Emslie GJ, Kratochvil C, Vitiello B, et al: Treatment for Adolescents with Depression Study (TADS): Safety results. J Am Acad Child Adolesc Psychiatry 45:1440-1455, 2006.

Fluoxetine Bulimia Nervosa Study Group: Fluoxetine in the treatment of bulimia nervosa. A multicenter, placebo-controlled, double-blind trial. Arch Gen Psychiatry 49:139-147, 1992.

Frey KA, Albin RL: Neuroimaging of Tourette syndrome. J Child Neurol 21:672-677, 2006.

Geller B, Cooper TB, Sun K, et al: Double-blind and placebo-controlled study of lithium for adolescent bipolar disorders with secondary substance dependency. J Am Acad Child Adolesc Psychiatry 37:171-178, 1998.

Geller DA, Wagner KD, Emslie G, et al: Paroxetine treatment in children and adolescents with obsessive-compulsive disorder: A randomized, multicenter, double-blind, placebo-controlled trial. J Am Acad Child Adolesc Psychiatry 3:1387-1396, 2004.

Gibbons RD, Hur K, Bhaumik DK, et al: The relationship between antidepressant prescription rates and rate of early adolescent suicide. Am J Psychiatry 163:1898-1904, 2006.

Gilbert DL, Dure L, Sethuraman G, et al: Tic reduction with pergolide in randomized controlled trial in children. Neurology 60:606-611, 2003.

Gilbert DL, Batterson JR, Sethuraman G, et al: Tic reduction with risperidone versus pimozide in a randomized, double-blind crossover trial. J Am Acad Child Adolesc Psychiatry 43:206-214, 2004.

Gittelman-Klein R, Klein DF: Controlled imipramine treatment of school phobia. Arch Gen Psychiatry 25:204-207, 1971.

Gittelman-Klein R, Klein DF, Katz S, et al: Comparative effects of methylphenidate and thioridazine in hyperactive children: I. Clinical results. Arch Gen Psychiatry 33:1217-1231, 1976.

Goodyer I, Dubicka B, Wilkinson P, et al: Selective serotonin reuptake inhibitors (SSRIs) and routine specialist care with and without cognitive behaviour therapy in adolescents with major depression: Randomized controlled trial. BMJ 335:142, 2007.

Graae F, Miller J, Rizzotto L, et al: Clonazepam in childhood anxiety disorders. J Am Acad Child Adolesc Psychiatry 33:372-376, 1994.

Grant P, Lougee L, Hirschtritt BA, et al: An open label trial of riluzole, a glutamate antagonist, in children with treatment-resistant obsessive-compulsive disorder. J Child Adolesc Psychopharmacol 17:761-767, 2007.

Greenhill L, Kollins S, Abikoff H, et al: Efficacy and safety of immediate-release methylphenidate treatment for preschoolers with ADHD. J Am Acad Child Adolesc Psychiatry 45:1284-1293, 2006.

Gross H, Ebert MH, Faden VB, et al: A double-blind controlled trial of lithium carbonate primary anorexia nervosa. J Clin Psychopharmacol 1:376-381, 1981.

Gross H, Ebert MH, Faden VB, et al: A double-blind trial of delta 9-tetrahydrocannabinol in primary anorexia nervosa. J Clin Psychopharmacol 3:165-171, 1983.

Günther T, Herpertz-Dahlmann B, Jolles J, et al: The influence of risperidone on attentional functions in children and adolescents with attention-deficit/hyperactivity disorder and co-morbid disruptive behavior disorder. J Child Adolesc Psychopharmacol 16:725-735, 2006.

Halmi KA, Eckert ED, LaDu TJ: Anorexia nervosa: Treatment efficacy of cyproheptadine and amitriptyline. Arch Gen Psychiatry 43:177-181, 1986.

Hamilton BE , Miniño AM, Martin JA, et al: Annual summary of vital statistics: 2005. Pediatrics 119:345-360, 2007.

Hazell P, O'Connell D, Heathcote D, et al: Tricyclic drugs for depression in children and adolescents. Cochrane Database Syst Rev 2: CD002317, 2002.

Heiligenstein JH, Hoog SL, Wagner KD, et al: Fluoxetine 40-60 mg versus fluoxetine 20 mg in the treatment of children and adolescents with a less-than-complete response to nine-week treatment with fluoxetine 10-20 mg: A pilot study. J Child Adolesc Psychopharmacol 16:207-217, 2006.

Hollander E, Phillips A, Chaplin W, et al: A placebo controlled crossover trial of liquid fluoxetine on repetitive behaviors in childhood and adolescent autism. Neuropsychopharmacology 30:582-589, 2005.

Jensen PS, Hinshaw SP, Swanson JM, et al: Findings from the NIMH multimodal treatment study of ADHD (MTA): Implications and applications for primary care providers. J Dev Behav Pediatr 22:60-73, 2001.

Jensen PS, Arnold LE, Swanson JM, et al: 3-year follow-up of the NIMH MTA study. J Am Acad Child Adolesc Psychiatry 46:989-1002, 2007.

Kowatch RA, Suppes T, Carmody TJ, et al: Effect size of lithium, divalproex sodium, and carbamazepine in children and adolescents with bipolar disorder. J Am Acad Child Adolesc Psychiatry 39:713-720, 2000.

Kowatch RA, Sethuraman G, Hume JH, et al: Combination pharmacotherapy in children and adolescents with bipolar disorder. Biol Psychiatry 53:978-984, 2003.

Kowatch RA, Fristad M, Birmaher B, et al: Treatment guidelines for children and adolescents with bipolar disorder. J Am Acad Child Adolesc Psychiatry 44:213-235, 2005.

Kratochvil CJ, Newcorn JH, Arnold LE, et al: Atomoxetine alone or combined with fluoxetine for treating ADHD with comorbid depressive or anxiety symptoms. J Am Acad Child Adolesc Psychiatry 44:915-924, 2005.

Kumra S, Frazier JA, Jacobsen LK, et al: Childhood-onset schizophrenia. A double-blind clozapine-haloperidol comparison. Arch Gen Psychiatry 53:1090-1097, 1996.

Lask B, Fosson A, Rolfe U, et al: Zinc deficiency and childhood-onset anorexia nervosa. J Clin Psychiatry 54:63-66, 1993.

Lerner A, Bagic A, Boudreau EA, et al: Neuroimaging of neuronal circuits involved in tic generation in patients with Tourette syndrome. Neurology 68:1979-1987, 2007.

Levy SE, Hyman SL: Novel treatments for autistic spectrum disorders. Ment Retard Dev Disabil Res Rev 11:131-142, 2005.

Libby AM, Brent DA, Morrato EH, et al: Decline in treatment of pediatric depression after FDA advisory on risk of suicidality with SSRIs. Am J Psychiatry 164:884-891, 2007.

Liebenluft E, Charney DS, Towbin KE, et al: Defining clinical phenotypes of juvenile mania. Am J Psychiatry 160:430-437, 2003.

Linde K, Mulrow CD, Berner M, et-al: St John's wort for depression. Cochrane Database Syst Rev 2:CD000448, 2005.

Llorca PM, Spadone C, Sol O, et al: Efficacy and safety of hydroxyzine in the treatment of generalized anxiety disorder: A 3-month double-blind study. J Clin Psychiatry 63:1020-1027, 2002.

Luby JL, Heffelfinger AK, Mrakotsky C, et al: Preschool major depressive disorder: Preliminary validation for developmentally modified DSM-IV criteria. J Am Acad Child Adolesc Psychiatry 41:928-937, 2002.

Malone RP, Delaney MA, Luebbert JF, et al: A double-blind placebo-controlled study of lithium in hospitalized aggressive children and adolescents with conduct disorder. Arch Gen Psychiatry 57:649-654, 2000.

March JS, Wells K: Combining pharmacotherapy and psychotherapy: An evidence-based approach. *In* Martin A, Scahill L, Charney DS, Lechman JF(eds): Pediatric Psychopharmacology: Principles and Practice, New York, Oxford, 2003, pp 426-443.

March JS, Biederman J, Wolkow R, et al: Sertraline in children and adolescents with obsessive-compulsive disorder: A multicenter randomized controlled trial. JAMA 280:1752-1756, 1998.

March JS, Silva S, Petrycki S, et al: Fluoxetine, cognitive-behavioral therapy, and their combination for adolescents with depression: Treatment for Adolescents with Depression Study (TADS) randomized controlled trial. JAMA 292:807-820, 2004.

March JS, Silva S, Petrycki S, et al: The Treatment for Adolescents with Depression Study (TADS): Long-term effectiveness and safety outcomes. Arch Gen Psychiatry 64:1132-1143, 2007.

McClellan J, Kowatch R, Findling RL: the Work Group on Quality Issues: Practice parameter for the assessment and treatment of children and adolescents with bipolar disorder. J Am Acad Child Adolesc Psychiatry 46:107-125, 2007.

McCracken JT, McGough J, Shah B, et al: Risperidone in children with autism and serious behavioral problems. N Engl J Med 347:314-321, 2002.

McDougle CJ, Scahill L, Aman M, et al: Risperidone for the core symptom domains of autism: Results from the study of the autism network of the Research Units on Pediatric Psychopharmacology. Am J Psychiatry 162:1142-1148, 2005.

McGrath MJ, Campbell KM, Parks CR, et al: Glutamatergic drugs exacerbate symptomatic behavior in a transgenic model of comorbid Tourette's syndrome and obsessive-compulsive disorder. Brain Res 877:23-30, 2000.

Michelson D, Faries D, Wernicke J, et al: Atomoxetine in the treatment of children and adolescents with attention-deficit/hyperactivity disorder: A randomized, placebo-controlled, dose-response study. Pediatrics 108:1-9, 2001.

Mink JW, Walkup J, Frey KA, et al: Patient selection and assessment recommendations for deep brain stimulation in Tourette syndrome. Mov Disord 21:1831-1838, 2006.

Monuteaux MC, Spencer TJ, Faraone SV, et al: A randomized, placebo-controlled clinical trial of bupropion for the prevention of smoking in children and adolescents with attention-deficit/hyperactivity disorder. J Clin Psychiatry 68:1094-101, 2007.

Mufson L, Dorta KP, Wickramaratne P, et al: A randomized effectiveness trial of interpersonal psychotherapy for depressed adolescents. Arch Gen Psychiatry 61:577-584, 2004.

National Institute of Mental Health: Abnormal Involuntary Movement Scale(AIMS).2000.Availableat:http://www.atlantapsychiatry.com/forms/AIMS.pdf.

National Institute of Mental Health: Child and Adolescent Anxiety Disorders (CAMS). 2007. Available at: http://www.clinicaltrials.gov/ct/show/NCT00052078?order=1.

Nemets H, Nemets B, Apter A, et al: Omega-3 treatment of childhood depression: A controlled, double-blind pilot study. Am J Psychiatry 163:1098-1100, 2006.

Olfson M, Shaffer D, Marcus SC, et al. Relationship between antidepressant medication treatment and suicide in adolescents. Arch Gen Psychiatry 60:978-982, 2003.

Olvera RL, Pliszka SR, Luh J, Tatum R: An open trial of venlafaxine in the treatment of attention-deficit/hyperactivity disorder in children and adolescents. J Child Adolesc Psychopharmacol 6:241-250, 1996.

Parker G, Gibson NA, Brotchie H, et al: Omega-3 fatty acids and mood disorders. Am J Psychiatry 163:969-978, 2006.

Pavone P, Parano E, Rizzo R, et al: Autoimmune psychiatric disorders associated with streptococcal infection: Sydenham chorea, PANDAS, and PANDAS variants. J Child Neurol 21:727-736, 2006.

Pediatric OCD Treatment Study (POTS) Team: Cognitive-behavior therapy, sertraline, and their combination for children and adolescents with obsessive-compulsive disorder: The Pediatric OCD Treatment Study (POTS) randomized controlled trial. JAMA 292:1969-1976, 2004.

Perrin JM, Friedman RA, Knilans TK, et al: Cardiovascular monitoring and stimulant drugs for attention-deficity/hyperactivity disorder. Pediatrics 122:451-453, 2008.

Pliszka SR; AACAP Work Group on Quality Issues: Practice parameter for the assessment and treatment of children and adolescents with attention-deficit/hyperactivity disorder. J Am Acad Child Adolesc Psychiatry 46:894-921, 2007.

Plioplys AV: Autism: Electroencephalogram abnormalities and clinical improvement with valproic acid. Arch Pediatr Adolesc Med 148:220-222, 1994.

Popper CW: Combining methylphenidate and clonidine: Pharmacologic questions and new reports about sudden death. J Child Adolesc Psychopharmacol 5:157-166, 1995.

Reyes M, Buitelaar J, Toren P, et al: A randomized, double-blind, placebo-controlled study of risperidone maintenance treatment in children and adolescents with disruptive behavior disorders. Am J Psychiatry 163:402-410, 2006.

Riddle MA, Scahill L, King RA, et al: Double-blind, crossover trial of fluoxetine and placebo in children and adolescents with obsessive-compulsive disorder. J Am Acad Child Adolesc Psychiatry 31:1062-1069, 1992.

Riddle MA, Reeve EA, Yaryura-Tobias JA, et al: Fluvoxamine for children and adolescents with obsessive-compulsive disorder: A randomized, controlled, multicenter trial. J Am Acad Child Adolesc Psychiatry 40:222-229, 2001.

RUPP: Fluvoxamine for the treatment of anxiety disorders in children and adolescents. The Research Unit on Pediatric Psychopharmacology Anxiety Study Group. N Engl J Med 344:1279-1285, 2001.

Rynn MA, Siqueland L, Rickels K: Placebo-controlled trial of sertraline in the treatment of children with generalized anxiety disorder. Am J Psychiatry 158:2008-2014, 2001.

Safer DJ, Zito JM, dosReis S: Concomitant psychotropic medication for youths. Am J Psychiatry 160:438-449, 2003.

Sallee FR, Kurlan R, Goetz CG, et al: Ziprasidone treatment of children and adolescents with Tourette's syndrome: A pilot study. J Am Acad Child Adolesc Psychiatry 39:292-299, 2000.

Samuels JA, Franco K, Wan F, Sorof JM: Effect of stimulants on 24-h ambulatory blood pressure in children with ADHD: A double-blind, randomized, cross-over trial. Pediatr Nephrol 21:92-95, 2006.

Sandor P: Pharmacologic management of tics in patients with TS. J Psychosom Res 55:41-48, 2003.

Scahill L, Aman MG, McDougle CJ, et al: A prospective open trial of guanfacine in children with pervasive developmental disorders. J Child Adolesc Psychopharmacol 16:589-598, 2006.

Seeman P, Tallerico T: Antipsychotic drugs which elicit little or no parkinsonism bind more loosely than dopamine to brain D_2 receptors, yet occupy high levels of these receptors. Mol Psychiatry 3:123-134, 1998.

Seidel L, Walkup JT: Selective serotonin reuptake inhibitor use in the treatment of the pediatric non–obsessive-compulsive disorder anxiety disorders. J Child Adolesc Psychopharmacol 16:171-179, 2006.

Shea S, Turgay A, Carroll A, et al: Risperidone in the treatment of disruptive behavioral symptoms in children with autistic and other pervasive developmental disorders. Pediatrics 114:634-641, 2004.

Sikich L, Frazier JA, McClellan J, et al: Double-blind comparison of first- and second-generation antipsychotics in early-onset schizophrenia and schizoaffective disorder: Findings from the Treatment of Early-Onset Schizophrenia Spectrum Disorders (TEOSS) study [published online ahead of print, September 15, 2008]. Am J Psychiatry.

Sikich L, Hamer RM, Bashford RA, et al: A pilot study of risperidone, olanzapine, and haloperidol in psychotic youth: A double-blind, randomized, 8-week trial. Neuropsychopharmacology 29:133-145, 2004.

Silva RR, Munoz DM, Alpert M: Carbamazepine use in children and adolescents with features of attention-deficit hyperactivity disorder: A meta-analysis. J Am Acad Child Adolesc Psychiatry 35:352-358, 1996.

Simeon JG, Dinicola DF, Ferguson HB, et al: Adolescent depression: A placebo-controlled fluoxetine treatment study and follow-up. Prog Neuropsychopharmacol Biol Psychiatry 14:791-795, 1990.

Simeon JG, Ferguson HB, Knott V, et al: Clinical, cognitive, and neurophysiological effects of alprazolam in children and adolescents with overanxious and avoidant disorders. J Am Acad Child Adolesc Psychiatry 31:29-33, 1992.

Singer HS, Wendlandt J, Krieger M, et al: Baclofen treatment in Tourette syndrome: A double-blind placebo-controlled, crossover trial. Neurology 56:599-604, 2001.

Steiner H, Remsing L; Work Group on Quality Issues: Practice parameter for the assessment and treatment of children and adolescents with oppositional defiant disorder. J Am Acad Child Adolesc Psychiatry 46:126-141, 2007.

Still GF: Some abnormal psychical conditions in children. Lancet 1:1077-1082, 1902.

Swanson J, Greenhill L, Wigal T, et al: Stimulant-related reductions of growth rates in the PATS. J Am Acad Child Adolesc Psychiatry 45:1304-1313, 2006.

Swanson JM, Elliott GR, Greenhill LL, et al: Effects of stimulant medication on growth rates across 3 years in the MTA study follow-up. J Am Acad Child Adolesc Psychiatry 46:1015-1027, 2007.

Swedo SE, Leonard HL, Rapoport JL: The pediatric autoimmune neuropsychiatric disorders associated with streptococcal infection (PANDAS) subgroup: Separating fact from fiction. Pediatrics 113:907-911, 2004.

Szmukler GI, Young GP, Miller G, et al: A controlled trial of cisapride in anorexia nervosa. Int J Eat Disord 17:347-357, 1995.

The Tourette's Syndrome Study Group: Treatment of ADHD in children with tics: A randomized controlled trial. Neurology 58:527-536, 2002.

U.S. FDA: 2002. http://www.fda.gov/cder/foi/esum/2004/20031s037_paxil_Clincal_BPCA_FIN.pdf.

U.S. FDA: 2003. http://www.fda.gov/cder/foi/esum/2003/20151se5-024BPCA.pdf.

U.S. FDA: 2004a. http://www.fda.gov/cder/foi/esum/2004/20415SE5_011_Mirtazapine %20MO%20ReviewFIN.pdf.

U.S. FDA: 2004b. http://www.fda.gov/cder/drug/antidepressants/SSRIPHA200410.htm.

U.S.FDA:2006.http://www.fda.gov/cder/foi/esum/2007/019908s022_Zolpidem_ Clinical_BPCA.pdf.

U.S. FDA: 2007a. http://www.fda.gov/cder/pediatric/labelchange.htm#New-listings.

U.S. FDA: 2007b. http://www.fda.gov/cder/foi/esum/2007/020272s046s047,020588s006s037,021444s020s021_risperidone_clinical_BPCA.pdf.

U.S. FDA: 2007c. http://www.fda.gov/cder/foi/esum/2007/021436_S017_Aripiprazole_.Clinical_BPCA.pdf.

U.S. FDA: 2008. http://www.fda.gov/cder/foi/ped_review/2008/021436S017_Aripiprazole_.Statistical_BPCA.pdf.

Vetter VL, Elia J, Erickson C, et al: Cardiovascular monitoring of children and adolescents with heart disease receiving medications for attention deficit/hyperactivity disorder. Circulation 117:2407-2434, 2008.

Vitiello B, Jensen PS: Medication development and testing in children and adolescents; current problems, future directions. Arch Gen Psychiatry 54:871-876, 1997.

Wagner KD, Ambrosini P, Rynn M, et al: Efficacy of sertraline in the treatment of children and adolescents with major depressive disorder. JAMA 290:1033-1041, 2003.

Wagner KD, Berard R, Stein MD, et al: A multicenter, randomized, double-blind, placebo-controlled trial of paroxetine in children and adolescents with social anxiety disorder. Arch Gen Psychiatry 61:1153–1162, 2004a.

Wagner KD, Robb AS, Findling RL, et al: A randomized, placebo-controlled trial of citalopram for the treatment of major depression in children and adolescents. Am J Psychiatry 161:1079–1083, 2004b.

Wagner KD, Jonas J, Findling RL, et al: A double-blind, randomized, placebo-controlled trial of escitalopram in the treatment of pediatric depression. J Am Acad Child Adolesc Psychiatry 45:280-288, 2006.

Waizer J, Hoffman SP, Polizos P, et al: Outpatient treatment of hyperactive school children with imipramine. Am J Psychiatry 131:587-591, 1974.

Walkup JT, Albano AM, Piacentini J, et al: Cognitive behavioral therapy, sertraline, or a combination in childhood anxiety [published online ahead of print October 30, 2008]. N Engl J Med doi: 10.1056/NEJMoa0804633.

Walsh BT, Kaplan AS, Attia E, et al: Fluoxetine after weight restoration in anorexia nervosa: A randomized controlled trial. JAMA 295:2605-2612, 2006.

Wassink TH, Hazlett HC, Epping EA, et al: Cerebral cortical gray matter overgrowth and functional variation of the serotonin transporter gene in autism. Arch Gen Psychiatry 64:709-717, 2007.

Wilens TE, Faraone SV, Biederman J, et al: Does stimulant therapy of attention-deficit/hyperactivity disorder beget later substance abuse? A meta-analytic review of the literature. Pediatrics 111:179-185, 2003.

91 PEDIATRIC SELF-REGULATION

Dale Sussman Gertz and Timothy Culbert

Self-regulation refers to the exercise of control over oneself by the self. In child language, this translates to "be the boss of your body" (Culbert and Kajander, 2007). It involves the process of increasing internal awareness of the mind and body and gaining some measure of conscious control of selected psychological and physiologic functions. Self-regulation skills give children the means to help themselves manage a variety of biobehavioral problems and can also be used proactively to maintain optimal health and to manage stress. Self-regulation techniques, such as hypnosis, biofeedback and meditation, provide the opportunity for pediatric patients to participate actively in achieving a desired level of health and wellness. Table 91-1 provides a list of self-regulation strategies used with pediatric patients.

Self-regulation treatment strategies facilitate a child's natural, developmental drives for mastery and autonomy. Learning self-regulation empowers patients to focus their minds in a way that positively affects their bodies. Self-regulation includes myriad activities, such as the following:

- voluntary modulation of selected physiologic functions;
- directed use of mental imagery and therapeutic suggestion;
- self-monitoring;
- learning to discriminate between states of arousal and relaxation;
- development of positive self-talk skills;
- heightened awareness of mind-body connections; and
- healthy lifestyle choices (diet, exercise, stress management).

Through the use of self-regulation, children are encouraged to acknowledge and to take "ownership" of their problem and to be an active participant in improving their health.

Behavioral modification, environmental manipulations, and psychopharmacologic interventions are important and proven treatment strategies that approach biobehavioral problems from an *external* standpoint. Through the use of self-regulation strategies, children and adolescents develop an *internal* sense of control over problems and symptoms. They feel less helpless and become involved in their own care.

In the last 25 years, self-regulation techniques have been widely used and increasingly appreciated as valid and effective treatments of a wide variety of biobehavioral problems (Astin et al, 2003; Olness and Kohen, 1996). The literature documenting the efficacy of self-regulation techniques, as the sole treatment of or as an adjunct to mainstream medical therapy for a variety of medical and behavioral problems, continues to grow (Astin et al, 2003; Wolsko et al, 2004). Self-regulation techniques can serve as an excellent complement to conventional therapies and in some cases be used as a primary intervention. Table 91-2 identifies pediatric disorders responsive to self-regulation techniques.

IMPORTANT CONSIDERATIONS IN MIND-BODY INTERVENTIONS

Children must be encouraged to actively participate in their treatment process. It is important to start with an interactive discussion of the mind-body relationship so that the child can visualize and create positive intention. As pediatric patients are taught a specific technique, the therapist serves as a coach and facilitator. Pediatric patients are guided through the process as they personalize their experience. The patient helps determine which type of self-regulation strategies are best for his or her individual treatment plan and learning style. Children of all ages are expected to participate in daily self-monitoring of symptoms and are responsible for daily practice of the skills that they have been taught.

The intimate connection between the mind and body is discussed in a developmentally appropriate manner so that the pediatric patient gains an appreciation of the physiologic responses of the body in relation to different feelings and situations. The impact of thoughts and emotions on certain symptoms (e.g., headaches, shortness of breath, and muscle tension) and overt behaviors (e.g., aggression, crying, and withdrawal) is explored with each child. The idea that a change in thinking and feeling can result in a change in a physiologic process is interesting and exciting for most children.

Studies during the past 50 years have clearly documented the ability of adults and children to modulate voluntarily a number of physiologic processes, many of which were previously thought to be exclusively under autonomic control (Bakal, 1999). Experts in the fields of hypnosis and biofeedback have noted children's

Table 91-1. Some Examples of Pediatric Self-Regulation Techniques

Self-hypnosis	An altered state of awareness usually involving relaxation, during which individuals experience heightened suggestibility
Biofeedback	The use of electronic or electromechanical instruments to measure and then feed back physiologic processes, which then can be altered by an individual in a desirable direction
Relaxation or "diaphragmatic" breathing	Adopting an effortless, slow, and deep rhythmic breathing pattern, typically in the range of 5 to 7 breaths/minute
Progressive muscle relaxation	Alternately tightening and then relaxing specific muscle groups throughout the body
Autogenics	Employing self-administered, repetitive suggestions involving sensations of warmth, heaviness, and relaxation throughout the body
Cognitive-behavioral therapy	Use of positive self-talk and the development of problem solving strategies
Self-monitoring	Keeping an accurate record of mind, body, and symptom changes over time
Mind-body education	Explaining in a developmentally appropriate manner how body systems work to provide a logical understanding of disease and optimal health. In addition, it is important to explore how changes in thinking cause changes in physiologic processes, and vice versa.
Meditation	Cultivation of the mind through quieting and observing inner thoughts, emotions, and sensations
Yoga	An ancient science and philosophy of the mind, body, and soul that includes body movement, posture, and breathing techniques

Table 91-2. Pediatric Problems Responsive to Self-Regulation Techniques

These pediatric disorders positively respond to self-regulation strategies used as primary or adjunctive modalities in the overall treatment plan.

- Chronic or recurrent pain
  - Recurrent abdominal pain, headaches
- Acute pain
  - Medical procedures, trauma, burns
- Anxiety and stress disorders
- Trichotillomania
- Disorders of elimination
  - Enuresis, encopresis
- Sleep disorders
- Autonomic nervous system dysregulation
  - Raynaud syndrome, complex regional pain syndrome, hypertension
- Neuromuscular rehabilitation
- Habit disorders
  - Thumb sucking, bruxism, habit cough, nail biting
- Tics and Tourette syndrome
- Symptom management
  - Pruritus, nausea
- Warts
- Attention and disruptive behavior disorders
- Learning disorders
- Seizure disorders
- Feeding and swallowing problems
  - Dysphagia, cyclic vomiting, anorexia, bulimia
- Chronic illness
  - Asthma, juvenile rheumatoid arthritis, sickle cell anemia, malignant neoplasms, diabetes mellitus
- Dysfluencies
  - Stuttering

superior self-regulatory abilities (Culbert et al, 1994). For example, as a group, children appear to be more hypnotically susceptible than adults are (Olness and Kohen, 1996). Despite certain developmental differences, children make excellent biofeedback subjects as well (Attanasio et al, 1985). They note that compared with adult subjects:

- Children are more enthusiastic.
- Children learn more quickly.
- Children are less skeptical about self-control procedures.
- Children have more confidence in special abilities.
- Children have more psychophysiologic lability.
- Children enjoy practice sessions.
- Children are more reliable at symptom monitoring.

Although there are few absolute contraindications, biofeedback training and self-hypnosis should be approached with caution for children with depression, post-traumatic stress disorder, or severe emotional problems and children who have experienced abuse (Wester and Sugarman, 2007).

A child's age, developmental strengths and weaknesses, and natural talents and interests are all taken into account in crafting a self-regulation treatment plan. In many instances, mind-body therapies are integrated with other therapies for successful pain or symptom management. For example, biofeedback games can be used initially as a comfortable, fun, and tangible way to begin treatment. Self-hypnosis may be introduced later with other relaxation methods, including diaphragmatic breathing, progressive muscle relaxation, and autogenics. After the initial consultation, most children are able to learn several self-regulation strategies and to achieve good symptom control within four to six 30- to 40-minute sessions.

When a child is referred for self-regulation training, it is important to complete a comprehensive assessment and to identify treatable organic disease and psychiatric comorbidity. A patient's family and cultural context should be taken into consideration during the evaluation. In one group of 80 children with behavioral symptoms who were referred specifically for hypnotherapy, 20 of those children were found to have an undiagnosed medical problem that explained their symptoms (Olness and Libbey, 1987).

Biofeedback

Biofeedback is the use of electronic or electromechanical equipment (usually computer based) to measure and then to feed back information about physiologic

Table 91-3. Biofeedback Modalities and Explanations

Modality	Explanation
Peripheral temperature (thermography)	Measures finger temperature, which serves as an indirect measurement of autonomic nervous system balance; the more stress activity (reflecting increased sympathetic arousal), the less peripheral blood flow and the lower the finger temperature. Relaxation improves peripheral vasodilation and increases finger temperature.
Breathing (pneumography)	Measures abdominal or thoracic movement during respiration by a "stretch" sensor.
Exhaled carbon dioxide level (capnometry)	Measures exhaled carbon dioxide. During hyperventilation, carbon dioxide levels drop below the normal range.
Heart rate (photoplethysmography)	Measures heart rate by finger pulse.
Heart rate variability	Measures heart rate changes and related parameters and then uses mathematical calculations to evaluate the balance of the autonomic nervous system as reflected in heart rate acceleration and deceleration phenomena. Mediators of heart rate variability include emotional state and breathing pattern.
Muscle tension (electromyography)	Measures muscle electrical activity.
Skin conductance, electrodermal activity	Reflects sympathetic nervous system arousal by measuring relative skin surface electrical conductance or resistance (which is a function of the number of sweat glands open or closed).
Electroencephalographic biofeedback or neurofeedback	Measures the amount of delta, theta, alpha, and beta waves in various geographic locations on the brain with scalp surface electrodes.

processes. The goal of biofeedback is to help patients become aware of different states of physiologic arousal and their ability to control physiologic changes in their bodies. Goals of biofeedback treatment also commonly include improvement of the pediatric patient's ability to discern and cultivate lowered levels of sympathetic nervous system arousal and achieve a balanced state of mind-body "relaxation." Patients are coached in a variety of techniques including the awareness and control of breathing, the discrimination and modulation of muscle tension levels, and the modulation of peripheral (finger) temperature (Table 91-3).

Biofeedback equipment can be used to measure a number of physiologic parameters either one at a time or in combination. Studies have clearly demonstrated children's ability to control a variety of physiologic responses, including finger temperature, breathing rate and rhythm, and electrical brain wave activity. Research has also indicated consistent and dramatic changes in parameters such as heart rate and electrodermal activity associated with children's use of specific types of mental imagery (Culbert et al, 1996; Lee and Olness, 1996).

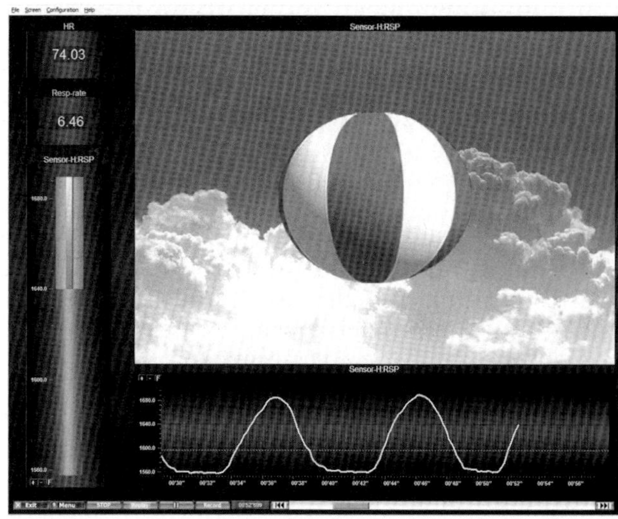

Figure 91-1. A biofeedback game in which the child is instructed to breathe with good abdominal movement and has a stretch sensor or "pneumograph" belt attached around the abdomen. As the child breathes, the balloon animation increases and decreases in size, matching the abdominal movements. *(Copyright Nexus and Stens Corporation.)*

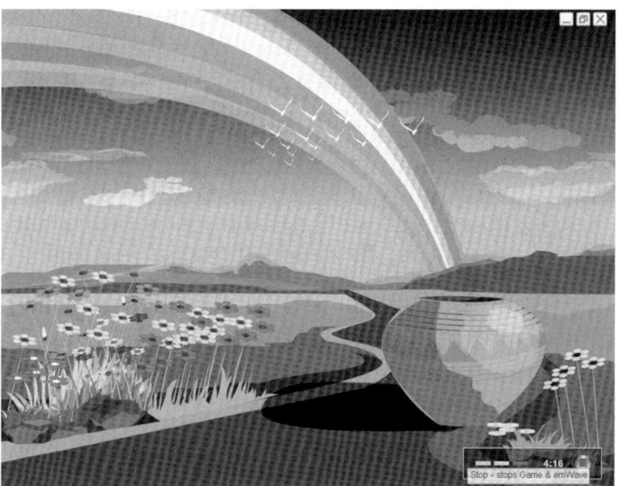

Figure 91-2. This animation displays a rainbow that eventually leads to a pot of gold. The activity on the screen is controlled by the patient's heart rate variability pattern. *(Copyright HeartMath, LLC.)*

The current availability of computerized biofeedback equipment with game-display type formats is culturally syntonic with present-day youth and offers an attractive and engaging treatment vehicle. Biofeedback display formats that are set up as games offer intrinsically motivating elements that can enhance the patient's engagement in the treatment process. Patients can be coached to achieve desired therapeutic outcomes (e.g., decreased muscle tension, slow diaphragmatic breathing) through participation in games that challenge them and that also hold their attention with high-quality graphics and audio (Figs. 91-1 and 91-2).

Hypnosis (Relaxation and Mental Imagery)

Hypnosis is an altered state of consciousness or awareness usually but not always involving relaxation, within which individuals experience heightened suggestibility. This state of consciousness is different from both the various stages of sleep and the normal waking state. During everyday activities, children move readily in and out of "altered" states. Fantasy, imagery, and intensely focused or absorbed attention are common experiences and reflect natural, developmental tendencies for children. Hypnotherapy refers to the use of self-hypnosis by an individual to achieve a therapeutic goal. Self-hypnosis is usually associated with a sensation of relaxation, well-being, and enhanced self-control abilities.

> *The goal of hypnotherapy is always to teach the patient an attitude of hope in the context of mastery. The patient learns to be an active participant in his or her own behalf, to focus on creating a solution rather than on enduring a problem, and to discover and use resources for inner control as much as possible.*
>
> OLNESS AND KOHEN (1996)

There are a number of common myths and misperceptions about hypnosis. Hypnosis is not a sleeplike state. Individuals in hypnotic states cannot be forced to do things against their will. In fact, there is usually heightened awareness of physical sensations and increased self-control in a hypnotic trance. Pediatric practitioners hold that all hypnosis is self-hypnosis and therefore the therapist can facilitate and influence but not "control" those experiences for pediatric patients. The process of engaging in self-hypnosis typically involves discrete steps including induction, deepening, therapeutic suggestion, re-alerting, and de-briefing (Table 91-4).

Self-hypnosis has a wide variety of valuable applications (see Table 91-2). It is highly personalized for each child, with particular consideration given to his or her developmental status. Most practitioners agree that a child should have at least a developmental age equivalent of 5 to 6 years for hypnotherapy to be effective. Children are readily susceptible to hypnosis, with hypnotic susceptibility increasing markedly in middle childhood.

Table 91-4. The Stages of Hypnosis

Stage	Description
Induction	Initiation of the experience of hypnosis, typically by practicing a procedure or activity that narrows and focuses attention, evokes curiosity, or facilitates relaxation
Deepening	Intensification of the trance experience by various strategies, such as imagery, sensory awareness, relaxation
Therapeutic suggestion	Suggestions—direct, indirect, metaphorical—about creating desired therapeutic change
Re-alerting	The client returns to the usual state of awareness
De-briefing	Discussion of the experience, planning for the ongoing practice of self-hypnosis and arranging follow-up

Self-hypnosis can be modified for treatment of those children with particular sensory impairments as well.

Hypnotherapy facilitates children's innate creative and imaginative skills to construct helpful solutions to their problems. Pediatric patients describe various mental images; some prefer visual and others create more auditory images. Individual differences might also include olfactory or kinesthetic imaginative preferences. Through the use of carefully selected and developmentally appropriate language, the practitioner encourages children's imaginative abilities to explore and to create unique ways to help themselves.

Cognitive-Behavioral Therapy

Cognitive-behavioral therapy is a therapeutic technique that emphasizes a person's awareness of internal positive and negative self-talk patterns and behavioral habits and helps that person develop effective problem solving strategies. Children are coached in the self-directed development of positive coping strategies and in enhanced perceptions of self-efficacy. They are encouraged to identify problematic situations and to respond with acceptable adaptive behavior. Selecting age- and reading level–appropriate self-help books can be an effective part of cognitive-behavioral therapy as well (www.freespirit.com). Cognitive-behavioral therapy can be very beneficial with impulse control problems, anxiety, and acute and chronic pain.

Diaphragmatic Breathing

Breathing control is a seemingly simple skill but one with extremely powerful and widespread applications. Diaphragmatic breathing, also called belly breathing, is useful for many different pediatric problems, including sleep disturbance, rumination, panic and performance anxiety symptoms, somatic complaints including headache and recurrent abdominal pain, anger management, chronic conditions such as asthma, and disorders related to autonomic nervous system dysregulation. It can be particularly helpful for children undergoing painful medical procedures such as venipuncture, bone marrow aspiration, and laceration repair. The basic technique involves coaching children in the development of a relaxed, rhythmic breathing pattern that results in a controlled, deep state of relaxation. Often, encouraging younger children to blow bubbles facilitates their use of breath control.

Progressive Muscle Relaxation

There are other self-guided techniques that cultivate states of decreased muscle tension, lower sympathetic nervous system arousal, and facilitate the subjective sense of relaxation and comfort. Progressive muscle relaxation is a technique in which the client is taught to alternately tighten and then relax specific muscle groups throughout the body to improve the ability to discriminate and to control areas of muscle tension (Jacobson, 1977).

Autogenics

Autogenics training teaches the use of a number of self-administered, repetitive suggestions involving one's awareness and experience of sensations of warmth, heaviness, and relaxation throughout various regions of the body (Linden, 1990). Progressive muscle relaxation and autogenics are particularly beneficial in the treatment of sleep onset problems, headaches, myofascial pain, and anxiety-related symptoms in children.

Yoga

Yoga is a physical activity that has been shown to reduce stress, to increase self-awareness and flexibility and strength, and to help create a positive body image. It works in part by affecting brain γ-aminobutyric acid levels (Streeter et al, 2007). There are several different types of yoga that use a combination of posture, breath control, concentration, and self-restraint as the basis for therapy. Yoga has been shown to be beneficial for treatment of children with respiratory conditions (Jain et al, 1991), "risk indices associated with the insulin resistance syndrome" (Innes et al, 2005), stress-related conditions, hypertension, menstrual problems, carpal tunnel syndrome, and insomnia. A particular method of yoga called Sonia Sumar is designed to be used by specially trained professionals with children who have special needs, including Down syndrome, cerebral palsy, autism, attention-deficit/hyperactivity disorder, and learning disabilities (*www.specialyoga.com*). Yoga also appears to be a promising intervention in teens with irritable bowel syndrome (Kuttner et al, 2006).

Meditation

Meditation is a conscious mental process in which a person learns to focus attention and to suspend his or her normal stream of thoughts to achieve a state of greater physical relaxation and mental calmness. There are three basic kinds of meditation (concentrative, mindfulness, and expressive) that have four basic elements in common: quiet location, specific comfortable posture, focus of attention, and open attitude (National Center for Complementary and Alternative Medicine). Meditation has been used successfully to treat hypertension in adolescents, irritable bowel syndrome, stress-related issues, headaches, asthma, and pain conditions and to reduce seizure frequency in patients with epilepsy.

Psychoneuroimmunology

Psychoneuroimmunology can be defined as the study of interactions between behavior, neural and endocrine function, and immune processes (Ader et al, 1995). Ongoing research suggests that the mind and body share bidirectional influences (Hidderley et al, 2004), and the science of psychoneuroendoimmunology (or psychoneuroimmunology and neuroendocrinology) identifies specific mechanisms by which these mind-body changes are mediated. The mind and body communicate bidirectionally continuously through chemical messengers. Positive and negative affective states probably create different neuroimmune responses in the body and thus influence health and recovery from illness (Cohen and Herbert, 1996; Olness, 1990). Two competing responses, the stress response (Selye, 1965) and the relaxation response (Lazar et al, 2000), counterbalance each other on an ongoing basis.

Under stressful conditions the body produces excess cortisol, which has been shown to affect the immune system (Lengacher et al, 1998). When the relaxation response is elicited, health-promoting chemicals including dehydroepiandrosterone (DHEA) and homeostatic physiologic changes are produced. Use of self-regulation techniques to calm the mind reduces the sympathetic nervous system's response to stress and enables an inner healing process. In addition to enhancing treatment of medical problems or procedures, mind-body strategies have also been shown to prevent advancement of disease. Lengacher and colleagues demonstrated in 1998 that the use of mental imagery is associated with improvement in cancer disease progression. Children can modulate several immunologic functions, and this may have implications in preventing viral illness (Hewson-Bower and Drummon, 1996; Olness et al, 1989).

CLINICAL APPLICATIONS

Self-regulation strategies (see Table 91-1) are commonly used sequentially or simultaneously in an integrated or "layered" behavioral treatment plan. These self-regulation techniques have several common characteristics. Perhaps the most important and generic component of these strategies is the "emphasis on mastery, coping and control achieved by the child or adolescent." Children are often taught several self-regulation techniques either alone or in combination and are encouraged to choose the therapeutic strategies that they find most effective and enjoyable to use in home practice.

Portable, low-cost biofeedback devices, such as biodots, can be used at home independently so that a child can see tangible results of a practice. Biodots are small adhesive discs that change color as skin temperature changes and are placed somewhere on the hands. An individual can track temperature readings before and after practicing a mind-body technique. A positive temperature change is usually observed after the body is in a relaxed state for 10 to 15 minutes, and the success of changing peripheral temperature serves as reinforcement for the child to continue the daily self-regulation practices. Other home training devices, such as the em-Wave from HeartMath (*www.heartmath.com*) and the Wild Divine (*www.wilddivine.com*) biofeedback game products for kids, are also useful (see Fig. 91-2).

Nocturnal Enuresis

Self-regulation techniques can be very useful in treating children with disorders of elimination, such as enuresis and encopresis. Self-hypnosis has been well described as a helpful strategy for children with primary nocturnal enuresis (Banerjee et al, 1993; Olness, 1975). Conditioning alarms, which are considered to be biofeedback devices, are also very effective (Glazener et al, 2003).

In the following vignette, Laura achieved 100% nighttime dryness after only one meeting. Pediatric patients are introduced to self-hypnosis on the first or second visit. During the next three or four follow-up appointments, they review and practice their skills and typically achieve increasing dryness. Although some children become dry after only one visit, many children require several visits before resolving their problem. The drawing of the urinary system and the mind-body connections depicted in Figure 91-3 was done by an 8-year-old boy at a follow-up visit for nocturnal enuresis.

Vignette

Laura, a 9½-year-old girl, wet the bed almost every night. She had been diagnosed with primary nocturnal enuresis and was treated unsuccessfully during the last few years. Laura had tried medications including imipramine and desmopressin for this problem but achieved no long-term success. She had used an alarm system, but the alarm was used inconsistently and awakened everyone in the house except Laura. In addition, Laura's parents had intermittently restricted her fluids and taken her to the bathroom to urinate in the middle of the night. Laura had become increasingly anxious because she was afraid that her younger siblings would tell her friends about "her problem" or discover the pull-ups that were hidden in the house. She had more recently felt left out because she could not participate in sleepovers with her friends. It was clear that Laura was motivated to resolve her problem.

During the initial meeting, Laura was taught the normal anatomy and physiology of the urinary tract system. The discussion emphasized the mind-body connections, specifically how her brain instructs her "bladder gate" to stay shut except when she sits on the toilet. Laura was encouraged to engage in self-hypnosis (review the discussion of her mind-body connections in relation to the urinary system) for 5 to 10 minutes just before bed each evening. She would imagine or visualize in her thinking that it was the middle of the night and her bladder was full. Her bladder gate would send the message to her brain, which would then decide whether to wake her body up to go to the bathroom or to send a message back down to the bladder gate to stay shut for the remainder of the night. The daily practice would enable her to "reprogram" her brain to keep her bladder gate shut at night just as she has it programmed to do during the day. Laura was also encouraged to keep a daily calendar to monitor her dry beds. Laura was responsible for practicing her self-hypnosis each night. After the initial meeting, Laura had all dry beds after 2 weeks of the self-regulation program, and after 4 months, she had been on three sleepovers and "her problem" was considered only a part of her past.

Sleep Disorder

Children with sleep onset difficulties and parasomnias can benefit greatly from learning relaxation strategies and self-hypnosis. Coaching children to fall asleep with a positive emotional attitude and to calm the "nervous system" by self-hypnosis and positive self-talk can help them achieve a restful, uninterrupted night's sleep. Diaphragmatic breathing and muscle relaxation strategies can help children cultivate a low level of sympathetic nervous system arousal and assist them in an easier transition from a waking to a sleep state. Relaxation helps counteract the potential disruptive impact of stress on sleep-wake cycles. Autogenics training is one technique that works well with children who describe that their mind is "too busy" and full of thoughts and "won't shut off" at bedtime.

Vignette

Davis, a bright 6½-year-old boy, was having frequent nightmares. His dreams about snakes woke him up and made it very difficult for him to fall back asleep. He had these nightmares two to three times each week. When Davis woke up with a bad dream, he yelled out fearfully to his parents. His parents comforted him after the nightmares, but Davis was too frightened to return to his room and slept the rest of the night in his parents' bed. His younger sisters were woken by the noise as well, and this was causing significant disruption to the whole family's ability to get a good night's sleep.

Davis' parents followed a consistent bedtime routine, and he had a night-light in his room. He was doing well academically and socially in his first-grade class, and he was healthy except for occasional colds. Davis was generally a happy child. He had some anxiety in kindergarten, and his family had recently moved, but the anxiety quickly resolved with individual counseling.

On Davis' first visit, he appeared comfortable and readily discussed the fearful nightmares that he had involving snakes. He admitted that the nightmares made it difficult for him to go to sleep by himself and expressed enthusiasm in learning a way to make it easier for him to get to sleep alone after a bad dream. He was invited to imagine a favorite place in his thinking. He readily engaged in favorite-place mental imagery and described "being in the woods." He spontaneously explained that he was wearing a "blue shirt and green pants" and playing alone. He was encouraged to notice how happy and content he was while engaged in mental imagery (self-hypnosis). It was suggested that he practice the self-hypnosis before going to sleep each night so that if he woke up in the middle of the night, he would be able to help himself get back to sleep. Davis was then asked to talk about his "nightmares" and to create an ending to those dreams in which he would "win" and feel good. Davis described how he had "switch power" and could shift his thinking to remove himself from the place with the snakes and just be in the woods he preferred as a favorite, safe place. He easily followed through with this suggestion and left the meeting feeling enabled and confident. Follow-up from his parents weeks later revealed that Davis quickly learned to do the self-hypnosis on his own and reportedly used it effectively to help him fall asleep. Soon after the initial visit, Davis no longer had frequent nightmares and no further problems with sleep.

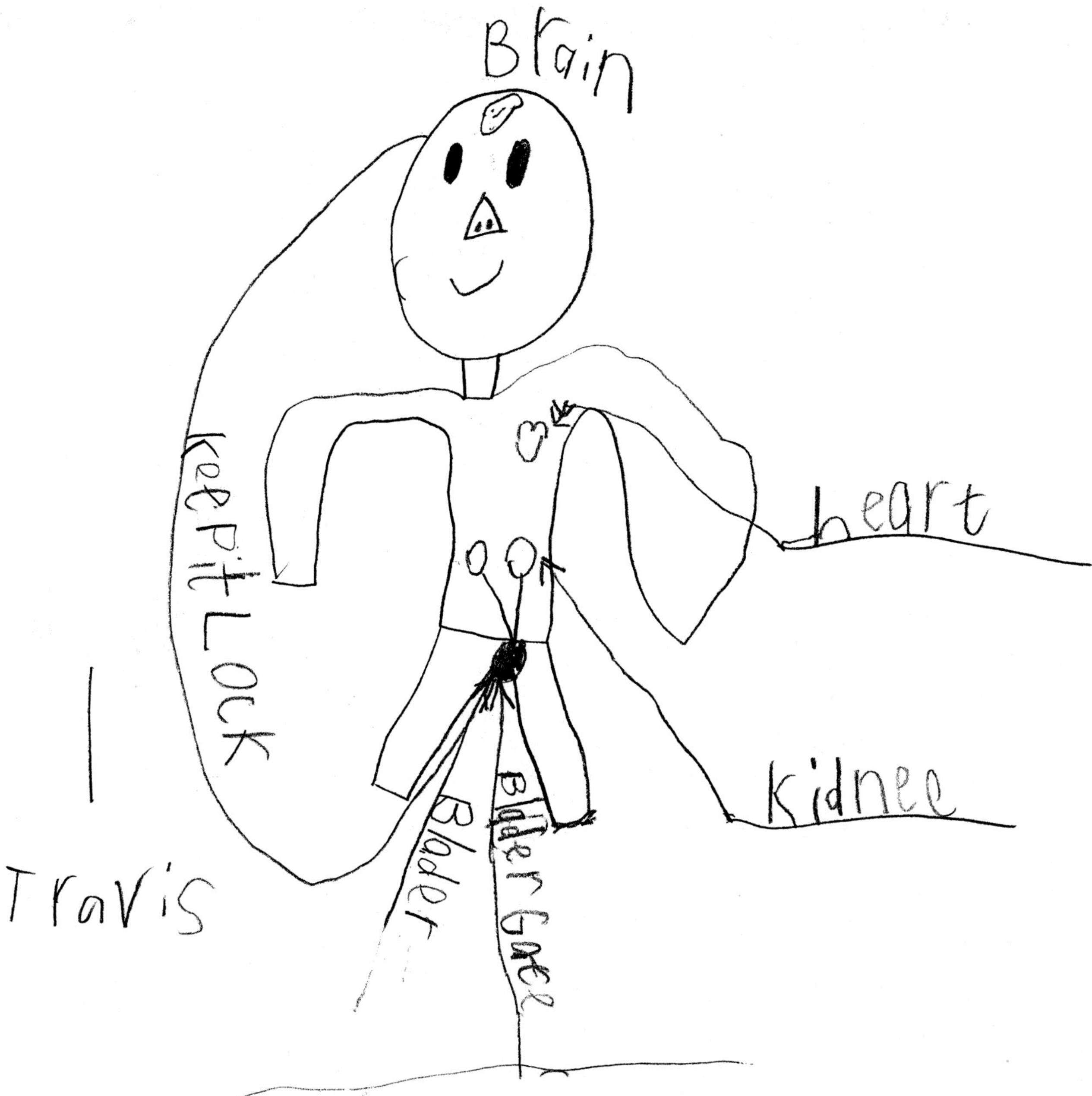

Figure 91-3. A drawing by an 8-year-old boy describing the connections between his brain and his bladder.

Recurrent Pain

Self-regulation strategies are particularly effective when they are applied to pediatric pain management. Studies of chronic, recurrent pain like migraine headaches and recurrent abdominal pain have clearly documented the effectiveness of self-regulation strategies. One prospective study compared propranolol, placebo, and self-hypnosis in the treatment of pediatric migraine and found that self-hypnosis was most effective in reducing the frequency of migraine headaches (Olness et al, 1987). Multiple studies have documented the effectiveness of biofeedback training (surface electromyography and also peripheral temperature) in the long-term management of pediatric headache, both tension-type and migraine headaches (Andrasik and Schwartz, 2006).

Studies (Anbar, 2001) have demonstrated the effectiveness of using self-hypnosis to treat recurrent abdominal pain. A study by Weydert and colleagues (2006) also supports the usefulness of self-hypnosis for recurrent abdominal pain. Recurrent abdominal and related functional gastrointestinal problems may be mediated by stress (increased sympathetic nervous arousal) for many children and teens. Therefore, biofeedback may also be a useful tool in addressing functional gastrointestinal disorders.

Vignette

Kara, a 12½-year-old, presented with chronic stomachaches and sore throats. Since her initial complaints 3 to 4 months ago, she had three negative throat cultures, two courses of antibiotics, a normal complete blood cell count, a normal urinalysis, and an upper gastrointestinal tract study that showed nonspecific findings. Kara was given a short course of an H_2 blocker, but her stomachaches continued. She had missed several days of school until arrangements were made for her to spend time as needed with the school nurse instead of being sent home. Kara spent approximately one third of her school day lying down in the nurse's office. Kara was being seen by a psychologist, weekly, for anxiety thought to be related to school. Further history revealed occasional headaches, no weight loss, and no vomiting or bowel problems; findings on physical examination were normal.

Kara described two types of abdominal pain: a sharp constant, epigastric pain that she believed was "a virus," and a lower abdominal pain that occurred intermittently when she was nervous. On a scale of 0 (no pain) to 12 (worst pain), Kara rated her stomachache as 9 on the initial visit (the worst that it had been was 11, and the best that it had been was 7). Further laboratory testing determined no organic cause of the stomachaches. When asked how her life would be different when she no longer had the pain, Kara tearfully replied that she "wouldn't have to go to the school nurse" and that she would "eat and feel better."

Kara was given examples of how she gets signals from her body when she has different feelings and the specific physiologic changes of the body in response to being nervous or scared versus relaxed. Kara was encouraged to hear that many children with problems like hers improve by learning how to use their mind to help their body. She was given a calendar and asked to monitor her stomachaches. On the second visit, Kara was taught diaphragmatic breathing and introduced to biofeedback. Electromyogram sensors were placed on her trapezius muscles bilaterally to monitor muscle tension during breathing, while an abdominal stretch sensor (pneumography) was used to track stomach movement with relaxation breath training. Through self-regulation training, she quickly learned to control her breathing pattern and slow its rate. At the end of the first session, she had lowered her stomachache to a rating of 4, the lowest that it had been! She recognized that her stomachache bothered her less when she slowed her breathing rate and relaxed. She agreed to practice the "belly breathing" at home each night before bed. Kara had five subsequent biofeedback sessions in which she mastered the physiologic self-regulation of her peripheral temperature (an indirect measure of sympathetic nervous system activity), muscle activity, and sweat gland response in a video game format.

After 5 weeks, Kara's stomachaches had improved dramatically (down to a rating of 1 to 2), with only one visit to the school nurse each day. At follow-up 8 weeks after the initial visit, Kara no longer had any somatic complaints and visited the school nurse only to say hello.

Tic Disorder

Self-regulation strategies have been applied successfully to treat repetitive behaviors including habits, tics, obsessive-compulsive disorder, and Tourette syndrome (Kohen, 1995). A significant number of patients who present to developmental-behavioral pediatricians with mild to moderate tics improve with self-regulation techniques alone. It is important to discuss with the patient the significant impact that anxiety and stress may have on the repetitive behaviors, that is, that heightened autonomic nervous arousal tends to "drive" tic behaviors. During treatment, self-awareness of behavior patterns and an enhanced sense of self-control are emphasized.

Vignette

Nick, a 17-year-old boy with a chronic motor tic disorder, was referred for self-regulation training. Nick had recently been on a psychotropic medication trial to help with the tics, but he did not respond optimally to the medication and did not want to consider alternative medication options. Nick has had difficulties with motor tics since he was 10 years old. At that time, he developed facial tics, which seemed to come and go during the next several years but did not impair him functionally. However, within the last 18 to 24 months, the tics had worsened considerably and had become widespread (occurring in muscle groups all over his body), more frequent, and quite intense. He had been seen several times by a pediatric neurologist, who had established the diagnosis of chronic motor tics and had prescribed a medication trial.

Nick described tics of his wrists and ankles that were so repetitive and severe that his joints would become sore. At the time of referral, he also noticed that his eye-blink and head-throw tics were interfering with his reading. Nick reported that the tics occurred daily, and he felt that they were exacerbated by stress. Despite the severity of the tics, Nick was well adjusted and had a very close and supportive group of friends at school. Nick was a well-rounded and highly successful high-school student. Not only was he doing well academically and on the honor role, but also he was a key player on the football team. In addition, Nick had a part-time job.

Nick's facial tics were evident throughout the first visit. Initially, the potential triggers of the tic flare-ups and the role of stress and anxiety on the tic exacerbations were discussed. Nick was then coached through a progressive muscle relaxation exercise and encouraged to let go of any muscle tension that he felt in his body. His tics stopped abruptly. Nick spontaneously closed his eyes and was encouraged to enjoy his choice of pleasant mental imagery. Particular attention was given to Nick's experience of a sense of warmth, heaviness, and comfort in his facial muscle groups. Nick was excited and surprised at how his tics had stopped so suddenly while using the relaxation technique. The session concluded with teaching Nick the basic diaphragmatic breathing techniques. Nick was encouraged to practice the progressive muscle relaxation and breathing techniques at least twice a day for 5 minutes and also at times when he felt stressed or anxious. He was also encouraged to self-monitor through the use of a symptom diary.

Nick returned to the clinic 2 weeks later. At this visit, further discussion focused on the connection between stress (or increased sympathetic nervous system arousal) and the role that played in increased tic frequency and severity. Nick was additionally introduced to the technique of heart rate variability biofeedback. His ability to achieve balanced autonomic nervous activity was reflected in a symmetric, high-amplitude "rolling wave" pattern (also called coherence) that he could visualize in real time on the biofeedback computer monitor. He was taught a technique engaging in "effortless" breathing combined with positive emotional imagery as a way to shift from negative emotional or "stress" states to a state of calm, positive balance—emotionally and physiologically. He was instructed in home practice and provided written support information.

Nick returned as scheduled for a follow-up visit 1 month later. He reportedly used the relaxation techniques regularly every day with great success, and he was excited to share the noticeable decrease in his motor tic activity that he had experienced. He described the use of very vivid and colorful mental imagery as part of his practices. The application of self-hypnosis was discussed in more explicit terms, and the progressive muscle relaxation and diaphragmatic breathing strategies were reviewed. A peripheral temperature sensor was attached to Nick's left index finger before the practice session. Nick once again demonstrated the ability to very quickly and deeply relax soon after the practice began. He did an excellent job and raised his peripheral temperature 12 degrees during the 20-minute relaxation session. Nick stated that he felt quite confident that he had good control over his tics by using the self-regulation strategies that he had learned in real-life settings. In addition, he was provided with some temperature-sensitive adhesive "dots" that changed color as his hands got warmer. These were used during the day at home and school as a way to monitor his relative stress level.

At a final follow-up visit 1 month later, Nick exhibited only mild facial tics at the beginning of the session. Since his last visit, he had been chosen for one of the lead roles in his school play. Self-hypnosis strategies, including an imagined "rehearsal" of his performance in the play, were reviewed. Once again, while actively involved in the relaxation techniques, Nick's facial tics completely resolved. He stated that he had been using diaphragmatic breathing and progressive muscle relaxation between scenes in the play when he was performing and had continued excellent symptom control.

Acute Procedural Pain and Distress

In acute pain associated with trauma and related medical procedures, a variety of behavioral and self-regulatory strategies have been shown to be successful in alleviating discomfort and allowing treatment to proceed easily (Kuttner, 1996). Butler and associates (2006) found in a randomized controlled trial that self-hypnosis significantly reduced the distress and resistance to voiding cystourethrography procedures for children and their families. In another randomized controlled study, self-hypnosis was shown to be more effective than midazolam on preoperative anxiety (Calipel et al, 2005). The research is also very supportive on the positive effects of self-hypnosis and biofeedback in the management of pediatric procedure-related cancer pain (Liossi et al, 2006).

Vignette

Brooke, an 8-year-old girl, was being managed by the developmental-behavioral pediatrician for treatment of her attention-deficit/hyperactivity disorder symptoms. She also had a diagnosis of premature adrenarche and was being observed every 3 months by the endocrinologist. Brooke's inattention and impulsivity were well controlled with stimulant medication, but Brooke was having significant anxiety and stress around the blood draws for her hormone levels required once every 2 to 3 months to monitor her precocious puberty. Brooke's grandmother, her primary caregiver, and the technicians have had to hold Brooke down for each venipuncture.

First, the discomfort of having to be held down and to have a needle stick was acknowledged and discussed. Then, Brooke was asked if she would like to learn some skills so that the blood draws would not bother her so much. She was told how she gets signals from her body when she has different feelings and that there are specific physiologic changes of the body in response to being nervous or scared versus relaxed. Brooke was interested to hear that many children have been helped to go through difficult procedures by learning how to use their mind to help their body. Brooke agreed that her grandmother would be her coach for her daily practices and during her venipunctures.

(Continued)

Brooke was advised to go to her favorite place in her thinking. She responded that she was playing in the park and spontaneously answered questions describing the sun shining, her clothes, and the people around her. Although her eyes were open and she was moving around, Brooke was deeply engaged in visual imagery. She was complimented several times on her ability and encouraged to notice how relaxed she felt. After 5 to 10 minutes, the practice was over. Brooke and her grandmother were then shown the technique of diaphragmatic breathing. It was suggested that practicing these two self-regulation skills daily and rehearsing the blood draw would make venipunctures much less bothersome in the future.

Follow-up was obtained by telephone 2 weeks later when Brooke's grandmother called for a medication refill. According to Brooke's grandmother, they continued to practice the self-regulation skills, and the subsequent blood draw was much easier. Brooke was very proud of herself!

Applications for the General Pediatrician in a Busy Practice

Vignette

Four-year-old Evie is sitting at the edge of the examination table blowing intently on the bubble wand her mother is holding in front of her mouth. At the same time, the nurse is supporting Evie's arm while the pediatrician gives her two immunizations in each deltoid muscle. Evie is excited and a little sore when it is over, but she is empowered with her ability to cooperate with the process.

In a general pediatrician's office, a busy practitioner has many opportunities to incorporate self-regulation skills into routine medical practice (Wester and Sugarman, 2007). The first step is to focus on the child being seen for a specific issue rather than attending solely to the presenting problem or procedure. This will encourage an alliance between the clinician and the child, establishing the basis of good therapeutic treatment. Including the child as an active participant in his or her care allows the child to have some control in an otherwise powerless situation (Olness and Kohen, 1996). Use of self-regulation techniques empowers a child and encourages a child's natural inclination for health and wellness.

In children younger than 10 years, use of breath control exercises by having a child blow bubbles focuses his or her attention on the quality of the bubble in front of the child and makes the child less aware of the pain of an immunization or blood draw. Also, pain perception may be reduced when a child is relaxed and more in control of a situation. Use of favorite-place imagery while blood pressure is taken or an abdominal examination is performed is easy and fun and offers an appropriate attentional shift away from any unpleasant sensations.

It is important to get a child's "buy-in" into the process. Here are a few examples of useful phrases:

Is it OK if we work together so that the needle stick does not bother you so much?

If you could be any place right now, where would you be? How does it look? Are there other people with you? Is it warm? What are you wearing?

Isn't it great that you can be the boss of your body and feel any way you want to!

In older children, it would be beneficial to explain in more detail the mind-body connections and controls before making suggestions. Explaining how thoughts and feelings affect body temperature and heart rate, for example, may challenge an adolescent and allow greater independence and self-sufficiency. After learning a self-regulation strategy, an older child can be encouraged to practice the techniques and to use them in other situations. This can lead to increased self-confidence and a greater comfort with anxiety-provoking situations.

TRAINING AND CERTIFICATION

Child health care professionals who would like to acquire and to apply these techniques should have appropriate training and experience. Self-regulation techniques are not viewed as a separate discipline or profession but are meant to be used in the context of the practice of medicine, nursing, dentistry, psychology, child life, and social work. Therefore, competency and licensure in a defined medical or mental health–related discipline are required before training or certification in self-regulation techniques. Hypnosis and biofeedback, in particular, have strong professional organizations, training opportunities, and formal testing and certification standards.

Child health care professionals who desire training in hypnosis methods would be advised to take a basic workshop sponsored by the Society for Developmental and Behavioral Pediatrics, the American Society of Clinical Hypnosis, and the Society for Clinical and Experimental Hypnosis or through an appropriate academic offering usually found in a university medical or psychology department. After adequate training, supervision, and clinical experience, individuals seeking formal certification of hypnosis training can contact the American Society of Clinical Hypnosis, the American Board of Medical Hypnosis, the American Board of Psychological Hypnosis, the American Board of Dental Hypnosis, or the American Board of Hypnosis in Clinical Social Work for information.

Training in biofeedback techniques is offered at meetings of the Association for Applied Psychophysiology and Biofeedback and the Biofeedback Foundation of Europe. Board certification in biofeedback is available through the Biofeedback Certification Institute of America. Table 91-5 contains the names and addresses of the organizations referred to in this section.

Table 91-5. Organization and Resource Guide

Hypnosis Certification and Training
- Society for Clinical and Experimental Hypnosis
  Massachusetts School of Professional Psychology
  221 Rivermoor Street
  Boston, MA 02132
  www.sceh.us
- American Society of Clinical Hypnosis
  140 N. Bloomingdale Road
  Bloomingdale, IL 60108
  www.asch.net
- Society for Developmental and Behavioral Pediatrics
  6728 Old McLean Village Drive
  McLean, VA 22101
  www.sdbp.org
- American Board of Medical Hypnosis
  c/o Steven F. Bierman, MD
  143 8th Street
  Del Mar, CA 92014

Biofeedback Certification and Training
- Association for Applied Psychophysiology and Biofeedback
  10200 West 44th Avenue, Suite 304
  Wheat Ridge, CO 80033
  www.aapb.org
- Biofeedback Certification Institute of America
  10200 West 44th Avenue, Suite 310
  Wheat Ridge, CO 80033
  www.bcia.org
- Biofeedback Foundation of Europe
  www.bfe.org

THE FUTURE

Growing literature and successful clinical experience support the utility and cost-efficacy of the self-regulation strategies described in this chapter and underscore the increasing importance of these techniques in the armamentarium of the developmental-behavioral pediatrician and other pediatric health professionals. They can be useful in both inpatient and outpatient clinical settings. It is also clear that parents are increasingly interested in nonpharmacologic treatment modalities for their children with biobehavioral problems as concerns grow about the potential serious side effects of conventional medications. Biofeedback, hypnosis, and the other mind-body techniques offer children the option acquiring "skills" to replace "pills" (Wickramasekera, 1988). Once children learn self-regulation strategies, they commonly apply the techniques to other challenging situations that they encounter and continue to use these techniques throughout their lives. One would hope to see these techniques become part of all child health care providers' curricula, including medical and nursing schools, child-life programs, and pediatric residency programs.

Pioneering research in pediatric self-regulation supports the ability of children to voluntarily modulate certain aspects of immune system function (Olness et al, 1989). Research in this area documents children's ability to eradicate warts, to change levels of salivary immunoglobulins, and to influence the activity of certain white blood cell types (Olness, 1990). Researchers are exploring the role of relaxation, directed mental imagery, and related mind-body strategies in children with cancer, autoimmune disorders, and infectious processes. The links of mental imagery and emotions to learned physiologic response patterns are also being clarified.

Practitioners in this field look forward to the day when biofeedback computers, hypnotherapy, and breathing control training are part of the general pediatrician's daily office practice. The idea of proactive stress management or stress "inoculation" for the pediatric population by training in mind-body skills is also timely and consistent with the Bright Futures guidelines for anticipatory guidance. The idea that early training in self-regulation techniques may help certain at-risk populations in reducing morbidity from conditions such as asthma, hemophilia, migraine headache, irritable bowel syndrome, sleep disturbances, and Tourette syndrome is very promising. A preventive approach to these disorders employing hypnosis, biofeedback, diaphragmatic breathing, and related skills could result in huge savings in medical costs over time.

With the advance of computer graphics technology, children can learn and practice these self-regulation skills in interactive multimedia formats—playing a "video game for your body" in a way that is both therapeutic and enjoyable for pediatric patients.

It would seem likely, given the studies and clinical experiences to date, that biofeedback, self-hypnosis, and related self-regulation techniques will become the primary "treatments of choice" for a variety of biobehavioral problems of childhood, including headaches, somatization disorders, anxiety spectrum problems, enuresis, sleep disorders, and disorders of autonomic nervous system dysregulation.

REFERENCES

Ader R, Cohen N, Felten D: Psychoneuroimmunology: Interactions between the nervous system and the immune system. Lancet 345:99-103, 1995.

Anbar R: Self hypnosis for the treatment of functional abdominal pain in childhood. Clin Pediatr 40:447-451, 2001.

Andrasik F, Schwartz M: Behavioral assessment and treatment of pediatric headache. Behav Modif 30:93-113, 2006.

Astin JA, Shapiro SL, Eisenberg DM, Forys KL: Mind-body medicine: State of the science, implications for practice. J Am Board Fam Pract 16:131-147, 2003.

Attanasio V, Andrasik F, Burke E, et al: Clinical issues in utilizing biofeedback with children. Clin Biofeedback Health 8:134-141, 1985.

Bakal D: Minding the Body: Clinical Uses of Somatic Awareness. New York, Guilford, 1999, pp 1-43.

Banerjee S, Srivastav A, Palan B: Hypnosis and self-hypnosis in the management of nocturnal enuresis: A comparative study with imipramine therapy. Am J Clin Hypnosis 36:113-119, 1993.

Butler LD, Symons BK, Henderson SL, et al: Hypnosis reduces distress and duration of an invasive medical procedure for children. Pediatrics 115:77-85, 2006.

Calipel S, Lucas-Polomeni MM, Wodey E, Ecoffey C: Premedication in children: Hypnosis versus midazolam. Pediatr Anesth 15:275-281, 2005.

Cohen S, Herbert T: Health psychology: Psychological factors and physical disease from the perspective of human psychoneuroimmunology. Annu Rev Psychol 47:113-142, 1996.

Culbert T, Kajander R: Be the Boss of Your Stress. Minneapolis, Freespirit Publishing, 2007.

Culbert T, Rearney J, Kohen D: Cyberphysiologic strategies for children: The clinical hypnosis, biofeedback interface. Int J Clin Exp Hypnosis 442:17-97, 1994.

Culbert T, Kajander R, Reaney J: Biofeedback with Children and Adolescents: Clinical Observations and Patient Perspectives. J Dev Behav Pediatr 17:342-350, 1996.

Glazener CM, Evans JH, Peto RE: Alarm interventions for nocturnal enuresis in children. Cochrane Database Syst Rev 2: CD002911, 2003.

Hewson-Bower B, Drummon P: Secretory immunoglobulin A increases during relaxation in children with and without recurrent upper respiratory infection. J Dev Behav Pediatr 17:311-316, 1996.

Hidderley M, Holt M: A pilot randomized trial assessing the effects of autogenic training in early stage cancer patients in relation to psychological status and immune system responses. Oncol Nurs 8:61-65, 2004.

Innes KE, Bourguignon C, Brooke AG: Risk indices associated with the insulin resistance syndrome, cardiovascular disease, and possible protection with yoga: A systematic review. J Am Board Fam Pract 18:491-519, 2005.

Jacobson E: The origins and development of progressive relaxation. J Behav Ther Exp Psychiatry 8:119-123, 1977.

Jain SC, Rai L, Valecha A, et al: Effect of yoga training on exercise tolerance in adolescents with childhood asthma. J Asthma 28:437-442, 1991.

Kuttner L, Chambers CT, Hardial J, et al: A randomized trial of yoga for adolescents with irritable bowel syndrome. Pain Res Manag 11:217-223, 2006.

Kohen DP: Ericksonian communication and hypnotic strategies in the management of tics and Tourette syndrome in children and adolescents. *In* Lankton S, Zeig I (eds): Difficult Contexts for Therapy. New York, Brunner/Mazel, 1995, pp 116-138.

Kuttner L: A Child in Pain, How to Help, What to Do. Vancouver, Hartley and Marks, 1996.

Kuttner L, Chambers CT, Hardial J, et al: A randomized trial of yoga for adolescents with irritable bowel syndrome. Pain Res Manag 11:217-223, 2006.

Lazar SW, Bush G, Gollub RL, et al: Functional brain mapping of the relaxation response and meditation. Neuroreport 11:1581-1585, 2000.

Lee L, Olness K: Effects of self-induced mental imagery on autonomic reactivity in children. J Dev Behav Pediatr 17:323-327, 1996.

Lengacher CA, Bennett M, Gonzalez L, et al: Psychoneuroimmunology and immune system link for stress, depression, health behaviors, and breast cancer. Alternative Health Practitioner 4:95-108, 1998.

Lengacher CA, Bennett M, Gonzalez L, et al: The effects of relaxation guided imagery on natural killer (NK) cell and cytokine IL-2 induced NK cytotoxicity in breast cancer patients. Breast Cancer Res Treat 100:345, 2006.

Linden W: Autogenic Training: A Clinical Guide. New York, Guilford, 1990.

Liossi C, White P, Hatira P: Randomized clinical trial of local anesthetic versus combination of local anesthetic with self-hypnosis in the management of pediatric procedure-related pain. Health Psychol 25:307-315, 2006.

Olness K: The use of self-hypnosis in the treatment of childhood nocturnal enuresis: A report on forty patients. Clin Pediatr 14:273-279, 1975.

Olness K: Pediatric psychoneuroimmunology: Hypnosis as a mediator. Potentials and problems. *In* Van Dyck R: Hypnosis: Current Theory, Research and Practice. Amsterdam, The Netherlands, VU University Press, 1990.

Olness K: Hypnosis and biofeedback with children and adolescents; clinical, research, and educational aspects. Introduction. J Dev Behav Pediatr 17:299, 1996.

Olness K, Culbert T, Uden D: Self-regulation of salivary immunoglobulin A by children. Pediatrics 83:66-71, 1989.

Olness K, Kohen DP: Hypnosis and Hypnotherapy with Children, 3rd ed. New York, Guilford Press, 1996.

Olness K, Libbey P: Unrecognized biologic basis for behavioral symptoms in children referred for hypnotherapy. Am J Clin Hypnosis 30:1-8, 1987.

Olness K, MacDonald J, Uden D: Comparison of self-hypnosis and propranolol in the treatment of juvenile migraine. Pediatrics 79:593-597, 1987.

Selye H: The stress syndrome. AJN Am J Nurs 65:97-99, 1965.

Streeter C, Jensen J, Perlmutter R, et al: Yoga Asana sessions increase brain GABA levels: A pilot study. J Altern Complement Med 13:419-426, 2007.

Wester W, Sugarman L: Therapeutic Hypnosis with Children and Adolescents. Bethel, CT, Crown House Publishing, 2007.

Weydert J, Shapiro DE, Acra SA, et al: Evaluation of guided imagery as treatment for recurrent abdominal pain in children: A randomized controlled trial. BMC Pediatr 6:26, 2006.

Wickramasekera I: Clinical Behavioral Medicine: Some Concepts and Procedures. New York, Plenum, 1988.

Wolsko PM, Eisenberg DM, Davis RB, Phillips RS: Use of mind-body medical therapies: Results of a national survey. J Gen Intern Med 19:43-50, 2004.

92 EARLY INTERVENTION SERVICES

PENNY HAUSER-CRAM AND MARJI ERICKSON WARFIELD

WHAT ARE EARLY INTERVENTION SERVICES?

Early intervention (EI) services are designed to benefit the development from birth to the age of 3 years of children who have or are at risk of having disabilities or special needs that substantially delay development and to support the adaptation of their families. In general, the goals of EI are to facilitate service provision and coordination and, when necessary, to provide direct services. The services vary according to the nature of the child's special needs. Direct services include speech and language therapy, occupational therapy, physical therapy, special instruction, and family education and counseling, although other services, such as assistive technology, nutrition instruction, and audiology services, may also be provided. Both the frequency and the intensity of EI direct services are low compared with other early education services, such as preschool or Head Start; the actual hours of EI service provided to families average less than 2 hours a week (Shonkoff et al, 1992; U.S. Department of Education, 2003). Therefore, EI services are designed to coordinate other services and to support parents and other caregivers in optimizing child development and family adaptation.

A BRIEF HISTORY OF EARLY INTERVENTION

The history of EI is embedded in a larger history of dual national commitments to serving young children at risk of poor developmental (including health) outcomes and their families and to providing services for individuals with disabilities within typical settings rather than in settings specialized only for those with disabilities. The federal responsibility for the well-being of children and their mothers was affirmed by the Social Security Act of 1935, Title V, which established the framework for Maternal and Child Health Services, Services for Crippled Children, and Child Welfare Services. Through Title V legislation, financial assistance to the states is provided to establish prenatal care, well-child clinics, and services to prevent infant mortality and disabilities that limit children's health and development. In 1991, the Maternal and Child Health Bureau began supporting Healthy Start, an initiative to stimulate community-based services to reduce infant mortality and low birth weight and to eliminate racial disparities in perinatal outcomes.

In addition to public health services, federal support for children with disabilities emerged from educational services. Stimulated by the War on Poverty in the 1960s, Head Start was established as a means of providing early education experiences for children and support for their families. Related programs (e.g., the Abecedarian Project, the Brookline Early Education Project, and the High/Scope Education Perry Preschool Project) were initiated as randomized experiments or quasi-experiments to evaluate educational interventions in the early childhood years, largely for children living in poverty. Evaluations of such early childhood programs indicate that they have had positive effects on children, especially in the domain of cognitive development and long-term health and functional outcomes (Anderson et al, 2003; Palfrey et al, 2005).

Programs focusing on children with developmental disabilities were stimulated by the passage by Congress of the Handicapped Early Education Program in 1968, which provided federal funding for the development of a series of model programs. A more comprehensive federal role in supporting the development of programs and services for young children with disabilities took several decades. In 1975, the landmark legislation Education of All Handicapped Children Act (Public Law 94-142) was passed and guaranteed the right to free and appropriate education for school-age children with disabilities. Although this legislation also provided incentives for states to serve children aged 3 to 5 years with disabilities, it did not address the needs of infants and toddlers. In 1986, however, in amendments to the Education of the Handicapped Act (PL 99-457), states were required to provide services for children aged 3 to 5 years with disabilities in order to qualify for federal special education funding. That legislation also provided incentives to states to create programs to address the needs of infants and toddlers with disabilities. Reauthorized under a new title, the Individuals with Disabilities Education Act (IDEA) in 1991 (PL 101-476), the legislation determined specific activities required of the states (described in the

Partial support for this chapter was provided by Grant R40MC00333 from the Maternal and Child Health Bureau (Title V, Social Security Act), Health Resources and Services Administration, U.S. Department of Health and Human Services.

next section) should they decide to set up a statewide system of EI services and thus participate in the federal program.

HOW DOES FEDERAL LEGISLATION GUIDE CURRENT EARLY INTERVENTION SERVICES?

A national commitment to the provision of EI services is codified by Part C of the current reauthorization of the Individuals with Disabilities Education Act (IDEA 2004) (PL 108-446). All states have elected to participate in Part C. According to IDEA, the goal of such services is "to enhance the development of infants and toddlers with disabilities" and "to enhance the capacity of families to meet the special needs of their infants and toddlers" (20 USC 1431, as amended by the IDEA amendments of 2004). Several key components of EI services are required by IDEA. Among these are (1) the construction of an early identification and referral program (often referred to as child find activities), (2) the development of an individualized family service plan (IFSP), (3) the stipulation that EI services be provided in "natural environments" to the maximum extent possible, and (4) the construction of an interagency coordinating council. Each is described briefly.

Children and families may be referred to EI services by parents or by professionals, but current data indicate that in most states, the majority of referrals are made by pediatricians or other health care personnel. Although parents are often the source of referral in suburban communities, they rarely are in urban centers. States have indicated that their child find efforts have faced numerous obstacles. In general, public service campaigns including television, radio, and newspaper advertisements and distribution of information to health and medical settings are used, but these are often not produced in multiple languages or distributed sufficiently, especially in rural areas (U.S. Government Accountability Office, 2005). Therefore, a screening questionnaire completed by parents and reviewed by pediatricians or other health care providers can serve a critical function in locating children and families for whom EI services may be warranted.

Although participation in EI services is optional and services are subject to family approval, once a family decides to participate, the target child is provided with a comprehensive, multidisciplinary assessment. This assessment generally involves measurement of a child's skills in all areas of development but also should focus on the child's abilities within family-identified activities and routines. After the assessment, parents are asked to participate in the development of an IFSP, which includes the components listed in Table 92-1. Part C further mandates that families must be informed of their rights and must receive a review of the IFSP every 6 months.

A wide range of services can be specified on the IFSP (including, for example, speech and language therapy, occupational therapy, physical therapy, educational support, social services, audiology, assistive technology), but health services are included only to the extent that they are deemed "necessary for the infant or toddler to benefit from other early intervention services" (20 USC 1432). The service provided most frequently is speech and language therapy, followed by special instruction, physical therapy, and occupational therapy (U.S. Government Accountability Office, 2005).

Table 92-1. Components of the Individualized Family Service Plan

The individualized family service plan (IFSP) contains a description of the following:
The child's current functioning and skills
The family's strengths, resources, priorities, and concerns
The major expected outcomes (including measures, criteria, and timeline)
The specific services the child and family will receive, including their initiation and duration
The natural environments in which EI services will be provided
A named service coordinator
Plans for a successful transition from EI to preschool services

EI, early intervention.

Another requirement of Part C is that services be provided in natural environments. Natural environments are interpreted as those contexts in which children typically learn, play, and are nurtured. The child's home, the childcare home or center, and the settings of other activities in which a family participates (e.g., religious services, community-based athletics) are considered natural environments. The most frequent setting in which services are provided is the home, followed by the childcare setting. Although a parent usually participates in EI services when they occur at home, a parent is less likely to do so when the services are provided in a childcare setting. Therefore, the Council for Exceptional Children recommends that EI service providers consult with teachers and childcare providers as well as with parents to maximize continuity in approaches to enhancing the child's development.

Consideration of the transition from services provided through Part C to those provided by Part B of IDEA (i.e., preschool services) has also been placed in the legislation. Children can receive Part C EI services until they turn 3 years of age. Although a provision has been made for Part C funds to be used to continue to provide services from the age of 3 years to the beginning of the next school year, only 14 states have adopted this policy. In the most recent reauthorization, states have also been given the option of providing children and families with Part C services until the child is eligible for kindergarten (U.S. Government Accountability Office, 2005).

Finally, each state is required to develop an interagency coordinating council (ICC), which is a statewide, coordinated multidisciplinary and interagency system. In general, the ICC is composed of members from public health, mental health, education, and social services. The composition of the ICC differs by state, but all states are required to have parents on the ICC, which is consistent with the family focus of EI services.

STATE VARIATIONS IN EARLY INTERVENTION SERVICES

Much state discretion has been built into the federal legislation relating to EI services. In particular, states vary considerably in three dimensions of EI services: lead agency, service eligibility criteria, and service intensity. States are required to designate a lead agency, which will be responsible for ensuring public awareness about EI services as well as for defining eligibility criteria and establishing the process of service delivery. In 23 states, a combination of health and human service departments serves as the lead agency, whereas 16 states have designated health departments and 11 states have designated education departments as the lead agency (U.S. Government Accountability Office, 2005).

EI services are provided to children younger than 3 years who are developmentally delayed, but the definitions of such delay and how to measure it vary widely across states. These variations in turn influence eligibility. Some states (e.g., Georgia) base the definition of delay on standard deviation units, others (e.g., Arizona) on percent delay. Hawaii differs from other states by basing eligibility on the judgment of a multidisciplinary team. States also vary in whether they serve children who do not have a documented delay but who are at risk of having a substantial delay because of biologic or medical risk (e.g., low birth weight, chronic lung disease) or because of environmental risk associated with the caregiving and family situation (e.g., homelessness, parental developmental disability, parental age). In some states (e.g., Massachusetts), families of children with low birth weight are eligible for services; in others, (e.g., Hawaii), families in which a parent is younger than 16 years may qualify. Other states (e.g., Florida) do not serve children who are "at risk" through Part C programs but monitor such children through other programs.

The most recent reauthorization indicates that states need to put in place policies and procedures of referral to EI services for children who have been victims of substantiated abuse or neglect or affected by illegal substance abuse (Danaher et al, 2006). The link between social service agencies and EI services optimally will be strengthened by this requirement, but so too should the relationship between physicians and EI. Once states embark on this new policy, an additional population will enter the EI service system regardless of a state's decision about including children "at risk."

Nationwide, about 2.1% of the total population of children in the United States are served by EI (U.S. Department of Education, 2003), although it is estimated that EI currently serves less than the estimated 15% of children who will eventually be eligible for special education services (Bailey et al, 1999). States vary in terms of the percent of the 0-3 population served, from a low of 1.6% in Oregon to a high of 7.1% in Hawaii. Funding sources also seem to vary by state. Although all states receive funding under IDEA Part C, some use additional public or private funding sources. For example, Medicaid, Child Care and Development Block Grants, Temporary Assistance for Needy Families, Early Head Start, and Maternal and Child Health Title V are other sources of funds used in some states to support the provision of EI services. At least one state (New Jersey) charges a sliding monthly fee that depends on family size and income related to federal poverty guidelines (U.S. Government Accountability Office, 2005), although in most states, EI services are provided without charge to families regardless of their socioeconomic status.

WHO PARTICIPATES IN EARLY INTERVENTION SERVICES?

Although there is no one typical child or family who participates in EI services, data from the National Early Intervention Longitudinal Study (NEILS) (Scarborough et al, 2004) yielded findings about important demographic trends in EI participation. The authors of this national survey reported that a higher proportion of African American and a lower proportion of white infants and toddlers were being served in EI in relation to the U.S. population for the 0-3 age group. Families also appeared to be disproportionately poor and mothers were less likely to be employed, although families of all employment and income groups are eligible to participate. Children were less likely to be living in a family with two parents and were more likely to have a sibling with special needs. About 40% of children had spent time in the neonatal intensive care unit. In addition, a relatively higher proportion of children in foster care (7%) were in EI services compared with those in foster care in the general population of infants and toddlers (0.8%). It is not clear if children in foster care represent a new demographic trend in participation in EI services or if they have been overlooked in prior investigations. Regardless, the reauthorization of IDEA Part C now includes an emphasis on locating infants and toddlers in foster care who meet the criteria for participating in EI. In summary, EI services are used by a large range of families, and trends indicate that future increases in EI enrollment will be composed of children in foster care and children who have been abused or neglected. Currently, EI services are reaching fewer young children with special needs than the number that is estimated to exist in the U.S. population (3.4%), and not all eligible children are being served (U.S. Government Accountability Office, 2005).

It has been noted that some children who could potentially benefit from EI services, such as those with socioemotional disorders, are not systematically tracked (U.S. Government Accountability Office, 2005) and therefore may not be receiving services. Children with socioemotional disorders appear to be a group that has been overlooked in referrals to EI services. Despite data indicating that 10% of kindergarteners arrive at school with problematic behavior (West et al, 2000), children with challenging behaviors are seldom identified in the infant and toddler years. This is a critical oversight as young children with severe behavior problems are likely to exhibit continuing difficulties with self-regulation, and their families are likely to experience increasing levels of stress (Fox et al, 2002). Some of these children may be referred to EI because of speech and language delays and consequent poor skills in verbal self-regulation. Others, however, may be overlooked because the "typical toddler" is often seen as having difficulties with self-regulation.

Children with autism spectrum disorder (ASD) are another group with socioemotional difficulties. The

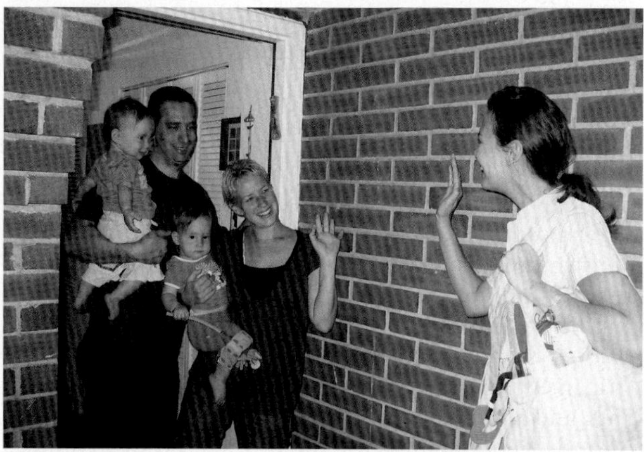

Figure 92-1. An EI educator leaves a home visit with twins and their parents.

prevalence rate of children with ASD appears to have been underestimated according to a study funded by the Centers for Disease Control and Prevention (Yeargin-Allsop et al, 2003). As the ability to diagnose children with ASD during the infant and toddler years increases, it is likely that children with ASD will be a growing population in EI. Moreover, pediatricians will be asked to screen for ASD and refer young children who may show signs of this disorder.

THE PRINCIPLES OF EARLY INTERVENTION

The principles of EI emerge primarily from the scientific research base on child development, family systems, and human ecology. EI services have transformed from placing primary focus on providing therapeutic services to the child alone to a broader focus on providing services to the child as an integral part of a family, neighborhood, and community. This represents a move away from a deficit "fix the child" model to a relationship-based model in which the family with its social network is considered the main source of intervention and support for the young child's development (Fig. 92-1). During the last 2 decades, the field of child development has increasingly recognized the importance of an ecologic perspective of the child as a part of the family, community, and culture (Bronfenbrenner, 1986), with a broader understanding that the child with disabilities, like all children, lives within multiple interacting systems (Guralnick, 2005b). EI is one of those systems, but it also has the concomitant responsibility of organizing other systems through service coordination.

One important principle of EI is that earlier provision of services is better for children and families. This is based on evidence that developmental trajectories can potentially be changed during the early years and that the development of secondary disabilities can be prevented by the provision of services when a child is very young. A comprehensive review of the science of development in early childhood suggests two critical findings about the role of experience in brain development (Shonkoff and Phillips, 2000). First, although few in number, some studies suggest that gene-environment interaction may explain differences in children's reaction to patterns of parenting and child rearing events. Second, studies indicate that much brain development is experience dependent and that such development can change behavioral functioning. Although the early years are not the exclusive domain of such transformations, they often set the course of developmental trajectories.

Another critical principle is the importance of the family, especially of relationships within the family, as both a context and conduit for children's optimal development. Parents and caregivers are central sources of support for the child's learning and emotional well-being, but family relationships can also create the context in which parent-child and sibling interactions occur. The results of our research study on children and families who have participated in EI services, the Early Intervention Collaborative Study (EICS), indicate that children with disabilities have more positive developmental trajectories when they reside in cohesive families, regardless of the marital or socioeconomic status of the family (Hauser-Cram et al, 2001).

Families hold and pass on values and beliefs that are both distinct and culturally derived. Some values and beliefs are demonstrated through family rituals, such as family dinners and bedtime routines. Such rituals and routines require modification whenever a new individual joins the family, but when that individual is a child with disabilities, a larger number of accommodations are often required. These can include attending many appointments, gathering information from a range of sources, and changing employment schedules. Core values about parenting, the meaning of disability, and the appropriate role of service systems in assisting the family are situated within cultural belief systems that even in the absence of being fully articulated need to be acknowledged and respected by EI and other service providers. For example, parents are not the sole decision makers about a child's well-being in some cultures in which grandparents' views are given much weight (Garcia Coll and Magnuson, 2000). Moreover, the cause of a problem may be perceived differently across cultural groups. For example, Fadiman (1997) describes how the etiology of a child's seizure disorders is viewed in distinctly different ways by her Hmong parents in comparison to her Western physicians. Such differences may result in cultural clashes about appropriate preventive and ongoing treatment. In addition, intervention that is meaningful to a family is bound to cultural theories of change. Such theories may be consonant with or differ significantly from those of Western service providers. The potential for cultural mismatch exists at many levels of belief systems, encompassing perspectives on how children best develop, the role of family members in supporting that development, and the ways in which services can effect developmental change.

EI often serves as a catalyst in helping the family build on the learning potential of the young child (Fig. 92-2). Through EI services, parents can be guided in ways to scaffold the child's learning and can develop strategies to help the child participate in family and community activities. Parents in our study (i.e., EICS) have indicated that through EI, they have learned new routes to their

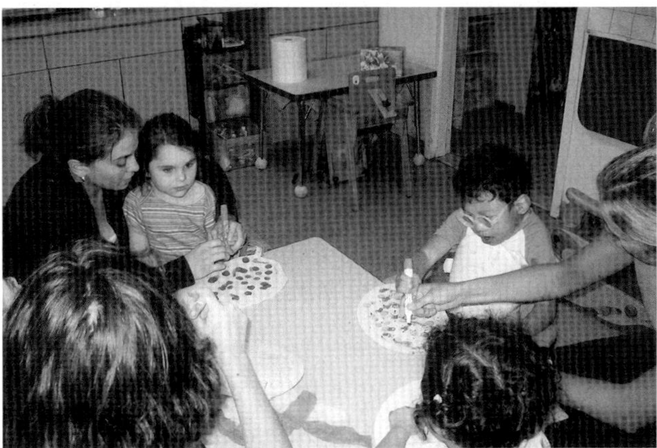

Figure 92-2. Children work on art projects as part of a group experience.

child's learning by, for example, positioning the child appropriately, being patient by waiting for a child's delayed response to a stimulus before responding, breaking down tasks into smaller and more manageable chunks, encouraging task persistence, and providing activities that are slightly but not overly advanced for the child. Through these accommodations, parents discover their child's approach to learning and reaffirm their own role in the learning partnership.

Such a partnership, supported by EI services, can enhance the positive perceptions parents have of their child's strengths and accomplishments. Although parents are often distressed at the time of their child's diagnosis, EI services can help parents discover the unique ways their child with disabilities contributes to their life and the life of their family as a whole. In EICS, we found that mothers who had received more hours of EI service from entry to discharge reported positive changes in family cohesion (Warfield et al, 2000). In cohesive families, the child with disabilities is an integral and respected member of the overall family. For some families, the support and culture of EI can help them become more cohesive units.

Related findings have been reported by the researchers conducting NEILS (2007). They indicate that one benefit of EI is in helping families be hopeful about their child's future. Optimism is likely to be an important ingredient in the parent-child partnership as well as in the relationships within the family. Indeed, the posited family strengths built into the culture of EI provide an attitude essential to the development of a strong parent-child relationship.

An additional aspect of parental and child benefits of EI is based on the importance of parents becoming advocates for their child. The difficulty of negotiating multiple systems of care has been highlighted in many studies of families with young children with special health care needs and developmental disabilities. Such negotiation is often a lifelong demand on families. The NEILS study found that a large majority of parents considered their sense of efficacy and skills related to child advocacy among the benefits they gained from EI services (Bailey et al, 2005). Parents also are an excellent source of assistance to other parents in becoming advocates. When we

Table 92-2. Parents' Advice to Families Entering Early Intervention Services

Always ask questions. You are the one who knows your child the best.
Don't wait for people to call you, call them.
Learn as much as you can about the ability and disability of your child.
Be an advocate and ask about what resources are available.
Link up early with other parents who have already gone through this experience.
No one really knows how your child will progress, so be patient.
Ask for documentation. The EI program had all this documentation that said "3 weeks ago he couldn't do this" and now he's doing it. They helped us see all the small milestones.
Professionals need to know that they are not just dealing with an illness or delay, they are dealing with the whole child and the whole family.
Understand that things don't have to be cheerful all the time.
Don't make too many exceptions for your child. At the same time, keep in mind her or his limitations and special needs.
Remember to take some breaks for your own well-being.
This is not the end of your life; it may even be the beginning.

asked our EICS parents about advice they would give to families entering EI services, they provided a wide range of useful and practical suggestions but mainly focused on three themes: gather information, take care of yourself, and be patient with your child (Table 92-2).

A third critical principle of EI services is that systems need to work together on behalf of the child. This is accomplished through the ICC at the state level but requires effort on the part of service providers at the individual level. This principle is consistent with selected goals from Healthy People 2010 and recommendations from the Institute of Medicine (Anderson et al, 2003). Both entities indicate that multiple levels of influence (e.g., individual, interpersonal, institutional, community, and policy) need to be linked so that early childhood programs can best promote optimal child and family outcomes. All ICCs include parents and have a chairperson from an agency that is not the lead agency in the state. The goals of the ICCs are to collaboratively plan, implement, and evaluate EI services and to serve as a model for systems integration at all levels of service.

The need for such interagency collaboration exists at the program level as well, and some findings from an evaluation of Early Head Start indicate that links between that program and EI services can be made productively (Wall et al, 2005). Collaboration also needs to occur within the program as many types of service providers, with varying backgrounds and expertise in different domains of information and skills, need to function together on behalf of children and families. Such collaboration is rarely taught in university domain-specific programs yet is essential to service provision in EI.

Systems often become taxed during times of transition, and the federal law has some provisions to prevent gaps in services when families move from EI (Part C) to preschool services (Part B). Nevertheless, such gaps exist, and even when a smooth transition is enacted, families are likely to experience a difference between the family focus of EI and the child focus of preschool programs.

Preparation for this transition requires collaboration at all levels of service from the state ICCs to the individual EI and preschool programs.

EFFECTIVENESS OF EARLY INTERVENTION SERVICES

Given the legislation that has pushed the development of state and local level EI systems and the general proliferation of programs and services under the EI umbrella, it is reasonable to ask what research evidence exists to support this national commitment. This section presents a brief review of past and current evaluations of EI, highlighting both the challenges and opportunities in conducting evaluation research in the EI field. An assessment is made of how the four key components of EI service systems operate and to what extent they have an impact on the children and families who are served. Directions for future EI evaluations are also discussed, with an emphasis on outlining opportunities for pediatricians to share their expertise in the continuing development and implementation of the EI service system.

Past Evaluations of Early Intervention

Guralnick (2005b) has divided evaluations of EI programs and services into two phases based roughly on whether they assessed EI before or after the passage of the original legislation, PL 99-457, in 1986. First-generation studies, defined as those conducted primarily before PL 99-457, assessed whether EI was effective in terms of whether child functioning improved as a result of the intervention. Consistent evidence has been found for the positive although modest impact of EI on children with disabilities, including those at environmental risk, those at biologic risk, children with autism, and children with Down syndrome (Guralnick, 2005a).

In addition to addressing the question of the overall effectiveness of EI, one prominent analysis selected the 31 highest quality evaluations of EI for children with biologic concerns to assess whether effectiveness varied for children with different characteristics and which selected program characteristics had a greater impact on child outcomes (Shonkoff and Hauser-Cram, 1987). Greater cognitive gains were found for children characterized as developmentally delayed in comparison to children with intellectual disabilities. Children with orthopedic disabilities experienced the smallest gains in cognition. In terms of severity, infants identified as mildly impaired experienced better outcomes if they entered an EI program before they were 6 months of age versus after 6 months of age, whereas age at entry had no influence on the outcomes for children with more severe disabilities. Two program characteristics were also found to be associated with greater child effects. Programs with well-defined curriculums versus those with less well defined curriculums and programs that had high levels of parent involvement versus those with little parent involvement were more effective. Although the studies selected for this analysis were the best available for children with biologic disabilities, there was not enough data to assess effectiveness in terms of outcomes other than child cognition, such as social competence, behavior, or motivation. Further, even fewer data were available to evaluate effectiveness relative to family functioning.

Despite these overall positive findings, the first-generation studies were based primarily on model EI programs with considerable resources and highly trained staff. EI programs operating under Part C legislation, however, are more varied and serve a more diverse population. To help guide the development and implementation of effective EI service systems under Part C, therefore, evaluations must address a greater number of more specific questions.

Current Evaluations of Early Intervention

Second-generation evaluations of EI have focused on assessing what types of interventions work best for whom, under what conditions, and toward what ends. Thus, second-generation evaluations are seen as a potential source for development of evidence-based practices (i.e., practices that have been identified by empiric research as influencing desired outcomes for children, families, professionals, and systems) (Odom and Wolery, 2003).

Evaluation Challenges and Opportunities

Two key methodologic challenges face researchers who want to conduct second-generation evaluations. First, traditional experimental designs, using random assignment to create a treatment group that gets the intervention and a control group that does not, have been promoted as the best way to attribute the benefits participants get from an intervention to the treatment itself (Weiss, 1998). Now that EI services are mandated for all eligible children and families who want to participate, however, denying services to a child and family for the purposes of placing them in a control group is unethical and illegal. Second, services under Part C are to be individualized to fit with the needs and goals of each child and family. The treatment can no longer be a "one size fits all" intervention with predefined types of services provided at a set level of intensity for a selected time aimed at one common set of outcomes.

Fortunately, evaluation science has moved away from a strict focus on experimental designs, random assignment, predetermined interventions, and impact studies and has embraced the use of a broader set of evaluation questions and methods (Warfield and Hauser-Cram, 2005). No one standard evaluation strategy is considered appropriate for all programs, services, or interventions. Rather, individualized plans need to be developed for each situation to maximize the fit between the program's or system's capacity for evaluation and the goals of the evaluation. Evaluation plans should encourage input from all stakeholders (i.e., not only EI administrators and staff but also current collaborators and potential collaborators such as pediatricians and social workers).

Three main foci of evaluations can produce data needed by EI administrators and providers seeking to institute evidence-based practices. First, EI evaluations must address questions of accountability. Evaluations can document accountability by presenting data on the extent to which the program is identifying and serving those who are entitled to services, providing the range of services it is mandated to provide, and establishing some reasonable match between participant need and service receipt. In addition, evaluations that measure participant satisfaction can show how a program is being accountable to its constituents. Second, EI evaluations need to address questions of system and service quality. These studies must seek to develop ways to assess the quality of the services delivered (i.e., to what extent services go beyond the minimum standards required by law) and measure the perceived (as opposed to the objective) effects of the intervention. These analyses are useful for providing feedback that can be used to reform or to improve the system, program, or service being evaluated. Third, EI evaluations must still address impact questions, particularly to understand the nature of the relation between the mandated components of EI services (i.e., child find and referral activities, individualized services, the provision of services in the natural environment, and service coordination) and a series of appropriate outcomes, which depending on the nature of the evaluation could be focused on child development, family adaptation and empowerment, or system operation and efficiency.

Complementing these expanded evaluation questions are a broader array of qualitative and quantitative methods available to address them. A wide range of qualitative methodologies are now encouraged because of their ability to ask questions and to probe for answers not easily obtained by quantitative strategies. These approaches include focus groups, case studies, and observation studies (Patton, 1987) as well as mixed method approaches that integrate quantitative and qualitative methods (Hauser-Cram et al, 2000). Further, sophisticated multilevel data analysis techniques are now widely available that allow evaluators to assess the influence of community-level characteristics on individual children and families as well as to track changes in measures of child development and family adaptation over time and test whether child, family, or program characteristics are significant predictors of those changes (e.g., Hauser-Cram et al, 2001).

The following sections review selected evaluation studies that have sought to assess accountability, quality, and impact questions relative to the implementation of each of the four key components of EI outlined in the legislation.

Child Find and Referral Services

Three main strategies have been identified as useful in making states and localities more accountable for identification and referral. First, five types of risk registries have been identified as useful for child find purposes (Dunst et al, 2004). These include birth defects surveillance programs, newborn medical screening programs, newborn hearing programs, child protective services registries, and population-based registries. Second, pilot studies have been conducted to understand the processes and relationships that must be built between systems to use these information sources not only to increase identification but to set up procedures for the consistent referral of children to EI. For example, a pilot program in Massachusetts built linkages between the Department of Social Services that handles cases of child abuse and neglect and the Department of Public Health that is the lead agency for Part C EI. These linkages increased the number of children in substantiated cases of abuse and neglect who were referred to and assessed by EI. More than two thirds of these children were found eligible for EI and subsequently received services (Lippitt, 2003). Third, physician training and pediatric resident training programs that promote an understanding of the value and benefit of EI have facilitated referrals by physicians (Shapiro et al, 2003).

Individualized, Family-Centered Services

Many barriers to implementation of individualized family-centered EI services have been identified. These often involve dilemmas around matching resources and needs. For example, although ideally families are to list their needs and goals and the types of services they require to meet those needs and to reach their goals, providers may emphasize the use of those services that are reimbursable under Part C (Shannon, 2004). The match between resources and needs also must consider the number and duration of visits that insurance companies will cover. One model for better equalizing the involvement of families and professionals in developing and implementing family-centered services has been to use parents of young children with disabilities as parent educators in the Part C system (Gallagher et al, 2004). In Georgia, parent educators work with families new to EI to help identify family needs, inform families about parent resources, help train EI providers, and serve on local and state ICCs. During the years, families have consistently rated the parent educators as most helpful in terms of disseminating information, encouraging families to become involved in EI, and helping families feel like an important member of the EI team (Shannon, 2004).

Services in the Natural Environment

The requirement to provide early interventions in natural learning environments is a tremendous test for providers because the traditional service delivery models do not fit easily into this new approach. One indicator of the challenge in making this shift was demonstrated by a study in which the content of IFSPs from EI programs in eight states was examined in relation to how they referenced activities in natural environments (Dunst et al, 1998). More than 3000 IFSP outcome statements were evaluated and only 1.3% of the outcome statements were described in terms of everyday family activities; even fewer (0.4%) were described with reference to everyday community activities. Despite these findings, some limited evidence exists on the effectiveness of natural learning environments to improve child functioning. Dunst, Bruder, and Trivette (2001) described how parents can identify goals for their child to achieve and activities that their child enjoys. In consultation with an EI provider, a match between a favorite activity (e.g., playing in the sandbox at a local playground) and a desired outcome (e.g., improved social interactions with other children) can be achieved by encouraging parents to increase the frequency with which their children participate in their favorite activity over time and giving them strategies for reducing negative behaviors (e.g., throwing sand) and increasing positive behaviors (e.g., sharing sand shovels). The use of these natural learning opportunities has been associated with reductions in behavior problems.

Service Coordination

In a review of studies assessing the benefits of service coordination in EI, the impact was found to vary by the type of outcome evaluated (Dunst and Bruder, 2002). In these studies, the implementation of service coordination was demonstrated by an improved flow of resources, supports, and services. Although increased coordination was not associated with improved parenting and child functioning, it was consistently associated with higher levels of parent satisfaction and reports of greater parental well-being and quality of life. The status of implementing service coordination policies and procedures at the state level has been examined in a national survey of state Part C coordinators. Harbin and colleagues (2004) found that in general, most states do not yet have a sufficient policy infrastructure (e.g., specific interagency agreements) to support the implementation of effective service coordination. However, some progress has been made. For example, although only about one quarter of states specify the authority of the service coordinator to integrate services across agencies, when authority is specified in detailed interagency agreements, service coordinators have authority to direct personnel in multiple agencies and thereby increase integration.

Future Evaluations of Early Intervention

Guralnick (2005a) outlines three key areas for future evaluation studies in EI. First, greater specificity is required that matches intervention strategies, child and family needs, and improved outcomes. This requires well-defined subgroups of children and families as well as better defined interventions. Second, given that 25% to 30% of children with disabilities experience behavioral difficulties, evaluation studies need to incorporate mental health issues in part by including socioemotional development as an outcome. Third, more evaluations focused at the system level are needed to assess and better understand the variation in program quality across community-based EI programs.

Pediatricians can facilitate the future development of EI services and systems by developing closer ties with the EI programs in their area and lending their clinical expertise in the creation of IFSPs. Pediatricians can also consider ways to more closely screen and monitor their young patients for socioemotional difficulties that may warrant an EI referral. Finally, pediatricians have some experience referring their patients to specialists and setting up associated mechanisms for coordinating care. This expertise could be very helpful to local and state ICCs, where much work is needed to implement the service coordination envisioned in the IDEA legislation.

PEDIATRICIANS AND EARLY INTERVENTION SERVICES

The role that pediatricians take in relation to EI services is variable and still evolving, but pediatricians are a central part of the multidisciplinary team serving the child and family and often act as the gateway for referrals to other services like EI. Pediatricians also provide continuity for the family across the span from early childhood through adolescence, when children and families are entering and exiting other services including EI and various school settings. The American Academy of Pediatrics Committee on Children with Disabilities (1999) has identified nine services that have direct relevance for the EI experience of children and families. By ensuring that children with disabilities in their practices have access to these services, pediatricians can fulfill the roles outlined for them by IDEA. These services are listed in Table 92-3.

Across these services, pediatricians must perform three critical tasks: identification, collaboration, and management. These tasks make it possible for infants and toddlers with disabilities and delays to benefit fully from EI services. Identification supports child find activities by using medical expertise to indicate at an early age whether a child might benefit from EI. Making a diagnosis or supplying information relevant to an eligibility determination can enhance the ability of EI providers to serve children with a variety of needs. The results of one study indicate that pediatricians are likely to refer a child with an established diagnosis but disinclined to refer children to EI because of speech and language delays or because of parental concerns about a child's inappropriate behavior (Silverstein et al, 2006). Thus, children and families who might benefit from EI are not consistently referred.

Collaboration involves building relationships with EI providers so that the pediatric office and EI agency are able to create an intervention plan best suited for each individual child and family. Although such collaboration would be useful for all children, it is essential for children with special health care needs. Research has identified practices that facilitate building of collaboration among physicians and EI providers (Buck et al, 2001). For example, the Richmond Infant Council, one of 40 ICCs in Virginia, established working relationships with key personnel in physician offices, such as

Table 92-3. Pediatric Services Relevant to Children and Families in Early Intervention

Establish a medical home.
Be knowledgeable of criteria for referral to EI.
Provide screening, surveillance, and diagnosis.
Make referrals.
Participate in assessments.
Provide counsel and advice to parents.
Assist in the creation of the IFSP.
Provide coordinated medical services.
Advocate for the child and family.

EI, early intervention; IFSP, individualized family service plan.
Summarized from the American Academy of Pediatrics, Committee on Children with Disabilities.

referral coordinators and nurses. From this work came the development and posting of a Web site designed for use by physicians that includes eligibility information, referral forms, and links to other related Web sites. Training in use of the Web site was provided to physicians and nurse practitioners. As a result, referrals from physicians for infants and toddlers in need of EI services in Richmond have grown (Buck et al, 2001).

Finally, management refers to coordination of services across systems for individual children and families but also to identification of areas where changes in policy could facilitate EI service delivery for all children and families. One way in which this could occur is by having pediatricians participate in local and state early intervention ICCs. At the individual level, pediatricians need to routinely ask parents about their experiences in EI and to educate service providers as well as parents about a child's health concerns and needs.

SUMMARY

EI services, authorized under IDEA, are now part of the service network in every state. These services, although modest in intensity, are designed to help coordinate resources for infants and toddlers with disabilities and their families as well as to provide some direct services, such as speech and language therapy, occupational therapy, and physical therapy. The services aim to be individualized and family focused as indicated by the development of an IFSP for each family that has been created by both providers and family members. Pediatricians and other health care providers serve a critical role in identifying infants and toddlers who warrant such services as well as in providing information to parents and, when appropriate, to EI service providers about a child's health care needs in relation to EI services. By learning about available EI services and making direct connections with local EI providers, the pediatrician can provide an essential link between health care needs and optimal child and family functioning.

REFERENCES

American Academy of Pediatrics: The pediatrician's role in development and implementation of an individual education plan (IEP) and/or an Individual Family Service Plan (IFSP). Pediatrics 104:124-127, 1999.

Anderson LM, Shinn C, Fullilove MT, et al: The effectiveness of early childhood development programs: A systematic review. Am J Prev Med 24:32-46, 2003.

Bailey DB, Aytch LS, Odom SL, et al: Early intervention as we know it. Ment Retard Developmental Disabilities 5:11-20, 1999.

Bailey DB, Hebbeler KJ, Spiker D, et al: Thirty-six-month outcomes for families of children who have disabilities and participated in early intervention. Pediatrics 116:1346-1352, 2005.

Bronfenbrenner U: Ecology of the family as a context for human development: Research perspectives. Dev Psychol 22:723-742, 1986.

Buck DM, Cox AW, Shannon P, et al: Building collaboration among physicians and other early intervention providers: Practices that work. Infants Young Children 13:11-20, 2001.

Danaher J, Armijo C, Lazara A (eds): Part C Updates, 8th ed. Chapel Hill, NC, The University of North Carolina, FPG Child Development Institute, National Early Childhood Technical Assistance Center, 2006.

Dunst CJ, Bruder MB: Valued outcomes of service coordination, early intervention, and natural environments. Except Child 68:361-375, 2002.

Dunst CJ, Bruder MB, Trivette CM, et al: Increasing Children's Learning Opportunities Through Families and Communities Early Childhood Research Institute: Year 2 Progress Report. Asheville, NC, Orelena Hawks Puckett Institute, 1998.

Dunst C, Bruder MB, Trivette CM, et al: Characteristics and consequences of everyday natural learning opportunities. Topics Early Childhood Special Educ 21:68-92, 2001.

Dunst CJ, Fromework J, Lucas SM: Sources of information on risk registries useful for Child Find. Milemarkers 1:1-5, 2004.

Fadiman A: The Spirit Catches You and You Fall Down: A Hmong Child, Her American Doctors, and the Collision of Two Cultures. New York, Farrar, Straus and Giroux, 1997.

Fox L, Dunlap G, Cushing L: Early intervention, positive behavior support and transition to school. J Emot Behav Dis 10:149-157, 2002.

Gallagher PA, Rhodes CA, Darling SM: Parents as professionals in early intervention: A parent educator model. Topics Early Childhood Special Educ 24:5-13, 2004.

Garcia Coll C, Magnuson K: Cultural differences as sources of developmental vulnerabilities and resources. *In* Shonkoff JP, Meisels SJ (eds): Handbook of Early Childhood Intervention. New York, Cambridge University Press, 2000, p 94-114.

Guralnick MJ: Early intervention for children with intellectual disabilities: Current knowledge and future prospects. J Appl Res Intellect Disabil 18:313-324, 2005a.

Guralnick MJ: The Developmental Systems Approach to Early Intervention. Baltimore, Paul H. Brookes, 2005b.

Harbin GL, Bruder MB, Whitbread K, et al: Early intervention service coordination policies: National policy infrastructure. Topics Early Childhood Special Educ 24:89-97, 2004.

Hauser-Cram P, Warfield ME, Upshur CC, et al: An expanded view of program evaluation in early childhood intervention. *In* Shonkoff JP, Meisels SJ (eds): Handbook of Early Childhood Intervention. New York, Cambridge University Press, 2000, pp 487-509.

Hauser-Cram P, Warfield ME, Shonkoff JP, et al: Children with disabilities: A longitudinal study of child development and parent well-being. Monogr Soc Res Child Dev 66:3, 2001.

Hebbeler K, Spiker D, Bailey D, et al: Final report of the National Early Intervention Longitudinal Study (NEILS). Menlo Park, CA, SRI International, 2007.

Lippitt J: The Massachusetts Early Childhood Linkage Initiative. Zero to Three 24:46, 2003.

Odom SL, Wolery M: A unified theory of practice in early intervention/early childhood special education: Evidence-based practices. J Special Educ 37:164-173, 2003.

Palfrey J, Hauser-Cram P, Bronson MB, et al: The Brookline Early Education Project: A 25-year follow-up study of a family-centered early health and development intervention. Pediatrics 116:144-152, 2005.

Patton MQ: How to Use Qualitative Methods in Evaluation. Thousand Oaks, CA, Sage, 1987.

Scarborough AA, Spiker D, Mallik S, et al: A national look at children and families entering early intervention. Exceptional Children 70:469-483, 2004.

Shannon P: Barriers to family-centered services for infants and toddlers with developmental delays. Social Work 49:301-308, 2004.

Shapiro B, Derrington T, Smith B: Educating the health community: Selling early intervention to primary care physicians. Calif J Health Promotion 1:105-124, 2003.

Shonkoff JP, Hauser-Cram P: Early intervention for disabled infants and their families: A quantitative analysis. Pediatrics 80:650-658, 1987.

Shonkoff JP, Phillips DA: Neurons to Neighborhood: The Science of Early Childhood Development. Washington, DC, National Research Council and Institute of Medicine, 2000.

Shonkoff JP, Hauser-Cram P, Krauss MW, et al: Development of infants with disabilities and their families. Monogr Soc Res Child Dev 57:6, 1992.

Silverstein M, Sand N, Glascoe P, et al: Pediatric practices regarding referral to early intervention services: Is an established diagnosis important? Ambul Pediatr 6:105-109, 2006.

Spiker D, Hebbeler K, Wagner M, et al: A framework for describing variations in state early intervention systems. Topics Early Childhood Special Educ 20:195-207, 2000.

U.S. Department of Education, Office of Special Education and Rehabilitation Services: 25th Annual Report to Congress on the Implementation of the Individuals with Disabilities Education Act. Washington, DC, 2003.

U.S. Government Accountability Office: Individuals with disabilities education act: Education should provide additional guidance to help states smoothly transition children to preschool. Washington, DC, 2005 (GAO-06–26).

Wall SM, Taylor NE, Liebow H, et al: Early Head Start and access to early intervention services: A qualitative investigation. Topics Early Childhood Special Educ 25:218-231, 2005.

Warfield ME, Hauser-Cram P: Monitoring and evaluation in early intervention programs. *In* Guralnick MJ (ed): The Developmental Systems Approach to Early Intervention. Baltimore, Paul H. Brookes, 2005, pp 351-372.

Warfield ME, Hauser-Cram P, Krauss MW, et al: The effect of early intervention services on maternal well-being. Early Educ Dev 11:499-517, 2000.

Weiss, CH: Evaluation, 2nd ed. Upper Saddle River, NJ, Prentice Hall, 1998.

West J, Denton K, Germino-Hausken E: America's kindergartener: Findings from the early childhood longitudinal study: Kindergarten class of 1998-99. Washington, DC, U.S. Department of Education, National Center for Education, 2000.

Yeargin-Allsopp M, Rice C, Karapurkan T, et al: Prevalence of autism in a U.S. metropolitan area. JAMA 289:49-55, 2003.

93 SPECIAL EDUCATION SERVICES

LOUISE KACZMAREK AND DIEGO CHAVES-GNECCO

Vignettes

Mateo

Mateo Gonzalez, a 9-year-old Hispanic boy, was born in the United States of immigrant parents. He acquired Spanish quite typically at about the same age as his siblings did, but he did not start to learn English formally until he began school. Although Mateo's mother was never concerned about his development as a young child, she is concerned now about his difficulties learning to read and write in school. Mrs. Gonzalez does not speak English and cannot read or write in either English or Spanish, but she feels that Mateo, who has repeated second grade twice, is having more difficulty in school than his siblings had (see Fig. 93-1). Even Mateo's 6-year-old brother seems to do better than Mateo at reading and writing. At first, Mateo's teachers thought his problems were related to learning English as a second language, but recently they have expressed concern that he may have a learning disability. Mateo's physical and neurologic examination findings have been normal. Following the recommendations of Mateo's pediatrician, Mrs. Gonzalez requested a multidisciplinary evaluation through the school system. She also learned about her son's rights to an appropriate education and was encouraged to be an advocate for him within the school system with the help of her pediatrician.

Mateo had a multidisciplinary evaluation at school in both Spanish and English that included an IQ test in which he scored 70. Mrs. Gonzalez, who attended an individualized educational program (IEP) meeting for Mateo with an interpreter provided by the school district, helped to write Mateo's goals and his educational plan. Mateo started to receive specialized instruction and speech-language therapy in his third-grade classroom in accordance with his IEP. Mrs. Gonzalez now works with Mateo on his reading and writing at home as she also is now learning to speak, read, and write English through courses offered by a local organization.

Ashley

Ashley Smith is an 8-year-old girl who was recently diagnosed with attention-deficit/hyperactivity disorder (ADHD), inattentive type, by her pediatrician. She has considerable difficulty maintaining attention to schoolwork and other similar tasks that require concentration, resulting often in incomplete or poor work. Her overall school performance is marginally satisfactory, although she sometimes achieves higher grades. After the diagnosis, the pediatrician prescribed 18 mg of methylphenidate extended release. Ashley did not have any side effects from this stimulant medication; her appetite, blood pressure, and sleeping patterns remained normal, and she did not demonstrate any abnormal movements or headaches. However, her symptoms did not respond to the medication, and her behavior at school got worse.

Ashley was then seen by a developmental-behavioral pediatrician who had her parents and third grade teacher complete the Vanderbilt surveys (Leslie et al, 2004; Wolraich et al, 1998). After her developmental-behavioral evaluation, Ashley's diagnosis of ADHD inattentive type was confirmed and her dose of methylphenidate extended release was increased to 36 mg. Through his conversation with Mrs. Smith, the developmental-behavioral pediatrician learned that after her mother shared the diagnosis with the teacher, Ashley was seated in the last row of the classroom with other children who apparently have the same condition. The other children, who were fidgety and unable to sit still most of the time, distracted Ashley (see Fig. 93-2). The developmental-behavioral pediatrician's report was shared with Ashley's parents, her pediatrician, and her school. In this report, accommodations for Ashley were requested from the school, including preferential seating next to the teacher and reduction in length of her class and homework assignments. The use of checklists for Ashley to remember her chores both at home and in school and the use of a log at school to help her remember what she needed to do for homework were also recommended. The developmental-behavioral pediatrician provided

(Continued)

Mrs. Smith with information about Ashley's educational rights based on IDEA and Section 504. A couple of weeks later, Ashley saw her developmental-behavioral pediatrician on a follow-up visit. At this time, she was doing much better both at home and in school. The school implemented the recommended educational accommodations for Ashley. The absence of side effects from her methylphenidate continues, and her Vanderbilt scores continue to support her progress.

Today, more than 6.5 million children, like Mateo, receive special education and related services (U.S. Department of Education, 2006). Other children, like Ashley, have medical conditions that do not necessarily qualify them for special education but may require schools to make accommodations or to provide health-related supports. With the large number of children affected, most pediatric practices encounter children who are either eligible for or are receiving special education, parents who need information about school services, and cases in which direct interaction by a physician with a school might be advisable.

Being familiar with special education, its laws and regulations, and the school resources available for children and parents provides the clinician with additional tools when learning and development are compromised. In addition, pediatricians and clinicians may find parents expecting them to serve as resources for their children's special education. This chapter examines the legislative underpinnings of education for children with disabilities, describes the special education process, proposes how pediatricians might play a role in that process, and highlights the current trends and issues in special education.

THE LEGISLATIVE UNDERPINNINGS OF EDUCATION FOR CHILDREN WITH DISABILITIES

The modern era of education for children with disabilities began with two important class action suits in the early 1970s that ruled that schools must provide a free appropriate education to children with disabilities regardless of their functioning levels (Office of Special Education Programs, n.d.). Within a few short years after these court rulings, landmark legislation called PL 94-142 mandated special education services in 1975. The law has been reauthorized six times, most recently in 2004.

The Individuals with Disabilities Education Act

The Education of All Handicapped Children Act of 1975 (PL 94-142) mandated special education services, ensuring that all handicapped children between the ages of 3 and 21 years receive a free and public education in the "least restrictive environment." This law, which was reauthorized as the Individuals with Disabilities Education Act (IDEA) in 1990, defined four essential features of special education (Office of Special Education Programs, n.d.): (1) a free appropriate public education for all children; (2) education in the least restrictive environment, in other words, to the maximum extent possible in classrooms with children without disabilities; (3) an individualized education program (IEP), which a team of professionals in conjunction with a child's parents develops and which outlines the details of a child's special education; and (4) procedural safeguards to ensure the rights of children and their families under the law and due process procedures if parents have a complaint. Mateo in the vignette received these considerations when he was enrolled in special education services.

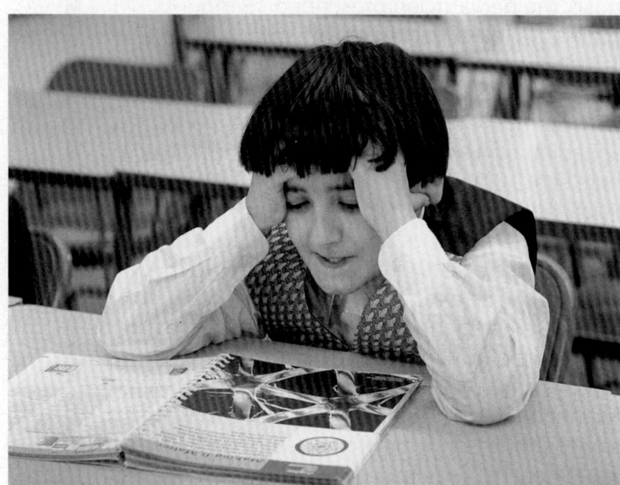

Figure 93-1. Aboy experiencing difficulty with reading. Over 6.5 million children in the United States receive special education and related services (U.S. Department of Education, 2006). Some of these children carry the diagnosis of learning disability. (Courtesy of Robert Louis and the Hispanic/Latino Community of Southwestern Pennsylvania.)

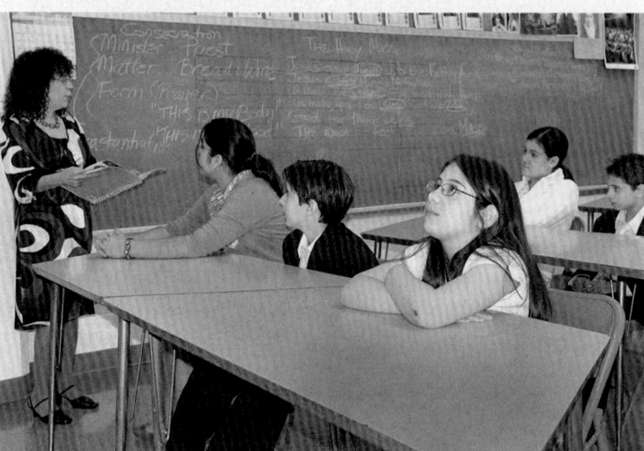

Figure 93-2. A girl with attention deficit daydreaming while her classmates are paying attention to the teacher. Some children have medical conditions that do not necessarily qualify them for special education but may require schools to make accommodations or provide health-related supports based on IDEA and Section 504. An example of these medical conditions is the diagnosis of ADHD, predominantly inattentive type. (Courtesy of Robert Louis and the Hispanic/Latino Community of Southwestern Pennsylvania.)

Since 1975, these essential features of special education and related services in the schools have remained unchanged, despite many critical modifications in response to identified needs (National Dissemination Center for Children with Disabilities, n.d.). Among the most dramatic modifications was the provision of early childhood special education for children between the ages of 3 and 5 years in 1986. In that same year, states were offered financial incentives for developing systems for serving infants and toddlers. Other changes have included strengthening the role and supports for parents; increasing sensitivity to children of ethnic, racial, and linguistic diversity; and adding new services and disability categories (see Figure 93-3 for details). Mateo's mother, for example, was able to receive the services of a Spanish-speaking interpreter at his IEP meeting because of the modifications in the law.

During the years, the inclusion of children in learning environments with their age-matched peers has been strengthened. In the early legislation, the amount of time spent in regular classrooms had to be noted on the IEP; today, IEPs must provide justification if children are removed from classrooms with typical children, and the IEP notes the amount of time in special settings.

The Individuals with Disabilities Education Improvement Act

The 2004 reauthorization of IDEA initiated significant modifications in special education policy (Committee on Education and the Workforce, 2005), marked by a change in title that underscores it as an "improvement." These sweeping changes have brought the law into alignment with the reforms advanced in the general education law, entitled No Child Left Behind, and shifted the focus of special education from process to outcomes.

No Child Left Behind (U.S. Department of Education, 2003) was passed in 2002 to improve the level of basic achievement of the nation's children in general education, especially those from disadvantaged backgrounds, by requiring stronger accountability for results, highly qualified teachers in every classroom, and the use of proven educational practices. This law requires schools to show a measure of annual yearly progress based on children's aggregated scores on state-level tests. Those schools that do not meet their annual yearly progress criterion are required to provide supplemental services to children, including free tutoring, after-school assistance, and summer school. If a school consistently fails to meet its annual yearly progress goals, parents are

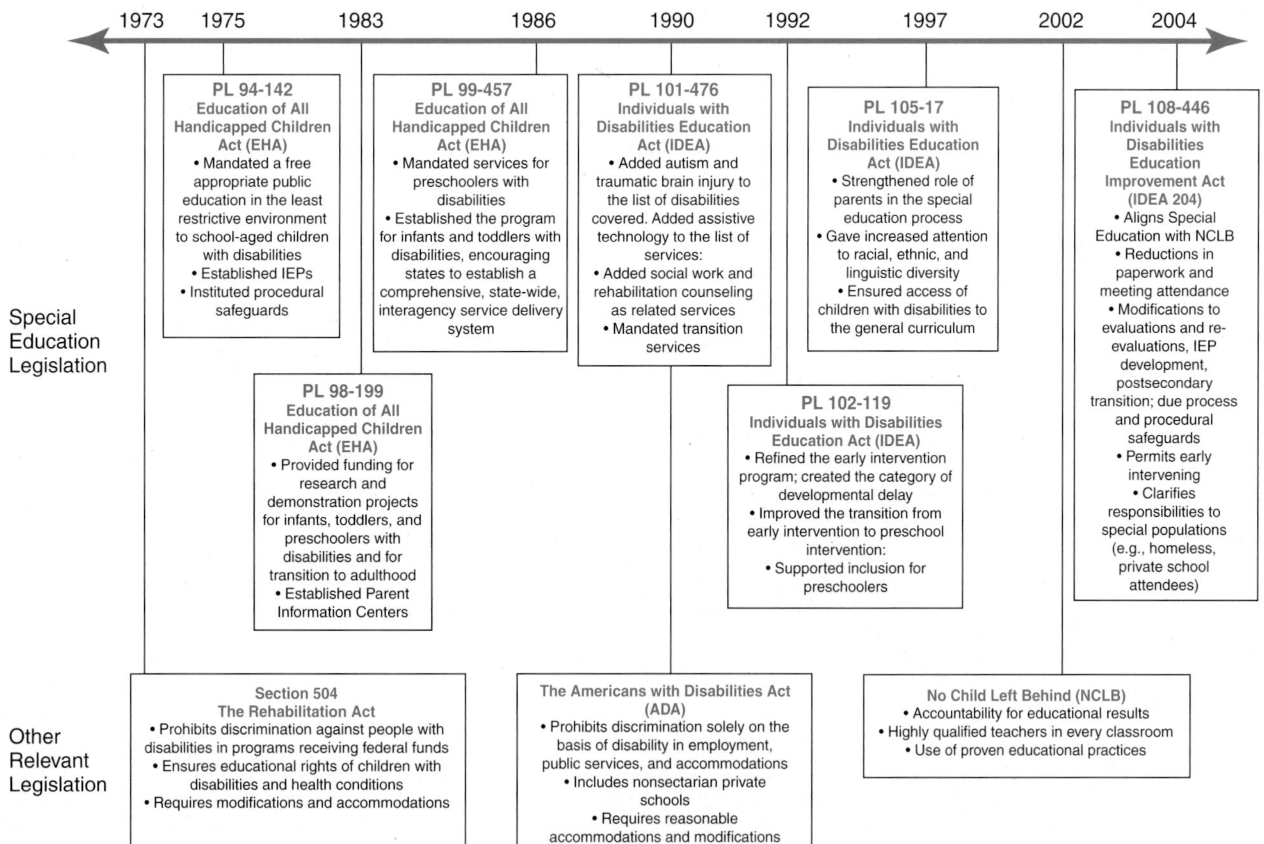

Figure 93-3. Time line of changes in special education and other relevant legislation. (Data from National Dissemination Center for Children with Disabilities, n.d.; Office of Special Education Programs, n.d.; Committee on Education and the Workforce, 2005; U.S. Department of Education, 2003; Office of Civil Rights, 2005)

entitled to transfer their children to better performing schools, including alternative charter schools. No Child Left Behind also spells out specific criteria for high-qualified teachers and requires that teachers use educational practices that have been proven effective. These same themes are echoed in the Individuals with Disabilities Education Improvement Act (IDEA 204).

IDEA 204 also has made changes to the evaluation of children, IEPs, and procedural safeguards. The themes within these modifications include reduction in paperwork, greater flexibility in meeting attendance by professionals, and reducing adversarial relationships with parents. The statute allows money for special education to be used for preventive "early intervening," so that children who are evidencing initial signs of educational risk can receive additional academic and behavioral support to succeed in the general education environment. The provision of special education services to nonpublic schools is also clarified.

Civil Rights Legislation

Two other major laws that affect the education of children with disabilities are Section 504 of the Rehabilitation Act of 1973 and the Americans with Disabilities Act of 1990 (Office of Civil Rights, 2005). Section 504 outlaws discrimination against individuals with disabilities in public or private programs that receive federal assistance. It ensures that children with disabilities and medical conditions receive equal access to education through the provision of necessary supports. Section 504 plans, which may be identified by other names, describe the unique supports, modifications, and accommodations needed for a child to participate in education or outline the medical needs of a child as determined by the health care provider. Because an IEP may serve the purpose of a Section 504 plan for a child receiving special instruction, Section 504 plans, as such, are written primarily to accommodate those children whose disabilities do not require special instruction, such as children with diabetes, asthma, and seizures. Ashley in the vignette, for example, does not qualify for special education services under IDEA 204 because her school performance has been acceptable, but she would qualify for protections under Section 504 because of her diagnosis of ADHD. Table 93-1 compares Section 504 and IDEA.

The Americans with Disabilities Act strengthens the protections provided under Section 504, protecting the civil rights of individuals with disabilities in employment, access to public facilities, transportation, telecommunication, and government services. Equal opportunities for people with disabilities are guaranteed, requiring that "reasonable accommodations" be made. Under this law, children with disabilities have access

Table 93-1. **Comparison of IDEA and Section 504 of the Rehabilitation Act**

	IDEA	**Section 504**
Overview	An education law to provide special education and related services to children with disabilities; applies to state and local educational agencies	A civil rights law to prevent discrimination on the basis of disability; applies to educational and noneducational programs and activities that receive or benefit from federal assistance; provides and guarantees access to education
Eligibility	Children are determined through evaluation to be eligible for services; specific categories of disability are defined; disability must affect the child's educational performance	Broadly defined as any person with a physical or mental impairment limiting one or more life activities, having a record of such impairment, or regarded as having an impairment; includes children who need specialized instruction as well as those who do not (e.g., children with asthma, temporary disabilities)
Funding	Federal funding assists states in meeting the mandate; state and local funding is also applied in the implementation of the law	No federal funding is provided; law is under state and local jurisdiction
Evaluation	Requires a comprehensive evaluation by a multidisciplinary team, including the collection of information from a variety of sources; requires parents to provide written consent; re-evaluation required every 3 years	Requires the compilation of information from a variety of sources; does not require testing; requires parents to be notified; re-evaluation required periodically
Free appropriate public education	Requires an IEP that is appropriate to the child's unique educational needs and designed to help the child receive educational benefit; provided at no cost to parents	Requires a plan that identifies accommodations to permit equal access to education and its benefits compared with nondisabled peers; provided at no cost to parents
Placement	Requires placement be made by a knowledgeable team made up of specific types of personnel; requires parents to be a part of the decision making process	Requires placement to be determined by a knowledgeable committee but does not prescribe membership; parents are not required to be on the committee; placement is usually in regular education
Procedural safeguards and due process	Required and describes specific procedures for written consent, impartial hearings, pendency; requires notice to parents before a change in placement; enforced by the U.S. Department of Education, Office of Special Education	Requires procedural safeguards for notice, access to records, and impartial hearings; local education agencies may develop their own or adopt IDEA procedural safeguards; does not require parent notice *before* a change in placement but does require notice; enforced in schools by U. S. Department of Education, Office of Civil Rights

Data from Council for Exceptional Children, 2002; Henderson, 2007; Rosenfeld, 2006.

to all types of childcare, including center-based care, family childcare homes, and after-school care. The only exception is childcare administered by religious organizations. Although the Americans with Disabilities Act does not focus directly on education, it does cover nonsectarian private schools and aspects of special education that may bring children out into the community, such as community-based job preparation programs.

THE SPECIAL EDUCATION PROCESS

Federal and state regulations specify how the special education process is to be carried out. The process consists of child find and referral, assessment and eligibility, development of the IEP, implementation of services, and evaluation of services (Office of Special Education and Rehabilitative Services, 2000). Federal laws and regulations establish broad requirements that state laws and regulations use as a framework. Aspects not federally regulated may differ across states. Details of the process also may differ between preschool and school-aged programs within states.

Child Find and Referral

Child find refers to materials and activities typically sponsored by schools or other agencies to inform the general public, particularly parents, about behaviors or developmental deviations that may suggest that a child has a disability. Such activities take the form of television advertisements and videos, pamphlets posted in public places, and events that heighten the public awareness of disabilities. Local contact information is provided for follow-up if one suspects that a child may have a problem. School districts and other agencies may hold screening events in malls or schools to identify young children in need of more in-depth assessment.

Requests to evaluate a child, especially those younger than school age, may come from parents. Once a child is in school, direct referrals are also made by teachers or other school professionals. Written parental consent is always required before an evaluation can take place. With the passage of IDEA 204, the evaluation must occur within 60 calendar days after written parental consent is given.

Assessment and Eligibility

A child with a suspected disability must be assessed by qualified professionals in the areas of the suspected disability. Assessments, at no charge to the parents, may include tests to determine a child's strengths and weaknesses, observations of the child in the school setting, and information provided by parents. Children must be tested in their native languages and in ways that do not put them at a disadvantage because of ethnic, racial, or cultural diversity. Recall that Mateo was assessed in both Spanish and English to facilitate complete understanding of his abilities in both languages. Assessment information from outside the school system (such as a report from a physician) may also be used in the determination of whether a child has one of the disabilities specified under IDEA and requires special education. If parents disagree with a school's evaluation of their child, they may request an outside evaluation at the school's expense. The evaluation results, typically provided in a written report, are examined by a team of qualified professionals to determine whether the child has a disability and is eligible to receive special education services.

Development of the Individualized Education Program

Within 30 calendar days of a child's determination of eligibility for special education, an IEP is developed at a meeting by the IEP team, consisting of the child's parents, a general education teacher, a special education teacher, a representative of the school district, someone who is able to interpret the assessment results, and anyone else who the parents and school district think appropriate to attend, including a parent advocate. Children may also attend their own IEP meetings, especially as they get older and when planning begins for the transition to adulthood. An IEP meeting should be scheduled sufficiently in advance and at a time and place agreed on by parents and the school. Parents must be notified in writing of the purpose of the meeting and of its time, location, and attendees, and they are informed that they may invite others who know their child.

The IEP includes sections about the child's current performance, specific annual goals, special education and related services, plans for participation with peers without disabilities, decisions regarding participation in state and district-wide tests, and the nature of progress monitoring. Consideration must be given to the supports and accommodations that may be necessary for the child to be involved and make progress in the general curriculum as well as extracurricular and nonacademic activities. For children at the preschool level, there is usually an additional section for parents to indicate what needs they have in relation to facilitating their child's development. Once the plan addressing the child's needs is completed, the nature, frequency, location, and providers of services are specified. In some states, the placement is determined as part of the IEP meeting immediately after the development of the educational program; in other states, another team makes the determination of placement. In either case, the parents must be involved in the decision making.

School districts must offer a continuum of alternative placements for children with disabilities. The "least restrictive environment" is considered to be the regular education classroom in the child's neighborhood school. Mateo, for example, was receiving specialized instruction and speech-language therapy in his third-grade classroom. If the IEP team determines that the child's needs cannot be met in that setting with supplemental aids and services, alternative placements may be represented. Other placements on this continuum in increasing levels and restriction include a special class for part of the school day; a special class all day; and placement in a special school, home, hospital, residential placement, or some other setting as determined by the team. If a district is unable to meet the needs of a child, it may contract with other agencies or districts or make any other arrangement consistent with IDEA so that the child's needs are met. Parents must provide written consent for their child to receive special education and related services *for the first time*. The parents must be given a copy of the IEP, and it is to be made available to all school personnel involved in implementing it.

Parents may disagree with an IEP or their child's placement, and they may try to negotiate an agreement on such issues with the IEP team. If agreement cannot be reached, the parent may request or the school may offer mediation. If mediation fails or if mediation is not pursued, parents may file a complaint with the state, requesting a due process hearing. The pre-hearing conference is the first step in due process, followed by a hearing if the pre-hearing conference fails to resolve the issue. A child's program cannot be changed by the school without parental agreement once due process proceedings are initiated.

There have been some significant changes to the IEP process with the passage of IDEA 2004, primarily to improve the efficiency of the process by reducing paperwork and consolidating, reducing, or allowing alternatives to meetings. In the current iteration, not all members need attend the IEP meeting if parents and school agree in writing that a member may be excused. However, the written contribution of an excused member may be required. The development of short-term objectives is now required only for those children who do not take the standard state assessment required by No Child Left Behind, that is, the children who have the most severe cognitive disabilities. Transition planning need not be considered in the IEP process until a child is 16 years old, replacing the requirement under the previous reauthorization that it start at 14 years. In addition, safeguards for program continuation for students transferring within or outside of a state have been included. There also have been a number of changes in due process with the passage of IDEA 2004 in an effort to encourage resolution of disagreements more quickly and with less acrimony than previously.

Implementation of Services

It is expected that the IEP will be carried out as written. A child's annual progress on the IEP goals must be measured in accordance with the measurement parameters identified in the IEP. Schools must provide parents with regular reports of a child's progress at least as often as parents receive reports for children without disabilities in the school.

Individualized Educational Program Review and Re-evaluation

A child's IEP must be reviewed at least annually, although a review may occur more frequently if it is requested by parents or the school. The purpose of the review, which involves the full participation of the parents, is to determine whether the child is achieving the annual goals and if the child is making expected progress in the general curriculum. The meeting may result in modifications to the IEP. A request to revise the IEP may be made by the parents or school at any time. The reauthorization of IDEA in 2004 makes face-to-face meetings for changing IEPs no longer necessary. Rather, with the agreement of the parent and school, such changes may be made in writing or by video or telephone conferencing.

A child must be re-evaluated every 3 years to determine whether there is still a need for special education and related services. With the 2004 reauthorization, this re-evaluation need not occur at all if both parents and school agree that it is unnecessary. Re-evaluation may also not occur more frequently than once a year unless both parents and school concur.

ROLE OF THE PEDIATRICIAN

Pediatricians and clinicians play an important role in the educational life of a child (Committee on Children with Disabilities, 1999) by identifying and evaluating learning and developmental-behavioral concerns and helping families to find resources (Table 93-2). The role of the pediatrician or clinician includes screening for disabilities and referral to the school system for evaluation. If findings support the need, pediatricians also may refer for accommodations and educational support, communicate with the family and the school so that all involved (parents, health care providers, school) function as a team with common goals, serve as a support to the family as they navigate the school system, and advocate for the child while helping parents to become advocates themselves. Recall that copies of the developmental-behavioral pediatric evaluation were sent with the parents' consent to all parties involved in Ashley's case.

Screening

The role of the pediatrician is to recognize possible disabilities and to identify the source of the problem. When general pediatricians who fulfill the role of primary care providers see children whose parents raise concerns about learning problems and poor school performance, the pediatrician may address the concerns directly and find ways to help the family and the child. However, parents do not always recognize the learning difficulties of their children or, more importantly, the home or health factors that may underlie a child's learning problems. A problem may come to light only after developmental screening results are analyzed in context with the review of systems and the social history. In either case, screening tools such as the Vanderbilt surveys (Leslie et al, 2004; Wolraich et al, 1998), which you may remember were completed by Ashley's parents and teacher to assist in her diagnosis, are available to assist the pediatrician in identifying the specific problem. In addition, the role of the general pediatrician or clinician is also to rule out other causes that may affect learning and school performance, such as poor sleeping habits, including snoring; hearing and vision difficulties; problems with relationships at home or school; and changes in life circumstances (e.g., moving or divorce).

Referral

Once the living habits and the environment of the child have been ruled out as a source of the problem, the pediatrician or clinician can discuss referral to the

Table 93-2. **Contributions of Educational Professionals and Pediatricians to the Early Intervention, Special Education, and Section 504 Processes**

	Educational Professionals	**Pediatricians**
Child find and referral	Offer public screenings for developmental delays and disabilities Provide referral information about early intervention to parents Refer school-age children presenting with learning problems for multidisciplinary evaluations or Section 504 consideration	Screen and monitor children regularly for developmental delays and disabilities Provide parents with information about accessing early intervention, special education, and Section 504 services and their rights under IDEA and Section 504
Assessment and eligibility	Secure appropriate parental consent Advise parents of their due process rights Conduct multidisciplinary evaluations for early intervention and special education Collect information for Section 504 consideration Determine eligibility for early intervention, special education, and Section 504 accommodations based on state requirements	Conduct evaluations that can be used in the determination of eligibility for early intervention, special education, and Section 504 services Participate as appropriate in the multidisciplinary assessment team through written correspondence, conference calls, or other means Advise parents of state requirements for multidisciplinary assessments
Plan development	Develop IEPs and IFSPs with parents as part of the team Consider parents' issues and concerns in the development of IFSPs and IEPs Develop Section 504 plans in conjunction with parents	Participate on IFSP, IEP, and Section 504 teams as appropriate Review IFSPs, IEPs, and Section 504 plans, offering comments and advice about health and medically related issues Counsel and advise parents about the IFSP, IEP, or Section 504 process
Plan implementation	Implement the educational program as specified in the IFSP or IEP Measure and monitor the child's progress Report the child's performance to parents Implement the Section 504 plan	Discuss the child's progress and program implementation with the child's parents
Plan review and re-evaluation	Conduct reviews and evaluations in accordance with federal and state laws	Participate as appropriate in the ongoing processes Continue monitoring child Continue advising and counseling parents

IDEA, Individuals with Disabilities Education Act; IEP, individualized educational program; IFSP, individual family service plan.

school for a comprehensive evaluation. Included in the role of the health professional is the obligation to explain how to request an evaluation from the school system and how the special education process works, including such details as how long the school can take to answer a request for evaluation and the possibilities of a non-school evaluation. The pediatrician in Mateo's case gave Mrs. Gonzalez this type of information.

Under other circumstances, the pediatric or clinician subspecialist (e.g., developmental-behavioral pediatrician, neurodevelopmental disabilities pediatrician, neurologist) will see children with specific diagnoses, such as learning disabilities, autism, and intellectual disability, or conditions that interfere with the learning process, such as ADHD. Here, the professional's chief concerns are the services that a child may or may not be receiving, often requiring more detailed information and specific responses on the pediatrician's part about children's and parents' rights, additional evaluations, and school and learning accommodations. Recall that it was the pediatrician who provided recommendations for Ashley's classroom accommodations that led to her more successful performance.

Providing printed information is a useful strategy to assist parents once they leave the health care provider's office. This may include pamphlets, brochures, booklets, and papers that describe specific disabilities or identify national, regional, and local resources such as Web sites, organizations, agencies, and list serves. It is also useful to hand parents materials that provide information about the special education process, including contact numbers within local school districts and sample letters requesting an evaluation or special accommodations. This kind of information is often available with minimal or no charge from advocacy organizations for specific disabilities, professional organizations, and local and state educational agencies. For example, the American Academy of Pediatrics, as part of its ADHD tool kit, provides clinicians with a sample letter that can be handed to the parents as a template to request special accommodations from the school.

Advocacy

The role of the health care professional not only should be to inform and to provide written information to families but also should include being a companion to them in the special education process that they are initiating with the school. It is understandable that the schedules of clinicians and pediatricians at present are busier than ever. However, the presence of the pediatrician or the clinician either in person or by phone at an IEP meeting, for example, can mean a lot to the family and the educators and often enhances the personal and professional experience of the clinician. Being a companion to the family and playing the part of an active member of a special education team, the clinician not only serves as advocate but also helps the parents to become better advocates for their own children.

ISSUES AND TRENDS

Role of Families

By law, parents must be involved in the special education process. They give permission for evaluation, participate in the development of the IEP, sign off on placement decisions and the IEP, receive progress reports, and may exercise their due process rights. Parents of preschoolers may also request services from schools to assist them in supporting their child's development (e.g., information about handling challenging behaviors at home, training in how to use assistive technology). Parent involvement is predicated on the belief that parents are partners in the process. However, the way in which parents are treated as they engage in the process often determines the extent to which they feel they are partners. IEP meetings, for example, can be very intimidating. Parents may enter a room with as many as 10 professionals, many of whom they have never met, and be expected to participate equally in the deliberations about their child's education program. For even the most extraverted, confident parents, this situation can be overwhelming. Parents are more likely to participate in the process if they have prior knowledge of how the meeting will proceed, opportunities to meet and talk to the professionals in advance, someone to help them prepare their contributions to the meeting, and at least one other person of their choosing at the meeting (Turnbull and Turnbull, 2001).

Transitions to new educational settings can be particularly difficult for children with disabilities because transitions to new service delivery systems, placements, or services often occur more frequently than with typically developing children. Transitioning usually means new surroundings, new peers, and new teachers for the children. For parents, in addition to worrying about their children's adjustment, it means getting used to working with new personnel. As children age within the system of special education services, one typical difference for parents is the amount of support they receive from educational personnel (Kaczmarek et al, 2004). For parents whose children are identified as infants and toddlers, family support is an integral part of the service delivery system. Services are usually home based, and parents establish close relationships with their services providers. Each family also has a service coordinator to assist them in negotiating the maze of services available in a community. The transition to preschool services is often accompanied by a shift to less intimate relationships with service providers as the teaching context changes from homes to classrooms. Parents may have less direct and frequent contact with professionals because children may take the bus to school. Although classroom professionals at the preschool level usually do attend to the needs of parents through notes, phone calls, e-mails, and conferences, many parents keenly feel the differences in support. Once children transition to school-aged programs, parents may again feel a further drop in support and communication.

Inclusion

Inclusion refers to educating children with and without disabilities in the same educational settings. The term *inclusion* means that children with disabilities have a right to be educated with their nondisabled peers in age-appropriate classrooms in their neighborhood schools. *Mainstreaming* was the word used before *inclusion*. Although the terms are similar and may sometimes be used interchangeably, *mainstreaming* as applied historically implied that children needed to demonstrate academic and social readiness before being placed in the "mainstream." Today, children are included in the same classrooms as their typical peers for all or part of the school day without having to "earn" it, as you may recall was the case for both Ashley and Mateo. The amount of time that children are included in regular classrooms will vary, depending on their IEPs. For example, some may be included only for so called "specials," such as art and music classes, or activities with minimum academic focus, such as recess, homeroom, and lunch. Others may leave the regular classroom for a resource room for special instruction in just one or two subjects. When children are in regular educational settings for the entire school day, they are considered to be "fully included," and all support services prescribed on the IEP are then received in the regular classroom. In 2002, 96% of all special education students were educated in regular school buildings, with nearly 50% spending at least 79% of their day inside the regular classroom; the percentages spending this amount of time in regular classrooms has increased steadily since 1993 (U.S. Department of Education, 2006).

Empirical evidence demonstrates that inclusion is beneficial to children with disabilities and also their peers, school programs, and teachers (Hunt et al, 2003). Benefits, which have been identified for children with mild disabilities as well as for those with severe disabilities, include increased social interaction and friendships; learning of new cognitive, social, sensory, and motor behaviors; improvement in standardized test scores; higher quality IEPs; and better preparation for adulthood. Other research has yielded more equivocal outcomes for children with disabilities in which improvements in inclusive settings have been no better or only marginally better than those in segregated settings. Outcomes for children without disabilities have included greater understanding and acceptance of human differences; improved sensitivity, empathy, and caring for others; and enhanced self-esteem. There is also some evidence that low-achieving students who do not qualify for special education benefit from the specialized instructional strategies used in the classroom. Ultimately, inclusion in schools is viewed as benefiting society generally because as children grow up understanding, knowing, and befriending children with diverse abilities, society as a whole will be more likely to create physical and social environments within communities that are designed universally for all.

Challenges to inclusion fall into three categories (Kochhar et al, 2000): knowledge, organizational, and attitudinal. Although many teachers, both regular and special, feel that they have not had sufficient training for inclusion, state and local educational agencies often provide staff development to assist teachers in addressing the needs of inclusion, and under current law, teacher education programs are gearing up to ensure that all teachers are highly qualified. Organizational barriers refer to the manner in which schools are structured, staffed, and managed. Most agree that successful inclusion requires changes in traditional professional roles. No longer is one teacher responsible for a classroom of children; rather, the principal teacher in a classroom either may share the teaching responsibilities with a special educator (i.e., co-teaching) or may receive consultative services within a collaborative context from the special educator or such related service providers as speech-language pathologists, occupational therapists, and physical therapists. Lack of appropriate training and the aforementioned organizational modifications often lead to attitudinal barriers on the part of teachers and administrators. However, teachers who embrace a more collaborative approach often find themselves shifting their attitudes when they find the experience more rewarding than the traditional classroom.

Collaborative Teaming

Children in special education generally receive services from multiple service providers, just as Mateo did in the vignette; minimally, this is a regular educator and a special educator, and often it also includes various therapists, requiring a level of coordination and collaboration generally atypical of traditional educational service delivery. There are a variety of models of how regular and special educators or related service personnel work together (McWilliam, 1995). The most traditional model is for the child to be pulled out of the regular classroom for special services in resource rooms or other isolated locations. Sometimes other children either with or without disabilities might accompany the child, providing opportunities for social interaction as part of the special session. Other options maintain the special services within the classroom environment, with the special educator or related service provider delivering the services one-on-one or in small groups somewhere within the classroom. Special service providers may also work within the regular curriculum by teaching a group of children that includes one or more children with disabilities (e.g., a speech-language pathologist conducting reading lessons for a group that includes several children who may have language problems) or by assisting one or more children who need support or assistance during the routine schedule of lessons (e.g., an occupational therapist who assists individual children during their daily writing period). Specialists may also consult with teachers without providing services directly (e.g., a special education teacher who guides a regular education teacher in dealing with a child's challenging behaviors by observing, offering recommendations, and monitoring the child's progress). Co-teaching is another model that might be used in which a regular educator and a special educator are both responsible for all the children in a classroom. Such arrangements, like many of the others, require the personnel involved to understand and respect each other's contributions, to work out job responsibilities clearly, and to communicate and plan together regularly.

Issues Related to Culture

The overrepresentation of minority students and English language learners in special education has been a continuing concern since the 1960s (DeValenzuela et al, 2006). The data reported in the IDEA Report to Congress for 2004 (U.S. Department of Education, 2006) compared the percentage of school-age children from specific ethnic or racial groups with that of the IDEA total student population. Trends indicated overrepresentation for blacks in the categories of emotional disturbance and intellectual disability; for Hispanics in specific learning disabilities and hearing impairment; for Asian/Pacific Islanders in hearing impairment and autism; and for American Indian/Alaska Native in specific learning disabilities and developmental delay.

Overrepresentation of an ethnic or racial group in special education is problematic if it represents inequities in how the special education process is applied across groups. Consequently, it is possible that children are being misidentified and that cultural differences underlie the problem, perhaps reflecting the ethnic and racial biases of our society generally. Damaging effects may result from being unnecessarily identified as a special education student (Hosp and Reschly, 2003). For example, receiving a special education label might be stigmatizing, further limiting the expectations that teachers and others have for a child's ability, reducing the positive educational experiences and opportunities that a child receives, and restricting satisfactory social experiences with peers. African American special education students, for example, have been disproportionately placed in more segregated than inclusive settings because children with labels of intellectual disability and emotional disturbance in general are more likely to be placed in segregated settings and African American children are overrepresented in these categories (Serwatka et al, 1995).

The disproportionate representation of minorities in special education is clearly a complex problem in which there are no immediate or easy solutions. In addition to the parental involvement already mentioned, IDEA builds into the special education process some safeguards. These include nondiscriminatory, multifaceted assessment, testing in the dominant language, notifications to parents in their native language, and provision of an interpreter for meetings. The National Center for Culturally Responsive Educational Systems (*http://www.nccrest.org/*), a project funded by the U.S. Department of Education's Special Educations Programs, proposes to address the problem by developing culturally responsive educational systems (Klingner et al, 2005). The Center offers a range of trainings and products appropriate for parents and professionals to this end.

One aspect of the remedy proposed by the National Center for Culturally Responsive Educational Systems is the development of culturally responsive teachers and school administrators; others have referred to this as cultural or cross-cultural competence. Such efforts seek to improve the understanding that all teachers have of their own culture, sensitize them to how their own culture affects their worldview and actions, and teach them to approach children and their families in a responsive or culturally competent manner. Such competence goes well beyond developing multicultural curricula to include learning how to interact respectfully, reciprocally, and responsively with those from other cultural and linguistic groups (Lynch and Hanson, 1998). The use of evidenced-based practices and early intervening services are two other strategies included in the 2004 reauthorization of IDEA that look promising in addressing this issue.

Evidence-Based Practices

As in the health care field, the importance of basing practice on scientifically derived evidence and research has gained prominence, largely because No Child Left Behind requires teachers to use scientifically proven practices in their classrooms. However, understanding what type of scientific information is acceptable as evidence is a complex question when it is applied to education generally but even more so when it is applied to special education (Odom et al, 2005). Some have suggested that a single methodology, namely, randomized clinical trials, should be the gold standard for education, whereas others argue for multiple methodologies. The variability in special education populations and the contexts in which children with disabilities are educated make randomized clinical trials very difficult. Four basic research designs have been identified for special education: (1) experimental group, (2) correlational, (3) single subject, and (4) qualitative. These multiple methodologies have worked historically in identifying effective special education practices. Presently, professional organizations play a pivotal role in identifying evidence-based practices in special education by proposing guidelines and writing compendiums of effective practices.

Early Intervening

Early intervening, which should not be confused with early intervention, refers to providing additional academic and behavioral support to children in general education who have not been identified for special education services. The intent of these services is to allow school staff to give children specialized assistance with research-based strategies as soon as they start to fall behind to prevent school failure. With the passage of IDEA 2004, up to 15% of a local educational agency's IDEA funds may be used for early intervening services for children in kindergarten through grade 12, with heavy emphasis on the primary grades. School districts that have a significant overrepresentation of minorities in special education must use the maximum amount allowed for this purpose. Had this provision been in place when Mateo was in the earlier grades, he would probably have received help with his reading and writing much sooner.

Because many states have current definitions of learning disabilities that require a discrepancy between intelligence and achievement, children with learning difficulties are often not identified for special education services until they experience school failure, usually not until the second or third grade. In addition to creating circumstances for children that predispose them to behavioral, self-esteem, and peer relationship problems, this discrepancy model of learning disabilities is considered to be at least partially responsible for the overrepresentation of children from minority and linguistically diverse groups in special education. To circumvent these problems, researchers have developed what is called response to intervention, a model of pre-referral and prevention of learning disabilities. Response to intervention consists of three components (National Association of State Directors of Special Education, 2005): (1) a three-tiered intervention hierarchy, representing core instruction for all children (general education) as Tier 1, targeted group interventions as Tier 2, and intensive individualized intervention (special education) as Tier 3; (2) a step-by-step problem solving approach for educators to identify problems and plan, implement, and monitor interventions; and (3) an assessment and data collection system for each level of the hierarchy. The model, which is loosely based on a public health model of care, appears to be gaining recognition as an empirically validated approach for preventing or ameliorating learning disabilities. This type of model is also being given consideration for use with preschool children (Coleman et al, 2006).

SUMMARY

Both Mateo and Ashley, whose stories were told at the beginning of this chapter, realized better outcomes because of the support provided by physicians. Although traditionally education and health care have been viewed as separate and distinct entities, it is imperative to acknowledge, as with Mateo and Ashley, their emerging relationship in the delivery of services to children and youth with disabilities. Physicians can play an important role in supporting children with disabilities by providing information to parents about school services, communicating with school personnel when necessary, and recommending appropriate accommodations and modifications. The recent shift in the legislative foundation of special education from process to outcomes potentially enhances the role that medical professionals can play in bridging health care and education. Sensitivity to parental concerns about the developmental and school performance of their children, knowledge of available school services as well as educational trends and issues, and willingness to expediently create this bridge for parents are invaluable in maximizing the positive outcomes of children with disabilities.

REFERENCES

Coleman MR, Buysse V, Neitzel J: Recognition and Response: An Early Intervening System for Young Children At-Risk for Learning Disabilities. 2006. Available at: http://www.fpg.unc.edu/products/. Accessed September 9, 2006.

Committee on Children with Disabilities: The pediatrician's role in the development and implementation of an Individualized Education Plan (IEP) and/or an Individual Family Service Plan (IFSP). Pediatrics 104:124–127, 1999. Available at: http://pediatrics.aappublications.org/cgi/content/full/l04/1/124. Accessed February 2, 2007.

Committee on Education and the Workforce: Individuals with Disabilities Education Act (IDEA): Guide to Frequently Asked Questions. 2005. Available at: http://www.house.gov/ed_work force/issues/109th/education/idea/ideafaq.pdf#search=%22IDEA%20guide%20freguently%22. Accessed September 7, 2006.

Council for Exceptional Children: Understanding the Differences Between IDEA and Section 504. 2002. Available at: http://www.ldonline.org/article/6086. Accessed February 1, 2007.

DeValenzuela JS, Copeland SR, Qi CH, Park M: Examining educational equity: Revisiting the disproportionate representation of minority students in special education. Exceptional Children 72:425-441, 2006.

Henderson K: Overview of ADA, IDEA, and Section 504. 2007. Available at: http://www.kidsource.com/kidsource/content3/ada.idea.html. Accessed February 1, 2007.

Hosp J, Reschly DJ: Referral rates for intervention or assessment: A meta-analysis of racial differences. J Special Educ 37:67-80, 2003.

Hunt P, Soto G, Maier J, Doering K: Collaborative teaming to support students at risk and students with severe disabilities in general education classrooms. Exceptional Children 69:315-332, 2003.

Kaczmarek L, Goldstein H, Florey JD, et al: Supporting families: A preschool Model. Topics Early Childhood Special Educ 24:213-226, 2004.

Klingner JK, Artiles AJ, Kozleski E, et-al: Addressing the disproportionate representation of culturally and linguistically diverse students in special education through culturally responsive educational systems. Education Policy Analysis Archives, 13(38), 2005. Available at: http://epaa.asu.edu/epaa/v13n38/. Accessed September 10, 2006.

Kochhar CA, West LL, Taymans JM: Successful Inclusion: Practical Strategies for a Shared Responsibility. Upper Saddle River, NJ, Prentice-Hall, 2000.

Leslie LK, Weckerly J, Plemmons D, et al: Implementing the American Academy of Pediatrics attention-deficit/hyperactivity disorder diagnostic guidelines in primary care settings. Pediatrics 114: 129-140, 2004.

Lynch E, Hanson M: Developing Cross-Cultural Competence: A Guide for Working with Young Children and Their Families. Baltimore, Paul Brookes, 1998.

McWilliam R: Integration of therapy and consultative special education: A continuum in early intervention. Infants Young Children 7:29-38, 1995.

National Association of State Directors of Special Education: Response to Intervention: Policy Considerations and Implementations. Alexandria, VA, Author, 2005.

National Dissemination Center for Children with Disabilities: Module 3: The History of IDEA. n.d. Available at: http://www.nichcy.org/ideatrai.htm. Accessed August 18, 2006.

Odom SL, Brantlinger E, Gersten R, et al: Research in special education: Scientific methods and evidence-based practices. Exceptional Children 71:137-148, 2005.

Office of Civil Rights: Protecting Students with Disabilities. 2005. Available at: http://www.ed.gov/about/offices/list/ocr/504faq.html#interrelationship. Accessed September 4, 2006.

Office of Special Education and Rehabilitative Services: A Guide to the Individualized Education Program. 2000. Available at: http://www.ed.gov/parents/needs/speced/iepguide/index.html. Accessed August 18, 2006.

Office of Special Education Programs: History: Twenty-five Years of Progress in Educating Children with Disabilities Through IDEA. n.d. Available at: http://www.ed.gov/policy/speced/leg/idea/history.html. Accessed August 15, 2006.

Rosenfeld SJ: Section 504 and IDEA: Basic Similarities and Differences. 2006. Available at: http://www.wrightslaw.com/advoc/articles/504_IDEA_Rosenfeld.html. Accessed February 1, 2007.

Serwatka TS, Deering S, Grant P: Disproportionate representation of African Americans in emotionally handicapped classes. J Black Studies 25:492-506, 1995.

Turnbull A, Turnbull R: Families, Professionals, and Exceptionality: Collaboration for Empowerment. 4th ed, Upper Saddle River, NJ, Merrill, 2001.

U.S. Department of Education: No Child Left Behind: A Parent's Guide. 2003. Available at: http://www.ed.gov/parents/academic/involve/nclbguide/parentsguide.html. Accessed September 1, 2006.

U.S. Department of Education: The Twenty-Sixth Annual Report to Congress on the Implementation of the Individuals with Disabilities Education Act. 2006. Available at: http://www.ed.gov/about/reports/annual/osep/2004/index.html. Accessed September 20, 2006.

Wolraich ML, Feurer ID, Hannah JN, et al: Obtaining systematic teacher reports of disruptive behavior disorders utilizing DSM-IV. J Abnormal Child Psychol 26:141-152, 1998.

94 THE ARTS THERAPIES

Donna Madden Chadwick

All parents and health care professionals strive to assist children in reaching their highest potential—to understand them intimately, to encourage them toward mastery, and to comfort them in difficult situations and conditions. We seek to nurture resilient children who possess self-respect and strategies to cope with life's challenges. The arts therapies (art therapy, dance/movement therapy, poetry, drama, and music therapy) stand among an arsenal of treatments that help children to prevail regardless of emotional or physical circumstances.

From the first lullaby, the first soothing, rocking parent's embrace, a baby is receptive to sound and movement. With each annual "happy birthday" and holiday song, the social ritual incorporating elements of the arts is experienced and becomes a familiar presence. "Art is a human invariant; people in all times and in all places sing, draw, and dance" (Hodges, 1996).

THE ARTS THERAPIES IN INTEGRATIVE MEDICINE

For decades, consumers have augmented allopathic medicine with complementary treatments that address their physical, emotional, and spiritual selves as a whole.

There is no doubt that appreciation of or engagement with the arts enhances one's quality of life. The approaches of performing arts medicine (a medical specialty devoted to the prevention and treatment of performance-caused physical and psychological conditions), Arts in Health Care Settings (providing live performances for patients in hospitals), and Kindermusik and Music Together (musicians providing curriculum-designed music experiences for preschool children and their parents) seek to accomplish this. Valuable though they may be, these applications are not arts therapies. It is important to distinguish the arts therapies from all other uses of the arts, both credible and questionable.

Statements of the arts' "healing" abound. Some companies, authors, and Internet sites proclaim curative properties of sound and color at which responsible, science-based clinicians look askance. We should be skeptical of unsubstantiated claims. Since their foundation in the mid-20th century, national arts therapy associations have worked toward differentiating the clinical professions from other arts endeavors and disseminating accurate information on accomplishments of clinical efforts.

The arts therapies are art, dance/movement, music, poetry, and drama. Each practitioner is highly educated and clinically trained; they are nationally credentialed and, in many cases, state licensed.

- Art therapy is the therapeutic use of art making, within a professional relationship, by people who experience illness, trauma, or challenges in living to express feelings and to increase emotional well-being.
- Dance/movement therapy is the psychotherapeutic use of movement as a process that furthers the emotional, cognitive, and physical integration of the individual.
- Music therapy is the clinical, evidence-based use of music interventions to accomplish individual emotional, cognitive, social, and physical goals within a therapeutic relationship.
- Poetry therapy is the use of self-reflective writing for expression and personal growth. Journaling, interacting with literature, and therapeutic storytelling are components of this discipline.
- Drama therapy is an experiential modality that uses theater techniques and processes to facilitate personal growth and to promote health.

All arts therapies, also known as creative arts therapies, share the common belief that artistic involvement and the clinical relationships experienced within the arts are life affirming and beneficial across many human domains.

Each year brings increasing use of the arts therapies in hospitals, special education collaboratives, public schools, and private clinics. It is now recognized that arts therapists are uniquely skilled clinicians, capable of treating children in any subspecialty area. These incomparable modalities are increasingly sought after in the team model of service delivery because they provide viable treatment options that cultivate children's resilience in nonthreatening and, in fact, joy-filled ways.

The 21st century integrative medicine movement recognizes the importance of evidence-based complementary therapies. Never before has there been such intense inquiry into the effects of the arts on the lives of human beings.

Creative arts clinicians meet criteria as psychotherapists and can act as a child's primary therapist. Art, dance/movement, and music therapy practice in the scientific model and are accountable for assessment, treatment, and evaluation of the patient. The arts therapies use effective clinical techniques and are well documented in research journals. They fare well under scientific scrutiny and promote self-validating studies.

THE ARTS AS A CLINICAL TOOL

Unique among the helping professions, the creative arts therapies bring vitality and creativity to assessment and treatment that are not generally delivered through other disciplines. Art, dance/movement, and music therapies share a fundamental core of characteristics that set them apart as distinctive interventions.

1. Natural childhood behavior: Children thrive in the arts because they incorporate the familiar, enjoyable acts of drawing, pretending, moving the body, singing, and exploring interesting instruments and media. Uninhibited expressions emerge easily through these intrinsically inviting channels.
2. Fail-safe context: In arts therapy, the child functions in a safe haven. All judgment is suspended and failure is prevented. The child is supported as he or she self-explores, takes risks, and assumes power.
3. Creative process: The essence of the therapy lies in creative expression and the insight and relationships that develop as a result of them. Artistic acts can be satisfying and transformative. They access and nourish the "well" part of the child. The pride of creation is innately vitalizing and ignites self-esteem.
4. Nonverbal quality: Use of one's body, instruments, or art media can stand alone and "speak for itself." The art form is a metaphor, a surrogate voice. This gives the child a valid new avenue of communication free from verbal vulnerability.
5. Improvisation: Therapists use no rigid formulas. Rather, they apply art to mirror the child's emotional state continuously and spontaneously. The treatment is entirely child centered and constantly evolving—the clinical relationship exists within the present moment of the art.
6. Aesthetic reception: Experience in beauty invests in the heart of the child. Identifying with the arts develops the capacity to be deeply moved, more balanced, and fully human.

KNOWING THE CHILD

Assessment

Assessment is the process by which the therapist strategically observes the child and, on the basis of findings, makes recommendations for treatment planning. Formal and informal prescriptive assessments, achieved within the context of the art itself, can be accomplished according to many theoretical constructs. The clinician arranges art opportunities in which to observe the child's responses and initiations as well as symbolic behavior.

Assessments are performed as part of general intake before planning treatment, or they are called for to pursue a specific area of inquiry, for instance, eligibility for music therapy in an individual education plan or appraisal of self-image.

The therapist chooses the proper instrument from among many published models in the field's literature. A comprehensive assessment yields a complete profile of the child, reporting on sensory, developmental, receptive, and expressive communication and cognitive, motor, and social-emotional abilities. Domain-specific or diagnosis-specific assessments investigate a sole functional area, such as communication (Wigram, 2000), or diagnosis, such as depression (Silver, 2002).

What most arts therapy assessments have in common is that they bypass language yet nonetheless receive an abundance of information about the essence of the child's self in nonverbal (painting, music making, movement) forms. This is precisely why these modalities are able to successfully draw the child in. The clinician expertly translates the meaning of the child's process and product into traditional educational and psychological terminology. Team members, especially parents, have remarked that the novel information sparks a more positive view of the child "patient" as arts receptive.

Gardner (1999) put forth the theory of multiple intelligences. Named among these special aptitudes are musical intelligence, visual-spatial intelligence, and body-kinesthetic intelligence, which relate directly to music, art, and dance/movement therapy. Children's strengths in these areas are more readily identified through creative arts therapy assessments than by other means.

Each creative art therapy offers a wealth of assessment potential. Each is capable of gently investigating multiple aspects and contributing unique information to the team's complete knowledge of the child. His or her arts responsivity is a prominent factor in planning how to best treat the educational, emotional, physical, and spiritual whole.

In Early Life

The arts therapies can make effective contributions at any stage during the years of childhood. Parents and other caregivers included in much pediatric creative arts therapy work acquire skills for lifelong productive interaction with their children.

Dance/movement therapy conducts programs in which expectant mothers learn techniques that promote healthy bonding. Sensitivity to child movement communication begins in utero, when mothers are taught through touch attunement. Working with the movement repertoire of the fetus, the mother can learn to accommodate it and become watchful for and responsive to physical cues both before and after birth (Loman, 1994). Dance/movement therapy increases sensory and nonverbal skills of new mothers as they interact with their young infants. Using touch, body shaping, and other techniques, they become proficient in observing interpersonal physical action and reaction and discerning the meaning of their infant's body language.

The recent discovery by neuroscientists of mirror neurons substantiates the fact that there is a physiologic basis for intimate movement and emotive synchronicity. "Studies are revealing that the identical sets of neurons can be activated in an individual who is simply witnessing another person performing a movement as the one actually engaged in the action or the expression of some emotion or behavior" (Berrol, 2006).

Application of music for preterm infants is used to assist neonates with feeding skills, in turn leading to weight gain and timely hospital discharge. Positive benefits for infants in the neonatal intensive care unit have been reported; those who listened to lullabies lost less weight and were released from isolettes, the neonatal intensive care unit, and the hospital sooner (Caine, 1991). Standley (2003), designer of the Pacifier Activated Lullaby, found that participating infants who used nonnutritive sucking to activate recorded music increased nipple feeding competency.

Early intervention, a legally mandated program of treatment for children aged 0 to 3 years who have special needs, is the perfect place to introduce the arts therapies. Music therapists are particularly adept at engaging the young child's attention and tuning it into external expression and active developmental learning.

Vignette

Mirembe is a beautiful 9-month-old girl who was born full term with no complications. She developed well until 6 months of age, when she had a massive seizure episode that left her legally blind with continuing seizures and a severe developmental setback in all areas. She could no longer roll, raise her head, or make sound. With music therapy, Mirembe is beginning to localize to sound, pick up her head, reach for chimes, and relearn how to smile. Her grandmother, who came from Uganda to help with her care, joins in the singing, clapping for Mirembe as she achieves each little milestone. The soft strumming of the guitar and the clinician's voice singing, "Mirembe, play your own song," encourage Mirembe to reconnect with her caregivers and continue to work so hard to regain the skills she has lost.

TREATING THE CHILD

Individual Therapy

When a child is not socially ready or sensorially capable of a group experience, individual treatment is recommended. In addition, this is the choice for children who experience complex emotional or physical involvements, perhaps the child who is in a hospital bed, someone who travels by wheelchair and benefits from maximal physical assistance, or the child who is fresh with trauma. The therapist is able to establish a trusting alliance in a shorter time and center all attention on one child's process. Depth of treatment is enhanced by this private work. Quantification of changes in a child's status is also optimally accurate.

Vignette

Kelly, a personable adolescent with developmental disabilities, could speak a few intelligible words after prompts. She loves music. Communication erupts in a music context. In individual music therapy (MT), Kelly added to her vocabulary by learning new approximations that reflect her own milieu. When "carried" on melody, new words flowed in improvised songs about boys, dances, and fun activities. When MT commenced, she could not verbally produce a name for either of her parents. In song, she worked on using the new words Ma and Da; then she progressed to singing an approximation of her first short sentence: I love you. Intelligibility improved; over time, the music was faded and Kelly could combine both her parents' names and the sentence. After 3 years of MT, Kelly proudly made a tape recording for her parents on which she said, "I love you Ma. I love you Da."

Individual music therapy is a treatment of choice for girls who have Rett syndrome. *The Rett Syndrome Handbook* states, "Girls with Rett syndrome are very motivated by music. It calms them when they are anxious, and allows them to communicate feelings they cannot otherwise express" (Hunter, 2007). Recommending that girls with Rett syndrome receive music therapy as often as they can, Hunter goes on to say that music alone is not enough. It is the therapist who makes music experiences meaningful by acknowledging the girls' feelings and opening them to learning opportunities. The *Handbook* lists 14 specific areas of potential gain through music therapy, among them cognition, relaxation, freedom of movement and expression, purposeful hand use, and improved self-esteem (Fig. 94-1).

Group Therapy

The aims of all group work are in general agreement—for members to gain self-awareness, to understand and relate to others, to contribute to the whole, and to develop a sense of mutuality and cohesion.

The art therapies work well in dyads, trios, and other manageable configurations with a reasonable therapist-to-child ratio. Members can create a whole product such as a mural, dance, or music ensemble while simultaneously achieving group and individual goals. Sharing fun and process in creative arts therapies can be a source of community, friendship, and belonging for children who have an otherwise limited social network. The art itself becomes the child's ally.

HELPING THE CHILD COPE

For centuries, society has processed collective experience through the arts. The terrorist attacks that occurred on September 11, 2001, deeply affected the United States. In the aftermath emerged a body of poetry, literature, film, dance, art, and music that reflects the creators' feelings about the event. News reports speak of the "healing" benefits of transforming despair into a creative product.

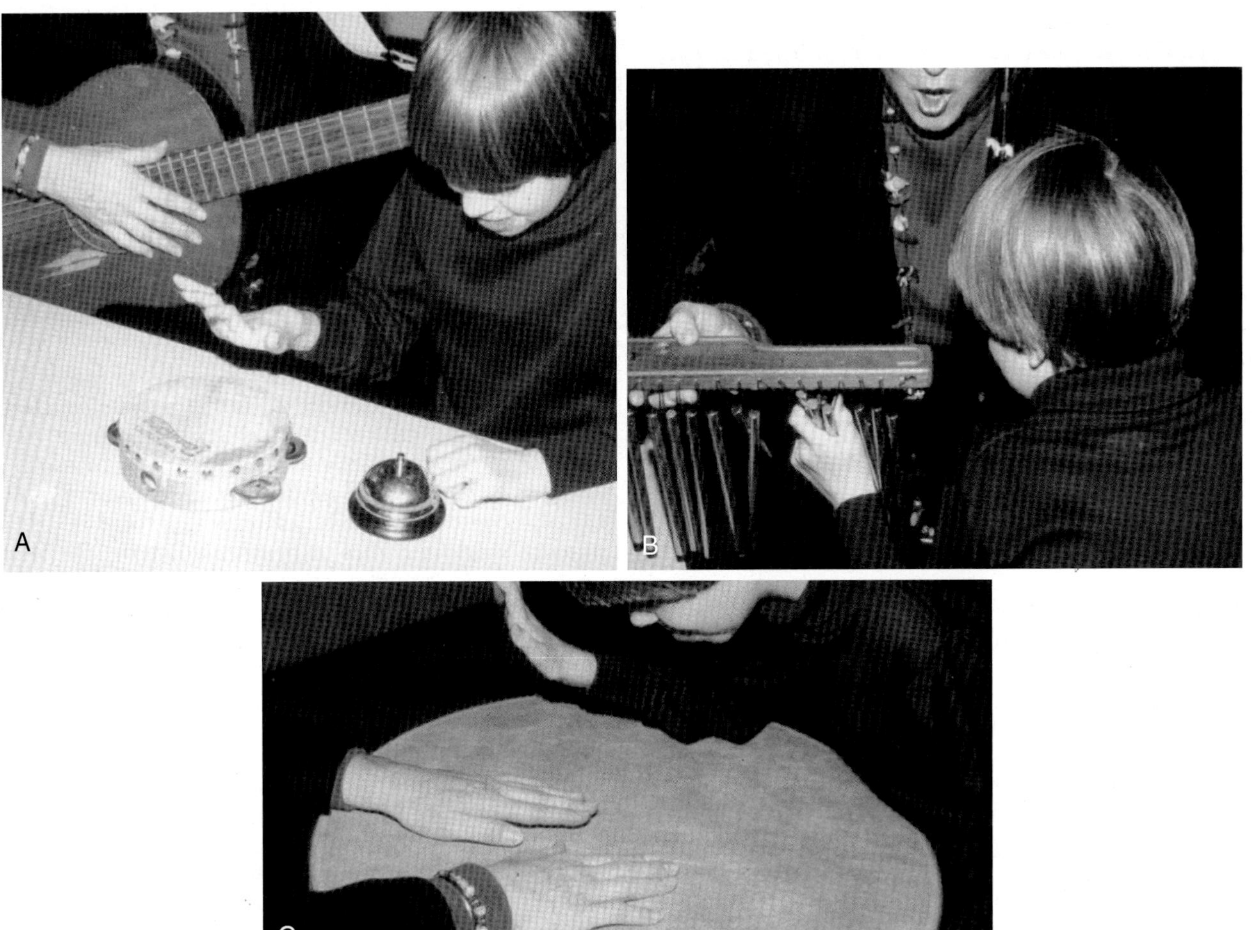

Figure 94-1. A-C, Girls who have Rett syndrome are so motivated by music that they can often separate their hands to contact instruments. *(Courtesy of Kim Abrano, 2006.)*

9-11 altered the lives of many American children. Living in the overwhelming trauma, they have generally increased feelings of fear and vulnerability in addition to lack of hope and trust. Responses to this and other catastrophic events vary, depending on the child's coping skills and the level of loss and trauma. Some may be depressed and emotionally shut down, unable to disclose the terror they carry. Others, equally hurting, present as disorganized, angry, and aggressive.

The creative arts therapies tap into deeply buried emotions. Because they travel along an alternate route in accessing the unspeakable, they often succeed where traditional therapies have failed. They use the creative process as a catalyst to call forth, explore, and reframe the child's response to horrific occurrences. When experiences are too painfully, personally "real" to be acknowledged in words, the arts therapies offer a safe context. The child's truth can be stated through the arts' surrogate voice.

The arts provide a location for even the darkest truth to go—to be concretely placed outside of the self and into sculpture, song lyrics, dances, and plays. Once released, the child is distanced from the life-changing event and can develop control over feelings about it. The stability of form and structure and the regularity of rhythm in the arts provide predictability that can help the child regain boundaries and order and lead to the child's own reorganization.

This is often the need of children who have experienced sexual abuse. Being in control of choosing projects and media and determining whether to keep or to destroy art products address these needs. Often the art object itself or style of image discloses helplessness, secrecy, low self-esteem, self-blame, or unexpectedly precocious sexual symbology of the child who made them.

Art therapy has set precedent by being qualified in the state of New Jersey as expert witness in child sexual abuse litigation. Art therapy was recognized as a mental health profession and proven to have a scientific or other credible basis. The testifying clinician qualified as an expert and her opinion was valid "by virtue of her knowledge, skill, experience, training, and education" (Cohen-Liebman, 1994).

Drawings made during the forensic interview process give children an indirect way to depict descriptions and feelings they may have difficulty comprehending. They stimulate the exploration of both manifest and latent material and are admissible as judiciary aids (Cohen-Liebman, 1999).

Successful treatment through the arts therapies also gives children tools for applying self-soothing behaviors. The child is supported and assisted in identifying preferred, optimally comforting self-care habits and learns to independently apply them when needed. The clinician teaches parents new ways to employ natural techniques, such as reading, coloring, and crooning at bedtime. They can be used when an unanticipated trigger reactivates fear or regularly as a ritual to ease into a gentle night's sleep.

Vignette

Seven-year-old Mateo, diagnosed with an anxiety disorder, experiences panic attacks. With his music therapist, he composed a song titled "You Can Still be Safe," which names his stressors (peers teasing, Mom leaving, school tests). The song also identifies his coping strategies (think of your room, get warm and cozy, tell your favorite story in your head). An evening talk with Mom followed by listening to a tape recording of the song empowers proactivity in Mateo and assures him of his competency in self-protection.

Certain differently abled children are endowed with a strong affinity for music. This attraction is universally recognized in individuals who have Down syndrome and those who have Williams syndrome. A magnetism drives them to seek out and achieve in music experience. The child with Williams syndrome may even demonstrate a level of music ability higher than that in the general population. Receptive and expressive musicality is part of their essential makeup. Capitalizing on this positive natural attribute in the child's education program is highly desirable. In a music-brightened mood, the child opens to learning; music techniques can extend attention, smooth transitions, and be an aid to memory.

ACCESSING SERVICES

The creative arts therapies are accessed through traditional means of funding for children who have special needs. The primary source is their home community if the creative arts therapy is included in the individual education plan (IEP). To get an art therapy on the IEP, the process begins with referral. The parent, physician, or other treater who works with the child is entitled to contact the town's director of special education and request an assessment by an art, dance/movement, or music therapist. The school administration then secures the assessment at public expense, and the resulting information is considered by team members, including parents. Some directors of special education are unfamiliar with creative arts therapies and require a legal as well as clinical rationale for adding a new discipline to the treatment team.

The legal basis for inclusion of creative arts therapies in a child's IEP is stated in the reauthorization of the Individuals with Disabilities Education Act (IDEA), now titled the Individuals with Disabilities Education Improvement Act of 2004 (PL 108-446). The creative arts therapies are not directly named in IDEA, but they are considered to be related services. When the team determines any related service to be necessary, it is legally mandated to become part of the education plan. Arts therapies have been established as related services in communities across the United States.

Most creative arts therapists, licensed at the master's degree level, qualify as mental health counselors or psychotherapists in the state where they practice. Massachusetts, New York, Pennsylvania, Texas, and Wisconsin currently feature licensure for practitioners who meet particular criteria. Moreover, these therapies may be reimbursable by health maintenance organizations. In 2005, a well-established health insurer, Blue Cross/Blue Shield of Massachusetts, through a credentialing vendor, WholeHealth Networks Incorporated, began offering music therapy to providers within their affinity program.

Many short-term arts therapies are grant funded through community service agencies, hospital outreach programs, and college campus schools. Some client groups who need creative arts therapy the most, such as children in shelters, are funded in this manner. Families can also contract privately, as many therapists in private practice work in clinics or provide home or school visits. Each professional organization has a reimbursement specialist who will guide consumers toward obtaining funding.

RESOURCES

The professional organizations maintain high standards for their discipline by establishing the code of ethics and standards of best practice, providing information on education and training requirements, and producing publications and conferences. On request, they supply referrals from their annual membership directory according to location and clinical specialty.

In addition to these associations, there may be an independent credentialing organization, for example, the Certification Board for Music Therapists or the Art Therapy Credentials Board, which have a complete international list of certified practitioners (Table 94-1).

SUMMARY

Evidence-based art therapy, dance/movement therapy, and music therapy as well as drama and poetry therapy have inherent advantages in pediatric assessment and treatment (Table 94-2). Distinctive because they employ natural childhood behavior and bypass verbal language, these disciplines externalize feelings and expression through relationships in the creative process. Practitioners usually meet criteria as psychotherapists. Applied early in life, dance/movement therapy can assist expectant and new mothers to attune to their infant's movement communication. Music therapy has benefited preterm infants in the neonatal intensive care unit by decreasing weight loss and increasing nipple feeding competency. It is also notably effective in early intervention programs with children who have Down syndrome or Williams syndrome and with girls who have Rett syndrome. Art therapy not only aids in treatment of children who have been sexually abused but is diagnostically used during the forensic interview; drawings are admissible as evidence in litigation. All the arts therapies offer techniques that can be taught to the child, parents, and caregivers for soothing use at home. It is desirable for an art therapy to be named on the child's IEP because it is then funded by the school district and the clinician becomes a treatment team member. The national associations can assist consumers in locating therapists and surveying funding sources.

Table 94-1. National Arts Therapy Associations

Art Therapy

American Art Therapy Association
5999 Stevenson Avenue
Alexandria, VA 22304
888-290-0878
http://www.arttherapy.org

Art Therapy Credentials Board
3 Terrace Way, Suite B
Greensboro, NC 27403
877-213-2822
http://www.atcb.org

Dance/Movement Therapy

American Dance Therapy Association
2000 Century Plaza, Suite 108
10632 Little Patuxent Parkway
410-997-4040
Columbia, MD 21044
http://www.adta.org

Music Therapy

American Music Therapy Association
8455 Colesville Road, Suite 1000
Silver Spring, MD 20910
301-589-3300
http://www.musictherapy.org

Certification Board for Music Therapists
506 East Lancaster Avenue, Suite 102
Downingtown, PA 19335
800-765-2268
http://www.cbmt.org

Poetry Therapy

National Association for Poetry Therapy
Center for Education, Training and Holistic Approaches, Inc.
777 E. Atlantic Avenue, #243
Delray Beach, FL 33483
866-844-NAPT
www.poetrytherapy.org

Drama Therapy

National Association for Drama Therapy
15 Post Side Lane
Pittsford, NY 14534
585-381-5618
www.nadt.org

Table 94-2. Areas of Special Interest

Early intervention
Autism spectrum disorders
Emotional needs: children who have experienced abuse or trauma
Multiple physical challenges: cerebral palsy
Developmental disabilities
Chronic and terminal illness
Traumatic brain injury
Down syndrome, Rett syndrome, Williams syndrome

REFERENCES

Berrol CF: Neuroscience meets dance/movement therapy: Mirror neurons, the therapeutic process and empathy. The Arts in Psychotherapy 33:302-315, 2006.

Caine J: The effects of music on the selected stress behaviors, weight, caloric and formula intake, and length of hospital stay of premature and low birth weight neonates in a newborn intensive care unit. J Music Therapy 18:180-192, 1991.

Cohen-Liebman MS: The arts therapist as expert witness in sexual abuse litigation. Art Therapy 11:260-265, 1994.

Cohen-Liebman MS: Draw and tell: Drawings within the context of child sexual abuse investigations. The Arts in Psychotherapy 26:185-194, 1999.

Gardner H: Intelligence Reframed: Multiple Intelligences for the Twenty First Century. New York, Basic Books, 1999.

Hodges DA (ed): Handbook of Music Psychology. San Antonio, TX, The University of San Antonio, 1996.

Hunter K: The Rett Syndrome Handbook, 2nd ed. Clinton, MD, International Rett Syndrome Association, 2007.

Loman S: Attuning to the fetus and young child: Approaches from dance/movement therapy. Zero to Three August/September:20-26, 1994.

Silver R: Three Art Assessments. New York, Brunner-Routledge, 2002.

Standley J: The effects of music-reinforced non-nutritive sucking on feeding rate of premature infants. J Pediatr Nurs 18:169-173, 2003.

Wigram T: A method of music therapy assessment for the diagnosis of autism and communication disorders in children. Music Therapy Perspectives 18:13-22, 2000.

95 ALTERNATIVE THERAPIES

THOMAS D. CHALLMAN

Vignette

Tyler was diagnosed with autism at 30 months of age when he presented for the evaluation of significant impairments in receptive and expressive communication, limited social reciprocity, and a variety of repetitive behaviors. Intensive interventions, including applied behavior analysis strategies, were initiated. Through other parents they met in a local support group, Tyler's parents heard about various vitamins and supplements that are supposed to help children with autism. They also read on the Internet that some people believe exposure to certain heavy metals causes autism and that chelation therapy would help their son by removing these toxins from his body. They want to know if they should be pursuing any of these treatments. How should you counsel Tyler's parents?

H. L. Mencken made the observation that "there is always a well-known solution to every human problem: neat, plausible, and wrong" (Mencken, 1920, p 158). It is not uncommon for people facing medical problems that defy easy treatment to use unproved therapies that fall outside the boundary of conventional medicine. Nonstandard therapy use is common in children with developmental disorders, as it is in many areas of health care in which standard treatment approaches are not dramatically effective or curative. During the past few decades, a diverse group of unconventional therapies arising from disparate traditions and theories have come to be viewed under the conceptual umbrella of complementary and alternative medicine (CAM).

Parents and caregivers of children with developmental and behavioral disorders may be inclined to pursue almost any treatment that they feel presents some hope of benefit for their children. They are also certain to encounter questionable therapies that are at best ineffective and at worst can cause either direct or indirect harm. It can be difficult for even savvy caregivers to differentiate among therapies with an acceptable evidence base, those that are potentially plausible but untested, and those that are purely pseudoscientific. Advancements in information technology and the ease with which dubious theories and practices can spread by the Internet have compounded this problem. Caregivers need the appropriate tools to help them sort through and interpret the myriad potential treatments promoted by various individuals and groups. Health care providers who treat children with developmental and behavioral disorders must recognize that their patients often use nonstandard therapies and that it is essential to adopt a stance that demands the rational analysis of therapeutic claims so that children can be appropriately protected from those interventions that are ineffective or potentially harmful.

DEFINITIONS AND CONCEPTUALIZATION OF COMPLEMENTARY AND ALTERNATIVE MEDICINE

The boundary between therapies considered conventional and those viewed as nonstandard can be poorly delineated, and some writers have rightfully argued that the concept of "alternative medicine" is nonsensical—there is only medicine that works and medicine that does not (Angell and Kassirer, 1998). In common usage, the term *complementary medicine* (or *integrative medicine*) has been used to refer to nonstandard practices used in concert with accepted medical interventions, whereas *alternative medicine* describes interventions used in lieu of conventional medicine. The National Center for Complementary and Alternative Medicine (NCCAM), which defines CAM as diagnostic or therapeutic practices "not presently considered an integral part of conventional medicine" (NCCAM, 2000, p 10), organizes CAM practices into five domains: mind-body medicine, manipulative and body-based practices, energy medicine, biologically based practices, and a fifth domain composed of alternative medical "systems" that may use therapies found in the other domains (Table 95-1). This classification was created in an effort to provide some organization to a concept that suffered from shifting borders and inexact terminology.

The diversity of practices included under the CAM umbrella, however, highlights the difficulty we face in conceptualizing CAM as a single entity. Therapies not presently accepted as part of conventional medicine

This chapter is adapted and expanded with permission from earlier works by the same author (Challman et al, 2007; Challman, 2008), published by Paul H. Brookes Publishing Co., Inc.

Table 95-1. **National Center for Complementary and Alternative Medicine Classification of Complementary and Alternative Practices**

Alternative medical systems	Homeopathy, naturopathy, traditional Chinese medicine, Ayurvedic medicine
Mind-body medicine	Meditation, biofeedback, prayer, hypnosis, yoga
Manipulative and body-based practices	Sensory integration therapy, massage, auditory integration therapy, music therapy
Energy medicine	Therapeutic touch, Qigong, Reiki, magnet therapy, acupuncture
Biologically based practices	Vitamins and other supplements, herbs, diets, chelation

but in which testable claims are made usually fall into one of several categories that themselves have imprecise boundaries: therapies that are potentially plausible (based on current knowledge) but are insufficiently tested; those that have very weak (or nonexistent) plausibility; and those that should be more properly viewed as part of religion, spirituality, or cultural practice and not be considered part of science or medicine. A particular intervention may also be considered either CAM or conventional, depending on the context in which it is being used. For instance, vitamin therapies are accepted treatments for specific deficiency states but should be considered nonstandard when they are promoted for the treatment of developmental disorders.

There has been a dramatic rise in federal research funding directed toward alternative therapies during the past 15 years, largely as a result of strong political forces. The U.S. Congress created the Office of Alternative Medicine within the National Institutes of Health (NIH) in 1991, with an initial annual budget of $2 million. This office evolved into NCCAM, an NIH Center created in 1999 with a primary mission to investigate CAM practices by more rigorous scientific methodology. Despite substantial funding (the NCCAM appropriation for fiscal year 2006 was more than $122 million), there has been extremely slow progress toward proving or disproving the value of specific CAM therapies. Although CAM use in children with developmental disorders is widespread, the NIH has funded few studies to evaluate the safety or efficacy of these therapies in this population.

PREVALENCE AND COSTS OF COMPLEMENTARY AND ALTERNATIVE MEDICINE USE

In 1997, annual out-of-pocket expenditures for CAM services in the U.S. population were estimated to be $27 billion (Eisenberg et al, 1998). Although surveys suggest that there is widespread use of these practices among adults in the United States, increasingly inclusive interpretation of what should be considered CAM has led to inflation in these estimates. In the 2002 National Health Interview Survey, 62% of U.S. adults reported using at least one CAM therapy (including spiritual practices such as prayer) during the previous year (Barnes et al, 2004). Although elevated rates of CAM use (as high as 50%) have been reported in some general pediatric samples, much lower estimates in children and young adults in the United States have been derived from population-based data (Davis and Darden, 2003). Children with chronic medical conditions do use CAM at higher rates than the general population does. Increased rates of CAM use have been reported in children with various developmental disabilities, including autism, attention-deficit/hyperactivity disorder (ADHD), cerebral palsy, Down syndrome, and spina bifida. Higher levels of parental education as well as parental CAM use have been consistently identified in multiple studies as factors that predict pediatric CAM use.

THE USE OF COMPLEMENTARY AND ALTERNATIVE MEDICINE IN DEVELOPMENTAL-BEHAVIORAL PEDIATRICS: AN OVERVIEW

Although therapies that fall under the NCAAM definition of complementary and alternative medicine are used frequently in children with developmental-behavioral disorders, much of the evidence used to promote these therapies remains anecdotal in nature (Challman et al, 2007).

Alternative Medical Systems

Alternative medical systems are entire systems of health theory and practice (including traditional Chinese medicine, Ayurvedic medicine, naturopathy, and homeopathy) that developed separately from conventional medicine. These systems typically use a variety of methods that fall under the CAM umbrella (herbal remedies, manipulative practices). Traditional Chinese medicine relies heavily on the use of "energy"-based practices such as acupuncture and Qigong, based on the belief that the uninterrupted flow of energy through 20 meridians is necessary for the maintenance of health (a view that still lacks supporting experimental evidence). The quality of clinical trials performed to evaluate traditional Chinese medicine has generally been poor (Tang et al, 1999). There have been a number of studies of traditional Chinese medicine in the treatment of various developmental disabilities, including cerebral palsy, intellectual disability, and ADHD, although significant methodologic shortcomings and biases in these studies preclude any conclusion about whether such methods are truly beneficial. Ayurvedic medicine, which originated on the Indian subcontinent, is based on Hindu philosophy and uses dietary or herbal remedies and various mind-body therapies. There are no published controlled trials indicating efficacy for any Ayurvedic practice in the treatment of developmental-behavioral disorders. Caregivers of children with developmental disorders should actively avoid naturopathy, which comprises a number of suspect diagnostic and therapeutic approaches that lack experimental validation and often do not have acceptable biologic plausibility. There have been some efforts to study homeopathy (which is based on the theory that "like cures like" and that disease can be treated by the administration of extremely dilute solutions of various compounds) in ADHD and traumatic brain injury, although there is no replicated experimental evidence showing that these methods are effective in treating these or any other medical conditions.

Mind-Body Medicine

Techniques such as meditation, biofeedback, hypnosis, and prayer have all been used to try to treat disease or to improve physical and mental functioning. Electroencephalographic biofeedback has been promoted predominantly for the treatment of children with ADHD. In this technique, children try to learn to use brain electrical activity to control a video game–like interface, with the hope that this will improve attention in other settings. Although some early studies showed apparent effectiveness of this technique, criticisms have been raised about certain methodologic deficiencies. Electroencephalographic biofeedback remains under investigation, but it is not currently a recommended treatment approach for children with ADHD. Studies investigating relaxation training or other meditation techniques in children with ADHD, cerebral palsy, or intellectual disability have largely been equivocal or limited by methodologic issues, although short-term improvements in certain behavioral measures have been observed in some studies. Hypnosis has been proposed as a treatment modality for certain behavioral or learning disorders but has not been validated as an effective therapeutic approach.

Manipulative and Body-Based Practices

Body-based methods, including sensory integration therapy, massage, auditory integration training, and chiropractic manipulation, rely on physical manipulation or the application of other forces (such as sound) in an effort to achieve a specific therapeutic effect. The concept of sensory integration dysfunction, proposed by Jean Ayres in the 1970s, postulates that abnormal or inefficient functioning in various central nervous system sensory pathways lies at the root of many developmental and behavioral disorders. Although a variety of "sensory integration" techniques are commonly used by occupational therapists in the treatment of children with developmental and behavioral disorders (particularly autism spectrum disorders), there is a minimal body of research that supports their clinical utility (Schaaf and Miller, 2005). Better designed studies that clarify the role of these interventions are needed. Perhaps not surprisingly, massage may be associated with short-term behavioral benefits in children with various developmental disorders. There is not, however, convincing evidence that there are measurable developmental benefits of massage in preterm or low-birth-weight infants (Vickers et al, 2004). Auditory integration training is based on a theory that abnormal auditory perception is a cause of various behavioral features in children with autism. There have been several trials of auditory integration training in children with autism, but there is insufficient evidence to support its use (Sinha et al, 2006). Music therapy has some evidence of effectiveness in improving communication skills in children with autism, although the precise role of this therapy in clinical practice remains unclear (Gold et al, 2006). There is extremely scant evidence to support the use of optometric visual training as a treatment for learning or behavior disorders, and the ophthalmology and pediatric communities do not endorse this approach. Craniosacral therapy and chiropractic manipulation (which may be particularly risky in children with certain conditions, such as Down syndrome) have highly questionable scientific bases and have no role in developmental-behavioral pediatrics.

Energy Medicine

Energy therapies are based on the theory that energy fields ("biofields") are present around all living organisms and that a disruption in these fields is a cause of disease. Manipulation of these fields by use of various techniques restores "balance" and therefore health. Ancient practices such as acupuncture, Qigong, and Reiki as well as practices of more recent origin (such as therapeutic touch) are based in these beliefs. Although there is limited evidence that acupuncture is effective in the treatment of certain pain syndromes in adults, studies of acupuncture in children with developmental disorders have typically been uncontrolled or have had ill-defined or unreliable outcome measures. Therapeutic touch, which involves a practitioner's purportedly manipulating the "biofield" by performing smoothing movements above the body, is meant to balance the nonphysical "life energy" and restore the body to a state of good health. There is no experimental evidence supporting the existence of biofields that can be manually detected and manipulated, and any measurable benefit of these therapies is likely to be derived from various expectancy effects. Therapeutic touch and other forms of energy medicine are good examples of pseudoscientific therapies, largely because of their significant lack of connection to other areas of scientific knowledge.

Biologically Based Therapies

Biologic interventions constitute the largest group of CAM therapies that have been used in children with developmental and behavioral disorders. Although these approaches are inherently more plausible than many CAM therapies (and there is a long tradition in medicine of effective pharmaceuticals being derived from botanical agents), experimental evidence of effectiveness is weak for most of these interventions.

The use of vitamins, minerals, and other supplements (so-called orthomolecular treatments) in the treatment of various disorders became popular in the 1970s. In children with ADHD, placebo-controlled trials of various supplements have not confirmed the initially positive results reported in anecdotes and uncontrolled studies. Various vitamins, minerals, probiotics, antifungals, and immunologic agents have also been used widely in children with autism (Levy and Hyman, 2005). A number of trials of vitamin B_6 and magnesium treatment have been published, although most had significant methodologic shortcomings. The best available data do not support the combined use of vitamin B_6 and magnesium in the treatment of autism (Nye and Brice, 2006). Melatonin has been used as a treatment for sleep disorders in children with developmental disabilities, and there is some evidence to support this use (Jan and Freeman, 2004). Open label trials suggest that melatonin may be effective in shortening sleep latency in children with autism, although controlled trials are not available in this population. Omega-3 fatty acids have also received considerable interest as a supplement in both typically developing children and in children with developmental disorders. There is no conclusive evidence to suggest a beneficial effect of omega-3 fatty acids on developmental outcome in children or in the treatment of specific psychiatric conditions (Lewin et al, 2005; Schachter et al, 2005), although this area remains under investigation. There are no supplements currently accepted as safe and effective in the treatment of autism spectrum disorders (American Academy of Pediatrics, Committee on Children with Disabilities, 2001b).

Dietary interventions also have a long history in the field of developmental disabilities. The diet that has gained the most popularity in children with autism has been the gluten- and casein-free diet. This approach is based on the unproved and improbable hypothesis that peptides derived from gluten and casein cross into the bloodstream from the gastrointestinal tract and exert a central nervous system effect that leads to the behavioral features seen in autism. There have been several trials of this diet in children with autism (Millward et al, 2006). One controlled trial of this diet had certain methodologic limitations, including the fact that parents were not blinded to group assignment (Knivsberg et al, 2002). The gluten- and casein-free diet is currently not a validated treatment for children with autism, although an NIH-funded study is in progress. Controlled trials of the Feingold diet, which is based on the hypothesis that various food additives are the cause of hyperactive behavior, have not shown consistent benefit in children with ADHD. Oligoantigenic diets, which arose from a theory that ADHD is caused by a food allergy–mediated mechanism, have also been promoted as a therapeutic option. There are six clinical trials of oligoantigenic diets in ADHD between 1985 and 1997 in the Cochrane Central Register of Controlled Trials—any observed positive effect of this dietary approach does not appear to be robust and may occur only in a subset of children.

Hyperbaric oxygen therapy for children with cerebral palsy and other disorders developed a great deal of popularity in the 1990s and remains popular in some geographic locales. Promoters of this intervention contend that oxygen delivered at high concentration and pressure can revive dormant brain tissue adjacent to areas of previous injury. There is insufficient evidence to determine whether hyperbaric oxygen treatment improves functional outcome in children with cerebral palsy (McDonagh et al, 2003), and its use in the treatment of developmental-behavioral disorders cannot be endorsed.

Concern about the possibility of a toxic environmental trigger in the etiology of developmental disorders (primarily autism) has led to an increase in the use of chelation therapy, in which various drugs are used to remove heavy metals from the body. The contention that heavy metals play any causal role in autism is based on exceedingly flimsy evidence, and there have been no published clinical trials of chelation in autism. An NIH study of chelation in children with autism was recently suspended due to safety concerns. As potentially serious risks of toxicity are known (Brown et al, 2006), chelation should be actively avoided in the absence of a valid indication (such as lead poisoning).

PLACEBO AND OTHER EXPECTANCY EFFECTS

In 1998, following the publication of a small case series that reported improvement in certain language and social features in three children with autism who had undergone endoscopy, a sudden and explosive interest developed in the gastrointestinal hormone secretin as a therapeutic agent for the treatment of autism. Fueled by uncritical Internet and mainstream media hype, thousands of children with autism were treated with secretin prior to any organized attempts to demonstrate its safety and efficacy. The medical research community was compelled to establish an evidence base after the use of secretin had already become widespread. Numerous randomized controlled trials subsequently failed to show that secretin is any more effective than placebo in improving language or behavioral functioning in children with autism (Sturmey, 2005).

Why would a parent believe that secretin is responsible for improving a child's developmental and behavioral functioning when evidence of this cannot be demonstrated in a controlled trial? Why do many people believe in the power of various nonstandard therapies when there is a similar lack of objective evidence of effectiveness? Questions such as these have led to resurgence in interest in the placebo response and other expectancy effects as topics of legitimate scientific inquiry.

The "placebo effect" should not be viewed as a single phenomenon, as a number of diverse psychological and nonpsychological factors can contribute to the false appearance of treatment efficacy. Multiple factors associated with treatment response have been subsumed under the umbrella of placebo effects, including patient and clinician attributes, expectancy effects, participation effects, conditioning phenomena, and biologic effects (Sandler, 2005). Although the reality of an inherent placebo effect has been challenged (Hrobjartsson and Gotzsche, 2004), notable responses to placebo have consistently been observed in clinical trials for disorders in which outcome measures are often subjective (such as depression or pain). An additional layer of complexity is introduced in trials of children with developmental disabilities, as often the outcomes are being measured indirectly (i.e., through caregiver report of behavior change). Consequently, the phenomena considered part of the placebo "effect" have the potential to operate on parental behavior and perception, in addition to any effect on the child. CAM therapies, which have rarely been subject to rigorous scientific scrutiny, are likely to acquire the appearance of effectiveness as a result of these expectancy effects. Open label trials of any therapy in children with conditions such as autism are likely to overestimate the true efficacy of the intervention, and the results should be viewed with caution. The randomized, blinded, controlled trial remains the best tool we have for determining whether a therapy has specific beneficial effects.

Although the value of placebos in the research setting is widely accepted, it is much less clear whether placebos have any therapeutic role in modern clinical medicine. Some proponents of nonstandard therapies suggest that it does not matter if a treatment is biologically inert; what matters is that benefits are realized. Can family- and patient-centered care be based on a fundamental deception? Should children be subjected to ineffective therapies if the main benefit resides in parental perception of improvement in some aspect of the child's functioning? An argument has been made that a role for placebos in the treatment of children with developmental disorders might be possible (Sandler, 2005), although the scientific merits and ethical implications of this idea will require further analysis and debate.

In one of the first published controlled trials of secretin in children with autism (Sandler et al, 1999), 30% of the participants in both the secretin and placebo groups exhibited improvement (by parent and teacher observation) in several behavioral and communication features. Amazingly, a high percentage of parents continued to express an interest in secretin as a therapy for their children even after they were informed of the negative results of the study. When belief is strong in the potential power of a therapy, or if the treatment simply provides some hope of benefit, caregivers may dismiss even overwhelming contrary evidence. In Bronislaw Malinowski's anthropologic study of Trobriand Islanders, environmental conditions that resulted in increased danger or uncertainty (and higher levels of anxiety) led to an increase in magical thinking (Malinowski, 1954, p 139). In developmental disorders, causes can be obscure and outcomes uncertain—contributing to an environment in which caregivers are susceptible to the development of beliefs concerning causes and treatments that might be viewed as unscientific. Priority should therefore be given to interventions that reduce caregiver anxiety and uncertainty, through appropriate psychosocial supports as well as education about what is truly known about the etiology, potential outcomes, and best treatments of a developmental disorder.

COUNSELING FAMILIES ABOUT COMPLEMENTARY AND ALTERNATIVE THERAPIES

All consumers of health care should be able to evaluate evidence critically, understand the methods of science, and recognize pseudoscience. Parents of children with developmental and behavioral disorders need to be particularly adept at analyzing treatment claims to determine whether a particular therapy is valid. Pediatricians and other health care providers have an obligation to provide families with practical approaches they can use to interpret the multitude of theories and therapies they will encounter on the Internet and in the media—surely this should be a fundamental element of family-centered care. Although an appropriate amount of respect has to be accorded to the choices that parents make about the interventions they pursue for their children, health care providers have a responsibility to provide accurate, evidenced-based guidance to help shape their decisions.

When counseling families of children with disabilities about complementary and alternative therapies, providers need to be informed about various nonstandard practices, critically analyze the merits of specific therapies, identify potential risks of different treatments, provide education about different therapeutic options, and stress the importance of studying nonstandard practices by rigorous scientific methodology (American Academy of Pediatrics, Committee on Children with Disabilities, 2001a). Providers should avoid criticizing particular practices in a manner that suggests a lack of concern about the family's perspective and beliefs. However, these guidelines should not be interpreted as a mandate for health care practitioners to adopt a neutral stance when discussing CAM with families. Parents are often bombarded with misinformation from multiple directions, and health care providers should not abdicate their responsibility to fight just as vigorously to educate families with use of information based in science. Those who aspire to practice scientific medicine should also not be afraid to challenge promoters of unproved and implausible remedies to produce evidence to support their claims.

Although the most philosophically defensible position to take in the discussion of CAM practices with families is one of unwavering skepticism, care must be taken to preserve the provider-family relationship and remain compassionate. Certain adjustments in the counseling approach may need to be made, depending on which specific therapy is being considered and in what context. Therapies that are potentially plausible but insufficiently tested should not be endorsed but may merit more rigorous scientific testing to prove or disprove their worth. There is always the possibility that a therapy currently viewed as CAM will acquire sufficient evidence to be considered safe and effective—such a therapy should move into the realm of accepted medical practice (although history suggests that this is truly an uncommon occurrence). "N of 1" trials (blinded, single-patient controlled trials with multiple crossovers) have been suggested as a means of exploring the value of nonstandard treatments in individual patients in a more rational fashion, although these can be difficult to perform with the appropriate rigor within the constraints of a typical clinical practice. Strongest opposition should be directed against implausible remedies that are being promoted as medicine but are fundamentally pseudoscientific. A more tolerant approach is acceptable in regard to those practices that are more appropriately viewed as part of a religious belief or cultural tradition important to the family and pose low risk.

Health care providers need to remain informed about the evidence base for various CAM therapies and potential risks that might be associated with particular treatments. That a therapy is generally safe is not, by itself, sufficient justification to support its use. Likewise, the fact (often used in fallacious *tu quoque* arguments by CAM proponents) that adverse effects can occur in conventional medical interventions does not diminish the direct and indirect risks that are recognized for some nonstandard therapies. Even a small chance of harm is unacceptable if a treatment is worthless. Risks of CAM therapies can include toxic effects of biologic agents or manipulative techniques, interference with appropriate nutrition, and interruption or postponement of valid therapies as well as the indirect hazards of financial and time burdens (which can be substantial). Alternative medicine practitioners may also foster attitudes against medical practices, such as vaccination, that are known to be effective. Health care providers need to be aware that there may be liability implications if they endorse unsubstantiated therapies known to be potentially harmful or develop supervisory relationships with CAM providers (Cohen and Kemper, 2005).

The distinction between "science" and "pseudoscience" can be ill-defined and is best viewed as a continuum that has as much to do with the approach (or lack thereof) practitioners of the therapy take in building an evidence base as it does with the nature of the therapy itself. As such, it is not always easy for families, health care providers, and other professionals to distinguish between a potentially valid therapy and one that is pseudoscientific. Skepticism and critical thinking skills should be fostered in all those who are concerned with the welfare of children. These skills can be as helpful in the analysis of mainstream medical practices as they are in the evaluation of CAM therapies. At the same time, care should be taken to guard against the reflexive rejection of all new ideas (itself a stance that can be as detrimental as uncritical acceptance).

A number of characteristic features can be recognized as warning signs that a particular therapy is questionable. The following questions can help families and health care providers recognize treatment claims that may be pseudoscientific (adapted from Nickel, 1996, and Lilienfeld et al, 2003):

Is the therapy based on an overly simplistic theory, or is it reported to be curative? Developmental disorders are complex in causality and neurobiology, and we should be rightfully suspicious of treatments that are promoted as quick fixes or magic bullets.

Is the treatment reported to have no potential side effects? Such a claim (which can be misleading) is often a marketing tool used to promote generally innocuous but ineffective therapies.

Is the treatment claim testable? Do proponents attempt to explain away contradictory evidence and try to preserve an original theory by using layers of additional hypotheses, without efforts to consider alternative (and simpler) explanations? A claim that is not potentially falsifiable falls outside the realm of science.

Has the treatment evolved over time in response to new evidence? Therapies that remain unchanged for decades or centuries (a characteristic viewed as desirable by the promoters of some therapies) have not undergone the process of self-correction that is an essential element of scientific medicine.

Have studies of the treatment been published in the peer-reviewed medical literature? What is the quality of these studies? Purported evidence of effectiveness of a therapy must be available for scrutiny by members of the scientific community; this is one of the fundamental error-correcting mechanisms of science.

Do proponents of the treatment selectively seek evidence that confirms the effectiveness of the therapy and ignore contradictory data? This confirmation bias is a common feature of pseudoscientific claims. Science is a double-edged sword—we must be as willing to reject treatments and theories in the face of appropriate evidence as we are to accept them.

Do proponents suggest that it is acceptable to assume the treatment is effective until proven otherwise? As shown by the example of secretin, widespread use of a therapy before the development of evidence of effectiveness does occur and represents an unnatural reversal in the normal direction of the scientific process.

Does the treatment appear to be disconnected from knowledge in other scientific disciplines? Is the treatment based on new forces or principles that are inconsistent with our current understanding of the natural world? Therapies that are based on such unverified forces (therapeutic touch) have extremely low *prima facie* plausibility; a high level of evidence should be demanded before such claims are believed.

Is the treatment promoted primarily through the use of anecdotes and testimonials as opposed to a body of evidence from controlled trials? The high rate of placebo response in trials of autism therapies shows that we should not make broad extrapolations from the observation of a single child's response to a treatment. Therapies that are supported only by anecdote should be viewed with skepticism.

Is the treatment described in scientific-sounding jargon that on closer analysis is very imprecise or meaningless? Such language is commonly used to hide the fact that a true scientific basis for the therapy is lacking.

Are claims made that the treatment is effective for a wide range of conditions? A single intervention can rarely if ever effectively treat diverse conditions with disparate pathophysiologic mechanisms.

Are claims made that the treatment can be viewed only as part of a larger package of interventions and practices? This can be a ploy used to obstruct the scientific analysis of a claim or to explain away evidence of ineffectiveness.

SUMMARY

Nonstandard therapies are commonly used in children with various chronic health conditions, particularly in those disorders in which conventional treatment approaches are not dramatically effective. Currently, there is no accepted role for virtually any CAM therapy in developmental-behavioral pediatrics. Health care providers and families must recognize that various expectancy effects can contribute to the appearance of CAM treatment efficacy, and all proposed therapies must be held to high standards of scientific evidence before being accepted as worthwhile. Parents of children with developmental and behavioral disorders should be encouraged to evaluate evidence critically and learn to recognize the characteristic features that indicate a particular theory or therapy may be pseudoscientific.

REFERENCES

American Academy of Pediatrics, Committee on Children with Disabilities: Counseling families who choose complementary and alternative medicine for their child with chronic illness or disability [published erratum appears in Pediatrics 108:507, 2001]. Pediatrics 107:598-601, 2001a.

American Academy of Pediatrics, Committee on Children with Disabilities: The pediatrician's role in the diagnosis and management of autistic spectrum disorder in children. Pediatrics 107:1221–1226, 2001b.

Angell M, Kassirer JP: Alternative medicine—the risks of untested and unregulated remedies. N Engl J Med 339:839-841, 1998.

Barnes PM, Powell-Griner E, McFann K, Nahin RL: Complementary and alternative medicine use among adults: United States, 2002. Advance Data 343:1-19, 2004.

Brown MJ, Willis T, Omalu B, Leiker R: Deaths resulting from hypocalcemia after administration of edetate disodium: 2003-2005. Pediatrics 118:e534-536, 2006.

Challman TD: Complementary and alternative medicine in autism—promises kept? *In* Shapiro BK, Accardo PJ (eds): Autism Frontiers. Baltimore, Brookes, 2008, pp 177-190.

Challman TD, Voigt RG, Myers SM: Nonstandard therapies. *In* Accardo PJ (ed): Capute and Accardo's Neurodevelopmental Disabilities in Infancy and Childhood, 3rd ed. Baltimore, Brookes, 2007, pp 721-741.

Cohen MH, Kemper KJ: Complementary therapies in pediatrics: A legal perspective. Pediatrics 115:774-780, 2005.

Davis MP, Darden PM: Use of complementary and alternative medicine by children in the United States. Arch Pediatr Adolesc Med 157:393-396, 2003.

Eisenberg DM, Davis RB, Ettner SL, et al: Trends in alternative medicine use in the United States, 1990-1997: Results of a follow-up national survey. JAMA 280:1569-1575, 1998.

Gold C, Wigram T, Elefant C: Music therapy for autistic spectrum disorder. Cochrane Database Syst Rev 2: CD004381, 2006.

Hrobjartsson A, Gotzsche PC: Placebo interventions for all clinical conditions. Cochrane Database Syst Rev 3: CD003974, 2004.

Jan JE, Freeman RD: Melatonin therapy for circadian rhythm sleep disorders in children with multiple disabilities: What have we learned in the last decade? Dev Med Child Neurol 46:776-782, 2004.

Knivsberg AM, Reichelt KL, Hoien T, Nodland M: A randomised, controlled study of dietary intervention in autistic syndromes. Nutr Neurosci 5:251-261, 2002.

Levy SE, Hyman SL: Novel treatments for autistic spectrum disorders. Ment Retard Dev Disabil Res Rev 11:131-142, 2005.

Lewin GA, Schachter HM, Yuen D, et al: Effects of omega-3 fatty acids on child and maternal health. Evid Rep Technol Assess (Summ) 118:1-11, 2005.

Lilienfeld SO, Lynn SJ, Lohr JM: (eds): Science and Pseudoscience in Clinical Psychology. New York, Guilford, 2003.

Malinowski B: Magic, Science, and Religion: And Other Essays. Garden City, NY, Doubleday Anchor Books, 1954.

McDonagh M, Carson S, Ash J: Hyperbaric Oxygen Therapy for Brain Injury, Cerebral Palsy, and Stroke. Evidence Report/Technology Assessment No. 85. Rockville, MD, Agency for Healthcare Research and Quality, 2003. AHRQ publication 04-E003.

Mencken HL: Prejudices: Second Series. New York, Knopf, 1920.

Millward C, Ferriter M, Calver S, Connell-Jones G: Gluten- and casein-free diets for autistic spectrum disorder. Cochrane Database Syst Rev 2: CD003498, 2006.

National Center for Complementary and Alternative Medicine: Expanding horizons of healthcare: Five year strategic plan 2001-2005. Washington, DC, U.S. Department of Health and Human Services, 2000.

Nickel R: Controversial therapies for young children with developmental disabilities. Infants Young Child 8:29-40, 1996.

Nye C, Brice A: Combined vitamin B_6–magnesium treatment in autism spectrum disorder. Cochrane Database Syst Rev 4: CD003497, 2006.

Sandler A: Placebo effects in developmental disabilities: Implications for research and practice. Ment Retard Dev Disabil Res Rev 11:164-170, 2005.

Sandler AD, Sutton KA, DeWeese J, et al: Lack of benefit of a single dose of synthetic human secretin in the treatment of autism and pervasive developmental disorder. N Engl J Med 341:1801-1806, 1999.

Schaaf RC, Miller LJ: Occupational therapy using a sensory integrative approach for children with developmental disabilities. Ment Retard Dev Disabil Res Rev 11:143-148, 2005.

Schachter HM, Kourad K, Merali Z, et al: Effects of omega-3 fatty acids on mental health. Evid Rep Technol Assess (Summ) 116: 1-11, 2005.

Sinha Y, Silove N, Wheeler D, Williams K: Auditory integration training and other sound therapies for autism spectrum disorders: A systematic review. Arch Dis Child 91:1018-1022, 2006.

Sturmey P: Secretin is an ineffective treatment for pervasive developmental disabilities: A review of 15 double-blind randomized controlled trials. Res Dev Disabil 26:87-97, 2005.

Tang JL, Zhan SY, Ernst E: Review of randomised controlled trials of traditional Chinese medicine. BMJ 319:160-161, 1999.

Vickers A, Ohlsson A, Lacy JB, Horsley A: Massage for promoting growth and development of preterm and/or low birth-weight infants. Cochrane Database Syst Rev 2: CD000390, 2004.

96 TRANSITION TO ADULTHOOD FOR YOUTH WITH DEVELOPMENTAL DISABILITIES

MELISSA THINGVOLL AND STEPHEN SULKES

Vignette

Elmer, a 19-year-old man with athetotic cerebral palsy and mild intellectual disability, is brought to the pediatrician by his parents because he is increasingly having emotional outbursts at home with his family. They became extremely concerned when he pushed his sister through a first-floor window. Elmer had left his self-contained school program a year before and has been working in a supported employment setting, making cardboard boxes. His health has been stable, with no seizures or other chronic medical problems and no sleep or appetite problems. He uses no medications, tobacco, alcohol, or other drugs. He is ambulatory but with fine and gross motor coordination limitations related to his athetosis.

As part of the evaluation, the pediatrician asks the parents to leave the room so he can speak in private with Elmer. Once confidentiality is ensured, the youth reveals that his closest relationships are with staff members at his workplace and family friends without disabilities. He socializes only with his family. He describes having strong attractions for several female workplace staff. He obtained their phone numbers and called them often and then was disappointed when they didn't reciprocate his affections. He becomes agitated in describing these frustrations and confirms that his outbursts at home had been in relation to them. Elmer also has sexually related frustrations. When asked about masturbation, he blushed deeply and said, "You can't do that, you make a mess!" He explains that on one occasion, when masturbating in bed, he had experienced a bowel movement at the moment of orgasm, and he assumed that this would happen every time in the future. On physical examination, he is a slim young man with several days' growth of beard. His speech is dysarthric, and he has difficulty with saliva overflow.

How can the pediatrician assist Elmer and his family with his outbursts and also support his transition to adulthood?

Transition from childhood to adulthood can be exciting, confusing, and stressful for all adolescents and their families, but this process is often more difficult for adolescents and young adults with developmental disabilities and special health care needs. The adolescent not only must deal with the increase in responsibility and the expectation for autonomy that come with this rite of passage, but he or she must do so in the context of a physical or cognitive disability. This move into the adult community occurs across many different areas, as the adolescent moves from the pediatric to adult-oriented health care system, from school to workplace, and from home to community living.

Transition has become an increasingly important topic during the last several years as the number of adolescents and young adults with developmental disabilities has grown. With advances in neonatal intensive care and medical technology and greater understanding of their health needs, children who were previously expected to die before adolescence now live long into adult years. Currently, nearly 90% of children with special health care needs survive to adulthood (Betz and Redcay, 2002). Changes in disability culture, exemplified by the passage of the Americans with Disabilities Act (ADA) in 1990, have increased expectations for community participation by young adults with disabilities. As described in Chapter 1, our society has moved from isolation and institutionalization of people with disabilities to integration into the schools, the workforce, the health care setting, and the community at large.

This chapter reviews current practices and issues of transition from adolescence to adulthood for individuals with developmental disabilities. In providing an outline of the various aspects of transition, with some examples of successful transition practices, this chapter can help professionals create a systematic, comprehensive, and interdisciplinary transition plan for those adolescents and families under their care who need guidance during a time of significant change and new experiences in their lives.

HEALTH CARE TRANSITION

As individuals enter adulthood, their health care services need to change to remain age appropriate as part of the expected developmental progress that all adolescents must make. However, this transition is often far more difficult for those with special health care needs (Scal, 2002). As the number of adolescents with developmental disabilities and special health care needs has grown dramatically during the last few decades, the importance of the process of moving from pediatric to adult-centered health care has increased as well.

Conferences in 1989 and 1999 began to characterize the need for developmentally and medically appropriate health care for the growing population of young adults with special health care needs, to outline the issues facing young adults during their move into the adult medical world, and to develop an action plan for successful transition (Reiss and Gibson, 2002). The Maternal and Child Health Bureau has established health care transition as one of its priorities to ensure that "comprehensive community-based service systems are in place for all children and youth with special health care needs" by the year 2010 (Blum, 2002).

As they approach transition, adolescents and their families face several barriers and challenges, outlined in Table 96-1. Young adults with special health care needs require developmentally appropriate health services commensurate with their age and emerging autonomy. Pediatricians, who lack knowledge of adult health care issues and who are attempting to aid the transition of their young adult patients, report not knowing to whom to refer them for knowledgeable ongoing care (Betz and Redcay, 2002). Adult health care providers may lack knowledge of the developmental disabilities system, specific disability conditions, and available services to provide adequate care to meet the needs of youth with special health care needs (Reiss and Gibson, 2002). Individuals and families feel "lost in the shuffle," needing to find and personally coordinate care from multiple service providers in several different settings.

Services for children with special health care needs are often family centered and interdisciplinary, coordinating care across service systems. Adult health care is comparatively more individual focused, presuming that individuals will advocate and coordinate services for themselves. Families may feel ignored or unnecessary, and individuals may feel confused or insecure (Reiss et al, 2005). Adult providers cite lack of time and poor reimbursement as barriers to their accepting these patients into their practices (Scal, 2002). Adult mental health providers may also be ill prepared to provide care and counseling to young adults with disabilities (see Chapter 49). Shared training, communication, and expertise between pediatric and adult health care providers is often limited, particularly when subspecialty expertise for pediatric patients is housed in separate children's hospitals (Reiss and Gibson, 2002). Individuals and families (Reiss et al, 2005) and pediatricians (Reiss and Gibson, 2002) are reluctant to sacrifice the comfort and familiarity of their relationship and are apprehensive about and lack confidence in new, unfamiliar physicians. Youths with developmental disabilities and their families report feeling "dropped" by their pediatric providers when they turn 21. Families unprepared for transition report anxiety and reluctance to take the next step.

Access to health insurance is another crucial aspect of the transition to adult-centered health care for youth with special health care needs. Family-based insurance coverage available to children and adolescents is typically age limited, ending at the age of 19 to 23 years, depending on the state, and one in five young adults aged 19 to 29 years with a disability is uninsured (White, 2002). Aging out may lead to a change to a less comprehensive plan or loss of coverage altogether, in turn creating barriers to individuals seeking necessary health care and their ability or willingness to comply with suggested treatment plans because of lack of financial means. Eighty percent of adults with severe disabilities younger than 65 years use Medicaid or Medicare for their health insurance. Although some children with disabilities also receive Supplemental Security Income (SSI), up to 74% of children with severe medical conditions on Medicaid do not receive it. Low-income children with disabilities may lose their Medicaid coverage once they become adults if they do not also meet SSI criteria. Moreover, youths who received SSI as children must requalify for benefits at the age of 18 years; up to 30% of these individuals lose SSI and Medicaid eligibility at this time (White, 2002). Medicare may also be an insurance resource for people with disabilities, but a waiting period is required before coverage begins, and plans are usually more restrictive for covered services. Private insurance covers about two thirds of children with disabilities, although many are "underinsured" in that their plans are limited in the scope of coverage. Children with special health care needs, covered under their parents' private insurance plans, may lose coverage as adults. Although insurance laws in most states require ongoing coverage for adults with developmental disabilities under their parents' policies if desired, families have to make (and often re-make) the case of their members' lack of independent insurability to access coverage. Moreover, many young adults with special health care needs are unemployed, work part time, or work for small employers whose insurance premiums are prohibitively expensive. Individuals with disabilities can attempt to obtain insurance coverage from the unregulated individual insurance market but may encounter coverage

Table 96-1. Barriers to Successful Health Care Transition

Barrier	Contributing Cause	Response
Provider Factors		
Lack of pediatric provider knowledge of generic adult health problems	Limited training of pediatricians	Enhance residency and continuing medical education training on transition
Pediatric provider resistance to "letting go"	Same as above	Same as above
Lack of pediatric provider knowledge of adult resources	Lack of resource knowledge	Developmental disabilities system supports
Lack of adult provider knowledge of generic issues of developmental disabilities	Limited training of adult-focused providers	Specific residency and continuing medical education training activities
Adult provider confusion on age-appropriate versus developmentally appropriate care (support versus autonomy)	Same as above	Same as above
Lack of adult provider knowledge of specific conditions with childhood onset	Same as above	Same as above
Lack of interdisciplinary supports in adult health care environments (e.g., social work)	"Individual-focused" care, limited to health issues in isolation	Developmental disabilities system supports
Relative lack of coordinated care as found in pediatric settings	Same as above	Same as above
Family and Developmental Disabilities Service System Factors		
Family and staff desire for ongoing involvement in care	Perceived needs of patient; persistent infantilization of individual	Counseling and support of families and staff about self-determination
Perceived lack of individual autonomy or self-direction ability, leading to difficulty "letting go"	Same as above	Same as above
Paperwork demands	Governmental regulations	Standardized forms and rules across providers
Bureaucratic impediments	Same as above	Same as above
Individual Factors		
Communication barriers	Disability-specific needs	Spend extra time needed to allow adequate communication, incorporate others in appointments, use simplified educational materials, and code for time
Anxiety and health care environment behavior problems	Unfamiliarity with new environments	Same as above
Lack of personal health care knowledge	Cognitive limitations, previous lack of involvement in personal health care	Same as above
Health Care Environment Factors		
Need for extra time	Need to adapt to above individual factors	Current Procedural Terminology (CPT) coding based on time
Limited reimbursement: "graduation" from family-based insurance coverage to only Medicaid or lack of insurance	Limited reimbursements	Code based on time, consider managed care programs
Need for physical accessibility in health environment	Traditional expectation of individual skills (should not be a problem if geriatric accessibility adaptations are in place)	Americans with Disabilities Act accessibility consultation and residence visit models

denial (sometimes because their disability conditions are characterized as "preexisting"), benefit limits, and high surcharges (White, 2002).

Strategies to overcome some of these challenges have been found, and work is needed to overcome additional barriers. Transition processes should start early in adolescence, encouraging youths and their families to think about goals and expectations for adulthood long before transition age approaches. Medical independence and self-advocacy should be promoted at each visit (Reiss et al, 2005). Anticipating changes in medical care, insurance coverage, and services before they occur in young adulthood removes anxiety and helps people to feel prepared and comfortable. Although age often determines when transition occurs, not every person is prepared to move on at the same time. It is important to assess the readiness of the individual and family before successful transition can occur. Ideally, people should clearly understand their disabilities and medical needs and have a functional knowledge of the health care system and how to access necessary services. Planning visits specifically to provide education about the person's disability condition and medications and an instructional physical examination are ideal opportunities to foster independence and self-advocacy skills.

Lack of communication between pediatric and adult providers has often been cited as a major barrier to transition. Organized, comprehensive health history summaries can help adult providers feel comfortable in taking on new patients with complex needs. A team meeting including the individual, family, and pediatric and adult health care providers to review this health summary promotes a smooth transition. One sample document, equally applicable in childhood and adult life, has been created by the American Academies of Pediatrics and Emergency Medicine (*www.aap.org/advocacy/eif.doc*). The special demands of health care for the person with functional limitations can be more adequately reimbursed by coding based on time rather than on tasks performed.

Health care transitions should be recognized and celebrated as rites of passage marking important milestones in young adults' lives. Termination of the relationship between the patient and pediatrician is an emotional and often difficult process for all involved. "Graduation" ceremonies, certificates of completion, and opportunities to say good-bye are important measures that can help affirm young adults' feelings of maturity and personal responsibility, allow therapeutic closure, and create a positive sense of confidence as they move on to the adult health care system.

Finally, major policy changes will be necessary to provide adequate health insurance coverage to youth with developmental disabilities and special health care needs.

SEXUALITY

Like all adolescents, teens with disabilities want to marry, have children, and experience healthy and fulfilling adult sex lives. However, sexuality issues are often overlooked or ignored for them (see Chapter 43). People with disabilities are often viewed as childlike or asexual or, alternatively, as inappropriate or uncontrollably hypersexual, leading to misconceptions or misinformation (Murphy and Elias, 2006). Sexuality is often inappropriately considered inaccessible for individuals with physical disabilities.

For many youths with developmental and physical disabilities, barriers exist to discussion of the age-appropriate topics listed in Table 96-2. Physicians may need to spend a majority of health visits addressing the more complex functional or medical issues facing the person with a disability, leaving little time to explore issues of sexuality. Many special education curricula, unlike those of general education programs, do not include formal sexual education as required components (Stinson et al, 2002). When sex education is provided, the specific learning characteristics of the adolescent may not be considered, resulting in poor comprehension of the material and information presented. Material must be explained concretely and specifically, without "medicalization" of information. Teachers may be embarrassed by having to be more graphic and to use more vernacular terminology than usual in their presentations. Parents who infantilize their adolescent with a disability, especially if there is continued need for support in basic self-care, may also ignore or minimize the importance of sexuality, hindering necessary education (Murphy and Elias, 2006). It is therefore key for health care providers to ask questions about sexuality in the confidential setting of the health care interaction. Questions must be raised frankly, concretely, and without value judgment.

The capacity for sexual consent must be determined in an individual with a disability. It is prudent for an adolescent with a disability to undergo psychological evaluation to explore this as part of the transition process into adulthood. No formal guidelines are established, but many factors are considered, including cognitive and problem solving abilities, reasoning skills, functional and adaptive skills, and "knowledge about the consequences and potential risks of specific sexual activity, understanding one's choice about whether or not to engage in sexual activity, and the ability to say 'no' or respond appropriately when someone else says 'no'" (Stinson et al, 2002).

Unfortunately, people with disabilities, especially women, are easy targets and are at a higher risk for sexual abuse than their typically developing peers. Nearly 80% of women with developmental disabilities report being sexually assaulted in their lifetimes, but fewer than half seek assistance from legal or treatment services (Murphy, 2005). Dependence on others for intimate care, multiple caregivers, limited self-advocacy ability, and relative weaknesses in judgment and social skills all contribute to this statistic.

Young women with disabilities need appropriate, accessible gynecologic care. However, health care providers may lack understanding and training in the field of developmental disabilities or be uncomfortable in providing care to this population. Some young women with disabilities may require sedation for gynecologic examinations, carrying additional risk and expense (Stinson et al, 2002).

Specific contraception issues must be considered in young adults with disabilities. Numerous medications, including antiepileptics and some psychotropics, may interfere with the efficacy of hormonal contraception, requiring adaptation of dosing regimens. Oral hormonal contraceptives may be beneficial in allowing predictable hormonal cycling when a young woman has behavioral symptoms associated with specific parts of the menstrual cycle. For others, suppression of ovulation by injected contraceptives such as medroxyprogesterone (Depo-Provera) or leuprolide (Lupron) can minimize the self-care and behavioral challenges sometimes associated with menstruation. However, ovulatory suppression is associated with long-term deficiencies in bone density, and appropriate monitoring should be in place. Longer acting oral preparations such as Seasonale provide estrogen-progesterone cycling but reduce frequency of menstruation to every 3 months. Individuals' fine motor skill deficits may limit the utility of barrier methods. People with latex allergy or sensitivity require alternative, non-latex barrier contraceptives, which may

Table 96-2. **Sexuality Topics to Discuss During Primary Care Visits**

Understanding of sexual development
Gender identity and orientation
Fantasy and masturbation
Social behavior
Contraception and pregnancy planning thoughts
Understanding and prevention of sexually transmitted disease
Recognition and prevention of victimization and sexual abuse
Physical disability and sexual function
Special needs in gynecologic care

not be as effective in preventing pregnancy or sexually transmitted disease.

Families, seeking to "protect" their members with developmental disabilities from the pregnancy consequences of unprotected intercourse, sometimes seek surgical sterilization. Although it is an option for rare individuals, sterilization is not reimbursable under Medicaid regulations and demands careful consideration. Nonbarrier contraception methods, including surgical sterilization, do not protect the individual from sexually transmitted disease and are not a substitute for "safe sex" teaching. Decision making should include individuals at whatever level possible, considering their attitudes and desires with regard to pregnancy and parenting (Murphy, 2005). Although there may be roles for contraceptive vasectomy or tubal ligation, contraception is not an indication for hysterectomy, oophorectomy, or orchiectomy. The associated surgical risks and hormonal impacts of these procedures far outweigh any benefits in the absence of usual indications for their use in nondisabled populations.

EDUCATION

In contrast to health care, procedures for planning for educational transition are well established, even if inconsistently applied. Chapter 93 outlines the Individuals with Disabilities Education Act (IDEA), which specifically identifies procedures for transition planning as students move out of school-based services at adulthood. Recent amendments to IDEA specifically pertain to the post-graduation transition, requiring involvement of the student in the general education curriculum, if possible; cooperative decision making and support among the student, parents, and school staff; and preparation of the student with a disability for employment and other post–high school outcomes. IDEA requires transition planning to begin by the age of 14 years, and individualized education program (IEP) documents must include statements of transition service needs from this age forward, creating an individualized high-school curriculum to help the student prepare for transition and achieve goals after graduation. By the age of 16 years, a statement of transition service needs is added, encompassing instructional services, community experiences, vocational evaluation, employment, and other adult-living activities that the student will need to ensure success on entering the adult world (NCSET 1, n.d.).

Transition planning works best with a team approach. The most important member of the team is the student, who should be as actively engaged as possible and who must be specifically invited to attend any IEP meetings in which transition will be discussed. Involving students in transition planning gives them opportunities to learn about their skills and the challenges they may face with learning, career, relationships, and independence in the context of their disability. They can gain necessary information about accommodations they will require and learn how to speak up and advocate for their own needs (NCSET 1, n.d.). IDEA also requires notification and invitation of parents and other agencies that will be serving the student. Parents contribute their long-term, intimate knowledge of their child's behaviors, interests, medical and developmental history, and family values. Other transition team members include general and special educators and service agencies outside of the school system, such as adult agency representatives, physicians, mental health workers, case managers, vocational rehabilitation counselors, employers, and residential facility staff (Johnson et al, 2005).

Under the requirements of IDEA and the No Child Left Behind Act of 2001, schools are experiencing increasing pressure to improve graduation rates for all students, including those with disabilities. Many states currently offer several diploma options as alternative means of graduating from high school. Beyond standard diplomas, these may include certificates of completion or achievement, IEP diplomas, and occupational diplomas (NCSET 2, 2002). For many students whose disabilities prevent their meeting the criteria for standard diplomas, alternative diplomas may be their only feasible route to graduation.

Many students with disabilities progress to postsecondary education (i.e., college). Students with disabilities who engage in formal transition planning are more likely to pursue postsecondary education than are those who have not (Halpern et al, 1995). Disability knowledge, knowledge of postsecondary support services, knowledge of disability legislation, and self-advocacy ability all facilitate effective college transition planning (Milsom and Hartley, 2005). Colleges and universities increasingly try to accommodate students with disabilities, in response to ADA concerns. Students with physical disabilities are more often provided physical access alterations than are students with cognitive or social disabilities, but even these are now becoming more common (Heath Center, 2002).

Several postsecondary education models, outlined in Table 96-3, exist to allow students with disabilities to achieve their goals of college participation (Stodden

Table 96-3. College Participation Education Models for Students with Developmental Disabilities (Stodden and Whelley, 2004)

Model	Learning Focus	Staffing	Limitation
Substantially separate	Functional life skills	Special education	Separate from general curriculum and social milieux
Mixed	Life skills and integrated college coursework	Special education and college staff	Increased interaction with individualized functional training
Individualized support	Regular college curriculum with IEP-like adaptations	College staff and developmental disabilities support	Maximal academic and social integration

IEP, individualized education program.

and Whelley, 2004). Unfortunately, financing of a postsecondary education is often even more difficult for students with disabilities than it is for other college students. Financial aid packages often require a minimum number of credits per semester, and work-study opportunities may be limited. Coordination of the many required supports and services from the institute of higher education and multiple other agencies is often a confusing and complicated task once IDEA entitlement ends (Stodden and Whelley, 2004).

VOCATIONAL TRANSITION

The school-to-work transition should be smooth because IDEA requires that vocational planning and prevocational training be built into all individualized educational planning. In fact, such planning is highly variable. Adolescents with more severe intellectual and physical disabilities may have school programs that focus well on self-care goals and provide some rudimentary prevocational skills but often do not prepare individuals for specific vocational tasks. Inclusive programs that emphasize academics for individuals with more functional skills may give short shrift to practical vocational independence.

Vocational rehabilitation is a state/federal program designed to empower individuals with disabilities to achieve employment consistent with their strengths, resources, and personal goals (Dowdy, 1996). The federal Rehabilitation Services Administration works with state vocational rehabilitation agencies to provide direct assistance to individuals with disabilities through local offices. Vocational rehabilitation counselors elicit information about the person's work history, education, training, strengths, interests, and goals to help the individual develop an individualized written rehabilitation program similar to a school-based IEP in its content and objectives. Vocational rehabilitation services may include counseling and work-related placement services, vocational and training services, transportation, assistive technology, and supported employment services. Collaboration between special education and vocational education personnel during high school can provide students with disabilities with comprehensive curricula that will help them achieve their adult goals (Stodden and Whelley, 2004). The Maternal and Child Health Bureau's Healthy and Ready to Work program has developed tools that incorporate input from school, health, family, workplace, and the individual to ensure appropriate vocational transitions (Maternal and Child Health Bureau, 2007; *www.hrtw.org/tools/check.html*). Other laws that affect the workplace for people with disabilities include the ADA and Section 504 of the federal Rehabilitation Act; both ensure accommodation and prevent discrimination (U.S. Department of Justice, 2005). Each state has its own system of vocational rehabilitation evaluation and placement agencies, listed by state at *https://secure.ssa.gov/apps10/oesp/providers.nsf/bystate*. A broad array of state-run agencies, publicly licensed nonprofit providers, and private employers exist in each community. Schools often work closely with such employers to provide their staffing needs, and public councils often exist to support employers in including individuals with disabilities in their work settings. The Ticket to Work Employment Network serves SSI recipients aged 18 to 64 years with employability services, supports, and incentives and provides schools supplemental school-to-work transition funds for students up to the age of 21 years (*www.socialsecurity.gov/work/youth.html*).

WHERE TO LIVE?

As young adults with developmental disabilities move toward graduation from IDEA-supported educational programs and into employment, questions arise for families about residential options. With the past decades' experience of community inclusion and noninstitutional care, families have become used to having their children with developmental disabilities continue to live at home with community help from health, educational, social services, and other support systems. Out-of-home residential placement for a child with developmental disabilities has become sufficiently stigmatized that when it occurs, it may carry an implication of parental inadequacy or of physical or behavioral challenge of such severity that parents should not be expected to be able to manage the child's care. Whereas in many cultures it is common for many generations to continue to live together throughout life, it is the widely held norm in industrialized nations for young adults to move into independent living as they pass into adulthood. In an effort to provide "normal" experiences and expectations for youth with developmental disabilities, discussion of plans to move to a new living environment and the supports needed to carry this out should be part of transition planning starting in the early teen years.

Although many individuals with developmental disabilities continue to live with their families (Braddock et al, 2001), a spectrum of residential options exists, with much variation among government entities, because most such facilities in the United States are either managed or licensed by state governments. Large residential institutions are fading from the scene, being replaced by community residences, small intermediate care facilities, supervised apartments, and other individualized living alternatives, extending even to home ownership. In some communities, groups of families work with public or private nonprofit agencies to establish staffed residences for their young adult members. Factors to consider in determining a person's level of residential independence include complexity of health and associated support needs, self-care skills, transportation skills, mobility, and other factors. Adult service coordinators help to individualize placement recommendations.

SELF-DETERMINATION AND AUTONOMY

People with developmental disabilities, like all other citizens, are considered legal adults at the age of 18 years. However, when families have grown used to providing supports for their children with developmental disabilities, they may have difficulty recognizing that it is normal for young adults to begin making decisions for themselves. Education laws like IDEA that allow

Table 96-4. **Legally Appointed Representative Models**

Model	Individual Capabilities and Needs	Legal Formalities	Individual and Partner Decision Making
Joint account/co-signator	Mostly independent; needs occasional help with finances	Simple forms through bank	Individual and supporter have equal say
Trusts	Mostly independent, needs help with long-term financial management	Legal forms through attorney	Unless written otherwise, trust rules supersede individual desires. Trustees do not necessarily have close relationships with individuals.
Health care proxy	Needs help with health care decisions	Legal forms through attorney	Proxy invoked when individual cannot make wishes known
Durable power of attorney	Needs help with almost all financial and contractual decisions	Legal forms through bank or attorney	Individual and supporter have equal say; supporter may act without individual's consent
Legal guardian	Needs help with almost all decisions	Court appointed	Guardian's opinion supersedes individual's; no guarantee of self-determination

young adults to continue to receive public school–based educational services through the age of 21 years compound this confusion. An analogy is that of the college student who depends on parents for support but is increasingly independent in behavior and self-care. The "helicopter parent," hovering over the young adult, overly ready to take care of problems, also applies to the family of the young adult with developmental disabilities. It is normal to make mistakes and learn from them; it is often particularly hard for parents of youth with developmental disabilities to allow this to happen.

Wehmeyer (2001) defines self-determination in people with developmental disabilities as "the attitudes and abilities required to act as the primary causal agent in one's life and to make choices regarding one's actions free from undue external influence or interference." Self-determination implies that individuals act autonomously and in a "self-realizing" manner and that behaviors are self-initiated, goal-oriented, and self-regulated. For youth with more severe cognitive disabilities, attempts to ensure self-determination may seem to create conflict with supportive, well-intentioned family members. This becomes particularly relevant when family members and individuals disagree, such as when educational, residential, social, and health care choices arise.

Although emerging from educational, vocational, and philosophical fields, self-determination affects medical decision making. Reflecting the ethical principle of autonomy, it implies that individuals should, if possible, make decisions for themselves. Assessing the capacity of people with developmental disabilities to make health care decisions based on adequate information can be frustrating for providers. Limitations in language, cognition, and understanding of the causes and implications of disease and issues of long-term benefit versus short-term inconvenience or discomfort can affect decisions. However, individuals should be assumed to be able to participate in health care decision making on their own behalf. Appropriate supports should be provided to support this except in the most urgent emergency situations. Health care proxy laws in most states allow specific designation of preferred health care decision makers (Powers et al, 1996).

Family members may want to consider pursuing court-appointed legal guardianship for the youth with developmental disabilities as the 18th birthday approaches. Protection and advocacy agencies for individuals with developmental disabilities exist in each state and territory under federal law. They can ensure free legal representation for individuals with developmental disabilities and their families to help negotiate the legal processes around guardianship and other self-determination issues. Particularly with regard to guardianship proceedings, it is desirable for the individual to have personal legal representation to ensure that his or her rights are being considered separately from those of even the most well meaning families. A list of federally funded protection and advocacy agencies in each state for additional support can be found at *http://www.acf.hhs.gov/programs/add/states/pas.html*. Variations on legally appointed representatives for individuals with developmental disabilities are described in Table 96-4.

Each state defines guardianship differently, but usually court-appointed guardians can make all official decisions on behalf of individuals. Ideal guardians make decisions honoring individuals' wishes based on good communication; but legally, appointment of a guardian eliminates guarantees of self-determination. Families may establish trusts or other financial instruments as financial supports for their members with developmental limitations, assigning contingent trustees to serve if family members cannot fulfill these responsibilities as the person with disability matures. The family's philosophy and the goal of optimizing the individual's self-determination should be made clear to all. Families should seek legal and financial counsel about laws and procedures in their state, given their needs, resources, and desires.

VIGNETTE OUTCOME

The pediatrician decides to handle some of the issues at the current visit and to then help the family plan a transition to an adult health care provider. The pediatrician counsels Elmer in private that masturbation can take place on the toilet, or he can evacuate his bowels before masturbating. He also discusses drooling with Elmer and gains Elmer's consent to discuss this issue with his parents. The pediatrician deems it inappropriate to advise him on whom he should choose for friends but encourages him to find social friends with whom he shares interests. Although Elmer likes to make friends at his workplace, the pediatrician gets him to recognize that his supervisors are friendly to him but might be prohibited by company rules from developing more intimate relationships.

With the parents back in the room, the pediatrician briefly counsels about Elmer's outbursts as related to emerging adult issues and then focuses the discussion on the need for Elmer to find an adult health care provider. A final visit at the pediatric clinic for children and adolescents with cerebral palsy may be a good place for Elmer to discuss shaving, other self-help issues, sexuality, and socialization. For cosmetic purposes, his salivary overflow can be treated with anticholinergic medications and, later, if necessary, surgically. Elmer is encouraged to share questions and concerns about his body with his physicians and to visit regularly in the early days to establish a meaningful relationship.

SUMMARY

Transition-age youth with developmental disabilities face many challenges as they move from organized and supportive systems in place in school and pediatric health care systems to those focused on adults. Although developmental disabilities services offer residential, advocacy, and self-determination supports, community-based vocational services and particularly health services are less coordinated. A thoughtfully articulated plan for transition, incorporating all relevant systems and a documented transition packet outlining functional strengths and needs, health concerns, and self-direction abilities, should be developed well before the young person reaches legal adulthood at the age of 18 years or leaves school at the age of 22 years. Professionals with relationships with the young person should frankly explore understanding of sexuality and personal relationship issues to ensure safety and optimal social adjustment.

REFERENCES

A consensus statement on health care transitions for young adults with special health care needs. Pediatrics 110(pt 2):1304-1306, 2002.

Betz CL, Redcay G: Lessons learned from providing transition services to adolescents with special health care needs. Issues Compr Pediatr Nurs 25:129-149, 2002.

Blum RW: Introduction. Improving transition for adolescents with special health care needs from pediatric to adult-centered health care. Pediatrics 110(pt 2):1301-1303, 2002.

Braddock D, Emerson E, Felce D, Stancliffe RJ: Living circumstances of children and adults with mental retardation or developmental disabilities in the United States, Canada, England and Wales, and Australia. Ment Retard Dev Disabil Res Rev 7:115-121, 2001.

Dowdy CA: Vocational rehabilitation and special education: Partners in transition for individuals with learning disabilities. J Learn Disabil 29:137-147, 1996.

Halpern AS, Yovanoff P, Doren B, Benz MR: Predicting participation in postsecondary education for school leavers with disabilities. Exceptional Children 62:151-164, 1995.

Heath Center: 2001 College Freshmen with Disabilities: A Biennial Statistical Profile. Washington, DC, George Washington University, 2002. Available at: www.heath.gwu.edu/PDFs/collegefreshmen.pdf.

Johnson DR, Thurlow M, Cosio A, Bremer C: Diploma issues for students with disabilities. Addressing Trends and Developments in Secondary Education and Transition. Minneapolis, MN, National Center on Secondary Education and Transition (NCSET), Vol. 4, 2005. Available at: http://www.ncset.org/publications.

Milsom A, Hartley MT: Assisting students with learning disabilities transitioning to college: What school counselors should know. Professional School Counseling 8:431-436, 2005.

Murphy N: Sexuality in children and adolescents with disabilities. Dev Med Child Neurol 47:640-644, 2005.

Murphy NA, Elias ER: Sexuality of children and adolescents with developmental disabilities. Pediatrics 118:398-403, 2006.

National Center on Secondary Education and Transition (NCSET 1): IEP & Transition Planning: Frequently Asked Questions. n.d. Available at: http://www.ncset.org/topics/ieptransition.

National Center on Secondary Education and Transition (NCSET 2): Parent Brief: IDEA 1997 Transition Issues. The IEP for Transition-Aged Students. July 2002. Available at: http://www.ncset.org/publications.

Powers LE, Sowers J, Turner A, et al: A model for promoting self-determination among adolescents with challenges. *In* Powers LE, Singer GHS, Sowers JE (eds): On the Road to Autonomy: Promoting Self-Competence for Children and Youth with Disabilities. Baltimore, Paul H. Brookes, 1996, pp 69-92.

Reiss J, Gibson R: Health care transition: Destinations unknown. Pediatrics 110(pt 2):1307-1314, 2002.

Reiss JG, Gibson RW, Walker LR: Health care transition: Youth, family, and provider perspectives. Pediatrics 115:112-120, 2005.

Scal P: Transition for youth with chronic conditions: Primary care physicians' approaches. Pediatrics 110(pt 2):1315-1321, 2002.

Stinson J, Christian L, Dotson LA: Overcoming barriers to the sexual expression of women with developmental disabilities. Res Pract Persons Severe Disabil 27:18-26, 2002.

Stodden RA, Whelley T: Postsecondary education and persons with intellectual disabilities: An introduction. Education Training Dev Disabil 39:6-15, 2004.

U.S. Department of Justice, Civil Rights Division, Disability Rights Section: A Guide to Disabilities Rights Laws, 9-2005. Available at: http://www.usdoj.gov/crt/ada/cguide.pdf.

Wehmeyer ML: Self-determination and mental retardation. Int Rev Res Ment Retard 24:1-48, 2001.

White PH: Access to health care: Health insurance considerations for young adults with special health care needs/disabilities. Pediatrics 110(pt 2):1328-1335, 2002.

Part XI LEGAL, ADMINISTRATIVE, AND ETHICAL ISSUES

97 LEGAL ISSUES

MARY ANN CHIRBA-MARTIN

Medicine is inevitably practiced within a framework of legal and ethical obligations affecting the physician-patient relationship. When the patient is a child, the physician faces additional concerns and responsibilities because the parent and various governmental authorities may also play a role in directing the course of treatment. This is especially true for the child with developmental-behavioral issues whose "medical" needs typically require an array of interventions and supports from the educational and social service sectors. Consequently, the health care provider needs a basic understanding of the workings of the legal system as it pertains to treatment of the child with developmental-behavioral disabilities.

"The law" may be imposed by the state or federal government. Both state and federal law derive from the following sources:

Constitutions are the foundational documents of a government and its legal system. In addition to the U.S. Constitution, states have their own constitutions.

Statutes are codified laws enacted by the U.S. Congress and state legislatures.

Case law or *judicial precedent* consists of judicial opinions interpreting and applying federal and state constitutions, statutes, and agency regulations as well as the "common law" derived from prior court cases and long-standing legal traditions.

Agency regulations are promulgated by government agencies to interpret and enforce statutes and administer programs that have been established by federal and state legislatures. Agency regulations assume the force of law unless and until they are overturned in court or rejected by the legislature.

Additional ethical obligations may be imposed by professional codes of conduct. However, this chapter focuses primarily on the legal aspects of treating children in general and those with developmental-behavioral concerns in specific, but it provides only a basic introduction to health care law as it pertains to this particular pediatric population. The health care system, including institutional and individual providers, is among the most heavily regulated sectors in the United States today. Like medicine, law, especially health care law, is extremely complex; and like medical issues, legal concerns are usually treated most effectively and efficiently with a proactive, "preventive" approach. Accordingly, the health care professional should err on the side of consulting an attorney sooner rather than later. Many hospitals have their own attorneys or "general counsel" on-call who would welcome the opportunity to consult as soon as the provider senses the need for legal clarification or guidance.

To provide a basic introduction to the complexities of the extensive governmental oversight and wide-ranging legal obligations of the health care provider, this chapter organizes the material in terms of the health care provider's direct obligations to the patient and the provider's obligations to, or interactions with, external authorities on the patient's behalf (excluding the juvenile justice system, which is covered elsewhere in this book).

For the most part, the legal obligations discussed herein apply equally to the physician and other health care providers. Thus, the terms *provider* and *physician* are used interchangeably to refer to all persons involved in the direct provision of medical care to the pediatric patient.

THE PHYSICIAN'S DIRECT OBLIGATIONS TO THE PATIENT

Parties to the Relationship

Unlike the typical binary relationship between the physician and adult patient, the pediatric relationship is usually a triad of physician, patient, and parent or guardian. For children already in state custody, the relationship may also involve representatives from various agencies, such as the Department of Social Services or Child Protection.

Duty of Confidentiality

The provider-patient relationship and, in this context, the provider-patient-parent relationship is one of trust and confidence. The patient or the patient's representative (typically the parent; *Parham v. J. R.*, 442 U.S.C. 584 [1979]), not the physician, decides when and with whom information will be shared. With few exceptions, the physician may not disclose confidential information to anyone outside the relationship without the patient's permission. A school's request for information, for example, cannot be granted without a prior release from the patient or the patient's representative.

Several federal statutes deal with specific issues regarding the confidentiality of records, and state law may impose additional or more stringent requirements. The federal Health Insurance Privacy and Portability Act (42 U.S.C. §300gg *et seq* [1996]) applies to health plans, health insurers, hospitals, and other health care providers and, in general, permits patient-identifiable information to be shared with a health insurer. The Federal Education Records Privacy Act (20 U.S.C. §1232g [1974]) would not permit such disclosure to a public school system that is paying for services absent a signed waiver from the parent. Under both the Health Insurance Privacy and Portability Act and the Federal Education Records Privacy Act, the patient/student has a right to obtain the record and also to amend the record if it is believed to be inaccurate. To maximize compliance with the various state and federal laws governing confidentiality, the provider should make it a practice to obtain written consent from the patient or patient's representative before disclosing confidential information.

Confidentiality Exceptions

Whereas parents typically have full access to their child's information, special statutory exceptions may exist to protect the confidentiality of an adolescent's information in matters involving sexual activity as well as substance abuse treatment (Morrissey et al, 1986). Thus, a provider may be free to discuss most aspects of a child's health status with the parent but be restricted from disclosing information pertaining to birth control, pregnancy, abortion, human immunodeficiency virus infection status, sexually transmitted disease, and the like. Another exception to the duty of confidentiality occurs when the physician sees the patient as posing a genuine risk of serious physical harm to a third party. In such cases, the patient's right to confidentiality is trumped by the need to avert imminent harm. Although the physician may have a duty to warn in such circumstances, the courts are not in agreement as to whom should be warned. Some courts will permit the physician to warn the target of the threat. Other courts insist that efforts should still be made to preserve patient confidences, and therefore warning of law enforcement authorities may be all that is permitted (*Tarasoff v. Regents of the University of California,* 551 P.2d 334, 343-344 [Cal. 1976]).

Medical Decision Making: Who Decides?

A health care provider commonly holds definite opinions about a patient's course of treatment. However, although the physician can inform, advise, and even strongly recommend, the ultimate decision belongs to the patient. In the large majority of cases, a patient younger than 18 years lacks the legal capacity to consent to his or her own medical treatment. Thus, decisions about medical treatment will be made by the parent or guardian, who has a legal right to consent to, withdraw, or compel medical care on behalf of the child (*Parham v. J. R.,* 442 U.S. 584 [1979]).

Legal Competence

The person charged with making treatment decisions for the child must be legally competent to do so. Competence exists if the person is capable of making a reasonable decision, can understand the information conveyed, and is voluntarily deciding on the child's behalf (i.e., not unduly influenced by other persons or conflicting interests). Although the decision maker must be "capable" of making a reasonable decision, the law does not require that the ultimate decision be reasonable as long as the decision is informed by adequate disclosure of material information (see later discussion of informed consent) and voluntary. When the patient is not making her or his own decisions, as in the case of a child or other person lacking legal competency, a court may require that the decision fall within a range of objectively reasonable choices that would promote the child's best interests.

Exceptions to the general rule of parent as primary decision maker may be made in the case of parental disagreement, guardianship, and parental incompetence as well as for legally emancipated and mature minors. When separated or divorced parents disagree about a child's health care, the physician should make the best effort to facilitate a consensus. Should disagreement persist or should the child be living in an informal custodial setting, the person with actual physical custody typically has the right to decide. Courts generally recognize that the legal intricacies of a custodial arrangement must yield to the practical demands of treating a child's medical needs in a timely manner to minimize the risk of serious harm (*Campbell v. Campbell,* 441 S.W.2d 658 [Tex. 1969]).

Guardianship

A parent makes medical decisions for a child because the child, by virtue of his or her immaturity, is legally incompetent to do so. However, a parent's own competence may be in question when the parent seems incapable of understanding information or acting in the child's interests. If parental competency is in question, the provider may need to seek court appointment of a guardian. A guardian may fulfill the role of the parent in medical decision making when a parent is unavailable because of death, disease, prolonged absence, legal incompetence, or termination of parental rights. A guardianship may exist through a formal court appointment or an informal family arrangement. Because third parties can initiate guardianship proceedings, a health care provider (usually the hospital) may seek to have a guardian appointed in instances in which the parent is believed either to lack mental competency or to be basing the decision on interests that conflict with those of the child. Because the guardian stands in the position of a parent, the term *parent* is used hereafter as including the guardian as well.

Emancipated Minors

A minor who has been legally emancipated from parental control (pursuant to a judicial decree or statutory exception for marriage or military enlistment) may direct the course of his or her medical treatment without parental control or participation. When a minor obtains a judicial declaration of independence from the parents, a parent has no right to consent to or otherwise participate in treatment decisions. The parent typically has no financial obligation to pay for treatment.

The Mature Minor Doctrine

Through statute or common law, most states permit "mature" minors to consent to at least some forms of treatment even if the minor has not reached the age of legal majority or become a legally emancipated minor. Courts employ a case by case evaluation of factors such as age, maturity, severity of condition, and significance of decision to determine whether the minor evidences sufficient maturity and reasoning ability to make medical decisions on his or her own behalf (*Bellotti v. Baird,* 443 U.S. 662 [1979]). When parent and child conflict over the decision, a court will usually defer to the parent if the child is younger than 16 years (*Parham v. J. R.,* 442 U.S. 584 [1979]). The judiciary presumes that parents act in the best interest of the child and that children are not fully capable of making important decisions, especially medical ones (*Parham v. J. R.,* 442 U.S. 584 [1979]). Once the patient turns 16 years of age, however, a court may be more willing to defer to the patient. For example, in *In re E. G.* (549 N.E.2d 322 [Ill. 1990]), a 17-year-old minor diagnosed with acute nonlymphatic leukemia was allowed to reject blood transfusions on religious grounds. Plus, a court is likely to give weight to the opinion of child who is not a mature minor but is still old enough to have some understanding of the medical situation. A parent who is at odds with an older child may petition the court to compel the child to submit to medical treatment. A parent did just that in *In re Thomas B.* (574 NYS2d 659 [1991]) to obtain a court order compelling a 15-year-old boy to submit to a biopsy.

Additional Statutory Exceptions to Parental Decision Making

Recognizing that parental consent requirements can discourage minors from seeking certain kinds of health care, most states have enacted laws allowing wider discretion for adolescents to direct their own medical care, especially in the areas of sexual activity, even though they may not qualify as mature minors. However, state regulation of adolescent reproductive issues varies significantly and is ever changing. Many states permit a "judicial bypass" for certain kinds of decisions in which the adolescent can seek court approval of a procedure in lieu of obtaining parental consent. Such statutes typically require the minor to demonstrate to the court that she or he is sufficiently mature and informed to make the decision (*Bellotti v. Baird,* 443 U.S. 622 [1979]). An important caveat should be respected, however. Even if a patient is deemed a mature minor and therefore legally competent to direct his or her own medical care, a practitioner must remain mindful of and sensitive to the parent-child dynamic as well as parental concern and influence over the child.

Medical Decision Making and the Doctrine of Informed Consent

Absent an emergency in which the child faces an imminent threat of serious or permanent physical harm, a health care provider must obtain a patient's informed consent before rendering treatment. When the patient is a child, the provider must obtain the informed consent of the parent or guardian. Informed consent exists when the physician has communicated all "material information" to the parent/guardian or mature minor regarding

- diagnosis;
- risks and benefits of the recommended tests and treatment; and
- risks and benefits of alternatives, including risks and benefits of no treatment.

Despite some variability between jurisdictions, information is deemed material if a reasonable patient would consider it to be a significant factor in reaching a decision.

Failure to obtain a parent's informed consent before treating a child can expose the physician to civil liability for battery (basically, intentionally touching another's person without consent) or, more commonly, negligent failure to obtain informed consent. Negligence constitutes a failure to exercise reasonable care that causes harm to the patient. In the context of informed consent, the patient would basically claim that she or he did not receive adequate information about the risks and benefits of the treatment and its alternatives and would have chosen a different course of treatment had the information been communicated. A more detailed discussion of negligence liability appears later with regard to the physician's duty of reasonable care.

The doctrine of informed consent is primarily controlled by state "common" law (i.e., nonstatutory, judicially made case law). In recent years, however, some states have begun to legislate the content of information to be communicated about certain treatment decisions. Practice guidelines also may address what information needs to be disclosed. Even if practice guidelines are not legally binding, they may serve as evidence of what reasonable care would require in a given circumstance.

For an adult patient, a decision may be legally "informed" even if it is patently unreasonable as long as (1) the patient was legally competent and adequately informed of material information and (2) the decision itself poses no risk of serious harm to third parties. Thus, an adult may refuse a low-risk, lifesaving procedure because the only one harmed would be the patient.

Nevertheless, the person could be compelled to undergo treatment for a contagious disease that threatens the public health.

When the patient is a minor, however, courts are far more willing to override a parent's decision that places the child at risk of serious harm, especially when the risk and intrusiveness of the recommended treatment are outweighed by the risk of harm to the child in the absence of treatment. The most common scenario involves parental denial of consent to a blood transfusion for religious reasons. Courts routinely override such parental objections, reasoning, "Parents may be free to become martyrs themselves. But it does not follow they are free, in identical circumstances, to make martyrs of their children before they have reached the age of full and legal discretion when they can make that choice for themselves" (*Prince v. Massachusetts,* 321 U.S. 158, 170 [1944]).

A threat to the child's physical health is the most common trigger for court-ordered treatment, but a risk to emotional well-being can also warrant judicial intervention. In the psychiatric context, a court would probably require objective evidence of psychosis or severe emotional, developmental, or social difficulty and would probably defer to the parent who had made at least some effort to obtain professional help for the child (e.g., Brandow, 1999). When a child's disabilities have adverse behavioral manifestations, a school or health care provider might believe that medication is required, particularly when the diagnosis is attention-deficit/hyperactivity disorder. To date, however, courts have been reluctant to override a parent's refusal to medicate the child in this context (Komoroski, 2001).

Although a parent's effort to withhold potentially lifesaving treatment is the more typical ground for a court order, excessive or unusual treatment that jeopardizes the child's well-being can also prompt judicial intervention. For example, a court may intervene when the psychological disorder of Munchausen syndrome by proxy causes the parent to invent or even to induce medical conditions in the child (Perman, 1998). Parental behavior of this kind can elicit a range of state intervention, including termination of parental rights as well as criminal prosecution.

For experimental treatment, parental decisions typically control, and there is no need for court approval unless the degree of risk seems excessive in light of the child's prognosis and available treatment alternatives. In such circumstances, consultation with the Institutional Review Board may also be wise. Parental consent to extremely risky treatment is likely to be respected when death or serious harm is otherwise likely. Court approval should be sought, though, when a medical procedure is being pursued for the benefit of a third party and not the child. As explained before with regard to legal competency, decisions must focus on the patient's best interests and not on potentially conflicting third-party objectives.

State Law Duty of Reasonable Care

A physician owes the patient a legal duty to exercise reasonable care in rendering treatment. What constitutes reasonable or "due" care is typically governed by state negligence law. A physician deemed to have breached this duty of care may be civilly liable for negligence if the breach actually caused harm to the patient. The A, B, C, D of a successful negligence claim must establish that

- A duty of care existed,
- it was Breached, and
- the breach Caused
- foreseeable harm or Damage.

All four elements must be satisfied, and the absence of even one will relieve the provider of liability. A successful negligence action may result in an award of money "damages" to provide financial compensation for the patient's harm, including pain and suffering. State and federal malpractice reform initiatives typically cap the dollar amount of damage awards.

Despite some variability from state to state, the standard of reasonable care is generally that of the reasonably prudent professional. This is intended to be an objective standard that may exceed or fall short of an individual provider's personal or subjective best efforts. Thus, reasonable or "due" care need not be the "best" care or involve the level of skill of the most accomplished expert. In contrast, a practitioner's subjective best efforts may fall short of what is objectively and legally required. Because the law requires only reasonable care, it does not guarantee a successful or accurate result. For this reason, an inaccurate diagnosis or an unwanted side effect or complication is not necessarily negligent as long as adequate warnings were provided in obtaining informed consent.

The Americans with Disabilities Act

The Americans with Disabilities Act (ADA) of 1990 (42 USC §§12101-12213 [1994 & Supp. IV 1998]) protects all persons with mental and physical disabilities from discrimination in both the public and private sectors. Under the ADA, a person has a "mental disability" if the person has an actual mental impairment, is regarded as having an impairment, or is perceived as impaired on the basis of a history of mental impairment. Some examples of actual mental impairment are intellectual disability, dementia, and cognitive deficits. In evaluating the existence of a disability, courts are sometimes guided by the *Diagnostic and Statistical Manual of Mental Disorders* but may be less inclined to do so for pediatric patients because its suitability for this group has been questioned. The ADA may offer grounds to oppose denials of coverage by managed care organizations or other health insurance programs, especially with regard to mental health treatment. Whether a patient is disabled or not, several courts have found that physicians have a duty to advocate on their patient's behalf when payment has been denied for care deemed "medically necessary" by the treating physician.

Disability cannot be used as a basis for denying a disabled child either services or inclusion in medical, social, or other programs when the disabling condition does not conflict with eligibility requirements. For example, a child with a congenital heart defect cannot be excluded from a cardiac rehabilitation program because the child has Down syndrome. The rehabilitation program may need to be adapted to the child's needs (i.e., a reasonable accommodation must be made), but it must be as available to that child as it is to children without Down syndrome. Similarly, a provider generally may not refuse to treat a disabled child simply because that provider prefers not to. However, the ADA does not require a program or provider to render services to such a child that would not be made available to nondisabled children. In deciding whether and how to treat a disabled child, the provider need not exceed genuine limitations on the nature and scope of expertise but may have a duty to refer the child for more specialized care.

Federal Due Process and Equal Protection Requirements

The fifth and fourteenth amendments to the U.S. Constitution require federal and state actors, respectively, to respect an individual's legal rights to due process and equal protection of law. In the health care context, these protections most typically arise in the provision of services that are either administered or funded by the government. Due process requires that a patient facing a denial or change in access to government benefits (such as Social Security or state children's health insurance programs) be given notice of the proposed change and an opportunity to challenge the decision. The equal protection clause basically prohibits government agents or federally funded private actors from treating similarly situated people differently. Consequently, denying a qualified patient access to a social service program may be unlawful on the basis of disparate treatment of similarly qualified patients. Driven in part by the scope and application of these constitutional protections, Congress has enacted numerous laws to prevent discrimination based on disability. These are explained in greater detail below; in general, they prevent a provider from treating a disabled child any differently from a nondisabled child unless the disability necessitates this difference.

Due Process, Least Restrictive Alternatives, Aversive Interventions, and Unconventional Treatments

When treatment involves a program or method that restricts the child's physical or personal liberty, federal due process protections insist that the least restrictive alternative be employed. The term *least restrictive* refers to the degree of curtailment of personal liberty and duration of use compared with appropriate and effective alternatives. Thus, if a residential treatment facility is needed, it should be as close to a child's normal home and school as possible while still being adequate to address the child's particular needs and seek to release the child as soon as would be medically indicated. Special concerns arise when the proposed treatment involves restraints, aversives, congregate living arrangements, or unconventional treatments.

Restraints, Seclusion, and Aversive Interventions

The U.S. Constitution and a growing body of federal and state disability laws make clear that a disabled child has the same right as any person to be free from unreasonable restraint or abuse. Unfortunately, horror stories still frequent the headlines in which a disabled child sustains serious injury or dies after being subjected to aversive forms of discipline or behavior modification. A long and very sad list of incidents can be found at *www.neurodiversity.com/restraints.html.* In response, lawmakers have acted to make restraints, seclusion, and other nonemergency aversive interventions illegal under virtually all federal and state laws.

Pursuant to the federal Children's Health Act of 2000 (42 U.S.C. §595), the Center for Medicaid and Medicare Services prohibits the use of nonemergency restraints in federally funded facilities. Specifically, individuals younger than 21 years may not be subjected to "restraint or seclusion, *of any form,* used as a means of coercion, *discipline,* convenience, or retaliation" (42 C.F.R. §483.356 [emphasis added]). Restraint or seclusion may be used only as an "emergency safety intervention" and must strictly adhere to rigorous federal safeguards. For example, restraint or seclusion can be used only for genuine safety emergencies, can never be used simultaneously, and must be terminated as soon as the emergency subsides (42 C.F.R. §482.13). An order for restraint or seclusion must be written by a physician (or other licensed practitioner permitted by the state) for that particular emergency; standing or "as needed" orders are invalid. The intervention must be closely monitored and "performed in a manner that is safe, proportionate, and appropriate to the severity of the behavior, and the resident's chronological and developmental age; size; gender; physical, medical, and psychiatric condition; and personal history (including any history of physical or sexual abuse)" (see, generally, 42 C.F.R. §§482.356-482.370).

In publicly funded school settings, whether residential or not, the federal Individuals with Disabilities Education Act (IDEA) requires "positive behavioral intervention" in place of the negative interventions of restraint, seclusion, and other aversives. IDEA states that when a disabled child's behavior impedes his or her learning or the learning of others, the educational team must "consider, if appropriate, strategies, including positive behavioral interventions, strategies, and supports to address that behavior" [20 U.S.C. §1414(d)(3)(B)(i); 34 C.F.R. §300.346(a)(2)(i)]. The U.S. Department of Education's Office of Special Education Programs (OSEP) provides technical assistance for development of appropriate behavioral and disciplinary strategies in the form of functional behavior assessments and positive behavioral interventions and support (PBIS). According to OSEP's Technical Assistance Center (*www.pbis.org/english/About_the_Center.htm*), PBIS involves use of "procedures based on understanding why challenging behavior occurs." The Technical Assistance Center states that a significant body of research has "demonstrated the efficacy of PBIS in addressing the challenges of behaviors that are dangerous, highly disruptive, and/or impede learning and result in social or educational exclusion," such as self-injury, aggression, and property damage. PBIS is "first and foremost an ongoing problem-solving process" involving assessment geared to designing effective, proactive approaches to reducing impeding behaviors, teaching new skills, and implementing "supports" to help the child maintain positive behavioral changes. OSEP states, "Interventions that result in humiliation, isolation, injury and/or pain would not be considered appropriate."

THE PHYSICIAN'S OBLIGATIONS TO EXTERNAL AUTHORITIES

Mandatory Reporting to Law Enforcement Authorities

As required by the federal Child Abuse Prevention and Treatment and Adoption Reform Act (42 U.S.C. §5101 *et seq.*, as amended, 42 U.S.C. §6301 *et seq.* [2003]), all states have enacted some form of mandatory child abuse and neglect reporting law. Today, most "mandated reporter" statutes have been expanded to include physicians, nurses, and other health care, social service, and educational professionals who have regular contact with children. Whereas only about 30% of reports receive significant intervention, reports may remain in a confidential state registry to identify patterns of abuse. Reporting laws grant immunity to mandated reporters and other reporters of suspected abuse. Some states provide protection only for those who report in good faith and may deny immunity if a reporter discloses to a private party rather than the proper public authorities. Although these statutes are often criticized for dissuading minors from seeking health care, mandated reporters may be held civilly or criminally liable for *not* reporting abuse!

State Intervention

State statutes usually authorize law enforcement officials or physicians to take a child into protective custody in an emergency situation. State officials who enter the child's home for investigative purposes are subject to the U.S. Constitution's fourth amendment search and seizure requirements. Thus, a warrant is typically required absent emergency. In determining the permissibility and extent of intervention, a court will weigh the state's *parens patriae* authority to protect the child with the parents' right to direct the child's upbringing. A court will be guided by state statutory law regarding (1) what the state must show in terms of the degree of actual or threatened harm before it may intervene and (2) how much the state must do to assist the family in resolving the risk before it actually removes the child from the home.

In general, the state's interest in intervention is sufficiently compelling to justify intervention only when the child faces serious physical illness, injury, or immediate physical danger. When intervention is justified, a court will still insist on the least restrictive alternative. Thus, removal of a child from home would be a last resort.

Medical Neglect

As discussed earlier regarding medical decision making, a court order may be sought when a parent "abuses" a child by failing to seek or to permit needed medical treatment of a child. Typically, medical neglect arises in two types of cases: (1) the refusal to provide medical care is part of a pattern of neglect or (2) the children are well cared for but there is a disagreement between the parents and the state on certain medical care. Courts hesitate to recognize a spiritual treatment exception for decisions that might otherwise qualify as neglect. A parent's refusal to provide medical care consequently may qualify as neglect even if it is based on religious grounds. The courts reason that parents may be free to reject treatment for themselves on religious grounds but cannot do so when it comes to the child (*Prince v. Massachusetts,* 321 U.S. 158 [1944]).

The Individuals with Disabilities Education Act and the Health Care Provider's Obligations Regarding the Child's Education

The Individuals with Disabilities Education Improvement Act was initially enacted in 1997 to clarify the obligations owed by public schools and school systems to disabled children (20 U.S.C. §1400 *et seq.* [2006]). Discussed in greater detail elsewhere in this text, it basically requires a public school system to provide a "free appropriate education" to a student with a disability who, by virtue of that disability, is unable to make effective progress in the general curriculum. IDEA protects all children, including those who are homeless, in private schools, or in state custody. Although it is properly characterized as an "educational" statute, the IDEA gives health care providers a critical role in diagnosing a disability, describing the ways in which it may impede progress, identifying needed accommodations, and providing ongoing evaluation of effective progress. In addition to these evaluative services, a second role for the health care professional is to be the direct provider of a "related service" such as speech-language therapy, occupational therapy, or physical therapy as well as mental health or behavioral counseling.

Given the importance of outside experts in securing needed services for a child on an individualized education program, the physician often must transcend the role of medical professional to act as both sentinel and advocate. *The provider must realize that educational and related services will not necessarily be provided simply because the health provider documents the need for them.* Consequently, evaluators must be both explicit and comprehensive in detailing *what* a child needs and *why* the child needs it. Like it or not, the health care provider's evaluations and communications are essential tools for securing the educational and related services required by IDEA.

Educational advocates and attorneys are often needed to help the child and family navigate the special education gauntlet. However, the child needs the health care professional to play two essential roles by (1) providing emotional, diagnostic, documentary, and other support to the child and parent in what is often a very difficult struggle to obtain an appropriate education and (2) providing the powerful and effective advocacy needed to secure the services to which the child is legally entitled.

SUMMARY

Too often, the health care professions view the law as an annoyance at best and, at worst, a barrier to the ability to practice one's profession with excellence and effectiveness. Treating a child with developmental-behavioral disabilities can be complicated enough; having to attend to so many legal obligations and concerns may seem completely overwhelming. What this chapter has tried to accomplish, however, is to show how a basic understanding of the law can enable the provider to fulfill the direct obligations to the patient in a way that minimizes liability exposure. Most important, it has endeavored to empower the provider, who genuinely wants to help the child whose needs are so enormously complex, to advocate to those gatekeepers who would otherwise deny life-changing if not lifesaving services. Toward this end, this discussion has tried to make clear that the law as well as lawyers can be the provider's allies in obtaining the care that these children need and so clearly deserve.

REFERENCES

Brandow MA: Spoonful of Sugar Won't Help This Medicine Go Down: Psychotropic Drugs for Abused and Neglected Children, 72 S Cal L Rev 1151 (1999).

Komoroski AL: Stimulant Drug Therapy for Hyperactive Children: Adjudicating Disputes Between Parents and Educators, 11 BU Pub Int LJ 97 (2001).

Morrissey JM, Hofmann AD, Thorpe JC: Consent and Confidentiality in the Health Care of Children and Adolescents: A Legal Guide. New York, Free Press, 1986.

Perman CM: Diagnosing the Truth: Determining Physician Liability in Cases Involving Munchausen Syndrome by Proxy, 54 Wash UJ Urb & Contemp L 267 (1998).

98 LEGISLATION FOR THE EDUCATION OF CHILDREN WITH DISABILITIES

Judith S. Palfrey

Since the landmark passage of PL 94-142 in 1975, special education legislation has greatly benefited many American children and youth with disabilities and special health care needs. Whereas some children and families have fared better than others under the implementation of the legislation, the existence of special education provisions ensures a level of community accountability and scrutiny that keeps the issues of inclusion and opportunity squarely on the agenda of policymakers and government officials. The rights afforded by the legislation protect against serious backsliding during years of retrenchment and, as important, allow improvement of services during times of public innovation.

FAMILY-PROFESSIONAL PARTNERSHIP

There are few stories that attest as strongly to the power of collaboration between families and professionals than that of the passage of special education legislation. The story of special education legislation is a 30-year tale of an evolving relationship between families and professionals. Drawn together by common goals to improve the life chances of children with disabilities, parents and child health care providers have learned that there is increased leverage when the two groups work in concert.

This combined constituency has achieved a number of remarkable legislative victories that have resulted in substantial legal protections and programmatic advances for children with disabilities. No legislation is free from attack and no program is immune from the vagaries of inadequate funding and inept implementation. Nonetheless, the existence of strong legislative underpinnings for special education attests to the power of family-professional collaboration.

In the United States, education is an entitlement. This fact makes the schools fundamentally different from most other institutions. Recognizing that every child has a right to education, advocates, including parents and pediatricians, have pushed for legislative assurance that all children with disabilities will have access to proper school programs. In the late 1960s and early 1970s, parent groups, child-helping professionals, and lawyers joined together in an effective lobby to establish legal precedents clarifying the rights of all children and youth with disabilities. Two landmark cases, *Pennsylvania Association for Retarded Citizens v Commonwealth of Pennsylvania* (334 F Supp 1257 [ED Pa 1971] and 343 F Supp [ED Pa 1972]) and *Mills v Board of Education of the District of Columbia* (348 F Supp 866 [DDC 1972]), provided that bulwark. Through these two court cases, the right to a free appropriate public education for children with developmental disabilities was upheld.

Advocacy moved rapidly in the 1970s into policy formation and legislative initiatives. The time was right and the mood of state legislators and the U.S. Congress was receptive to the advocates' message. As a result, one of the most extensive programs affecting children in the United States, namely, the Education for All Handicapped Children Act (PL 94-142), was passed by large majorities in Congress in 1975.

During the ensuing 30 years, the legislation has been added to, modified, and refined on the basis of experience at the state and local levels (Horne, 1991; Smith et al, 2000). Currently, the legislation is entitled the Individuals with Disabilities Education Act (IDEA).

INDIVIDUALS WITH DISABILITIES EDUCATION ACT

In 1991, two federal initiatives, PL 99-457, the early intervention legislation, and PL 94-142, the Education for All Handicapped Children Act, were combined into the Individuals with Disabilities Education Act (PL 101-476). This comprehensive act covers children with disabilities from birth to 21 years of age (Table 98-1). In 2004, IDEA was again reauthorized as the Individuals with Disabilities Improvement Act of 2004 and is generally referred to as IDEA 2004 (Wright, 2006).

Early Intervention

Families and professionals have argued persuasively for the value of early intervention services for children with a wide range of physical and developmental disabilities. Early intervention encompasses identification at the time of diagnosis, direct services for the disabling condition, and preventive services to avoid secondary disability. The services should be provided in the community and, whenever possible, at home. Parents should be involved at every level of the planning, including their participation in the individualized family service plan (IFSP).

Table 98-1. Individuals with Disabilities Education Act: Key Components

Early Intervention (birth to 3 years)
Identification of children with disabilities or at risk
Evaluation
Individualized family service plan (IFSP)
Special Education (3 to 21 years)
Identification
Individualized education plan (IEP)
Least restrictive environment
Related services
Parental due process
Transition services

Eligibility for IDEA services is met by children from birth to 3 years of age with developmental delays or diagnosed with a physical or medical condition (e.g., cerebral palsy, Down syndrome) and those who are at risk of having substantial developmental delays if early intervention services are not provided (e.g., low birth weight, mother addicted to cocaine). Because this latter particular criterion is at the discretion of each state, there is wide national variation in early intervention coverage for children "at risk" for developmental disabilities.

The services covered under early intervention include family training, counseling and home visits, special instruction, speech therapy and audiology, occupational therapy, physical therapy, case management, diagnostic medical services, health services, social work, vision services, assistive technology, transportation, and psychological services. States vary in whether these are discretionary or mandated services.

The process for obtaining early intervention services for a child requires referral to the appropriate state agency. This may be public health, education, the state's department of human services, or another special agency. Each state must have an interagency coordinating council that ensures that multidisciplinary services are available no matter which state agency is in the lead position. If a clinician is unaware of how to make a referral, the best first place to call is the public education authority that can steer the family to the proper agency, if it is not the schools.

Once a child is identified as eligible for early intervention, assessments are carried out to determine the extent of needs, and then all concerned parties (including family members and professionals) prepare an IFSP. The F in IFSP acknowledges the central role of the family in the process of early intervention.

Special Education for Children and Youth Aged 3 to 21 Years

When parents and professionals forged the original bonds to enact special education legislation, it was recognized that the legislation would need to be broad enough to accomplish three major goals. First, uniform standards for appropriate educational services were seriously wanted. Second, a concerted shift toward community and school system responsibility was essential if children with disabilities were to receive the most appropriate services. Third, the legislation must ensure the entitlement that previously had systematically been withheld from children with disabilities. To attain these goals, the authors of the federal legislation created a program that is comprehensive in scope and specific in detail.

Under the regulations of IDEA, states are required to provide "a full appropriate public education" for all children with disabilities. The law applies to children who are intellectually disabled, hard of hearing, deaf, speech impaired, visually limited, or seriously emotionally impaired and those who have other health impairments or multiple disabilities as well as children with specific learning disabilities.

The state education agencies are required to identify, locate, and evaluate all children with disabilities and to prepare and implement individualized education plans (IEPs) for these children. They are further required to ensure placement of children in the least restrictive environment possible and to uphold procedural safeguards for children in public schools. "Related services" needed by students to benefit from special education are also to be provided. These include transportation, counseling, physical therapy, occupational therapy, speech and hearing therapy, school nurse services, and diagnostic health services. Finally, states must provide in-service training for special and regular education teachers.

The pediatric role in special education is implied rather than delineated. Because pediatricians care for children with a wide range of disabilities, special educational services are either a resource for families or the bane of everyone's day. To work with school systems in the most effective manner, it is helpful for pediatricians to understand and engage in all aspects of the special education program, especially evaluation, services, and parent advocacy.

Individual diagnostic evaluation is the pivotal component of IDEA. Individual evaluations are required for every child receiving special education. The basic planning team consists of the child's teacher, a representative of special education, one or both parents, and other individuals at the discretion of parents or agencies as well as the child when appropriate. IDEA 2004 has further clarified that the evaluation team should include only those professionals whose input is most germane to the needs of the student.

Although IDEA does not specifically require physician input in regard to the individualized education plan, pediatricians are frequently asked by parents and schools to participate in the planning and evaluation of children with a range of disabilities from severe retardation and physical disability to emotional disorders to sensory problems and learning disabilities. It is important for clinicians to recognize the issues and questions that are foremost in the minds of the educators and parents (Porter et al, 1992; Walker, 1984). When children are referred to pediatricians for a medical component of the IEP, it is likely that the evaluation team wants a number of issues to be addressed. First, there is the lingering hope that somehow the physician can determine the cause of the child's problem and that then the child can be cured. It is thus extremely important that the physician document the efforts that have been made to establish a cause or cure for the disorder and spend some time explaining what is and is not understood about the child's problem, treatment, and prognosis. Second, educators wish to know the behavioral consequences of the child's disorder. Will the child be experiencing seizures in the classroom? Is he or she likely or unlikely to interact with other children? Are there any safety considerations? Third, the team will probably want as full an exploration of the child's history, current neurodevelopmental status, and attention-activity modulation as possible.

Although assessment of some of these areas will undoubtedly be covered by other specialists, the pediatrician is often in a good position to synthesize many issues, adding the longitudinal perspective derived from history taking or from a long-term relationship with the child. To have a better personal understanding of the developmental, functional, and behavioral issues under team consideration, the physician may wish to obtain some observational data (American Academy of Pediatrics, 1996; Levine et al, 1980). This process can help the pediatrician concentrate the medical reports on issues of highest relevance for the evaluation team.

The major service to be provided under IDEA and state laws is special education. However, the law also calls for the provision of "related services" needed by the student to benefit from special education. The related services aspect of the law challenges school systems to work with community health and mental health agencies to ensure that no barriers to special education remain unaddressed. A variety of systems have been established by school districts across the United States to meet the related services section of the law. Although many of these have worked well, there have been persistent problems in a number of areas, including counseling, supervision, and the extent to which school systems should be involved in the diagnosis of and therapy for certain mental and physical conditions (Palfrey, 1994).

For pediatricians, one of the most important developments in special education has been the increasing call on schools to provide health-related services and school-based nursing care. Because of advances in medical knowledge and technology availability, more and more severely ill children are living longer lives, depending on devices such as tracheostomies, oxygen administrators, respirators, suctioning, gastric feeding lines, central venous lines, ostomies, ureteral or urethral catheterization, and dialysis (Office of Technology Assessment, 1987). Most of these children are well enough to attend school if the necessary nursing support programs are available. In 1984, the Supreme Court heard *Tatro v Irving Independent School District,* which involved a young girl with myelomeningocele who required clean intermittent catheterization during school. The court ruled that clean intermittent catheterization should be seen as a related service that must be provided to remove the barrier to the child's education.

The Tatro case has extensive ramifications. Schools now must provide any nursing service required by a child in special education. Guidelines are available on the care of children with health technologic needs in the classroom (Porter et al, 1997). Payment remains the ultimate responsibility of the state (*Cedar Rapids Community School District v Garret F.*, 119 SCt 992 [1999]). During the past few years, significant clashes and controversies have revolved around this issue. Pediatricians with patients who are assisted by medical technology are advised that the state does, in fact, have the final fiscal responsibility for such services. As a result of the OBRA legislation of 1989 (PL 100-360, Medicare Catastrophic Coverage Act), schools can turn to the Medicaid agency for coverage of such services for children who are Medicaid eligible (Fox Health Policy Consultants, 1991).

Central to the concept of special education is parent participation. IDEA is in many ways a "consumer law." The position of parents vis-à-vis the educational system is protected by the due process clauses within the law. Physicians are in a position to help parents share actively in the decision making process. For many parents, this is a new role. They often want to have a helping professional available for consultation and advice. This is particularly true for parents of low socioeconomic status and ethnic minority background (Palfrey et al, 1989). Pediatricians can play a major advocacy role for families by acquainting them with their rights and coaching them in ways to approach school systems. Pediatricians who have strong partnerships with parent-to-parent support groups can help their patient families enormously by referring them to other parents who have blazed the special education trail before them.

Parents also frequently want a second opinion, and IDEA allows them to seek this from their physicians. When this happens, physicians should consider the request a call for mediation by the parents between themselves and the school. They should therefore obtain as much educational information as possible while maintaining some distance from the school. In addition, physicians should try to avoid preconceived biases toward one or another specialty. They should try to interpret the specialists' reports within the context of the whole child.

As advocates for children, physicians can join with parents to monitor their state education laws to see that these conform to IDEA. This is especially important in times of federal and state funding cutbacks, when compromise of quality and standards may be the consequence. In Massachusetts in 2005, for instance, a coalition of parents and professionals who were concerned about evaluation and services for children with autism were able to craft and shepherd legislation through the state legislature that clarified the process for evaluation and enhanced the opportunities for children with autism to receive timely and appropriate services (see *http://www.mass.gov/legis/laws/seslaw06/sl060057.htm*).

ONGOING CHALLENGES

Several serious ongoing issues hamper the special education systems and keep them from reaching their ultimate promise. Four of these are less than effective early identification systems, disparities in the quality of education afforded to children of different racial and ethnic backgrounds, poorly articulated transition programs into adulthood, and lack of full federal funding for the mandated services. IDEA 2004 links special education with No Child Left Behind legislation with the stated intent of identifying all children with disabilities by kindergarten, improving the standards of education for all children, and bridging the gap for children from low performing schools. In practice, the schools are feeling the effects of monitoring rather than of support. Schools and other agencies are also struggling with providing their older transition-age students with the services they need to move into the world of secondary education or work. Students with learning disabilities are still dropping out of school in high numbers before high-school completion. This problem is disproportionately felt by students of color from low resource backgrounds and poor schools. Students with cognitive and physical disabilities are still not receiving the types of training that will prepare them best to succeed in the world of work and adulthood. These problems are recognized and clearly acknowledged in IDEA 2004, and only time will tell how well they are addressed. What is clear, however, is that schools will have a very difficult time meeting the requirements of IDEA 2004 and No Child Left Behind unless the mandates are fully funded as originally intended by Congress. At the time of this writing, full funding has not been accomplished.

FUTURE DIRECTIONS

Legislation provides a foundation on which people build living, working structures. The outcomes depend on many factors, including the resources allotted, the commitment and support provided, and the presence or absence of competing demands. Some chapters of the IDEA saga delineate successes for children with severe physical disabilities and sensory impairments. Others document tragedies of promises half fulfilled for high school–aged youngsters from minority backgrounds who have learning disabilities. Monitoring, vigilance, and advocacy are warranted to ensure that high-quality services are furnished at every level and that providers have adequate training and support to carry out their assignments (Palfrey, 2006).

Such monitoring is best carried out by professionals and families working in concert. Several vehicles for such collaboration exist. One of the most accessible is Family Voices, a membership organization that provides information on a reliable and timely basis to parents and professionals so that, if need be, a combined voice can speak out to protect and advance special education services for children with disabilities.

REFERENCES

American Academy of Pediatrics: The Classification of Child and Adolescent Mental Diagnoses in Primary Care (DSM-PC); Wolraich M (ed). Elk Grove Village, IL, American Academy of Pediatrics, 1996.

Fox Health Policy Consultants, Lewin and Associates: Medicaid Coverage of Health-Related Services for Children Receiving Special Education: An Examination of Federal Policies. Washington, DC, U.S. Government Printing Office, 1991.

Horne RL: The education of children and youth with special needs: What do the laws say? NICHCY News Digest 1:1, 1991.

Individuals with Disabilities Education Act (PL 101-476). 20 USC, Chapter 33, §1400-1485 (1990).

Levine MD, Brooks R, Shonkoff J: A Pediatric Approach to Learning Disorders. New York, John Wiley & Sons, 1980.

Massachusetts Special Education Law: Chapter 57 of the Acts of 2006. An Act addressing the special education needs of children with the autism spectrum disorder. Available at: http://www.mass.gov/legis/laws/seslaw06/sl060057.htm.

Office of Technology Assessment: Technology-Dependent Children: Hospital vs. Homecare. Washington, DC, U.S. Government Printing Office, 1987.

Palfrey JS: Health care needs of children in special education programs. *In* Rubin L, Crocker A (eds): Developmental Disabilities: Delivery of Medical Care for Children and Adults. Philadelphia, Lea & Febiger, 1989, pp 23-29.

Palfrey JS: Community Child Health: An Action Plan for Today. Westport, CT, Praeger, 1994.

Palfrey JS: Child Health in America: Making a Difference Through Advocacy. Baltimore, Johns Hopkins University Press, 2006.

Palfrey JS, Walker DK, Butler JA, Singer JD: Patterns of family response to raising a child with chronic disabilities: An assessment in five metropolitan school districts. Am J Orthopsychiatry 59:94, 1989.

Porter S, Burkley J, Bierle T, et al: Working Toward a Balance in Our Lives: A Booklet for Families of Children with Disabilities and Special Health Care Needs. Boston, MA, Project School Care, The Children's Hospital, 1992.

Porter S, Haynie M, Bierle T, et al (eds): Children and Youth Assisted by Medical Technology in Educational Settings: Guidelines for Care. Baltimore, Paul H. Brooks, 1997.

Smith PJ, Mathews KS, Hehir T, Palfrey JS: Educating children with disabilities: How pediatricians can help. Contemp Pediatr 9:102, 2000.

Walker DK: Care of chronically ill children in schools. Pediatr Clin North Am 31:221, 1984.

Wright PD. Available at: http:www.wrightslaw.com/idea/law.htm. Accessed September 25, 2006.

SOME USEFUL WEB SITES

Our Children Left Behind (parent advocacy organization). www.OurChildrenLeftBehind.com.
http://p078.ezboard.com/fourchildrenleftbehindfrm17.showMessage?topicID=300.
http://p078.ezboard.com/fourchildrenleftbehindfrm17.showMessage?topicID=301.topic.

National PTA.http://www.pta.org/ptawashington/issues/idea.asp

USA Today. http://www.usatoday.com/news/washington/2004-05-13-special-education_x.htm.

Project Vote Smart (Jeffords' speech). http://www.vote-smart.org/speech_detail.php?speech_id=36067&keyword=&phrase=&contain=&PHPSESSID=a4e2f2e47f450c1723c3d099d4fbd9e6.

National Down Syndrome Society. http://capwiz.com/ndss/issues/bills/?bill=4319161&size=full.

Federation for Children with Special Needs. http://www.fcsn.org/idea/idea.html.

Learning Disabilities Association of America. http://www.ldanatl.org/legislative/nfw/04june.asp.

99 HEALTH CARE SYSTEMS

John B. Moeschler

Vignette

Duncan is a 2-year-old boy referred by his family physician in rural New England to rule out "a mucopolysaccharide storage disease." Duncan's mother has an acquaintance whose son was diagnosed with Hunter syndrome. After several conversations and some searching on the Internet, Duncan's mother has come to the conclusion that her son has this same disorder. She approached Duncan's family physician, who agreed to collect a urine sample that indeed demonstrated marked elevation of mucopolysaccharides (814 mg/mmoL). Duncan has been experiencing normal development aside from expressive language delay. He has had recurrent episodes of otitis media and snoring with sleep. Consults to otolaryngology and audiology specialists were set. Duncan, his parents, and older brother came to the local children's hospital, where his diagnosis was suspected by clinical examination. Urine electrophoresis showed the presence of a large amount of dermatan sulfate and trace of heparan sulfate. The plasma study for lysosomal storage diseases demonstrated deficient activity of α_2-sulfatase, supporting a diagnosis of Hunter syndrome. Sequencing of the gene encoding iduronate-2-sulfatase identified a C>T change at nucleotide 1122 (c.1122C>T), which creates a cryptic splice site known to be pathologic. Within a few weeks of Duncan's being seen in the clinic, his family's suspicions were confirmed, and his clinical diagnosis of Hunter syndrome was established without question. His mother, while awaiting laboratory confirmation, had arranged conversations with specialists in stem cell transplantation experimental treatment protocols and in enzyme replacement therapy protocols (otolaryngology). By the time the laboratory results returned, Duncan's mother had made arrangements to travel to the site of the enzyme replacement treatment research coordinating center in a state distant from her home for evaluation and treatment discussion.

Duncan's multispecialty baseline evaluations by specialists in neurology, audiology, otolaryngology, orthopedics, and developmental psychology revealed that he was experiencing mild to moderate conductive hearing loss, normal development aside from significant delays in expressive language, and no significant medical complication. His skeletal survey demonstrated mild "dysostosis multiplex"; he had significant hepatosplenomegaly and no other complications. The Food and Drug Administration had approved enzyme replacement therapy for Hunter syndrome, and within weeks Duncan began his weekly infusions at the children's hospital infusion center. Within 6 months, Duncan's parents noted that his hepatosplenomegaly had resolved and the irregularity of his craniofacial features had lessened subjectively. Early intervention services and family supports were in place. The state Medicaid program had enrolled Duncan in its children's state insurance plan as a secondary source for those expenses of treatment after his family's private insurance coverage maximum was reached. Duncan's treatment continues. His otolaryngologic problems have been treated surgically successfully by tonsillectomy and adenoidectomy and tympanostomy tube placement. His hearing loss has been addressed with hearing aids. His development remains age appropriate a year later; his speech delays persist. Weekly infusion of the enzyme replacement product has gone well with no significant adverse events; one medication error requiring institutional reporting has occurred.

This account reminds us of the astounding capacities of modern health care for children in America. Those who work in children's health care are dedicated to serving such patients and come to work every day to do the best possible for all patients every time health care is delivered. Much of the work is "from the heart," from the dedication to the well-being of children and families. This family was particularly effective at identifying resources after only a few hours at their desk computer in rural America. It is truly amazing the care one can obtain in the American health care system. All health professionals work within a "health system" that can both facilitate and serve as a barrier to professionals who desire to provide the best possible health care to every patient every time.

This chapter begins broadly with a discussion of the American health care system to set the context of those elements of particular interest to children with developmental and behavioral needs who look to health care professionals for care, guidance, support, and services. It then turns to the delivery of health care to children with special health care needs and their families and the requirements for training programs to bring knowledge of health care systems to residency and fellowship training programs.

> *The purpose of the health care system is to reduce continually the burden of illness, injury, and disability, and to improve the health status and function of the people of the United States.*
>
> PRESIDENT'S ADVISORY COMMISSION ON CONSUMER PROTECTION AND QUALITY IN THE HEALTH CARE INDUSTRY (1998)

AMERICAN HEALTH CARE SYSTEM

Research on the quality of American health care documents that often there are shortfalls in the ability to translate the tremendous recent advancements in the medical sciences and technology into practice. In 2001, the Institute of Medicine published *Crossing the Quality Chasm: A New Health System for the 21st Century* in response to growing evidence that health care often is not what the patients want (or need), is not available when they want (or need) it, nor is delivered in a way that addresses their cultural particularities. Americans "should be able to count on receiving care that meets their needs and is based on the best scientific evidence" (Institute of Medicine, 2001, p 1), but often that is not the case. For many Americans, the health care system is inaccessible and bewildering, and for some even dangerous.

In 1998, three major reports detailed questions about the health care system in America. The first was the literature review by Schuster and colleagues (1998) of the quality of health care in America. Schuster and colleagues established three categories of quality health care problems, defined as underuse, overuse, and misuse of health care in the United States. *Underuse* was defined as those health care services for which benefits are documented but had not been provided to patients (necessary care that is not provided). *Overuse* indicated the reverse—the provision of health care services in which the risks outweighed the potential benefits to the patient (i.e., inappropriate care). *Misuse* was defined as otherwise appropriate health care that is provided in a way that leads to or could lead to avoidable complications. One example of misuse is the prescription of the appropriate antibiotic to treat a minor infection but one to which the patient has a documented allergy. This literature review of 73 such articles described errors of each kind in health care services. One surprise was not that there were publications describing each kind of problem in quality health care services but that there were so few published studies of the quality of health care delivered in the United States, given the huge industry that health care represents. The predominant finding by this literature review was the large gap between the health care services patients should receive and the care they do receive, whether one examines preventive, acute, or chronic care services. Such findings were true for all health care settings and all age groups. An example of such a problem is the use of childhood vaccine, an essential pediatric preventive service; only 75% of those who should be fully vaccinated actually are (Centers for Disease Control and Prevention, 2007).

The second report was the Institute on Medicine's Roundtable on Health Care Quality that documented further the problems of underuse, overuse, and misuse of health care. That report stated that "the burden of harm conveyed by the collective impact of all of our health care quality problems is staggering. It requires the urgent attention of all the stakeholders: the health care professions, health care policymakers, consumer advocates and purchasers of health care. The challenge is to bring the full potential benefit of effective health care to all Americans while avoiding unneeded and harmful interventions and eliminating preventable complications of care" (Institute of Medicine, 2001, p 23).

The third key report of this watershed year of 1998 was that of the Advisory Commission on Consumer Protection and Quality. It concluded: "Exhaustive research documents the fact that today, in America, there is no guarantee that any individual will receive high-quality health care for any particular health problem. The health care industry is plagued with overutilization of services, underutilization of services and errors in health care practice" (Advisory Commission on Consumer Protection and Quality in the Health Care Industry, 1998).

These reports led, in part, to the Institute of Medicine reports *To Err Is Human: Building a Safer Health System* (2000) and *Crossing the Quality Chasm: A New Health System for the 21st Century* (2001). In the first Institute of Medicine report, the review of the literature regarding medical errors substantiated serious and widespread errors in care services that resulted in frequent and avoidable injuries to patients (Institute of Medicine, 2000). Both of these reports highlighted that the problems typically occur not because of a failure of goodwill, knowledge, effort, or resources but because of "fundamental shortcomings in ways care is organized. The nation's current health care system often lacks the environment, the processes, and the capabilities" needed to ensure that health care is what it should be (Institute of Medicine, 2001, p 25). They identified four key reasons for inadequate quality of health care:

1. Growing complexity of science and technology. In essence, no one clinician can retain all the information necessary for sound, evidence-based practice.
2. Increase in chronic conditions. One result of the advances and successes in medical science is that more Americans are living longer with chronic medical conditions. This increase in the prevalence and incidence of chronic conditions challenges the required collaborative process of health care services, with much of the care provided by the patients themselves and their families. This collaboration adds a level of complexity to health care services that must be managed properly for optimal outcomes.
3. Poorly organized delivery system. The health care system feels less like a system than a "confusing, expensive, unreliable, and often impersonal disarray" with overly complex series of steps and handoffs that are inefficient and leave gaps in care and waste resources (Picker Institute and the American Hospital Association, 1996).

4. Constraints on exploiting the revolution in information technology. Large numbers of patients are turning to the Internet and World Wide Web for health care information and health care services. Our children will expect to receive health care in the same way we make airline reservations and they create social networks. Tapping into the potential of information technology to inform health care systems will require a transformation of health care. The Committee on Quality of Health Care in America (2001) identified five key areas in which information technology could contribute to an improved health care delivery system:
    - Access to the medical knowledge base. See *www.genereviews.org* for an example of easily accessible reviews of clinical genetic conditions.
    - Computer-aided decision support systems for clinicians. See *http://www.dhmc.org/shared_decision_making.cfm* as an example of shared decision making efforts at one medical center.
    - Collecting and sharing of clinical information. Coordination of care of patients with chronic conditions with multiple providers requires many "handoffs" or potential barriers to health care quality.
    - Reduction in errors. Systems might standardize certain decisions, such as medication use or online prescription writing with built-in dosing safeguards and allergy information, for example.
    - Enhanced patient and clinician communication. E-mail and online scheduling offer opportunities for improved communication and efficiencies.

The Institute of Medicine report (2001) established six aims for the 21st-century American health care systems that it believes all health care systems would do well to adopt and to implement. These six aims address the key areas of health care that could be improved immediately. They propose that health care should be the following:

Safe, avoiding injuries to patients from care that is intended to help them.

Effective, providing services based on scientific knowledge to all who could benefit and refraining from providing services to those not likely to benefit.

Patient centered, providing care that is respectful and responsive to individual patient preferences, needs, and values and ensuring that patient values guide all decisions.

Timely, reducing waits and sometimes harmful delays for both those who receive and those who give care.

Efficient, avoiding waste, including waste of equipment, supplies, ideas, and energy.

Equitable, providing care that does not vary in quality because of personal characteristics such as gender, ethnicity, geographic location, and socioeconomic status.

A health care system that achieves and maintains major gains in each of these six domains would serve well the needs of the patients and the health care professionals.

In his article "A User's Manual for the IOM's 'Quality Chasm' Report," Berwick (2002) delineated the underlying framework for change needed to address the challenges ahead in American health care at four different levels:

1. the experience of patients (level A);
2. the functioning of small front-line units of care delivery ("microsystems") (level B);
3. the functioning of the organizations that house or otherwise support front-line health care teams (level C); and
4. the environment of policy, payment, regulation, accreditation, and other such factors (level D) that shape the behavior, interests, and opportunities of the organizations at level C.

The model is hierarchical because it asserts that the quality of actions at levels B, C, and D ought to be defined as the effects of those actions at level A, and in no other way. "'True north' in the model lies at level A, in the experience of patients, their loved ones, and the communities in which they live" (Berwick, 2002). We should judge the quality of professional work, delivery systems, organizations, and policies first and only by the cascade of effects back to the individual patient and to the relief of suffering, the reduction of disability, and the maintenance of health. He reviews the "old rules" and "new rules" of health care (Table 99-1).

Table 99-1. **Old Rules Versus the New Rules of Health Care**

Old Rules	New Rules
Care based on visits	Care based on continuous healing relationships
Professional autonomy drives variability in care	Customization based on patient needs and values
Professionals control care	The patient as the source of control
Information is a record	Shared knowledge and free flow of information
Decision making is based on training and experience	Evidence-based decision making
Do no harm is individual responsibility	Safety as a system property
Secrecy is necessary	The need for transparency
System reacts to needs	Anticipation of needs
Cost reduction is sought	Continuous decrease in waste
Preference is given to professional roles over the system	Cooperation among clinicians

Compiled from Institute of Medicine: Crossing the Quality Chasm: A New Health System for the 21st Century. Washington, DC, National Academy Press, 2001; and Berwick DM: A user's manual for the IOM's "Quality Chasm" report. Health Affairs 21:80-90, 2002.

DELIVERY OF HEALTH CARE TO CHILDREN

The health care system can be viewed as systems embedded in systems or as a series of concentric circles with the patient or, in pediatric health care, the patient and parent at the center. That infant's, child's, or adolescent's health is affected by ever-increasing surrounding concentric rings of the health care delivery system. There are also surrounding social circles that include characteristics of the individual child and the child's family, dwelling, neighborhood, communities, cities, and states (Shonkoff and Phillips, 2000). This is not the chapter in which there will be a discussion of such social characteristics that have an impact on child health and well-being. Rather, it is here that we discuss the characteristics of the formal health care systems for all children (which is a relatively small component of the whole health care system) and, in particular, for those with developmental and behavioral concerns.

In the center is the child and whomever is immediately responsible for the health and well-being of that child (e.g., parents). The center is the "self-care system" in which the family and the individual carry out their day-to-day health promotion or illness prevention habits based on their customs, beliefs, and desires. It is here, too, that the child, family, and social variables have an impact on child health and well-being. The patient is literally at the center of the health care system. The next circle is the individual interacting with a single physician or other health care provider. This reflects the interactions between that individual health care provider and the child and the child's parent. It is here that the special relationship between an individual and the health care professional develops, leading to interactions and actions aimed to improve health outcomes. It is here that family-centered care is created. This professional, however, is embedded in the next circle, the front-line health care team that Nelson and colleagues (2007) have named the "clinical microsystem" in health care delivery systems. This front-line team is the place where patients, families, care teams, and information technology come together to make health care. It is the place where quality, safety, outcomes, satisfaction, and staff morale are created. This clinical microsystem is defined as a population of patients, providers, and their support staff, core and supporting processes of care information, and information technology with a common purpose or aim. The clinical microsystem provides a framework to organize, measure, and improve the delivery of care. It has clinical and business aims, linked processes, and shared information environment and produces performance outcomes. It involves patients and families as meaningful members of the health system. Microsystems evolve over time and are embedded in larger organizations. The microsystem is nested within the mesosystem of health care, that is, departments (e.g., nursing, medicine) or special service lines (e.g., mental health care). The mesosystem is nested, in turn, in the macrosystem or the larger institution. Health systems leadership is required from each of these systems to ensure quality health care services. Finally, the community, market, and social policy system have an impact on health care and provide systems of care (Fig. 99-1). Characteristics of each of these circles determine the quality of health care and health outcomes any one patient or family might experience. It is only by recognizing and improving these health care systems that one can achieve improved health outcomes (Batalden et al, 1998, Berwick, 2002).

All health care systems must address all health care needs of all patients all the time to be considered high performing and successful. This includes preventive care, acute health care, care for those who have chronic conditions, and palliative care. To address the long-term needs of all children, and especially those children with special health care needs, the American Academy of Pediatrics, with key partners like the Maternal and Child Health Bureau, has established the concept of a medical home for all children and has actively supported efforts to implement changes in health care delivery systems to become transformed to medical homes. The American Academy of Pediatrics first defined the medical home as a concept and method of service delivery, rather than a specific location, in 1992 (American Academy of Pediatrics, 1992). Later, it expanded and implemented the definition, stating that "medical care of infants, children, and adolescents ideally should be accessible, continuous, comprehensive, family centered, coordinated, compassionate, and culturally effective" (American Academy of Pediatrics, 2002). The principles of the medical home can be effective only if they are embedded in a living clinical microsystem that has embraced attention to quality and outcomes as integral to

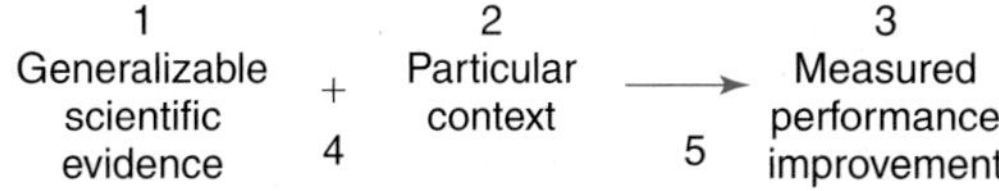

Figure 99-1. Health care implementation and improvement. Each of the five elements in this equation is driven by a different knowledge system. The generalizable scientific knowledge we need (element 1) is constructed from empiric studies that work to control context as a variable, thus minimizing or eliminating its effect on what is being studied. A knowledge of particular contexts (element 2) is developed by inquiry into the identity of local care settings—their processes, habits, and traditions. Knowledge of the effect of improvements on system performance (element 3) requires special types of measurement, techniques that include time in the analysis, as all improvement involves change over time; gaining this knowledge also requires the use of balanced measures that accurately reflect the richness and complexity of the phenomena under scrutiny. The + symbol (element 4) represents knowledge about the many modalities, including standardization, forcing functions, academic detailing, and so on, that are available for applying and adapting generalizable evidence to particular contexts. The → symbol (element 5) represents the knowledge required for execution—what you need to know to "make things happen," the drivers of change, in a particular place. It requires knowing where power resides and how it is asserted; it requires knowledge of the strategic aims, the usual ways of conducting work in that setting, the ways in which people are recognized and rewarded, and the ways in which they are held accountable for their work. Most developmental and behavioral pediatrics fellowship specialty training focuses on element 1, the clinical knowledge, skills, and attitudes, based on peer-reviewed published science, to practice this specialty. *(From Batalden P, Nelson EC, Gardent PB, Godfrey MM: Leading the macrosystem and mesosystem for microsystem peak performance. In From Front Office to Front Line: Essential Issues for Health Care Leaders. Joint Commission Resources, Oakbrook Terrace, IL, 2005.)*

the system/medical home. It is within the medical home that health care is coordinated for all children, including those children with special health care needs (Antonelli and Antonelli, 2004; Cooley and McAllister, 2004). The transformation of primary pediatric health care to the principles of the medical home optimizes circumstances for improved health outcomes. It is, in essence, a microsystem that is locally defined and might consist of pediatrician, nurse, scheduler, care coordinator, medical assistance, billing office staff, and information system specialists who are working together to meet the needs of a population of patients, a subset of which are children with special health care needs. This team addresses the preventive, acute, chronic, and palliative care of all those in their practice. The medical home is constructed from the transformation of this group of people. It consists of place, patients, professionals, and processes designed to meet the needs of all patients served and requires constant attention to improvement (Cooley and McAllister, 2004). Unfortunately, many children do not have access to a medical home. For example, Mulvihill and colleagues (2007) examined data from the 2003 National Survey of Children's Health to assess access to the medical home by children in Alabama and found that 51% of children with special health care needs and 48% of non–children with special health care needs have access to a medical home. These data are similar to other national measures of 47% and 44%, respectively (American Academy of Pediatrics, 2002). Although these recent American Academy of Pediatrics policy statements and interpretations have added clarity to the definition of the medical home, measurement issues persist. For example, the 2002 definition of the medical home contains 7 components covering at least 37 specific topics. This definition challenges efforts to address how to measure the processes of the medical home and link those to improved health outcomes.

The aim of the medical home methodology is to improve the health care and health of all patients served. For those children with special health care needs, the medical home must interact successfully with the specialty care providers and systems to ensure quality health care and health care outcomes. This system-to-system interaction adds complexity to the health care delivery system and challenges both the medical home and the specialty provider in meeting the needs of children and families.

"The core issue is fragmentation [of care], and the solution lies in forms of assembly and cooperation that the prevailing structures in health care cannot achieve. Disciplines divide from disciplines, organizations from organizations, events from events. Patients cross over these boundaries time and again, and their needs get lost in the disorder" (Berwick, 2002).

The medical home–medical specialist interaction is often addressed by methods of care coordination or shared care between specialist and medical home. Shared care and co-management are not new concepts. Co-management is shown to enhance access to needed services. It can be distinguished from a strictly "consultative model" because it emphasizes mutual education and shared and delineated responsibilities. It optimizes use of specialist resources and, together with care coordination, is reimbursable to both the specialist and the primary care provider. The individual interactions between the primary care provider and the specialist lead to a "shared learning" that improves access and communication that leads to sustainable relationships. Antonelli and colleagues (2005) have written extensively on the problems—and potential solutions—facing those who share care between the medical home and specialty care providers. They described different successful models for sharing of responsibility for care. Antonelli suggests adapting the Wagner model (Wagner, 1998) for conceptualizing the needs of those with special health care needs (Fig. 99-2). There are several models for collaborative care of children with special health care needs, and use of a model may depend on (1) the severity and complexity of the child's condition; (2) the expertise, interest, and availability of each type of provider; (3) the access of families to the various providers; and (4) the comfort of families and providers with different care situations (Hack, 1997). One example of collaborative care is the generalist as manager model, in which physician and family feel comfortable in implementing a comprehensive care plan with easy access to the medical home for a child with relatively straightforward clinical issues. Another model is the co-management model, in which the generalist manages all acute and some chronic medical conditions and may call on a specialist to manage a more complicated condition (e.g., diabetes care). A third model is the specialist as manager model, which might work best for children with complicated specialist management needs, such as the child with an inborn error of metabolism or an adolescent with cystic fibrosis. In this model, the specialist takes on many of the functions of the medical home. Ongoing and explicit conversations between families and generalist provider will lead to the best model for the particular situation. The medical home and the medical home–specialist interactions have specific benefits for health care (Tables 99-2 and 99-3) and specific challenges in achieving quality health care and substantial satisfaction for families and professionals.

There are macrosystem challenges as well. Chung and Schuster (2004) discuss "voltage drops" experienced by children in attempting to access quality health care. Just as an electrical system loses voltage when current passes through resistance (voltage drops), the health care system loses children as they confront barriers in six areas: access to insurance coverage, enrollment in available insurance plans, access to covered services and providers, consistent access to primary care, access to referral services, and delivery of high-quality care.

Voltage drop 1: access to insurance coverage. Lack of insurance is a major barrier to health services. Approximately 12% of U.S. children younger than 18 years lacked insurance between 2003 and 2005. Uninsured children are half as likely as privately insured children to have well-child visits, office visits, or hospitalizations (Yu et al, 2002).

Voltage drop 2: enrollment in available insurance plans. Even when they have access to insurance, many parents do not enroll their children in a plan. In

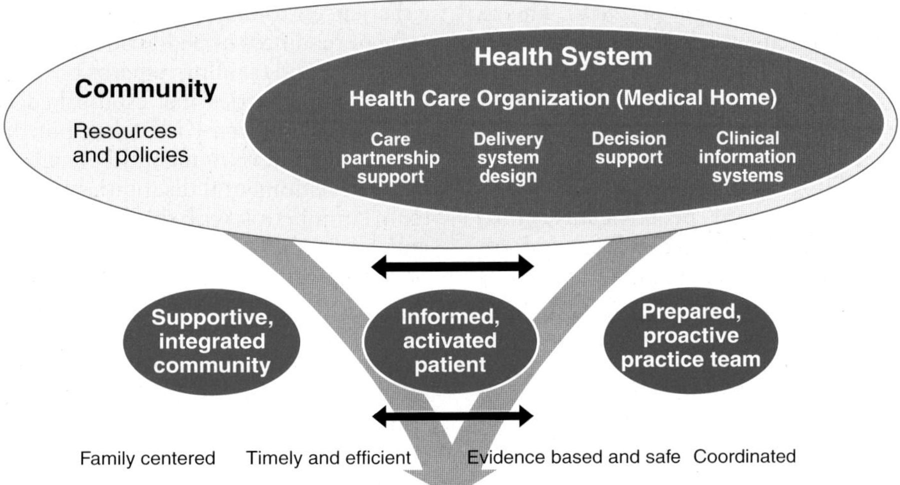

Figure 99-2. Model for child health care in a medical home. Bodenheimer and colleagues (2002) write that chronic care takes place in three overlapping "galaxies": (1) the entire community with its resources and public and private policies; (2) the health care system, including but not limited to its payment structures; and (3) the provider organization, no matter large or small. Within these three galaxies, the chronic care model identifies six essential elements: community resources and policies, health care organization, self-management support, delivery system design, decision support, and clinical information systems. Antonelli and coworkers (2005) and others have adapted this conceptual model for children with special health care needs in an effort to improve health care systems and health outcomes. *(Adapted from Wagner E: Chronic disease management: What will it take to improve care for chronic illness? Eff Clin Pract 1:2-4, 1998.)*

Table 99-2. Specialist-PCP Collaborative Care of Children with Special Health Care Needs: What Families Need

Preparation for the visit with the new provider
Timely and ongoing communication between the PCP and specialist
Specialist to receive all medical information before the visit
PCP follow-up and interpretation after specialist visit
PCP provides decision support, particularly if there are divergent opinions from specialists
A bedside visit from the PCP when the specialist hospitalizes the patient
Help with insurance (and other) barriers to referrals to specialists

PCP, primary care provider.
Adapted from Antonelli R, Stille C, Freeman L: Enhancing Collaboration Between Primary and Subspecialty Care Providers for Children and Youth with Special Health Care Needs. Washington, DC, Georgetown University Center for Child and Human Development, 2005.

Table 99-3. The Benefits of Collaborative Care Provided Within a Medical Home

Benefits to families	Care system that is easily accessible
	Care that is coordinated across health care providers, including primary and tertiary care
	Care that is family centered
	Families accepted as true partners in the care for their children
Benefits to physicians	Less redundancy
	Fewer errors
	Higher satisfaction
	Greater efficiency and productivity
	More appropriate use of physician expertise
Benefits to payers	Enhanced cost efficiency
Benefits to community organizations	Closer collaboration with health care providers and families
	Resources focused on filling gaps with less redundancy

From Antonelli R, Stille C, Freeman L: Enhancing Collaboration Between Primary and Subspecialty Care Providers for Children and Youth with Special Health Care Needs. Washington, DC, Georgetown University Center for Child and Human Development, 2005.

2001, 20% of children within typical income limits for Medicaid/SCHIP (state children's health insurance plans) were uninsured all year; 64% of uninsured children met income eligibility criteria for Medicaid or SCHIP but were not enrolled (Bhandari and Gifford, 2003). There are many potential barriers to enrollment that parents might experience: lack of awareness of Medicaid or SCHIP eligibility; lack of perceived value of insurance; and administrative obstacles (e.g., complicated application process), non–English-speaking parents enrolled, and confusion about eligibility for children whose parents are not citizens.

Voltage drop 3: access to covered services and providers. Enrollment in insurance plans may be "necessary but not sufficient" to guarantee access to needed health services. Both public and private insurance vary widely in what services are covered by the health plan. Even SCHIP rules allow states wide latitude in what is a covered service (Rosenbaum and Budetti, 2003). When services are covered, there can be substantial cost sharing by families, which suggests that cost is a significant barrier for many (Newacheck et al, 2000).

Voltage drop 4: access to a consistent source of primary care. Many families, in particular those who are nonwhite, non–English speaking, less educated, and poor, have drastically limited access to well-child care. Children in private or managed care plans are more likely than other children to have high continuity of primary care (Inkelas et al, 2004).

Voltage drop 5: access to referral services. This is particularly true for children with special health care needs whose needs exceed their use of services. They are twice as likely to delay care because of cost and to have an unmet health need, most of which are for referral services (Silver and Stein, 2001).

Voltage drop 6: delivery of high-quality health care services. In a survey of general pediatricians, most thought that treatment guidelines were helpful and improved outcomes but failed to use them in their practices (Flores et al, 2000). Health care services are beneficial only when the quality of such services is high. The study of quality of children's health services remains sparse but appears to mirror that for adults. The problems of overuse, underuse, and misuse appear to be as true for children's health care as for that of adults.

For each of these voltage drops in children's health care, Chung and Schuster propose incremental policy solutions, assuming that a comprehensive national solution providing universal access is not in the immediate future for the American health system. Their report reiterates the independence of access and quality, and they note that one does not guarantee the other and both are necessary to improve child health.

REQUIREMENTS FOR TRAINING PROGRAMS

The general pediatrician and those who specialize in developmental-behavioral pediatrics or neurodevelopmental pediatrics will be expected to contribute to improving the performance of the American health system. This expectation has been codified in the residency training program requirements recently. The American College of Graduate Medical Education revised the common program and institution requirements beginning July 2007 to include "systems-based practice," which addresses the changes needed in workforce development to address the challenges the American health care system faces. The new requirements state that residents must "demonstrate an awareness of and responsiveness to the larger context and system of health care, as well as the ability to call effectively on other resources in the system to provide optimal health care." Residents are expected to

1. work effectively in various health care delivery settings and systems relevant to their clinical specialty;
2. coordinate patient care within the health care system relevant to their clinical specialty;
3. incorporate considerations of cost awareness and risk-benefit analysis in patient or population-based care, as appropriate;
4. advocate for quality patient care and optimal patient care systems;
5. work in interprofessional teams to enhance patient safety and to improve patient care quality; and
6. participate in identifying system errors and implementing potential systems solutions.

All faculties and residency program directors are challenged now to develop meaningful educational experiences to meet these specific requirements. The state of readiness of pediatric training programs for such education and training remains uncertain. The American Board of Pediatrics has established two subspecialties relevant to children with developmental and behavioral disabilities: developmental-behavioral pediatrics and neurodevelopmental disabilities (*www.abp.org*), the latter in conjunction with the American Board of Psychiatry and Neurology (*www.abpn.com*). The American Board of Pediatrics content outline for the sub-board in developmental-behavioral pediatrics (*www.apd.org*) indicates that approximately 3% of board certification examination questions are on "law, policy, and ethics," including the following about "health care structures and processes":

- Understand the impact of various health care financing arrangements on the quality of services for children with special health care needs.
- Appreciate the financial incentive for insurance companies to discourage enrollment of children with special health care needs.
- Know the ethical implications of financial disincentives to specialty referrals within managed care systems and the differential impact on children with special health care needs.
- Be familiar with issues relating to the impact of mental health carve-outs on the quality of and access to mental health services for children.

The content outline for neurodevelopmental pediatrics examination does not list questions related to health care systems in its 2007 publication (*www.abpn.com*).

SUMMARY

The American health care system can be the best in the world, but often it is viewed as inaccessible, bewildering, frustrating, and even dangerous for patients. In this chapter, I have reviewed the means by which children and families are served by the health care systems as they exist, the efforts to improve care for children with special health care needs, and the need for constant tending of the system for optimal outcomes for our patients. At a policy level, the "voltage drops" in children's health care are complex and demand different answers to enhance and to ensure access to quality health care for all children. Tending to the challenges of the health care system for children requires a new set of skills and knowledge that soon will be integrated into residency training programs. Improvement in child health services systems will occur only with the explicit integration of systems knowledge and health care improvement knowledge into the medical home and care coordination methods for children with developmental and behavioral health needs.

Vignette

Irwin is a 13-year-old boy with Down syndrome whose parents have been asked to consider "out of district placement" by his school team because of self-injurious and aggressive behaviors for the last 2 years. The school has been unsuccessful in managing Irwin's behaviors and thinks that he would be served better in a specialized school for students with challenging behaviors. Irwin presented at birth with duodenal atresia and cyanosis along with the physical features of Down syndrome. Surgical repair was done on day 4 of life at the local children's hospital. At 6 months of age, Irwin traveled to the cardiac center at another children's hospital for correction of his atrial septal defect and ventricular septal defect when medical management was not successful at addressing his poor growth. He had been receiving supports and services since infancy. At school age, he attended elementary school with his siblings and neighbors and participated in the school play and in soccer. The transition to middle school was inconsequential, though by December of sixth grade, Irwin's behavior began to deteriorate with verbal outbursts at first and later physical aggression toward other students and a teacher. On one occasion, he was expelled from school because he was considered dangerous.

Irwin was brought to his pediatrician at the time of the expulsion, and the pediatrician intervened on Irwin's behalf with the promise that he would refer Irwin to child psychiatry for a behavioral health consultation. Psychiatry suggested that Irwin try risperidone, 0.5 mg, each morning and increase gradually to 0.5 mg each morning and evening, which appeared to lessen his verbal and physical striking out, and Irwin was able to return to school. However, behavioral outbursts persisted, and the following year his behavior deteriorated and out-of-district placement was suggested to his parents. Irwin was seen by his pediatrician again and noted to have lost 5 pounds. He was not experiencing any side effects of his medication and "appeared flat" in his affect. His pediatrician ordered a complete blood cell count, thyroid function studies, and a comprehensive metabolic profile, the results of all of which were unremarkable. Because he had read recently about the association of Down syndrome and celiac disease and because of his weight loss, he ordered a total serum immunoglobulin A determination, which was normal, and transglutaminase antibody assay, which was elevated. Irwin was started on a gluten-free diet and 6 months later had gained 10 pounds and "seemed better."

He was still presenting problems at school. Consultation with developmental pediatrics was arranged. After a comprehensive assessment, including a school visit and IEP meeting, the developmental pediatrician noted several contributors to Irwin's behavioral changes and suggested the school team consider arranging for a functional behavioral assessment and plan and that the recommendations from that be incorporated into Irwin's IEP. It was noted that at the time of transition to middle school, Irwin lost contact with his classmates because of his placements in self-contained classes and the loss of his classroom aide who had been with Irwin for 4 years. The developmental pediatrician also noted that Irwin's older sister had entered college at the same time Irwin transitioned to middle school. Together, they arranged for Irwin to identify a "big brother" who shared Irwin's interest in soccer. Also, the school agreed to ask for an integration facilitator to help support Irwin in the typical classroom so he might re-establish relationships with those students he had known for years. With the changes in his diet, the development of a positive behavioral support plan in school, and the technical assistance to his classroom teachers on including Irwin in the regular classroom, within another 6 months Irwin's school was delighted with their success with Irwin. Irwin was also able to stop the risperidone. Together, Irwin's family, pediatrician, and developmental pediatrician joined together to improve the quality of Irwin's life.

REFERENCES

Accreditation Council on Graduate Medical Education: Available at: www.acgme.org. Accessed April 1, 2007.

Advisory Commission on Consumer Protection and Quality in the Health Care Industry, 1998. Available at: www.hcqualitycommission.gov/final/. Accessed April 4, 2007.

American Academy of Pediatrics, Task Force on Definition of the Medical Home: The medical home. Pediatrics 90:774, 1992.

American Academy of Pediatrics, Medical Home Initiatives for Children With Special Needs Project Advisory Committee: The medical home. Pediatrics 110:184-186, 2002.

American Board of Pediatrics: Available at: www.abp.org. Accessed April 2007.

American Board of Psychiatry and Neurology: Available at: www.abpn.com. Accessed April 2007.

Antonelli R, Antonelli D: Providing a medical home: The cost of care coordination services in a community-based, general pediatric practice. Pediatrics 113(Suppl):1522-1528, 2004.

Antonelli R, Stille C, Freeman L: Enhancing Collaboration Between Primary and Subspecialty Care Providers for Children and Youth with Special Health Care Needs. Washington, DC, Georgetown University Center for Child and Human Development, 2005.

Batalden P, Berwick D, Bisognano M, et al: Knowledge Domains for Health Professional Students Seeking Competency in the Continual Improvement and Innovation of Health Care. Boston, MA, Institute for Healthcare Improvement, 1998.

Batalden P, Nelson EC, Gardent PB, Godfrey MM: Leading the macrosystem and mesosystem for microsystem peak performance. *In* From Front Office to Front Line: Essential Issues for Health Care Leaders. Joint Commission Resources, Oakbrook Terrace, IL, 2005.

Berwick DM: A user's manual for the IOM's "Quality Chasm" report. Health Affairs 21:80-90, 2002.

Bhandari S, Gifford E: Children with Health Insurance: 2001, Current Population Reports. Washington, DC, U.S. Census Bureau, 2003.

Bodenheimer T, Wagner EH, Grumbach K: Improving primary care for patients with chronic illness. JAMA 288:1775-1779, 2002.

Center for Medical Home Improvement: Available at: http://www.medicalhomeimprovement.org. Accessed March 2007.

Centers for Disease Control and Prevention: Available at http://www.cdc.gov/vaccines/stats-surv/imz-coverage.htm. Accessed October 20, 2008.

Chassin MR, Galvin RM; National Roundtable on Health Care Quality: The urgent need to improve health care quality. JAMA 280:1000-1005, 1998.

Chung BJ, Schuster MA: Access and quality in child health services: Voltage drops. Health Affairs 23:77-87, 2004.

Committee on Identifying Priority Areas for Quality Improvement, Institute of Medicine: Priority Areas for National Action: Transforming Health Care Quality. Washington, DC, National Academy Press, 2003.

Committee on Quality of Health Care in America, Institute of Medicine: Crossing the Quality Chasm: A New Health System for the 21st Century. Washington, DC, National Academy Press, 2001.

Cooley WC, McAllister JW: Building medical homes: Improvement strategies in primary care for children with special health care needs. Pediatrics 113(Suppl):1499-1506, 2004.

Flores G, Lee M, Bauchner H, Kastner B: Pediatricians' attitudes, beliefs, and practices regarding clinical practice guidelines: A national survey. Pediatrics 105(pt 1):496-501, 2000.

Hack CH: Paradigms of care for children with special healthcare needs. Pediatr Ann 26:674-678, 1997.

Inkelas M, Schuster MA, Olson LM, et al: Continuity of primary care clinician in early childhood. Pediatrics 113(Suppl):1917-1925, 2004.

Institute of Medicine: To Err is Human. Building a Safer Health System; Kohm LT, Corrigan JM, Donaldson MS (eds). Washington, DC, National Academy Press, 2000.

Institute of Medicine: Crossing the Quality Chasm: A New Health System for the 21st Century. Washington, DC, National Academy Press, 2001.

Mulvihill BA, Altarac M, Swaminathan S, et al: Does access to a medical home differ according to child and family characteristics, including special-health-care-needs status, among children in Alabama? Pediatrics 119:107-113, 2007.

Nelson EC, Batalden PB, Godfrey MM: Quality by Design: A Clinical Microsystems Approach. San Francisco, CA, Jossey-Bass, 2007.

Newacheck PW, Hughes DC, Hung YY, et al: The unmet health needs of America's children. Pediatrics 105(pt 2):989-997, 2000.

Picker Institute and American Hospital Association: Eye on Patient Reports. 1996.

Rosenbaum S, Budetti P: Low-income children and health insurance: Old news and new realities. Pediatrics 112(pt 2):551, 2003.

Schuster MA, McGlynn EA, Brook RH: How good is the quality of health care in the United States? Millbank Q 76:517-563, 1998.

Shonkoff J, Phillips DA: From Neurons to Neighborhoods: The Science of Early Childhood Development. National Research Council and Institute of Medicine. Washington, DC, National Academy Press, 2000.

Silver EJ, Stein RE: Access to care, unmet health needs, and poverty status among children with and without chronic conditions. Ambul Pediatr 1:314-320, 2001.

Wagner EH: Chronic disease management: What will it take to improve care of chronic illness? Eff Clin Pract 1:2-4, 1998.

Wagner EH: Quality improvement in chronic illness care. Jt Comm J Qual Improv 27:63-80, 2001.

Yu SM, Bellamy HA, Kogan MD, et al: Factors that influence receipt of recommended preventive pediatric health and dental care. Pediatrics 110:e73, 2002.

100 ETHICS

PETER J. SMITH AND JOHN J. HARDT

This chapter consists of two parts: an overview of the classical roots that bring together medicine and ethics and a survey of mainstream moral methodologies that contribute to contemporary bioethics. Its authors write from the perspective in which they have lived and trained, namely, that of the Western intellectual tradition. This is not to imply that this particular perspective is necessarily superior to others. Rather, limitations of space and the need to ground any discussion of ethics in a particular history, culture, and worldview both shape and constrain our contribution.

MEDICINE AND ETHICS: ANCIENT ROOTS, PERSISTENT THEMES

The Hippocratic Collection

Bioethics is as old as the practice of medicine itself. As Albert Jonsen notes in his synopsis, *A Short History of Medical Ethics*, bioethics' ancient roots reveal moral sensitivities and concerns that continue to shape the field today. These roots take geographic hold in ancient Greece and Rome and find personal impetus in the Greek physician Hippocrates (460-370 BC) and the Roman physician Galen (AD 129-216) (Jonsen, 2000). A conglomeration of some 70 treatises, first attributed to Hippocrates, that deliberate over the nascent identity of the classical physician is referred to as the Hippocratic Collection. It constitutes the originating impulse of what Jonsen describes as the "literate shape" of this "new medicine."

Contemporary scholarship indicates that the Hippocratic Collection was assembled during 5 centuries and authored by a variety of sources. Five of the treatises pay particular attention to the behavior of physicians in the application of their medical skills. They are entitled *Precepts, Art, Law, Decorum, Physician,* and *Oath.* Whereas the practice of novice physicians' taking the Hippocratic Oath as a symbolic entrance into the profession is a common aspect of medical training today, of more substantive importance to the foundations of contemporary bioethics is the Hippocratic Collection's identification of moral sensitivities that persist in their influence today, namely, reflection on the duties and character of the physician in practice. In the 2 millennia that follow, these moral inclinations of duty and character evolve into the moral methodologies of deontologic ethics and virtue ethics, both of which remain today as highly developed moral theories that, among others, bear on bioethics as a practice.

Duty

The ethical watermark of the treatise Oath is its repeated admonition against harm. The physician has an obligation, or duty (*deon* in Greek), not to harm one's patients. This admonition constitutes a primary deontologic component within the Oath. An ethic that depends on the proper identification and fulfillment of moral duties is a deontologic ethic. The duty neither to harm nor to treat one's patients unjustly is affirmed and reaffirmed in the Hippocratic Collection. This primary duty persists today as a cornerstone of bioethics and is commonly referred to as the principle of non-malfeasance. Moreover, deontologic ethics, especially in the work of the 19th-century moral philosopher Immanuel Kant, has become a well-regarded and highly nuanced moral methodology (Kant, 1964).

Character

The second moral impulse embodied in the Hippocratic Collection touches on the character development of the physician. Whereas discussion of moral character appears in multiple treatises within the Hippocratic Collection, it is most prominent in *Decorum* and *Physician.* Among other seemingly mundane matters, the author treats physician appearance, communication style, and determination of fee, but with special attention paid to what will be of most benefit to the patient. "If you begin by discussing fees," reads the *Decorum,* "you will suggest to the patient that you will go away… if no agreement is reached, or that you will neglect him and not prescribe any immediate treatment" (Jonsen, 2000).

The importance of the character of the physician found no better champion than the Roman physician Galen, who is credited with preserving and extending the Hippocratic tradition in the classical world. In his best known work entitled "The Best Doctor Is Also a Philosopher," Galen promotes virtuous actions as the foundation of good patient care. It is, to a considerable extent, the portrait of the Galenic physician that remains the template for the formation of the contemporary physician, one that stresses the cultivation of respect between the physician and the patient in the practice of medicine. The attention paid to physician behavior and character in ancient Greece and Rome has won renewed interest in moral theory as many now work to recover and to build on the work of the ancients and others in constructing what is now described as an ethic of virtue, another moral methodology that contributes to the varied terrain of contemporary bioethics.

Conclusion

In their early reflections on the developing practice of medicine, classical sources yield two moral compass points that remain influential in contemporary bioethical reflection on the formation of a good physician: duty and character. Hippocrates, Galen, and countless unknown others laid the foundation on which moral reflection would build for 2 millenia as reflection on the role of the physician in the practice of medicine developed.

ETHICAL SYSTEMS

Contemporary bioethics has been informed by a variety of moral theories, each of which has had its historical moment during the course of 2 millennia. Each of these theories continues to contribute to the ongoing dialogue within the field, some more prominently than others. Here, we survey four of the more influential moral methodologies at play today. They are deontologic ethics, utilitarian ethics, virtue ethics, and principlism.

Deontologic Ethics

The central tenant of a deontologic ethic is that some actions are obligatory, right or wrong, *regardless of their consequences.* The most famous proponent of deontologic ethics is the 18th-century philosopher Immanuel Kant (1724-1804). Kant argued that the moral life is based on reason alone. According to Kant, human emotions, desires, sympathies, or intuitions are a poor substitute for a rightly attuned sense of obligation in determining a proper course of action. Ultimately, according to Kant, one must identify a duty or rule that steers a course of action regardless of its outcome.

Although remaining a viable and influential moral methodology in bioethics—Edmund Pellegrino, the current Chairman of the President's Council on Bioethics, is one of its proponents (Pellegrino and Thomasma, 1993)—deontologic ethics is not without its critics (Beauchamp and Childress, 2001). An ethic that holds to the identification and enactment of universal obligations has a difficult time accommodating conflicting obligations. Whereas one might hold to a universal duty to keep promises, how should a person adjudicate conflicting promises, for example, promises to teach medical students and promises to care for patients? In the world of bioethics, such conflicting obligations occur with some frequency. One can imagine a physician's obligation to preserve life coming into conflict with a physician's obligation to adequately treat pain at the risk of unintentionally hastening death.

Deontologic ethics is also criticized for failing to adequately attend to the moral significance of relationship at the expense of rules and obligations. There are elements of our moral life that seem resistant to being reduced into a maxim or universal law. The moral commitments that tie us to family and friends and our experience of empathy, sympathy, and love call into question the feasibility of living solely by a deontologic ethic. In its abstractness and absolutism, deontologic ethics seems, sometimes, at some distance from our moral lives.

Utilitarian Ethics

The central tenant of a utilitarian holds that actions should be chosen to achieve the greatest balance of good consequences over bad consequence (Sugarman and Sulmasy, 37). In stark contrast to deontologic ethics, utilitarian ethics judges acts *solely on the basis of their consequences.* For this reason, utilitarian ethics is also commonly described as "consequentalist" ethics. The consequences sought in such an ethic are either happiness or pleasure or other, depending on which variant of a utilitarian ethic one endorses. The most famous proponents of utilitarianism were the 18th- and 19th-century philosophers Jeremy Bentham (1996) and John Stuart Mill. Utilitarianism also remains a vibrant and influential moral resource for contemporary bioethics.

Critics of utilitarianism have leveled two main complaints against it. Utilitarianism requires a moral judgment of the utility of consequences, which is not easily achieved within a morally plural society. For example, philosopher and bioethicist Peter A. D. Singer (1979) has been criticized for inappropriately judging individuals with cognitive disabilities as having a life not worth living (Reinders, 2000). In a morally plural world, who determines the measure of human happiness, pleasure, or value? A second, common critique of utilitarianism is that it encourages persons to distance themselves from their actions. Utilitarian calculations can have a corrosive effect both on the individual's personal character development and on society as a whole insofar as it fails to adequately account for the significance of the particular moral commitments that come with relationships among families, friends, and communities. It consistently runs the risk of sacrificing the well-being of the individual or minority interest for the sake of the whole.

Virtue Ethics

The central tenant of virtue ethics holds that the moral life is best promoted by attending to the moral agent herself or himself. Whereas deontologic ethics identifies and follows duties or obligations and utilitarian ethics attempts to maximize the good for the greatest number, virtue ethics seeks the moral formation of persons rather than the valuation of actions by paying attention to human virtue, friendship, moral wisdom, and discernment. As noted before, virtue ethics has deep roots in the classical world, and its philosophical origins are found in the Hippocratic Collection. Virtue ethics emphasizes the dynamic nature of ethical decisions, recognizing that individuals both shape and are shaped by what they choose to do in any given situation. Whereas virtue ethics flourished in the classical, philosophical world (Aquinas, 1920), its influence waned during the enlightenment. Virtue ethics has more recently experienced a revival in the 20th century in the work of moral philosopher Alasdair MacIntyre (1981) and others who have creatively recovered the work of their predecessors.

Critics of virtue ethics argue that it, like deontology and utilitarianism, cannot function within a morally plural society because of the lack of agreement on what virtues are actually worthy of promotion. Who decides what constitutes the good life and the good person among our ongoing disagreements about morality and value? Furthermore, the person-centered nature of this ethical system, insofar as it focuses on the moral agent rather than on obligations or principles, makes its content difficult to translate into codes, regulations, policies, or laws (Jonsen and Toulmin, 1988).

Principlism

Within the contemporary discussions of bioethical issues in Western liberal society, there is no doubt that the dominating system of thought is framed by considerations of basic "principles," which are understood to be universal, by thoughtful and preferably disinterested actors. The rise to preeminence of principlism as the dominant paradigm is due in large part to its clarity and ease of use in communication (to other professionals, students, and the general public). In addition, its deductive nature suggests its similarity to empiric sciences, and therefore it is often seen as "more true" than inductive or "softer" sciences. Most important, it is often tremendously helpful in confused situations with many conflicting actors with divergent views of "what is important" and several important outcomes in the balance. The ethical paradigm in medicine that immediately precedes principlism is now often referred to as benevolent paternalism, a term usually with negative connotations. Principlism has supplanted paternalism and now is the primary method that is currently taught at professional schools for health care clinicians. The most influential text used for teaching the system, *Principles of Biomedical Ethics* by Beauchamp and Childress (2001), has certainly evolved with time and in response to critics. However, the central claims remain the same: "The common morality contains a set of moral norms that includes principles that are basic for biomedical ethics. Most classical ethical theories include these principles in some form, and traditional medical codes presuppose at least some of them. The four clusters [of moral principles] are (1) respect for autonomy (a norm of respecting the decision-making capacities of autonomous persons), (2) non-malfeasance (a norm of avoiding the causation of harm), (3) beneficence (a group of norms for providing benefits and balancing benefits against risks and costs), and (4) justice (a group of norms for distributing benefits, risks, and costs fairly)."

In theory, these four principles ought to be weighed equally when they are seen as being in conflict in any given dilemma. However, in reality, given the underlying assumptions of the liberal society into which they have been promoted, the first principle, autonomy, consistently and effectively trumps all of the others. This has been so obviously the case that Beauchamp and Childress felt compelled in their most recent edition to highlight that this state of affairs was not their original attempt: "Although we begin our discussion of principles of biomedical ethics with respect for autonomy, our order of presentation does not imply that this principle has priority over all other principles" (Beauchamp and Childress, 2001).

Their frustrations with the current use of their system, and the problems that ensue from this interpretation, suggest that their system may be "inadequate" to the contemporary situation. Ironically, this inadequacy is not due to the fact that their system has assumptions that are different from those of the larger society (the problem with the earlier systems that they criticize); rather, it fits all too well into the orientations and desires of the larger society. In other words, their proposals were initially an important corrective to a system that had lost its vitality, but now it seems that their system has become a product of society (rather than a corrective to it). In addition, whereas principlism has clearly shown remarkable skill at abstracting generalities from particulars, it has proven much less adept when working in the opposite direction (i.e., when attempting to provide guidance regarding particular situations by drawing on generalities). The current situation has become one in which principlism reigns because it suits the needs and purposes of teachers, journals, and institutions while offering little succor to actual patients, family members, and clinicians.

Finally, the greatest problem with principlism, especially regarding the purposes of this chapter, is that it fails to include appropriate provisions for individuals who are unable to exercise independent autonomy and therefore is inadequate for anyone interested in a bioethic that considers individuals who are disabled, especially if their disability affects their cognition. "People or potential people with intellectual disability are most likely to be rendered, even on biological determination alone, profoundly irrelevant or disqualified within bioethical conversations because they are deemed incapable of being rational, competent, independent beings" (Clapton, 2002). Clearly, this is inadequate, yet it has its roots in Beauchamp and Childress: "Personal autonomy, [which] is, at a minimum, self-rule that is free from both controlling interference by others and from limitations. The autonomous individual acts freely in accordance with a self-chosen plan, analogous to the way an independent government manages its territories and sets its policies" (Beauchamp and Childress, 2001).

It is critical to note that this framework is based on the definition that personhood is determined by an ability to choose. This conception will encounter its greatest difficulties in that situation in which ability to choose becomes disenabled or is intrinsically limited: "People with mental disabilities are lacking to a greater or lesser extent the powers of reasons and free will. Since these are the powers that bring substance to the core values of the liberal view on public morality, mentally disabled people never acquire full moral standing in this view. This is because its moral community is constituted by "persons" and these, in turn, are constituted by the powers of reason and free will" (Reinders, 2000).

In addition, one of the foundational assumptions of principlism is that individuals are usually in competition and do not share world views (except for the core principles). Consequently, it is particularly adept at helping to referee disputes that arise within a competitive, pluralistic community comprising articulate individuals who are included within liberal society's definition of citizenship. However, another consequence is that it (like utilitarianism) can foster a breakdown in a communitarian spirit. Because of its primary and exalted emphasis on individual liberties, it has no room for defining or promoting a "common good." Rather, its emphasis on individual liberty has led to the convention that any person is free to act in any way that does not impinge on the freedom of another individual or group of individuals, like the image of protecting the boundaries of a country.

SUMMARY

Contemporary bioethics has roots in ancient traditions, particularly that tradition as transmitted through Galen. This ancient tradition especially emphasized the duty and character of the physician. Current systems of ethics include deontology (which judges actions regardless of consequences), utilitarianism (which judges action solely on consequences), virtue ethics (which judges the actor rather than actions), and principlism (which assumes a set of core principles that are shared universally). Principlism is currently dominant. However, as currently construed, it places its primary emphasis on autonomy (narrowly defined as related to the ability to make conscience decisions), which makes it cumbersome (at best) and troublesome (at worst) when it is used in situations including individuals with inability to make decisions. Therefore, its hegemonic position seems to be under threat (especially as a greater percentage of the population has direct contact with individuals with cognitive impairments).

REFERENCES

Aquinas T; literally translated by Fathers of the English Dominican Province: Summa Theologica, 2nd ed, revised. London, Burns Oates & Washbourne, 1920.

Beauchamp TL, Childress JF: Principles of Biomedical Ethics, 5th ed. New York, Oxford University Press, 2001, p 12.

Bentham J: An Introduction to the Principles of Moral Legislation. New York, Oxford University Press, 1996.

Clapton J: Tragedy and Catastrophe: Contentious Discourse of Ethics and Disability. Newslett Network Ethics Intellectl Disabil 6:1, 3-4, 2002.

Jonsen AR: A Short History of Medical Ethics. New York, Oxford University Press, 2000.

Jonsen AR, Toulmin S: The Abuse of Casuistry. Berkeley, University of California Press, 1988.

Kant I: Groundwork of the Metaphysic of Morals. New York, Harper and Row Publishers, 1964.

MacIntyre A: After Virtue [2nd ed, 1984; 3rd ed, 2007]. Notre Dame, IN, University of Notre Dame Press, 1981.

Pellegrino ED, Thomasma DC: The Virtues in Medical Practice. New York, Oxford University Press, 1993.

Reinders HS: The Future of the Disabled in Liberal Society: An Ethical Analysis. Notre Dame, IN, University of Notre Dame Press, 2000.

Singer PAD: Practical Ethics [2nd ed, 1993]. Cambridge, UK, Cambridge University Press, 1979.

Sugarman J, Sulmasy DP: Methods in Medical Ethics. Washington, DC, Georgetown University Press, 2001.

101 THE RIGHT TO BE DIFFERENT

The Editors

The work of developmental-behavioral pediatrics often involves evaluating children who are different from their peers in terms of their developmental skills, behavioral profile, physical appearance, or a combination of these features. Some of these children receive a clinical formulation of temperamental differences (Chapter 7); others are diagnosed with neurodevelopmental conditions, such as attention-deficit/hyperactivity disorder (Chapter 54) or genetic disorders (Chapter 26). Management and treatments in this field are often designed to help the child to function better in the family, school, or community. We discussed counseling to parents of difficult children (Chapter 86), psychopharmacologic interventions for children with psychiatric illness (Chapter 90), and cognitive-behavioral therapy for anxiety and depression (Chapter 87). Indeed, a casual reading of this book might suggest that the professionals in this field seek to normalize children to an implicit idealized version. In this final chapter, we, the editors, want to set the record straight. As in the previous editions of the book, we reaffirm "the right to be different."

We recognize that despite and sometimes because of continued advances in science, medicine, and technology, the variation among individuals remains enormous. In so many ways, human society benefits from such diversity. After all, some of us become rocket scientists and others farmers, plumbers, chefs, teachers, and pediatricians. Some of us focus on raising the children and others focus on earning a living. Some prefer to work the day shift and others like the night shift. Yet, there remains a great tension between societal appreciation for human diversity and the expectations that people will conform in appearance, ability, attitudes, and beliefs. Reduced options, lack of social acceptance, and outright hostility are among the high costs incurred by being different. Even in the United States of America, where respect for pluralism was an essential element of our nation's founding, differences among individuals may invoke profound social isolation.

RESPONSES TO VARIATION: PRIVATE AND PUBLIC

Impatience and intolerance are common responses to human variation, even to children. Even though we think of ourselves as a child-centered society, we are particularly critical of children who are different from the norm. Adults are allowed to design a family life to their liking, to pick the place where they want to live, and to choose their own occupation. Children are expected to fit in with their family, to attend the school that their caregivers choose for them, and to learn to read at the same age and grade as all other children do. Moreover, we expect that they will learn to read with a single educational approach, without regard to their distinctive temperaments, learning styles, and cognitive abilities. We educate children within large and often noisy classrooms with hardly any individual attention. We expect them to learn without any consideration of the vast differences in their social situations, including the amount of food they have available, the warmth of their homes, the relationships among their family members, and the ability of their parents or siblings to help them with homework.

Children who are different suffer as a result of social ostracism by peers and adults. Friendships occur less readily. We know that they face bullying and aggression (Chapter 40) and often develop low self-esteem (Chapter 44). This social isolation is often more of a reflection on limited understanding, not necessarily the individual's degree of difference from the norm. Being out of synchrony with one's peers robs that child of needed positive feedback and is destructive of self-image.

Parents feel the impact of differences in their children as well. Recently released data from the National Survey of Children with Special Health Care Needs reveal that a large number of children with special needs are underinsured and that they have unmet needs. Parents report that they often must cut back their work hours or quit their jobs to meet the high needs of their children. This sacrifice results in reduced family income. Parents often find themselves in the role of service coordinator in addition to the roles of advocate, nurse, and care provider. Parents may also be coping with the emotional consequences of having a child with differences, including sadness and isolation. These emotions can sometimes adversely affect the relationship between the parents and their children (Chapter 10) or parents and the medical and service providers. They can also clearly have effects on other family members, particularly sisters and brothers (Chapter 11).

In earlier times, society often visited on children and adults with substantial differences lasting segregation (Chapter 1). Thankfully, in the current era, there are protections against prejudice and isolation (Chapter 97). The Universal Declaration of Human Rights, adopted on December 10, 1948, by the General Assembly of the United Nations, proclaims that "all human beings are born free and equal in dignity and rights. They are endowed with reason and conscience and should act towards one another in a spirit of brotherhood." The 30 articles of this impressive document remain the standard for human rights and serve as the foundation for national legislation in many countries, protecting children and adults who are different. We in the United States have incorporated such rights into federal legislation (Chapters 1 and 97). Public Law 101-336, commonly known as the Americans with Disabilities Act (ADA), prohibits discrimination against individuals with disabilities in the workplace and allows accessibility in public transportation and in public accommodations (places such as stores, restaurants, and public buildings). The legal foundation for a free and public education for all is the Individuals with Disabilities Education Act, or IDEA (Chapter 93). It mandates a free and public education for all children with disabilities in the "least restrictive environment."

The legal protections in the workplace and public accommodations and the right to a free and public education in the least restrictive environment remain subject to the political will of the nation. Threats to these laws arise regularly. Special education, for example, is sometimes presented as an unnecessary financial burden on the society rather than as a civil right. This attitude is particularly short-sighted. Although approximately 10% to 20% of schoolchildren receive special education, the fact is that these supports are far less costly than the outcomes of limited opportunity and neglect, including underemployment, incarceration, institutionalization, and the cycle of poverty. Moreover, public programs, including public education, remain underfunded.

CHANGING CHILDREN

We in developmental-behavioral pediatrics and related fields must become cautious and self-reflective when we design management plans and treatments. We must remain aware that attempts to remedy variation can result from a complex of motivations. In general, the focus of management and treatment is on enhancement of a child's functioning rather than on correction of a difference. That broad goal, enhancement of function, may encompass one or more domains of function: learning and academic performance, ability to handle tasks and demands, mobility, communication, self-care, and social relationships. Even then, however, it is difficult to determine what is appropriate and what is not an appropriate target of treatment. The use of psychoactive medications, for example, to quickly alleviate the burden of raising or educating a child with atypical behavior may be a substitute for a more penetrating, child-focused program of primary assistance in behavioral adaptation.

Even counseling (Chapter 86) and therapy (Chapter 89) can raise significant ethical questions. To what extent is the therapeutic counseling designed primarily to edge the child toward uniformity and conformity? Is there a danger that the therapist or counselor will superimpose his or her own values on a naive child? Should parents and therapists press the development of social skills for a youngster who prefers to be alone? If a child has gross motor delays or is clumsy and shows little or no interest in sports, is the adult world privileged to insist on physical therapy and physical education for the child? Even among children with minimal differences from the norm, should they be allowed to determine academic and recreational direction?

Although we may provide management and treatments to improve a child's functioning, at the same time children should be afforded the right to "specialize." When families were large, it was not unusual for each child to assume a different adult role: one a doctor, one a religious leader, one a farmer, and maybe one a ne'er-do-well. We could tolerate one going off to explore a distant country because many stayed close to home for their entire lifetime. In an era of small family size, we want our one or two children to successfully fill many different roles and expectations. Children may need help in resisting the overriding drive of adults to make them good at almost everything. We must modulate our zeal to help children to function in a complex society. We must balance encouragement of exploration, excellence, and change with support and acceptance.

The inadequacies of services, fiscal resources, and social supports for families caring for children who are different may prompt a great desire for change. The pressure for change in a setting of severe disabilities was highlighted in a highly controversial approach to management called Ashley's Treatment, named for a child with significant neurologic disabilities from Washington State. This child underwent removal of her uterus, ovaries, and breast buds as well as hormonal treatment so that she could remain very small and therefore easier to care for. Although the family had considered this approach only after much medical consultation and discussion with the ethics committee at the local institution, the reaction to the treatment once it was publicized was quite vehement. The rights of the child with disabilities must be balanced with the interests of the adults who take care of the child. The sterilization of a person with disabilities who could not express her own will was a violation of her human rights. At the same time, there was sympathy and understanding for the plight of the parents and the realization that parents must often make difficult decisions for their child and try to come to a decision in the child's best interest. In many situations, like this one, the "right thing to do" is not straightforward. Open dialogue among all parties, including an impartial representative of the child, might help with difficult decisions.

INTEGRATION VERSUS PERSONAL CHOICE

The same tension between acceptance of difference and push for change can affect entire groups as well as individuals. Some groups resist the pull toward integration and normalization. Take, for example, the Deaf Community. The Deaf Community appreciates the resources and protections it has received under ADA regarding telecommunications. Special communication devices, such as teletypewriter machines (TYY), were mandated for individuals who are deaf or hard of hearing, making communication with others far easier than it had been. Recent advances in computer and cell phone technology, especially text messaging, have further improved how individuals who are deaf can communicate with each other and with their hearing peers. In the medical arena, cochlear implantation became available (Chapter 70). This technology is akin to a prosthesis that can either restore or allow some degree of hearing in individuals whose hearing impairment was previously considered permanent. Whether or not to have a child with congenital deafness get a cochlear implant has become a highly contentious issue. The Deaf Community, the capital letters here very important, does not conceptualize hearing impairment as a disability. Rather, it defines deafness as a community or culture, with its own language (American Sign Language), history, humor, values, and beliefs. Thus, many individuals who are deaf choose not to have cochlear implantation for themselves or their children. We can ask, Who should decide about the cochlear implant for a deaf child of deaf parents?

Likewise, individuals with skeletal dysplasias have come together and formed a vibrant group known as the Little People of America. They advocate for accessibility in the workplace and in the community. They welcome modifications that allow them to drive and to work within the community. However, like members of the Deaf Community, they often choose to have children with other members of their group with short stature, a decision that often results in another generation with skeletal dysplasia who also require accommodations at home and in the workplace.

Similar issues arise within education. The least restrictive environment is usually interpreted to mean that children with learning disorders and other educational needs receive their education alongside typically developing children in a regular educational environment. The positive effects of IDEA on children with developmental disabilities has been incalculable in terms of minimizing differences on many levels. Moreover, typically developing children who grow up with children with special needs alongside them in the classroom become more accepting of differences and more able to see the "person" with a disability, rather than the disability itself, compared with peers without this educational experience. However, some parents insist on placing their children with learning problems or disabilities in specialized classrooms or programs. Some worry that their children will not be adequately educated if they are a minority of the classroom. Others have seen their children ridiculed or bullied in those regular education settings. It challenges us when two of our fundamental beliefs, inclusion and personal choice, conflict with one another. How should we come to a decision about placement in cases in which the parents push for a segregated program? Who should decide?

A FINAL WORD

We, the editors of this text, remain committed to a pluralistic society. We believe that diversity brings vitality and enrichment. We believe that all individuals deserve respect and belonging. On that basis, we believe that there is indeed "the right to be different." We note that slowly this belief is becoming accepted by a wider range of citizens. We welcome the many changes we have seen in the course of our careers.

- The movement for assistance in adoption of "hard to place" children (e.g., those who have developmental disabilities or behavioral disorders) has been strikingly successful. Adoption of children with special needs has transformed a once rejected child into an avidly chosen child. Many hundreds of adoptions of children with Down syndrome have now taken place, and in most major cities there is a waiting list of couples for adoption of infants and young children with Down syndrome. Again, these children are raised at home and get all the benefits accrued on that basis.
- Families of children with disabilities are now raising their children in their homes. The benefits of this decision have become obvious to those in the field. Children with disabilities have better social, linguistic, and academic skills than they had in the past. They are ultimately working in the community, sometimes in competitive and sometimes in supported employment positions.
- "Deinstitutionalization" is bringing persons with serious disabilities into community living. In some states, all of the large state hospitals and institutions have now been shuttered. Deinstitutionalization has led to substantial victories. Major functional gains are commonplace when individualized programs are provided to those who reenter the community.
- New technologies are igniting the excitement of learning in children and adults who would have been written off. The child who is nonverbal but then speaks with the use of augmentative communication, the young child with autism who is able to be established in a regular class after home parent training, the atypical youth who receives reimbursement for graded accomplishments in a vocational training program—these are victories of the social revolution.
- Children who are dependent on technology who used to live within the hospital are now being raised at home. Nursing services in the home, although a real cost, are usually lower than an endless hospital stay. In many instances, individuals living at home are less susceptible to secondary complications and nosocomial infection.
- Children with learning differences are able to get support within the regular classroom rather than attend specialized programs in isolated settings. The distinction between regular and special education is blurring in some areas, benefiting the children whose learning differences are not labeled as well as those who carry a diagnosis.

We are also beginning to see changes in the attitudes, beliefs, and practices of the professionals who work with children and adults with differences. Here are a few of the promising trends.

- Pediatricians and other primary health care clinicians are increasing the rates of screening for developmental delays and behavioral differences. Their willingness to do so reflects a push by the American Academy of Pediatrics and other professional and advocacy organizations. It also reflects the changing nature of primary care for children, moving away from a focus on infectious and other acute disorders to early identification and management of chronic conditions, including delays and disabilities.
- Professionals are broadening their concepts to accommodate the complexity of the human condition. Intelligence is no longer just how well you do on the traditional IQ test but how capable you are in several spheres, such as learning and social understanding (Chapter 81). Learning differences and disabilities are increasingly being recognized as issues requiring respect and specialized care.
- Professionals have developed a better understanding than they previously had about gender differences and sexual preferences. No longer are the preferences of a minority viewed as a mental disorder (Chapter 43).
- The variations of behavioral style or temperament are increasingly recognized. This shift is enriching our appreciation for the wide range of normal that must be accepted as such and not reduced to a pathologic state or a simplistic diagnosis (Chapters 7 and 78).
- Many in psychiatry and developmental-behavioral pediatrics are starting to move beyond the static categorical diagnostic system of the *Diagnostic and Statistical Manual of Mental Disorders* to one that is dimensional and contextual, as suggested by Jensen and colleagues (2006), which should advance the recognition and respect for differences in normal behavior.

In conclusion, the vast variations in human presentation delineated in this book can be considered the products of the array of phenotypic, genotypic, sociocultural, and individual circumstances that characterize our species. The concept of "normal" or "average" is statistically perceivable but often subject to political inducement, and it is assuredly irrelevant on many occasions. We have much to learn from a far broader view. We seek to celebrate the diversity of the human experience. We wish to include all individuals as equal members of our community. We will continue to work to promote equality and acceptance.

REFERENCES

Jensen PS, Knapp P, Mrazek DA: Toward a New Diagnostic System for Child Psychopathology: Moving Beyond the DSM. New York, Guilford, 2006.

The "Ashley Treatment." Available at: http://ashleytreatment.spaces.live.com/blog.

U.S. Department of Justice: Americans with Disabilities Act home page. Available at: http://www.usdoj.gov/crt/ada/adahom1.htm.

U.S. Department of Education: Twenty-five Years of Progress in Educating Children with Disabilities Through IDEA. Available at: http://www.ed.gov/policy/speced/leg/idea/history.pdf.

U.S. Department of Health and Human Services and Health Resources and Services Administration; Maternal and Child Health Bureau: The National Study on Children with Disabilities Chartbook 2005-6. Rockville, MD, U.S. Department of Health and Human Services, 2007.

INDEX

Note: Page numbers followed by b indicate boxed material; those followed by f indicate figures; those followed by t indicate tables.

A

B

C

E

F

G

H

I

M

N

O

P

S

W

X

Y